W9-AFS-469

Kirklin/Barratt-Boyes

Cardiac Surgery

Morphology, Diagnostic Criteria, Natural History, Techniques, Results, and Indications

Volume 2

Kirklin/Barratt-Boyes

Cardiac Surgery

Morphology, Diagnostic Criteria, Natural History, Techniques, Results, and Indications

Fourth Edition

Nicholas T. Kouchoukos, MD
Attending Cardiothoracic Surgeon
Division of Cardiovascular and Thoracic Surgery
Missouri Baptist Medical Center
St. Louis, Missouri

Eugene H. Blackstone, MD
Head, Clinical Investigations, Heart and Vascular Institute
Staff, Departments of Thoracic and Cardiovascular Surgery and Quantitative Health Sciences
Professor of Surgery
Cleveland Clinic Lerner College of Medicine of Case Western Reserve University
Cleveland Clinic
Cleveland, Ohio
Professor of Surgery, University of Toronto
Toronto, Ontario, Canada

Frank L. Hanley, MD
Professor of Cardiothoracic Surgery
Stanford University
Executive Director, Pediatric Heart Center
Lucile Packard Children's Hospital
Stanford, California

James K. Kirklin, MD
Professor and Director
Division of Cardiothoracic Surgery
University of Alabama at Birmingham
Birmingham, Alabama

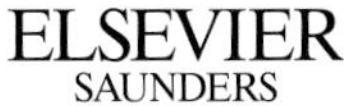

ELSEVIER
SAUNDERS

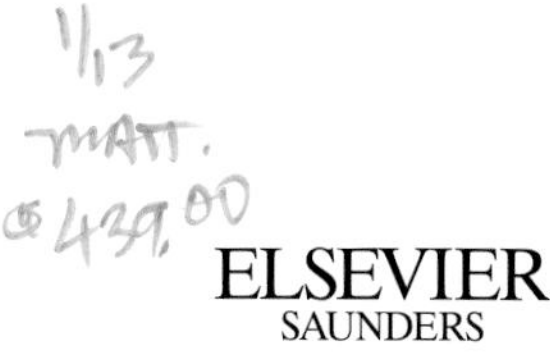

ELSEVIER
SAUNDERS

1600 John F. Kennedy Blvd.
Ste 1800
Philadelphia, PA 19103-2899

KIRKLIN/BARRATT-BOYES CARDIAC SURGERY

ISBN: 978-1-4160-6391-9
Volume 1 Part Number: 9996060306
Volume 2 Part Number: 9996060365

Notices

Knowledge and best practice in this field are constantly changing. As new research and experience broaden our understanding, changes in research methods, professional practices, or medical treatment may become necessary.

Practitioners and researchers must always rely on their own experience and knowledge in evaluating and using any information, methods, compounds, or experiments described herein. In using such information or methods they should be mindful of their own safety and the safety of others, including parties for whom they have a professional responsibility.

With respect to any drug or pharmaceutical products identified, readers are advised to check the most current information provided (i) on procedures featured or (ii) by the manufacturer of each product to be administered, to verify the recommended dose or formula, the method and duration of administration, and contraindications. It is the responsibility of practitioners, relying on their own experience and knowledge of their patients, to make diagnoses, to determine dosages and the best treatment for each individual patient, and to take all appropriate safety precautions.

To the fullest extent of the law, neither the Publisher nor the authors, contributors, or editors assume any liability for any injury and/or damage to persons or property as a matter of products liability, negligence or otherwise, or from any use or operation of any methods, products, instructions, or ideas contained in the material herein.

Library of Congress Cataloging-in-Publication Data
Kirklin/Barratt-Boyes cardiac surgery: morphology, diagnostic criteria, natural history, techniques, results, and indications / Nicholas T. Kouchoukos ... [et al.]. – 4th ed.
p. ; cm.
Cardiac surgery
Includes bibliographical references and index.
ISBN 978-1-4160-6391-9 (hardcover) – ISBN 978-9996060304 (hardcover: v. 1) – ISBN 9996060306 (hardcover: v. 1) – ISBN 978-9996060366 (hardcover: v. 2) – ISBN 9996060365 (hardcover: v. 2)
I. Kouchoukos, Nicholas T. II. Kirklin, John W. (John Webster). Cardiac surgery. III. Title: Cardiac surgery.
[DNLM: 1. Cardiac Surgical Procedures–methods. 2. Cardiovascular Diseases–surgery. WG 169]
617.4'12059–dc23

2012007384

Global Content Development Director: Judy Fletcher
Content Development Manager: Maureen Iannuzzi
Publishing Services Manager: Anne Altepeter
Project Manager: Cindy Thoms
Design Direction: Steven Stave

Printed in China

Last digit is the print number: 9 8 7 6 5 4 3 2 1

Contributors

Colleen Koch, MD, MS
Vice Chair of Research and Education
Department of Cardiothoracic Anesthesia
Cardiothoracic Anesthesia
Cleveland Clinic
Cleveland, Ohio
Anesthesia for Cardiovascular Surgery

Chandra Ramamoorthy, MBBS, FRCA
Professor of Anesthesiology
Stanford University Medical Center
Director, Division of Pediatric Cardiac Anesthesia
Lucile Packard Children's Hospital
Palo Alto, California
Anesthesia for Cardiovascular Surgery

Acknowledgments

The authors gratefully acknowledge the assistance of the following individuals and organizations whose contributions made publication of this textbook possible:

St. Louis, Missouri:	Catherine F. Castner, RN, BSN; Sandra E. Decker; John H. Niemeyer, MD; John D. Brooks, CCP; Elizabeth White The Missouri Baptist Health Care Foundation
Cleveland, Ohio:	Michelle Haywood; Luci Mitchin; Tess Parry; Kristin Purdy; Gina Ventre Cleveland Clinic
Stanford, California:	Sam Suleman; V. Mohan Reddy, MD; Frandics Chan, MD; and Norman Silverman MD, for their expertise and contributions
Birmingham, Alabama:	Dr. David McGiffin for his expertise and contributions Ms. Peggy Holmes for her expert editorial assistance

Preface to Fourth Edition

The fourth edition of *Cardiac Surgery* has been prepared without contributions from two of the authors of the third edition, Drs. Robert B. Karp and Donald B. Doty. Dr. Karp was fatally injured in an automobile accident in 2006. Dr. Doty retired from the practice of cardiothoracic surgery in 2004. We are extremely grateful to both of them for their outstanding contributions, many of which remain in the fourth edition. We are equally pleased to welcome as a contributor to the fourth edition, Dr. James K. Kirklin, son of Dr. John W. Kirklin, co-author with Sir Brian Barratt-Boyes of the first two editions of *Cardiac Surgery*.

Except for Dr. Frank Hanley, we received our cardiothoracic surgical education at the University of Alabama Medical Center under the tutelage of John Kirklin, and we were privileged to serve as faculty members in the Department of Surgery at the University of Alabama at Birmingham School of Medicine during his tenure as chair of the department and director of the Division of Cardiothoracic Surgery. James Kirklin currently serves as director of that division.

We have all, including Dr. Hanley, been profoundly influenced by the teachings of John Kirklin, and by his intellect, vision, and clinical skills. His commitment to improving the quality of cardiac surgery through rigorous clinical and laboratory investigations and providing superb clinical care and disciplined training of young surgeons was truly exemplary. Although our interactions with Sir Brian Barrett-Boyes were less frequent and less intense, he possessed these same attributes and was an inspiration to us as well. In the last year of his life, he was engaged in updating the echocardiographic and structural valve deterioration data of the entire Green Lane Hospital experience of aortic allografts, with the intent of transmitting these data for analysis by one of us (EHB).

The systematic approach to cardiac surgery developed and promulgated by these two pioneering surgeons, who both died between publication of the third and this fourth edition of *Cardiac Surgery*, has been a major fixture in our professional careers. The decision to author the third and now fourth editions of *Cardiac Surgery* was in large part influenced by our desire to perpetuate their philosophical approach to this discipline. Thus, the general format of the three previous editions has been maintained.

All chapters present in the third edition have been revised. They have been rearranged so that every chapter relating to surgical treatment of congenital heart disease (except for Chapter 29, "Congenital Heart Disease in the Adult") has been placed in Volume 2. Each chapter was rewritten with input from at least two of the four authors. Chapter 4 ("Anesthesia for Cardiovascular Surgery") was revised by Drs. Colleen G. Koch and Chandra Ramamoorthy. The content, and in some instances the titles, of several chapters have been altered to reflect current knowledge and practice. As an example, the chapter "Heart Failure" in the third edition has been expanded into three chapters in the fourth edition: "Cardiomyopathy," "Cardiac Transplantation," and "Mechanical Circulatory Support." New illustrations and new echocardiographic, computed tomographic, and magnetic resonance images have been added to reflect important advances in the diagnosis and management of congenital and acquired diseases of the heart and great vessels.

We recognize the potential limitation of four authors writing separate portions of this textbook. This challenge was met, in part at least, by dual authorship of each chapter, and by author meetings and correspondence. It was also met by a process of universal review. Specifically, as with the third edition, Dr. Blackstone was designated as the final arbiter. After completion of the revision of each chapter by the primary author, copyedited material was forwarded to Dr. Blackstone in Cleveland, where he and his assistant, Tess Muharsky Parry, reviewed, edited, reorganized, questioned, and adjudicated the entire content of each chapter. It is our hope that this intensive process has improved the accuracy and comprehensiveness of each chapter.

As in the previous editions, Part I of Volume 1 discusses basic concepts of cardiac surgery: anatomy, support techniques, myocardial management, anesthesia, postoperative care, and methodology for generating new knowledge from previous experience. These core chapters are applicable to the broad audience of medical professionals who care for patients with cardiac disease. The remaining chapters of Volume 1 (Parts II to V) discuss specific acquired diseases of the heart and great vessels, and congenital heart disease in adults. This edition has retained, in these later sections and in all of the chapters in Volume 2, presentation of "Indications for Operation" at the end of each chapter, because the indications are the derivatives of comparison of various outcomes (results) of alternative forms of treatments, including no treatment (natural history).

The abbreviation *UAB* has been retained, and is used to identify data and illustrations from the University of Alabama at Birmingham; similarly, *GLH* identifies those from Green Lane Hospital in Auckland, New Zealand. The bibliographic references are again designated using the first letter of the surname of the first author and a number (e.g., L4), rather than simply a number. This convention is simple and convenient, and allows the reader to easily locate a given author's publication among the alphabetically arranged references. The abbreviation *CL* is used throughout to denote 70% confidence limits around the point estimate. The reasons for presenting 70% rather than 95% or 50% confidence limits are presented in Chapter 6.

The fourth edition is written at a time of great change for the specialty of cardiac surgery. Percutaneous catheter-based interventions are being increasingly used to treat patients with coronary arteriosclerotic heart disease, aortic valve stenosis, mitral valve regurgitation, hypertrophic obstructive cardiomyopathy, diseases of the thoracic aorta, and congenital cardiac lesions such as patent ductus arteriosus, coarctation of the aorta, atrial and ventricular septal defects, and pulmonary valvar stenosis and regurgitation. Less invasive techniques are rapidly being incorporated into cardiac surgical practice for many conditions that continue to require open surgical repair. These advances must be acknowledged and embraced if cardiac surgery is to thrive in the future.

It is our hope that this textbook will be of value to cardiac surgeons who care for patients with congenital and acquired heart disease and with disorders of major blood vessels in the chest, as well as to cardiologists and interventional cardiologists who treat children and adults with these conditions, anesthesiologists, intensivists, pulmonologists, imaging specialists, cardiovascular nurses, trainees in all of these disciplines, and others.

— *Nicholas T. Kouchoukos, MD*
— *Eugene H. Blackstone, MD*
— *Frank L. Hanley, MD*
— *James K. Kirklin, MD*

Contents

PART VII

Congenital Heart Disease

30 Atrial Septal Defect and Partial Anomalous Pulmonary Venous Connection

DEFINITION

An *atrial septal defect* (ASD) is a hole of variable size in the atrial septum. A patent foramen ovale that is functionally closed by overlapping of limbic tissue superiorly and the valve of the fossa ovalis inferiorly (in response to the normal left-to-right atrial pressure gradient) is excluded. ASDs generally permit left-to-right shunting at the atrial level. *Partial anomalous pulmonary venous connection* (PAPVC) is a condition in which some but not all pulmonary veins connect to the right atrium or its tributaries, rather than to the left atrium. The term *connection* is preferred to the term "return," because *connection* is anatomic and return is governed by hemodynamic factors. PAPVCs may occur as isolated anomalies or may be combined with ASDs.

These two groups of anomalies are considered together in this chapter because they manifest similar physiology and result in similar clinical findings. *Total* anomalous pulmonary venous connection is considered in Chapter 31. ASDs typically occur in association with other cardiac anomalies, and these are considered in chapters dealing with those anomalies.

HISTORICAL NOTE

Clinical recognition of an ASD has been possible only in about the past 70 years. Among the 62 recorded autopsy cases of ASD analyzed by Roesler in 1934, only one had been correctly diagnosed during life.[R6] By 1941, Bedford and colleagues were able to make the diagnosis clinically in a number of patients.[B3] When cardiac catheterization came into general use during the late 1940s and early 1950s, secure diagnosis became possible. The first descriptions of PAPVC are attributed to Winslow in 1739[B15] and Wilson in 1798.[M11] The first diagnosis of PAPVC during life was reported by Dotter and colleagues in 1949.[D7]

A number of ingenious closed methods for repair of ASDs and related conditions were proposed and studied experimentally in the productive and expansive surgical era following the end of World War II in 1945. In 1948 in Toronto, Murray reported closing an ASD in a child by external suturing.[M18] Several other closed methods had clinical application, including Bailey and colleagues' "atrioseptopexy" and Søndergard's purse-string suture closure.[B2,S12] However, limited applicability of these methods was always apparent, and they were soon abandoned.

Hypothermia, induced by surface cooling, and inflow occlusion for repair of ASDs was introduced during the early 1950s (see Historical Note in Section I of Chapter 2). Lewis and Taufic reported the first successful open repair of an ASD with this method in 1953.[L5] At about the same time, Gross invented the ingenious atrial well technique, a semi-open approach in which a rubber open-bottomed well or cone was sutured to an incision in a clamp-exteriorized portion of the right atrial wall.[G11,K6] When the clamp was released, the blood rose into the well, and through this pool of blood, the surgeon could place sutures under digital control for direct or patch closure of the defect. Gibbon started the era of open heart surgery in 1953 when he successfully repaired an ASD in a young woman using a pump-oxygenator.[G9] Although these three methods—hypothermia and inflow occlusion, atrial well, and cardiopulmonary bypass (CPB)—were all used during the late 1950s and provided similar early results,[K8] by the late 1960s almost all surgeons used CPB exclusively for these repairs. Percutaneous catheter techniques for closing a fossa ovalis ASD using a polyester double umbrella device were introduced by King and Mills in 1974.[K4]

The first reported treatment for a type of PAPVC was lobectomy in 1950.[D9] In 1953, Neptune and colleagues reported repair using a closed technique in 17 patients with PAPVC of the right lung to the right atrium associated with ASD.[N5] It is not certain who first repaired the sinus venosus syndrome, but the malformation was clearly illustrated by Bedford and colleagues in 1957.[B4] Repair of PAPVC to the inferior vena cava was performed by Kirklin and colleagues at Mayo Clinic in 1960 and was also subsequently reported by Zubiate and Kay in 1962.[M17,Z2] Correction of anomalous connection of the left pulmonary veins to the left brachiocephalic vein and other forms of PAPVC was reported from the Mayo Clinic in 1953[G6,K5] and later in 1956.[K7]

MORPHOLOGY

Types of Atrial Septal Defect

As viewed from the right atrial side (see Fig. 1-2 in Chapter 1), the normal atrial septum may have defects in almost any location (Box 30-1). Although the morphology of these defects has been known since the early descriptions by Robitansky in 1875,[R5] the advent of open heart surgery emphasized their surgically important aspects[B4,L6] (Fig. 30-1).

Fossa Ovalis Defect

The most common ASD is the *fossa ovalis type,* also called *foramen ovale type* or *ostium secundum defect.* This defect lies within the perimeter inscribed by the limbus anteriorly, superiorly, and posteriorly (Fig. 30-2). The smallest defects are

Box 30-1 Types of Atrial Septal Defect[a]

- Fossa ovalis defect[b]
- Posterior defect
- Coronary sinus defect
- Sinus venosus defect
- Confluent defect
- Ostium primum defect (absence of atrioventricular septum)

[a]Fossa ovalis, posterior, and most confluent defects can be classified as *secundum type*.
[b]Varies in size from small valvar-incompetent foramen ovale ASD to complete absence of septum primum tissue with resultant ASD extending to inferior vena cava.

essentially valvar incompetent foramina ovale that occur beneath the superior limbus, between it and the valve (floor) of the fossa ovalis. The floor of the fossa ovalis (remnant of septum primum) may in this situation have multiple fenestrations of various sizes (Fig. 30-3). When more of the floor of the fossa ovalis is absent, a larger fossa ovalis defect is present. When all fossa ovalis tissue is absent, the ASD is confluent with the orifice of the inferior vena cava (IVC). The eustachian valve of the IVC then overhangs the ASD and must not be mistaken for its inferior edge at operation. Size of this type of ASD is also affected by any hypoplasia of the limbus that may be present. When the limbus is quite hypoplastic anteriorly, there is only a thin rim of tissue above the atrioventricular (AV) valves (formerly this was called an *intermediate defect* and was sometimes confused with an ostium primum defect). The limbus may also be hypoplastic superiorly or posteriorly.

Normally the IVC–right atrial junction is partly to the left of the plane of the limbus, so that when the floor of the fossa ovalis is absent and an ASD of fossa ovalis type extends to the IVC, the caval ostium overrides (or straddles) the defect onto the left atrium.[V1] This defect results in some right-to-left shunting of IVC blood to the left atrium in virtually all patients with a large fossa ovalis–type ASD (as documented in experimental studies[K9,M5,S10]) and severe shunting with cyanosis in a few patients.[W5] Also, the position of the normally connected right pulmonary veins next to the atrial septal remnant results in preferential left-to-right shunting of their venous drainage.[B12,S10]

Posterior Defect

A defect in the most posterior and inferior part of the atrial septum, with absence, hypoplasia, or anterior displacement of the posterior limbus, is termed a *posterior ASD*. The orifices of the right pulmonary veins usually open directly into the area of the defect, but true anomalous pulmonary venous connection of the right lung frequently coexists. In the pure form of this type of ASD, the tissue of the fossa ovalis (including the posterior limbus) is present, and the ASD is an oval defect posterior to this tissue (Fig. 30-4).

Sinus Venosus Defect

The ASD that occurs in sinus venosus syndrome (subcaval defect, superior vena caval defect) is located immediately beneath the orifice of the superior vena cava (SVC), superior to the limbic tissue, and is usually associated with anomalous pulmonary venous connection of the right superior pulmonary vein to the SVC near or at the SVC–right atrial junction. The lower margin of the defect is a sharply defined crescentic edge of atrial septum, whereas its upper margin is devoid of septum, being continuous with the posterior SVC wall, which in turn is continuous with the upper edge of the left atrium. The SVC usually overrides the atrial septum onto the left atrium to some extent (see "Sinus Venosus Malformation [Syndrome]" later in this chapter).

Coronary Sinus Defect

Coronary sinus ASDs are part of *unroofed coronary sinus syndrome*. When the sinus is completely unroofed and no partition is present to separate it from the left atrium, the ostium of the coronary sinus is a hole in the atrial septum that permits free communication between left and right atria (see Chapter 33). Occasionally a fenestration may exist in this partition in the midportion of the coronary sinus, particularly in hearts with tricuspid atresia, or rarely the fenestration may be almost at the ostium of the coronary sinus[R9] (Fig. 30-5).

Confluent Defect

Large ASDs may represent a confluence of two of the defects already described. Thus, a fossa ovalis defect coexisting with absence of the posterior limbus can present as a very large ASD with no septal remnant posteriorly. Another confluent defect occasionally seen is a combination of coronary sinus and fossa ovalis ASDs.

Ostium Primum Defect

An ASD occurs anterior to the fossa ovalis (and the anterior limbus) when the AV septum is absent. Such defects are called *AV septal defects, AV canal defects,* or *ostium primum atrial septal defects* and are considered in Chapter 34. When essentially the entire atrial septum is absent (common atrium), the defect includes absence of the AV septum (see "Atrial Septal Deficiency and Interatrial Communications" under Morphology in Chapter 34).

Types of Partial Anomalous Pulmonary Venous Connection

Sinus Venosus Malformation

The most common type of PAPVC is the defect present in sinus venosus malformation, in which PAPVC coexists with a superior caval ASD. In sinus venosus malformation, the right upper and middle lobe pulmonary veins (right superior pulmonary vein) attach to the low SVC or the SVC–right atrial junction, an arrangement present in about 95% of patients with a superior caval ASD.[C6,L4,S20] Most often, the anomalous pulmonary venous connection is through two anomalous veins from upper and middle lobes, one superior to the other, but there may be three or rarely four veins, with the uppermost entering the SVC near the azygos vein entry. Infrequently, only part of the right superior vein connects anomalously, with the inferior (right middle lobe) portion of that vein connecting to the left atrium. Rarely, both the right superior and right inferior pulmonary veins connect anomalously to the low SVC or SVC–right atrial junction (Fig. 30-6).

The lowermost part of the SVC that receives the anomalous veins is usually wider than normal, although it may be relatively small, particularly when there is also a well-formed left SVC, which is not uncommon.[T6] The SVC typically overrides the atrial septum to some extent and enters partly into

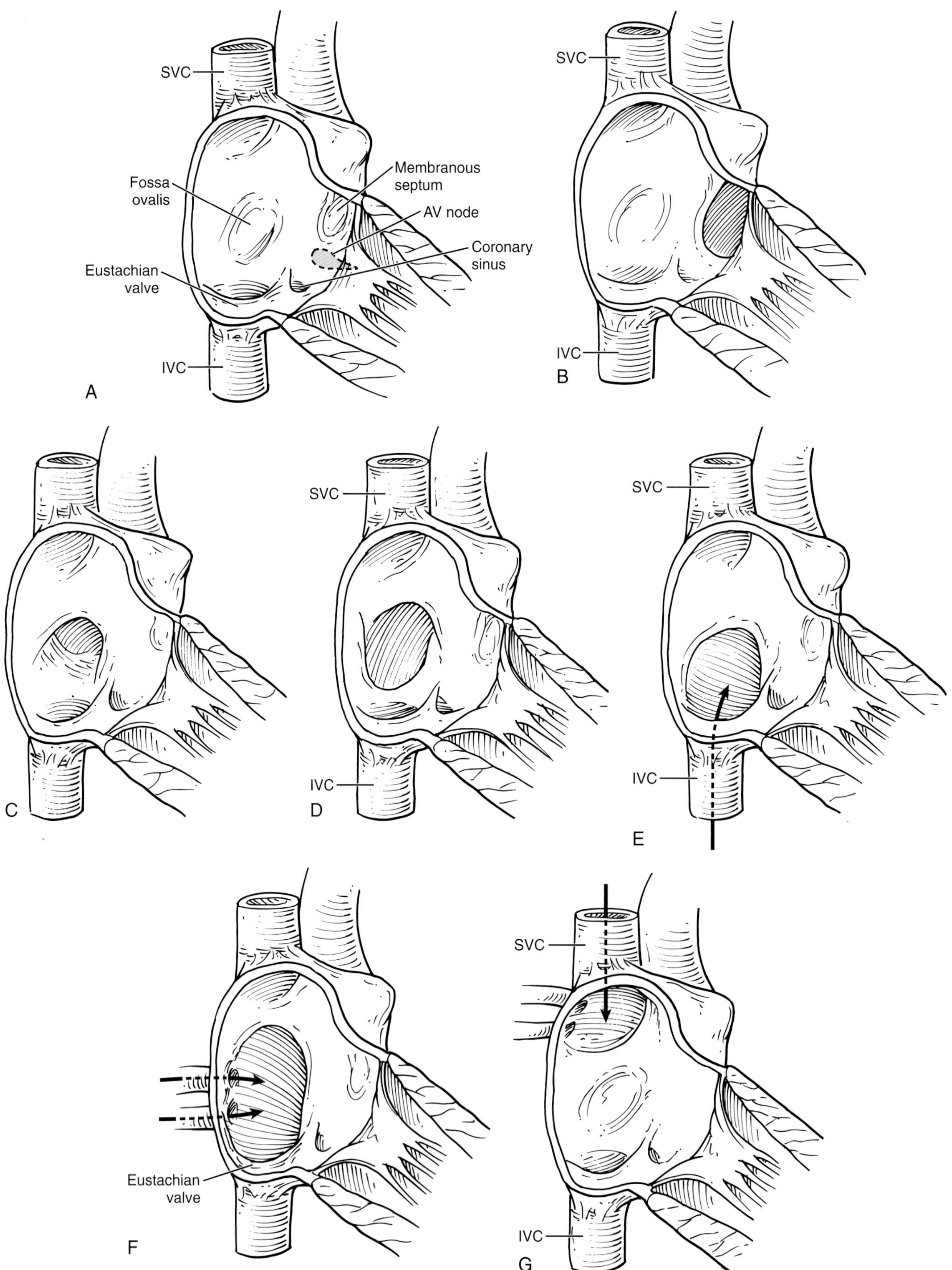

Figure 30-1 Anatomy of atrial septal defect (ASD), viewed from right atrium. **A,** Normal atrial septum. **B,** Atrioventricular (primum) type of ASD. **C,** Widely patent foramen ovale. **D,** Fossa ovalis defect with complete septal rim (secundum). **E,** Low fossa ovalis ASD astride inferior caval orifice with large eustachian valve. **F,** Large fossa ovalis ASD without posterior rim, with pseudoanomalous right pulmonary veins. **G,** Sinus venosus defect. Key: *AV,* Atrioventricular; *IVC,* inferior vena cava; *SVC,* superior vena cava.

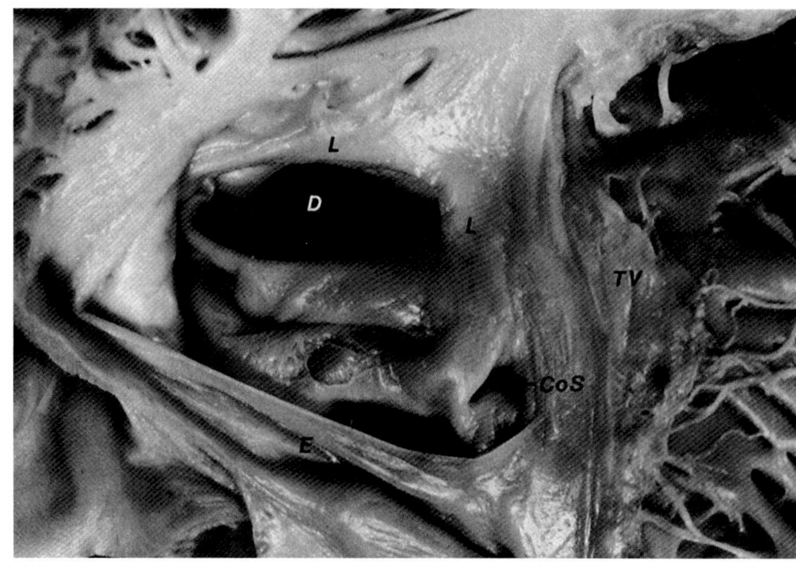

Figure 30-2 Specimen with fossa ovalis atrial septal defect, viewed in anatomic orientation with superior vena cava above and inferior vena cava and its eustachian valve below. Limbus forms anterior, superior, and posterior rim of defect, and remnants of the floor (valve) of fossa ovalis form inferior rim. Key: *CoS,* Coronary sinus; *D,* atrial septal defect; *E,* eustachian valve; *L,* limbus; *TV,* septal leaflet of tricuspid valve.

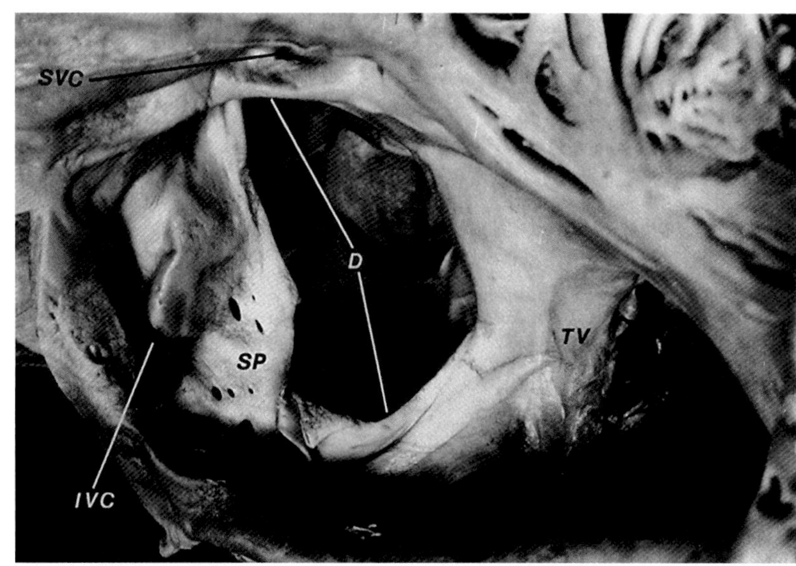

Figure 30-3 Specimen with large fossa ovalis atrial septal defect viewed from opened right atrium in same orientation as Fig. 30-2. Thin remnant of septum primum (floor of fossa ovalis) shows numerous perforations. Key: *D,* Atrial septal defect; *IVC,* inferior vena cava; *SP,* septum primum; *SVC,* superior vena cava; *TV,* tricuspid valve.

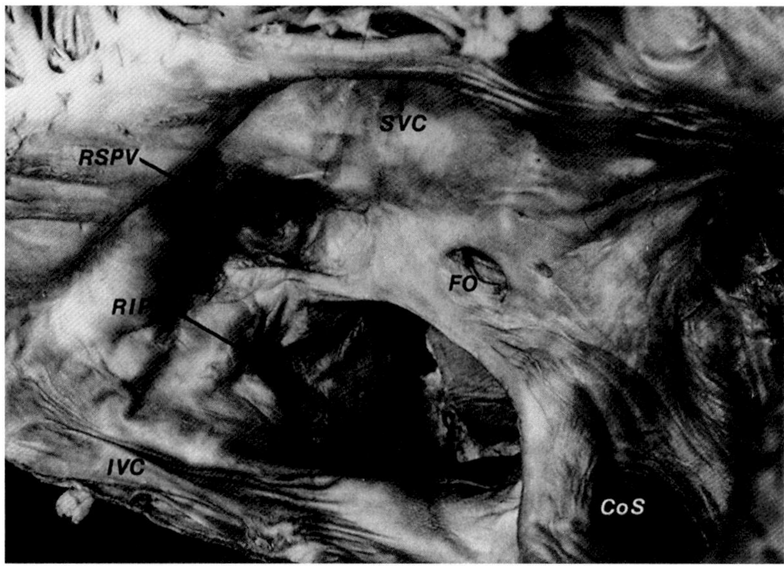

Figure 30-4 Specimen with large posterior atrial septal defect, viewed from opened right atrium. Orientation is as in Fig. 30-2. Fossa ovalis is intact, but there is a patent foramen ovale. Right inferior pulmonary vein certainly drains anomalously, but is probably normally connected. Right superior pulmonary vein is anomalously connected to right atrium. Key: *CoS,* Coronary sinus; *D,* atrial septal defect; *FO,* fossa ovalis; *IVC,* inferior vena cava; *RIPV,* right inferior pulmonary vein; *RSPV,* right superior pulmonary vein; *SVC,* superior vena cava.

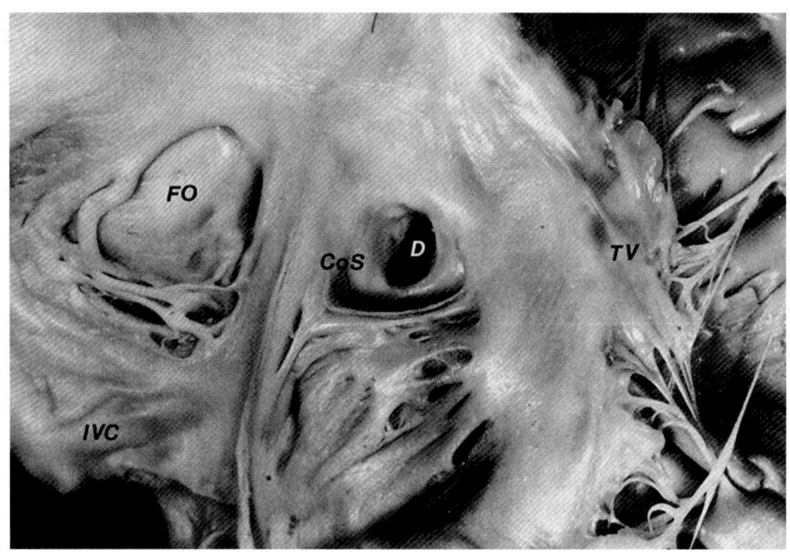

Figure 30-5 Unusual example of small coronary sinus atrial septal defect near ostium. Other anomalies include patent foramen ovale, ventricular septal defect, mild aortic regurgitation, and possible mitral regurgitation. Key: *CoS,* Coronary sinus; *D,* atrial septal defect; *FO,* fossa ovalis; *IVC,* inferior vena cava; *TV,* tricuspid valve.

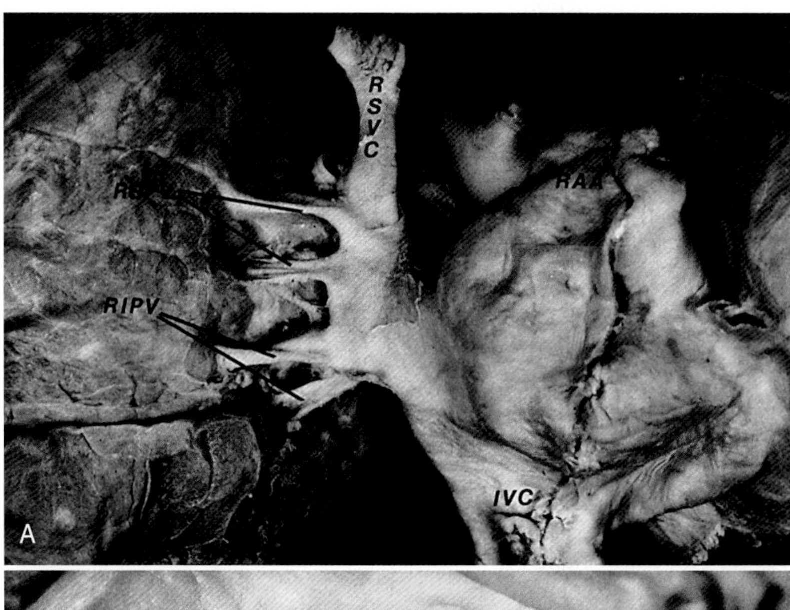

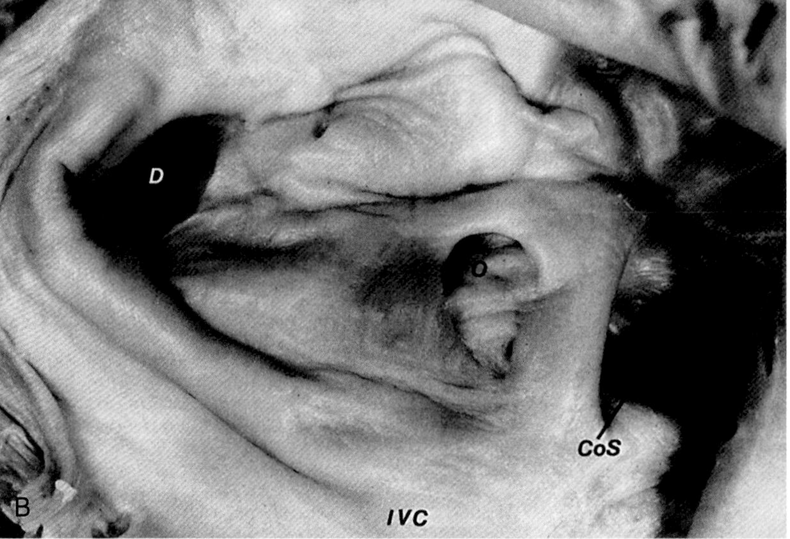

Figure 30-6 Unusual example of sinus venosus malformation. **A,** Specimen with typical subcaval atrial septal defect (ASD), but with both right superior and right inferior pulmonary veins entering superior vena caval–right atrial junction. In addition, the left pulmonary veins form a common channel connected to left atrium and right superior vena cava. Left superior vena cava and mitral atresia were also present. **B,** Interior of right atrium showing the subcaval ASD high in the septum and enlarged coronary sinus ostium to which is connected the left superior vena cava. Key: *CoS,* Coronary sinus; *D,* atrial septal defect; *FO,* fossa ovalis; *IVC,* inferior vena cava; *RAA,* right atrial appendage; *RIPV,* right inferior pulmonary vein; *RSPV,* right superior pulmonary vein; *RSVC,* right superior vena cava.

the left atrium, resulting in a right-to-left shunt of some SVC blood to the left atrium. In a few patients, SVC overriding is severe enough to produce a large right-to-left shunt and marked cyanosis.[S6] The overriding may also be complete, so that the SVC drains directly and completely into the left atrium.[B8,P2]

The relationship between anomalous connection of the SVC to the left atrium without an ASD and sinus venosus ASD is indicated by connection of pulmonary veins from the right upper lobe to the cardiac end of the SVC in some patients with PAPVC.[B14,K9,P2] This relationship also occurs in patients with no ASD but in whom the pulmonary veins from the right upper lobe are connected to the cardiac end of the SVC, with the SVC connected to the left atrium by a large opening, and to the right atrium by a small opening.[B8,S6]

Rarely, a typical high superior caval ASD is present without anomalous pulmonary venous connection; right pulmonary veins connect to the left atrium but more superiorly than normal.

Right Superior Pulmonary Vein to Superior Vena Cava

Occasionally the entire right superior pulmonary vein connects to the SVC without an associated superior caval ASD. The connection is then usually well above (superior to) the SVC–right atrial junction, and the lower part of the SVC is not dilated. Rarely, even when no superior caval ASD is present, the connection may be in the typical low position of sinus venosus syndrome. At times, only a *portion* of the right superior pulmonary vein draining one or two segments of the right upper lobe connects directly to the SVC. The PAPVC may be isolated or associated with a fossa ovalis ASD.

Right Pulmonary Veins to Right Atrium

Right pulmonary veins may connect directly to the right atrium, either in toto, where they may connect as two or three separate veins, or only through the superior (or rarely inferior) right pulmonary vein. This anomaly may exist as an isolated defect, without an ASD or with only a patent foramen ovale, with the plane of the atrial septum altered from coronal to near-sagittal because of leftward displacement of its lateral attachment. The plane of the right pulmonary vein is actually altered minimally from normal. Because the posterior limbus is present in such defects, the veins are clearly anomalously connected to the right atrium. In ASDs with absence of posterior limbus (posterior ASD), and at times in large fossa ovalis ASDs, the plane of division between right and left atria posteriorly can be questionable, and thus the atrial connection of the right pulmonary veins in this area is debatable. In such defects, however, true anomalous connection of the right pulmonary veins may be present[M6,S19] (see Fig. 30-4).

Right Pulmonary Veins to Inferior Vena Cava (Scimitar Syndrome)

An anomalous right pulmonary vein, generally draining the entire right lung but occasionally only the middle and lower lobes, may descend in a cephalad-to-caudad direction toward the diaphragm, more or less parallel to the pericardial border but with a crescentic (scimitar) shape, and then curve sharply to the left just above or below the IVC–right atrial junction.[K3] The anomalous pulmonary venous trunk usually passes anterior to the hilum of the right lung but occasionally is posterior to it. Entrance into the IVC is just superior to the hepatic vein orifices. The atrial septum may be intact, or a fossa ovalis ASD may be present. Occasionally the anomalous vein also connects to *left* atrium,[G5,M11] and rarely scimitar syndrome can exist with connection of the anomalous vein *only* to left atrium.[M13] Pulmonary venous *drainage* is then normal. (Rarely, the left lung may connect via a scimitar-shaped vein to the IVC.[D1,M2])

Right-sided scimitar syndrome occurs as an isolated malformation in a minority of cases. In most patients, anomalies of the right lung are also present.[N1] The most common anomaly is *right lung hypoplasia,* which is associated with a marked mediastinal shift and dextroposition of the heart, and in its severe form with the entire heart lying in the right side of the chest. Blood supply to the hypoplastic right lung comes mainly from a branch of the abdominal aorta in the region of the celiac axis, which ascends through the inferior pulmonary ligament to supply the lower lobe, or more often the entire right lung. A small pulmonary artery may be present, but often the central and hilar portions of the right pulmonary artery are absent. Occasionally a true right lower lobe bronchopulmonary sequestration may exist, with secondary intrapulmonary cyst formation.

Associated cardiac anomalies are often present in scimitar syndrome. In one study, for example, 11 of 13 infants had associated malformations, seven of whom had left-sided hypoplastic conditions.[G2] Diaphragmatic anomalies occurred in about 20% of the cases reviewed by Kiely and colleagues.[K3] These defects included herniation of the right lung through the foramen of Bochdalek and abnormal attachments of the diaphragm.

Rare Connections of Right Pulmonary Veins

Rarely, right pulmonary veins connect anomalously to the azygos vein or coronary sinus, with or without a fossa ovalis ASD.

Left Pulmonary Venous Connections

Left pulmonary veins may connect to the left brachiocephalic vein by way of an anomalous vertical vein.[S11] Anomalous drainage is usually from the entire left lung, but may be only from the left upper lobe.[B15] A fossa ovalis ASD coexists in some patients, and in others the atrial septum is intact.[H7] Rarely, left pulmonary veins connect anomalously to the coronary sinus, a right-sided SVC, or the right atrium.

Bilateral Partial Pulmonary Venous Connection

Partial but bilateral anomalous pulmonary venous connection is rare. The most common variant is probably the defect in which the atrial septum is intact, the left superior pulmonary vein attaches to the left brachiocephalic vein by way of an anomalous vertical vein, and the right superior pulmonary vein attaches to the SVC–right atrial junction. In another form, a common pulmonary venous chamber is present (see "Pulmonary Venous Anatomy" under Morphology in Chapter 31 for definition), and some veins from both lungs connect to it. All but one lobe or only one lobe from each side may connect to the sinus. The common venous sinus may connect to the right atrium or brachiocephalic vein.

Cardiac Chambers in Atrial Septal Defect and Related Conditions

Typically in ASD and related conditions, the right atrium is greatly enlarged (at least grade 3 or 4 on a scale of 1 to 6) and thick walled. The left atrium is not enlarged. This discrepancy occurs in the absence of any flow or pressure restriction between the two, speculatively because the right atrial wall is more distensible than the left.

Right ventricular (RV) diastolic size is increased, often greatly, because of volume overload imposed by the left-to-right shunt. Whereas normal RV diastolic dimensions are between 0.6 and 1.4 cm · m^2, in patients with large left-to-right shunts at atrial level they average 2.66 cm · m^2 and may be as large as 4 cm · m^2.[P3] Consequently, the cardiac apex is often formed by the RV.

Morphologically, the left ventricle (LV) is normal or slightly decreased in size. However, important LV dynamic abnormalities are present in most patients (see "Mitral Prolapse").

Mitral Valve and Atrial Septal Defects

Mitral Prolapse

Mitral valve prolapse occurs in association with fossa ovalis ASD, sinus venosus syndrome,[T6] and probably other types of ASDs and related conditions that result in left-to-right shunts at the atrial level. Prevalence of true prolapse is about 20%,[L2] increasing with age and with magnitude of the pulmonary-to-systemic blood flow ratio ($\dot{Q}p/\dot{Q}s$).[L2,S3]

Schreiber and colleagues have clarified a previously confused subject by relating mitral valve prolapse to abnormalities of LV shape[S3] in patients with ASD.[L3,L9,W3] Alteration in LV configuration results from leftward shift of the ventricular septum, a process that begins as a slight decrease in the normal rightward convexity and progresses with time to flattening and then reversal, with a resultant central bulge into the LV. This process is a response to RV enlargement, which is secondary to volume overload. This etiologic basis of mitral valve prolapse is supported by its decreased degree or elimination in most cases by ASD closure, with return of LV geometry to normal.[A5,S3]

Mitral Regurgitation

Mitral prolapse in ASD can lead to mitral regurgitation, as does ordinary mitral prolapse. True prevalence of regurgitation in unselected patients varies because older patients and those with larger pulmonary blood flows have a higher prevalence of this abnormality and prolapse. Prevalence of mitral regurgitation severe enough to require correction at the time of ASD repair is about 5% or less. The data of Leachman and colleagues strongly suggest that this type of mitral prolapse can also precipitate chordal rupture, as it can in Barlow syndrome.[L2]

Cleft Mitral Leaflets

Cleft anterior or posterior mitral leaflets that cause mitral regurgitation are reported to occur occasionally in patients with ASD.[D4,G10,H3] However, judging from some of the illustrations of such "clefts," they may simply be *spaces* between commissural and main leaflets in prolapsed valves.

Lungs and Pulmonary Vasculature

Pulmonary arteries are considerably dilated and elongated when pulmonary blood flow is increased. This dilatation involves even the smallest branches, which tend to compress the smaller airways, with resultant retention of secretions and bronchiolitis.

Hypertensive pulmonary vascular disease develops infrequently in patients with ASD, and then usually not until the third or fourth decade of life (see "Pulmonary Vascular Disease" under Morphology in Section I of Chapter 35). This contrasts sharply with ventricular septal defects (VSDs), complete AV septal defects, and patent ductus arteriosus, in which pulmonary vascular disease may be present early in life. In ASD, pulmonary vascular disease is caused mainly by secondary thrombosis in the dilated pulmonary artery branches, with changes in the intima and media of vessels usually playing a minor role. Haworth has suggested, however, that an increase in pulmonary arterial smooth muscle may be the only finding.[H6]

Associated Cardiac Conditions

ASDs and related conditions may coexist with almost all varieties of congenital heart disease, but such cases are not considered here unless the left-to-right shunt at atrial level is the dominant hemodynamic lesion. A wide spectrum of cardiac anomalies coexist with ASD as the dominant lesion (Table 30-1).

Valvar heart disease may coexist with hemodynamically important ASDs. Six cases with moderate or severe rheumatic mitral stenosis and a hemodynamically significant ASD (Lutembacher syndrome) were observed among 443 patients with an ASD at GLH (1957-1983). Eleven cases of moderate or severe mitral regurgitation were observed; in three, regurgitation was rheumatic in origin. Both mitral stenosis and regurgitation increase left-to-right shunting.

Tricuspid regurgitation of variable severity frequently complicates ASDs in older patients with heart failure, the mechanism generally being RV and tricuspid anular dilatation.

Related Conditions

Rarely, ASD may occur in patients with Marfan, Turner, Noonan, or Holt-Oram syndromes.

Table 30-1 Associated Cardiac Anomalies in Patients with Atrial Septal Defect or Partial Anomalous Pulmonary Venous Connection[a]

Anomaly	No.	% of 443
Left superior vena cava	24	5
Mild or moderate pulmonary artery stenosis	16	4
Peripheral pulmonary artery stenosis	4	1
Azygos extension of inferior vena cava	4	1
Small ventricular septal defect	2	0.01
Small patent ductus arteriosus	2	0.01
Mild coarctation of aorta	2	0.01
Small coronary artery–pulmonary trunk fistula	2	0.01
Anomalous right subclavian artery	2	0.01
Dextrocardia (isolated)	1	0.005

[a]Data from 443 patients undergoing repair at GLH from 1957 to 1983. Some patients had more than one anomaly, so the figures are not cumulative.

CLINICAL FEATURES AND DIAGNOSTIC CRITERIA

Symptoms, clinical features, and signs in ASD and related conditions producing left-to-right shunting at the atrial level are related largely to size of the left-to-right shunt. Thus, in general, when $\dot{Q}p/\dot{Q}s$ is less than 1.5, there are neither signs nor symptoms of the shunt, and this is often true with a $\dot{Q}p/\dot{Q}s$ up to 1.8. When $\dot{Q}p/\dot{Q}s$ is larger than this, signs of the shunt are usually present, and symptoms appear eventually (see "Changes in Pulmonary/Systemic Blood Flow Over Time" later under Natural History). Infants present an exception to these generalizations. Their clinical features are often atypical; for example, splitting of the second heart sound is unrelated to $\dot{Q}p/\dot{Q}s$.[H9]

Determinants of Interatrial Shunting

Left-to-right shunting across a nonrestrictive (>2 cm in an adult) ASD under ordinary circumstances is a function of the relative compliance (reflected in the diastolic pressures) of RVs and LVs. RV compliance in particular is unpredictable and is one factor causing variability in $\dot{Q}p/\dot{Q}s$. A compliant distensible RV (in association with a normal pulmonary vascular bed) will permit a large shunt; a less compliant one (such as may result from pulmonary hypertension or from morphologic RV changes occurring later in life[J1,P4]) permits a more modest shunt. LV compliance tends to decrease with age, which tends to increase $\dot{Q}p/\dot{Q}s$ as patients become older. Shunting is increased by systemic hypertension when this results in decreased LV compliance.

Mitral regurgitation or stenosis increases $\dot{Q}p/\dot{Q}s$. When the ASD is small and flow is restrictive, left-to-right shunting is limited. Even then, mitral stenosis may elevate left atrial pressure sufficiently that a large left-to-right shunt through all phases of the cardiac cycle results, leading to a soft continuous murmur.

Symptoms

Symptoms may be absent for several decades, but when they occur, they consist of effort breathlessness and a tendency toward recurrent respiratory tract infections. Palpitation from paroxysmal atrial tachycardia or atrial fibrillation may occur later in life. Older adults may present with chronic heart failure with fluid retention, hepatomegaly, and severe cardiac cachexia. Occasionally an infant with ASD and a large left-to-right shunt, often in association with PAPVC, may have heart failure with tachypnea, but this is uncommon. In such infants, other associated malformations may contribute to the heart failure.

Atypical presentations occur. Rarely, an unequivocal history of cyanosis may bring a patient with an uncomplicated ASD to medical attention.[J1,M14,M15] For example, a large fossa ovalis ASD extending to the IVC may cause streaming of blood from the IVC into the left atrium, with resultant cyanosis. This coincides with occasional bidirectional shunting in patients with otherwise uncomplicated ASDs,[G1] usually older patients.[G1] For the same anatomic reasons (see Morphology, earlier), patients may present with paradoxical emboli or cerebral infarctions. This presentation occurred in 9 (2%) of a Mayo Clinic series of 546 patients.[R1] Infrequently the presentation may be modified by presence of severe pulmonary hypertension, in which case cyanosis, effort intolerance, and hemoptysis may be present.

Signs

Clinical signs diagnostic of a large shunt at the atrial level ($\dot{Q}p/\dot{Q}s$ > 1.8 to 2.0) are:

- Overactive left parasternal systolic lift
- Fixed splitting of the second heart sound throughout the respiratory cycle (absent when large $\dot{Q}p/\dot{Q}s$ is from PAPVC with an intact atrial septum)
- A soft pulmonary midsystolic flow murmur (in second and third left intercostal spaces)
- A mid-diastolic tricuspid flow murmur (in fourth and fifth left intercostal spaces) present in borderline situations only on inspiration

This last sign is occasionally absent, however, particularly in older patients and in those with a larger shunt.

In addition, an extremely large shunt produces a more marked left-sided precordial RV lift, occasionally some prominence of the left anterior chest wall, and leftward displacement of the cardiac apex. Many such patients are short and thin. When heart failure is present, jugular venous pressure is elevated, the liver is enlarged, and there is gross cardiomegaly.

Tricuspid regurgitation produces systolic liver pulsation and a greater tendency to ascites and peripheral edema. Important pulmonary hypertension is evident clinically by accentuation of the second heart sound and a more marked RV and pulmonary artery lift. A pulmonary regurgitation murmur may be heard, as well as a murmur of tricuspid regurgitation.

Chest Radiography

Chest radiography reflects the large $\dot{Q}p/\dot{Q}s$. The right atrium and right ventricle are large. The pulmonary trunk shadow in the upper left portion of the cardiac silhouette is enlarged, and right and left pulmonary arteries are enlarged to the periphery of the lung field. In general, pulmonary vascular markings are increased, or plethoric. The shadow of the transverse aortic arch is abnormally small. Patients with heart failure may have interstitial pulmonary edema and areas of pulmonary consolidation and atelectasis. These signs are probably secondary to compression of smaller airways by enormously enlarged small pulmonary vessels.

The chest radiograph may suggest the specific anatomic diagnosis. Occasionally the right superior pulmonary vein can be identified lying more superiorly than normal (Fig. 30-7), leading to suspicion of sinus venosus syndrome. A crescentic shadow more or less parallel to the right-sided heart border (Fig. 30-8) suggests the diagnosis of anomalous pulmonary venous connection of right pulmonary veins to IVC (scimitar syndrome).

Electrocardiography

Electrocardiogram (ECG) almost always shows the pattern of incomplete right bundle branch block and a clockwise frontal loop. Left axis deviation and a counterclockwise loop strongly suggest an AV septal defect, although this pattern occurs in about 10% of patients with fossa ovalis ASDs.

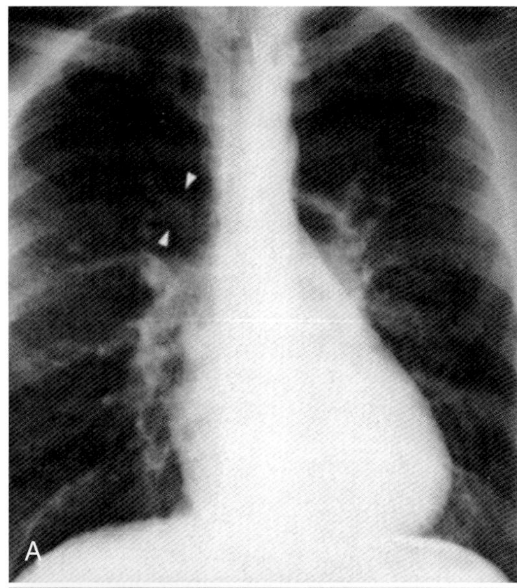

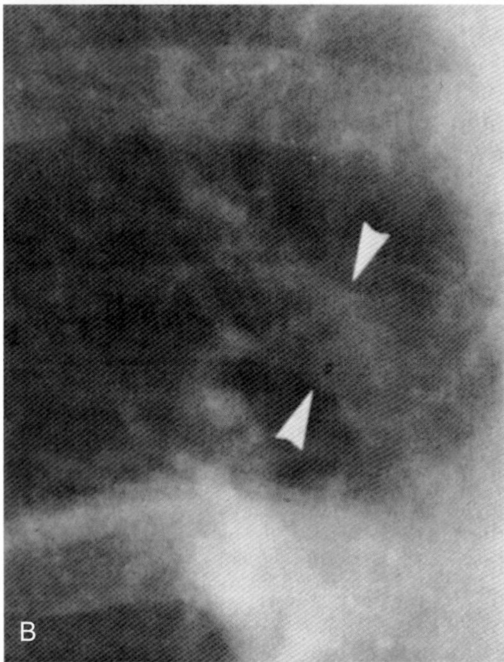

Figure 30-7 Chest radiograph of sinus venosus malformation. **A,** Usual view. **B,** Magnification copy. Arrowheads indicate right superior pulmonary vein.

Echocardiography

Clinical diagnosis of ASD, particularly of the foramen ovale type, can be confirmed by visualizing the defect directly using two-dimensional echocardiography[F4,L9,S7] (Fig. 30-9). Echocardiography also gives indirect evidence of ASD in demonstrating RV volume overload, which includes increased RV diastolic size and abnormal (flat or paradoxical) septal motion.[M9,T1] However, two-dimensional echocardiography has been unreliable (<75% sensitivity) in detecting anomalous connection of right pulmonary veins to SVC. More often these sinus venosus defects can be detected by *transesophageal echocardiography* (TEE). TEE also can localize fossa ovalis defects to the high, low, or posterior septum. AV septal defects can be separated from secundum defects, and localization of subcaval defects and anomalous pulmonary venous connection is usually possible. Addition of Doppler color flow interrogation allows a reasonable estimate of $\dot{Q}p/\dot{Q}s$.

Magnetic Resonance Imaging

Limitations of echocardiography in delineating anomalous pulmonary venous connection can be largely overcome with magnetic resonance imaging (MRI). Anatomic detailing of pulmonary venous connection and calculation of $\dot{Q}p/\dot{Q}s$ are generally reproducible.[D5,F1,R4]

Cardiac Catheterization and Cineangiography

When diagnosis of a typical and apparently uncomplicated ASD has been made by noninvasive methods in children, adolescents, and young adults, cardiac catheterization is not required.[S8] The surgeon then becomes responsible for confirming the type of ASD at operation and presence or absence of any anomalous pulmonary venous connections. Cardiac catheterization and appropriate cineangiography are indicated in infants (because of possible associated anomalies), in many adults (for assessing possible pulmonary hypertension and status of mitral valve), and in any patient in whom noninvasive tests suggest PAPVC. Coronary angiography is performed in patients older than 35 to 40 years.

Assessment of operability in patients with pulmonary hypertension is particularly challenging. Even in Eisenmenger syndrome with shunt reversal at atrial level, pulmonary artery pressure (PPA) is rarely more than two thirds that of systemic pressure. (There is no transmission of systemic pressure across the defect, as is the case with large defects at ventricular or ductus levels; see "Cardiac Catheterization" under Clinical Features and Diagnostic Criteria in Chapter 35.)

The most reliable criterion of inoperability is the absolute level of pulmonary vascular resistance normalized to body surface area (RpI) and calculated when possible using measured, rather than assumed, oxygen uptake.[N6] $\dot{Q}p/\dot{Q}s$ or resistance ratios are much less discriminating. In fact, precise criteria have not been established as accurately for ASD as for VSD. Using VSD criteria (with no reason to believe these are not equally applicable to ASD), a resting RpI of 8 U · m^2 or more may preclude complete operative closure. In this event, RpI must also be calculated while using a pulmonary vasodilator (isoproterenol,[N6] tolazoline,[M12] or 100% oxygen[M4]).

If arterial desaturation (<97%) exists when measured by the usual finger sensor, cardiac catheterization is indicated in both adults and children. Interventions such as 100% O_2, exercise, and nitric oxide (NO) are appropriate to gauge pulmonary vascular reactivity, response of pulmonary vascular resistance, and reversion to a strictly left-to-right shunt condition. If arterial oxygen saturation (SaO_2) increases to normal levels and pulmonary vascular resistance falls, operation can be done even in the presence of intermittent arterial desaturation (right-to-left shunt).

A vasodilator must produce a fall in RpI to below 7 U · m^2 before the patient can be considered operable,[M12,N6] because only then can pulmonary vascular disease be expected to regress. Otherwise, disease is likely to progress despite closure of the ASD. Progressive pulmonary vascular disease is less well tolerated when the atrial septum is intact, because the right side of the heart is then unable to decompress

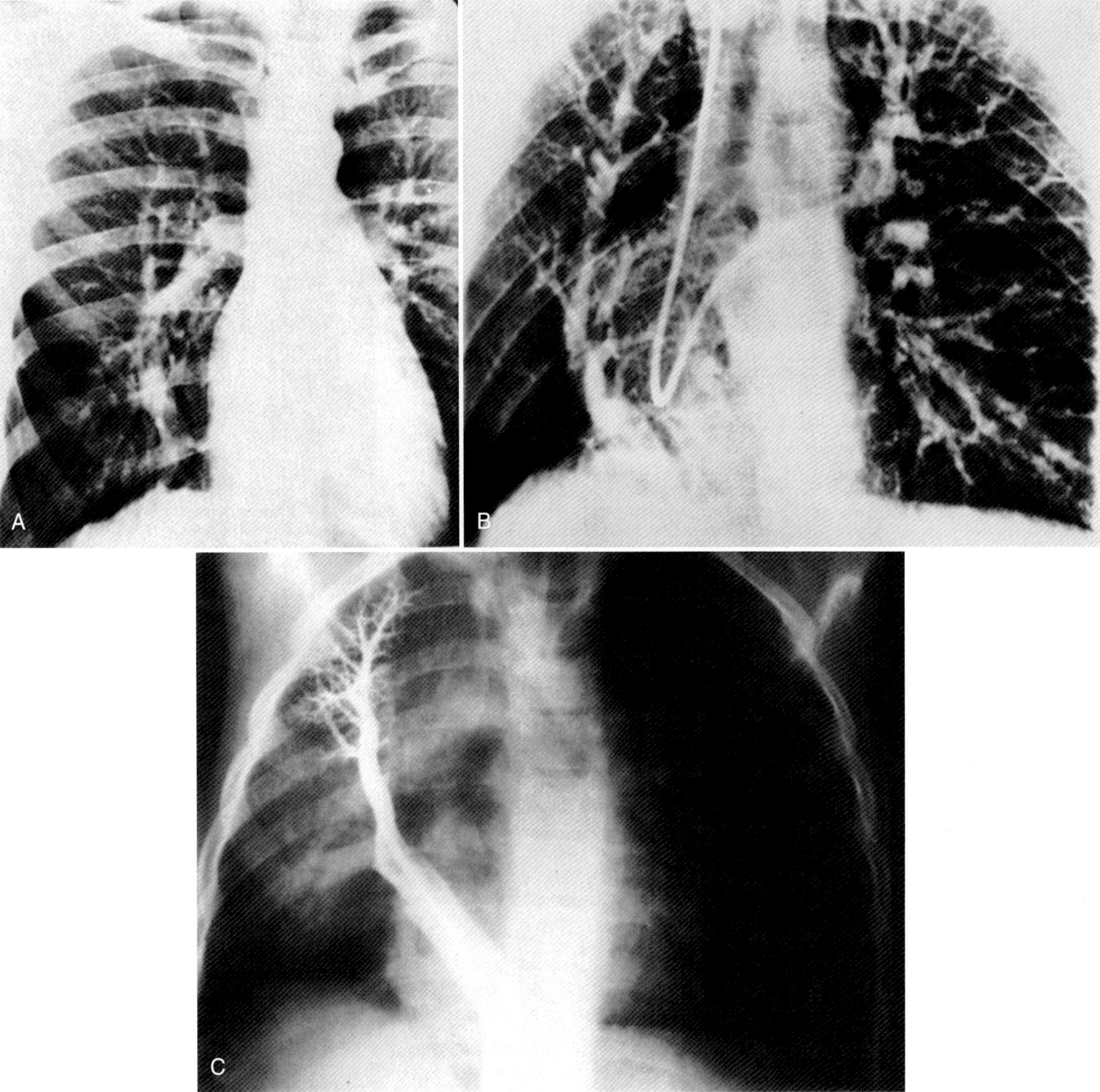

Figure 30-8 Partial anomalous pulmonary venous connection of right pulmonary veins to inferior vena cava in patient with scimitar syndrome. **A,** Plain chest radiograph, frontal view, showing crescentic shadow of anomalous pulmonary vein. **B,** Levophase of pulmonary angiogram showing anomalous pulmonary vein draining into inferior vena cava. **C,** Selective angiogram into anomalous pulmonary vein.

through a right-to-left shunt at atrial level; thus, ASD closure under such circumstances usually decreases life expectancy.

Cardiac catheterization and angiography are also useful in defining anatomic details of related conditions that can cause shunting at the atrial level. Increased SaO_2 in the low SVC provides presumptive evidence of sinus venosus syndrome, and this becomes virtually certain if the catheter can be passed through a subcaval ASD into the left atrium. An indicator dilution curve obtained after injecting dye into the SVC may show some right-to-left shunting, which is generally completely absent in patients with a fossa ovalis ASD (who may have right-to-left shunting from the IVC). In addition, curves obtained after injection into the right pulmonary artery generally show a much larger left-to-right shunt, a result of the anomalously draining right pulmonary veins, than curves obtained after injection into the left pulmonary artery.

Identification of the specific anatomic details of sinus venosus syndrome is best accomplished by angiography after right pulmonary artery injection, because the typical location and drainage of the right superior pulmonary vein can then be seen. Pulmonary artery injection may confirm anomalous connection of the right pulmonary veins to the right atrium or IVC (see Fig. 30-8), of left veins to brachiocephalic or other veins, or of bilateral anomalous pulmonary venous connections. When anomalous connection of the right pulmonary veins to the IVC is demonstrated, *aortography* should

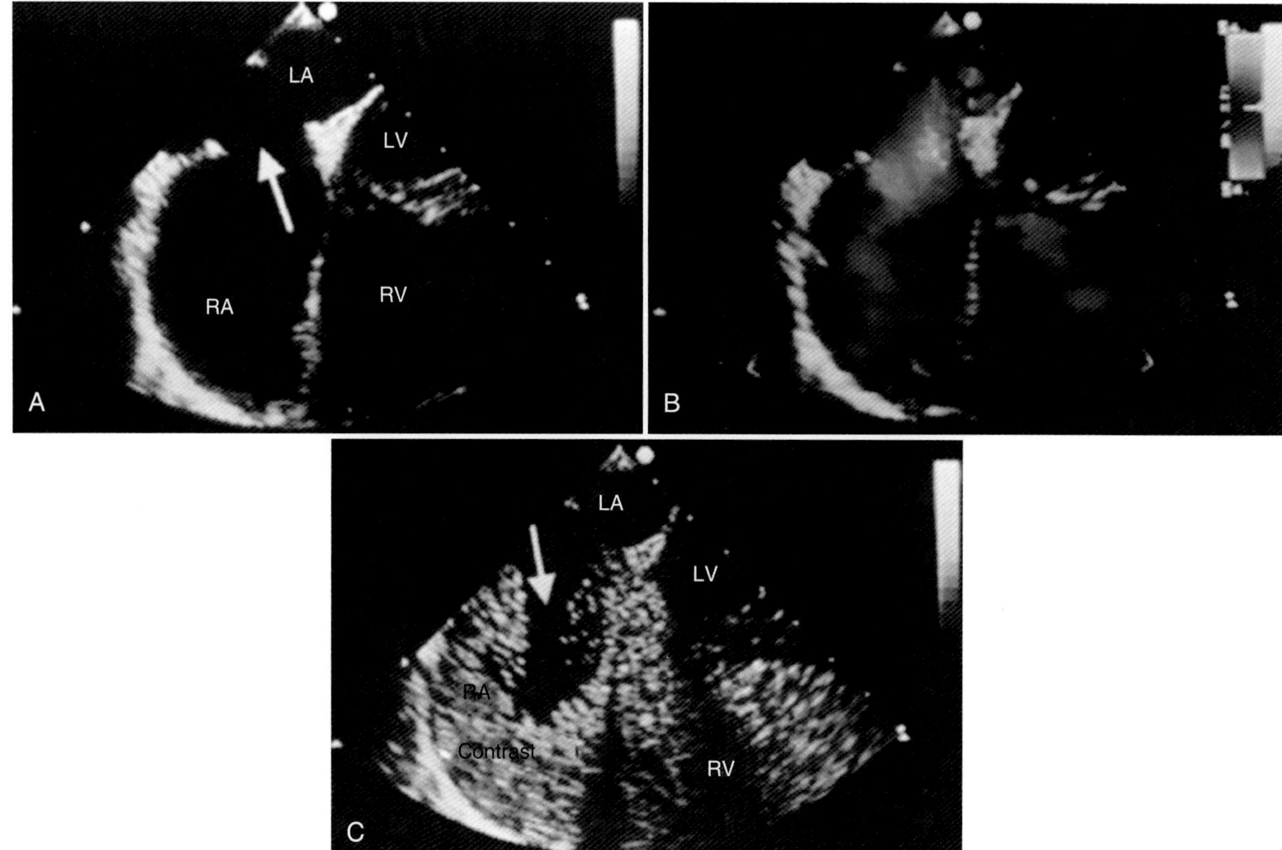

Figure 30-9 Transesophageal echocardiogram of fossa ovalis atrial septal defect. **A,** Arrow indicates dropout of atrial septum with clear evidence of tissue superiorly and inferiorly (above atrioventricular valves), diagnostic of fossa ovalis (secundum) defect. **B,** Blood flow is directed through the defect left to right from left to right atrium. **C,** Negative image of left-to-right flow during injection of saline (as contrast). Key: *LA,* left atrium; *LV,* left ventricle; *RA,* right atrium; *RV,* right ventricle. (From Lang and Marcus.[L1])

also be done to identify any anomalous systemic arteries from the abdominal or thoracic aorta to the right lower lobe. If the right lung is small, if the right lower lobe is contracted or seems otherwise abnormal on chest radiography, or if the patient gives a history of hemoptysis or recurrent pulmonary infections, *bronchoscopy* or *bronchography* is also indicated.

Calculations of $\dot{Q}p/\dot{Q}s$ are of particular importance in patients with isolated PAPVC of only part of one lung. An operation is not indicated when the ratio is less than 1.8 (see Indications for Operation later in this chapter). This approach is especially relevant with isolated connection of some of the right upper lobe veins to the high SVC, because diversion or transfer to the left atrium is quite difficult (and probably needless). Even when only the right superior pulmonary vein is involved and the atrial septum is intact, the shunt may be greater than this, presumably because right atrial and caval pressures are distinctly lower than left atrial pressures, producing a larger-than-usual pulmonary venous gradient.[H5]

NATURAL HISTORY

The natural history of persons born with ASDs and related conditions producing left-to-right shunts at atrial level is not known precisely, but its general characteristics have been described.[C1,C7]

Survival

In 1970, Campbell published the most detailed study available on survival of patients with ASD treated nonsurgically.[C1] Transformation of these findings into conventional survival format and comparison with life expectancy of the general population provide good insight into the life expectancy of patients with ASD (Fig. 30-10). Campbell's data support the idea that only 0.1% of individuals born with a large ASD and no other important cardiac anomaly die in infancy, and that few who are unrepaired die in the first or second decade. About 5% to 15% die in the third decade, usually with pulmonary hypertension and Eisenmenger syndrome.[C7] Premature late death with heart failure occurs in an increasing proportion after the fifth decade. Even so, probably no more than 25% of persons born with a large ASD die from the defect, because lethal manifestations of the disease tend to occur so late in life that other unrelated conditions cause death first.

The natural history of patients with sinus venosus syndrome[H7] and most other types of PAPVC and ASD[B1,S1] is similar to that of patients with large fossa ovalis ASD. Patients with sinus venosus syndrome in the fourth to sixth decades present with heart failure or severe pulmonary hypertension from pulmonary vascular disease. The natural history of scimitar syndrome is not clear. Presumably, patients

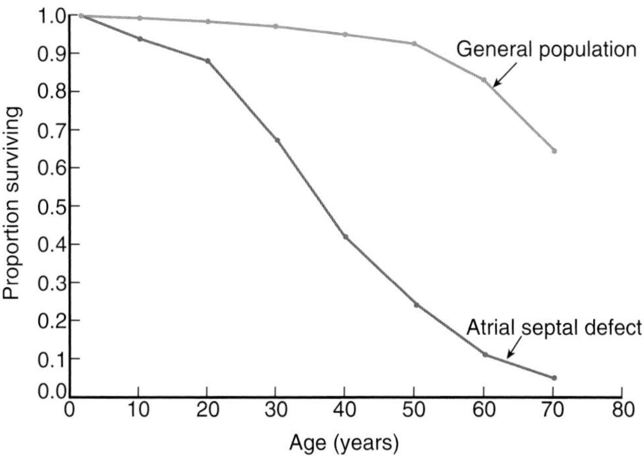

Figure 30-10 Plot of Campbell's survival computations of life expectancy for surgically untreated patients with atrial septal defects (ASD) who reach age 1 year, based on three sets of collected data. Spread among the data sets indicates confidence limits of modest width around point estimates (confidence limits cannot be calculated from data). Life expectancy of the general population at age 1 year is also from Campbell and is close to that computed from U.S. life tables. Data suggest that 99.9% of patients born with ASD reach the first year of life unless unrelated conditions cause their death. (From Campbell.[C1])

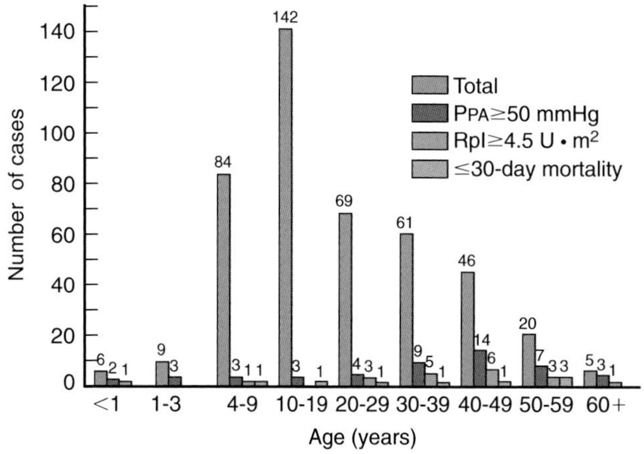

Figure 30-11 Histogram showing frequency of pulmonary hypertension and increased pulmonary vascular resistance in a series of surgically treated patients with atrial septal defects (data set is same as in Table 30-1). Of these patients, 372 were catheterized, and in the remaining 71, pulmonary artery systolic pressure was assumed to be less than 50 mmHg and Rpl less than 4.5 U · m^2. Key: *PPA,* Pulmonary artery systolic pressure, *Rpl,* pulmonary vascular resistance index.

without important anomalies of the right lung and with a large left-to-right shunt have a life history similar to patients with a large fossa ovalis ASD. Those with right lung hypoplasia, however, often have a life history dominated by their pulmonary pathology, including hemoptysis and recurrent pulmonary infections. When there is isolated PAPVC of part of one lung and $\dot{Q}p/\dot{Q}s$ is less than 1.8, life expectancy may be normal. Rarely, paradoxical emboli occur in patients with sinus venosus syndrome (from SVC) as well as in those with fossa ovalis ASDs (from IVC).

Pulmonary Hypertension

In a UAB surgical series, 14% of patients catheterized had pulmonary hypertension with mean PPA greater than 25 mmHg. In a GLH surgical series, systolic PPA was greater than 50 mmHg in 13% of catheterized patients and 11% of the total series (Fig. 30-11). Prevalence of elevated RpI (≥4 U · m^2) was 4.5%, and rare (1%) in patients younger than 20 years of age. In a few high-altitude locations, however, prevalence of pulmonary hypertension is greater. Cherian and colleagues reported that in their region of India, pulmonary hypertension was present in 13% of patients younger than age 10.[C3] Pulmonary hypertension is particularly prevalent in patients with scimitar syndrome, partly due to increased pulmonary blood flow but also to stenosis of the anomalous vein, presence of systemic arterial collaterals to the right lung, or reduction of the pulmonary vascular bed on the right side.[N1]

Functional Status

Probably only about 1% of patients born with a large ASD have symptoms during the first year.[A1,D6,H4,N3,S14] Most are asymptomatic through the first and second decades, although many are short and thin. Effort intolerance and easy fatigability may develop in the second or third decade or as late as the fifth or sixth decade. These symptoms progress gradually to fluid retention, hepatomegaly, and elevated jugular venous pressure, leading to gradually increasing disability. These phenomena are well exemplified in the surgical experience, in which preoperative New York Heart Association (NYHA) functional class and age at operation are moderately well correlated ($r = .61$, $P < .05$) (Table 30-2). When heart failure becomes advanced, both mitral and tricuspid regurgitation are likely to have developed.

Table 30-2 Relationship between New York Heart Association Functional Class and Age at Operation[a]

Preoperative NYHA Class	Age (Years) Mean	Median	Range
I	16	12	3.3-63
II	32	30	4.2-72
III	50	54	0.9-68
IV	51	57	2.2-66

[a]Data from 340 patients undergoing repair of atrial septal defect at UAB, 1967 to 1979.
Key: *NYHA,* New York Heart Association.

Spontaneous Closure

Spontaneous closure of a hemodynamically significant isolated ASD occasionally occurs in the first year.[M18] Cockerham and colleagues found closure in 22% of 87 patients,[C5] and Ghisla and colleagues in 14%.[G7] Smaller left-to-right shunts were present in patients whose defects spontaneously closed than in those whose did not.[C5] Spontaneous closure is uncommon after the first year,[C2,G8,H7,H8,M7,M10] although Ghisla and colleagues found that closure occasionally occurred in the second year.[G7]

Changes in Pulmonary/Systemic Blood Flow Over Time

As already noted, decreasing LV compliance increases $\dot{Q}p/\dot{Q}s$ in patients with ASD, and this may develop during the fifth and sixth decades. Systemic arterial hypertension accelerates this process and may unmask an ASD that was not an important shunt before onset of decreased LV compliance. It is also likely that most ASDs increase in size as time passes; this has been clearly demonstrated in the case of patent foramen ovale.[H2] The direct relationship between $\dot{Q}p/\dot{Q}s$ and the tendency toward mitral valve prolapse also support the concept that the shunt increases with age.[S3] These increases in $\dot{Q}p/\dot{Q}s$ with time do not occur when the shunt is due to anomalous pulmonary venous connection without ASD. $\dot{Q}p/\dot{Q}s$ decreases when pulmonary hypertension develops, a result of decreased RV compliance that accompanies RV hypertrophy (see "Determinants of Interatrial Shunting" under Clinical Features and Diagnostic Criteria).

Right Ventricular Function

RV volume overload and consequent increased RV diastolic dimensions are characteristic of patients with a hemodynamically significant ASD or PAPVC. The ventricular septum is displaced posteriorly and leftward under such circumstances,[W3] but systolic anterior motion of the septum occurs.[H1,P6] These features are well tolerated by the RV for many years, much longer than for the volume-overloaded *left* ventricle and probably longer than for volume overload produced by acute tricuspid or pulmonary valve regurgitation. RV failure eventually occurs, however, with decreased RV ejection fraction and hypokinesia. Doty and colleagues demonstrated loss of coronary reserve in patients with ASD and volume-induced RV hypertrophy,[D8] which contributes further to development of RV failure. Associated signs and symptoms of elevated systemic venous pressure then develop (peripheral edema, elevated jugular venous pressure, hepatomegaly, and finally ascites), often with tricuspid regurgitation.

These RV phenomena have been documented by several studies. Liberthson and colleagues found increased RV volume but normal (64%) ejection fraction in 9 asymptomatic patients with a mean age of 25 years. However, 11 symptomatic patients with a mean age of 52 years had diffuse RV hypokinesia and ejection fraction averaging 36%, in addition to increased RV volume.[L7] In a possibly related finding, adult patients with ASD but without pulmonary hypertension occasionally have marked pulmonary valve regurgitation,[L8] which disappears after ASD repair.

Left Ventricular Function

Most adult patients with hemodynamically significant ASD or PAPVC have normal LV systolic dimensions but subnormal diastolic dimensions.[B11,P6,T2] Some loss of LV functional reserve is present in most adult patients and in some children with ASD. In contrast to normal persons, such individuals do not increase LV ejection fraction during maximal exercise[B11] (Fig. 30-12), although resting ejection fraction is usually within normal limits.[B11,P6] These preoperative LV abnormalities likely result from effects of the volume-overloaded *right* ventricle.[B11] Even in the absence of symptoms of systemic venous hypertension from RV failure, LV structure and function are influenced by increased RV volume rather than changes in LV compliance.[K2,L3,W3]

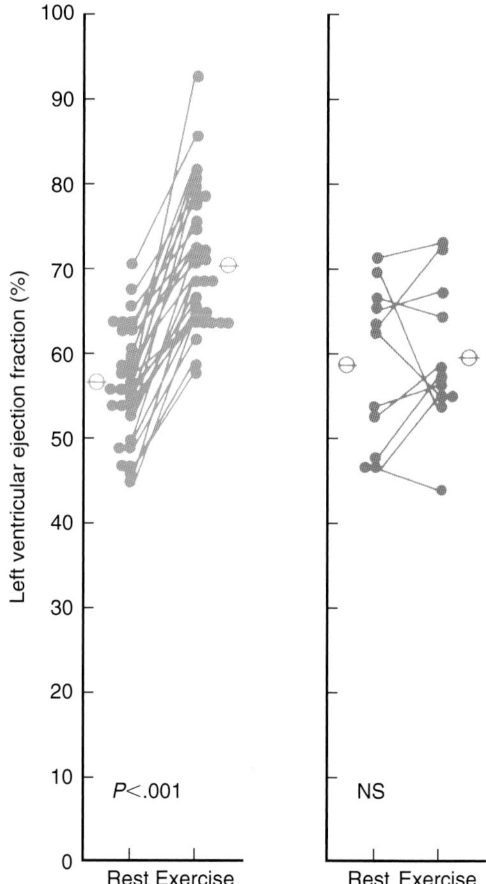

Figure 30-12 *Left,* Normal response of increased left ventricular ejection fraction with maximal exercise. *Right,* In contrast, adult patients with atrial septal defects generally do not increase ejection fraction with maximal exercise. Key: *NS,* Not significant. (From Bonow and colleagues.[B11])

Atrioventricular Valvar Dysfunction

As discussed earlier, important mitral regurgitation is present in 2% to 10% of adults with large ASDs,[H11] and both mitral and tricuspid regurgitation may become prominent in older patients who develop heart failure. When viewed at operation, the tricuspid valve does not appear to be intrinsically abnormal. Presumably, regurgitation develops because of anular dilatation and lack of proper shortening of the tricuspid anulus during systole, secondary to RV enlargement resulting from long-standing volume overload.[T4,T5]

Supraventricular Arrhythmias

After the third decade, supraventricular arrhythmias complicate the natural history of patients with large ASDs and related conditions in increasing numbers over time. Most often this begins with paroxysmal atrial fibrillation, which gradually becomes permanent. Atrial fibrillation was present in 15 (20%; CL 15%-26%) of 75 patients over age 40 operated on by Magilligan and colleagues.[M11] Of 19 patients preoperatively in NYHA class III or IV, 47% (CL 34%-64%) had this arrhythmia, compared with 11% (CL 6%-17%) of 56 patients in class I or II. St. John Sutton and colleagues found that 56% of their patients over age 60 had atrial fibrillation at operation.[S15]

In addition, more subtle abnormalities of conduction system function develop. Benedini and colleagues found concealed sinus node dysfunction in 17 (65%; CL 53%-76%) of 26 adult patients with fossa ovalis ASD, which became evident only with electrophysiologic testing.[B5] Such abnormalities are less common in children with ASDs.[R8]

Systemic Arterial Hypertension

Adult patients with hemodynamically important ASDs are likely to have systemic arterial hypertension. In a Mayo Clinic study, 25 (38%) of 66 patients had systemic arterial blood pressure above 150/90, a higher proportion ($P < .01$) than an age-matched general population.[S15] As noted, this relationship may result partly from the effect of hypertension on shunt size.

TECHNIQUE OF OPERATION

Fossa Ovalis Atrial Septal Defect

Anesthetic management, positioning and preparation of the patient, median sternotomy, and preparations for CPB are discussed in detail in Section III of Chapter 2 and in Chapter 4. An alternative to the midline skin incision may be used for cosmetic reasons; in this approach, a bilateral fourth interspace submammary skin incision is made and a skin flap raised superiorly and inferiorly before the sternum is incised vertically in the usual way. However, some surgeons have expressed concern regarding breast development and symmetry late following right submammary incisions in females. Alternatively, a right anterolateral fifth intercostal space incision may be used if the patient expresses concern about the cosmetic effects of a midline scar. Repair of ASD may also be accomplished using the small lower sternotomy approach and also a small vertical right parasternal incision. Each requires modification of the setup for caval cannulation (see Section III in Chapter 2).

In children and young adults with uncomplicated ASDs, routine placement of a left atrial pressure monitoring catheter is usually unnecessary, but such monitoring should be done routinely in older patients, whose left atrial pressure may be considerably higher than right atrial pressure after repair.

After the incision is made and pericardial stay sutures are placed, intrapericardial anatomy is assessed. The characteristically large right atrium and RV of ASD are noted, as well as the normal-sized left atrium and LV. A left SVC in the fold of Marshall is sought. The external position and connections of the right and left superior and inferior pulmonary veins are noted. Optimally, TEE is available to establish the position of the ASD, relationship of the pulmonary veins, and function of the mitral and tricuspid valves.

The patient is heparinized and arterial cannula inserted. Direct caval cannulation with two angled cannulae is generally employed. CPB is established, with the perfusate temperature at 34°C. The cardioplegic needle or aortic root catheter is now placed in the ascending aorta, the aorta clamped, and cold cardioplegic solution injected. Rewarming of the patient with the perfusate is begun once the heart is cold and isolated. The caval tapes are "snugged," and the right atrium is opened obliquely (Fig. 30-13). A left atrial suction catheter is *not* inserted through the left atrial wall in fossa ovalis ASD, because it is unnecessary and imposes a remote risk of cerebral air embolism.

A few fine stay sutures are placed on the edges of the atriotomy incision. Blood in the left atrium is suctioned only enough to clearly expose the edges of the ASD; evacuation of more blood than this from the left side of the heart needlessly exposes the patient to risk of air entrapment and subsequent air embolization. An exception to this policy is presence of mitral valve pathology.

The entire right atrial internal anatomy is examined, particularly identifying the limbus and defining any rim of the ASD. The relationship of the defect to the ostium of the

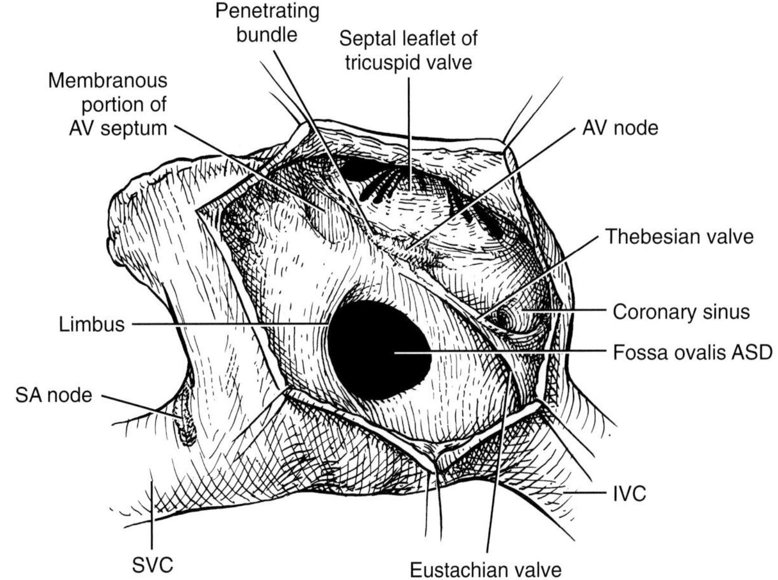

Figure 30-13 Internal anatomy of a fossa ovalis (secundum) atrial septal defect as seen through usual atrial incision. Sinus node is lateral at cavoatrial junction at superior aspect of crista terminalis. Anterior inferior rim of defect lies near atrioventricular *(AV)* node, which lies in the muscular portion and just inferior to membranous portion of AV septum. Key: *ASD,* Atrial septal defect; *IVC,* inferior vena cava; *SA,* sinoatrial; *SVC,* superior vena cava.

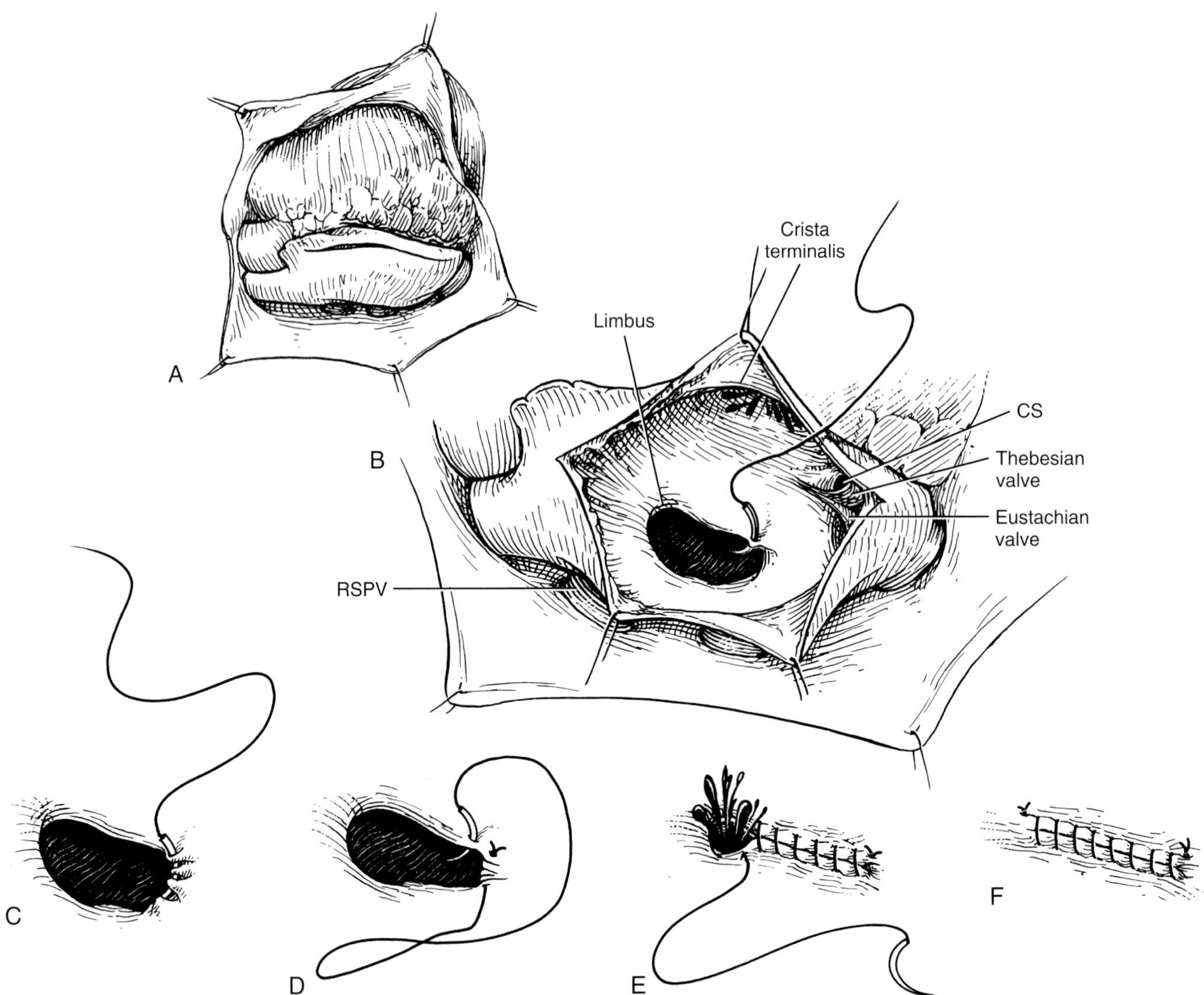

Figure 30-14 Repair of fossa ovalis atrial septal defect (ASD). **A,** Usual oblique right atriotomy is made and retracting sutures placed. **B-C,** After exposure is arranged and all structures examined (orifices of pulmonary veins, valve of inferior vena cava [eustachian] coronary sinus), the first sutures are taken as a half purse-string stitch. If ASD extends to inferior vena cava (IVC), initial sutures are placed in floor of the IVC; eustachian valve of the IVC must be noted so that it is not erroneously included. **D,** After first set of stitches is tied, ASD becomes slitlike. **E,** Before last stitch is tied, anesthesiologist places positive pressure on lung to express air from left atrium. **F,** Completed repair. Key: *CS,* Coronary sinus; *RSPV,* right superior pulmonary vein.

coronary sinus, membranous portion of the AV septum, and commissural area between the septal and anterior tricuspid leaflets is studied because these features serve as guides to the location of the AV node and penetrating portion of the bundle of His (see Fig. 30-13).

Possible fenestrations in the valve (floor) of the fossa ovalis are sought; these are usually between the fossa ovalis and limbus anteriorly or near the IVC inferiorly. When present in thin tissue, fenestrations may be joined to the main defect by excising sufficient tissue to create an edge strong enough to hold sutures well, or the fenestrated tissue simply may be imbricated into the suture line.

Usually the fossa ovalis ASD is closed directly (see "Direct Suture versus Patch Repair" under Special Situations and Controversies later in this chapter). The suturing is begun at the inferior angle by placing a half purse-string stitch. Care is taken to catch good, substantial anterior and posterior limbic tissue with the first and last bites of this stitch (Fig. 30-14), which must be inferior to any remaining fenestrations. Great care is taken to avoid confusing the eustachian valve of the IVC with the remnant of the floor of the fossa ovalis. Such an error results in connecting the IVC to the *left* atrium, which can occur when the operation is done under circulatory arrest and there is no IVC cannula, or when direct caval cannulation is used. After this half purse-string stitch is tied, the ASD assumes a slitlike appearance. The suture line is now carried superiorly, catching tough limbic tissue anteriorly and posteriorly. To avoid damaging the AV node, the sutures must not be placed too far from the edge anteriorly.

Before the last few stitches are pulled up, a clamp or tissue forceps is placed in the aperture, and the anesthesiologist inflates the lung to expel any air from the left atrium. The suture line is snugged while lung inflation is maintained, and

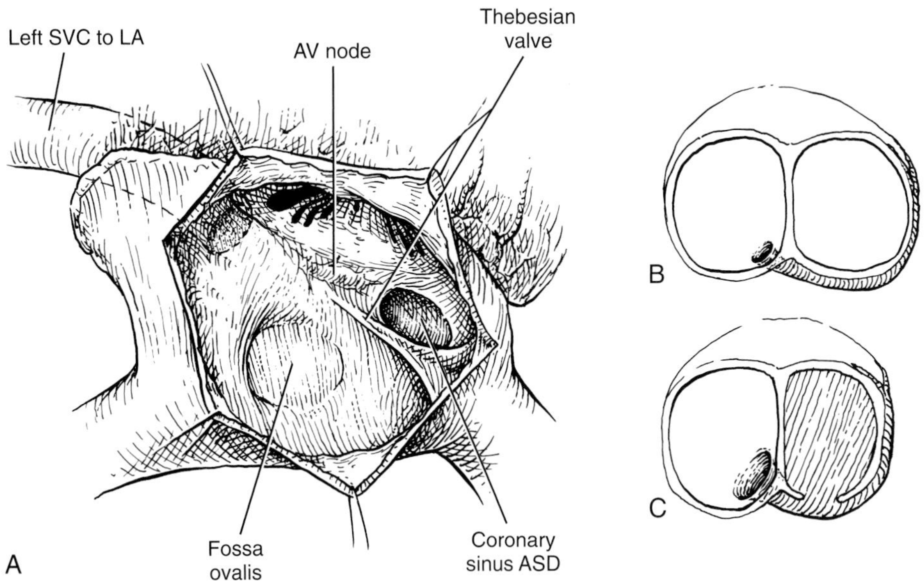

Figure 30-15 Repair of coronary sinus atrial septal defect *(ASD)*. **A,** Anatomy of coronary sinus ASD showing its proximity to atrioventricular *(AV)* node. ASD is closed with a patch sutured to edges of defect to avoid AV node, but only after surgeon is assured there is no unroofing of coronary sinus. If sinus is unroofed, a different type of repair is done by opening the atrial septum for better access (see Technique of Operation in Chapter 33). **B,** Normal coronary sinus without ASD, diagrammed in transverse section. **C,** Coronary sinus ASD associated with unroofed coronary sinus allowing left-to-right (and obligatory right-to-left) shunt. A large coronary sinus defect suggests an unroofed coronary sinus, whereas a small defect indicates an ASD. Key: *LA,* Left atrium; *SVC,* superior vena cava.

an additional bite is taken with the stitch, which is then tied. After the right atrium is sucked dry, once again the lungs are inflated to drive through left atrial blood and thus identify any defects in the suture line. If seen, defects are closed with interrupted sutures. Generally the clamp has been in place about 10 minutes or less for this procedure. Strong suction is placed on the aortic needle vent, and the aortic clamp is removed. The right atrium is then closed. The caval tapes are released.

After good cardiac action has developed, usual de-airing procedures are carried out (see "De-Airing the Heart" in Section III of Chapter 2). Atrial wires are placed routinely or may be omitted in young patients. CPB is now discontinued, with care taken not to overdistend the left side of the heart in the process. Even when a left atrial catheter is not left for the postoperative period, left atrial pressure is measured at this time (or estimated by palpation of the pulmonary artery) and noted to be 5 to 15 mmHg higher than right atrial pressure. This increase is related to small size and decreased compliance of the LV compared with that of the RV (see "Determinants of Interatrial Shunting" under Clinical Features and Diagnostic Criteria in this chapter and "Relative Performance of Left and Right Ventricles" under Cardiac Output and Its Determinants in Section I of Chapter 5). Remainder of the operation is completed as usual.

Posterior Atrial Septal Defect

If the anomaly is a pure posterior ASD, closure by direct suture is possible in a manner similar to that described in the previous text. If the posterior ASD is confluent with a fossa ovalis ASD, the defect may be too large for direct closure. Then a patch of pericardium, knitted polyester velour, or polytetrafluoroethylene (PTFE) is used.

Coronary Sinus Atrial Septal Defect

Because coronary sinus ASDs are close to the AV node (Fig. 30-15), stitches must be placed near the edge of the defect superiorly in tissue that may not be strong. For these reasons, patch closure is generally advisable. Additionally, when a coronary sinus ASD is identified, presence of a completely or partially unroofed coronary sinus must be ruled out (see Chapter 33). These defects are often associated with a left SVC. Inappropriate simple closure of the defect may result in a right-to-left shunt.

Sinus Venosus Atrial Septal Defect

Preparation and positioning of the patient are as usual. After sternotomy, the pericardium is cleared of pleural reflections bilaterally, and a large pericardial piece is removed and set aside between moist towels or in 0.6% glutaraldehyde. After the remaining pericardium is widely opened, stay sutures are placed and the anatomy examined. The right superior pulmonary vein is easily seen attached to the low SVC or SVC–right atrial junction. At this point, the pulmonary vein (or veins) should be differentiated from the azygos vein, which is slightly more cephalad and directed more medially. Size of the SVC is noted, as is the possible presence of a left SVC, in which case the right-sided SVC is likely to be small. The right atrium and RV are usually considerably enlarged.

Purse-string sutures are inserted, including those for direct caval cannulation. Sutures for SVC cannulation are placed on the anterior aspect of the SVC cephalad to the area of abnormal connection of the right superior pulmonary vein. Alternatively, the brachiocephalic vein can be cannulated with a right-angle cannula directed toward the left and small enough to allow flow around it. CPB is then established, the aorta clamped, and cold cardioplegia infused (see "Cold Cardioplegia, Controlled Aortic Root Reperfusion, and [When Needed] Warm Cardioplegic Induction" in Chapter 3). The caval tapes are secured. In infants, repair may be done with a single venous cannula and hypothermic circulatory arrest. When the aorta is clamped, the perfusate temperature is stabilized at 25°C to 32°C.

When configuration of the superior pulmonary vein is usual and the SVC–right atrial junction is wide, the right atrium is opened through the usual oblique incision beginning at the base of the right atrial appendage and extending down toward the IVC cannula (Fig. 30-16). This does not damage the sinoatrial node or its artery. Stay sutures are placed. A pump sump-sucker is placed across the foramen ovale into the left atrium (or through a stab wound), or no left atrial vent may be used. The repair directs pulmonary venous drainage through the ASD into the left atrium while closing the interatrial communication (see Fig. 30-16). A pericardial baffle forms approximately the anterior half of this internal conduit. Width of the pericardial patch should be about 1.5 times the diameter of the ASD, and length about 1.25 times the estimated length of the distances from the superior edge of the anomalous vein to the inferior edge of the ASD. This ensures an adequate pulmonary venous pathway and does not obstruct the SVC.

After the ASD repair is repaired, the sump (if used) is removed and the created defect closed. Rewarming is begun, and with suction on the needle vent in the ascending aorta, the aortic clamp is released. The right atriotomy is closed, and the operation is completed as usual (see "Completing Cardiopulmonary Bypass" in Section III of Chapter 2).

When the right superior pulmonary veins enter more cephalad in the SVC (more than about 2 cm above the cavoatrial junction)[S5] or when the SVC is small (as in the presence of bilateral SVCs), the single patch technique described above may require a long tunnel or create possible SVC obstruction, or both. Because of concerns about the potential for sinus node dysfunction with incisions across the cavoatrial junction,[S5,S18] the Warden operation may be used[W2] (Fig. 30-17). After extensive mobilization and division of the azygos vein, the SVC is divided cephalad to the anomalously connected right pulmonary veins. The central end is closed, and as a final step the distal end is anastomosed to the right atrial appendage. Particular care is needed to completely excise all trabeculated muscle within the appendage and the associated pathway into the right atrial chamber. From within the right atrium, the inferior lip of the subcaval ASD is joined to the right atrial wall, anterior and lateral to the caval orifice. This closes the interatrial communication and diverts pulmonary venous drainage from the anomalously connected right pulmonary veins to the left atrium.

Another alternative is the V-Y–plasty technique. A vertical atriotomy is made posteriorly and extended into the SVC posterior to the sinus node and just in front of the anomalous veins (Fig. 30-18) in preparation for a V-Y–plasty enlargement of the SVC.

Others have recommended near-routine use of a two-patch technique, in which the original incision is extended across the cavoatrial junction below the sulcus terminalis and just anterior to insertion of the anomalous pulmonary veins.[A4] After placing the internal baffle, the incision is closed with an autologous or bovine pericardial patch.

Anomalous Connection of Right Pulmonary Veins to Right Atrium

The operation begins exactly as described for sinus venosus malformation, including opening the right atrium through the usual oblique incision. The interior of the right atrium is examined, anomalous connections of the right pulmonary veins and normal connections of the left pulmonary veins to the left atrium are confirmed, and any defects in the atrial septum are identified.

When the atrial septum is intact, repair can often be accomplished by making a longitudinal incision in it next to the atrial wall posteriorly and resuturing it to the lateral right atrial wall in front of the right pulmonary vein orifices. Alternatively, and particularly when geometry in the right atrium does not lend itself to this simple repair, the fossa ovalis and posterior limbic tissue may be excised and a pericardial, PTFE, or knitted polyester patch used for baffle reconstruction (Fig. 30-19).

When an ASD is present, repair is similar. When the defect is large and of the fossa ovalis or confluent type, a patch similar to the one shown in Fig. 30-19 is used. Occasionally, and particularly when the associated ASD is posterior, repair by direct suture is possible.

Anomalous Connection of Right Pulmonary Veins to Inferior Vena Cava (Scimitar Syndrome)

Initial stages of the operation for scimitar syndrome proceed as described for sinus venosus malformation. An internal conduit is then constructed within the right atrium to conduct the right pulmonary venous blood from its entrance into the IVC across the atrial septum into the left atrium.

In small infants, the entire repair may be done during hypothermic circulatory arrest. In older patients, part of the repair can be performed during hypothermic circulatory arrest; alternatively, the entire repair can be performed during conventional CPB at 20°C to 28°C. In the latter approach, the IVC tape may be passed inferior (caudad) to the entrance of the anomalous pulmonary vein into the IVC, and a right-angled metal cannula can be used to cannulate the IVC inferior to this point. This possibility depends on whether the anomalous vein enters at the IVC–right atrial junction. Alternatively, the common femoral or external iliac vein can be cannulated for IVC return.

In any case, CPB is established with two venous cannulae, and if part of the repair is to be made with circulatory arrest, the IVC tape is placed on the cardiac side of the IVC entrance of the anomalous vein. The aorta is clamped and cold cardioplegic solution infused. After caval tapes have been tightened, the right atrium is opened with the usual oblique incision and carried down to the IVC. If present, the valve of the fossa ovalis is completely excised to create a large ASD (Fig. 30-20). The pericardial patch is trimmed according to the measurements made, and stay sutures are applied at the four corners.

Circulatory arrest is established with the patient's nasopharyngeal temperature at 18°C when this modality is used, and the IVC cannula is removed. Otherwise, repair proceeds during CPB. The pericardial patch is sewn into place so as to form the anterior wall of a conduit between the entrance of the anomalous vein and the defect created in the atrial septum (see Fig. 30-20). If repair has been done during circulatory

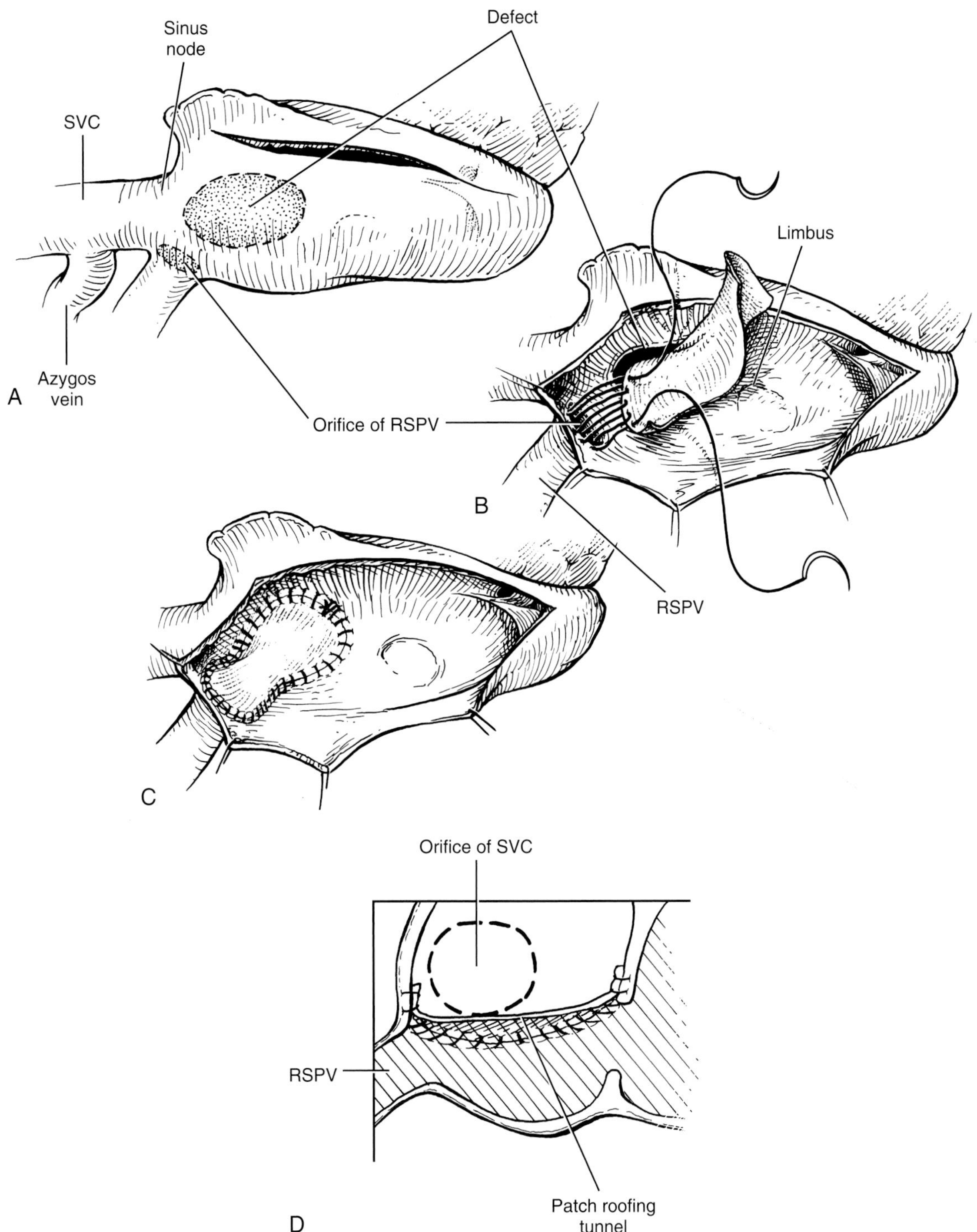

Figure 30-16 Repair of sinus venosus malformation, which typically consists of subcaval atrial septal defect (ASD) associated with partial anomalous pulmonary venous connection of right superior pulmonary vein *(RSPV)* to low superior vena cava *(SVC)*. **A,** Usual atriotomy is away from sinus node. **B,** Incision can be extended superiorly and medially to sinoatrial node. Subcaval ASD is superior to limbus. At times the SVC overrides the defect to drain in part directly into left atrium. ASD is far removed from tricuspid valve and atrioventricular node. First stitches for inserting pericardial patch are shown at right lateral edge of SVC orifice at its junction with laterally placed orifice of RSPV. Patch is sewn into place with continuous 4-0 or 5-0 polypropylene suture. Suture line continues medially in an anterior and posterior direction to form a tunnel or roof leading the anomalous RSPV through ASD. **C,** Convex roof of tunnel has been completed, and blood from anomalously connected RSPV drains beneath this roof into left atrium. Pathway from SVC to right atrium is unobstructed. When SVC is cannulated directly, exposure is good through this incision, and augmentation of the atrial closure is not necessary. **D,** Transverse section through repair seen from below.

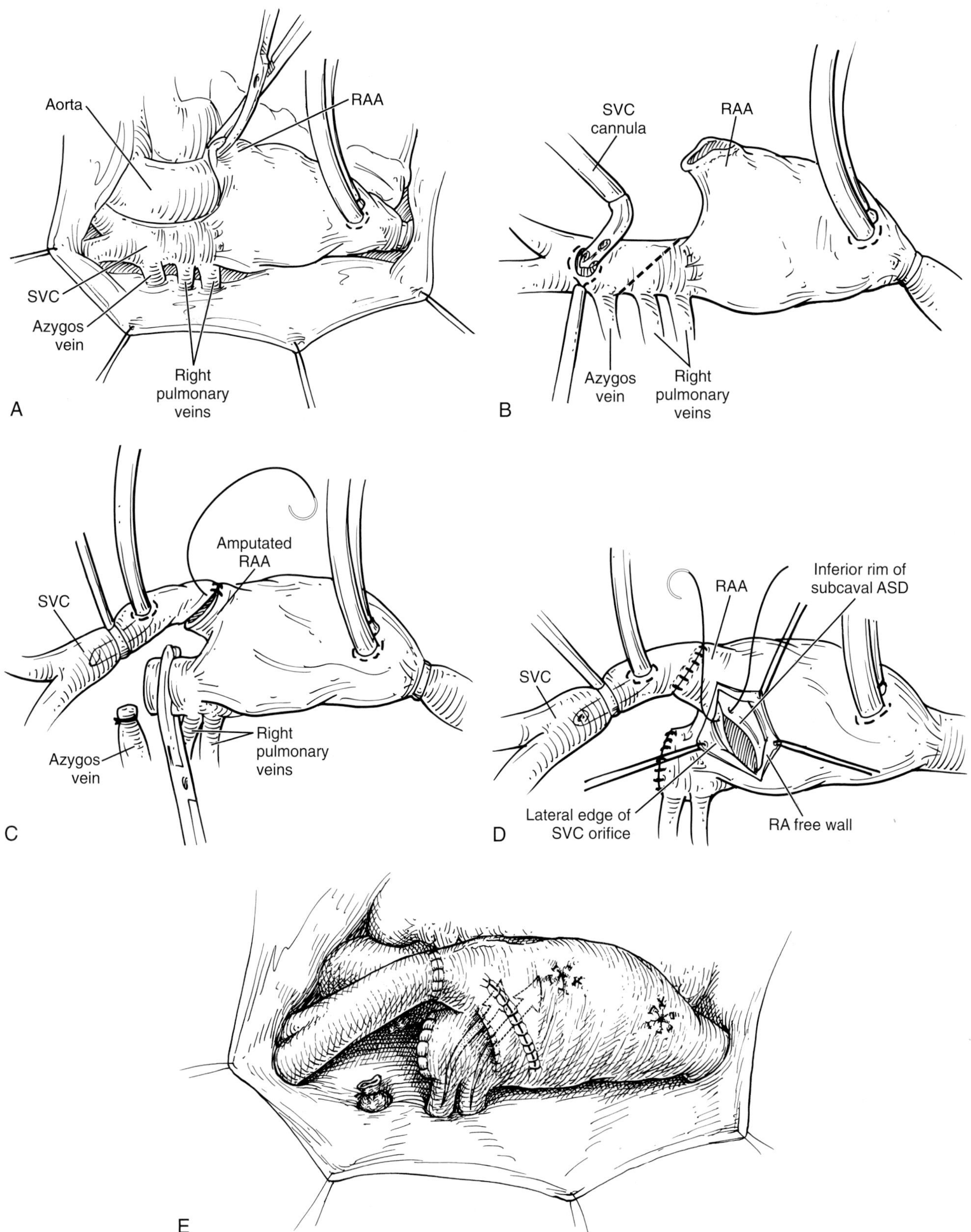

Figure 30-17 Warden operation for sinus venosus malformation with right upper and middle lobe pulmonary veins entering superior vena cava *(SVC)*. **A,** Right upper and middle pulmonary veins entering SVC. Right atrial appendage is amputated. **B,** High SVC or innominate vein is cannulated. Dashed line indicates the transecting incision in SVC. **C,** Cephalad end of transected SVC is anastomosed to amputated right atrial appendage. For mobilization, azygos vein is divided. **D,** Small incision is made in right atrial wall. Lateral edge of SVC orifice is sutured to lower rim of subcaval atrial septal defect (ASD), or the pathway is completed with a pericardial or polytetrafluoroethylene patch. Cardiac end of transected SVC is closed. **E,** Right pulmonary vein blood now flows *(arrows)* across the roofed ASD into left atrium. Key: *RA,* Right atrium; *RAA,* right atrial appendage. (From Warden and colleagues.[W2])

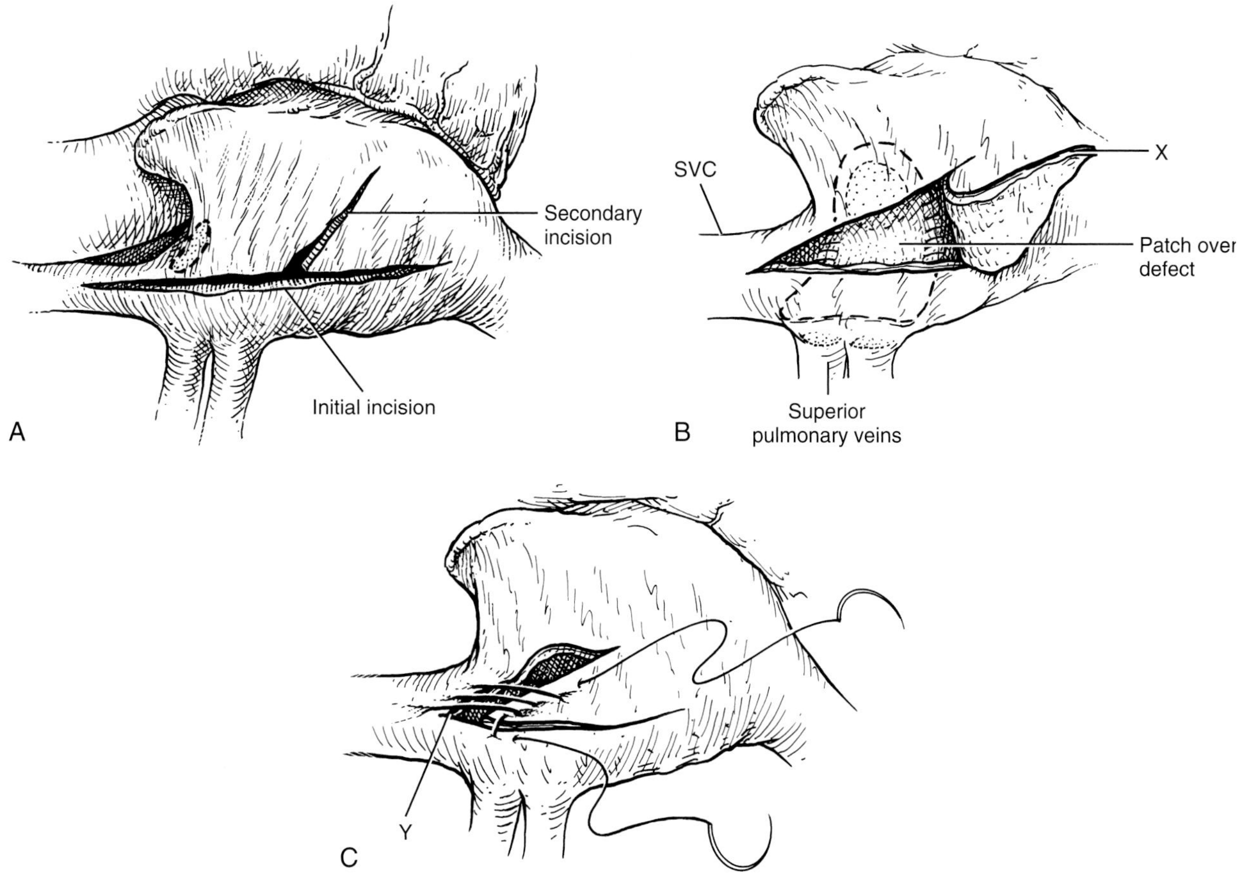

Figure 30-18 V-Y atrioplasty technique for enlarging superior vena cava *(SVC)*. **A,** Initial incision is longitudinal and does not cross SVC–right atrial junction unless SVC enlargement is believed to be required. In such cases, a secondary incision is then added to create a V flap of right atrial wall. **B,** SVC is enlarged by advancing tip of V flap to apex of SVC incision. **C,** Augmentation is completed with a continuous suture line (X in **B** is brought to Y in **C**).

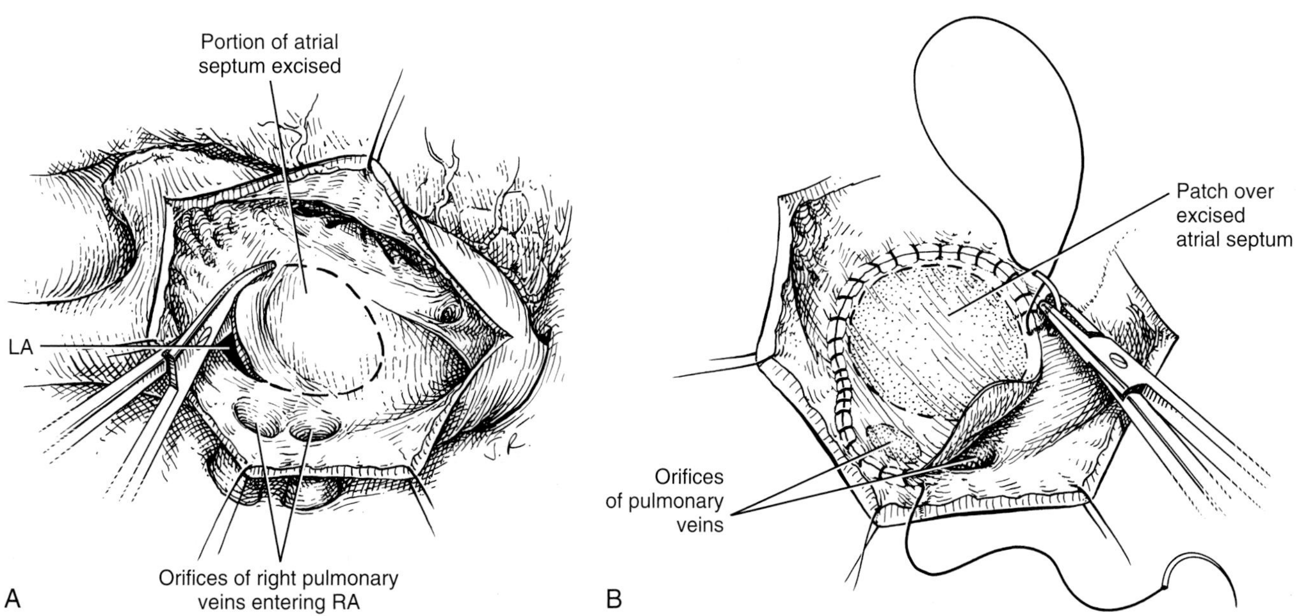

Figure 30-19 Repair of anomalous connection of right superior and inferior pulmonary veins to right atrium without atrial septal defect. **A,** Right atrial incision is the usual oblique transverse one, and fossa ovalis and posterior limbus are excised. **B,** Repair is made by replacing excised portion of atrial septum with a patch, sewn to right of (anterior to) the right pulmonary vein orifices. Key: *LA,* Left atrium; *RA,* right atrium.

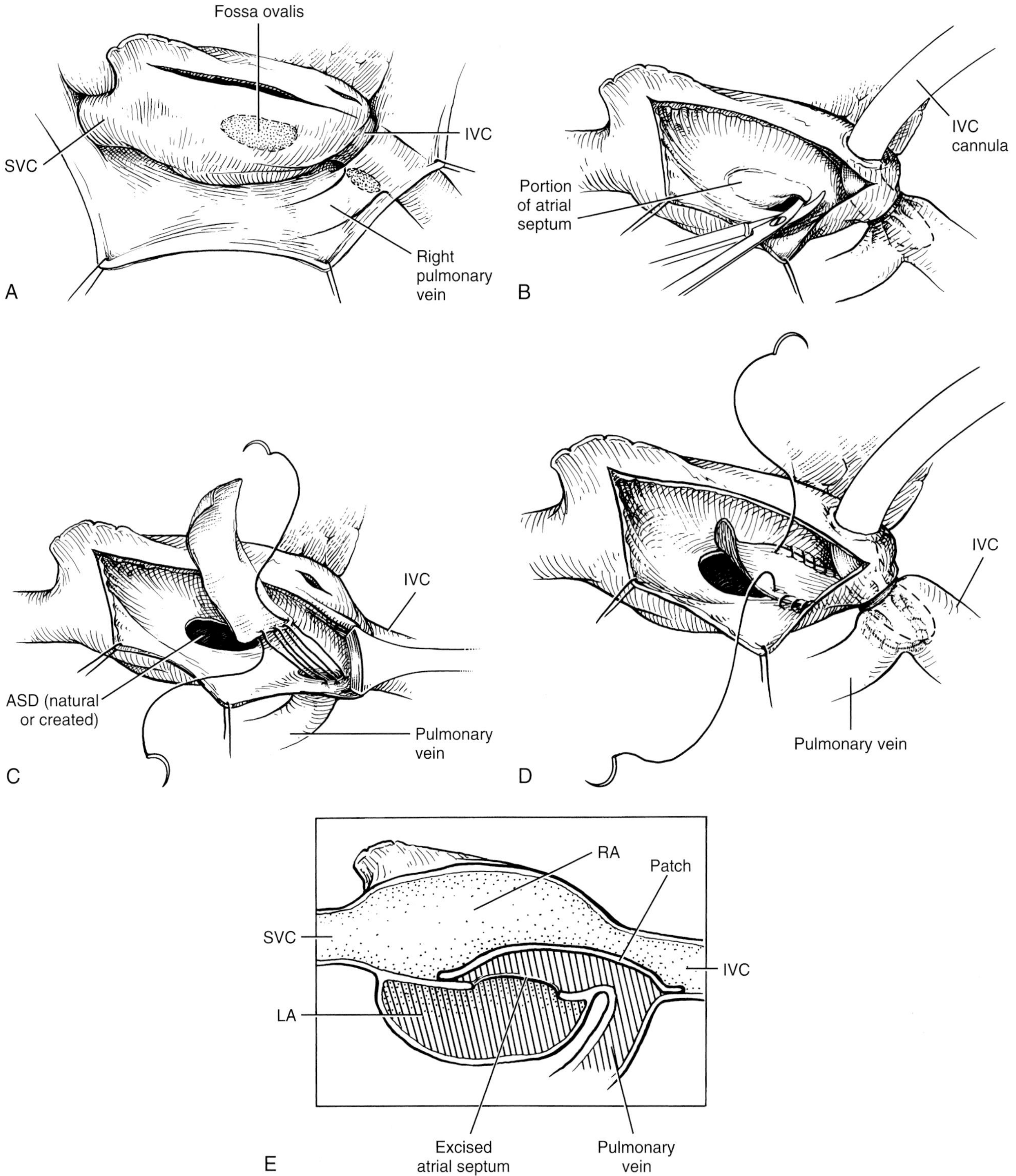

Figure 30-20 Repair of partial anomalous pulmonary venous connection, right pulmonary veins to inferior vena cava (scimitar syndrome). **A,** Usual oblique right atriotomy is made, extending it to inferior vena cava *(IVC)*. **B,** Valve (floor) of fossa ovalis (septum primum) is excised, creating an atrial septal defect that extends almost to IVC. **C,** During a short period of circulatory arrest or with sucker trickle flow, IVC cannula is removed. Distance between inferior aspect of orifice of anomalous vein entrance into IVC and superior limbus is measured, as is width of fossa ovalis. Pericardial patch is trimmed in a rectangular shape, with length about 1.25 times the measured length and width about 1.5 times the width of the fossa ovalis. Using a continuous polypropylene suture, patch insertion is begun at inferior aspect of orifice of anomalous pulmonary vein in IVC, after this orifice and that of the hepatic vein are positively identified. Suture line between patch and floor of IVC is carried to patient's left and then up toward and onto anterior limbus, where it is held. With the other arm of original suture, patch is attached above orifice of anomalous vein as suture line is carried superiorly. IVC cannula is reinserted, and cardiopulmonary bypass is resumed at usual flow. **D,** Patch is then attached successively to posterior limbus, superior limbus, and anterior limbus, and tied there to other end of suture. **E,** Patch now forms approximately half of an intraatrial internal conduit conducting right pulmonary vein blood across defect created in the fossa ovalis into the left atrium. This is drawn in parasagittal section. Key: *ASD,* Atrial septal defect; *LA,* left atrium; *RA,* right atrium; *SVC,* superior vena cava.

arrest, the IVC cannula is reinserted, caval tape retightened, CPB reestablished, and rewarming with the perfusate begun. The anomalous vein is observed from time to time to ensure pressure in it is not elevated, because its drainage is now temporarily obstructed by the IVC tape. The right atrium is closed and the caval tapes promptly released. With suction on the aortic needle vent, the aortic clamp is released.

Alternatively, the anomalous pulmonary vein can be disconnected from its low insertion at the cavoatrial junction and reimplanted higher on the right atrial wall with connection via a baffle to the left atrium.[B16,S9,T3] As a third option, after disconnection, the anomalous vein can be implanted directly onto the left atrial wall at its rightmost aspect because this area is "bare" (having no natural entrance of right pulmonary veins).[H9]

Usually, repair of the anomalous venous connection should be complemented by interrupting the aberrant systemic subphrenic arterial collateral supply to the right lower lobe. This can be accomplished by surgical ligation or catheter intervention. In neonates, it may be sufficient simply to interrupt the aberrant arterial supply and leave the anomalous venous connection intact.

Anomalous Connection of Left Pulmonary Veins to Brachiocephalic Vein

When the atrial septum is intact or there is only a valve-competent foramen ovale, operation is performed using a closed technique. The left chest is entered through a posterolateral incision (Fig. 30-21). The left groin should be prepared and draped for possible surgical access in case cannulation of the left femoral artery and vein are needed for CPB bypass. The anomalous left vertical vein is dissected up to the brachiocephalic vein. Left superior and inferior veins are dissected and mobilized as much as possible. A tape is placed around the left pulmonary artery.

The pericardium is opened, usually behind the phrenic nerve, and a large window is made. A clamp is placed across the very base of the left atrial appendage, and most of the appendage is amputated. The left pulmonary artery is temporarily occluded, the left vertical vein is ligated flush with the brachiocephalic vein, a clamp is placed across its proximal portion, and it is divided as near the ligature as safety allows. The vein is positioned with great care to avoid any rotation and is anastomosed to the base of the left atrial appendage. At least part of the anastomosis is made with interrupted sutures to avoid any possible purse-string effect. Before releasing the clamps, care is taken that no air is in the vein.

When there is an associated fossa ovalis ASD, both the left anomalous pulmonary venous connection and ASD should be repaired. (The first patient undergoing repair of this type of anomalous pulmonary venous connection, reported by the Mayo Clinic in 1953, required later closure of the ASD, at which time the previously made anastomosis was functioning well.[K5]) This repair can all be accomplished through a median sternotomy with CPB. The anastomosis between the vertical vein and left atrial appendage can be modified when CPB is used. Ports and colleagues make a long incision in the lateral aspect of the left atrial appendage, carrying it down onto the left atrium.[P7] The anomalous vein is cut transversely, then a T extension is made posteriorly. The end-to-side anastomosis is thus extremely wide. Alternatively, a side-to-side vertical vein–left atrial anastomosis is made, ligating the vertical vein at its junction with brachiocephalic vein.

Other Anomalous Pulmonary Venous Connections

Bilateral PAPVCs and rare right or left anomalous connections require individual techniques using principles described for standard repairs.

Treatment of Associated Mitral or Tricuspid Valve Disease

Mitral stenosis is treated by valvotomy. Mitral and tricuspid regurgitation are treated by anuloplasty when possible (see "Repair of Mitral Regurgitation" under Technique of Operation in Chapter 11). If mitral valve replacement is necessary, great care is required because the anulus tends to be friable.

SPECIAL FEATURES OF POSTOPERATIVE CARE

Convalescence of most children and adolescents who have had repair of an uncomplicated ASD, as well as most adults operated on before they have reached NYHA functional class IV, is uneventful. They are extubated in the operating room or within a few hours of leaving it. Arterial blood pressure is monitored until the next morning via an arterial catheter, and the atrial pressures via any polyvinyl catheters placed at operation.

Occasionally, older patients have unusually high left atrial pressures (20 to 25 mmHg) in the early hours after repair, presumably because systolic and diastolic LV functions are more impaired than usual by the aging process or by coexisting coronary artery disease, systolic arterial hypertension, or residual important mitral regurgitation that has been underestimated preoperatively. In contrast to a few examples reported in the literature,[B6,B7] in which urgent reoperation was performed and the ASD reopened because of severe left-sided heart failure with pulmonary edema, in 35 years of experience with this malformation at GLH, Mayo Clinic, and UAB, no ASD has been reopened. A partial explanation for this may be that ASD closure has not been recommended when the *primary* problem was LV cardiomyopathy. However, because of these considerations, left atrial pressure is routinely monitored intraoperatively and for about 24 hours postoperatively in older patients.

Occasionally, when mitral regurgitation has been underestimated preoperatively and there are signs of severe pulmonary venous hypertension postoperatively, an urgent echocardiographic study may be required. If important residual mitral regurgitation is detected, reoperation may be necessary to repair or replace the mitral valve.

All patients over age 35 years at operation receive sodium warfarin prophylactically beginning on the evening of the second postoperative day and continuing for 8 to 12 weeks after repair. The rationale is that both pulmonary and systemic arterial embolization occur after repair in patients older than 35 years.[H5] Occurrence is particularly high in elderly patients in atrial fibrillation (see Results in text that follows), in whom permanent anticoagulation is usually warranted.

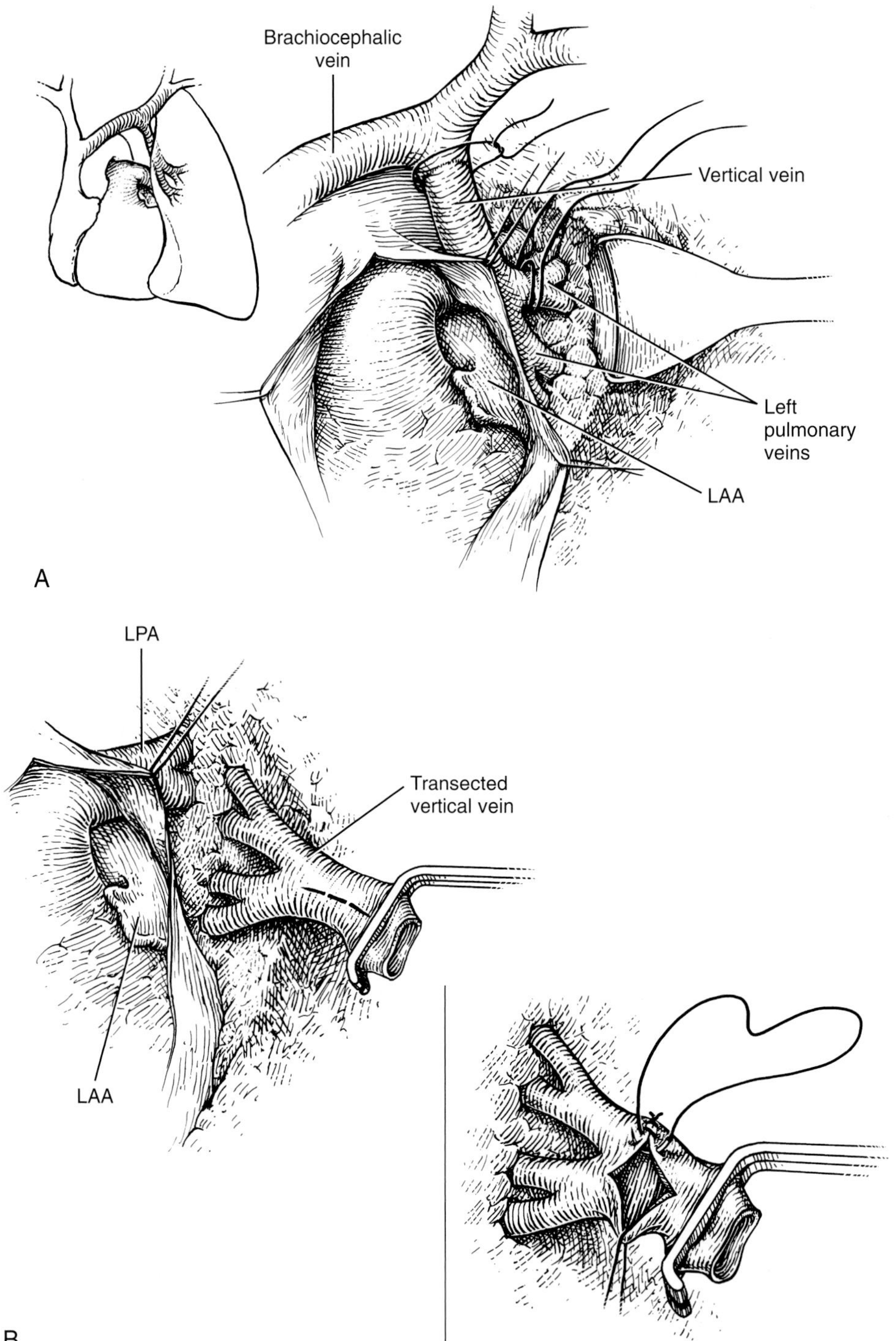

Figure 30-21 Repair of partial anomalous pulmonary venous connection of left pulmonary veins to brachiocephalic vein. **A,** Often, veins of left lung drain anomalously through a vertical vein into brachiocephalic vein. Through a left thoracotomy and without cardiopulmonary bypass, the vertical vein is connected to left atrial appendage *(LAA)*. **B,** Left pulmonary artery *(LPA)* and left pulmonary veins are temporarily occluded, and vertical vein is divided near its insertion into brachiocephalic vein. *Inset,* Occasionally a counterincision is made in the vertical vein to widen it.

RESULTS

Early (Hospital) Death

Hospital mortality for repair of ASDs and related conditions has approached zero for many years in most cardiac surgical centers throughout the world. In the presence of pulmonary hypertension in the elderly, the imponderables are greater in predicting expected early mortality, but in any case it is generally less than about 3%.

Time-Related Survival

Time-related survival of patients with ASD or PAPVC repaired during the first few years of life is that of the matched general population. When operation is performed later in childhood

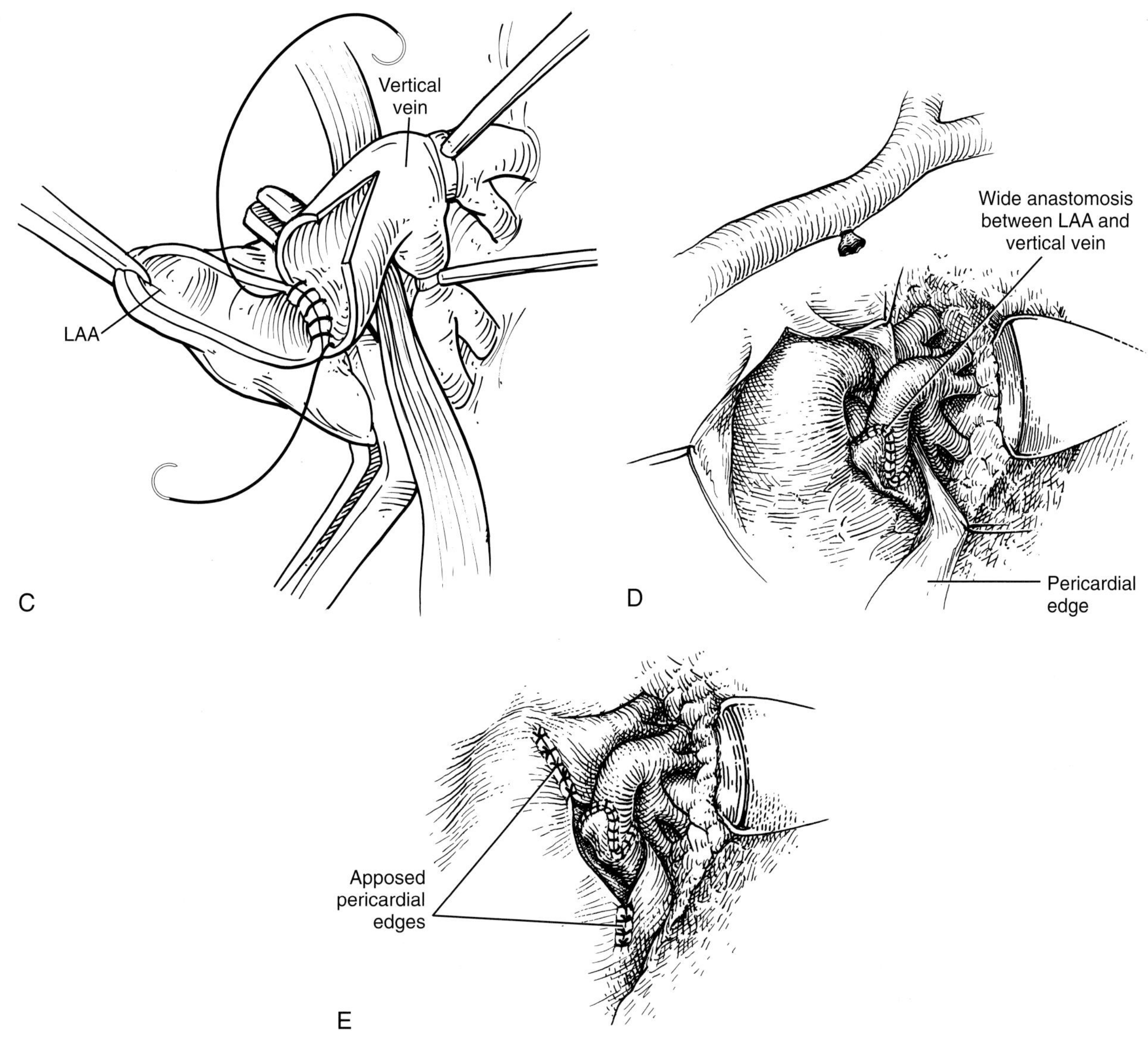

Figure 30-21, cont'd **C,** Spatulated vertical vein is sewn to a trapdoor opening near base of left atrial appendage. **D,** Wide opening at this anastomosis must result. **E,** Pericardium is closed loosely to prevent herniation.

or in early adult life, survival is nearly as good.[F5] In older patients, repair of ASD improves life expectancy,[M1] but survival is lower than in the matched population.[M16] In an observational study, Konstantinides and colleagues compared surgical closure of ASD to medical treatment in 179 patients over age 40 (mean age 56 ± 9 years). Ten-year survival of the surgically treated patients was 95% vs. 84% for those treated medically.[K10]

Modes of Death

The rare patient who dies in hospital after repair of an ASD or PAPVC usually has a serious coexisting condition such as pulmonary vascular disease or old age. The exception is the rare occurrence of death from air embolization, which is about the only risk in repair of ASDs and the reason for using the particular surgical techniques described (see Technique of Operation earlier in this chapter). Premature late death likewise occurs infrequently and almost exclusively in the types of patients just described. Horvath and colleagues found that premature late death occurred more often in patients undergoing surgery in adulthood when preoperative systolic PPA was 30 mmHg or greater than when it was less (survival 85% ± 1% vs. 99% ± 6% at 10 years; $P < .0002$).[H10] Neurologic failure from cerebral embolization or hemorrhage is the most common mode of late death in elderly patients, most of whom have hypertension. Heart failure is the next most common mode of death, again in elderly patients.[S15] In rare instances, late death results from severe supraventricular arrhythmias.

Incremental Risk Factors for Death

In contrast to most types of congenital heart disease, patients with ASD or PAPVC rarely have serious important coexisting cardiac anomalies. Therefore, this incremental risk factor is absent. Likewise, neither morphology of the ASD nor morphology of most types of PAPVC is a risk factor for death. Again, in contrast to most types of congenital and acquired heart disease, preoperative functional class is not a confirmed risk factor for death, probably because the operation is relatively atraumatic and requires only a short duration of CPB and global myocardial ischemia.

Pulmonary Vascular Disease

Preoperative pulmonary hypertension severe enough to indicate important pulmonary vascular disease is a risk factor for death, and if severe enough, death may occur early after operation.[F2,S16] This risk factor appears in various forms in different analyses; in the study by Murphy and colleagues, for example, pulmonary vascular disease appears as the level of systolic PPA.[M16] Elevation of RpI becomes a major risk factor when greater than 6 U · m^2 and may be an irreversible risk when it reaches about 12 U · m^2 (see Special Situations and Controversies later in this chapter).

Older Age at Operation

Neither older age at operation nor young age at operation is a risk factor for hospital death. Older age is a risk factor for premature late death, identifiable after the first decade and becoming progressively more powerful as age increases.[M16] Patients in the first decade have about a 98% chance of surviving at least 25 years after repair, those in the third decade a 93% chance, and those in the fourth decade an 84% chance; patients older than about 40 years have even less probability of long-term survival.[G4] St. John Sutton and colleagues found that 10-year survival was 64% after repair of ASD in patients older than age 60, importantly better than that of similar patients treated nonsurgically but not as good as that of a matched general population[S15] (Fig. 30-22). It remains uncertain whether age at operation in the first decade has an effect on long-term outcome. Cardiomegaly before repair in a 5-year-old patient often remains late postoperatively, suggesting that repair ideally should be performed in the first few years of life.

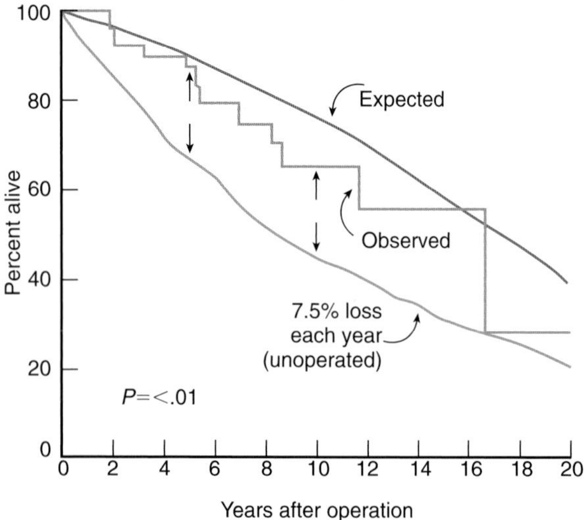

Figure 30-22 Late survival of patients over age 60 years after undergoing repair of atrial septal defect (hospital survivors only) compared with survival of an age-gender–matched general population ("Expected") and with that of patients of the same age treated nonsurgically ("Unoperated"). (From St. John Sutton and colleagues.[S15])

Anatomic Type of Interatrial Communication

The anatomic type of interatrial communication or PAPVC does not appear to affect survival.[D2,H5,K11,S15,T6] An exception may be scimitar syndrome, with the right pulmonary veins connecting anomalously to the IVC. Increased risk is caused primarily by abnormalities in the right lung rather than by PAPVC itself.

Functional Status

Asymptomatic children have no symptoms after operation, but symptomatic infants undergoing repair of ASD may also experience complete relief of symptoms.[P5] Older symptomatic patients typically show improvement.[D3,R3,S2] Forfang and colleagues found that ASD closure in patients over age 40 improved symptomatic state by one NYHA functional class in every patient.[F3] Both Konstantinides and Gatzoulis and their colleagues reported improved functional status in their surgically treated groups that were over age 40.[G3,K10] Even patients undergoing surgery after age 60 showed striking functional and symptomatic improvement[N4,P1]: 87% improved at least one NYHA functional class.

Among the 31 patients preoperatively in NYHA class III or IV in the study by St. John Sutton and colleagues, only two (6%) remained severely disabled.[S15] This striking symptomatic improvement, even in older patients whose cardiomegaly does not always regress, has been documented by Pearlman and colleagues.[P3] Excellent treadmill exercise performance and normal maximal oxygen consumption were found in all 14 consecutive patients studied late after repair of ASD, despite 9 with persistently large RV diastolic dimensions.

Hemodynamic Results

Important hemodynamic changes occur immediately after closure of an uncomplicated ASD. Mean pressure in the ascending aorta increases, as does mean aortic blood flow.[S13] There is an immediate reduction in pulmonary blood flow.[L11] Right atrial pressure decreases and left atrial pressure increases; Søndergard and Paulsen found an average immediate rise of 8 mmHg.[S13] The small amount of available information indicates that in older patients, RpI drops negligibly late after operation.

Ventricular Function

RV diastolic dimensions are strikingly decreased after operation[B11] but are still above normal in many patients[L7,M8,S3] (Fig. 30-23). This finding is consistent with Young's early observation that some children had important residual cardiomegaly years after complete repair of their ASD, which he correctly ascribed to the secondary cardiomyopathy resulting from chronic RV volume overload.[Y1] Pearlman and colleagues showed an effect of older age at operation in this regard; 7 (64%; CL 44%-81%) of 11 patients aged 10 years or younger at operation had normal or near-normal RV diastolic volumes late postoperatively, whereas only 3 (21%; CL 10%-38%) of 14 patients older than age 25 displayed this finding (P [Fisher] for difference = .04).[P3]

In adult patients with preoperatively decreased RV wall motion and ejection fraction, most of whom have elevated right atrial pressure and are importantly symptomatic,

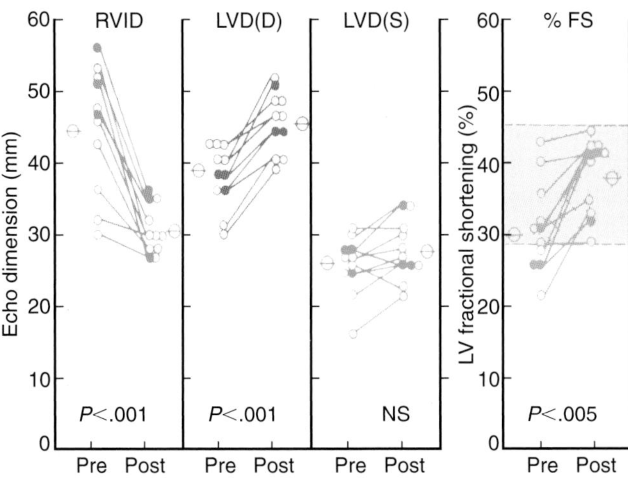

Figure 30-23 Effect of atrial septal defect repair on echocardiographic right ventricular internal dimension *(RVID)* at end-diastole, left ventricular dimension *(LVD)* at end-diastole *(D)* and end-systole *(S)*, and left ventricular fractional shortening *(FS)*. *Shaded area,* Normal range of fractional shortening (29%-45%); *open circles with bars,* mean values; *solid symbols,* three symptomatic patients with marked drop in ejection fraction during exercise. Key: *LV,* Left ventricular; *NS,* not significant; *Pre,* preoperative; *Post,* postoperative. (From Bonow and colleagues.[B11])

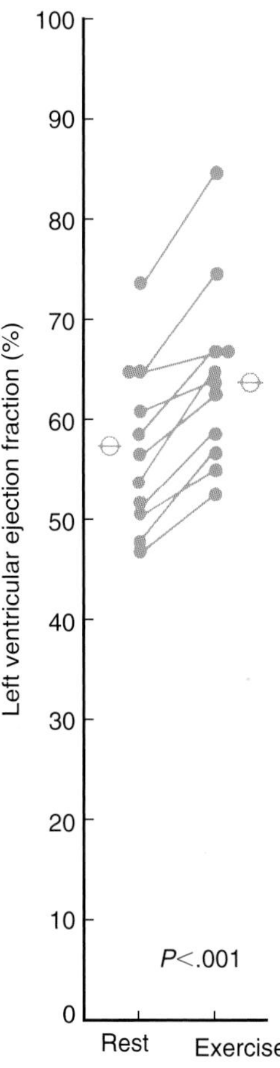

Figure 30-24 Left ventricular ejection fraction at rest and during exercise after repair of atrial septal defect. *Open circles with bars,* Mean values. (From Bonow and colleagues.[B11])

reduction in RV size after surgical repair is less, and ejection fraction, although higher than preoperatively, remains abnormally low (47% in the experience of Liberthson and colleagues[L7]). These patients are improved by operation but do not become asymptomatic. Analogies between this and response to surgery of the volume-overloaded LV are apparent (see "Left Ventricular Structure and Function" under Results in Chapter 12).

Postoperatively, in contrast to the preoperative condition, LV ejection fraction increases normally with maximal exercise (Fig. 30-24). Even in patients who have undergone repair in adult life, exercise ejection fraction is usually normal. This favorable change is the result of ablation of the RV volume overload by closure of the ASD. Also, LV diastolic dimensions, when abnormally small preoperatively, increase to normal within 6 months of operation.[B11,W1] The abnormalities of LV geometry present preoperatively are also corrected by repair of the ASD.

Arrhythmic Events

Closure of ASDs in children has been shown to improve AV conduction, decrease AV nodal refractory periods, and improve sinus node function in most patients early postoperatively.[B10,K1] Presumably this improvement results from reduction in RV and right atrial volume after ablation of the left-to-right shunt at the atrial level. However, Bolens and Friedli found loss of sinus node function after operation and an atrial ectopic rhythm.[B10] Although possibly the result of direct surgical damage to the sinus node, these effects may represent the unmasking of preoperatively concealed sinus node dysfunction.[B5]

Little specific information is available on arrhythmias late after repair of ASDs in infants and children, but presumably these are uncommon. Forfang and colleagues, as well as other groups, found that arrhythmic symptoms regress less frequently than other symptoms.[F3] Thus, most adult patients with atrial fibrillation preoperatively continue to experience it late postoperatively.[B13] Shah and colleagues, however, as well as Konstantinides, noted a persistent occurrence of new arrhythmias and thromboembolic events in adults followed long term after surgical repair.[K10,S4] Furthermore, at least in patients over about age 40, almost half of those not in atrial fibrillation preoperatively develop it late postoperatively.[H5,M11] This tendency to atrial fibrillation or flutter late postoperatively may be less when venous cannulation is directly into the venae cavae rather than through the right atrial appendage.[B9]

These same findings apply after repair of PAPVC, particularly of sinus venosus malformation, so the pessimistic view expressed by Clark and colleagues is not justified.[C4] Twenty-three (79%; CL 69%-87%) of the 29 patients followed by Trusler and colleagues after repair of sinus venosus malformation were in sinus rhythm late postoperatively, and 6 were in junctional rhythm (one of whom had it preoperatively).[T6]

Also, prevalence of changed heart rhythms after repair is similar in patients with fossa ovalis ASDs and those with sinus venosus malformation. Twenty-six (84%; CL 74%-91%) of 31 patients undergoing repair of sinus venosus malformation had no change in their preoperative rhythm during the first 7 days after operation, compared with 190 (92%; CL 89%-94%) of 207 such patients undergoing repair of fossa ovalis defects ($P[\chi^2] = .16$) (Rouse RG, MacLean WH, Kirklin JW;

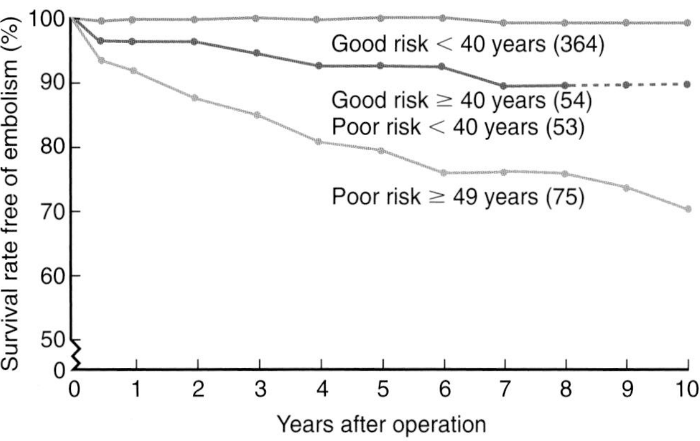

Figure 30-25 Estimates of survival in hospital patients who were free of embolization after repair of atrial septal defect. "Good-risk" patients did not have preoperative embolization, preoperative pulmonary hypertension, or postoperative atrial fibrillation. "Poor-risk" patients had one or more of these conditions. Good-risk patients age 40 or older and poor-risk patients younger than age 40 are combined in a single line because their curves were similar. Numbers in parentheses represent number of patients in the group initially. (From Hawe and colleagues.[H5])

unpublished study, 1979). Trusler and colleagues reported similar findings; 4 of 29 children had sick sinus syndrome or junctional rhythm late postoperatively, and all 4 had an atriotomy across the cavoatrial junction.[T6]

Thromboembolism

Both systemic and pulmonary emboli tend to occur in patients with ASDs. Among 587 hospital survivors of ASD repair at Mayo Clinic between 1953 and 1963, Hawe and colleagues found postoperative embolization as late as 11 years after repair.[H5] A higher incidence was found in patients over age 40, especially those with atrial fibrillation (Fig. 30-25).

Reintervention

Recurrent ASD has required reoperation in about 2% of patients. Recurrence of ASD is more likely in older patients with heart failure preoperatively. Reoperation is likewise rarely necessary after repair of PAPVC. In the UAB experience, 1 of 56 hospital survivors required reoperation for partial patch dehiscence resulting in partial SVC obstruction and diversion of the SVC largely to the left atrium. At reoperation an entirely new patch was placed with a good result. Two of 12 patients required reoperation after repair of scimitar syndrome because of stenosis of the surgically created channel. Both had right lung hypoplasia with a $\dot{Q}p/\dot{Q}s$ of 1.6. Reoperation carries negligible risk. When occurring beneath a pericardial or polyester tunnel, however, stenosis may be difficult to relieve.

INDICATIONS FOR OPERATION

Presence of an uncomplicated ASD or of PAPVC with evidence of RV volume overload is an indication for operation. The indication can be restated as a $\dot{Q}p/\dot{Q}s$ of 1.8 or more and at times, if the anomaly is uncomplicated, of greater than 1.5. An exception is patients with scimitar syndrome who have severe hypoplasia of the right lung and a $\dot{Q}p/\dot{Q}s$ of less than 1.8; operation, usually lobectomy or pneumonectomy with ligation of the anomalous arterial supply, may be required in these patients because of complications of bronchopulmonary sequestration. Isolated PAPVC of a part of one lung without an ASD is not an indication for operation when $\dot{Q}p/\dot{Q}s$ is less than 1.8, particularly because the shunt under such circumstances does not increase with age. Isolated PAPVC of a whole lung is an indication for repair; whenever an entire lung drains anomalously and the atrial septum is intact, only the opposite, correctly draining lung can return oxygenated blood to the systemic circuit. If this normal lung is importantly compromised (e.g., by pneumonia, pneumothorax, or atelectasis from inhaled foreign body or tumor), potentially fatal hypoxia occurs.

Optimal age for operation is 1 to 2 years because of the deleterious effects of longer periods of RV volume overload. However, opportunity to intervene surgically as early as age 1 year is not always present, because diagnosis is often made later in life. Very young or very old age is not a contraindication to operation. Mainwaring and colleagues, however, caution that infants presenting with major symptoms and large fossa ovalis defects may not benefit from ASD closure.[M3] The inference is that these young patients' failure to thrive is not related to presence of the defect.

Pulmonary vascular disease of sufficient severity to raise Rpl to 8 to 12 U · m^2 at rest and to prevent its decrease to less than 7 with a pulmonary vasodilator is a contraindication to operation (see "Cardiac Catheterization and Cineangiography" earlier in this chapter). Such conditions are usually present with a resting $\dot{Q}p/\dot{Q}s$ of less than 1.5 in patients with elevated PPA, but may be present with a $\dot{Q}p/\dot{Q}s$ of 2.0. These ideas are inferential and based on postoperative studies in patients with VSDs and elevated RpI.[N6] Of considerable importance is the interaction of pulmonary and systemic vascular resistance with exercise. As a practical consideration, a marked decrease in peripheral pulse oximetry with exercise strongly suggests sufficient increase in pulmonary vascular resistance to cause right-to-left shunting at the atrial level with exertion. This finding indicates need for extreme caution in proceeding with repair, because loss of the "pop-off" hole during exertion could induce syncope or sudden death.

Associated tricuspid or mitral regurgitation, which occurs especially in older patients, is not a contraindication to operation. If important, such conditions are repaired at closure of the ASD. Grading of mitral regurgitation by angiography and echocardiography may be misleading when major runoff occurs from left to right atrium through the ASD, and the regurgitation becomes more important when the ASD is closed. For these reasons, moderate mitral regurgitation is usually an indication for mitral valve repair.

SPECIAL SITUATIONS AND CONTROVERSIES

Closure of Atrial Septal Defects by Percutaneous Techniques

At least some ASDs can be closed with transcatheter techniques and a device known as the "clam shell," introduced and manipulated percutaneously.[R7] The procedure has been successfully performed on an outpatient basis. Currently, 60% to 70% of patients with a fossa ovalis ASD are treated by percutaneous techniques at institutions with the necessary devices and experienced operators. The procedure is limited

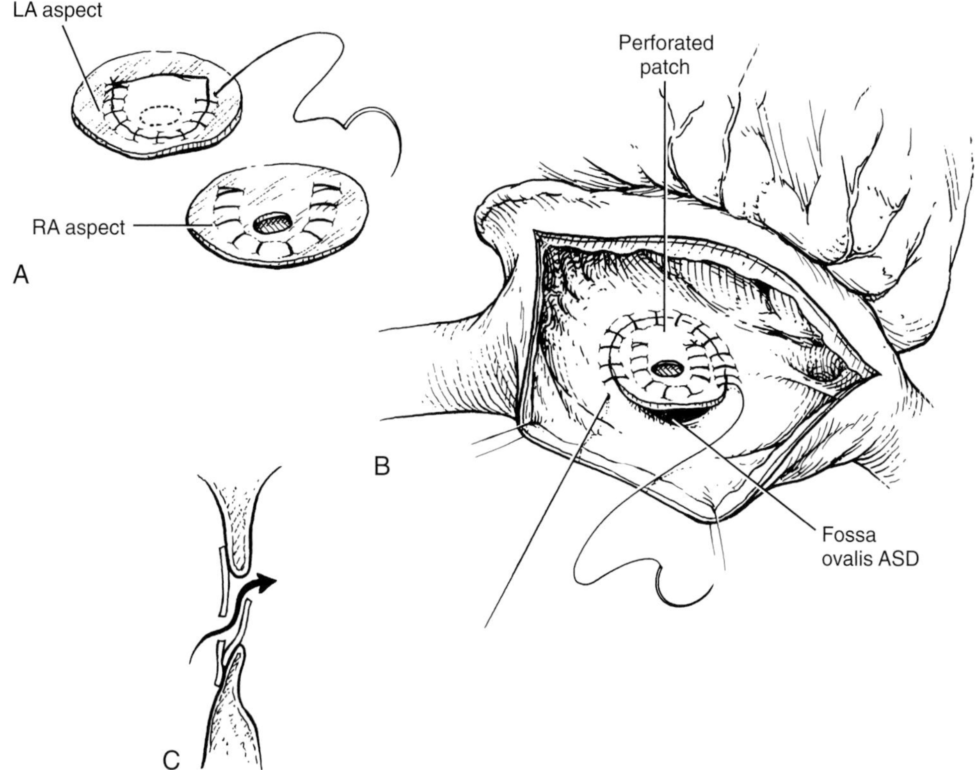

Figure 30-26 Operation for patients with atrial septal defect and high pulmonary vascular resistance. **A,** Suggested operation using perforated flap-valve patch. **B,** Complex patch is created such that higher right atrial *(RA)* pressure opens flap leftward. Thus, flap is placed on left atrial *(LA)* side of patch. **C,** Coronal section through repaired atrial septum. Key: *ASD,* Atrial septal defect.

to "central" defects with well-defined margins and size of 5 to 20 mm. Potential complications of percutaneous ASD closure include device migration, embolization requiring urgent operation, and residual shunts. With experience, these complications are rare.[L10,R2] Simple foramen ovale defects permitting right-to-left shunting and a paradoxical embolus in elderly patients are ideally managed by transcatheter closure.[E1]

Direct Suture versus Patch Repair

Cardiac surgeons vary as to the frequency with which they use a patch (usually pericardium, PTFE, or knitted polyester velour) to close ASDs. For example, this approach was used in 17% of patients in a Mayo Clinic experience,[H5] approximately 30% of those in a GLH experience, and 3% of those at UAB. Provided a patch is used when the defect is particularly large or the tissues are unduly friable, there appears to be no difference in end results, including early or late thromboembolic complications.[H5] Under such circumstances, the ease and simplicity of direct suturing support its use in most patients.

Patch Material in Atrial Septum

Pericardium is the material of choice for interatrial patches (1) when a regurgitant jet may strike the patch, such as after repair of AV septal defects (prosthetic patches may produce severe hemolysis under these circumstances); (2) when pericardium forms part of the wall of an intracardiac conduit, the precise contour (position) of which is primarily determined by pressures on the two sides; and (3) when the patch is sewn to a very delicate area. In other situations, knitted polyester and PTFE patches are suitable alternatives.

Complications after Repair of Sinus Venosus Malformation

When the SVC is normal or enlarged and the pulmonary veins enter at or near the cavoatrial junction, late postoperative narrowing of the SVC is rare after repair of sinus venosus malformation by the techniques described.[S18] For this reason, minimal information is available to recommend more complex repairs.[W2,W4]

In the unusual situations of a small right SVC (usually in the setting of bilateral SVC) or right pulmonary veins entering well above the cavoatrial junction, controversy exists regarding the optimal repair technique. Evidence exists to implicate occasional SVC stenosis when an autologous pericardial patch has been placed across the cavoatrial junction, and early and late sinus node dysfunction may be more likely secondary to disruption of blood supply to the sinoatrial node.[S18,T5,T6] However, several experienced groups report good results with "two-patch" techniques.[A4] Others prefer the Warden procedure in this setting (see Technique of Operation earlier in this chapter). Sinus node dysfunction is rare with this technique,[S5,S17] but occasional stenosis at the SVC–right atrial connection has been reported.[N2,S5] Thus, currently the standard one-patch technique (see Fig. 30-16) appears optimal for the most common variant of sinus venosus ASD with PAPVC to the cavoatrial junction and a normal or enlarged SVC. Long-term data have not generated a consensus about the optimal technique in the setting of a small SVC or pulmonary veins entering well above the cavoatrial junction.

Pulmonary Venous Obstruction after Repair of Scimitar Syndrome

The long intracardiac baffle often required to repair anomalous connection of right pulmonary veins to the IVC carries a greater risk of late baffle obstruction compared with other forms of PAPVC.[A4] Baffle length, relative stasis caused by the sudden change in direction of blood entering the baffle, and other factors may contribute to this complication. In a series of 15 patients with a baffle repair of scimitar syndrome, Alsoufi and colleagues from Toronto reported pulmonary venous stenosis in 7 of 10 undergoing late cardiac catheterization.[A4] Insufficient follow-up data are available to conclude whether alternative techniques, such as direct reimplantation of the anomalous vein, will yield better long-term results.[B16]

Repair in Presence of Increased Pulmonary Vascular Resistance

Some information indicates that a few patients with high RpI (>6 U · m^2) may benefit from closure of an ASD using a flap-valve patch[A1,A2,A3,Z1] (Fig. 30-26). The flap opens right to left, such that if right atrial pressure exceeds left atrial pressure in severe pulmonary hypertension, the right atrium will decompress to the left atrium, supporting systemic cardiac output (see "Lateral Tunnel Fontan Operation with Deliberately Incomplete Atrial Partitioning" in Section IV of Chapter 41). It is inferred that as PPA and RpI decrease late postoperatively, the flap valve will close by cicatrix.

REFERENCES

A

1. Ad N, Barak J, Birk E, Diamant S, Vidne BA. A one-way, valved, atrial septal patch in the management of postoperative right heart failure: an animal study. J Thorac Cardiovasc Surg 1994;108:134.
2. Ad N, Barak J, Birk E, Snir E, Vidne BA. Unidirectional valve patch. Ann Thorac Surg 1996;62:626.
3. Ad N, Birk E, Barak J, Diamant S, Snir E, Vidne BA. A one-way valved atrial septal patch: a new surgical technique and its clinical application. J Thorac Cardiovasc Surg 1996;111:841.
4. Alsoufi B, Cai S, Van Arsdell GS, Williams WG, Caldarone CA, Coles JG. Outcomes after surgical treatment of children with partial anomalous pulmonary venous connection. Ann Thorac Surg 2007;84:2020-6.
5. Angel J, Soler-Soler J, Garcia del Castillo H, Anivarro I, Batlle-Diaz J. The role of reduced left ventricular end diastolic volume in the apparently high prevalence of mitral valve prolapse in atrial septal defect. Eur J Cardiol 1980;11:341.

B

1. Babb JD, McGlynn TJ, Pierce WS, Kirkman PM. Isolated partial anomalous venous connection: a congenital defect with late and serious complications. Ann Thorac Surg 1981;31:540.
2. Bailey CP, Nichols HT, Bolton HE, Jamison WL, Gomez-Almedia M. Surgical treatment of forty-six interatrial septal defects by atrio-septopexy. Ann Surg 1954;140:805.
3. Bedford DE, Papp C, Parkinson J. Atrial septal defect. Br Heart J 1941;3:37.
4. Bedford DE, Sellors TH, Somerville W, Belcher JR, Besterman EM. Atrial septal defect and its surgical treatment. Lancet 1957;272:1255.
5. Benedini G, Affatato A, Bellandi M, Cuccia C, Niccoli L, Renaldini E, et al. Preoperative sinus node function in adult patients with atrial septal defect (ostium secundum type). Eur Heart J 1985;6:261.
6. Beyer J. Atrial septal defect: acute left heart failure after surgical closure. Ann Thorac Surg 1978;25:36.
7. Beyer J, Brunner L, Hugel W, Kreuzer E, Reichart B, Sunder-Plassmann L, et al. Acute left heart failure following repair of atrial septal defects. Thoraxchir Vask Chir 1975;23:346.
8. Bharati S, Lev M. Direct entry of the right superior vena cava into the left atrium with aneurysmal dilatation and stenosis at its entry into the right atrium with stenosis of the pulmonary veins: a rare case. Pediatr Cardiol 1984;5:123.
9. Bink-Boelkens MT, Meuzelaar KJ, Eygelaar A. Arrhythmias after repair of secundum atrial septal defect: the influence of surgical modification. Am Heart J 1988;115:629.
10. Bolens M, Friedli B. Sinus node function and conduction system before and after surgery for secundum atrial septal defect: an electrophysiologic study. Am J Cardiol 1984;53:1415.
11. Bonow RO, Borer JS, Rosing DR, Bacharach SL, Green MV, Kent KM. Left ventricular functional reserve in adult patients with atrial septal defect: pre- and postoperative studies. Circulation 1981; 63:1315.
12. Bowes DE, Kirklin JW, Swan HJ. Effect of large atrial septal defects in dogs. Am J Physiol 1954;179:620.
13. Brandenburg RO Jr, Holmes DR Jr, Brandenburg RO, McGoon DC. Clinical follow-up study of paroxysmal supraventricular tachyarrhythmias after operative repair of a secundum type atrial septal defect in adults. Am J Cardiol 1983;51:273.
14. Braudo M, Beanlands DS, Trusler G. Anomalous drainage of the right superior vena cava into the left atrium. Can Med Assoc J 1968;99:715.
15. Brody H. Drainage of the pulmonary veins into the right side of the heart. Arch Pathol 1942;33:221.
16. Brown JW, Ruzmetov M, Minnich DJ, Vijay P, Edwards CA, Uhlig PN, et al. Surgical management of scimitar syndrome: an alternative approach. J Thorac Cardiovasc Surg 2003;125:238-45.

C

1. Campbell M. Natural history of atrial septal defect. Br Heart J 1970;32:820.
2. Cayler GG. Spontaneous functional closure of symptomatic atrial septal defects. N Engl J Med 1967;276:65.
3. Cherian G, Uthaman CB, Durairaj M, Sukumar IP, Krishnaswami S, Jairaj PS, et al. Pulmonary hypertension in isolated secundum atrial septal defect: high frequency in young patients. Am Heart J 1983;105:952.
4. Clark EB, Rolad JM, Varghese PJ, Neill CA, Haller JA. Should the sinus venosus type ASD be closed? A review of the atrial conduction defects and surgical results in twenty-eight children (abstract). Am J Cardiol 1975;35:127.
5. Cockerham JT, Martin TC, Gutierrez FR, Hartmann AF Jr, Goldring D, Strauss AW. Spontaneous closure of secundum atrial septal defect in infants and young children. Am J Cardiol 1983; 52:1267.
6. Cooley DA, Ellis PR, Bellizi ME. Atrial septal defects of the sinus venosus type: surgical considerations. Dis Chest 1961;39:158.
7. Craig RJ, Selzer A. Natural history and prognosis of atrial septal defect. Circulation 1968;37:805.

D

1. D'Cruz IA, Arcilla RA. Anomalous venous drainage of the left lung into the inferior vena cava: a case report. Am Heart J 1964;67:539.
2. Daicoff GR, Brandenburg RO, Kirklin JW. Results of operation for atrial septal defect in patients forty-five years of age and older. Circulation 1967;35:I143.
3. Dave KS, Pakrashi BC, Wooler GH, Ionescu MI. Atrial septal defect in adults. Am J Cardiol 1973;31:7.
4. Davies RS, Green DC, Brott WH. Secundum atrial septal defect and cleft mitral valve. Ann Thorac Surg 1977;24:28.
5. Dellegrottaglie S, Pedrotti P, Pedretti S, Mauri F, Roghi A. Atrial septal defect combined with partial anomalous pulmonary venous return: complete anatomic and functional characterization by cardiac magnetic resonance. J Cardiovasc Med (Hagerstown) 2008;9:1184-6.
6. Dimich I, Steinfeld L, Park SC. Symptomatic atrial septal defect in infants. Am Heart J 1973;85:601.

7. Dotter CT, Hardisty NM, Steinberg I. Anomalous right pulmonary vein entering the inferior vena cava: two cases diagnosed during life by angiocardiography and cardiac catheterization. Am J Med Sci 1949;218:31.
8. Doty DB, Wright CB, Hiratzka LF, Eastham CL, Marcus ML. Coronary reserve in volume-induced right ventricular hypertrophy from atrial septal defect. Am J Cardiol 1984;54:1059.
9. Drake EH, Lynch JP. Bronchiectasis associated with anomaly of the right pulmonary vein and right diaphragm. J Thorac Surg 1950;19:433.

E

1. Ende DJ, Chopra PS, Rao PS. Transcatheter closure of atrial septal defect or patent foramen ovale with the buttoned device for prevention of recurrence of paradoxic embolism. Am J Cardiol 1996;78:233.

F

1. Festa P, Ait-Ali L, Cerillo AG, De Marchi D, Murzi B. Magnetic resonance imaging is the diagnostic tool of choice in the preoperative evaluation of patients with partial anomalous pulmonary venous return. Int J Cardiovasc Imaging 2006;22:685-93.
2. Fiore AC, Naunheim KS, Kessler KA, Pennington DG, McBride LR, Barner HB, et al. Surgical closure of atrial septal defect in patients older than 50 years of age. Arch Surg 1988;123:965.
3. Forfang K, Simonsen S, Andersen A, Efskind L. Atrial septal defect of secundum type in the middle-aged. Am Heart J 1977;94:44.
4. Forfar JC, Godman MJ. Functional and anatomical correlates in atrial septal defect. An echocardiographic analysis. Br Heart J 1985;54:193.
5. Friedli B, Guerin R, Davignon A, Fouron JC, Stanley P. Surgical treatment of partial anomalous pulmonary venous drainage: a long-term follow-up study. Circulation 1972;45:159.

G

1. Galve E, Angel J, Evangelista A, Anivarro I, Permanyer-Miralda G, Soler-Soler J. Bidirectional shunt in uncomplicated atrial septal defect. Br Heart J 1984;51:480.
2. Gao YA, Burrows PE, Benson LN, Rabinovitch M, Freedom RM. Scimitar syndrome in infancy. J Am Coll Cardiol 1993;22:873.
3. Gatzoulis MA, Redington AN, Somerville J, Shore DF. Should atrial septal defects in adults be closed? Ann Thorac Surg 1996;61:657.
4. Gault JH, Morrow AG, Gay WA Jr, Ross J Jr. Atrial septal defect in patients over the age of 40 years: clinical and hemodynamic studies and the effects of operation. Circulation 1968;37:261.
5. Gazzaniga AB, Matloff JM, Harken DE. Anomalous right pulmonary venous drainage into the inferior vena cava and left atrium. J Thorac Cardiovasc Surg 1969;57:251.
6. Geraci JE, Kirklin JW. Transplantation of left anomalous pulmonary vein to left atrium: report of case. Mayo Clin Proc 1953;28:472.
7. Ghisla RP, Hannon DW, Meyer RA, Kaplan S. Spontaneous closure of isolated secundum atrial septal defects in infants: an echocardiographic study. Am Heart J 1985;109:1327.
8. Giardina AC, Raptoulis AS, Engle MA, Levin AR. Spontaneous closure of atrial septal defect with cardiac failure in infancy. Chest 1979;75:395.
9. Gibbon JH. Application of a mechanical heart-lung apparatus to cardiac surgery. Minn Med 1954;37:171.
10. Goodman DJ, Hancock EW. Secundum atrial septal defect associated with a cleft mitral valve. Br Heart J 1973;35:1315.
11. Gross RE, Pomeranz AA, Watkins E Jr, Goldsmith EI. Surgical closure of defects of the interauricular septum by use of an atrial well. N Engl J Med 1952;247:455.

H

1. Hagan AD, Francis GS, Sahn DJ, Karliner JS, Friedman WF, O'Rourke RA. Ultrasound evaluation of systolic anterior septal motion in patients with and without right ventricular volume overload. Circulation 1974;50:248.
2. Hagen PT, Scholz DG, Edwards WD. Incidence and size of patent foramen ovale during the first 10 decades of life: an autopsy study of 965 normal hearts. Mayo Clin Proc 1984;59:17.
3. Hara M, Char F. Partial cleft of septal mitral leaflet associated with atrial septal defect of the secundum type. Am J Cardiol 1966;17:282.
4. Hastreiter AR, Wennemark JR, Miller RA, Paul MH. Secundum atrial septal defects with congestive heart failure during infancy and early childhood. Am Heart J 1962;64:467.
5. Hawe A, Rastelli GC, Brandenburg RO, McGoon DC. Embolic complications following repair of atrial septal defects. Circulation 1969;39:I185.
6. Haworth SG. Pulmonary vascular disease in secundum atrial septal defect in childhood. Am J Cardiol 1983;51:265.
7. Hickie JB, Gimlette TM, Bacon AP. Anomalous pulmonary venous drainage. Br Heart J 1956;18:365.
8. Hoffman JI, Rudolph AM, Danilowicz D. Left-to-right atrial shunts in infants. Am J Cardiol 1972;30:868.
9. Honey M. Anomalous pulmonary venous drainage of right lung to inferior vena cava (scimitar syndrome): clinical spectrum in older patients and role of surgery. Q J Med 1977;46:463.
10. Horvath KA, Burke RP, Collins JJ Jr, Cohn LH. Surgical treatment of adult atrial septal defect: early and long-term results. J Am Coll Cardiol 1992;20:1156.
11. Hynes KM, Frye RL, Brandenburg RO, McGoon DC, Titus JL, Giuliani ER. Atrial septal defect (secundum) associated with mitral regurgitation. Am J Cardiol 1974;34:333.

J

1. Joffe HS. Effect of age on pressure flow dynamics in secundum atrial septal defect. Br Heart J 1984;51:469.

K

1. Karpawich PP, Antillon JR, Cappola PR, Agarwal KC. Pre- and postoperative electrophysiologic assessment of children with secundum atrial septal defect. Am J Cardiol 1985;55:519.
2. Kelly DT, Spotnitz HM, Beiser GD, Pierce JE, Epstein SE. Effects of chronic right ventricular volume and pressure loading on left ventricular performance. Circulation 1971;44:403.
3. Kiely B, Filler J, Stone S, Doyle EF. Syndrome of anomalous venous drainage of the right lung to the inferior vena cava. Am J Cardiol 1967;20:102.
4. King TD, Mills NL. Nonoperative closure of atrial septal defects. Surgery 1974;75:383.
5. Kirklin JW. Surgical treatment of anomalous pulmonary venous connection (partial anomalous pulmonary venous drainage). Mayo Clin Proc 1953;28:476.
6. Kirklin JW, Ellis FH Jr, Barratt-Boyes BG. Technique for repair of atrial septal defect using the atrial well. Surg Gyn Obst 1956;103:646.
7. Kirklin JW, Ellis FH Jr, Wood ED. Treatment of anomalous pulmonary venous connections in associations with interatrial communications. Surgery 1956;39:389.
8. Kirklin JW, Swan HJ, Wood EH, Burchell HB, Edwards JE. Anatomic, physiologic, and surgical considerations in repair of interatrial communications in man. J Thorac Surg 1955;29:37.
9. Kirsch WM, Carlsson E, Hartmann AF Jr. A case of anomalous drainage of the superior vena cava into the left atrium. J Thorac Cardiovasc Surg 1961;41:550.
10. Konstantinides S, Geibel A, Olschewski M, Gornandt L, Roskamm H, Spillner G, et al. A comparison of surgical and medical therapy for atrial septal defect in adults. N Engl J Med 1995;333:469.
11. Kyger ER 3rd, Frazier OH, Cooley DA, Gillette PC, Reul GJ Jr, Sandiford FM, et al. Sinus venosus atrial septal defect: early and late results following closure in 109 patients. Ann Thorac Surg 1978; 25:44.

L

1. Lang RM, Marcus RH. Images in clinical medicine. Ostium secundum atrial septal defect. N Engl J Med 1995;332:1337.
2. Leachman RD, Cokkinos DV, Cooley DA. Association of ostium secundum atrial septal defects with mitral valve prolapse. Am J Cardiol 1976;38:167.
3. Levin AR, Liebson PR, Ehlers KH, Diamant B. Assessment of left ventricular function in secundum atrial septal defect: evaluation by determination of volume, pressure and external systolic time indices. Pediatr Res 1975;9:894.
4. Lewis FJ. High defects of the atrial septum. J Thorac Cardiovasc Surg 1958;36:1.
5. Lewis FJ, Taufic M. Closure of atrial septal defects with the aid of hypothermia: experimental accomplishments and the report of the one successful case. Surgery 1953;33:52.

6. Lewis FJ, Taufic M, Varco RL, Niazi S. The surgical anatomy of atrial septal defects: experiences with repair under direct vision. Ann Surg 1955;142:401.
7. Liberthson RR, Boucher CA, Strauss HW, Dinsmore RE, McKusick KA, Pohost GM. Right ventricular function in adult atrial septal defect. Am J Cardiol 1981;47:56.
8. Liberthson RR, Buckley MJ, Boucher CA. Pulmonary regurgitation in large atrial shunts without pulmonary hypertension. Circulation 1976;54:966.
9. Lieppe W, Scallion R, Behar VS, Kisslo JA. Two-dimensional echocardiographic findings in atrial septal defect. Circulation 1977; 56:447.
10. Lloyd TR, Rao PS, Beekham RH 3rd, Mendelsohn AM, Sideris EB. Atrial septal defect occlusion with the buttoned device (a multi-institutional U.S. trial). Am J Cardiol 1994;73:286.
11. Lucas CL, Wilcox BR, Coulter NA. Pulmonary vascular response to atrial septal defect closure in children. J Surg Res 1975;18: 571.

M

1. Magilligan DJ Jr, Lam CR, Lewis JW Jr, Davila JC. Late results of atrial septal defect repair in adults. Arch Surg 1978;113:1245.
2. Mardini MK, Sakati NA, Nyhan WL. Anomalous left pulmonary venous drainage to the inferior vena cava and through the pericardiophrenic vein to the innominate vein: left-sided scimitar syndrome. Am Heart J 1981;101:860.
3. Mainwaring RD, Mirali-Akbar H, Lamberti JJ, Moore JW. Secundum-type atrial septal defects with failure to thrive in the first year of life. J Card Surg 1996;11:116.
4. Marshall HW, Swan HJ, Burchell HB, Wood EH. Effect of breathing oxygen on pulmonary artery pressure and pulmonary vascular resistance in patients with ventricular septal defect. Circulation 1961;23:241.
5. Marshall HW, Helmholz HF, Wood EH. Physiologic consequences of congenital heart disease. In Hamilton WF, ed. Handbook of physiology: circulation, vol. 1. Washington, DC: American Physiologic Society, 1962, p. 417.
6. McCormack RJ, Pickering D. A rare type of atrial septal defect. Thorax 1968;23:350.
7. Menon VA, Wagner HR. Spontaneous closure of secundum atrial septal defect. N Y State J Med 1975;75:1068.
8. Meyer RA, Korfhagen JC, Covitz W, Kaplan S. Long-term follow-up study after closure of secundum atrial septal defect in children: an echocardiographic study. Am J Cardiol 1982;50: 143.
9. Meyer RA, Schwartz DC, Benzing G 3rd, Kaplan S. Ventricular septum in right ventricular volume overload: an echocardiographic study. Am J Cardiol 1972;30:349.
10. Mody MR. Serial hemodynamic observations in secundum atrial septal defect with special reference to spontaneous closure. Am J Cardiol 1973;32:978.
11. Mohiuddin SM, Levin HS, Runco V, Booth RW. Anomalous pulmonary venous drainage: a common trunk emptying into the left atrium and inferior vena cava. Circulation 1966;34:46.
12. Momma K, Takao A, Ando M, Nakazawa M, Takamizawa K. Natural and postoperative history of pulmonary vascular obstruction associated with ventricular septal defect. Jpn Circ J 1981;45: 230.
13. Morgan JR, Forker AD. Syndrome of hypoplasia of the right lung and dextroposition of the heart: "scimitar sign" with normal pulmonary venous drainage. Circulation 1971;43:27.
14. Morishita Y, Yamashita M, Yamada K, Arikawa K, Taira A. Cyanosis in atrial septal defect due to persistent eustachian valve. Ann Thorac Surg 1985;40:614.
15. Morrison JG, Merrill WH, Friesinger GC, Bender HW Jr. Cyanosis, interatrial communication, and normal pulmonary vascular resistance in adults. Am J Cardiol 1986;58:1128.
16. Murphy JG, Gersh BJ, McGoon MD, Mair DD, Porter CJ, Ilstrup DM, et al. Long-term outcome after surgical repair of isolated atrial septal defect. Follow-up at 27 to 32 years. N Engl J Med 1990; 323:1645.
17. Murphy JW, Kerr AR, Kirklin JW. Intracardiac repair for anomalous pulmonary venous connection of right lung to inferior vena cava. Ann Thorac Surg 1971;11:38.
18. Murray G. Closure of defects in cardiac septa. Ann Surg 1948; 128:843.

N

1. Najm HK, Williams WG, Coles JG, Rebeyka IM, Freedom RM. Scimitar syndrome: twenty years' experience and results of repair. J Thorac Cardiovasc Surg 1996;112:1161.
2. Nakahira A, Yagihara T, Kagisaki K, Hagino I, Ishizaka T, Koh M, et al. Partial anomalous pulmonary venous connection to the superior vena cava. Ann Thorac Surg 2006;82:978-82.
3. Nakamura FF, Hauck AJ, Nadas AS. Atrial septal defect in infants. Pediatrics 1964;34:101.
4. Nasrallah AT, Hall RJ, Garcia E, Leachman RD, Cooley DA. Surgical repair of atrial septal defect in patients over 60 years of age. Long-term results. Circulation 1976;53:329.
5. Neptune WB, Bailey CP, Goldberg H. The surgical correction of atrial septal defects associated with transposition of the pulmonary veins. J Thorac Cardiovasc Surg 1953;25:623.
6. Neutze JM, Ishikawa T, Clarkson PM, Calder AL, Barratt-Boyes BG, Kerr AR. Assessment and follow-up of patients with ventricular septal defect and elevated pulmonary vascular resistance. Am J Cardiol 1989;63:327.

P

1. Paolillo V, Dawkins KD, Miller GA. Atrial septal defect in patients over the age of 50. Int J Cardiol 1985;9:139.
2. Park HM, Summerer MH, Preuss K, Armstrong WF, Mahomed Y, Hamilton DJ. Anomalous drainage of the right superior vena cava into the left atrium. J Am Coll Cardiol 1983;2:358.
3. Pearlman AS, Borer JS, Clark CE, Henry WL, Redwood DR, Morrow AG, et al. Abnormal right ventricular size and ventricular septal motion after atrial septal defect closure. Am J Cardiol 1978; 41:295.
4. Perloff JK. Ostium secundum atrial septal defect: survival for 87 and 94 years. Am J Cardiol 1984;53:388.
5. Phillips SJ, Okies JE, Henken D, Sunderland CO, Starr A. Complex of secundum atrial septal defect and congestive heart failure in infants. J Thorac Cardiovasc Surg 1975;70:696.
6. Popio KA, Gorlin R, Teichholz LE, Cohn PF, Bechtel D, Herman MV. Abnormalities of left ventricular function and geometry in adults with an atrial septal defect. Am J Cardiol 1975;36:302.
7. Ports TA, Turley K, Brundage BH, Ebert PA. Operative correction of total left anomalous pulmonary venous return. Ann Thorac Surg 1979;27:246.

R

1. Rahimtoola SH, Kirklin JW, Burchell HB. Atrial septal defect. Circulation 1968;38:V2.
2. Rao PS, Sideris EB, Hausdorf G, Rey C, Lloyd TR, Beekman RH, et al. International experience with secundum atrial septal defect occlusion by the buttoned device. Am Heart J 1994;128:1022.
3. Richmond DE, Lowe JB, Barratt-Boyes BG. Results of surgical repair of atrial septal defects in the middle-aged and elderly. Thorax 1969;24:536.
4. Riesenkampff EM, Schmitt B, Schnackenburg B, Huebler M, Alexi-Meskishvili V, Hetzer R, et al. Partial anomalous pulmonary venous drainage in young pediatric patients: the role of magnetic resonance imaging. Pediatr Cardiol 2009;30:458-64.
5. Robitansky CF. Die Defect der Scheidewande des Herzens. Vienna: Wilhelm Braumuller, 1875, p. 153.
6. Roesler H. Interatrial septal defect. Arch Intern Med 1934;54:339.
7. Rome JJ, Keane JF, Perry SB, Spevak PJ, Lock JE. Double umbrella closure of atrial defects. Circulation 1990;82:751.
8. Ruschhaupt DG, Khoury L, Thilenius OG, Replogle RL, Arcilla RA. Electrophysiologic abnormalities of children with ostium secundum atrial septal defect. Am J Cardiol 1984;53:1643.
9. Russell GA, Stovin PG. Coronary sinus type atrial septal defect in a child with pulmonary atresia and Ebstein's anomaly. Br Heart J 1985; 53:465.

S

1. Saalouke MG, Shapiro SR, Perry LW, Scott LP 3rd. Isolated partial anomalous pulmonary venous drainage associated with pulmonary vascular obstructive disease. Am J Cardiol 1977;39:439.
2. Saksena FB, Aldridge HE. Atrial septal defect in the older patient. Circulation 1970;42:1009.
3. Schreiber TL, Feigenbaum H, Weyman AE. Effect of atrial septal defect repair on left ventricular geometry and degree of mitral valve prolapse. Circulation 1980;61:888.

4. Shah D, Azhar M, Oakley CM, Cleland JG, Nihoyannopoulos P. Natural history of secundum atrial septal defect in adults after medical or surgical treatment: a historical prospective study. Br Heart J 1994;71:224.
5. Shahriari A, Rodefeld MD, Turrentine MW, Brown JW. Caval division technique for sinus venosus atrial septal defect with partial anomalous pulmonary venous connection. Ann Thorac Surg 2006;81:224-30.
6. Shapiro EP, Al-Sadir J, Campbell NP, Thilenius OG, Anagnostopoulos CE, Hays P. Drainage of right superior vena cava into both atria. Circulation 1981;63:712.
7. Shub C, Dimopoulos IN, Seward JB, Callahan JA, Tancredi RG, Schattenberg TT, et al. Sensitivity of two-dimensional echocardiography in the direct visualization of atrial septal defect utilizing the subcostal approach: experience with 154 patients. J Am Coll Cardiol 1983;2:127.
8. Shub C, Tajik AJ, Seward JB, Hagler DJ, Danielson GK. Surgical repair of uncomplicated atrial septal defect without "routine" preoperative cardiac catheterization. J Am Coll Cardiol 1985;6:49.
9. Shumacker HB Jr, Judd D. Partial anomalous pulmonary venous return with reference to drainage into the inferior vena cava and to an intact atrial septum. J Cardiovasc Surg (Torino) 1964;5:271-8.
10. Silver AW, Kirklin JW, Wood EH. Demonstration of preferential flow of blood from inferior vena cava and from right pulmonary veins through experimental atrial septal defects in dogs. Circ Res 1956;14:413.
11. Snellen HA, Van Ingen HC, Hoefsmit EC. Patterns of anomalous pulmonary venous drainage. Circulation 1968;38:45.
12. Søndergard T. Closure of atrial septal defects: report of three cases. Acta Chir Scand 1954;107:492.
13. Sondergard T, Paulsen PK. Some immediate hemodynamic consequences of closure of atrial septal defects of the secundum type. Circulation 1984;69:905.
14. Spangler JG, Feldt RH, Danielson GK. Secundum atrial septal defect encountered in infancy. J Thorac Cardiovasc Surg 1976;71:398.
15. St. John Sutton MG, Tajik AJ, McGoon DC. Atrial septal defect in patients ages 60 years or older: operative results and long-term postoperative follow-up. Circulation 1981;64:402.
16. Steele PM, Fuster V, Cohen M, Ritter DG, McGoon DC. Isolated atrial septal defect with pulmonary vascular obstructive disease—long-term follow-up and prediction of outcome after surgical correction. Circulation 1987;76:1037.
17. Stewart RD, Bailliard F, Kelle AM, Backer CL, Young L, Mavroudis C. Evolving surgical strategy for sinus venosus atrial septal defect: effect on sinus node function and late venous obstruction. Ann Thorac Surg 2007;84:1651-5.
18. Stewart S, Alexson C, Manning J. Early and late results of repair of partial anomalous pulmonary venous connection to the superior vena cava with a pericardial baffle. Ann Thorac Surg 1986;41:498.
19. Sturm JT, Ankeney JL. Surgical repair of inferior sinus venosus atrial septal defect. J Thorac Cardiovasc Surg 1979;78:570.
20. Swan HJ, Kirklin JW, Becu LM, Wood EH. Anomalous connection of right pulmonary veins to superior vena cava with interatrial communications: hemodynamic data in eight cases. Circulation 1957;16:54.

T

1. Tajik AJ, Gau GT, Ritter DG, Schattenberg TT. Echocardiographic pattern of right ventricular diastolic volume overload in children. Circulation 1972;46:36.
2. Tikoff G, Schmidt AM, Kuida H, Hecht HH. Heart failure in atrial septal defect. Am J Med 1965;39:533.
3. Torres AR, Dietl CA. Surgical management of the scimitar syndrome: an age-dependent spectrum. Cardiovasc Surg 1993;1:432.
4. Tsakiris AG, Mair DD, Seki S, Titus JL, Wood EH. Motion of the tricuspid valve annulus in anesthetized intact dogs. Circ Res 1975;36:43.
5. Tsakiris AG, Sturm RE, Wood EH. Experimental studies on the mechanisms of closure of cardiac valves with use of roentgen videodensitometry. Am J Cardiol 1973;32:136.
6. Trusler GA, Kazenelson G, Freedom RM, Williams WG, Rowe RD. Late results following repair of partial anomalous pulmonary venous connection with sinus venosus atrial septal defect. J Thorac Cardiovasc Surg 1980;79:776.

V

1. Van Praagh R, Van Praagh S. Does connection of the IVC with the LA exist? (letter.) Pediatr Cardiol 1987;8:151.

W

1. Wanderman KL, Ovsyshcher I, Gueron M. Left ventricular performance in patients with atrial septal defect: evaluation with noninvasive methods. Am J Cardiol 1978;41:487.
2. Warden HE, Gustafson RA, Tarnay TJ, Neal WA. An alternative method for repair of partial anomalous pulmonary venous connection to the superior vena cava. Ann Thorac Surg 1984;38:601.
3. Weyman AE, Wann S, Feigenbaum H, Dillon JC. Mechanism of abnormal septal motion in patients with right ventricular volume overload: a cross-sectional echocardiographic study. Circulation 1976;54:179.
4. Williams WH, Zorn-Chelton S, Raviele AA, Michalik RE, Guyton RA, Dooley KJ, et al. Extracardiac atrial pedicle conduit repair of partial anomalous pulmonary venous connection to the superior vena cava in children. Ann Thorac Surg 1984;38:345.
5. Winters WL Jr, Cortes F, McDonough M, Tyson RR, Baier H, Gimenez J, et al. Venoarterial shunting from inferior vena cava to left atrium in atrial septal defects with normal right heart pressures. Am J Cardiol 1967;19:293.

Y

1. Young D. Later results of closure of secundum atrial septal defect in children. Am J Cardiol 1973;31:14.

Z

1. Zhou Q, Lai Y, Wei H, Song R, Wu Y, Zhang H. Unidirectional valve patch for repair of cardiac septal defects with pulmonary hypertension. Ann Thorac Surg 1995;60:1245.
2. Zubiate P, Kay JH. Surgical correction of anomalous pulmonary venous connection. Ann Surg 1962;156:234.

31 Total Anomalous Pulmonary Venous Connection

DEFINITION

Total (totally) anomalous pulmonary venous connection (TAPVC) is a cardiac malformation in which there is no direct connection between any pulmonary vein and the left atrium; rather, all the pulmonary veins connect to the right atrium or one of its tributaries. Although not part of the malformation, a patent foramen ovale or atrial septal defect is present in essentially all persons with TAPVC and is necessary for survival after birth.

This chapter concerns TAPVC in hearts with concordant atrioventricular and ventriculoarterial connections without other major cardiac anomalies except patent ductus arteriosus. TAPVC can occur in hearts with a wide range of other cardiac anomalies, ranging from ventricular septal defect to tetralogy of Fallot to functional single ventricle. TAPVC in hearts with atrial isomerism is considered in Chapter 58.

HISTORICAL NOTE

TAPVC was apparently first described by Wilson in 1798.[W4] In 1951, Muller, while at the University of California Medical Center in Los Angeles, reported the first successful surgical approach.[M6] His correction was partial, achieved by anastomosing the common pulmonary venous sinus to the left atrial appendage using a closed technique. In 1956, Lewis, Varco, and colleagues[L5] at the University of Minnesota reported successful open repair of this malformation, using moderate hypothermia induced by surface cooling and temporary occlusion of venous inflow to the heart. The same year, Burroughs and Kirklin reported successful repair of TAPVC using cardiopulmonary bypass (CPB).[B19] Their report also described a successful operation several years earlier using the atrial well technique of Gross and colleagues.[G9] Subsequently, it became apparent that mortality in infants following repair of TAPVC using CPB was strikingly higher than in older patients, but attempts to improve results by staged operation or palliative measures were generally unsuccessful.[B6,C8,M7,M8,S10] Success was reported from time to time, however, even for critically ill infants with infracardiac connection.[W5] Eventually, improvement in intraoperative techniques substantially improved results in infants. In 1967, Dillard and colleagues achieved good results using hypothermic circulatory arrest without CPB,[D7] and in 1971, Malm, Gersony, and colleagues reported success in a small group of young infants using standard normothermic CPB.[G3] Hypothermic circulatory arrest and limited CPB were used in 1969 with strikingly improved results.[B3,B5] However, refinements in intraoperative techniques developed over the last 2 decades now allow excellent outcomes using continuous CPB.

MORPHOLOGY

Pulmonary Venous Anatomy

TAPVC is supracardiac in about 45% of cases, cardiac in about 25%, infracardiac in about 25%, and mixed in about 5% to 10% (Fig. 31-1).[B9,B15,C5,D1,D5] The connection in *supracardiac TAPVC* is usually to a left vertical vein draining into the left brachiocephalic vein, less often to the superior vena cava, usually at its junction with the right atrium, and rarely to the azygos vein. In *cardiac TAPVC,* the connection is usually to the coronary sinus and less often to the right atrium directly. Connection to the supradiaphragmatic inferior vena cava also has been reported.[S6] The most common sites of connection in patients with *infracardiac (infradiaphragmatic) TAPVC* are the portal vein (65% of cases, according to Duff and colleagues[D10]) and ductus venosus; less common are the gastric vein, right or left hepatic vein, and inferior vena cava. Uncommonly, the pulmonary venous drainage may be through two connections.[A5] Also, part of the pulmonary venous drainage may be to one site and part to another in what is termed *mixed TAPVC.* At least 15 different morphologic mixed variants have been identified. In the most common form, the left upper lobe of the lung drains to a left vertical vein, and the remainder of both lungs drains to the coronary sinus. In the next most common form, the right lung drains to the coronary sinus, and the left lung drains to a vertical vein.[C5] Chowdhury and colleagues have categorized this wide assortment of mixed TAPVC into three general groups: the 2+2 pattern, the 3+1 pattern, and the bizarre pattern.[C6]

No matter what the final connection or termination may be, individual right and left pulmonary veins usually converge to form a *common pulmonary venous sinus,* which in turn connects to the systemic venous system in one of the ways noted earlier. It is usually posterior to the pericardium. Its long axis is usually oriented transversely, with the pulmonary veins of the left lung converging to form its left extremity and those from the right lung to form its right extremity. When the drainage is infracardiac, the right and left pulmonary veins slope downward to converge into a vertical sinus, with the entire arrangement having a Y, T, or tree shape.[C7,K3,T5] Rarely, there are two vertical veins that are not confluent until below the diaphragm.[W6] Two vertical veins have also been identified in supracardiac TAPVC.[G10]

A common pulmonary venous sinus may be absent in some cases with cardiac or mixed connections. Its apparent absence in some patients may be an illusion attributable to a defect in the anterior wall of the sinus. That defect is the orifice connecting it to the coronary sinus or right atrium. Pulmonary venous obstruction is a severe associated condition usually resulting from a stenosis involving the vein connecting the common pulmonary venous sinus to the systemic venous system. A localized stenosis may occur at the junction of the left vertical vein with either the left brachiocephalic vein or the common pulmonary venous sinus, or at the junction of a connecting vein that joins the superior vena cava. Severe obstruction may be due to the so-called vascular vice, in which the left vertical vein passes posterior rather than anterior to the left pulmonary artery and is compressed between it and the left main bronchus.[S7]

When TAPVC is to the coronary sinus, a stenosis may occur where the common pulmonary venous sinus joins the coronary sinus or (rarely) at the coronary sinus ostium.[A4,J2] In infracardiac connection, the connecting vein may be similarly narrowed at its junction with the portal vein or ductus venosus, or it may be compressed where it penetrates the diaphragm. In those varieties of infracardiac connection in which the ductus venosus is not available to bypass the liver, the portal sinusoids offer additional important obstruction to venous return. Finally, pulmonary venous obstruction may result simply from the length of a comparatively narrow connecting vein. Rarely, associated cor triatriatum is present and serves as the cause of obstruction.[T1,V2]

Important pulmonary venous obstruction of these various types exists in nearly all patients with infracardiac connection and in almost all with connections to the azygos vein, in 65% of those with connections to the superior vena cava, in 40% of those with connections to the left brachiocephalic vein, and in 40% with connections of the mixed type.[D5] It is less common in patients with a cardiac connection, although it has been found in 20% of patients in whom the connection is to the coronary sinus.[J2] Rarely, pulmonary venous obstruction is the result of stenoses of individual pulmonary veins at or close to their connections to the common pulmonary venous sinus.[G2] Functional pulmonary venous obstruction arguably occurs in patients having a patent foramen ovale rather than an atrial septal defect, although this occurrence may be limited to those with a small orifice at the foramen ovale.

Cardiac Chamber and Septal Anatomy

For survival after birth, a communication between systemic and pulmonary circulations must exist. Nearly always, an atrial septal defect or patent foramen ovale is present. However, in the review of Delisle and colleagues, one of 93 autopsy cases was an 11-year-old with an intact atrial septum and multiple ventricular septal defects, and Hastreiter and colleagues reported a 6-week-old patient with TAPVC to the ductus venosus, a patent ductus, and a closed foramen ovale.[D9,H3] Atrial communication in TAPVC is usually of adequate size and not obstructive,[B6,G2] although the GLH group reported that the defect was small in about half the infants operated on.[W3] There is frequently no pressure gradient between the two atria even when the defect is small.[E2,W3]

The right atrium is enlarged and thick walled in patients with TAPVC, and the left atrium is abnormally small.[B9,B18] Cineangiographic studies by Mathew and colleagues have shown left atrial volume to be 53% of predicted normal.[M3]

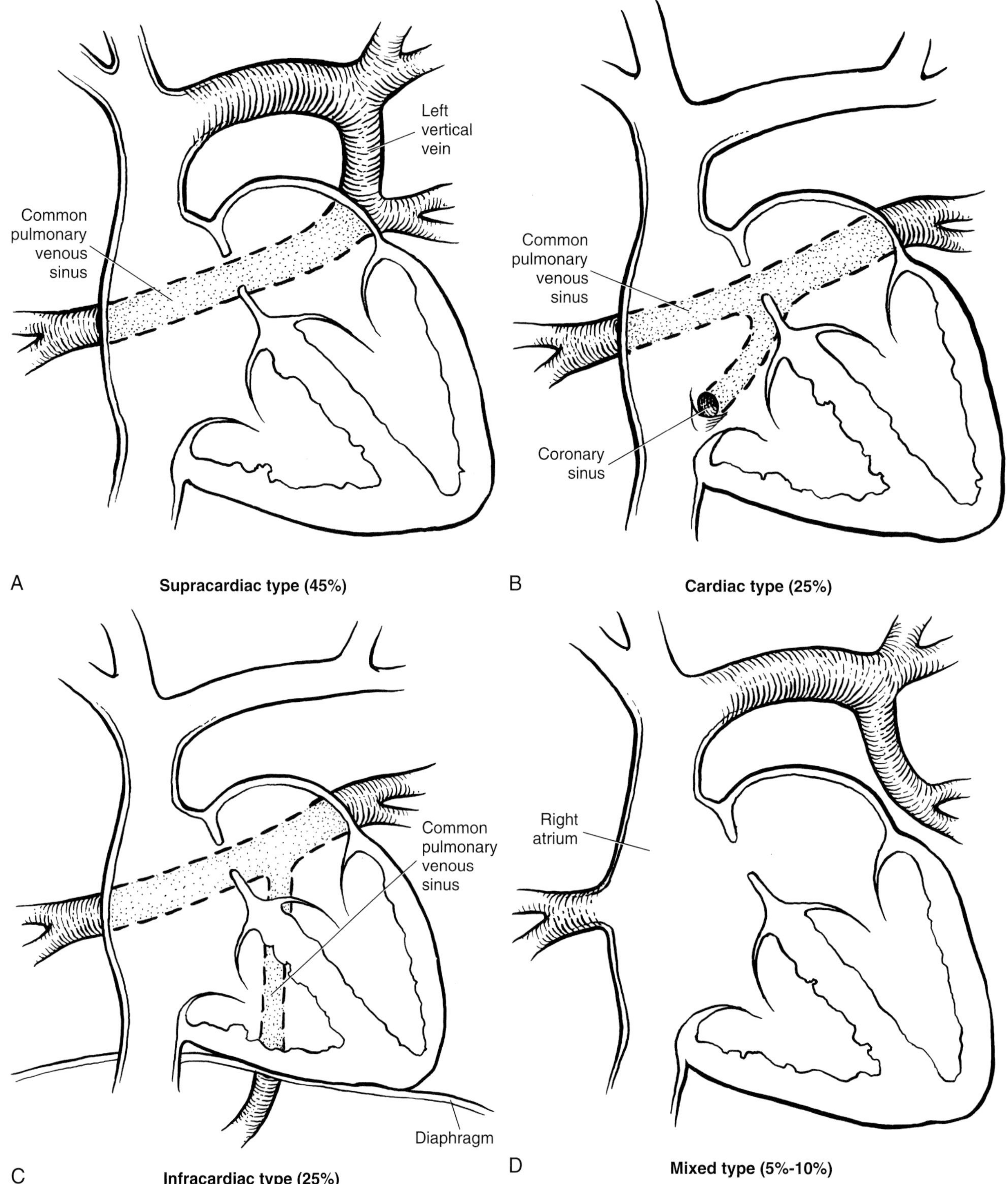

Figure 31-1 Classification of total anomalous pulmonary venous connection. **A,** Supracardiac type (45% of cases), in which the common pulmonary venous sinus connects by a vertical vein on the left side to left brachiocephalic vein. **B,** Cardiac type (25% of cases), in which the common pulmonary venous sinus connects to the coronary sinus in right atrium. **C,** Infracardiac type (25% of cases), in which the common pulmonary venous sinus connects to the portal vein or ductus venosus below the diaphragm. **D,** Mixed type (5%-10% of cases), in which there is no common pulmonary venous sinus, and pulmonary veins connect randomly to the heart.

These investigators noted that the left atrial appendage was normal in size and believed that left atrial smallness could be explained by absence of the pulmonary vein component. In addition, in patients with TAPVC to the right atrium, the posterior attachment of the atrial septum is shifted to the left, so the septum lies nearer to the sagittal than the usual coronal plane. Anatomic studies have shown that the left ventricle (LV) is usually normal in size.[B9,R5] Haworth and Reid's quantitative study showed that inflow measurements of the LV were normal in eight of nine infants dying with TAPVC.[H5]

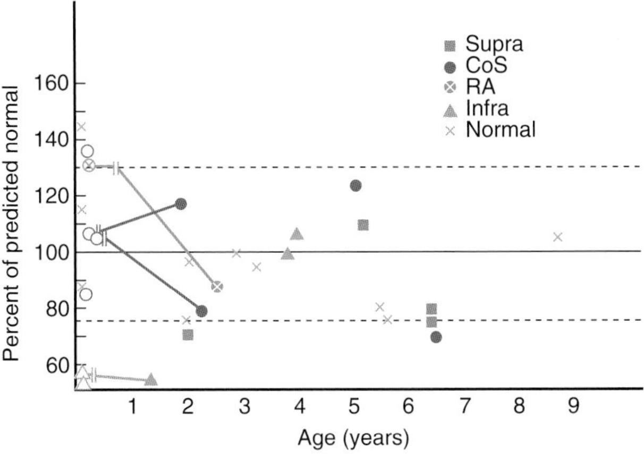

Figure 31-2 Preoperative left ventricular end-diastolic volume, expressed along vertical axis as percent of predicted normal according to age and cardiac morphology. Dashed horizontal lines enclose ±2 SD from mean normal value. Open symbols represent preoperative values in seven patients, and closed symbols represent postoperative values. When both values were measured in the same patient, symbols are connected by solid lines, with two short vertical parallel lines indicating time of repair. X represents values in normal patients. Key: *CoS,* Coronary sinus total anomalous pulmonary venous connection (TAPVC); *Infra,* infracardiac TAPVC; *RA,* right atrial cardiac TAPVC; *Supra,* supracardiac TAPVC. (From Whight and colleagues.[W3])

In one infant, however, LV inflow measurements were abnormally small, and weight of the free LV wall plus the septum was less than that of a normal fetus at full term. In all nine infants, LV free-wall thickness was normal. In a quantitative autopsy study of infants with TAPVC, Bove and colleagues found LV mass to be normal as well.[B12] However, they found the LV cavity was small because of leftward displacement of the septum secondary to right ventricular (RV) pressure-volume overload (see "Mitral Prolapse" under Morphology in Chapter 30). Correspondingly, Nakazawa and colleagues reported that angiographically determined LV end-diastolic volume (LVEDV) was 79% less than normal ($P = .009$) in a group of infants with TAPVC and severe pulmonary hypertension.[N2] Hammon and colleagues also reported small LVEDV in infants with TAPVC.[H1] These findings are all compatible with those of Whight and colleagues[W3] (Fig. 31-2).

The RV varies in size, depending on the magnitude of pulmonary blood flow, presence or absence of pulmonary venous stenosis, and the point at which anomalous pulmonary veins connect. When connection was infracardiac, Haworth and Reid found that the RV was neither hypertrophied nor dilated.[H5] When venous connection was supradiaphragmatic, the septum and RV were hypertrophied and the RV dilated.

Pulmonary Vasculature

Because most infants with TAPVC have marked pulmonary hypertension, structural changes are usually found in the lungs of even the youngest infants dying with the malformation.[N3] Haworth and Reid demonstrated increased pulmonary arterial muscularity in all infants dying with TAPVC, including an 8-day-old neonate, as shown by increased arterial wall thickness and extension of muscle into smaller and more peripheral arteries than normal.[H5] Vein wall thickness was increased in all but the youngest child.

Associated Conditions

Except for an atrial communication, most infants presenting with severe symptoms from TAPVC have either no associated condition or a small or large patent ductus arteriosus. Patent ductus arteriosus is present in nearly all infants coming to operation in the first few weeks of life with pulmonary venous obstruction and, overall, in about 15% of cases. Ventricular septal defects occasionally occur. However, more than one third of cases coming to autopsy, few of which are infants, have other major associated cardiac anomalies.[D5] These include tetralogy of Fallot, double-outlet RV, interrupted aortic arch,[B4] and other lesions.[D4] The combination of TAPVC with other major cardiac anomalies is especially likely to occur when there is atrial isomerism[B9,D5,S15] (see Chapter 58). Other associations have been identified. Esophageal varices can occur in obstructed TAPVC, and these are likely caused by obstructed veins.[C2,E1,E3,K6,P2,R4] Hypoplasia of the small pulmonary arteries has recently been identified in obstructive TAPVC.[M1]

CLINICAL FEATURES AND DIAGNOSTIC CRITERIA

Presentation

Patients with TAPVC present as seriously and often critically ill neonates, especially when a component of obstruction is present.[C1] The diagnosis can be missed when obstruction is absent, because of lack of florid signs and symptoms. TAPVC must be suspected in any neonate who has unexplained tachypnea, the cardinal sign of this anomaly. During the first 2 weeks of life, there are other causes of tachypnea that may be impossible to distinguish clinically from TAPVC, particularly a diffuse pneumonic process and retention of fetal lung fluid.[S17] Meconium aspiration and myocarditis may also confound the diagnosis. Respiratory distress syndrome should not be difficult to differentiate, because of its classic radiologic features, prematurity, and intercostal and sternal indrawing. Cyanosis is usually unimpressive in TAPVC unless there is marked pulmonary venous obstruction or a widely open ductus arteriosus that permits right-to-left shunting. Both LV and RV functions are depressed compared with normal ($P < .001$ in both instances) in infants presenting when seriously ill with obstructed TAPVC and marked pulmonary hypertension.[H1,N2] Severe metabolic acidosis develops soon after birth when pulmonary venous obstruction is severe, rapidly leading to myocardial necrosis. Some neonates are so critically ill that they require intubation immediately upon hospital admission and before evaluation is begun.

Examination

In neonates and infants, the heart is not particularly overactive on examination. There may be an unimpressive precordial systolic murmur and gallop sound (the latter often proves to be a tricuspid flow murmur). The second heart sound is usually single or narrowly split. In older children, the signs are those of a large atrial septal defect unless there is increased pulmonary vascular resistance.

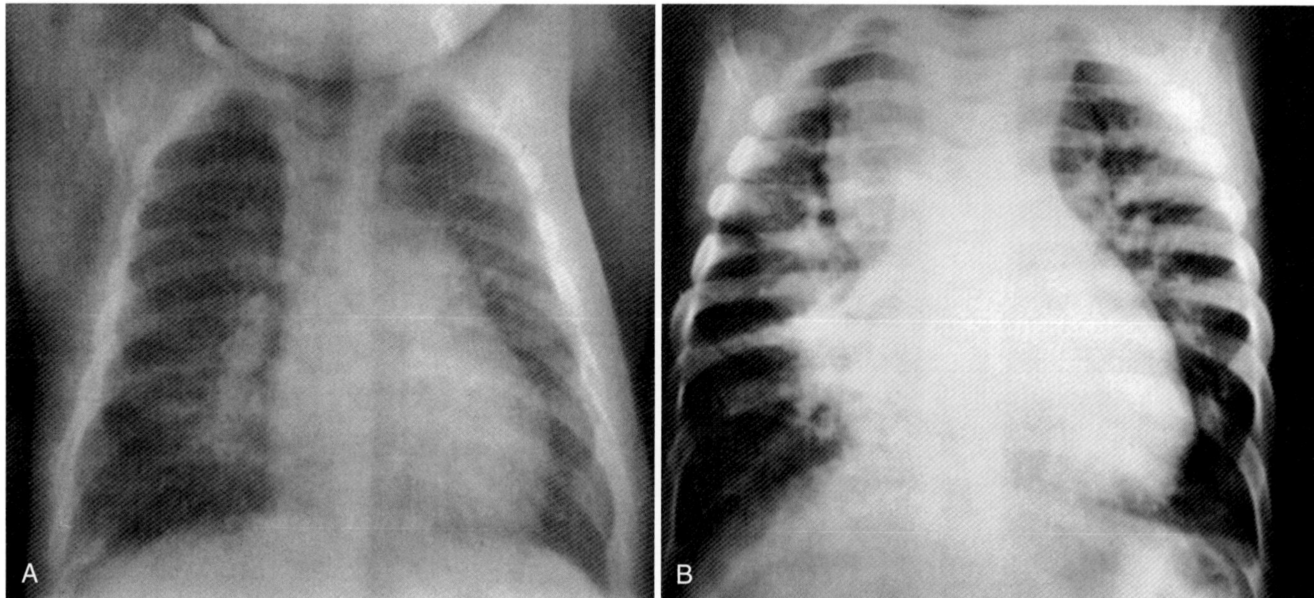

Figure 31-3 Chest radiographs of patients with total anomalous pulmonary venous connection (TAPVC). **A,** A 2.5-month-old infant with infracardiac TAPVC. Note mild cardiac enlargement and evidence of pulmonary venous hypertension. Even less radiologic change is seen in neonates. **B,** "Snowman" or "figure-of-eight" configuration in a 1-year-old patient with TAPVC to left brachiocephalic vein. Shadow on left above the heart is large left vertical vein. Shadow on right is cast by large superior vena cava.

Chest Radiography

On chest radiography, heart size is usually near normal if there is pulmonary venous obstruction, but it may be large when there is increased pulmonary blood flow. The latter is associated with plethora (Fig. 31-3, *A*), but the more common pulmonary venous obstruction is evident as a diffuse haziness or, in its severe forms, a "ground glass" appearance. This sign is reduced when the pulmonary circuit can decompress via a patent ductus arteriosus. Older infants with TAPVC to the left brachiocephalic vein have a characteristic "figure-of-eight" or "snowman" configuration on the chest radiograph[S17] (Fig. 31-3, *B*).

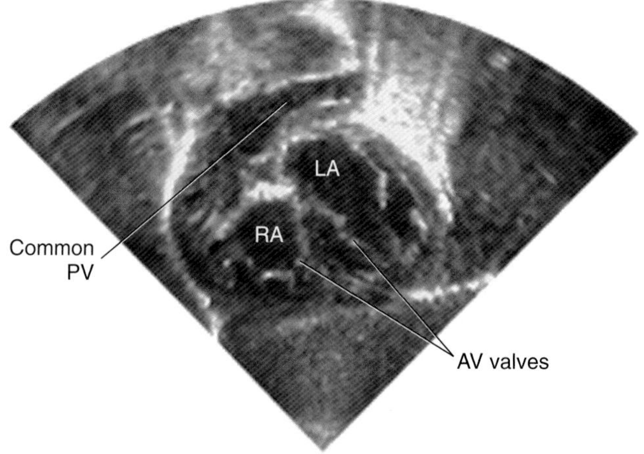

Figure 31-4 Two-dimensional echocardiogram of an infant with total anomalous pulmonary venous connection. There is no connection of common pulmonary vein to left atrium. Key: *AV,* Atrioventricular; *LA,* left atrium; *PV,* pulmonary venous sinus; *RA,* right atrium.

Echocardiography

Two-dimensional (2D) echocardiography is remarkably accurate in assessing the morphology of TAPVC[S12] (Fig. 31-4). Along with Doppler color flow interrogation, it is almost always diagnostic.[C3,G6,H8] Echocardiographic features include criteria for RV diastolic overload and an echo-free space posterior to the left atrium.[P3] However, a second drainage site might be overlooked.[C3] Echocardiography is commonly accepted as a definitive diagnostic procedure in neonates with important pulmonary venous obstruction, because contrast medium is not required.[S13,W1] Cardiac catheterization delays operation and exacerbates myocardial failure and pulmonary edema.

Cardiac Catheterization and Cineangiography

Angiograms obtained by pulmonary artery or pulmonary vein injections define the malformation, identify the site of drainage, and often localize the site of pulmonary venous obstruction. This procedure is nearly always diagnostic.[G2] However, it should not be used in seriously ill neonates (see previous discussion). When the connection is to a left vertical vein, the common pulmonary venous sinus and vertical vein can usually be demonstrated (Fig. 31-5, *A*). When the anomalous connection is to the coronary sinus, it appears as an ovoid opacification over the left side of the spine within the right atrial contour.[R6] When it is infracardiac, the descending vein can usually be demonstrated, although its precise infradiaphragmatic connection may not be seen (Fig. 31-5, *B*).

Tynan and colleagues have pointed out that in neonates, umbilical vein catheterization permits direct injection of contrast medium into the anomalously connecting infradiaphragmatic vein and an accurate diagnosis of its connections.[T5] Presence of pulmonary venous obstruction is established by demonstrating a gradient between left atrial and pulmonary

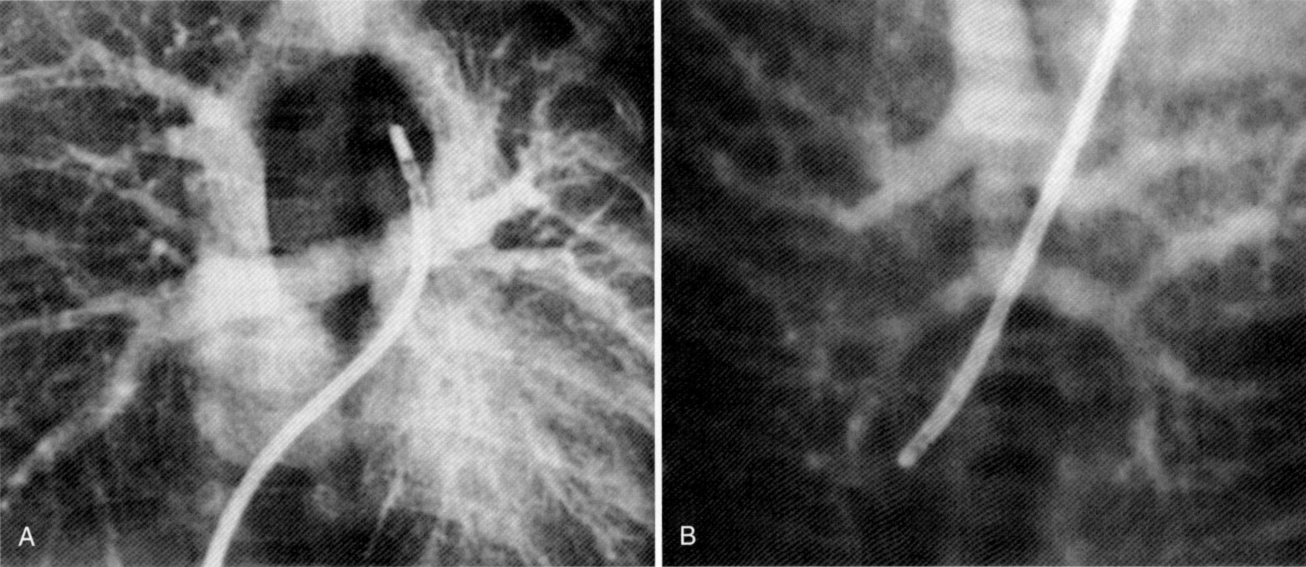

Figure 31-5 Angiograms of infants with total anomalous pulmonary venous connection (TAPVC). **A,** TAPVC to left brachiocephalic vein. **B,** TAPVC draining infradiaphragmatically.

artery wedge pressures. Greene and colleagues employ superimposition digital subtraction angiography to define pulmonary venous anatomy, relationship of common pulmonary vein to left atrium, and size of left atrium.[G7]

Magnetic Resonance Imaging and Computed Tomography

Because of diagnostic limitations of echocardiography in complex cases and morbidity associated with cardiac catheterization in gravely ill patients, both magnetic resonance imaging (MRI) and computed tomography (CT) have become increasingly important in diagnosing TAPVC. Both modalities should be used selectively, primarily in patients in whom echocardiography is not definitive. When compared with both catheterization and echocardiography, numerous studies have demonstrated the accuracy of MRI and CT in diagnosing TAPVC.[C4,F1,G8,K5,M2,S14,U1] Several demonstrate improved accuracy of diagnosis using both helical CT angiography, with and without three-dimensional (3D) reconstruction,[K5] and gadolinium-enhanced 3D cardiac magnetic resonance (CMR) angiography.[F1,G8]

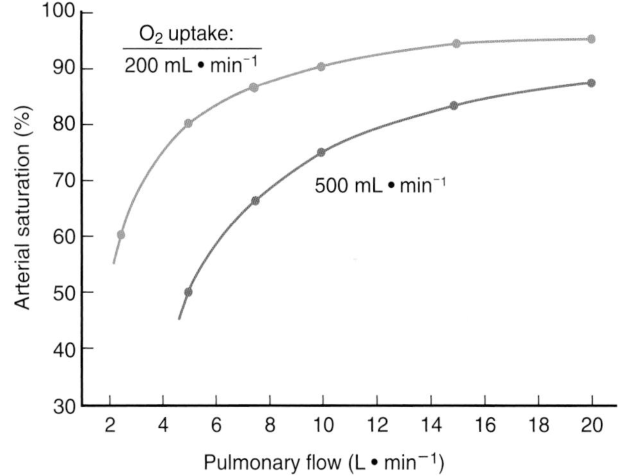

Figure 31-6 Relation between percent arterial oxygen saturation and pulmonary blood flow in persons with common mixing chambers, formulated on theoretical grounds by Burchell.[B17] The upper curve is at rest; the lower is at moderate exercise. Systemic blood flow is assumed to be 25 L · min^{-1}. (From Burchell.[B17])

Physiology of Common Mixing Chamber

In TAPVC, the right atrium is theoretically a common mixing chamber.[B17] This situation is reflected in the frequent finding of close similarity of oxygen content and saturations from the right atrium, left atrium, pulmonary artery, and systemic artery.[F4] There is considerable deviation from this pattern, however, because of streaming of systemic venous return in the right atrium, directing inferior vena caval blood through the foramen ovale to the mitral valve, and superior vena caval blood through the tricuspid valve. Thus, in infracardiac TAPVC, systemic arterial saturation is typically higher than pulmonary artery saturation.

Because TAPVC has this common mixing chamber, in most patients who live beyond infancy, a direct relationship exists between the magnitude of pulmonary blood flow and arterial oxygen saturation, assuming a constant oxygen consumption and blood hemoglobin level. This relationship was formulated into a nomogram by Burchell[B17] (Fig. 31-6). Because the pulmonary/systemic blood flow ratio ($\dot{Q}p/\dot{Q}s$) in such patients is determined primarily by magnitude of the pulmonary blood flow, and because their pulmonary vascular resistance is inversely related to pulmonary blood flow, arterial oxygen saturation in children (not in seriously ill neonates and young infants) is a rough guide to the patient's operability vis-à-vis pulmonary vascular disease. When, in children and adults, arterial oxygen saturation is less than about 80%, the $\dot{Q}p/\dot{Q}s$ is likely to be less than 1.4 and pulmonary vascular resistance greater than 10 U · m^2.

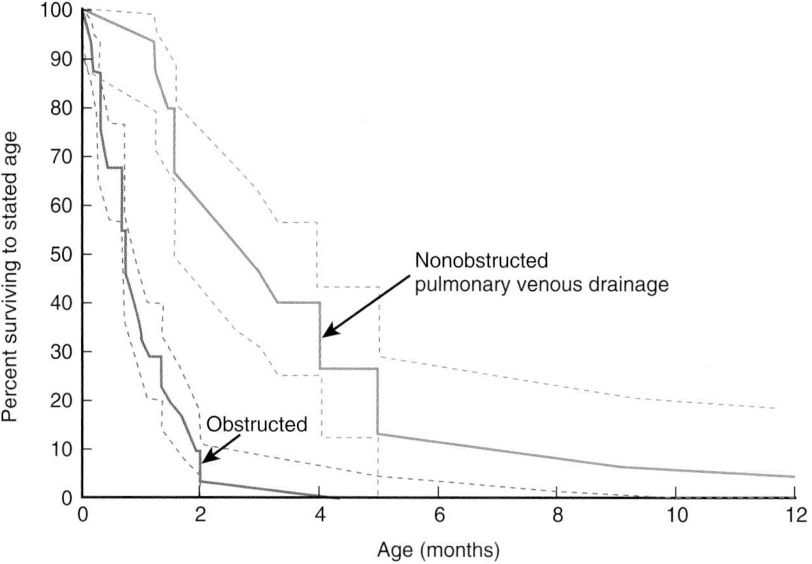

Figure 31-7 Survival of surgically untreated persons with total anomalous pulmonary venous connection, according to clearly present or clearly absent obstruction to pulmonary venous drainage; based on 31 cases among 183 in which the autopsy protocol was clear in this regard. Dashed lines represent 70% confidence limits (P for difference < .0001). (From Hazelrig and colleagues.[H6])

NATURAL HISTORY

TAPVC is relatively uncommon, accounting for only about 1.5% to 3% of cases of congenital heart disease.[B9] Infants born with TAPVC have a generally unfavorable prognosis, with only about 20% surviving the first year of life.[B18,K4] Only about 50% survive beyond 3 months, with death occurring during the first few weeks or months of life in most neonates in whom tachypnea, cyanosis, and clinical evidence of low cardiac output develop. Such infants usually have pulmonary venous obstruction, long pulmonary venous pathways, and a small patent foramen ovale.[B18] Survival past the critical first few weeks and months does not portend a favorable prognosis, because only about half the patients surviving to age 3 months survive to 1 year. Infants who survive the first few weeks of life usually have cardiomegaly and a large pulmonary blood flow, with mild cyanosis. Most have some degree of pulmonary artery hypertension.[G2] Their clinical syndrome includes tachypnea, recurrent episodes of severe pulmonary congestion, failure to thrive, fluid retention, and hepatomegaly.

Those with TAPVC who survive the first year of life without surgical treatment usually have a large atrial septal defect. Characteristically, they exhibit important physical underdevelopment similar to that of patients with other kinds of large left-to-right shunts, mild cyanosis, and mild exercise intolerance (see "Survival" under Natural History in Chapter 30). Like patients with isolated large atrial septal defects, they tend to have a stable hemodynamic state for 10 to 20 years, with little change in pulmonary vascular resistance and thus little change in pulmonary artery pressure, blood flow, and arterial oxygen levels.[G2] In the second decade of life, pulmonary vascular disease develops in some patients, and there is increasing cyanosis as pulmonary blood flow diminishes (Eisenmenger complex).[S5]

To quantify the natural history, Hazelrig and colleagues analyzed data from 183 autopsied cases of surgically untreated TAPVC reported in the literature.[H6] Median survival was 2 months, with the shortest survival being 1 day and the longest 49 years; 90% of deaths occurred in the first year of life. Obstruction of the pulmonary venous pathway importantly reduced median survival (P < .0001) (Fig. 31-7) from 2.5 months in the nonobstructed group to 3 weeks in the obstructed group. Patients with supracardiac and cardiac connections had a similar history, with median survival of 2.5 and 3 months, respectively, whereas those with infracardiac connections had a worse prognosis, with median survival of 3 weeks (Fig. 31-8). Only three patients had mixed connections; two died at 5 months and one at 3.3 months. Presence of an atrial septal defect (rather than a patent foramen ovale) was associated with increased survival, particularly when the connection was not infracardiac (see Fig. 31-8).

TECHNIQUE OF OPERATION

Operation should be undertaken as an emergency immediately after diagnosis by 2D echocardiography in neonates and infants who enter the hospital critically ill. Preoperative preparation and stabilization should be brief. In stable patients, typically non-neonates without obstruction, the operation can be scheduled electively. Approach is via median sternotomy. The CPB technique can vary depending on surgeon preference, ranging from continuous CPB with either moderate or deep hypothermia to limited CPB with deep hypothermic circulatory arrest. Cardiac arrest using cardioplegia is essential for repair (see Chapters 2 and 3 for a detailed discussion of these techniques).

The ductus arteriosus must be dissected and closed routinely in infants, even if not visualized in preoperative studies.[B11,F2] This is usually accomplished just after CPB is established and before cooling is begun. Also, at some point in the operation, the foramen ovale or atrial septal defect must be closed. This is usually done after correcting the anomalous veins. Regardless of the type of TAPVC or type of technical repair, anastomosis of the pulmonary venous sinus to the left atrium is performed with a continuous suture technique using fine polypropylene or polydioxanone suture.

Following completion of the operation, regardless of technical approach to the repair, careful consideration should be given to placing fine polyvinyl pressure catheters into the right atrium, left atrium, and RV or pulmonary trunk for appropriate postoperative monitoring.

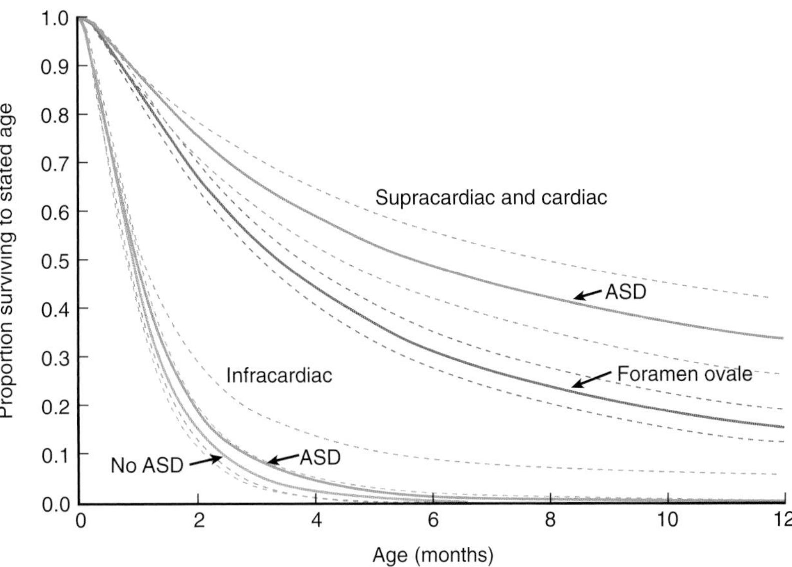

Figure 31-8 Nomogram of multivariable equation relating survival of surgically untreated persons with total anomalous pulmonary venous connection ($n = 183$) to type of connection and presence or absence of an atrial septal defect (ASD). Survival was not different for supracardiac and cardiac types. Solid lines represent probabilities; dashed lines represent 70% confidence limits. The separation into ASD and foramen ovale groups was based simply on words used in autopsy protocol, under the presumption that *atrial septal defect* denoted larger holes. (From Hazelrig and colleagues.[H6])

Total Anomalous Pulmonary Venous Connection to Left Brachiocephalic Vein

After sternotomy and anterior pericardotomy, the common pulmonary venous sinus, lying behind the pericardium, is identified after lifting up the apex of the heart for a moment to visualize the retrocardiac portion of the pericardium. The right pulmonary artery, running parallel and just cephalad to the sinus, is also identified to avoid confusing it with the common pulmonary venous sinus. The vertical vein connecting the common pulmonary venous sinus to the left brachiocephalic vein can sometimes be seen inside the pericardium, but in most cases the pericardium on the left must be retracted toward the patient's right and the persistent left vertical vein identified beneath the mediastinal pleura. The vein is isolated after carefully freeing the left phrenic nerve. A ligature is tied to the tip of the left atrial appendage for leftward retraction.

CPB and cardiac arrest are established using the techniques described in the previous section. The ductus arteriosus (if patent) and persistent vertical vein are ligated. The common pulmonary venous sinus can be exposed in several ways. One method approaches the common pulmonary venous sinus from the right side of the heart. The posterior pericardial reflection is opened (Fig. 31-9, *A*), and the common pulmonary venous sinus is mobilized and opened (Fig. 31-9, *B-C*). The posterior left atrial wall is opened, and the anastomosis is then made between the common pulmonary venous sinus and left atrium (Fig. 31-9, *D-F*). The continuous suture line must not be pulled up so tightly as to purse-string the anastomosis and narrow it. The right atrium is opened, the foramen ovale closed, and the atrium closed. The remainder of CPB and reestablishment of myocardial perfusion are completed (see Chapters 2 and 3).

A second method of repairing TAPVC is similar to that just described, but the common pulmonary venous sinus is exposed from the left side of the heart by lifting the cardiac mass out of the pericardial sac by retracting the cardiac apex anteriorly and rightward. This is best achieved by placing a retracting suture into the apical myocardium (Fig. 31-10, *A*). This avoids the warming effect on the myocardium that occurs when the surgical assistant's finger or hand is used to directly retract the heart. The pericardial sac is now essentially vacant, and the incision in the common pulmonary venous sinus is made under direct vision (Fig. 31-10, *B*). The back of the left atrium is also exposed by this maneuver and is incised. The anastomosis is then made in a fashion similar to that described in the preceding text (Fig. 31-10, *C*).

A third method of repairing TAPVC to the left brachiocephalic vein is via a right atrial approach.[D8] This method has the advantage of allowing the anastomosis of the common pulmonary venous sinus to the left atrium to be performed in precise anatomic relationships, because there is no retraction or displacement of critical structures to gain exposure. The right atrium is incised parallel to the atrioventricular groove (Fig. 31-11, *A*), exposing the atrial septum. The membrane of the foramen ovale is excised to gain entry to the left atrium. The posterior wall of the left atrium is incised transversely (Fig. 31-11, *B*) into the free pericardial space behind the atrium. The common pulmonary venous sinus is identified lying beneath the pericardium directly behind the incision in the left atrium. An incision is made in the common pulmonary venous sinus, which extends from the bifurcation on the left side to the bifurcation on the right side (see Fig. 31-11, *C*). A large anastomosis is constructed between the common pulmonary venous sinus and left atrium (Fig. 31-11, *D*). This anastomosis has little chance for distortion because it is performed without displacing anatomically adjacent structures. Repair is completed by closing the foramen ovale with a pericardial patch (Fig. 31-11, *E*). The patch serves both to repair the atrial septum and enlarge the left atrial filling capacity.

Total Anomalous Pulmonary Venous Connection to Superior Vena Cava

A common pulmonary venous sinus is usually present in the rare anomaly of TAPVC to the superior vena cava, providing free communication between right and left pulmonary veins. After the presence of this sinus is confirmed by direct

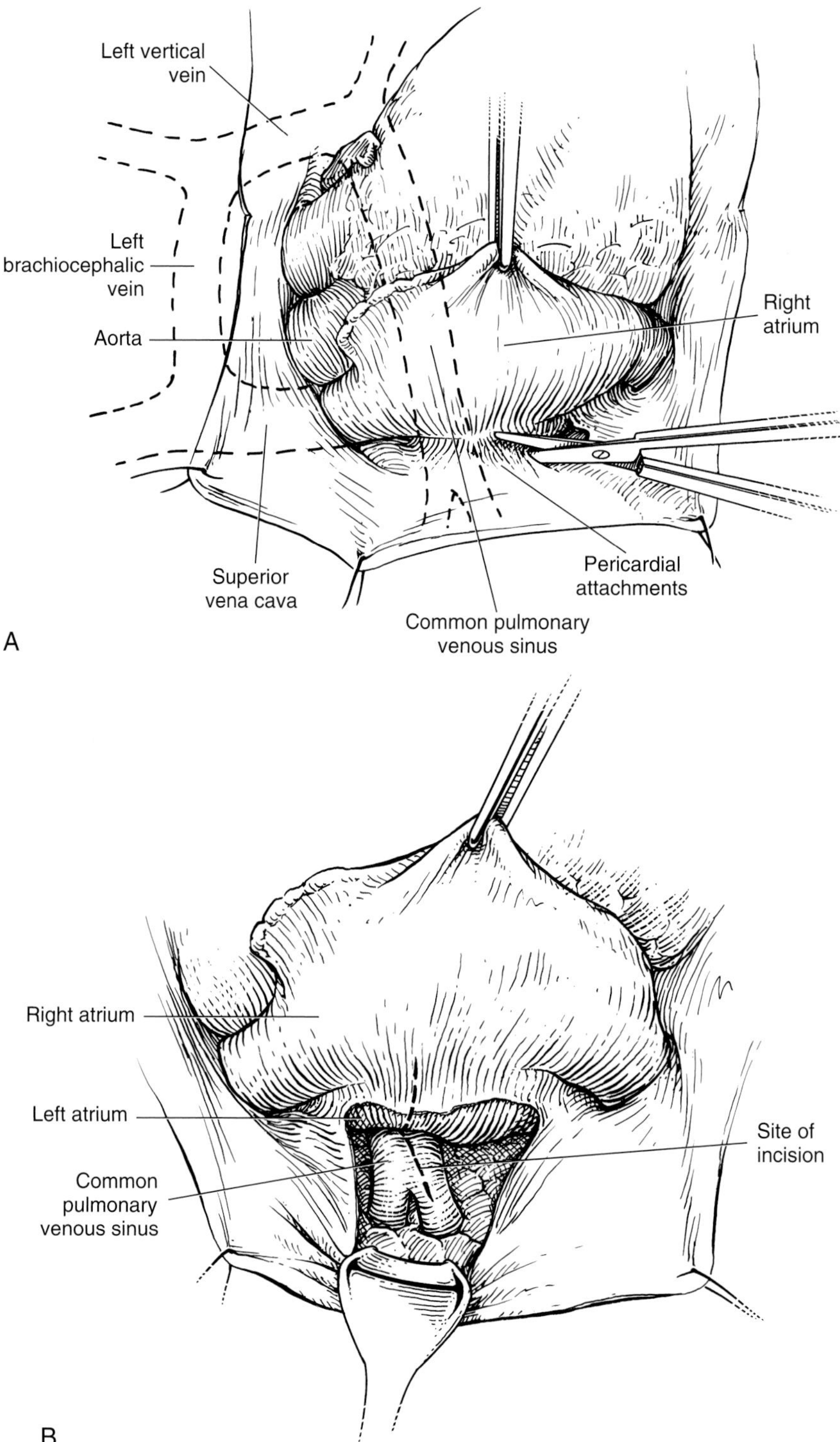

Figure 31-9 Repair of total anomalous pulmonary venous connection (TAPVC) to left brachiocephalic vein, right lateral approach. **A,** Posterior pericardial attachments of heart are cut, allowing cavae and atria to be lifted completely free of common pulmonary venous sinus, which is behind the pericardium. Left vertical vein is exposed, preferably from within the pericardium. If extrapericardial exposure is required, the phrenic nerve is elevated off the pericardium and vein. This dissection must be done sharply and with perfect exposure and visibility, because damage to this vein might necessitate its premature ligation. In this case, the common pulmonary venous sinus would have to be opened immediately to prevent severe pulmonary venous hypertension. Also, the dissection must identify the site of connection of the uppermost left pulmonary vein so that the vertical vein may be ligated superior to that point. **B,** With ventricles in normal position in the pericardium, exposure for repair (and for repair of other types of TAPVC) is obtained by elevating atria up and to the left.[K8] Posterior pericardium over common pulmonary venous sinus and anterior wall of the sinus are opened parallel to long axis of the sinus.

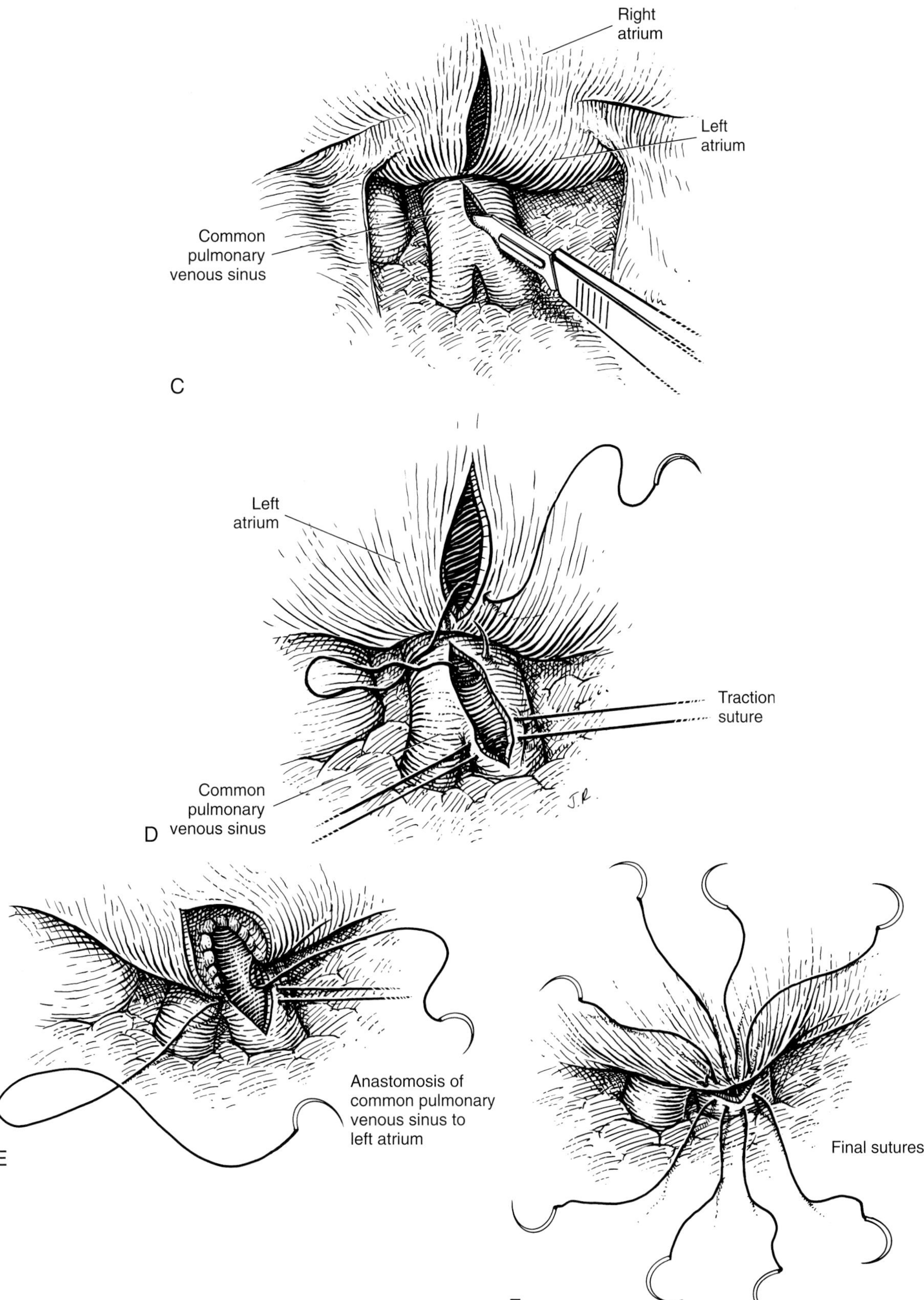

Figure 31-9, cont'd **C,** Incision should be made over full length of sinus. Orifices of left and right pulmonary veins are located and inspected, and care is taken to avoid damaging them. A corresponding incision is made more or less transversely in the back wall of left atrium. The incision may need to be carried onto the base of the left atrial appendage to gain sufficient length. It is carried to the atrial septum on the right, but care is taken not to enter the septum itself. When in doubt about initial placement of the left atrial incision, it is helpful to pass a small curved clamp through an incision in the right atrial wall and through the foramen ovale so that its tip tents the back wall of the left atrium outward. **D,** Traction sutures of 5-0 polypropylene are placed on inferior and superior lips of the incision into the common pulmonary venous sinus; both the sinus wall and posterior pericardium are caught with these sutures and with the suture line. Anastomosis is begun at the point shown, with the first stitch placed from outside to inside in the atrial wall, allowing suture line to be made from inside the vessels. **E,** Suture line is carried toward and around the left-sided angle of the incisions and along most of the superior side. The previously held other end of the double-armed 6-0 or 7-0 polypropylene or polydioxanone stitch is then used to approximate, in similar fashion, the inferior edge. Here the stitches are placed from outside to inside on the sinus and from inside to outside on the atrial wall. Suture line is carried nearly to the right-sided angle. **F,** Suture line is then completed, either with a few interrupted stitches or as a continuous stitch.

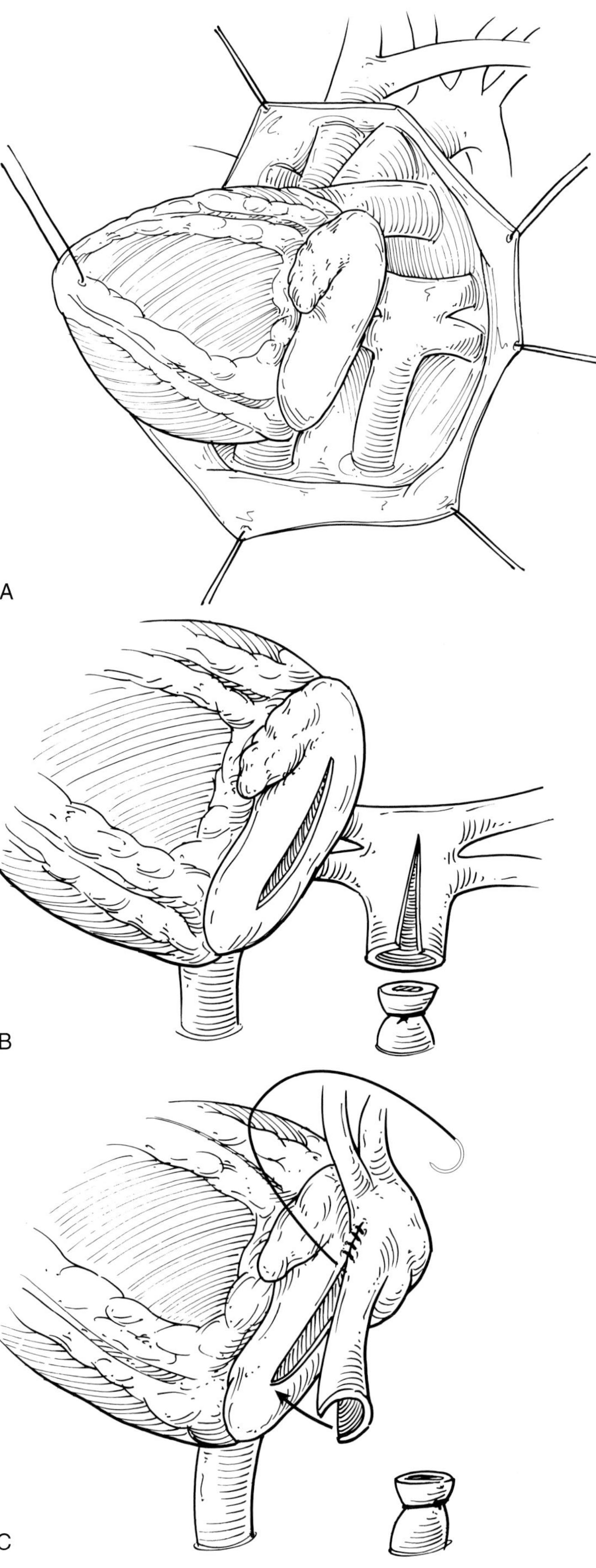

Figure 31-10 **A,** A retraction suture is placed into the myocardium at the apex and is used to retract the cardiac mass, elevating it superiorly and to the right, out of pericardial space, exposing posterior parietal pericardium. This allows visualization of pulmonary venous sinus lying behind pericardium. **B,** Cardiac mass is raised and lowered in and out of pericardial sac using retraction suture to identify region of left atrial free wall that lies directly against pulmonary venous sinus. Identifying this region of left atrium is necessary to plan the left atrial incision so that there is no distortion of pulmonary veins after anastomosis. Parallel incisions of equal length are made in the left atrial free wall and pulmonary venous sinus. Incisions are made as large as possible, but the pulmonary venous sinus incision does not extend into individual pulmonary veins. **C,** Anastomosis is performed using a continuous suture technique.

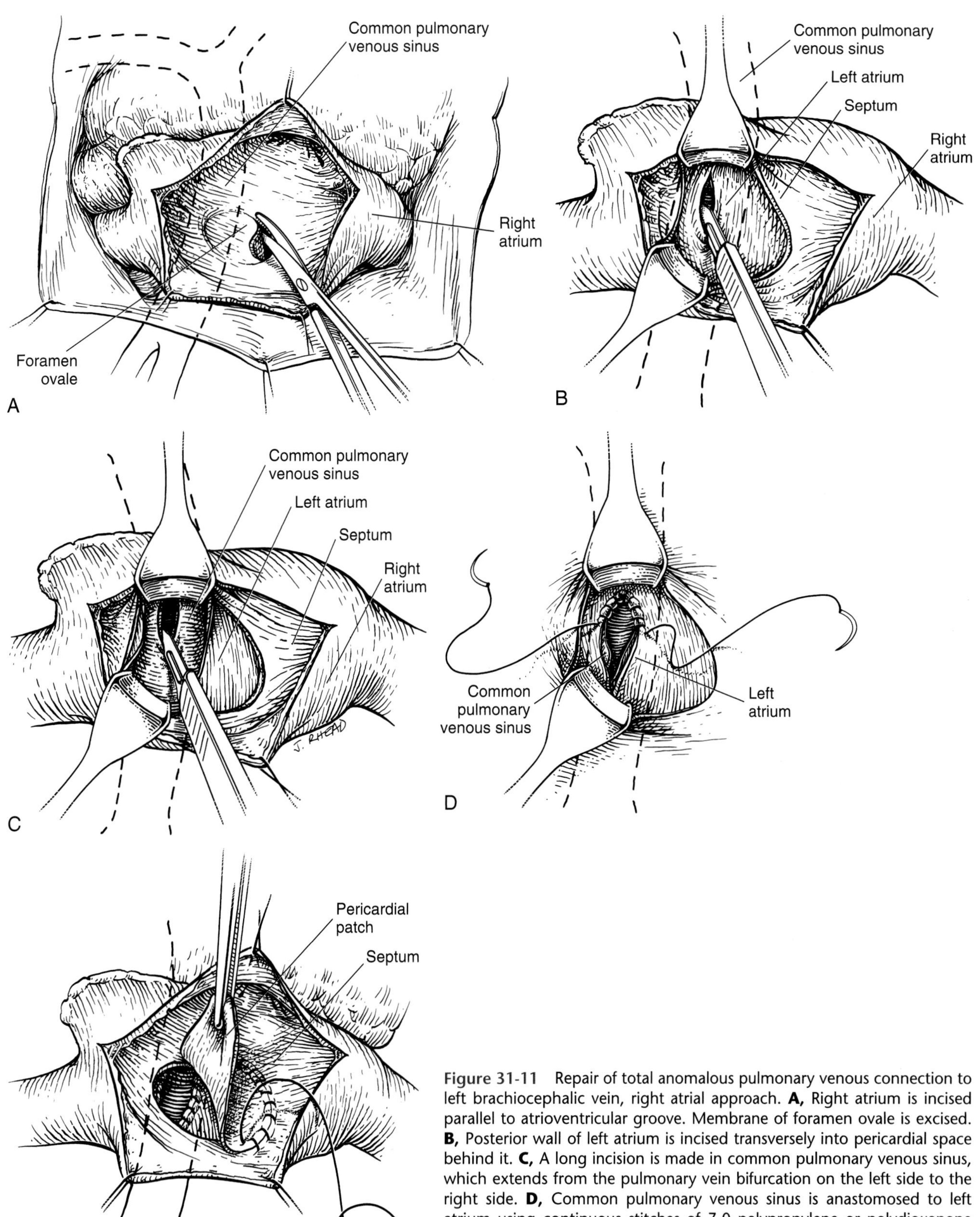

Figure 31-11 Repair of total anomalous pulmonary venous connection to left brachiocephalic vein, right atrial approach. **A,** Right atrium is incised parallel to atrioventricular groove. Membrane of foramen ovale is excised. **B,** Posterior wall of left atrium is incised transversely into pericardial space behind it. **C,** A long incision is made in common pulmonary venous sinus, which extends from the pulmonary vein bifurcation on the left side to the right side. **D,** Common pulmonary venous sinus is anastomosed to left atrium using continuous stitches of 7-0 polypropylene or polydioxanone suture. Suture line is started at apex of pulmonary venous sinus incision on the left side, placing stitches from inside the pulmonary vein. **E,** Foramen ovale is closed with pericardial patch to increase capacity of left atrium.

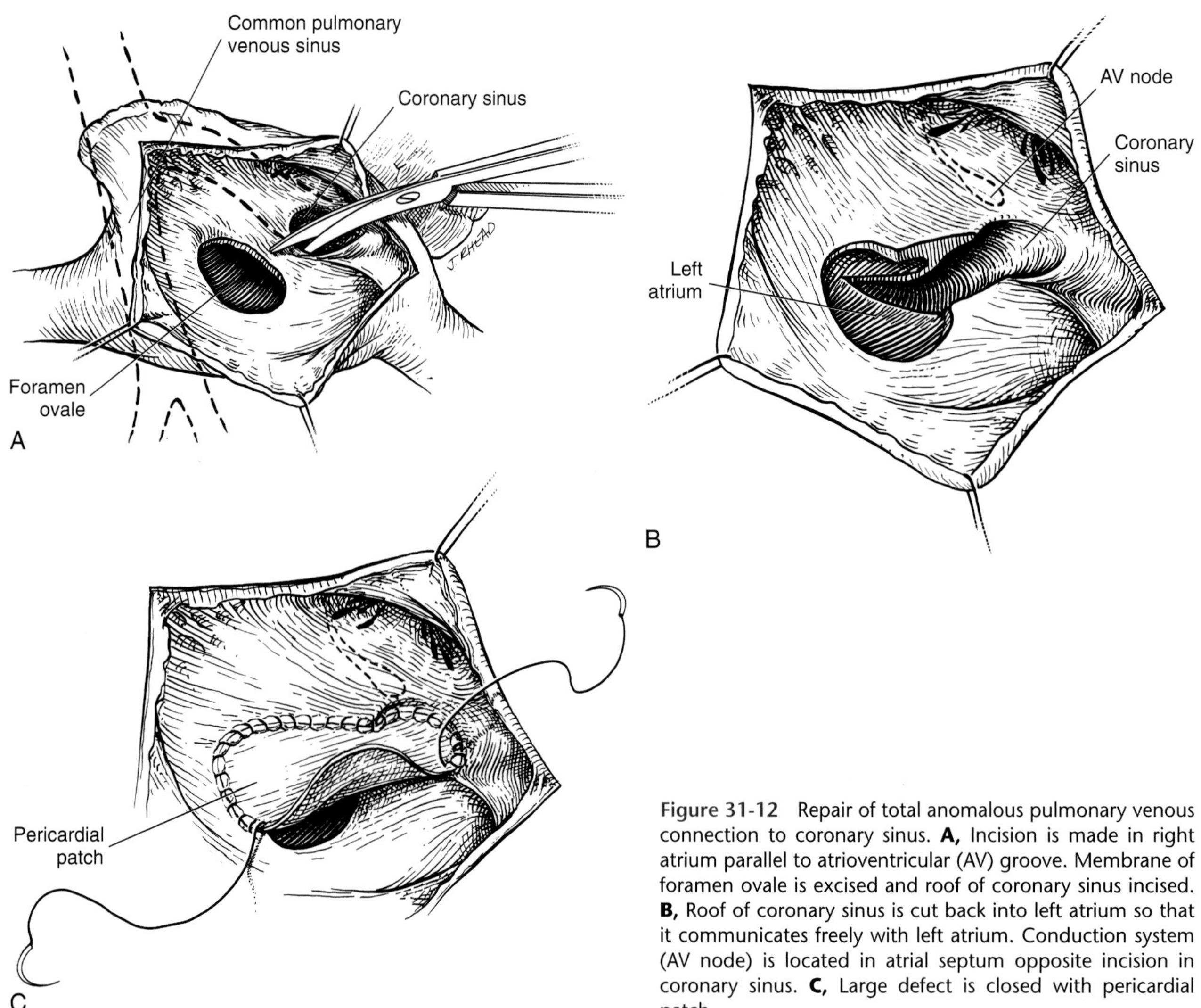

Figure 31-12 Repair of total anomalous pulmonary venous connection to coronary sinus. **A,** Incision is made in right atrium parallel to atrioventricular (AV) groove. Membrane of foramen ovale is excised and roof of coronary sinus incised. **B,** Roof of coronary sinus is cut back into left atrium so that it communicates freely with left atrium. Conduction system (AV node) is located in atrial septum opposite incision in coronary sinus. **C,** Large defect is closed with pericardial patch.

inspection (see "Total Anomalous Pulmonary Venous Connection to Left Brachiocephalic Vein" earlier), the operation proceeds in the same manner as described for patients with TAPVC to the left brachiocephalic vein, using the right atrial approach. The connection into the lower part of the superior vena cava is identified, and palpation is performed with a right-angled clamp to confirm the anatomic details. The sinus is disconnected from the superior vena cava by cutting across the connection. The resultant opening in the sinus is extended in both directions and the sinus-to–left atrial anastomosis made. The site of connection into the superior vena cava is then easily closed from within the right atrium, using a pericardial patch. The right atrium is then closed, rewarming begun, and the remainder of the operation completed as described for patients with connection to the left brachiocephalic vein.

Total Anomalous Pulmonary Venous Connection to Coronary Sinus

The right atrial approach described in the preceding text is used. The right atrium is opened by the usual oblique incision. The repair most commonly used includes excising both the roof of the coronary sinus, so that it communicates freely with the left atrium, and the fossa ovalis (Fig. 31-12, *A-B*). The resulting large defect, made up of a confluence between the rim of the fossa ovalis and the coronary sinus ostium, is then closed with a pericardial patch (Fig. 32-12, *C*).

However, occurrence of stenosis at the repair site late after operation has prompted use of the technique described by Van Praagh and colleagues.[V1] The foramen ovale is enlarged to obtain an adequate exposure within the left atrium (Fig. 31-13, *A*). The wall between the coronary sinus and left atrium is incised (Fig. 31-13, *B*), and the incision is enlarged as much as possible in both directions. The foramen ovale and coronary sinus ostium are closed separately (Fig. 31-13, *C*). The pulmonary veins then drain into the left atrium through the surgically unroofed coronary sinus (Fig. 31-13, *D*). The remainder of the operation is completed as described for other types of TAPVC.

Obstructed pulmonary venous drainage can occur in patients with TAPVC to the coronary sinus. Thus, the surgeon must be prepared to abandon usual approaches if a stenosis is proximal to the coronary sinus itself, and proceed to anastomose the common pulmonary venous sinus, which

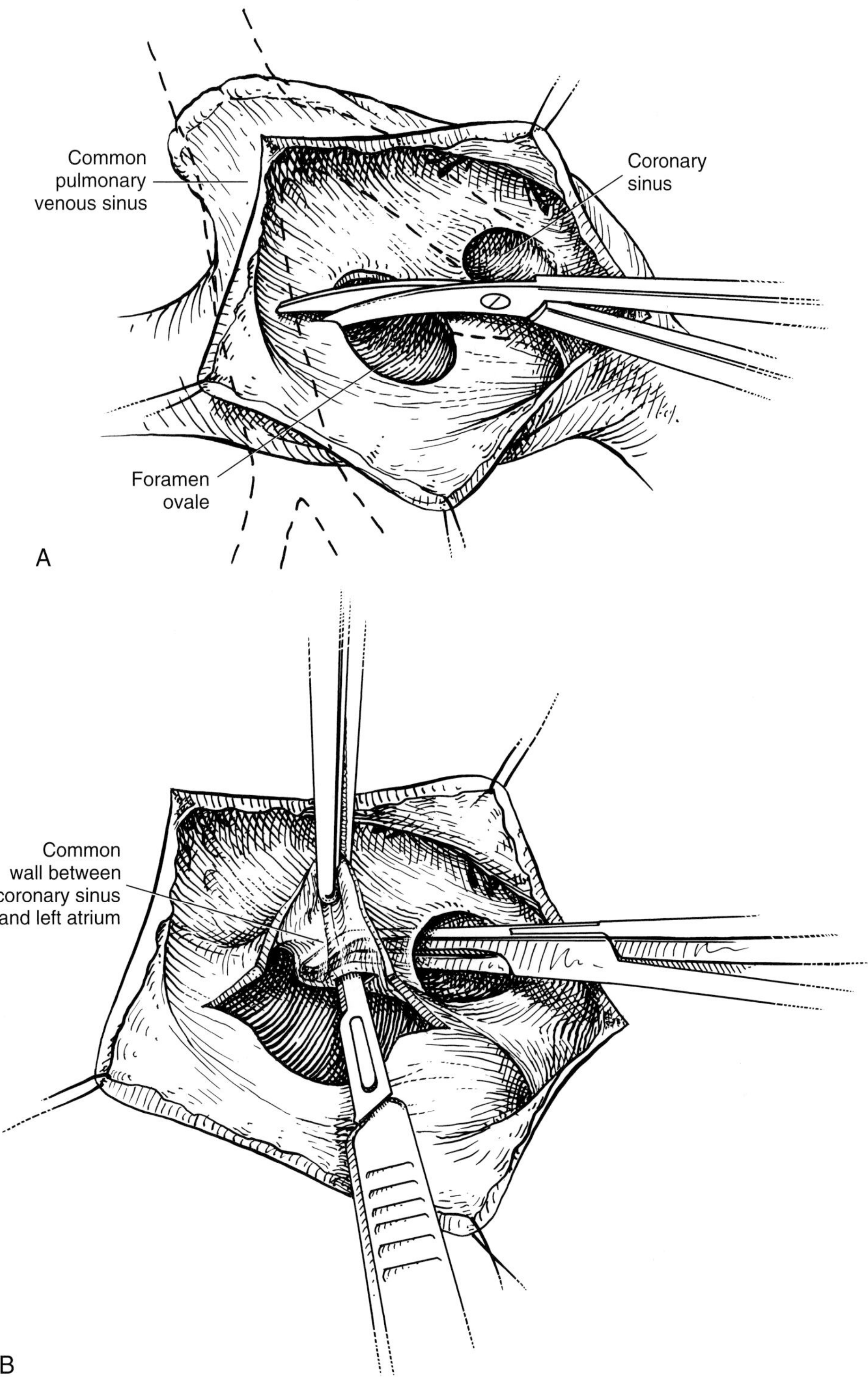

Figure 31-13 Repair of total anomalous pulmonary venous connection to coronary sinus, Van Praagh method.[V1] **A,** After usual preparations, right atrium is opened obliquely and exposure arranged. Foramen ovale is enlarged cephalad and at times caudad to attain adequate visibility within left atrium. **B,** An opening is made in the common wall between coronary sinus and left atrium after wall has been tented with right-angle forceps. This opening is enlarged downward and to the left; care must be taken not to go outside the heart in the process. (If this occurs, the opening must be closed at this point from within the heart by a few sutures, because the area is difficult to expose from outside the heart.) The incision is carried anteriorly and to the right to within a few millimeters of the ostium of the coronary sinus.

Continued

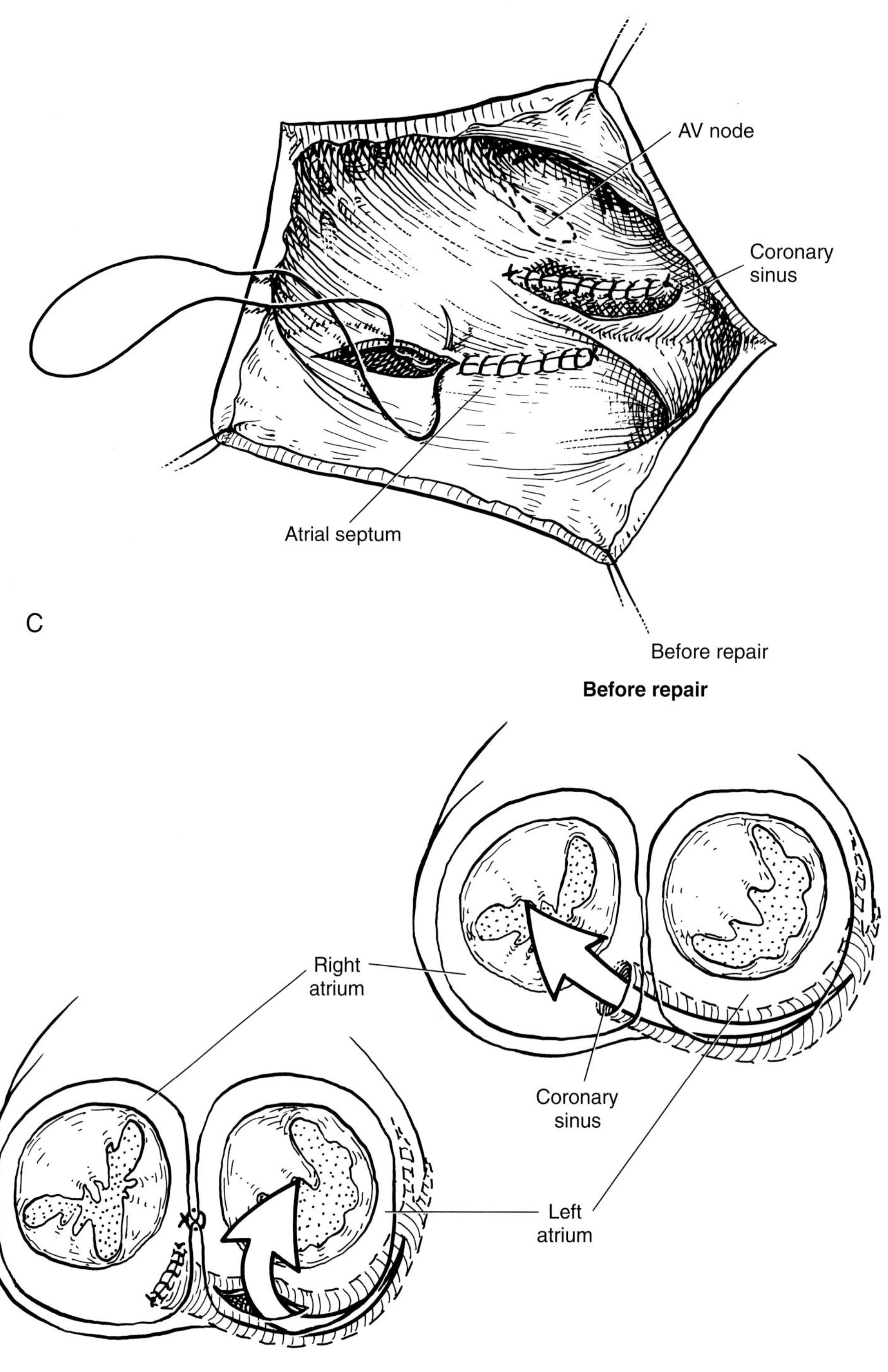

Figure 31-13, cont'd **C,** Foramen ovale and ostium of coronary sinus are closed, usually individually, with interrupted or continuous suture. Suture line should start inferiorly just below the last tiny coronary vein entering the sinus and, as it proceeds superiorly, should be made with shallow bites and preferably kept within the coronary sinus ostium to avoid the atrioventricular (AV) node. **D,** Arrow indicates path of blood flow through the coronary sinus to the right atrium before repair. After repair, blood flow from the coronary sinus is to the left atrium above the mitral valve through the unroofed coronary sinus.

is actually the junction of the right and left pulmonary veins, to the back of the left atrium.[J2]

Total Anomalous Pulmonary Venous Connection to Right Atrium

Initial stages of the operation are as described for other types of TAPVC using the right atrial approach. The right atrium is opened obliquely. The anomalous connection into the right atrium is explored with an instrument to verify the presence of a confluent pulmonary venous sinus. The foramen ovale is then enlarged, and working through it, an incision is made in the posterior left atrial wall. The common pulmonary venous sinus is visualized through this incision, and the anterior wall of the sinus is incised. This opening is enlarged and anastomosed to the left atrial incision, still working from within the atria. The enlarged foramen ovale is closed by direct suture. The original connection of the common pulmonary venous sinus to the right atrium is closed with a relatively small pericardial patch; it must be remembered that the pulmonary venous pathway from the right lung is beneath the patch.

Alternatively, as described for the repair of TAPVC to the superior vena cava, the common pulmonary venous sinus can be detached from the right atrium, the opening in the sinus enlarged and used for anastomosis to the left atrium, and the resulting defect in the posterior atrial wall closed. The remainder of the operation is completed as usual.

Total Anomalous Pulmonary Venous Connection to Infradiaphragmatic Vein

In TAPVC to an infradiaphragmatic vein, the distal (inferior) portion of the common pulmonary venous sinus is vertical, and proximally (superiorly) it forms a Y or T connection with the left and right pulmonary veins. Therefore, after initial stages of the operation have been performed as described for other types of TAPVC, a decision is made about the approach, which may be similar to that for other types, through the opened right atrium, or through the back of the left atrium directly after tilting the apex of the heart up and to the right. Good results have been obtained by all approaches. The approach using retraction of the cardiac mass out of the pericardial sac is described. The heart is freed from its posterior attachments and the back of the left atrium exposed (Fig. 31-14, *A*). The common pulmonary venous sinus and left atrium are incised (Fig. 31-14, *B*). The common pulmonary venous sinus is anastomosed to the back of the left atrium (Fig. 31-14, *C*) and is ligated (Fig. 31-14, *D*) and may be divided to allow the anastomosis to conform better.[P4,T4]

Miscellaneous Types of Total Anomalous Pulmonary Venous Connection

Some rare types of TAPVC occur, such as connection to the azygos vein or inferior vena cava, or dual connection from the common pulmonary venous sinus.[G10,S6,T1,V2] These connections can usually be sorted out using MRI or CT. In the rare event that the connection cannot readily be found or dissected out at operation, the common pulmonary venous sinus is opened and the connection(s) identified from within it. After the connection is closed, the usual anastomosis is made between the common pulmonary venous sinus and left atrium.

Mixed Total Anomalous Pulmonary Venous Connection

Patients with mixed TAPVC present a diagnostic as well as surgical challenge. MRI or CT is almost always used to supplement echocardiographic imaging and to provide an accurate characterization of the morphologic details.[F1,G8,K5,M2,S14,U1] Chowdhury and colleagues have recently categorized the spectrum of mixed TAPVC into five major groups.[C5,C6] Each group is characterized by a set of similar general morphologic patterns, but many variations occur from case to case.

Management of each patient must be individualized based on analysis of the mixture presented. A variety of techniques must be used, including many of those already described for TAPVC to the left brachiocephalic vein, right atrium, superior vena cava, and structures below the diaphragm. Combining these techniques with others, such as construction of a right atrial intracardiac baffle for isolated veins to the superior vena cava (similar to repair of partial anomalous pulmonary venous connection) or direct anastomosis of isolated left upper pulmonary vein to the left atrial appendage, will usually allow complete repair.[B7,C9,D6,I1,S8] In some small babies in whom an extensive operation would be required for complete one-stage repair, subtotal repair can be successful, leaving unrepaired, for example, anomalous connection of the left upper lobe to the left brachiocephalic vein.

SPECIAL FEATURES OF POSTOPERATIVE CARE

Overall management of patients after correction of TAPVC is accomplished in the usual way (see Chapter 5). The relationship between left and right atrial pressures is of particular importance. Left atrial pressure may be considerably higher than right when pulmonary artery pressure decreases immediately after repair, particularly when a small and noncompliant left atrium acts more like a conduit than a reservoir.[P1] The left atrial pressure pulse after operation is then characterized by a steep *y* descent (Fig. 31-15). A small or borderline-sized LV contributes to this situation.

In infants, particularly neonates, who present for operation in critical condition with pulmonary venous obstruction, pulmonary artery pressure and resistance may remain high early postoperatively, which in part may reflect the damaging effects of CPB (see Chapter 2), preoperative lung injury, and postoperative acidemia. Because of this, continuous monitoring of pulmonary artery pressure for at least 48 hours after repair is essential.[S9] When pulmonary artery systolic pressure remains elevated to two thirds or more of systemic arterial systolic pressure, right atrial and RV end-diastolic pressures are usually higher than left atrial pressure, and RV stroke volume is likely to be reduced. When this situation is present, acidemia must be vigorously treated; in addition, $PaCO_2$ should be kept low (25-30 mmHg) by hyperventilation.[D9]

Fentanyl should be continued for at least 36 hours postoperatively, and all features of the regimen to minimize occurrence of paroxysmal pulmonary hypertension employed (see "Pulmonary Hypertensive Crises" under Pulmonary Subsystem in Section I of Chapter 5). Use of inhaled nitric oxide may be particularly helpful in this setting and has essentially replaced other pulmonary vasodilatory drugs that have important side effects such as systemic hypotension.

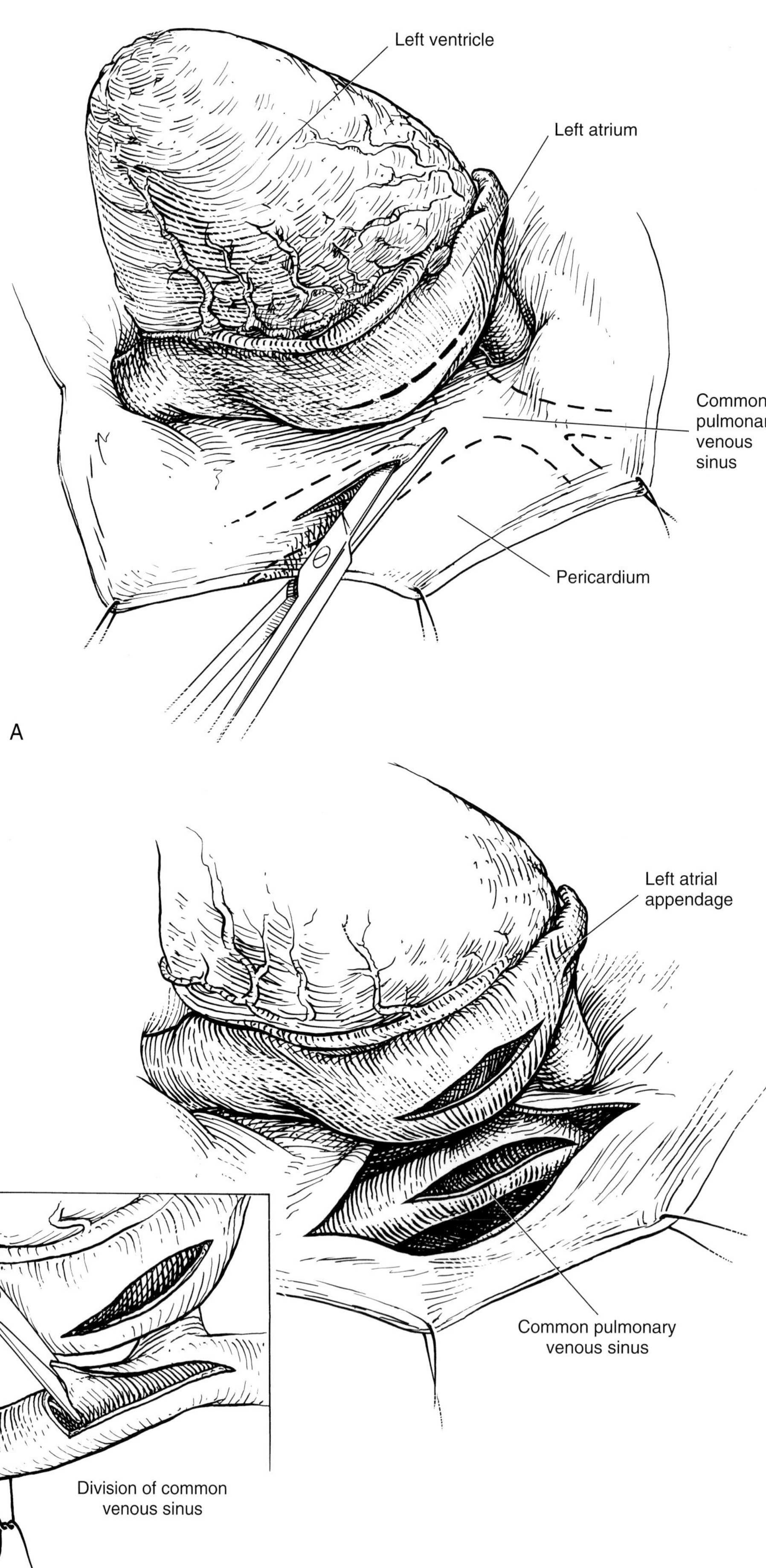

Figure 31-14 Repair of total anomalous pulmonary venous connection draining infradiaphragmatically. **A,** Exposure of common pulmonary venous sinus and posterior wall of the left atrium is obtained by tilting the heart superiorly and to the right. Pulmonary venous sinus is identified behind the pericardium posteriorly. **B,** Posterior wall of left atrium is incised beginning at base of the appendage and somewhat more vertically than for other types of repair of total anomalous pulmonary venous connection (TAPVC). A long incision is made in common pulmonary venous sinus. Alternatively, common pulmonary venous sinus may be ligated and divided *(inset)*.

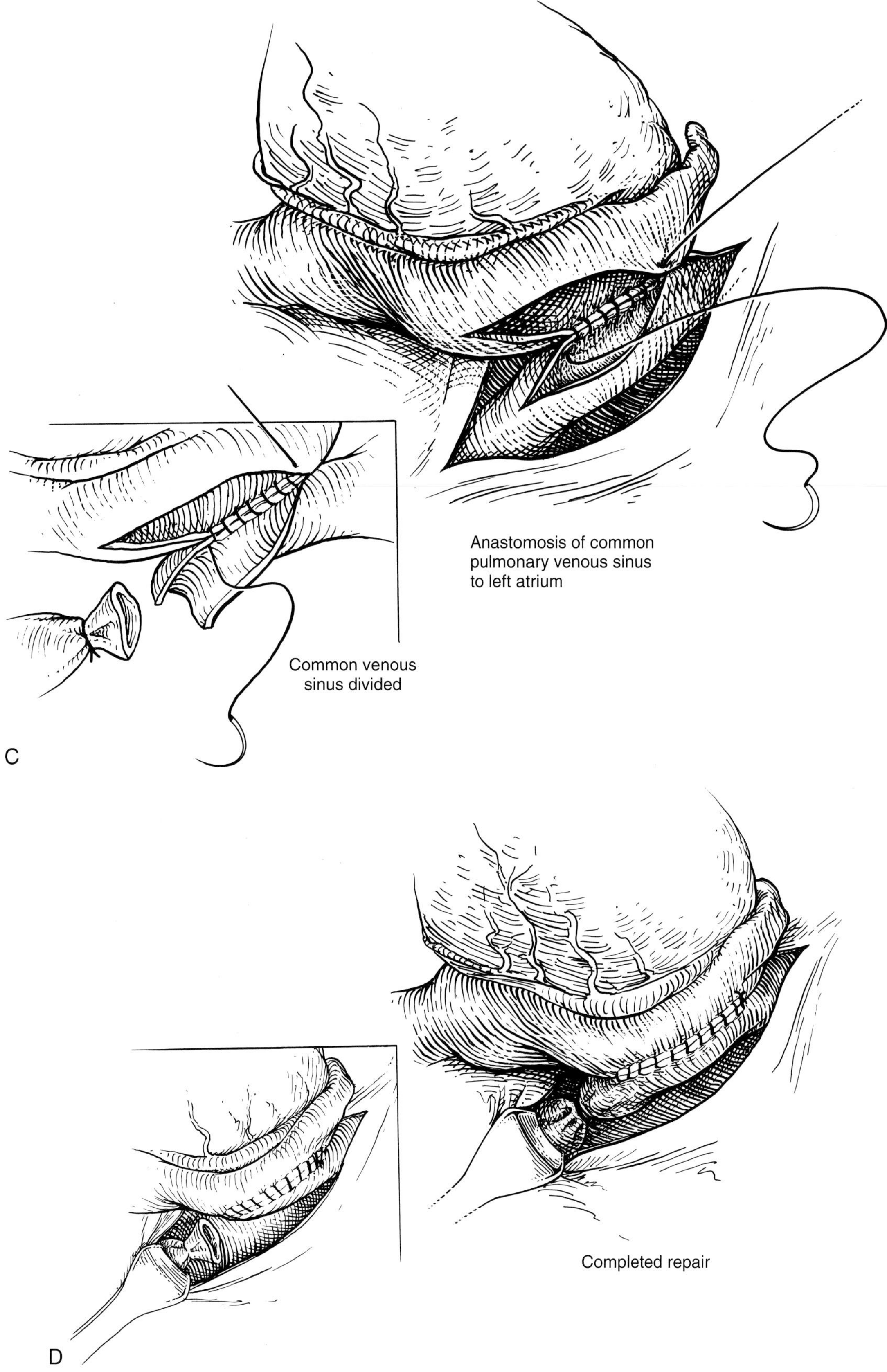

Figure 31-14, cont'd **C,** Anastomosis of common pulmonary venous sinus to left atrium is constructed using 6-0 or 7-0 polypropylene or polydioxanone suture. Anastomosis is started at the apex superiorly, working from within the left atrium and pulmonary venous sinus. The technique with the venous sinus divided is also shown *(inset)*. **D,** Common pulmonary venous sinus is ligated below the anastomosis, with care taken to place ligature below any pulmonary vein branch. The sinus may be divided to allow the anastomosis to conform better *(inset)*.

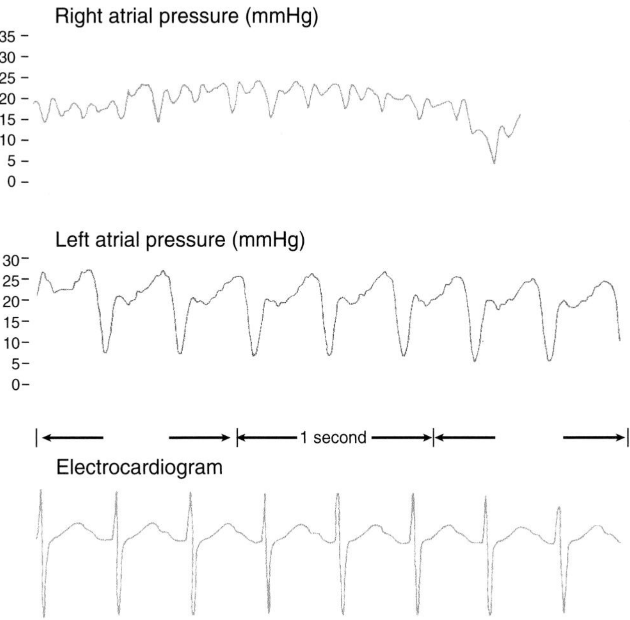

Figure 31-15 Left and right atrial pulses and electrocardiogram in an infant a few hours after repair of total anomalous pulmonary venous connection (TAPVC). Left atrial pressure pulse is characterized by a rapid *y* descent, probably because of low left atrial compliance. Right atrial pressure pulse has an essentially normal contour, because of its large size and normal compliance. Electrocardiogram shows that the *y* descent coincides with opening of the mitral valve. (From Parr and colleagues.[P1])

RESULTS

Results of operation for TAPVC can be excellent, but three types of complication still occur and can be fatal: (1) consequences of severe preoperative cardiopulmonary instability in neonates with obstruction, (2) a strong tendency to early postoperative paroxysms of pulmonary hypertension (described earlier), and (3) delayed development and progression of pulmonary vein stenosis.

Survival

Early (Hospital) Death

Hospital mortality following surgery for TAPVC has been low for patients aged 1 year or more since the early days of cardiac surgery.[C8] For neonates and infants undergoing operation before 1970, however, mortality was high.[D10] Since 1970, hospital mortality for neonates and infants has steadily improved, but considerable variability remains in single-institution reports, with mortality ranging from 2% to 20%.[A2,B16,G1,J2,K11,L3,O1,R1,S1,T4,Y1] Data from the Society of Thoracic Surgeons database, which includes combined outcomes of 32 institutions, show that for 226 cases of TAPVC repair performed between 2002 and 2004, early mortality was 12%: 9.9% for infants within the normal weight range, but 29% for infants weighing less than 2.5 kg.[H2]

Time-Related Survival

Long-term survival is determined primarily by early mortality. Late deaths occur, but at a much lower rate than early deaths. In the study by Ando and colleagues, survival was unchanged at 90% from 2.3 months to 10 years of follow up.[K1] Kirshbom and colleagues reported similar findings.[A2] Other studies indicate a slight drop in survival at mid- to late follow-up. The study by Hancock Friesen and colleagues shows 1-month survival of 90% and 3-year survival of 87%.[K11] Karamlou and colleagues reported that most deaths occurring outside the perioperative period occurred within a few months of surgery, with essentially no late events.[B1] In patients with mixed TAPVC, Chowdhury and colleagues demonstrated late mortality of 4.3%, with follow-up of 42 months (median).[C5]

Table 31-1 Incremental Risk Factors for Mortality after Repair of Mixed TAPVC

Risk Factor	Odds Ratio (CL, %)	*P*
Age ≤2 months	5.2 (1.2-22)	.02
Obstructive TAPVC	13 (2.5-75)	.01
Pulmonary hypertensive crises	10 (1.5-57)	.02
Complex anatomy	5.8 (1.5-36)	.02

Data from Chowdhury and colleagues.[C5]
Key: *CL,* 95% confidence limits; *TAPVC,* total anomalous pulmonary venous connection.

Modes of Death

The most common modes of hospital death after repair are cardiac failure and hypertensive pulmonary artery crises. Postoperative pulmonary hypertensive crisis can occur in neonates and infants who go into surgery with severe cardiopulmonary instability, even though an adequate vein repair has been achieved, or in patients with postoperative pulmonary venous obstruction. In the modern era, most early and late deaths are associated with some combination of pulmonary venous obstruction, complex mixed TAPVC morphology, and low birth weight.[A2,C5,H2,K11,S1]

Incremental Risk Factors for Death

Risk factors for early death have been identified. These include earlier year of operation, single-ventricle intracardiac morphology, mixed TAPVC morphology, infradiaphragmatic TAPVC morphology, pulmonary venous obstruction, poor preoperative physiologic state, and lower weight at operation.[B2,B11,C5,C6,C9,D6,H1,H2,K7,K11,M4,T4] Importantly, the many studies cited here are not uniform in identifying all these risk factors. This variability reflects variations in analysis from study to study and also acknowledges that many or most of these risk factors are mutable. For example, Bove and colleagues found severe acidosis on admission to be the most important risk factor for hospital death after repair of infracardiac TAPVC.[B11] Other studies indicate that preoperative pulmonary venous obstruction is not a risk factor unless accompanied by single-ventricle intracardiac morphology.[K11] Studies by Bando and colleagues[H9] and Hyde and colleagues[M5] argue that preoperative pulmonary venous obstruction and infradiaphragmatic connection have been neutralized as risk factors for death. Risk factors for death in mixed TAPVC have been defined[C5] (Table 31-1).

Risk factors for late death are difficult to define because late deaths occur so infrequently. Most deaths outside the perioperative period involve recurrent or persistent pulmonary venous obstruction. Possibly, preoperatively small pulmonary veins predispose patients to develop the lethal postoperative complication of pulmonary vein stenosis.[J1] Therefore, this finding may also be a risk factor for death after repair, as may small size of the coronary sinus in cardiac TAPVC.[B8]

In older patients presenting for surgical correction, a mild or moderate increase in pulmonary vascular resistance increases the risk of operation,[G4,L4] and severe elevation makes older patients inoperable. The situation in these older patients is analogous to that in patients with atrial septal defect (see Indications for Operation in Chapter 30). There may be a few patients with TAPVC in which the LV is so small that it per se represents an incremental risk factor. However, this is rare. More commonly, preoperative LV volume calculations are falsely reduced because of the ventricular septal shift that occurs with pulmonary hypertension. Fortunately, major associated cardiac anomalies in this condition are rare as well.

Functional Status

McBride and colleagues have shown that compared with healthy children, peak oxygen consumption (88% ± 16% of predicted) and ventilatory anaerobic threshold (91% ± 21% of predicted) were mildly reduced in a group of 27 patients with a mean age of 11 years. Chronotropic impairment was observed in seven patients (32%).[K10] Neurodevelopmental outcome has been evaluated. Kirshbom and colleagues assessed 30 patients, mean age 11 years, who had undergone TAPVC repair in the neonatal period or infancy. All patients underwent repair using hypothermic circulatory arrest. Microcephaly was present in 28%, and abnormal neuromuscular examination in 27%. Performance IQ, motor skills, and attention were below normal, while full and verbal IQ and memory were normal.[A1] In another study of 34 patients at 18 to 24 months of age, all of whom underwent repair using hypothermic circulatory arrest, Mental Developmental Index (87 ± 16) and Psychomotor Developmental Index (89 ± 13) were at the low end of normal.[R3]

Hemodynamic Result

Pulmonary artery pressure is normal in patients recatheterized after repair unless there is abnormal cardiac rhythm, and cardiac index is normal, ranging from 2.9 to 5.2 L · min^{-1} · m^{-2} (average 3.7 L · min-1 · m^{-2}) in the study of Whight, Barratt-Boyes, and colleagues.[W3]

Postoperative cineangiographic studies of infants have shown that left atrial volumes are mostly within normal range, with the exceptions more often large than small. Incorporation of the pulmonary venous sinus, and the coronary sinus in some types of TAPVC, probably increases left atrial size (which was small before repair) to normal for age postoperatively. Some functional left atrial abnormality is present early and late postoperatively, perhaps based on abnormally low compliance of part of the atrium, because left atrial pressure tracings are often abnormal both early[P1] and late postoperatively.[W3]

RV volume, variable but often increased preoperatively, is normal or only mildly enlarged late postoperatively.[H1] LVEDV, abnormally small preoperatively, increases to normal late postoperatively.[H1] LV systolic function, often markedly depressed before operation, returns to normal late postoperatively[H1] (Fig. 31-16). Part of the explanation for this may be

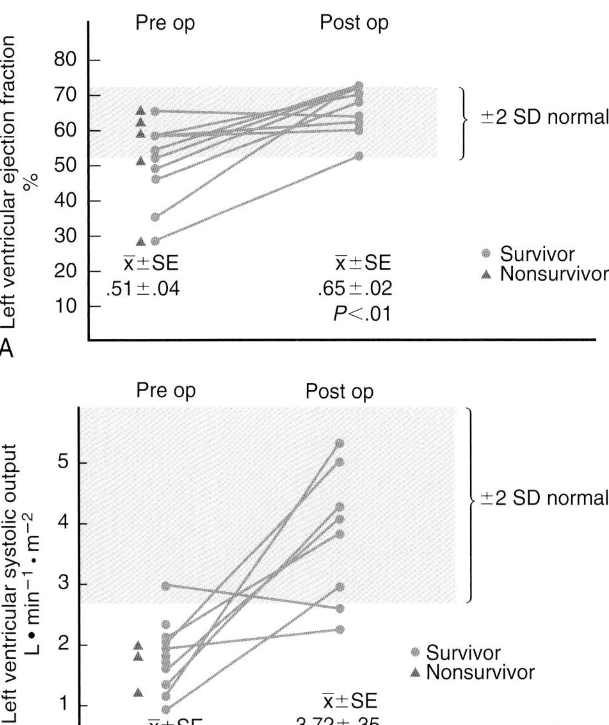

Figure 31-16 Depressed preoperative left ventricular (LV) systolic function returning to normal late after repair of total anomalous pulmonary venous connection (TAPVC) in infancy. **A,** Changes in LV ejection fraction. **B,** Changes in LV systolic output. Key: *Pre op,* Preoperative; *Post op,* postoperative; *SD,* standard deviation; *SE,* standard error. (From Hammon and colleagues.[H1])

the improved LV geometry resulting from reduction in RV size (see "Ventricular Function" under Results in Chapter 30).

Cardiac Rhythm

Normal sinus rhythm is present in nearly all patients unless there is rhythm abnormality preoperatively. However, at least some of the preferential pathways of conduction from the sinus node to the atrioventricular node (see "Internodal Pathways" under Conduction System in Chapter 1) could be damaged by the repair.[D3] Thus, Holter monitoring after repair demonstrates that asymptomatic ectopic atrial pacemaker activity and other abnormalities are present in most patients.[B12,S3] To date, these conditions appear not to have handicapped patients. McBride and colleagues reported that of 22 patients achieving peak aerobic capacity during late evaluation, 7 (32%) had an attenuated heart rate response (168 ± 14 beats · min^{-1}).[K10]

Reoperation and Development of Postoperative Pulmonary Venous Obstruction

Reoperations are performed for two reasons: *severe anastomotic stenosis* and *pulmonary vein stenosis.* They have been necessary in every experience.[G1,J2,L3,O1,R2,S4,W3,Y1] In an early unpublished study by Kirklin, essentially all patients with restenosis required reoperation within the first 6 to 12 months of repair (Fig. 31-17). Karamlou and colleagues, who reviewed 377 cases over a 60-year span, confirmed this

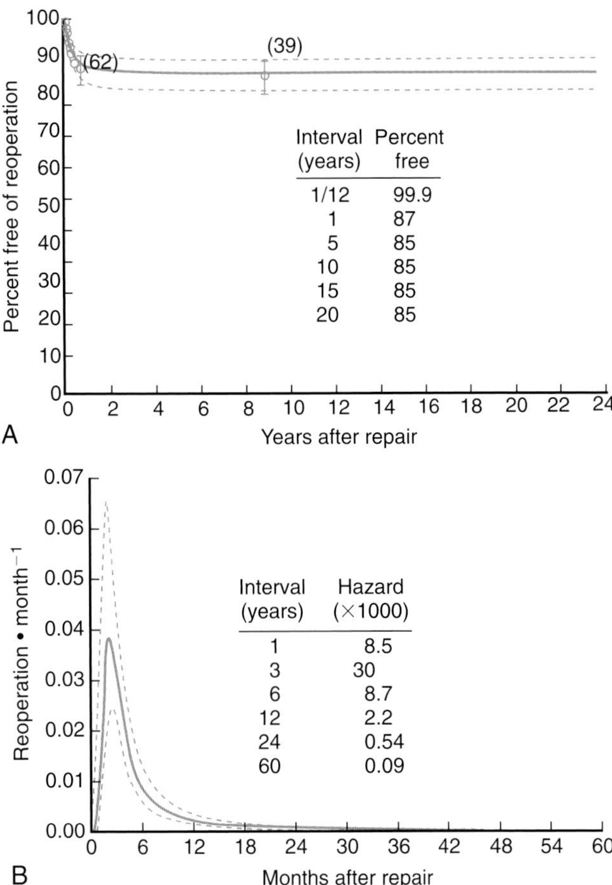

Figure 31-17 Freedom from reoperation after repair of total anomalous pulmonary venous connection in 112 patients at UAB, 1967 to 1991. **A,** Freedom from reoperation. **B,** Hazard function for reoperation. Note that hazard function for reoperation peaks within 6 months of repair and declines rapidly thereafter.

finding.[B1] However, other studies imply that need for reoperation may develop later. An analysis from Great Ormand Street Hospital showed that only one third of reoperations (7/20) occurred within 6 months of initial repair.[L1]

Patients usually become symptomatic with development of recurrent dyspnea and signs of pulmonary venous congestion, but ideally the diagnosis should be made before that stage. Risk factors for developing recurrent pulmonary venous obstruction include an original diagnosis of infracardiac[L1] or mixed[B1] TAPVC, and obstructed TAPVC.[L1]

A powerful tool for evaluating patients after repair of pulmonary venous obstruction but before hospital discharge is 2D pulsed Doppler echocardiography.[S11] Ideally, it should be repeated on several occasions during the first postoperative year. High-velocity turbulent flow at either the anastomosis or the pulmonary vein orifices suggests stenosis. Prompt angiographic restudy may further clarify the anatomic point of stenosis. The pulmonary veins are entered retrogradely from the left atrium to make a direct pulmonary vein angiogram and to determine pressure gradient across the anastomotic site.

MRI and CT are also useful imaging modalities for defining morphology of the obstruction. According to Ricci and colleagues,[L1] about half (10/20) of all cases of recurrence are due to anastomotic stenosis, about one third to combined anastomotic and ostial (6/20) stenosis, and a minority (3/20)

Table 31-2 Prevalence of Anastomotic Strictures after Repair of Total Anomalous Pulmonary Venous Connection[a]

		Anastomotic Stricture		
Source	**n**	**No.**	**%**	**CL (%)**
Whight et al., 1969-1977[W3]	8	0	0	0-21
Applebaum et al.[A3] and Katz et al.[K2]	32	3	9	4-18
Behrendt et al., 1963-January 1970[B6]	11	1	9	1-33
Breckenridge et al.[B13]	11	2	18	6-38
Cooley et al., 1995-1964[C8]	16[b]	1	6	1-20
Hawkins et al., 1982-1988[H4]	23[c]	4	17	9-29
Hawkins et al., 1989-1994[H4]	32[d]	1	3	0.4-10
Hancock Freisen et al., 1989-2000[K11]	84	5	6	3-10
TOTAL	217	17	9	6-10
$P(\chi^2)$			.4	

[a]The variable *n* refers to number of hospital survivors. Except in the GLH (Whight et al.) patients, in whom routine postoperative cardiac catheterization was performed, the data concern patients dying or requiring reoperation for stricture formation. The 70% confidence limits of the individual proportions all overlap; this overlap and the *P* value make institutional differences in prevalence unlikely.
[b]This may include some infants with a cardiac connection.
[c]These patients had anastomosis with polypropylene suture.
[d]These patients had anastomosis with polydioxanone suture.
Key: *CL,* 70% CLs.

to ostial stenosis alone. Risk factors for death following reoperation are earlier age at recurrence and persistence of pulmonary hypertension after reoperation.[L1]

Anastomotic Stenosis

In up to 10% of patients, strictures appear to develop at the anastomosis (Table 31-2), usually within a few months of repair. However, results of reoperation are occasionally disappointing, with an important chance of a subsequent restenosis, as reported by Breckenridge and colleagues.[B13] Despite theoretical considerations favoring use of interrupted sutures,[S2] there is no correlation between stricture formation and method of suturing. It is likely, however, that the open technique of anastomosis is preferable to use of clamps.[B13,D2] Suture material may influence formation of anastomotic stricture. Absorbable polydioxanone suture as a continuous stitch has been recommended by Hawkins and colleagues for constructing the left atrium–to–common pulmonary venous sinus anastomosis.[H4] Late anastomotic stricture occurred in 1 (3.2%; CL 0.4%-10%) of 32 survivors having anastomosis with polydioxanone compared with 4 (17%; CL 9%-29%) of 23 patients having anastomosis with nonabsorbable suture. However, groups compared in this series were not concurrent. Based on complete absence of this complication late postoperatively, it is likely that anastomoses grow appropriately as patients grow.

Pulmonary Vein Stenosis

Compared with anastomotic stenosis, pulmonary vein stenosis tends to occur later[K11] and is less common.[K11,L1] In most instances, the stenosis is due to diffuse fibrosis and thickening of the vein wall and often to localized narrowing at the vein–left atrial junction.[F2,F3,G2,L6,T4] Pulmonary vein stenosis may or may not be accompanied by anastomotic stenosis.[K11,L1] Karamlou and colleagues report recurrent obstruction in

5.7% of 377 patients undergoing TAPVC repair but do not make a distinction between anastomotic and pulmonary vein stenosis.[B1]

Pulmonary vein stenosis is usually lethal, even with reoperation and extensive attempts at revision or repair. This lack of success has led to alternative treatment such as balloon dilatation and stenting, but these do not appear to provide additional benefit. In 1996, Lacour-Gayet and colleagues described the sutureless repair technique, using in situ autologous pericardium, for recurrent pulmonary vein stenosis following initial TAPVC repair.[N1] Subsequent reports emphasize the utility of this technique in selected cases.[L2,Y2] Following their initial description of the sutureless technique, Lacour-Gayet and colleagues reported that of 178 patients undergoing correction of TAPVC, progressive obstruction developed in 16 (9%) within a median interval of 4 months (range 5 weeks to 12 years) after operation.[L2] Only 4 of these 16 had isolated pulmonary vein stenosis, with the remaining 12 having either isolated anastomotic stenosis or combined anastomotic and pulmonary vein stenosis. The obstruction was bilateral in 7 patients. Fifteen of the 16 patients underwent reoperation, and 4 (27%) died afterward. The authors used the in situ pericardial patch technique to relieve the stenosis in 7 of the 16 patients.

Despite interest in the sutureless technique, there is little firm evidence that it provides a benefit over conventional techniques. Yun and colleagues[Y2] used a retrospective analysis to compare the outcomes of death and restenosis after conventional and sutureless techniques. Patients in this series were heterogeneous, and only 17 of the 60 had a history of previous TAPVC repair. By multivariable analysis, there was no statistically significant difference between the conventional and sutureless techniques, although a trend for better outcome using the sutureless technique was observed when all 60 patients were considered.

Development of pulmonary vein stenosis many years after repair is exceedingly rare but has been reported. Kveselis and colleagues reported successful repair of infracardiac TAPVC in a 17-day-old infant who had a demonstrated absence of pulmonary vein obstruction when recatheterized 3.7 years after operation. This patient continued to be healthy without limitations until 12 years of age, at which time he became symptomatic, and important obstruction was demonstrated at the anastomosis.[K12] Reoperation successfully corrected the problem.

INDICATIONS FOR OPERATION

Investigation must be undertaken promptly in any neonate or infant, no matter how young, who develops signs and symptoms suggestive of TAPVC. Procrastination leads to death in babies with obstructive TAPVC (and in some without it) or to hospital admission in a semimoribund state, which importantly increases operative mortality.

Once the diagnosis is made, operation should be undertaken immediately in any neonate or infant importantly ill with TAPVC. This policy should lead to surgical intervention during the first few days or week of life, frequently in the first month of life, and usually before 6 months of age. In infants in whom the diagnosis is made between 6 and 12 months of age, operation should be undertaken promptly because risk of operation is low, and even infants who appear to be doing well are at risk of dying before age 1 year.[B10,K4]

Rarely, individuals survive into childhood or early adult life with TAPVC and are first seen for surgical consideration at that time. Operation is advisable if severe pulmonary vascular disease has not developed; the criteria for operability are the same as for patients with atrial and ventricular septal defects (see Indications for Operation in Chapters 30 and 35. In TAPVC, degree of cyanosis is not helpful because of the common mixing chamber, nor is height of mean pulmonary artery pressure relative to systemic pressure, because the shunt is not at systemic level.

When pulmonary vascular disease is suspected clinically, measurement of pulmonary vascular resistance is required at preoperative cardiac catheterization. Using the Fick principle, the patient's response to 100% oxygen and to inhaled nitric oxide is determined. If pulmonary vascular resistance is less than 8 U · m^2 using these maneuvers, operation is undertaken. If resistance is higher than 8 U · m^2, chronic pulmonary vasodilatory therapy, both pre- and postoperatively, can be considered in an attempt to increase operability.

SPECIAL SITUATIONS AND CONTROVERSIES

Pulmonary Vein Stenosis

Pulmonary vein stenosis may be either a postoperative complication (as discussed previously) or a primary congenital anomaly.[H7] Congenital lesions are classified as (1) diffuse hypoplasia, (2) long-segment (tubular) focal stenosis, and (3) ostial (discrete) stenosis. Diffusely hypoplastic pulmonary veins extending into the lung parenchyma usually require heart-lung or lung transplantation, and prognosis is poor. Long-segment tubular stenoses of pulmonary veins with normal-caliber intraparenchymal pulmonary veins may be treated, but prognosis is also poor.

Treatment includes operative patch venoplasty, the sutureless technique, catheter dilatation and stent placement, or a combination of therapies. Currently, balloon dilatation and stent placement are not considered effective therapies, because rapid restenosis is the rule. Short-segment discrete stenoses located at or near the left atrial ostium of the pulmonary vein have the best chance for success following surgery. In general, congenital pulmonary vein stenosis has a poor prognosis because of development of pulmonary venous hypertension, followed by pulmonary arterial hypertension.

Delayed Operation

In critically ill neonates and young infants whose obstruction is primarily at the atrial level (an unusual situation), balloon atrial septostomy (with a blade if necessary) and delay of operation for *1 to 2 days* are reasonable approaches.[W2] Preoperative preparation of the critically ill neonate by infusion of prostaglandin E_1 combined with low-dose dopamine for a few hours has been advised by Serraf and colleagues.[S9] However, such treatment may shunt blood away from the lungs and increase cyanosis in neonates with severe pulmonary venous obstruction and pulmonary venous hypertension.

Operative Exposure

Tucker and colleagues described exposing the structures for anastomosis of the common pulmonary venous sinus to the left atrium through the transverse sinus between the aorta and superior vena cava.[T3] This approach can occasionally be helpful if the pulmonary venous sinus is positioned superiorly.

Surgical Enlargement of Left Atrium

Trusler and colleagues found that in dogs, a decrease in atrial volume of more than 50% resulted in an important reduction in cardiac output.[T2] Brighton and colleagues, using a mechanical model, obtained substantial improvement in cardiac output by adding a flexible atrium to the inlet of their artificial heart.[B14] In studying the effect of atrial compliance on cardiac performance with a mathematical electrical analog, Suga found that cardiac performance was markedly improved by increasing atrial compliance while maintaining constant ventricular contractility.[S16] Analysis suggested that increased atrial compliance facilitated the reservoir function of the atrium and maintenance of a relatively high mean atrial pressure during ventricular filling. These facts, combined with the preoperatively observed small left atrium in patients with TAPVC, have made its enlargement by shifting the atrial septum to the right attractive.[D8,G5,K9]

Katz and colleagues, on the other hand, found similar survival with and without left atrial enlargement.[K2] This may be because surgical efforts to improve left atrial size are not effective, or because adequate left atrial enlargement may result from incorporating the common pulmonary venous sinus into the left atrium.[M3,W3] Also, lack of left atrial reservoir function may rarely be critical early or late postoperatively if other aspects of the situation favor survival. Nonetheless, the repair must be done in a manner that *does not decrease* size of the left atrium.

REFERENCES

A

1. Alton GY, Robertson CM, Sauve R, Divekar A, Nettel-Aguirre A, Selzer S, et al. Early childhood health, growth, and neurodevelopmental outcomes after complete repair of total anomalous pulmonary venous connection at 6 weeks or younger. J Thorac Cardiovasc Surg 2007;133:905-11.
2. Ando M, Takahashi Y, Kikuchi T. Total anomalous pulmonary venous connection with dysmorphic pulmonary vein: a risk for postoperative pulmonary venous obstruction. Interact Cardiovasc Thorac Surg 2004;3:557-61.
3. Applebaum A, Kirklin JW, Pacifico AD, Bargeron LM Jr. The surgical treatment of total anomalous pulmonary venous connection. Israel J Med 1975;11:89.
4. Arciniegas E, Henry JG, Green EW. Stenosis of the coronary sinus ostium. J Thorac Cardiovasc Surg 1980;79:303.
5. Arciprete P, McKay R, Watson GH, Hamilton DI, Wilkinson JL, Arnold RM. Double connections in total anomalous pulmonary venous connection. J Thorac Cardiovasc Surg 1986;92:146.

B

1. Bando K, Turrentine MW, Ensing GJ, Sun K, Sharp TG, Sekine Y, et al. Surgical management of total anomalous pulmonary venous connection: thirty-year trends. Circulation. 1996;94(suppl):II12-16.
2. Barratt-Boyes BG. Corrective surgery for congenital heart disease in infants with the use of profound hypothermia and circulatory arrest techniques. Aust N Z J Surg 1979;47:737.
3. Barratt-Boyes BG. Primary definitive intracardiac operations in infants: total anomalous pulmonary venous connection. In Kirklin JW, ed. Advances in cardiovascular surgery. Orlando, Fla.: Grune & Stratton, 1973, p. 127.
4. Barratt-Boyes BG, Nicholls TT, Brandt PW, Neutze JM. Aortic arch interruption associated with patent ductus arteriosus, ventricular septal defect and total anomalous pulmonary venous connection: total correction in an eight day old infant using profound hypothermia and limited cardiopulmonary bypass. J Thorac Cardiovasc Surg 1972;63:367.
5. Barratt-Boyes BG, Simpson M, Neutze JM. Intracardiac surgery in neonates and infants using deep hypothermia with surface cooling and limited cardiopulmonary bypass. Circulation 1971;43:I25.
6. Behrendt DM, Aberdeen E, Waterston DJ, Bonham-Carter RE. Total anomalous pulmonary venous drainage in infants. I. Clinical and hemodynamic findings, methods, and results of operation in 37 cases. Circulation 1972;46:347.
7. Berdat PA, Pfammatter JP, Genyk I, Carrel TP. Modified repair of mixed total anomalous pulmonary venous connection. Ann Thorac Surg 2001;71:723-5.
8. Bhan A, Saxena A, Sharma R, Venugopal P. Coronary sinus size a determinant of outcome in cardiac TAPVC (letter). Ann Thorac Surg 1996;62:940.
9. Bharati S, Lev M. Congenital anomalies of the pulmonary veins. Cardiovasc Clin 1973;5:23.
10. Bonham-Carter RE, Capriles M, Noe Y. Total anomalous pulmonary venous drainage. Br Heart J 1969;31:45.
11. Bove EL, de Leval MR, Taylor JF, Macartney FJ, Szarnicki RJ, Stark J. Infradiaphragmatic total anomalous pulmonary venous drainage: surgical treatment and long-term results. Ann Thorac Surg 1981;31:544.
12. Bove KE, Geiser EA, Meyer RA. The left ventricle in anomalous pulmonary venous return. Arch Pathol Lab Med 1975;99:522.
13. Breckenridge IM, de Leval M, Stark J, Waterston DJ. Correction of total anomalous pulmonary venous drainage in infancy. J Thorac Cardiovasc Surg 1973;66:447.
14. Brighton JA, Wade ZA, Pierce WS, Phillips WM, O'Bannon W. Effect of atrial volume on the performance of a sac-type artificial heart. Trans Am Soc Artif Intern Organs 1973;19:567.
15. Brody H. Drainage of the pulmonary veins into the right side of the heart. Arch Pathol Lab Med 1942;33:221.
16. Buckley MJ, Behrendt DM, Goldblatt A, Laver MB, Austin WS. Correction of total anomalous pulmonary venous drainage in the first month of life. J Thorac Cardiovasc Surg 1972;63:269.
17. Burchell HB. Total anomalous pulmonary venous drainage: clinical and physiologic patterns. Mayo Clin Proc 1956;31:161.
18. Burroughs JT, Edwards JE. Total anomalous venous connection. Am Heart J 1960;59:913.
19. Burroughs JT, Kirklin JW. Complete surgical correction of total anomalous pulmonary venous connection: report of three cases. Mayo Clin Proc 1956;31:182.

C

1. Carter RE, Capriles M, Noe Y. Total anomalous pulmonary venous drainage: a clinical and anatomical study of 75 children. Br Heart J 1969;31:45.
2. Chen HY, Chen SJ, Li YW, Wu MH, Wang JK, Tsai YF, et al. Esophageal varices in congenital heart disease with total anomalous pulmonary venous connection. Int J Card Imaging 2000;16:405-9.
3. Chin AJ, Sanders SP, Sherman F, Lang P, Norwood WI, Castaneda AR. Accuracy of subcostal two-dimensional echocardiography in prospective diagnosis of total anomalous pulmonary venous connection. Am Heart J 1987;113:1153.
4. Choe YH, Lee HJ, Kim HS, Ko JK, Kim JE, Han JJ. MRI of total anomalous pulmonary venous connections. J Comput Assist Tomogr 1994;18:243.
5. Chowdhury UK, Airan B, Malhotra A, Bisoi AK, Saxena A, Kothari SS, et al. Mixed total anomalous pulmonary venous connection: anatomic variations, surgical approach, techniques, and results. J Thorac Cardiovasc Surg 2008;135:106-16.
6. Chowdhury UK, Malhotra A, Kothari SS, Reddy SK, Mishra AK, Pradeep KK, et al. A suggested new surgical classification for mixed totally anomalous pulmonary venous connection. Cardiol Young 2007;17:342-53.
7. Cooley DA, Balas PE. Total anomalous pulmonary venous drainage into the inferior vena cava: report of successful surgical correction. Surgery 1962;51:798.
8. Cooley DA, Hallman GL, Leachman RD. Total anomalous pulmonary venous drainage: correction with the use of cardiopulmonary bypass in 62 cases. J Thorac Cardiovasc Surg 1966;51:88.
9. Curzon CL, Milford-Beland S, Li JS, O'Brien SM, Jacobs JP, Jacobs ML, et al. Cardiac surgery in infants with low birth weight is associated with increased mortality: analysis of the Society of

Thoracic Surgeons Congenital Heart Database. J Thorac Cardiovasc Surg 2008;135:546-51.

D

1. Darling RC, Rothney WB, Craig JM. Total pulmonary venous drainage into the right side of the heart. Lab Invest 1957;6:44.
2. Davignon A. Cure du retour veineux anormal total du nourisson: pont de vue de medicin. Journees de Cardiologie Pediatrique. Chateau de Feillac. October 7, 1972.
3. Davis JT, Ehrlich R, Hennessey JR, Levine M, Morgan RJ, Bharati S, et al. Long-term follow-up of cardiac rhythm in repaired total anomalous pulmonary venous drainage. Thorac Cardiovasc Surg 1986;34:172.
4. DeLeon SY, Gidding SS, Ilbawi MN, Idriss FS, Muster AJ, Cole RB, et al. Surgical management of infants with complex cardiac anomalies associated with reduced pulmonary blood flow and total anomalous pulmonary venous drainage. Ann Thorac Surg 1987; 43:207.
5. Delisle G, Ando M, Calder AL, Zuberbuhler JR, Rochenmacher S, Alday LE, et al. Total anomalous pulmonary venous connection: report of 93 autopsied cases with emphasis on diagnostic and surgical considerations. Am Heart J 1976;91:99.
6. Delius RE, de Leval MR, Elliott MJ, Stark J. Mixed total pulmonary venous drainage: still a surgical challenge. J Thorac Cardiovasc Surg 1996;112:1581-8.
7. Dillard DH, Mohri H, Hessel EA II, Anderson HN, Nelson RJ, Crawford EW, et al. Correction of total anomalous pulmonary venous drainage in infancy utilizing deep hypothermia with total circulatory arrest. Circulation 1967;35:I105.
8. Doty DB. Cardiac surgery: operative technique. St Louis: Mosby-Yearbook, 1997, p. 74.
9. Drummond WH, Gregory GA, Heymann MA, Phibbs RA. The independent effects of hyperventilation, tolazoline and dopamine on infants with persistent pulmonary hypertension. J Pediatr 1981;98:603.
10. Duff DF, Nihill MR, McNamara DG. Infradiaphragmatic total anomalous pulmonary venous return: review of clinical and pathological findings and results of operation in 28 cases. Br Heart J 1977;39:619.

E

1. Elias-Jones AC, Cordner SV. Infra-diaphragmatic total anomalous pulmonary venous drainage presenting with rectal bleeding. Arch Dis Child 1983;58:637-9.
2. el-Said GM, Mullins CE, McNamara DG. Management of total anomalous pulmonary venous return. Circulation 1972;45:1240.
3. Eyskens B, Cilliers A, Dumoulin M, Veereman G, Gewillig M. Oesophageal varices in a child after neonatal correction of an infradiaphragmatic total anomalous pulmonary venous return. Eur J Pediatr 1999;158:1009-10.

F

1. Festa P, Ait-Ali L, Cerillo AF, De Marchi D, Murzi B. Magnetic resonance imaging is the diagnostic tool of choice in the preoperative evaluation of patients with partial anomalous pulmonary venous return. Int J Cardiovasc Imaging 2006;22:685-93.
2. Fleming WH, Clark EB, Dooley KJ, Hofschire PJ, Ruckman RN, Hopeman AR, et al. Late complications following surgical repair of total anomalous pulmonary venous return below the diaphragm. Ann Thorac Surg 1979;27:435.
3. Friedli B, Davignon A, Stanley P. Infradiaphragmatic anomalous pulmonary venous return: surgical correction in a newborn infant. J Thorac Cardiovasc Surg 1971;62:301.
4. Friedlich A, Bing RJ, Blount SG Jr. Physiological studies in congenital heart disease. IX. Circulatory dynamics in the anomalies of venous return to the heart including pulmonary arteriovenous fistula. Bull Johns Hopkins Hosp 1950;86:20.

G

1. Galloway AC, Campbell DN, Clarke DR. The value of early repair for total anomalous pulmonary venous drainage. Pediatr Cardiol 1985;6:77.
2. Gathman GE, Nadas AS. Total anomalous pulmonary venous connection: clinical and physiologic observations of 75 pediatric patients. Circulation 1970;42:143.
3. Gersony WM, Bowman FO Jr, Steeg CN, Hayes CJ, Jesse MJ, Malm JR. Management of total anomalous pulmonary venous drainage in early infancy. Circulation 1971;43:I19.
4. Gomes MM, Feldt RH, McGoon DC, Danielson GK. Total anomalous pulmonary venous connection: surgical considerations and results of operation. J Thorac Cardiovasc Surg 1970;60:116.
5. Goor DA, Yellin A, Frand M, Smolinsky A, Neufeld N. The operative problem of small left atrium in total anomalous pulmonary venous connection: report of 5 patients. Ann Thorac Surg 1976;72:245.
6. Goswami KC, Shrivastava S, Saxena A, Dev V. Echocardiographic diagnosis of total anomalous pulmonary venous connection. Am Heart J 1993;126:433.
7. Greene CA, Case CL, Oslizlok P, Gillette PC. "Superimposition" digital subtraction angiography: evaluation of total anomalous pulmonary venous connection. Pediatr Cardiol 1993;14:47.
8. Greil GF, Powell AJ, Gildein HP, Geva T. Gadolinium-enhanced three-dimensional magnetic resonance angiography of pulmonary and systemic venous anomalies. J Am Coll Cardiol 2002;39: 335-41.
9. Gross RE, Watkins E Jr, Pomeranz AA, Goldsmith EL A method for surgical closure of interauricular septal defects. Surg Gynecol Obstet 1953;96:1.
10. Grosse-Wortmann L, Friedberg MK. Images in cardiovascular medicine. Bilateral vertical veins from a common confluence in supracardiac total anomalous pulmonary venous connection. Circulation 2008;118:e103-4.

H

1. Hammon JW Jr, Bender HW Jr, Graham TP Jr, Boucek RJ Jr, Smith CW, Erath HG Jr. Total anomalous pulmonary venous connection in infancy: ten years' experience including studies of postoperative ventricular function. J Thorac Cardiovasc Surg 1980; 80:544.
2. Hancock Friesen CL, Zurakowski D, Thiagarajan RR, Forbess JM, del Nido PJ, Mayer JE, et al. Total anomalous pulmonary venous connection: an analysis of current management strategies in a single institution. Ann Thorac Surg 2005;79:596-606.
3. Hastreiter AR, Paul MH, Molthan ME, Miller RA. Total anomalous pulmonary venous connection with severe pulmonary venous obstruction. Circulation 1962;25:916.
4. Hawkins JA, Minich LL, Tani LY, Ruttenberg HD, Sturtevant JE, McGough EC. Absorbable polydioxanone suture and results in total anomalous pulmonary venous connection. Ann Thorac Surg 1995;60:55.
5. Haworth SG, Reid L. Structural study of pulmonary circulation and of heart in total anomalous pulmonary venous return in early infancy. Br Heart J 1977;39:80.
6. Hazelrig JB, Turner ME Jr, Blackstone EH. Parametric survival analysis combining longitudinal and cross-sectional-censored and interval-censored data with concomitant information. Biometrics 1982;38:1.
7. Herlong JR, Jaggers JJ, Ungerleider RM. Congenital heart surgery nomenclature and database project: pulmonary venous anomalies. Ann Thorac Surg 2000;69:S56.
8. Huhta JC, Gutgesell HP, Nihill MR. Cross sectional echocardiographic diagnosis of total anomalous pulmonary venous connection. Br Heart J 1985;53:525.
9. Hyde JA, Stumper O, Barth MJ, Wright JG, Silove ED, de Giovanni JV, et al. Total anomalous pulmonary venous connection: outcome of surgical correction and management of recurrent venous obstruction. Eur J Cardiothorac Surg. 1999;15:735-40.

I

1. Imoto Y, Kado H, Asou T, Shiokawa Y, Tominaga R, Yasui H. Mixed type of total anomalous pulmonary venous connection. Ann Thorac Surg 1998;66:1394-7.

J

1. Jenkins KJ, Sanders SP, Coleman L, Mayer JE Jr, Colan SD. Individual pulmonary vein size and survival in infants with totally anomalous pulmonary venous connection. J Am Coll Cardiol 1993;22:201.
2. Jonas RA, Smolinsky A, Mayer JE, Castaneda AR. Obstructed pulmonary venous drainage with total anomalous pulmonary venous connection to the coronary sinus. Am J Cardiol 1987;59:431.

K

1. Karamlou T, Gurofsky R, Al Sukhni E, Coles JG, Williams WG, Caldarone CA, et al. Factors associated with mortality and reoperation in 377 children with total anomalous pulmonary venous connection. Circulation 2007;115:1591-8.
2. Katz NM, Kirklin JW, Pacifico AD. Concepts and practices in surgery for total anomalous pulmonary venous connection. Ann Thorac Surg 1978;25:479.
3. Kawashima Y, Matsuda H, Nakano S, Miyamoto IC, Fujino M, Kozaka T, et al. Tree-shaped pulmonary veins in intracardiac total anomalous pulmonary venous drainage. Ann Thorac Surg 1977; 23:436.
4. Keith JD, Rowe RD, Vlad P, O'Hanley JH. Complete anomalous pulmonary venous drainage. Am J Med 1954;16:23.
5. Kim TH, Kim YM, Suh CH, Cho DJ, Park IS, Kim WH, et al. Helical CT angiography and three-dimensional reconstruction of total anomalous pulmonary venous connections in neonates and infants. AJR Am J Roentgenol. 2000;175:1381-6.
6. King DR, Marchildon MB. Gastrointestinal hemorrhage. An unusual complication of total anomalous pulmonary venous drainage. J Thorac Cardiovasc Surg 1977;73:316-8.
7. Kirklin JK, Blackstone EH, Kirklin JW, McKay R, Pacifico AD, Bargeron LM Jr. Intracardiac surgery in infants under age 3 months: incremental risk factors for hospital mortality. Am J Cardiol 1981;48:500.
8. Kirklin JW. Surgical treatment of total anomalous pulmonary venous connection in infancy. In Barratt-Boyes BG, Neutze JM, Harris EA, eds. Heart disease in infancy: diagnosis and surgical treatment. Edinburgh: Churchill Livingstone, 1973, p. 89.
9. Kirklin JW. Corrective surgical treatment of cyanotic congenital heart disease. In Bass AD, Moe GK, eds. Congenital heart disease. Washington, DC: American Association for the Advancement of Science, 1960, p. 329.
10. Kirshbom PM, Flynn TB, Clancy RR, Ittenbach RF, Hartman DM, Paridon SM, et al. Late neurodevelopmental outcome after repair of total anomalous pulmonary venous connection. J Thorac Cardiovasc Surg 2005;129:1091-7.
11. Kirshbom PM, Myung RJ, Gaynor JW, Ittenbach RF, Paridon SM, DeCampli WM, et al. Preoperative pulmonary venous obstruction affects long-term outcome for survivors of total anomalous pulmonary venous connection repair. Ann Thorac Surg 2002; 74:1616-20.
12. Kveselis DA, Chameides L, Diana DJ, Ellison L, Rowland T. Late pulmonary venous obstruction after surgical repair of infradiaphragmatic total anomalous pulmonary venous return. Pediatr Cardiol 1988;9:175.

L

1. Lacour-Gayet F, Rey C, Planché C. Pulmonary vein stenosis: Description of the sutureless surgical procedure using the pericardium in situ (in French). Arch Mal Coeur Vaiss 1996;89:633-6.
2. Lacour-Gayet F, Zoghbi J, Serraf AE, Belli E, Piot D, Rey C, et al. Surgical management of progressive pulmonary venous obstruction after repair of total anomalous pulmonary venous connection. J Thorac Cardiovasc Surg 1999;117:679.
3. Lamb RK, Qureshi SA, Wilkinson JL, Arnold R, West CR, Hamilton DI. Total anomalous pulmonary venous drainage. J Thorac Cardiovasc Surg 1988;96:368.
4. Leachman RD, Cooley DA, Hallman G, Simpson JW, Dear WE. Total anomalous pulmonary venous return: correlation of hemodynamic observations and surgical mortality in 58 cases. Ann Thorac Surg 1969;7:5.
5. Lewis FJ, Varco RL, Taufic M, Niazi SA. Direct vision repair of triatrial heart and total anomalous pulmonary venous drainage. Surg Gynecol Obstet 1956;102:713.
6. Lucas RV, Anderson RC, Amplatz K, Adamas P Jr, Edwards JE. Congenital causes of pulmonary venous obstruction. Pediatr Clin North Am 1963;10:781.

M

1. Maeda K, Yamaki S, Yokota M, Murakami A, Takamoto S. Hypoplasia of the small pulmonary arteries in total anomalous pulmonary venous connection with obstructed pulmonary venous drainage. J Thorac Cardiovasc Surg 2004;127:448-56.
2. Masui T, Seelos KC, Kersting-Sommerhoff BA, Higgins CB. Abnormalities of the pulmonary veins: evaluation with MR imaging and comparison with cardiac angiography and echocardiography. Radiology 1991;181:645-9.
3. Mathew R, Thilenius OG, Replogle RL, Arcilla RA. Cardiac function in total anomalous pulmonary venous return before and after surgery. Circulation 1977;55:361.
4. Mazzucco A, Rizzoli G, Fracasso A, Stellin G, Valfre C, Pellegrino P, et al. Experience with operation for total anomalous pulmonary venous connection in infancy. J Thorac Cardiovasc Surg 1983; 85:686.
5. McBride MG, Kirshbom PM, Gaynor JW, Ittenbach RF, Wernovsky G, Clancy RR, et al. Late cardiopulmonary and musculoskeletal exercise performance after repair for total anomalous pulmonary venous connection during infancy. J Thorac Cardiovasc Surg 2007;133:1533-9.
6. Muller WH. The surgical treatment of transposition of the pulmonary veins. Ann Surg 1951;134:683.
7. Mustard WT, Keith JD, Trusler GA. Two-stage correction for total anomalous pulmonary venous drainage in childhood. J Thorac Cardiovasc Surg 1962;44:477.
8. Mustard WT, Keon WJ, Trusler GA. Transposition of the lesser veins (total anomalous pulmonary venous drainage). Prog Cardiovasc Dis 1968;11:145.

N

1. Najm HK, Caldarone CA, Smallhorn J, Coles JG. A sutureless technique for the relief of pulmonary vein stenosis with the use of in situ pericardium. J Thorac Cardiovasc Surg 1998;115:468-70.
2. Nakazawa M, Jarmakini JM, Gyepes MT, Prochazka JV, Yabek SM, Marks RA. Pre- and postoperative ventricular function in infants and children with right ventricular volume overload. Circulation 1977;55:479.
3. Newfeld EA, Wilson A, Paul MH, Reisch JS. Pulmonary vascular disease in total anomalous pulmonary venous drainage. Circulation 1980;61:103.

O

1. Oelert H, Schafers HJ, Stegmann T, Kallfelz HC, Borst HG. Complete correction of total anomalous pulmonary venous drainage: experience with 53 patients. Ann Thorac Surg 1986; 41:392.

P

1. Parr GV, Kirklin JW, Pacifico AD, Blackstone EH, Lauridsen P. Cardiac performance in infants after repair of total anomalous pulmonary venous connection. Ann Thorac Surg 1974;17:561.
2. Park JA, Lee HD, Ban JE, Jo MJ, Sung SC, Chang YH, et al. Supracardiac type total anomalous pulmonary venous connection (TAPVC) with oesophageal varices. Pediatr Radiol 2008;38: 1138-40.
3. Paquet M, Gutgesell H. Electrocardiographic features of total anomalous pulmonary venous connection. Circulation 1975; 51:599.
4. Phillips SJ, Kongtahworn C, Zeff RH, Skinner JR, Chandramouli B, Gay JH. Correction of total anomalous pulmonary venous connection below the diaphragm. Ann Thorac Surg 1990;49:738.

R

1. Raisher BD, Grant JW, Martin TC, Strauss AW, Spray TL. Complete repair of total anomalous pulmonary venous connection in infancy. J Thorac Cardiovasc Surg 1992;104:443.
2. Reardon MJ, Cooley DA, Kubrusly L, Ott DA, Johnson W, Kay GL, et al. Total anomalous pulmonary venous return: report of 201 patients treated surgically. Tex Heart Inst J 1985;12:131.
3. Ricci M, Elliott M, Cohen GA, Catalan G, Stark J, de Leval MR, et al. Management of pulmonary venous obstruction after correction of TAPVC: risk factors for adverse outcome. Eur J Cardiothorac Surg 2003;24:28-36.
4. Ritter S, Tani LY, Shaddy RE, Pagotto LT, Minich LL. An unusual variant of total anomalous pulmonary venous connection with varices and multiple drainage sites. Pediatr Cardiol 2000;21: 289-91.
5. Rosenquist GC, Kelly JL, Chandra R, Ruckman RN, Galioto FM Jr, Midgley FM, et al. Small left atrium and change in contour of the ventricular septum in total anomalous pulmonary venous connection: a morphometric analysis of 22 infant hearts. Am J Cardiol 1985;55:777.

6. Rowe RD, Glass IH, Keith JD. Total anomalous pulmonary venous drainage at cardiac level: angiocardiographic differentiation. Circulation 1961;23:77.

S

1. Sano S, Brawn WJ, Mee RB. Total anomalous pulmonary venous drainage. J Thorac Cardiovasc Surg 1989;97:886.
2. Sauvage LR, Harkins HN. Growth of vascular anastomoses: an experimental study of the influence of suture type and suture method with a note on certain mechanical factors involved. Bull Johns Hopkins Hosp 1952;91:276.
3. Saxena A, Fong LV, Lamb RK, Monro JL, Shore DF, Keeton BR. Cardiac arrhythmias after surgical correction of total anomalous pulmonary venous connection: late follow-up. Pediatr Cardiol 1991;12:89.
4. Schafers HJ, Luhmer I, Oelert H. Pulmonary venous obstruction following repair of total anomalous pulmonary venous drainage. Ann Thorac Surg 1987;43:432.
5. Schamroth CL, Sareli P, Klein HO, Davidoff R, Barlow JB. Total anomalous pulmonary venous connection with pulmonary venous obstruction: survival into adulthood. Am Heart J 1985;109:1112.
6. Seale AN, Uemura H, Sethia B, Magee AG, Ho S, Daubeney PE. Total anomalous pulmonary venous connection to the supradiaphragmatic inferior vena cava. Ann Thoracic Surg 2008;85:1089-92.
7. Seo JW, Lee HJ, Choi JY, Choi YH, Lee JR. Pulmonary veins in total anomalous pulmonary venous connection with obstruction: demonstration using silicone rubber casts. Pediatr Pathol 1991;11:711.
8. Serraf A, Belli E, Roux D, Sousa-Uva M, Lacour-Gayet F, Planché C. Modified superior approach for repair of supracardiac and mixed total anomalous pulmonary venous drainage. Ann Thorac Surg 1998;65:1391-3.
9. Serraf A, Bruniaux J, Lacour-Gayet F, Chambran P, Binet JP, Lecronier G, et al. Obstructed total anomalous pulmonary venous return. Towards neutralization of a major risk factor. J Thorac Cardiovasc Surg 1991;101:601.
10. Sloan H, Mackenzie J, Morris JD, Stern A, Sigmann J. Open heart surgery in infancy. J Thorac Cardiovasc Surg 1962;44:459.
11. Smallhorn JF, Burrows P, Wilson G, Coles J, Gilday DL, Freedom RM. Two-dimensional and pulsed Doppler echocardiography in the postoperative evaluation of total anomalous pulmonary venous connection. Circulation 1987;76:298.
12. Smallhorn JF, Sutherland GR, Tommasini G, Hunter S, Anderson RH, Macartney FJ. Assessment of total anomalous pulmonary venous connection by two-dimensional echocardiography. Br Heart J 1981;46:613.
13. Sreeram N, Walsh K. Diagnosis of total anomalous pulmonary venous drainage by Doppler color flow imaging. J Am Coll Cardiol 1992;19:1577.
14. Sridhar PG, Kalyanpur A, Suresh PV, John C, Sharma R, Maheshwari S. Total anomalous pulmonary venous connection: helical computed tomography as an alternative to angiography. Indian Heart J 2003;55:624-7.
15. Stanger P, Rudolph AM, Edwards JE. Cardiac malpositions. Circulation 1977;56:159.
16. Suga H. Importance of atrial compliance in cardiac performance. Circ Res 1974;35:39.
17. Swischuk LE, ed. Radiology of the newborn and young infant. Baltimore: Williams & Wilkins, 1973, p. 40.

T

1. Tachibana K, Takagi N, Osawa H, Takamuro M, Yokozawa M, Tomita H, et al. Cor triatriatum and total anomalous pulmonary venous connection to the coronary sinus. J Thorac Cardiovasc Surg 2007;134:1067-9.
2. Trusler GA, Bull RC, Hoeskema T, Mustard WT. The effect on cardiac output of a reduction in atrial volume. J Thorac Cardiovasc Surg 1963;46:109.
3. Tucker BL, Lindesmith GG, Stiles QR, Meyer BW. The superior approach for correction of the supracardiac type of total anomalous pulmonary venous return. Ann Thorac Surg 1976;22:374.
4. Turley K, Tucker WY, Ullyot DJ, Ebert PA. Total anomalous pulmonary venous connection in infancy: influence of age and type of lesion. Am J Cardiol 1980;45:92.
5. Tynan M, Behrendt D, Urquhart W. Portal vein catheterization and selective angiography in diagnosis of total anomalous pulmonary venous connection. Br Heart J 1974;36:115.

U

1. Uçar T, Fitoz S, Tutar E, Atalay S, Uysalel A. Diagnostic tools in the preoperative evaluation of children with anomalous pulmonary venous connections. Int J Cardiovasc Imaging 2008;24:229-35.

V

1. Van Praagh R, Harken AH, Delisle G, Ando M, Gross RE. Total anomalous pulmonary venous drainage to the coronary sinus: a revised procedure for its correction. J Thorac Cardiovasc Surg 1972;64:132.
2. Vouhe PR, Baillot-Vernant F, Fermont L, Bical O, Leca F, Neveux JY. Cor triatriatum and total anomalous pulmonary venous connection: a rare, surgically correctable anomaly. J Thorac Cardiovasc Surg. 1985;90:443-5.

W

1. Wang JK, Lue HC, Wu MH, Young ML, Wu FF, Wu JM. Obstructed total anomalous pulmonary venous connection. Pediatr Cardiol 1993;14:28.
2. Ward KE, Mullins CE, Huhta JC, Nihill MR, McNamara DG, Cooley DA. Restrictive interatrial communication in total anomalous pulmonary venous connection. Am J Cardiol 1986;57:1131.
3. Whight CH, Barratt-Boyes BG, Calder L, Neutze JM, Brandt PW. Total anomalous pulmonary venous connection: long-term results following repair in infancy. J Thorac Cardiovasc Surg 1978;75:52.
4. Wilson J. A description of a very unusual formation of the human heart. Philos Trans R Soc Lond 1798;88:346.
5. Woodwark GM, Vince DJ, Ashmore PG. Total anomalous pulmonary venous return to the portal vein: report of a case of successful surgical treatment. J Thorac Cardiovasc Surg 1963;45:662.
6. Wyttenbach M, Carrel T, Schupbach P, Tschappeler H, Triller J. Total anomalous pulmonary venous connection to the portal vein. Cardiovasc Intervent Radiol 1996;19:113.

Y

1. Yee ES, Turley K, Hsieh WR, Ebert PA. Infant total anomalous pulmonary venous connection: factors influencing timing of presentation and operative outcome. Circulation 1987;76:III83.
2. Yun TJ, Coles JG, Konstantinov IE, Al-Radi OO, Wald RM, Guerra V, et al. Conventional and sutureless techniques for management of the pulmonary veins: evolution of indications from postrepair pulmonary vein stenosis to primary pulmonary vein anomalies. J Thorac Cardiovasc Surg 2005;129:167-74.

32 Cor Triatriatum

DEFINITION

Classic (or typical) cor triatriatum, or *cor triatriatum sinister,* is a rare congenital cardiac anomaly in which the pulmonary veins typically enter a "proximal" left atrial chamber separated from the "distal" left atrial chamber by a partition in which there are one or more restrictive ostia.[1] In the Congenital Heart Surgery Nomenclature and Database Project, cor triatriatum is classified as a pulmonary venous anomaly, with subclassifications as described in Box 32-1.

HISTORICAL NOTE

Cor triatriatum was apparently first described in 1868 by Church.[C2] The name *cor triatriatum* was applied to the malformation by Borst in 1905.[B3] The angiographic diagnosis seems first to have been made at Mayo Clinic and described by Miller and colleagues in 1964.[M3] Echocardiographic diagnosis of this cardiac anomaly was described by Ostman-Smith and colleagues in 1984 and by Wolf in 1986.[O3,W2] The first surgical correction is believed to have been performed by Vineberg and Gialloreto in 1956; the second by Lewis and colleagues followed shortly thereafter.[L1,V5]

MORPHOLOGY

It is unfortunate that cor triatriatum was first defined as "an abnormal septum in the left auricle"[C2] and has been described as resulting in a "subdivided left atrium,"[R1,T1] because these terms obscure surgically important concepts about cor triatriatum.

[1] *Cor triatriatum dexter* is a term used to describe the partially divided right atrium present in some cardiac malformations. This condition is considered in the chapter on tricuspid atresia (see Morphology in Chapter 41) and is unrelated to cor triatriatum sinister.

Morphology of Classic Cor Triatriatum

Typically, the proximal (common pulmonary venous) chamber is somewhat larger than the distal (left atrial) chamber. The common wall partitioning them ("diaphragm" or "membrane"), which may have one or more openings (apertures), is usually thick and fibromuscular (Fig. 32-1). The aperture is typically two dimensional, meaning it has no length, but occasionally it is three dimensional, exhibiting a tubular or tunnel-like configuration.[M1,R1]

The proximal chamber contains all pulmonary vein connections and is usually thick-walled, whereas the distal chamber always contains the left atrial appendage, leads into the mitral valve, and is thin-walled (Fig. 32-2). Despite high pressure in the proximal chamber, the pulmonary veins are not dilated. Entry of the right pulmonary veins into the proximal chamber usually bears the same relationship to the right atrium and superior vena cava as in the normal heart (Fig. 32-3).

The right ventricle is usually enlarged, but this enlargement depends on the presence and degree of left-to-right shunting at the atrial level. The left ventricle is usually normal in size or small. The fossa ovalis may be in the septum between the proximal chamber and right atrium, but occasionally it is in the septum between the distal chamber and right atrium.[N1] The foramen ovale is usually patent and stretched.

Relationship of Cor Triatriatum to Partial and Total Anomalous Pulmonary Venous Connection

In classic cor triatriatum, the right and left pulmonary veins can be considered as not joining the left atrium but rather as entering a chamber, generally posterior and a little superior or medial to the left atrium, that is analogous to the common pulmonary venous sinus found in many patients with total anomalous pulmonary venous connection (TAPVC; see

Box 32-1 Proposed Classification of Pulmonary Venous Anomalies

I. Primary Anomalies of Pulmonary Venous Connection

A. Partially (or partial) anomalous pulmonary venous connection (or return or drainage) (PAPVC, PAPVR)
   1. Non-scimitar
   2. Scimitar (right pulmonary vein[s] draining to inferior vena cava)

B. Totally (or total) anomalous pulmonary venous connection (or return or drainage) (TAPVC, TAPVC)
   1. Supracardiac (supradiaphragmatic, type I)
   2. Cardiac (supradiaphragmatic, type II)
   3. Infracardiac (infradiaphragmatic, type III)
   4. Mixed (type IV)

II. Atresia of the Common Pulmonary Vein

III. Cor Triatriatum (Stenosis of the Common Pulmonary Vein, Triatrial Heart, Cor Triatriatum Sinister)

A. Accessory atrial chamber receives all pulmonary veins and communicates with left atrium
   1. No other connections (classic cor triatriatum)
   2. Other anomalous connections
      a. To right atrium directly
      b. With TAPVC

B. Accessory atrial chamber receives all pulmonary veins and does not communicate with left atrium
   1. Anomalous connection to right atrium directly (cardiac TAPVC with all pulmonary veins first draining to a venous confluence)
   2. With TAPVC (supracardiac or infracardiac TAPVC)

C. Subtotal cor triatriatum
   1. Accessory atrial chamber receives part of the pulmonary veins and connects to left atrium
      a. Remaining pulmonary veins connect normally
      b. Remaining pulmonary veins connect anomalously (partial cor triatriatum with PAPVC)
   2. Accessory atrial chamber receives part of the pulmonary veins and connects to right atrium
      a. Remaining pulmonary veins connect normally (PAPVC with anomalously connected pulmonary veins first draining to a venous confluence)
      b. Remaining pulmonary veins connect anomalously (mixed TAPVC)

IV. Stenosis of Individual Pulmonary Veins

A. Congenital

B. Acquired
   1. Postoperative
   2. Other

From Herlong and colleagues.[H1]

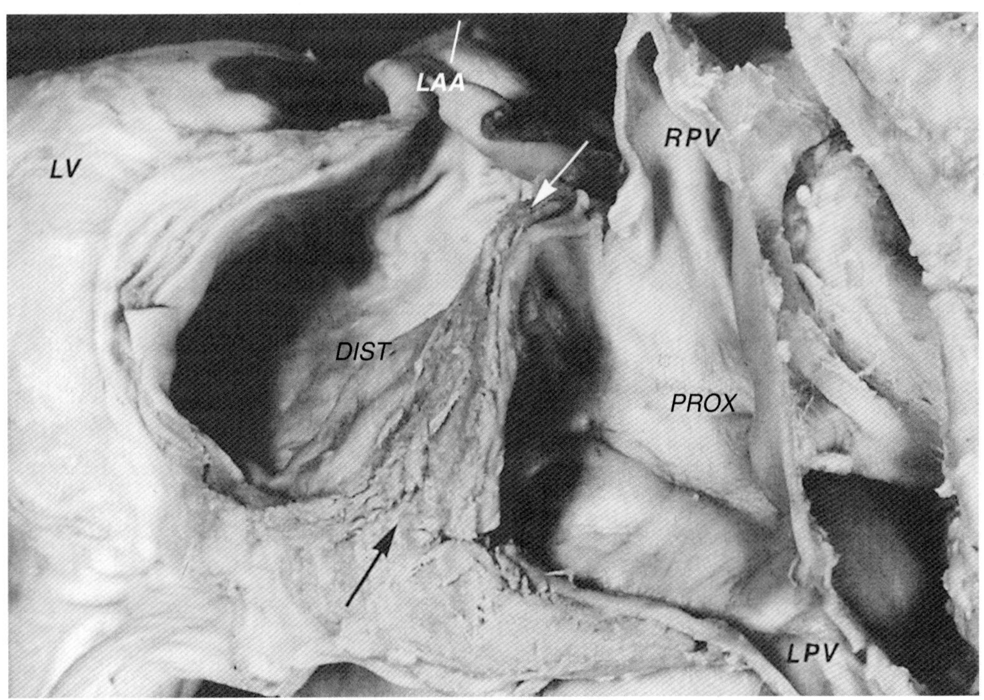

Figure 32-1 Autopsy specimen of cor triatriatum showing opened proximal chamber separated by thick partition *(between arrows)* from opened distal chamber. The partition has a restrictive aperture (not illustrated here) in its center. The relationship of this anomaly to total anomalous pulmonary venous connection is evident from this specimen. Key: *DIST,* Distal chamber; *LA,* left atrium (distal chamber); *LAA,* left atrial appendage; *LPV,* left pulmonary veins; *LV,* left ventricle; *PROX,* proximal; *RPV,* right pulmonary veins.

Chapter 31). Indeed, Van Praagh and Corsini did not use the term *proximal left atrial chamber,* but called it the *common pulmonary vein chamber of cor triatriatum.*[V2] Marin-Garcia and colleagues used similar terminology.[M1]

From an embryologic standpoint, the confluence of the pulmonary veins is completely incorporated into the left atrium in a normal heart, is not incorporated into the left atrium in TAPVC, and is partially incorporated into the left atrium in cor triatriatum. Just as TAPVC does not always involve all pulmonary veins connecting to a single pulmonary venous sinus (i.e., mixed TAPVC), cor triatriatum does not always involve all pulmonary veins draining to the proximal chamber. There are several examples of cor triatriatum in which some of the pulmonary veins drain to the

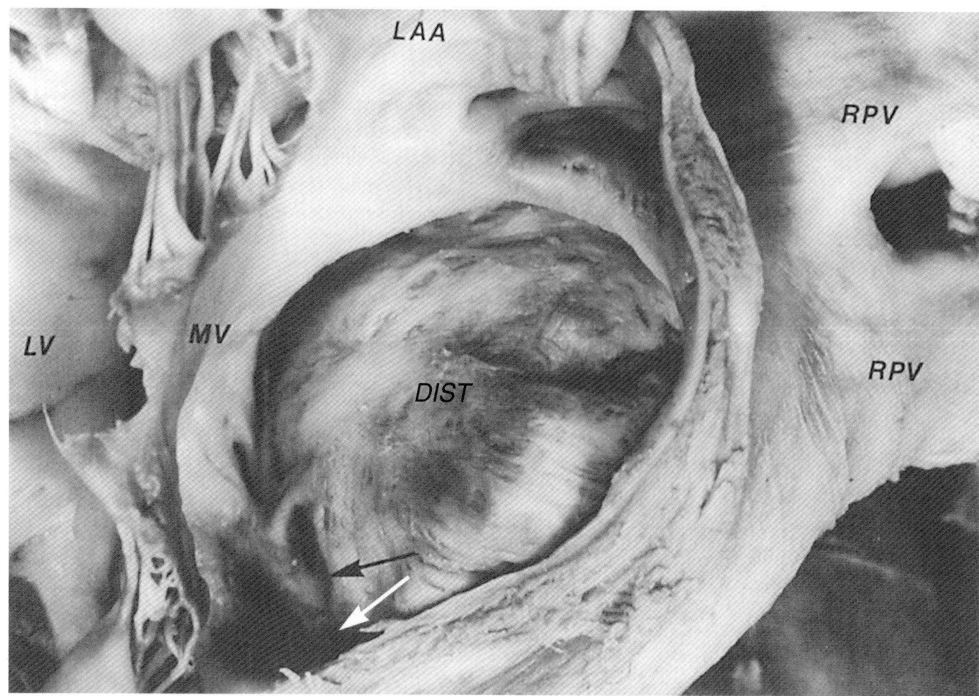

Figure 32-2 Autopsy specimen of cor triatriatum in which only the distal chamber and left ventricle have been opened. Arrows indicate two small apertures in the partition that communicate with the proximal chamber, to which all pulmonary veins are attached. Key: *DIST,* Distal chamber; *LAA,* left atrial appendage; *LV,* left ventricle; *MV,* mitral valve; *RPV,* right pulmonary veins.

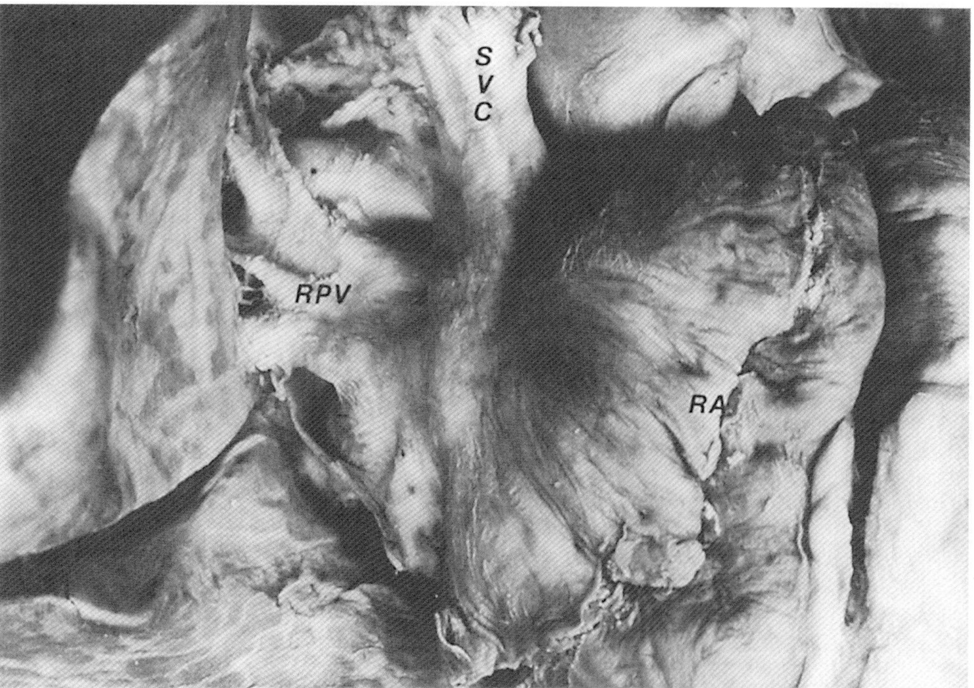

Figure 32-3 Same specimen as in Fig. 32-2, oriented anatomically with the great vessels at the top. Specimen is viewed from the front, and an incision made in the right atrium has been closed. Note normal relationship between right pulmonary veins and superior vena cava and right atrium. Key: *RA,* Right atrium; *RPV,* right pulmonary veins; *SVC,* superior vena cava.

proximal chamber, and the remainder have classic anomalous drainage.

Partial anomalous left pulmonary venous connection (from left upper lobe only or from entire left lung) may connect to a left vertical vein that connects to the left brachiocephalic vein, with all other pulmonary veins entering the proximal chamber.[R1,S3,V2] Partial anomalous venous connection may consist of all left pulmonary veins connecting to the coronary sinus, with the proximal chamber receiving only the right pulmonary veins and connecting through the usual small orifice into the distal left atrial chamber.[G1] Comparisons to partial anomalous pulmonary venous connection (PAPVC) also exist. In these examples, some pulmonary veins connect to the proximal chamber, and the remainder connect normally to the left atrium.

In "partial" cor triatriatum, the right pulmonary veins alone may connect to the proximal chamber, with the left pulmonary veins connecting normally to the left atrium.[T1] Other unusual variants have been documented. The proximal chamber, receiving all pulmonary veins, may have an imperforate portion between it and a typical distal chamber and instead connect to the *right* atrium, whereas the right and left atria are in communication through a coronary sinus atrial septal defect, with the coronary sinus itself being completely unroofed (see Chapter 33). In another example, all pulmonary veins may fail to join an otherwise typical proximal chamber separated from the distal chamber by a perforated partition, and instead connect to a common pulmonary venous sinus behind the heart that may connect to the coronary sinus, superior vena cava, or infradiaphragmatically.[K3,V6]

Relationship of Cor Triatriatum to a Left Superior Vena Cava

A left superior vena cava coexists with cor triatriatum considerably more frequently than with other types of congenital heart disease.[A5,G1,O2] One proposed pathogenesis of cor triatriatum is impingement of a left superior vena cava on the developing left atrium.[G2] Ascuitto and colleagues reported cases in which a persistent left superior vena cava joining a dilated coronary sinus impinged on the posterior wall of the left atrium and divided it into two chambers, both of which had defects that communicated with the right atrium.[A6] It seems clear that a relationship exists between these two anomalies, at least in some patients.

Associated Anomalies

In addition to PAPVC and unroofed coronary sinus with a left superior vena cava joining the left atrium, other associated anomalies include ventricular septal defect, coarctation of the aorta, atrioventricular septal defect, tetralogy of Fallot, and (rarely) asplenia and polysplenia.[M1]

CLINICAL FEATURES AND DIAGNOSTIC CRITERIA

Infants with classic cor triatriatum, with a small aperture between the proximal and distal chambers, usually present with evidence of low cardiac output, including pallor, tachypnea, poor peripheral pulses, and growth failure.[W1] When there is associated left-to-right shunting due to connection of the proximal chamber to the right atrium or because of associated PAPVC, evidence of pulmonary overcirculation and venous obstruction may be present in the chest radiograph, and right ventricular enlargement is prominent. In children and young adults, the classic presentation is with signs and symptoms of pulmonary venous hypertension. However, like mitral stenosis, cor triatriatum may present with less classic symptoms.[S3]

Diagnosis is usually made by echocardiography[M5,S2] (Fig. 32-4). Transesophageal echocardiography has also proven useful in selected cases.[M4] Recently, three-dimensional echocardiography has been used to identify complex morphology in cor triatriatum.[A5,B1] Magnetic resonance imaging with three-dimensional reconstruction provides excellent delineation of both simple and complex morphology in cor triatriatum and is the imaging study of choice if standard two-dimensional echocardiography is not definitive.[L2] Cardiac catheterization and cineangiographic studies are no longer considered necessary unless major associated cardiac anomalies are suspected. However, further evidence may be obtained from selective cineangiographic studies and pressure measurements in the proximal and distal chambers. If the catheter cannot be manipulated into the proximal and distal chambers from the right atrium, sometimes an arterial catheter can be advanced into the left ventricle and retrogradely across the mitral valve and into the distal and then proximal chamber.[V1] Gradients of 20 to 25 mmHg have been demonstrated between the two chambers.[V1]

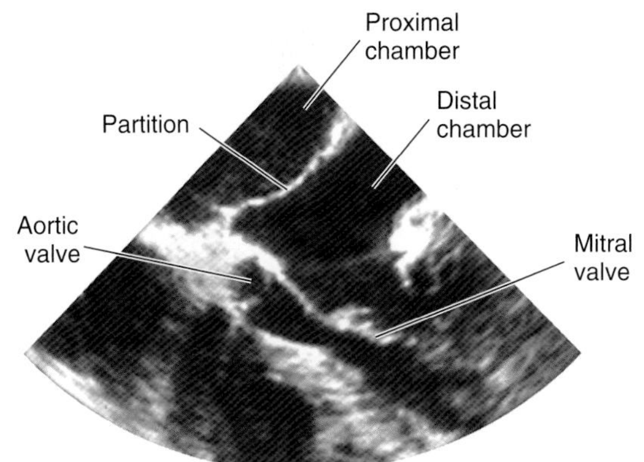

Figure 32-4 Two-dimensional echocardiogram of cor triatriatum. Computer-enhanced image shows partition subdividing the left atrium into proximal and distal chambers.

NATURAL HISTORY

Natural history depends on the effective size of the aperture in the partition between the proximal and distal chambers. When it is small, the infant becomes critically ill during the early months of life, with signs of pulmonary venous obstruction (Fig. 32-5, *A*). Without surgical treatment, such patients die at that young age.[J1,O1,P1,W1] If the aperture is larger, the patient presents in childhood or young adulthood with the signs, symptoms, and prognosis of mitral stenosis.[B2]

In most patients, the aperture is severely restrictive, and approximately 75% of persons born with classic cor triatriatum die in infancy. However, when the proximal chamber communicates with the right atrium through a fossa ovalis atrial septal defect, the prognosis is better because the proximal chamber decompresses into the right atrium (Fig. 32-5, *B*). These patients present with signs of a large left-to-right shunt and generally survive longer than those with an obstructive aperture. Rarely, cor triatriatum may be discovered in an adult.[A2,M1,M2,M3] Delay in diagnosis may be accounted for by a lesser degree of obstruction by the partition or by a unilateral pulmonary venous obstruction.[K1]

TECHNIQUE OF OPERATION

Classic Cor Triatriatum

Treatment of cor triatriatum is primarily by operation. In small infants, approach through the right atrium is preferable. In older patients, especially when the proximal chamber is

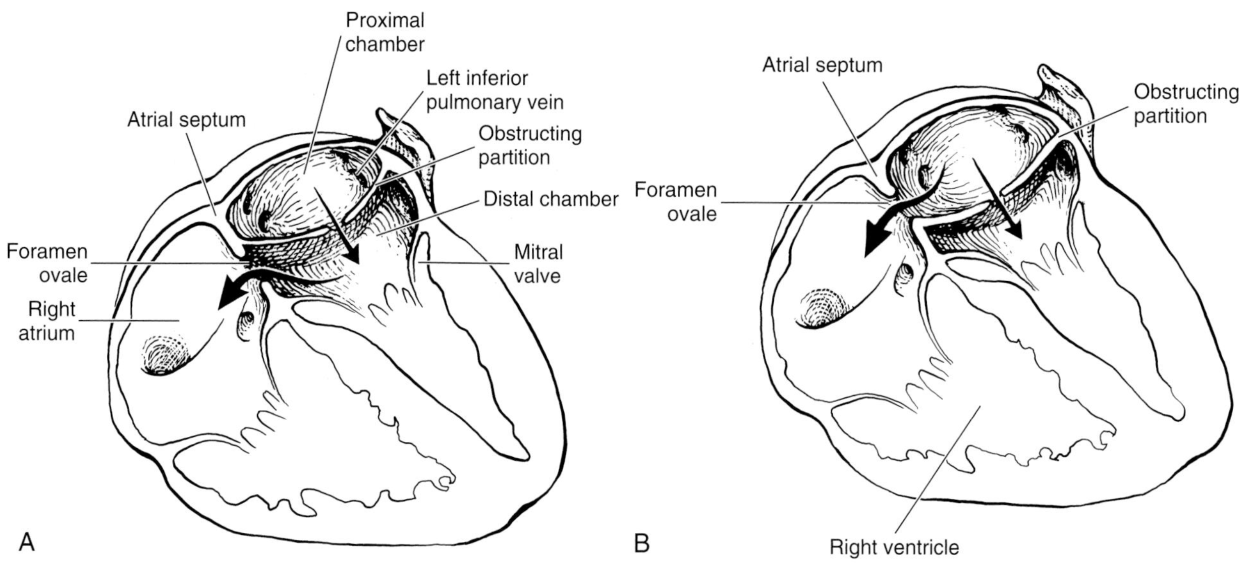

Figure 32-5 Morphology of cor triatriatum. **A,** Cor triatriatum with patent foramen ovale below obstructing partition. Proximal chamber is separated from distal chamber by an obstructing partition. Partition is attached to the atrial septum medially and immediately below left inferior pulmonary vein laterally. The lateral attachment is also closely related to the mitral valve. Left atrial appendage is in the distal chamber. Clinical presentation is that of pulmonary venous obstruction (like mitral valve stenosis) when the aperture in the partition is small. Distal chamber communicates with right atrium through foramen ovale, but left-to-right shunt is small. **B,** Cor triatriatum with patent foramen ovale above obstructing partition, through which the proximal chamber may communicate with the right atrium. Clinical presentation in this situation is that of a large left-to-right shunt or may mimic total anomalous pulmonary venous connection. Right ventricle may be enlarged.

enlarged and no other cardiac anomalies exist, approach through an incision in the right side of this chamber is recommended.

After usual preparations, moderately hypothermic cardiopulmonary bypass (CPB) using two venous cannulae is established (see Section III of Chapter 2). Alternatively, hypothermic circulatory arrest may be employed according to surgeon preference. Cold cardioplegia is established as usual after clamping the aorta (see "Cold Cardioplegia, Controlled Aortic Root Reperfusion, and [When Needed] Warm Cardioplegic Induction" in Chapter 3).

When the approach is through the proximal chamber, a vertical incision is made in the chamber anterior to the right pulmonary veins (Fig. 32-6, *A*) exactly as for mitral valve surgery (see Technique of Operation in Chapter 11). After insertion of an appropriately sized Richardson retractor or similar instrument, the diaphragm is exposed and apertures in it identified. A preliminary incision out from the apertures improves exposure for the definitive excision (Fig. 32-6, *B*). Orifices of the pulmonary veins on both sides are located. Position of the atrial septum is also identified, if necessary, by opening the right atrium and inserting a curved clamp to displace the atrial septum into either the distal or proximal chamber. Most of the partition between these chambers is then excised to make as large an opening as possible (Fig. 32-6, *C*). This procedure is usually easily and quickly done.

When an approach through the right atrium is used, its free wall is incised as in atrial septal defect closure. The right side of the atrial septum is examined and the fossa ovalis identified. If a foramen ovale or atrial septal defect is present, this is enlarged by incision to gain access into the left-sided chamber with which it communicates, either proximal or distal. If there is no atrial septal defect, the septum primum within the fossa ovalis is incised. The partition between the proximal and distal chambers is then identified. In Fig. 32-7, the exposure provided by an atrial septal incision leading into the proximal chamber is shown (Fig. 32-7, *A*). The partition is easy to identify and expose by this approach (Fig. 32-7, *B*). The procedure described for the left-side approach is carried out and the opening in the atrial septum closed with a pericardial patch (Fig. 32-7, *C*). The cardiotomy is closed, the heart having been filled with blood or saline solution before the last few sutures were placed. The remainder of the operation is completed in the usual fashion (see "Completing Cardiopulmonary Bypass" in Section III of Chapter 2).

In the rare case in which there is a specific contraindication to CPB, percutaneous balloon dilatation is possible using a double balloon technique similar to that proposed for mitral valve stenosis.[K2] Relief of symptoms is good, but follow-up is too short (3 months) to establish confidence in this treatment.

Atypical Cor Triatriatum

As noted earlier under Morphology, patients occasionally present for treatment with atypical forms of cor triatriatum, or other important cardiac anomalies may coexist. A persistent left superior vena cava may be present, connecting to the coronary sinus or directly to the upper left atrium, with "unroofing" of the coronary sinus.[V3] Because almost any number of specific combinations may be encountered, the general surgical approach is described rather than a detailed description of each possible combination.

Before operation, the surgeon must determine with reasonable certainty the connections and drainage of all pulmonary and systemic veins, including the possible presence and connection of a left superior vena cava. The possible presence

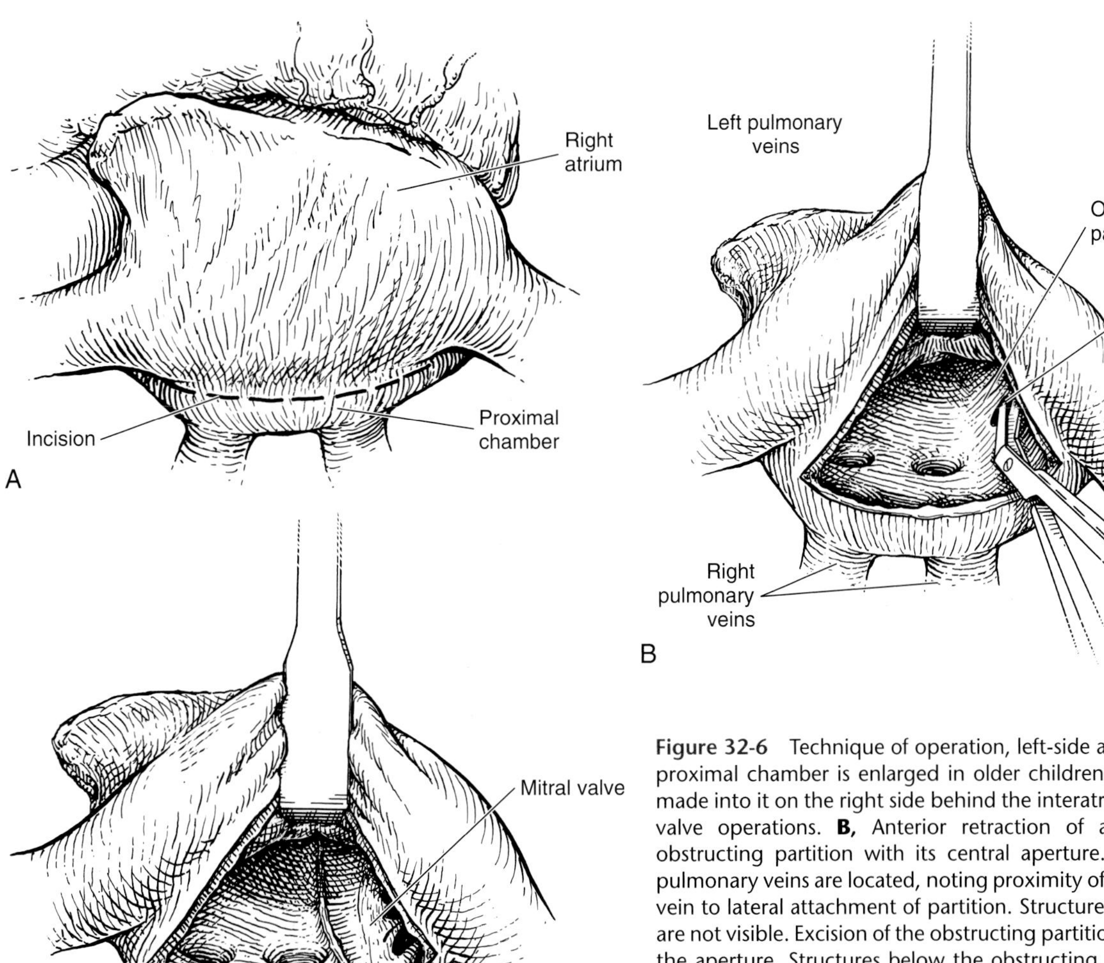

Figure 32-6 Technique of operation, left-side approach. **A,** When the proximal chamber is enlarged in older children and adults, incision is made into it on the right side behind the interatrial groove, as for mitral valve operations. **B,** Anterior retraction of atrial septum exposes obstructing partition with its central aperture. Positions of the four pulmonary veins are located, noting proximity of left inferior pulmonary vein to lateral attachment of partition. Structures in the distal chamber are not visible. Excision of the obstructing partition is started by opening the aperture. Structures below the obstructing partition are identified as opening is enlarged. **C,** Excision of obstructing partition proceeds to the left once its position relative to the left inferior pulmonary vein and mitral valve is clarified. Partition is completely excised, taking care not to penetrate free wall of left atrium. Foramen ovale and left atriotomy are closed to complete the repair.

of both a confluence of all (or some of) the pulmonary veins behind the heart *and* a proximal left atrial chamber should be investigated. The possible connections, through apertures in the wall, of the proximal chambers with both the distal chamber *and* right atrium are determined. Initially, the largest "atrial" chamber appearing on the right side of the heart should be opened. If this is not the right atrium, the right atrium often should be opened subsequently to complete a thorough examination of the morphologic details, all of which must be verified at operation. The repair itself is usually some combination of the repair of typical cor triatriatum, PAPVC and TAPVC (see Technique of Operation in Chapters 30 and 31), and unroofed coronary sinus syndrome (see Chapter 33).

SPECIAL FEATURES OF POSTOPERATIVE CARE

Postoperative care is as usual (see Chapter 5), with special attention given to support of the respiratory system, which may be compromised by pulmonary venous obstruction existing before operation.

RESULTS

Early (Hospital) Death

Hospital deaths are uncommon after repair of *classic* cor triatriatum. Those that occur are in critically ill infants and should be considered to be related to inadequate myocardial management.[R2] Seven separate single-institution retrospective studies constitute a combined total of 96 surgical cases of classic cor triatriatum with six early deaths (6.2%; CL 4.1%-9.4%)[A3,A4,C1,G3,R2,S1,V4] (Table 32-1).

Atypical cor triatriatum can also be successfully repaired. Many of the studies documented in Table 32-1 report successful repairs in patients in this more complex subset but also emphasize that mortality is higher than for classic cor triatriatum.

Time-Related Survival and Functional Status

Life expectancy after repair of classic cor triatriatum approaches that of the general population, especially when the operation is done in infancy.[S1] Richardson and colleagues

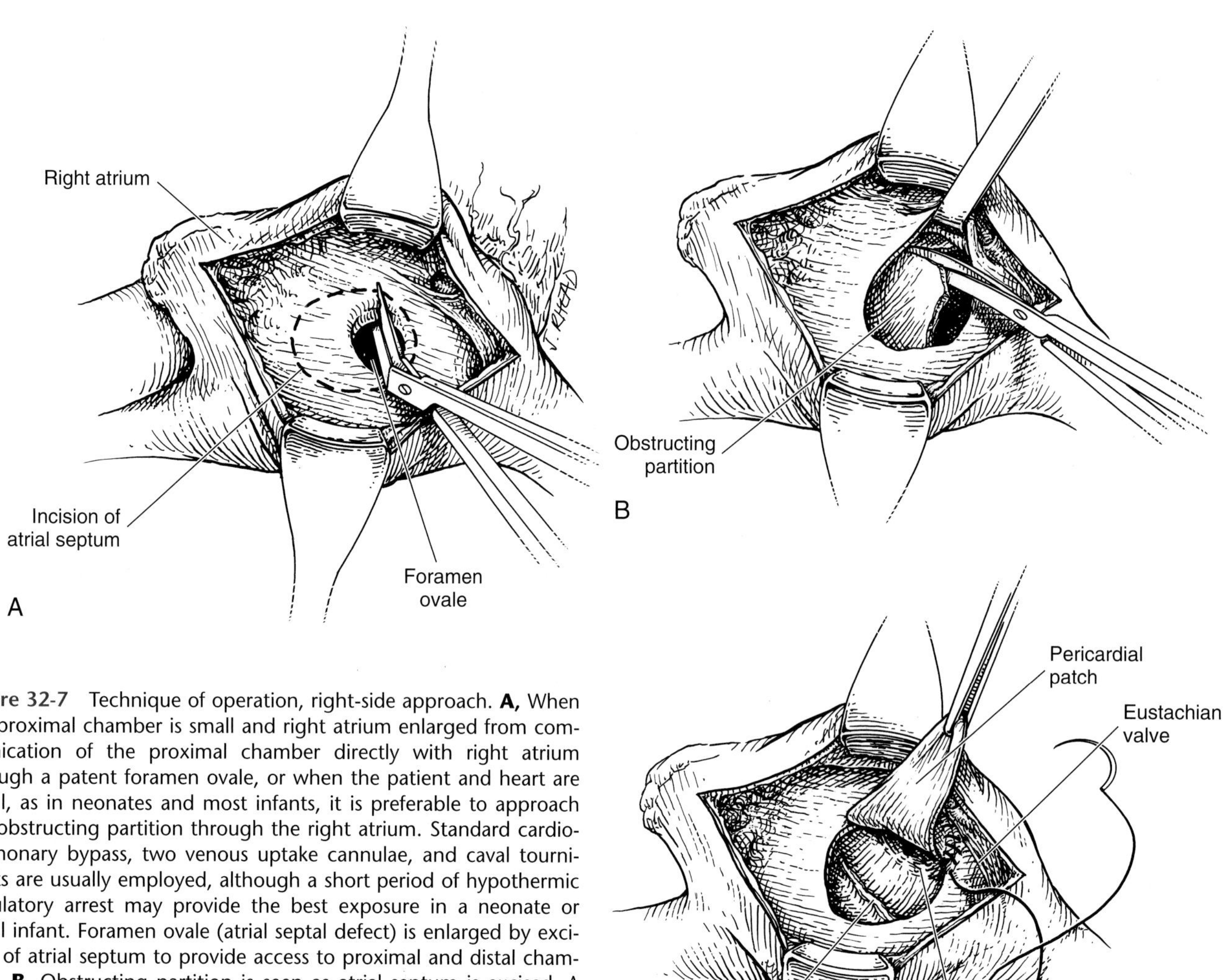

Figure 32-7 Technique of operation, right-side approach. **A,** When the proximal chamber is small and right atrium enlarged from communication of the proximal chamber directly with right atrium through a patent foramen ovale, or when the patient and heart are small, as in neonates and most infants, it is preferable to approach the obstructing partition through the right atrium. Standard cardiopulmonary bypass, two venous uptake cannulae, and caval tourniquets are usually employed, although a short period of hypothermic circulatory arrest may provide the best exposure in a neonate or small infant. Foramen ovale (atrial septal defect) is enlarged by excision of atrial septum to provide access to proximal and distal chambers. **B,** Obstructing partition is seen as atrial septum is excised. A retractor placed anteriorly on the septum provides exposure for identifying the left inferior pulmonary vein and mitral valve. **C,** Obstructing partition is completely excised. Atrial septum is repaired using a pericardial patch.

Table 32-1 Hospital Mortality after Repair of Classic Cor Triatriatum

			Hospital Deaths		
Source	**Year**	***n***	**No.**	**%**	**CL (%)**
Van Son et al.[V4]	1993	11	1	9.0	
Gheissari et al.[G3]	1992	7	1	14	
Rodefeld et al.[R2]	1990	11	0	0	
Carpena et al.[C1]	1974	4	0	0	
Alphonso et al.[A4]	2005	28	1	3.6	
Al Qethamy et al.[A3]	2006	20	0	0	
Salomone et al.[S1]	1991	15	3	20	
TOTAL		96	6	6.2	4.1-9.4

reported one late death attributed to pulmonary vein stenosis in their group of eight hospital survivors.[A1,R1] Qethamy and colleagues[A3] reported no late deaths in 20 patients with a mean follow-up of 31 months. Alphonso and colleagues[A4] reported 27 patients with a mean follow-up of 98 months; survival was 96% at 5 years and 88% at 15 years. The association of pulmonary vein stenosis with cor triatriatum reinforces the interrelationship between cor triatriatum and TAPVC (see "Pulmonary Vein Stenosis" under Reoperation and the Development of Pulmonary Venous Obstruction in Chapter 31). Another unfavorable late event is restenosis of the orifice between the proximal chamber and left atrium.[J1] This may be the result of an inadequate original operation in which the common wall between the two chambers was incompletely resected. Most follow-up studies suggest that essentially all patients are either described as asymptomatic or are documented to be in New York Heart Association functional class I.[A1,A4,R2,S1]

INDICATIONS FOR OPERATION

Classic cor triatriatum with a restrictive aperture in the partition between the proximal and distal chambers is an urgent indication for operation, because 75% of patients with such malformations die in infancy. When older patients present with chronic symptoms, operation is also urgently indicated.

In atypical cor triatriatum, when the proximal chamber opens into the right atrium, a restrictive opening or no opening is present between the proximal and distal chambers, and only a small patent foramen ovale exists between the right atrium and distal chamber, physiologic instability will be present. A large left-to-right shunt combined with restricted left atrial and left ventricular inflow produces severe symptoms during the early months of life, and operation is urgently indicated.

REFERENCES

A

1. Abadir S, Acar P. Live 3D Transthoracic echocardiography for assessment of cor triatriatum sinister. Echocardiography 2008;25:1147-8.
2. al-Abdulla HM, Demany MA, Zimmerman HA. Cor triatriatum: preoperative diagnosis in an adult patient. Am J Cardiol 1970;26:310.
3. Al Qethamy HO, Aboelnazar S, Al Faraidi Y, et al. Cor triatriatum: operative results in 20 patients. Asian Cardiovasc Thorac Ann 2006;14:7-9.
4. Alphonso N, Nørgaard MA, Newcomb A, et al. Cor triatriatum: presentation, diagnosis and long-term surgical results. Ann Thorac Surg 2005;80:1666-71.
5. Arciniegas E, Farooki ZQ, Hakimi M, Perry BL, Green EW. Surgical treatment of cor triatriatum. Ann Thorac Surg 1981;32:571.
6. Ascuitto RJ, Ross-Ascuitto NT, Kopf GS, Fahey J, Kleinman CS, Hellenbrand WE, et al. Persistent left superior vena cava causing subdivided left atrium: diagnosis, embryological implications, and surgical management. Ann Thorac Surg 1987;44:546.

B

1. Baweja G, Nanda NC, Kirklin JK. Definitive diagnosis of cor triatriatum with common atrium by three-dimensional transesophageal echocardiography in an adult. Echocardiography 2004;21:303-6.
2. Belcher JR, Somerville W. Cor triatriatum (stenosis of the common pulmonary vein): successful treatment of a case. Br Med J 1959; 1:1280.
3. Borst H. Ein Cor triatriatum. Zentralbl Allg Pathol 1905;16:812.

C

1. Carpena C, Colokathis B, Subramanian S. Cor triatriatum. Ann Thorac Surg 1974;17:325.
2. Church WS. Congenital malformation of the heart: abnormal septum in left auricle. Trans Pathol Soc Lond 1867/1868;19:188.

G

1. Geggel RL, Fulton DR, Chernoff HL, Cleveland R, Hougen TJ. Cor triatriatum associated with partial anomalous pulmonary venous connection to the coronary sinus: echocardiographic and angiocardiographic features. Pediatr Cardiol 1987;8:279.
2. Gharagozloo F, Bulkley BH, Hutchings GM. A proposed pathogenesis of cor triatriatum: impingement of the left superior vena cava on the developing left atrium. Am Heart J 1977;94:618.
3. Gheissari A, Malm JR, Bowman FO Jr, Bierman FZ. Cor triatriatum sinistrum: one institution's 28-year experience. Pediatr Cardiol 1992;13:85-8.

H

1. Herlong JR, Jaggers JJ, Ungerleider RM. Congenital Heart Surgery Nomenclature and Database Project: pulmonary venous anomalies. Ann Thorac Surg 2000;69:S56-69.

J

1. Jorgensen CR, Ferlic RM, Varco RL, Lillehei CW, Eliot RS. Cor triatriatum: review of the surgical aspects with a follow-up report on the first patient successfully treated with surgery. Circulation 1967;36:101.

K

1. Kerensky RA, Bertolet BD, Epstein M. Late discovery of cor triatriatum as a result of unilateral pulmonary venous obstruction. Am Heart J 1995;130:624.
2. Kerkar P, Vora A, Kulkarni H, Narula D, Goyal V, Dalvi B. Percutaneous balloon dilatation of cor triatriatum sinister. Am Heart J 1996;132:888.
3. Kirk AJ, Pollock JC. Concomitant cor triatriatum and coronary sinus total anomalous pulmonary venous connection. Ann Thorac Surg 1987;44:203.

L

1. Lewis FJ, Varco RL, Taufic M, Niazi SA. Direct vision repair of triatrial heart and total anomalous pulmonary venous drainage. Surg Gynecol Obstet 1956;102:713.
2. Locca D, Hughes M, Mohiaddin R. Cardiovascular magnetic resonance diagnosis of a previously unreported association: cor triatriatum with right partial anomalous pulmonary venous return to the azygos vein. Int J Cardiol 2009;135:e80-2.

M

1. Marin-Garcia J, Tandon R, Lucas RV Jr, Edwards JE. Cor triatriatum: study of 20 cases. Am J Cardiol 1975;35:59.
2. McGuire LB, Nolan TB, Reeve R, Dammann JF. Cor triatriatum as a problem of adult heart disease. Circulation 1965;30:263.
3. Miller GA, Ongley PA, Anderson MW, Kincaid OW, Swan HJ. Cor triatriatum: hemodynamic and angiocardiographic diagnosis. Am Heart J 1964;68:298.
4. Modi KA, Senthilkumar A, Kiel E, Reddy PC. Diagnosis and surgical correction of cor triatriatum in an adult: combined use of transesophageal and contrast echocardiography, and review of literature. Echocardiography 2006;23:506-9.
5. Muhiudeen-Russell IA, Silverman NH. Images in cardiovascular medicine. Cor triatriatum in an infant. Circulation 1997;95:2700.

N

1. Niwayama G. Cor triatriatum. Am Heart J 1960;59:291.

O

1. Oelert H, Breckenridge IM, Rosland G, Stark J. Surgical treatment of cor triatriatum in a 4½-month-old infant. Thorax 1973;28:242.
2. Oglietti J, Cooley DA, Izquierdo JP, Ventemiglia R, Muasher I, Hallman GL, et al. Cor triatriatum: operative results in 25 patients. Ann Thorac Surg 1983;35:415.
3. Ostman-Smith I, Silverman NH, Oldershaw P, Lincoln C, Shinebourne EA. Cor triatriatum sinistrum: diagnostic features on cross sectional echocardiography. Br Heart J 1984;51:211.

P

1. Perry LW, Scott LD, McClenathan JE. Cor triatriatum: preoperative diagnosis and successful repair in a small infant. J Pediatr 1967;71:840.

R

1. Richardson JV, Doty DB, Siewers RD, Zuberbuhler JR. Cor triatriatum (subdivided left atrium). J Thorac Cardiovasc Surg 1981;81:232.
2. Rodefeld MD, Brown JW, Heimansohn DA, King H, Girod DA, Hurwitz RA, et al. Cor triatriatum: clinical presentation and surgical results in 12 patients. Ann Thorac Surg 1990;50:562.

S

1. Salomone G, Tiraboschi R, Crippa M, Ferri F, Bianchi T, Parenzan L. Cor triatriatum. Clinical presentation and operative results. J Thorac Cardiovasc Surg 1991;101:1088.
2. Shuler CO, Fyfe DA, Sade R, Crawford FA. Transesophageal echocardiographic evaluation of cor triatriatum in children. Am Heart J 1995;129:507.
3. Somerville J. Masked cor triatriatum. Br Heart J 1966;28:55.

T

1. Thilenius OG, Bharati S, Lev M. Subdivided left atrium: an expanded concept of cor triatriatum sinistrum. Am J Cardiol 1976;37:743.

V

1. van der Horst RL, Gotsman MS. Cor triatriatum: angiographic diagnosis by retrograde catheterization of the dorsal accessory chamber. Br J Radiol 1971;44:273.
2. Van Praagh R, Corsini I. Cor triatriatum: pathologic anatomy and a consideration of morphogenesis based on 13 postmortem cases and

a study of normal development of the pulmonary vein and atrial septum in 83 human embryos. Am Heart J 1969;78:379.

3. van Son JA, Autschbach R, Mohr FW. Repair of cor triatriatum associated with partially unroofed coronary sinus. Ann Thorac Surg 1999;68:1414.
4. van Son JA, Danielson GK, Schaff HV, Puga FJ, Seward JB, Hagler DJ, et al. Cor triatriatum: diagnosis, operative approach, and late results. Mayo Clin Proc 1993;68:854.
5. Vineberg A, Gialloreto O. Report of a successful operation for stenosis of common pulmonary vein (cor triatriatum). Can Med Assoc J 1956;74:719.
6. Vouhe PR, Baillot-Vernant F, Fermont L, Bical O, Leca F, Neveus JY. Cor triatriatum and total anomalous pulmonary venous connection: a rare, surgically correctable anomaly. J Thorac Cardiovasc Surg 1985;90:443.

W

1. Wolf RR, Ruttenberg HD, Desilets DT, Mulder DE. Cor triatriatum. J Thorac Cardiovasc Surg 1968;56:114.
2. Wolf WJ. Diagnostic features and pitfalls in the two-dimensional echocardiographic evaluation of a child with cor triatriatum. Pediatr Cardiol 1986;6:211.

33 Unroofed Coronary Sinus Syndrome

DEFINITION

Unroofed coronary sinus syndrome is a spectrum of cardiac anomalies in which part or all of the common wall between the coronary sinus and left atrium is absent. Hearts with atrial isomerism and a left-sided superior vena cava (LSVC) entering a left-sided atrium are included in this chapter, despite the controversy concerning proper classification of such anomalies (see "Atrial Isomerism" under Morphology later in this chapter; see also Chapter 58).

HISTORICAL NOTE

Unroofed coronary sinus syndrome was unknown to cardiac pathologists before the era of cardiac catheterization and cardiac surgery. In 1954, Campbell and Deuchar referred to instances of LSVC attached to the left atrium.[C1] Although they did not have such an example in their own series of LSVC, they appreciated that in such cases there was no true coronary sinus. That same year, Winter, a radiologist at Hahnemann Hospital in Philadelphia, published a report that identified persistent LSVC attached to the left atrium, and 2 years later, Friedlich and colleagues identified by cardiac catheterization LSVC entering the left atrium in four patients.[F3,W1] An isolated case was also reported by Tuchman and colleagues in 1956.[T3] However, true understanding of the morphology of the syndrome awaited the classic paper by Raghib, Edwards, and colleagues in 1965.[R1] The descriptive phrase "unroofed coronary sinus" was first used by Helseth and Peterson in 1974.[H2]

In cyanotic patients with a communication between the left and right SVC, the LSVC was first ligated (appropriately) by Hurwitt and colleagues in 1955 and then by Davis and colleagues in 1959.[D1,H3] In 1965, Taybi and colleagues reported a ligation and mentioned "transferring the left SVC to the right atrium," but presumably this was unsuccessful, because no further details were given.[T1] The first report of successful repair was from the Mayo Clinic in 1963.[R2] In this case, a tunnel was constructed from the posterior wall of the left atrium. In a second case, a large pericardial atrial baffle was constructed that corrected the anomalous connection of both the SVC and the inferior vena cava (IVC) to a left-sided atrium.[M2] This procedure was also described by Helseth and Peterson in 1974.[H2]

MORPHOLOGY

Completely Unroofed Coronary Sinus with Persistent Left Superior Vena Cava

In one form of unroofed coronary sinus syndrome, the coronary sinus does not exist, because the common wall between it and the left atrium is absent. A persistent LSVC, which usually becomes continuous with the coronary sinus, connects to the left upper corner of the left atrium.[S4] The site of connection of the LSVC to the left atrium appears to be constant and lies between the opening of the left atrial appendage anteriorly and slightly superiorly, and the opening of the left pulmonary veins posteriorly and inferiorly. The pulmonary veins may enter the left atrium more superiorly than usual in this form of the syndrome.

A coronary sinus atrial septal defect (ASD) is present in the posteroinferior region of the atrial septum in the usual position of the ostium of the coronary sinus (see Chapter 30, Fig. 30-5). The ASD is separated from the atrioventricular (AV) valve ring by a remnant of atrial septum (in contrast to an ostium primum ASD), and its posterior margin is formed by the atrial wall where it joins the IVC. There may be a separate foramen ovale ASD or a single large ASD formed by the confluence of both defects. The coronary sinus ASD may be confluent with an ostium primum ASD, or there may be a common atrium. Because the coronary sinus does not exist, individual coronary veins connect separately to the inferior aspect of the left atrium. Some also connect to the right atrium.

Of considerable surgical importance is the fact that the left brachiocephalic vein is absent in 80% to 90% of cases of unroofed coronary sinus syndrome and LSVC.[Q1,R2] The right SVC is frequently small and may be absent. The IVC not infrequently crosses to the left side below the diaphragm to enter the left hemiazygos vein, which joins the LSVC. The hepatic veins usually enter the inferior aspect of the right atrium, but they too may enter the inferior wall of the left atrium. When all the systemic veins enter a morphologically left atrium, total anomalous systemic venous connection is present (see Chapter 31).

Completely Unroofed Coronary Sinus without Persistent Left Superior Vena Cava

In some cases, the syndrome is characterized by a completely unroofed coronary sinus without a persistent LSVC. Such cases consist of a coronary sinus type of ASD and total absence of the coronary sinus because of absence of the partition between it and the left atrium.

Partially Unroofed Midportion of Coronary Sinus

Another form of the syndrome is characterized by a partially unroofed midportion of the coronary sinus (also called *biatrial opening of coronary sinus* or *coronary sinus to left atrial window* or *fenestration*). In this anomaly, an aperture is present in the midportion of the wall between the coronary sinus and left atrium. Through this aperture, a left-to-right or right-to-left shunt occurs, depending on whether obstruction is present to left atrial or right atrial outflow.[F2] When this rare form of unroofed coronary sinus syndrome occurs as an isolated lesion, there may be a large left-to-right shunt.[A1,M1] It has also been reported as a major cardiac anomaly associated with tricuspid atresia, recognized only after the Fontan repair has elevated the right atrial pressure and produced a right-to-left shunt.[F2,R5,R6]

When midportion unroofing occurs in the presence of LSVC, there is a right-to-left shunt into the left atrium.

Partially Unroofed Terminal Portion of Coronary Sinus

Particularly in the presence of an atrioventricular septal defect (see "Completely Unroofed Coronary Sinus with Left Superior Vena Cava" under Morphology in Chapter 34), the coronary sinus ostium may open into the left atrium rather than the right. Also, a localized unroofing of the sinus may occur just before it enters the ostium of the coronary sinus, resulting in a coronary sinus ASD with preservation of the coronary sinus (see "Coronary Sinus Defect" under Morphology in Chapter 30). Such anomalies can be considered to be unroofing (or absence) of the terminal portion of the coronary sinus.

Relationship of Unroofed Coronary Sinus Syndrome to Cor Triatriatum and Atrioventricular Septal Defect

As indicated, when a completely unroofed coronary sinus with persistent LSVC is present, both the left and right pulmonary veins may enter the left atrium more superiorly than usual. Sometimes this condition is accompanied by a mild or moderate narrowing between the portion of the left atrium to which the pulmonary veins are attached (the common pulmonary venous chamber) and that to which the LSVC, left atrial appendage, and mitral valve are attached (see "Relationship of Cor Triatriatum to a Left Superior Vena Cava" under Morphology in Chapter 32).

Unroofed coronary sinus syndrome has as its most common major associated cardiac anomaly an atrioventricular septal defect, not infrequently with a common atrium (see Chapter 34). Interestingly, atrioventricular septal defects are more commonly associated with persistent LSVC than are other types of ASD.

Atrial Isomerism

Many patients with an LSVC connecting to a left-sided atrium have atrial isomerism (see Chapter 58), and the majority of such patients have an atrioventricular septal defect. In an unpublished autopsy series from GLH of 26 hearts with the LSVC connecting to the left-sided atrium, only 3 were examples of classic unroofed coronary sinus syndrome; 23 hearts had atrial isomerism, 17 with bilateral morphologically right atria (most with asplenia) and 6 with bilateral morphologically left atria (most with polysplenia). Of the 23, 20 had an atrioventricular septal defect in addition to numerous other cardiac anomalies. When bilateral morphologically right atria are present, the LSVC enters the left-sided right atrium behind a typical crista terminalis and is not therefore an example of unroofed coronary sinus, even though the coronary sinus is usually absent. When bilateral morphologically left atria are present, the LSVC may or may not be part of an unroofed coronary sinus syndrome. In such cases, however, the coronary sinus is frequently absent.

CLINICAL FEATURES AND DIAGNOSTIC CRITERIA

In most cases, diagnosis of unroofed coronary sinus syndrome is made by two-dimensional echocardiography and confirmed at operation[A2] (Fig. 33-1). Demonstration of an LSVC by catheter passage into the vein or by cineangiography suggests the diagnosis, which is confirmed at operation if the LSVC can also be shown to drain into the left atrium. Diagnosis of a partially unroofed midportion of the coronary sinus can be made by cineangiography after injection into the right atrium, when right atrial pressure is higher than left (e.g., after the Fontan operation). Konstam and colleagues have pointed out that radionuclide angiography can be diagnostic, because intravenous injections into the left arm show much larger right-to-left shunting than those into the right arm.[K1] Diagnosis sometimes can be made by cross-sectional, contrast, and

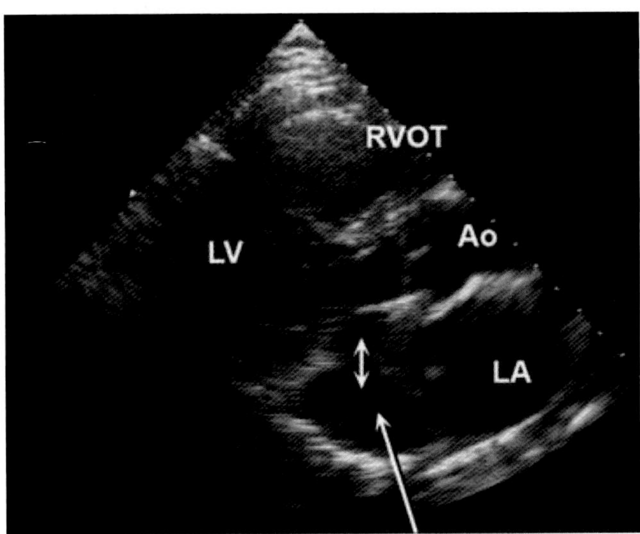

Figure 33-1 Transthoracic echocardiogram showing a dilated coronary sinus *(long arrow)* and small communication between the coronary sinus and left atrium *(small double-headed arrow)*. Key: *Ao,* Aorta; *LA,* left atrium; *LV,* left ventricle; *RVOT,* right ventricular outflow tract. (From Attenhofer Jost and colleagues.[A2])

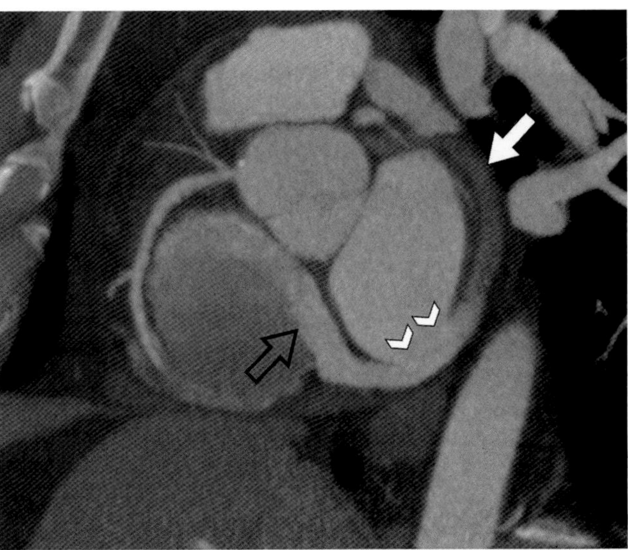

Figure 33-2 Contrast-enhanced gated multidetector computed tomography image of a 53-year-old man with unroofed coronary sinus. Multiplanar reformat image in valve plane shows coronary sinus partially unopacified *(white arrow)*, site of unroofing and communication with the left atrium *(arrowheads)*, and jet of dense contrast entering the right atrium through the Thebesian valve *(open arrow)*. (From Thangaroopan and colleagues.[T2])

transesophageal echocardiography.[K2,S2] Contrast-enhanced gated multidetector computed tomography is also useful for diagnosis (Fig. 33-2). Often, however, the diagnosis is made by the surgeon viewing external and internal morphology of the heart at operation.

NATURAL HISTORY

Cyanosis from right-to-left shunting dominates the clinical picture of isolated completely unroofed coronary sinus with persistent LSVC and determines its natural history. In the series of Quaegebeur and colleagues, cyanosis was mild (all patients were younger than 17 years), but it was severe in some older patients in other series.[Q1]

Cerebral embolization manifested by transient ischemic attacks or stroke and brain abscess complicate the life history in 10% to 25% of patients[Q1,R1] (Table 19-1). This situation is similar to that in other types of right-to-left shunting. Presumably, life expectancy is considerably reduced by these complications and by other problems associated with increasing cyanosis and polycythemia.

TECHNIQUE OF OPERATION

Isolated Completely Unroofed Coronary Sinus with Persistent Left Superior Vena Cava

Anesthesia and preparation of the patient for repair of isolated completely unroofed coronary sinus with persistent LSVC are as described in Section III of Chapter 2. When the diagnosis is known preoperatively, the anesthesiologist inserts a pressure-monitoring line into the *left* external or, preferably, internal jugular vein.

Operation may be done with cardiopulmonary bypass (CPB) at 25°C and the usual direct caval cannulation (see "Clinical Methodology of Cardiopulmonary Bypass" in Section III of Chapter 2); venous blood from the LSVC is collected with a sump sucker connected to the pump oxygenator. Alternatively in infants, a single venous cannula and repair during hypothermic circulatory arrest may be used. Myocardial management is conducted as for other cardiac operations (see "Methods of Myocardial Management during Cardiac Surgery" in Chapter 3).

Intracardiac Repair

After sternotomy, a large piece of pericardium is excised and set aside (see Chapter 30). Following aortic clamping and infusion of cardioplegic solution, the right atrium is opened through the usual oblique incision. Orifices of the three vena cavae are identified with certainty. Repair can be accomplished satisfactorily using one of two methods (the original method of "reroofing the coronary sinus"[Q1,R2,S3] is no longer used because of its technical difficulty and because the left pulmonary veins are at risk of obstruction by the baffle).

One method consists of excising the entire atrial septum except for the anterior limbus, which is preserved to protect the AV node and bundle of His.[C3,M2] A pericardial patch is sutured into place as a repositioned atrial septum, and all three caval orifices are positioned on the right side of this septum (Figs. 33-3 and 33-4). This method is particularly useful when a common atrium is part of the cardiac anomaly.

A second method, described by Sand and colleagues, consists of "rerouting the coronary sinus" to the roof of the left atrium (Fig. 33-5) and then reconstructing the atrial septum.[S1]

After the right atriotomy is closed, the caval tapes are released and aortic clamp removed. Usual de-airing maneuvers are performed (see "De-airing the Heart" in Section III of Chapter 2), and the operation is completed.

Extracardiac Repair

A third method involves extracardiac correction of the unroofed coronary sinus in combination with the associated intracardiac repair. If the brachiocephalic vein is absent, the LSVC is divided at its junction with the left atrium, and the

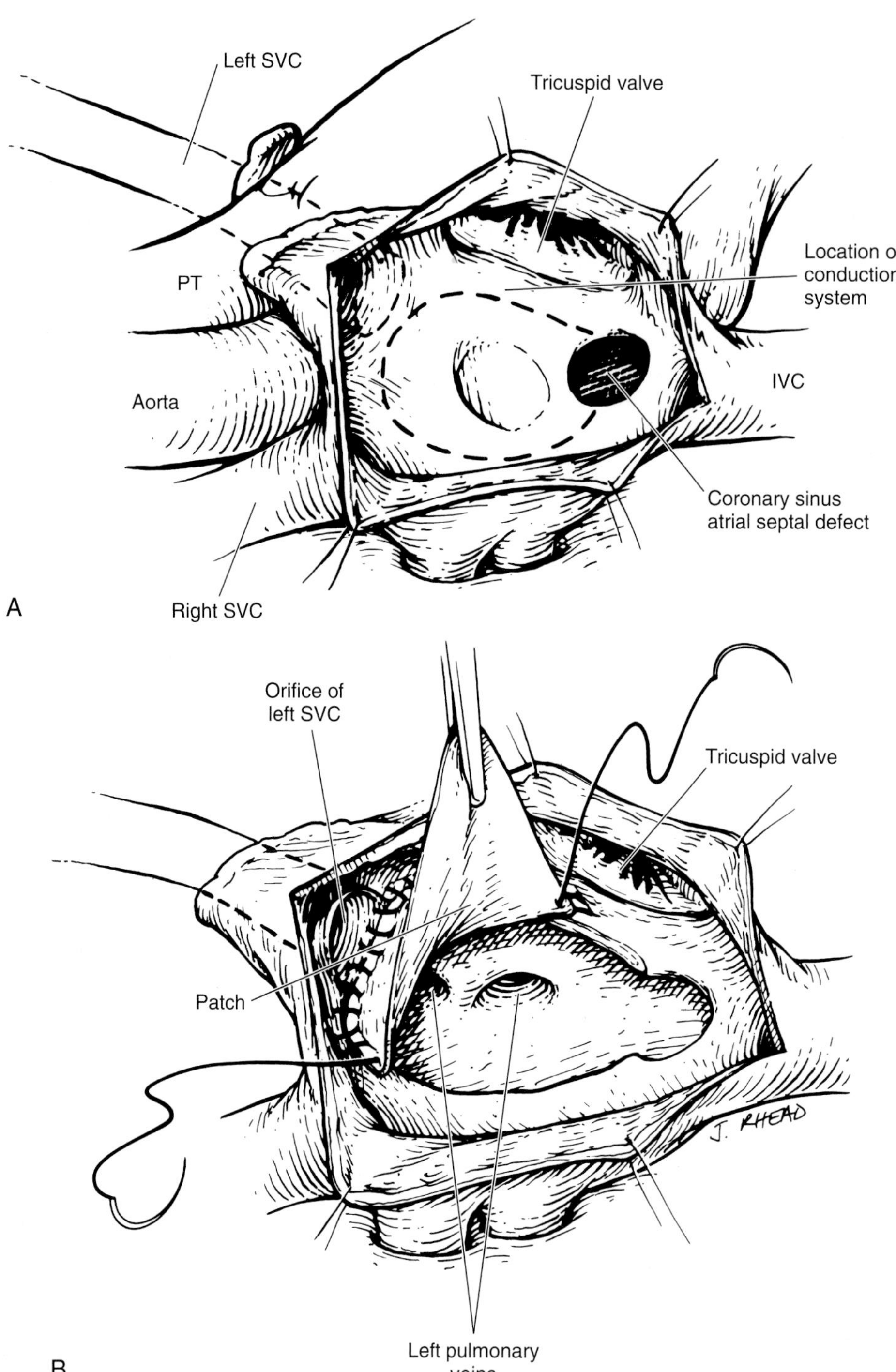

Figure 33-3 One technique for repair of unroofed coronary sinus with large persistent left superior vena cava (LSVC) entering the upper left corner of left atrium. **A,** Exposure is through an oblique right atriotomy. Dashed circle represents line of incision in atrial septum. **B,** Atrial septum has been excised, with care taken to preserve anterior limbus to protect atrioventricular node and bundle of His. Orifices of left pulmonary veins are visible. Anterosuperior to these orifices is the orifice of the LSVC, and just anterior to that is the left atrial appendage. A pericardial patch is sutured to the posterior rim of the LSVC using a continuous 4-0 or 5-0 polypropylene suture.

opening in the left atrium is oversewn. The divided end of the LSVC is anastomosed to the side of the right SVC either anterior or posterior to the aorta.[R3,V3] Alternatively, the LSVC can be anastomosed to the right atrial appendage or left pulmonary artery as a bidirectional superior cavopulmonary shunt.[F1,R3,S4,T1,V4] A continuous 6-0 or 7-0 absorbable monofilament suture is used for these anastomoses.

If the brachiocephalic vein is present but restrictive, it can be enlarged with a patch of autologous pericardium.[V2] The LSVC is then divided at its junction with the left atrium, and both ends are oversewn.

These extracardiac techniques eliminate the need for constructing an intraatrial baffle or tunnel. They can be performed during the period of rewarming after correction of

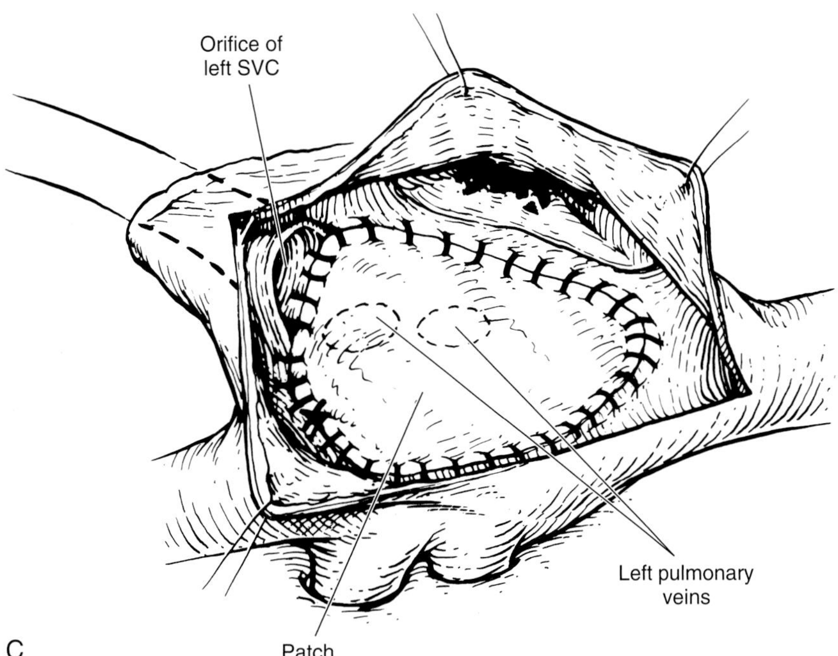

Figure 33-3, cont'd C, Suture line is continued along rim of the atrial septum and rim of coronary sinus atrial septal defect. Key: *IVC,* Inferior vena cava; *PT,* pulmonary trunk; SVC, superior vena cava.

associated intracardiac anomalies, thus reducing the durations of myocardial ischemia and CPB. They also eliminate the potential for creating a small left atrium with reduced compliance and reduce the potential for developing pulmonary venous obstruction.

Partially Unroofed Midportion of Coronary Sinus

Repair of a partially unroofed midportion of the coronary sinus is made through a right atrial approach. The important step is defining the aperture, which is accomplished by passing a small forceps or clamp into the coronary sinus, through the defect, and into the left atrium, verifying that the tip has in fact entered the left atrium. Closure can usually be made from within the coronary sinus, whether there is an LSVC or not. Alternatively, repair can be made from the left atrial side, approaching the defect through an opening in the atrial septum.

Partially Unroofed Terminal Portion of Coronary Sinus

A partially unroofed terminal portion of the coronary sinus occurs primarily in association with atrioventricular septal defects. The coronary sinus ostium is simply left to drain into the left atrium by the repair (see Chapter 34).

Unroofed Coronary Sinus Syndrome with Left Superior Vena Cava and Atrioventricular Septal Defect

For unroofed coronary sinus syndrome with LSVC and atrioventricular septal defect, repair is made exactly as described for uncomplicated cases, except that rather than being attached to the limbus, the pericardial baffle is attached to the crest of the ventricular septum and AV valves (partial atrioventricular septal defect) or to the top of the polyester patch used to close the interventricular communication (complete atrioventricular septal defect) (see Fig. 33-4; see also Chapter 58 and Fig. 58-6).

Completely Unroofed Coronary Sinus Associated with Other Complex Cardiac Anomalies

No simple description can be given of repairing complex anomalies in which unroofed coronary sinus syndrome is but a part. Such cases are often unique, and the surgeon must study the malformation in detail and plan the repair according to the findings. General comments concerning atypical cor triatriatum may be applicable (see Chapter 32). The types of procedures performed in two large surgical series of uncomplicated unroofed coronary sinus are shown in Tables 33-1 and 33-2.[A2,Q1]

RESULTS

Early (Hospital) Death

Risk associated with repair of simple unroofed coronary sinus syndrome is low. No deaths occurred among 18 patients (0%; CL 0%-10%) reported by Quaegebeur and colleagues[Q1] (Table 33-3). In two subsequent series reported by Ootaki and colleagues[O1] and Attenhofer Jost and colleagues,[A2] early mortality was 0% (0 of 11 patients; CL 0%-16%) and 4.3% (1 of 23 patients; CL 0.7%-14%), respectively.

When the syndrome is part of a complex anomaly associated with atrial isomerism, risk has been much higher. Three of six patients (50%; CL 24%-76%) reported by Quaegebeur and colleagues died[Q1] (see Table 33-3). A similar experience was reported by Cherian and Rao.[C2] Better understanding of morphology and improved operative methods, including avoidance of intracardiac repair, should result in improved outcomes (for further details, see Chapter 58).

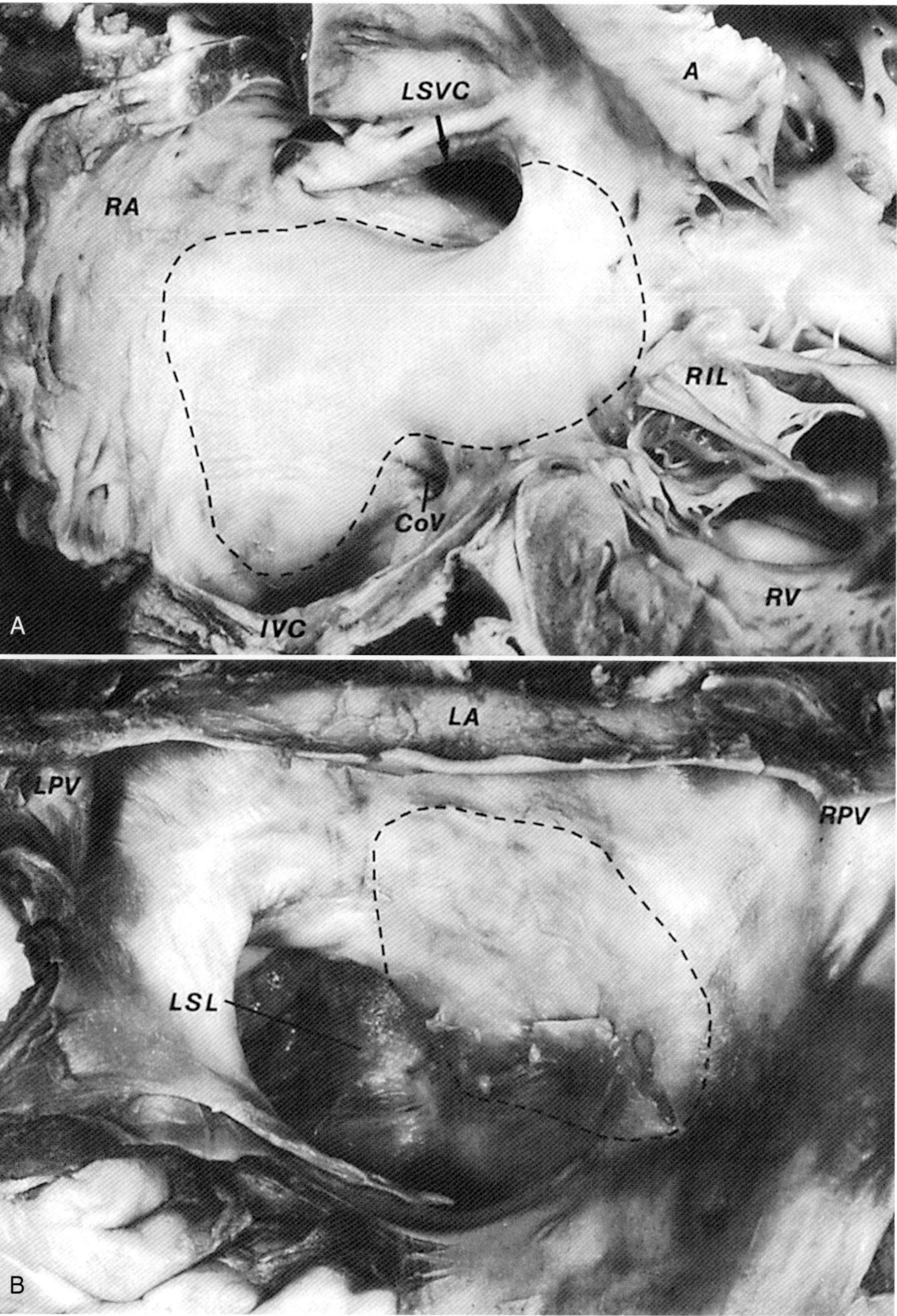

Figure 33-4 Autopsy specimen showing a pericardial baffle that corrects an unroofed coronary sinus syndrome (left superior vena cava [LSVC] to left atrium) in association with a common atrium and partial atrioventricular septal defect. Operation was performed on a patient 20 months of age; the child died at 13 years of age, probably from arrhythmia. In both views, the pericardial baffle suture line is identified by a dashed line. **A,** Exposure from opened right atrium and right ventricle. Baffle suture line passes behind the LSVC ostium to reach the ventricular septal crest between right and left atrioventricular valves and then behind inferior vena caval ostium. There is no right superior vena cava in this heart. **B,** Viewed from opened left atrium. Key: *A,* Anterior leaflet of right atrioventricular valve; *CoV,* opening of large coronary vein into atrium; *IVC,* inferior vena cava; *LA,* left atrium; *LPV,* left pulmonary veins; *LSL,* left superior atrioventricular valve leaflet; *RA,* right atrium; *RIL,* right inferior atrioventricular valve leaflet; *RPV,* right pulmonary veins; *RV,* right ventricle.

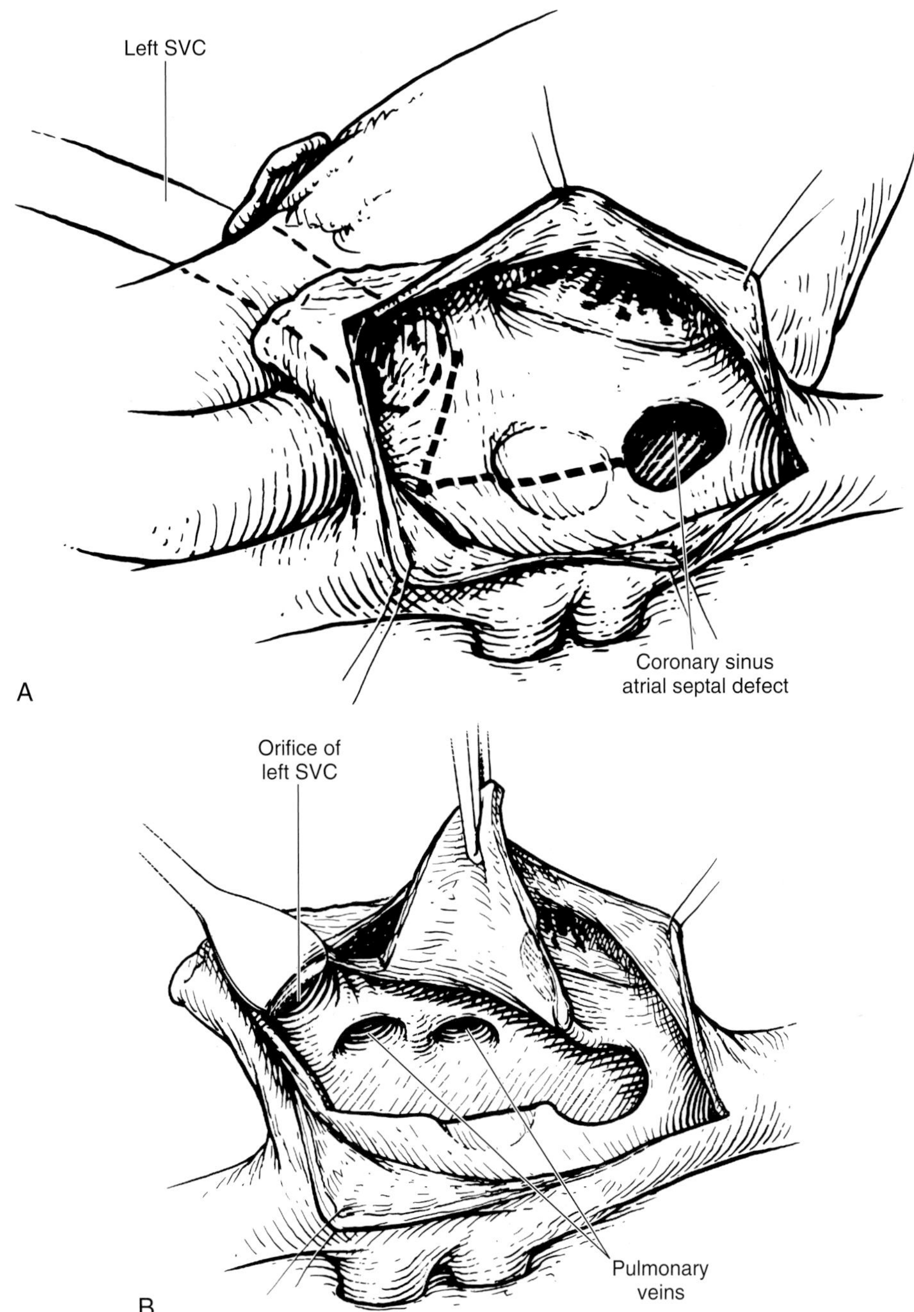

Figure 33-5 Another technique for repair of left superior vena cava (LSVC) entering left atrium. **A,** In a patient with only a small coronary sinus atrial septal defect (completely unroofed coronary sinus), an incision is made in the atrial septum as shown by angled dashed lines. **B,** Atrial septal incision has been made and the flap retracted. Orifice of entrance of LSVC into left atrium is shown in its usual position just anterior and superior to the orifices of the pulmonary veins.

Continued

Time-Related Survival and Functional Status

No late deaths occurred after repair of simple unroofed coronary sinus syndrome in the series of Quaegebeur and colleagues, but one patient required reoperation after 8 years because of tunnel obstruction.[Q1] No late deaths occurred among the patients reported by Ootaki and colleagues[O1] (mean duration of follow-up, 85.5 months), and one late death occurred among 22 hospital survivors (mean duration of follow-up, 85 months) in the series of Attenhofer Jost and colleagues.[A2] In the series of Cherian and Rao, one of eight hospital survivors required reoperation for closure of a coronary sinus ASD.[C2] At the time of the reports, surviving patients in all series were without symptoms, including the ones who required reoperation.

INDICATIONS FOR OPERATION

When diagnosis of isolated completely unroofed coronary sinus with persistent LSVC is made, operation is advisable because of arterial desaturation, risk of cerebral emboli, and satisfactory results of operation. Indications for repair of the rare isolated completely unroofed coronary sinus without persistent LSVC (coronary sinus ASD) are the same as for other

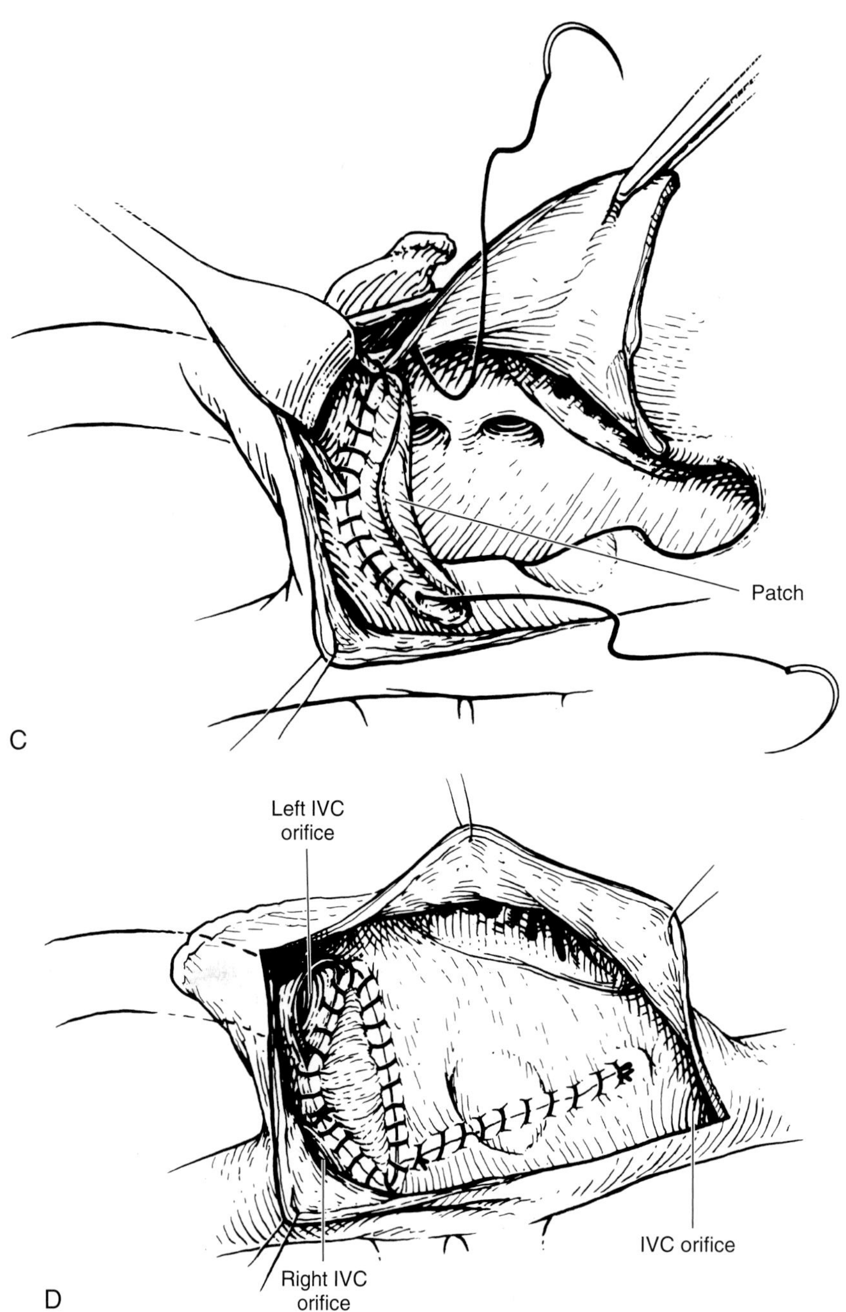

Figure 33-5, cont'd **C,** Elliptical contoured patch (of pericardium, polyester, or polytetrafluoroethylene) is sutured into place posteriorly to begin creating a pathway for diverting blood from LSVC to right atrium. Care is taken to avoid encroachment of suture line or patch on orifice of left superior pulmonary vein. **D,** Atrial flap has been laid back into position. Posteriorly and inferiorly, it is resutured to remnant of atrial septum to close the coronary sinus atrial septal defect. Superiorly, the flap is sewn to the other edge of contoured patch; before this, the patch is trimmed to be as narrow as possible to avoid any encroachment on pulmonary veins. Note free access of all three caval orifices to the right atrium. Key: *IVC,* Inferior vena cava; *SVC,* superior vena cava.

types of ASD[L1] (see Chapter 30). When unroofed coronary sinus is associated with complex cardiac anomalies, the associated anomaly usually presents a clear indication for operation.

SPECIAL SITUATIONS AND CONTROVERSIES

Ligation of Left Superior Vena Cava

When the brachiocephalic vein is absent or restrictive, some surgeons ligate the LSVC in this and other conditions even when the jugular venous pressure goes as high as 30 mmHg after temporary occlusion of the LSVC. No ill effects have been reported late postoperatively, although venous engorgement, facial edema, and chylothorax may be early complications.[D2]

We do not recommend ligation in this circumstance, because the other methods described are safe and widely applicable. An alternative practice, when correction of unroofed coronary sinus may complicate intracardiac repair of a coexisting condition and extracardiac repair is not possible, involves temporarily occluding the LSVC and ligating it if the increase in left jugular venous pressure does not

Table 33-1 Some Details of Eight Patients with Isolated Completely Unroofed Coronary Sinus with Left Superior Vena Cava

Data	No. of Patients[a]
Age	
1-11 years	8
History	
Brain abscess or TIA	2
Mild arterial desaturation	8
Anatomy	
LSVC to upper corner of left atrium	8
LSVC to brachiocephalic vein	1
Coronary sinus–type ASD:	4
Isolated	2
With foramen ovale	2
Confluent ASD (coronary sinus plus fossa ovalis type)	4
Management	
Ligation of LSVC and closure of ASD	1
Roofing of coronary sinus:	
With posterior wall of left atrium	4
With pericardium	2
With opened polyester tube	1

Data from Quaegebeur and colleagues.[Q1]
[a]Numbers are not cumulative.
Key: *ASD,* Atrial septal defect; *LSVC,* left superior vena cava; *TIA,* transient ischemic attack.

Table 33-2 Methods of Repair for Partially Unroofed Coronary Sinus and Persistent Superior Caval Vein in 23 Patients

Type of Procedure[a]	No. of Patients
Intraatrial Baffle (n = 7)	
CS drainage:	
To left atrium	6
To right atrium	1
Repair of CS Fenestration (n = 6)	
Suture closure	5
Patch closure	1
CS Ostium Closure (n = 10)	
Suture closure	6
Patch closure	4
TOTAL	**23**

Modified from Attenhofer Jost and colleagues.[A2]
[a]PSVC ligated in 5 patients (4 left, 1 right) and anastomosed to LPA in 1 patient.
Key: *CS,* Coronary sinus; *LPA,* left pulmonary artery; *PSCV,* persistent superior caval vein.

exceed 15 to 20 mmHg. Even in this setting, however, creating an LSVC–to–left pulmonary artery anastomosis (bidirectional Glenn) would seem preferable to ligating the LSVC. This procedure is technically simple and is feasible in essentially all circumstances except in the presence of pulmonary hypertension. Increasing experience with the bidirectional pulmonary shunt as part of a two-ventricle repair (the

Table 33-3 Repair of Unroofed Coronary Sinus Syndrome

Category	*n*	No. of Hospital Deaths
Pure, with LSVC	**8**	0
With Simple Cardiac Malformations	**10**	0
With LSVC	5	
Common atrium with partial AVSD	4	
Tetralogy of Fallot	1	
Without LSVC	5	
Partial AVSD (partially unroofed)	3	
Complete AVSD (partially unroofed)	1	
Tetralogy of Fallot	1	
With Complex Cardiac Malformations[a]	**6**	3
Common atrium, complete AVSD, DORV, polysplenia	2	
Common atrium, complete AVSD, DORV, PS, TASVC, hypoplastic LV, asplenia	1[b]	
TAPVC, polysplenia	1[b]	
Dextroversion, isolated ventricular inversion, polysplenia	1[b]	
Situs inversus totalis, complete AVSD, DORV, PS	1[b]	
TOTAL	**24**	3

Data from Quaegebeur and colleagues.[Q1]
[a]Atrial situs ambiguous or inversus.
[b]Patient died.
Key: *AVSD,* Atrioventricular septal defect; *DORV,* double outlet right ventricle; *LSVC,* left superior vena cava; *LV,* left ventricle; *PS,* pulmonary stenosis; *TAPVC,* total anomalous pulmonary venous connection; *TASVC,* total anomalous systemic venous connection.

"one-and-a-half ventricle repair") has shown that this physiologic arrangement is well tolerated when applied to a variety of morphologic conditions (see Chapters 34, 40, 41, and 55).[H1,R4,V1]

REFERENCES

A

1. Allmendinger P, Dear WE, Cooley DA. Atrial septal defect with communication through the coronary sinus. Ann Thorac Surg 1974;17:193.
2. Attenhofer Jost CH, Connolly HM, Danielson GK, Dearani JA, Warnes CA, Jamil Tajik A. Clinical features and surgical outcome in 25 patients with fenestrations of the coronary sinus. Cardiol Young 2007;17:592-600.

C

1. Campbell M, Deuchar DC. The left-sided superior vena cava. Br Heart J 1954;16:423.
2. Cherian KM, Rao SG. Surgical correction of the unroofed coronary sinus syndrome. Indian Heart J 1994;46:91.
3. Chiu IS, Hegerty A, Anderson RH, de Leval M. The landmarks to the atrioventricular conduction system in hearts with absence or unroofing of the coronary sinus. J Thorac Cardiovasc Surg 1985;90:297.

D

1. Davis WH, Jordaan FR, Snyman HW. Persistent left superior vena cava draining into the left atrium, as an isolated anomaly. Am Heart J 1959;57:616.

2. de Leval MR, Ritter DG, McGoon DC, Danielson GK. Anomalous systemic venous connection. Surgical considerations. Mayo Clin Proc 1975;50:599.

F

1. Foster ED, Baeza OR, Farina MF, Shafer RM. Atrial septal defect associated with drainage of the left superior vena cava to left atrium and absence of the coronary sinus. J Thorac Cardiovasc Surg 1978;76:718.
2. Freedom RM, Culham JA, Rowe RD. Left atrial to coronary sinus fenestration (partially unroofed coronary sinus). Morphological and angiocardiographic observations. Br Heart J 1981;46:63.
3. Friedlich A, Bing RJ, Blount SG Jr. Circulatory dynamics in the anomalies of venous return to the heart including pulmonary arteriovenous fistula. Bull Johns Hopkins Hosp 1956;86:20.

H

1. Hanley FL. The one and a half ventricular repair—we can do it, but should we do it? J Thorac Cardiovasc Surg 1999;117:659.
2. Helseth HK, Peterson CR. Atrial septal defect with termination of left superior vena cava in the left atrium and absence of the coronary sinus. Recognition and correction. Ann Thorac Surg 1974;17:186.
3. Hurwitt ES, Escher DJ, Citrin LI. Surgical correction of cyanosis due to entrance of left superior vena cava into left auricle. Surgery 1955;38:903.

K

1. Konstam MA, Levine BW, Strauss HW, McKusick KA. Left superior vena cava to left atrial communication diagnosed with radionuclide angiocardiography and with differential right to left shunting. Am J Cardiol 1979;43:149.
2. Kuhn A, Hauser M, Eicken A, Vogt M. Right heart failure due to an unroofed coronary sinus in an adult. Int J Cardiol 2006; 113:248-9.

L

1. Lee ME, Sade RM. Coronary sinus septal defect. Surgical considerations. J Thorac Cardiovasc Surg 1979;78:563.

M

1. Mantini E, Grondin CM, Lillehei CW, Edwards JE. Congenital anomalies involving the coronary sinus. Circulation 1966;33:317.
2. Miller GA, Ongley P, Rastelli GC, Kirklin JW. Surgical correction of total anomalous systemic venous connection: report of a case. Mayo Clin Proc 1965;40:532.

O

1. Ootaki Y, Yamaguchi M, Yoshimura N, Oka S, Yoshida M, Hasegawa T. Unroofed coronary sinus syndrome: diagnosis, classification, and surgical treatment. J Thorac Cardiovasc Surg 2003;126:1655-6.

Q

1. Quaegebeur J, Kirklin JW, Pacifico AD, Bargeron LM Jr. Surgical experience with unroofed coronary sinus. Ann Thorac Surg 1979; 27:418.

R

1. Raghib G, Ruttenberg HD, Anderson RC, Amplatz K, Adams P Jr, Edwards JE. Termination of left superior vena cava in left atrium, atrial septal defect, and absence of coronary sinus. Circulation 1965;31:906.
2. Rastelli GC, Ongley PA, Kirklin JW. Surgical correction of common atrium with anomalously connected persistent left superior vena cava: report of a case. Mayo Clin Proc 1965;40:528.
3. Reddy VM, McElhinney DB, Hanley FL. Correction of left superior vena cava draining to the left atrium using extracardiac techniques. Ann Thorac Surg 1997;63:1800.
4. Reddy VM, McElhinney DB, Silverman NH, Marianeschi SM, Hanley FL. Partial biventricular repair for complex congenital heart defects: an intermediate option for complicated anatomy or functionally borderline right complex heart. J Thorac Cardiovasc Surg 1998;116:21.
5. Rose AG, Beckman CB, Edwards JE. Communication between coronary sinus and left atrium. Br Heart J 1974;36:182.
6. Rumisek JD, Pigott JD, Weinberg PM, Norwood WI. Coronary sinus septal defect associated with tricuspid atresia. J Thorac Cardiovasc Surg 1986;92:142.

S

1. Sand ME, McGrath LB, Pacifico AD, Mandke NV. Repair of left superior vena cava entering the left atrium. Ann Thorac Surg 1986;42:560.
2. Schmidt KG, Silverman NH. Cross-sectional and contrast echocardiography in the diagnosis of interatrial communications through the coronary sinus. Int J Cardiol 1987;16:193.
3. Sherafat M, Friedman S, Waldhausen JA. Persistent left superior vena cava draining into the left atrium with absent right superior vena cava. Ann Thorac Surg 1971;11:160.
4. Shumacker HB Jr, King H, Waldhausen JA. The persistent left superior vena cava. Surgical implications, with special reference to caval drainage into the left atrium. Ann Surg 1967;165:797.

T

1. Taybi H, Kurlander GJ, Lurie PR, Campbell JA. Anomalous systemic venous connection to the left atrium or to a pulmonary vein. Am J Roentgenol Radium Ther Nucl Med 1965;94:62.
2. Thangaroopan M, Truong QA, Kalra MK, Yared K, Abbara S. Images in cardiovascular medicine. Rare case of an unroofed coronary sinus: diagnosis by multidetector computed tomography. Circulation 2009;119:e518-20.
3. Tuchman H, Brown JF, Huston JH, Weinstein AB, Rowe GC, Crumpton CW. Superior vena cava draining into left atrium. Am J Med 1956;21:481.

V

1. Van Arsdell GS, Williams WG, Maser CM, Streitenberger KS, Rebeyka IM, Coles JG, et al. Superior vena cava to pulmonary artery anastomosis: an adjunct to biventricular repair. J Thorac Cardiovasc Surg 1996;112:1143.
2. van Son JA, Falk V, Mohr FW. Pericardial patch augmentation of restrictive innominate vein and division of left superior vena cava in unroofed coronary sinus syndrome. J Thorac Cardiovasc Surg 1997;114:132.
3. van Son JA, Hambsch J, Mohr FW. Repair of complex unroofed coronary sinus by anastomosis of left to right superior vena cava. Ann Thorac Surg 1998;65:280.
4. Vargas FJ, Rozenbaum J, Lopez R, Granja M, De Dios A, Zarlenga B, et al. Surgical approach to left ventricular inflow obstruction due to dilated coronary sinus. Ann Thorac Surg 2006;82:191-6.

W

1. Winter FS. Persistent left superior vena cava. Angiology 1954;5:90.

34 Atrioventricular Septal Defect

DEFINITION

Atrioventricular (AV) septal defects are characterized by a deficiency or absence of septal tissue immediately above and below the normal level of the AV valves, including the region normally occupied by the AV septum, in hearts with two ventricles. The AV valves are abnormal to a varying degree.

These defects have also been called *AV canal defects, AV defects, endocardial cushion defects, ostium primum atrial septal defects* (when there is no interventricular communication), and *common AV orifice* (when there is only a single AV valve orifice).[B8]

HISTORICAL NOTE

Morphology

Abbott apparently recognized ostium primum atrial septal defect (ASD) and common AV canal defect, but it was Rogers and Edwards who in 1948 recognized their morphologic similarity.[A1,R10] This concept was further elaborated by Wakai and Edwards in 1956 and 1958.[W1,W2] The terms *partial* and *complete atrioventricular canal defects* were introduced by these investigators, who realized nonetheless that not all cases fit their definitions. During this period, Lev was formulating his concepts of ostium primum ASD (or partial AV canal) and common AV orifice (or complete AV canal), and he described the position of the AV node and bundle of His in these malformations.[L5] Wakai and Edwards and later Bharati and Lev became dissatisfied with trying to compress all cases into two categories and added the terms *intermediate* and *transitional*.[B14,W1,W2] During this period, Van Mierop's scholarly studies added a great deal of knowledge about the overall anatomic features of AV septal defects.[V4]

By the early 1960s, surgical treatment of these defects provided a stimulus to further morphologic studies. In 1966, Rastelli and colleagues at the Mayo Clinic described in more detail the morphology of AV valve leaflets in cases with common AV orifice.[R1] The error made in this study was to compress into the designation *common anterior leaflet* a leaflet that was in fact divided in two by a commissure (i.e., the divided common anterior leaflet of type A). The description of AV valve leaflets by Rastelli and colleagues was accepted for some years, but in 1976 a publication by Ugarte and colleagues emphasized the idea of leaflets *bridging* the ventricular septum, a concept also held by Lev.[U1] Meanwhile, based on anatomic and cineangiographic studies and in accordance with the description of Baron and colleagues and Van Mierop and colleagues, it was recognized in the late 1960s that the basic defect in these malformations was *absence of the AV septum*.[B4,B20,V4] This concept is particularly important because the AV septum can be imaged by echocardiography and in the left ventriculogram in the right anterior oblique projection. These concepts were further expanded by Piccoli and colleagues under the direction of Anderson, who further emphasized that all the variations of the defect were part of a spectrum[P6,P8] (Fig. 34-1).

Surgical Treatment

In 1952 at the University of Minnesota Hospital in Minneapolis, after a long period of laboratory investigation, Dennis and Varco attempted for the first time a cardiac operation in a human using a pump-oxygenator. The preoperative diagnosis was ASD, and at operation the defect was thought to be closed. The patient died, and autopsy showed the true diagnosis to be partial AV septal defect (Edwards JE: personal communication, 1980). The first successful repair of a complete AV septal defect was performed by Lillehei and colleagues in 1954, using cross-circulation and direct suture of the atrial rim of the septal defect to the crest of the ventricular septum.[L10] In 1954, Kirklin and colleagues successfully repaired a partial AV septal defect through the atrial well of Watkins and Gross, and in 1955 began repairing AV septal defects by open cardiotomy and use of the pump-oxygenator.[K12,K13,R6,W3]

Early experiences with complete AV septal defects were all associated with a high hospital mortality, often related to complete heart block, postrepair left AV valve regurgitation, or creation of subaortic stenosis.[C12,E7,L7,S3] Interestingly, in many of these early operations, a two-patch technique was used (see "Two-Patch Technique" under Technique of Operation later in this chapter). In 1958, Lev's description of the location of the bundle of His provided the basis for repair techniques that avoid heart block.[L5] In 1959, Dubost and Blondeau reported their early experience and emphasized that the "cleft" in the "mitral leaflet" need not be sutured in repairing partial AV septal defects, a concept currently challenged.[D8] In 1962, Maloney and colleagues described two cases in which a single patch was used to close both

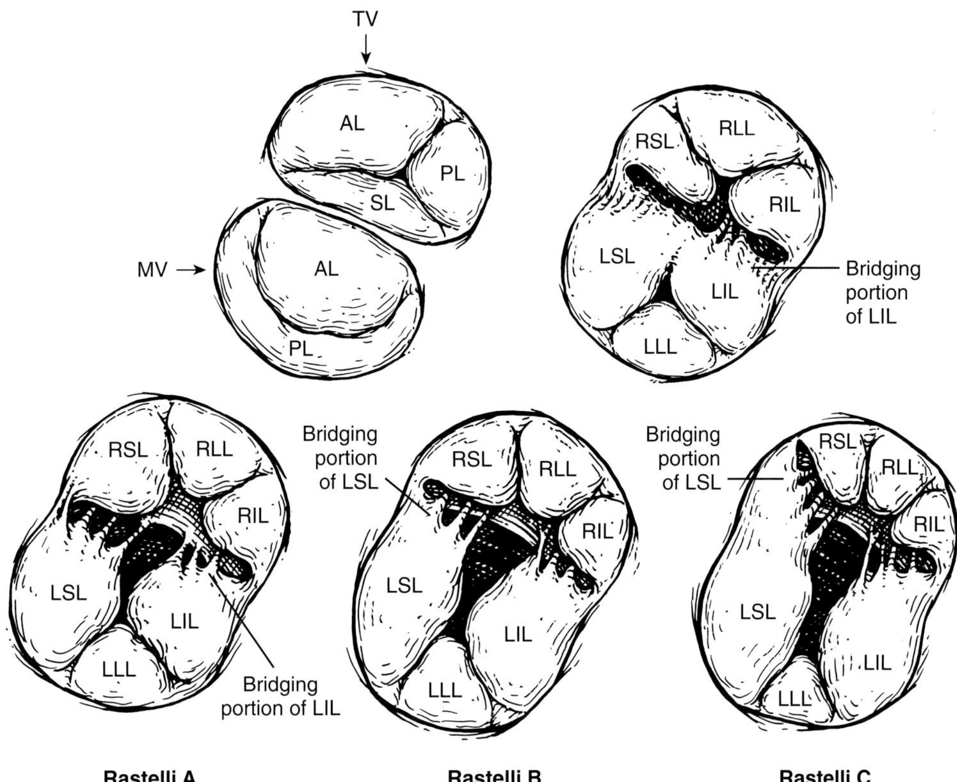

Figure 34-1 Diagrammatic representation of atrioventricular (AV) valves viewed from atrial side (surgical orientation). **A,** Normal, with anterior and posterior mitral valve *(MV)* leaflets and septal, anterior, and posterior tricuspid valve *(TV)* leaflets. **B,** Leaflets in partial AV septal defects. Left superior *(LSL)*, left inferior *(LIL)*, and left lateral *(LLL)* leaflets form left AV valve; right superior *(RSL)*, right inferior *(RIL)*, and right lateral *(RLL)* leaflets form right AV valve. **C,** Leaflets in complete AV septal defects, or common AV orifice, are similar to those in **B**. However, LSL and LIL are not connected. LIL usually bridges a little (grade 1 or 2, based on 1 to 5) across crest of ventricular septum. LSL may bridge slightly or not at all (grade 0 or 1, Rastelli type A), moderately (grade 2 or 3, Rastelli type B), or markedly (grade 4 or 5, Rastelli type C). Key: *AL,* Anterior leaflet; *PL,* posterior leaflet; *SL,* septal leaflet.

defects and with the valve tissue suspended from the patch.[M5] This technique was again described by Gerbode in 1962 and was associated with decreased in-hospital mortality.[R3] McGoon recognized the importance of "taking from the tricuspid valve" to leave sufficient tissue from which to create an adequate left AV valve. These technical advances allowed repair of even the more complex variants of the defect.[P1,R4] Subsequently, good results were obtained in patients older than about 2 years of age, but results in infants remained relatively poor.[B1,B9,G1,H2,K3,M9,M12,R3,V2] Between 1968 and 1971, Barratt-Boyes successfully repaired this anomaly in four severely ill infants[B5]; subsequently, improved results in infants were reported by many others.[A5,B1,B12,C13,C17,M3,M11,N1]

In 1978, Carpentier again emphasized (as did Dubost and Blondeau[D8]) that generally, the left AV valve functions best when repaired as a three-leaflet valve.[C2] As a result of these advances, risks of operation for nearly all types of AV septal defect are now low.[C6,S15]

MORPHOLOGY

General Morphologic Characteristics

AV septal defects have as defining characteristics a deficiency or absence of the AV septum, resulting in an ostium primum defect immediately above the AV valves and a deficiency (or scooped-out area) in the inlet (basal) portion of the ventricular septum immediately below the AV valves.

Patients with partial AV septal defects have a normal length of atrial septum, and the ostium primum ASD is the result of absence of the relatively small AV septum plus some deficiency in the inlet portion of the ventricular septum.[G5] The deficiency in the inlet portion of the ventricular septum is variable, but on average is greater in patients with complete AV septal defects than in those with partial defects.[G5,P5]

These septal deficiencies may or may not result in interatrial or interventricular communications, depending on configuration and attachments of the AV valves (Tables 34-1 and 34-2). Whereas the basic defect in these malformations is absence of the AV septum, whether the ventricular septal or atrial septal deficiency or the AV valve abnormality is the result only of AV septal absence is still debated.[B4,B20,V4]

Five or more AV valve leaflets of variable size are usually present (see Fig. 34-1), but there is often variability in completeness of commissures and prominent crenations in the leaflets (Fig. 34-2). For example, among the 43 hearts with all types of AV septal defects and 2 ventricles in the GLH autopsy series in which the number of leaflets could be accurately assessed, 10 (23%) had 4 leaflets, 18 (42%) had 5 leaflets, 14 (33%) had 6 leaflets, and 1 (2%) had 7 leaflets. When a large interventricular communication was present (complete AV septal defect), the most common number of leaflets was 5 (16 of 28, or 57%).

Table 34-1 Size of Interatrial Communication in Atrioventricular Septal Defects[a]

Size	Prevalence No.	Prevalence % of 310
0[b]	2	0.6
1	2	0.6
2	27	8.7
3	35	11.3
4	223	71.9
5[c]	21	6.8

Data from Studer and colleagues.[S15]
[a]Study is based on data from 310 surgical patients.
[b]Condition in which the characteristic atrioventricular (AV) septal deficiency is present, but the AV valves are adherent on their atrial side to the edge of the defect, resulting in no interatrial communication.
[c]Common atrium.

Table 34-2 Size of Interventricular Communication in Atrioventricular Septal Defects

	Beneath Left Superior Leaflet		Beneath Left Inferior Leaflet	
Size	No.	% of 310	No.	% of 309[a]
0[b]	158	51	176	57
1	3	1.0	3	1.0
2	9	2.9	9	2.9
3	4	1.3	16	5.2
4	9	2.9	22	7.1
5[c]	127	41	82	27

Data from Studer and colleagues.[S15]
[a]Data not available for one patient.
[b]Condition in which the characteristic atrioventricular (AV) septal deficiency is present, but the AV valves are adherent on their ventricular side to the crest of the ventricular septum, resulting in no interventricular communication (if this occurs under both left AV valve leaflets, it is commonly called *partial AV septal defect*. If size greater than 1 occurs under both AV valve leaflets, the condition is commonly called *complete AV septal defect*).
[c]Very large communication but not common ventricle.

The left superior leaflet (LSL) and left inferior leaflet (LIL) are particularly variable in size, connections one to another (Table 34-3), and degree of bridging across the crest of the ventricular septum (Table 34-4; see Figs. 34-1 and 34-2). There may be one or two AV valve orifices (Table 34-5).

Hearts with AV septal defects are also characterized by absence of the usual wedged position of the aortic valve above the AV valves. Instead, it is elevated and deviated anteriorly.[P6,V3,V4] Details of the aortic-mitral fibrous continuity often differ from those in the normal heart. Thus, continuity was abnormal in more than half of 21 specimens with normally related great arteries in the GLH autopsy series; continuity was to the base of the noncoronary cusp in only 5 (24%) and to both the noncoronary and right coronary cusps in 7 (33%). In addition, the left ventricular (LV) inflow tract is shortened in relationship to length of the outflow portion, and there is a related reduction in length of the diaphragmatic wall of the LV.[G3,P6,V3,V4] The LV outflow tract is also narrowed, although rarely is the narrowing sufficient to be of hemodynamic importance in the unrepaired heart.[P7]

AV septal defects include a spectrum of malformations. At one end is the simplest type, in which there is an interatrial communication but no interventricular communication and a connection of variable width between the LSL and LIL; this is called a *partial AV septal defect* or *ostium primum defect*. At the other end of the spectrum is the most extreme form, with large deficiencies in atrial and ventricular septa, a common AV valve orifice, and large interatrial and interventricular communications; this is called a *complete AV septal defect*. Because a continuous spectrum of gradations lies between these extremes, some anomalies have been grouped

Table 34-3 Left Superior and Left Inferior Leaflet Connections in Atrioventricular Septal Defects

Degree of LSL-LIL Connection[a]	No Interventricular Communication (*n* = 154) No.	No Interventricular Communication (*n* = 154) % of 154	Interventricular Communication (*n* = 156) No.	Interventricular Communication (*n* = 156) % of 156
0	2	1.3	139	89
1	55	36	11[b]	7
2	82	53	5[b]	3
3	9	6	0	—
4	5	3	0	—
5	1	0.6	0	—
Connected, unknown degree	0	0	1[b]	0.6

Data from Studer and colleagues.[S15]
[a]0, Separate LSL and LIL, such as in common AV orifice; 1 and 2, narrow connections (deep cleft in "anterior mitral leaflet"); 3 and 4, broad connection (shallow cleft or notch); 5, no cleft, anterior mitral leaflet.
[b]Among these 17, in four the LSL and LIL were connected but free-floating, with large interventricular communications beneath them and their connections (Bharati type C[B16]). In 11, very small interventricular communications were present beneath the LSL and/or LIL. In two, no interatrial communication was present.
Key: *LIL*, Left inferior leaflet; *LSL*, left superior leaflet.

Table 34-4 Left Superior Leaflet Bridging in Atrioventricular Septal Defects

Degree of LSL Bridging	Without Interventricular Communication (*n* = 154) No.	Without Interventricular Communication (*n* = 154) % of 153[a]	With Interventricular Communication (*n* = 156) No.	With Interventricular Communication (*n* = 156) % of 154[b]	
0	150	98	65	42	Rastelli type A
1	3	2.0	23	15	
2			5	3.2	Rastelli type B
3			10	6.5	
4			8	5.2	Rastelli type C
5			43	28	

Data from Studer and colleagues.[S15]
[a]Data not available for one patient.
[b]Data not available for two patients.
Key: *LSL*, Left superior leaflet.

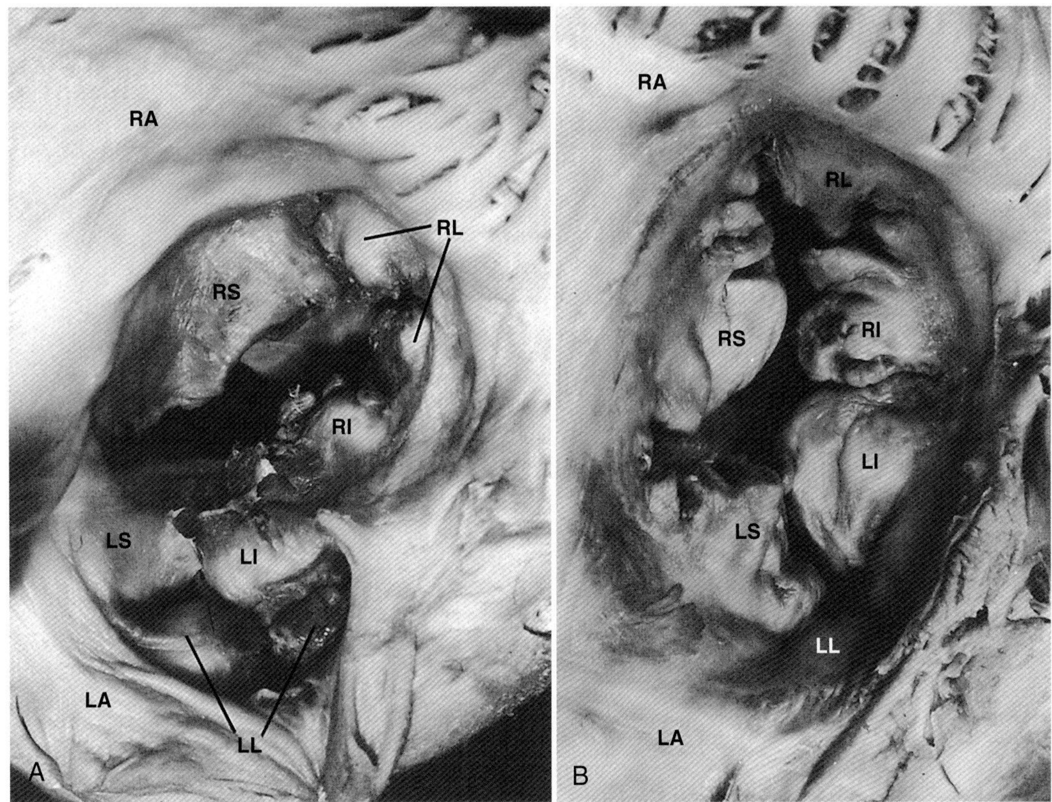

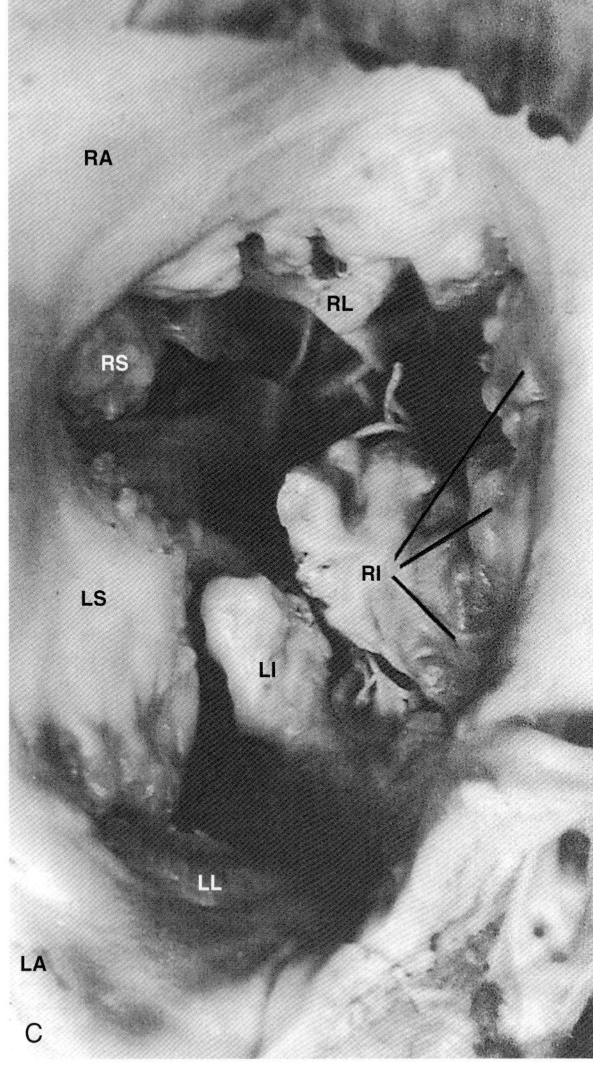

Figure 34-2 Atrioventricular (AV) valves in AV septal defects viewed from atrial aspect in a series of fixed specimens. **A,** Specimen with partial AV septal defect in which left superior *(LS)* and left inferior *(LI)* leaflets are adherent to crest of ventricular septum and there is no interventricular communication. Arrow marks line of closure between LS and LI leaflets, formerly called the "cleft in the anterior mitral leaflet." Note that as usual, LS leaflet does not bridge septum (there is no leaflet tissue in the position of the superior portion of the normal tricuspid septal leaflet). In this heart, as is not uncommon, there are two left lateral and two right lateral leaflets. **B,** Specimen with complete AV septal defect in which there are interventricular communications beneath LS and LI leaflets. LS leaflet does not bridge crest of septum. Right superior *(RS)* leaflet is characteristically large. LI leaflet is bridging (grade 2) and very distinct from right inferior *(RI)* leaflet. **C,** Specimen of a complete AV septal defect in which LS leaflet markedly bridges crest of septum. Correspondingly, RS leaflet is small. LS leaflet is characteristically larger than LI leaflet. Key: *LA,* Left atrium; *RA,* right atrium.

as *intermediate* or *transitional AV septal defects.* Definitions of these intermediate types have varied but usually include presence of two AV valve orifices and a restrictive inlet ventricular septal defect (VSD), with dense chordal attachments to the ventricular septum (see "Unusual Atrioventricular Combinations" under Morphology).[M13] Added complexity is provided by occurrence of a large variety of major and minor associated cardiac anomalies (Tables 34-6 and 34-7). In addition, Down syndrome is common, particularly in patients with an interventricular communication.

Because it is virtually impossible to subdivide the spectrum of AV septal defects into satisfactory noncontroversial subgroups, this chapter describes cases based on morphologic and functional variables rather than categorizing them into subgroups.[S15] The older imprecise terms continue to be useful as shorthand, and in this chapter, *partial AV septal defect* refers to a malformation with two AV valve orifices and no interventricular communication, whereas *complete AV septal defect* refers to a malformation with a common AV valve orifice and large (grade 2 or more) nonrestrictive interventricular communication.

Table 34-5 Type of Atrioventricular Valve Orifices in Atrioventricular Septal Defects[a]

Type	No.	% of 310
Two AV valves	171[b]	55
Common AV valve	139	45

Data from Studer and colleagues.[S15]
[a]Database is same as in Table 34-1.
[b]Includes the 154 patients without interventricular communications; 11 with small interventricular communications beneath the left superior (LSL) and/or inferior leaflets (LIL); four with connected but free-floating and connected LSL and LIL (see Table 34-3); and two with no interatrial communication but large interventricular communication (not inlet atrioventricular septal-type ventricular septal defects).
Key: *AV,* Atrioventricular.

Table 34-6 Major Associated Cardiac Anomalies in Atrioventricular Septal Defects

Anomaly	No.	% of 310
None	237	76
Patent ductus arteriosus	31	10.0
Tetralogy of Fallot	20	6.5
Completely unroofed coronary sinus with left SVC	9	2.9
Situs ambiguus	7	2.3
DORV without PS	6	1.9
Additional VSDs	5	1.6
DORV + PS	3	1.0
Situs inversus totalis	3	1.0
TAPVC	2	0.6
Left ventricular outflow obstruction	2	0.6
Transposition of the great arteries	1	0.3
PS, supravalvar mitral stenosis, Ebstein malformation, coarctation, isolated dextrocardia	1 each	0.3

Data from Studer and colleagues.[S15]
Key: *DORV,* Double outlet right ventricle; *PS,* pulmonary stenosis; *SVC,* superior vena cava; *TAPVC,* total anomalous pulmonary venous connection; *VSD,* ventricular septal defect.

Table 34-7 Minor Associated Cardiac Anomalies in Atrioventricular Septal Defects

	Without Interventricular Communication (*n* = 154)			With Interventricular Communication (*n* = 156)		
Anomaly	**No.**	**% of 154**	**CL (%)**	**No.**	**% of 156**	**CL (%)**
(Sizable) ASD[a]	17	11	8-14	32	21	17-24
Left SVC without unroofed coronary sinus	10	6	4-9	7	4	3-7
Partially unroofed coronary sinus	5	3	1-5	2	1	0.4-3
Azygos extension of IVC	4	3	1-5	3	1	0.6-3
IVC to lower left common atrium				1	1	0.1-2
Bilateral IVCs	1	1	0.1-2			
TASVC to common atrium				1	1	0.1-2
Right PVs to RA	1	1	0.1-2			
Anomalous origin LAD from RCA (TF)				1	1	0.1-2
Origin stenosis LPA (not TF)	1	1	0.1-2			
Wolff-Parkinson-White syndrome	1	1	0.1-2			
Spontaneous heart block	1	1	0.1-2			
Coronary artery disease requiring CABG	1	1	0.1-2			

Data from Studer and colleagues.[S15]
[a]Does not include patent foramen ovale.
Key: *ASD,* Atrial septal defect; *CABG,* coronary artery bypass grafting; *CL,* 70% confidence limits; *IVC,* inferior vena cava; *LAD,* left anterior descending coronary artery; *LPA,* left pulmonary artery; *PV,* pulmonary vein; *RA,* right atrium; *RCA,* right coronary artery; *SVC,* superior vena cava; *TASVC,* total anomalous systemic venous connection; *TF,* tetralogy of Fallot.

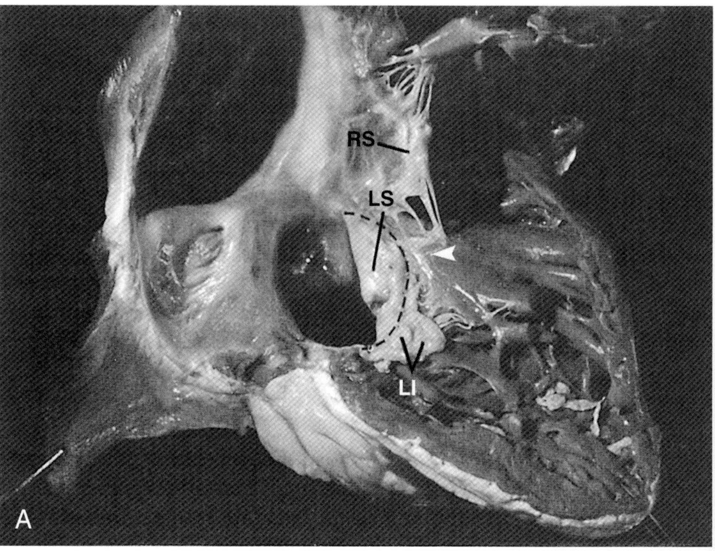

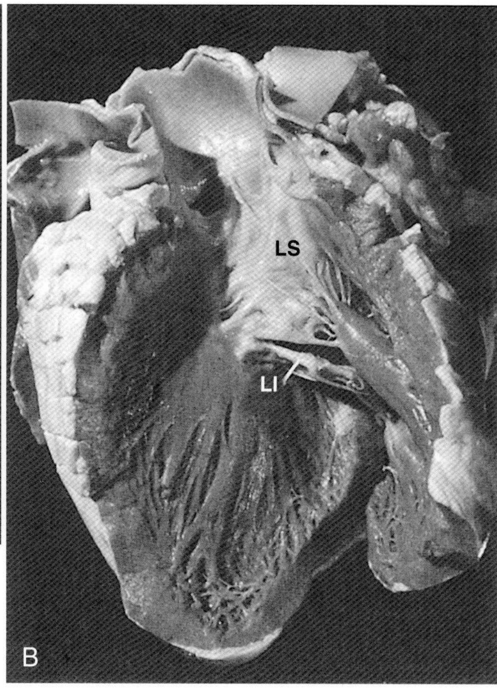

Figure 34-3 Partial atrioventricular (AV) septal defect. **A,** View from right atrium and right ventricle. Large ostium primum atrial septal defect is seen above AV valve leaflets. No interventricular communication is present beneath the leaflets. However, deficiency of basal (inlet) portion of ventricular septum is apparent. Left superior *(LS)* leaflet is attached firmly by fibrous tissue to crest of septum *(dashed line)* and does not bridge onto right ventricular side. There is thus a bare area on right side of superior aspect of ventricular septum *(arrow)*. Left inferior *(LI)* leaflet bridges on right ventricular side. Right superior *(RS)* leaflet is clearly visible, but right lateral and inferior leaflets are not in photograph. **B,** Left ventricular outflow view. LS and LI leaflets are firmly attached to crest of ventricular septum. Narrowing and elongation of left ventricular outflow tract are apparent. This figure makes clear why, in describing position of the two leaflets attached to the ventricular crest, the terms *superior* and *inferior* are preferable to *anterior* and *posterior,* terms that lead to confusion with normal mitral leaflets. (Courtesy Dr. Maurice Lev.)

Atrial Septal Deficiency and Interatrial Communications

Partial Atrioventricular Septal Defect

Usually there is an interatrial communication related to *deficiency of the AV septum,* the so-called *ostium primum ASD* (Fig. 34-3). The defect is bounded below by the inferiorly displaced AV valve leaflets and above by a crescentic ridge of atrial septum that fuses with the AV valve anulus only at its extremities.

Generally, there is little atrial septal tissue at the superior point of fusion of the atrial septum with the valve anulus adjacent to the aorta, but more tissue is usually present inferiorly adjacent to the coronary sinus (Fig. 34-4). The distance between the crescentic atrial margin of the defect and the AV valves (and thus the size of the interatrial communication) is variable. In most cases, the fossa ovalis is normally formed and there is a patent foramen ovale or an associated fossa ovalis ASD. Usually the interatrial communication through the ostium primum defect is moderate in size. When the interatrial communication is small, the atrial septal deficiency is restricted to the area normally occupied by the AV septum.[V12] The communication may be still smaller due to fusion of the base of the LSL or LIL to the edge of the adjacent portion of the atrial septum. Rarely, there may be an accessory "parachute" of fibrous tissue that narrows or obstructs the defect. Under such circumstances, a pressure difference exists between the two atria.

Common Atrium

Deficiencies in the anterior limbus or fossa ovalis may be associated with AV septal defects, resulting in a larger interatrial communication. Occasionally the entire limbus and fossa ovalis are absent, along with the AV septum. The condition is then termed *common atrium*[E6,G2,R2,R5] (see Table 34-1).

Absence of Interatrial Communication

Rarely, AV valve tissue is attached completely to the edge of the atrial septum, and no interatrial communication exists despite the deficiency in the septum[P6,S15] (see Table 34-1). In this unusual variant, the characteristic deficiency of the inlet (basal) portion of the ventricular septum is also present and associated with a large interventricular communication beneath the leaflets. The functionally left AV valve, consisting only of those portions of the LSL and LIL on the *left side* of their attachment to the atrial septum, tends to be competent. As seen from a right atrial approach, part of the right AV valve may have chordal attachments across the ventricular defect to the left side of the septum—that is, it is straddling. When viewed from the ventricular side, the appearance is typical of a complete AV septal defect. It is distinct from an inlet type of perimembranous VSD that is sometimes called *inlet septal, AV septal,* or *AV canal type of VSD,* which is unrelated to deficiency of the AV septum (see "Inlet Septal Ventricular Septal Defect" under Morphology in Chapter 35

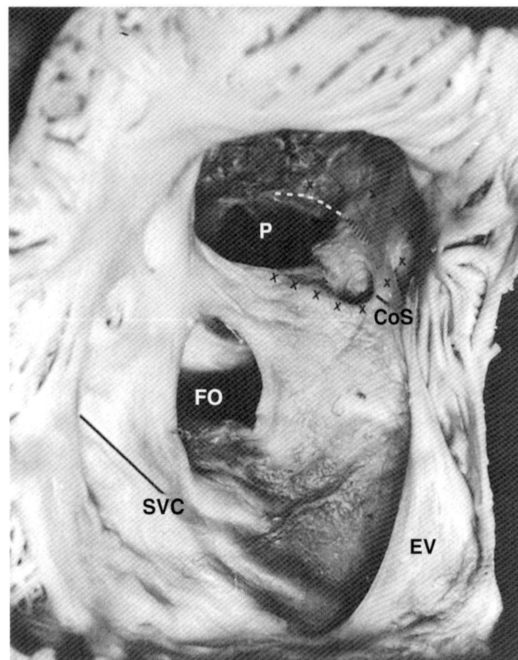

Figure 34-4 Right atrial view of a specimen of a partial atrioventricular (AV) septal defect. Coronary sinus ostium *(CoS)* is seen inferior and posterior to ostium primum *(P)* defect in atrial septum. Approximate position of AV node and bundle of His is shown as a dashed line. Placement of inferior part of patch suture line is shown by the line of x's. Key: *EV,* Eustachian valve of inferior vena cava; *FO,* fossa ovalis; *SVC,* superior vena cava.

and "Inlet Septal Type of Ventricular Septal Defect" in text that follows).

Ventricular Septal Deficiency and Interventricular Communications

Partial Atrioventricular Septal Defect

Some degree of deficiency of the inlet portion of the ventricular septum immediately beneath the AV valves is a constant finding. Thus, the inlet portion of the ventricular septum is shortened. There is usually no interventricular communication when the LSL and LIL are connected and attached to the downwardly displaced crest of the septum throughout its length (Fig. 34-5; see also Fig. 34-3), the situation described as a *partial AV septal defect.* Occasionally, one or several small interventricular communications are present beneath the attachment of the AV valve to the septum (Fig. 34-5, *B*).

Complete Atrioventricular Septal Defect

With ventricular septal deficiency generally greater than that in a partial AV septal defect, a moderate or large interventricular communication may be present, and usually the LSL and LIL are separate. This anomaly is described as a *complete AV septal defect* (Fig. 34-5, *C*). Deficiency of the inlet portion of the ventricular septum (the "scoop") is generally deeper in hearts with complete AV septal defects than in those with partial AV septal defects.[A10,E1,F2] Often the communication is particularly large beneath the LSL and smaller beneath the LIL (see Table 34-2), whereas in about 5% of cases there is a larger interventricular communication beneath the LSL and none beneath the LIL. Rarely, there is no VSD beneath the LSL and a large one beneath the LIL.

A remnant of the membranous ventricular septum may be present (see Fig. 34-5, *B*). This was the case in 8 of 27 (30%) GLH autopsy specimens of AV septal defect with normally related great arteries; in 19 specimens the membranous septum could not be identified.

Atrioventricular Valves

Attachments of the AV valves to the crest of the ventricular septum in partial AV septal defects, as well as their chordal attachments in complete AV septal defects, are displaced toward the apex of the heart because of deficiency of the inlet (basal) portion of the septum. This alters orientation of the AV orifices relative to the aortic orifice (i.e., the aortic valve is no longer wedged between the AV valves) and provides an important diagnostic imaging criterion of this malformation.[A9,B3,B20]

Two Atrioventricular Valve Orifices

Typically when two AV valve orifices are present, as in partial AV septal defects, the LSL and LIL are joined together to a variable extent anteriorly by leaflet tissue near the crest of the ventricular septum (see Figs. 34-1 and 34-3). Together they resemble an anterior (septal) mitral leaflet with a cleft, but in fact the left AV valve is tricuspid and oriented differently from the normal valve (see Figs. 34-1 and 34-2). The connection between the LSL and LIL may be only a thin strand of tissue (complete cleft), but more commonly it is 2 to 4 mm or more deep (see Table 34-3). This connection, too, is usually fused to the crest of the ventricular septum in partial AV septal defects. Occasionally, chordae pass from opposing edges of the LSL and LIL to the muscular ventricular septum beneath.[E5] Yilmaz and colleagues identify a difference in this area of separation and distinguish between a commissure supported by chordal apparatus on either side of the gap and a cleft that is relatively unsupported and bereft of chordae at its edges.[Y2] In addition, the chordae that originate from the central edges of the LSL and LIL attach to different papillary muscles, which can cause a distracting force on the leaflets during closure. This contrasts with the normal commissure in which the chordae from adjacent leaflet edges attach to a single papillary muscle, encouraging coaptation. Rarely, separation into LSL and LIL is represented only by a notch in the center of the free edge of a nearly normal "anterior mitral leaflet." The left lateral leaflet (LLL) is usually smaller than the other two leaflets and is triangular.

In aggregate, these left AV valve leaflet anomalies may make the valve regurgitant to a variable degree, sometimes severely (Table 34-8). When LSL and LIL are nearly completely separated (connection grades 1 and 2; see Table 34-3), an appreciable gap may occur during systole, producing regurgitation. When there is failure of valve coaptation at this site, leaflet tissue forming the margin usually becomes thickened and rolled. In other cases, regurgitation appears to be due to deficiency of leaflet tissue, particularly in the LIL.[B16,M10] The mechanism of severe left AV valve regurgitation is, however, not evident in some cases. The jet of regurgitation is usually directed into the right atrium. Rarely, the left AV valve is stenotic, but this usually is associated with hypoplasia of the LV.[B18]

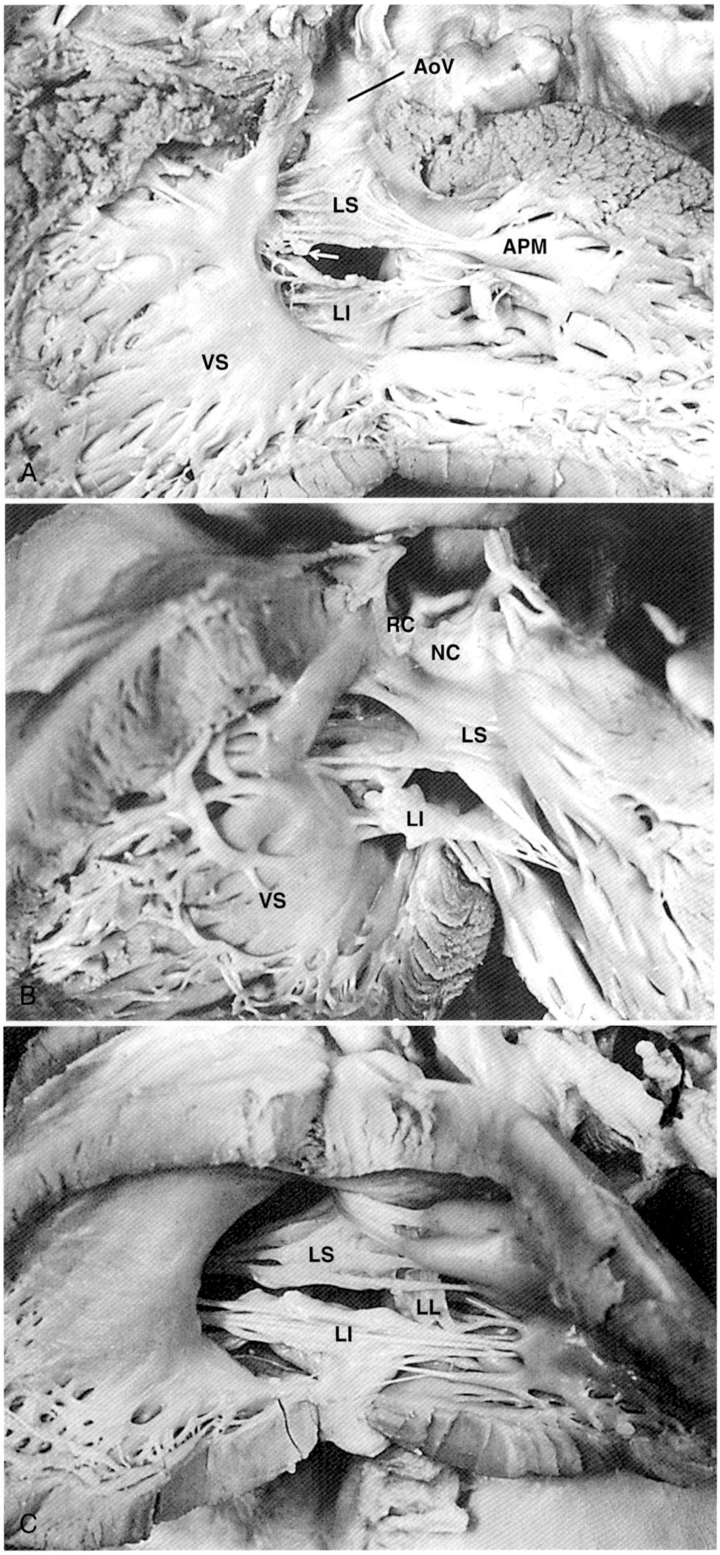

Figure 34-5 Left ventricular aspect of atrioventricular (AV) septal defects. **A,** Partial AV septal defect viewed from opened left ventricle. Left superior *(LS)* and left inferior *(LI)* leaflets are completely attached to crest of a deficient ventricular septum *(VS)*. Area of contact or closure between left superior and left inferior leaflets is indicated by arrow. In this specimen, only the anterior papillary muscle *(APM)* is present ("parachute" mitral valve). **B,** Intermediate type of AV septal defect from left ventricular view. Numerous small interventricular communications are present between thick, short chordae that tether both LS and LI leaflets to ventricular crest. Fibrous tissue extending from superior leaflet to below right coronary aortic cusp *(RC)* represents remnant of membranous septum. **C,** Complete AV septal defect viewed from left ventricular aspect. LS and LI bridging leaflets are free floating, and there is a large interventricular communication between them and the underlying crest of the ventricular septum. This specimen also has double outlet right ventricle. Key: *AoV,* Aortic valve; *LL,* left lateral leaflet; *NC,* noncoronary aortic cusp.

Table 34-8 Preoperative Atrioventricular Valve Regurgitation in Patients with Atrioventricular Septal Defect without Major Associated Cardiac Anomalies

Magnitude of AV Valve Regurgitation	Total		Without Interventricular Communication			With Interventricular Communication		
	No.	% of 305[a]	No.		% of 154	No.		% of 151[a]
0	29	10	15		10	14		9
1	39	13	26		17	13		9
2	85	28	48		31	37		25
3	98	32	41	65/154 (42%)[b]	27	57	87/151 (58%)[b]	38
4	43	14	16		10	27		18
5	11	4	8		5	3		2
TOTAL	305		154			151		

Data from Studer and colleagues.[S15]
[a]No information on five patients.
[b]$P(\chi^2)$ for difference = .007.

The right AV valve is also abnormal when there are two AV orifices, although less attention has been paid to it. It may consist of three leaflets—right superior leaflet (RSL), right lateral leaflet (RLL), and right inferior leaflet (RIL)—or of two or four leaflets (see Figs. 34-1 and 34-2). Leaflet tissue attached directly or by chordae to the crest or right side of the crest of the septum, and thus contributing to closure of the right AV valves, is considered to represent bridging of the LSL or LIL (see Fig. 34-1).

Usually in cases without an interventricular communication, the LSL does not bridge at all (previously, this finding was interpreted as absence or hypoplasia of the superior part of the tricuspid septal leaflet) and the LIL bridges moderately (see Fig. 34-2, *A*). Even with abnormalities of the right AV valve, regurgitation is rare (unless right heart failure develops).

Common Atrioventricular Orifice

When the AV valve orifice is a common one and the interventricular communication is large (complete AV septal defect), the LSL and LIL are separate, and a bare area is exposed on the crest of the ventricular septum (Fig. 34-6; see Figs. 34-1 and 34-5, *C*). The LSL may be entirely on the LV side of the septum or may, to a variable degree, bridge the septum and extend onto the right ventricular side (see Fig. 34-2, *B-C* and Table 34-4). This variability formed the basis for the classification by Rastelli and colleagues into types A, B, and C.[R1] Chordal attachments of the right ventricular extremity of the LSL vary according to degree of bridging[P8] (Fig. 34-7). When there is no bridging, chordal attachments are to the ventricular crest (Fig. 34-7, *A*). With mild bridging, they are to the medial papillary muscle in the right ventricle; with moderate bridging, to an accessory (often large) apical papillary muscle (Fig. 34-7, *B*); and with marked bridging, to the normally positioned (although often bifid) anterolateral papillary muscle of the right ventricle (Fig. 34-7, *C*). When the LSL bridges the septum moderately or markedly and extends into the right ventricle, it is usually unattached to the underlying ventricular crest (free-floating), but it may occasionally be attached by chordae (tethered). Length of the chordal or fibrous attachments to the right side or crest of the ventricular septum varies according to size of the interventricular communication or the position of the leaflet.

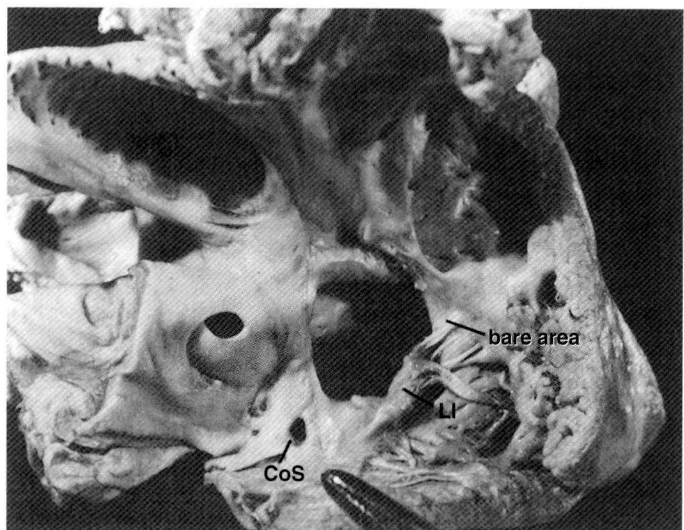

Figure 34-6 Complete atrioventricular septal defect viewed from right ventricular side in a specimen in which left inferior leaflet bridges over crest of septum onto right ventricular side. Left superior leaflet (poorly seen) does not bridge, resulting in a bare area of crest of ventricular septum on right ventricular side, where in a normal heart, superior aspect of septal leaflet touches septum. A small fossa ovalis atrial septal defect is also present. Key: *CoS,* Coronary sinus; *LI,* left inferior leaflet.

The LIL typically bridges moderately, but it too varies in this respect. It is not uncommon for a bridging LIL to be attached to the underlying ventricular crest either completely or by short, thick chordae with interchordal spaces.

Chordal attachments of the leftward components of the common AV valve in the LV are usually relatively normal, although the posterior papillary muscle is displaced more laterally than normal and a third papillary muscle may be present.[C2] There may be only one papillary muscle, producing a parachute-type valve that is difficult to repair.[C2] This was true in 7 of 53 (13%) cases in the GLH autopsy series, in 14% of the specimens described by David and colleagues, and in 4% of 155 surgical cases reported by Ilbawi and colleagues.[D2,I1]

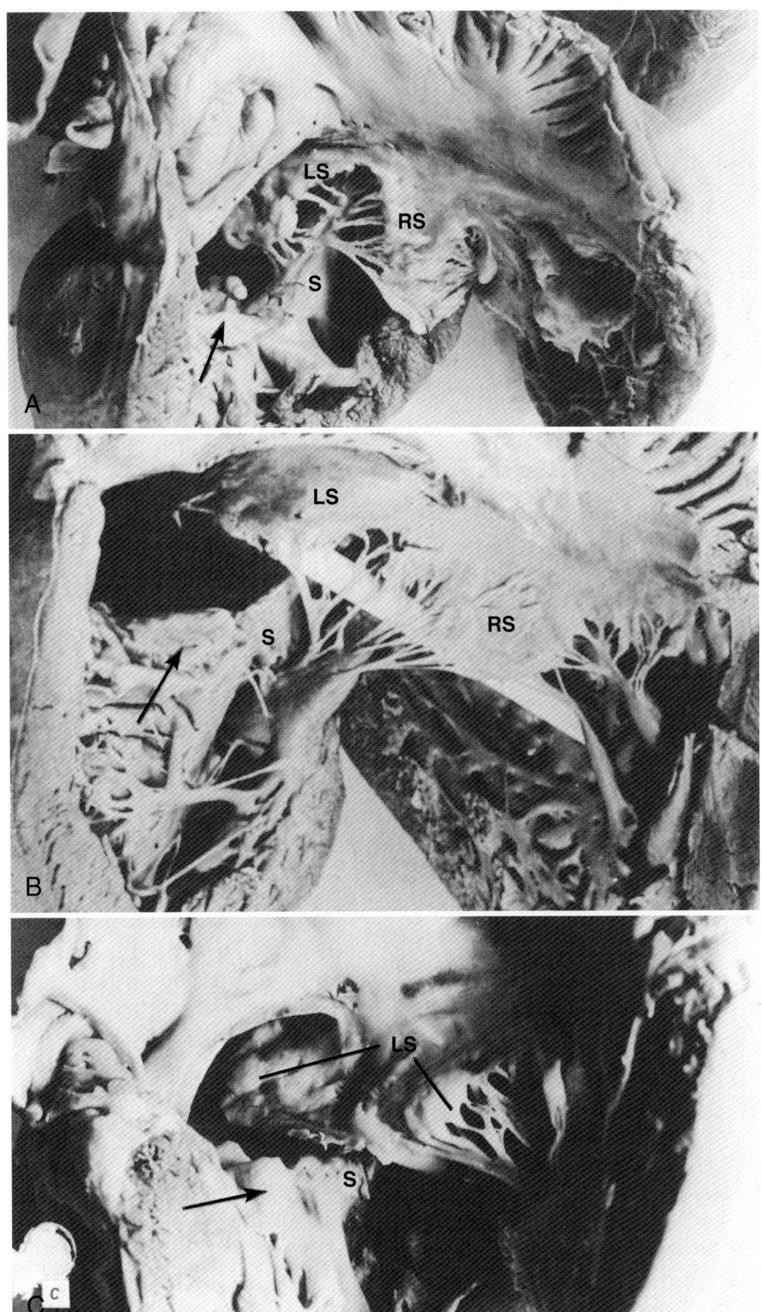

Figure 34-7 Complete atrioventricular septal defects with varying degrees of bridging of left superior *(LS)* leaflet. **A,** Nonbridging (bridging grade 0) LS leaflet (Rastelli type A). This surgical specimen (the patch having been removed) is viewed from right atrium. Arrow marks mildly bridging left inferior (LI) leaflet. **B,** Moderate (grade 2 or 3) bridging of LS leaflet. Chordae from its right ventricular extremity go to a papillary muscle in right ventricle. Arrow indicates bridging portion of LI leaflet. (Rastelli and colleagues termed this *type B,* but it is just part of the spectrum of bridging.) **C,** Marked (grade 5) bridging of LS leaflet (Rastelli type C). Arrow marks bridging part of LI leaflet. Key: *RS,* Right superior leaflet; *S,* ventricular septal crest. (From Rastelli and colleagues.[R1])

The right ventricular portion of the common AV valve has superior, lateral, and inferior leaflets, but as in partial AV septal defects, they vary considerably in number and size (see Fig. 34-2). When bridging of the LSL is absent or mild, the RSL is large, whereas with more extensive bridging, it is smaller.[P8]

When leaflets of the common AV valve close appropriately during ventricular systole, AV valve regurgitation is absent or mild. However, important left AV valve regurgitation may be present (see Table 34-8). The mechanism of the regurgitation is often not clearly understood.

Anatomic studies by Kanani and colleagues have emphasized the marked valvar abnormalities in this malformation, not only of the anular component but also of the subvalvar apparatus (with deficiency of chordal arrangement) and leaflet tissue (which is often deficient in coaptation surface and pliability following repair).[K5]

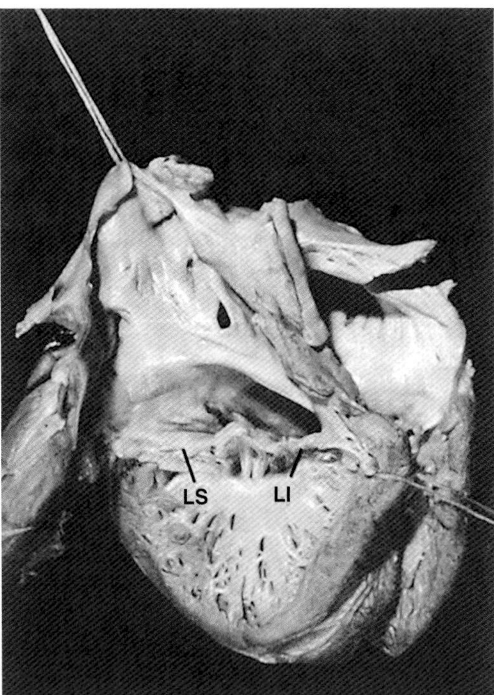

Figure 34-8 Intermediate type of atrioventricular (AV) septal defect viewed from left ventricular aspect. Left superior *(LS)* leaflet is connected to left inferior *(LI)* leaflet by leaflet tissue, resulting in two AV valve orifices; yet there are interventricular communications between short, thick chordae connecting leaflets and their connection to scooped-out underlying ventricular septum. LS and LI leaflets, particularly the latter, are deficient. (From Bharati and colleagues.[B16])

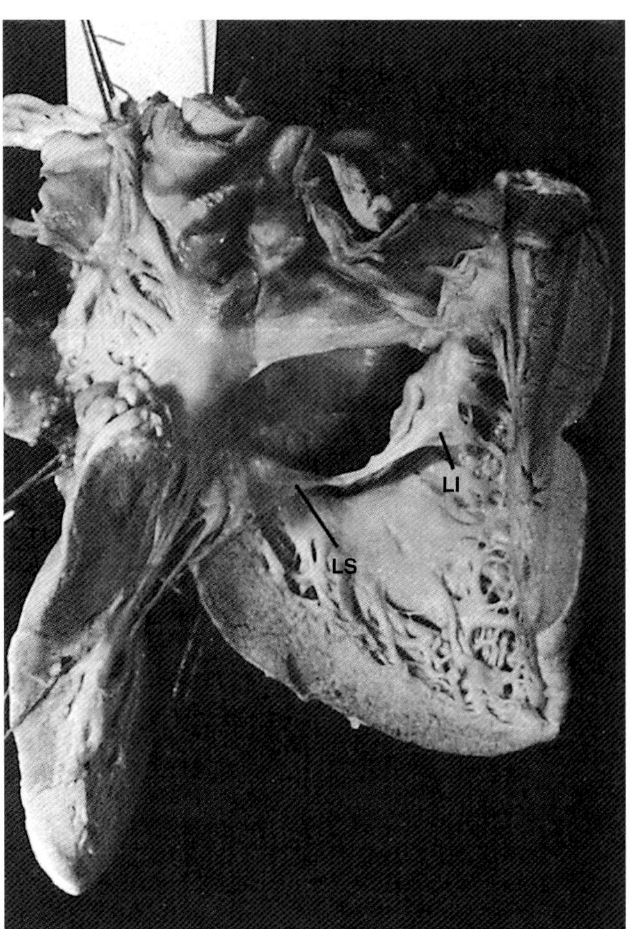

Figure 34-9 Intermediate type of atrioventricular septal defect viewed from left ventricular aspect. Left superior *(LS)* and left inferior *(LI)* leaflets are connected by leaflet tissue, and thus two AV valve orifices are present. However, the interventricular communication is large, and neither connection nor leaflets are attached to scooped-out underlying ventricular septum. (From Bharati and colleagues.[B16])

Unusual Atrioventricular Combinations

Other unusual combinations of size, connections, attachments, and degree of bridging of AV valve leaflets in the spectrum of AV septal defects prompted Wakai and Edwards, Bharati and colleagues, and others to use a *transitional* or *intermediate category*.[B16,W1,W7] Rarely in patients with two AV valve orifices with no interventricular communication beneath the LSL and LIL, these leaflets are connected only by a fibrous strand adherent to the ventricular septal crest (see Tables 34-3 and 34-5), forming what Bharati and colleagues have called a "pseudomitral leaflet," rather than an "anterior mitral leaflet with a complete cleft."[B16]

In such patients, deficiency of LIL tissue and severe left AV valve regurgitation are common. Occasionally when the LSL and LIL are connected (and thus two AV valve orifices are present), one or multiple small interchordal interventricular communications are present beneath the leaflets (see Tables 34-2 and 34-5), and occasionally one or two larger holes may be present (Fig. 34-8; see Fig. 34-5, *B*). In about 1% of cases, the connected LSL and LIL have large interventricular communications beneath them; in these patients, the connection is a thin strand of valve tissue beneath which there is also a large interventricular communication (Fig. 34-9), but two AV valve orifices can be said to be present (see Table 34-5). Bharati and colleagues have referred to this as *intermediate type C*.[B16]

Table 34-9 Left Atrioventricular Valve Orifice in Atrioventricular Septal Defect

Left AV Valve Orifice	Without Interventricular Communication ($n = 154$)		With Interventricular Communication ($n = 156$)	
	No.	% of 154	No.	% of 156
Single	149	97	147	94
Double	5	3[a]	9	6[a]

Data from Studer and colleagues.[S15]
[a]$P(\chi^2)$ for difference = .3.

Accessory Orifice

An accessory orifice (double left AV valve orifice) is present in the commissure on one side, usually the inferior side, of the LLL in about 5% of cases[I1,L4,M10,W2] (Table 34-9). A ring of chordae surrounds the orifice, and a very small papillary muscle is usually beneath it.[B2,E2] The accessory orifice may be conceptualized as an incomplete commissure, and the fibrous tissue "bridge" between the accessory orifice and main orifice

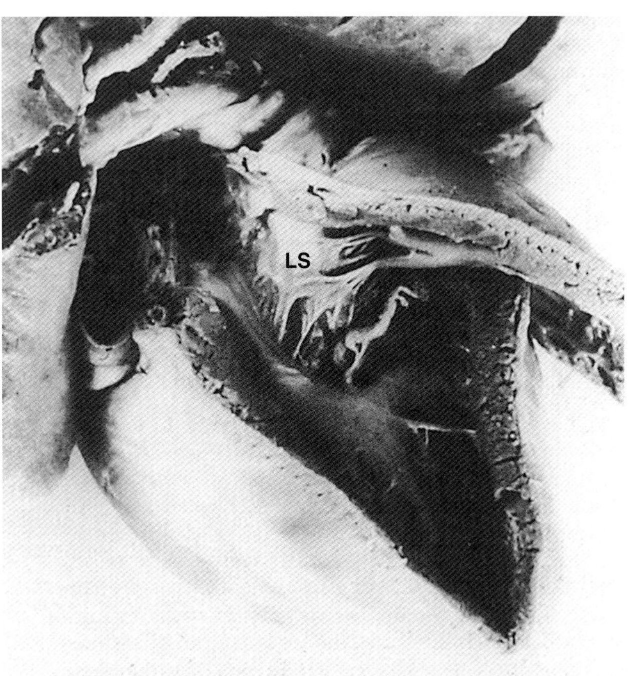

Figure 34-10 Left ventricular aspect of a complete atrioventricular septal defect with no bridging of left superior *(LS)* leaflet and connection of leaflet to underlying ventricular septum by long chordae. Narrowness of left ventricular outflow tract is apparent. (From Rastelli and colleagues.[R1])

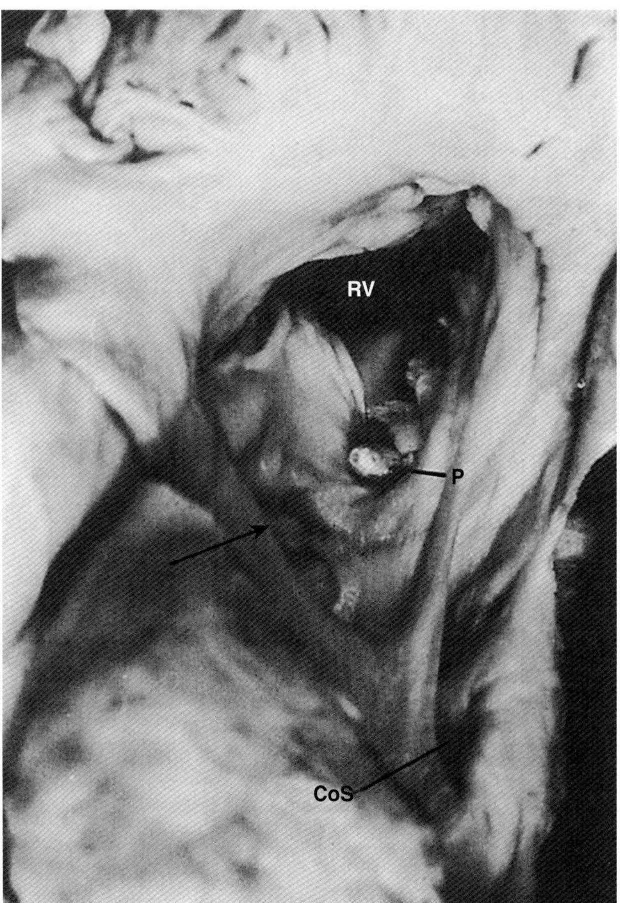

Figure 34-11 Complete atrioventricular (AV) septal defect with hypoplasia of left ventricle and a dominant right ventricle *(RV)*. Specimen is viewed from its right atrial aspect, and a probe *(P)* passes into left ventricular cavity. The common AV valves open almost entirely into right ventricle. Arrow indicates superior margin of the ostium primum atrial septal defect. Key: *CoS*, Coronary sinus.

consists of valvar tissue and chordae.[B2] This emphasizes the danger of producing regurgitation by cutting the bridge. The LLL is often underdeveloped when an accessory orifice is present.[D7] Accessory orifices predispose patients to stenosis after repair.

Single Papillary Muscle

A single papillary muscle in the LV uncommonly (about 5% of cases) complicates AV septal defects, most commonly the complete type.[D2,T2] All chordae of the left AV valve leaflets insert into this single papillary muscle, which is usually situated anteriorly in the LV. In complete AV septal defect with a free-floating and bridging LSL, no LV inflow obstruction results. Otherwise, or after repair, the situation is entirely analogous to a true "parachute mitral valve" (see "Papillary Muscle Anomalies" under Morphology in Chapter 50), and inflow obstruction can complicate intracardiac repair.[D2,D7,I1,T2]

Ventricles

The LV outflow tract is characteristically elongated and narrowed (Fig. 34-10) in all types of AV septal defect (see "General Morphologic Characteristics" under Morphology earlier in this chapter).

In AV septal defect with large interventricular communications, the LV may be abnormally large, but its size is variable, both absolutely and in relation to the right ventricle.[B14,C10,J1,S19] In the severely right-dominant type of AV septal defect, the LV is severely hypoplastic[S15] (Fig. 34-11). In such cases, the atrial septum may be displaced leftward in relation to the plane of the ventricular septum, in which case it overrides the left AV valve to a varying degree and may be associated with hypoplasia of the left atrium.[T4,U1] This variant is therefore sometimes included in "hypoplastic left heart physiology" (see Chapter 49).

The right ventricle has no specific anomalies, but is usually enlarged secondary to the left-to-right shunt. Its size is also variable, and occasionally it is importantly hypoplastic.

The LV or right ventricle is severely hypoplastic in about 7% of patients born with complete AV septal defect.[C8] Prevalence of the two types is similar. Presence of severe ventricular hypoplasia can increase risk of surgical correction and may demand a Fontan-type repair, alone or with a technique for correcting the hypoplastic left heart physiology[C8,J1,S15] (see Special Situations and Controversies later in this chapter and Chapter 41).

Septal Malalignment

Usually the two AV valves or common AV valve orifice lies in proper proportion over the two ventricles. When one ventricle is hypoplastic, the ventricular septum is malaligned and lies more to the side of the hypoplastic ventricle (see Fig. 34-11).

Less commonly, the atrial septal remnant is malaligned, and then usually leftward. When this is severe, both AV valves (or common AV valve orifice) are accessible only from the right atrium, and blood exists from the left atrium only through the ostium primum defect (so-called double outlet right atrium).[A6,C15,W5]

Left Ventricular Outflow or Inflow Obstruction

Important LV outflow tract obstruction occurs rarely in unoperated hearts (about 1% of cases) in all types of AV septal defect.[C8,P7,S3,S15,T4] It more often becomes apparent as a postoperative complication. It is surprising that it is not more frequent, in view of the elongation and narrowing of this area in affected hearts.[D6,E4]

Part of the elongation and narrowing is due to the more extensive area of direct fibrous continuity between the aortic valve and the LSL than is present normally between the aortic and mitral valves.[E3] This is caused in part by the short, thick chordae that often anchor the LSL to the crest of the ventricular septum.[C5,V6] Also, the anterolateral muscle bundle of the LV (muscle of Moulaert) bulges more into the LV outflow tract in hearts with AV septal defects than in normal hearts, contributing to the tendency to outflow obstruction after repair.[D6] In addition to these basic arrangements tending to narrow the LV outflow tract, LV obstruction may be contributed to by morphologically discrete subaortic stenosis or by excrescences of AV valve tissue heaped up in the LV outflow tract.[B10,P7,S11,T3] It may also result from abnormally positioned papillary muscles.[P7] Occasionally, its presence is overlooked preoperatively, and it becomes apparent or develops only after operation.

Important LV inflow obstruction may occur rarely.[P7] This may be from simple narrowing of the AV valve entrance into the LV, usually associated with marked right ventricular dominance. It may be related to presence of an accessory AV valve orifice on the left side, or it may result from cor triatriatum (see Chapter 32) or a supravalvar fibrous ring.[T6] These associated cardiac anomalies appear to be more prevalent in patients without Down syndrome.[D3,V5]

Conduction System

The defect in the AV septum often displaces the coronary sinus ostium inferiorly, which may appear to lie in the left atrium, especially when the ostium primum atrial defect is particularly large. The AV node is also displaced inferiorly (caudally) and lies in the posterior right atrial wall between the orifice of the coronary sinus and ventricular crest[L5] (Fig. 34-12) in what has been termed the *nodal triangle*.[T5] The bundle of His passes forward and superiorly from the node to the ventricular crest, reaching it where the crest fuses posteriorly with the AV valve anulus.[B15] It then courses along the top of the ventricular septum beneath the bridging portion of the LIL, giving off the left bundle branches. As it reaches the midpoint of the crest of the ventricular septum, it becomes the right bundle branch, which continues along the crest a little farther before it descends toward the muscle of Lancisi and moderator band. These anatomic findings have been supported by electrophysiologic studies at operation.[K4,K17] This morphology of the conduction system is a determinant of the electrocardiographic pattern usually seen in AV septal defects.[F1,T5]

Major Associated Cardiac Anomalies

Table 34-6 presents the prevalence of the major cardiac anomalies associated with AV septal defects.

Patent Ductus Arteriosus

A patent ductus arteriosus is present in about 10% of patients with AV septal defects. It is particularly common in those with an interventricular communication.

Tetralogy of Fallot

Typical tetralogy of Fallot is present in about 5% of patients with complete AV septal defects, and about 1% of patients with tetralogy of Fallot have associated complete AV septal defects.[B13,K11,N1] The LSL bridges markedly and is free-floating over the crest of the ventricular septum, and the interventricular communication beneath it is large and juxtaaortic.[D1,L6] An interventricular communication beneath the LIL is present in only about half of cases.[V9] Rarely the LSL and LIL are connected by a fibrous (or valvar) band, beneath which also is a large interventricular communication. The right ventricular outflow tract has typical tetralogy morphology (see Chapter 38) that may be so severe that pulmonary atresia is present. Localized narrowing occasionally occurring in that portion of the LV outflow tract just upstream from the recess formed by the subaortic deficiency of the ventricular septum further complicates the situation in rare cases.

Double Outlet Right Ventricle

Double outlet right ventricle (DORV) without pulmonary stenosis complicates complete AV septal defect in about 2% of cases.[B6,B13,R1,S12,S15] As in tetralogy of Fallot, usually

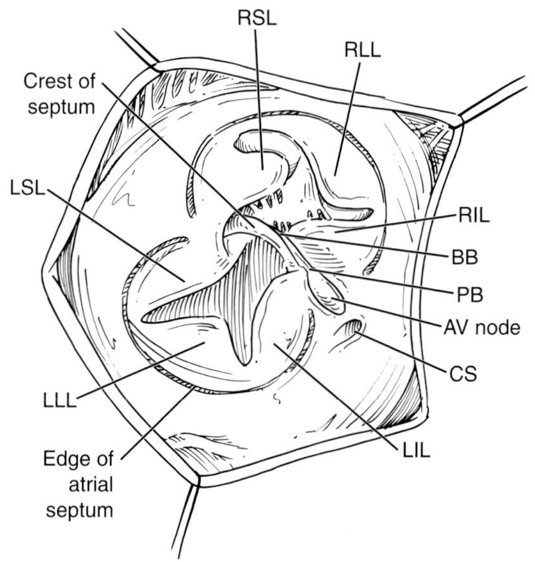

Figure 34-12 Location of conduction system in atrioventricular septal defect. See text for further details. AV, Atrioventricular; BB, branching portion of bundle of His; CS, coronary sinus orifice; LIL, left inferior leaflet; LLL, left lateral leaflet; LSL, left superior leaflet; PB, penetrating portion of bundle of His; RIL, right inferior leaflet; RLL, right lateral leaflet; RSL, right superior leaflet.

deficiency of the ventricular septum is large and juxtaaortic beneath the extensively bridging and free-floating LSL. However, occasionally the interventricular communication is far from the aortic and pulmonary valves and is "non-committed."[B6] Rarely, Taussig-Bing type of DORV is present.[B13,S12] DORV combined with severe pulmonary stenosis coexists with complete AV septal defects in about 1% of cases.[S15] These combinations of DORV and AV septal defect with large interventricular communication frequently also have atrial isomerism or situs inversus, common atrium, completely unroofed coronary sinus with left superior vena cava, azygos extension of the inferior vena cava, or total anomalous pulmonary venous connection.[P2,S12]

Transposition of the Great Arteries

Very rarely, transposition of the great arteries (discordant ventriculoarterial connection) is associated.[B13]

Completely Unroofed Coronary Sinus with Left Superior Vena Cava

Completely unroofed coronary sinus with persistent left superior vena cava (see Chapter 33) attached to left atrium occurs in about 3% of patients with an interventricular communication and in about 3% without, and is more frequent when common atrium is present.[Q1] A partially unroofed distal end of the coronary sinus resulting in drainage of the coronary sinus into the left atrium occasionally occurs, but is a minor and unimportant associated anomaly.[Y3] When complete AV septal defect is associated with persistent left superior vena cava and unroofed coronary sinus, atrial isomerism is also frequent (see Chapter 58).[A4]

Minor Associated Cardiac Anomalies

Table 34-7 lists minor cardiac anomalies associated with AV septal defects.

Pulmonary Vascular Disease

In partial AV septal defects, as in other types of ASDs, pulmonary vascular disease is uncommon, whereas in complete AV septal defects, as with large VSDs, pulmonary vascular disease usually appears early in life and progresses.[H3]

Morphologically, pulmonary vascular disease associated with complete AV septal defects is similar to that associated with large VSDs (see "Pulmonary Vascular Disease" under Morphology in Section I of Chapter 35). However, it tends to progress more rapidly in patients with complete AV septal defects. Correlation between histologic findings and pulmonary vascular resistance is similar in the two conditions.[F3] The pulmonary vascular changes probably are more frequent and occur at an earlier age in patients with Down syndrome with complete AV septal defects compared with patients without Down syndrome.[C9,Y1]

Down Syndrome

Down syndrome is rare in patients with partial AV septal defects but common (about 75%) in those with complete AV septal defects.[W9] Left-sided obstructive lesions are 10 times less common in Down syndrome patients[D3,V5]; other associated anomalies are probably also less common,[P5] whereas advanced pulmonary vascular disease may be more frequent.[F3]

Inlet Septal Type of Ventricular Septal Defect

It is important to note that an isolated inlet (AV septal) type of VSD (see Morphology in Section I of Chapter 35) occurs without any of the features of an AV septal defect as defined in this chapter, except that it involves the inflow portion of the ventricular septum beneath the septal tricuspid valve leaflet and usually also the area of the membranous ventricular septum. The AV septum, however, is intact, and the mitral and tricuspid anuli and aortic orifice lie in normal positions. This feature allows these VSDs to be readily differentiated echocardiographically and angiographically from AV septal defects. Interestingly, in isolated inlet VSD, the anterior mitral leaflet is occasionally cleft.

CLINICAL FEATURES AND DIAGNOSTIC CRITERIA

Pathophysiology

Left-to-right shunting is present in AV septal defects unless severe pulmonary vascular disease has developed or important right ventricular outflow tract obstruction or pulmonary valve stenosis coexists. When there is no interventricular communication, the shunt is at atrial level and usually large, but it may be small or moderate; in such cases, a pressure gradient can be demonstrated between left and right atria. When the shunt is large and left AV valve regurgitation is mild or absent, the hemodynamic state of the patient is identical to that in isolated ASD (see Clinical Features and Diagnostic Criteria in Chapter 30); only right ventricular stroke volume is increased. When important left AV valve regurgitation is present, the left-to-right shunt becomes much larger; in fact, the regurgitation jet usually goes directly from LV to right atrium. Left as well as right ventricular stroke volume is increased, and marked cardiomegaly and heart failure develop early in life.

When a large interventricular communication is also present (complete AV septal defect), the left-to-right shunt is large, and right ventricular and pulmonary artery pressures approach or equal systemic pressures (Table 34-10). Pulmonary vascular resistance rises rapidly and is usually importantly elevated after age 6 to 12 months and sometimes before.[N2]

Table 34-10 Preoperative Pulmonary Artery–Aortic Pressure Ratios in Patients without Major Associated Cardiac Anomalies

PPA/PAO			Without Interventricular Communication ($n = 140$)			With Interventricular Communication ($n = 97$)		
≤	Ratio	<	No.	% of 97[a]		No.	% of 74[b]	
		.03	65	67	87/97	5	7	12/74
.03		.05	20	21	(88%)	7	9	(16%)
.05		.07	5	5		10	14	
.07		.09	6	6	7/97	29	39	52/74
.09			1	1	(7%)	23	31	(70%)

Data from Studer and colleagues.[S15]
[a]Data not available for 43 patients.
[b]Data not available for 23 patients.
Key: *AO*, Aortic; *PA*, pulmonary artery.

When present, AV valve regurgitation adds greatly to ventricular volume overload. For some reason, however, the overload usually seems to enlarge the right ventricle more than the left.

Atrioventricular Valve Regurgitation

Prevalence of regurgitation at the left AV valve or common AV valve is considered to be less than before echocardiographic studies were available. Probably 10% to 15% of patients with partial AV septal defect have important regurgitation, not 40% as was estimated earlier (see Table 34-8). Moderate AV valve regurgitation is present in about 20% of infants with complete AV septal defects and severe regurgitation in only about 15%.[A3,C6,W4] AV valve regurgitation may be considerably more common in older patients with complete AV septal defects.

A not-uncommon site of regurgitation is through the gap between the LSL and LIL, particularly near the leaflet hinge or base; partly for this reason, regurgitant flow frequently goes directly into the right atrium. Under such circumstances, the left atrium remains small and the right becomes large; but when the interatrial communication is smaller or the regurgitation is sited elsewhere, regurgitation may enter the left atrium, which enlarges.

Although the precise mechanism of AV valve regurgitation is often unclear, it apparently varies considerably, as would be expected from variations in the number, size, and configuration of the leaflets and their chordal attachments. In patients with partial AV septal defects and important left AV valve regurgitation, the LIL is commonly severely hypoplastic.

Symptoms and Physical Findings

Patients without an interventricular communication (partial AV septal defect) and with absent or mild left AV valve regurgitation often present in the first decade of life but may remain asymptomatic well beyond that age. Their clinical presentation is virtually identical to that of patients with the more common fossa ovalis ASD (see "Fossa Ovalis Defect" under Morphology in Chapter 30), except that they may have an apical systolic murmur when mild left AV valve regurgitation is present, and left axis deviation and a counterclockwise frontal plane loop.[O1,T7]

Moderate or severe (grade 3, 4, or 5) left AV valve regurgitation in patients with partial AV septal defects may produce symptoms earlier, and progressive severe heart failure may require treatment in infancy.[B5] In addition to the usual signs of ASD, the heart is more active in association with a loud apical pansystolic murmur, and the apex of the LV may be palpable. Tachypnea and hepatomegaly are often evident.

In patients with complete AV septal defect, presentation is usually in the first year of life, frequently during the first months, as a result of progressive severe heart failure, which may not be controllable medically. There is associated tachypnea, poor peripheral perfusion, and failure to thrive. Occasionally, heart failure is minimal early in life, and presentation may be delayed until some years later, by which time there is almost always severe hypertensive pulmonary vascular disease and Eisenmenger complex (see "Clinical Findings" under Clinical Features and Diagnostic Criteria in Section I of Chapter 35). On physical examination, cardiomegaly with increased ventricular activity is apparent. The second heart sound at the base is split and usually fixed, with accentuation of the second component caused by elevated pulmonary artery pressure. A systolic murmur is audible over the left precordium from the shunt at ventricular level and is increased in intensity and nearer the apex when there is important AV valve regurgitation. A mid-diastolic flow murmur is characteristically widely heard both over the lower left precordium and at the apex secondary to the large diastolic flow across the malformed AV valve leaflets (depending on both the left-to-right shunt and any AV valve regurgitation).

In those patients with morphology intermediate between the partial and complete AV septal defects, clinical features depend on size of the interventricular communication and severity of left AV valve regurgitation.

Chest Radiograph

In patients without an interventricular communication or important left AV valve regurgitation, the chest radiograph is the same as in other large ASDs. When moderate or severe left AV valve regurgitation is present, the radiograph usually shows marked cardiomegaly with evidence of LV, right ventricular, and right atrial enlargement and marked pulmonary plethora. Left atrial enlargement is not apparent unless the ostium primum defect is restrictive.

In complete AV septal defect, cardiomegaly and pulmonary plethora are evident in infants and young children presenting with heart failure. In patients who survive beyond this age, severely increased pulmonary vascular resistance usually dominates, and the heart is less enlarged, central pulmonary arteries are large, and lung fields are clear.

Electrocardiogram

Electrocardiographic findings are rather specific.[D9] They usually indicate marked right ventricular hypertrophy and may show LV hypertrophy as well. The PR interval is frequently prolonged. Of considerable diagnostic importance is the vectorcardiogram.[T7] Ongley and colleagues conclude that a counterclockwise frontal plane loop anterior and to the right strongly suggests, but does not prove, the diagnosis.[O1]

Two-Dimensional Echocardiogram

In AV septal defects without an interventricular communication or important left AV valve regurgitation, two-dimensional echocardiography, together with clinical presentation, chest radiograph, and electrocardiogram, is diagnostic, and cardiac catheterization with cineangiography is not necessary.[L11,S8] Two-dimensional echocardiography, particularly with Doppler color flow imaging and, when possible, with a transthoracic window, can also provide full information for complete AV septal defects.[C4,S7]

The common AV orifice is easily seen in the four-chamber view (Fig. 34-13). Characteristically, left and right AV valves (separated or common) exist at the same level, in contrast to the cephalad displacement of the normal mitral valve. The elongated outflow septum and unwedged position of the aortic valve are also identifiable. Chordal attachment and degree of leaflet bridging can also be assessed. Finally, the degree of AV valve regurgitation is assessed with color flow.

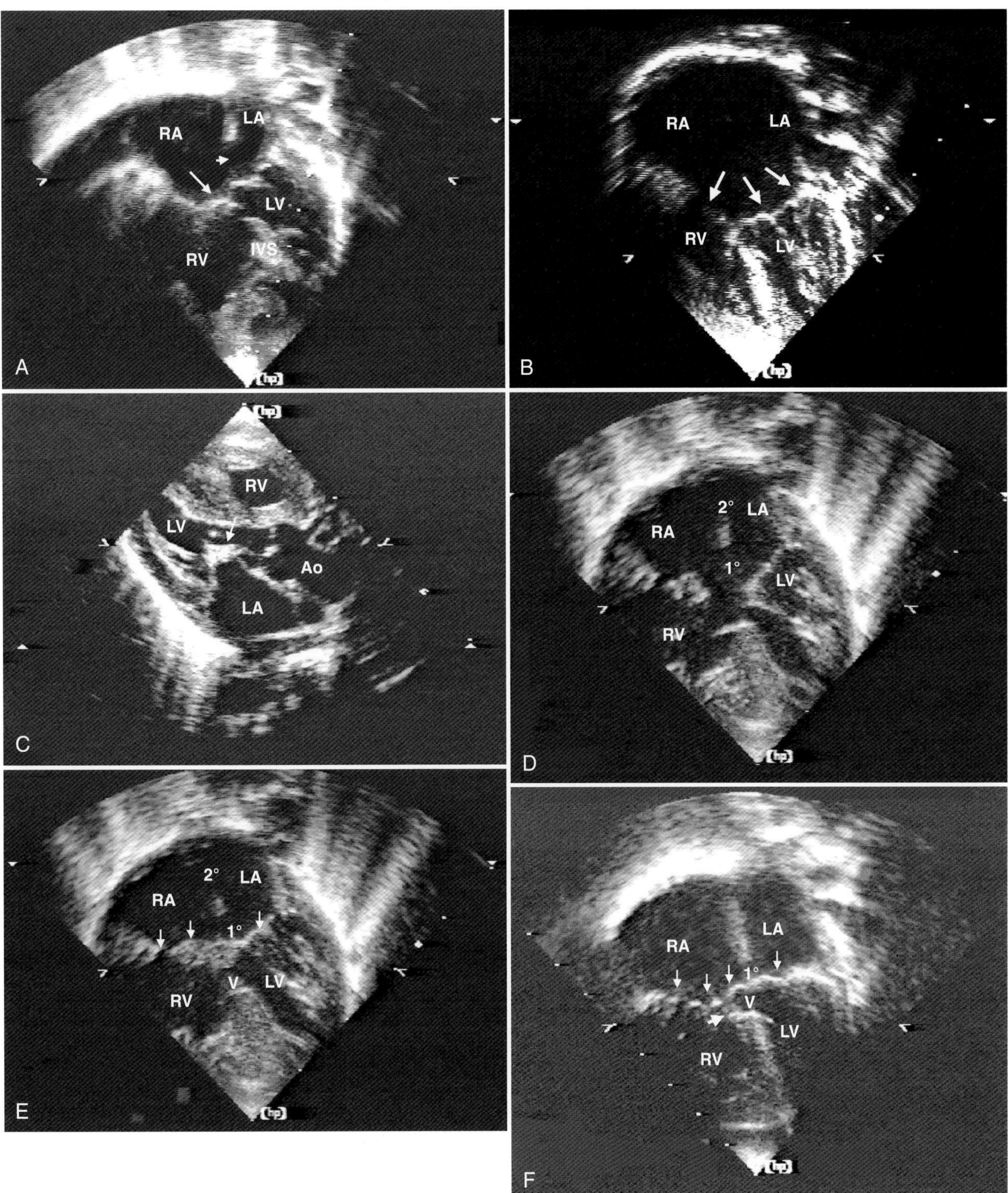

Figure 34-13 Echocardiograms of atrioventricular (AV) septal defects. **A,** Apical four-chamber view of a heart with an unbalanced AV septal defect. In this figure, the common AV valve *(arrow)* is positioned such that there is malalignment between interatrial septum and interventricular septum and a disproportionate size of the ventricles. Smaller arrow shows primum atrial septal defect. **B,** Apical four-chamber view showing common AV valve *(arrows)* with virtual absence of interatrial septum. **C,** Parasternal long axis view showing a "gooseneck" appearance of left ventricular outflow tract caused by displacement of left-sided portion of a common AV valve *(arrow).* **D,** Coronal image of heart as viewed from apex (apical four-chamber view). This heart has a complete AV septal defect. There are both primum and secundum atrial septal defects. **E,** Coronal image of a heart with a complete AV septal defect as viewed from the apex (apical four-chamber view). Arrows point to the common AV valve. There are both primum and secundum atrial septal defects. **F,** Coronal image of a heart with a partial AV septal defect as viewed from the apex (apical four-chamber view). Thin arrows point to common AV valve. Thick arrow points to tissue occluding the inlet ventricular septal defect right AV valve pouch formation. Key: *Ao,* Aorta; *IVS,* interventricular septum; *LA,* left atrium; *LV,* left ventricle; *RA,* right atrium, *RV,* right ventricle; *V,* inlet ventricular septal defect; *1°,* primum; *2°,* secundum.

With subcostal views, the degree of balance in the commitment of the common AV orifice to right and left ventricles can be ascertained (see "Unbalanced Atrioventricular Septal Defects" under Special Situations and Controversies).

Limitations of echocardiography include lack of sensitivity for double orifice left AV valve and inability to assess quantitatively pulmonary vascular resistance and reactivity.

Cardiac Catheterization and Cineangiogram

Direction and magnitude of shunting; pulmonary and systemic pressures, resistances, and flows; and right and left ventricular pressures can be measured and calculated from data obtained at cardiac catheterization (see "Cardiac Catheterization" under Clinical Features and Diagnostic Criteria in Section I of Chapter 35).[P4] However, these studies are now required only when major cardiac anomalies coexist and when operability is questioned because of evidence of pulmonary vascular disease.

Angiocardiographic features of AV septal defects were well described by Baron and colleagues in 1964 and further refined by the work of Brandt and colleagues, Bargeron and colleagues, and Macartney and colleagues.[B3,B4,B20,M1,S10] Both oblique and axial views are used.[B3,B20] They demonstrate absence of the AV septum and deficiency of the inlet portion of the ventricular septum, elongation of the LV outflow tract in relationship to the inflow tract, elevation and anterior displacement of the aortic valve vis-à-vis the AV valves, and the anomalous relationship of anterior components of the left AV valve to the aorta. These are well portrayed by the line drawings of Baron and colleagues and representative cineangiograms[B4] (Figs. 34-14 through 34-16). The anomalous left AV valve's relationship to the aorta results in change in direction of left AV valve movement. Interatrial and interventricular shunting can also be demonstrated, as can presence of one or two AV valve orifices. With high-quality studies, leaflets of the left AV valve often can be visualized in motion to delineate the degree, location, and mechanism of valvar regurgitation.

The relative size of the two ventricles and of AV orifices must be determined by whatever technique—echocardiography or angiography—is preferred. Severe hypoplasia of one or the other ventricle must be identified preoperatively, because such hypoplasia makes it less likely anatomic correction will be successful.[C8,J1]

Special Situations and Associated Defects

Presence of *common atrium* generally can be identified preoperatively by echocardiography or a cineangiogram, which show nearly complete absence of both atrial and AV septum (see Fig. 34-13). Finding mild arterial desaturation in a patient with clinical findings of an AV septal defect, but without an interventricular communication or pulmonary artery hypertension, suggests presence of common atrium.[D9,M18,R2,R5] Presence of a left superior vena cava in such a setting suggests both unroofed coronary sinus syndrome and common atrium, because they frequently coexist.[Q1,R5] In patients with common atrium and atrial isomerism, even more complex associations occur, including DORV, partial or total anomalous pulmonary venous connection, and azygos extension of the inferior vena cava[D7,K16,P2,S13,T1] (see Morphology in Chapter 58).

A patent ductus arteriosus can be identified on aortography. Likewise, associated malformations such as tetralogy of Fallot, DORV, transposition of the great arteries, and additional VSDs are identified by a combination of echocardiography and cineangiography.

It is essential to recognize functionally important *LV outflow tract obstruction*. Narrowing of this tract is inherent in AV septal defects but rarely results in a systolic pressure gradient. Distortion results from the shortened inflow axis of the LV and anterior displacement of the left AV valve complex[V1] (Fig. 34-17). Thus, LV outflow obstruction is most prevalent in patients with Rastelli type A valve morphology.[P7,S17] This distortion is rarely evident preoperatively as LV outflow obstruction. More frequently, important obstruction becomes evident postoperatively, both early and later. Usually it takes the form of subaortic discrete membranous stenosis, but the process may be relatively diffuse along the outflow tract. Infrequently, it occurs as a result of the ventricular patch component pulling the left AV valve apically and anteriorly such that the new "mitral" valve apparatus narrows the outflow tract. Thus, the initial AV septal repair must place the left AV valve at the appropriate level: caudad toward the apex may result in LV outflow tract obstruction; cephalad toward the atria may result in left AV valve regurgitation.

NATURAL HISTORY

The life history of patients with surgically untreated AV septal defects depends on morphologic and functional details of their malformation. When there is a *partial AV septal defect*, only *mild left AV valve regurgitation*, and *no major associated cardiac anomaly*, life history without surgical treatment is similar to that of patients with large fossa ovalis ASDs (see Natural History in Chapter 30). Important pulmonary vascular disease develops in a small number of patients in their 20s, 30s, and 40s.[P4] As in other types of large ASD, symptomatic deterioration of patients in adult life often coincides with development of atrial fibrillation[S9] (Fig. 34-18).

Patients with a *partial AV septal defect* and *moderate or severe left AV valve regurgitation* have a different natural history. Because of a nonrestrictive interatrial communication, severe left atrial and pulmonary venous hypertension are absent, but the left-to-right shunt is large and pulmonary artery pressure usually at least moderately elevated. Probably at least 20% of such individuals are severely symptomatic in infancy, and without surgical treatment, many would die in the first decade of life.

Patients with a *complete AV septal defect* have a still more unfavorable natural history. Because no group of infants known to have this malformation has been followed from birth without surgical intervention, the ideal database for delineation of their natural history does not exist. The closest approach is the prospective study of 56,109 live births by Mitchell and colleagues that included 10 infants judged to have isolated complete AV septal defect (excluding four stillbirths with the malformation), 4 of whom died within the first 3 years of life.[M15] This information is inconclusive, however, because of the small number of patients involved; failure to obtain a positive diagnosis by surgery, autopsy, or cardiac catheterization in all patients in the study; use of surgical intervention in some cases; and nonreporting of specific ages of the six survivors.

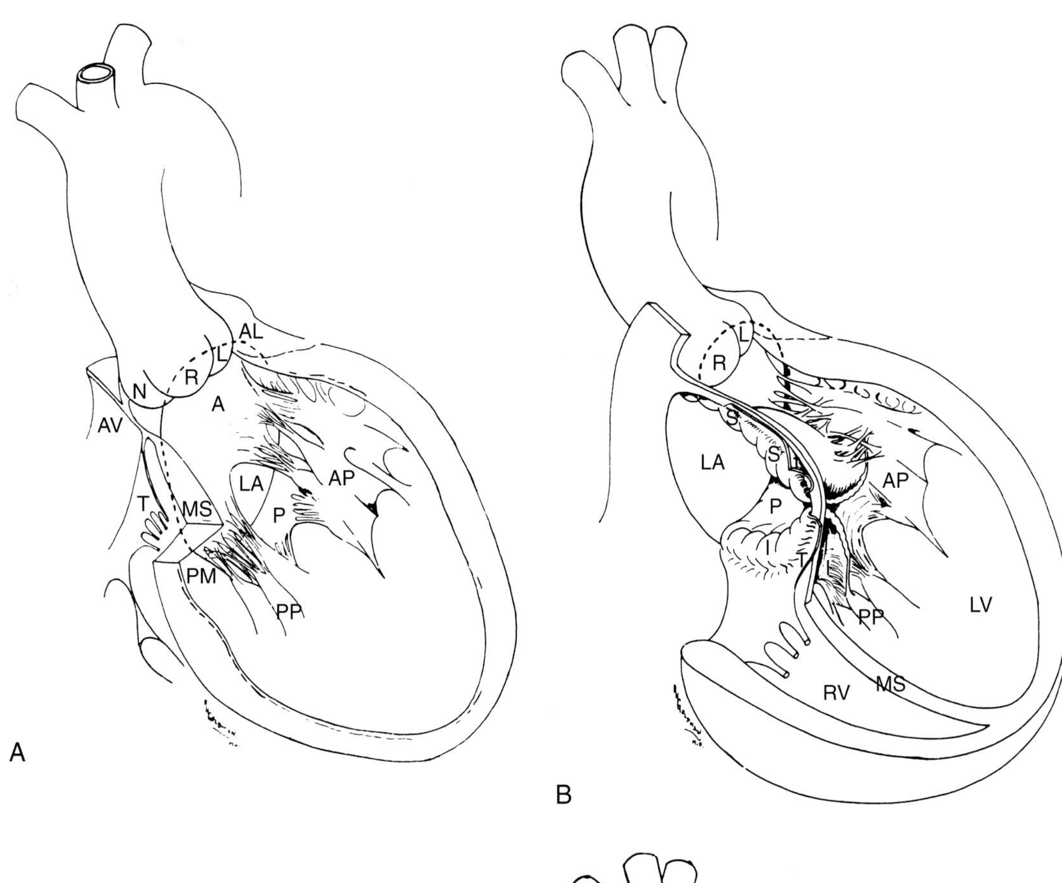

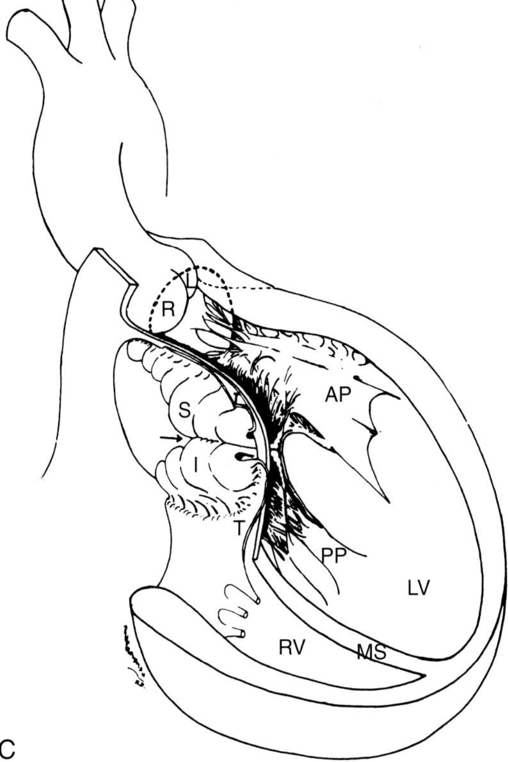

Figure 34-14 Diagrams of altered attachment of left atrioventricular *(AV)* valve leaflets in AV septal defect compared with normal heart. Heart is shown in its in vivo position as seen in a frontal angiogram. Right ventricle *(RV)* and most of the ventricular septum and right atrium have been removed. Dashed line indicates portion of line of attachment of left AV valve hidden by other structures. **A,** Normal heart. Attachment of anterior mitral leaflet *(A)* begins at anterolateral commissure *(AL)* and runs anteriorly for a short distance along free wall of left ventricle *(LV)*. It is then continuous with root of aorta in relation to adjacent portion of left coronary *(L)* and noncoronary *(N)* aortic cusps. Line of attachment proceeds downward along AV septum to posteromedial commissure *(PM)*. Attachment of mitral valve to AV septum is profiled in right anterior oblique view (see Fig. 34-15). **B-C,** Partial AV septal defect shown in diastole **(B)** and systole **(C)**. Scooped-out crest of basal portion of ventricular septum is shown considerably thinner than it actually is. Right AV valve leaflets are shown only at their sites of attachment. Diastolic figure **(B)** depicts left superior and left inferior leaflets as open; their line of attachment to aortic root is nearly normal, but it then passes along the superior rim of the scooped-out ventricular septal crest. Left superior leaflet is displaced upward into the left ventricular outflow tract, narrowing it. Left inferior leaflet is folded back against left ventricular aspect of sinus septum. In systolic figure **(C),** left superior and inferior leaflets are closed. Increased left ventricular pressure balloons them toward the atria. Arrow marks their point of coaptation. Key: *AP,* Anterior papillary muscle; *AV,* atrioventricular septum; *I,* left inferior leaflet of atrioventricular valve; *LA,* left atrium; *MS,* muscular ventricular septum; *P,* posterior mitral leaflet; *PP,* posterior papillary muscle; *R,* right aortic cusp; *S,* left superior leaflet of atrioventricular valve; *T,* tricuspid valve. (From Baron and colleagues.[B4])

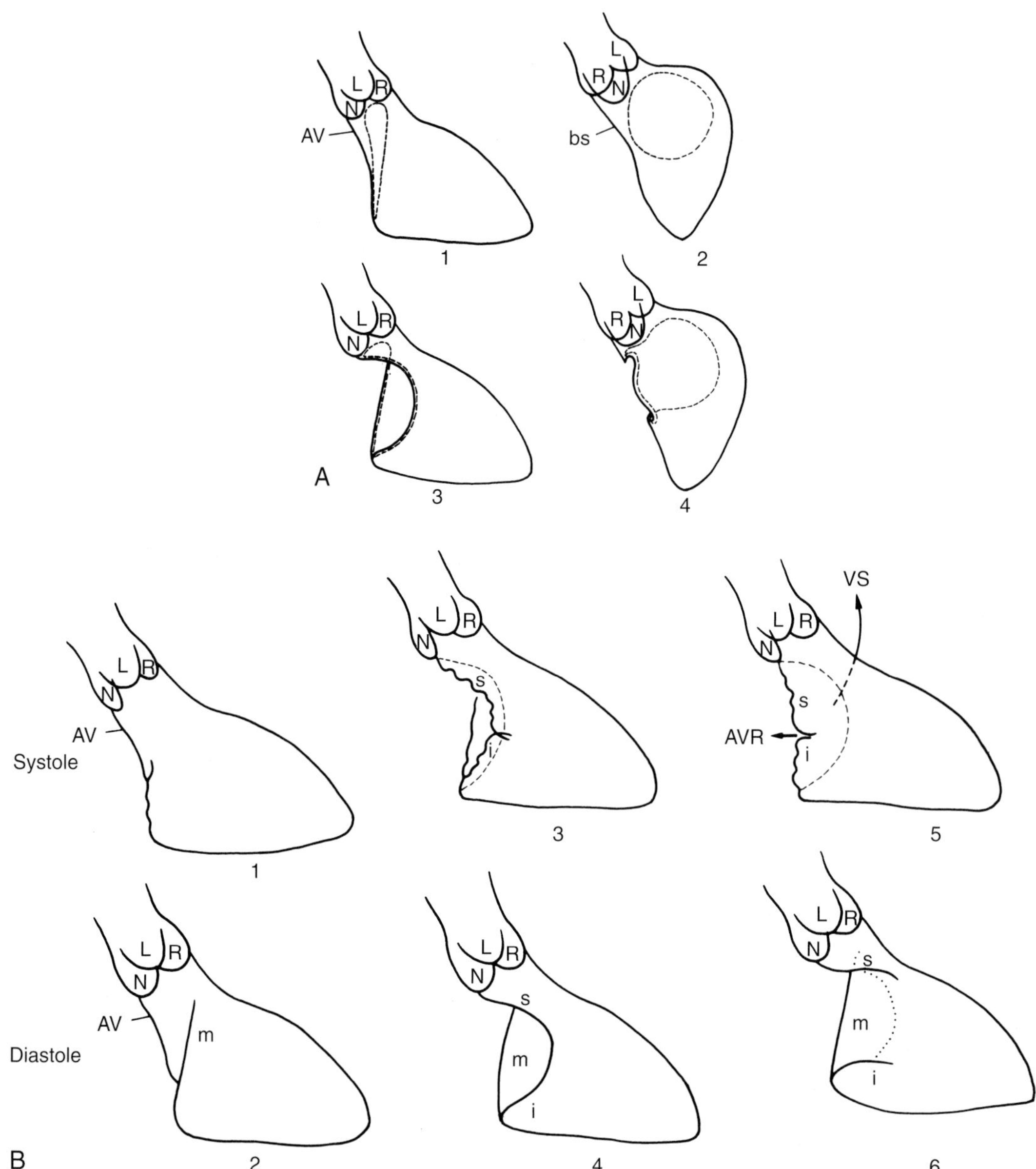

Figure 34-15 Diagrammatic representations of cineangiograms of a normal heart and hearts with atrioventricular *(AV)* septal defects, in oblique and axial views. **A,** Mitral valve orifice and leaflet attachments *(interrupted line)* in right anterior oblique (RAO) and left anterior oblique (LAO) projections. *(1)* Normal mitral orifice is approximately profiled in 40-degree RAO projection, but is overlapped by left ventricular (LV) outflow tract. Rightward posterior border of normal LV outflow tract is formed by AV septal tissue, not mitral valve. *(2)* In 50-degree LAO projections, the rightward anterior margin of the normal outflow tract consists of the basal ventricular sinus (inlet) septum: membranous above, muscular below. Mitral valve attachments do not reach the septal margin. *(3, 4)* In AV septal defects, absence of AV septum and adjacent deficiency of basal (inlet) ventricular septum modify left AV valve attachments and position and shape of left AV orifice and LV outflow tract. **B,** LV cineangiograms in 40-degree RAO projections. *(1, 2)* Normal features can be compared with those of typical partial *(3, 4)* and complete *(5, 6)* AV septal defect in systole and diastole. In the normal heart, mitral (left AV valve) leaflets contribute only to the lowest portion of rightward posterior LV outflow margin in systole, the relatively immobile AV septum forming the remainder of this margin throughout cardiac cycle in diastole. Line of attachment *(m)* of mural (posterior) leaflet of mitral valve can be identified, because contrast is trapped between leaflet and adjacent LV wall. In AV septal defects, rightward posterior margin of LV outflow tract consists of mobile leaflet tissue: left superior leaflet *(s)* above and left inferior leaflet *(i)* below. AV septum is absent. Mural leaflet attachment lies in relatively normal position. When there is complete attachment of left superior and inferior leaflets to septal crest *(dashed line)*, LV outflow tract deformity is well marked in systole, and position of septal crest can be identified in diastole, with contrast being trapped between open leaflets and septum. When there is a large interventricular communication with superior and inferior leaflets free-floating or attached to septal crest by thin chordae only *(5, 6)*, systolic deformity may be less marked and septal crest may be invisible, because contrast is washed away by non-radiopaque inflow. RAO view separates an AV regurgitant stream *(AVR)* from an interventricular shunt *(VS)*.

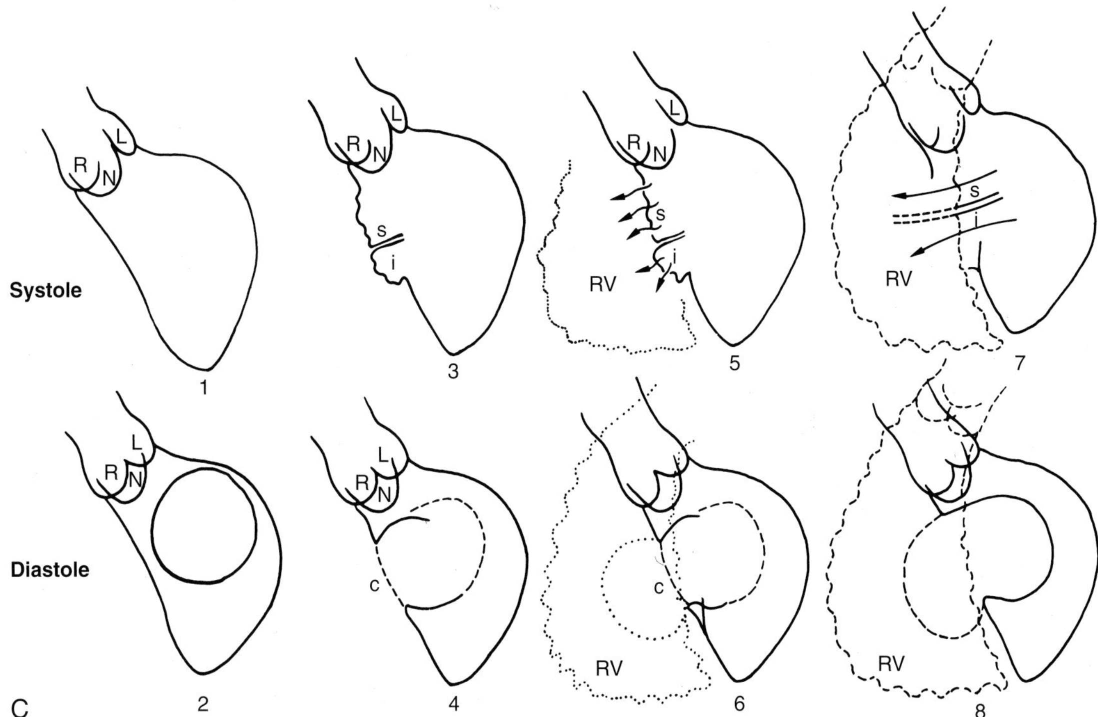

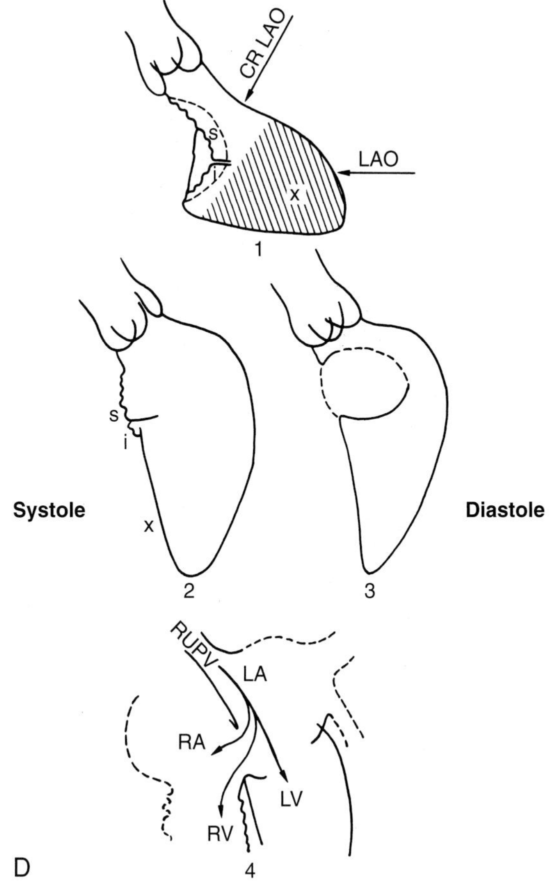

Figure 34-15, cont'd **C,** Left ventricular (LV) cineangiograms in 50-degree left anterior oblique (LAO) projection. *(1, 2)* In normal heart, septal margin of LV outflow tract is uninterrupted in systole and diastole. In AV septal defect *(3-8)*, septal margin is interrupted by defect in basal (inlet) ventricular septum, the defect being continuous with left AV orifice. *(3, 4)* When left superior *(s)* and inferior *(i)* leaflets are completely attached to septal crest, as in partial AV septal defect, leaflet tissue bulges into defect in systole, and position of septal crest *(c)* can be identified in diastole. *(7, 8)* When there is a large interventricular communication, systolic flow into right ventricle can be observed passing beneath left superior *(upper arrow)* or left inferior *(lower arrow)* leaflets. In diastole, a common AV orifice is identified. *(5, 6)* In some cases, attachments to septal crest are present but leave smaller interventricular communications. AV valve regurgitation tends to obscure valve detail as overlying atria opacify. **D,** LV or left atrial cineangiograms of AV septal defect in 50-degree LAO with cranial angulation (axial, hepatoclavicular, or four-chamber view). *(1)* Arrows in 40-degree RAO view illustrate why conventional LAO (part **C**) shows full height of the AV orifice, providing the best separation of left superior from left inferior leaflets. Cranially tilted version of LAO *(CR LAO)* foreshortens AV orifice and tends to superimpose these leaflets. *(2, 3)* However, the characteristic deformity of septal and AV orifice anatomy seen in conventional LAO view can be appreciated in axial LAO views, which are shown in both systole and diastole. In addition, midmuscular and apical parts of the sinus septum are better separated from basal defect so that additional muscular defects in cross-hatched area (e.g., at *x*) may be identified. AV valve regurgitation obscures detail, but partial separation of atria from ventricles improves differentiation of regurgitation from interventricular shunting. With a left atrial or right upper pulmonary venous injection in 50-degree LAO with cranial angulation *(4)*, contrast flow *(arrows)* early in the sequence shows position of atrial septal defect adjacent to AV valves. Contrast enters right atrium, right ventricle, and left ventricle. Cranial angulation rarely achieves a perfect profile of AV anulus, and ventricular opacification obscures detail later in the sequence. Key: *AV,* Atrioventricular septum; *AVR,* atrioventricular regurgitant stream; *bs,* basal (inlet) portion of ventricular septum; *c,* septal crest; *CR LAO,* cranial left anterior oblique; *i,* left inferior leaflet; *L,* left coronary sinus of aortic root, *LA,* left atrium; *LAO,* left anterior oblique; *LV,* left ventricle; *m,* line of attachment of posterior mitral leaflet; *N,* noncoronary sinus of aortic root; *R,* right coronary sinus of aortic root; *RA,* right atrium; *RUPV,* right upper pulmonary venous injection; *RV,* right ventricle; *s,* left superior leaflet; *VS,* ventricular shunt.

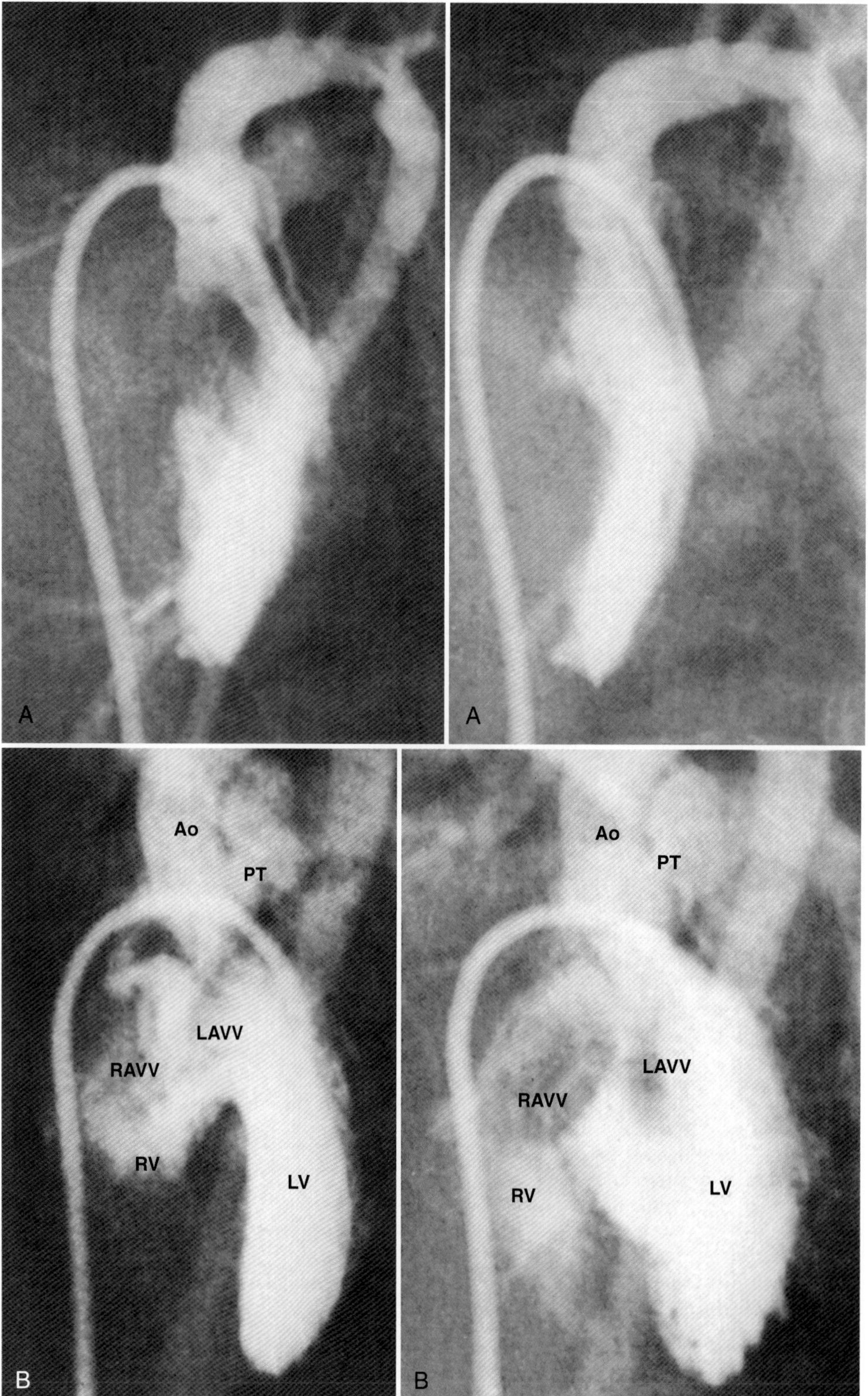

Figure 34-16 Cineangiograms of atrioventricular (AV) septal defects. **A,** Partial AV septal defect shown by left ventriculogram in four-chamber position: diastolic frame *(left)* and systolic frame *(right)*. Loss of straight line contour from aortic valve to crux cordis indicates absence of major part of AV septum. **B,** AV septal defect with two AV valve orifices and an interventricular communication.

An important event in the natural history is development of severe pulmonary vascular disease. This complication becomes apparent at 7 to 12 months of age in up to 30% of patients with complete AV septal defect and is probably present in 90% of such patients by age 3 to 5 years.[F3,N2] Thus, its prevalence in early life is higher in patients with complete AV septal defect than in those with large VSD.

In the absence of a definitive prospective study, approximation of natural history of complete AV septal defect has been constructed from 39 patients in two reports of

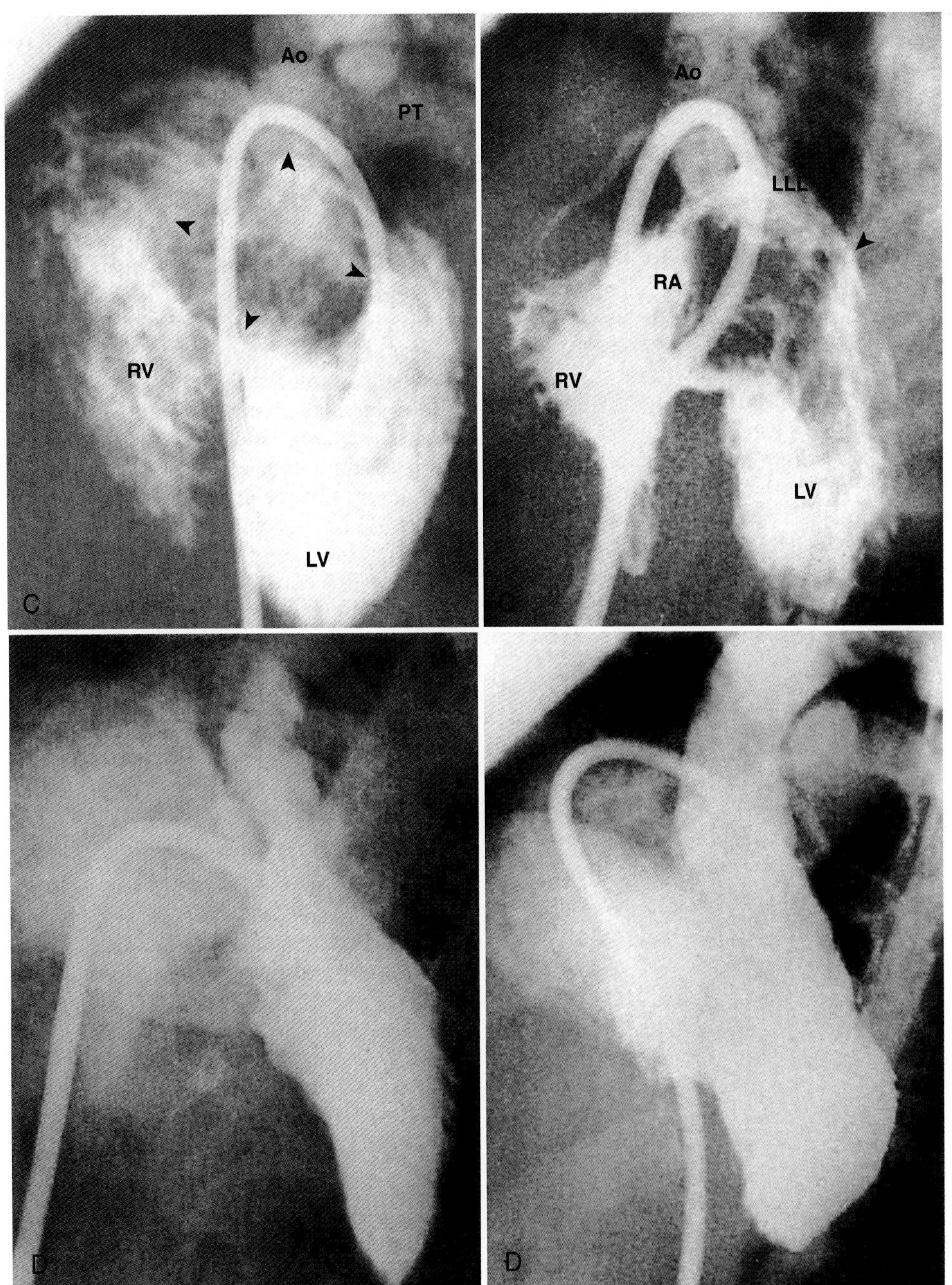

Figure 34-16, cont'd **C,** Complete atrioventricular (AV) septal defect shown by left ventriculogram in four-chamber view. Anulus of valve is seen as a negative shadow formed by accumulation of contrast medium between the leaflets and ventricular free wall *(arrowheads)*; it includes right *(RV)* and left ventricles *(LV)* in almost equal proportions. On right, contrast medium outlines left lateral leaflet *(LLL)*, which is related to aorta *(Ao)* and separated from left superior leaflet by a commissure *(arrowhead)* marking position of papillary muscle of conus. Outline of left superior leaflet is separated from left lateral leaflet by a commissure marking position of anterior papillary muscle of left ventricle. This represents an example of Rastelli type A defect. **D,** Partial AV septal defects with moderate *(left)* and severe *(right)* regurgitation of left AV valve. Contrast medium has passed from left ventricle into right atrium *(RA)* through regurgitant valve. Key: *LAVV,* Left atrioventricular valve; *PT,* pulmonary trunk; *RAVV,* right atrioventricular valve.

autopsies.[B11] This analysis indicates that about 80% of patients who do not undergo operation die by age 2 years (Fig. 34-19). A child surviving to age 1 year has only about a 15% chance of living to age 5. Those who die in the first 1 to 2 years of life usually do so with heart failure, with or without recurrent pulmonary infections, as a result of the large left-to-right shunt and moderate-to-severe AV valve regurgitation present in 60%.[S15] The high incidence of death in the first year of life has been confirmed by Samanek.[S1] Thereafter, valve regurgitation and increasing pulmonary vascular disease become dominant factors in the natural history. Newfeld and colleagues showed histologically that advanced pulmonary vascular disease (Heath-Edwards grade 3 and 4; see "Pulmonary Vascular Disease" under Morphology in Section I of Chapter 35) is occasionally present in such infants, even in the first year of life.[N2] However, it is

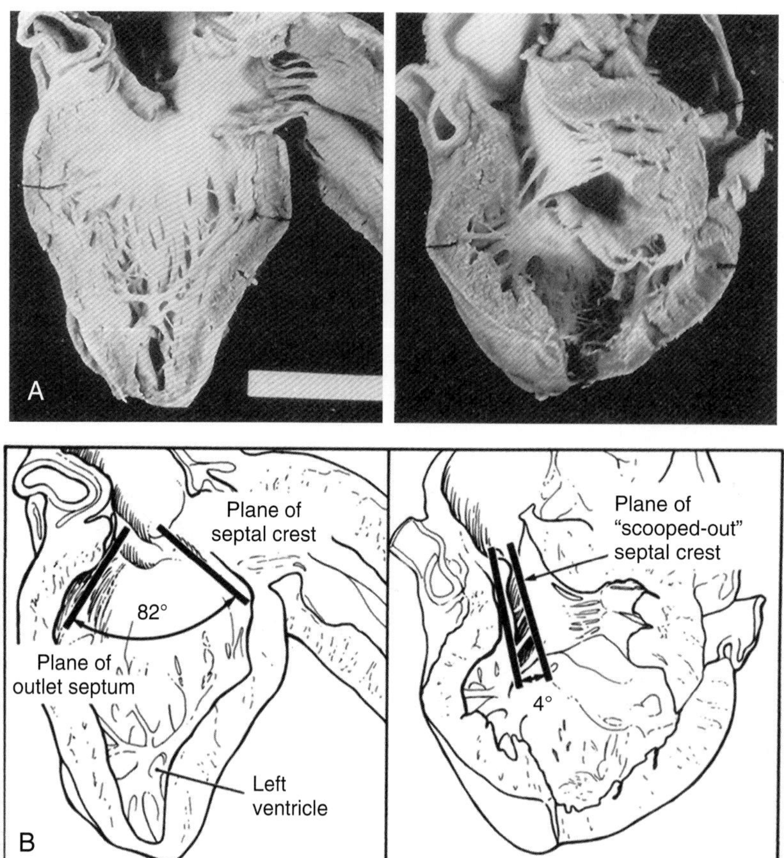

Figure 34-17 Anatomic specimens *(above)* and drawings of them *(below)* contrasting outflow angle in a normal heart compared with that in atrioventricular (AV) septal defect. **A,** Wide angle between plane of outlet septum and plane of septal crest (outflow angle) in a normal heart. **B,** Narrow angle in a heart with AV septal defect. Septal crest is scooped out, shortened, and anteriorly displaced; outflow axis is elongated. (From Van Arsdell and colleagues.[V1])

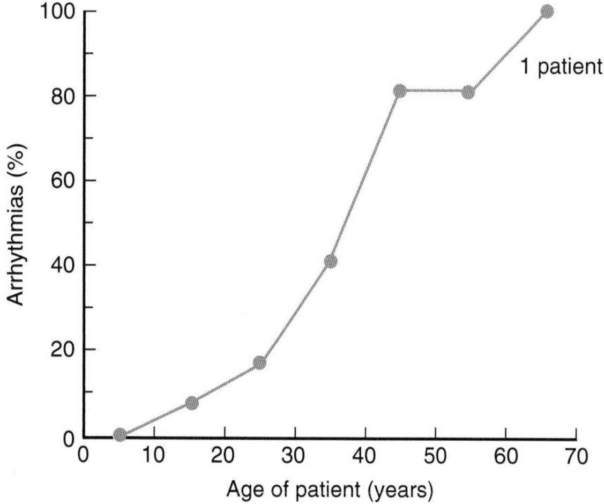

Figure 34-18 Cardiac arrhythmias in surgically untreated patients with a partial atrioventricular septal defect according to age. Increased prevalence in older patients is striking. (From Somerville.[S9])

present in nearly 90% of patients older than age 1 year (7 of their 8 specimens).

Bull and colleagues dispute these inferences and deduce a more favorable prognosis for infants with complete AV septal defects based on a study of patients with Down syndrome and this anomaly.[B21] Careful study of their report generates uncertainty as to the appropriateness of analyses underlying their inferences, however.[K8,W9]

Another aspect of the natural history of patients with AV septal defects is the tendency of their offspring to have similar defects or other congenital cardiac malformations. Emanuel and colleagues found that 14% of children of mothers with AV septal defects have congenital heart disease[E8]; half have tetralogy of Fallot, and half have AV septal defects. This prevalence is much higher than the 2% to 4% among children of parents with other types of congenital heart disease.[N4]

TECHNIQUE OF OPERATION

Surgical treatment of AV septal defects is directed toward (1) closing the interatrial communication, which is virtually always present; (2) closing the interventricular communication if one is present; (3) avoiding damage to the AV node and bundle of His; and (4) maintaining or creating two competent, nonstenotic AV valves.

Repair techniques vary considerably, but when used properly, all appear to provide good results.[E1,L1] For example:

- One or two patches may be used to repair the malformation when there is large interventricular communication.[R3]
- A markedly bridging LSL may be divided to facilitate the repair, or it may be left intact.[B17,R4,S15]

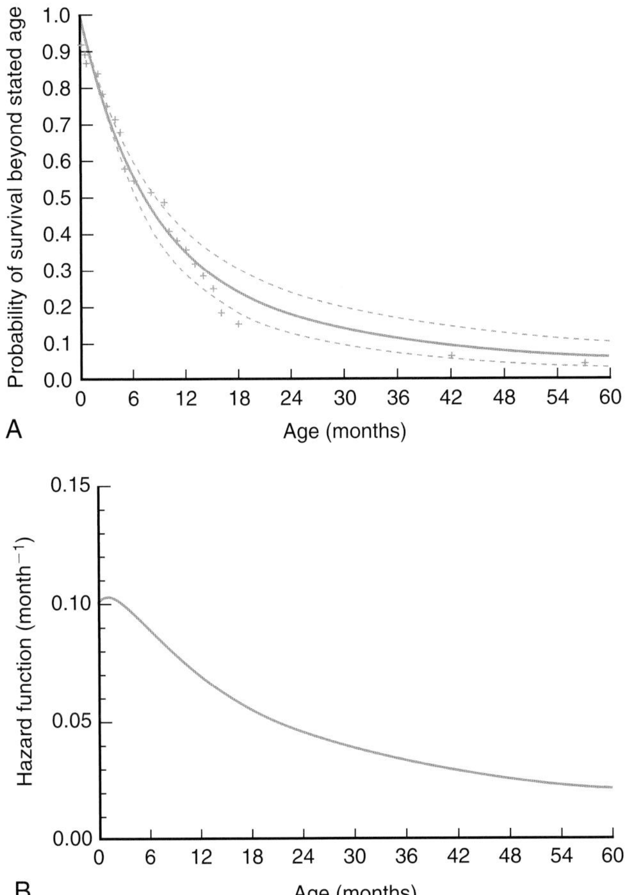

Figure 34-19 Life expectancy without surgery of patients with complete atrioventricular septal defects. **A,** Plus signs represent nonparametric survival estimates; solid line, with its 70% confidence limits *(dotted lines)*, represents parametric survival estimates. Note that probability of surviving beyond 6 months is 50%, and beyond a year is only 30%. **B,** Hazard function according to age. Note that risk of dying is highest in the first few months of life. (From Berger and colleagues.[B11])

- The AV node and bundle of His may be avoided by staying on the LV and left atrial side (McGoon DC: personal communication, 1978) or by staying on the right side of the septum.[S15]
- Contiguous surfaces of the LSL and LIL may be sutured together, or the left AV valve may be left as a tricuspid structure.[C2,R6]
- The patch may be attached to leaflet tissue by simple sutures or by pledgeted mattress sutures with some sort of sandwich method,[S15] with assortment of techniques employed to establish AV valve competence.[C2]

Methods described in this chapter are the product of experiences in several centers and have improved surgical results. They avoid functionally important damage to the conduction system, provide complete and permanent closure of interatrial and interventricular communications, and are suitable for the many variations across the spectrum of AV septal defects. They are well adapted to cases with major associated cardiac anomalies. They retain AV valve competence when it is present, minimize occurrence of valve repair dehiscence, and generally abolish or lessen AV valve regurgitation, although in this regard the results are imperfect, particularly in patients without interventricular communications.[K6,S15] The same improvements have been obtained while retaining the single-patch technique. Addition of intraoperative transesophageal echocardiography (TEE) to assess completeness of repair provides a further safeguard against an imperfect anatomic and functional result.[R9]

Repair of Complete Atrioventricular Septal Defect with Little or No Bridging of Left Superior and Left Inferior Leaflets: Rastelli Type A

Two-Patch Technique

After the usual preparations, a median sternotomy is made, a large piece of pericardium is removed and set aside, and pericardial stay sutures are applied. External cardiac anatomy is evaluated and a left superior vena cava sought. If one is present, there is a 50% chance of associated unroofed coronary sinus syndrome. Purse-string sutures are placed.

In patients weighing less than 5 kg, repair may be performed with limited cardiopulmonary bypass (CPB) with a single venous cannula and hypothermic circulatory arrest; in larger patients, standard CPB is used. Alternatively, in both infants and older children, hypothermic CPB at 20°C and cold cardioplegia may be used. In this method, the cavae are cannulated directly with thin-walled, right-angled metal cannulae (see "Venous Cannulation" in Section III of Chapter 2). CPB flow is reduced to about 1.2 $L \cdot min^{-1} \cdot m^{-2}$ when the patient's temperature reaches 20°C. Short periods of circulatory arrest or low flow perfusion are occasionally used if visibility is not excellent. As cooling proceeds, the aorta is clamped, and cold cardioplegic solution is injected. The right atrium is opened widely, and a sump sucker is passed through the foramen ovale into the left atrium. Stay sutures are applied.

The malformation is examined and each morphologic detail noted (Fig. 34-20). Morphology of the LSL and LIL is noted carefully with the leaflets in both the closed and open positions. Cold saline solution is injected once or twice through the valve and the closure pattern and any regurgitant leaks studied (Fig. 34-21, *A-C*). The most anterior point of LSL-LIL opposing edges is found, and a double-armed 6-0 or 7-0 polypropylene suture is placed through it. Leaflet stay and marking sutures are placed, measurements are made, and the polyester interventricular patch is trimmed.

The patch is sutured to the right side of the crest of the ventricular septum with continuous polypropylene suture (Fig. 34-21, *D* and *E*). Chordae of the RSL and RIL stay on the right ventricular side of the patch; those of the LSL and LIL stay on the LV side, and some may be cut if they interfere with the suturing, because the anterior edges of these leaflets will be sutured to the polyester patch.

When this phase is completed, the marking suture on the anterior edges of the coapting surfaces of the LSL-LIL complex is passed through the appropriate point of the edge of the polyester ventricular defect patch. The pericardial interatrial patch is then trimmed to appropriate shape and size, and the first part of its insertion is accomplished (Fig. 34-21, *F*). For this, interrupted mattress sutures of 5-0 or 6-0 polyester are placed to enclose anterior edges of the LSL and LIL between the polyester patch below and pericardial patch above. Alternatively, left-sided leaflet tissue is anchored as a separate maneuver to the polyester patch; the pericardial atrial

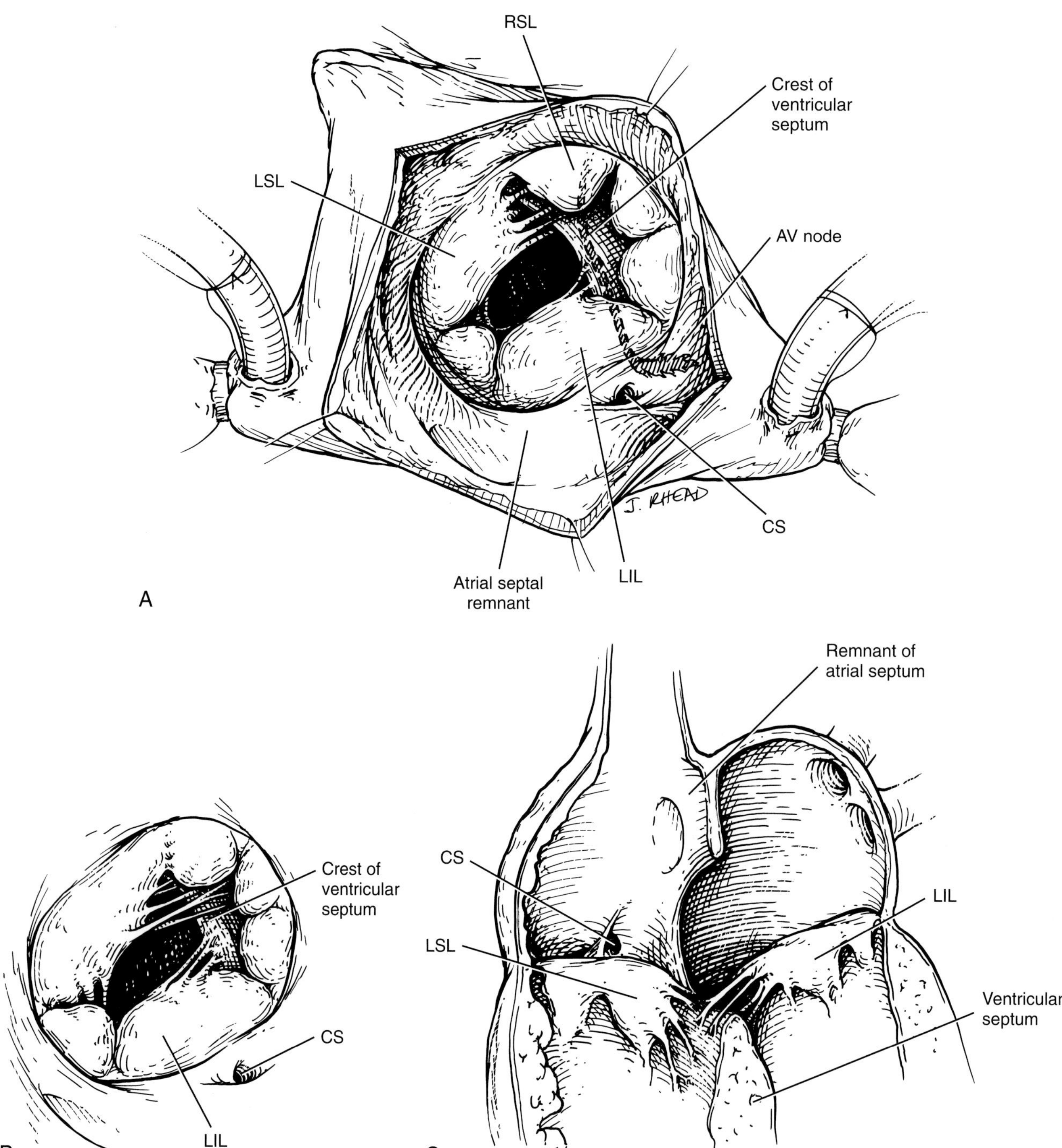

Figure 34-20 Repair of complete atrioventricular *(AV)* septal defect; right atrial view, showing two variations of bridging. **A,** Bridging grade 1. **B,** Bridging grade 4. In both there is a common AV orifice and interventricular communication. AV node lies on right side of inferior (caudad) atrial septal remnant at its junction with floor of right atrium over crux cordis. Node pierces abnormally formed central fibrous body to become the short penetrating portion of bundle of His. This structure immediately becomes the branching bundle, which gives off left bundle branches earlier than normal as it travels along crest of ventricular septum. **C,** Cross-section through AV septal defect with common AV valve orifice showing mild bridging of left inferior leaflet *(LIL)* and scooped-out crest of ventricular septum. View is anterior to posterior. Key: *CS,* Coronary sinus; *LSL,* left superior leaflet; *RSL,* right superior leaflet.

septal patch is then sewn to the leaflet-patch line of attachment. Great care is taken to ensure alignment of left AV valve leaflets is perfect and without distortion during this process.

Saline solution is again injected through the left-sided portion of the AV valves (two orifices are present once the interventricular patch is in place) to study its closure pattern and competence. A few additional "tailoring sutures" are placed without tension along the coapting surfaces of the LSL and LIL near the patch, if needed, to prevent systolic eversion or prolapse; usually they are not required. If a central leak (at the point of junction of LSL, LIL, and LLL) persists, an

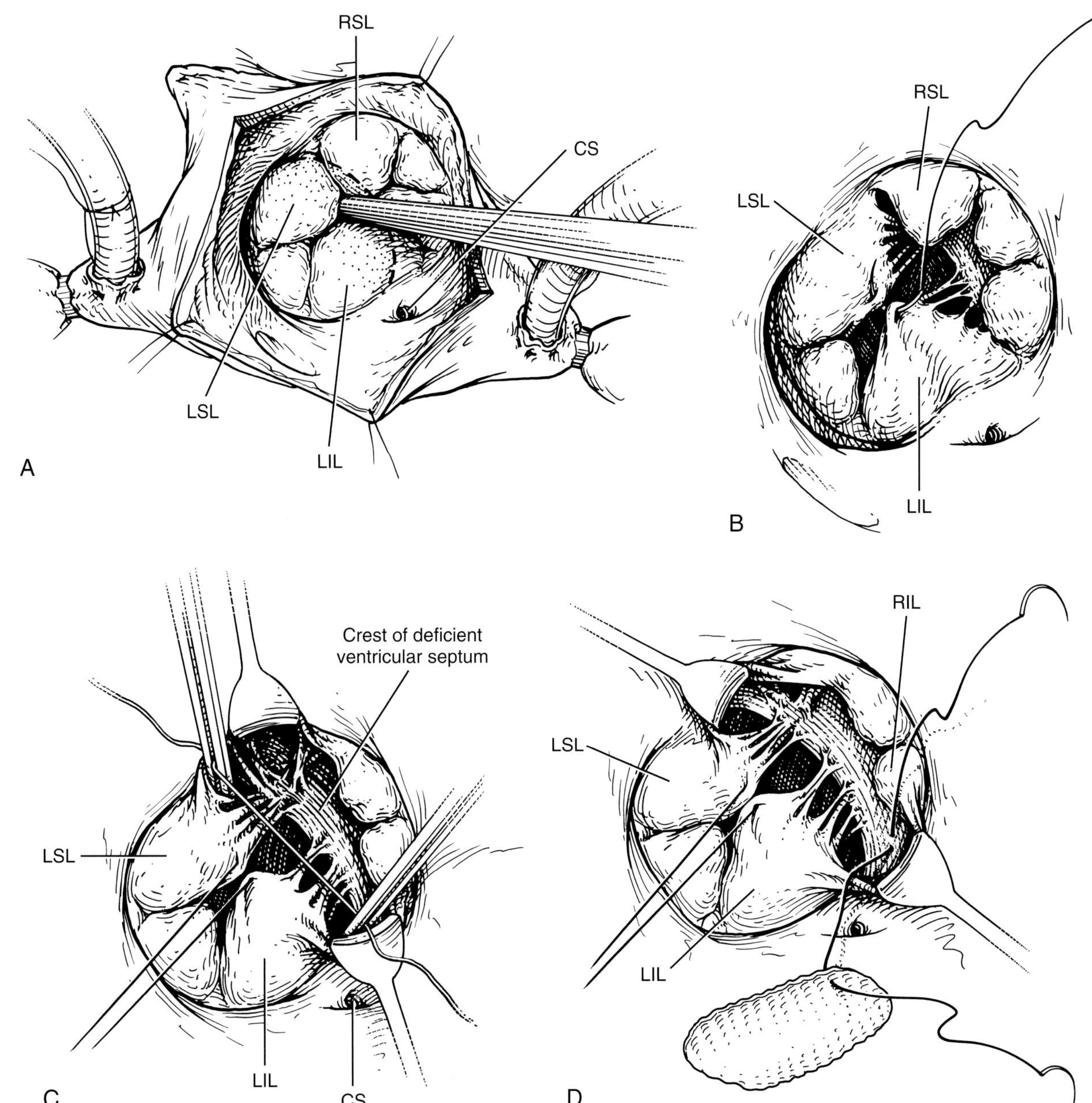

Figure 34-21 Repair of complete atrioventricular (AV) septal defect. **A,** After right atrium is opened, valve leaflets are often closed exactly as they are in systole. If, instead, they are open, saline is injected into left ventricle to close them. At this point, morphology of the leaflets, particularly their closure pattern, is studied and information obtained is used to plan repair of any regurgitation present or accommodate any lack of left AV valve tissue. **B,** A fine polypropylene suture is placed between left superior leaflet *(LSL)* and left inferior leaflet *(LIL)* in position shown (anterior aspect) and left loose. **C,** Leaflets are allowed to open, and details of atrial and ventricular septal deficiencies and of interatrial and interventricular communications are studied. Position of coronary sinus *(CS)* is noted, and course of the unseen AV node and bundle of His is conceptualized by surgeon from knowledge of the anatomy. Leaflets are retracted as much as possible and projected width (shown here) and depth of AV patch estimated. Planned suture line of interventricular patch to ventricular septum and free wall is thus visualized by surgeon. **D,** Polyester ventricular patch is trimmed to a flat, rectangular-pyramidal shape. Suture line may begin anywhere along ventricular septum, but it must be on the right ventricular side of all chordae from left-sided leaflets, including those from any bridging components of the LIL. Retractor in right inferior aspect of the common valve marks position in which base of right inferior leaflet *(RIL)* is sandwiched between ventricular and atrial patches. Suture line here stays well back from crest of interventricular septum and catches some of the base of the RIL to avoid the bundle of His. *Continued*

anuloplasty stitch is placed in the region of the commissure between the LSL and LLL. If necessary and if the orifice is large enough, a similar stitch can be placed at the LLL-LIL commissure, the surgeon being certain not to approach the AV node. This part of the operation is critically important and requires patience and ingenuity (see "Repair of Complete or Partial Atrioventricular Septal Defect with Moderate or Severe Left Atrioventricular Valve Regurgitation" under Technique of Operation).

Assessment of both the left and right AV valves at this point includes consideration of their size. The diameter of each is estimated with Hegar dilators and considered

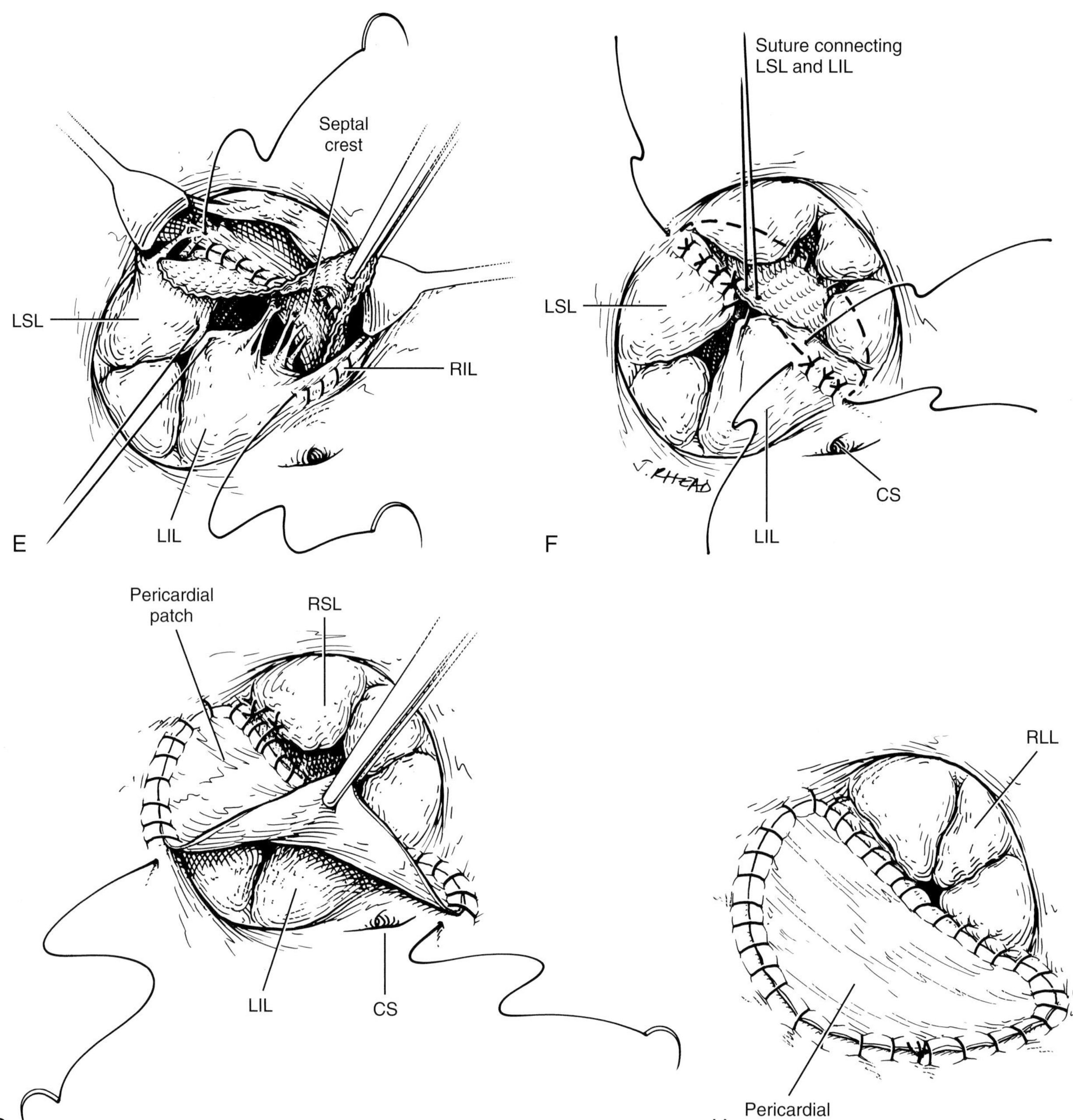

Figure 34-21, cont'd **E,** Suture line for interventricular patch is completed anteriorly, retracting defect posteriorly and elevating the RSL to expose the aspect of the defect closest to left ventricular outflow tract. Width of patch at the valve level will be less than its width deeper on ventricular septum level. **F,** Left superior leaflet *(LSL)* and left inferior leaflet *(LIL)* are precisely anchored to ventricular septal patch using fine interrupted simple or mattress sutures. It is here that care is taken to ensure that the left-sided valve apparatus at the patch is appropriately narrow so as not to create regurgitation and at the correct height so as not to produce left ventricular outflow tract narrowing (too low) or left AV valve regurgitation (too high). To provide accuracy, the previously placed fine stay suture joining LSL and LIL is positioned approximately at midpoint of the suture line. **G,** Pericardial patch for closure of the atrial defect is trimmed to size and a new suture line is begun with bites incorporating pericardial patch, left AV valve tissue (at its junction with the top of the polyester patch), and polyester patch, sandwiching delicate left AV valve tissue between pericardium and fabric. Initial suturing at crest of polyester patch can be done with the pericardial patch folded leftward toward left AV valve. Conduction system is avoided by extending the pericardium to the right of the coronary sinus, leaving its drainage to left atrium. Competence of left (and right) AV valve is next tested with saline injection. If necessary, small anuloplasty sutures can be placed between LSL and left lateral leaflet (LLL) and between LIL and LLL. **H,** Remainder of pericardial patch is sutured inferiorly and then superiorly to rim of atrial defect, often also incorporating closure of foramen ovale defect. Key: *RLL,* Right lateral leaflet; *RSL,* right superior leaflet.

acceptable if within 2 SD of normal for the size of the patient (z value is −2 or greater; see Chapter 1, Appendix 1D, Table 1D-2).

Repair is completed by suturing the rest of the pericardial interatrial patch in place, with the suture line passing *around* the AV node and bundle of His and not across them (Fig. 34-21, *G* and *H*). The right-sided leaflets are usually not sutured to the patch because they close competently without this. If any commissural tissue between the LSL and RSL or LIL and RIL is cut, the right side of this (as well as the left side) is sutured to the patch.

Rewarming of the patient is begun (see "Completing Cardiopulmonary Bypass" in Section III of Chapter 2). A few sutures are placed, but not pulled up or tied, for closure of the foramen ovale. Air is evacuated through the foramen ovale, and the aortic clamp is removed with suction on the needle vent.

The first stitch for closure of the right atriotomy is placed at its inferior angle, and closure of the right atriotomy is continued up to the midportion. Usually, cardiac action has begun by then, so the pump sump-sucker is removed from the right atrium and sutures closing the foramen ovale are tied, with care taken to avoid trapping air in the left atrium. The remainder of the right atrium is closed and caval tapes released. Assessment at this stage of the morphologic and functional result by two-dimensional color flow Doppler TEE is useful.[S7] If important abnormalities are present, CPB and cardioplegia are reestablished and corrections made. Otherwise, the remainder of the operation is completed in the usual manner (see "Completing Cardiopulmonary Bypass" in Section III of Chapter 2 and "Cold Cardioplegia, Controlled Aortic Root Reperfusion, and [When Needed] Warm Cardioplegic Induction" in Chapter 3). Left and right atrial and pulmonary artery pressure-monitoring catheters are placed.

Alternatively, when hypothermic circulatory arrest is used in infants, circulatory arrest is continued until the right atrium is closed, provided the procedure can be completed within 45 minutes (which is usually possible). The single venous cannula is then reinserted, the heart is de-aired, CPB for rewarming is begun, and the remainder of the procedure continues as usual. (For repair that requires more than 45 minutes, the sequence described in Chapter 2, Section IV, is adopted.)

Repair of Complete Atrioventricular Septal Defect with Bridging of Left Superior Leaflet: Rastelli Type B or C

Repair is similar to that just described, but special consideration is given to the LSL. Whether bridging is moderate (Rastelli type B) or marked (Rastelli type C), the commissure between it and the RSL is generally only slightly on the right ventricular side of the intersection of the atrial (and ventricular) septum with the anulus. This location is critically important because, again, suturing for insertion of the interventricular polyester patch usually begins in the anulus at the level of this commissural tissue. If suturing in the anulus is too far anterior—that is, too far on the right ventricular side of the junction of anulus with atrial septum—either by error or because the LSL-RSL commissure is far anterior, the right AV valve orifice will be too narrow. Narrowing of its orifice can also be produced by attaching the

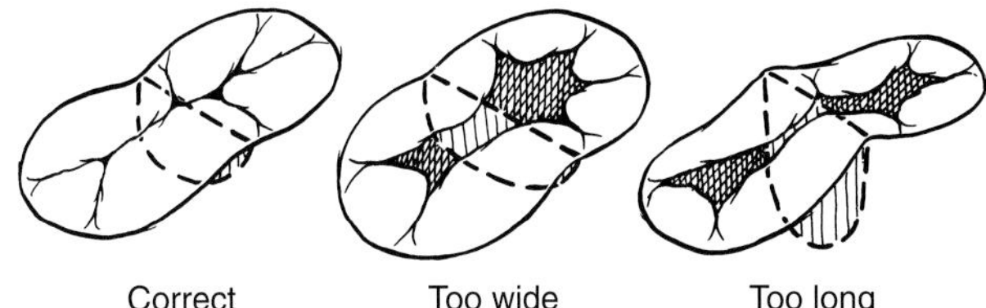

Figure 34-22 Depiction of ventricular septal portion of two-patch technique. If patch is too wide, theoretically left ventricular outlet flow obstruction may be produced. If patch is too long, with level of atrioventricular (AV) valves too high, there is a high probability of left AV valve regurgitation. (Modified from Lacour-Gayet and colleagues.[L1])

interventricular polyester patch too far to the right of the crest of the septum with the first few superior (cephalad) stitches. Compensation too far leftward narrows the LV outflow tract.

The interventricular patch is slid beneath the chordae going from the right extremity of the LSL to right ventricular papillary muscles. The interventricular patch must have appropriate dimensions and configuration (Fig. 34-22). If the patch is excessively wide (in a superior-inferior direction), there is greater likelihood of postoperative LV outflow tract obstruction. If the patch is excessively long (deep, in a caudad-cephalad direction), there is a greater likelihood of left AV valve regurgitation.

Incising the LSL from its free edge to the anulus is rarely necessary, although in extreme cases in which a small right AV valve would otherwise result, it may be done, with both divided edges later sutured onto the interventricular polyester patch.

Repair of Complete Atrioventricular Septal Defect with Single-Patch Technique

Repair using a single patch differs from the two-patch technique in the following ways: (1) the single patch is almost always pericardium, (2) tailoring the waist of the patch (at the level of the AV valves) is critical, and (3) both the LSL and RSL and the LIL and RIL are sutured to the patch. Setup using bicaval cannulation is the same as for the two-patch technique, making sure that the inferior vena cava cannula is placed well caudad at the cavoatrial junction. CPB is established at 20°C to 24°C, and antegrade cardioplegia is infused after aortic clamping. The right atrial incision is made and atrial exposure is arranged as for the two-patch technique. The most anterior point of LSL-LIL apposing edges is identified, and a 6-0 polypropylene suture is placed to retain that apposing relationship. Bridging leaflets superiorly and occasionally inferiorly are incised laterally to the valve anulus (Fig. 34-23, *A*). This maneuver allows easy later exposure for closing the intraventricular portion of the defect and accommodating the waist of the patch.

The patch for the ventricular septal closure is inserted using continuous polypropylene or interrupted synthetic braided mattress sutures. Generally the initial suture is placed at the midpoint of the ventricular defect and is continued upward anteriorly (Fig. 34-23, *B*). Posteriorly, the suture line stays behind the rim of the defect to avoid conduction fibers. Both left and right AV valve leaflets are then anchored to the waist of the patch using double-pledgeted horizontal mattress sutures (Fig. 34-23, *C*). Pledgets are

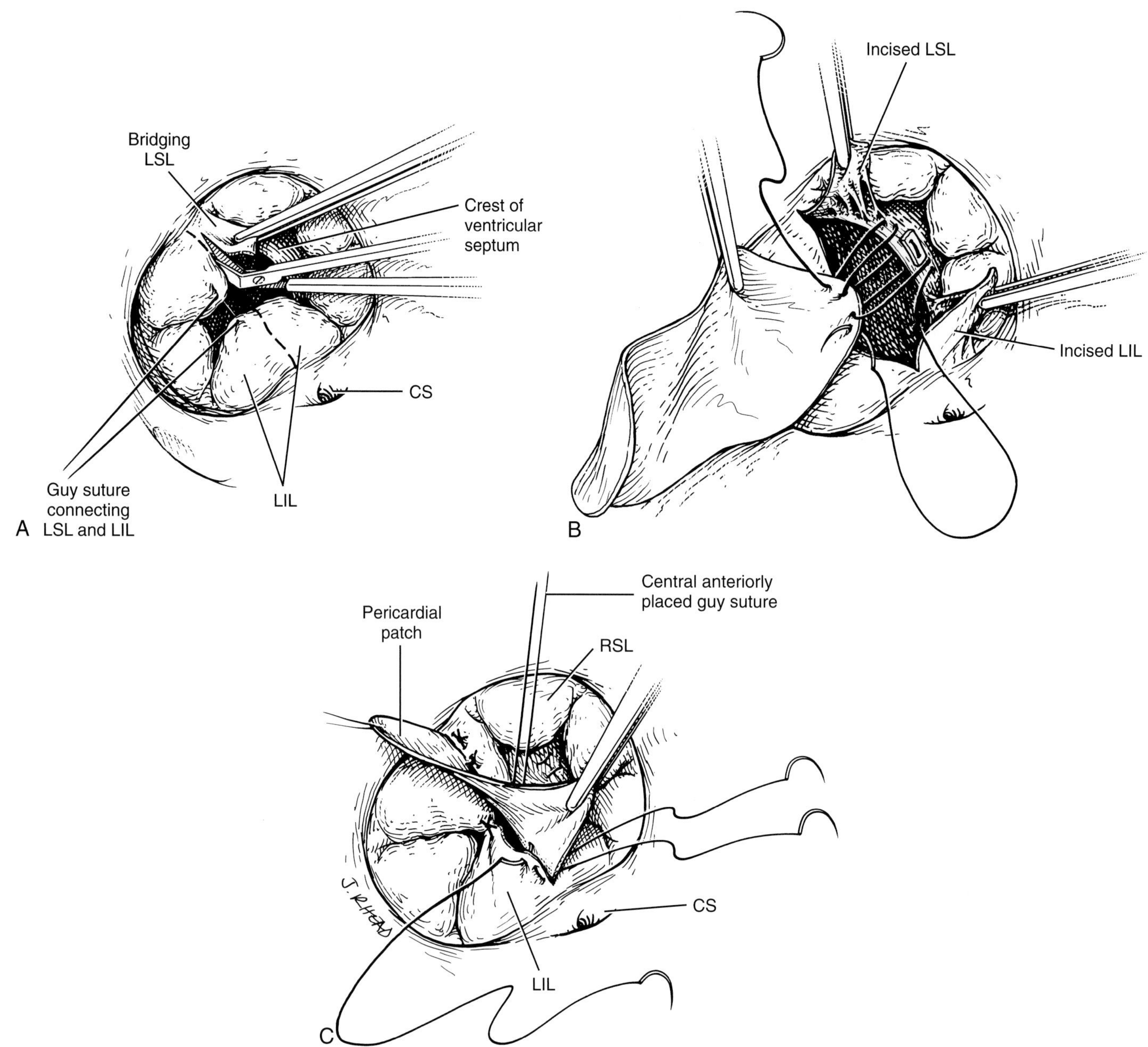

Figure 34-23 Complete atrioventricular (AV) septal defect repair, single-patch technique. **A,** Right atriotomy is made as for two-patch technique and AV valves are inspected. Saline is infused into ventricles as for two-patch technique, and apposition point of left superior leaflet *(LSL)* and left inferior leaflet *(LIL)* is identified as the leaflets float up to their systolic position. A fine guy suture is placed for alignment and left loose. Frequently, the bridging LSL or LIL is incised to gain access to the anterior portion of interventricular defect. Later, each cut edge of the superior leaflet will be attached to pericardial patch at its waist. **B,** Fresh or glutaraldehyde-treated pericardial patch is trimmed partially after measuring height and width of interventricular communication. Generally, ventricular portion of patch is attached to right side of crest of ventricular septum using a continuous suture initiated at the deepest aspect (midpoint) of the rim of the ventricular septal defect *(VSD)*. Usual precautions are taken as in the two-patch technique to avoid the bundle of His at posterior-inferior aspect of ventricular defect. **C,** AV leaflets, both left and right, are attached to pericardial patch at appropriate level. As in the two-patch technique, the central guy suture, which approximates the gap between LSL and LIL, helps position the AV valves at correct height and midpoint on the single pericardial patch. Interrupted horizontal mattress sutures incorporate bites of right-sided valve tissue, pass through pericardium, and end with bites of left-sided valve tissue. Small pledgets of pericardium may be used to buttress sutures on left and right AV valve tissue. Several additional sutures complete closure of gap between LSL and LIL.

generally of pericardium; often a single strip is used on the left-sided aspect. The strip is made a little shorter than the anteroposterior width of the anulus to somewhat narrow the anulus and contribute to AV valve competency. The level of this suture line (in a cephalad-caudad direction) must ensure that height of the AV valve anulus is such that left AV valve regurgitation is avoided (patch too high) and LV outflow obstruction is not produced (patch too low). At this point, the LV is loaded by saline injection to test valve competency and VSD closure. The left AV valve cleft is closed

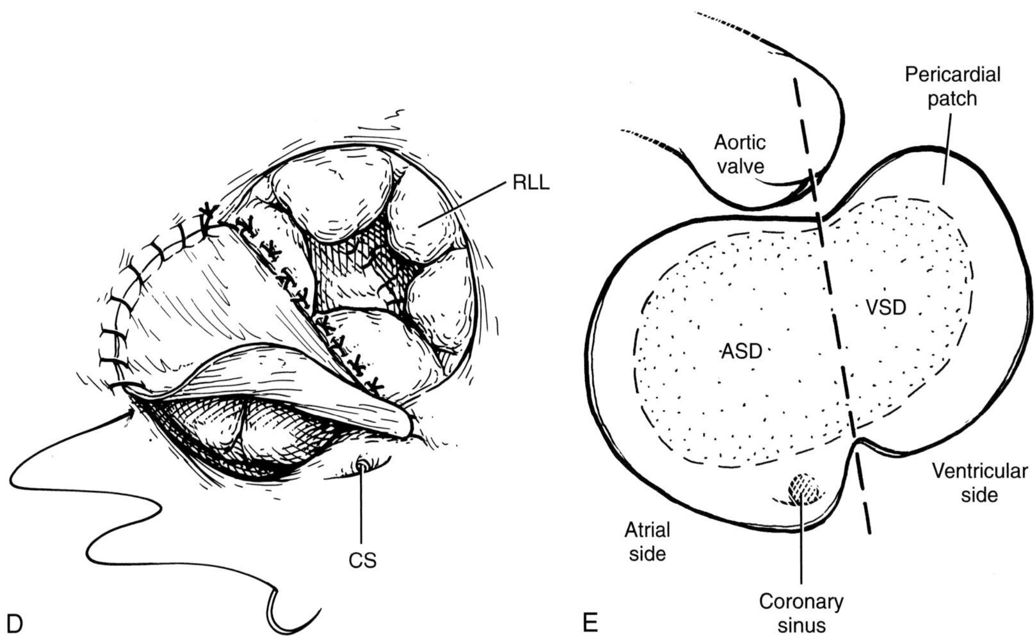

Figure 34-23, cont'd D, Atrial portion of patch is completed with continuous suture extending inferiorly and medially to place coronary sinus *(CS)* on left atrial side, incorporating any foramen ovale defect within superior rim of patch. Before completing atrial septal patch insertion, the atrioventricular valves are tested by saline infusion and anuloplasty is done as necessary. **E,** Approximate configuration of pericardial patch for single patch technique. Height and width of waist (indicated by *dashed line*) are critical. Key: *ASD,* Atrial portion of atrioventricular septal defect; *RSL,* right superior leaflet; *RLL,* right lateral leaflet.

with fine interrupted sutures at its opposing edges to the previously placed marking suture. At this point if necessary, anuloplasty sutures (horizontal mattress) are placed at the two lateral commissures. Repair of the remaining atrial defect proceeds as for the two-patch technique (Fig. 34-23, *D*), outside the rim of the coronary sinus and including the foramen ovale defect. The completed single pericardial patch has a lopsided, dumbbell-shaped configuration (Fig. 34-23, *E*).

Repair of Complete Atrioventricular Septal Defect with Modified Single-Patch Technique

In 1997, Wilcox and colleagues reported direct suturing of the AV valves to the ventricular septum in complete AV septal defects with a small ventricular component.[W6] Others extended the application of this technique to all forms of complete AV septal defects.[N3,N5] The advantages of this procedure are (1) simplicity by avoiding a separate patch for VSD closure, (2) no division of valve leaflets or chordae, and (3) reduced operative time.

Key features of the procedure are illustrated in Fig. 34-24. Interrupted pledgeted 5-0 braided sutures are placed on the right side of the interventricular septal crest (as in the ventricular septal suture line of the standard ventricular patch technique) and passed through the bridging LSL and LIL. These sutures are then passed through the edge of the autologous pericardial patch used to close the atrial defect and through a thin strip of polyester whose length is slightly shorter than the corresponding ventricular septum, with the intent of producing a central anuloplasty of the LSL and LIL. These sutures are tied, and the remainder of the operation proceeds as in the single- or two-patch techniques.

Nunn and colleagues reported uniform application for all patients with complete AV septal defects, 30-day mortality of less than 2%, no reoperations for residual VSDs, and no reoperations for LV outflow tract obstruction out to a median follow-up of 7.3 years.[N5] This procedure has now been widely applied in the setting of shallow ventricular defects. General acceptance of its wider application to all defects awaits analyses from other institutions.

Repair of Partial Atrioventricular Septal Defect with Little or No Left Atrioventricular Valve Regurgitation

Repair is similar to that described for complete AV septal defects, but no interventricular polyester patch is required. After CPB is established, intraatrial exposure is arranged, cold cardioplegic solution infused, and morphology studied. Attachments of the LSL and LIL to the crest of the ventricular septum are probed to be certain there are no small interventricular communications.

The "cleft" in the AV valve is then identified and its medial and septal extremities noted (Fig. 34-25, *A-C*). In the past, if there were no left AV valve regurgitation, nothing was done to the valve at the cleft (commissure). More recently, most surgeons obliterate this gap (close the cleft) using several interrupted simple sutures or pericardial pledgeted mattress sutures. The margins here are characterized by slightly thickened and rolled edges, and it is at these margins that sutures are based.

An anuloplasty stitch may also be placed at the LSL-LLL commissure. The intraatrial pericardial patch is sewn into place in the same way used for repairing complete AV septal defect (Fig. 34-25, *D*; see also Fig. 34-21). Small, pledgeted mattress sutures of 5-0 or 6-0 polyester are passed from the right ventricular side through the base of the RIL and the

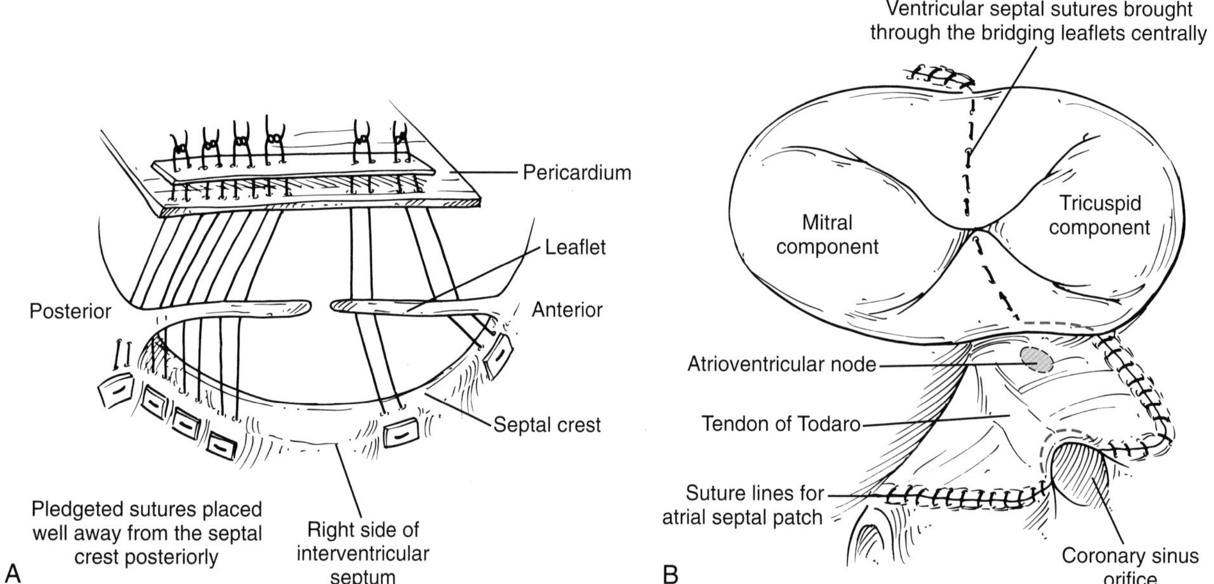

Figure 34-24 Repair of complete atrioventricular septal defect with modified single-patch technique. **A,** Cross-section through defect with atrial and ventricular communications. **B,** Interrupted pledgeted 5-0 braided sutures are placed on right side of interventricular septal crest (as in the ventricular septal suture line of standard ventricular patch technique) and passed through bridging left superior leaflet *(LSL)* and left inferior leaflet *(LIL)*. These sutures are then passed through edge of autologous pericardial patch used to close the atrial defect and through a thin strip of Dacron whose length is slightly shorter than the corresponding ventricular septum, with the intent of producing a central anuloplasty of the LSL and LIL. These sutures are tied, and remainder of operation proceeds as in single- or two-patch techniques. (From Nunn.[N5])

bridging part of the LIL and through the pericardial patch. More cephalad, the patch is sewn to fibrous valvar tissue attached to the crest of the ventricular septum in this reinforced manner, analogous to its suturing to the top of the polyester patch (see Fig. 34-21).

Repair of Atrioventricular Septal Defect with Small Interchordal Interventricular Communications (Intermediate Form)

When two AV valve orifices are present but small interventricular communications exist between thick, short chordae attaching the LSL to the crest of the ventricular septum, repair is simple. The interventricular communication is simply closed by taking the anterior portion of the pericardial patch just to the right side of the septal crest, catching the base of the LSL with each stitch.

When the interventricular communications are beneath the LIL, the same maneuver may be followed. However, because of the bundle of His, care must be taken to keep the suture line well away from the crest of the septum and to attach the patch in the same manner in which the interventricular patch is attached in repair of complete AV septal defects.

Repair of Atrioventricular Septal Defect with Common Atrium

When a common atrium is present, either with or without an interventricular communication, special effort is made to ensure that there is no left superior vena cava or, if one is present, that there is not a completely unroofed coronary sinus, which would change the repair (see Technique of Operation in Chapter 33).

Repair is accomplished by sewing an appropriately larger pericardial patch to the atrial wall on the left atrial side of the orifice of the inferior vena cava, to the right of the right pulmonary veins, and beneath the superior vena cava (where there is usually a small septal remnant).

Repair of Complete or Partial Atrioventricular Septal Defect with Moderate or Severe Left Atrioventricular Valve Regurgitation

For repair of an AV septal defect with moderate or severe left AV valve regurgitation, results seem to vary from one institution to another, even when the same techniques have apparently been used.

In the repair of complete AV septal defects, the primary determinant of left AV valve competence, particularly when preoperative AV valve regurgitation is moderate or less, is accurate sizing of the ventricular patch (or patch component) to produce an anuloplasty effect (width somewhat less than the combined width of the LSL and LIL) and avoiding elevation by the patch of the LSL and LIL above their pre-repair level (see Fig. 34-22). If the size and placement of the patch have been imperfect, this should be corrected.

If the patch and its placement are considered optimal, the basic options depend on observations about location and mechanism of regurgitation by filling the LV with saline:

- If the major leakage is between the LSL and LIL, the "cleft" is partially or completely closed with interrupted 5-0 polypropylene or braided sutures, which may be reinforced with small bovine pericardial pledgets if the leaflet tissue is fragile.

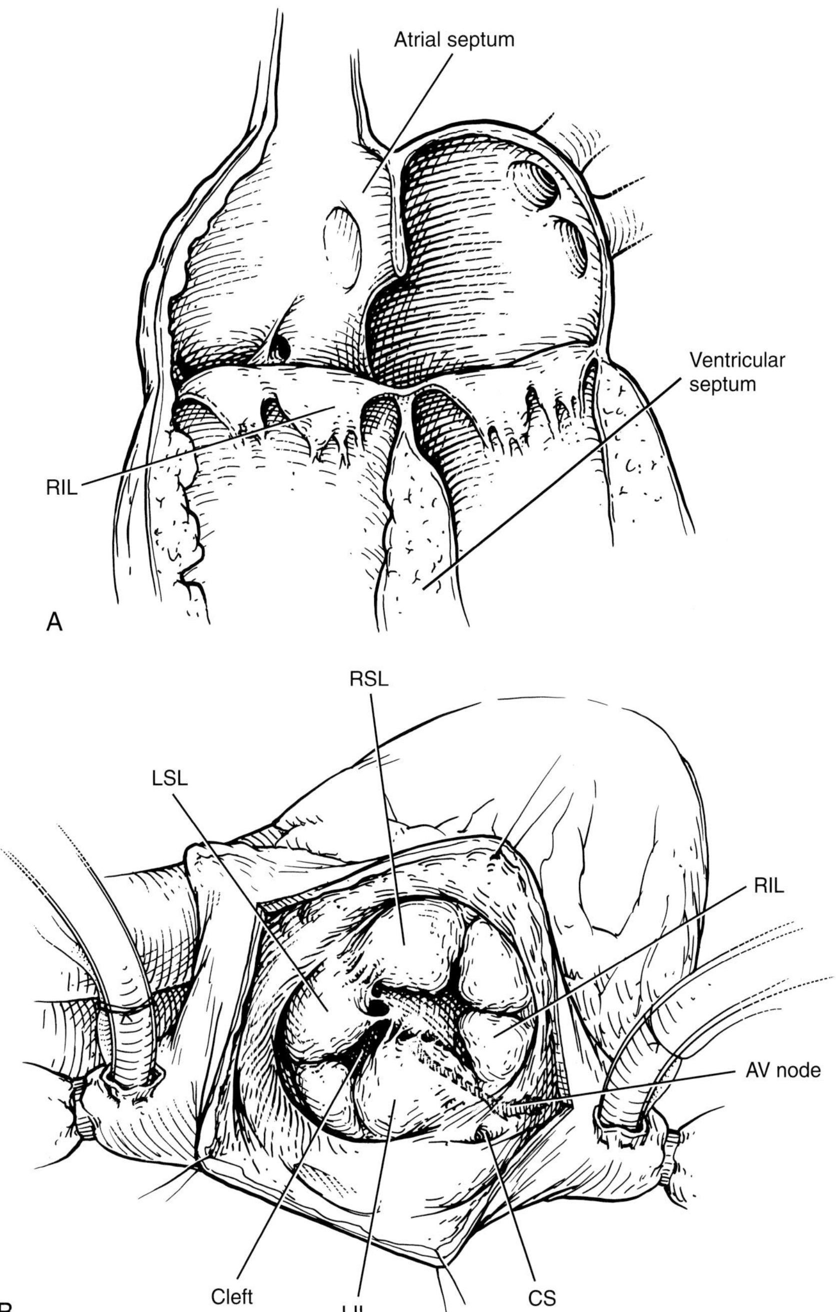

Figure 34-25 Repair of partial atrioventricular *(AV)* septal defect. **A,** Cross-section through defect with an atrial communication and intact ventricular septum. **B,** Right atrium is opened in a superior-to-inferior direction. (Inferior vena cava cannula is placed well caudal.) Atrial defect (primum ASD) is seen with its inferior border composed partially of AV valve tissue. A search is made for interventricular communications as the left-sided AV valve is tested for regurgitation by saline infusion. Extent of cleft is seen and any regurgitation through it identified. *Continued*

- If the leakage is central or at the commissure between the LLL and LSL or between the LLL and LIL, anuloplasty sutures (with or without pledgets) are placed to reduce anular circumference. In cases of marked central leakage and an enlarged orifice, a more extensive anuloplasty of the LLL and its commissures using a polytetrafluoroethylene band has been reported.[K5]
- If leakage is through accessory clefts, they may be partially closed. When the repair is completed and leakage is trivial or absent by saline injection, the remaining orifice is sized with Hegar dilators; a measured diameter yielding a z value of -2 or greater is generally adequate to avoid valve stenosis.

In the presence of persistent moderate to severe residual regurgitation (particularly in the reoperative setting) despite the maneuvers described above, two other more radical techniques may be applied:

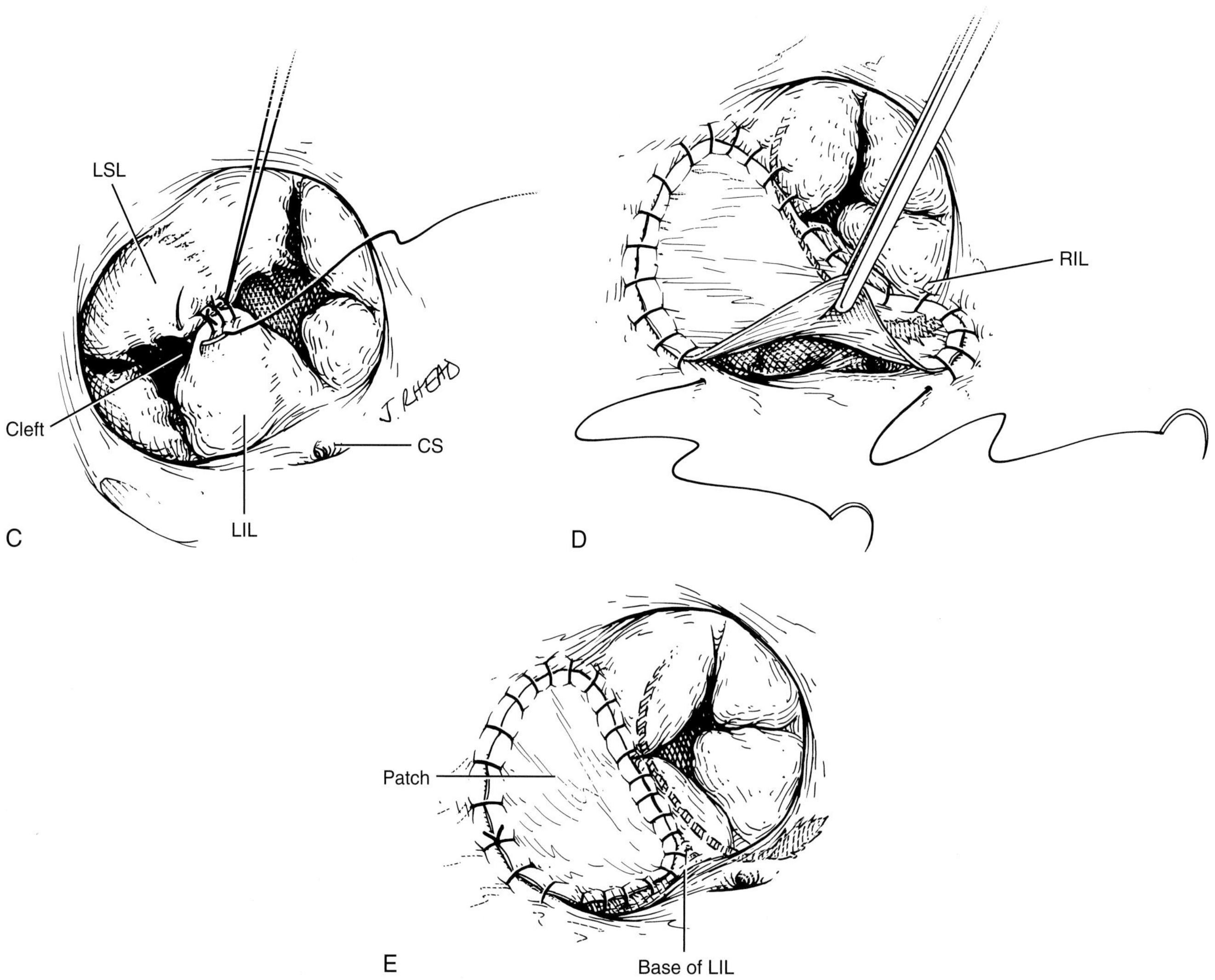

Figure 34-25, cont'd **C,** Cleft is closed with interrupted sutures; if necessary, anuloplasty sutures are added. **D,** Defect is closed with a pericardial patch, placed in a fashion similar to that used in the two-patch technique for repair of complete AV septal defect. It is inserted using fine continuous polypropylene suture. Suture line begins at the confluence of left- and right-sided AV valves over ventricular septum and passes rightward and caudally over right inferior leaflet to surround the coronary sinus *(CS)*, leaving coronary sinus draining to left atrium. **E,** An alternative to avoid the conduction system is the McGoon technique. Patch is sutured to base of left-sided valve tissue, and in area near conduction system, superficial bites are taken. Key: *LIL,* Left inferior leaflet; *LSL,* left superior leaflet; *RIL,* right inferior leaflet; *RSL,* right superior leaflet.

- When there is severe central regurgitation, particularly in the presence of leaflet prolapse, the LLL and the reconstructed anterior leaflet may be approximated with a pledgeted mattress suture, creating a double orifice valve[H6,L2,M2,M4,M14] (Fig. 34-26). To avoid physiologic stenosis, care must be taken that the orifice of the reconstructed "mitral" valve is somewhat larger than normal (probably a *z* value of +1 or larger) before placing the approximation suture.
- An additional procedure in the presence of leaflet deficiency that has reported short- and mid-term success[M14,P9,R11] (Fig. 34-27) is patch augmentation of the neoanterior leaflet.

If moderate or severe left AV valve regurgitation remains, repair should be immediately reassessed. If, in the surgeon's judgment, improvement by further repair is possible, the patient is returned to CPB. If no further repair is likely, valve

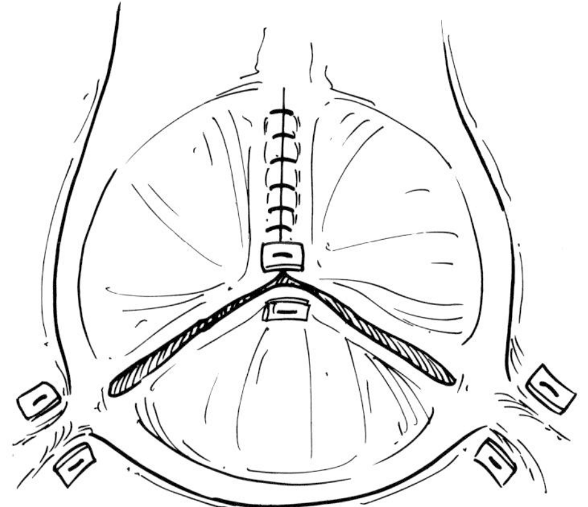

Figure 34-26 Creating a double orifice valve for persistent severe left ventricular valve regurgitation. Lateral leaflet and reconstructed anterior leaflet have been approximated. (From Mitchell and colleagues.[M14])

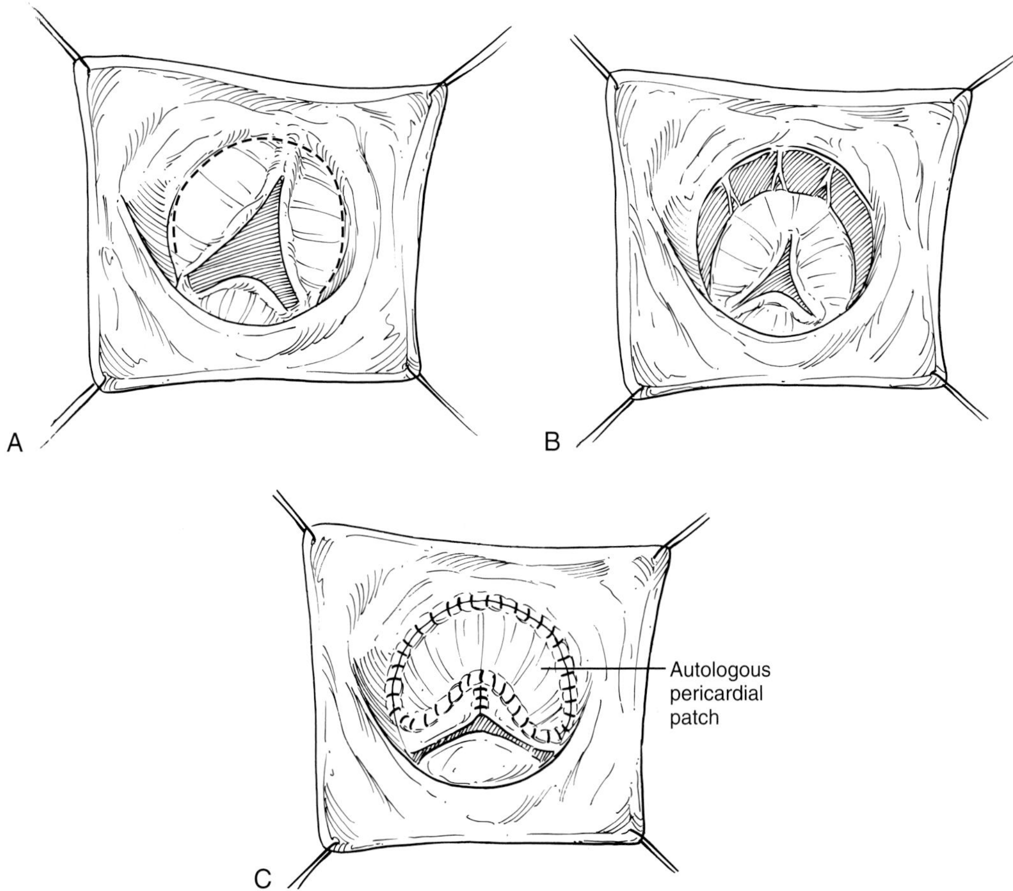

Figure 34-27 Leaflet augmentation technique using glutaraldehyde-treated autologous pericardium for severely dysplastic left atrioventricular valves. **A,** Radial incision adjacent to anulus is made in superior and inferior bridging leaflets from commissure to commissure. **B,** Abnormal secondary chords to ventricular side of leaflet are divided. **C,** Patch of autologous glutaraldehyde-treated pericardium is sutured in place, augmenting anterior leaflet. Tension-free closure of cleft is now possible. Key: *LIL,* Left inferior leaflet; *LLL,* left lateral leaflet; *LSL,* left superior leaflet.

replacement is performed. If the patient is small, no further intervention is feasible, and the infant is managed as well as possible postoperatively.

Right Atrioventricular Valve

In hearts with or without interventricular communications, the right AV valve usually does not require attention. Two-patch repair leaves this valve without a complete "septal leaflet," but in this and other situations, regurgitation does not result. The RSL and RIL (and the RLL) are well supported by chordae, and this, combined with their closure against the polyester patch or bare ventricular septum, generally results in adequate valve function. However, the right AV valve should be analyzed separately with saline injection and Hegar sizing (valve diameter should provide a z value of −2 or greater). If important leakage is identified, it should be surgically addressed. Often, attachment of the RIL to the VSD patch will correct the leakage.

Left Superior Leaflet–Right Superior Leaflet and Left Inferior Leaflet–Right Inferior Leaflet Commissures

Generally, repair of LSL-RSL and LIL-RIL commissures can be made without disturbing the commissural leaflet tissue in these areas. Occasionally, however, these commissural leaflet areas are larger than usual and handicap exposure. Then they may be incised back to the anulus, *once it is certain that this is commissural tissue!* Tissue on the LV side is incorporated into the repair along with the LSL or LIL. That on the right side should be reattached to the patch with a few sutures at the end of the repair.

Replacement of Left Atrioventricular Valve

When severe left AV valve regurgitation cannot be repaired, or when it persists or develops postoperatively, left AV valve replacement may be necessary.[C3] Because the left AV valve nearly always encroaches on the LV outflow tract (see Figs. 34-5, *A* and 34-10), valve replacement may accentuate or produce subaortic stenosis. The prosthesis must therefore be kept away from the subaortic area. This may be accomplished by attaching a rectangular piece of polyester to the anulus of the left AV valve in the subaortic area[M8,P8,P9] (Fig. 34-28). (Poirier and colleagues describe the outcome of eight patients in which similar augmentation was used at reoperation to increase deficient bridging leaflet coaptation without valve replacement.) The prosthesis is then sutured to this artificial mitral-aortic anulus and to the natural anulus for the rest of its circumference. To minimize the chance of damage to the AV node and bundle of His, particular care is taken anteriorly and inferiorly to sew only to the fringe of left AV

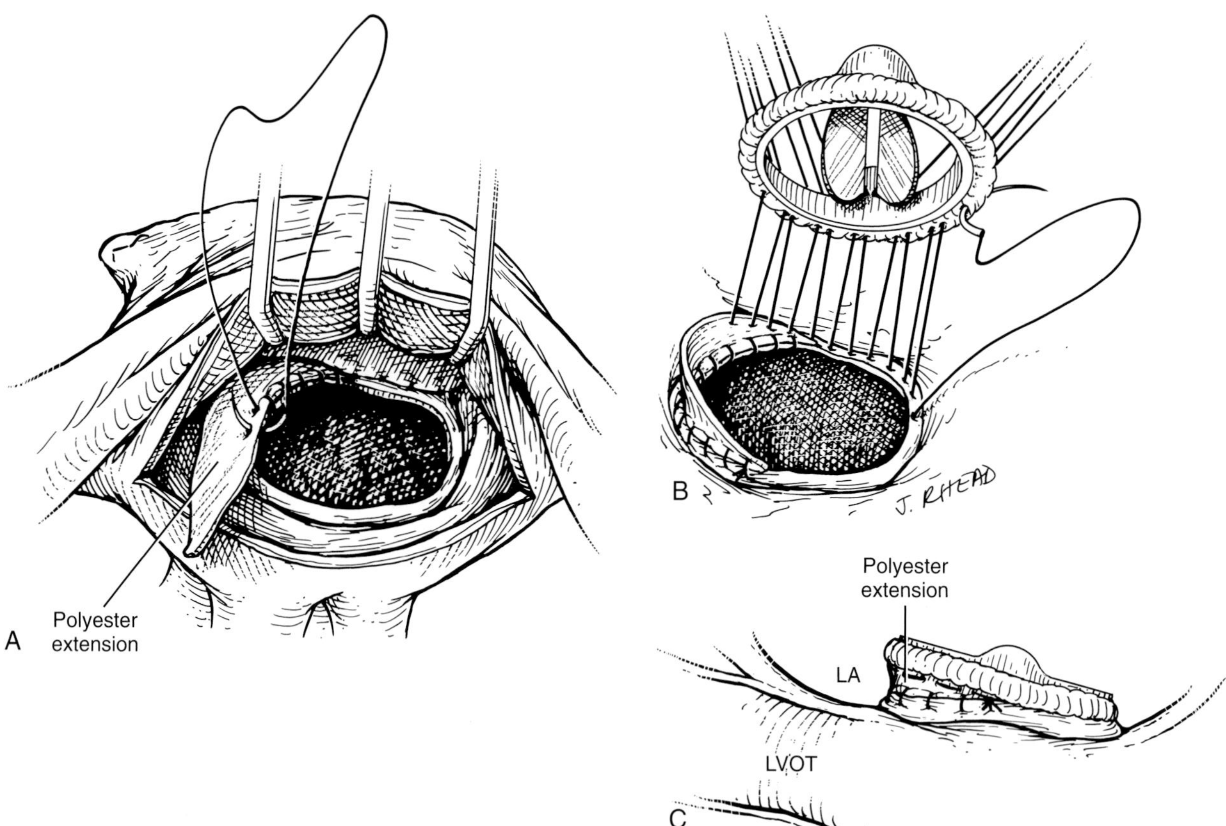

Figure 34-28 Left atrioventricular (AV) valve replacement for regurgitation late after repair of AV septal defect, with an approach through right side of left atrium *(LA)*. **A,** Crescent-shaped piece of polyester patch is sutured to superior aspect of left AV valve anulus, thereby lengthening or creating the "mitral"-aortic septum. Thus, the valve replacement device is well away from left ventricular outflow tract *(LVOT)*. **B,** Valve replacement device is inserted, sutured to free edge of polyester patch superiorly, anulus posteriorly, and undersurface of pericardial patch anteriorly. Using leaflet remnants in this region avoids damage to AV node and bundle of His. **C,** Prosthesis is positioned up out of left ventricular outflow tract and into left atrium.

valve that has been preserved. Alternatively, the prosthesis can be attached in a supraanular position using atrial wall to base the sewing ring. When possible, valve replacement should be deferred until childhood, when risk is less.[K1] This decision is particularly difficult in infants for whom no device of appropriate size is available. Then, even moderate or severe left AV valve regurgitation must be accepted.

Ebels and colleagues have suggested a somewhat different method for avoiding encroachment on the LV tract by the prosthesis.[E1,E3] Their technique involves resecting the atrial fold lying external to the area of fibrous continuity between the aortic leaflets and LSL, presumably along with part of the fibrous continuity. The prosthesis then lies against the aortic valve, rather than in a subvalvar, obstructing position. Clinical evaluation of this method is limited.

Repair of Complete Atrioventricular Septal Defect with Tetralogy of Fallot

In complete AV septal defect associated with tetralogy of Fallot, the large VSD is also juxtaaortic. The LSL bridges moderately (grade 3) or markedly (grades 4 or 5) and is not attached to the crest of the ventricular septum. Any of the types of right ventricular outflow tract obstruction associated with tetralogy of Fallot may be present (see "Convenient Morphologic Categories of Right Ventricular Outflow Obstruction" under Morphology in Section I of Chapter 38), and anterior deviation of the infundibular septum is always present and must be considered in the repair. Preoperative cineangiographic studies are often necessary to delineate the surgically important details of right ventricular outflow obstruction and morphology of the pulmonary arteries.

Operation is begun as for repair of any complete AV septal defect. Before heparinization, however, if a right ventricular outflow patch is required, an appropriately sized patch is prepared as described in Section I of Chapter 38 (see "Decision and Technique for Transanular Patching" under Technique of Operation). The VSD patch is trimmed with a wide superior aspect, which is important in preventing *left* ventricular outflow obstruction.

Usually the anteriorly deviated parietal extension of the infundibular septum (band) can be seen through the AV valve, and it is cut and mobilized (see "Repair of Uncomplicated Tetralogy of Fallot with Pulmonary Stenosis via Right Atrium" under Technique of Operation in Section I of Chapter 38). Other muscular infundibular obstructions can be visualized and resected. The pulmonary valve can be visualized and fused commissures opened. The right ventricular outflow tract is sized with Hegar dilators. At this point the surgeon may decide on a combined right atrial–right ventricular (RA-RV) approach. If so, a small vertical incision is made in the right ventricular outflow tract, and parietal and septal extensions are mobilized and partially resected. This incision is later closed with a small patch.

The interventricular communication is closed by suturing into place a polyester or pericardial patch from this right atrial approach, sequencing the repair exactly as described for other complete AV septal defects. This can be accomplished with a single- or two-patch technique. With either, the shape of the ventricular component of the patch must be modified to account for the anterior-superior extension of the interventricular communication. Familiarity with the atrial approach for repair of isolated VSD (see Technique of Operation in Section I of Chapter 35) and for repair of the VSD in simple tetralogy of Fallot (see "Repair of Uncomplicated Tetralogy of Fallot with Pulmonary Stenosis via Right Atrium" under Technique of Operation in Section I of Chapter 38), as well as familiarity with repair of uncomplicated complete AV septal defects, are important preparations for this procedure. Stay sutures are placed as usual for transatrial repair. Repair is begun at the AV valve anulus superiorly, where the atrial septal remnant meets the anulus.

Care must be taken that repair does not begin too far rightward, in which case the right side of the surgically partitioned AV valve orifice will be too small. Because of the dextroposed aorta, attachment of the VSD patch to tissue over the aortic root (and beneath the commissural tissue and RSL) is particularly important. The patch is generally beneath (on the *left* ventricular side of) chordae attached to the right extremity of the bridging LSL and beneath this leaflet itself. Because this leaflet will be attached to the VSD patch, some of these chordae may be cut to facilitate exposure. In the single-patch technique, the entire bridging leaflet is incised. The suture line is then carried around the interventricular communication and along the base of the RIL as described earlier for the usual complete AV septal defect. When the aorta overrides the interventricular septum to a considerable degree (and when DORV is present), the juxtaaortic portion of the repair may be completed through a small infundibular incision. Remainder of the AV septal defect is repaired as described earlier.

The right ventricular outflow tract is again sized with Hegar dilators. If it is adequate, nothing further is done. Otherwise, it is enlarged by an infundibular patch, or, if necessary, a transanular patch (see "General Plan and Details of Repair Common to All Approaches" under Technique of Operation in Section I of Chapter 38). Moderate or severe pulmonary regurgitation should be avoided because associated right ventricular dilatation may result in severe right AV valve regurgitation from deficiency of right-sided AV valve tissue. Therefore, the threshold for inserting a valve (monocusp or allograft) in the right ventricular outflow tract is lower than usual.

Repair of Complete Atrioventricular Septal Defect with Double Outlet Right Ventricle

When the interventricular communication is large and subaortic, configuration and insertion of the interventricular patch are similar to that just described for tetralogy of Fallot. Pulmonary stenosis, when coexisting, is also treated similarly.

When the interventricular communication is not subaortic and cannot be converted into one by septal excision (see "Intraventricular Tunnel Repair of Double Outlet Right Ventricle with Noncommitted Ventricular Septal Defect" under Technique of Operation in Chapter 53), a Fontan repair (see Technique of Operation in Section IV of Chapter 41) is necessary if pulmonary stenosis coexists.

Repair with Transposition of the Great Arteries

When size of the LV allows it, usual repair of the AV septal defect is carried out and an arterial switch operation is performed (see "Arterial Switch Operation" under Technique of Operation in Chapter 52).

SPECIAL FEATURES OF POSTOPERATIVE CARE

Usual care as described in Chapter 5 is accorded patients after repair of AV septal defects, but certain features require emphasis. Because of the complexity of repair and despite the generally good results now obtained, vigilance must be exercised to detect any important imperfections in the repair. Thus, TEE or transthoracic echocardiography (if the infant is small) is of great help in the operating room and a few hours after the patient's return to the intensive care unit to verify complete closure of the interatrial and interventricular communications and absence of important AV valve regurgitation. Left atrial pressure more than 6 mmHg higher than right atrial pressure raises the possibility of either severe left AV valve regurgitation or stenosis, although it can result simply from small size and low compliance of the LV (see Chapter 5). Height of the *v* wave is not helpful because, as in all circumstances, this correlates more with height of mean left atrial pressure than with degree of regurgitation. Usual prophylaxis is taken against pulmonary hypertensive crises. Generally this includes introducing a pulmonary artery catheter intraoperatively. Because average age at repair has decreased, this complication is seen less frequently now (see "General Care of Neonates and Infants," Section IV of Chapter 5).

If the patient's condition is not optimal and important residual left AV valve regurgitation is suspected—particularly if deterioration continues over several hours—repeat echocardiographic study in the intensive care unit is advisable. If results of this study are inconclusive, left ventriculographic studies (or some other reliable method of quantifying left AV valve regurgitation) should be considered. Indirect indications, both in the operating room and early postoperatively (including absence of a murmur), are unreliable. If severe regurgitation is demonstrated, reoperation is indicated. Likewise, if the patient's condition is unsatisfactory and a large residual left-to-right shunt is present, reoperation is indicated.

When the patient does not convalesce normally, echocardiographic and possibly left ventriculographic studies before hospital discharge are indicated. Because left AV valve repair failure predisposes the patient to death within the first year after operation, consideration should be given to early reoperation if severe regurgitation is found.

RESULTS

Survival

Early (Hospital) Death

Hospital mortality after repair of *partial AV septal defects* has been low for a long time, dating back to the early experience reported from the Mayo Clinic.[R6] In the current era, hospital mortality generally is 1% or less.[M13]

Hospital mortality after repair of uncomplicated *complete AV septal defects* was 30% to 50% during the early years of cardiac surgery, but has declined steadily in recent years. This has been the result of greatly improved understanding of the morphology of this complex malformation, better surgical techniques, and general improvements in cardiac surgery in infants.[G4,K10,M7,M17] These improvements are evident in most major pediatric cardiac surgical programs. Improvement in hospital mortality has been particularly evident in infants.

Major congenital heart disease centers report mortality of under 3% for patients with complete AV septal defects with balanced ventricles undergoing repair in the first 3 to 6 months of life.[C16,K14,S18,W4] As is often the case, results from individual centers of excellence are superior to results from unselected institutional studies. The Pediatric Cardiac Care Consortium reported results of 10 years of activity in 25 institutions within the United States.[M16] Overall operative mortality was 14% and did not differ between Down and non-Down patients. There were a total of 768 cases, averaging three cases per year per institution. This report should be contrasted with individual institutional reports demonstrating low mortality representing caseloads of 20 to 50 yearly.[C16,K14,S18]

Even when complete AV septal defect coexists with other major cardiac anomalies such as tetralogy of Fallot, hospital mortality remains generally low.[K9] However, other less common major associated anomalies with both partial and complete AV septal defects impose a considerable increase in hospital mortality.

Time-Related Survival

Late outcomes are generally good, with reported 15-year survival of 80% to 90%.[C16,H5]

Incremental Risk Factors for Premature Death

Earlier Date of Operation

An earlier date of operation as a risk factor in a surgical experience that covers a large number of years, such as that at UAB (Table 34-11), demonstrates that many risks of repair have been neutralized across the experience.[K8,S15] Others report similar experiences.[A3,C16,H1,H5] The effect of date of operation on outcome is just as evident in long-term events as it is in hospital mortality. This is dramatically evident in predicted 10-year survival after repair of partial and complete AV septal defects in patients operated on in 1967 versus 1977 and 1985 (Fig. 34-29).

Higher New York Heart Association Functional Class

As in most cardiac surgery, severe preoperative disability (higher New York Heart Association [NYHA] functional class) is a risk factor for premature death in both the early and constant hazard phases (see Table 34-11).

Important Pre-Repair Atrioventricular Valve Regurgitation

Important pre-repair regurgitation of either the left AV valve in partial AV septal defects or the common AV valve in complete AV septal defects increases risk of premature death, but only in the constant hazard phase (see Table 34-11). This suggests that post-repair moderate regurgitation, the prevalence of which is almost surely increased by severe preoperative regurgitation in patients with partial AV septal defects but probably less so in patients with complete AV septal defects, is reasonably well tolerated early postoperatively but becomes more serious several months later.[W4] However, severe left AV valve regurgitation is poorly tolerated in infants post-repair and is a risk factor for early mortality (see Table 34-11).

Table 34-11 Incremental Risk Factors (Hazard Function Domain) for Premature Death After Repair of Atrioventricular Septal Defects

Risk Factor	Hazard Phase: Early and Decreasing	Hazard Phase: Constant
Demographic Variables		
Prematurity	•	
Younger age	•	
Clinical Variables		
Higher NYHA class	•	•
Greater severity of preoperative AV valve regurgitation	•[a]	•
Morphologic Variables		
Single papillary muscle	•	
Accessory valve orifice		•
Major associated cardiac anomalies	•	
Severe LV hypoplasia	•	•
Surgical Variables		
Earlier date of operation	•	
Interaction with age	•	
Postoperative Variables		
Severe postoperative left AV valve regurgitation	•	•
Absence of sinus rhythm	•	
Higher left atrial, right atrial, or pulmonary artery pressure	•	
Reoperation Variables		
For pacemaker	•	
For VSD	•	
For left AV valve regurgitation	•	

Data from Kirklin and colleagues[K8] and Hanley and colleagues.[H1]
[a]If regurgitation is severe.
Key: *AV,* Atrioventricular; *LV,* left ventricular; *NYHA,* New York Heart Association; *VSD,* ventricular septal defect.

Interventricular Communication

An interventricular communication (complete AV septal defect) has been an important risk factor, but only in the early declining hazard phase. The effect of this aspect of morphology indicates that outcomes after repair of complete AV septal defects currently approximate those of partial AV septal defects, which have been excellent for many years[R6] (see Fig. 34-29). Residual interventricular communication after repair of complete AV septal defect may be an infrequent cause for reoperation and a risk factor for premature death. Early postoperative residual VSD should be suspected in the presence of "pulmonary hypertensive crisis" and low cardiac output.

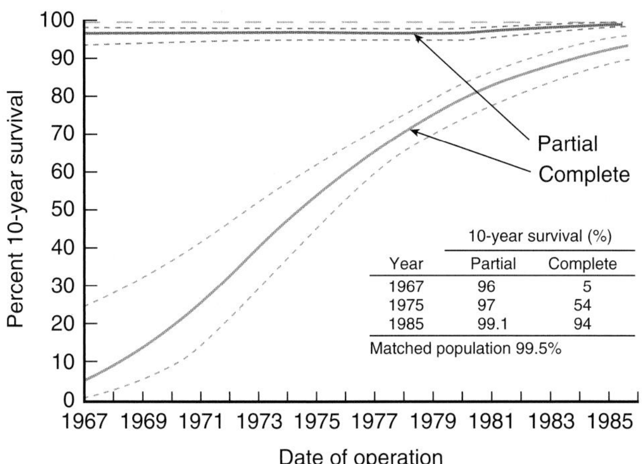

Figure 34-29 Nomogram representing predicted 10-year survival (including hospital deaths) after repair of partial and complete atrioventricular septal defects with or without major associated cardiac anomalies, according to year in which operation was performed. Solid lines are survival estimates, and dashed lines are 70% confidence limits. (See original publication for details, risk factors, coefficients, and *P* values of multivariable equation.) (From Kirklin and colleagues.[K8])

Accessory Valve Orifice

An accessory valve orifice is an incremental risk factor for premature death (see Table 34-11), almost surely because of its potentially adverse effect on function of the surgically created left AV valve[C6,C15,L4,S15] (see description under Morphology earlier in this chapter). Despite the realization that the accessory orifice should not be "tampered with," this risk factor has not been neutralized.[H1]

Major Associated Cardiac Anomalies

Included among important risk factors are major associated cardiac anomalies (see Table 34-11), but some of them, particularly tetralogy of Fallot, have been largely neutralized.

Young Age

Young age has been an incremental risk factor for death, usually hospital death, in all experiences that go back 30 years or so.[B12,H5] However, it has been virtually eliminated as a risk factor,[H1,K8,K14,P3,S18,W4] primarily because of overall improvement in knowledge and repair techniques, but also because of advances in intraoperative and early postoperative care of infants. However, despite low hospital mortality, lower weight among infants is associated with more frequent postoperative complications and longer hospital stay.[K14]

Down Syndrome

Risk-adjusted analysis does not show that Down syndrome affects risk of premature death early or late after repair, except when complete AV septal defect is associated with tetralogy of Fallot.[K8,K9,N1,S15] However, in view of the considerably decreased prevalence of LV inflow and outflow obstruction in patients with AV septal defects and Down syndrome, these patients may in fact have a better early and intermediate-term survival than patients without Down syndrome. The left AV valve may also be easier to repair, lessening the likelihood of late death from mitral regurgitation.[W5]

Need for Reoperation

The need for reoperation to insert a pacemaker, close a residual interventricular communication, or deal with important left AV valve regurgitation has been associated with added risk of death.[H1]

Other Risk Factors

Other incremental risk factors for premature death after repair have been reported. A single papillary muscle (see description under Morphology earlier in this chapter) becomes a serious problem after repair because of its tendency to result in LV inflow obstruction. It may therefore be a contraindication to typical two-ventricle repair. Severe ventricular hypoplasia is a risk factor for hospital death after a two-ventricle repair.[S15] Severe LV hypoplasia is more common in patients with complete AV septal defects than is severe right ventricular hypoplasia (see "Unbalanced Atrioventricular Septal Defects" under Special Situations and Controversies). Most hearts with severe LV hypoplasia are properly classified and treated as part of hypoplastic left heart syndrome (see Chapter 49).

Heart Block and Other Arrhythmias

Since Lev described the architecture of the conduction system in AV septal defects in 1958, prevalence of surgically induced permanent complete heart block has been approximately 1%.[L5] Avoiding heart block is generally facilitated by incorporating the coronary sinus on the left atrial side of the atrial patch. An equally low occurrence of heart block can also be accomplished by maintaining the coronary sinus on the right atrial side as long as appropriate attention is given to the anatomy of the conduction system (see also discussion under Special Situations and Controversies).[B7] Heart block is more frequent after repair of AV septal defect associated with tetralogy of Fallot and after AV valve replacement.[N1,S15]

First-degree AV block, present in about 30% of patients preoperatively, has been found in about 50% of patients after repair.[F2] Right bundle branch block is common after repair of complete AV septal defects but uncommon after repair of partial AV septal defects.[F2]

In an earlier UAB experience, when left AV valve replacement was required, heart block occurred in 4 of 20 patients (20%; CL 10%-33%).[S15] This is because sutures placed in the left AV valve anulus at about the 2-o'clock position overlie the AV node. A fringe of AV valve tissue must be left in this area so that valve replacement sutures can be placed there and more anteriorly in the interatrial pericardial patch, rather than along the ventricular septal crest. Placing the prosthesis in supraanular position is also helpful.[K2] With these precautions, complete heart block is minimized.

Functional Status

Most long-term survivors are in excellent health. In one center, 88% of surviving patients were in NYHA functional class I, and 11% were in class II.[K8,S15]

Atrioventricular Valve Function

Doppler color flow interrogation combined with two-dimensional echocardiography have increased the knowledge about postrepair left AV valve function considerably. Also,

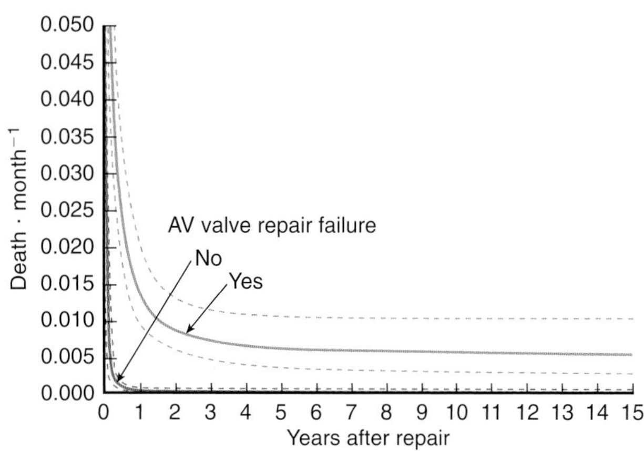

Figure 34-30 Hazard functions for death after repair of atrioventricular *(AV)* septal defects, one determined from analysis of those patients known to have had failure of the AV valve repair (n = 32; deaths = 19) and the other from analysis of those without valve repair failure (n = 278; deaths = 51). (From Kirklin and colleagues.[K8])

the reinforced leaflet method of repair has appeared to improve results.[S15,W4] Better techniques for repairing the left AV valve have played a major role in improving overall results, because patients whose repair fails are likely to have a considerably higher death rate in the intermediate and long term than are patients whose valve repair is good (Fig. 34-30). Left AV valve regurgitation is the major cause of reoperation.[A7,C16,S16]

After repair of *partial AV septal defects*, about 10% of patients have late severe left AV valve regurgitation, and such patients are more likely to have had severe regurgitation prior to the repair.[A1,C7,K7,L8,L12, M10,S15] Generally these patients have a deficiency of the LIL of the AV valve; to date, valve replacement has been the only certain method of achieving left AV valve competence in such patients.[B16,M10] Lesser degrees of regurgitation are present late postoperatively in about half of patients[A2,M10]; 30% to 40% have essentially no left AV valve regurgitation late postoperatively. Recent studies[M13] suggest that moderate or worse postoperative left AV valve regurgitation is more common in children repaired after about 4 years of age, possibly related to longer exposure to LV volume overload and anular dilatation induced by the regurgitation.

In patients undergoing repair of *complete AV septal defects*, there appears to be little relationship between preoperative severity of AV valve regurgitation and that present late postoperatively in some studies,[W4] but in others, an association is suggested.[A11,C16] Use of single- vs. two-patch technique of repair does not increase the likelihood of early or late postrepair left AV valve regurgitation.[K15]

More severe abnormalities of left AV valve morphology, including deficient LLL,[S18] papillary muscle abnormalities of the LLL, incomplete commissures, double orifice valve, and severe disparities in length of the LSL and LIL contributing to the "cleft," have been associated with a greater likelihood of postoperative left AV valve regurgitation.[A11] Absence of "cleft" closure has been identified as a risk factor for late reoperation for valve regurgitation.[H5]

About 10% to 20% of infants and older patients have important regurgitation late postoperatively, with the remainder having little or none.[S15,W4] Despite general improvements in surgical techniques, late reoperation for left AV valve regurgitation has remained a challenge.[C16,S16] When reoperation is necessary, left AV valve repair is possible in about half the patients; the rest require valve replacement.[A7,P9,S16] Stulak and colleagues at the Mayo Clinic found no difference in subsequent survival or freedom from additional operations according to whether valve repair or replacement was performed.[S16]

Repair of uncomplicated partial and complete AV septal defects uncommonly results in stenosis of the left AV valve. More often, this complication results when an accessory valve orifice or single papillary muscle coexists with the AV septal defect.

Important regurgitation or stenosis of the right AV valve is rare after repair of AV septal defects.

Left Ventricular Outflow Tract Obstruction

Uncommonly, LV outflow tract obstruction develops after repair of AV septal defects. As predicted on anatomic grounds by Ebels and colleagues, the AV septal defect has usually been the partial form.[E3] Prevalence of clinically significant late outflow obstruction is probably about 5% after repair of partial AV septal defect, which is up to three times more frequent than with the complete form.[K7,M6,P7]

When LV outflow obstruction develops, it may be associated with worsening left AV valve regurgitation; its relief usually permits regression of the regurgitation.

Prevalence of subaortic LV outflow tract obstruction late after repair of complete AV septal defect is not precisely known, but not negligible. Obstruction may have the appearance characteristic of discrete subaortic stenosis, with an "acquired fibromuscular ridge" (see "Resection of Localized Subvalvar Aortic Stenosis" in Section II of Chapter 47), or it may appear to result from the long, narrow LV outflow tract itself.[S4] In either case, simple resection rarely suffices. Extensive transaortic myectomy or the modified Konno operation, without aortic valve replacement, is indicated (see "Modified Konno Operation" in Section II of Chapter 47). Other techniques have been described that specifically address the scooped-out deficiency in the ventricular septum by detaching the LSL attachments to the crest of the ventricular septum and augmenting the anterosuperior aspect of the VSD patch or the LSL with a pericardial patch, followed by reattachment of the LSL. This moves the left AV valve farther into the left atrium during systole.[L3,M6,S14,V8]

Residual Pulmonary Hypertension

When important pulmonary hypertension is present preoperatively, it can be expected to regress postoperatively if pulmonary blood flow is large and the patient receives a timely operation, usually when younger than age 6 months.[C6,L9]

INDICATIONS FOR OPERATION

Presence of an AV septal defect indicates need for operation, because an important hemodynamic derangement is nearly always present, and spontaneous closure does not occur.

Partial Atrioventricular Septal Defects

In partial AV septal defects, pulmonary hypertension is usually absent, and the optimal age for operation is 1 to 2 years, assuming a competent left AV valve. If AV valve regurgitation is present, earlier operation is indicated to prevent further damage to valve tissue. Also, when heart failure or severe growth failure is evident earlier in life, operation is indicated at that time.

Complete Atrioventricular Septal Defects

Operation is indicated early in the first year of life. When the infant's general condition is good, repair can be delayed until about age 3 to 6 months. When refractory heart failure or severe growth failure is evident at an earlier age, repair at that time is indicated. Often in patients who are older than 1 year, and occasionally in those in the last part of the first year of life, pulmonary vascular disease may already be too severe to permit repair. Criteria of inoperability are the same as described for patients with VSD (see Indications for Operation in Section I of Chapter 35). Lung biopsy is not recommended as an aid in grading severity of pulmonary vascular disease because of its associated morbidity and mortality and because of the scatter between histopathologic findings and pulmonary vascular resistance.

Coexisting Cardiac Anomalies

Although certain major associated cardiac anomalies increase risk of repair of AV septal defects, their presence rarely alters the indication for operation. Thus, although a coexisting large patent ductus arteriosus has in the past increased risk of repair of complete AV septal defects, it increases the urgency of early repair rather than contraindicating it. When tetralogy of Fallot coexists, indication and timing of repair are similar to that for tetralogy of Fallot in general (see Indications for Operation in Section I of Chapter 38), although some favor elective operation for tetralogy of Fallot with complete AV septal defects at age 9 to 12 months. When complete AV septal defect with juxtaaortic VSD is combined with DORV without pulmonary stenosis, life history and indications for operation are the same as for isolated complete AV septal defect; in the past, risk of repair has been high, but in the current era, early risk has been much less and intermediate-term results good.[P2,P3]

SPECIAL SITUATIONS AND CONTROVERSIES

Pulmonary Trunk Banding

Pulmonary trunk banding has been used episodically as initial management for small infants with complete AV septal defects, and some excellent results have been reported.[E9] This approach has been used only sparingly in recent years. However, Silverman and colleagues, as well as Williams and colleagues, demonstrated in the early era that some very sick, small infants can be well managed initially by banding and deferral of repair for 6 to 18 months.[S5,W8] In the absence of other contraindications to repair (unbalanced ventricles, comorbid conditions), banding is not indicated, because age, left AV valve regurgitation, and many other risk factors have been neutralized, and overall results of complete repair are excellent. In the rare instances in which preliminary pulmonary banding is elected, a device that is adjustable by remote control has provided encouraging results.[B19,C14,D5]

Septal Patches

There have been several reports of near-fatal hemolysis from the regurgitant jet of a left AV valve striking a synthetic interatrial patch after repair of AV septal defect.[H4,S2,V10] Therefore, for maximal safety, the interatrial patch material should be pericardium.

Avoiding Heart Block

For years, McGoon and colleagues successfully used a method that involved keeping the suture line on the *left* and *superior sides* of the conduction tissue, rather than on the right side and inferiorly.[M7] Starr's group has used the same general method with good results.[A3] The patch is sutured to the LSL-LIL complex on the *left* ventricular side of its attachment to the crest of the ventricular septum. Inferiorly, the suture line then goes to the *edge* of the ostium primum defect, posterior and central to the AV node and bundle of His, and posteriorly along the atrial septal edge. This method keeps the suture line to the *left* of, and away from, the AV node and bundle of His (see Fig. 34-25, *E*).

Unbalanced Atrioventricular Septal Defects

In about 10% of patients with complete AV septal defects, the common AV valve is unequally balanced over the right ventricle or LV. The majority of cases are right dominant with associated LV hypoplasia.[M14,S6] The surgical options include biventricular repair or single-ventricle strategies. When one ventricle is severely hypoplastic, a repair resulting in a two-ventricle system frequently fails. Theoretically, a Fontan-type repair should be applicable to patients with this type of major associated cardiac anomaly. In the small number of patients treated in this manner, however, hospital mortality has been high.[C8,K8] This may be related to very early development of pulmonary vascular disease in patients with complete AV septal defects.

Echocardiographic analyses have been proposed that define the degree of "balance" of the AV valve over each ventricle. Using the subcostal view, the area of the common orifice can be divided into right and left AV valve orifices by a line drawn from the conal septum to the crest of the muscular septum.[C11,M14] Cohen and colleagues[C10,C11] (Fig. 34-31) used this method to calculate an AV valve index using the ratio of the left AV valve area divided by the right AV valve area in patients with a larger right AV valve (left/right valve area). In general, patients with a balanced complete AV septal defect have an area ratio greater than 0.67, and a value less than 0.67 indicates right ventricular dominance.

Approximately one third of patients with *right ventricular dominance* have Down syndrome.[C11] Patients with Down syndrome frequently have traits that increase the risk of single-ventricle palliations, such as lung hypoplasia, increased pulmonary vascular resistance, hypotonia with hypoventilation, and upper airway obstruction with nocturnal hypercarbia.[C1] Additional left-sided anomalies are also common in patients with right-dominant complete AV septal defects. Precise guidelines have not been established for the degree of RV dominance that is consistent with a successful two-ventricle repair. Available analyses are also confounded by the important additional risk imposed by additional major anomalies.[C11]

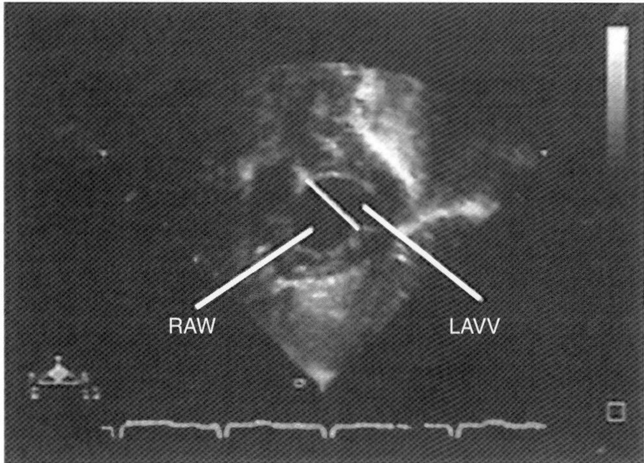

Figure 34-31 Subcostal view of a right-dominant unbalanced complete atrioventricular (AV) septal defect demonstrating unequal distribution of the common AV valve. A line bisects the valve from conal septum to crest of muscular septum. Relative valve areas can be used to calculate valve area index. Key: *LAVV,* Left AV valve; *RAVV,* right AV valve. (From Mitchell and colleagues.[M14])

In data from Cohen and colleagues on patients undergoing two-ventricle repairs with left AV valve/right AV valve ratio between 0.27 and 0.65, the specific ratio failed to predict survivors.[C10] Similarly, a study by Van Son and colleagues[V7] examined outcomes with two-ventricle repair among five patients with a diameter ratio (left/right valve diameter) of 0.23 to 0.39. All survived hospitalization, but one died late from left AV valve dysfunction.

Others have examined calculated LV volumes in decision making. Van Son and colleagues suggested that the actual LV volume may be underestimated in right ventricle–dominant AV septal defects secondary to leftward septal bowing, and they introduced the concept of "potential LV volume" to predict the volume of the LV post-repair that could be accomplished with only a change in shape.[V7] Patients with a potential volume of 15 mL · m^{-2} have survived repair. Individual reports have shown dramatic increases in LV size of twofold to threefold after repair.[V11] A small interventricular communication may be a favorable prognostic factor.

Another method of assessing dominance is the ratio of the left AV valve area to the total AV valve area.[J1] A ratio of 0.4 or less indicates right ventricular dominance, and a ratio of 0.6 or more indicates LV dominance. In a multicenter study from the Congenital Heart Surgeons Society, a ratio less than 0.2 (severe right ventricular dominance) uniformly predicted a single-ventricle strategy. A valve ratio of 0.4 to 0.6 indicated a "balanced" defect, and a two-ventricle repair was performed. A ratio of 0.2 to 0.4 represented the "gray zone" of moderately severe right ventricular dominance, in which either single- or two-ventricle strategies were applied, with a disproportionately high number of deaths in that range.[J1]

If biventricular repair is undertaken, placing a left atrial catheter for postoperative monitoring is advisable. A persistently elevated left atrial pressure and signs of low cardiac output, persistent pulmonary edema, or failure to wean from ventilator indicate need for reoperation and conversion to single-ventricle palliation. Unfortunately, outcomes after single-ventricle palliation in this setting are generally worse than for most other single-ventricle cohorts. Owens and colleagues noted a midterm survival of only 50% among 32 patients with severe right-dominant unbalanced AV septal defects, worse than that of a contemporary cohort of hypoplastic left heart syndrome patients.[O2] Thirty percent of the unbalanced AV septal defect patients required replacement or repair of their systemic AV valve.

Left-dominant unbalanced complete AV septal defect may be defined by a right AV valve area/left AV valve area less than 0.5 or a left AV valve area/total valve area greater than 0.6. Down syndrome has been reported in 80% of this subset.[D4] When the valve ratio is less than 0.5, risk of biventricular repair may carry an increased risk. De Oliveira and colleagues reported improved outcomes with a restrictive atrial fenestration intended to lower right atrial pressure and increase cardiac output with some degree of desaturation.[D4] The general surgical strategies in this patient group are similar to those for pulmonary atresia with intact ventricular septum (see Chapter 40). When right ventricular hypoplasia is severe and success of biventricular repair is in question, a "one-and-a-half ventricle repair," as suggested by Alvarado and colleagues and others, may be appropriate.[A8,V1] In this repair, the usual procedure to correct the AV septal defect is accompanied by a bidirectional cavopulmonary anastomosis. Pulmonary blood flow is augmented, and the right ventricle is unloaded. A potential but unusual problem is pulmonary artery–to–right atrial circular flow if superior vena cava–to–right atrium continuity is maintained.

Late Reoperation

The only residual condition that remains an important cause of late reoperation is left AV valve regurgitation. Najm and colleagues reported that 9.4% of 363 patients operated on for complete AV septal defect underwent subsequent repair or replacement of the left AV valve; 3 of 34 (8.8%; CL 3.9%-17%) patients died.[N1] Intraoperative echocardiography reduces the occurrence of residual important left AV valve regurgitation. The report of Reddy and colleagues is illustrative[R7]: 72 infants (median age 3 to 9 months) underwent repair of complete AV septal defect, and cleft closure or anuloplasty was done in 70. Based on TEE, 10 were returned to CPB for revision of the left AV valve. Among all 72 patients, there was 1 early death. There were 5 late reoperations with a median follow-up of 24 months; 2 were for AV valve regurgitation and 3 for subaortic obstruction. Although there may have been mild deterioration of AV valve function in patients with mild to moderate regurgitation early postoperatively, there was a 90% probability of not having severe late AV valve regurgitation at a mean follow-up of 45 months (range 3 to 169 months).[R8]

REFERENCES

A

1. Abbott ME. Atlas of congenital cardiac disease. New York: The American Heart Association, 1936, pp. 34 and 50.
2. Abbruzzese PA, Napoleone A, Bini RM, Annecchino FP, Merlo M, Parenzan L. Late left atrioventricular valve insufficiency after repair of partial atrioventricular septal defects: anatomical and surgical determinants. Ann Thorac Surg 1990;49:111.
3. Abruzzese PA, Livermore J, Sunderland CO, Nunley DL, Issenberg H, Khonsari S, et al. Mitral repair in complete atrioventricular canal: ease of correction in early infancy. J Thorac Cardiovasc Surg 1983;85:388.

4. Adatia I, Gittenbergerde Groot AC. Unroofed coronary sinus and coronary sinus orifice atresia. Implications for management of complex congenital heart disease. J Am Coll Cardiol 1995;25:948.
5. Alfieri O, Subramanian S. Successful repair of complete atrioventricular canal with undivided anterior common leaflet in a 6-month-old infant. Ann Thorac Surg 1975;19:92.
6. Alivizatos P, Anderson RH, Macartney FJ, Zuberbuhler JR, Stark J. Atrioventricular septal defect with balanced ventricles and malaligned atrial septum: double-outlet right atrium. Report of two cases. J Thorac Cardiovasc Surg 1985;89:295.
7. Alsoufi B, Al-Halees Z, Khouqeer F, Canver CC, Siblini G, Saad E, et al. Results of left atrioventricular valve reoperations following previous repair of atrioventricular septal defects. J Card Surg 2010;25:74-8.
8. Alvarado O, Sreeram N, McKay R, Boyd IM. Cavopulmonary connection in repair of atrioventricular septal defect with small right ventricle. Ann Thorac Surg 1993;55:729.
9. Anderson R, Baker E, Ho S, Rigley M, Ebels T. The morphology and diagnosis of atrioventricular septal defects. Cardiol Young 1991;1:291.
10. Anderson RH, Neches WH, Zuberbuhler JR, Penkoske PA. Scooping of the ventricular septum in atrioventricular septal defect. J Thorac Cardiovasc Surg 1988;95:146.
11. Ando M, Takahashi Y. Variations of atrioventricular septal defects predisposing to regurgitation and stenosis. Ann Thorac Surg 2010;90:614-21.

B

1. Bailey LL, Takeuchi Y, Williams WG, Trusler GA, Mustard WT. Surgical management of congenital cardiovascular anomalies with the use of profound hypothermia and circulatory arrest. Analysis of 180 consecutive cases. J Thorac Cardiovasc Surg 1976;71:485.
2. Bano-Rodrigo A, Van Praagh S, Trowitzsch E, Van Praagh R. Double-orifice mitral valve: a study of 27 postmortem cases with developmental, diagnostic and surgical considerations. Am J Cardiol 1988;61:152.
3. Bargeron LM Jr, Elliott LP, Soto B, Beam PR, Curry GC. Axial cineangiography in congenital heart disease. I. Concept, technical and anatomic considerations. Circulation 1977;56:1075.
4. Baron MG, Wolf BS, Steinfeld L, Van Mierop LH. Endocardial cushion defects. Specific diagnosis by angiocardiography. Am J Cardiol 1964;13:162.
5. Barratt-Boyes BG. Correction of atrioventricular canal defects in infancy using profound hypothermia. In Barratt-Boyes BG, Neutze JM, Harris EA, eds. Heart disease in infancy: diagnosis and surgical treatment. Edinburgh: Churchill Livingstone, 1973, p. 110.
6. Barratt-Boyes BG, Calder AL. Double outlet ventricle: classification and surgical management. In Davila JC, ed. Second Henry Ford Hospital International Symposium on Cardiac Surgery. East Norwalk, Conn.: Appleton & Lange, 1977, p. 285.
7. Baslaim G, Basioni A. Repair of complete atrioventricular septal defects: results with maintenance of the coronary sinus on the right atrial side. J Card Surg 2006;21:545-9.
8. Becker AE, Anderson RH. Atrioventricular septal defects: what's in a name? J Thorac Cardiovasc Surg 1982;83:461.
9. Bender HW Jr, Hammon JW Jr, Hubbard SG, Muirhead J, Graham TP. Repair of atrioventricular canal malformation in the 1st year of life. J Thorac Cardiovasc Surg 1982;84:515.
10. Ben-Shacher G, Moller JH, Castaneda-Zuniga W, Edwards JE. Signs of membranous subaortic stenosis appearing after correction of persistent common atrioventricular canal. Am J Cardiol 1981; 48:340.
11. Berger TJ, Blackstone EH, Kirklin JW, Bargeron LM Jr, Hazelrig JB, Turner ME Jr. Survival and probability of cure without and with operation in complete atrioventricular canal. Ann Thorac Surg 1979;27:104.
12. Berger TJ, Kirklin JW, Blackstone EH, Pacifico AD, Kouchoukos NT. Primary repair of complete atrioventricular canal in patients less than 2 years old. Am J Cardiol 1978;41:906.
13. Bharati S, Kirklin JW, McAllister HA Jr, Lev M. The surgical anatomy of common atrioventricular orifice associated with tetralogy of Fallot, double outlet right ventricle and complete regular transposition. Circulation 1980;61:1142.
14. Bharati S, Lev M. The spectrum of common atrioventricular orifice (canal). Am Heart J 1973;86:553.
15. Bharati S, Lev M, Kirklin JW. Cardiac surgery and the conduction system, 2nd Ed. Mount Kisco, N.Y.: Futura, 1992.
16. Bharati S, Lev M, McAllister HA Jr, Kirklin JW. Surgical anatomy of the atrioventricular valve in the intermediate type of common atrioventricular orifice. J Thorac Cardiovasc Surg 1980;79:884.
17. Binet JP, Losay J, Hvass U. Tetralogy of Fallot with type C complete atrioventricular canal: surgical repair in three cases. J Thorac Cardiovasc Surg 1980;79:761.
18. Bloom KR, Freedom RM, Williams CM, Trusler GA, Rowe RD. Echocardiographic recognition of atrioventricular valve stenosis associated with endocardial cushion defect: pathologic and surgical correlates. Am J Cardiol 1979;44:1326.
19. Bonnet D, Corno AF, Sidi D, Sekarski N, Beghetti M, Schulze-Neick I, et al. Early clinical results of the telemetric adjustable pulmonary artery banding FloWatch-PAB. Circulation 2004;110:II158-63.
20. Brandt PW, Clarkson PM, Neutze JM, Barratt-Boyes BG. Left ventricular cineangiocardiography in endocardial cushion defect (persistent common atrioventricular canal). Australas Radiol 1972;16:367.
21. Bull C, Rigby ML, Shinebourne EA. Should management of complete atrioventricular canal defect be influenced by coexistent Down syndrome? Lancet 1985;1:1147.

C

1. Campbell RM, Adatia I, Gow RM, Webb GD, Williams WG, Freedom RM. Total cavopulmonary anastomosis (Fontan) in children with Down's syndrome. Ann Thorac Surg 1998;66:523-6.
2. Carpentier A. Surgical anatomy and management of the mitral component of atrioventricular canal defects. In Anderson RH, Shinebourne EA, eds. Pediatric cardiology. London: Churchill Livingstone, 1978, p. 477.
3. Castaneda AR, Nicholoff DM, Moller JH, Lucas RV Jr. Surgical correction of complete atrioventricular canal utilizing ball-valve replacement of the mitral valve: technical considerations and results. J Thorac Cardiovasc Surg 1971;62:926.
4. Chan KY, Redington AN, Rigby ML. Color flow mapping in atrioventricular septal defects: does it have an important role in diagnosis and management? Cardiol Young 1991;1:315.
5. Chang CI, Becker AE. Surgical anatomy of left ventricular outflow tract obstruction in complete atrioventricular septal defect. A concept for operative repair. J Thorac Cardiovasc Surg 1987;94:897.
6. Chin AJ, Keane JF, Norwood WI, Castaneda AR. Repair of complete common atrioventricular canal in infancy. J Thorac Cardiovasc Surg 1982;84:437.
7. Chowdhury UK, Airan B, Malhotra A, Bisoi AK, Kalaivani M, Govindappa RM, et al. Specific issues after surgical repair of partial atrioventricular septal defect: actuarial survival, freedom from reoperation, fate of the left atrioventricular valve, prevalence of left ventricular outflow tract obstruction, and other events. J Thorac Cardiovasc Surg 2009;137:548-55.
8. Clapp SK, Perry BL, Farooki ZQ, Jackson WL, Karpawich PP, Hakimi M, et al. Surgical and medical results of complete atrioventricular canal: a ten year review. Am J Cardiol 1987;59:454.
9. Clapp S, Perry BL, Farooki ZQ, Jackson WL, Karpawich PP, Hakimi M, et al. Down's syndrome, complete atrioventricular canal, and pulmonary vascular obstructive disease. J Thorac Cardiovasc Surg 1990;100:115.
10. Cohen MS, Jacobs ML, Weinberg PM, Rychik J. Morphometric analysis of unbalanced common atrioventricular canal using two-dimensional echocardiography. J Am Coll Cardiol 1996;28: 1017-23.
11. Cohen MS, Spray TL. Surgical management of unbalanced atrioventricular canal defect. Semin Thorac Cardiovasc Surg Pediatr Card Surg Annu 2005:135-44.
12. Cooley DA. Results of surgical treatment of atrial septal defects: particular consideration of low defects including ostium primum and atrioventricular canal. Am J Cardiol 1960;6:605.
13. Cooper DK, de Leval MR, Stark J. Results of surgical correction of persistent complete atrioventricular canal. Thorac Cardiovasc Surg 1979;27:111.
14. Corno AF, Prosi M, Fridez P, Zunino P, Quarteroni A, von Segesser LK. The non-circular shape of FloWatch-PAB prevents the need for pulmonary artery reconstruction after banding. Computational fluid dynamics and clinical correlations. Eur J Cardiothorac Surg 2006;29:93-9.
15. Corwin RD, Singh AK, Karlson KE. Double-outlet right atrium: a rare endocardial cushion defect. Am Heart J 1983;106:1156.

16. Crawford FA Jr, Stroud MR. Surgical repair of complete atrioventricular septal defect. Ann Thorac Surg 2001;72:1621-9.
17. Culpepper W, Kolff J, Lin CY, Vitullo D, Lamberti J, Arcilla RA, et al. Complete common atrioventricular canal in infancy: surgical repair and postoperative hemodynamics. Circulation 1978;58:550.

D

1. D'Allaines C, Colvez P, Fevre C, Levasseur P, Facquet J, Dubost C. A rare congenital cardiopathy: association of tetralogy of Fallot and complete A-V canal. Arch Mal Coeur 1969;62:996.
2. David I, Castaneda AR, Van Praagh R. Potentially parachute mitral valve in common atrioventricular canal: pathological anatomy and surgical importance. J Thorac Cardiovasc Surg 1982;84:178.
3. De Biase L, Di Ciommo V, Ballerini L, Bevilacqua M, Marcelletti C, Marino B. Prevalence of left-sided obstructive lesions in patients with atrioventricular canal without Down's syndrome. J Thorac Cardiovasc Surg 1986;91:467.
4. De Oliveira NC, Sittiwangkul R, McCrindle BW, Dipchand A, Yun TJ, Coles JG, et al. Biventricular repair in children with atrioventricular septal defects and a small right ventricle: anatomic and surgical considerations. J Thorac Cardiovasc Surg 2005;130:250-7.
5. Dhannapuneni RR, Gladman G, Kerr S, Venugopal P, Alphonso N, Corno AF. Complete atrioventricular septal defect: outcome of pulmonary artery banding improved by adjustable device. J Thorac Cardiovasc Surg 2011;141:179-82.
6. Draulans-Noe HA, Wenink AC. Anterolateral muscle bundle of the left ventricle in atrioventricular septal defect: left ventricular outflow tract and subaortic stenosis. Pediatr Cardiol 1991;12:83.
7. Draulans-Noe HA, Wenink AC, Quaegebeur J. Single papillary muscle ("parachute valve") and double-orifice left ventricle in atrioventricular septal defect convergence of chordal attachment: surgical anatomy and result of surgery. Pediatr Cardiol 1990;11:29.
8. Dubost C, Blondeau P. Canal atrio-ventriculaire et ostium primum. J Chir 1959;78:241.
9. DuShane JW, Weidman WH, Brandenburg RO, Kirklin JW. Differentiation of interatrial communications by clinical methods: ostium secundum, ostium primum, common atrium, and total anomalous pulmonary venous connection. Circulation 1960;21:363.

E

1. Ebels T. Surgery of the left atrioventricular valve and of the left ventricular outflow tract in atrioventricular septal defect. Cardiol Young 1991;1:344.
2. Ebels T, Anderson RH, Devine WA, Debich DE, Penkoske PA, Zuberbuhler JR. Anomalies of the left atrioventricular valve and related ventricular septal morphology in atrioventricular septal defects. J Thorac Cardiovasc Surg 1990;99:299.
3. Ebels T, Ho SY, Anderson RH, Meijboom EJ, Eijgelaar A. The surgical anatomy of the left ventricular outflow tract in atrioventricular septal defect. Ann Thorac Surg 1986;41:483.
4. Ebels T, Meijboom EJ, Anderson RH, Schasfoort-van Leeuwen MJ, Lenstra D, Eijgelaar A, et al. Anatomic and functional "obstruction" of the outflow tract in atrioventricular septal defects with separate valve orifices ("ostium primum atrial septal defect"): an echocardiographic study. Am J Cardiol 1984;54:843.
5. Edwards JE. The problem of mitral insufficiency caused by accessory chordae tendineae in persistent common atrioventricular canal. Mayo Clin Proc 1960;35:299.
6. Ellis FH Jr, Kirklin JW, Swan HJ, DuShane JW, Edwards JE. Diagnosis and surgical treatment of common atrium (cor trilocularebiventriculare). Surgery 1959;45:160.
7. Ellis FH, McGoon D, Kirklin JW. Surgical management of persistent common atrioventricular canal. Am J Cardiol 1960;6:598.
8. Emanuel R, Somerville J, Inns A, Withers R. Evidence of congenital heart disease in the offspring of parents with atrioventricular defects. Br Heart J 1983;49:144.
9. Epstein ML, Moller JH, Amplatz K, Nicoloff DM. Pulmonary artery banding in infants with complete atrioventricular canal. J Thorac Cardiovasc Surg 1979;78:28.

F

1. Feldt RH, DuShane JW, Titus JL. The atrioventricular conduction system in persistent common atrioventricular canal defect. Circulation 1970;42:437.
2. Fournier A, Young ML, Garcia OL, Tamer DF, Wolff GS. Electrophysiologic cardiac function before and after surgery in children with atrioventricular canal. Am J Cardiol 1986;57:1137.
3. Frescura C, Thiene G, Franceschini E, Talenti E, Mazzucco A. Pulmonary vascular disease in infants with complete atrioventricular septal defect. Int J Cardiol 1987;15:91.

G

1. Gerbode F, Sanchez PA, Arguero R, Kerth WJ, Hill JD, DeVries PA, et al. Endocardial cushion defects. Ann Surg 1967;166:486.
2. Ghosh PK, Donnelly RJ, Hamilton DI, Wilkinson JL. Surgical correction of a case of common atrium with anomalous systemic and pulmonary venous drainage. J Thorac Cardiovasc Surg 1977;74:604.
3. Goor D, Lillehei CW, Edwards JE. Further observations on the pathology of the atrioventricular canal malformation. Arch Surg 1968;97:954.
4. Gunther T, Mazzitelli D, Haehnel CJ, Holper K, Sebening F, Meisner H. Long-term results after repair of complete atrioventricular septal defects: analysis of risk factors. Ann Thorac Surg 1998;65:754.
5. Gutgesell HP, Huhta JC. Cardiac septation in atrioventricular canal defect. J Am Coll Cardiol 1986;8:1421.

H

1. Hanley FL, Fenton KN, Jonas RA, Mayer JE, Cook NR, Wernovsky G, et al. Surgical repair of complete atrioventricular canal defects in infancy: twenty-year trends. J Thorac Cardiovasc Surg 1993;106:387.
2. Hardesty RL, Zuberbuhler JR, Bahnson HT. Surgical treatment of atrioventricular canal defect. Arch Surg 1975;110:1391.
3. Haworth SG. Pulmonary vascular bed in children with complete atrioventricular septal defect: relation between structural and hemodynamic abnormalities. Am J Cardiol 1986;57:833.
4. Hines GL, Finnerty TT, Doyle E, Isom OW. Near fatal hemolysis following repair of ostium primum atrial septal defect. J Cardiovasc Surg 1978;19:7.
5. Hoohenkerk GJ, Bruggemans EF, Rijlaarsdam M, Schoof PH, Koolbergen DR, Hazekamp MG. More than 30 years' experience with surgical correction of atrioventricular septal defects. Ann Thorac Surg 2010;90:1554-61.
6. Hori H, Yoshikawa K, Tayama E, Aoyagi S. Double-orifice repair for left atrioventricular valve regurgitation in atrioventricular septal defect: report of two cases. J Card Surg 2006;21:500-2.

I

1. Ilbawi MN, Idriss FS, DeLeon SY, Riggs TW, Muster AJ, Berry TE, et al. Unusual mitral valve abnormalities complicating surgical repair of endocardial cushion defects. J Thorac Cardiovasc Surg 1983;85:697.

J

1. Jegatheeswaran A, Pizarro C, Caldarone CA, Cohen MS, Baffa JM, Gremmels DB, et al. Echocardiographic definition and surgical decision-making in unbalanced atrioventricular septal defect: a Congenital Heart Surgeons' Society multiinstitutional study. Circulation 2010;122:S209-15.

K

1. Kadoba K, Jonas RA. Replacement of the left atrioventricular valve after repair of atrioventricular septal defect. Cardiol Young 1991;1:383.
2. Kadoba K, Jonas RA, Mayer JE, Castaneda AR. Mitral valve replacement in the first year of life. J Thorac Cardiovasc Surg 1990;100:762.
3. Kahn DR, Levy J, France NE, Chung KJ, Dacumos GC. Recent results after repair of atrioventricular canal. J Thorac Cardiovasc Surg 1977;73:413.
4. Kaiser GA, Waldo AL, Beach PM, Bowman FO Jr, Hoffman BF, Malm JR. Specialized cardiac conduction system: improved electrophysiologic identification at surgery. Arch Surg 1970;101:673.
5. Kanani M, Elliott M, Cook A, Juraszek A, Devine W, Anderson RH. Late incompetence of the left atrioventricular valve after repair of atrioventricular septal defects: the morphologic perspective. J Thorac Cardiovasc Surg 2006;132:640-6.
6. Katz NM, Blackstone EH, Kirklin JW, Bradley EL, Lemons JE. Suture techniques for atrioventricular valves: experimental study. J Thorac Cardiovasc Surg 1981;81:528.

7. King RM, Puga FJ, Danielson GK, Schaff HV, Julsrud PR, Feldt RH. Prognostic factors and surgical treatment of partial atrioventricular canal. Circulation 1986;74:I42.
8. Kirklin JW, Blackstone EH, Bargeron LM Jr, Pacifico AD, Kirklin JK. The repair of atrioventricular septal defects in infancy. Int J Cardiol 1986;13:333.
9. Kirklin JW, Blackstone EH, Jonas RA, Shimazaki Y, Kirklin JK, Mayer JE, et al. Morphologic and surgical determinants of outcome events after repair of tetralogy of Fallot and pulmonary stenosis: a two-institution study. J Thorac Cardiovasc Surg 1992;103:706.
10. Kirklin JK, Blackstone EH, Kirklin JW, McKay R, Pacifico AD, Bargeron LM Jr. Intracardiac surgery in infants under age 3 months: incremental risk factors for hospital mortality. Am J Cardiol 1981;48:500.
11. Kirklin JW, Blackstone EH, Pacifico AD, Brown RN, Bargeron LM Jr. Routine primary repair vs. two-stage repair of tetralogy of Fallot. Circulation 1979;60:373.
12. Kirklin JW, Daugherty GW, Burchell HB, Wood EH. Repair of the partial form of persistent common atrioventricular canal: so-called ostium primum type of atrial septal defect with interventricular communication. Ann Surg 1955;142:858.
13. Kirklin JW, DuShane JW, Patrick RT, Donald DE, Hetzel PS, Harshbarger HG, et al. Intracardiac surgery with the aid of a mechanical pump-oxygenator system (Gibbon type): report of eight cases. Mayo Clin Proc 1955;30:201.
14. Kogon BE, Butler H, McConnell M, Leong T, Kirshbom PM, Kanter KR. What is the optimal time to repair atrioventricular septal defect and common atrioventricular valvar orifice? Cardiol Young 2007;17:356-9.
15. Krasemann T, Debus V, Rellensmann G, Rukosujew A, Scheld HH, Vogt J, et al. Regurgitation of the atrioventricular valves after corrective surgery for complete atrioventricular septal defects—comparison of different surgical techniques. Thorac Cardiovasc Surg 2007;55:229-32.
16. Krayenbuhl CU, Lincoln JC. Total anomalous systemic venous connection, common atrium, and partial atrioventricular canal. A case report of successful surgical correction. J Thorac Cardiovasc Surg 1977;73:686.
17. Krongrad E, Malm JR, Bowman FO Jr, Hoffman BF, Waldo AL. Electrophysiological delineation of the specialized A-V conduction system in patients with congenital heart disease. II. Delineation of the distal His bundle and the right bundle branch. Circulation 1974;49:1232.

L

1. Lacour-Gayet F, Comas J, Bruniaux J, Serraf A, Losay J, Petit J, et al. Management of the left atrioventricular valve in 95 patients with atrioventricular septal defects and a common atrioventricular orifice—a ten year review. Cardiol Young 1991;1:367.
2. Lai YQ, Luo Y, Zhang C, Zhang ZG. Utilization of double-orifice valve plasty in correction of atrioventricular septal defect. Ann Thorac Surg 2006;81:1450-4.
3. Lappen RS, Muster AJ, Idriss FS, Riggs TW, Ilbawi M, Paul MH, et al. Masked subaortic stenosis in ostium primum atrial septal defect: recognition and treatment. Am J Cardiol 1983;52:336-40.
4. Lee CN, Danielson GK, Schaff HV, Puga FJ, Mair DD. Surgical treatment of double-orifice mitral valve in atrioventricular canal defect. J Thorac Cardiovasc Surg 1985;90:700.
5. Lev M. The architecture of the conduction system in congenital heart disease. I. Common atrioventricular orifice. AMA Arch Pathol 1958;65:174.
6. Lev M, Agustsson MH, Arcilla R. The pathologic anatomy of common atrioventricular orifice associated with tetralogy of Fallot. Am J Clin Pathol 1961;36:408.
7. Levy MJ, Cuello L, Tuna N, Lillehei CW. Atrioventricularis communis. Clinical aspects and surgical treatment. Am J Cardiol 1964;14:587.
8. Levy S, Blondeau P, Dubost C. Long-term follow-up after surgical correction of the partial form of common atrioventricular canal (ostium primum). J Thorac Cardiovasc Surg 1974;67:353.
9. Lillehei CW, Anderson RC, Ferlic RM, Bonnabeau RC Jr. Persistent common atrioventricular canal: recatheterization results in 37 patients following intracardiac repair. J Thorac Cardiovasc Surg 1969;57:83.
10. Lillehei CW, Cohen M, Warden HE, Varco RL. The direct-vision intracardiac correction of congenital anomalies by controlled cross circulation: results in thirty-two patients with ventricular septal defects, tetralogy of Fallot, and atrioventricularis communis defects. Surgery 1955;38:11.
11. Lipshultz SE, Sanders SP, Mayer JE, Colan SD, Lock JE. Are routine preoperative cardiac catheterization and angiography necessary before repair of ostium primum atrial septal defect? J Am Coll Cardiol 1988;11:373.
12. Losay J, Rosenthal A, Castaneda AR, Bernhard WH, Nadas AS. Repair of atrial septal defect primum: results, course, and prognosis. J Thorac Cardiovasc Surg 1978;75:248.

M

1. Macartney FJ, Rees PG, Daly K, Piccoli GP, Taylor JF, de Leval MR, et al. Angiocardiographic appearances of atrioventricular defects with particular reference to distinction of ostium primum atrial septal defects from common atrioventricular orifice. Br Heart J 1979;42:640.
2. Mace L, Dervanian P, Houyel L, Chaillon-Fracchia E, Piot D, Lambert V, et al. Surgically created double-orifice left atrioventricular valve: a valve-sparing repair in selected atrioventricular septal defects. J Thorac Cardiovasc Surg 2001;121:352-64.
3. Mair DD, McGoon DC. Surgical correction of atrioventricular canal during the first year of life. Am J Cardiol 1977;40:66.
4. Maisano F, Torracca L, Oppizzi M, Stefano PL, D'Addario G, La Canna G, et al. The edge-to-edge technique: a simplified method to correct mitral insufficiency. Eur J Cardiothorac Surg 1998;13:240-6.
5. Maloney JV Jr, Marable SA, Mulder DG. The surgical treatment of common atrioventricular canal. J Thorac Cardiovasc Surg 1962;43:84.
6. Manning PB. Partial atrioventricular canal: pitfalls in technique. Semin Thorac Cardiovasc Surg Pediatr Card Surg Annu 2007:42-6.
7. McGoon DC, McMullan MH, Mair DD, Danielson GK. Correction of complete atrioventricular canal in infants. Mayo Clin Proc 1973;48:769.
8. McGrath LB, Kirklin JW, Soto B, Bargeron LM Jr. Secondary left atrioventricular valve replacement in atrioventricular septal (AV canal) defect: a method to avoid left ventricular outflow tract obstruction. J Thorac Cardiovasc Surg 1985;89:632.
9. McMullan MH, Wallace RB, Weidman WH, McGoon DC. Surgical treatment of complete atrioventricular canal. Surgery 1972;72:905.
10. Meijboom EJ, Ebels T, Anderson RH, Schasfoort-van Leeuwen MJ, Deanfield JE, Eijgelaar A, et al. Left atrioventricular valve after surgical repair in atrioventricular septal defect with separate valve orifices ("ostium primum atrial septal defect"): an echo-Doppler study. Am J Cardiol 1986;57:433.
11. Midgley FM, Galioto FM, Shapiro SR, Perry LW, Scott LP. Experience with repair of complete atrioventricular canal. Ann Thorac Surg 1980;30:151.
12. Mills NL, Ochsner JL, King TD. Correction of type C complete atrioventricular canal. Surgical considerations. J Thorac Cardiovasc Surg 1976;71:20.
13. Minich LL, Atz AM, Colan SD, Sleeper LA, Mital S, Jaggers J, et al. Partial and transitional atrioventricular septal defect outcomes. Ann Thorac Surg 2010;89:530-6.
14. Mitchell ME, Litwin SB, Tweddell JS. Complex atrioventricular canal. Semin Thorac Cardiovasc Surg Pediatr Card Surg Annu 2007:32-41.
15. Mitchell SC, Korones SB, Berendes HW. Congenital heart disease in 56,109 births: incidence and natural history. Circulation 1971;43:323.
16. Moller JH. Perspectives in pediatric cardiology, Vol. 6. Surgery of congenital heart disease. Armonk, N.Y.: Futura Publishing, 1998.
17. Moreno-Cabral RJ, Shumway NE. Double-patch technique for correction of complete atrioventricular canal. Ann Thorac Surg 1982;33:88.
18. Munoz-Armas S, Gorrin JR, Anselmi G, Hernandez PB, Anselmi A. Single atrium: embryologic, anatomic, electrocardiographic and other diagnostic features. Am J Cardiol 1968;21:639.

N

1. Najm HK, Coles JG, Endo M, Stephens D, Rebeyka IM, Williams WG, et al. Complete atrioventricular septal defects: results of repair, risk factors, and freedom from reoperation. Circulation 1997;96:II311.

2. Newfeld EA, Sher M, Paul MH, Nikaidoh H. Pulmonary vascular disease in complete atrioventricular canal defect. Am J Cardiol 1977;39:721.
3. Nicholson IA, Nunn GR, Sholler GF, Hawker RE, Cooper SG, Lau KC. Simplified single patch technique for the repair of atrioventricular septal defect. J Thorac Cardiovasc Surg 1999;118:642-6.
4. Nora JJ, Nora AH. The evolution of specific genetic and environmental counseling in congenital heart diseases. Circulation 1978;57:205.
5. Nunn GR. Atrioventricular canal: modified single patch technique. Semin Thorac Cardiovasc Surg Pediatr Card Surg Annu 2007: 28-31.

O

1. Ongley PA, Pongpanich B, Spangler JG, Feldt RH. The electrocardiogram in atrioventricular canal. In Feldt RH, ed. Atrioventricular canal defects. Philadelphia: WB Saunders, 1976, p. 51.
2. Owens GE, Gomez-Fifer C, Gelehrter S, Owens ST. Outcomes for patients with unbalanced atrioventricular septal defects. Pediatr Cardiol 2009;30:431-5.

P

1. Pacifico AD, Kirklin JW. Surgical repair of complete atrioventricular canal with anterior common leaflet attached to an anomalous right ventricular papillary muscle. J Thorac Cardiovasc Surg 1973;65:727.
2. Pacifico AD, Kirklin JW, Bargeron LM Jr. Repair of complete atrioventricular canal associated with tetralogy of Fallot or double-outlet right ventricle: report of 10 patients. Ann Thorac Surg 1980;29:351.
3. Pacifico AD, Ricchi A, Bargeron LM Jr, Colvin EC, Kirklin JW, Kirklin JK. Corrective repair of complete atrioventricular (AV) canal defects (CAV) and major associated cardiac anomalies. Circulation 1987;76:IV72.
4. Park JM, Ritter DG, Mair DD. Cardiac catheterization findings in persistent atrioventricular canal. In Feldt RH, ed. Atrioventricular canal defects. Philadelphia: WB Saunders, 1976, p. 76.
5. Penkoske PA, Neches WH, Anderson RH, Zuberbuhler JR. Further observations on the morphology of atrioventricular septal defects. J Thorac Cardiovasc Surg 1985;90:611.
6. Piccoli GP, Gerlis LM, Wilkinson JL, Lozsadi K, Macartney FJ, Anderson RH. Morphology and classification of atrioventricular defects. Br Heart J 1979;42:621.
7. Piccoli GP, Ho SY, Wilkinson JL, Macartney FJ, Gerlis LM, Anderson RH. Left-sided obstructive lesions in atrioventricular septal defects: an anatomic study. J Thorac Cardiovasc Surg 1982;83:453.
8. Piccoli GP, Wilkinson JL, Macartney FJ, Gerlis LM, Anderson RH. Morphology and classification of complete atrioventricular defects. Br Heart J 1979;42:633.
9. Poirier NC, Williams WG, Van Arsdell GS, Coles JG, Smallhorn JF, Omran A, et al. A novel repair for patients with atrioventricular septal defect requiring reoperation for left atrioventricular valve regurgitation. Eur J Cardiothorac Surg 2000;18:54-61.

Q

1. Quaegebeur J, Kirklin JW, Pacifico AD, Bargeron LM Jr. Surgical experience with unroofed coronary sinus. Ann Thorac Surg 1979; 27:418.

R

1. Rastelli GC, Kirklin JW, Titus JL. Anatomic observations on complete form of persistent common atrioventricular canal with special reference to atrioventricular valves. Mayo Clin Proc 1966;41:296.
2. Rastelli GC, Ongley PA, Kirklin JW. Surgical correction of common atrium with anomalously connected persistent left superior vena cava. Mayo Clin Proc 1965;40:528.
3. Rastelli GC, Ongley PA, Kirklin JW, McGoon DC. Surgical repair of complete form of persistent common atrioventricular canal. J Thorac Cardiovasc Surg 1968;55:299.
4. Rastelli GC, Ongley PA, McGoon DC. Surgical repair of complete atrioventricular canal with anterior common leaflet undivided and unattached to ventricular septum. Mayo Clin Proc 1969;44:335.
5. Rastelli GC, Rahimtoola SH, Ongley PA, McGoon DC. Common atrium: anatomy, hemodynamics, repair and surgery. J Thorac Cardiovasc Surg 1968;55:834.
6. Rastelli GC, Weidman WH, Kirklin JW. Surgical repair of the partial form of persistent common atrioventricular canal, with special reference to the problem of mitral valve incompetence. Circulation 1965;31:31.
7. Reddy VM, McElhinney DB, Brook MM, Parry AJ, Hanley FL. Atrioventricular valve function after single patch repair of complete atrioventricular septal defect in infancy: how early should repair be attempted? J Thorac Cardiovasc Surg 1998;115:1032.
8. Rhodes J, Warner KG, Fulton DR, Romero BA, Schmid CH, Marx GR. Fate of mitral regurgitation following repair of atrioventricular septal defect. Am J Cardiol 1997;80:1194.
9. Roberson DA, Muhiudeen IA, Silverman NH, Turley K, Haas GS, Cahalan MK. Intraoperative transesophageal echocardiography of atrioventricular septal defect. J Am Coll Cardiol 1991;18:537.
10. Rogers HM, Edwards JE. Incomplete division of the atrioventricular canal with patent interatrial foramen primum (persistent common atrioventricular ostium): report of five cases and review of the literature. Am Heart J 1948;36:28.
11. Roman KS, Nii M, Macgowan CK, Barrea C, Coles J, Smallhorn JF. The impact of patch augmentation on left atrioventricular valve dynamics in patients with atrioventricular septal defects: early and midterm follow-up. J Am Soc Echocardiogr 2006;19:1382-92.

S

1. Samanek M. Prevalence at birth, "natural" risk and survival with atrioventricular septal defect. Cardiol Young 1991;1:285.
2. Sayed HM, Dacie JV, Handley DA, Lewis SM, Cleland WP. Haemolytic anaemia of mechanical origin after open heart surgery. Thorax 1961;16:356.
3. Sellers RD, Lillehei CW, Edwards JE. Subaortic stenosis caused by anomalies of the atrioventricular valves. J Thorac Cardiovasc Surg 1964;48:289.
4. Silverman NH, Gerlis LM, Ho SY, Anderson RH. Fibrous obstruction within the left ventricular outflow tract associated with ventricular septal defect: a pathologic study. J Am Coll Cardiol 1995;25:475.
5. Silverman N, Levitsky S, Fisher E, DuBrow I, Hastreiter A, Scagliotti D. Efficacy of pulmonary artery banding in infants with complete atrioventricular canal. Circulation 1983;68:II148.
6. Sittiwangkul R, Ma RY, McCrindle BW, Coles JG, Smallhorn JF. Echocardiographic assessment of obstructive lesions in atrioventricular septal defects. J Am Coll Cardiol 2001;38:253-61.
7. Smallhorn JF, Perrin D, Musewe N, Dyck J, Boutin C, Freedom RM. The role of transesophageal echocardiography in the evaluation of patients with atrioventricular septal defect. Cardiol Young 1991;1:324.
8. Smallhorn JF, Tommasini G, Anderson RH, Macartney FJ. Assessment of atrioventricular septal defects by two dimensional echocardiography. Br Heart J 1982;47:109.
9. Somerville J. Ostium primum defects: factors causing deterioration in the natural history. Br Heart J 1965;27:413.
10. Soto B, Bargeron LM Jr, Pacifico AD, Vanini V, Kirklin JW. Angiography of atrioventricular canal defects. Am J Cardiol 1981;48:492.
11. Spanos PK, Fiddler GI, Mair DD, McGoon DC. Repair of atrioventricular canal associated with membranous subaortic stenosis. Mayo Clin Proc 1977;52:121.
12. Sridaromont S, Feldt RH, Ritter DG, Davis GD, McGoon DC, Edwards JE. Double-outlet right ventricle associated with persistent common atrioventricular canal. Circulation 1975;52:933.
13. Stanger P, Rudolph AM, Edwards JE. Cardiac malpositions. An overview based on study of sixty-five necropsy specimens. Circulation 1977;56:159.
14. Starr A, Hovaguimian H. Surgical repair of subaortic stenosis in atrioventricular canal defects. J Thorac Cardiovasc Surg 1994; 108:373-6.
15. Studer M, Blackstone EH, Kirklin JW, Pacifico AD, Soto B, Chung GK, et al. Determinants of early and late results of repair of atrioventricular septal (canal) defects. J Thorac Cardiovasc Surg 1982;84:523.
16. Stulak JM, Burkhart HM, Dearani JA, Schaff HV, Cetta F, Barnes RD, et al. Reoperations after initial repair of complete atrioventricular septal defect. Ann Thorac Surg 2009;87:1872-8.
17. Suzuki K, Ho SY, Anderson RH, Becker AE, Neches WH, Devine WA, et al. Morphometric analysis of atrioventricular septal defect with common valve orifice. J Am Coll Cardiol 1998;31:217.

18. Suzuki T, Bove EL, Devaney EJ, Ishizaka T, Goldberg CS, Hirsch JC, et al. Results of definitive repair of complete atrioventricular septal defect in neonates and infants. Ann Thorac Surg 2008;86:596-602.
19. Szwast AL, Marino BS, Rychik J, Gaynor JW, Spray TL, Cohen MS. Usefulness of left ventricular inflow index to predict successful biventricular repair in right-dominant unbalanced atrioventricular canal. Am J Cardiol 2011;107:103-9.

T
1. Takanashi Y, Anzai N, Okada T, Sano A, Ando M, Konno S. Common atrium associated with anomalous high insertion of the inferior vena cava. J Thorac Cardiovasc Surg 1975;69:912.
2. Tandon R, Moller JH, Edwards JE. Single papillary muscle of the left ventricle associated with persistent common atrioventricular canal: variant of parachute mitral valve. Pediatr Cardiol 1986;7: 111.
3. Taylor NC, Somerville J. Fixed subaortic stenosis after repair of ostium primum defects. Br Heart J 1981;45:689.
4. Tenckhoff L, Stamm SJ. An analysis of 35 cases of the complete form of persistent common atrioventricular canal. Circulation 1973;48:416.
5. Thiene G, Wenink AC, Frescura C, Wilkinson JL, Gallucci V, Ho SY et al. Surgical anatomy and pathology of the conduction tissues in atrioventricular defects. J Thorac Cardiovasc Surg 1981; 82:928.
6. Thilenius OG, Vitullo D, Bharati S, Luken J, Lamberti JJ, Tatooles C, et al. Endocardial cushion defect associated with cor triatriatum sinistrum or supravalve mitral ring. Am J Cardiol 1979;44:1339.
7. Toscano-Barbosa E, Brandenburg RO, Burchell HB. Electrocardiographic studies of cases with intracardiac malformations of the atrioventricular canal. Mayo Clin Proc 1956;31:513.

U
1. Ugarte M, Enriquez de Salamanca F, Quero M. Endocardial cushion defects: an anatomical study of 54 specimens. Br Heart J 1976;38:674.

V
1. Van Arsdell GS, Williams WG, Boutin C, Trusler GA, Coles JG, Rebeyka IM, et al. Subaortic stenosis in the spectrum of atrioventricular septal defects: solutions may be complex and palliative. J Thorac Cardiovasc Surg 1995;110:1534.
2. Vanetti A, Dumet. Surgical treatment of severe forms of atrioventricular canal. Arch Mai Coeur Vaiss 1975;68:719.
3. Van Mierop LH, Alley RD. The management of the cleft mitral valve in endocardial cushion defects. Ann Thorac Surg 1966;2: 416.
4. Van Mierop LH, Alley RD, Kausel HW, Stranahan A. The anatomy and embryology of endocardial cushion defects. J Thorac Cardiovasc Surg 1962;43:71.
5. Van Praagh S, Antoniadis S, Otero-Coto E, Leidenfrost RD, Van Praagh R. Common atrioventricular canal with and without conotruncal malformations. An anatomic study of 251 postmortem cases. In Nora JJ, Ta Kao A, eds. Congenital heart disease. Causes and processes. Mount Kisco, N.Y: Futura, 1984, p. 599.
6. Van Praagh R, Corwin RD, Dahlquist EH Jr, Freedom RM, Mattioli L, Nebesar RA. Tetralogy of Fallot with severe left ventricular anomalous attachment of the mitral valve to the ventricular septum. Am J Cardiol 1970;26:93.
7. van Son JA, Phoon CK, Silverman NH, Haas GS. Predicting feasibility of biventricular repair of right-dominant unbalanced atrioventricular canal. Ann Thorac Surg 1997;63:1657-63.
8. van Son JA, Schneider P, Falk V. Repair of subaortic stenosis in atrioventricular canal with absent or restrictive interventricular communication by patch augmentation of ventricular septum, resuspension of atrioventricular valves, and septal myectomy. Mayo Clin Proc 1997;72:220-4.
9. Vargas FJ, Coto EO, Mayer JE Jr, Jonas RA, Castaneda AR. Complete atrioventricular canal and tetralogy of Fallot: surgical considerations. Ann Thorac Surg 1986;42:258.
10. Verdon TA Jr, Forrester RH, Crosby WH. Hemolytic anemia after open-heart repair of ostium-primum defects. N Engl J Med 1963; 269:444.
11. Vida VL, Sanders SP, Milanesi O, Stellin G. Biventricular repair of right-dominant complete atrioventricular canal defect. Pediatr Cardiol 2006;27:737-40.
12. Virdi IS, Keeton BR, Shore DF. Atrioventricular septal defect with a well developed primary component of the atrial septum ("septum primum"). Int J Cardiol 1985;9:243.

W
1. Wakai CS, Edwards JE. Development and pathologic considerations in persistent common atrioventricular canal. Proc Mayo Clin 1956;31:487.
2. Wakai CS, Edwards JE. Pathologic study of persistent common atrioventricular canal. Am Heart J 1958;56:779.
3. Watkins E Jr, Gross RE. Experiences with surgical repair of atrial septal defects. J Thorac Cardiovasc Surg 1955;30:469.
4. Weintraub RG, Brawn WJ, Venables AW, Mee RB. Two-patch repair of complete atrioventricular septal defect in the first year of life. J Thorac Cardiovasc Surg 1990;99:320.
5. Westerman GR, Norton JB, Van Devanter SH. Double-outlet right atrium associated with tetralogy of Fallot and common atrioventricular valve. J Thorac Cardiovasc Surg 1986;91:205.
6. Wilcox BR, Jones DR, Frantz EG, Brink LW, Henry GW, Mill MR, et al. Anatomically sound, simplified approach to repair of "complete" atrioventricular septal defect. Ann Thorac Surg 1997;64: 487-94.
7. Williams RG, Rudd M. Echocardiographic features of endocardial cushion defects. Circulation 1974;49:418.
8. Williams WH, Guyton RA, Michalik RE, Plauth WH Jr, Zorn-Chelton S, Jones EL, et al. Individualized surgical management of complete atrioventricular canal. J Thorac Cardiovasc Surg 1983;86:838.
9. Wilson NJ, Gavalaki E, Newman CG. Complete atrioventricular canal defect in presence of Down syndrome (letter). Lancet 1985;2:834.

Y
1. Yamaki S, Yasui H, Kado H, Yonenaga K, Nakamura Y, Kikuchi T, et al. Pulmonary vascular disease and operative indications in complete atrioventricular canal defect in early infancy. J Thorac Cardiovasc Surg 1993;106:398.
2. Yilmaz AT, Arslan M, Kuralay E, Demrkilic U, Ozal E, Tatar H, et al. Repair of the left AV valve in atrioventricular septal defect in adults. J Card Surg 1996;11:363.
3. Yokoyama M. The location of the coronary sinus orifice in endocardial cushion defects. Kyobu Geka 1973;26:35.

35 Ventricular Septal Defect

Section I Primary Ventricular Septal Defect

DEFINITION

Ventricular septal defect (VSD) is a hole or multiple holes in the interventricular septum. This chapter discusses VSDs that occur as the primary lesion, recognizing that hearts with primary VSDs may have minor coexisting morphologic abnormalities.[O9]

VSD may be part of another major cardiovascular anomaly, such as tetralogy of Fallot (see Chapter 38), complete atrioventricular (AV) septal defect (see Chapter 34), anatomically corrected malposition of the great arteries (see Chapter 57), truncus arteriosus (see Chapter 43), tricuspid atresia (see Chapter 41), sinus of Valsalva aneurysm (see Chapter 36), and interrupted aortic arch (see Chapter 48). VSDs also may be acquired, as discussed in Chapters 9 and 17.

HISTORICAL NOTE

In 1954, Lillehei, Varco, and colleagues at the University of Minnesota in Minneapolis began to repair VSDs using normothermic, low-flow, controlled cross-circulation based on the so-called azygos flow principle,[A17,C16] with an adult human as the oxygenator (see Historical Note in Section II of Chapter 2).[W4] This was the beginning of the era of cardiac surgery using *cardiopulmonary bypass* (CPB), a term coined by Cooley a few years later. Five of the first eight patients were in their first year of life, and only two (40%; CL 14%-71%) of the five died, a tribute to surgical skill, lack of cardiac ischemia (the aorta was not clamped), and quality of their human oxygenator. The dramatic weight gain of the surgically cured infants with large VSDs was documented. Three older patients, aged 4, 5, and 5 years, also survived, one of whom had multiple VSDs.

In 1956, DuShane and colleagues reported 20 patients who had undergone intracardiac repair of large VSDs with a mechanical pump-oxygenator at the Mayo Clinic beginning in March 1955.[D11] Normothermic flow of 70 mL · kg^{-1} · min^{-1} (about 2.1 L · min^{-1} · m^{-2}) was used, along with a pump-sucker system to return intracardiac blood to the machine. Duration of CPB varied from 10 to 45 minutes. Four (20%; CL 10%-33%) of the 20 patients died in hospital, a mortality considered low in that era.

Truex described the location of the specialized conduction tissue in hearts with VSD.[T12] In a more detailed study, Lev expanded on this topic,[L9] and his work was the basis on which

Table 35-1 Morphologic Classification of Ventricular Septal Defect

Classification	% of VSDs	Location/Borders
Perimembranous	80	Borders tricuspid valve Conduction system in posterior rim
Muscular	5	Borders all muscle Frequently multiple Conduction system remote
Doubly committed subarterial	5-10	Borders both semilunar valves Conduction system remote
Inlet septal	<5	Atrioventricular septal type Posterior position Conduction system in posterior rim

Key: *VSD*, Ventricular septal defect.

Kirklin and DuShane developed a surgical technique that avoided producing heart block during VSD repair.[C9,K20]

Lillehei showed the feasibility of an atrial approach to VSD in 1957.[S26] The technique of hypothermic circulatory arrest, with rewarming by a pump-oxygenator, was applied successfully to infants with VSD by Okamoto.[O4] Kirklin and DuShane (1961) and Sloan's group (1967) reported the feasibility of primary repair of VSD in infants.[K13,S11]

Barratt-Boyes and colleagues (1969-1971) found that routine primary repair of VSD in sick, small infants was superior to pulmonary artery banding.[B4]

MORPHOLOGY

Although this chapter considers VSD that occurs as the primary lesion, the method of morphologic description is applied in other chapters to VSDs that are part of other major cardiac malformations. The morphologic classification described here represents an attempt to simplify VSD classification by encompassing all variations of the lesion while conforming to other systems of classification (Table 35-1). This classification conforms generally with the consensus of the Congenital Heart Surgery Nomenclature and Database Project[J1] and includes many of the concepts of Anderson and Wilcox.[A13,A14]

Size

VSDs are highly variable in size, and their division into size groups is arbitrary but useful. The echocardiographic criteria for VSD size are discussed in "Two-Dimensional Echocardiography" under Clinical Features and Diagnostic Criteria.

Large VSDs are approximately the size of the aortic orifice or larger. They offer little resistance to flow, and thus their VSD resistance index[1] is less than 20 units · m^2 in situations in which the calculation of the index is valid.[H13,S3] Right ventricular (RV) systolic pressure approximates left ventricular (LV) pressure, and the pulmonary to systemic blood flow ratio ($\dot{Q}p/\dot{Q}s$) is increased to a degree dependent on the level of pulmonary vascular resistance (Rp).

Moderate-sized VSDs, although still restrictive, are of sufficient size to raise RV systolic pressure to approximately half LV pressure and $\dot{Q}p/\dot{Q}s$ to 2.0 or greater.

Small VSDs are of insufficient size to raise RV systolic pressure, and $\dot{Q}p/\dot{Q}s$ is not increased above 1.75. Small VSDs have a VSD resistance index greater than 20 units · m^2.[H13] Multiple small defects behave in aggregate as a large defect.

Location in Septum and Relationship to Conduction System

VSDs can occur in all portions of the ventricular septum[2] (Fig. 35-1). VSDs with entirely muscular borders (muscular VSDs) may occupy several areas of the ventricular septum; other VSDs have one or several nonmuscular borders consisting of spaces or structures against which they are juxtaposed (Table 35-2). These nonmuscular borders may be a semilunar valve, an AV valve, or the crux cordis (intersection of the posterior aspect of the interventricular septum and AV junction). Some VSDs in the periphery of the ventricular septum are bordered by the ventricular free wall, but such VSDs are conventionally considered to be muscular. VSDs in the category of subarterial may be (1) *juxta-aortic,* (2) *juxtapulmonary,* (3) *juxta-arterial* (bordered by both pulmonary and aortic valves), or (4) *juxtatruncal* (bordered by the valve of a common arterial trunk). Subarterial VSDs are typically associated with some degree of overriding of the related arterial trunk, and the margin of the VSD is actually a space over which is a semilunar valve(s).[A9]

Many VSDs are associated with malalignment of portions of the ventricular septum or atrial septum relative to the interventricular septum, in which case an AV valve usually overrides the VSD. *Malalignment VSD terminology* results from two-dimensional (2D) echocardiographic examination of the heart regarding alignment of the trabecular and the outlet (conal) septum. In some cardiac anomalies, the aorta seems displaced relative to the VSD. The malalignment is referred to as *anterior* when the outlet septum appears anterior to the trabecular septum, with the VSD interposed. Tetralogy of Fallot–type defects are considered anterior malalignment types, with the aorta "overriding" the VSD (see Fig. 35-18, *C*). Malalignment is *posterior* when the outlet septum appears posterior to the trabecular septum in anomalies such as interrupted aortic arch and severe coarctation of the aorta. There may also be a *rotational* malalignment in anomalies characterized under the broad category of Taussig-Bing heart.

Anatomic location of the VSD determines its relation to the conduction system.

VSDs may also be characterized according to their *commitment to the great arteries* (Lev and colleagues[L10]): *subaortic, subpulmonary, doubly committed,* and *noncommitted.*

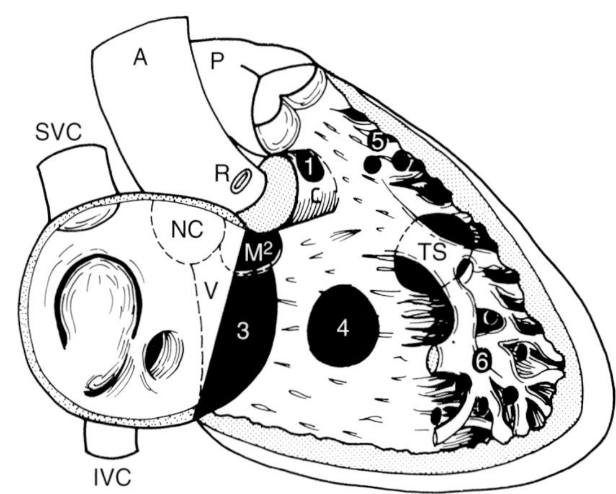

Figure 35-1 Schematic representation of position of ventricular septal defect *(VSD)* as seen from right ventricular *(RV)* side of septum. Front of right ventricle, right atrium, and tricuspid valve have been removed. Shown are *(1)* doubly committed subarterial (juxta-arterial) VSD; *(2)* a perimembranous (conoventricular) VSD, which is juxta-aortic and juxtatricuspid; *(3)* an inlet septal VSD, which is juxtatricuspid and juxtamitral and, in this instance, juxtacrucial, a defect generally associated with atrial and ventricular septal malalignment and overriding tricuspid valve; and *(4, 5, 6)* trabecular VSDs. In positions 5 and 6, VSDs tend to be small and multiple, and when most of this trabeculated area and midmuscular septum are peppered with holes, the term *Swiss cheese defect* is used. Position 5 would be classified *muscular, outlet type*; position 6 is *muscular, apical.* Key: *A,* Aorta; *c,* conal (outlet, infundibular) septum; *IVC,* inferior vena cava; *M,* membranous septum with ventricular and atrioventricular portions; *NC,* noncoronary aortic cusp; *P,* pulmonary trunk and valve; *R,* right coronary artery cut off at its origin; *SVC,* superior vena cava; *TS,* trabecula septomarginalis (septal band); *V,* muscular portion of atrioventricular septum.

Table 35-2 Expanded Morphologic Classification of Ventricular Septal Defect

Classification	Extension
Perimembranous	Inlet Anterior Outlet
Muscular	Outlet (conal) Trabecula Inlet Anterior Apical
Doubly committed subarterial	—
Inlet septal	Atrioventricular septal type
Malalignment	Anterior (tetralogy of Fallot) Posterior (interrupted arch or coarctation) Rotational (Taussig-Bing)

[1] $$\text{VSD resistance index} = \frac{P_{LV}\ (\text{peak}) - P_{RV}\ (\text{peak}) \times BSA}{\dot{Q}p - \dot{Q}s}$$
where *BSA* is body surface area, P_{LV} is left ventricular systolic pressure, P_{RV} is right ventricular systolic pressure, $\dot{Q}p$ is pulmonary blood flow, and $\dot{Q}s$ is systemic blood flow.

[2] The location is described in words that are relevant to the RV aspect of the VSD (see "Right Ventricle" under Cardiac Chambers and Major Vessels in Chapter 1), because most reparative procedures are performed from that aspect.

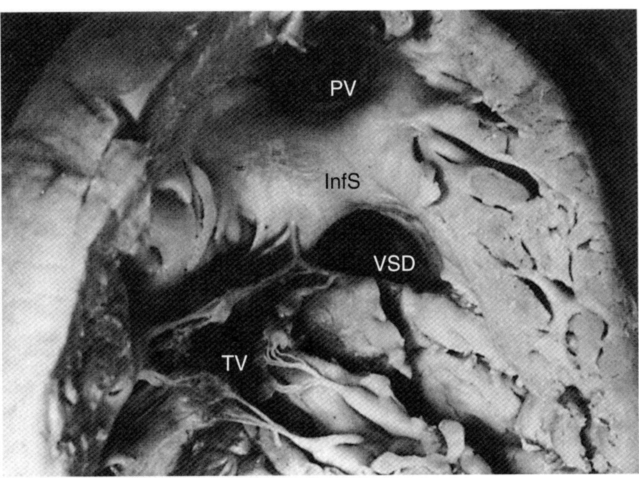

Figure 35-2 Perimembranous ventricular septal defect *(VSD)* viewed from right ventricle. VSD borders anteroseptal commissure of tricuspid valve (juxtatricuspid) and has anterior extension to VSD and midportion of muscular septum. Key: *InfS,* Infundibular (outlet) septum; *PV,* pulmonary valve; *TV,* tricuspid valve.

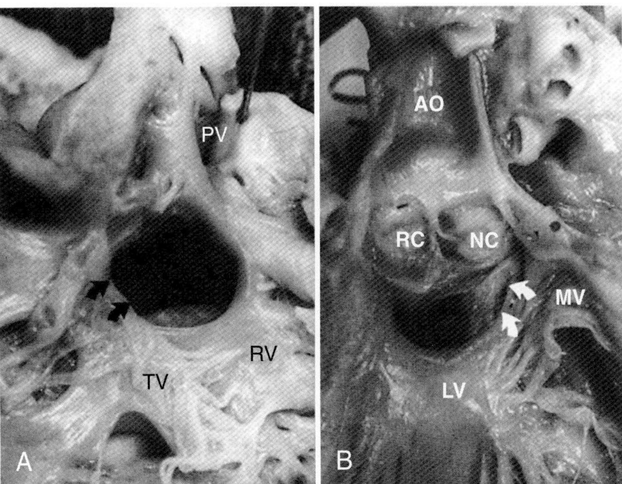

Figure 35-3 Large perimembranous ventricular septal defect, viewed from right ventricle *(RV)* **(A)** and left ventricle **(B)**. In **A**, septal tricuspid leaflet was folded back into right atrium after its chordae were cut. Arrows indicate areas of tricuspid-mitral continuity, and defect borders tricuspid valve; it is juxtatricuspid, juxtamitral, and juxta-aortic. This defect, viewed from RV, lies far to the right in aortic margin of ventricular septum and thus is beneath the commissure between noncoronary and right coronary cusps. Defect is perimembranous, and no muscle is between it and anterior septal tricuspid commissure. Conal septum is hypoplastic but not malaligned. Key: *AO,* Aorta; *LV,* left ventricle; *MV,* mitral valve; *NC,* noncoronary cusp; *PV,* pulmonary valve; *RC,* right coronary cusp; *TV,* tricuspid valve. (From Soto and colleagues.[S16])

This type of characterization—which is relational, not morphologic—preferably is restricted to hearts with double outlet ventricles, because its use in other situations has resulted in considerable confusion.

All these features of the location of VSDs should be included in descriptions of these defects.

Perimembranous Ventricular Septal Defect

Approximately 80% of patients operated on for primary VSD have a perimembranous VSD.[S14,S16,V3] These defects could be called *junctional VSDs* because they are in the junctional area between the trabecular (sinus) and outlet (conal) portions of the ventricular septum (Fig. 35-2) and usually appear to be between the posterior and anterior divisions of the trabecula septomarginalis (septal band). Thus, these VSDs are between the outlet (conus) and inlet (ventricular) portions of the *right* ventricle, but characteristically they are in the outlet portion of the *left* ventricle.

Perimembranous VSDs are often associated with anomalies of the outlet septum[O9] and other adjacent structures, although when small, they may be truly isolated anomalies. Some perimembranous VSDs are *juxtatricuspid* (abutting the tricuspid valve), *juxtamitral,* and *juxta-aortic.*[B5] These perimembranous VSDs are also conoventricular (conotruncal)[S15] (Fig. 35-3). Such defects abut the commissural area between the noncoronary and right coronary cusps of the aortic valve. Others are only juxtatricuspid (Fig. 35-4), and in hearts with these as well as in hearts with perimembranous VSDs, the bundle of His passes along the posteroinferior border of the defect.[B5,K16,L5,S15] Some perimembranous VSDs abut none of these valvar structures and are separated from the tricuspid anulus posteriorly by a band of muscle that is part of the posterior division of the trabecula septomarginalis joining with the ventriculoinfundibular fold. The bundle of His is not in this muscular band but is in its usual position more posteriorly. Technically, although this type of defect is located in a perimembranous position, it is better classified as *muscular inlet–type VSD* because all borders are muscle.

VSDs have also been described in the past as *typically high, infracristal, membranous,* or *perimembranous,* without the original specific description.[B5,B7,S14,S15]

As already indicated, the AV node and penetrating portion of the bundle of His are in their normal position in hearts with perimembranous VSDs. As the bundle penetrates the fibrous right trigone of the central fibrous body at the base of the noncoronary cusp of the aortic valve, it lies along the posteroinferior border of perimembranous and inlet-type VSDs. As the bundle continues along the inferior border of the VSD (at times slightly to the left or right of the free edge), the left bundle branch fascicles emerge from the branching portion. Only the right bundle branch remains when the bundle reaches the level of the muscle of Lancisi.

Abnormalities of the ventricular portion of the membranous septum are often associated with perimembranous VSDs. The membranous septum may be absent or nearly so, and then the right trigone (beneath the nadir of the noncoronary aortic valve cusp) and base of the septal and anterior leaflets of the tricuspid valve are exposed and form the posteroinferior rim of the VSD (see Fig. 35-3). The bundle of His, as it penetrates the fibrous right trigone at the base of the noncoronary cusp, is intimately related to the posteroinferior angle of such a defect. This is associated with a deficiency in the posterior limb of the trabecula septomarginalis.[K27] Rarely the ventricular portion of the membranous septum may be well developed, thickened, and perforated by one or many holes, forming an *aneurysm of the membranous septum* that bulges toward the right in systole. This so-called aneurysm is simulated on angiography by the much more common tethered anterior leaflet and the involved and usually fused chordae. Accessory fibrous tissue not part

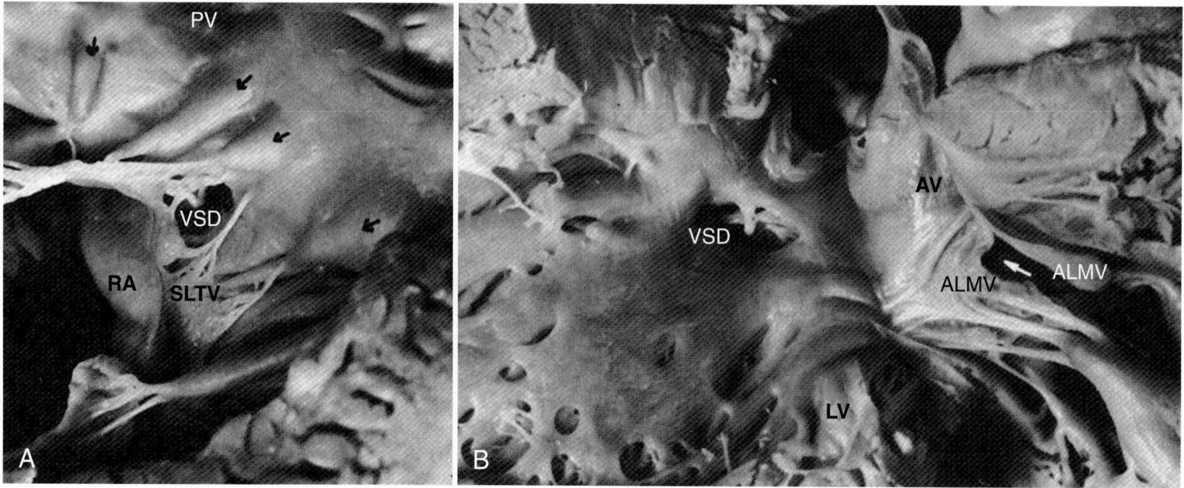

Figure 35-4 Perimembranous ventricular septal defect *(VSD)* of moderate size. **A,** VSD in region of anteroseptal commissure of tricuspid valve, viewed from right ventricle. VSD extends inferiorly beneath septal leaflet of tricuspid valve and abuts commissural area between anterior and septal tricuspid leaflets (juxtatricuspid) and remnant of membranous septum. Numerous tricuspid chordae and papillary muscles *(arrows)* are present. **B,** Same defect viewed from left ventricle. VSD lies below noncoronary cusp of aortic valve and is not juxta-aortic. Arrow indicates cleft in anterior mitral leaflet. Key: *ALMV,* Anterior leaflet of mitral valve; *AV,* aortic valve; *LV,* left ventricle; *PV,* pulmonary valve; *RA,* right atrium; *SLTV,* septal leaflet of tricuspid valve.

of the tricuspid valve mechanism may lie along the posterior or superior margin of the defect. This phenomenon is most marked in the *flap valve VSD.*

Not surprisingly, in hearts with perimembranous VSDs, still other adjacent structures may be abnormal. The medial papillary muscle characteristically joins the anteroinferior angle of the defect and receives chordae from adjacent portions of the tricuspid anterior and septal leaflets. These chordae may be increased in number and abnormally positioned around the edges of a perimembranous VSD, attached to the posterior edge, superior edge (Fig. 35-5), or most often anterior edge.[U1] A thick leash of chordae joining the center of the anterior edge of a large defect may produce an appearance on angiography or even at operation of a double defect. Chordae from the anterior leaflet may attach to all three margins, and the anterior leaflet then limits the shunt from left to right through the defect, as well as hinder its repair.

Close association of some perimembranous VSDs with the commissure between anterior and septal tricuspid leaflets sometimes results in adherence of leaflet tissue to edges of the defect and shunting directly from LV into right atrium[B13,L8] (Fig. 35-6). This so-called LV–right atrial defect,[G6,P5,S18] which constitutes fewer than 5% of perimembranous VSDs in this region, rarely involves the AV septum. Adherence of tricuspid leaflet and chordal tissue is also an important mechanism of spontaneous closure of these VSDs.

Ventricular Septal Defect in Right Ventricular Outlet (Doubly Committed Subarterial Ventricular Septal Defect)

Some 5% to 10% of patients treated operatively have a single VSD, usually of moderate or large size, within the outlet portion of the RV. VSDs in this location are also in the outlet portion of the LV and, in contrast to perimembranous VSDs, are more beneath the right aortic cusp than the commissure between it and the noncoronary cusp. In the past, these have also been termed *conal, infundibular, supracristal,* and *intracristal* defects. The complex morphology of the ventricular septum in the outlet portion of the RV and many controversies concerning the term "outlet septum" support use of a simple descriptive terminology for this group of VSDs.

VSDs in this general location are bordered in part by a space over which lie the pulmonary and aortic valves[S15] (Fig. 35-7). As such, these VSDs are subarterial. VSDs of this type are more common in Asians than in white or black races.[T5] Subarterial VSDs may be circular, diamond shaped, or oval with the long axis lying transversely (Fig. 35-8). When viewed from the LV aspect, these defects are in the outflow portion of the ventricular septum (see Fig. 35-7, *B*), beneath the right coronary cusp (or commissure between it and the left cusp). The aortic and pulmonary valve cusps are separated by only a thin rim of fibrous tissue. The right aortic cusp and (less often) noncoronary cusp may prolapse into the upper margin of the defect, with or without aortic regurgitation (see Section II later in this chapter).

The posteroinferior margin of RV outlet VSDs is usually well separated from the tricuspid valve anulus by a band of muscle and is consequently well above the bundle of His. Occasionally, however, a particularly large confluent VSD may be both subarterial and perimembranous (Fig. 35-9). The conduction system is related to such a VSD as it is to other perimembranous defects. This particular type of VSD is sometimes associated with severe overriding of the aorta, and the cardiac anomaly is then termed *double outlet right ventricle* (DORV) *with doubly committed VSD.* The same type of VSD may also be seen in double outlet left ventricle (DOLV), in which the pulmonary artery severely overrides the VSD.

Morphology of these subarterial VSDs has been well elucidated by 2D echocardiography and color Doppler examinations.[G11,S4] Despite the potential confusion of using Lev's *relational* terminology in a morphologic sense, in the echocardiographic literature, subarterial defects are usually referred to as *doubly committed VSDs.* Thus, it is useful to

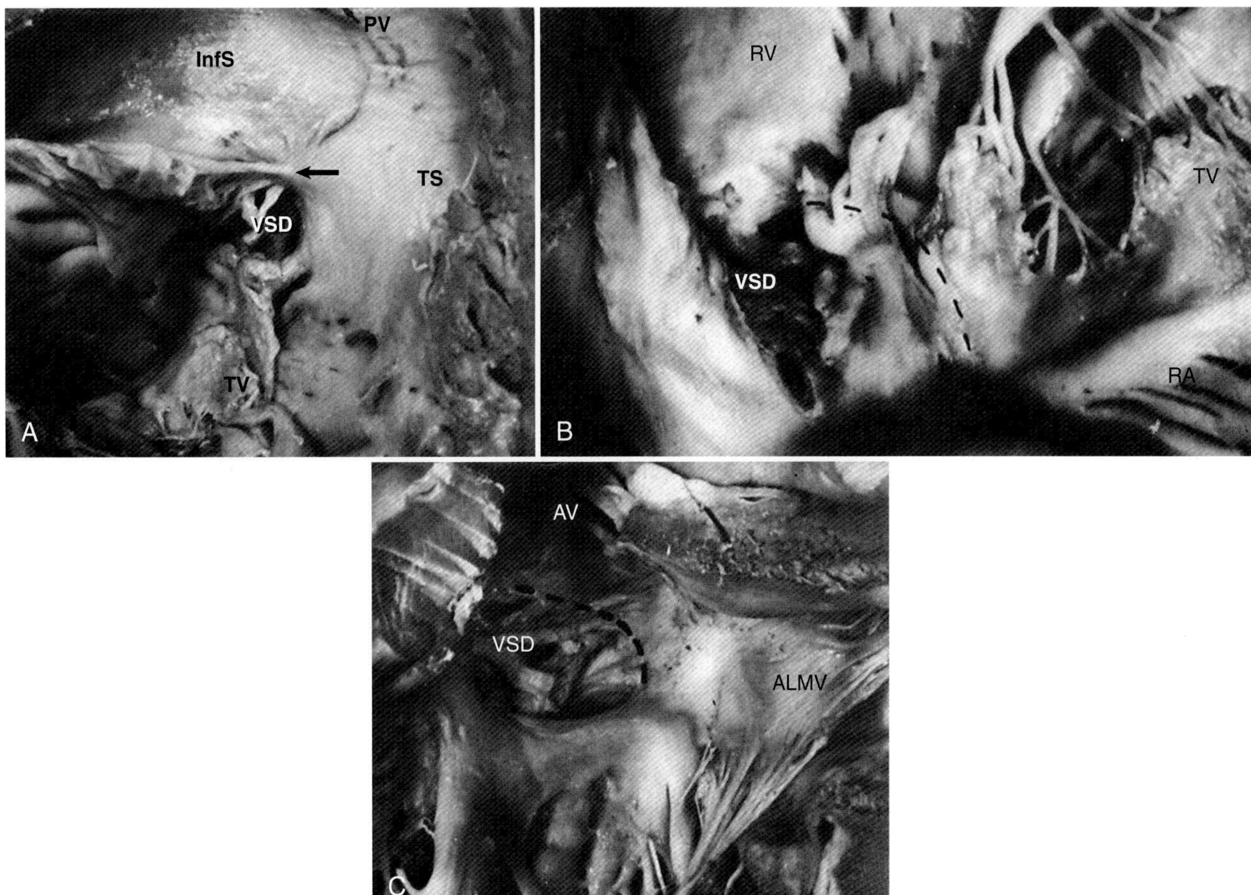

Figure 35-5 Perimembranous ventricular septal defect *(VSD)* associated with anomalous leaflet tissue. **A,** VSD viewed from right ventricle. Note chordal attachment *(arrow)* of anterior tricuspid leaflet to anterosuperior margin of defect. Normal position of infundibular (outlet) septum between two limbs of trabecula septomarginalis (septal band) is well seen. **B,** Same defect viewed from right atrium. VSD is partly obscured by tricuspid leaflet tissue, but its extent is indicated by dashed line. **C,** Same defect viewed from left ventricle. VSD is immediately beneath aortic valve (juxta-aortic), and its extent is indicated by dashed line. Abnormal tricuspid valve attachments are obvious and on an angiocardiogram are indistinguishable from an aneurysm of the membranous ventricular septum. Key: *ALMV,* Anterior leaflet of mitral valve; *AV,* aortic valve; *InfS,* infundibular (outlet) septum; *PV,* pulmonary valve, *RA,* right atrium; *RV,* right ventricle; *TS,* trabecula septomarginalis (septal band); *TV,* tricuspid valve.

combine morphologic and echocardiographic descriptions to characterize these VSDs occurring in the RV outlet as *doubly committed subarterial VSDs*. Echocardiography has demonstrated that aortic and pulmonary valves are frequently at the same level in the presence of subarterial (or doubly committed) VSDs, rather than the pulmonary valve being elevated above (cephalad to) or offset relative to the aortic valve, seemingly by the RV infundibulum.[G11] This description often provides a diagnostic tool useful in both echocardiography and angiography, along with the finding that the outlet septum appears to be absent and the subpulmonary infundibulum deficient. Echocardiography has also demonstrated the frequently associated prolapse of an aortic cusp and aortic regurgitation present in up to half of patients with this type of VSD.[S4] Aortic cusp prolapse may nearly close the VSD during diastole. At times the fibrous raphe between the arterial valves is displaced relative to the ventricular septum, resulting in overriding of one arterial valve and narrowing of the other.[G11]

Some VSDs in the RV outlet are only *juxta-aortic* and abut the nadir of the right coronary cusp. The cusp typically prolapses through this type of VSD, and aortic regurgitation frequently develops.[S16] Rarely, VSDs in the RV outlet are only juxtapulmonary and lie far to the left.

Some defects in the outlet portion of the septum have *muscular* borders and lie in the substance of the infundibular septum (muscular VSD, outlet type), with a muscle bridge of infundibular septum superior to the defect. The superior muscular bridge may be malaligned and displaced leftward into the aortic outflow tract (posterior malalignment type of VSD), producing muscular subaortic stenosis that lies above the VSD.[M11] This anomaly occasionally occurs in association with interrupted aortic arch and with coarctation,[A10,D4,F4] although perimembranous VSDs are more common in both settings.

Inlet Septal Ventricular Septal Defect

Five percent or less of surgical patients have *inlet septal VSD* (or *AV septal type* or *AV canal type* of VSD).[N4] This defect involves the RV *inlet septum* beneath the tricuspid septal leaflet and LV *outlet septum.* Its posterior margin is formed by the exposed AV valve anulus (juxtatricuspid), and its

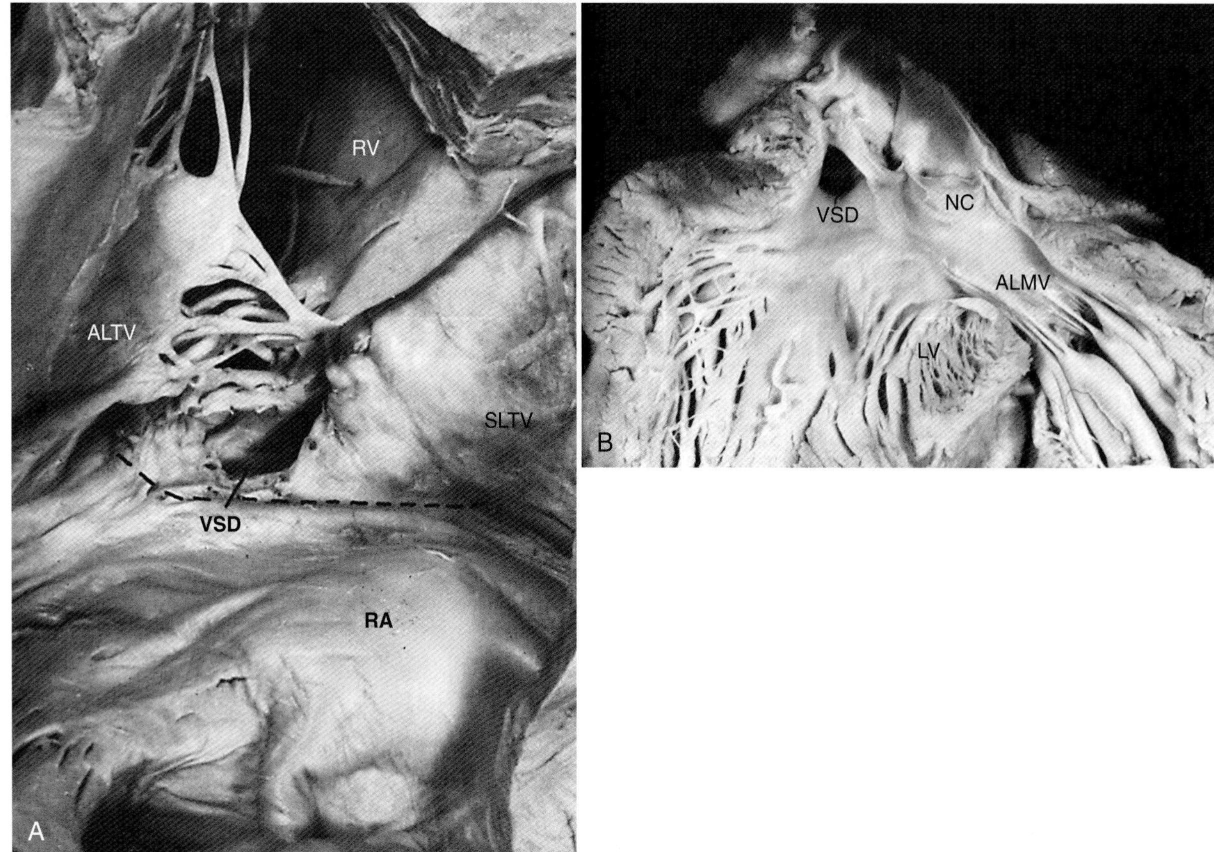

Figure 35-6 Type of perimembranous ventricular septal defect *(VSD)* that ejects directly into right atrium, a so-called left ventricular–right atrial defect. **A,** VSD viewed from right atrium. Posterior part of tricuspid anulus is marked by dashed line. Tricuspid septal leaflet is anomalously adherent to underlying ventricular septum and edges of VSD, which is juxtatricuspid. Intact atrioventricular septum lies on atrial side of tricuspid anulus (beneath letters *VSD*). Bundle of His is along posterior angle of defect. **B,** Same defect viewed from left ventricle. VSD is juxta-aortic and beneath commissure between right and noncoronary aortic cusps. Key: *ALMV,* Anterior leaflet of mitral valve; *ALTV,* anterior leaflet of tricuspid valve; *LV,* left ventricle; *NC,* noncoronary aortic cusp; *RA,* right atrium; *RV,* right ventricle; *SLTV,* septal leaflet of tricuspid valve.

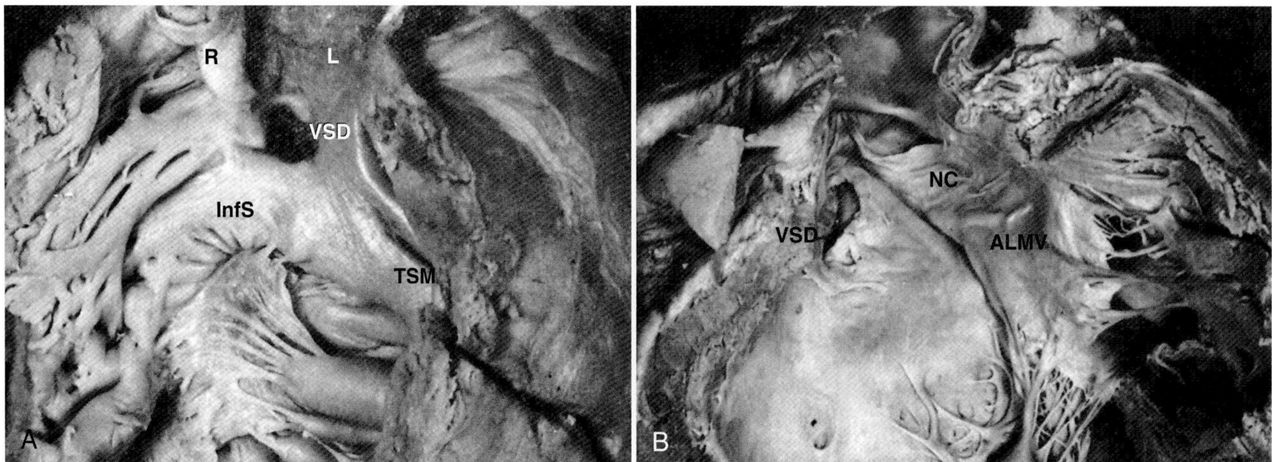

Figure 35-7 Doubly committed subarterial ventricular septal defect *(VSD)* in outlet portion of ventricular septum. **A,** VSD viewed from right ventricle. Its inferior margin is formed of thick septal tissue and its superior margin by confluent right pulmonary and right aortic cusps, which are separated by a thin ridge of fibrous tissue. **B,** Same defect viewed from left ventricle. VSD is beneath right coronary cusp of aortic valve and more anterior than a conoventricular VSD. Key: *ALMV,* Anterior leaflet of mitral valve; *InfS,* infundibular (outlet) septum; *L,* left pulmonary cusp; *NC,* noncoronary aortic cusp; *R,* right pulmonary cusp; *TSM,* trabecula septomarginalis (septal band).

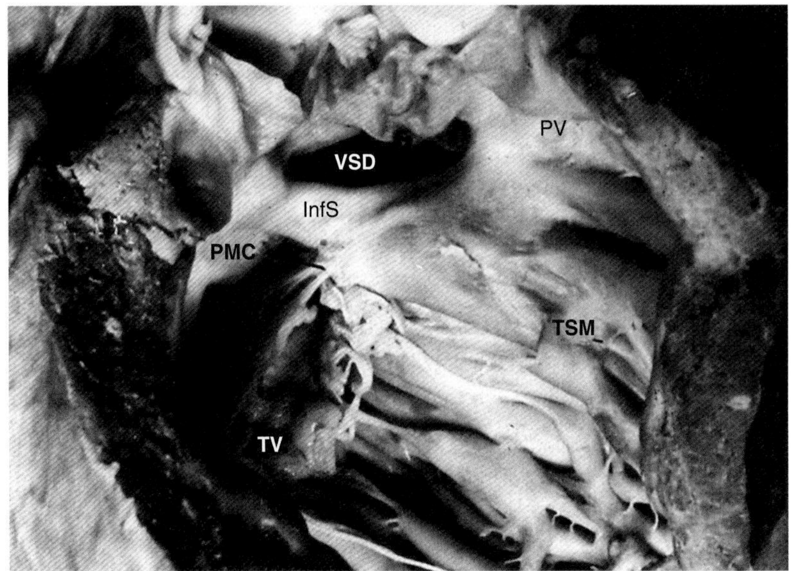

Figure 35-8 Doubly committed subarterial ventricular septal defect *(VSD)* viewed from right ventricle. VSD lies immediately beneath pulmonary valve (and, although it is unseen, aortic valve). Inferior to defect are infundibular septum and trabecula septomarginalis (septal band). Tricuspid valve, papillary muscle of conus, and bundle of His are far from defect. Key: *InfS,* Infundibular septum; *PMC,* papillary muscle of Lancisi; *PV,* pulmonary valve; *TSM,* trabecula septomarginalis (septal band); *TV,* tricuspid valve.

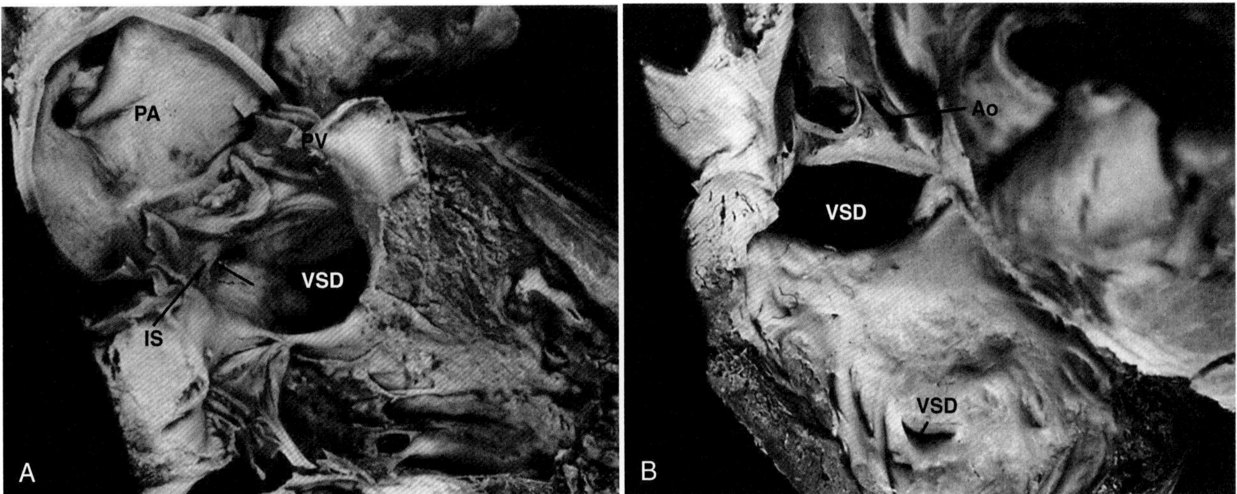

Figure 35-9 Large confluent ventricular septal defect *(VSD)* that is both subarterial and perimembranous, extending downward to reach tricuspid anulus. This type of VSD is also seen in double outlet right ventricle with doubly committed VSD and in double outlet left ventricle. **A,** VSD viewed from right ventricle. At superior margin of VSD, pulmonary and aortic cusps are in fibrous continuity. Arrow points toward aortic valve. **B,** Same defect viewed from left ventricle. Note additional small trabecular muscular defect. Key: *Ao,* Aorta; *IS,* infundibular septum; *PA,* pulmonary artery; *PV,* pulmonary and aortic cusps.

anterior margin is muscular and crescentic (Fig. 35-10). Superiorly, inlet septal defects usually extend to the membranous septum. The AV septum is intact, in contrast to the situation in hearts with AV canal septal defects (see Morphology in Chapter 34). The anterior (septal) mitral leaflet occasionally may be cleft, either partially or completely, with associated mitral regurgitation. Rarely, VSDs in the inlet portion of the septum extend completely to the crux cordis and thus are also *juxtacrucial* in position. The tricuspid valve is overriding and usually straddling.

In inlet septal VSDs, the AV node lies more laterally and anteriorly along the tricuspid anulus than normal and at the point at which the tricuspid anulus meets the underlying ventricular septum, because of straddling of the tricuspid valve.[H17] The bundle of His lies along the *posteroinferior* rim of the inlet septal VSD, slightly on the LV side, as in juxtatricuspid VSDs.

A *muscular VSD* can occur in the inlet portion of the ventricular septum beneath the tricuspid septal leaflet (Fig. 35-11). The posterior margin of such a defect is separated from the tricuspid ring by muscle. A muscular VSD must be distinguished from the inlet septal type of VSD because the conducting tissue runs superior and anterior to a muscular defect.

Muscular Ventricular Septal Defect

VSDs in other locations are generally muscular VSDs. Such defects are frequently multiple and may be associated with perimembranous or subarterial VSDs. Single or multiple muscular defects in the trabecular septum are more common

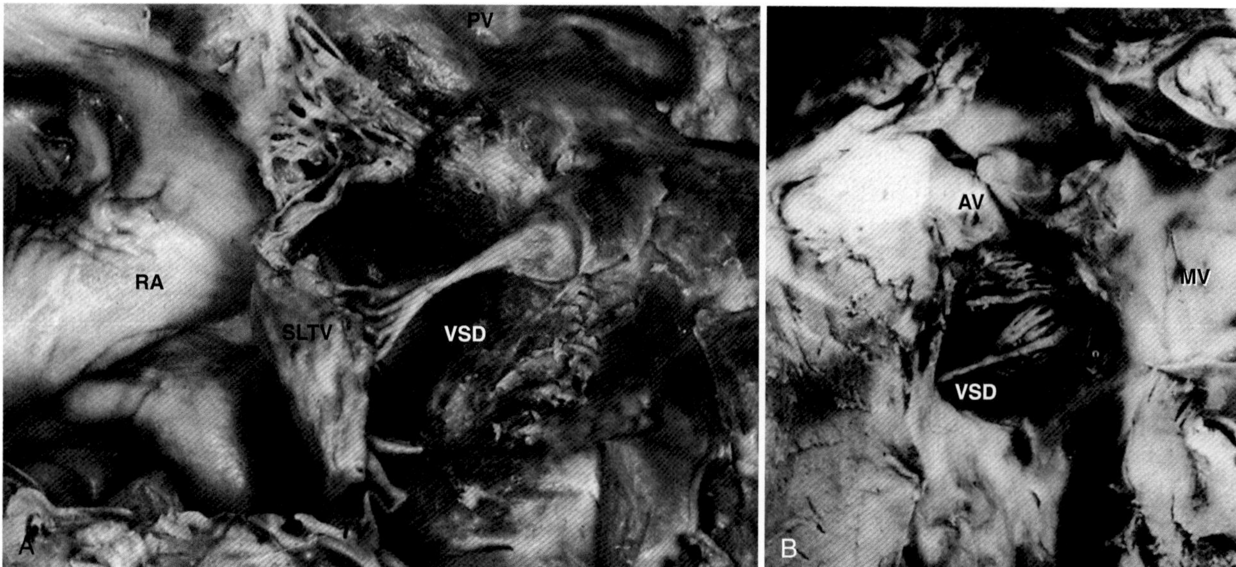

Figure 35-10 Inlet septal ventricular septal defect *(VSD)* beneath septal leaflet of tricuspid valve. Posterior margin of defect is formed by tricuspid anulus. VSD is juxtatricuspid. **A,** VSD viewed from right ventricle. Note crescentic anterior margin of defect. (A previously placed polyester patch has been removed.) **B,** Same defect viewed from left ventricle. Superiorly, defect reaches almost to aortic valve; posteriorly, it extends to mitral valve. Key: *AV,* Aortic valve; *MV,* mitral valve; *PV,* pulmonary valve; *RA,* right atrium; *SLTV,* septal leaflet of tricuspid valve; *TV,* tricuspid valve.

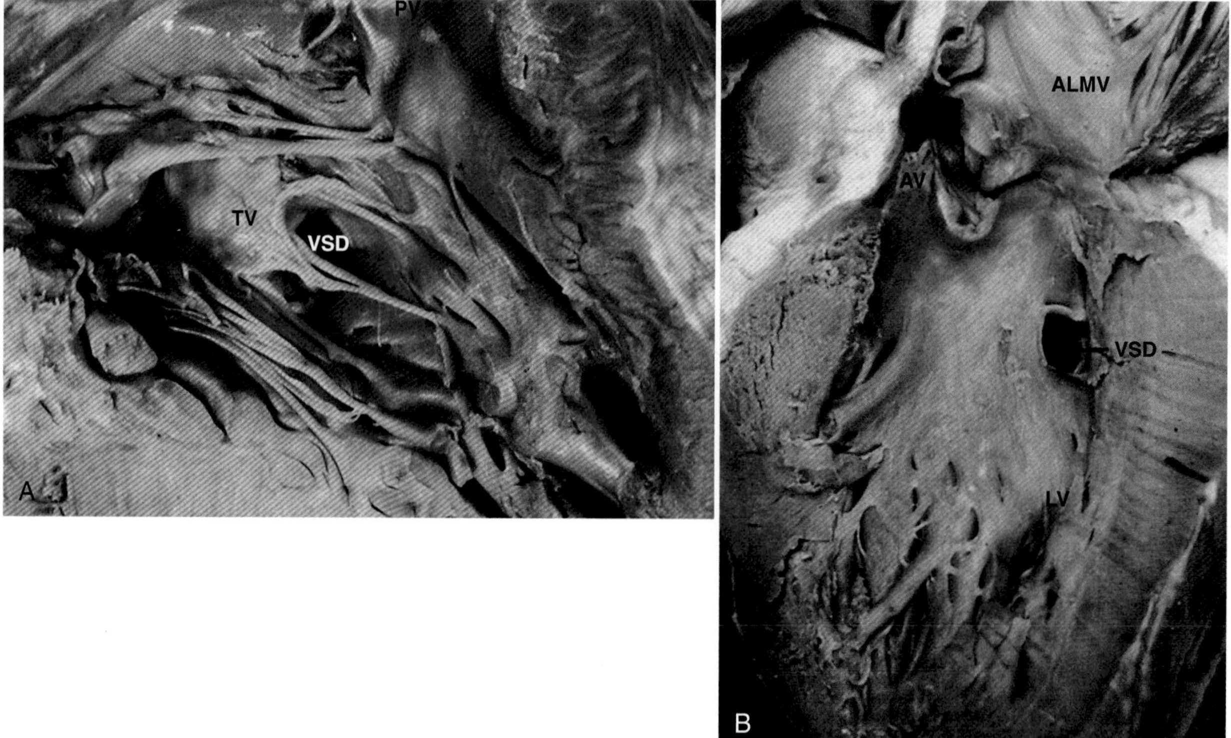

Figure 35-11 Single, moderate-sized, muscular inlet septal ventricular septal defect *(VSD)* lying beneath tricuspid septal leaflet. **A,** VSD viewed from right ventricle. Note septal muscle between VSD and tricuspid valve. Bundle of His lies superior to VSD. This defect can easily be closed from a right atrial approach. **B,** Same defect viewed from left ventricle. VSD is in posterior part of nontrabeculated portion of left side of ventricular septum. Key: *ALMV,* Anterior leaflet of mitral valve; *AV,* aortic valve; *LV,* left ventricle; *PV,* pulmonary valve; *TV,* tricuspid valve.

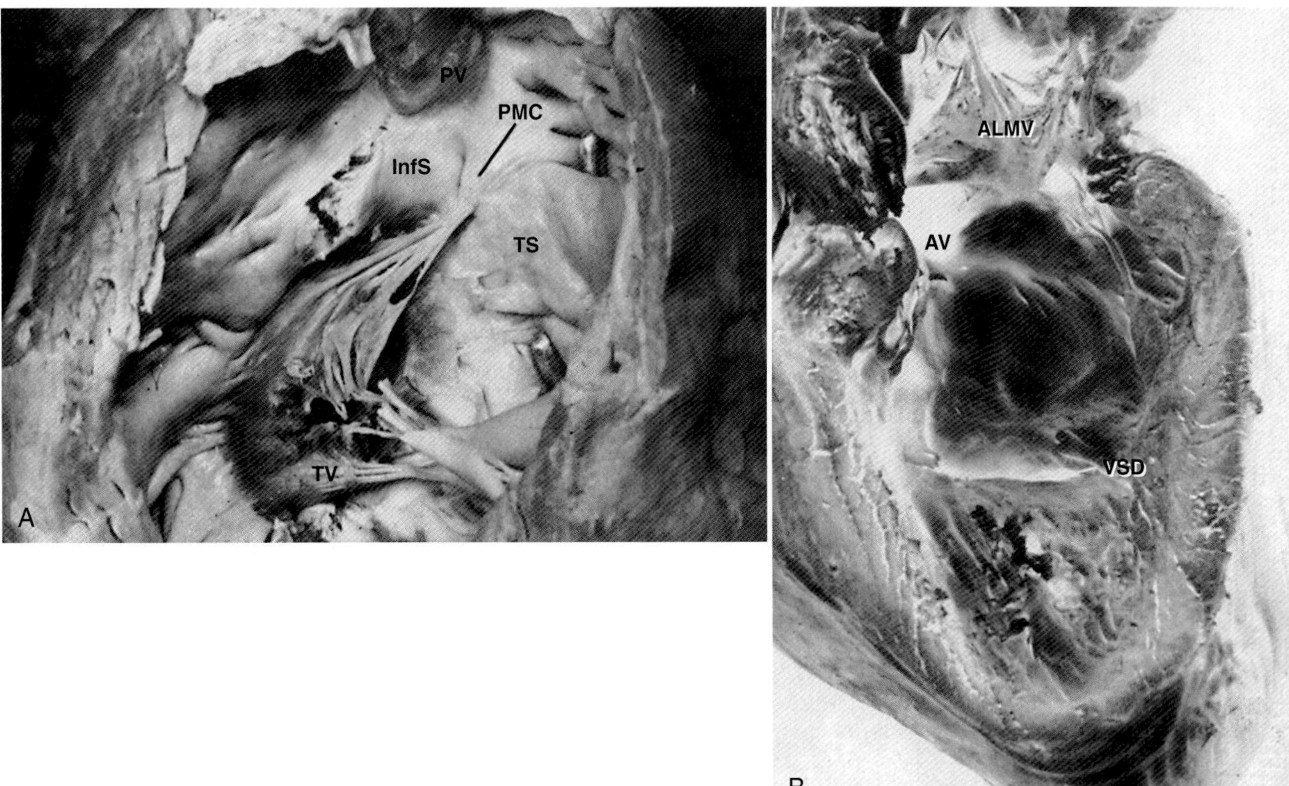

Figure 35-12 Muscular trabecular septal ventricular septal defect *(VSD)*. **A,** VSD viewed from right ventricle (RV). VSD is actually a single one, but is covered by trabecula septomarginalis (septal band) and therefore has two openings into right ventricle (see probes). **B,** Same defect viewed from left ventricle. VSD, appearing more slitlike than it actually is, lies at junction of smooth and trabeculated portions of septum. This defect can be closed from RV, provided lower end of septal band is detached. Key: *ALMV,* Anterior leaflet of mitral valve; *AV,* aortic valve; *InfS,* infundibular septum, or crista supraventricularis; *PMC,* papillary muscle of Lancisi; *PV,* pulmonary valve; *TS,* trabecula septomarginalis (septal band); *TV,* tricuspid valve.

in infants requiring operative treatment than in older children.

Muscular defects can occur anywhere in the ventricular septum (see Fig. 35-1). Those in the middle portion of the trabecular septum are the most common (Fig. 35-12) and may be overlaid by the trabecula septomarginalis; thus, even when single on the LV side, these defects have at least two openings on the RV side. Anterior muscular defects are usually multiple and most often in the apical and outlet portions of the septum. They may extend all along the anterior part of the septum from apex to outlet septum. Typically there are more openings on the RV than LV side.

A particularly important group of patients are those with *Swiss cheese defects* (Fig. 35-13), many defects of variable size, not only along the anterior portion of the septum but throughout the midportion as well. These defects often pass obliquely through the septum to appear on both sides of the trabecula septomarginalis or in the anterior part of the septum. They may be associated with large or small perimembranous or subarterial defects. Major associated cardiac anomalies are common, especially severe coarctation of the aorta.

The bundle of His is not closely related to the borders of any muscular VSD.

Confluent Ventricular Septal Defect

Some unusually large, single confluent VSDs involve more than one area of the septum. Rarely a confluent VSD may involve most of the septum (Fig. 35-14), but hearts with such defects should not be classified as having a single ventricle.

Ventricular Septal Defect with Straddling or Overriding Tricuspid Valve

In rare instances, tricuspid valve chordae may *straddle* the ventricular septum in association with a large inlet septal defect resembling an inlet septal–type VSD but extending to the crux cordis[L12,M10,R3] (Fig. 35-15). The tricuspid valve usually *overrides* both ventricles. When overriding is severe, the tricuspid anulus is usually very large, and many chordae from it are attached to the LV side of the septum (a combination of straddling and overriding).[B8] The atrial septum is malaligned relative to the ventricular septum. The RV is often hypoplastic. The tricuspid valve may be regurgitant.

Associated Lesions

Nearly half of patients undergoing surgical treatment for a primary VSD have an associated cardiac anomaly.[B10,G9] A moderate-sized or large *patent ductus arteriosus* (PDA) is

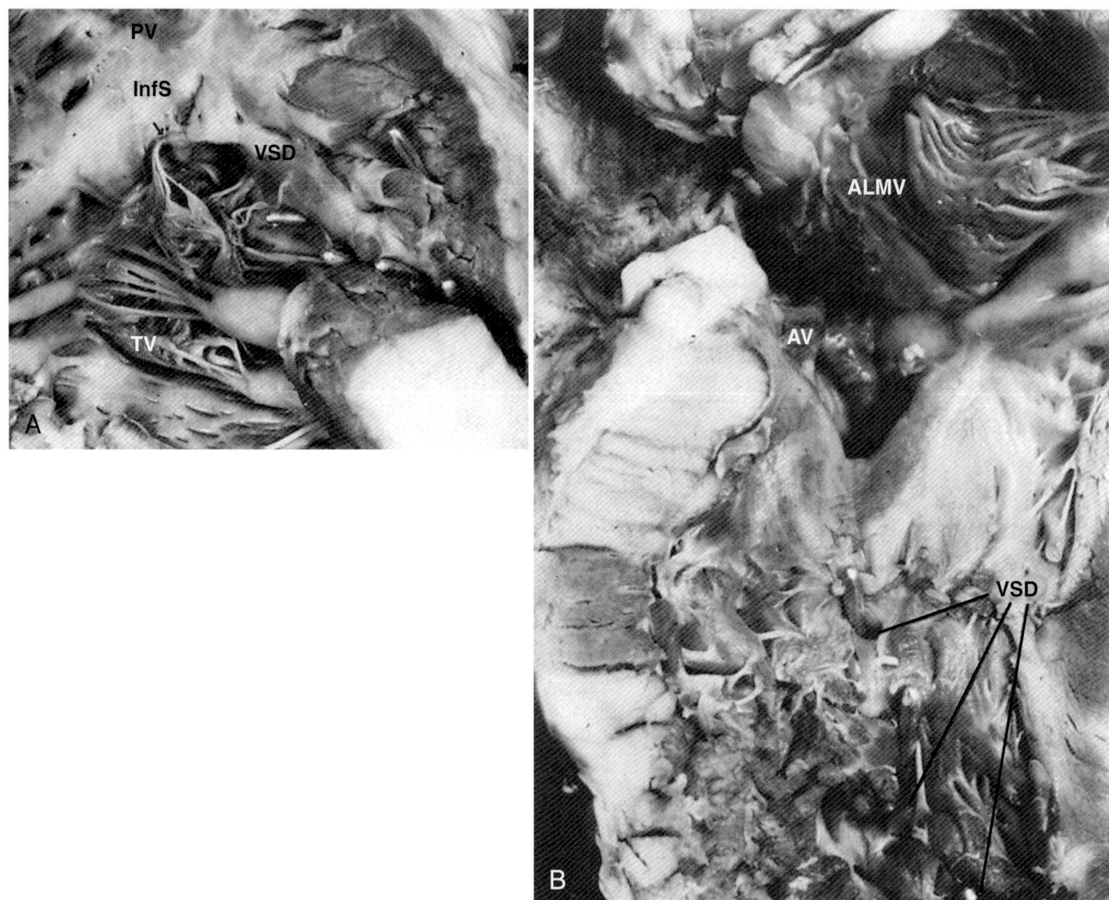

Figure 35-13 "Swiss cheese" type of multiple ventricular septal defect *(VSD)* associated with a large perimembranous VSD. **A,** VSDs viewed from right ventricle. Perimembranous defect shows anomalous chordal attachment from tricuspid valve to posterosuperior margin of defect *(arrow)*. Probes demonstrate five separate openings of small defects, one above and four below trabecula septomarginalis (septal band). **B,** Same defects viewed from left ventricle. Perimembranous defect is seen. Probes demonstrate three separate openings of Swiss cheese defects, but many more lie in grossly trabeculated lower portion of septum. Key: *ALMV,* Anterior leaflet of mitral valve; *AV,* aortic valve; *InfS,* infundibular septum; *PV,* pulmonary valve; *TV,* tricuspid valve.

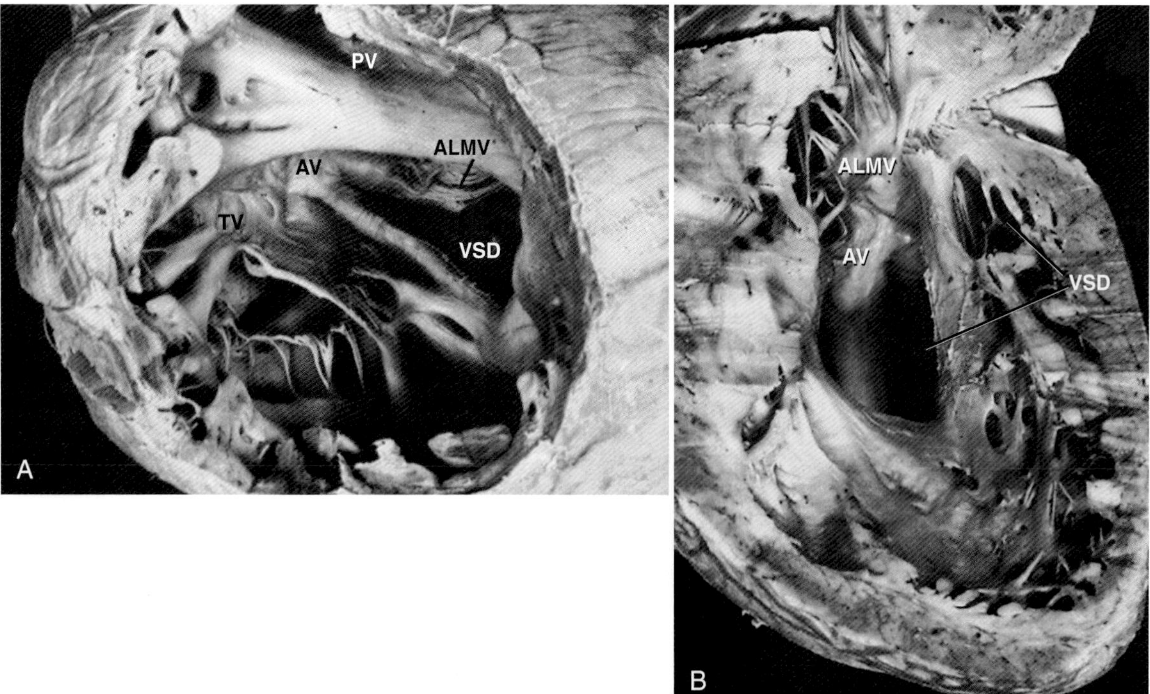

Figure 35-14 Large confluent ventricular septal defect *(VSD)* is perimembranous and occupies upper half of muscular septum beneath infundibular septum (anterior extension). It is associated with Swiss cheese VSDs. **A,** VSD viewed from right ventricle. Surgeon's initial impression would be that patient had a single ventricle. **B,** Same defect viewed from left ventricle. Malformation is clearly not a single ventricle. Key: *ALMV,* Anterior leaflet of mitral valve; *AV,* aortic valve; *PV,* pulmonary valve; *TV,* tricuspid valve.

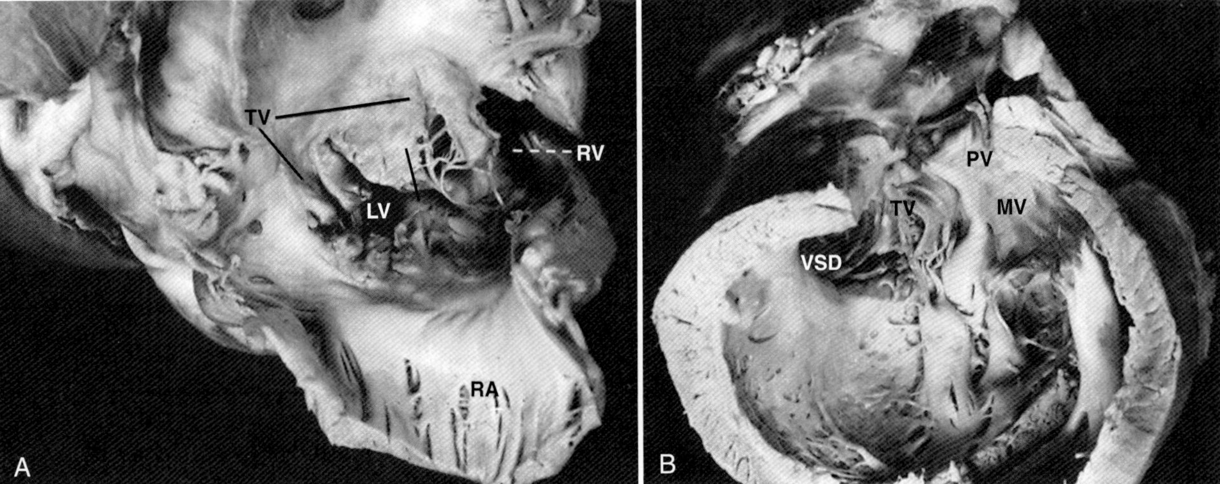

Figure 35-15 Inlet septal type of ventricular septal defect *(VSD)* with posterior extension and straddling tricuspid valve. **A,** VSD viewed from right atrium. Crest of ventricular septum forming lower boundary of defect *(black arrow)* crosses almost beneath center of large tricuspid orifice, indicating severe malalignment of atrial and ventricular septa. **B,** Same defect viewed from left ventricle. Chordal attachments of tricuspid valve cross VSD to attach to septal surface of left ventricle. This heart also exhibits transposition of the great arteries, with pulmonary trunk above left ventricle. Key: *LV,* Left ventricle; *MV,* mitral valve; *PV,* pulmonary valve; *RA,* right atrium; *RV,* right ventricle; *TV,* tricuspid valve orifice.

present in about 6% of patients of all ages, but about 25% of infants in heart failure. VSD occurs in combination with moderate or severe *coarctation of the aorta* in about 5% of patients. This combination is also much more common among infants with large VSD coming to operation younger than age 3 months.

Congenital *aortic stenosis* occurs in about 2% of patients requiring operation for VSD. Subvalvar stenosis is more common than valvar[L4] and may also occur in association with infundibular pulmonary stenosis. *Subvalvar stenosis* can be due to (1) a discrete fibromuscular bar lying inferior (caudad or upstream) to the VSD; (2) a discrete fibromuscular bar located distal (downstream) to the VSD, often consisting of displacement of infundibular septal muscle into the LV outflow tract (posterior malalignment), and often associated with aortic coarctation and interrupted arch[A10,D6,M14] (see "Morphology" in Sections I and II of Chapter 48); (3) pulmonary artery banding[F3]; and (4) excrescences of AV valvar tissue.[N2]

Congenital *mitral valve disease* occurs in about 2% of patients.[B10] One of the *pulmonary arteries* may be absent or severely stenotic. Severe peripheral pulmonary artery stenoses occur rarely.

Although *atrial septal defects* in general are not considered major associated anomalies, they may coexist with a large VSD in small infants and may be important lesions.

Severe positional cardiac anomalies (e.g., isolated dextrocardia, situs inversus totalis) are *uncommon* in patients with VSD.

Pulmonary Vascular Disease

The classic description of the pathology of hypertensive pulmonary vascular disease is that of Heath and Edwards[H4] (Box 35-1).

Box 35-1 Heath-Edwards Classification of Pulmonary Vascular Disease Pathology

Grade 1
Medial hypertrophy without intimal proliferation

Grade 2
Medial hypertrophy with cellular intimal reaction

Grade 3
Medial hypertrophy with intimal fibrosis and possibly early generalized vascular dilatation

Grade 4
Generalized vascular dilatation, areas of vascular occlusion by intimal fibrosis, and plexiform lesions

Grade 5
Other dilatation plexiform lesions such as cavernous and angiomatoid lesions

Grade 6
Necrotizing arteritis in addition to characteristics of grade 5 changes

Rp in patients with large VSD (and those with large PDA) is positively correlated with histologic severity of the hypertensive pulmonary vascular disease, classified by Heath and colleagues[H5] (Fig. 35-16). A close positive correlation also exists between lowest Rp at rest or with isoproterenol infusion and Heath-Edwards grade of vascular disease. Heath-Edwards grades above 3 were not found in patients with Rp index less than 7 units · m^2, whereas those with Rp greater than 8.5 units · m^2 showed changes characteristic of grade 4 or greater.[B17] Similarly, Fried and colleagues found a rather close negative correlation ($P = .001$) between magnitude of left-to-right shunt and Heath-Edwards grade in infants and children coming to VSD repair.[F5] Variability in these matters[B17] is not unexpected because Heath-Edwards classification is based on the most severe lesion seen, regardless of its frequency. As noted by Wagenvoort and colleagues[W1,W2] and

Yamaki and Tezuka,[Y3] grading should include assessment of the number of vessels affected. In addition, calculation of Rp is open to errors.[H12]

Hislop and colleagues provide a different view of hypertensive pulmonary vascular disease in infants with large VSD.[H10] Other investigators had noted earlier that intimal proliferation (and thus Heath-Edwards changes of grade 2 or greater) rarely develops in patients with large VSD until 1 or 2 years of age,[D2,W1] despite infants occasionally having severely elevated Rp. Hislop and colleagues found that infants dying at 3 to 6 months of age with large VSD and high (>8 units $\cdot$ m^2) Rp with intermittent right-to-left shunting have marked medial hypertrophy affecting both large and small pulmonary arteries, including those less than 200 μm in diameter.[H10] The usual number of intraacinar vessels was present. By contrast, these investigators found that infants 3 to 10 months of age with large VSDs dying with a history of large $\dot{Q}p$ and heart failure and normal or slightly elevated Rp have medial hypertrophy affecting mainly arteries larger than 200 μm. The intraacinar vessels were fewer than usual, so-called lessened arterial density. These histologic features have been shown by Rabinovitch and colleagues to correlate with pulmonary hemodynamic findings after repair of VSDs.[R1] Fried and colleagues have emphasized that Heath-Edwards grade and arterial density are the best correlates of fall in pulmonary artery pressure after repair.[F5]

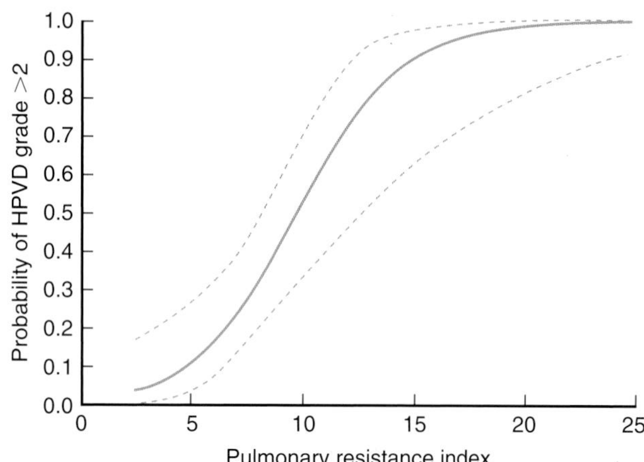

Figure 35-16 Probability of hypertensive pulmonary vascular disease (HPDV) greater than grade 2 in patients with ventricular septal defect, given total pulmonary resistance index (units $\cdot$ m^2). Dotted lines enclose 70% confidence limits (P = .07). (From Heath and colleagues.[H5])

Histologic reversibility of pulmonary vascular disease after closure of VSD has not been documented. Favorable results in infants may be from an increase in arterial density as growth proceeds. Presumably, pulmonary vascular disease of Heath-Edwards grade 3 or greater severity is not reversible.

CLINICAL FEATURES AND DIAGNOSTIC CRITERIA

Clinical Findings

In infants, signs and symptoms of heart failure include tachypnea and liver enlargement, often associated with poor feeding and growth failure, and physical findings of a precordial pansystolic or more abbreviated systolic murmur and a hyperactive heart. These findings suggest the diagnosis of a large VSD. An apical diastolic murmur suggests large flow across the mitral valve during diastole, the result of a large $\dot{Q}p$. Cardiomegaly and evidence of large $\dot{Q}p$ are seen on the chest radiograph (Fig. 35-17). The electrocardiogram (ECG) usually shows biventricular hypertrophy. In older patients with large VSD, the history is often nonspecific, but

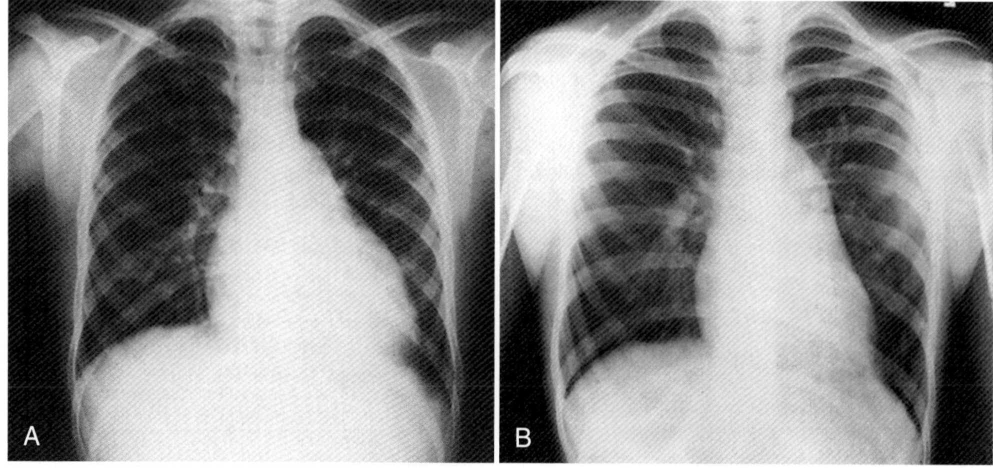

Figure 35-17 Chest radiographs of children with ventricular septal defect (VSD). **A,** Large VSD in 11-year-old girl with large left-to-right shunt, severe pulmonary hypertension, and low pulmonary vascular resistance. Cardiac enlargement and increased pulmonary vascularity are evident. Pulmonary trunk is enlarged and aortic arch small. Examination revealed an overactive heart with a systolic thrill and a loud (grade 4), long systolic murmur extending from lower left sternal border to apex and an apical diastolic murmur. Electrocardiogram (ECG) showed evidence of left ventricular overwork. **B,** Large VSD in 10-year-old girl with severe pulmonary hypertension, pulmonary/systemic flow ratio of 1.2, and pulmonary vascular resistance of 11 units $\cdot$ m^2. Cardiac size is normal, but pulmonary trunk is enlarged. Pulmonary vascularity is not increased. Examination revealed a quiet heart, no thrill, a soft (grade 2) systolic murmur, and no apical diastolic murmur; closure of pulmonic valve was loud and palpable. ECG demonstrated right ventricular hypertrophy without evidence of left ventricular overwork. (From Kirklin and DuShane.[K14])

examination also shows evidence of LV and RV enlargement and a systolic murmur usually best heard in the third and fourth left interspaces. In patients with doubly committed subarterial VSDs, the systolic murmur is maximal in the second and third interspaces, and in defects shunting mainly into the right atrium, in the fourth and fifth interspaces.

A high Rp from severe pulmonary vascular disease changes the hemodynamic state and clinical findings in patients with large VSDs. A large left-to-right shunt is no longer present because output resistances of the two pathways for LV emptying are similar, and the shunt is bidirectional and of about equal magnitude in both directions. The heart is not enlarged or hyperactive. A systolic murmur (produced by the large flow across the VSD) is soft or absent, and no apical diastolic murmur is heard. The pulmonary component of the second sound at the base is loud and sometimes palpable. Chest radiography reflects these features (see Fig. 35-17). ECG shows severe RV hypertrophy rather than combined ventricular hypertrophy, and evidence of LV volume overload. When pulmonary vascular disease is even more advanced, cyanosis develops *(Eisenmenger complex)* because the shunt across the VSD becomes right to left as RV output resistance through the pulmonary vascular bed becomes higher than that through the VSD and aorta.

Patients with *small* VSDs have small shunts and often no abnormal signs or symptoms other than a pansystolic murmur. Chest radiography and ECG both may be normal. When the defect is *moderate* in size, the LV is mildly or moderately enlarged (shown by physical examination, chest radiography, and ECG), and the volume of the RV is increased.

When there is associated *pulmonary or aortic stenosis,* diagnostic features are changed. Thus, with important pulmonary stenosis, $\dot{Q}p$ is reduced, and the shunt may even be right to left. RV hypertrophy is increased. With important aortic stenosis, the load on the LV is increased, and if the obstruction is cephalad to the VSD, left-to-right shunt is also greater, resulting in more than the expected degree of LV hypertrophy on ECG. Coarctation of the aorta may also produce these features in older children.

Two-Dimensional Echocardiography

Two-dimensional echocardiography imaging of the VSD with color Doppler flow evaluation of shunt flow by proximal isovelocity surface area (PISA)[K28] has changed traditional views about preoperative studies. Thus, cardiac catheterization and cineangiography are not necessary before closure of primary VSDs when (1) the clinical syndrome in neonates and infants indicates a large $\dot{Q}p/\dot{Q}s$; (2) noninvasive imaging clearly defines the morphology, including that of the aortic arch and ductus arteriosus; and (3) the surgeon is experienced in surgical identification and repair of congenital heart disease.[C2]

For identifying a large single perimembranous VSD, combined 2D echocardiography and Doppler flow interrogation is highly reliable in combination with clinical criteria[B9,O10] (Fig. 35-18). Echocardiography adds to anatomic clarification, particularly in the case of doubly committed subarterial VSDs.[G11] Particularly for small VSDs and multiple muscular defects, 2D Doppler color flow echocardiographic imaging increases the sensitivity of echocardiography[L18] (Fig. 35-18, *A* and *B*). However, and particularly in the presence of a single large VSD, multiple muscular defects can go undetected even with refined techniques of echocardiography.[L18] Because perimembranous VSDs are infrequently (<3%[C8]) accompanied by additional muscular VSDs, this does not contraindicate proceeding to repair in infants without cardiac catheterization. Malalignment VSD is diagnosed by 2D echocardiography by the appearance of the alignment of the RV trabecular septum with the outlet septum. Malalignment may be *anterior* as in tetralogy of Fallot (Fig. 35-18, *C*), *posterior* as in interrupted aortic arch, or *rotational* as in Taussig-Bing heart.

Size of a VSD is generally categorized echocardiographically as small, moderate, or large for purposes of decisions regarding surgery (see Morphology and Indications for Operation later in this chapter).[H16] A *large* defect has a diameter of 75% or greater of the aortic anulus and low-velocity flow by Doppler, measuring no more than 1 $m \cdot s^{-1}$. A *moderate* defect has a diameter of 33% to 75% of the aortic anulus and flow velocity of 1 to 4 $m \cdot s^{-1}$, indicating moderate flow restriction. (By the modified Bernoulli equation, gradient across the defect is calculated by multiplying velocity squared times 4.) A *small* defect has a diameter less than 33% of the aortic anulus and a flow velocity of 4 $m \cdot s^{-1}$ or greater. When considering Rp, it is important to note that as resistance (or obstructions in the RV outflow tract) increases, flow velocity across the VSD decreases.

Other Noninvasive Diagnostic Methods

Other noninvasive imaging modalities may come into use. At present, only magnetic resonance imaging (MRI) has shown promise to provide accurate information about the morphology of all types of VSDs.[B1] Dynamic three-dimensional echocardiographic reconstructions may refine ability to image and portray VSDs spacially.[T3]

Cardiac Catheterization

When surgical intervention is under consideration in older children, cardiac catheterization and angiography are generally indicated to assess Rp and precisely identify location, size, and number of VSDs and any associated anomalies. Furthermore, preoperative sizing of VSDs is often important in arriving at management decisions. Sizing can be especially difficult when the VSD is associated with another lesion such as coarctation or pulmonary stenosis. The most reliable way to size the defect is to measure its diameter either by 2D color flow Doppler echocardiography or cineangiography. With cineangiography, the VSD must be accurately profiled and the measurement either corrected to allow for magnification or compared with aortic root diameter. In applying this method to perimembranous VSDs, the defect is smaller in a cranially tilted left anterior oblique (LAO) projection than in the conventional LAO position.

Cardiac catheterization should include both right-sided and left-sided heart studies, the latter mainly to obtain LV angiograms. Basic data obtained at cardiac catheterization should include oxygen consumption ($\dot{V}o_2$); systolic, diastolic, and mean pulmonary arterial, pulmonary artery wedge, and systemic arterial pressures; oxygen content and saturation in right atrial, pulmonary arterial, aortic, or peripheral arterial blood and, when possible, left atrial blood. Pulmonary ($\dot{Q}p$) and systemic ($\dot{Q}s$) blood flows and $\dot{Q}p/\dot{Q}s$

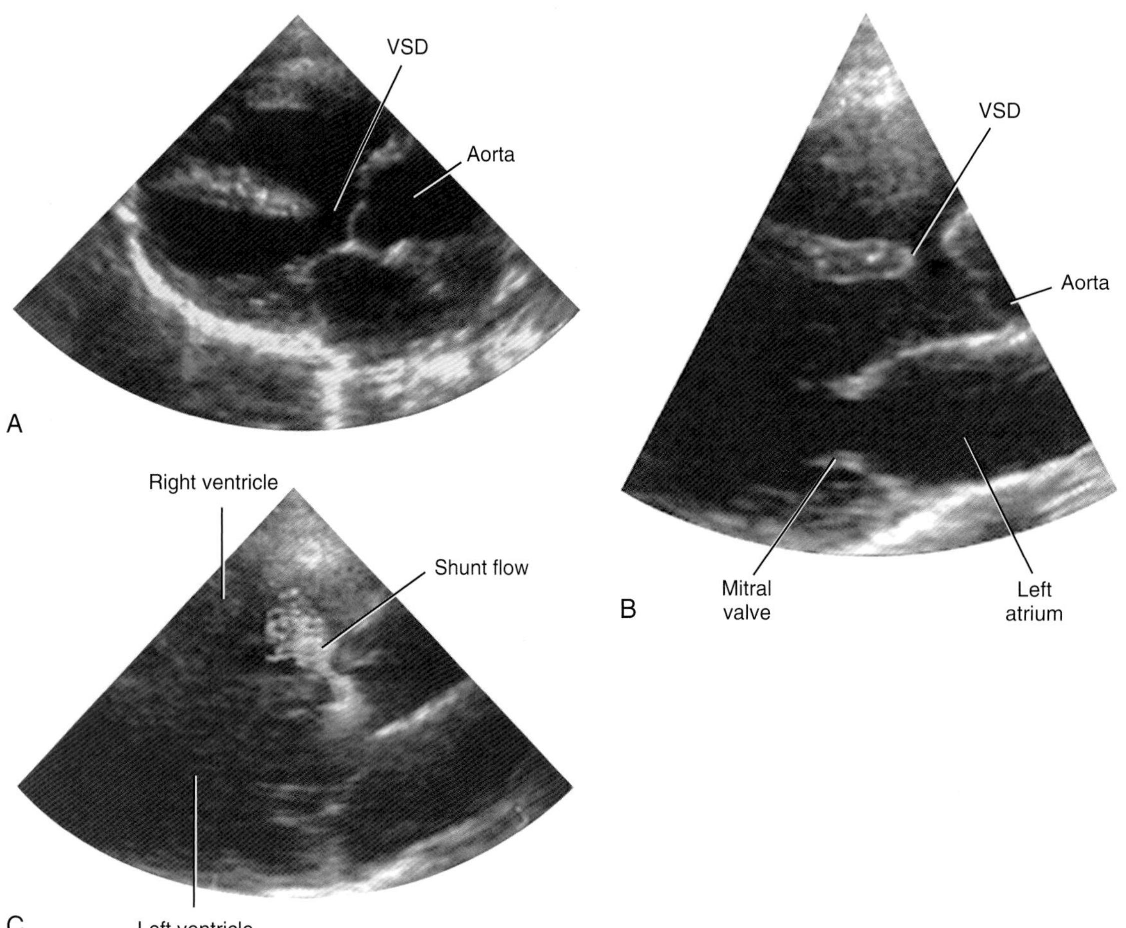

Figure 35-18 Two-dimensional echocardiograms with Doppler directional flow velocity in perimembranous ventricular septal defect *(VSD)*. **A,** Four-chamber view demonstrating VSD as gap in ventricular septum between right ventricle and left ventricle. **B,** Magnified view of VSD. **C,** Turbulent blood flow through VSD is directed from left ventricle to right ventricle.

are calculated[3] with Rp (Table 35-3). When left atrial (or pulmonary arterial wedge) pressure is not available, only total pulmonary resistance (TPR)[4] can be calculated. Rp in absolute units × body surface area is of more value in predicting operability than is the ratio of resistances in pulmonary and systemic circuits.[N5] When Rp is elevated, further information concerning operability should be obtained by assessing response to exercise and to isoproterenol (see Indications for Operation later in this chapter).

Table 35-3 Pulmonary Vascular Resistance

Resistance		
≤ units · m²	<	Description
	4	Normal
4	5	Mildly elevated
5	8	Moderately elevated
8		Severely elevated

Angiography

Angiographic assessment of VSD is best performed using biplane techniques in appropriate projections.[B2,E4] Whereas cardiologists and radiologists carry primary responsibility for these studies, appreciation of their findings and limitations is essential to the surgeon, who must also understand when the study is incomplete.[B12]

Fig. 35-19 summarizes the surgically important features of angiograms of VSD by diagram. Fig. 35-20 presents representative angiograms of the various types of VSDs.

NATURAL HISTORY

Spontaneous Closure

VSDs tend to close spontaneously.[E6] This is relevant to decisions about operation and explains, for the most part, the infrequency with which large VSDs are encountered in adults.[C17] Spontaneous closure can be complete by 1 year of

[3] $\dot{Q}p = \dot{V}O_2 / (Cp\bar{v}O_2 - CpaO_2)$ in $L \cdot min^{-1}$
where *pv* is pulmonary vein and *pa* is pulmonary artery. $\dot{Q}p$ may be expressed as index ($L \cdot min^{-1} \cdot m^{-2}$) by dividing by body surface area (BSA) expressed in square meters.
$\dot{Q}s = \dot{V}O_2 / (CaO_2 - C\bar{v}O_2)$ in $L \cdot min^{-1}$
where *a* is aorta or arterial and $\bar{v}$ is mixed venous.
$\dot{Q}p / \dot{Q}s = (CaO_2 - C\bar{v}O_2) / (Cp\bar{v}O_2 - CpaO_2)$
Note that total oxygen consumption is not needed for this calculation.
$Rp = [(Ppa - Pla) / \dot{Q}p] \cdot BSA$; Rp is expressed in units $\cdot m^2$.
[4] $TPR = [Ppa / \dot{Q}p] \cdot BSA$; TPR is expressed in units $\cdot m^2$.

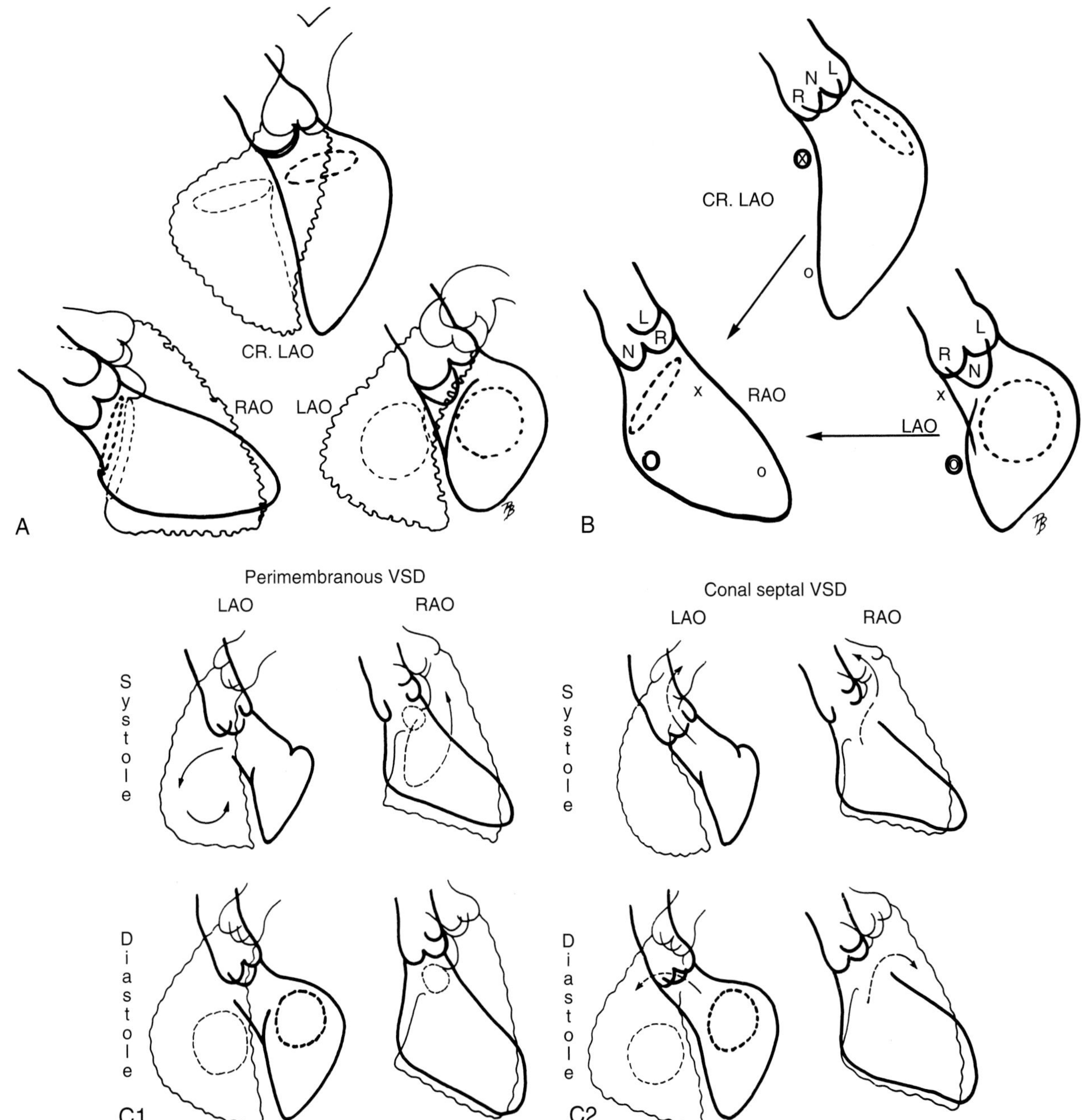

Figure 35-19 Line drawings of angiographic projections for assessment of ventricular septal defect *(VSD)*. **A,** Interrelationships of left ventricle (LV) and aortic root *(thick line)* with right ventricle (RV) and pulmonary trunk *(thin line)* in 40-degree right anterior oblique *(RAO)*, 50-degree left anterior oblique *(LAO)*, and 40-degree cranially tilted *(CR. LAO)* projections. RAO view profiles infundibular (conal) and high anterior portions of RV outlet septum below and in front of right coronary sinus and profiles atrioventricular (AV) septum beneath noncoronary sinus of aortic root. Both LAO views profile apical trabecular portion of septum. LAO view also partly profiles RV outlet septum but superimposes it on LV outflow tract and aortic root. CR. LAO projection views RV outlet septum en face and superimposes it on LV. Because orientation shows a horizontally lying heart, LAO view depicts full length (cranial to caudal) of apical and anterior trabecular portion of ventricular septum and AV valve anuli *(interrupted lines)*, whereas CR. LAO view depicts full length of sinus portion of trabecular septum from base to apex. **B,** Both cranially tilted *(CR. LAO)* and conventional LAO views are required for a complete assessment of sinus septum. Basal (inlet) *(O, x)* VSDs are separated from more apical *(o)* VSDs by CR. LAO projection, whereas high *(x)* VSDs are separated from low *(O)* VSDs by LAO view. **C,** Anatomic and hemodynamic features of VSDs shown by LV angiograms. LAO diagrams show a compromise between conventional and cranially tilted options. LV and aorta are shown by thick lines, RV and pulmonary trunk by thin lines, and AV valves and nonprofiled VSDs by interrupted lines. **C1,** Perimembranous VSD. LAO view profiles VSD just beneath parietal band (ventriculoinfundibular fold) at upper margin of inlet septum. Flow enters base of RV above tricuspid valve, filling base before reaching infundibulum. Tricuspid valve is well seen in diastole, and lower margin of defect can be accurately related to tricuspid anulus in LAO. RAO view does not profile defect unless it extends into outlet septum. Note intact AV septum beneath noncoronary sinus of aortic root. Shunt enters RV infundibulum, crossing but not interrupting intact superior margin of LV, indicating intact conal and high anterior septal regions. **C2,** Doubly committed subarterial VSD (labeled *conal septal VSD*). LAO view shows an intact septum from aortic valve to apex. RV sinus usually fills only faintly by diastolic mixing from infundibular region, and tricuspid valve may not be seen. Defect is superimposed on aortic root. RAO view profiles defect beneath contiguous parts of aortic and pulmonary valves. Systolic streaming through RV infundibulum to pulmonary trunk is well shown, with some mixing to more anterior part of RV in diastole, but high anterior septal region is intact.

Continued

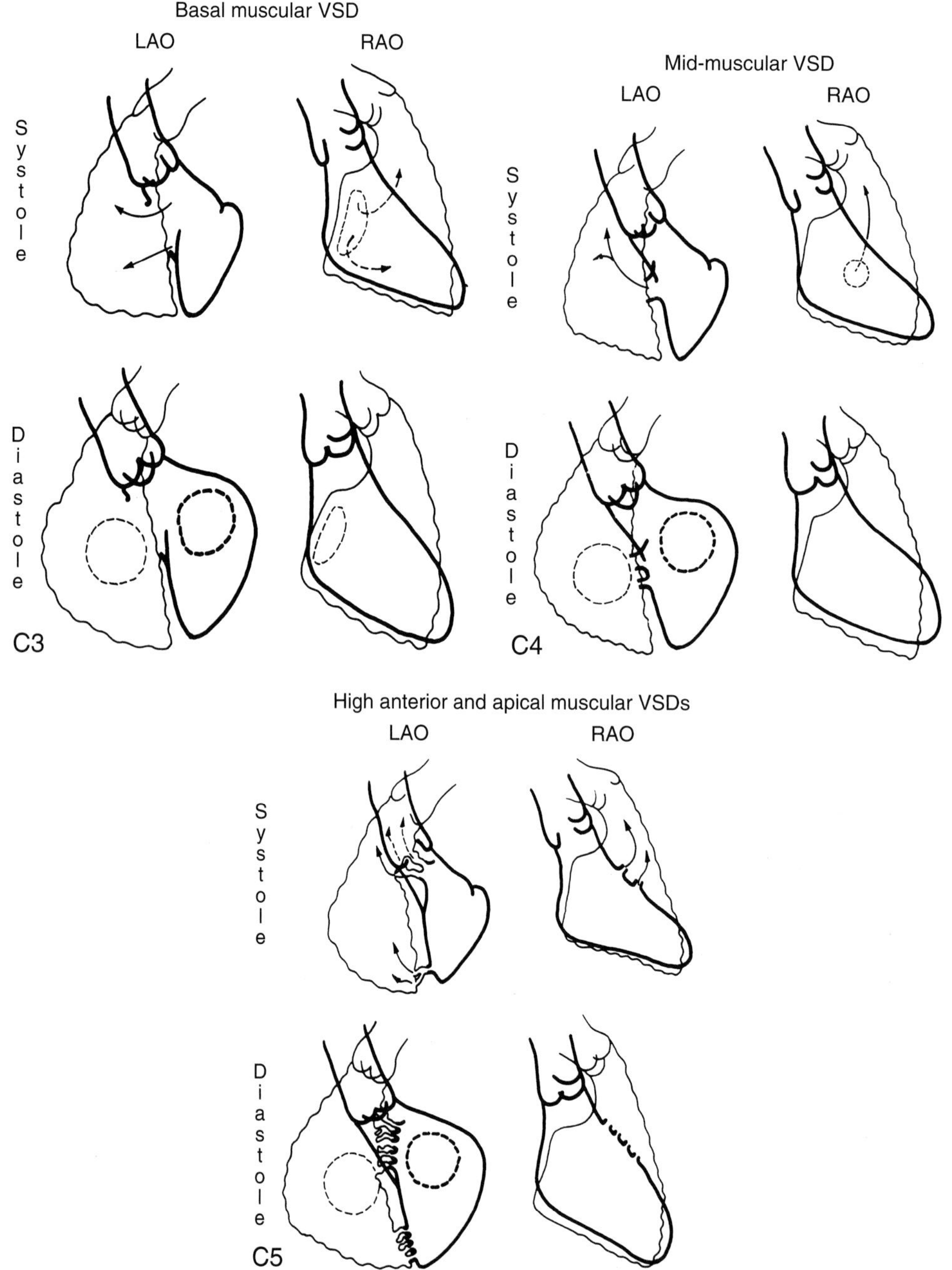

Figure 35-19, cont'd **C3,** Inlet septal VSD (labeled *basal muscular VSD*). VSD is adjacent to tricuspid valve (AV septal type) or separated from it by a rim of muscle (muscular VSD). These two types of VSDs are not readily distinguished radiologically. In LAO view, defect is profiled between AV valves, replacing full height of basal septum (conventional LAO view), perhaps extending into adjacent middle portion of ventricular septum but not into apical region (cranially tilted LAO view). Contrast medium streams directly into base of RV sinus in systole, providing a good depiction of tricuspid orifice in diastole. Separate AV valves are present, in contrast to the finding in a complete AV septal defect (see Chapter 34). In RAO view, VSD is not profiled. Intact AV septum distinguishes this defect from a true AV septal defect. Note intact conal and high anterior septal regions. **C4,** Muscular, trabecular VSD (labeled *mid-muscular VSD*). LAO views show an intact inlet septum and no extension into apical region, although a small additional defect is seen in diastole, closing in systole. Some of the contrast medium streams directly into RV outflow during systole. Height of defect from floor of ventricle (bottom of AV valve) is appreciated in LAO view, and separation from basal and apical regions in cranially tilted LAO view. RAO features are as in parts **C1** and **C3. C5,** Multiple muscular anterior and apical VSDs. Muscular VSDs in these regions frequently coexist and, if numerous, form a continuous series throughout trabeculated septum from high in RV infundibulum to apical sinus septum. For clarity, only highest and lowest are shown here. In LAO view, intact basal and middle septal regions are profiled. Apical defects are profiled, but high anterior defects are superimposed on LV outflow region. Contrast medium tends to stream to RV outflow tract without filling basal parts. In RAO view, high anterior defects are profiled, interrupting superior margin of LV anterior to intact outlet septum. More defects are open in diastole than in systole. Key: *CR.LAO,* Cranial left anterior oblique; *L,* left coronary; *LAO,* left anterior oblique; *LV,* left ventricle; *N,* noncoronary; *R,* right coronary; *RAO,* right anterior oblique; *RV,* right ventricle. (From Brandt.[B11])

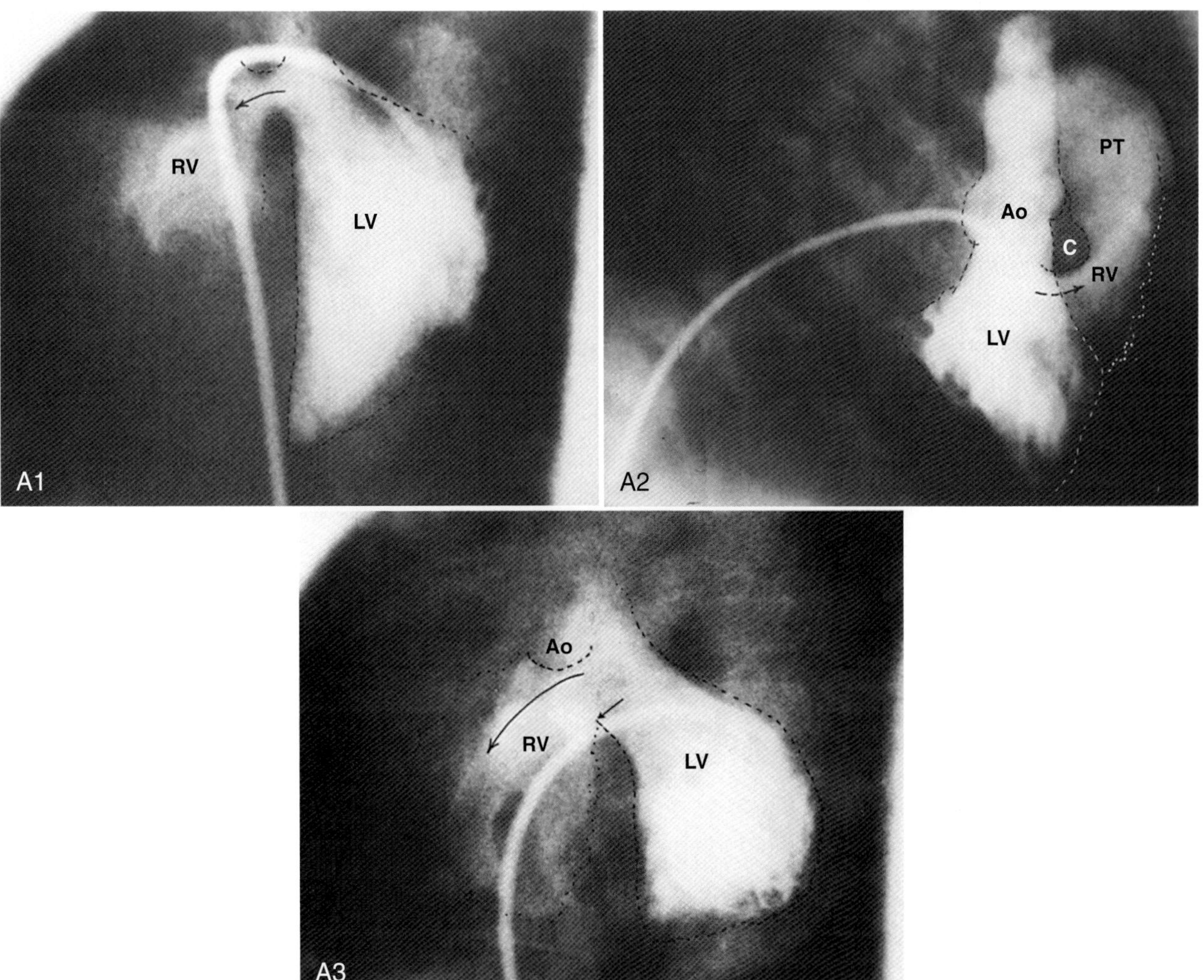

Figure 35-20 Angiograms of patients with ventricular septal defect (VSD). **A,** Left ventricular *(LV)* angiograms of a perimembranous VSD. **A1,** 40-degree cranially tilted 60-degree left anterior oblique (LAO) projection, systolic frame, early in perimembranous angiographic sequence. VSD *(arrow)* lies in basal part of ventricular septum adjacent to aortic root. No additional defects are seen in middle and apical portions of septum (catheter to LV through atrial septum and mitral valve). **A2,** 30-degree right anterior oblique (RAO) projection, systolic frame, slightly later than **A1** in sequence. Patient was positioned to achieve cranial tilting of simultaneously exposed LAO view shown in **A1.** Note intact atrioventricular septum beneath noncoronary aortic sinus and intact outlet septum *(C)*. Contrast medium from shunt through nonprofiled VSD fills right ventricular *(RV)* outflow tract, crossing *(arrow)* but not interrupting high anterior margin of LV. **A3,** 50-degree LAO projection, systolic frame early in sequence (second injection). Perimembranous VSD is profiled as in **A1** beneath aortic root. Large arrow indicates flow into base of RV above tricuspid valve (identified in diastole but not illustrated). Downward extent of VSD *(small arrow)* is accurately shown, and there are no additional defects lower in septum. Perimembranous defects are frequently small, of dimensions profiled in cranially tilted LAO projection in **A1,** compared with LAO.

Continued

age, or the defect may have only narrowed by then, with complete closure taking considerably longer. An inverse relation exists between the probability of eventual spontaneous closure and age at which the patient is observed[A6,B10,H13,K24] (Fig. 35-21). About 80% of patients with large VSDs seen at age 1 month experience eventual spontaneous closure, as do about 60% of those seen at age 3 months, about 50% of those seen at age 6 months, and about 25% of those seen at age 12 months. This decreasing tendency for spontaneous closure of a VSD as the patient grows older has also been confirmed by Beerman and colleagues,[B6] and spontaneous closure has been documented to occur in only one patient between age 21 and 31 years.[H19] Onat and colleagues studied 106 children with VSD and concluded that these patients should be followed closely through adolescence because the defects may decrease in diameter, shunt flow may diminish, and spontaneous closure may be expected in 23% of patients.[O8]

The mechanism of narrowing or closure of perimembranous VSDs is usually adherence of tricuspid leaflet or chordal tissue to the edges of the VSD.[C1,S30] Closure has erroneously been related to echocardiographic diagnosis of aneurysm of the membranous septum.[R2] Aneurysm of the membranous septum is usually considered benign and functionally reduces the size of the VSD. It has the potential consequence of promoting tricuspid regurgitation and RV outflow tract obstruction and is a nidus for infective endocarditis.[Y5]

Perimembranous VSDs, as well as VSDs that are juxta-aortic and inlet VSDs of the AV septal type, are less likely to

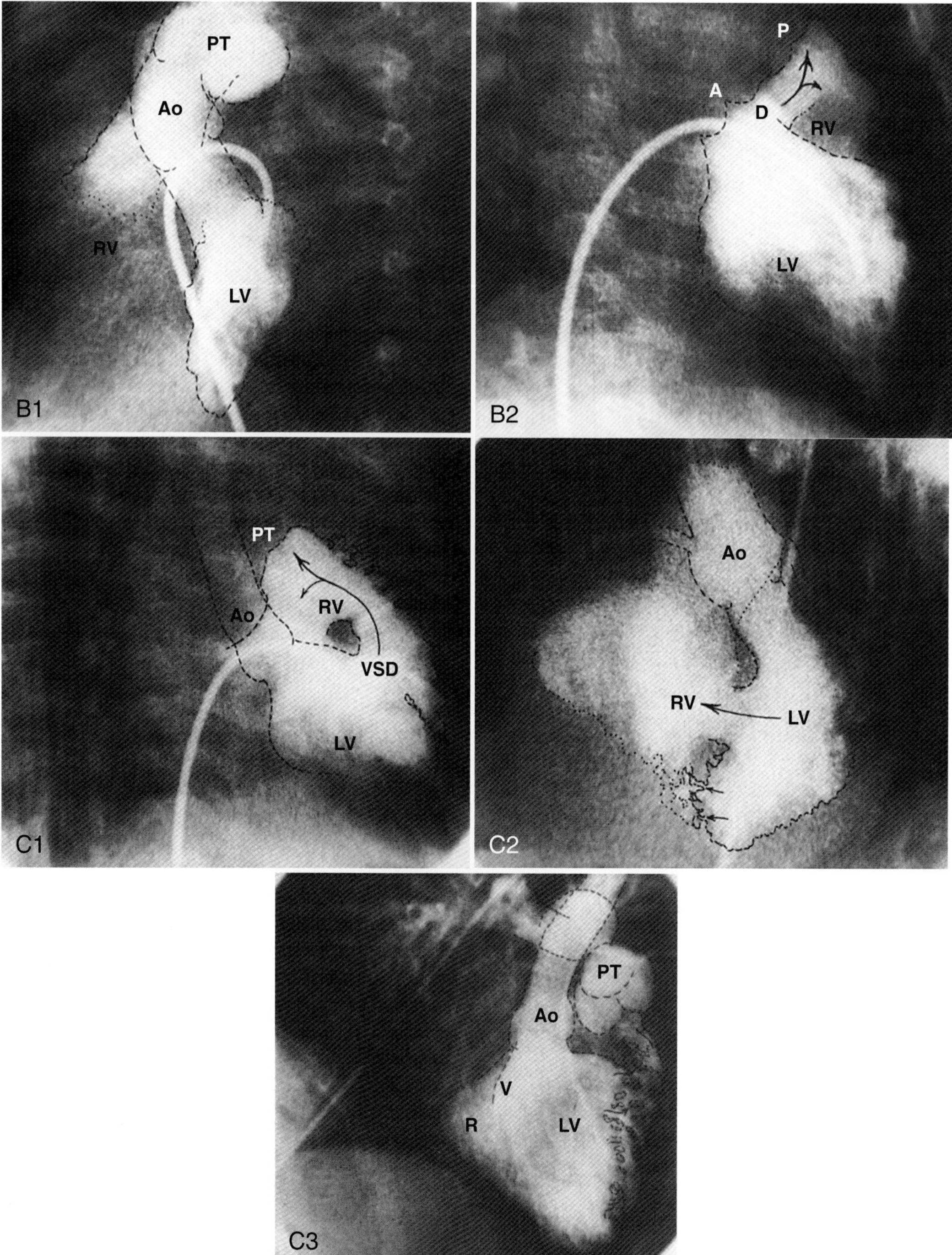

Figure 35-20, cont'd **B,** LV angiograms of doubly committed subarterial VSD. **B1,** 60-degree LAO projection, systolic frame early in sequence. Pulmonary arteries are filled by shunt through RV outlet defect superimposed on LV outflow tract. Only slight contrast medium is seen in RV sinus, and whole of sinus septum is shown to be intact. **B2,** 30-degree RAO projection, diastolic or very early systolic frame early in sequence. Doubly committed subarterial VSD is profiled immediately beneath contiguous parts of aortic and pulmonary valves, still closed. Arrows show streaming from VSD toward pulmonary valve, with some filling of remainder of RV infundibulum, but high anterior LV margin is intact. **C,** LV angiocardiograms of muscular VSDs. **C1,** Muscular anterior VSD. 30-degree RAO projection, diastolic or very early systolic frame early in sequence. Shunt through large, high-anterior muscular VSD fills anterior part of RV infundibulum. Arrows show the main stream toward pulmonary valve, which is still closed. There is a little mixing in RV sinus, but outlet septum is intact. **C2,** Multiple muscular VSDs (Swiss cheese septum); 40-degree cranially tilted 60-degree LAO projection, systolic cine frame. Large muscular trabecular VSD *(large arrow)*, accompanied by numerous small muscular apical defects *(small arrows)*, is profiled, but basal part of ventricular septum beneath aortic root is intact. In diastole (not shown), more numerous apical defects were apparent. **C3,** 30-degree RAO projection, diastolic frame in same patient as in **C2.** Numerous muscular anterior VSDs *(arrows)* interrupt LV margin. Note intact outlet septal margin of LV near aortic valve. Earlier in sequence, intact atrioventricular septum was identified, but base of filled RV overlaps base of LV in this frame. Note that position of large muscular VSD is incompletely evaluated (trabecular); an LAO view would be necessary. Note surgically banded pulmonary trunk. Key: *A,* Aortic valve; *Ao,* Aorta; *C,* septum; *D,* subarterial ventricular septal defect; *P,* pulmonary valve; *PT,* pulmonary trunk; *R,* right ventricle; *V,* atrioventricular septum.

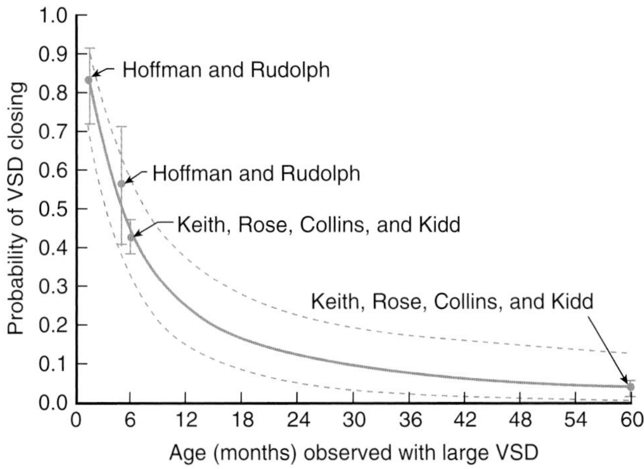

Figure 35-21 Probability of eventual spontaneous closure of a large ventricular septal defect *(VSD)* according to age at which patient is observed. Dotted lines enclose 70% confidence limits. Specific ratios, with 70% confidence limits, reported by Hoffman and Rudolph[H13] and Keith and colleagues[K7] are shown centered on mean or assumed ages of patients in their reports. *P* for age < .0001. See original sources for equations and statistics. (From Blackstone and colleagues.[B10])

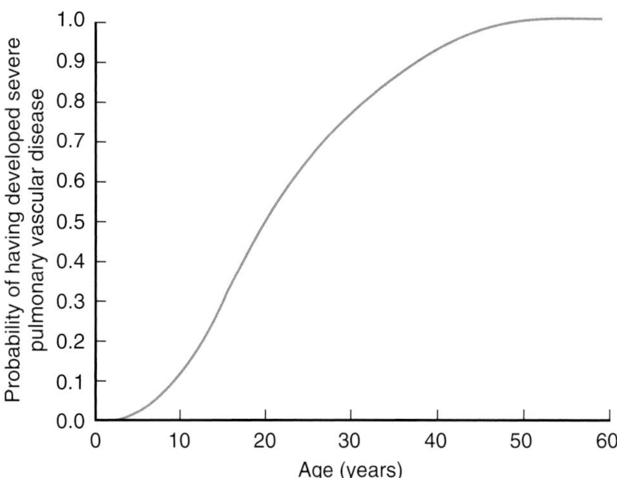

Figure 35-22 Estimated (not calculated) probability of developing severe pulmonary vascular disease (pulmonary vascular resistance 8 units · m^2 or greater) in patients with large ventricular septal defects, according to age. (From Keith and colleagues.[K7])

close than juxtatricuspid or subarterial muscular VSDs.[C1] Perimembranous VSD with LV-to–right atrial shunt (Gerbode defect) in infancy is also associated with less chance of spontaneous closure.[K8,K21,S19,W6]

Inferences about the tendency toward spontaneous closure seem to be in disagreement with the results of some studies. Hoffman and Rudolph's data (one of the sources for Fig. 35-21) indicate that 80% of infants aged 6 weeks with large VSDs will experience spontaneous closure or reduction in size of the VSD.[H13] Rowe found that none of 11 infants (mean age 46 days) with a VSD 80% or greater in diameter than that of the aorta showed subsequent reduction in size during the period of observation.[R8] These apparent discrepancies may be explained by lack of information about location or size of VSDs.

Pulmonary Vascular Disease

A large VSD exposes the patient to risk of developing increased Rp from hypertensive pulmonary vascular disease, which tends to worsen with age.[A19,L17] Thus, the proportion of patients with large VSDs who have severely elevated Rp is directly related to age (Fig. 35-22). The statement that some infants younger than 2 years of age with large VSDs have severely elevated Rp is doubted by some, but its occurrence is well documented.

Some infants and children with severely elevated Rp have not undergone the usual fall in Rp a few weeks to a few months after birth. Others have undergone this decrease,[J6] but later in the first 2 years of life, they have developed a rapid increase in Rp.[H14]

Some infants with large VSDs and most of those with moderate-sized VSDs have normal or mildly elevated Rp and retain this through the first decade of life. Then, if their VSD is still large, more severe pulmonary vascular changes may or may not develop as they age. In infants with small VSDs, pulmonary vascular disease does not develop.[K14]

Infective Endocarditis

Infective endocarditis is rare in patients with VSD, occurring at a rate of about 0.15% to 0.3% per year.[C1,C21,G7,S9] Its prevalence is greater in males and individuals older than 20 years of age.[G7] Infective endocarditis is more common in small and moderate VSDs than in large VSDs. Often a pulmonary process is the presenting feature, presumably developing from emboli secondary to right-sided bacterial vegetations or bacteria carried to the lungs by left-to-right–directed flow through the VSD. Prognosis with modern antibiotic treatment regimens is good.

Premature Death

Past experience and reports in the literature indicate that without surgical treatment, about 9% of infants with *large* VSDs die from them in the first year of life.[A18] Death may result from heart failure, which may develop very early but usually occurs at about age 2 to 3 months, presumably because at that time the left-to-right shunt increases as the medial hypertrophy present in the small pulmonary arteries at birth regresses.[D2] Death may also result from recurrent pulmonary infections, often viral in origin, secondary to pulmonary edema from high pulmonary venous pressure. Death is most likely to occur in those infants with large VSDs who have associated conditions of major anatomic or functional importance, such as PDA, coarctation of the aorta, or large atrial septal defect.

After the age of 1 year, few if any patients die of their VSD until the second decade of life. By then, many patients whose VSDs have remained large have pulmonary vascular disease and ultimately die with complications of Eisenmenger complex[C15] (Fig. 35-23). These include hemoptysis, polycythemia, cerebral abscess or infarction, and right-sided heart failure.

Patients with *small* VSDs die very rarely as a result of bacterial endocarditis. However, in common with patients with larger VSDs, some of these patients may develop disturbed systolic function and increased compliance in both ventricles.[O11]

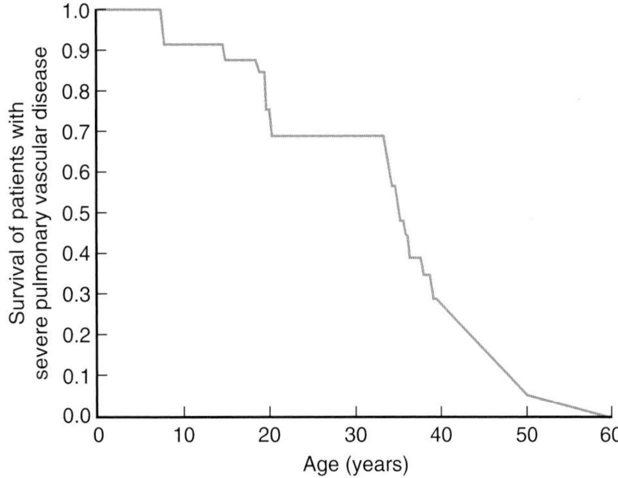

Figure 35-23 Survival after diagnosis of patients with large ventricular septal defects who had proven elevation of pulmonary vascular resistance to a level that made them inoperable (10 units · m^2 or greater), as demonstrated at cardiac catheterization at various ages. Note that fatalities begin to occur in the second decade of life, about half the patients were dead by age 35, and a few survived until 50 years of age. (Modified from Clarkson and colleagues.[C15])

Clinical Course

Patients with small VSDs rarely have symptoms related to the defect. Those with large VSDs may have symptoms of intractable heart failure in the first few months of life, with poor peripheral pulses, inability to feed, sweating, and chronic pulmonary edema. About half the patients coming to operation in the first 2 years of life do so because of intractable heart failure. During early life, rapid and labored respiration and recurrent pulmonary infections may occur secondary to high pulmonary venous pressure and chronic pulmonary edema. Lobes of the lung may become chronically hyperinflated because of pressure of the large and tense pulmonary arteries on the bronchi, preventing complete escape of air during expiration.[O2] All this causes many babies with large VSDs to be small and physically underdeveloped. Symptomatic patients who fail to respond well to medical management are at particular risk of dying in the first year of life. Some babies who survive through the first year of life with large VSDs have controlled heart failure and failure to thrive in the second year of life as well.

Children and young adults with large VSDs are usually symptomatic and tend to be small in both height and weight. As pulmonary vascular disease develops, symptoms may regress.

Development of Aortic Regurgitation

See Section II: Ventricular Septal Defect and Aortic Regurgitation

Development of Infundibular Pulmonary Stenosis

A small proportion (5%-10%) of patients with large VSDs and large left-to-right shunt in infancy develop infundibular pulmonary stenosis.[G3,H15] The mild and moderate infundibular pulmonary stenoses in patients operated on for primary VSD, as well as some of the more important pulmonary stenoses, probably develop in this way. Stenosis may become severe enough to produce shunt reversal and cyanosis, and the condition then can properly be termed *tetralogy of Fallot* (see Chapter 38). Those who undergo the transformation probably are born with a mild degree of anterior displacement of the infundibular septum and its extensions.

TECHNIQUE OF OPERATION

VSDs are repaired either through the right atrium, RV, or in special circumstances, LV or pulmonary trunk.[K15] Currently, RV and LV approaches are rarely used. Repair is done on conventional CPB at 20°C to 28°C, with direct caval cannulation and brief periods of low flow perfusion or (rarely) total circulatory arrest (see Sections III and IV of Chapter 2). For infants weighing less than about 3 kg, a single venous cannula may be used, and the repair is performed during hypothermic circulatory arrest (see Section IV of Chapter 2). Cold cardioplegia is used in all cases.

After the usual anesthetic and surgical preparations (see Chapter 4), a median sternotomy is made. Presence of anomalies of pulmonary or systemic venous return is determined. It should be known from preoperative study whether the ductus arteriosus is open or closed. An open ductus during open cardiotomy, particularly during hypothermic circulatory arrest, allows air to enter the aorta and later migrate to the brain; during CPB an open ductus increases intracardiac return and overdistends the pulmonary circulation. A patent ductus is ligated from the anterior approach, usually during cooling. In neonates and infants undergoing hypothermic circulatory arrest, the ductus is ligated as a routine procedure.

Repair of Perimembranous Ventricular Septal Defect

After CPB (with or without circulatory arrest) has been established, the aorta is occluded, cold cardioplegic solution injected, and the right atrium opened obliquely. A suction device is placed across the naturally present or surgically created foramen ovale (Fig. 35-24). Before repair is started, the defect is carefully examined to establish that all margins can be seen and reached. In rare circumstances in which this is not possible because of chordal arrangement, an incision is made to disconnect a portion of the tricuspid valve from the anulus, and the VSD is exposed through the resulting aperture. Particular attention is directed toward determining whether the VSD is juxtatricuspid, in which case it abuts the tricuspid valve in the region of the commissure between septal and anterior leaflets. If the VSD has a bar of muscle of varying width between it and the tricuspid valve, it is not juxtatricuspid. Relationship of the bundle of His to the posterior and inferior margins of the defect must be clearly understood (see Morphology earlier in this section) to accomplish a safe repair (Fig. 35-24, *A*).

In older infants and children, the VSD is repaired with a polyester patch sewn in place with continuous polypropylene sutures (Fig. 35-24, *B*), a technique confirmed to be entirely adequate in such patients. In neonates and small infants, the technique may not be adequate because of the delicate nature and friability of the structures. In these patients, the patch may be sewn into place using a combination of continuous and interrupted pledgeted mattress sutures or, alternatively,

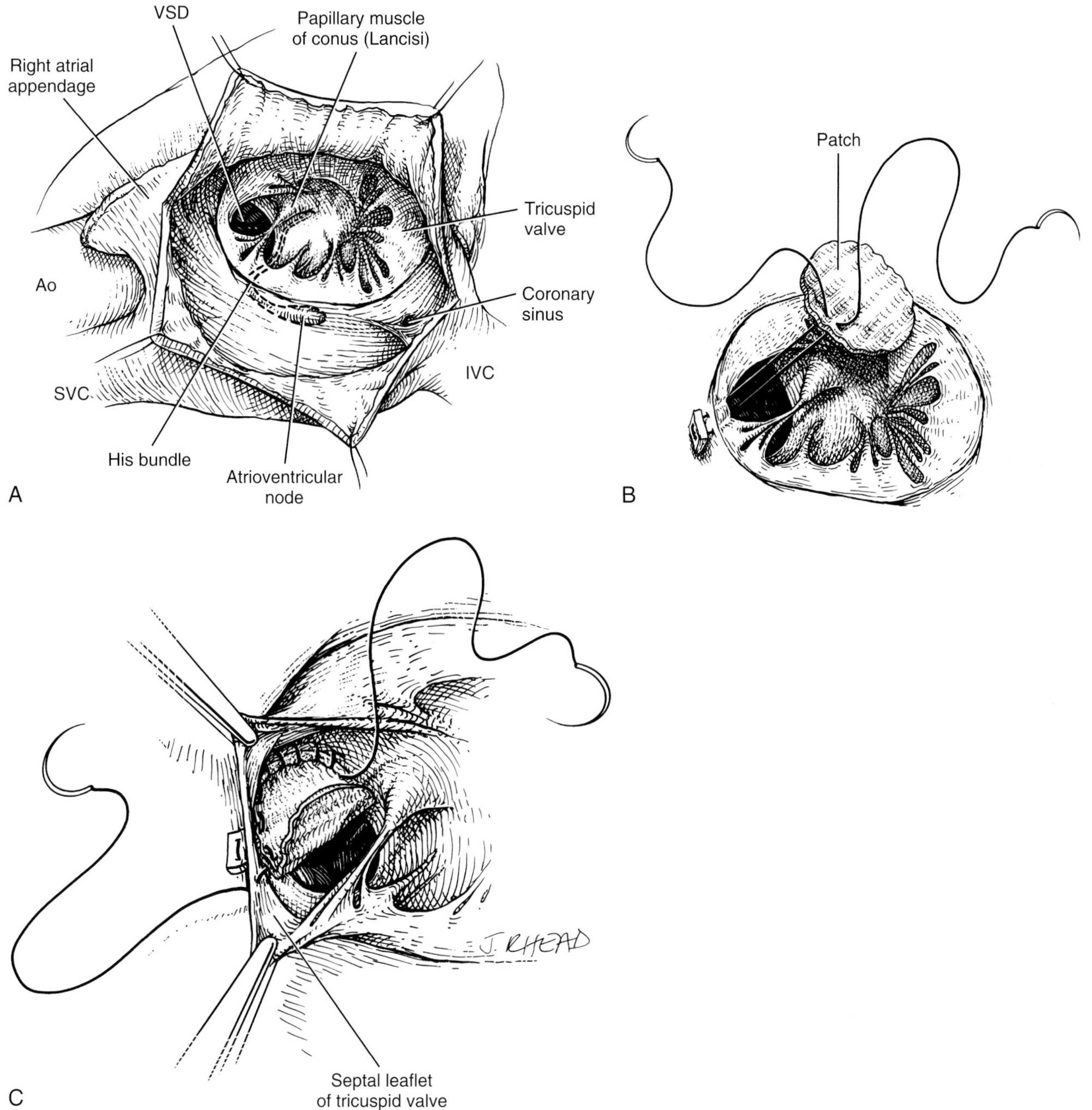

Figure 35-24 Repair of perimembranous ventricular septal defect *(VSD)* from right atrium, continuous suture technique. **A,** Right atriotomy is parallel to atrioventricular groove from right atrial appendage toward inferior vena cava. Stay sutures are placed to expose tricuspid orifice. Superior edge of VSD is not visible because of overlying anterior leaflet of tricuspid valve. Atrioventricular node lies within triangle of Koch, with bundle of His penetrating to ventricular septum at posterior angle of VSD, where it is particularly vulnerable to injury. **B,** Repair of VSD is started at junction of septal with anterior leaflets of tricuspid valve. A pledget-reinforced 4-0 polypropylene suture is placed as a mattress stitch through tricuspid anulus, with pledget on atrial side of tricuspid valve. Suture is passed through a knitted double-velour polyester patch trimmed to slightly larger than size of VSD. Alternative patch material could be pericardium or polytetrafluoroethylene. **C,** Continuous stitches are placed along right side of superior rim of defect to approximate patch to ventricular septum. Simultaneous traction on suture and on patch exposes next area to be stitched and provides good visibility. Aortic valve is located to left side of septum in this area (ventriculoinfundibular fold) and must be protected from inclusion of cusp tissue in suture line. Opposite end of suture is then passed through septal leaflet of tricuspid valve as a continuous mattress stitch working inferiorly. Bundle of His crosses beneath this portion of suture line. Stitches must not penetrate tricuspid anulus or into atrial myocardium, to preserve integrity of conduction system.

Continued

employing exclusively interrupted mattress sutures reinforced with small pledgets.

A ventricular approach may be used when the VSD cannot be well visualized from the right atrium. An RV approach is performed through a transverse incision. The patch is sewn into place with continuous or interrupted sutures (Fig. 35-25). Technique of repair and sequence for suturing shown in Fig. 35-25 are slightly different from those shown for the atrial approach. Suturing begins at the transition point between the septal leaflet of the tricuspid valve and the

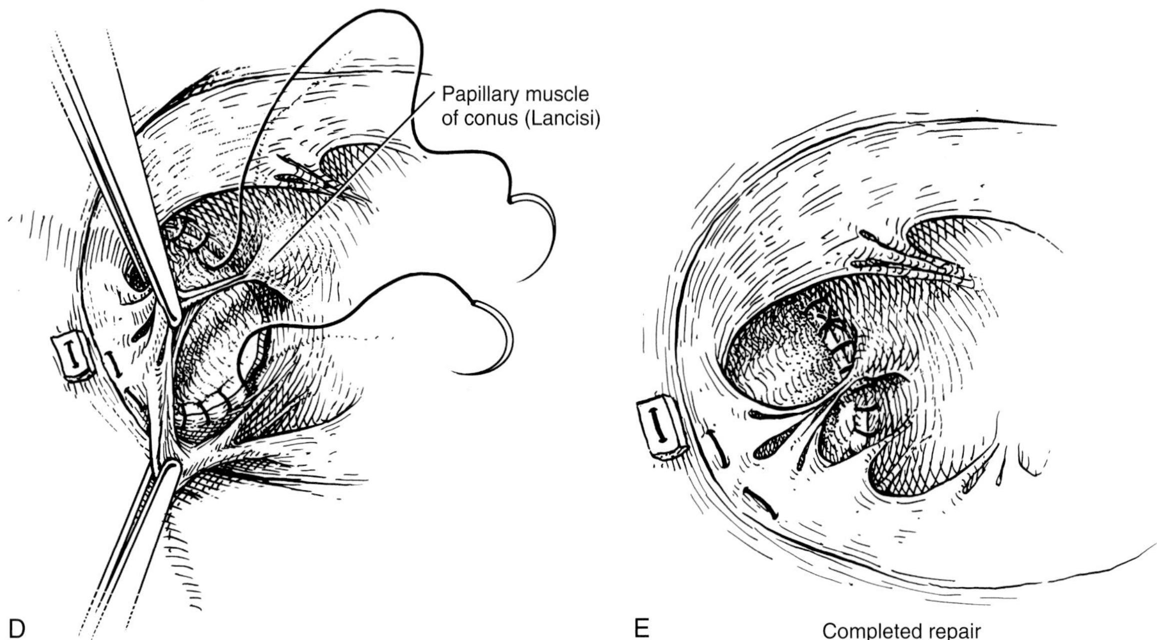

Figure 35-24, cont'd **D,** At a point 5 to 7 mm below inferior margin of VSD, suture line is transitioned from septal leaflet onto ventricular septum. Stitching continues along inferior rim of VSD, with stitches placed 5 to 7 mm below rim until reaching muscle of Lancisi. An alternative technique uses interrupted pledgeted mattress sutures for very thin portions of the septal leaflet and posteroinferior edge of defect (conduction system) to facilitate secure suture placement while avoiding conduction system. Remainder of suture line employs a continuous suture technique. **E,** Suture line may come to edge of VSD anterior to muscle of Lancisi and is continued until meeting previously completed superior suture line. Suture ends are joined to complete repair. Alternatively, repair may begin at point described here as end point.[D8] Initial suture line proceeds along superior edge of defect to junction of anterior and septal leaflet of tricuspid valve. Second part of suture line is carried along septum inferiorly, 5 to 7 mm below edge of defect, transitions to septal leaflet, then proceeds as a continuous mattress stitch along septal leaflet superiorly to join other end of suture to complete repair. Key: *Ao,* Aorta; *IVC,* inferior vena cava; *SVC,* superior vena cava.

ventricular septum, 5 to 7 mm below the edge of the septal defect. This critical point is given attention by all experienced surgeons.[D8]

Usual de-airing procedures are performed, and the remainder of the operation is completed as usual.

Repair of Doubly Committed Subarterial Ventricular Septal Defect

Transverse incision in the RV infundibulum is the classic approach for repair of doubly committed subarterial VSDs[D4] (Fig. 35-26). These defects should always be closed with a patch to reduce the possibility of distorting the semilunar valves. A continuous stitch technique is employed. When pledgeted sutures are used, they are placed from just above the pulmonary valve leaflets, and pledgets come to lie in the pulmonary valve sinuses. Care is taken not to damage the left main coronary artery. An approach through the pulmonary trunk is also convenient for repairing doubly committed subarterial VSDs.

Repair of Inlet Septal Ventricular Septal Defect

Inlet septal (AV septal type) VSD is most easily repaired through the right atrium (see Technique of Operation in Chapter 34). Such defects are always repaired with a patch. The defect lies beneath the septal leaflet of the tricuspid valve, and care is taken to avoid damage to the leaflet or its chordae and to tailor the patch such that it is not too bulky beneath the leaflet. One method of avoiding damage to the leaflet and improving exposure is to temporarily detach the base of the septal leaflet and a portion of the anterior leaflet of the tricuspid valve and retract the leaflet anteriorly.[H20]

Repair of Muscular Ventricular Septal Defect

A right-sided approach is used for repair of muscular VSDs. Left ventriculotomy provides excellent exposure,[A1] and although it has been reported not to be disadvantageous in infants,[M6,S13] it can produce ventricular aneurysm and important LV dysfunction early and late postoperatively.[G12] Therefore, use of left ventriculotomy is not recommended. Defects in the lower part of the muscular septum may be obscured by trabeculations and thus difficult to visualize, resulting in incomplete closure. Wollenek and colleagues found that an apical left ventriculotomy was a useful approach in 23 patients, and in follow-up over 3 to 18 years (mean 11 years), echocardiography showed no residual VSD, normal LV shortening, no regional wall motion abnormality, and small LV aneurysm in only two patients.[W8]

Single or multiple muscular defects in the inlet and trabecular septum (see Figs. 35-1 and 35-12) are approached through the right atrium. When a single defect is slitlike or oval, direct suture (often in part at least with pledgeted mattress sutures) is satisfactory, but when it is large and circular, a patch is used. A cluster of defects can be closed with a single patch or individually.

Division of RV trabeculations can aid exposure of the defects, which may be difficult to close because of multiple

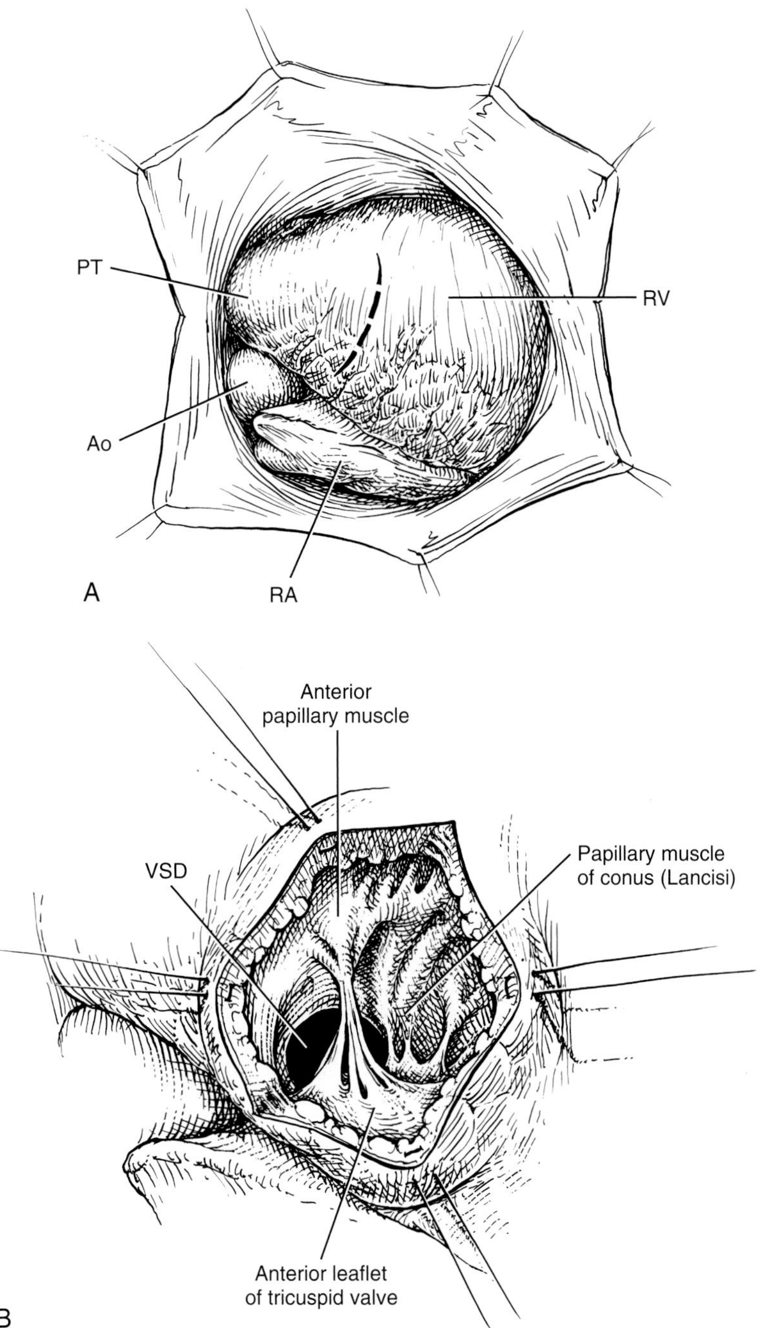

Figure 35-25 Repair of perimembranous ventricular septal defect *(VSD)* from right ventricle *(RV)*, interrupted suture technique. **A,** Transverse ventriculotomy is made low in outflow tract. A right atriotomy has been made previously to examine atrial septum for defect, with a vent device placed across patent or surgically made foramen ovale, which will be closed later. **B,** Retraction stitches are placed through myocardium superiorly and inferiorly to expose interior of RV. VSD is partially obscured by anterior leaflet of tricuspid valve, which must be retracted to expose septal leaflet.

Continued

sites of jet penetration. A heavy traction stitch passed through the defect and back through the left side of the defect may improve exposure. A single patch of autologous pericardium supported by pledget-reinforced sutures covering an extensive portion of the trabecular septum is useful when there are multiple defects.[S25] Kitagawa and colleagues described resection of trabeculations to expose the defect and attaching an oversized patch to the left side of the ventricular septum by sutures passed through the septum from the left side.[K18] They also described placing pledget-supported sutures through the rim of an anterior muscular defect, passing the sutures to the outside and tying down on the epicardial surface.[5]

When a muscular VSD coexists with a perimembranous VSD, a single patch may be used to avoid damaging the bundle of His.

VSDs with a single LV opening but two or more openings into the RV on both sides of the trabecula septomarginalis

[5]The pledget is a "firm" polyester mini-pledget, $\frac{1}{12}$ inch × $\frac{1}{8}$ inch × $\frac{1}{16}$ inch.

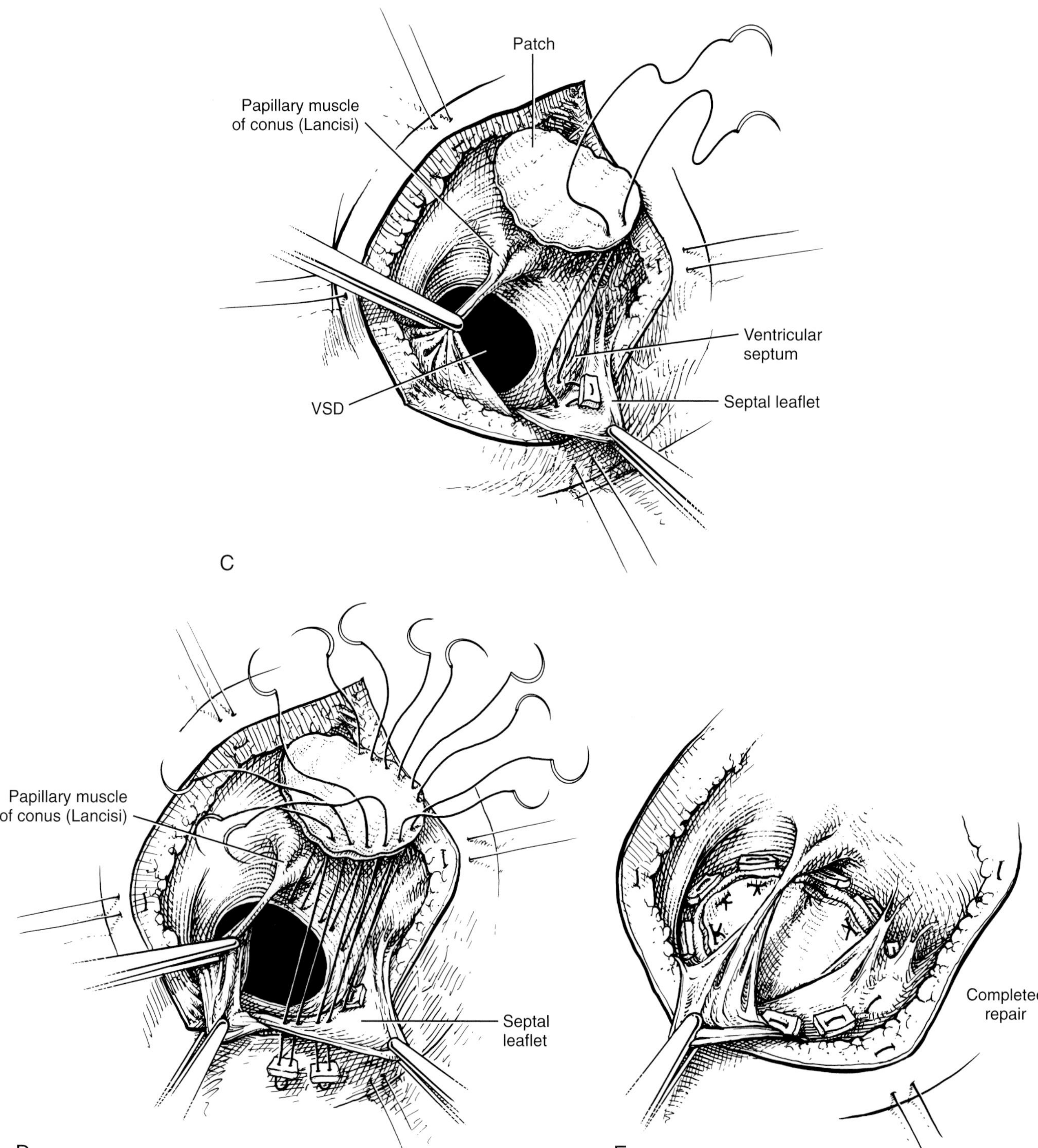

Figure 35-25, cont'd **C,** Septal leaflet of tricuspid valve is retracted to expose junction of tricuspid anulus with ventricular septum. A pledget-reinforced mattress stitch of 4-0 polypropylene suture is placed to create a transition from septal leaflet to ventricular septum. One arm of suture is placed entirely on septal leaflet, and other arm is placed into ventricular septum at hinge point of septal leaflet on ventricular septum. Stitch is at least 5 to 7 mm below rim of VSD. Suture is passed through a knitted double-velour polyester patch fashioned to be somewhat larger than VSD. Alternative patch material could be pericardium or polytetrafluoroethylene. **D,** Several pledget-reinforced mattress stitches are placed around perimeter of VSD. Stitches are placed entirely in septal leaflet tissue between transition stitch and junction of septal and anterior leaflets of tricuspid valve. Stitches are placed 5 to 7 mm below rim of defect between transition stitch and papillary muscle of Lancisi, which demarcates anterior extent of specialized conduction system. Rest of stitches may be placed in rim of septal defect. All stitches are placed through ventricular septum and septal leaflet of tricuspid valve before approximating patch to ventricular septum. **E,** Patch is attached securely to ventricular septum by tying all sutures. Key: *Ao,* Aorta; *PT,* pulmonary trunk; *RA,* right atrium.

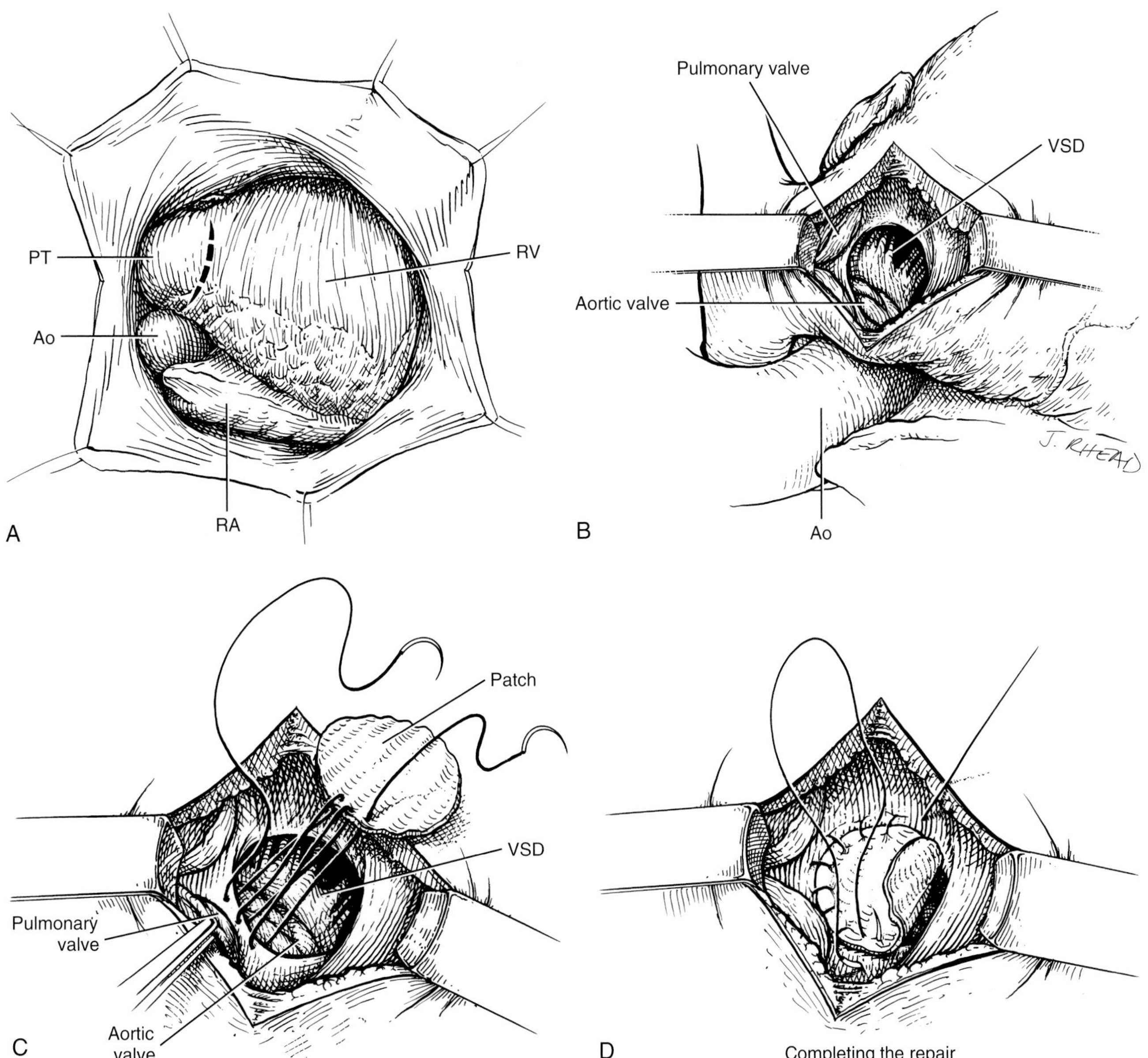

Figure 35-26 Repair of doubly committed subarterial ventricular septal defect *(VSD)*. **A,** Transverse incision is made in outflow tract of right ventricle *(RV)* near ventriculopulmonary arterial junction. VSD could also be approached via pulmonary trunk *(PT)*. **B,** VSD is subarterial, meaning that it is directly below valves of both great arteries. Superior border of VSD is pulmonary and aortic valves, and both valves are committed equally to defect. **C,** Initial stitches of 4-0 or 5-0 polypropylene suture are placed through narrow fibrous rim separating pulmonary valve anteriorly from aortic valve posteriorly. Stitches are passed through a patch (knitted double-velour polyester, polytetrafluoroethylene, or pericardium) that is slightly larger than VSD. Each stitch in this area must be placed with aortic valve in view to avoid damaging its cusps. Cardioplegic solution may be infused into aortic root for better visualization of aortic valve while placing stitches in this area. **D,** Remainder of defect is closed by placing stitches through rim of VSD and through patch. Bundle of His is located far posterior and is unrelated to posterior rim of VSD. Key: *Ao,* Aorta; *RA,* right atrium.

are also approached through the right atrium.[S7] The defect is converted into a single LV orifice by detaching the lower end of the trabecula septomarginalis and moderator band from the septum and retracting them (see Fig. 35-12). The VSD is closed with a patch. The trabecula septomarginalis then falls back into place.

Multiple defects in the anterior portion of the septum may be closed through a high transverse ventriculotomy. At times, VSDs may be considered too numerous to close individually; these VSDs are simply compressed and often totally closed by interrupted mattress sutures between a felt strip on the anterior ventricular wall (away from the left anterior descending coronary artery) and pledgets inside the RV and inferior to the VSDs.[B14] This repair may be done from the right atrium or through a right ventriculotomy.

Apical muscular VSDs can be exposed through the right atrium and tricuspid valve or through a low vertical right ventriculotomy.[S25] This can be extended around the apex for a short distance onto the posterior wall.

The rare Swiss cheese septum, with features resembling ventricular noncompaction (spongy ventricular septum) and defects involving all components of the ventricular septum, may not be correctable through the right side. Its repair requires an LV approach, and a patch over the entire muscular septum may be necessary. An associated perimembranous defect should be repaired through the right atrium because its repair from the LV side increases risk of heart block. Incisions into both ventricles are avoided whenever possible. Great care is used in making and closing the left ventriculotomy incision so as not to damage coronary artery branches. A continuous mattress suture over fine polytetrafluoroethylene (PTFE) felt strips plus an over-and-over stitch give a secure closure. Mace and colleagues used a right atrial approach and inserted a single large patch to cover the right side of the trabecular septum, adding several intermediate fixation stitches to prevent septal bulging.[M1] Regardless of the approach employed, these patients often have poor LV function after repair and may ultimately require transplantation for heart failure.[K18] This group of patients may be better served by pulmonary trunk banding with the hope that some of these defects may close as a result of ventricular hypertrophy.[S6]

Although it is important to avoid residual shunts, multiple incisions and a prolonged search for a few small additional muscular VSDs are generally not advisable. Preoperative echocardiography should accurately delineate the size as well as position of all the defects.

Closure of Associated Patent Ductus Arteriosus

Dissection of the ductus arteriosus is done after establishing CPB; this reduces the risk of hemorrhage should an error in dissection occur because of exposure, which can be difficult. After establishing CPB with the perfusate temperature at about 34°C, with caval tapes still unsnugged (so the heart will not distend) and right atrial pressure at zero, the ductus is dissected. The heart must continue to beat; otherwise a large shunt will rapidly overdistend the right side of the heart and lungs as it steals from the systemic and cerebral circulation. If the heart does fibrillate, CPB flow is immediately reduced while the dissection is rapidly completed. With downward traction on the pulmonary trunk[K17] (see Technique of Operation in Chapter 37), the ductus can usually be seen through its pericardial reflection and surrounding adventitial tissue. The left pulmonary artery and undersurface of the aorta—both proximal and distal to the ductus—are clearly identified to prevent these structures from being damaged or ligated after being mistaken for the ductus. The delicate pericardial reflection and adventitial tissue on both sides of the ductus are sharply dissected from it. The adventitia of the ductus itself and of the adjacent pulmonary artery and aorta must not be entered. The recurrent laryngeal nerve is not seen. Only when the dissection is complete, the left pulmonary artery visualized, and the ductus identified with absolute certainty is a right-angled clamp passed behind it to grasp the 2-0 silk ligature. One ligature, tied on the ductus while CPB flow is reduced to lower intravascular pressure, is sufficient to close it. A surgical clip may be used instead. The operation then proceeds as usual.

Pulmonary Trunk Banding

Banding of the pulmonary trunk may be performed through a small left anterolateral thoracotomy. However, now that pulmonary trunk banding is reserved for special situations, often to be followed by a Fontan operation (see "Pulmonary Trunk Banding" in Section II of Chapter 41) or use of a valved conduit, avoiding distortion of the pulmonary trunk bifurcation by the band is crucial. To ensure this, placement of the pulmonary trunk band via median sternotomy is the best approach because it permits accurate dissection, placement, and anchoring of the band on both the left and right sides of the pulmonary trunk.

According to *Trusler's rule*,[A5,T14] in the case of patients with a two-ventricle circulation, the pulmonary trunk band is marked to a length of 20 mm, plus the number of millimeters corresponding to the child's weight in kilograms, to indicate the ultimate tightness of the band. If the banding is done for a complex cardiac anomaly with mixed circulation, the length is 24 mm plus the child's weight. A 3- to 4-mm-wide tape is used. The preferred material for the band is silicone or silicone-impregnated polyester, which minimizes erosion into the pulmonary trunk and allows easy removal.

When a left anterolateral thoracotomy is used, a small incision is made in the pericardium, generally anterior to the phrenic nerve. When a median sternotomy is used, the pericardium is opened in the midline. To minimize subsequent adhesions, the pericardial incision should be limited to the area needed to expose the great vessels. The pulmonary trunk is separated from the aorta by dissecting close to the *aorta*. A right-angled clamp is passed around and behind the aorta to grasp one end of the band and pull it through. The other end of the band is retrieved by a clamp passed through the transverse sinus. Small angiocatheters are placed in the aorta and left pulmonary artery for pressure monitoring. Transesophageal echocardiography (TEE) may be useful during the procedure to estimate gradient across the band.

With the band now safely around the proximal portion of the pulmonary trunk, the marked points on the band are joined temporarily with a hemoclip to produce the desired circumference. With proper band tightening in patients with a two-ventricle circulation, systolic and mean blood pressures rise, but systemic oxygen saturation should remain at 100%. If systemic oxygen saturation drops below 100%, the $\dot{Q}p/\dot{Q}s$ will be less than 1, and the band is too tight. The distal pulmonary artery systolic pressure should be less than 50% of systemic systolic blood pressure. In cases of complete mixing, arterial oxygen saturation will vary with band tightening and should be set at 80% to 85% by pulse oximetry with F_{IO_2} of 50%. This implies a $\dot{Q}p/\dot{Q}s$ of about 1 (see "Pulmonary Trunk Banding in Section II of Chapter 41). If bradycardia or cyanosis develops, the band must be slightly loosened by placing a hemoclip more distally and removing the initial clip. If the narrowing is insufficient, as judged by the criteria mentioned earlier, it is tightened by adding a hemoclip more proximally.

When the ideal diameter is obtained, the band is joined by sutures. It is essential that stitches be placed between the band and the pulmonary trunk adventitia to prevent migration of the band. The pericardium is loosely closed to facilitate dissection at subsequent operation.

Pulmonary Trunk Debanding

When a pulmonary trunk band has been properly applied for 6 months or less, simple band removal may be all that is necessary. When the band must remain in place longer, reconstruction of the pulmonary trunk is usually required.

The band can almost always be cut and removed without damaging the underlying artery. The tip of the left atrial appendage actually is more likely to be damaged, because it is always adherent to the banded area. Dissection is usually delayed until CPB has been established, when if necessary, CPB flow can be reduced to facilitate exposure and dissection.

The VSD is usually closed after repair of the pulmonary trunk. The pulmonary trunk is usually reconstructed. The most satisfactory technique is local excision of the short, narrowed, scarred segment of artery and reanastomosis of the divided pulmonary trunk using a continuous polypropylene suture.[D6] This technique can usually be employed even when the band lies close to the pulmonary valve, by extending the incision vertically into the most anterior sinus between the valve commissures to enlarge the diameter of the proximal end. A similar technique can be used to enlarge an orifice stenosis involving only one branch of the pulmonary trunk. When the pulmonary valve cusps have become excessively thick, their edges may require excision. If an adequate diameter is unobtainable by the technique of excision and end-to-end anastomosis, an oval-shaped patch is inserted. To adequately enlarge the stenotic area, the patch (autologous pericardium, bovine pericardium, pulmonary allograft, or thin PTFE) should extend from within the sinus of Valsalva of the pulmonary trunk proximally and across the anastomosis to the distal trunk. Extensive reconstruction (see "Repair of Tetralogy of Fallot with Bifurcation Stenosis of Pulmonary Trunk" in Section I of Chapter 38) is required when the band constricts the origin of the pulmonary arteries.

SPECIAL FEATURES OF POSTOPERATIVE CARE

General measures and management of complications described in Chapter 5 are used for postoperative care of patients undergoing repair of primary VSD.

Hemodynamic state typically is good early postoperatively after closure of VSD. In the unusual situation of poor hemodynamic performance, the possibility of residual left-to-right shunting must be considered, particularly if left atrial pressure is considerably higher than right atrial pressure.[6] Also, the finding of a considerably higher oxygen content or saturation in blood from the pulmonary artery than that from the right atrium establishes existence of a shunt.[V4] Two-dimensional Doppler color flow echocardiography can be used to settle the matter.[L18] Although some shunting may occur for 12 to 24 hours after VSD closure with a porous patch, the usual cause of poor hemodynamic state from a left-to-right shunt is patch dehiscence. Thus, if the hemodynamic state is poor or a large left-to-right shunt is present, prompt reoperation is probably indicated. Intraoperative echocardiography at the original operation, if done, will usually have indicated residual shunting,[S27] as confirmed by postoperative echocardiography, which may be done transesophageally for greatest resolution and quality of images.

It is prudent to place temporary pacing wires on the RV after VSD repair. Complete AV dissociation is often present for a short time intraoperatively. Even if this resolves promptly to normal sinus rhythm, it is advisable to leave pacing wires in place and have an external pacemaker available while the patient is hospitalized, because AV dissociation may occur temporarily.

RESULTS

Early (Hospital) Death

Hospital mortality is low for repair of single large VSDs, most of which are now repaired in early infancy. In the current era in experienced centers, hospital mortality for isolated VSD closure is 1% or less.[S5] Risk is higher when VSDs are multiple and when major associated cardiac anomalies coexist.

Mode of Early Death

The most common mode of death after repair of a primary VSD is acute cardiac failure.[R6] This may be related to failure of intraoperative myocardial protection in the face of myocardial dysfunction, often present in sick small patients coming to operation. Occasionally, paroxysms of pulmonary arterial hypertension (see "Pulmonary Hypertensive Crises" under Pulmonary Subsystem in Section I of Chapter 5) precipitate acute cardiac failure.[S21] Persisting severe pulmonary dysfunction, often from viral pneumonitis present before operation, characterizes death of a few infants after repair of VSD.

Incremental Risk Factors for Hospital Death

Studies of experiences extending back a number of years permit identification of incremental risk factors. With death after repair now less common, risk factors are now more difficult to identify.

Risk of repair has decreased, and thus *early date of operation* is an incremental risk factor.[S20,S22,S28] Improvement from an original risk of hospital death of 20% began in the experience at the Mayo Clinic during the early 1960s. This type of improvement has been demonstrated in other centers.[C18,R7]

In previous eras, *young age* increased the risk of operation.[R7,Y4] However, in the current era at experienced centers, this risk factor has been neutralized.[J5,S5] Young age may still be an incremental risk factor when major associated anomalies coexist.

Multiple VSDs increased risk of operation in the past,[F1,F7,K12] but risk has declined considerably in the current era. However, multiple VSDs complicated by additional cardiac anomalies impose a higher risk of hospital death than do uncomplicated ones.[R7] This again may not be an immutable risk and may be improved by better myocardial management, avoidance of ventricular incisions, and device closure.[S7]

[6]When the two ventricles have equal stroke volumes (i.e., no shunts or valvar regurgitation are present), left and right atrial pressures are determined by the relative contractility, distensibility, and volume at zero pressure of the two ventricles.[B7] The greater each of these values is for a given ventricle, the better its performance and the lower its end-diastolic and (if the AV valves are not stenotic) atrial pressures tend to be relative to those of the other ventricle. (For a more detailed discussion of these matters, see "Cardiac Output and Its Determinants" in Section I of Chapter 5.) After complete repair of a large VSD through the right atrium in a patient who preoperatively had a large left-to-right shunt and a large $\dot{Q}p/\dot{Q}s$, the atrial pressures are similar, or right is slightly higher than left. When repair is through a right ventriculotomy, right atrial pressure may be 20% to 30% higher than left. Unless repair has been done through a left ventriculotomy and in the absence of other left heart lesions (e.g., aortic stenosis, coarctation), a left atrial pressure considerably greater than right (>6 mm Hg) suggests a residual left-to-right shunt. The high left atrial pressure under such circumstances is related to large LV stroke volume.

Major associated cardiac anomalies increased risk of hospital death in the past and continue to do so to some extent, particularly when they are associated with multiple VSDs.[R7] Coexisting PDA and coarctation of the aorta have not increased risk of repair of VSD to the extent that occurs with more serious anomalies such as congenital mitral valve disease. Again, better surgical techniques for managing complex anomalies and current methods of myocardial management (see Chapter 3) may neutralize much of the increased risk formerly imposed by major associated cardiac anomalies.

Neither location of the VSD nor surgical approach affects risk of operation. Previous pulmonary trunk banding and associated lesions (e.g., aortic regurgitation, sinus of Valsalva aneurysm) likewise do not increase surgical risk.

Preoperative PPA and Rp are not determinants of early mortality at present, although they affect late results.[B10] This current situation is different from earlier experiences,[C4,C15] no doubt because the upper limit of operable Rp is better understood, and perioperative management (including surgical techniques and myocardial management) has improved.

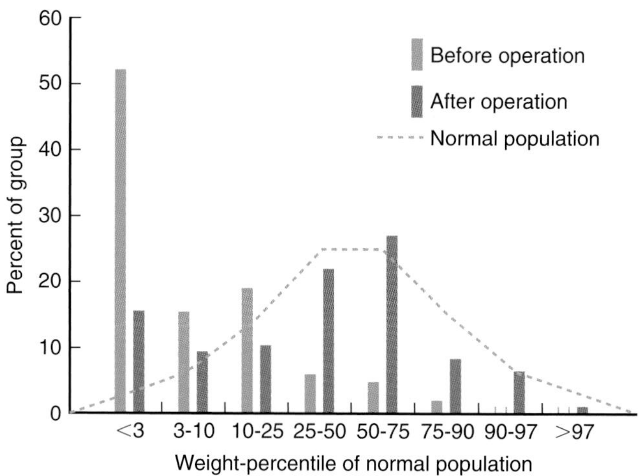

Figure 35-27 Changes in weight after repair of ventricular septal defect in 96 patients aged 10 years or less, with ratio of pulmonary and systemic pressures greater than 0.45 and ratio of pulmonary and systemic resistances less than 0.75 preoperatively. (From Cartmill and colleagues.[C4])

Survival

Premature late death occurs in less than 2.5% of patients when Rp is low preoperatively. Presumably, the few deaths in this setting are from arrhythmias, either ventricular fibrillation or sudden development of heart block late postoperatively. Patients with a high Rp preoperatively often die from progression of pulmonary vascular disease.

Repair of VSD during the first 1 or 2 years of life is curative for most patients, resulting in full functional activity and normal or near-normal life expectancy.

Physical Development

A prominent feature of the late postoperative course after repair of large VSDs in infants is improved physical development, and an impressive increase in weight may also be seen, as Lillehei and colleagues first showed in 1955. There is a less impressive increase in length and head circumference.[C14] This improved physical development is usually associated with complete relief of symptoms. Postoperative weight increase also occurs in children in whom a large VSD is repaired later in the first decade of life[C4] (Fig. 35-27).

These generalizations were refined by Weintraub and Menahem in a definitive study.[W5] They confirmed that repair of a large VSD in the first 6 months of life results in near-normal long-term growth in most patients, so that by age 5 years, weight, length, and head circumference are normal. Low-birth-weight infants were an exception, and catch-up occurred only in their weight.

Conduction Disturbances

Conduction disturbances are frequent after repair of VSDs.

Right Bundle Branch Block

Right bundle branch block (RBBB) is present late postoperatively in many patients in whom VSDs are repaired via right ventriculotomy. In one series of infants, prevalence was 80% (CL 72%-86%). Based on their studies, Gelband and colleagues concluded that the cause is the ventriculotomy.[G5] However, Weidman and colleagues at Mayo Clinic reported that 44% (CL 35%-54%) of 36 patients undergoing repair of perimembranous VSDs through a right atriotomy developed new RBBB.[O6] Rein and colleagues reported RBBB in 34% (CL 26%-43%) of infants undergoing repair via right atriotomy. Thus, in some patients, RBBB must result from damage to the right bundle by sutures along the inferior border of perimembranous VSDs. In any event, RBBB is less prevalent when the right atrial approach is used for VSD repair.[H18,O6] Although an adverse effect on late ventricular function has not been established, at least one study has associated RBBB with increased risk of late diastolic dysfunction.[P4]

Right Bundle Branch Block and Left Anterior Hemiblock

A small proportion of patients develop the ECG pattern of RBBB and left anterior hemiblock after repair of VSD. Prevalence was 8% (CL 4%-14%) in patients repaired through right ventriculotomy and 10% (CL 6%-16%) in another group of 68 patients.[Z2] Prevalence was 17% (CL 11%-25%) in Rein and colleagues' patients repaired via right atriotomy and 12% (CL 7%-19%) in Lincoln and colleagues' patients, 72% of whom were repaired through the right atrium.[L15] Such a combination of disturbances has not yet proved to be a poor prognostic finding, but concern and some controversy have been expressed.[K25,Z2] Wolff and colleagues reported that this combination was associated with important development of late complete heart block and sudden death after repair of tetralogy of Fallot.[W7] However, Downing and colleagues, who found this combination in 6% (CL 4%-10%) of 109 patients undergoing repair of isolated VSD, observed no late complications of any kind in patients followed 1 to 10 years.[D9] The controversy may relate in part to heterogeneity[S24]; that is, RBBB can result from damage to the main right bundle branch during repair, in which case its combination with left anterior hemiblock might be more hazardous than when RBBB results from disruption of a peripheral branch of the right bundle arborization secondary to a right ventriculotomy.[K23] Intracardiac recording techniques at cardiac catheterization may distinguish between these two groups and be helpful prognostically.[S29]

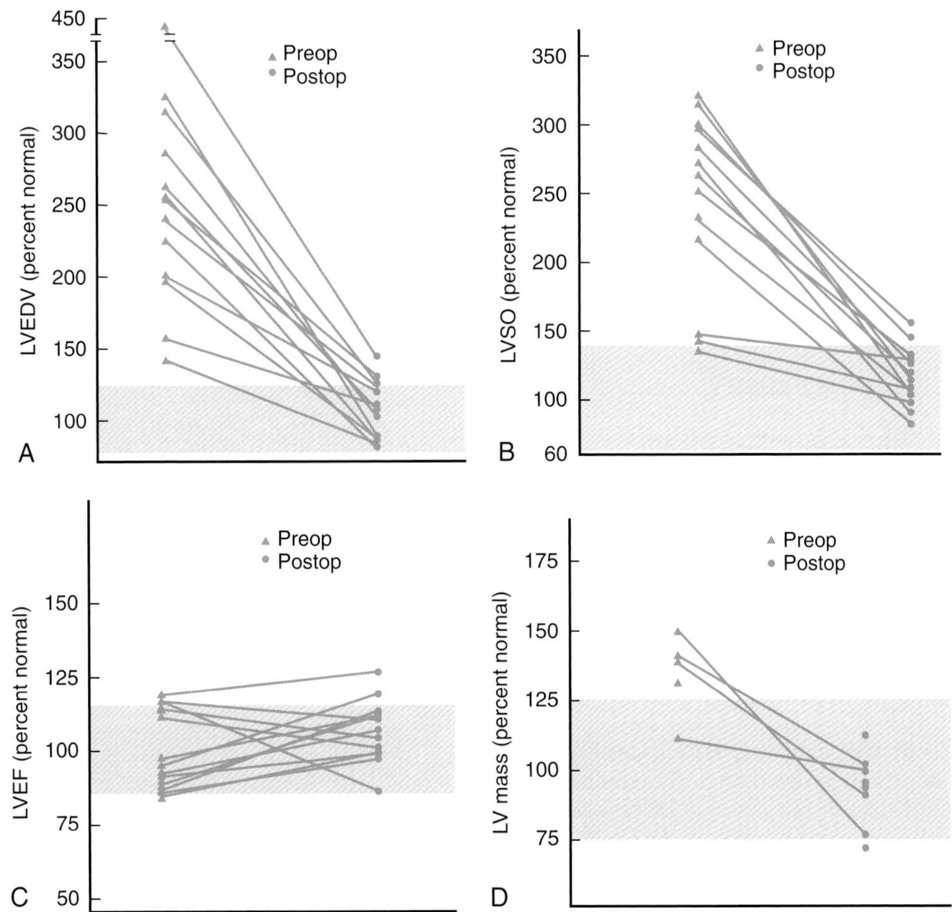

Figure 35-28 Preoperative and postoperative cardiac function 1 year after repair of large ventricular septal defect in infants. Shaded areas represent 95% confidence limits around normal value. **A,** Left ventricular end-diastolic volume *(LVEDV)*, large preoperatively, returns to normal. **B,** Left ventricular systolic output *(LVSO)* returns to normal with ablation of shunt. **C,** Ejection fraction is normal preoperatively and postoperatively. **D,** Left ventricular mass returns to normal. Key: *LVEF,* Left ventricular ejection fraction; *LV,* left ventricle; *Preop,* preoperative; *Postop,* postoperative. (From Cordell and colleagues.[C20])

Ventricular Arrhythmias

Serious ventricular arrhythmias and sudden death late after repair of VSDs have been rare. In a group of children aged 4 to 5 years at repair of the VSD, ventricular premature beats were identified by Holter monitoring late postoperatively in about 40%.[H18] All patients were asymptomatic, and no instances of ventricular tachycardia were observed. Prevalence was lower when an atrial rather than a ventricular approach to repair had been used and also in patients who were younger at time of repair.

Permanent Heart Block

Occurrence of permanent heart block (complete atrioventricular dissociation, with independent atrial activity not conducted to the ventricles) after repair of single VSD approaches zero with present techniques.[A8,S5] Prevalence is slightly higher in patients undergoing repair of multiple VSDs. Inlet VSDs extending posteriorly to the crux, associated with straddling tricuspid valve, also have increased prevalence of heart block after repair.

Cardiac Function

Late postoperative cardiac function is essentially normal when repair is done during the first 2 years of life by modern techniques through the right atrium or RV[C20,J2,J3] (Fig. 35-28). Others have found persisting abnormalities of LV size and function after repair of large VSDs at an older age, although all patients were asymptomatic.[M5] This information suggests that in general, patients with large VSDs should be operated on before they reach 2 years of age, preferably during the first year of life.

Experience with LV function after left ventriculotomy for repairing VSDs in infants has been sobering; in some patients, cardiac output has been low and left atrial pressure high despite absence of a shunt. False aneurysm has occurred after closure of VSD through a left ventriculotomy.

Residual Shunting

Postoperative left-to-right shunts large enough to require reoperation are uncommon when proper techniques are used. In experienced centers, reoperation for residual VSD should be 2% or less.[B10,S5]

Small but hemodynamically unimportant residual VSDs cannot be entirely ignored; theoretically, the possibility of infective endocarditis at such sites exists. Accurate estimation of their prevalence would require routine postoperative left ventriculography, however, and this has not been done. With near-routine intra- and postoperative assessment of cardiac

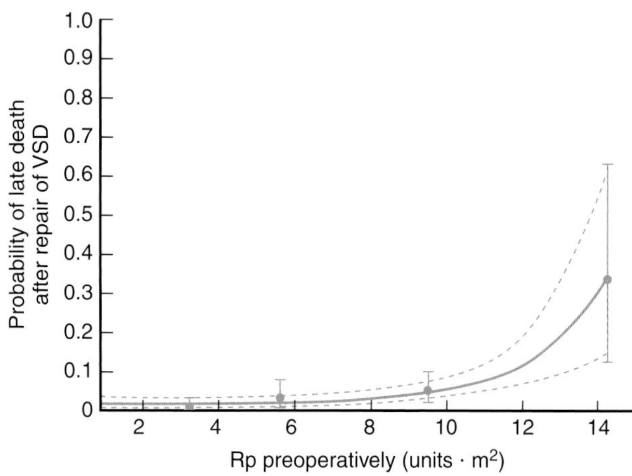

Figure 35-29 Probability of late death (within 5 years of operation) in patients who have survived early postoperative period, according to pulmonary vascular resistance *(Rp)* preoperatively. Dashed lines enclose 70% confidence limits. Actual proportions of death obtained from Cartmill and colleagues[C4] are shown with their 70% confidence limits (*P* for Rp = .0002). See Blackstone and colleagues for data, equations, and statistics.[B10] Key: *VSD,* Ventricular septal defect.

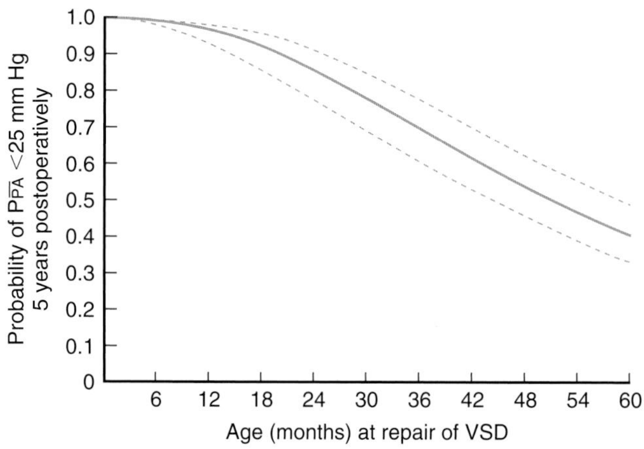

Figure 35-30 Probability of good late results (mean pulmonary artery pressure of <25 mm Hg 5 years after repair) in patients leaving hospital alive after operation and surviving 5 years, according to age (months) at repair of a large ventricular septal defect *(VSD).* Dashed lines enclose 70% confidence limits (*P* for age <.0001). Equations and statistics are based on data of DuShane and Kirklin.[D10] Key: *PPA,* Mean pulmonary artery pressure.

repairs by echocardiography, detection of even small residual defects late after operation is uncommon.[H3] Among early residual defects of less than 2 mm detected by echocardiography, greater than 80% are undetectable at 1 year.[D7]

Pulmonary Hyperinflation Syndrome

When pulmonary hyperinflation syndrome is present in infants before VSD repair, it usually resolves within 1 to 2 months after repair.[O2]

Surgically Produced Aortic or Tricuspid Regurgitation

As complications of repair of primary VSD, surgically produced aortic and tricuspid regurgitation are rare.

Rarity of surgically induced tricuspid regurgitation is surprising considering how often abnormal chordae are attached around the defect. Aortic valve regurgitation occurring after patch closure of doubly committed subarterial VSD may be a special problem. Tomita and colleagues reported that aortic valve regurgitation was detected by echocardiography in 6 of 23 patients (26%; CL16%-39%) having neither aortic valve prolapse nor regurgitation before operation.[T11] Aortic valve regurgitation in these patients was silent and asymptomatic.

Pulmonary Hypertension

When severe pulmonary hypertension persists after operation, it may worsen with passage of time and may cause premature late death.[D10,F6,H2] About 25% of patients with preoperative pulmonary hypertension and high Rp (at least 10 units · m^2) die with pulmonary hypertension within 5 years of operation[B10] (Fig. 35-29). However, some patients with pulmonary hypertension and elevated Rp late postoperatively have neither progression nor regression of their disease for as long as 20 years, although they have some limitation in exercise tolerance.[D10,H1]

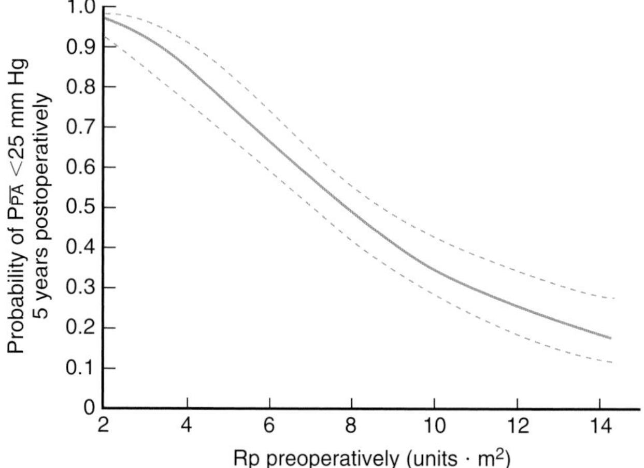

Figure 35-31 Probability of good late results (mean pulmonary artery pressure of <25 mm Hg 5 years after repair) in patients leaving hospital alive after operation and surviving 5 years, according to preoperative pulmonary vascular resistance *(Rp).* Dashed lines enclose 70% confidence limits (*P* for Rp < .001). Equations and statistics are based on data of DuShane and Kirklin.[D10] Key: *PPA,* Mean pulmonary artery pressure.

In general, the younger the child at time of repair, the better are the chances of surviving and having an essentially normal PPA 5 years and more later[C5,D10,H14,L13,M4,S10,Y2] (Fig. 35-30). The lower the Rp at repair, the better the chances of having normal pressure late postoperatively (Fig. 35-31). These two factors, age and preoperative Rp, interact in determining late postoperative PPA.

A more specific correlate of survival and good outcome in patients with important preoperative pulmonary hypertension is preoperative response to infusion of a pulmonary vascular dilator such as isoproterenol.[L21,M12,N5] Generally, outcome is good in patients of all ages when preoperative Rp is only mildly or moderately elevated (<8 units · m^2; see Table 35-3). Outcome is good in patients with severely elevated Rp only

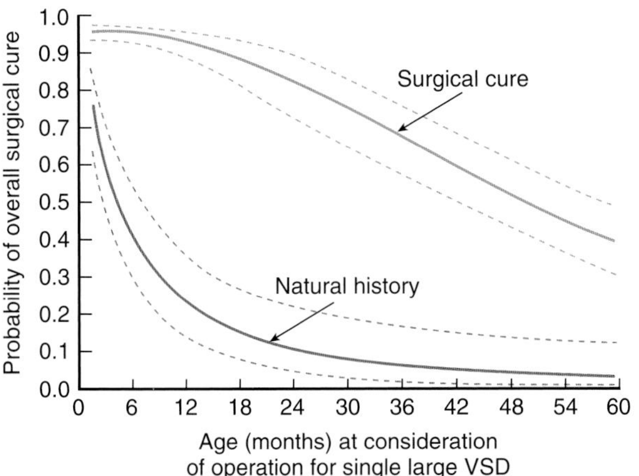

Figure 35-32 Probability of overall surgical cure (survival at least 5 years postoperatively with a mean pulmonary artery pressure of <25 mm Hg) according to age (months) at repair for all patients with single large ventricular septal defects *(VSD)*. Dashed lines enclose 70% confidence limits. Analysis is based on data of DuShane and Kirklin.[D10] Natural history is also shown, with vertical axis the probability of long-term survival and ultimate spontaneous closure of the defect and horizontal axis the age at observation of a patient with a large VSD. (From Blackstone EH, Kirklin JW: Unpublished study, 1982.)

when it drops below 7.0 units · m^2 with preoperative infusion of isoproterenol.[N5] Sodium nitroprusside infusion or nitric oxide may also be used and has the advantage of not producing tachycardia.

Surgical Cure

Combining data on PPA late postoperatively with the proportion of patients dying early and late postoperatively, chances of "surgical cure" (defined as surviving the early postoperative period and being alive late postoperatively with essentially normal PPA) can be estimated for an individual patient (Fig. 35-32). If repair of a large VSD is performed in a patient at 6 months of age, there is at least a 95% chance of surgical cure, unless preoperative Rp is greater than about 8 units · m^2 and does not fall to less than 7 units · m^2 with infusion of isoproterenol (which is rare at that age). This is supported by studies by Rabinovitch and colleagues, in which it was also found that surgical cure is likely to result in any infant in whom the VSD is repaired before age 6 to 9 months, irrespective of degree of pulmonary vascular disease.[R1] In a 2-year-old patient, chances of cure are this good only if preoperative Rp is less than about 5 units · m^2. In a patient operated on for repair of large VSD at age 4 years, chances are that good only if Rp is normal preoperatively (which is unusual). This unfavorable effect of older age has been confirmed by John and colleagues.[J4] This finding supports the practice of repair of large defects at least by age 12 months and can be used to predict results of operation in individual patients.

INDICATIONS FOR OPERATION

In earlier eras, great emphasis was placed on details of calculated Rp and $\dot{Q}p/\dot{Q}s$ in determining appropriate timing of surgical intervention or whether continued observation was advisable. In the current era in which hospital mortality after surgical closure of isolated VSD approaches 1% or less, and the majority of infants and children undergo transthoracic echocardiography (without cardiac catheterization) as the definitive diagnostic study, the decision-making process has evolved away from these hemodynamic measurements.

Decisions regarding operation vary somewhat among experienced institutions, but generally relate to size of the defect as assessed echocardiographically (see "Two-Dimensional Echocardiography" under Clinical Features and Diagnostic Criteria), morphologic characteristics related to likelihood of spontaneous closure (see Fig. 35-32), estimated Rp, and presence or absence of Down syndrome.

Infants with an isolated large VSD are rarely truly asymptomatic in the absence of elevated Rp, which results in lower $\dot{Q}p$. In addition to overt signs of heart failure or failure to thrive, the experienced pediatric cardiologist will note subtle signs of failure such as isolated tachypnea or decrease in the slope of the growth curve even with adequate feeding. Left atrial enlargement detected echocardiographically supports the presence of LV volume overload secondary to increased $\dot{Q}p$. In the presence of a large defect and absence of such symptoms or signs, specific echocardiographic interrogation for signs of elevated Rp or associated obstructive lesions in the RV outflow tract is warranted. In infants with a large VSD and major symptoms of heart failure or failure to thrive, operation is advisable irrespective of age. In the presence of mild symptoms, elective repair of isolated large VSD is advisable during the first 6 months of life or at the time of diagnosis if older. Infants with Down syndrome and large VSD are likely at increased risk for developing pulmonary vascular disease; therefore, operation should be undertaken within the first few months of life.

Infants with a moderate or large perimembranous VSD associated with aneurysm of the membranous system or a VSD partially covered by accessory tricuspid valve tissue have increased likelihood of spontaneous closure, and operation can be deferred for 6 to 12 months in the absence of symptoms, with planned reevaluation for signs of decreasing size. A VSD of moderate size still carries an ongoing risk of pulmonary vascular disease, and surgical closure is recommended by 12 months of age (or at the time of diagnosis if older) unless there are signs of decreasing defect size. Appearance of decreasing flow velocity in the absence of decreasing size suggests increasing Rp, although such findings may appear transiently in the face of bronchiolitis or other self-limited reasons for increased Rp. If increasing Rp is identified, prompt surgical closure is advisable.

Exceptions to this general practice are made for rare infants with Swiss cheese septum, who present a special problem because of higher risk of surgery. In this setting during the first 3 months of life, pulmonary trunk banding may be indicated; when there are no complications from the band, repair of the Swiss cheese septum and debanding are postponed until age 2 to 4 years. This general plan is also followed when Swiss cheese septum coexists with coarctation of the aorta. Other exceptions to primary repair during the first 3 months of life include infants with straddling tricuspid valve.

In patients with evidence of important elevation of Rp by echocardiography, cardiac catheterization is advisable.[K14] When Rp is truly and precisely measured at preoperative cardiac catheterization and is only mildly or moderately elevated (<8 units · m^2), operation can be undertaken with near certainty that the early and late outcome will be good[N5] (Fig. 35-33). Such patients usually have a large $\dot{Q}p/\dot{Q}s$.

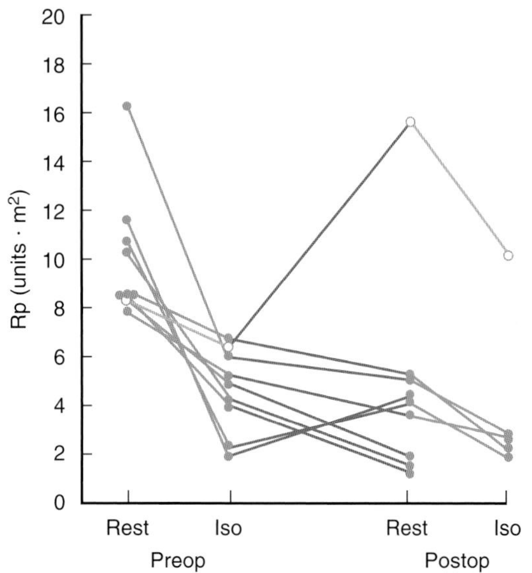

Figure 35-33 Preoperative *(Preop)* and late postoperative *(Postop)* pulmonary arteriolar resistance in patients with preoperatively severely elevated pulmonary vascular resistance *(Rp)*, responsive to isoproterenol *(Iso)* infusion. Tan lines represent a patient whose ventricular septal defect repair dehisced postoperatively. (From Neutze and colleagues.[N5])

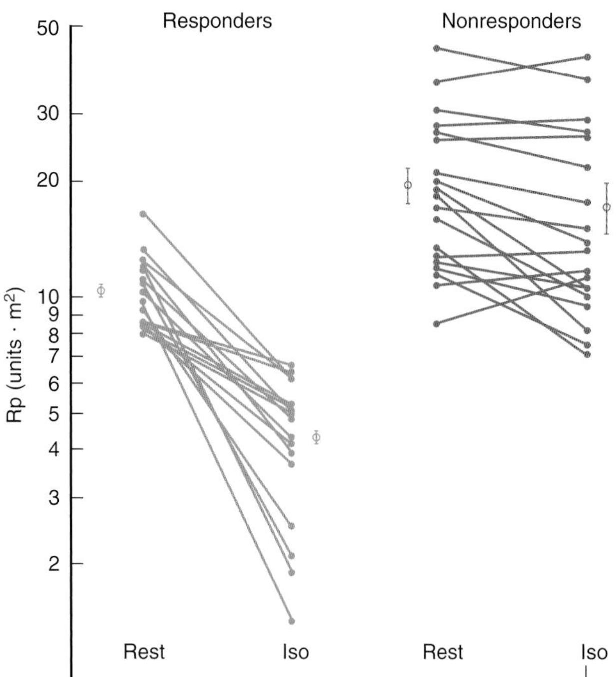

Figure 35-34 Pulmonary arteriolar resistance in patients with severe elevation of resistance (resting resistance 8 units · m^2 or greater) at rest and with infusion of isoproterenol *(Iso)*. Responders experienced a fall in resistance to less than 7 units · m^2; nonresponders did not. Key: *Rp*, Pulmonary vascular resistance. (From Neutze and colleagues.[N5])

When Rp is severely elevated (>8 units · m^2), pulmonary vasodilator challenge is performed during cardiac catheterization (ensuring adequate ventilation or hyperventilation, 100% inspired oxygen, plus nitric oxide or other specific pulmonary vasodilator), and Rp is remeasured. If it falls to 7 units · m^2 or less, the response is considered favorable and operation is advised (Fig. 35-34). Otherwise, closure of the VSD is inadvisable. In fact, VSD closure under these circumstances would prevent right-to-left shunting during exercise, resulting in a lower exercise capacity and life expectancy with the defect closed than with it open.

In older patients, operation is generally advisable with a $\dot{Q}p/\dot{Q}s$ above 1.5 in the absence of additional major operative risk factors. However, in patients with a large VSD, a $\dot{Q}p/\dot{Q}s$ of 1.5 to 1.8 at rest that becomes 1.0 or less during moderate exercise (from systemic peripheral vasodilatation, increased $\dot{Q}s$, and a fixed and high Rp preventing increased $\dot{Q}p$) is an indication of probable inoperability. An important fall in SaO_2 during exercise (from right-to-left shunting across the VSD for the reasons described) also suggests inoperability, but a more complete investigation with determination of response to nitric oxide is required for a final decision. Response of Rp to inhalation of mixtures high in oxygen alone is not useful in determining operability in borderline situations.

Children with small VSDs can be safely observed unless other cardiac anomalies (e.g., aortic regurgitation from aortic cusp prolapse, subaortic stenosis, subpulmonary stenosis) are observed. Periodic reevaluation is advisable to verify that observed clinical and echocardiographic findings are compatible with safe continued observation.

Doubly committed subarterial and juxta-aortic VSDs constitute a special situation.[R4] Even though apparently small, they should not be left untreated if there is any aortic cusp deformity on 2D echocardiography or cineangiography; development of aortic regurgitation must be prevented (see Section II). These defects should be repaired promptly if an aortic diastolic murmur develops.

SPECIAL SITUATIONS AND CONTROVERSIES

Ventricular Septal Defect and Patent Ductus Arteriosus

Combination of large VSD and moderate-sized or large PDA is particularly likely to cause severe symptoms and require operation early in infancy. During the first 6 to 8 weeks of life in patients with a very large ductus and only a moderate-sized or small VSD, the PDA alone may be repaired because the VSD may narrow or close spontaneously. If this does not occur, the VSD is closed at an appropriate time. When the VSD is large, both it and the PDA are closed simultaneously if operation is required in early life. Risk of operation should not be higher than that for isolated VSD.

Ventricular Septal Defect and Coarctation of Aorta

Combination of VSD and aortic coarctation frequently causes severe symptoms in infancy. Both coarctation and VSD are variable in severity. Clearly, the worst combination is a large VSD and severe coarctation, but even a small VSD in association with important coarctation may produce heart failure early in life.[T9]

Management options for this combination of defects include simultaneous repair of both lesions,[T8] sequential single-stage repair through separate incisions,[K25,K26] initial repair of the coarctation alone,[N3] initial coarctation repair and pulmonary trunk banding, or initial VSD closure alone.[R9] With a large VSD and severe coarctation, repairing the VSD first has certain theoretic advantages[R9] but has been practiced rarely under such circumstances. *Repair of the coarctation only* as the initial operation has the advantage of reducing afterload on the LV and, theoretically at least, reducing shunt through the defect. It also avoids a second operation if the VSD closes spontaneously.[N3] Mortality with repair of aortic coarctation in this setting has been high in the past,[N3] but more recent experience has been good.[M3,P2] The results have also been good with *initial coarctation repair with pulmonary trunk banding.*

Simultaneous repair of both the coarctation and a large VSD in early infancy in the current era in experienced institutions carries a low risk, with hospital mortality of about 5%.[G4,W3] The operation is generally performed via a median sternotomy and combined regional perfusion and circulatory arrest. Alternatively, the operation can be performed as a single stage with repair of coarctation through a left thoracotomy followed by repair of a VSD via median sternotomy using standard CPB. Kanter and colleagues have reported excellent survival with this method.[K1,K2] In the current era, the following practice can be recommended:

1. When the VSD is large, the coarctation is severe, and the infant presents with severe heart failure, a single-stage repair of coarctation and VSD is advisable, using one of the techniques described previously. When multiple VSDs or Swiss cheese septum is present, the pulmonary trunk is banded, and debanding and repair are delayed if possible until the patient is about age 3 years.
2. When the coarctation is severe and VSD small or moderate-sized, only the coarctation is repaired, and subsequent repair of the VSD is performed according to standard indications.
3. When the coarctation is moderately severe and VSD large, the VSD may be repaired initially and the coarctation repaired either at the same operation or as a second procedure within a few months. Techniques of CPB are standard, with perfusion of the lower body satisfactory in this situation.

Pulmonary Trunk Banding

Civin and Edwards noted good prognosis and freedom from pulmonary vascular disease in patients with single ventricle and moderate pulmonary stenosis.[C13] Based on that observation, Muller and Dammann performed pulmonary trunk banding in 1952.[M16] For many years thereafter, this procedure was used by many for infants who required operation for large VSD, thereby allowing deferral of the intracardiac repair until an older age.[M9,O7,P3]

For several reasons, banding is seldom indicated for primary isolated large VSDs. Hospital mortality of patients with pulmonary trunk banding has been substantial, and a second operation, which carries additional mortality, is always required.[G8,H6,H21] Early mortality is independent of type of VSD. It is difficult to adjust the tightness of the band perfectly, and reentry a few days later may be needed to modify the tightness. Furthermore, good palliation is not always achieved by banding, and there may be important intermediate mortality before second-stage repair. Complications result from banding in some patients, including development of infundibular and valvar pulmonary stenosis, subaortic stenosis,[F3] and migration of the band to the pulmonary trunk bifurcation (Fig. 35-35). Although hospital

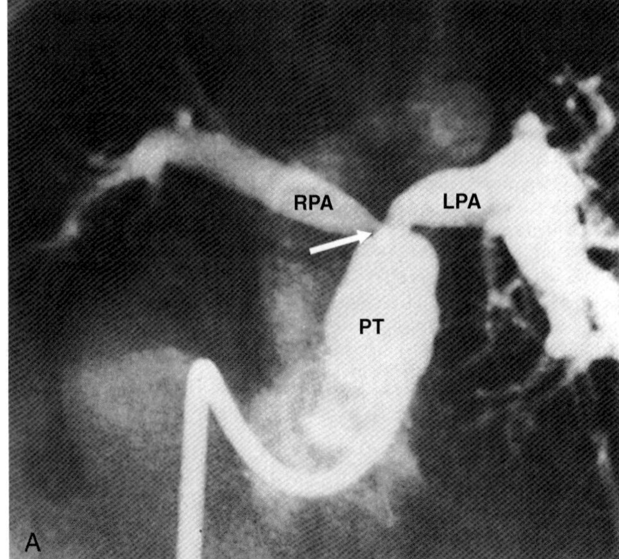

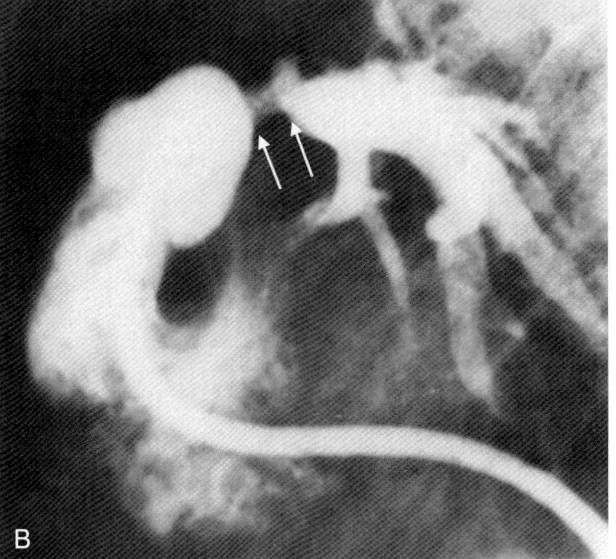

Figure 35-35 Angiograms of 4-year-old patient who had previously undergone pulmonary trunk banding. **A,** Pulmonary artery injection in frontal view of sitting-up position. Arrow indicates position of band at bifurcation of pulmonary trunk and narrowing of origin of right and left pulmonary arteries. **B,** Lateral view. Width of pulmonary band is indicated by two arrows as well as by its migration to bifurcation. Key: *LPA,* Left pulmonary artery; *PT,* pulmonary trunk; *RPA,* right pulmonary artery.

mortality from pulmonary trunk debanding and VSD repair is low, combined mortality of the banding procedure and subsequent debanding and VSD closure is at least as high as primary VSD repair. Furthermore, restenosis of the pulmonary trunk may follow debanding and VSD repair, necessitating a third operation.[K11]

Pulmonary trunk banding as an initial palliative procedure in very young or very small patients with refractory heart failure may still be appropriate in some centers.[S2] For a number of years, however, there have been only two standard indications for pulmonary trunk banding in infants with primary VSD: (1) severe heart failure from Swiss cheese septum and (2) associated severe coarctation of the aorta and severe heart failure during the first few months of life. The second is no longer an indication for banding.

Right Atrial versus Right Ventricular Approach for Perimembranous Ventricular Septal Defect

The RV approach may be used for repair of perimembranous VSDs and results in low hospital mortality even in patients with high Rp. The RV approach has the advantage that the nadir of the noncoronary cusp of the aortic valve, which is the area of the right trigone and bundle of His, can be accurately visualized, which may be helpful in choosing the suture technique that will minimize prevalence of heart block (see Fig. 35-25). The RV approach has the disadvantages of (1) leaving a scar in the RV, (2) being associated with a higher prevalence of complete RBBB than with an atrial approach, and (3) possibly resulting in more ventricular arrhythmias late postoperatively.

The right atrial approach may be used almost exclusively, a practice begun in about 1960 at the Mayo Clinic.[C4] An accurate repair can be obtained through a right atrial approach in nearly all cases. Associated infundibular pulmonary stenosis can be excised. An RV scar is avoided, and occurrence of RBBB is lower than with the transventricular approach.[H11] With the right atrial approach, however, techniques must be accurate to avoid damaging the tricuspid valve leaflets or chordae.

Closure of Ventricular Septal Defect Through Less Invasive Approaches

Smaller incisions (less invasive approaches) have been used for closure of VSDs.[B16,L14] Although it is technically feasible to close a VSD successfully through a variety of these techniques, no advantages have been demonstrated other than the smaller incision.[A15]

Percutaneous Closure of Ventricular Septal Defects

In selected cases, especially in patients with complex cardiac anomalies (e.g., multiple muscular VSDs) and those with overlooked VSDs after surgical repair of a large defect, transcatheter closure of the VSD by a percutaneously placed double umbrella can be considered.[B15,L16] This may be particularly advantageous in apical muscular defects.[K26] This method in general should be considered only when surgery is contraindicated or has unusually high risks and when suitable skill and equipment are available.

A current perception is that primary multiple muscular VSDs, particularly those near the apex, are more suitably closed by a percutaneous catheter technique than by operation. This remains unproven, however, particularly for multiple muscular VSDs that can be closed from the right atrium after taking down the trabecula septomarginalis.[P2] The technique is a promising one, but additional experience and information are required for definitive evaluation.

These devices may also be deployed intraoperatively.[A7,G1,M17,Q1]

Closure of Ventricular Septal Defect When Pulmonary Resistance Is High

Patients with VSD in which pulmonary hypertension is severe, with PPA at or above systemic blood pressure, have traditionally been thought to be inoperable because of the high risk of operation. Zhou and colleagues reported use of unidirectional valve patch closure of cardiac septal defects with severe pulmonary hypertension.[Z1] There was a VSD in 22 of 24 patients in the series, all with marked elevation of PPA (80 ± 12 mm Hg) and increased $\dot{Q}p/\dot{Q}s$ (1.1 ± 0.11). SaO_2 was reduced to 88% ± 4%. The patch consisted of polyester fabric with a 0.5- to 1.0-cm hole covered by a pericardial patch left open at one side to function as a one-way valve, placed on the systemic side of the defect. Two patients died after operation (8.3%). PPA fell to 56 ± 19 mm Hg and $\dot{Q}p/\dot{Q}s$ to 0.7 ± 0.1, while SaO_2 rose to 96% ± 1%. Excellent improvement of functional state was noted. These results were corroborated by Ad and colleagues while claiming earlier right of discovery of this method (see Fig. 30-26 in Chapter 30).[A2,A3,A4]

Section II Ventricular Septal Defect and Aortic Regurgitation

DEFINITION

Ventricular septal defect and aortic regurgitation (VSD-AR) syndrome includes hearts in which AR is of congenital origin, although rarely present at birth, and caused by cusp prolapse or a bicuspid aortic valve.[K5] The VSD is doubly committed subarterial, perimembranous (with outlet extension or simply juxta-aortic), or rarely, outlet muscular. These locations are in fact a continuum, with the subarterial VSD lying farthest to the patient's left (and anteriorly), the perimembranous VSD with outlet extension lying more rightward (and slightly inferior) than the subarterial, and the perimembranous juxta-aortic VSD lying still more rightward (and inferiorly).

VSD-AR syndrome is related to congenital sinus of Valsalva aneurysm (see Chapter 36) and tetralogy of Fallot with AR (see Chapter 38).

HISTORICAL NOTE

Initial description of VSD-AR syndrome due to aortic cusp prolapse is attributed to Laubry and Pezzi's publication in 1921.[L3] First reports of operative correction were those of Garamella and Starr and their colleagues in 1960.[G2,S23]

Experience at Mayo Clinic began about the same time.[K6] On review of this experience in 1963, of the 30 patients in whom the aortic valve cusps were reconstructed and repaired, 10 (33%; CL 24%-44%) still had important AR.[E5] This and other reports in which results of cusp reconstruction were equally unsatisfactory[T4] led to adoption of aortic valve replacement using either an allograft[G10] or prosthetic valve. During this period, operations were delayed beyond childhood whenever possible to avoid valve replacement at a young age. Renewed interest in use of cusp reconstruction dates from publications of Spencer and Trusler and their colleagues in 1973, which followed the work of Frater.[F2,S18,T13]

Tatsuno and colleagues in Japan have done much to elucidate the nature of the anomaly and document the good results obtained by VSD closure alone when AR is mild.[T5,T6,T7]

MORPHOLOGY AND MORPHOGENESIS

Perimembranous VSDs are most prevalent among predominantly white patients with VSD and AR.[L7,M2] Among Asians with VSD and AR, VSDs are more prevalent in the RV outlet, particularly doubly committed subarterial VSDs.[H8,O5] Rarely, the defect may be a muscular outlet (also called "intracristal") defect in which the superior rim is formed by the remnant of a deficient subpulmonary infundibulum. The posteroinferior margin of the defect is formed by fusion of the posteroinferior rim of the trabecula septomarginalis with the ventriculoinfundibular fold.[A8] AR is most often caused by prolapse of the right cusp of the aortic valve (about two thirds of patients); the remaining third have prolapse of the noncoronary cusp or of both noncoronary and right coronary cusps, with about equal prevalence. The common feature of all these defects associated with AR is that the affected cusp or cusps lack the normal muscular support provided by attachment of the sinus of Valsalva to the muscular ventricular septum. Infrequently, no cusp is prolapsing, but the aortic valve is bicuspid and regurgitant.

Variable degrees of RV outflow obstruction are present in many patients. The infundibular septum may be underdeveloped and displaced anteriorly and leftward[V1] (malaligned as in tetralogy of Fallot), a feature responsible for mild infundibular stenosis that may be present. Occasionally, RV trabeculae near the junction of the infundibular septum and free wall may contribute to infundibular stenosis, as may hypertrophy of the moderator band at a lower level. Typical low-lying infundibular pulmonary stenosis (double-chambered RV) accounts for the gradient in some patients.[K4]

The aortic root and valve exhibit a variety of anomalies. Cusps may prolapse not only into but at times through the VSD. Protrusion through the VSD increases during diastole and effectively plugs the defect, limiting the shunt even when the defect is large. Extensive cusp prolapse through a large VSD can also produce some obstruction to RV outflow. In advanced cases, the center of the prolapsed free margin of the cusp is thickened and retracted, a feature that makes resuspension of the leaflet less effective.[A16] Some patients have additional damage produced by endocarditis.

The sinus of Valsalva adjacent to the prolapsed leaflet is enlarged, often considerably. This enlarged sinus is associated with asymmetric splaying and dilatation of the aortic "anulus," a feature aggravated by severe AR and volume changes in the LV. It is virtually impossible to distinguish the junction between the prolapsed cusp and dilated sinus at cineangiography and at times at operation. The wall of the enlarged sinus may be thinned and aneurysmal adjacent to the cusp hinge line and rarely may protrude into the RV immediately above the prolapsed cusp. Such a finding indicates the close similarity between this condition and that of ruptured congenital sinus of Valsalva aneurysm with VSD.

Mechanism of Aortic Regurgitation

The mechanism for cusp prolapse remains speculative; multiple theories have been proposed. Prolapse may result in part from lack of support of the aortic sinus of Valsalva and "anulus" by the infundibular septum,[T6,V1] although because most large perimembranous defects are closely adjacent to the aortic "anulus" and very few have associated regurgitation, this cannot be the entire explanation.[S1] A structural defect in the base of the sinus itself may also play a role, particularly when the VSD is small.[E2] Loss of continuity of the aortic media from the aortic "anulus" and the ventricular septum has also been proposed.[Y1] Hemodynamic influences during both systole and diastole aggravate the tendencies toward AR.[T6] Such influences are more marked once AR develops, resulting in progressive prolapse and distortion.

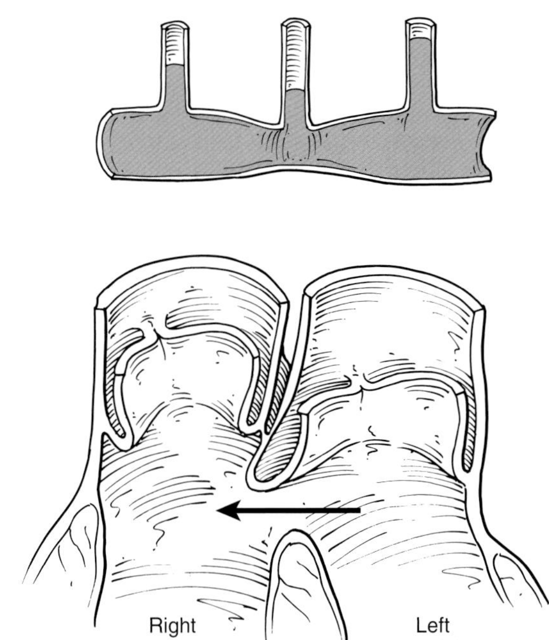

Figure 35-36 Proposed pathophysiology of aortic regurgitation in ventricular septal defect (VSD) with aortic regurgitation by Venturi effect. *Top,* As fluid passes through conduits of varying diameter, changes in velocity and pressure occur. As caliber of the conduit decreases, fluid velocity increases and pressure decreases. *Bottom,* This low-pressure zone within a restrictive VSD can affect adjacent cusp of aortic valve. (From Tweddell and colleagues.[T16])

The most widely accepted predominant mechanism of cusp prolapse is the *Venturi effect,*[K9] which describes changes in velocity and pressure that occur when fluid passes through conduits of varying diameter. As conduit caliber decreases, fluid velocity increases and pressure decreases. If there is restriction to flow through a VSD and an aortic valve cusp is adjacent to the defect, it is vulnerable to being drawn into the high-velocity, low-pressure jet[T5] as blood shunts left to right through the restrictive VSD (Fig. 35-36). This tends to displace the unsupported "anulus" outward and downward into the RV. Later in systole, the aortic cusp prolapses into the VSD and is acted upon by direct pressure from the cavity of the LV, displacing both "anulus" and cusp into the RV. During diastole, the high pressure in the aortic root distends the dilated sinus, with further displacement of the aortic "anulus" toward the RV. As the sinus dilates, the distending force becomes greater from increase in wall tension.

Observations supporting the Venturi effect as the predominant cause of aortic cusp prolapse and subsequent AR include:

- The Venturi effect requires a restrictive VSD. Previous studies in the era of near-routine cardiac catheterization indicate that with occasional exceptions, most such defects are restrictive, and PPA is usually near normal.[C7,C11,K21,L20] In a study from Taiwan, Chiu and colleagues found that among patients who developed aortic valve prolapse, mean $\dot{Q}p/\dot{Q}s$ for perimembranous VSDs was 1.7; for subarterial defects, 1.6; and for muscular outlet VSDs, 1.45.[C11]

- There appears to be a minimum shunt size required to induce sufficient cusp distortion for development of prolapse. The lower limit of $\dot{Q}p/\dot{Q}s$ among patients with VSD and aortic valve prolapse or AR appears to be about 1.4.[C11,R4,T10]
- AR in association with VSD is an acquired lesion. AR or prolapse with VSD is not present at birth and is rarely diagnosed in infancy.[C11,T15]
- The nadir of the affected leaflet would be expected to lie within the stream of the shunt. This is consistent with observations that overriding of the involved cusp is commonly noted,[C11] and override of the aortic cusp in perimembranous VSDs has been identified as a risk factor for developing cusp prolapse and subsequent AR.[E1]

CLINICAL FEATURES AND DIAGNOSTIC CRITERIA

Potential for development of AR can be assessed by noting the possible presence of aortic cusp prolapse at echocardiography or cineangiography. Studies in such patients should include 2D echocardiography with Doppler flow velocity evaluation. Anatomic relationships of the aortic valve and VSD should be easily demonstrated. AR is estimated qualitatively. Aortic root dimensions are measured accurately. Usually, echocardiography provides sufficient information on which to base clinical decisions.

In some patients, it is desirable to have cardiac catheterization, which should include (1) right-sided heart catheterization (for calculating shunt and measuring pressures in the pulmonary artery and RV), (2) right ventriculography (for studying possible infundibular pulmonary stenosis), (3) left ventriculography (for identifying location and size of VSD), and (4) aortography (for estimating magnitude of AR and morphology of aortic root). Finding a normal aortic root diameter without cusp prolapse suggests that AR is caused by a bicuspid valve and may not be amenable to repair. Anatomic size of the VSD cannot be demonstrated angiographically when, as often occurs, it is occluded throughout the cardiac cycle by the prolapsed aortic cusp.

In patients with mild AR (e.g., younger patients), signs of the VSD dominate the clinical picture, but as AR increases, the shunt decreases.[P6] Such patients characteristically have a to-and-fro murmur that may simulate the continuous murmur of PDA, but occasionally may be mistaken for that of isolated AR or combined AR and stenosis.

NATURAL HISTORY

Among all patients with VSD, the prevalence of aortic valve prolapse and AR is reported to be 4% to 9% and 2% to 6%, respectively.[N1] Prevalence is also related to type of VSD. The reported prevalence of aortic cusp prolapse in subarterial VSD exceeds 40%,[T5] with over half demonstrating progression of AR. Eroglu and colleagues reported a prevalence of aortic cusp prolapse of 12% and aortic regurgitation of 7% among patients with perimembranous VSD.[E7] Aortic cusp prolapse and AR are more frequently reported with VSD among Asian populations[T3] because of the greater prevalence of subarterial VSD in China[L19] and Japan.[K3,T5,T10]

Prevalence is related in part to age at which the population is studied. AR is rarely present at birth but develops during the first decade of life (after age 2 years), then gradually worsens, such that by the end of the second decade it is usually severe.[C12,D5] This rate of progression is similar whether the VSD is subarterial or perimembranous. At repair, the AR is mild to moderate in about half of patients and severe in about half.

As regurgitation increases, VSD shunt flow often decreases from occlusion of the VSD by the prolapsed aortic cusp. If the defect remains open through adolescence, about 10% of patients develop aortic valve prolapse or AR.[O8]

Secondary effects of AR on the LV are at least as marked as those of rheumatic AR and may be more severe because of additional volume load from the VSD. Rp is seldom if ever elevated, presumably because functionally the VSD is usually not large. Risk of infective endocarditis is high.[R4]

Aneurysms of the sinuses of Valsalva also may develop as part of the natural history of patients with doubly committed subarterial VSD or perimembranous VSD with outlet extension. This is a slower process than development of AR, and Momma and colleagues did not observe sinus of Valsalva aneurysms before age 10 years in patients with perimembranous VSDs.[M13] Most often the aneurysm is observed during the third decade, when it may be present in 10% of patients whose VSDs of these types are still open.[M13]

TECHNIQUE OF OPERATION

In patients in whom AR is trivial or absent, only the VSD is repaired. When AR is moderate or severe and often when it is mild, the aortic valve is repaired.[M15] The aortic valve is usually replaced in adults, and this is done only when AR is moderate or severe.

TEE is performed after induction of anesthesia and before incision for a final analysis of the aortic valve and VSD. For myocardial protection, operation is performed on CPB with cold cardioplegia. A transverse aortotomy is made. Dimensions of the aortic root are measured at the ventriculoaortic junction ("anulus") and sinutubular junction. These dimensions are compared with normal valves adjusted for size of the patient (see "Dimensions of Normal Cardiac and Great Artery Pathways" in Chapter 1). The aortic valve is examined to assess feasibility of repair rather than replacement. If the cusp edge is retracted and thickened or the valve bicuspid, repair is usually not possible.

One or more leaflets may be repaired by the Trusler method of plication[T13] (Fig. 35-37). This procedure is carried out at the commissure adjacent to the prolapsed cusp (usually the right or noncoronary cusp). A 5-0 or 6-0 polypropylene suture is placed through the fibrous lacunae at the midpoint of each cusp. Cusps can then be assessed for elongation and attenuation. Cusp plication is performed at the elongated free edges of the aortic valve cusps. A 5-0 or 6-0 PTFE suture is woven between the right and noncoronary cusps to adjust the excessive length of the prolapsed cusp to the adjacent aortic wall. Repair may be reinforced by pledgets (pericardial or felt) or a small cap of polyester secured as a pledget over both affected cusps adjacent to the commissure. Hisatomi and colleagues proposed pledget stitch aortoplasty to make

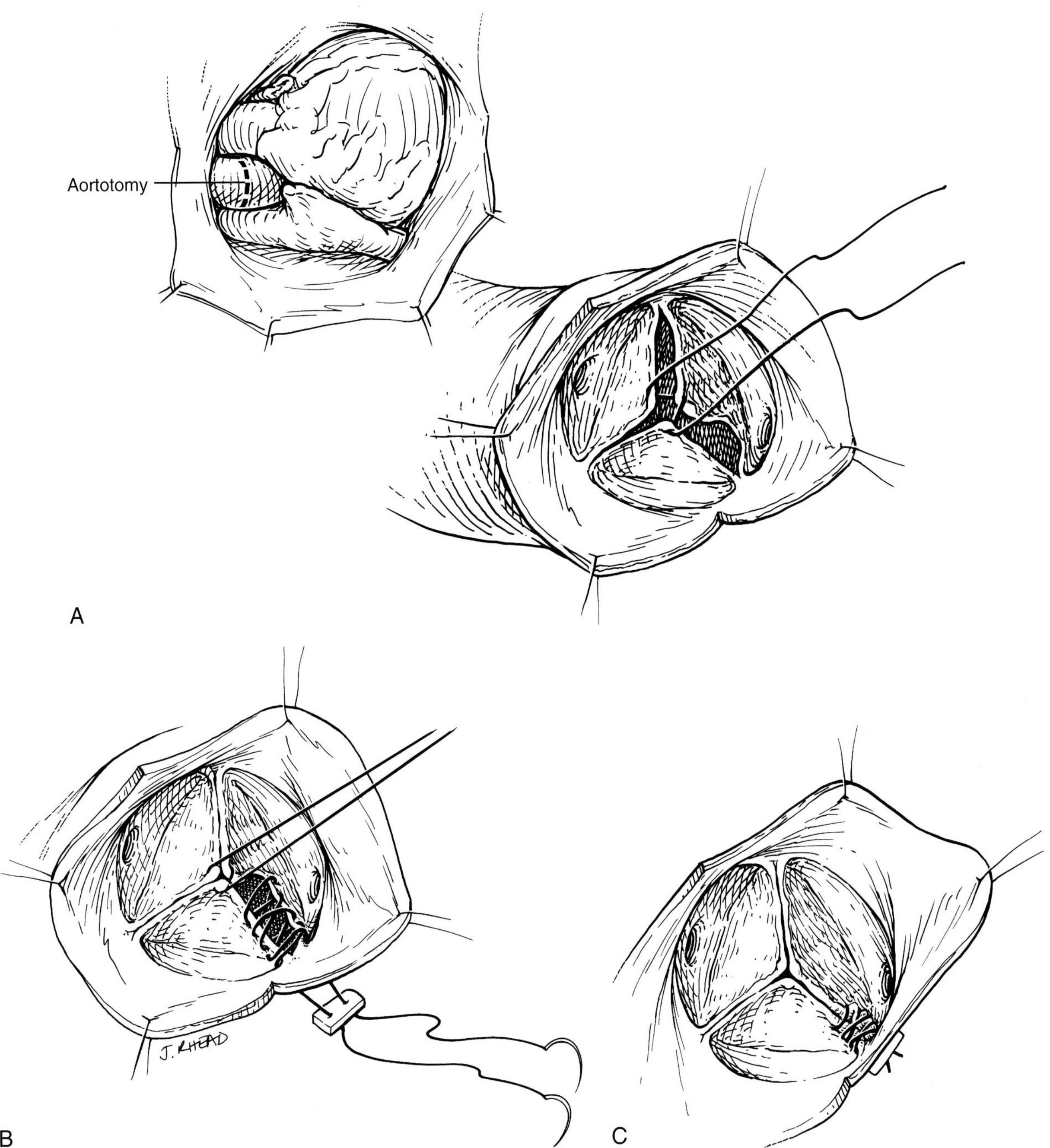

Figure 35-37 Repair of prolapsed aortic valve cusp by Trusler technique in patients with ventricular septal defect and aortic valve regurgitation. **A,** Transverse aortotomy is made at a level just downstream from commissural attachments of aortic valve. **B,** A stitch of 5-0 or 6-0 polypropylene is placed through midpoint of each cusp. Traction on this stitch allows identification of redundant or elongated free edges of a cusp, as shown here in the case of right coronary cusp near its commissure with noncoronary cusp. **C,** A 5-0 or 6-0 polytetrafluoroethylene suture is used to "reef up" redundant and attenuated portions of aortic valve. Double row of reefing stitches is used to bring ends of suture to outside of aorta at commissures. Pledget is added to strengthen repair.

the aortic cusps protrude for even greater aortic cusp coaptation.[H7,H9] The stitch at the center of the valve is removed after VSD repair.

Approach to the VSD is appropriate to the location of the defect and may be transaortic if the defect is accessible. Any infundibular stenosis is relieved by excising trabecular muscle bands between the infundibular septum and free wall of the RV and, when necessary, by mobilizing and excising parietal and septal extensions of the infundibular septum and portions of the moderator bands.

An entirely different technique has been successfully used by Carpentier, Chauvaud, and colleagues.[C3,C6] Its basic feature is triangular excision and reconstruction of the prolapsing cusp. Combined with this is an anuloplasty of the left ventriculoaortic junction. They also recommend that the VSD be repaired through the aortic root, using a glutaraldehyde-treated pericardial patch.

Yacoub and colleagues have proposed another alternative repair (Fig. 35-38) that addresses the basic morphologic defect more completely.[Y1] All anatomic components of the

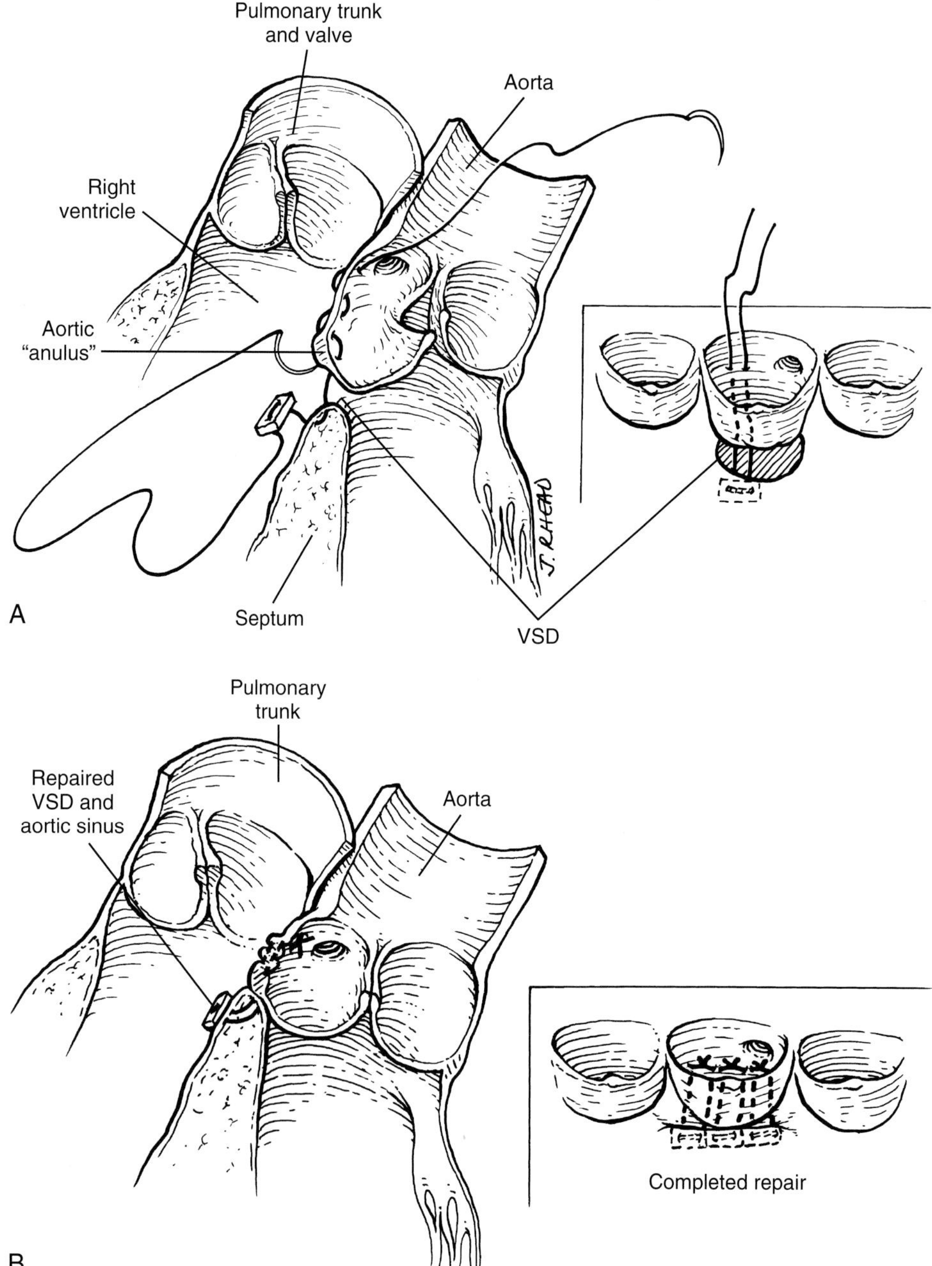

Figure 35-38 Repair of aortic valve in syndrome of ventricular septal defect *(VSD)* and aortic valve regurgitation by Yacoub technique. **A,** Aortic valve and VSD are approached through a transverse aortotomy. Morphologic defect causing lack of coaptation of aortic cusps is considered to be discontinuity between aortic media and "anulus" of aortic valve, resulting in lack of support to "anulus" and sinus of Valsalva, with downward and outward displacement of "anulus" into right ventricle. VSD is closed by plication suture, which elevates crest of septum to aortic media and plicates unsupported sinus of Valsalva. A series of interrupted mattress stitches using 4-0 braided polyester suture with pericardial pledgets are placed from crest of ventricular septum slightly toward its right ventricular aspect. Stitches are passed through "anulus" of aortic valve and reefed through unsupported sinus of Valsalva to strong tissue of aortic media. **B,** Stitches are tied down (knots inside aortic sinus), elevating ventricular crest to aortic valve "anulus" to close VSD as well as displacing "anulus" and aortic valve cusp centrally to achieve greater aortic cusp coaptation, restoring valve competence. (Modified from Yacoub and colleagues.[Y1])

defect are corrected by a simple transaortic repair. A transverse aortotomy is made (Fig. 35-38, *A*). Extent of dilatation of the right coronary sinus and exact definition of the thin area of sinus resulting from discontinuity between aortic valve "anulus" and media of aorta are accurately defined. A series of pledget-reinforced mattress sutures are placed through the crest of the ventricular septum slightly on the RV side to avoid injuring the conduction system. Sutures are passed through the "anulus" of the aortic valve and then used to plicate the thin portion of the sinus of Valsalva and continued until strong aortic tissue supported by aortic media is reached. Tying of sutures results in closing the VSD, elevating the right coronary anulus and cusp, and reducing the size of the right coronary sinus and RV outflow tract bulge (Fig. 35-38, *B*). Repair of the defect is possible in all cases regardless of VSD size, which is usually slitlike, because there are always redundant tissues in the septum and aortic sinus in the vertical plane. Plication of redundant tissues toward the media of the

Table 35-4 Grade of Aortic Regurgitation (AR) Late after Repair of Ventricular Septal Defect and AR, According to Preoperative AR Grade[a]

		Postoperative AR Grade											
		None		Mild		Mild to Moderate		Moderate		Moderate to Severe		Severe	
Preoperative AR Grade	*n*	No.	%	No.	%	No.	%	No.	%	No.	%	No.	%
Mild	10	2	20	1	10	6	60	1	10	0	0	0	0
Mild to moderate	4	0	0	1	25	1	25	1	25	0	0	1[b]	25
Moderate	12	4	33	4	33	2	17	0	0	1	8	1[b]	8
Moderate to severe	9	3	33	4	44	1	11	1	11	0	0	0	0
Severe	1	0	0	0	0	0	0	1	100	0	0	0	0
TOTAL	36	9	25	10	28	10	28	4	11	1	3	2	6

Data from Maehera and colleagues.[M2]
[a]Data from 36 patients operated on from 1967 to 1987. Three patients who had aortic valve replacement at the original operation after failure of Trusler repair and two other patients who had missing values for postoperative aortic regurgitation are not included.
[b]These two patients received late postoperative aortic valve replacement.

aortic sinus elevates the aortic valve cusp and anulus, displacing them centrally toward the aortic lumen. This results in increased aortic valve coaptation and restored aortic valve competence. This operation can be applied to patients with doubly committed subarterial VSDs with AR and thus may apply to the Asian population, in whom these types of defects are common.

If the valve requires replacement, the RV (or pulmonary trunk) should be opened before valve insertion, the VSD repaired, the RV closed, and then the aortic valve replaced. This sequence is advised because occasionally it may be necessary to place sutures from the prosthetic valve ring across the upper margin of the VSD patch where it extends between the base of the right and noncoronary cusps (in the region normally occupied by the membranous septum). Sutures in this area should be securely buttressed with pledgets. Although a freehand allograft has been used successfully for valve replacement under such circumstances,[G10] degree of distortion of the aortic sinuses often makes accurate placement difficult.[B3] Allograft aortic root replacement or aortic valve replacement with a pulmonary autograft (Ross procedure) is probably a better choice (see "Autograft Pulmonary Valve" under Technique of Operation in Chapter 12).

When there is also a true thin-walled aneurysm of the sinus of Valsalva at the base of the right aortic cusp and a VSD, repair is more difficult because the sinus must also be repaired. If the aortic valve requires excision and replacement, excision should include the base of the cusp and the thinned area of the sinus wall, which becomes continuous with the VSD and is incorporated into its closure. Again, under such circumstances, the prosthetic valve suture line will cross the polyester patch. Aortic root replacement may be a simpler solution. When the valve is suitable for plication, the base of the cusp is preserved and sutured back to the patch.

RESULTS

Survival

Only 1 of 76 patients operated on by the UAB and GLH groups died in hospital (1.3%; CL 0.2%-4.4%); at last follow-up, no late deaths had occurred, an experience similar to that of Okita and colleagues over an 18-year follow-up and Yacoub and colleagues over 24 years with a mean follow-up of 8.4 years.[O5,Y1] Thus, in the current era, risk of operation should approach 1%.

Heart Block

Heart block rarely occurs, even though operation is in the region of the conduction system. In Yacoub and colleagues' series of 38 patients, there were no cases of conduction abnormality, and ECG remained normal.[Y1]

Relief of Aortic Regurgitation

When AR is mild, VSD closure alone usually prevents progression of regurgitation. When AR is moderate before repair, about two thirds of patients have no or trivial AR after repair using the Trusler technique[E3,H6,H8,O1,T13,T15] (Table 35-4). Satisfactory late outcomes have also been reported with techniques described by Carpentier[C3] and Yacoub.[Y1] Infrequently, AR is severe preoperatively, and chances of a good result decrease in this setting.

Okita and colleagues have determined perimembranous VSD (rather than VSDs in the RV outlet) to be a risk factor for important residual AR, possibly because factors other than cusp prolapse are partly responsible for preoperative AR when the VSD is perimembranous.[O5] Bicuspid aortic valves are less satisfactorily repaired than tricuspid ones.

Older age at operation also contributes to presence of important AR after repair.

Freedom from Aortic Valve Replacement

Some patients will probably require aortic valve replacement in later life, although freedom from aortic valve reoperation using the Trusler technique was 89% at 8 years in the UAB group's series; parametrically predicted freedom at 20 years was 81%[M2] (Fig. 35-39). Elgamal and colleagues confirmed these data, reporting 15-year freedom from reoperation of 81% ± 19% after Trusler repair of the aortic valve.[E3] Adequacy of repair at operation was the most important determinant of long-term results. Yacoub and colleagues reported 5 valve replacements among 38 patients 8 to 11 years after operation.[Y1]

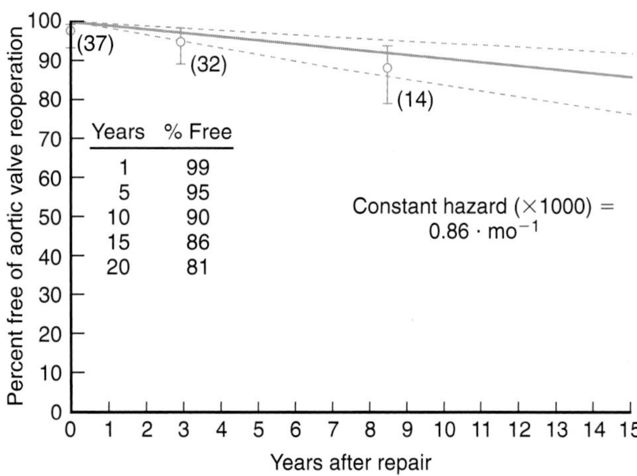

Figure 35-39 Nonparametric *(open circles)* and parametric estimates of freedom from aortic valve reoperation (one second repair, two valve replacements) after repair of ventricular septal defect and aortic regurgitation in 38 patients. (From Maehara and colleagues.[M2])

INDICATIONS FOR OPERATION

When the murmur of AR first develops in a child with a VSD, the VSD should be promptly repaired while the AR is still mild.[C10,K22,T5,T6] If cusp prolapse without AR is demonstrated by 2D echocardiography or on the aortogram in association with any perimembranous VSD, early repair is also indicated. Even if cusp prolapse has not occurred, doubly committed subarterial and moderate or large perimembranous VSDs with outlet extension should be closed before the patient is about 3 years of age to prevent cusp prolapse.[R4] Patients having doubly committed subarterial VSD should have prompt operation regardless of age if any aortic valve deformity or regurgitation is detected; anatomic and hemodynamic features of the VSD contribute greatly to development of aortic valve cusp deformity and subsequent AR.[K20,K21,O1,S12] When AR is moderate or severe and cusp prolapse is noted on the 2D echocardiogram or aortogram, operation should be undertaken promptly. Operation certainly should be done before the patient reaches age 10, because reconstruction of the valve is usually possible when operation is done during the first decade of life; thus, valve replacement is prevented or at least postponed. This fact is confirmed by the UAB experience, in which the average age of patients requiring replacement was 20 years, compared with 12 years for the remainder of the group.[M2]

When 2D echocardiography shows bicuspid aortic valve, or when the aortogram shows minimal enlargement of the sinuses and no cusp prolapse in the presence of severe AR, a bicuspid valve is probably present and valve replacement may be required. Operation should therefore be postponed until symptoms develop or LV enlargement indicates need for operation.

When operation is delayed until adult life, aortic valve replacement is usually required.[O3]

SPECIAL SITUATIONS AND CONTROVERSIES

Some surgeons prefer to visualize and repair VSDs through an aortotomy.[C19,L6] This practice can produce good results, but if the VSD is perimembranous rather than in the RV outflow tract, possibility of permanent damage to the bundle of His may be increased by this essentially LV approach to repair. Repair through the pulmonary trunk or RV is recommended for subarterial and anterior muscular defects, and through the right atrium or RV for perimembranous defects.

Section III Straddling and Overriding Tricuspid (or Mitral) Valve

A straddling and overriding tricuspid valve sometimes coexists with an otherwise isolated VSD, usually one that extends posteriorly to the crux. Straddling and overriding of an AV valve may also coexist with a VSD that is simply part of a congenital cardiac anomaly (e.g., transposition of the great arteries, congenitally corrected transposition of the great arteries, univentricular AV connection). The subject is considered in its entirety in this chapter, with reference to other chapters.

Straddling and overriding of an AV valve always occur in relation to a VSD close to the valve.[K10] When straddling or overriding of an AV valve is mild, surgical considerations are usually related primarily to associated anomalies. When straddling or overriding is severe, or when there is associated hypoplasia of the ventricle to which the AV valve is appropriately (see following text) connected, surgical considerations are usually based primarily on straddling and overriding and severity of any coexisting ventricular hypoplasia.

Hypoplasia of the ventricle guarded by the straddling or overriding valve (termed the ***appropriate ventricle***) usually coexists. Generally, the more severe the overriding, the greater the ventricular hypoplasia. Occasionally, a straddling or overriding AV valve has leaflets that differ from normal in number and morphology. Overriding and straddling AV valves may occasionally produce subpulmonary or subaortic obstruction.

DEFINITION

An AV valve is considered to be ***straddling*** when part of the tension apparatus of the valve crosses the VSD and the crest of the interventricular septum to attach to the septum or a papillary muscle in the opposite (inappropriate) ventricle. The tension apparatus is thus attached within both ventricles, and blood passing through the valve is directed into both ventricles. An AV valve is considered to be ***overriding*** when the AV junction to which the AV valve leaflets attach is connected to both ventricles. AV valve straddling and overriding usually occur in combination, and occasionally both AV valves are involved with these anomalies in the same heart.

HISTORICAL NOTE

Lambert in 1951 and Van Praagh and colleagues in 1964 appeared to be aware of AV valve straddling and overriding, although they were not explicit about it.[L2,V2] In 1966, Mehrizi and colleagues referred to overriding and straddling of the right AV valve onto the RV in hearts with double inlet left ventricle (DILV) and the LV lying posteriorly and to the left.[M8] Subsequently, de la Cruz and Miller in 1968 and Lev and colleagues in 1969 referred to this occurrence in hearts with various types of "single ventricle" (generally double inlet ventricles).[D3,L11]

Rastelli and colleagues reported "straddling right atrioventricular valves" in hearts with a large VSD, but the right AV valve in their cases appears to have been both overriding and straddling.[R3] These investigators identified malalignment of atrial and ventricular septa as the characteristic of hearts with overriding AV valves, along with cleft leaflets often present and juxtacrucial position of the VSD. Liberthson, one of whose coauthors was Lev, clearly distinguished between overriding and straddling AV valves in hearts with double inlet ventricles in 1971, although those terms were not used or defined.[L12] Again, in the context of double inlet ventricles, Tandon and colleagues discussed "straddling AV valves."[T2] Thereafter, ease of diagnosis provided by 2D echocardiography rapidly led to broader recognition and improved understanding of these AV valve abnormalities.[L1,S8]

Surgical management of straddling and overriding AV valves was first reported in 1979, independently by Pacifico and by Tabry and their colleagues.[D1,P1,T1] Surgical possibilities, rapidly expanding knowledge of morphology of congenital heart disease, and increased use of 2D echocardiography resulted in clear perception of the morphology and implications of these AV valve anomalies.

Clarifying terminology used in this section was evolved by Milo and Ho and their colleagues in studies of straddling and overriding AV valves.[H17,M10] Milo and colleagues described disposition of the conduction system in hearts with overriding AV valves,[M10] and Anderson and colleagues formulated the basis for categorizing these hearts as well as those with univentricular AV connections ("single ventricle").[A11]

MORPHOLOGY

Morphologic Syndromes

When atria are in usual (solitus) situs, ventricular topology is right-handed, and AV and ventriculoarterial (VA) connections are concordant (see "Terminology and Classification of Heart Disease" in Chapter 1), the right AV valve sometimes overrides or straddles. This anomaly is associated with a posteriorly placed (juxtacrucial) VSD in the inlet portion of the ventricular septum when viewed from the RV aspect. The interventricular septum does not attach to the crux cordis in this situation. The overriding tricuspid valve is associated with malalignment of the atrial and interventricular septa. The RV is usually somewhat hypoplastic.

When there is atrial situs solitus, ventricular right-handedness (D-loop), AV concordant connection, and discordant VA connection (complete transposition of the great arteries), the left AV valve may be overriding, in this case over a VSD in the anterior portion of the ventricular septum.

When there is atrial situs solitus, ventricular right-handedness, AV concordant connection, and DORV (one of the most common situations in which overriding and straddling of an AV valve occur[R5]), the right AV valve may be overriding and is usually straddling in hearts with a VSD that is juxta-aortic, and usually also perimembranous and juxtacrucial. When the VSD is juxtapulmonary and somewhat anterior (Taussig-Bing heart), the left AV valve may be straddling and overriding a VSD that does not extend to the crux cordis.[K19]

When there is atrial situs solitus, left-handed ventricular topology (L-loop), AV discordant connection, and VA discordant connection (congenitally corrected transposition of the great arteries), the right AV valve (which generally in this setting has two leaflets) may override an anteriorly situated VSD. The interventricular septum does reach the crux cordis. When overriding of the right AV valve in this setting is more than 50%, there is double inlet right ventricle (DIRV) with the RV lying to the left and more or less posterior, and an anterior, right-sided, and often hypoplastic and rudimentary (incomplete) LV.

In hearts with congenitally corrected transposition of the great arteries, the left-sided AV valve may override a posteriorly placed VSD; in these hearts, the interventricular septum does not reach the crux cordis. When overriding is more than 50%, the condition is DILV with left-sided and anteriorly placed hypoplastic and rudimentary (incomplete) RV, the most common type of double inlet ventricle. A special group of cases with AV discordant connection, usually with DORV, involves a VSD that is juxtacrucial and in which one or both AV valves are overriding and straddling. Ventricles in this setting are usually in an over-and-under position, and circulations appear to crisscross within the heart.

Similar patterns may occur with atrial situs inversus and with atrial situs ambiguous.

Conduction System

Knowledge of location of the AV node and bundle of His is required for satisfactory surgical treatment of cardiac malformations. When the AV valve is overriding or straddling a VSD that does not reach the crux cordis, the conduction system is usually unaffected by the overriding valve.[A12] Thus, the AV node is in its usual location in the AV septum when the ventricular topology is right-handed and the AV connection concordant. When the ventricular topology is left-handed and the AV connection discordant, the conduction system generally arises from an anomalous anterolateral node, and this is unaffected by the overriding valve.

When in hearts with AV concordant connection the AV valve (in this case the tricuspid valve) overrides a VSD that is juxtacrucial (such defects may be perimembranous as well), the AV node is situated anomalously.[A12] It lies at the point inferiorly at which the ventricular septum attaches to the anulus (or circumference) of the right AV valve.[M10]

When the VSD is juxtacrucial and the AV connection discordant, the left AV valve overrides and the AV node occupies an anterolateral position near the right AV valve anulus, as is usual in hearts with AV discordant connection.

CLINICAL FEATURES AND DIAGNOSTIC CRITERIA

Straddling and overriding of an AV valve are uncommon, occurring as an added anomaly in about 3% of patients with congenital heart disease. They seem to be more prevalent in hearts with AV discordant connection than in those with AV concordant connections (Table 35-5). Among hearts with AV concordant connections, straddling and overriding of an AV valve occur most often in hearts with DORV and in those with complete transposition of the great arteries.

Table 35-5 Cardiac Morphology and Mortality after Operation in Patients with Overriding and Straddling Atrioventricular Valves[a]

Cardiac Morphology	*n*	Hospital Deaths	Total Deaths
AV Concordant Connection			
VSD (RAVV)	6	0	0
VSD (LAVV)	1[b]	0	0
VSD and valvar PS (RAVV)	1	0	0
TF (RAVV)	3	0	0
TGA and PS (LAVV)	2	1	1
DORV			
Subaortic VSD and PS (RAVV)	3	2	2
Subpulmonary VSD and PS (LAVV)	4	0	2
Taussig-Bing heart (LAVV)	1	1	1
AV Discordant Connection			
CTGA (LAVV)			
PS	4	0	1
Without PS	3	0	2
TGA (RAVV) and PS	2	0	0
DORV with PS			
LAVV	2[c]	0	0
RAVV	2	1	1
AV Ambiguous Connection			
DORV, PS (RAVV)	1	0	0
Total	35	5	10

[a]Data from 35 patients operated on at UAB from 1967 to 1985. Total deaths include hospital deaths and those in follow-up period.
[b]Several cords from mitral valve straddled to insert on right ventricular side of septum near ventricular septal defect.
[c]One patient also had right atrioventricular valve atresia.
Key: *AV,* Atrioventricular; *CTGA,* corrected transposition of the great arteries; *DORV,* double outlet right ventricle; *LAVV,* left atrioventricular valve; *PS,* pulmonary stenosis; *RAVV,* right atrioventricular valve; *TF,* tetralogy of Fallot; *TGA,* transposition of the great arteries; *VSD,* ventricular septal defect.

Coexisting cardiac anomalies, not straddling and overriding of the AV valve, generally determine the clinical syndrome, natural history, and diagnostic features in patients with straddling or overriding of the AV valves.

Straddling and overriding AV valves are usually competent and have no features that permit their identification by history, physical examination, chest radiograph, or ECG. Echocardiography is the technique by which they are generally diagnosed, although overriding can often be diagnosed or inferred from the angiogram.[B15,S17]

TECHNIQUE OF OPERATION

When an AV valve is only overriding, repair of the associated VSD or other cardiac anomalies can usually be done in essentially the normal manner, except for some deviation of the patch to accommodate the overriding. Straddling presents a more severe surgical challenge, particularly when it is moderate or severe in degree and when the inappropriate ventricle into which the straddling cords enter is not the one the surgeon is working in which.[M7] For these reasons, the Fontan operation (see Section IV of Chapter 41) is often the most appropriate option when severe straddling or overriding is present.

Section of Straddling Cords

Rarely, a single straddling cord can be sectioned to permit repair of a VSD or an intraventricular tunnel repair, without rendering the AV valve regurgitant. This technique can probably be used only when straddling is mild.

Slotting of Repair Patch

Rarely, straddling cords can fit into a slot or cut made in the patch used to close the VSD or make an intraventricular tunnel. The slot is then closed by sutures. This technique is applicable only to mild or possibly moderate straddling involving just a few cords, and it probably results in loss of free motion of the cords.

Reattachment of Sectioned Tensor Apparatus

When straddling is mild or moderate, and when the straddling tensor apparatus attaches to only one papillary muscle or area of the muscular interventricular septum in the inappropriate ventricle, and when that muscle has no other cord attachments, the muscle may be sectioned at its base. Then, along with its straddling cords, the muscle is brought back into the appropriate ventricle. The VSD is closed with a patch, or if indicated, an intraventricular tunnel repair is performed. Finally, the muscle to which the straddling cords connect is reattached to the patch or tunnel.

This technique is used infrequently and is applicable only when surgery is being performed from within the appropriate ventricle, approached either through its atrium or a ventriculotomy. Probability of dehiscence of a reattached papillary muscle or tendinous cord has not been determined.

Minor Septation

The patch used to close a VSD or create an intraventricular tunnel may be deviated around the papillary muscle and septal attachments of a straddling AV valve so that they lie within the appropriate ventricle after repair (Figs. 35-40 and 35-41). This approach is most easily performed when straddling is *into* the ventricle the surgeon is working in, through its atrium or a ventriculotomy. This is usually the ventricle ejecting into the pulmonary trunk: the right-sided RV in DORV with concordant AV connection, or the right-sided LV in hearts with discordant AV connection. In some cases, however, the technique of minor septation can be applied when straddling is into the ventricle ejecting into the aorta (see Fig. 35-40).

Replacement of Straddling Atrioventricular Valve

When the straddling AV valve is regurgitant (a relatively unusual situation), operation usually includes valve replacement. In some cases, this approach may be used simply because of complexity and severity of the straddling. The valve replacement device may face onto the patch used for repair of the VSD or creation of an intraventricular tunnel, because of the malalignment of the atrial and ventricular septa. This possibility emphasizes the value of a low-profile device in this setting, and even with such a device, some functional impairment may result.

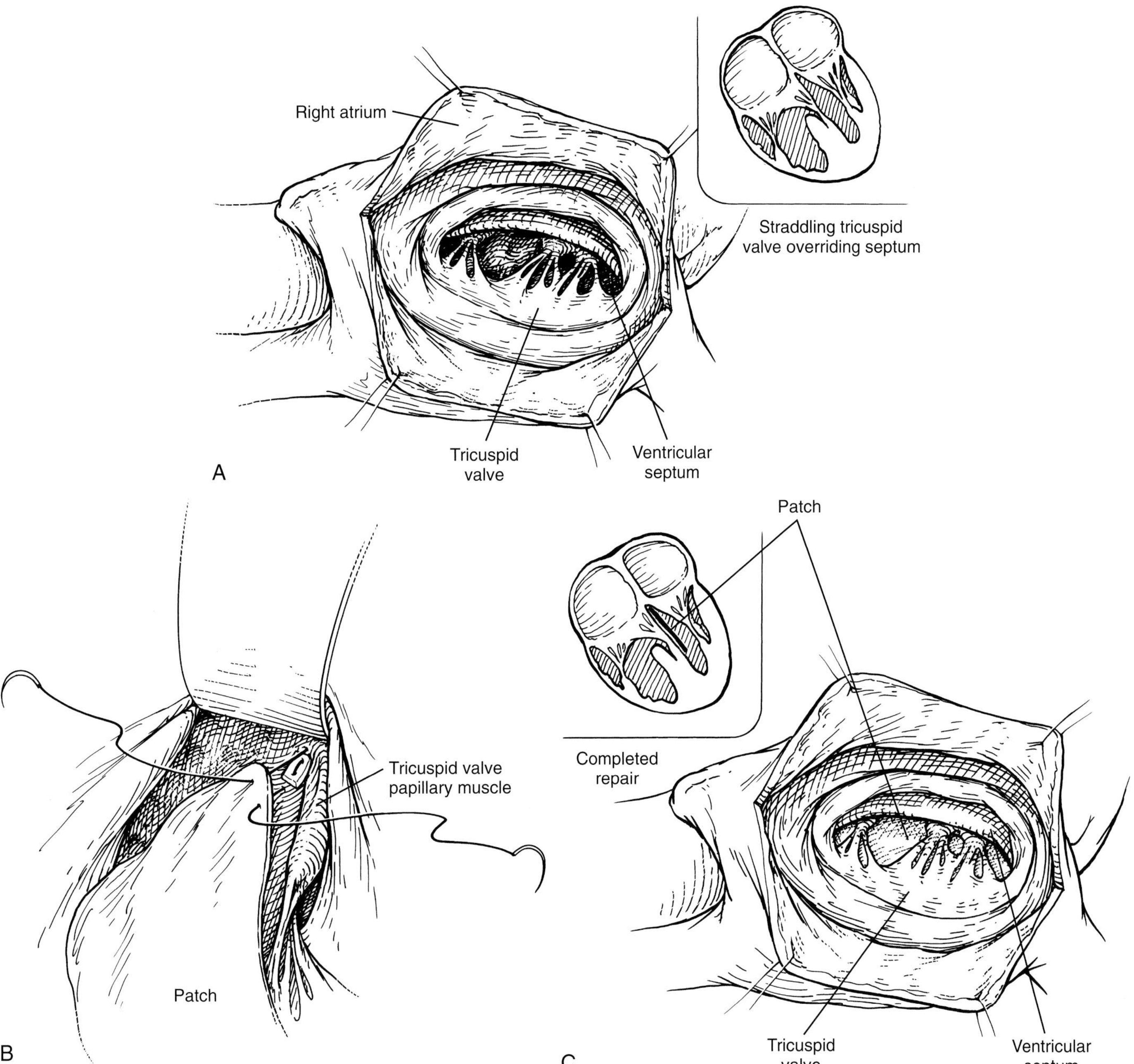

Figure 35-40 Minor septation for repair of a perimembranous, juxta-aortic, and juxtacrucial ventricular septal defect (VSD) associated with overriding and straddling of tricuspid valve in a patient with atrial situs solitus, ventricular D-loop, and atrioventricular and ventriculoatrial concordant connection. **A,** Approach is through usual oblique right atriotomy. Cords of septal leaflet straddle across VSD to attach anomalously to several papillary muscles within left ventricle; tricuspid valve also overrides 10% to 20% onto left ventricle. **B,** Repair is made through tricuspid valve. As shown, patch used for repair is placed on left side of septum and of papillary muscles to which tricuspid septal leaflet cords attach. **C,** Completed repair. (From Pacifico and colleagues.[P1])

Particular care and thoughtfulness are required when straddling or overriding occurs in the setting of ventricular L-loop, when valve replacement appears to be indicated. This situation, along with the sometimes associated complete heart block, may compromise long-term outlook sufficiently that a Fontan operation is preferable to a two-ventricle repair (see Chapter 41).

Fontan Operation

The Fontan operation is also the only method that can be used when moderate or severe hypoplasia of a ventricle is associated with straddling and overriding AV valves. Current information concerning early and intermediate-term results of this operation encourages its wider use when AV

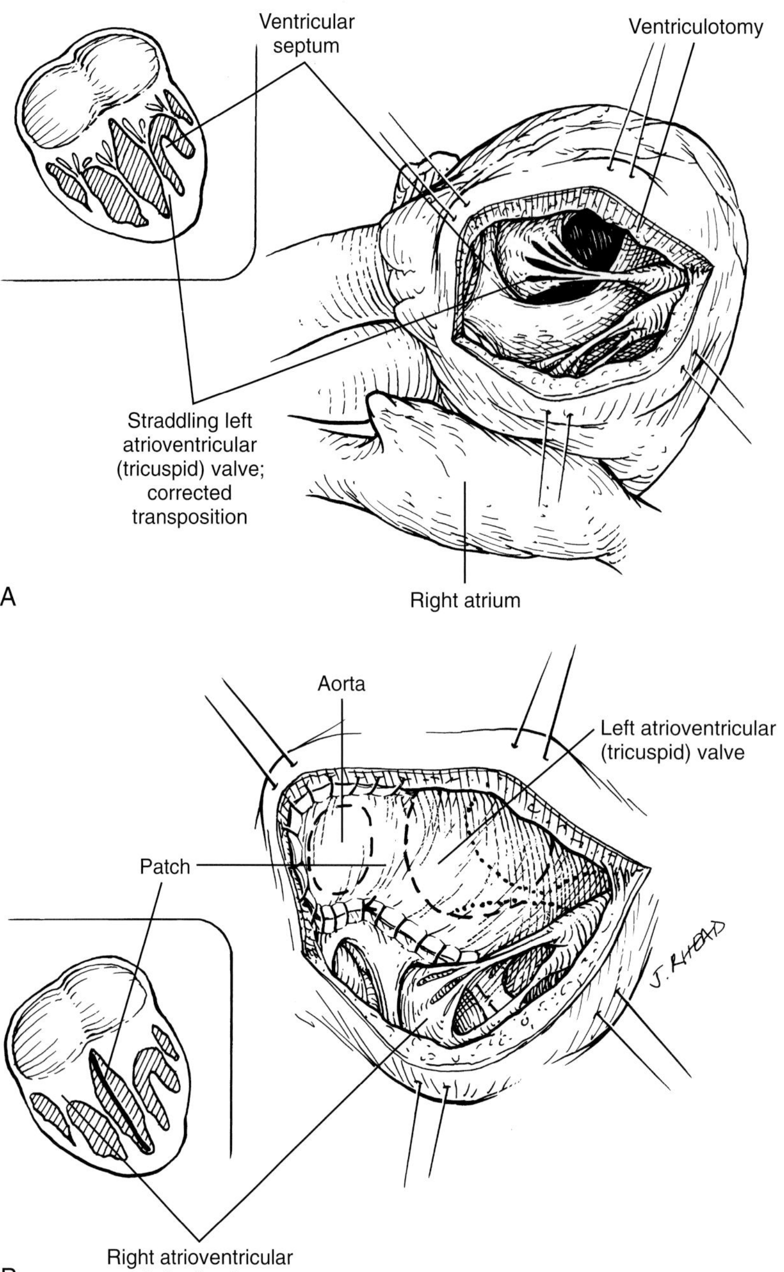

Figure 35-41 Intraventricular tunnel repair incorporating a minor septation for straddling and overriding left atrioventricular (AV) tricuspid valve in a patient with congenitally corrected transposition of the great arteries and about 40% overriding of aorta onto right-sided left ventricle. **A,** Vertical left (right-sided) ventriculotomy is shown, but an approach through right atrium is preferred. Straddling and overriding left AV (tricuspid) valve is shown, as well as ventricular septal defect and aortic overriding. **B,** Repair patch creates an intraventricular tunnel conducting systemic arterial blood flow from left-sided right ventricle to aorta and keeping entire left AV valve apparatus on appropriate side of patch. (From Pacifico and colleagues.[P1])

valve straddling or overriding is moderate or severe (see Chapter 41).

Cardiac Transplantation

Cardiac transplantation is reserved for patients with straddling and overriding AV valves in whom a severe secondary cardiomyopathy has developed (see Section II in Chapter 21).

RESULTS

Early and intermediate-term (5 to 15 years) survival after surgery in patients with straddling and overriding AV valves is determined primarily by the cardiac defect with which the AV valve anomaly is associated. However, survival is somewhat less satisfactory than that in general after repair of the primary cardiac defect. Exceptions are patients in whom the Fontan operation or cardiac transplantation is performed;

survival after these operations is unrelated to the cardiac anomaly for which the operation was done and is not lessened by presence of a straddling or overriding AV valve.

Heart block has occurred more frequently than usual after repair of hearts with concordant AV connection and overriding AV valves associated with a VSD extending to the crux cordis and in patients with discordant AV connection. Because position of the AV node and conduction system in such hearts is now known, heart block should now occur less frequently.

INDICATIONS FOR OPERATION

Indications for operation in patients with overriding and straddling AV valves lie with the coexisting anomalies rather than with the AV valve anomaly.

Strategy of operation is greatly influenced by the AV valve anomaly, and whenever possible that strategy should be decided in early life. If straddling is mild, the strategy can probably be that for the coexisting anomaly in general, and the AV valve anomaly can be managed by the technique of minor septation or an even lesser procedure.

When straddling is severe, these techniques seem likely to be associated with a relatively high early risk. Valve replacement in this setting carries more than the usual early and intermediate risks and imponderables. A Fontan operation probably is associated with better early and late results than these procedures and is the only type of procedure that can be considered when the patient has important ventricular hypoplasia. Therefore, diagnosis of AV valve straddling or overriding should be made in early infancy. If the patient has cyanosis from reduced pulmonary blood flow, a PTFE interposition systemic–pulmonary arterial shunt or a bidirectional cavopulmonary anastomosis should be performed (see Chapters 38 and 41). If there is a large left-to-right shunt, pulmonary trunk banding should be performed in early life. In either case, the Fontan operation is then performed in patients aged 1 to 2 years, before ventricular hypertrophy becomes marked (see Chapter 41).

REFERENCES

A

1. Aaron BL, Lower BR. Muscular ventricular septal defect repair made easy. Ann Thorac Surg 1975;19:568.
2. Ad N, Barak J, Birk E, Diamant S, Vidne BA. A one-way, valved, atrial septal patch in the management of postoperative right heart failure. An animal study. J Thorac Cardiovasc Surg 1994; 108:134.
3. Ad N, Barak J, Birk E, Snir E, Vidne BA. Unidirectional valve patch (letter). Ann Thorac Surg 1996;62:626.
4. Ad N, Birk E, Barak J, Diamant S, Snir E, Vidne BA. A one-way valved atrial septal patch: a new surgical technique and its clinical application. J Thorac Cardiovasc Surg 1996;111:84.
5. Albus RA, Trusler GA, Izukawa T, Williams WG. Pulmonary artery banding. J Thorac Cardiovasc Surg 1984;88:645.
6. Alpert BS, Cook DH, Varghese PJ, Rowe RD. Spontaneous closure of small ventricular septal defects: ten-year follow-up. Pediatrics 1979;63:204.
7. Amin Z, Berry JM, Foker JE, Rocchini AP, Bass JL. Intraoperative closure of muscular ventricular septal defect in a canine model and application of the technique in a baby. J Thorac Cardiovasc Surg 1998;115:1374.
8. Andersen HO, de Leval MR, Tsang VT, Elliott MJ, Anderson RH, Cook AC. Is complete heart block after surgical closure of ventricular septum defects still an issue? Ann Thorac Surg 2006;82: 948-56.
9. Anderson RH, Becker AE, Tynan M. Description of ventricular septal defects—or how long is a piece of string? Int J Cardiol 1986;13:267.
10. Anderson RH, Lenox CC, Zuberbuhler JR. Morphology of ventricular septal defect associated with coarctation of aorta. Br Heart J 1983;50:176.
11. Anderson RH, Macartney FJ, Tynan M, Becker AE, Freedom RM, Godman MJ, et al. Univentricular atrioventricular connection: single ventricle trap unsprung. Pediatr Cardiol 1983;4:273.
12. Anderson RH, Milo S, Ho SY, Wilkinson JL, Becker AE. The anatomy of straddling atrioventricular valves. In: Becker AE, Loosekoot G, Marcelletti C, Anderson RH, eds. Paediatric cardiology, Vol. 3. New York: Churchill Livingstone, 1981, p. 411.
13. Anderson RH, Wilcox BR. The surgical anatomy of ventricular septal defect. J Card Surg 1992;7:17.
14. Anderson RH, Wilcox BR. The surgical anatomy of ventricular septal defects associated with overriding valvar orifices. J Card Surg 1993;8:130.
15. Ando M, Takahashi Y, Kikuchi T. Short operation time: an important element to reduce operative invasiveness in pediatric cardiac surgery. Ann Thorac Surg 2005;80:631-5.
16. Ando M, Takao A. Pathological anatomy of ventricular septal defect associated with aortic valve prolapse and regurgitation. Heart Vessels 1986;2:117-26.
17. Andreasen AT, Watson F. Experimental cardiovascular surgery: "The azygos factor." Br J Surg 1952;39:548.
18. Ash R. Natural history of ventricular septal defects in childhood lesions with predominant arteriovenous shunts. J Pediatr 1964; 64:45.
19. Auld PA, Johnson AL, Gibbons JE, McGregor M. Changes in pulmonary vascular resistance in infants and children with left-to-right intracardiac shunts. Circulation 1963;27:257.

B

1. Baker EJ, Ayton V, Smith MA, Parsons JM, Ladusans EJ, Anderson RH, et al. Magnetic resonance imaging at a high field strength of ventricular septal defects in infants. Br Heart J 1989;62:305.
2. Bargeron LM Jr, Elliott LP, Soto B, Bream PR, Curry GC. Axial cineangiography in congenital heart disease: section I. Circulation 1977;56:1075.
3. Barratt-Boyes BG, Roche AH, Whitlock RM. Six year review of the results of freehand aortic valve replacement using an antibiotic sterilized homograft valve. Circulation 1977;55:353.
4. Barratt-Boyes BG, Simpson M, Neutze JM. Intracardiac surgery in neonates and infants using deep hypothermia with surface cooling and limited cardiopulmonary bypass. Circulation 1971;43:I25.
5. Becu LM, Fontana RS, DuShane JW, Kirklin JW, Burchell HB, Edwards JE. Anatomic and pathologic studies in ventricular septal defect. Circulation 1956;14:349.
6. Beerman LB, Park SC, Fischer DR, Fricker FJ, Mathews RA, Neches WH, et al. Ventricular septal defect associated with aneurysm of the membranous septum. J Am Coll Cardiol 1985;5:118.
7. Berglund E. Ventricular function. VI. Balance of left and right ventricular output: relation between left and right atrial pressures. Am J Physiol 1954;178:381.
8. Bharati S, McAllister HA Jr, Lev M. Straddling and displaced atrioventricular orifices and valves. Circulation 1979;60:673.
9. Bierman FZ, Fellows K, Williams RG. Prospective identification of ventricular septal defects in infancy using subxiphoid two-dimensional echocardiography. Circulation 1980;62:807.
10. Blackstone EH, Kirklin JW, Bradley EL, DuShane JW, Appelbaum A. Optimal age and results in repair of large ventricular septal defects. J Thorac Cardiovasc Surg 1976;72:661.
11. Brandt PW. Cineangiography of atrioventricular and ventriculoarterial connections. In: Godman MJ, ed. Paediatric cardiology, Vol. 4. Edinburgh: Churchill Livingstone, 1980, p. 191.
12. Brandt PW, Calder AL. Cardiac connections: the segmental approach to radiologic diagnosis in congenital heart disease. Curr Probl Diagn Radiol 1977;7:1.
13. Braunwald E, Morrow AG. Left-ventriculo–right atrial communication: diagnosis by clinical, hemodynamic, and angiographic methods. Am J Med 1960;28:913.
14. Breckenridge IM, Stark J, Waterston DJ, Bonham-Carter RE. Multiple ventricular septal defects. Ann Thorac Surg 1972;13:128.
15. Bridges ND, Perry SB, Keane JF, Goldstein SA, Mandell V, Mayer JE Jr, et al. Preoperative transcatheter closure of congenital muscular ventricular septal defects. N Engl J Med 1991;324:1312.

16. Burke RP. Minimally invasive techniques for congenital heart surgery. Semin Thorac Cardiovasc Surg 1997;9:337.
17. Bush A, Busst CM, Haworth SG, Hislop AA, Knight WB, Corrin B, et al. Correlations of lung morphology, pulmonary vascular resistance, and outcome in children with congenital heart disease. Br Heart J 1988;59:480.

C

1. Campbell M. Natural history of ventricular septal defect. Br Heart J 1971;33:246.
2. Carotti A, Marino B, Bevilacqua M, Marcelletti C, Rossi E, Santoro G, et al. Primary repair of isolated ventricular septal defect in infancy guided by echocardiography. Am J Cardiol 1997;79:1498.
3. Carpentier A. Cardiac valve surgery—the "French correction." J Thorac Cardiovasc Surg 1983;86:323.
4. Cartmill TB, DuShane JW, McGoon DC, Kirklin JW. Results of repair of ventricular septal defect. J Thorac Cardiovasc Surg 1966; 52:486.
5. Castaneda AR, Zamora R, Nicoloff DM, Moller JH, Hunt CE, Lucas RV. High-pressure, high-resistance ventricular septal defect: surgical results of closure through right atrium. Ann Thorac Surg 1971;12:29.
6. Chauvaud S, Serraf A, Mihaileanu S, Soyer R, Blondeau P, Dubost C, et al. Ventricular septal defect associated with aortic valve incompetence: results of two surgical managements. Ann Thorac Surg 1990;49:875.
7. Cheung YF, Chiu CS, Yung TC, Chau AK. Impact of preoperative aortic cusp prolapse on long-term outcome after surgical closure of subarterial ventricular septal defect. Ann Thorac Surg 2002; 73:622-7.
8. Chin AJ, Alboliras ET, Barber G, Murphy JD, Helton JG, Pigott JD, et al. Prospective detection by Doppler color flow imaging of additional defects in infants with a large ventricular septal defect. J Am Coll Cardiol 1990;15:1637.
9. Ching E, DuShane JW, McGoon DC, Danielson GK. Total correction of ventricular septal defect in infancy using extracorporeal circulation: surgical considerations and results of operation. Ann Thorac Surg 1971;12:1.
10. Chiu SN, Wang JK, Lin MT, Chen CA, Chen HC, Chang CI, et al. Progression of aortic regurgitation after surgical repair of outlet-type ventricular septal defects. Am Heart J 2007;153: 336-42.
11. Chiu SN, Wang JK, Lin MT, Wu ET, Lu FL, Chang CI, et al. Aortic valve prolapse associated with outlet-type ventricular septal defect. Ann Thorac Surg 2005;79:1366-71.
12. Chung KJ, Manning JA. Ventricular septal defect associated with aortic insufficiency: medical and surgical management. Am Heart J 1974;87:435.
13. Civin WH, Edwards JE. Pathology of the pulmonary vascular tree. I. A comparison of the intrapulmonary arteries in Eisenmenger's complex and in stenosis of ostium infundibuli associated with biventricular origin of the aorta. Circulation 1950;2:545.
14. Clarkson PM. Growth following corrective cardiac operation in early infancy. In: Barratt-Boyes BG, Neutze JM, Harris EA, eds. Heart disease in infancy: diagnosis and surgical treatment. London: Churchill Livingstone, 1973, p. 75.
15. Clarkson PM, Frye RL, DuShane JW, Burchell HB, Wood EH, Weidman WH. Prognosis for patients with ventricular septal defect and severe pulmonary vascular obstructive disease. Circulation 1968;38:129.
16. Cohen M, Lillehei CW. A quantitative study of the "azygos factor" during vena caval occlusion in the dog. Surg Gynecol Obstet 1954;98:225.
17. Collins G, Calder L, Rose V, Kidd L, Keith J. Ventricular septal defect: clinical and hemodynamic changes in the first five years of life. Am Heart J 1972;84:695.
18. Cooley DA, Garrett HE, Howard HS. The surgical treatment of ventricular septal defect: an analysis of 300 consecutive surgical cases. Prog Cardiovasc Dis 1962;4:312.
19. Cooley DA, Hallman GL, Wukasch DC, Sandiford FM. Transaortic repair of ventricular septal defect. Ann Thorac Surg 1973;16:99.
20. Cordell D, Graham TP Jr, Atwood GF, Boerth RC, Boucek RJ, Bender HW. Left heart volume characteristics following ventricular septal defect closure in infancy. Circulation 1976;54:294.
21. Corone P, Doyon F, Gaudeau S, Guerin F, Vernant P, Ducam H, et al. Natural history of ventricular septal defect: a study involving 790 cases. Circulation 1977;55:908.

D

1. Danielson GK, Tabry IF, Fulton FE, Hagler DJ, Ritter DG. Successful repair of straddling atrioventricular valve by technique used for septation of univentricular heart. Ann Thorac Surg 1979;28:554.
2. Davis Z, McGoon DC, Danielson GK, Wallace RB. Removal of pulmonary artery band. Isr J Med Sci 1975;11:110.
3. de la Cruz MV, Miller BL. Double inlet left ventricle: two pathological specimens with comments on the embryology and on its relation to single ventricle. Circulation 1968;37:249.
4. de Leval MR, Pozzi M, Starnes V, Sullivan ID, Stark J, Somerville J, et al. Surgical management of doubly committed subarterial ventricular septal defects. Circulation 1988;78:III40.
5. Dimich I, Steinfeld L, Litwak RS, Park S, Silvers N. Subpulmonic ventricular septal defect associated with aortic insufficiency. Am J Cardiol 1973;32:325.
6. Dirksen T, Moulaert AJ, Buis-Liem TN, Brom AG. Ventricular septal defect associated with left ventricular outflow tract obstruction below the defect. J Thorac Cardiovasc Surg 1978;75:688.
7. Dodge-Khatami A, Knirsch W, Tomaske M, Pretre R, Bettex D, Rousson V, et al. Spontaneous closure of small residual ventricular septal defects after surgical repair. Ann Thorac Surg 2007;83: 902-5.
8. Doty DB, McGoon DC. Closure of perimembranous ventricular septal defect. J Thorac Cardiovasc Surg 1983;85:781.
9. Downing JW Jr, Kaplan S, Bove KE. Postsurgical left anterior hemiblock and right bundle branch block. Br Heart J 1972;34:263.
10. DuShane JW, Kirklin JW. Late results of the repair of ventricular septal defect in pulmonary vascular disease. In: Kirklin JW, ed. Advances in cardiovascular surgery. Orlando, Fla: Grune & Stratton, 1973, p. 9.
11. DuShane JW, Kirklin JW, Patrick RT, Donald DE, Terry HR Jr, Burchell HB, et al. Ventricular septal defects with pulmonary hypertension: surgical treatment by means of a mechanical pump oxygenator. JAMA 1956;160:950.

E

1. Eapen RS, Lemler MS, Scott WA, Ramaciotti C. Echocardiographic characteristics of perimembranous ventricular septal defects associated with aortic regurgitation. J Am Soc Echocardiogr 2003;16: 209-13.
2. Edwards JE, Burchell HB. The pathologic anatomy of deficiencies between the aortic root and the heart including aortic sinus aneurysm. Thorax 1957;12:125.
3. Elgamal MA, Hakimi M, Lyons JM, Walters HL 3rd. Risk factors for failure of aortic valvuloplasty in aortic insufficiency with ventricular septal defect. Ann Thorac Surg 1999;68:1350.
4. Elliott LP, Bargeron LM Jr, Bream PR, Soto B, Curry GC. Axial cineangiography in congenital heart disease. II. Specific lesions. Circulation 1977;56:1048.
5. Ellis H Jr, Ongley PA, Kirklin JW. Ventricular septal defect with aortic valvular incompetence. Surgical considerations. Circulation 1963;27:789.
6. Eroglu AG, Oztunc F, Saltik L, Dedeoglu S, Ahunbay G. Evolution of ventricular septal defect with special reference to spontaneous closure rate, subaortic ridge and aortic valve prolapse. Pediatr Cardiol 2003;24:31-35.
7. Eroglu AG, Oztunc F, Saltik L, Dedeoglu S, Bakari S, Ahunbay G. Aortic valve prolapse and aortic regurgitation in patients with ventricular septal defect. Pediatr Cardiol 2003;24:36-9.

F

1. Fox KM, Patel RG, Graham GR, Taylor JF, Stark J, De Leval MR, et al. Multiple and single ventricular septal defect. A clinical and haemodynamic comparison. Br Heart J 1978;40:141.
2. Frater RW. The prolapsing aortic cusp: experimental and clinical observations. Ann Thorac Surg 1967;3:63.
3. Freed MD, Rosenthal A, Plauth WH Jr, Nadas AS. Development of subaortic stenosis after pulmonary artery banding. Circulation 1973;48:III7.
4. Freedom RM, Dische MR, Rowe RD. Pathologic anatomy of subaortic stenosis and atresia in the first year of life. Am J Cardiol 1977;39:1035.
5. Fried R, Falkovsky G, Newburger J, Gorchakova AI, Rabinovitch M, Gordonova MI, et al. Pulmonary arterial changes in patients

with ventricular septal defects and severe pulmonary hypertension. Pediatr Cardiol 1986;7:147.
6. Friedli B, Kidd BS, Mustard WT, Keith JD. Ventricular septal defect with increased pulmonary vascular resistance: late results of surgical closure. Am J Cardiol 1974;33:403.
7. Friedman WF, Mehrizi A, Pusch AL. Multiple muscular ventricular septal defects. Circulation 1965;32:35.

G

1. Gan C, Lin K, An Q, Tang H, Song H, Lui RC, et al. Perventricular device closure of muscular ventricular septal defects on beating hearts: initial experience in eight children. J Thorac Cardiovasc Surg 2009;137:929-33.
2. Garamella JJ, Cruz AB Jr, Heupel WH, Dahl JC, Jensen NK, Berman R. Ventricular septal defect with aortic insufficiency: successful surgical correction of both defects by the transaortic approach. Am J Cardiol 1960;5:266.
3. Gasul BM, Dillon RF, Vrla V, Hait G. Ventricular septal defects: their natural transformation into those with infundibular stenosis or into the cyanotic or non-cyanotic type of tetralogy of Fallot. JAMA 1957;164:847.
4. Gaynor JW, Wernovsky G, Rychik J, Rome JJ, DeCampli WM, Spray TL. Outcome following single-stage repair of coarctation with ventricular septal defect. Eur J Cardiothorac Surg 2000; 18:62-7.
5. Gelband H, Waldo AL, Kaiser GA, Bowman FO Jr, Malm JR, Hoffman BF. Etiology of right bundle-branch block in patients undergoing total correction of tetralogy of Fallot. Circulation 1971;44:1022.
6. Gerbode F, Hultgren H, Melrose D, Osborn J. Syndrome of left ventricular–right atrial shunt: successful surgical repair of defect in five cases, with observation of bradycardia on closure. Ann Surg 1958;148:433.
7. Gersony WM, Hayes CJ. Bacterial endocarditis in patients with pulmonary stenosis, aortic stenosis, or ventricular septal defect. Circulation 1977;56:I84.
8. Girod DA, Hurwitz RA, King H, Jolly W. Recent results of two-stage surgical treatment of large ventricular septal defect. Circulation 1974;50:II9.
9. Glen S, Burns J, Bloomfield P. Prevalence and development of additional cardiac abnormalities in 1448 patients with congenital ventricular septal defects. Heart 2004;90:1321-5.
10. Gonzalez-Lavin L, Barratt-Boyes BG. Surgical considerations in the treatment of ventricular septal defect associated with aortic valvular incompetence. J Thorac Cardiovasc Surg 1969;57:422.
11. Griffin ML, Sullivan ID, Anderson RH, Macartney FJ. Doubly committed subarterial ventricular septal defect: new morphological criteria with echocardiographic and angiocardiographic correlation. Br Heart J 1988;59:474.
12. Griffiths SP, Turi GK, Ellis K, Krongrad E, Swift LH, Gersony WM, et al. Muscular ventricular septal defects repaired with left ventriculotomy. Am J Cardiol 1981;48:877.

H

1. Hallidie-Smith KA, Edwards RE, Wilson R, Zeidifard E. Long-term cardiorespiratory assessment after surgical closure of ventricular septal defect in childhood (abstract). Br Heart J 1975;37:553.
2. Hallidie-Smith KA, Hollman A, Cleland WP, Bentall HH, Goodwin JF. Effects of surgical closure of ventricular septal defects upon pulmonary vascular disease. Br Heart J 1969;31:246.
3. Hanna BM, El-Hewala AA, Gruber PJ, Gaynor JW, Spray TL, Seliem MA. Predictive value of intraoperative diagnosis of residual ventricular septal defects by transesophageal echocardiography. Ann Thorac Surg 2010;89:1233-7.
4. Heath D, Edwards JE. The pathology of hypertensive pulmonary vascular disease: a description of six grades of structural changes in the pulmonary arteries with special reference to congenital cardiac septal defects. Circulation 1958;18:533.
5. Heath D, Helmholz HF Jr, Burchell HB, DuShane JW, Edwards JE. Graded pulmonary vascular changes and hemodynamic findings in cases of atrial and ventricular septal defect and patent ductus arteriosus. Circulation 1958;18:1155.
6. Henry J, Kaplan S, Helmsworth JA, Schreiber JT. Management of infants with large ventricular septal defects: results with two-stage surgical treatment. Ann Thorac Surg 1973;15:109.
7. Hisatomi K, Isomura T, Sato T, Kawara T, Kosuga K, Ohishi K, et al. Aortoplasty for aortic regurgitation with ventricular septal defect. J Thorac Cardiovasc Surg 1994;108:396.
8. Hisatomi K, Kosuga K, Isomura T, Akagawa H, Ohishi K, Koga M. Ventricular septal defect associated with aortic regurgitation. Ann Thorac Surg 1987;43:363.
9. Hisatomi K, Taira A, Oku S, Moriyama Y. New valid technique for ventricular septal defect associated with aortic regurgitation. J Thorac Cardiovasc Surg 1998;115:733.
10. Hislop A, Haworth SG, Shinebourne EA, Reid L. Quantitative structural analysis of pulmonary vessels in isolated ventricular septal defect in infancy. Br Heart J 1975;37:1014.
11. Hobbins SM, Izukawa T, Radford DJ, Williams WG, Trusler GA. Conduction disturbances after surgical correction of ventricular septal defect by the atrial approach. Br Heart J 1979;41:289.
12. Hoffman JI. Diagnosis and treatment of pulmonary vascular disease. Birth Defects 1972;8:9.
13. Hoffman JI, Rudolph AM. The natural history of ventricular septal defects in infancy. Am J Cardiol 1965;16:634.
14. Hoffman JI, Rudolph AM. Increasing pulmonary vascular resistance during infancy in association with ventricular septal defect. Pediatrics 1966;38:220.
15. Hoffman JI, Rudolph AM. The natural history of isolated ventricular septal defect with special reference to selection of patients for surgery. Adv Pediatr 1970;17:57.
16. Hornberger LK, Sahn DJ, Krabill KA, Sherman FS, Swensson RE, Pesonen E, et al. Elucidation of the natural history of ventricular septal defects by serial Doppler color flow mapping studies. J Am Coll Cardiol 1989;13:1111.
17. Ho SY, Milo S, Anderson RH, Macartney FJ, Goodwin A, Becker AE, et al. Straddling atrioventricular valve with absent atrioventricular connection. Br Heart J 1982;47:344.
18. Houyel L, Vaksmann G, Fournier A, Davignon A. Ventricular arrhythmias after correction of ventricular septal defects: importance of surgical approach. J Am Coll Cardiol 1990;16:1224.
19. Hu DC, Giuliani ER, Downing TP, Danielson GK. Spontaneous closure of congenital ventricular septal defect in an adult. Clin Cardiol 1986;9:587.
20. Hudspeth AS, Cordell AR, Meredith JH, Johnston FR. An improved transatrial approach to the closure of ventricular septal defects. J Thorac Cardiovasc Surg 1962;43:157.
21. Hunt CE, Formanek G, Levine MA, Castaneda A, Moller JH. Banding of the pulmonary artery: results in 111 children. Circulation 1971;43:395.

J

1. Jacobs JP, Burke RP, Quintessenza JA, Mavroudis C. Congenital Heart Surgery Nomenclature Database Project: ventricular septal defect. Ann Thorac Surg 2000;69:S25.
2. Jarmakani JM, Graham TP Jr, Canent RV Jr. Left ventricular contractile state in children with successfully corrected ventricular septal defect. Circulation 1972;45:I102.
3. Jarmakani JM, Graham TP Jr, Canent RV Jr, Capp MP. The effect of corrective surgery on left heart volume and mass in children with ventricular septal defect. Am J Cardiol 1971;27:254.
4. John S, Korula R, Jairaj PS, Muralidharan S, Ravikumar E, Babuthaman C, et al. Results of surgical treatment of ventricular septal defects with pulmonary hypertension. Thorax 1983;38:279.
5. Johnson DC, Cartmill TB, Celermajer JM, Hawker RE, Stuckey DS, Bowdler JD, et al. Intracardiac repair of large ventricular septal defect in the first year of life. Med J Aust 1974;2:193.
6. Juaneda E, Gittenberger de Groot A, Oppenheimer-Dekker A, Haworth SG. Pulmonary arterial development in infants with large perimembranous ventricular septal defects associated with overriding of the aortic valve. Int J Cardiol 1985;7:223.

K

1. Kanter KR. Management of infants with coarctation and ventricular septal defect. Semin Thorac Cardiovasc Surg 2007;19:264-8.
2. Kanter KR, Mahle WT, Kogon BE, Kirshbom PM. What is the optimal management of infants with coarctation and ventricular septal defect? Ann Thorac Surg 2007;84:612-8.
3. Kawashima Y, Danno M, Shimizu Y, Matsuda H, Miyamoto T, Fujita T, et al. Ventricular septal defect associated with aortic insufficiency: anatomic classification and method of operation. Circulation 1973;47:1057.

4. Keane JF, Fellows KE, Buckley L, Castaneda AR, Nadas AS. Ventricular septal defect with aortic regurgitation: a 33 year experience (abstract). In: Godman MJ, ed. World Congress of Paediatric Cardiology. Edinburgh: Churchill Livingstone, 1981, p. 292.
5. Keane JF, Plauth WH Jr, Nadas AS. Ventricular septal defect with aortic regurgitation. Circulation 1977;56:I72-7.
6. Keck EW, Ongley PA, Kincaid OW, Swan HJ. Ventricular septal defect with aortic insufficiency: a clinical and hemodynamic study of 18 proved cases. Circulation 1963;27:203.
7. Keith JD, Rose V, Collins G, Kidd BS. Ventricular septal defect: incidence, morbidity, and mortality in various age groups. Br Heart J 1971;33:81.
8. Kelle AM, Young L, Kaushal S, Duffy CE, Anderson RH, Backer CL. The Gerbode defect: the significance of a left ventricular to right atrial shunt. Cardiol Young 2009;19(Suppl 2):96-9.
9. Kent WG. An appreciation of two great workers in hydraulics. London: Blades, East & Blades; 1912.
10. Kirklin JW, Anderson RH, Pacifico AD, Kirklin JK, Bargeron LM Jr. Surgery for hearts with straddling and overriding atrioventricular valves. In: Baue AE, Geha AS, Hammond GL, Laks H, Naunheim KS, eds. Glenn's thoracic and cardiovascular surgery, 5th Ed. East Norwalk, Conn: Appleton & Lange, 1991, p. 1069.
11. Kirklin JW, Appelbaum A, Bargeron LM Jr. Primary repair versus banding for ventricular septal defects in infants. In: Kidd BS, Rowe RD, eds. The child with congenital heart disease after surgery. Mount Kisco, NY: Futura, 1976, p. 3.
12. Kirklin JK, Castaneda AR, Keane JF, Fellows KE, Norwood WI. Surgical management of multiple ventricular septal defects. J Thorac Cardiovasc Surg 1980;80:485.
13. Kirklin JW, DuShane JW. Repair of ventricular septal defect in infancy. Pediatrics 1961;27:961.
14. Kirklin JW, DuShane JW. Indications for repair of ventricular septal defects. Am J Cardiol 1963;12:79.
15. Kirklin JW, Harshbarger HG, Donald DE, Edwards JE. Surgical correction of ventricular septal defect: anatomic and technical considerations. J Thorac Surg 1957;33:45.
16. Kirklin JW, McGoon DC, DuShane JW. Surgical treatment of ventricular septal defect. J Thorac Cardiovasc Surg 1960;40: 763.
17. Kirklin JW, Silver AW. Technique of exposing the ductus arteriosus prior to establishing extracorporeal circulation. Proc Mayo Clin 1958;33:423.
18. Kitagawa T, Durham LA 3rd, Mosca RS, Bove EL. Techniques and results in the management of multiple ventricular septal defects. J Thorac Cardiovasc Surg 1998;115:848.
19. Kitamura N, Takao A, Ando M, Imai Y, Konno S. Taussig-Bing heart with mitral valve straddling: case reports and postmortem study. Circulation 1974;49:761.
20. Kobayashi J, Koike K, Senzaki H, Kobayashi T, Tsunemoto M, Ishizawa A, et al. Correlation of anatomic and hemodynamic features with aortic valve leaflet deformity in doubly committed subarterial ventricular septal defect. Heart Vessels 1999;14:240.
21. Komai H, Naito Y, Fujiwara K, Noguchi Y, Nishimura Y, Uemura S. Surgical strategy for doubly committed subarterial ventricular septal defect with aortic cusp prolapse. Ann Thorac Surg 1997; 64:1146-9.
22. Kostolny M, Schreiber C, von Arnim V, Vogt M, Wottke M, Lange R. Timing of repair in ventricular septal defect with aortic insufficiency. Thorac Cardiovasc Surg 2006;54:512-5.
23. Krongrad E, Hefler SE, Bowman FO Jr, Malm JR, Hoffman BF. Further observations on the etiology of the right bundle branch block pattern following right ventriculotomy. Circulation 1974; 50:1105.
24. Krovetz LJ. Spontaneous closure of ventricular septal defect. Am J Cardiol 1998;81:100.
25. Kulbertus HE, Coyne JJ, Hallidie-Smith KA. Conduction disturbances before and after surgical closure of ventricular septal defect. Am Heart J 1969;77:123.
26. Kumar K, Lock JE, Geva T. Apical muscular ventricular septal defects between the left ventricle and the right ventricular infundibulum: diagnostic and interventional considerations. Circulation 1997;95:1207.
27. Kurosawa H, Becker AE. Modification of the precise relationship of the atrioventricular conduction bundle to the margins of the ventricular septal defects by the trabecula septomarginalis. J Thorac Cardiovasc Surg 1984;87:605.
28. Kurotobi S, Sano T, Matsushita T, Takeuchi M, Kogaki S, Miwatani T, et al. Quantitative, noninvasive assessment of ventricular septal defect shunt flow by measuring proximal isovelocity surface area on colour Doppler mapping. Heart 1997;78:305.

L

1. LaCorte MA, Fellows KE, Williams RG. Overriding tricuspid valve. Echocardiographic and angiocardiographic features. Am J Cardiol 1976;37:911.
2. Lambert EC. Single ventricle with a rudimentary outlet chamber. Case report. Bull Johns Hopkins Hosp 1951;88:231.
3. Laubry C, Pezzi C. Traitedes maladies carpentales du coeur. In Laubry C, Routier D, Soulie P. Les souffles de (a maladie de Roger). Rev Med Paris 1933;50:439.
4. Lauer RM, DuShane JW, Edwards JE. Obstruction of left ventricular outlet in association with ventricular septal defect. Circulation 1960;22:110.
5. Lauer RM, Ongley PA, DuShane JW, Kirklin JW. Heart block after repair of ventricular septal defect in children. Circulation 1960;22:526.
6. Leao LE, Buffolo E, Coto AE, Maluf MA, Andrade JC. Transaortic approach has a role in the surgical treatment of ventricular septal defects. Cardiovasc Surg 1996;4:250.
7. Leung MP, Beerman LB, Siewers RD, Bahnson HT, Zuberbuhler JR. Long-term follow-up after aortic valvuloplasty and defect closure in ventricular septal defect with aortic regurgitation. Am J Cardiol 1987;60:890.
8. Leung MP, Mok CK, Lo RN, Lau KC. An echocardiographic study of perimembranous ventricular septal defect with left ventricular to right atrial shunting. Br Heart J 1986;55:45.
9. Lev M. The architecture of the conduction system in congenital heart disease. III. Ventricular septal defect. Arch Pathol 1960; 70:529.
10. Lev M, Bharati S, Meng CC, Liberthson RR, Paul MH, Idriss F. A concept of double-outlet right ventricle. J Thorac Cardiovasc Surg 1972;64:271.
11. Lev M, Liberthson RR, Kirkpatrick JR, Eckner FA, Arcilla RA. Single (primitive) ventricle. Circulation 1969;39:577.
12. Liberthson RR, Paul MH, Muster AJ, Arcilla RA, Eckner FA, Lev M. Straddling and displaced atrioventricular orifices and valves with primitive ventricles. Circulation 1971;43:213.
13. Lillehei CW, Anderson RC, Eliot RS, Wang Y, Ferlic RM. Pre- and postoperative cardiac catheterization in 200 patients undergoing closure of ventricular septal defects. Surgery 1968;63:69.
14. Lin PJ, Chang CH, Chu JJ, Liu HP, Tsai FC, Su WJ, et al. Minimally invasive cardiac surgical techniques in closure of ventricular septal defect: an alternative approach. Ann Thorac Surg 1998;65:165.
15. Lincoln C, Jamieson S, Joseph M, Shinebourne E, Anderson RH. Transatrial repair of ventricular septal defects with reference to their anatomic classification. J Thorac Cardiovasc Surg 1977;74: 183.
16. Lock JE, Block PC, McKay RG, Baim DS, Keane JF. Transcatheter closure of ventricular septal defects. Circulation 1988;78:361.
17. Lucas RV Jr, Adams P Jr, Anderson RC, Meyne NG, Lillehei CW, Varco RL. The natural history of isolated ventricular septal defect: a serial physiologic study. Circulation 1961;24:1372.
18. Ludomirsky A, Huhta JC, Vick GW 3rd, Murphy DJ Jr, Danford DA, Morrow WR. Color Doppler detection of multiple ventricular septal defects. Circulation 1986;74:1317.
19. Lue HC, Shen CT, Wang NK, Wu JR, Chu SH, Hung CR. Ventricular septal defect and coronary cusp prolapse: an assessment of some special features in Chinese (abstract). In Godman MJ, ed. World Congress of Paediatric Cardiology. Edinburgh: Churchill Livingstone, 1981, p. 291.
20. Lun K, Li H, Leung MP, Chau AK, Yung T, Chiu CS, et al. Analysis of indications for surgical closure of subarterial ventricular septal defect without associated aortic cusp prolapse and aortic regurgitation. Am J Cardiol 2001;87:1266-70.
21. Lupi-Herrera E, Sandoval J, Seoane M, Bialostozky D, Attie F. The role of isoproterenol in the preoperative evaluation of high pressure high resistance ventricular septal defect. Chest 1982;81:42.

M

1. Mace L, Dervanian P, Le Bret E, Folliguet TA, Lambert V, Losay J, et al. "Swiss cheese" septal defects: surgical closure using a single patch with intermediate fixings. Ann Thorac Surg 1999;67:1754.

2. Maehara T, Blackstone EH, Kirklin JW, Kirklin JK, Pacifico AD, Colvin EC. The results of the Trusler operation for ventricular septal defect and aortic valvar incompetence. In: Crupi G, Parenzan L, Anderson RH, eds. Perspectives in pediatric cardiology, Vol. 2: Pediatric cardiac surgery, Part 1. Mount Kisco, NY: Futura, 1989, p. 61.
3. Malm JR: Personal communication; 1989.
4. Maron BJ, Redwood DR, Hirschfeld JW Jr, Goldstein RE, Morrow AG, Epstein SE. Postoperative assessment of patients with ventricular septal defect and pulmonary hypertension: response to intense upright exercise. Circulation 1973;48:864.
5. Mason DT, Spann JF Jr, Zelis R, Amsterdam EA. Comparison of the contractile state of the normal, hypertrophied, and failing heart in man. In: Alpert N, ed. Cardiac hypertrophy. New York: Academic, 1971, p. 433.
6. McDaniel N, Gutgesell HP, Nolan SP, Kron IL. Repair of large muscular ventricular septal defects in infants employing left ventriculotomy. Ann Thorac Surg 1989;47:593.
7. McGoon DC, Danielson GK, Wallace RB, Puga FJ. Surgical implications of straddling atrioventricular valves. In: Becker AE, Loosekoot G, Marcelletti C, Anderson RH, eds. Paediatric cardiology, Vol. 3. New York: Churchill Livingstone, 1981, p. 431.
8. Mehrizi A, McMurphy DM, Ottesen OE, Rowe RD. Syndrome of double inlet left ventricle. Angiocardiographic differentiation from single ventricle with rudimentary outlet chamber. Bull Johns Hopkins Hosp 1966;119:255.
9. Menahem S, Venables AW. Pulmonary artery banding in isolated or complicated ventricular septal defects: results and effects on growth. Br Heart J 1972;34:87.
10. Milo S, Ho SY, Macartney FJ, Wilkinson JL, Becker AE, Wenink AC, et al. Straddling and overriding atrioventricular valves: morphology and classification. Am J Cardiol 1979;44:1122.
11. Moene RJ, Gittenbergerde Groot AC, Oppenheimer-Dekker A, Bartelings MM. Anatomic characteristics of ventricular septal defect associated with coarctation of the aorta. Am J Cardiol 1987;59:952.
12. Momma K, Takao A, Ando M, Nakazawa M, Takamizawa K. Natural and post-operative history of pulmonary vascular obstruction associated with ventricular septal defect. Jpn Circ J 1981;45:230.
13. Momma K, Toyama K, Takao A, Ando M, Nakazawa M, Hirosawa K, et al. Natural history of subarterial infundibular ventricular septal defect. Am Heart J 1984;108:1312.
14. Moulaert AJ, Bruins CG, Oppenheimer-Dekker A. Anomalies of the aortic arch and ventricular septal defects. Circulation 1976; 53:1011.
15. Moreno-Cabral RJ, Mamiya RT, Nakamura FF, Brainard SC, McNamara JJ. Ventricular septal defect and aortic insufficiency: surgical treatment. J Thorac Cardiovasc Surg 1977;73:358.
16. Muller WH Jr, Dammann JF Jr. The treatment of certain congenital malformations of the heart by the creation of pulmonic stenosis to reduce pulmonary hypertension and excessive pulmonary blood flow: a preliminary report. Surg Gynecol Obstet 1952;95:213.
17. Murzi B, Bonanomi GL, Giusti S, Luisi VS, Bernabei M, Carminati M, et al. Surgical closure of muscular ventricular septal defects using double umbrella devices (intraoperative VSD device closure). Eur J Cardiothorac Surg 1997;12:450.

N

1. Nadas AS, Thilenius OG, LaFarge CG, Hauck AJ. Ventricular septal defect with aortic regurgitation: medical and pathologic aspects. Circulation 1964;29:862-73.
2. Nanton MA, Belcourt CL, Gillis DA, Krause VW, Roy DL. Left ventricular outflow tract obstruction owing to accessory endocardial cushion tissue. J Thorac Cardiovasc Surg 1979;78:537.
3. Neches WH, Park SC, Lenox CC, Zuberbuhler JR, Siewers RD, Hardesty RL. Coarctation of the aorta with ventricular septal defect. Circulation 1977;55:189.
4. Neufeld HN, Titus JL, DuShane JW, Burchell HB, Edwards JE. Isolated ventricular septal defect of the persistent common atrioventricular canal type. Circulation 1961;23:685.
5. Neutze JM, Ishikawa T, Clarkson PM, Calder AL, Barratt-Boyes BG, Kerr AR. Assessment and follow-up of patients with ventricular septal defect and elevated pulmonary vascular resistance. Am J Cardiol 1989;63:327.

O

1. Ogino H, Miki S, Ueda Y, Tahata T, Morioka K, Sakai T, et al. Surgical management of aortic regurgitation associated with ventricular septal defect. J Heart Valve Dis 1997;6:174.
2. Oh KS, Park SC, Galvis AG, Young LW, Neches WH, Zuberbuhler JR. Pulmonary hyperinflation in ventricular septal defect. J Thorac Cardiovasc Surg 1978;76:706.
3. Ohkita Y, Miki S, Kusuhara K, Ueda Y, Tahata T, Komeda M, et al. Reoperation after aortic valvuloplasty for aortic regurgitation associated with ventricular septal defect. Ann Thorac Surg 1986; 41:489.
4. Okamoto Y. Clinical studies for open heart surgery in infants with profound hypothermia. Nippon Geka Hokan 1969;38:188.
5. Okita Y, Miki S, Kusuhara K, Ueda Y, Tahata T, Yamanaka K, et al. Long-term results of aortic valvuloplasty for aortic regurgitation associated with ventricular septal defect. J Thorac Cardiovasc Surg 1988;96:769.
6. Okoroma EO, Guller B, Maloney JD, Weidman WH. Etiology of right bundle-branch block pattern after surgical closure of ventricular septal defects. Am Heart J 1975;90:14.
7. Oldham HN Jr, Kakos GS, Jarmakani MM, Sabiston DC Jr. Pulmonary artery banding in infants with complex congenital heart defects. Ann Thorac Surg 1972;13:342.
8. Onat T, Ahunbay G, Batmaz G, Celebi A. The natural course of isolated ventricular septal defect during adolescence. Pediatr Cardiol 1998;19:230.
9. Oppenheimer-Dekker A, Gittenbergerde Groot AC, Bartelings MM, Wenink AC, Moene RJ, van der Harten JJ. Abnormal architecture of the ventricles in hearts with an overriding aortic valve and a perimembranous ventricular septal defect. Int J Cardiol 1985; 9:341.
10. Ortiz E, Robinson PJ, Deanfield JE, Franklin R, Macartney FJ, Wyse RK. Localisation of ventricular septal defects by simultaneous display of superimposed colour Doppler and cross sectional echocardiographic images. Br Heart J 1985;54:53.
11. Otterstad JE, Simonsen S, Erikssen J. Hemodynamic findings at rest and during mild supine exercise in adults with isolated, uncomplicated ventricular septal defects. Circulation 1985;71:650.

P

1. Pacifico AD, Soto B, Bargeron LM Jr. Surgical treatment of straddling tricuspid valves. Circulation 1979;60:655.
2. Park JK, Dell RB, Ellis K, Gersony WM. Surgical management of the infant with coarctation of the aorta and ventricular septal defect. J Am Coll Cardiol 1992;20:176.
3. Patel RG, Ihenacho HN, Abrams LD, Astley R, Parsons CG, Roberts KD, et al. Pulmonary artery banding and subsequent repair in ventricular septal defect. Br Heart J 1973;35:651.
4. Pedersen TA, Andersen NH, Knudsen MR, Christensen TD, Sorensen KE, Hjortdal VE. The effects of surgically induced right bundle branch block on left ventricular function after closure of the ventricular septal defect. Cardiol Young 2008;18:430-6.
5. Perry EL, Burchell HB, Edwards JE. Congenital communication between the left ventricle and the right atrium: coexisting ventricular septal defect and double tricuspid orifice. Mayo Clin Proc 1949;24:198.
6. Plauth WH Jr, Braunwald E, Rockoff SD, Mason DT, Morrow AG. Ventricular septal defect and aortic regurgitation: clinical, hemodynamic and surgical considerations. Am J Med 1965;39: 552.

Q

1. Quansheng X, Silin P, Zhongyun Z, Youbao R, Shengde L, Qian C, et al. Minimally invasive perventricular device closure of an isolated perimembranous ventricular septal defect with a newly designed delivery system: preliminary experience. J Thorac Cardiovasc Surg 2009;137:556-9.

R

1. Rabinovitch M, Keane JF, Norwood WI, Castaneda AR, Reid L. Vascular structure in lung tissue obtained at biopsy correlated with pulmonary hemodynamic findings after repair of congenital heart defects. Circulation 1984;69:655.
2. Ramaciotti C, Keren A, Silverman NH. Importance of (perimembranous) ventricular septal aneurysm in the natural history of

isolated perimembranous ventricular septal defect. Am J Cardiol 1986;57:268.

3. Rastelli GC, Ongley PA, Titus JL. Ventricular septal defect of atrioventricular canal type with straddling right atrioventricular valve and mitral valve deformity. Circulation 1968;37:816.
4. Rhodes LA, Keane JF, Keane JP, Fellows KE, Jonas RA, Castaneda AR, et al. Long follow-up (to 43 years) of ventricular septal defect with audible aortic regurgitation. Am J Cardiol 1990;66:340-5.
5. Rice MJ, Seward JB, Edwards WD, Hagler DJ, Danielson GK, Puga FJ, et al. Straddling atrioventricular valve: two-dimensional echocardiographic diagnosis, classification and surgical implications. Am J Cardiol 1985;55:505.
6. Richardson JV, Schieken RM, Lauer RM, Stewart P, Doty DB. Repair of large ventricular septal defects in infants and small children. Ann Surgery 1982;195:318.
7. Rizzoli G, Rubino M, Mazzucco A, Rocco F, Bellini P, Brumana T, et al. Progress in the surgical treatment of ventricular septal defect: an analysis of a twelve years' experience. Thorac Cardiovasc Surg 1983;31:382.
8. Rowe RD. Angiocardiography in the prognosis for young infants in congestive failure with ventricular septal defect: the value of defect/ascending aorta diameter ratio. In: Barratt-Boyes BG, Neutze JM, Harris EA, eds. Heart disease in infancy: diagnosis and surgical treatment. London: Churchill Livingstone, 1973, p. 119.
9. Rowe RD, Vlad P. Diagnostic problems in the newborn: origins of mortality in congenital cardiac malformations. In: Barratt-Boyes BG, Neutze JM, Harris EA, eds. Heart disease in infancy: diagnosis and surgical treatment. London: Churchill Livingstone, 1973, p. 3.

S

1. Saleeb SF, Solowiejczyk DE, Glickstein JS, Korsin R, Gersony WM, Hsu DT. Frequency of development of aortic cuspal prolapse and aortic regurgitation in patients with subaortic ventricular septal defect diagnosed at <1 year of age. Am J Cardiol 2007; 99:1588-92.
2. Sandrasagra FA, Hamilton DI, Wilkinson JL. Surgery of VSD in infancy (abstract). In: Godman MJ, ed. World Congress of Paediatric Cardiology. Edinburgh: Churchill Livingstone, 1981, p. 289.
3. Savard M, Swan JHC, Kirklin JW, Wood EH. Hemodynamic alterations associated with ventricular septal defects. In: Congenital heart disease. Washington, DC: American Association for the Advancement of Science, 1960, p. 141.
4. Schmidt KG, Cassidy SC, Silverman NH, Stanger P. Doubly committed subarterial ventricular septal defects: echocardiographic features and surgical implications. J Am Coll Cardiol 1988;12:1538.
5. Scully BB, Morales DL, Zafar F, McKenzie ED, Fraser CD Jr, Heinle JS. Current expectations for surgical repair of isolated ventricular septal defects. Ann Thorac Surg 2010;89:544-51.
6. Seddio F, Reddy VM, McElhinney DB, Tworetzky W, Silverman NH, Hanley FL. Multiple ventricular septal defects: how and when should they be repaired. J Thorac Cardiovasc Surg 1999;117:134.
7. Serraf A, Lacour-Gayet F, Bruniaux J, Ouaknine R, Losay J, Petit J, et al. Surgical management of isolated multiple ventricular septal defects. Logical approach in 130 cases. J Thorac Cardiovasc Surg 1992;103:437.
8. Seward JB, Tajik AJ, Ritter DG. Echocardiographic features of straddling tricuspid valve. Mayo Clin Proc 1975;50:427.
9. Shah P, Singh WS, Rose V, Keith JD. Incidence of bacterial endocarditis in ventricular septal defects. Circulation 1966;34:127.
10. Sigmann JM, Perry BL, Gehrendt DM, Stern AM, Kirsh MM, Sloan HE. Ventricular septal defect: results after repair in infancy. Am J Cardiol 1977;39:66.
11. Sigmann JM, Stern AM, Sloan HE. Early surgical correction of large ventricular septal defects. Pediatrics 1967;39:4.
12. Sim EK, Grignani RT, Wong ML, Quek SC, Wong JC, Yip WC, et al. Influence of surgery on aortic valve prolapse and aortic regurgitation in doubly committed subarterial ventricular septal defect. Am J Cardiol 1999;84:1445.
13. Singh AK, de Leval MR, Stark J. Left ventriculotomy for closure of muscular ventricular septal defects. Ann Surg 1977;186:577.
14. Smolinsky A, Castaneda AR, Van Praagh R. Infundibular septal resection: surgical anatomy of the superior approach. J Thorac Cardiovasc Surg 1988;95:486.
15. Soto B, Becker AE, Moulaert AJ, Lie JT, Anderson RH. Classification of ventricular septal defects. Br Heart J 1980;43:332.
16. Soto B, Ceballos R, Kirklin JW. Ventricular septal defects: a surgical viewpoint. J Am Coll Cardiol 1989;14:1291.
17. Soto B, Ceballos R, Nath PH, Bini RM, Pacifico AD, Bargeron LM Jr. Overriding atrioventricular valves. An angiographic–anatomical correlate. Int J Cardiol 1985;9:323.
18. Spencer FC, Doyle EF, Danilowicz DA, Bahnson HT, Weldon CS. Long-term evaluation of aortic valvuloplasty for aortic insufficiency and ventricular septal defect. J Thorac Cardiovasc Surg 1973;65:15.
19. Stahlman M, Kaplan S, Helmsworth JA, Clark LC, Scott HW Jr. Syndrome of left ventricular–right atrial shunt resulting from high interventricular septal defect associated with defective leaflet of the tricuspid valve. Circulation 1955;12:813.
20. Stark J, Hucin B, Aberdeen E, Waterston DJ. Cardiac surgery in the first year of life: experience with 1,049 operations. Surgery 1971;69:483.
21. Stark J, Sethia B. Closure of ventricular septal defect in infancy. J Cardiac Surg 1986;1:135.
22. Stark J, Tynan M, Aberdeen E, Waterston DJ, Bonham-Carter RE, Graham GR, et al. Repair of intracardiac defects after previous constriction (banding) of the pulmonary artery. Surgery 1970;67: 536.
23. Starr A, Menasche V, Dotter C. Surgical correction of aortic insufficiency associated with ventricular septal defect. Surg Gynecol Obstet 1960;111:71.
24. Steeg CN, Krongrad E, Davachi F, Bowman FO Jr, Malm JR, Gersony WM. Postoperative left anterior hemiblock and right bundle branch block following repair of tetralogy of Fallot: clinical and etiologic considerations. Circulation 1975;51:1026.
25. Stellin G, Padalino M, Milanesi O, Rubino M, Casarotto D, Van Praagh R, et al. Surgical closure of apical ventricular septal defects through a right ventricular apical infundibulotomy. Ann Thorac Surg 2000;69:597.
26. Stirling GR, Stanley PH, Lillehei CW. Effect of cardiac bypass and ventriculotomy upon right ventricular function. Surgical Forum 1957;8:433.
27. Stumper O, Fraser AG, Elzenga N, Van Daele M, Frohn-Mulder I, Van Herwerden LA, et al. Assessment of ventricular septal defect closure by intraoperative epicardial ultrasound. J Am Coll Cardiol 1990;16:1672.
28. Subramanian S, Wagner HR. Pulmonary artery banding and debanding in patients with ventricular septal defect. In: Barratt-Boyes BG, Neutze JM, Harris EA, eds. Heart disease in infancy: diagnosis and surgical treatment. London: Churchill Livingstone, 1973, p. 141.
29. Sung RJ, Tamer DM, Garcia OL, Castellanos A, Myerburg RJ, Gelband H. Analysis of surgically induced right bundle branch block pattern using intracardiac recording techniques. Circulation 1976;54:442.
30. Sutherland GR, Godman MJ, Keeton BR, Shore DF, Bain HH, Hunter S. Natural history of perimembranous ventricular septal defects: a prospective echocardiographic haemodynamic correlative study. Br Heart J 1984;51:682.

T

1. Tabry IF, McGoon DC, Danielson GK, Wallace RB, Tajik AJ, Seward JB. Surgical management of straddling atrioventricular valve. J Thorac Cardiovasc Surg 1979;77:191.
2. Tandon R, Becker AE, Moller JH, Edwards JE. Double inlet left ventricle. Straddling tricuspid valve. Br Heart J 1974;36:747.
3. Tantengco MV, Bates JR, Ryan T, Caldwell R, Darragh R, Ensing GJ. Dynamic three-dimensional echocardiographic reconstruction of congenital cardiac septation defects. Pediatr Cardiol 1997;18:184.
4. Tatooles CJ, Miller RA. Palliative surgery in infants with congenital heart disease. Prog Cardiovasc Dis 1973;15:331.
5. Tatsuno K, Ando M, Takao A, Hatsune K, Konno S. Diagnostic importance of aortography in conal ventricular septal defect. Am Heart J 1975;89:171.
6. Tatsuno K, Konno S, Ando M, Sakakibara S. Pathogenetic mechanisms of prolapsing aortic valve and aortic regurgitation associated with ventricular septal defect. Circulation 1973;48:1028-37.
7. Tatsuno K, Konno S, Sakakibara S. Ventricular septal defect with aortic insufficiency: angiocardiographic aspects and a new classification. Am Heart J 1973;85:13.
8. Tiraboschi R, Alfieri O, Carpentier A, Parenzan L. One stage correction of coarctation of the aorta associated with intracardiac defects in infancy. J Cardiovasc Surg 1978;19:11.

9. Tiraboschi R, Villani M, Bianchi T, Locatelli G, Vanini V, Crupi G, et al. Surgical management of ventricular septal defect and coarctation of the aorta. Observations on 40 cases, with particular references to infancy. G Ital Cardiol 1978;8:811.
10. Tohyama K, Satomi G, Momma K. Aortic valve prolapse and aortic regurgitation associated with subpulmonic ventricular septal defect. Am J Cardiol 1997;79:1285-9.
11. Tomita H, Arakaki Y, Ono Y, Yamada O, Tsukano S, Yagihara T, et al. Evolution of aortic regurgitation following simple patch closure of doubly committed subarterial ventricular septal defect. Am J Cardiol 2000;86:540.
12. Truex RC. The sinoatrial node and its connections with the atrial tissues. In: Wellens HJ, Lie KI, Janse MJ, eds. The conduction system of the heart. Philadelphia: Lea & Febiger, 1976, p. 209.
13. Trusler GA, Moes CA, Kidd BS. Repair of ventricular septal defect with aortic insufficiency. J Thorac Cardiovasc Surg 1973;66:394.
14. Trusler GA, Mustard WT. A method of banding the pulmonary artery for large isolated ventricular septal defect with and without transposition of the great arteries. Ann Thorac Surg 1972;13:351.
15. Trusler GA, Williams WG, Smallhorn JF, Freedom RM. Late results after repair of aortic insufficiency associated with ventricular septal defect. J Thorac Cardiovasc Surg 1992;103:276-81.
16. Tweddell JS, Pelech AN, Frommelt PC. Ventricular septal defect and aortic valve regurgitation: pathophysiology and indications for surgery. Semin Thorac Cardiovasc Surg Pediatr Card Surg Ann 2006;9:147-152.

U

1. Ueda M, Becker AE. Morphological characteristics of perimembranous ventricular septal defects and their surgical significance. Int J Cardiol 1985;8:149.

V

1. Van Praagh R, McNamara JJ. Anatomic types of ventricular septal defect with aortic insufficiency: diagnostic and surgical considerations. Am Heart J 1968;75:604-19.
2. Van Praagh R, Ongley PA, Swan HJ. Anatomic types of single or common ventricle in man: morphologic and geometric aspects of 60 necropsied cases. Am J Cardiol 1964;13:367.
3. Van Praagh R, Weinberg PM, Calder AL, Buckley LF, Van Praagh S. The transposition complexes: how many are there? In: Davila JC, ed. Second Henry Ford Hospital International Symposium on Cardiac Surgery. East Norwalk, Conn: Appleton & Lange, 1977, p. 207.
4. Vincent RN, Lang P, Chipman CW, Castaneda AR. Assessment of hemodynamic status in the intensive care unit immediately after closure of ventricular septal defect. Am J Cardiol 1985;55:526.

W

1. Wagenvoort CA, Neufeld HN, DuShane JW, Edwards JE. The pulmonary arterial tree in ventricular septal defect: a quantitative study of anatomic features in fetuses, infants, and children. Circulation 1961;23:740.
2. Wagenvoort CA, Wagenvoort N. Primary pulmonary hypertension: a pathological study of the lung vessels in 156 clinically diagnosed cases. Circulation 1970;42:1163.
3. Walters HL 3rd, Ionan CE, Thomas RL, Delius RE. Single-stage versus 2-stage repair of coarctation of the aorta with ventricular septal defect. J Thorac Cardiovasc Surg 2008;135:754-61.
4. Warden HE, Cohen M, Read RC, Lillehei CW. Controlled cross circulation for open intracardiac surgery. J Thorac Surg 1954;28:331.
5. Weintraub RG, Menahem S. Early surgical closure of a large ventricular septal defect: influence on long-term growth. J Am Coll Cardiol 1991;18:552.
6. Weng KP, Huang SH, Lin CC, Huang SM, Chien KJ, Ger LP, et al. Reappraisal of left ventricular to right atrial (LV-RA) shunt in pediatric patients with isolated perimembranous ventricular septal defect. Circ J 2008;72:1487-91.
7 Wolff GS, Rowland TW, Ellison RC. Surgically induced right bundle branch block with left anterior hemiblock: an ominous sign in postoperative tetralogy of Fallot. Circulation 1972;46:587.
8. Wollenek G, Wyse R, Sullivan I, Elliott M, de Leval M, Stark J. Closure of muscular ventricular septal defects through a left ventriculotomy. Eur J Cardiothorac Surg 1996;10:595.

Y

1. Yacoub MH, Khan H, Stavri G, Shinebourne E, Radley-Smith R. Anatomic correction of the syndrome of prolapsing right coronary aortic cusp, dilatation of the sinus of Valsalva, and ventricular septal defect. J Thorac Cardiovasc Surg 1997;113:253.
2. Yacoub MH, Radley-Smith R, de Gasperis C. Primary repair of large ventricular septal defects in the first year of life. G Ital Cardiol 1978;8:827.
3. Yamaki S, Tezuka F. Quantitative analysis of pulmonary vascular disease in complete transposition of the great arteries. Circulation 1976;54:805.
4. Yeager SB, Freed MD, Keane JF, Norwood WI, Castaneda AR. Primary surgical closure of ventricular septal defect in the first year of life: results in 128 infants. J Am Coll Cardiol 1984;3:1269.
5. Yilmaz AT, Ozal E, Arslan M, Tatar H, Ozturk OY. Aneurysm of the membranous septum in adult patients with perimembranous ventricular septal defect. Eur J Cardiothorac Surg 1997;11:307.

Z

1. Zhou Q, Lai Y, Wei H, Song R, Wu Y, Zhang H. Unidirectional valve patch for repair of cardiac septal defects with pulmonary hypertension. Ann Thorac Surg 1995;60:1245.
2. Ziady GM, Hallidie-Smith KA, Goodwin JF. Conduction disturbances after surgical closure of ventricular septal defect. Br Heart J 1972;34:1199.

36 Congenital Sinus of Valsalva Aneurysm and Aortico–Left Ventricular Tunnel

Section I Unruptured and Ruptured Sinus of Valsalva Aneurysms

DEFINITION

Congenital sinus of Valsalva aneurysms are thin-walled saccular or tubular outpouchings usually located in the right sinus or adjacent half of the noncoronary sinus. They generally have an intracardiac course but may protrude into the pericardial space. They may rupture into the right (or rarely the left) heart chambers to form an aortocardiac fistula, or into the pericardial cavity. Associated congenital cardiac anomalies are common.

HISTORICAL NOTE

The syndrome of acute rupture of a congenital sinus of Valsalva aneurysm was apparently first described by Hope in 1839.[H6] A year later, Thurman published the first important paper on the subject.[T4] He discussed Hope's case and added five of his own, none of which had ruptured. Eighty years later, Abbott reviewed the clinical features of acute rupture from eight previous cases and reported another case.[A1] At that time,[S7] and even as late as 1937,[S6] most ruptured and unruptured sinus of Valsalva aneurysms were considered syphilitic. Smith stated in 1914 that "the lesion, which is usually syphilitic, is not so rare as to be altogether devoid of clinical interest, but the diagnosis, perforating or otherwise, presents almost insurmountable difficulties."[S14] Jones and Langley reviewed congenital and acquired aneurysms in 1949.[J1] They accepted 25 cases as being of congenital origin and elucidated most of the important features of the condition. In 1951, Venning may have been the first to diagnose acute rupture during life,[V2] although Oram and East claimed this distinction in 1955,[O3] as did Brown and colleagues.[B11] In Oram and East's patients, cardiac catheterization confirmed the presence of a left-to-right shunt, although angiography was not performed. The earliest report of using aortography to diagnose an unruptured aneurysm was that of Falholt and Thomsen in 1953.[F1]

The first successful surgical repairs of sinus of Valsalva aneurysms were performed in 1956 at the Mayo Clinic and the University of Minnesota, using cardiopulmonary bypass (CPB).[B7,L3,M3] Spencer, Blake, and Bahnson[S16] and Morris and colleagues[M9] also reported early successful cases. In 1957, both Morrow and colleagues and Bigelow and Barnes successfully closed a ruptured congenital sinus of Valsalva aneurysm using mild hypothermia with inflow stasis,[B6,M8] but this technique was not subsequently employed. Numerous reports followed of one or two patients treated successfully using CPB. Dubost and colleagues reported eight cases in 1962,[D4] and Besterman and colleagues reported six cases in 1963.[B4] In a 1960 collective review, Kieffer and Winchell reported 78 surgical and nonsurgical patients, 59 of whom had rupture of the aneurysm into a cardiac chamber.[K5] Sakakibara and Konno noted the prevalence of this lesion in Japan and its association with ventricular septal defect (VSD) and aortic regurgitation (AR), and were among the first to provide a comprehensive classification.[S1,S2,S4] Their first patient underwent aneurysm repair in 1960.[S3]

MORPHOLOGY

The essential lesion of *congenital* sinus of Valsalva aneurysms is separation of the aortic media of the sinus from the media adjacent to the hinge line of the aortic valve cusp, as emphasized by Edwards and Burchell in 1957[E2] (Fig. 36-1). This defect may result from absence of normal aortic elastic tissue and media in this region.[E1,V2] The congenitally weak area gradually enlarges under aortic pressure to form an aneurysm, although the age at which this occurs is uncertain. Viewed from the aorta, the aneurysm appears as an excavation of the sinus of Valsalva that protrudes into the underlying cardiac chamber (Fig. 36-2).

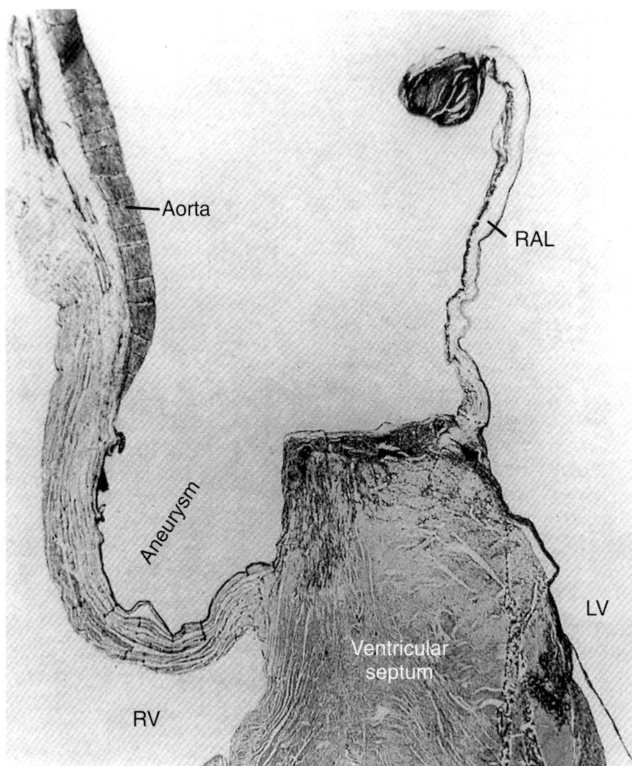

Figure 36-1 Unruptured right sinus of Valsalva aneurysm in a non-Asian patient. Low-power photomicrograph of a longitudinal section through the central portion of right aortic sinus shows separation of aortic media of the sinus from media adjacent to the hinge line of right aortic cusp. Aneurysm is walled by atrophic muscular tissue of right ventricular outflow tract. Key: *LV,* Left ventricle; *RAL,* right aortic leaflet (cusp); *RV,* right ventricle. (From Edwards and Burchell.[E2])

Precise location of this basic congenital abnormality, which may be accompanied by an adjacent separation of the ventricular septum from the aorta to form a VSD, tends to be different in Asians and non-Asians. In Asians, the basic abnormality is located leftward and toward the commissural area between the right and left coronary cusps, so compared with non-Asians, rupture occurs more often into the right ventricle than right atrium (94% vs. 77%, $P[\chi^2] = .0001$).[C5] The coexisting VSD in Asian patients is usually leftward and juxta-arterial, whereas in non-Asians it is usually rightward and only juxta-aortic (see Chapter 35 for definitions). The leftward tendency in Asians is also manifested by fewer aneurysms of the more rightward noncoronary sinus than in non-Asians (11% vs. 32%, $P < .0001$). Left sinus of Valsalva aneurysms are uncommon in both Asians (2%) and non-Asians (5%) ($P[\chi^2]$ for difference = .11).[C5]

Acquired sinus of Valsalva aneurysms caused by medionecrosis,[D1] syphilis,[S14] arteriosclerosis,[D2] endocarditis,[S11] Behçet disease,[K8,W1] or penetrating injuries[M9] are usually readily distinguishable from congenital forms. They are more diffuse, involving more of the sinus or multiple sinuses and often the ascending aorta, and therefore project into the pericardium outside the heart. A congenital aneurysm is frequently diagnosed by exclusion of other etiologies as well as by presence of associated congenital cardiac defects. Difficulties arise in establishing a diagnosis of mycotic aneurysms,[J1,V2] because endocarditis complicates about 5% to 10% of congenital aneurysms.[N1] Similarly, difficulty exists in diagnosing the presence of medionecrosis (cystic medial degeneration), because it and Marfan syndrome are both present in some patients with congenital sinus of Valsalva aneurysms.[A3,M2]

Rupture

In some patients, the aneurysm gradually develops a localized windsock, which ultimately ruptures into an adjacent low-pressure cardiac chamber (Fig. 36-3). The thin-walled, ruptured aneurysm characteristically has an intracardiac fistulous portion and a nipplelike projection into the cardiac chamber, with one or more points of rupture at its apex (Fig. 36-4). Rarely it projects outside the aortic root or heart. When the aneurysm coexists with a VSD, the windsock usually projects into the right ventricle through a thinned area of myocardium just downstream from the VSD; the aneurysm is separated from the VSD by the hinge line of the aortic valve cusp, at the septal portion of the left ventriculoaortic junction (Fig. 36-5; see also Fig. 36-2, *C*).

About one fourth of patients have no windsock or other suggestion of aneurysm formation, but rather have a direct fistulous communication between the aortic sinus and the heart.[N1,R3] This defect has been recognized in a few patients at or soon after birth.[D4,K5,P2,R3] Windsock deformity is typical in lesions originating from the right sinus and communicating with the right ventricle; a direct fistula is typical in those from the noncoronary sinus to the right atrium,[B7,R3] and an extracardiac aneurysm is typical[B3,K2,K5,N1,S16] in the rare cases of left sinus origin.[E3]

Although the prevalence of aneurysms of the sinus of Valsalva in various locations is different among Asians and non-Asians, in both groups the *sinus of origin* is the main determinant of the direction of protrusion and rupture of the aneurysm, and thus of the chamber into which it ruptures (Fig. 36-6). Also in both populations, but with differing

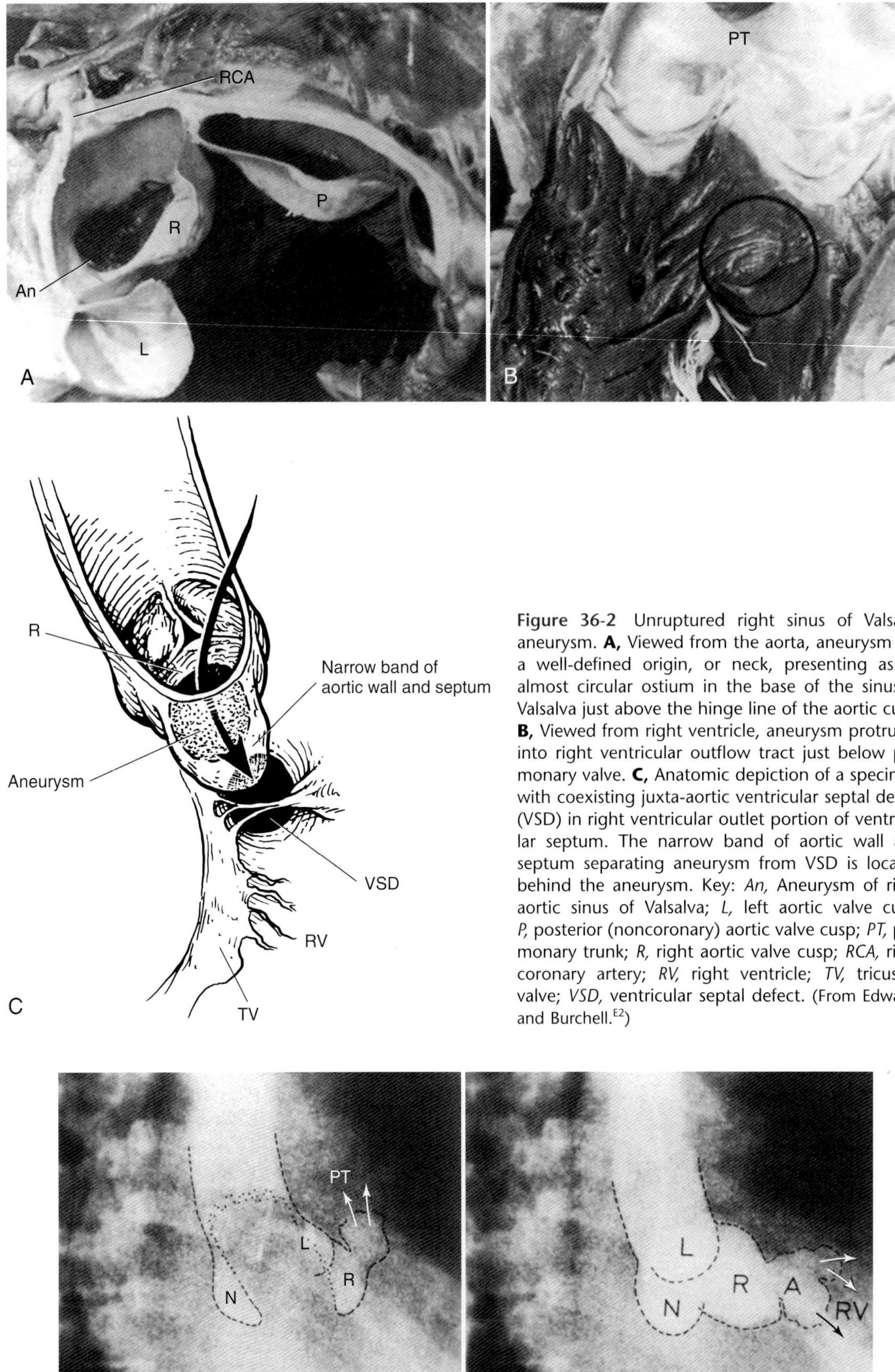

Figure 36-2 Unruptured right sinus of Valsalva aneurysm. **A,** Viewed from the aorta, aneurysm has a well-defined origin, or neck, presenting as an almost circular ostium in the base of the sinus of Valsalva just above the hinge line of the aortic cusp. **B,** Viewed from right ventricle, aneurysm protrudes into right ventricular outflow tract just below pulmonary valve. **C,** Anatomic depiction of a specimen with coexisting juxta-aortic ventricular septal defect (VSD) in right ventricular outlet portion of ventricular septum. The narrow band of aortic wall and septum separating aneurysm from VSD is located behind the aneurysm. Key: *An,* Aneurysm of right aortic sinus of Valsalva; *L,* left aortic valve cusp; *P,* posterior (noncoronary) aortic valve cusp; *PT,* pulmonary trunk; *R,* right aortic valve cusp; *RCA,* right coronary artery; *RV,* right ventricle; *TV,* tricuspid valve; *VSD,* ventricular septal defect. (From Edwards and Burchell.[E2])

Figure 36-3 Cineangiograms in right anterior oblique projection of a right sinus of Valsalva aneurysm ruptured into right ventricle in systole **(A)** and diastole **(B)**. Noncoronary and left coronary sinuses and cusps are normal. Right coronary sinus is enlarged, and there is an aneurysm (windsock) protruding into right ventricular infundibulum. Arrows indicate contrast medium shunting through holes in aneurysm and filling right ventricular infundibulum in diastole and pulmonary trunk in systole (when the aneurysm almost prolapses through the pulmonary valve). There is no aortic regurgitation, but the ruptured aneurysm is associated with a large conoventricular juxta-aortic ventricular septal defect. Key: *A,* Aneurysm; *L,* left coronary sinus; *N,* noncoronary sinus; *PT,* pulmonary trunk; *R,* right coronary sinus; *RV,* right ventricular infundibulum.

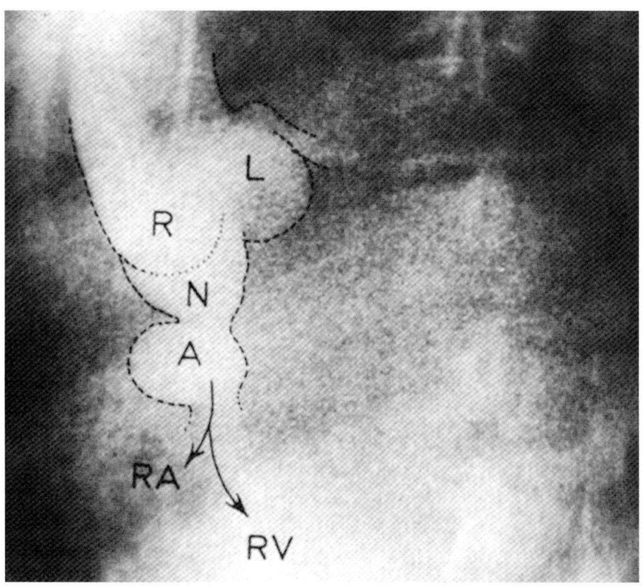

Figure 36-4 Cineangiogram in left anterior oblique projection of an aneurysm and fistula arising from the noncoronary sinus of Valsalva and rupturing into right atrium. Aneurysm fills from nadir of noncoronary sinus. There is shunting of contrast medium to the right atrium, through the tricuspid valve, and to the right ventricle. Right and left coronary sinuses appear normal. There is no aortic regurgitation and no ventricular septal defect. Key: *A,* Aneurysm; *L,* left coronary sinus; *N,* noncoronary sinus; *R,* right coronary sinus; *RA,* right atrium; *RV,* right ventricle.

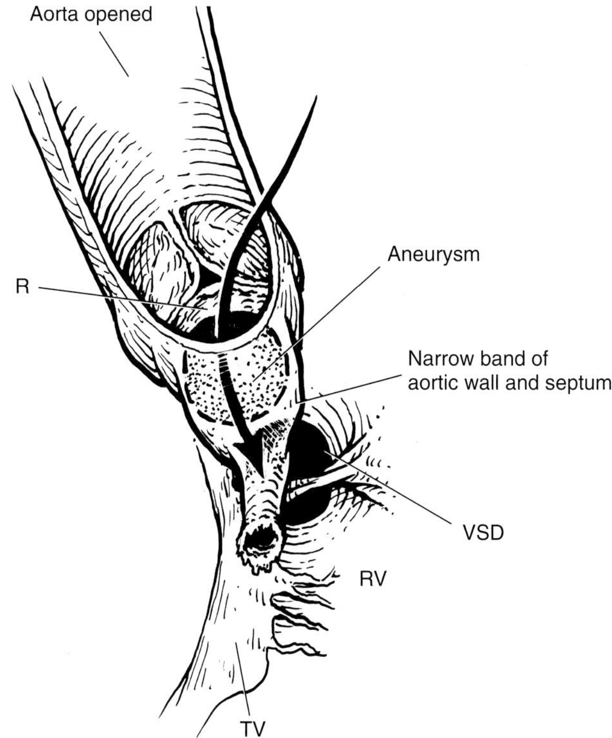

Figure 36-5 Anatomic depiction of a ruptured aneurysm of the rightward portion of right sinus of Valsalva associated with a conoventricular juxta-aortic ventricular septal defect (VSD). Rupture has occurred at apex of the windsock. Narrow band of aortic wall and septum separates aneurysm from VSD. Key: *R,* Right coronary cusp; *RV,* right ventricle; *TV,* tricuspid valve.

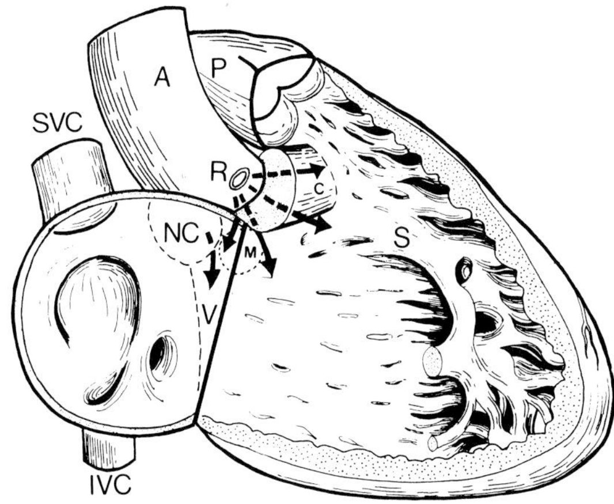

Figure 36-6 Diagrammatic representation of structures depicted in right anterior oblique view of heart. Arrows indicate common sites of rupture of sinus of Valsalva aneurysms. Key: *A,* Aorta; *C,* conal (infundibular) septum; *IVC,* inferior vena cava; *M,* membranous septum; *NC,* noncoronary sinus; *P,* pulmonary trunk; *R,* right coronary sinus; *S,* septal band; *SVC,* superior vena cava; *V,* atrioventricular septum.

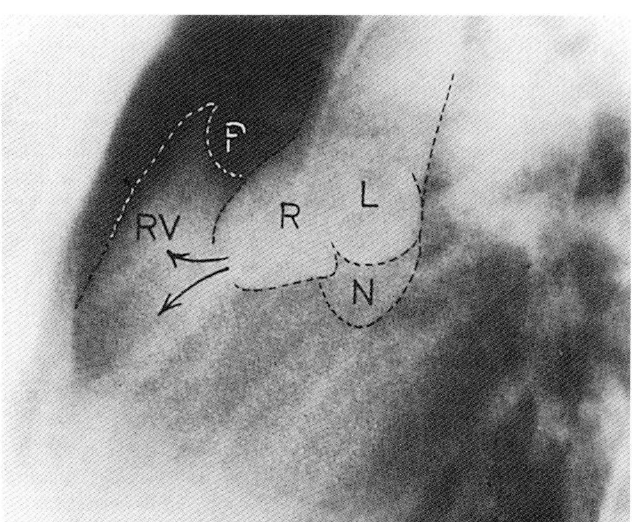

Figure 36-7 Cineangiogram in diastole (lateral projection) of an aneurysm of right coronary sinus that protrudes into right ventricular infundibulum, filled by contrast medium shunting through ruptured aneurysm. Pulmonary valve is still closed. Left coronary and noncoronary sinuses appear normal. There is no aortic regurgitation. At operation, aneurysm arose from center of right sinus, with a prominent windsock in the infundibular septum; immediately beneath it was a moderate-sized ventricular septal defect. Key: *L,* Left coronary sinus; *N,* noncoronary sinus; *P,* pulmonary valve; *R,* right coronary sinus; *RV,* right ventricular infundibulum.

prevalence, aneurysms of the right aortic sinus of Valsalva are most common.[C5,G3,J1,K5,N1,O3,S5] The aneurysm may arise from the leftward portion of this sinus, with the windsock projecting into the adjacent right ventricular outflow tract just below the pulmonary valve, termed *type I* by Sakakibara and Konno.[S1] It may also originate more centrally and project through the substance of the outlet portion of the right ventricular aspect of the ventricular septum (Fig. 36-7), or from the rightward portion of the sinus, entering the right ventricle beneath the parietal band (parietal extension of the

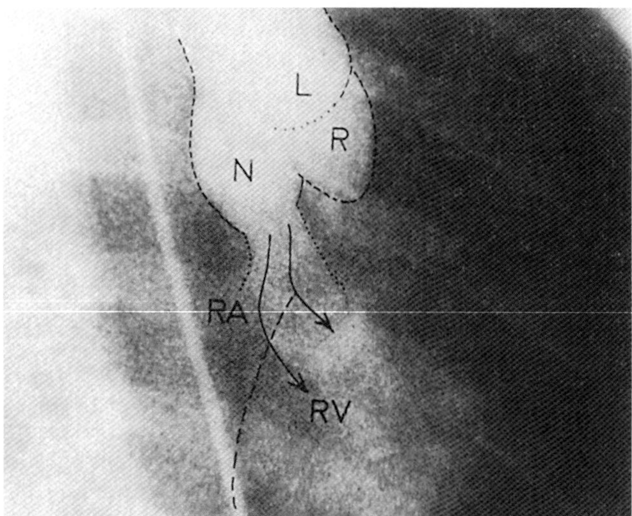

Figure 36-8 Cineangiogram in right anterior oblique projection (diastole) of a large aneurysmal connection of noncoronary sinus (N) to right atrium (RA). Contrast flow *(arrows)* was observed to enter RA close to tricuspid anulus *(dashed line)* before passing through tricuspid valve to right ventricle (RV). Right (R) and left (L) coronary sinuses appear normal. There is no aortic regurgitation and no ventricular septal defect. At operation a 15-mm-long windsock aneurysm was projecting into the right atrium adjacent to anteroseptal commissure of tricuspid valve.

infundibular septum) in the region of the membranous septum. Rarely the aneurysm may project into the pulmonary trunk.[S10]

Aneurysms from the noncoronary sinus usually originate from its anterior portion and project into the right atrium (Fig. 36-8), but in rare cases they project and rupture into the right ventricle. Rarely, rupture can occur simultaneously into the right ventricle and right atrium or into the muscular ventricular septum.[G5] Aneurysms arising from the posterior portion of the noncoronary sinus may rupture into the pericardium.[B9,F2,M10] Another rare occurrence is a right sinus or noncoronary sinus aneurysm that ruptures into the left ventricle.[H4,S12,W4] Rarity of rupture into the left ventricle may be related to the relatively thick wall and high pressure in that chamber. Aneurysms arising from the left coronary sinus may rupture into the left atrium, left ventricle, or rarely the pulmonary trunk or pericardium.[H3,K6]

Sinus of Valsalva aneurysms rupturing into areas adjacent to the tricuspid valve are also adjacent to the atrioventricular (AV) node and His bundle and may be a cause of heart block, bundle branch block, and ventricular fibrillation.[C3,H8,T1,W2]

Table 36-1 shows the overall distribution of the various sites of rupture, based on analysis by Chu and colleagues of 361 cases in the literature, including 57 from their own institution.[C5]

Table 36-1 Prevalence of Sites of Rupture for Sinus of Valsalva Aneurysms

Site of Rupture	Asian (% of 195)	Non-Asian (% of 166)	Total (% of 361)
Right atrium	13	35	23
Right ventricle	84	57	72
Right ventricle + right atrium	<1	1	<1
Left atrium	<1	1	<1
Left ventricle	<1	2	
Right atrium + left atrium + left ventricle	<1	<1	
Ventricular septum	1	1	<1
Pulmonary trunk	<1	<1	<1
Right ventricle + pulmonary trunk	<1	<1	<1
Pericardium	<1	2	<1

Data from Chu and colleagues.[C5]

Associated Cardiac Anomalies

Ventricular Septal Defect

A VSD is the most common coexisting cardiac anomaly and may arise from the same congenital anomaly that produced the aneurysm. VSDs occur in 30% to 50% of patients,[A5,C4,C5,N1,O1,S1,S2,V1] but prevalence is higher when the aneurysm arises from the right sinus.[C4,C5] When the aneurysm arises from the left third of the right aortic sinus, the VSD is *juxta-arterial*, with its upper margin formed by the confluent aortic and pulmonary valves. When the aneurysm arises from the central third of the right sinus, the VSD may be *juxta-aortic* or may lie within the muscle of the outlet portion of the septum. When the aneurysm arises from the right third of the right sinus (or rarely, the anterior portion of the noncoronary sinus),[E2,S2] the VSD is usually *conoventricular* and may be *perimembranous* as well (see Chapter 35 for definitions). Rarely, a conoventricular VSD occurs in association with an aneurysm arising from the central or leftward third of the right sinus. Sakakibara and Konno considered this a coincidental association between two independent malformations rather than a combined developmental anomaly.[S2]

Aortic Valve Abnormalities and Aortic Regurgitation

Aortic valve abnormalities and AR are common in patients with sinus of Valsalva aneurysms.[A5,C4,C5,V1] When a VSD is present, AR usually results from a prolapsed aortic cusp, similar to the finding in the syndrome of VSD and AR (see Section II of Chapter 35). When a VSD is not present, AR usually arises from other aortic valve abnormalities, including a bicuspid valve.

As in VSD and AR, when prolapse of the aortic cusp into a VSD is the cause, severity of AR progressively worsens.[S2] If the fibrous hinge line remains intact at the base of a prolapsed cusp, a sinus of Valsalva aneurysm projects toward the ventricle superior to the hinge line, and the cusp projects through the VSD inferior to it. When the hinge line does not retain its integrity, however, as in long-standing cases, both structures form a single sac.[S1,S2,S4] Taguchi and colleagues noted that prolonged AR produces a fixed fibrous deformity of the prolapsed cusp.[T1]

The frequency of aortic cusp prolapse in sinus of Valsalva aneurysms was undoubtedly underestimated in earlier reports, particularly when no aortograms or echocardiograms were obtained and the aorta was not opened at operation. Aortic cusp prolapse is also less common if only ruptured sinus aneurysm is considered. Thus, in the series of Taguchi and colleagues, which included unruptured cases, AR (although usually mild) was present in 75% of patients,[T1] whereas in the series of Okada and colleagues from Japan, which included only ruptured cases, the prevalence was 17%.[O1]

A complicating problem is the difficulty of determining what constitutes a true (unruptured) sinus aneurysm with combined VSD and AR. Aneurysmal enlargement of the aortic sinus is common in this setting, and the distinction from unruptured sinus aneurysm is difficult to delineate by aortography and even at operation or autopsy. However, 7 (15%) of 48 surgical patients with VSD and AR operated on at GLH from 1960 to 1982 had a distinct but unruptured sinus of Valsalva aneurysm.

Pulmonary Stenosis

Important pulmonary stenosis is uncommon in patients with congenital sinus of Valsalva aneurysms, but small gradients are common.[O1] The stenosis may be valvar but is usually caused by either a projection of the windsock in front of the infundibular septum[B7] or a developmental anomaly of the right ventricular outflow tract similar to that present in tetralogy of Fallot and VSD-AR syndrome.

Other Anomalies

Infrequently, other congenital cardiac anomalies coexist with sinus of Valsalva aneurysms, including aortic coarctation, patent ductus arteriosus, atrial septal defect, subaortic stenosis, and tetralogy of Fallot.[A5,C4,C5,V1]

CLINICAL FEATURES AND DIAGNOSTIC CRITERIA

Unruptured congenital sinus of Valsalva aneurysms are usually silent lesions; their diagnosis depends on echocardiograms or aortograms usually obtained to demonstrate associated symptomatic lesions such as VSD or AR. Diagnosis can be made incidentally during echocardiography or coronary angiography. Rarely, unruptured aneurysms produce tricuspid valve dysfunction or right ventricular outflow obstruction, bringing the patient to medical attention.[G4,K4] These aneurysms may also produce severe myocardial ischemia by compressing the right or left main coronary artery.[B3,B10,G1,G2,T2] Embolization from unruptured sinus of Valsalva aneurysms and complete heart block have also been reported.[R2,S18,W2,W6] Presence of this anomaly should be considered in men, who represent 80% of patients with sinus of Valsalva aneurysms.[J1,S5]

Acute symptoms occur in about 35% of patients with rupture of the aneurysm.[M6,N1,T1] In 45% of patients, surprisingly, rupture is associated only with gradual onset of effort dyspnea, and in 20%, no symptoms develop. Acute symptoms consist of sudden breathlessness and pain. The pain is usually precordial and may also be epigastric, probably because of acute hepatic congestion. Precordial pain may mimic myocardial infarction, although radiation of the pain beyond the substernal area is unusual.[O3] In a few patients, death occurs within days of rupture from right-sided heart failure, but most patients improve during the *latent period*,[O3] which may last for weeks, months, or years. This improvement may occur without specific medical therapy. The latent period is usually followed by recurrence of dyspnea and signs of right-sided heart failure. Characteristic features at this final stage are aortic and tricuspid regurgitation, an unusual combination.[O3,S5]

The infrequency of severe symptoms at rupture may be due to the initially small size of the rupture in many patients. Studies by Sawyers and colleagues in dogs indicate that symptoms are severe when the fistula is greater than 5 mm in diameter.[S5] However, in humans, Taguchi and colleagues found little correlation between size of the fistulous opening at operation and a history of acute symptoms.[T1] Acute symptoms at rupture may occur less often with a VSD[S2,T1] and more often with severe AR.

Acute symptomatic ruptures may be precipitated by heavy exertion, but they also occur after serious automobile accidents and at cardiac catheterization.[B7] Rarely, an episode of infective endocarditis may be the precipitating factor. Marfan syndrome may also predispose the aneurysm to rupture.[S19]

Rupture is heralded not only by pain and dyspnea but also by a characteristic murmur that is loud, harsh, superficial, and accompanied by a coarse thrill.[S8] The murmur is usually continuous with either systolic or diastolic accentuation, but it may be to and fro, similar to that present in the VSD-AR syndrome. In the past, this murmur has been mistaken for that of patent ductus arteriosus, but it is maximal at a lower site, usually the left second, third, or fourth intercostal space. With rupture into the sinus portion of the right ventricle or right atrium, the murmur tends to be maximal at a low level over the sternum or to the right of the lower sternum.[E4,M1,M7,S4] Rarely the murmur is systolic only,[B7] possibly because the communication is small.[H5] Alternatively, the murmur may be confined to diastole in those few cases when rupture occurs into the high-pressure left ventricle[N1,W4] or when right ventricular pressure is at systemic level, as in the neonate.[A3]

When the murmur is continuous, its timing and accentuation are a function of several factors including degree of associated AR, degree of aortic systolic murmur, functional size of the VSD, and size of the fistula.[T1] Morch and Greenwood assessed the various causes of murmurs that were believed to be continuous and associated with signs of rapid aortic runoff in their adult patients and found that ruptured sinus aneurysm (8 cases) was the second most common cause after patent ductus arteriosus (33 cases), followed by VSD and AR (3 cases), aortopulmonary window (3 cases), coronary arteriovenous fistula (1 case), and pulmonary arteriovenous fistula (1 case).[M6]

Other physical signs of ruptured aneurysm include widened aortic pulse pressure, suggesting mild to severe AR. An elevated jugular venous pressure with a prominent *v* wave, suggesting tricuspid regurgitation, may be caused by direct entrance of a fistula into the right atrium, but in most cases this sign is absent until onset of right-sided heart failure, when liver enlargement and pulsation also occur.[B4]

The chest radiograph does not show enlargement of the aortic root. Plethora may be present, although the left-to-right shunt through both the fistula and any associated VSD is usually small. The electrocardiogram shows either left ventricle or biventricular hypertrophy. Right bundle branch block may occur and may be more common in aneurysms with an intracardiac course close to the AV node and bundle of His. Complete heart block can also occur.[M5,W2]

Although the diagnosis is virtually certain on clinical grounds in patients with acute symptoms and sudden appearance of a continuous murmur, two-dimensional Doppler color flow echocardiography is used for verification (Fig. 36-9).[C2,T3,V3,W5] Cardiac catheterization and angiography are generally performed to study the site of origin and termination of the fistula and the presence of associated anomalies, particularly VSD, AR, and pulmonary stenosis (see Figs. 36-2, 36-4, 36-7, and 36-8). The true size of the VSD cannot be

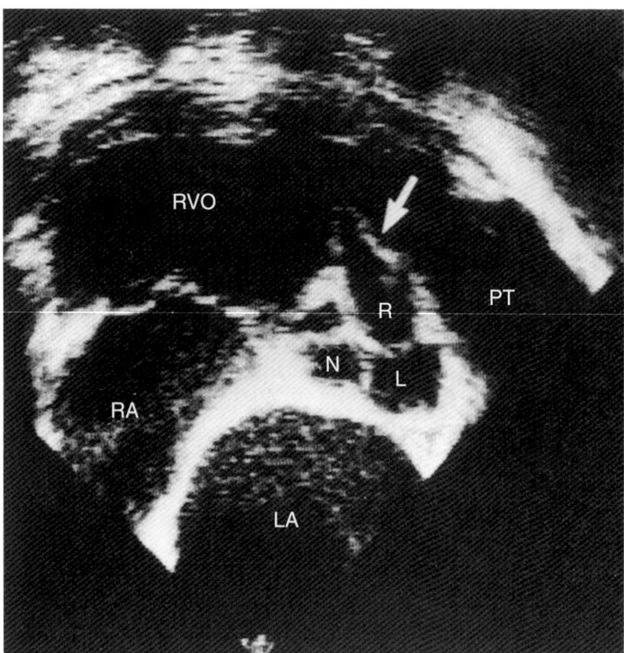

Figure 36-9 Transesophageal echocardiogram (short-axis view) of sinus of Valsalva aneurysm *(arrow)* that has ruptured into right ventricular outflow tract. Key: *L,* Left aortic sinus; *LA,* left atrium; *N,* noncoronary aortic sinus; *PT,* pulmonary trunk; *R,* right coronary sinus; *RA,* right atrium; *RVO,* right ventricular outflow tract. (From van Son and colleagues.[V1])

estimated angiographically when the right aortic cusp is prolapsed into the VSD. Degree of left-to-right shunting through the fistulous communication with the VSD is calculated, as is pulmonary vascular resistance (see "Cardiac Catheterization" under Clinical Features and Diagnostic Criteria in Section I of Chapter 35). Magnetic resonance imaging may establish the diagnosis of aneurysm in certain circumstances.[K1]

NATURAL HISTORY

In an era in which unruptured sinus of Valsalva aneurysms are being diagnosed with greater frequency (42% of those diagnosed by Chiang and colleagues were unruptured[C2]), it is unfortunate that the time-related probability of aneurysmal rupture is unknown. Such information would be useful not only in advising patients for or against operation, but also in managing an unruptured aneurysm at the time of surgical treatment of a coexisting cardiac anomaly. Occasionally, unruptured aneurysms of the sinuses of Valsalva cause important symptoms by protruding into either the right atrium, which causes tricuspid stenosis and regurgitation,[G4] or the right ventricle, which causes right ventricular outflow obstruction.[B12,K3,K4] Complete heart block and ventricular tachycardia may result from the sheer mass of a large and strategically located aneurysm of a sinus of Valsalva.[H8,M5,R1,W2]

When it ruptures, the aneurysm usually does so in the third or fourth decade of life. An exception is when there is already a small fistulous communication present at birth. This is generally well tolerated and is not a cause of early death.[A3,D4,S4] As already noted, in about 20% of patients, the time of rupture cannot be determined by history. Once symptoms develop, heart failure worsens, and without surgical treatment, most patients die within 1 year of rupture.[S5]

Although death after intracardiac rupture of a sinus of Valsalva aneurysm is usually from heart failure, infective endocarditis complicates heart failure in about 10% of patients[N1] and may itself be a cause of death.

When a VSD coexists with the aneurysm, the aortic valve is usually at least mildly regurgitant. The natural history then becomes similar to that of VSD and AR (see Section II of Chapter 35).[S2] The AR becomes progressively more severe, as does prolapse of the right aortic cusp and aneurysmal sac. This process gradually reduces the size of the VSD until even an anatomically large defect becomes functionally small. Pulmonary arterial hypertension and increased pulmonary vascular resistance therefore are rare.[N1] By the time most patients with this combination of anomalies reach age 15 to 20 years, a fixed fibrous deformity of the prolapsed cusp has developed.

TECHNIQUE OF OPERATION

The many types and variations of ruptured and unruptured sinus of Valsalva aneurysms, as well as the rarity of some, make detailed description of repair of each impractical. Instead, this section details repair of three of the most common varieties; from these, the techniques of repair for most other aneurysms can be deduced. For example, an aneurysm of the right sinus of Valsalva, without VSD, that has ruptured into the right ventricle is repaired much the same as described for this type of aneurysm that has ruptured into the right atrium, but substituting "ventricle" for "atrium." Some rare and difficult types may be most simply repaired through an aortic approach, closing the origin of the aneurysm from the sinus with a patch.

Unruptured sinus of Valsalva aneurysms are probably best repaired by excision or, occasionally, by exclusion of the aneurysm and reconstruction by the identical method used for a similar but ruptured aneurysm.

Ruptured Right Sinus of Valsalva Aneurysm, with Ventricular Septal Defect

Repair of a ruptured aneurysm at the midportion of the right sinus of Valsalva with coexisting juxta-aortic VSD is described first because the surgical principles are more easily appreciated in this setting. If the aneurysm is in the rightward portion of the right sinus, the VSD is probably conoventricular (perimembranous) and would be approached through the right atrium, often with detachment of the anterior and septal leaflets of the tricuspid valve. If the aneurysm is in the leftward portion of the right sinus of Valsalva, the associated VSD in the infundibular septum would be juxta-arterial, and the approach would be through the right ventricle or pulmonary trunk. In either case, operation is usually facilitated by a combined aortic and right ventricular, pulmonary trunk, or right atrial approach.[C5,M7,S3,S13,V1]

Initial preparations follow the usual routine (see Section III of Chapter 2). After median sternotomy, the pericardium is opened and complete external evaluation of the heart is made. The protruding nipple of the ruptured aneurysm may be palpated through the free wall of the right ventricle. It is important to note that no external evidence of the aneurysm itself is usually seen, and the aortic root appears to be normal on inspection. Intraoperative transesophageal echocardiography (TEE) is useful for defining the location of the aneurysm and the cardiac chamber into which it has ruptured (see Fig. 36-9), and for assessing completeness of the fistula and VSD repair and severity of AR before and after repair.

CPB is established after ascending aorta and direct caval cannulation, and body temperature is reduced. The aorta is clamped promptly, caval tapes are placed and secured, the right atrium is opened through a short oblique incision, and a sump suction catheter is placed across the foramen ovale. In most cases the aortic valve is at least mildly regurgitant. The aortic root is opened transversely (Fig. 36-10, *A*), and cold cardioplegic solution is infused directly into the left and right coronary ostia or retrogradely through the coronary sinus, which is cannulated directly through the opened right atrium (see Chapter 3).

Exposure is obtained by placing stay sutures on the edges of the aortotomy. The orifice of the aneurysm is visualized, and elevating the right aortic cusp reveals the underlying VSD. No attempt is made to determine the feasibility of

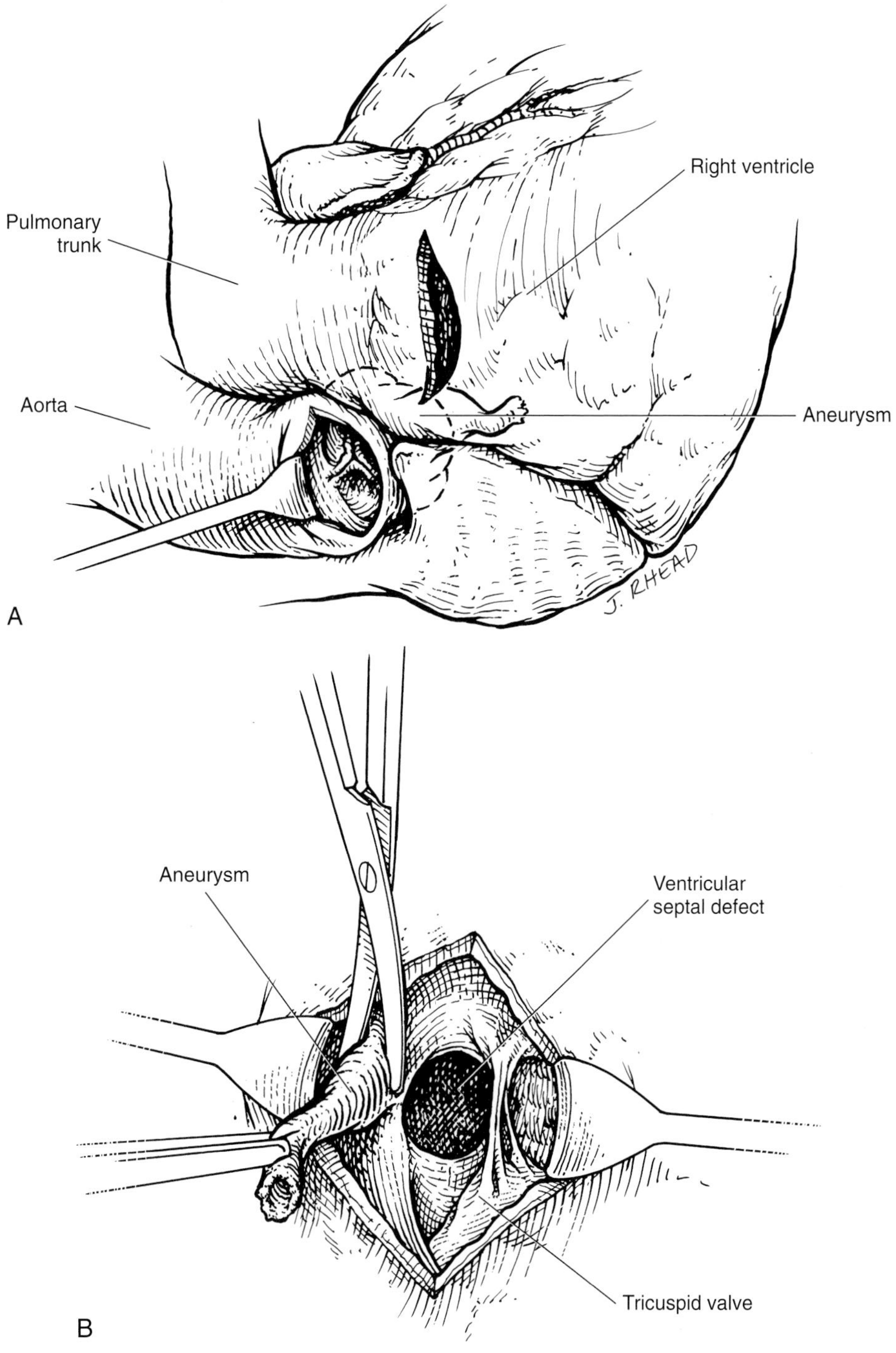

Figure 36-10 Repair of ruptured sinus of Valsalva aneurysm into right ventricle, with ventricular septal defect (VSD). **A,** Initial incision is a transverse aortotomy. The orifice of the aneurysm in the right sinus is visualized. The right ventricle is opened through a transverse incision. Care must be taken to ensure that the aortic incision does not extend into right coronary artery. **B,** Windsock of ruptured aneurysm is seen overlying VSD. The thinned-out portion of the windsock containing the perforation is excised, taking care not to damage the hinge line of the right aortic valve cusp.

Continued

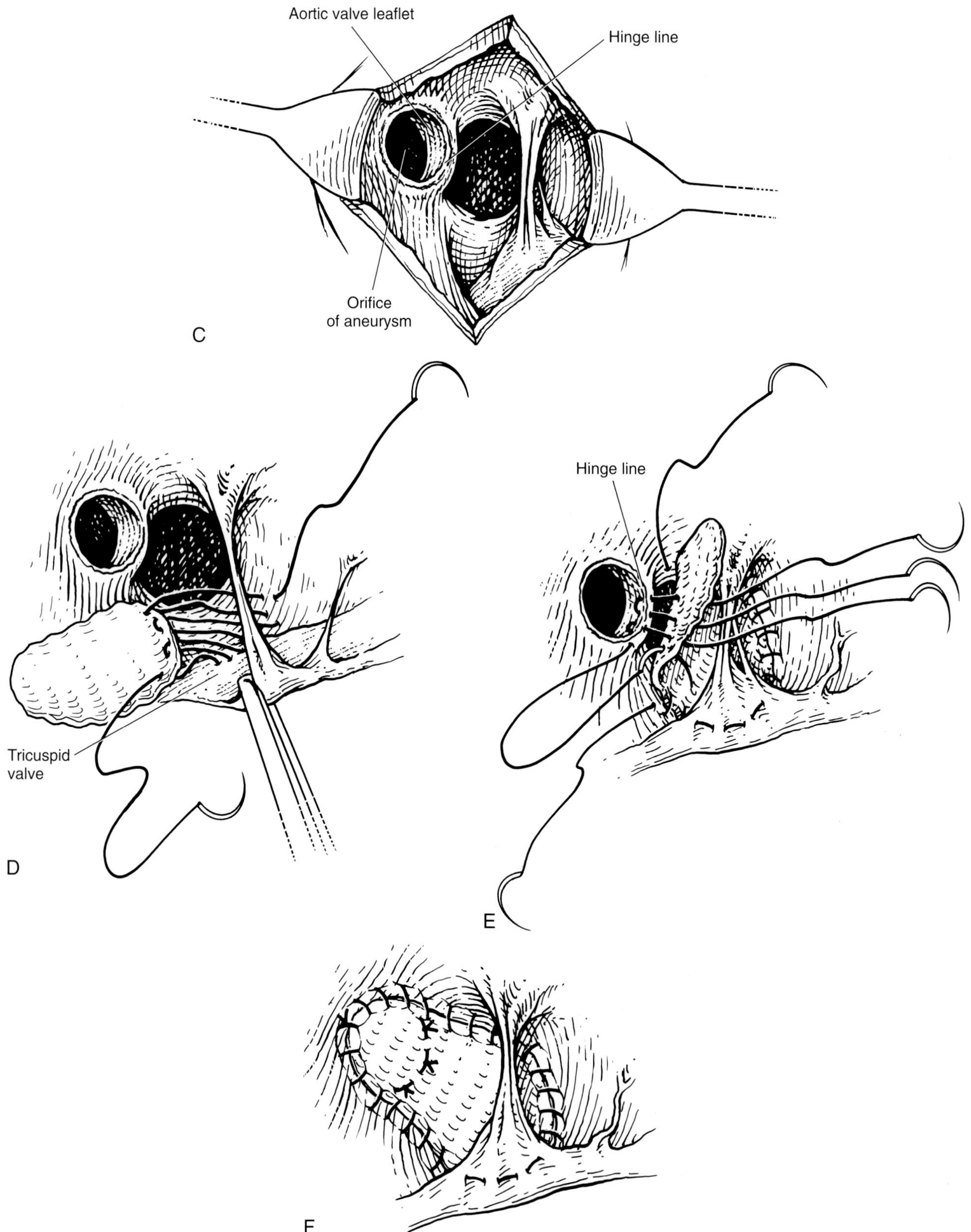

Figure 36-10, cont'd **C,** Hinge line is now visible between orifice of the aneurysm and VSD. **D,** Repair is performed using one patch and inserting it through right ventriculotomy. The patch is first sutured to inferior rim of VSD, incorporating septal leaflet of tricuspid valve and avoiding conduction system, using a continuous polypropylene suture. **E,** Midportion of patch is sutured to hinge line of right aortic cusp using interrupted polypropylene mattress sutures. This step is accomplished before remainder of patch is sewn into place. **F,** Superior aspect of patch is sewn into place over orifice of the aneurysm in the aortic sinus, completing the repair.

repairing the VSD through the aortic root; it may be difficult through the aortotomy to distinguish between a conoventricular VSD adjacent to the His bundle and a juxta-aortic VSD in the right ventricular outflow tract that does not border the His bundle. Any redundancy or tendency of the right coronary cusp to prolapse is noted, but its repair is deferred.

The right ventricle is opened through a transverse or vertical incision, depending on distribution of the branches of the right coronary artery. Alternatively, an approach is made through the pulmonary trunk. The anatomy is visualized (Fig. 36-10, *B*). The thinned-out windsock, often containing one or more perforations, is resected, creating a large defect in the right sinus of Valsalva. This defect is downstream (cephalad) from the VSD and separated from it by the hinge line of the right aortic cusp (Fig. 36-10, *C*). Most of the excised windsock is devoid of aortic media (see Fig. 36-1). A polyester or pericardial patch is sewn into place to close the VSD and the defect in the sinus of Valsalva, and the area of the hinge line of the right aortic cusp, which has been isolated by the resection, is sutured to the patch at an appropriate level (Fig. 36-10, *D-F*).

After closing the ventriculotomy (or pulmonary trunk) with polypropylene suture placed as a continuous stitch, the interior of the aortic root is again exposed through the aortotomy. When AR coexists and the patient is young with pathology limited to prolapse, all or part of a Trusler repair of the aortic valve is then performed (see Chapter 35, Figs. 35-37 and 35-38).[T5] In older patients with AR or when the aortic valve defect is more extensive, valve replacement is necessary (see “Cold Cardioplegia, Controlled Aortic Root Reperfusion, and [When Needed] Warm Cardioplegic Induction” in Chapter 12). Either before or after closing the aortic root, the controlled, initially hyperkalemic reperfusion is begun if indicated (see Chapter 3), the sump suction catheter is removed, and the foramen ovale and then the right atrium are closed. The remainder of the operation is completed in the usual manner (see Section III of Chapter 2). Alternatively, when it is certain that the VSD is *not* conoventricular, the entire repair can be performed through the aortic root. Attachment of the base of the right coronary cusp to the patch is more conveniently accomplished from this exposure than from the right ventricular approach.

Ruptured Sinus of Valsalva Aneurysm into Right Atrium, without Ventricular Septal Defect

When the sinus of Valsalva aneurysm, usually from the noncoronary sinus but occasionally from the right coronary sinus, ruptures into the right atrium, the approach may be through both aorta and right atrium. If AR and VSD can be securely excluded, the approach may be from the right atrium or aorta alone. Intraoperative TEE facilitates this assessment.

In either situation, CPB is established using direct caval cannulation, an aortic root cannula is inserted, and the aorta is clamped (see Section III of Chapter 2). After placing and securing caval tapes, the right atrium is opened obliquely and a sump suction catheter inserted across the foramen ovale. A clamp can be placed across the windsock, or it can be occluded with a finger. Infusion of cardioplegic solution into the aortic root is begun. If the aortic valve is not completely competent, the root infusion is stopped, a transverse aortotomy is made, and cardioplegic solution is infused directly into the coronary ostia (see “Perfusion of Individual Coronary Arteries” in Chapter 3). Alternatively, cardioplegic solution is administered retrogradely through the coronary sinus, which is cannulated directly (see “Technique of Retrograde Infusion” in Chapter 3).

A coexisting VSD is always sought because it may be overlooked during preoperative evaluation if it is plugged by a prolapsing aneurysm or valve cusp. The windsock is then excised, remembering the precise location of the hinge line of the valve cusp. When the windsock is narrow and the bordering edges of the sinus are of good quality, direct closure of the defect is safe. Usually, however, closure is made with a polyester or pericardial patch.

The remainder of the operation is completed in the usual manner (see Section III of Chapter 2).

Unruptured Sinus of Valsalva Aneurysm

Most unruptured sinus of Valsalva aneurysms can be repaired through the ascending aorta. CPB is established using a single cannula in the right atrium (see Section III of Chapter 2). A venting catheter is placed into the left atrium through the right superior pulmonary vein. A catheter is placed into the ascending aorta for delivery of cardioplegic solution; alternatively, a cannula can be placed into the coronary sinus for delivery of cardioplegic solution retrogradely. The ascending aorta is occluded and cardioplegic solution administered. The aorta is opened transversely and the site of origin of the aneurysm identified (Fig. 36-11, *A-B*). The orifice of the aneurysm is closed with a polyester or pericardial patch, avoiding injury to the aortic cusp and ostium of the coronary artery (Fig. 36-11, *C*). If the aneurysm is large with associated AR, valve replacement, aortic root replacement with a composite valve-graft or aortic allograft, or a valve-sparing procedure may be necessary.[G2,T2]

SPECIAL FEATURES OF POSTOPERATIVE CARE

The usual care is given to patients after repair of sinus of Valsalva aneurysm (see Chapter 5).

RESULTS

Survival

Most patients survive the early period after operation. Hospital mortality has not exceeded 5% in the largest reported series.[A5,C4,C5,H1,D3,H2,M11,O1,V1]

Long-term results are excellent, particularly when aortic valve replacement is not required.[M11] Abe and Komatsu reported 86% survival at 25 years in 31 surgical patients.[A2] All patients who died late after operation had undergone aortic valve replacement. In the report by van Son and colleagues of the entire Mayo Clinic experience, survival of 31 patients was 95% at 20 years.[V1] The single late death resulted from endocarditis 9 years after a subsequent aortic valve replacement.

Risk Factors for Premature Late Death

Severe AR accompanied by marked left ventricle enlargement is a risk factor for premature death in the late postoperative period.[M11] Aortic valve replacement appears to be a risk factor

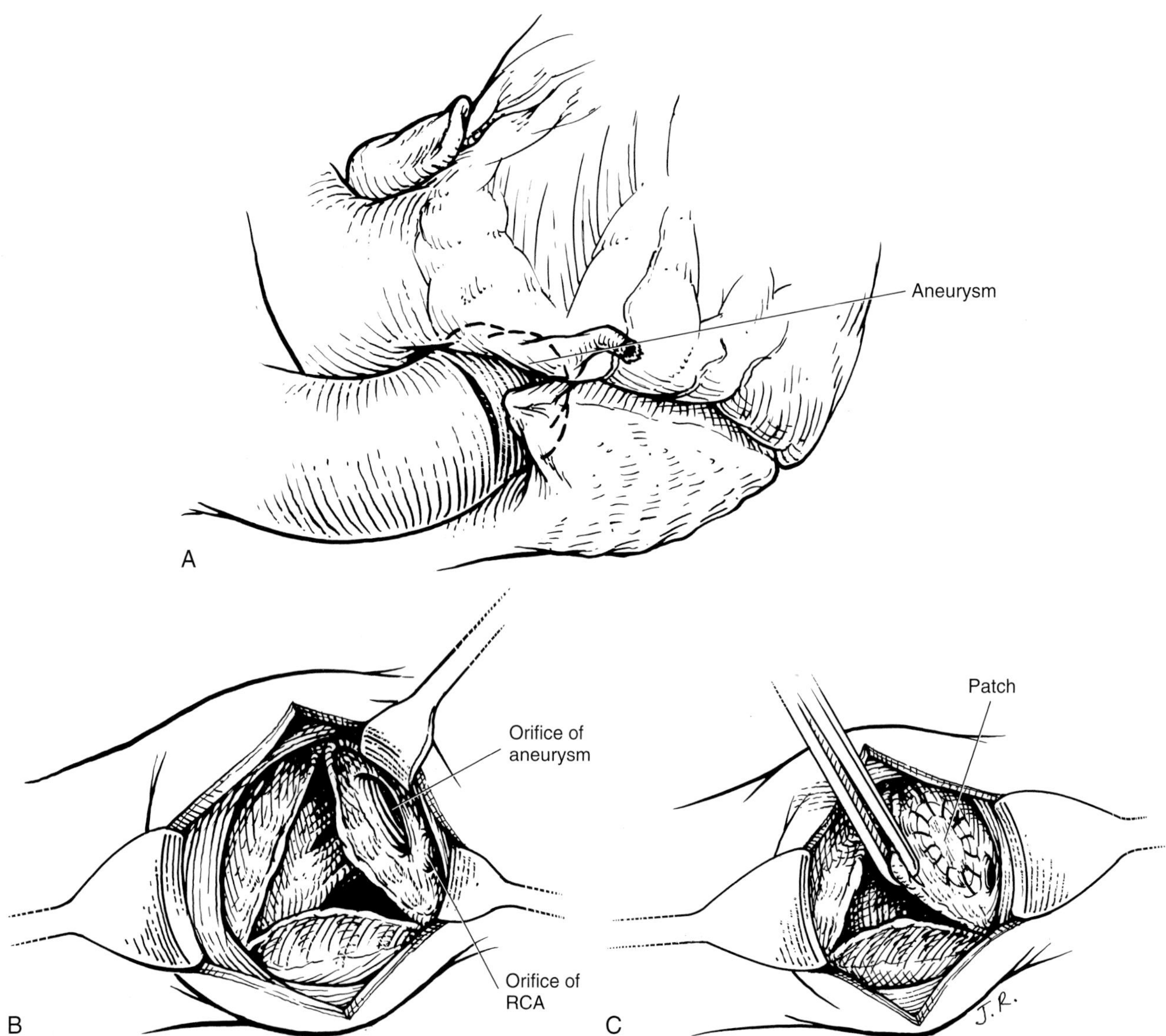

Figure 36-11 Repair of unruptured sinus of Valsalva aneurysm. **A,** Aneurysm is approached through a transverse aortotomy. **B,** Orifice of aneurysm in right coronary sinus is identified, noting its proximity to the right coronary artery (RCA) and hinge point of the aortic cusp. **C,** Orifice is closed with a polyester or pericardial patch using a continuous 5-0 or 6-0 polypropylene suture.

for late death,[A2] as does dehiscence of an aortic valve prosthesis.[A5]

Functional Status

Most surviving patients are asymptomatic.[T1] Abe and Komatsu found that 22 (86%) of 26 surviving patients were in New York Heart Association (NYHA) functional class I, and the other four were in class II.[A2] Similar results were observed in the Mayo Clinic series; 25 of 28 known surviving patients were in NYHA class I (89%), and the other three were in class II.[V1] Persistent or worsening AR accounted for most of the functional disability after operation.

Complications

Direct closure of the ruptured aneurysm, with or without repair of a coexisting VSD, has resulted in a 20% to 30% prevalence of reoperation for recurrence of the fistula.[A2,B1] Other groups have experienced a lower prevalence of reoperations.[B7,H10,V1] When the defect left by excision of the ruptured aneurysm is repaired with a patch, reoperation is rare.

Heart block occurs in 2% to 3% of patients postoperatively,[A5,C4,V1] occasionally late postoperatively.[B1,C4] This complication is not surprising given the proximity of the His bundle and its branches to the area of repair.

INDICATIONS FOR OPERATION

When congenital sinus of Valsalva aneurysm ruptures or is associated with VSD or with VSD and AR, prompt operation is advisable.

Unruptured sinus of Valsalva aneurysms that are (1) producing hemodynamic derangements and (2) enlarging should be repaired. Small and moderate-sized unruptured aneurysms probably should not be repaired surgically, at least with the present state of knowledge about the natural history of these lesions, although this issue is controversial.[M2]

SPECIAL SITUATIONS AND CONTROVERSIES

Transcatheter Closure of Ruptured Sinus of Valsalva Aneurysm

With improved cardiac imaging and advances in percutaneous interventional therapy, percutaneous closure of ruptured sinus of Valsalva aneurysms represents a therapeutic alternative. Percutaneous closure of a congenital ruptured sinus of Valsalva aneurysm was first described by Cullen and colleagues in 1994.[C7] Arora and colleagues employed percutaneous closure devices (Rashkind umbrella device, Amplatzer occluder) in eight patients with ruptured sinus of Valsalva aneurysms.[A4] One patient required surgical repair because of hemolysis, and one died of progressive cardiac failure. The remaining six patients were asymptomatic from 2 to 96 months following repair. Chang and colleagues subsequently reported successful treatment of four patients using the Amplatzer duct occluder in three and a Gianturco coil in one.[C1] One patient had a small residual shunt.

Section II Aortico–Left Ventricular Tunnel

DEFINITION

Aortico–left ventricular (LV) tunnel, or communication, is a short abnormal pathway that begins in an aneurysmal dilatation of the aortic root and upper portion of the right sinus of Valsalva (rarely the left), just to the left of the orifice of the right coronary artery. The defect then passes through the upper end of the ventricular septum to open into the LV cavity.

HISTORICAL NOTE

Aortico–LV tunnel, a rare congenital cardiac anomaly, was first described by Levy and colleagues in 1963.[L1]

MORPHOLOGY

In its most characteristic form, the aortic orifice of the aortico–LV tunnel is anterior and just downstream from the commissural level of the aortic valve and separated from the right sinus of Valsalva by a prominent transverse supravalvar ridge.[B8,C6,G6,L1,P1] The anomaly is visible externally, and the extracardiac bulge can often be seen on the chest radiograph. The tunnel passes directly downward, alongside the aortic valve and through the junction between the aorta and ventricular septum, to communicate with the LV. The tunnel may displace the outlet portion of the ventricular septum into the right ventricle and produce important subpulmonary stenosis.[K7,T7] A VSD may coexist.[B2] Rarely the tunnel may communicate with the infundibulum of the right ventricle rather than the left.

In one patient the orifice of the right coronary artery was shown to arise from the extracardiac portion of the tunnel.[B5] This finding, coupled with demonstration of elastic fibers in the extracardiac portion of some tunnels, suggests that some may actually be examples of coronary artery fistulae. However, most observers believe this anomaly is related to a congenital weakness in the region of the right sinus of Valsalva. In several patients the ostium and proximal portion of the right coronary artery were absent.[S15]

CLINICAL FEATURES AND DIAGNOSTIC CRITERIA

Patients with an aortico–LV tunnel usually have severe AR into the LV. They present with heart failure and marked cardiomegaly as well as symptoms and signs of severe AR.[L2,O2]

Diagnosis can usually be made with two-dimensional echocardiography and Doppler color flow imaging (Fig. 36-12).[B2,F3,H11,S17] Cardiac catheterization and angiography are usually performed to exclude uncommon associated cardiac anomalies.

NATURAL HISTORY

In view of the rarity of the condition, the natural history of patients with aortico–LV tunnel can be outlined only in general terms. Age at presentation and severity of symptoms are related to cross-sectional area of the tunnel and severity of AR. Some patients present as neonates with cardiomegaly and severe heart failure; others who have a smaller tunnel present in childhood without symptoms.[H7,H9] Patients rarely present beyond the second decade of life. When symptoms are present, marked LV enlargement has already occurred, and the natural history thereafter is that of severe AR (see Chapter 12). When symptoms are present in infancy and surgical repair is not accomplished, death usually occurs within a few months.

TECHNIQUE OF OPERATION

Repair is performed using CPB, and a single venous cannula may be used in most cases. In neonates and small infants, hypothermic circulatory arrest may be advantageous. The aorta must be clamped soon after cooling the patient with CPB to prevent LV distention from rapid aortic runoff. Cardioplegic solution must be infused directly into the coronary ostia or retrogradely via the coronary sinus (see "Perfusion of Individual Coronary Arteries" and "Technique of Retrograde Infusion" in Chapter 3).

A transverse aortotomy is made just downstream from the external bulge in the region of the right sinus of Valsalva. The ostium of the right coronary artery is identified and protected. Care is taken to avoid damaging the aortic cusps while visualizing the opening of the tunnel into the LV cavity through the aortic valve. If possible, both ends of the tunnel should be closed. The ventricular end is closed by sutures, usually pledgeted, or with a polyester or pericardial patch.[H7,K7,W3] The aortic end of the tunnel is closed by suturing a pericardial patch into place; direct suture closure distorts the sinus and may aggravate the tendency to develop AR postoperatively.[W3] If necessary, the ostium of the right coronary artery is excised before placing the patch and is reimplanted.[H7]

The aortotomy is closed, and the remainder of the operation is completed in the usual manner. Particular care is taken to avoid LV distention from residual AR, because the heart is recovering from the period of global myocardial ischemia.

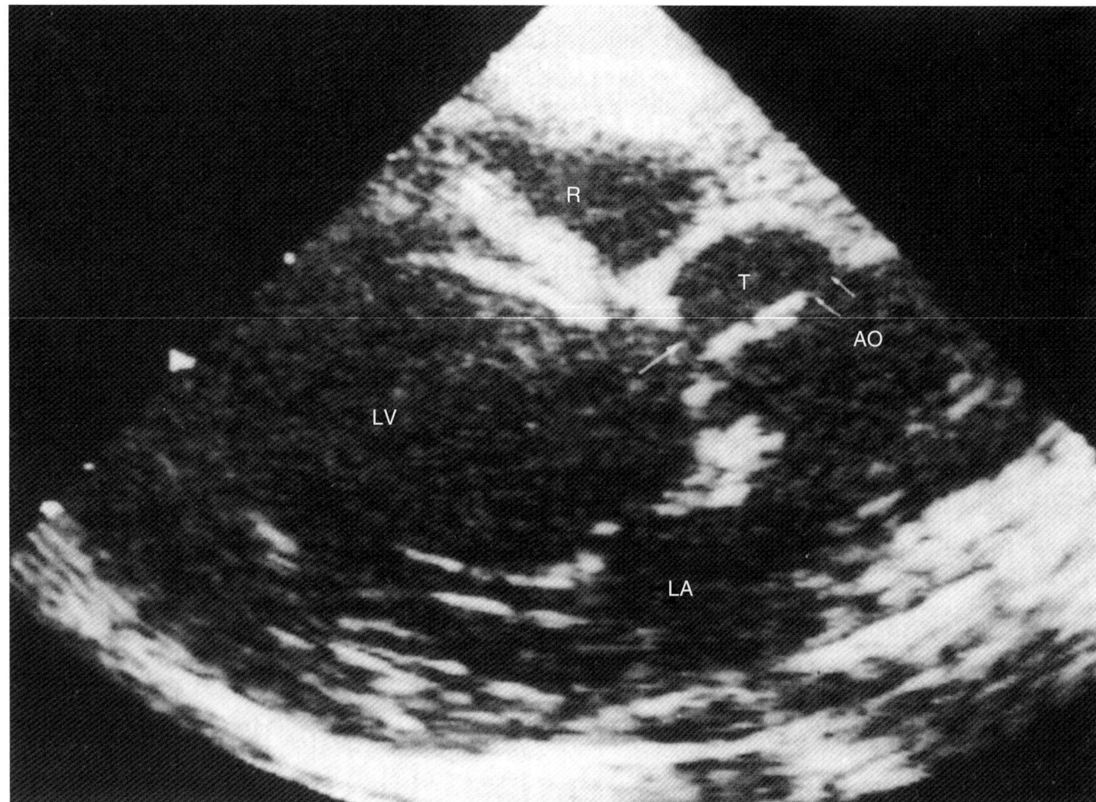

Figure 36-12 Two-dimensional echocardiogram in the parasternal long-axis view, demonstrating entire aortico–left ventricular tunnel and dilated aortic root. Aortic and ventricular ends of tunnel are defined by arrows. Key: *AO,* Aorta; *LA,* left atrium; *LV,* left ventricle; *R,* right ventricle; *T,* tunnel. (From Sreeram and colleagues.[S17])

SPECIAL FEATURES OF POSTOPERATIVE CARE

The usual care is given to patients after the repair (see Chapter 5).

RESULTS

Risk of hospital death has been 5% to 20%.[F3,H7,H9,T7] Most patients have at least mild AR after the operation,[M4,S9] and in about half of these the regurgitation becomes severe enough to require later aortic valve replacement.[M4,R4,S9,S15] The reason for postoperative AR is poorly understood,[T6] although in some patients it appears to be due to anuloaortic ectasia. Patients who do not require aortic valve replacement have excellent functional status.[H7,S17]

INDICATIONS FOR OPERATION

Diagnosis of aortico–LV tunnel is an indication for operation. Surgery should be performed as early in life as possible to minimize damage to the LV from chronic volume overload imposed by AR.

REFERENCES

A

1. Abbott ME. Clinical and developmental study of a case of ruptured aneurysm of the right anterior aortic sinus of Valsalva: contributions to medical and biological research, Vol. 2. New York: Hoeber, 1919, p. 899.
2. Abe T, Komatsu S. Surgical repair and long-term results in ruptured sinus of Valsalva aneurysm. Ann Thorac Surg 1988;46:520.
3. Ainger LE, Pate JW. Rupture of a sinus of Valsalva aneurysm in an infant: surgical correction. Am J Cardiol 1963;11:547.
4. Arora R, Trehan V, Rangasetty UM, Mukhopadhyay S, Thakur AK, Kalra GS. Transcatheter closure of ruptured sinus of Valsalva aneurysm. J Interv Cardiol 2004;17:53-8.
5. Au WK, Chiu SW, Mok CK, Lee WT, Cheung D, He GW. Repair of ruptured sinus of Valsalva aneurysm: determinants of long-term survival. Ann Thorac Surg 1998;66:1604.

B

1. Barragry TP, Ring WS, Moller JH, Lillehei CW. Fifteen- to 30-year follow-up of patients undergoing repair of ruptured congenital aneurysms of the sinus of Valsalva. Ann Thorac Surg 1988;46:515.
2. Bash SE, Huhta JC, Nihill MR, Vargo TA, Hallman GL. Aortico–left ventricular tunnel with ventricular septal defect: two-dimensional/Doppler echocardiographic diagnosis. J Am Coll Cardiol 1985;5:757.
3. Bashour TT, Chen F, Yap A, Mason DT, Baladi N. Fatal myocardial ischemia caused by compression of the left coronary system by a large left sinus of Valsalva aneurysm. Am Heart J 1996;132:1050.
4. Besterman EM, Goldberg MJ, Sellors TH. Surgical repair of ruptured sinus of Valsalva. Br Med J 1963;2:410.
5. Bharati S, Lev M, Cassels DE. Aortico–right ventricular tunnel. Chest 1973;63:198.
6. Bigelow WG, Barnes WT. Ruptured aneurysm of aortic sinus. Ann Surg 1959;150:117.
7. Bontils-Roberts EA, DuShane JW, McGoon DC, Danielson GK. Aortic sinus fistula: surgical considerations and results of operation. Ann Thorac Surg 1971;12:492.
8. Bove KE, Schwartz DC. Aortico–left ventricular tunnel: a new concept. Am J Cardiol 1967;19:696.
9. Brabham KR, Roberts WC. Fatal intrapericardial rupture of sinus of Valsalva aneurysm. Am Heart J 1990;120:1455.

10. Brandt J, Jogi P, Luhrs C. Sinus of Valsalva aneurysm obstructing coronary arterial flow: case report and collective review of the literature. Eur Heart J 1985;12:1069.
11. Brown JW, Heath D, Whitaker W. Cardioaortic fistula: a case diagnosed in life and treated surgically. Circulation 1955;12:819.
12. Bulkley B, Hutchins GM, Ross RS. Aortic sinus of Valsalva aneurysms simulating primary right-sided valvular heart disease. Circulation 1975;52:696.

C

1. Chang CW, Chiu SN, Wu ET, Tsai SK, Wu MH, Wang JK. Transcatheter closure of a ruptured sinus of Valsalva aneurysm. Circ J 2006;70:1043-7.
2. Chiang CW, Lin FC, Fang BR, Kuo CT, Lee YS, Chang CH. Doppler and two dimensional echocardiographic features of sinus of Valsalva aneurysm. Am Heart J 1988;116:1283.
3. Choudhary SK, Bhan A, Reddy SC, Sharma R, Murari V, Airan B, et al. Aneurysm of sinus of Valsalva dissecting into interventricular septum. Ann Thorac Surg 1998;65:735.
4. Choudhary SK, Bhan A, Sharma R, Airan B, Kumar AS, Venugopal P. Sinus of Valsalva aneurysms: 20 years' experience. J Card Surg 1997;12:300.
5. Chu SH, Hung CR, How SS, Chang H, Wang SS, Tsai CH, et al. Ruptured aneurysms of the sinus of Valsalva in Oriental patients. J Thorac Cardiovasc Surg 1990;99:288.
6. Cooley RN, Harris LC, Rodin AE. Abnormal communication between the aorta and left ventricle: aortico–left ventricular tunnel. Circulation 1965;31:564.
7. Cullen S, Somerville J, Redington A. Transcatheter closure of a ruptured aneurysm of the sinus of Valsalva. Br Heart J 1994;71: 479-80.

D

1. DeBakey ME, Diethrich EB, Liddocoat JE, Kinard SA, Garrett HE. Abnormalities of the sinuses of Valsalva. Experience with 35 patients. J Thorac Cardiovasc Surg 1967;54:312.
2. DeBakey ME, Lawrie GM. Aneurysm of sinus of Valsalva with coronary atherosclerosis: successful surgical correction. Ann Surg 1979;189:303.
3. Dong C, Wu QY, Tang Y. Ruptured sinus of valsalva aneurysm: a Beijing experience. Ann Thorac Surg 2002;74:1621-4.
4. Dubost C, Blondeau P, Piwnica A. Right aortaatrial fistulas resulting from a rupture of the sinus of Valsalva: a report on 6 cases. J Thorac Cardiovasc Surg 1962;43:421.

E

1. Edwards JE, Burchell HB. Specimen exhibiting the essential lesion in aneurysm of the aortic sinus. Mayo Clin Proc 1956;31:407.
2. Edwards JE, Burchell HB. The pathological anatomy of deficiencies between the aortic root and the heart, including aortic sinus aneurysms. Thorax 1957;12:125.
3. Eliott RS, Wolbrink A, Edwards JE. Congenital aneurysm of the left aortic sinus: a rare lesion and a rare cause of coronary insufficiency. Circulation 1963;28:951.
4. Evans JW, Harris TR, Brody DA. Ruptured aortic sinus aneurysm: case report, with review of clinical features. Am Heart J 1961;61:408.

F

1. Falholt W, Thomsen G. Congenital aneurysm of the right sinus of Valsalva, diagnosed by aortography. Circulation 1953;8:549.
2. Fealey ME, Edwards WD, McMaster KR 3rd, Carter JB. Congenital aortic sinus aneurysm causing sudden unexpected death in a 56-year-old woman. Am J Forensic Med Pathol 2009;30:195-7.
3. Fripp RR, Werner JC, Whitman V, Nordenberg A, Waldhausen JA. Pulsed Doppler and two-dimensional echocardiographic findings in aortico–left ventricular tunnel. J Am Coll Cardiol 1984;4:1012.

G

1. Gallet B, Combe E, Saudemont JP, Tetard C, Barret F, Gandjbakhch I, et al. Aneurysm of the left aortic sinus causing coronary compression and unstable angina: successful repair by isolated closure of the aneurysm. Am Heart J 1988;115:1308.
2. Garcia-Rinaldi R, Von Koch L, Howell JF. Aneurysm of the sinus of Valsalva producing obstruction of the left main coronary artery. J Thorac Cardiovasc Surg 1976;72:123.
3. Gerbode F, Osborne JJ, Johnston JB, Kerth WJ. Ruptured aneurysm of the aortic sinuses of Valsalva. Am J Surg 1961;102:268.
4. Gibbs KL, Reardon MJ, Strickman NE, de Castro CM, Gerard JA, Rycyna JL, et al. Hemodynamic compromise (tricuspid stenosis and insufficiency) caused by an unruptured aneurysm of the sinus of Valsalva. J Am Coll Cardiol 1986;7:1177.
5. Gibbs NM, Harris EL. Aortic sinus aneurysms. Br Heart J 1961; 23:131.
6. Goor DA, Lillehei CW. Congenital malformations of the heart. Orlando, Fla: Grune & Stratton, 1975, p. 301.

H

1. Hamid IA, Jothi M, Rajan S, Monro JL, Cherian KM. Transaortic repair of ruptured aneurysm of sinus of Valsalva: fifteen-year experience. J Thorac Cardiovasc Surg 1994;107:1464.
2. Harkness JR, Fitton TP, Barreiro CJ, Alejo D, Gott VL, Baumgartner WA, et al. A 32-year experience with surgical repair of sinus of Valsalva aneurysms. J Card Surg 2005;20:198-204.
3. Heilman KJ, Groves BM, Campbell D, Blount SG. Rupture of left sinus of Valsalva aneurysm into the pulmonary artery. J Am Coll Cardiol 1985;5:1105.
4. Heydorn WH, Nelson WP, Fitter JD, Floyd GD, Strevey TE. Congenital aneurysm of the sinus of Valsalva protruding into the left ventricle. J Thorac Cardiovasc Surg 1976;71:839.
5. Hong PW, Lee SS, Kim SW, Cha HD. Unusual manifestations of aneurysm of the aortic sinus: a report of 2 cases. J Thorac Cardiovasc Surg 1966;51:507.
6. Hope J. A treatise of disease of the heart and great vessels, 3rd Ed. London: Churchill, 1839.
7. Horvath P, Balaji S, Skovranek S, Hucin B, de Leval MR, Stark J. Surgical treatment of aortico–left ventricular tunnel. Eur J Cardiothorac Surg 1991;5:113.
8. Hoshino J, Naganuma F, Nagai R. Ventricular fibrillation triggered by a ruptured sinus of Valsalva aneurysm. Heart 1998;80:203.
9. Hovaguimian H, Cobanoglu A, Starr A. Aortico–left ventricular tunnel: a clinical review and new surgical classification. Ann Thorac Surg 1988;45:106.
10. Howard RJ, Moller J, Castaneda AR, Varco RL, Nicoloff DM. Surgical correction of sinus of Valsalva aneurysm. J Thorac Cardiovasc Surg 1973;66:420.
11. Humes RA, Hagler DJ, Julsrud PR, Levy JM, Feldt RH, Schaff HV. Aortico–left ventricular tunnel: diagnosis based on two-dimensional echocardiography, color flow Doppler imaging, and magnetic resonance imaging. Mayo Clin Proc 1986;61:901.

J

1. Jones AM, Langley FA. Aortic sinus aneurysms. Br Heart J 1949; 11:325.

K

1. Karaaslan T, Gudinchet F, Payot M, Sekarski N. Congenital aneurysm of sinus of Valsalva ruptured into right ventricle diagnosed by magnetic resonance imaging. Pediatr Cardiol 1999;20:212.
2. Kay JH, Anderson RM, Lewis RR, Reinberg M. Successful repair of sinus of Valsalva–left atrial fistula. Circulation 1959;20: 427.
3. Kerber RE, Ridges JD, Driss JP, Silverman JF, Anderson ET, Harrison DC. Unruptured aneurysm of the sinus of Valsalva producing right ventricular outflow obstruction. Am J Med 1972; 53:775.
4. Kiefaber RW, Tabakin BS, Coffin LH, Gibson RW. Unruptured sinus of Valsalva aneurysm with right ventricular outflow obstruction diagnosed by two-dimensional and Doppler echocardiography. J Am Coll Cardiol 1986;7:438.
5. Kieffer SA, Winchell P. Congenital aneurysms of the aortic sinuses with cardioaortic fistula. Dis Chest 1960;38:79.
6. Killen DA, Wathanacharoen S, Pogson GW Jr. Repair of intrapericardial rupture of left sinus of Valsalva aneurysm. Ann Thorac Surg 1987;44:310.
7. Knott-Craig CJ, van der Merwe PL, Kalis NN, Hunter J. Repair of aortico–left ventricular tunnel associated with subpulmonary obstruction. Ann Thorac Surg 1992;54:557.
8. Koh KK, Lee KH, Kim SS, Lee SC, Jin SH, Cho SW. Ruptured aneurysm of the sinus of Valsalva in a patient with Behcet's disease. Int J Cardiol 1994;47:177.

L

1. Levy MJ, Lillehei CW, Anderson RC, Arnplatz K, Edwards JE. Aortico–left ventricular tunnel. Circulation 1963;27:841.
2. Levy MJ, Schachner A, Blieden LC. Aortico–left ventricular tunnel: collective review. J Thorac Cardiovasc Surg 1982;84:102.
3. Lillehei CW, Stanley P, Varco RL. Surgical treatment of ruptured aneurysms of the sinus of Valsalva. Ann Surg 1957;146:460.

M

1. Magidson O, Kay JH. Ruptured aortic sinus aneurysms: clinical and surgical aspects of seven cases. Am Heart J 1963;65:597.
2. Mayer J, Wukasch DC, Hallman GL, Cooley DA. Aneurysm and fistula of the sinus of Valsalva. Ann Thorac Surg 1975;19:170.
3. McGoon DC, Edwards JE, Kirklin JW. Surgical treatment of ruptured aneurysm of aortic sinus. Ann Surg 1958;147:387.
4. Meldrum-Hanna W, Schroff R, Ross DN. Aortico–left ventricular tunnel: late follow-up. Ann Thorac Surg 1986;42:3904.
5. Metras D, Coulibalty AO, Outtra K. Calcified unruptured aneurysm of sinus of Valsalva with complete heart block and aortic regurgitation. Br Heart J 1982;48:507.
6. Morch JE, Greenwood WF. Rupture of the sinus of Valsalva: a study of eight cases with discussion on the differential diagnosis of continuous murmurs. Am J Cardiol 1966;18:827.
7. Morgan JR, Rogers AK, Fosburg RG. Ruptured aneurysms of the sinus of Valsalva. Chest 1972;61:640.
8. Morrow AG, Baker RR, Hanson HE, Mattingly TW. Successful surgical repair of a ruptured aneurysm of the sinus of Valsalva. Circulation 1957;16:533.
9. Morris GC Jr, Foster RP, Dunn RJ, Cooley DA. Traumatic aortico–ventricular fistula: report of two cases successfully repaired. Am Surg 1958;24:883.
10. Munk MD, Gatzoulis MA, King DE, Webb GD. Cardiac tamponade and death from intrapericardial rupture (corrected) of sinus of Valsalva aneurysm. Eur J Cardiothorac Surg 1999;15:100.
11. Murashita T, Kubota T, Kamikubo Y, Shiiya N, Yasuda K. Long-term results of aortic valve regurgitation after repair of ruptured sinus of Valsalva aneurysm. Ann Thorac Surg 2002;73:1466-71.

N

1. Nowicki ER, Aberdeen E, Friedman S, Rashkind WJ. Congenital left aortic sinus–left ventricle fistula and review of aortocardiac fistulas. Ann Thorac Surg 1977;23:378.

O

1. Okada M, Muranaka S, Mukubo M, Asada S. Surgical correction of the ruptured aneurysm of the sinus of Valsalva. J Cardiovasc Surg (Torino) 1977;18:171.
2. Okoroma EO, Perry LW, Scott LP 3rd, McClenathan JE. Aortico–left ventricular tunnel: clinical profile, diagnostic features, and surgical consideration. J Thorac Cardiovasc Surg 1976;71:238.
3. Oram S, East T. Rupture of aneurysm of aortic sinus (of Valsalva) into the right side of the heart. Br Heart J 1955;17:541.

P

1. Perez-Martinez V, Quero M, Castro C, Moreno F, Brito JM, Merino G. Aortico–left ventricular tunnel: a clinical and pathologic review of this uncommon entity. Am Heart J 1973;85:237.
2. Perloff JK. Sinus of Valsalva–right heart communications due to congenital aortic sinus defects. Am Heart J 1960;59:318.

R

1. Raizes GS, Smith HC, Vlietstra RE, Puga FG. Ventricular tachycardia secondary to aneurysm of sinus of Valsalva. J Thorac Cardiovasc Surg 1979;78:110.
2. Rajashekar D, Subramanyam G, Panchamukheswar R, Praveen M, Guruprasad S. Unruptured sinus of Valsalva aneurysms manifesting as complete heart block. Asian Cardiovasc Thorac Ann 2005;13:283-6.
3. Rosenberg H, Williams WG, Trusler GA, Smallhorn J, Rowe RD, Moes CA, et al. Congenital aortico–right atrial communications: the dilemma of differentiation from coronary cameral fistula. J Thorac Cardiovasc Surg 1986;91:841.
4. Ruschewski W, de Vivie ER, Kirchhoff PG. Aortico–left ventricular tunnel. J Thorac Cardiovasc Surg 1981;29:282.

S

1. Sakakibara S, Konno S. Congenital aneurysm of the sinus of Valsalva: anatomy and classification. Am Heart J 1962;63:405.
2. Sakakibara S, Konno S. Congenital aneurysm of the sinus of Valsalva associated with ventricular septal defect: anatomical aspects. Am Heart J 1968;75:595.
3. Sakakibara S, Konno S. Congenital aneurysm of the sinus of Valsalva: criteria for recommending surgery. Am J Cardiol 1963;12:100.
4. Sakakibara S, Konno W. Congenital aneurysms of sinus of Valsalva: a clinical study. Am Heart J 1962;63:708.
5. Sawyers JL, Adams JE, Scott HW Jr. Surgical treatment for aneurysms of the aortic sinuses with aortico atrial fistula: experimental and clinical study. Surgery 1957;41:26.
6. Schuster NH. Aneurysm of the sinus of Valsalva involving the coronary orifice. Lancet 1937;1:507.
7. Scott RW. Aortic aneurysm rupturing into the pulmonary artery: report of two cases. JAMA 1924;82:1417.
8. Segal BL, Likoff W, Novack P. Rupture of a sinus of Valsalva aneurysm. Am J Cardiol 1963;12:544.
9. Serino W, Andrade JL, Ross D, de Leval M, Somerville J. Aorto–left ventricular communication after closure: late postoperative problems. Br Heart J 1983;49:501.
10. Shiraishi S, Watarida S, Katsuyama K, Nakajima Y, Imura M, Nishi T, et al. Unruptured aneurysm of the sinus of Valsalva into the pulmonary artery. Ann Thorac Surg 1998;65:1458.
11. Shumacker HB Jr. Aneurysms of the aortic sinuses of Valsalva due to bacterial endocarditis, with special reference to their operative management. J Thorac Cardiovasc Surg 1972;63:896.
12. Shumacker HB Jr, Judson WE. Rupture of aneurysm of sinus of Valsalva into left ventricle and its operative repair. J Thorac Cardiovasc Surg 1963;45:650.
13. Shumacker HB Jr, King H, Waldhausen JA. Transaortic approach for the repair of ruptured aneurysms of the sinuses of Valsalva. Ann Surg 1965;161:946.
14. Smith WA. Aneurysm of the sinus of Valsalva with report of two cases. JAMA 1914;62:1878.
15. Somerville J, English T, Ross DN. Aorto–left ventricular tunnel: clinical features and surgical management. Br Heart J 1974;36:321.
16. Spencer FC, Blake HA, Bahnson HT. Surgical repair of ruptured aneurysm of sinus of Valsalva in two patients. Ann Surg 1960;152:963.
17. Sreeram N, Franks R, Arnold R, Walsh K. Aortico–left ventricular tunnel: long-term outcome after surgical repair. J Am Coll Cardiol 1991;17:950.
18. Stollberger C, Seitelberger R, Fenninger C, Prainer C, Slany J. Aneurysm of the left sinus of Valsalva. An unusual source of cerebral embolism. Stroke 1996;27:1424.
19. Szweda JA, Drake EH. Ruptured congenital aneurysms of the sinuses of Valsalva: a report of 2 cases treated surgically. Circulation 1962;25:559.

T

1. Taguchi K, Sasaki N, Matasuura Y, Mura R. Surgical correction of aneurysm of the sinus of Valsalva: a report of 45 consecutive patients, including 8 with total replacement of the aortic valve. Am J Cardiol 1969;23:180.
2. Takahara Y, Sudo Y, Sunazawa T, Nakajima N. Aneurysm of the left sinus of Valsalva producing aortic valve regurgitation and myocardial ischemia. Ann Thorac Surg 1998;65:535.
3. Terdjman M, Bourdarias JP, Farcot JC, Gueret P, Dubourg O, Ferrier A, et al. Aneurysms of sinus of Valsalva: two-dimensional echocardiographic diagnosis and recognition of rupture into the right heart cavities. J Am Coll Cardiol 1984;3:1227.
4. Thurman J. On aneurysms and especially spontaneous varicose aneurysms of the ascending aorta and sinuses of Valsalva, with cases. Med Chir Tr Lond 1840;23:323.
5. Trusler GA, Moes CA, Kidd BS. Repair of ventricular septal defect with aortic insufficiency. J Thorac Cardiovasc Surg 1973;66:394.
6. Tuna IC, Edwards JE. Aortico–left ventricular tunnel and aortic insufficiency. Ann Thorac Surg 1988;45:5.
7. Turley K, Silverman NH, Teitel D, Mavroudis C, Snider R, Rudolph A. Repair of aortico–left ventricular tunnel in the neonate: surgical, anatomic and echocardiographic considerations. Circulation 1982;65:1015.

V

1. Van Son JA, Danielson GK, Schaff HV, Orszulak TA, Edwards WD, Seward JB. Long-term outcome of surgical repair of ruptured sinus of Valsalva aneurysm. Circulation 1994;90:II20.
2. Venning GR. Aneurysms of the sinuses of Valsalva. Am Heart J 1951;42:57.
3. Vered Z, Rath S, Benjamin P, Motro M, Neufeld HN. Ruptured sinus of Valsalva: demonstration by contrast echocardiography during cardiac catheterization. Am Heart J 1985;109:365.

W

1. Wakabayashi Y, Tawarahara K, Kurata C. Aneurysms of all sinuses of Valsalva and aortic valve prolapse secondary to Behçet's disease. Eur Heart J 1996;17:1766.
2. Walters MI, Ettles D, Guvendik L, Kaye GC. Interventricular septal expansion of a sinus of Valsalva aneurysm: a rare cause of complete heart block. Heart 1998;80:202.
3. Warnke H, Bartel J, Blumenthal-Barby C. Aortico–ventricular tunnel. Thorac Cardiovasc Surg 1988;36:86.
4. Warthen RO. Congenital aneurysm of the right anterior sinus of Valsalva (interventricular aneurysm) with spontaneous rupture into the left ventricle. Am Heart J 1949;37:975.
5. Weyman AE, Dillon JC, Feigenbaum H, Chang S. Premature pulmonic valve opening following sinus of Valsalva aneurysm rupture into the right atrium. Circulation 1975;52:556.
6. Wortham DC, Gorman PD, Hull RW, Vernalis MN, Gaither NS. Unruptured sinus of Valsalva aneurysm presenting with embolization. Am Heart J 1993;125:896.

37 Patent Ductus Arteriosus

DEFINITION

Patent ductus arteriosus (PDA) is abnormal persistence of a patent lumen in the fetal ductus arteriosus, which usually connects the upper descending thoracic aorta with the proximal portion of the left pulmonary artery (LPA). When the aortic arch is right-sided, the ductus usually connects to the proximal right pulmonary artery. The ductus may at times connect to the adjacent subclavian or brachiocephalic artery rather than to the upper descending thoracic aorta.

This chapter is primarily concerned with isolated PDA. PDA associated with other anomalies is discussed briefly here and in more detail in other chapters (Coarctation of the Aorta and Interrupted Aortic Arch, Chapter 48; Ventricular Septal Defect, Chapter 35; and Ventricular Septal Defect with Pulmonary Stenosis or Atresia, Chapter 38).

HISTORICAL NOTE

The ductus arteriosus apparently was first described by Galen (born AD 129). It was rediscovered by Botallo in the 16th century, although some attribute the description of its postnatal closure to Acierno[A3,F6] and Harvey.[F5,H3] In 1888, Munro demonstrated in an infant cadaver the feasibility of dissecting and ligating a PDA.[M12] In 1900, Gibson described the characteristic continuous murmur of this anomaly.[G1] However, it was not until 1937 that Strieder in Boston attempted to close a PDA surgically in a patient with fulminating infective endarteritis; the patient died on the fourth postoperative day with gastric distention and aspiration of vomitus.[G8]

Cardiac surgery received a great impetus on August 26, 1938, when Gross successfully ligated the PDA of a 7-year-old girl at Boston Children's Hospital.[G13] Subsequently, he developed division rather than ligation as the surgical technique of choice.[G11,G12] The first successful repair of an infected PDA was reported in 1940 by Touroff and Vesell, who later reported successful division of an infected PDA.[T3,T4] Portsmann and colleagues reported catheter closure of this anomaly in 1971.[P6] The first successful catheter closure of a PDA in a neonate or infant was performed by Rashkind and Cuaso in 1977.[R2,R3] Thus, PDA is the anomaly that initiated not only the *surgical* treatment of congenital heart disease, but also its *transcatheter* treatment.

MORPHOLOGY AND MORPHOGENESIS

Morphology of Normal Ductal Closure

At birth, the fetal ductus arteriosus is patent, resembling, according to Gittenberger-de Groot and colleagues[G3]:

> *...a muscular artery with an intact, wavy internal elastic lamina, interrupted only underneath the intimal cushions. At those sites the elastic lamina is fragmented and is sometimes split up into several layers. The media is composed mainly of circularly arranged smooth muscle cells, with only minimal elastin fibers in between. The medial components may be widely separated, predominantly along the line of junction with intimal cushions, thereby creating large pools filled with a mucoid, slightly eosinophilic substance, the so-called mucoid lakes. In more advanced stages of anatomic closure, necrosis of cellular components of the media and a diffuse fibrous proliferation of the intima begin to appear.*

Postnatal closure occurs in two stages.[C4] The first stage is complete within 10 to 15 hours after birth in full-term infants; smooth muscle in the media of the ductal wall contracts, producing shortening and an increase in wall thickness. This functional closure is assisted by approximation of the intimal cushions. The *intimal cushions* (or mounds or pillows) are swellings composed of longitudinally oriented smooth muscle cells that protrude into the lumen and lie between the endothelium and internal elastic lamina and thus within the intima.[J2] They thicken as the duct matures and are most prominent at the pulmonary end. Muscle contraction occurs both circumferentially from the circularly arranged smooth muscle cells that fill almost the entire media, and longitudinally from one or more bands of muscle in the inner media.[S5]

The second stage of closure is usually completed by 2 to 3 weeks. It is the result of diffuse fibrous proliferation of the intima, sometimes associated with necrosis of the inner layer of the media, and hemorrhage into the wall. The latter may be due to intimal tears producing a limited dissection of the ductus wall; there may also be small thrombi within the lumen, but gross luminal thrombus is rare.[C1] These changes result in permanent sealing of the lumen and produce the fibrous *ligamentum arteriosum*.

Closure usually begins at the pulmonary end and may remain incomplete at the aortic end, leaving an aortic ampulla from which the ligamentum arteriosum arises. Less commonly, there may be a ductus diverticulum arising from the proximal LPA.

The ductus arteriosus is completely closed by 8 weeks of age in 88% of infants with a normal cardiovascular system.[C6] When the process is delayed, the term *prolonged patency* of the ductus arteriosus is appropriate; when the process ultimately fails, *persistent patency* of the ductus arteriosus is the appropriate term. Ductus closure or patency is mediated by release of vasoactive substances (acetylcholine, bradykinin, endogenous catecholamines, and probably others), by variations in pH, but chiefly by oxygen tension[M9] and prostaglandins (PGE_1, PGE_2, and prostacyclin PGI_2).[C9] Oxygen tension and prostaglandins act in opposite directions, with an increasing P_{O_2} constricting the ductus and prostaglandins relaxing it; the potency of each varies at different gestational ages.[H8] Thus, the ductus is considerably more sensitive to P_{O_2} in the mature fetus and to prostaglandins (specifically, PGE_1) in the immature fetus. The complex interplay of these factors is the reason prolonged patency of the ductus is more common in premature than term infants, particularly when there is associated respiratory distress syndrome (see Special Situations and Controversies later in this chapter). *Intermittent patency* of the ductus arteriosus has been documented, particularly when the ductus is long and narrow.[D5]

Position and Absence

At birth, usually in subjects with other cardiac anomalies, the ductus may be unilateral, bilateral, or (rarely) completely absent. It is absent in 35% of autopsy specimens with tetralogy of Fallot with pulmonary stenosis, in 40% of those with tetralogy of Fallot with pulmonary atresia, in almost all patients with tetralogy of Fallot and absent pulmonary valve (see Chapter 38), and in truncus arteriosus (see Chapter 43). It is rarely absent in patients with pulmonary atresia and intact ventricular septum (4%) (see Chapter 40) or in those with pulmonary atresia and other complex anomalies (15%).

Anatomic Details

Isolated Patent Ductus Arteriosus

The usual isolated PDA connects to the upper descending thoracic aorta 2 to 10 mm beyond the aortic origin of the left subclavian artery (Fig. 37-1).[C1] From the aorta, it passes centrally toward the origin of the LPA from the pulmonary trunk, either directly or angling superiorly and hugging the undersurface of the distal aortic arch. When, as in the normally developing heart, the ductus delivers approximately 55% of the combined ventricular output into the descending aorta, the ductus meets the aorta at a proximal acute angle (<40 degrees) and a distal obtuse angle (110 to 160 degrees, mean 134 degrees)[C1,H7,M3] (Table 37-1; see also Fig. 37-1).

The PDA is generally 5 to 10 mm in length (in autopsy specimens, 2.5-8 mm), with a wide aortic orifice (4-12 mm) and a considerably narrower pulmonary orifice, and it is restrictive to flow. The PDA may be longer or shorter than this and may have a wide pulmonary as well as aortic orifice.

Patent Ductus Arteriosus as a Coexisting Anomaly

When other cardiac anomalies are present, orientation of the ductus to the aortic arch varies, as does the flow pattern in fetal life.[C1] When there is pulmonary atresia and the pulmonary circulation is ductus dependent, with ductal flow in utero occurring from the aorta to the pulmonary artery, the ductus becomes a downwardly directed branch of the distal aortic arch. The proximal angle is much less acute and often

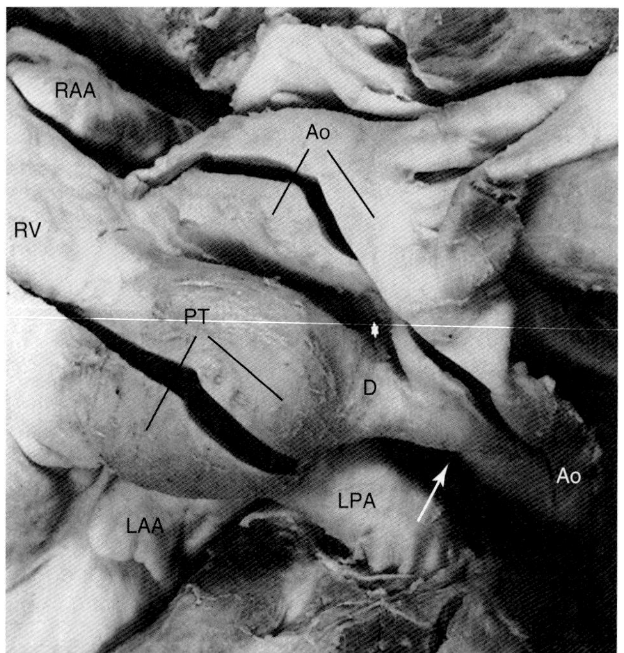

Figure 37-1 Specimen of isolated patent ductus arteriosus *(D)* in an infant. Ductus passes from junction of pulmonary trunk *(PT)* and left pulmonary artery *(LPA)* in an inferior and lateral direction to join descending aorta *(Ao)*. Angle between superior border of ductus *(asterisk)* and aorta (proximal angle) is acute, and that between the lower border and aorta *(arrow)* (distal angle) is obtuse. Key: *LAA,* Left atrial appendage; *RAA,* right atrial appendage; *RV,* right ventricle. (From Calder and colleagues.[C1])

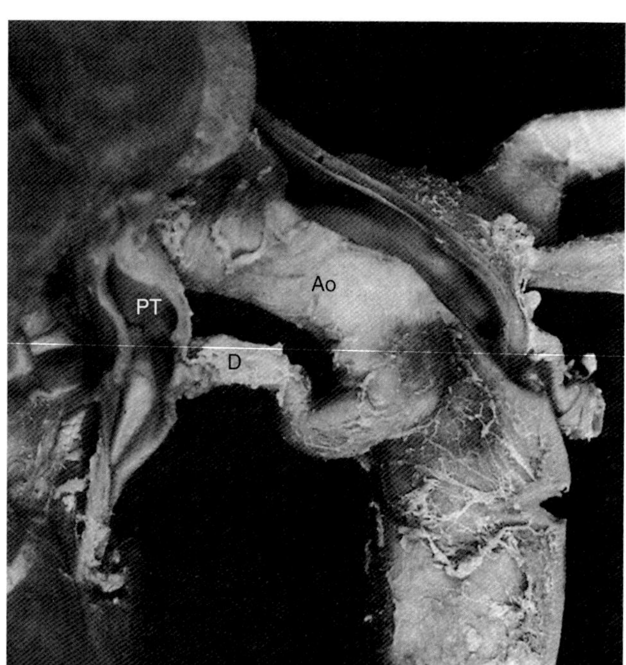

Figure 37-2 Specimen of patent ductus arteriosus *(D)* in an infant with pulmonary atresia. Compared with the ductus in Fig. 37-1, it is long and relatively narrow and joins the aorta *(Ao)* at a completely different angle: Proximal angle is obtuse and distal angle acute. Key: *PT,* Pulmonary trunk. (From Calder and colleagues.[C1])

Table 37-1 Morphologic Features of Ductus Arteriosus in Fixed Autopsy Specimens

		Age		Ductal Status					
Cardiac Diagnosis	*n*	Range	Median	Open	Closed	Average Length (mm)	Average Width (mm)	Average Prox Angle[a] (°)	Average Distal Angle[a] (°)
Normal[b]	13	SB-5 mo	2 d	10	3	8	5.9	29	134
Pulmonary atresia	32	SB-11 mo	8 d	13	19	9.7	3.7	83[c]	90[c]
Aortic atresia	13	2 d-11 wk	4 d	12	1	7.9	7.2	70[c]	127
Coarctation	14	3 d-6 mo	14 d	8	6	5.6	6.0	70[c]	139
Miscellaneous CHD	37	1 d-8 mo	23 d	18	19	7.1	4.6	52	124

Data from Calder and colleagues.[C1]
[a]Angle between ductus and descending aorta.
[b]Normal hearts except for open ductus arteriosus.
[c]Difference from normal: $P < .001$.
Key: *CHD,* Congenital heart disease; *d,* days; *mo,* months; *prox,* proximal; *SB,* stillborn; *wk,* weeks.

obtuse, and the distal angle is often acute[C1,R10] (Fig. 37-2; see also Table 37-1) (see "Aortic Arch and Ductus Arteriosus" under Morphology in Section I of Chapter 38). When this is not the case, pulmonary atresia likely developed late in pregnancy.[S1] The ductus is also usually narrower and longer (see Fig. 37-2).[C1] The lumen is usually narrower at the pulmonary end and wider at the aortic end, as in isolated PDA.

In aortic atresia and coarctation of the aorta, the distal angle is normal, but the proximal angle in these shorter, broader examples of PDA is much less acute, probably because ductal flow enters both the ascending and descending aorta.[C1]

Uncommonly, in the presence of a left aortic arch, the ductus may arise from an aortic diverticulum (thought to represent persistence of the most distal portion of the right fourth branchial arch) that projects from the medial aspect of the left arch just distal to the origin of the left subclavian artery.[G9] In rare cases in which the ductus is bilateral, the right-sided PDA connects the right pulmonary artery to the brachiocephalic artery.

In the presence of a right aortic arch, a left-sided ductus is still more common than a right-sided ductus. When there is mirror-image branching of the right arch, the left PDA arises from the distal brachiocephalic (or proximal left subclavian) artery (see Chapter 38). Much less commonly, the right PDA persists in mirror image to the normal, passing from the right arch beyond the right subclavian artery to the right pulmonary artery origin. A PDA (or ligamentum arteriosum) arising from an aortic diverticulum or from an aberrant left subclavian artery is one form of vascular ring (see Chapter 51).

Histology

Histology of a persistent PDA is different from that of simple prolonged patency of the ductus.[G2] It is also different from that of the adjoining great arteries. A persistent PDA has a relatively thick intima with an unfragmented elastic lamina separating it from the media, an additional and pronounced wavy unfragmented subendothelial elastic lamina, and variable mucoid material in the media where there is an intricate helicoid spiral muscular arrangement.[G2] The media contains variable amounts of elastic material that may form conspicuous lamellae, making the ductus wall resemble the wall of the aorta (aortification).

Aneurysms of Ductus Arteriosus

Aneurysms of the ductus arteriosus, which are rare lesions, appear to be of two types. One is the spontaneous infantile ductal aneurysm, which is present at birth or develops shortly thereafter.[H6] The other develops in childhood or adult life.

Presence of the first type may not be detected until autopsy after death from other causes.[D1] The aneurysm involves the entire length of the ductus arteriosus and is usually associated with occlusion of the pulmonary artery end and a relatively narrow but patent aortic end.[F8] It generally contains thrombus and is occasionally a site of infection and embolism. Rarely, it may be a true dissecting aneurysm of the ductal wall.[F1] This rare lesion manifests most often in newborns with a history of respiratory difficulties.[D6,H6] It produces a tumor-like shadow of variable size that projects beyond the mediastinum adjacent to the aortic knob in the posteroanterior chest radiograph. The aneurysm usually regresses spontaneously within weeks or months, presumably as a result of complete thrombosis and organization, but progressive enlargement or onset of hoarseness from recurrent laryngeal nerve involvement is an indication for surgical exploration and excision.[H6] Less marked dilatation of the ductus can be seen on the plain chest radiograph as a fusiform shadow between 6 and 18 hours after birth, disappearing by 24 to 48 hours of age.[B1] It has been called the *ductus bump.*

The second type of ductal aneurysm is thought to be unrelated to the infantile form. The ductus may be patent at both ends, but usually the pulmonary artery end is closed.[G5,T9] There is a tendency for progressive enlargement, and death may occur from rupture.[C13]

CLINICAL FEATURES AND DIAGNOSTIC CRITERIA

Symptoms and signs of a PDA are the consequence of left-to-right shunting, with the magnitude of the shunt dependent upon size of the communication and relationship between systemic and pulmonary vascular resistances. In this regard, it is similar to other types of high-pressure shunts, which include those across the ventricular septum and others from the aorta.

Large Patent Ductus Arteriosus

Aortic and pulmonary artery pressures are essentially equal when the PDA is large, and the magnitude and direction of shunting are dependent on changes in pulmonary vascular resistance, because systemic vascular resistance remains fairly constant after birth.[R9] As neonatal pulmonary vascular resistance decreases, left-to-right shunting increases and severe heart failure develops within a month or so of birth. There is tachypnea, tachycardia, sweating, irritability, poor feeding, and slow weight gain.[K4] Pulmonary edema and pneumonia or less severe, and recurrent respiratory infection may occur.

On examination, there is an overactive precordium, sometimes with a systolic thrill, and evidence of cardiac enlargement with a thrusting left ventricular apical impulse.[A5] The pulse is jerky or frankly collapsing, and the pulse pressure is correspondingly wide. These features become more obvious when heart failure is medically controlled. On auscultation, there is a systolic murmur maximal in the pulmonary area, with late systolic accentuation and minimal spillover into diastole.[R8] Occasionally the murmur is continuous, but sometimes with severe heart failure, no murmur is heard.[M8] The first and second heart sounds are accentuated, and there is a third sound at the apex or a prominent mid-diastolic mitral flow murmur.[R4] The liver enlarges and jugular venous pressure rises; frequently, rales are heard in the lung bases.

The electrocardiogram (ECG) shows left ventricular enlargement with deep Q and tall R waves in the left ventricular leads. There may be evidence of right ventricular hypertrophy with upright T waves in the right precordial leads and evidence of left atrial enlargement with widened P waves. The chest radiograph shows marked cardiomegaly and plethora with or without interstitial or alveolar pulmonary edema. The pulmonary trunk is enlarged, as is the ascending aorta. The echocardiogram shows left atrial enlargement. The ductus may be visualized with two-dimensional echocardiography.

In some infants with a large PDA, heart failure may be less marked, presumably because pulmonary vascular resistance does not fall to the usual level. Histologic changes of pulmonary vascular disease may develop within the first few months of life. These changes may occur in infants in whom heart failure is controlled medically and the ductus is not closed by intervention. These patients become asymptomatic, and the left-to-right shunt diminishes. The murmur becomes purely systolic, the pulmonary component of the second heart sound is markedly accentuated, the apical mid-diastolic murmur disappears, and the pulse loses its jerky quality. Right ventricular hypertrophy becomes dominant in the ECG, the heart becomes smaller on the chest radiograph, and pulmonary plethora disappears. Cyanosis develops as pulmonary vascular resistance increases above systemic vascular resistance (Eisenmenger syndrome), typically earlier than with ventricular septal defect (see Chapter 35).[E5] Differential cyanosis may be noted, with blueness of the feet and sometimes the left hand, but not of the face or right hand.

Moderate-Sized Patent Ductus Arteriosus

Left-to-right shunt in moderate-sized PDA is regulated by size of the ductus arteriosus. In this setting, pulmonary artery pressure is only moderately elevated. As neonatal pulmonary vascular resistance declines, the shunt increases and heart failure may occur. By the second or third month of life, however, compensatory left ventricular hypertrophy is usually associated with clinical improvement and stabilization of symptoms. Physical development may be somewhat retarded, and breathlessness and fatigue may occur, but many patients with moderate-sized PDA remain essentially asymptomatic until the second decade of life or later.

On examination, the pulse is jerky, the precordium is mildly overactive, and the left ventricle is palpable at the apex in association with some cardiac enlargement. The classic continuous murmur is usually heard by age 2 to 3 months, although it varies in intensity.[L3] The murmur is generally loud and often masks the heart sounds. It is maximal over the pulmonary artery and radiates upward beneath the mid-third of the clavicle. As described by Gibson in 1900, "it begins after the commencement of the first sound—it persists through the second sound and dies away gradually during the long pause. The murmur is rough and thrilling. It begins softly and increases in intensity so as to reach its acme at or immediately after the occurrence of the second sound, and from that point gradually wanes until its termination." [G1] Subnormal physical growth is common; Krovetz and Warden found body weight below the third percentile in 26% of 515 surgically proven cases.[K4] The ECG may be relatively normal during infancy, but some degree of left ventricular hypertrophy develops in older children. The chest radiograph shows moderate cardiac enlargement and plethora and a prominent ascending aorta (in contrast to findings in patients with a large ventricular or atrial septal defect). In adults, the PDA may be calcified. It is rare for pulmonary vascular resistance to increase, and Eisenmenger syndrome does not develop.

Small Patent Ductus Arteriosus

Left-to-right shunt is small in early life, and pulmonary vascular resistance decreases rapidly to normal after birth.

Left ventricular failure does not occur, and symptoms are absent in infancy and childhood. They may appear later in life, but usually attention is drawn to the condition by a murmur detected on physical examination.

Physical development is normal unless there is maternal rubella. The pulse is normal and the precordium not overactive. By age 2 to 3 months, a short systolic murmur is usually replaced by one that spills over into diastole, or it may be continuous in the second left intercostal space but less intense, and with less radiation than when the ductus is moderate in size. The continuous murmur varies greatly in intensity between patients and sometimes is detectable only when the patient is sitting or standing upright. The ECG and chest radiograph are normal or nearly so.

Special Investigations

Most children and young adults with a PDA and a continuous murmur that is maximal in the second left intercostal space do not need preoperative invasive studies unless other defects are suspected; such studies may be necessary for diagnosis in atypical cases. Instead, two-dimensional echocardiography is usually performed and will image the ductus arteriosus. It has identified so-called silent ductus (a PDA without auscultatory findings).[H11] Managing patients with isolated silent ductus remains controversial, although endarteritis has been reported and may be an indication for closure.[B2] Cardiac catheterization and angiography are indicated if the echocardiogram suggests elevated pulmonary vascular resistance or associated cardiac anomalies.

NATURAL HISTORY

Isolated PDA in term infants occurs in approximately 1 in 2000 live births and accounts for 5% to 10% of all types of congenital heart disease.[M10] It is twice as common in females[C2] and may occur in siblings, suggesting a genetic factor. It is particularly common when the mother contracts rubella during the first trimester of pregnancy and may then be associated with multiple peripheral pulmonary artery stenoses and renal artery stenosis.

Because of the early introduction of surgical treatment of PDA, which antedated methods for establishing the diagnosis, its natural history is not completely documented.

Spontaneous Closure

Campbell's study concluded that spontaneous closure of isolated PDA occurs in 0.6% of patients per year and that this rate is fairly constant through the first 4 decades of life.[C2] If this is accepted, it means that in approximately 20% of patients, the PDA will have closed by age 40. His study involved only patients diagnosed beyond age 12 months and was based entirely on clinical findings, closure being assumed to have occurred when a typical murmur was no longer audible, regardless of size of the ductus or initial right-to-left shunt. Other experience suggests that the closure rate is much lower, and it is generally agreed that spontaneous closure is uncommon beyond age 3 to 5 months in full-term infants. Delayed closure of the ductus arteriosus in preterm infants is, however, common (see Special Situations and Controversies later in this chapter).

Pulmonary Vascular Disease

Prevalence and type of pulmonary vascular disease in patients with large PDA are similar to those in patients with large ventricular septal defect (see "Pulmonary Vascular Disease" under Morphology in Section I of Chapter 35).

Rupture

Rupture of both non-aneurysmal and aneurysmal PDA has been reported.[C13,M5]

Death

Mortality with untreated PDA in infancy is high, and it has been estimated that, particularly in earlier eras, 30% of patients born with an isolated PDA died within the first year.[C2,H5] Risk of death is highest in the first few months of life (see "Patent Ductus Arteriosus in Preterm Infants" under Special Situations and Controversies later in this chapter).

After infancy, the annual death rate of patients with untreated PDA decreases dramatically to approximately 0.5% per year.[C2] By the third decade, the death rate has increased to about 1% per year; by the fourth decade, 1.8% per year; and in subsequent decades, as high as 4% per year.[C2] As a result, approximately 60% of patients with PDA die by age 45. Most of the deaths in older patients are related to development of intractable left ventricular failure secondary to long-standing volume overload.

Modes of Death

In infants with a large PDA, mode of death is usually heart failure. Recurrent respiratory infection terminating in pneumonia is a less common mode. In those with a large PDA who survive infancy, death is usually due to acute or chronic right heart failure secondary to development of severe pulmonary vascular disease by the second or third decade of life.

In patients with a moderate-sized PDA, mode of death from the third and fourth decades onward is heart failure. Excluding infants and deaths from pulmonary vascular disease, Campbell estimated that heart failure was the cause of death in 30% of patients.[C2]

Infective endarteritis occurs mainly as a complication of small and moderate-sized PDA. It rarely occurs when the ductus is large. In the preantibiotic era, endarteritis was responsible for approximately 45% of deaths in patients with surgically untreated PDA.[A2,C2,K2] After the advent of antibiotics, few patients died from this cause, although they remained subject to recurrent infection. In the current era, risk of infective endarteritis is extremely low.[F4]

TECHNIQUE OF OPERATION

Closure of Patent Ductus Arteriosus

Unless the patient is an infant in severe heart failure or elderly, an intraarterial monitoring catheter is usually unnecessary. After the usual induction of anesthesia and preparations for operation (see Chapter 4), the patient is positioned on the right side (Fig. 37-3, *A*). A small roll or pillow is placed under the mid-chest. The patient is positioned near the surgeon's side of the table, but not so much so that the first assistant across the table from the surgeon cannot see into the field well and work comfortably.

Posterolateral Thoracotomy

A curving skin incision is made, centered about 1 to 2 cm below the tip of the scapula. In infants and young children, the incision is really a lateral one, because only the latissimus dorsi and posterior part of the serratus anterior are divided. In older children, the incision is posterolateral, extending posterosuperiorly to overlie the lower 1 or 2 cm of the trapezius, which is also incised. In patients who are in the second decade of life or older, the incision extends from the anterior axillary line around the scapula and up midway between the spine and posterior scapular border over the lower 3 to 4 cm of the trapezius.

After incising the latissimus dorsi (and trapezius if indicated), the scapula is elevated with a retractor and the ribs are counted from the top down to the fifth rib. Identifying the appropriate rib or intercostal space requires an accurate point of reference. There are three possible points of reference (the second and third are often more reliable than the first):

- First rib: The surgeon passes his or her left hand under the serratus and identifies the first rib by palpation.
- Second rib: The serratus anterior attaches superiorly to the second rib. The surgeon identifies this attachment using upward traction on the scapular retractor, which makes the prominent posterior border of this muscle taut.
- Second intercostal space: This is usually appreciably wider than the third intercostal space.

Counting down from the reference point, the fifth rib is identified and scored. Only then are the posterior and mid-portions of the serratus anterior divided so that the muscle incision may be directly over the fifth rib. The fourth interspace may be opened with a knife or cautery or the chest may be entered through the superior part of the bed of the non-resected fifth rib. With the latter method, the periosteum over the rib is incised, and its superior portion is elevated from the front and back with a periosteal elevator.

After the incision in the rib cage is extended anteriorly and posteriorly, the rib retractor is placed with the ratcheted portion anteriorly (Fig. 37-3, *B*). The retractor is opened only partially at first, but as the operation proceeds, it is gradually opened further to obtain adequate exposure.

A retractor is gently placed on the lung, and a vertical incision is made in the mediastinal pleura over the proximal descending thoracic aorta (see Fig. 37-3, *B*).[1] Traction sutures are placed on the anterior and posterior pleural flaps. The lung retractor is removed, moist gauze is placed over the lung, and the anterior pleural traction sutures are pulled taut and anchored to the retractor or drapes. The vein that traverses the aorta obliquely on its anterior surface is divided. The PDA is completely dissected from the surrounding tissue (Fig. 37-3, *C-E*). In small infants, particular care is taken to be certain that the structure identified as the PDA connects the aorta and pulmonary artery, and that it is not the LPA or distal aortic arch. As dissection proceeds, the left recurrent laryngeal nerve is not isolated, although it should be clearly visualized behind the areolar tissue over the LPA, just inferior and posterior to the PDA (see Fig. 37-3, *C*).

When the PDA is an uncomplicated one, either division or ligation may be performed. Both techniques, when done properly, ensure complete closure with low risk.

Division When division is elected and the patient is an infant or young child, one straight and two angled fine-toothed Potts ductus clamps are selected. In teenagers and adults, longer-handled vascular clamps are used. At this time, and particularly in older children and adults, the anesthesiologist reduces arterial blood pressure (see Chapter 4) and maintains it below baseline level until the clamps are removed.

The straight clamp is placed completely across the aortic end of the PDA, making sure that its tip does not grasp the recurrent laryngeal nerve or other soft tissue posterior to the ductus. The clamp is placed in the surgeon's left hand and is gently pulled anteriorly. One angled ductus clamp is placed on the aortic side of the straight clamp and usually on the aorta contiguous with the PDA rather than on the ductus itself. The straight clamp is removed. With the clamp on the aortic origin of the PDA, which is held in the surgeon's right hand, the other angled clamp is placed with the left hand on

[1]Gross made an anterolateral thoracotomy incision, placed the pleural incision midway between the phrenic and vagus nerves, and retracted the vagus nerve posteriorly.[G11-G14] Exposure is probably less optimal with this approach, although it may be appropriate in small patients and those with variations of situs such as mesocardia and dextrocardia.

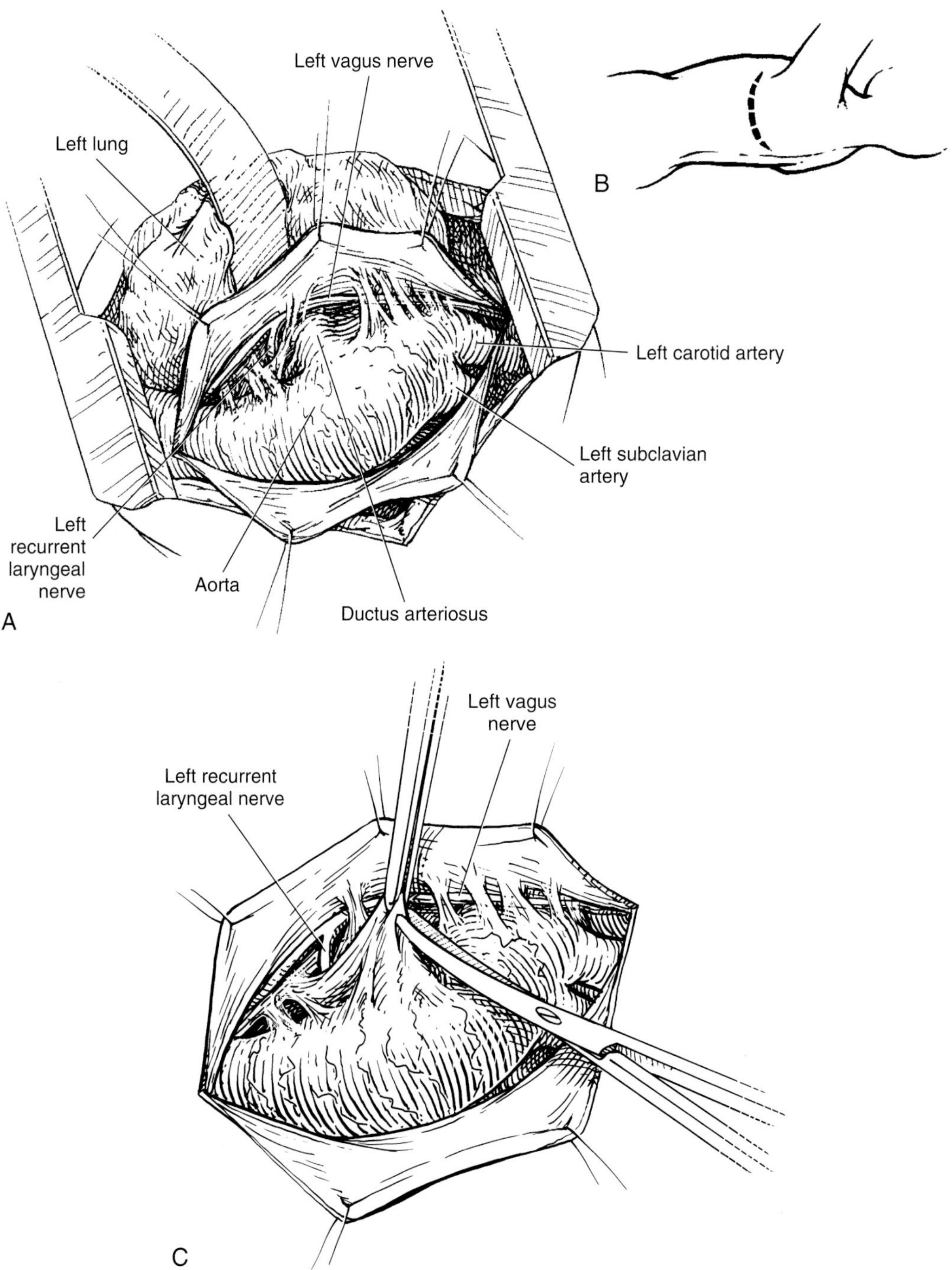

Figure 37-3 Closure of patent ductus arteriosus (PDA) by division. **A,** Posterolateral incision in a patient properly positioned for operation. **B,** Rib retractor has been placed and opened slowly to its final width. Lung is gently retracted anteriorly. Vertical incision is made in mediastinal pleura, and traction sutures are placed on pleural flaps. Left vagus and left recurrent laryngeal nerves are identified and protected. **C,** Areolar tissues and pericardial lappet anterior to ductus are elevated with forceps and sharply dissected free of it. Care is taken to leave the adventitial layer of ductus undisturbed.

the pulmonary end of the ductus. To avoid dislodgment from the clamp and retraction into the pericardial cavity, the clamp must grasp *only* the ductus and not any of the lappet of pericardium or other tissue. This clamp, like the one on the aortic end, is "squeezed" onto the pulmonary artery as much as possible when it is being placed to give added length to the ductus. The ductus is divided midway between these clamps by Potts scissors or a scalpel (Fig. 37-3, *F*).

The aortic end of the PDA is oversewn with two rows of 5-0 or 6-0 polypropylene suture placed as a whip stitch (Fig. 37-3, *G*). The pulmonary end is similarly closed. Although accurate suturing is of obvious importance, the key to a safe repair is separating the clamps widely enough so that a substantial cuff of ductus remains beyond them after the ductus is divided. This permits placing additional sutures for hemostasis.

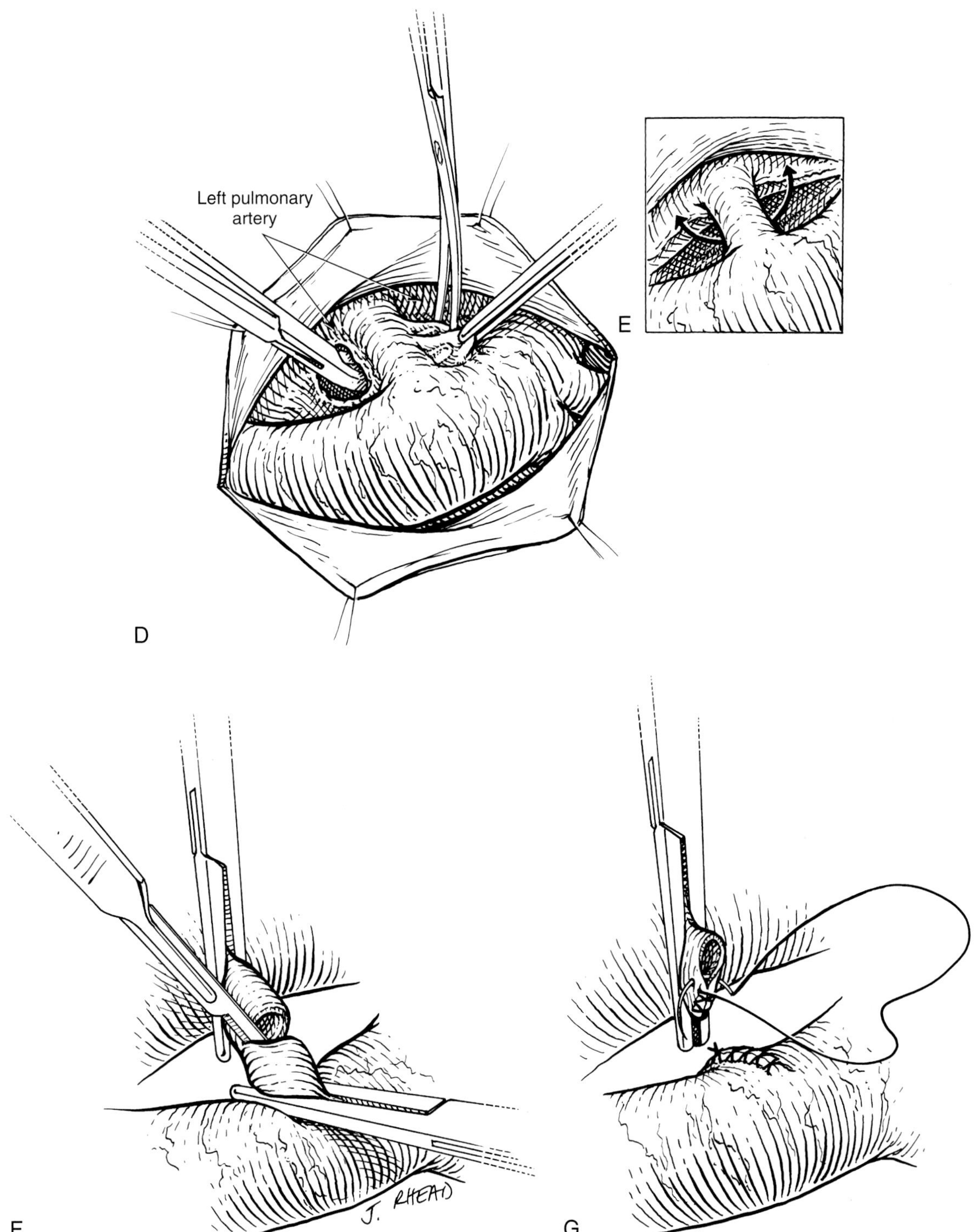

Figure 37-3, cont'd **D,** After anterior surface of ductus has been freed far enough medially so that junction of PDA with left pulmonary artery is visible, superior and inferior surfaces are similarly dissected. Right-angled clamp is passed behind ductus. Clamp stretches areolar tissue behind ductus, which is then grasped with forceps and cut away. **E,** This maneuver is repeated several times and creates a space behind ductus. **F,** Clamps are placed at aortic and pulmonary ends of ductus (see text), and it is divided midway between them. **G,** Aortic end of ductus is oversewn with two rows of 5-0 or 6-0 polypropylene suture. Clamp on aortic end of ductus is generally kept in place following closure and provides traction to expose pulmonary end, which is then oversewn in a similar fashion. Clamps are then released.

The clamp on the pulmonary end of the divided ductus generally is removed first. The clamp on the aortic end is then removed, and a sponge is placed between the divided ends and held in place with pressure for several minutes. Unless the original placement of the clamps has been faulty or the suture closure is inadequate, the bleeding that occurs when the clamps are released usually stops within this period. If not, and if there is no major bleeding that would require replacing one or both clamps, a 5-0 polypropylene suture approximating the adventitia from both sides of the suture line usually controls the bleeding. A pledget of absorbable porcine gelatin sponge is left between the divided ends of the ductus to prevent the suture lines from rubbing against each other.

Ligation If the situation is uncomplicated and the PDA is pliable, it may be ligated rather than divided. The technique is basically that described by Blalock in 1946.[B9] The operation proceeds exactly as described for ductal division until the PDA is completely dissected. Using a double-armed 5-0 or 6-0 polypropylene suture, adventitial stitches are placed into the accessible superior, inferior, and anterior aspects of the aortic wall contiguous with the PDA (Fig. 37-4, *A*). One end of the suture is passed beneath the ductus, and the ends are held. A similar stitch is placed on the pulmonary end of the ductus (Fig. 37-4, *B*). The aortic stitch is pulled up and snugly tied, and then the suture at the pulmonary end is tied. This leaves a long length of ductus between the tied sutures. Finally, a transfixion ligature of 5-0 or 6-0 polypropylene is placed at the middle of the ductus, and the ends are passed in the opposite direction around the ductus and tied to complete the ligation (Figs. 37-4, *C* to *F*).

The mediastinal pleura is closed with interrupted sutures, leaving a small opening at each end. In the unlikely event that there is substantial bleeding from the suture lines after operation, this closure will contain it and may be lifesaving.

The rib retractor is removed, a small catheter is inserted into the posterior part of the pleural space through a stab wound in the sixth or seventh intercostal space at the midaxillary line, and suction of 15 to 25 cm water is placed on it. The ribs on either side of the incision are approximated with interrupted sutures. The muscles are individually sutured with a slowly absorbable synthetic material (polyglycolic acid), and the skin edges are approximated with a subcutaneous stitch. In infants, the chest tube may be removed in the operating room.

Transaxillary Muscle-Sparing Lateral Thoracotomy

A 3- to 4-cm incision is made over the third intercostal space in the axilla. The serratus anterior is reflected inferiorly and laterally, and the pectoralis major is reflected anteriorly. The third intercostal space is entered and a rib retractor inserted. The lung is retracted anteriorly, and the pleura overlying the descending thoracic aorta is incised. The PDA is identified at its junction with the aorta, and the recurrent laryngeal nerve is identified and protected. The PDA is dissected circumferentially and is divided or ligated using the techniques just described. Alternatively, it may be occluded with a medium-sized surgical clip.[C5] The lung is inflated as the chest is closed.

Fluid and air can be aspirated as the chest wall is closed with interrupted pericostal sutures, making a chest tube unnecessary. The muscle and soft tissue layers are approximated with a slowly absorbable synthetic suture (polyglycolic acid), and the skin edges are approximated with a subcutaneous stitch. This technique is applicable to premature infants, neonates, older children, and adults.[G15,K1,M2,T5,T6]

Closure of Patent Ductus Arteriosus in Association with Repair of Intracardiac Lesions

Closure of a PDA may be required during operations to correct intracardiac anomalies that require the use of cardiopulmonary bypass (CPB). This occurs in two distinct clinical situations. When the PDA is an incidental finding and relatively small and restrictive, such as with a large ventricular septal defect, dissection of the ductus is usually performed after CPB has been established, because exposure of the adjacent aorta and pulmonary artery is facilitated when the heart is decompressed, and injury to the ductus or surrounding structures can be avoided. The technique for closure of the PDA under these circumstances is described in Technique of Operation in Chapter 35. In the second situation, as can occur in the neonate with transposition of the great arteries with intact ventricular septum, the ductus is large. It must be exposed and controlled before initiating CPB so that it can be ligated immediately after bypass is established.

Closure of Patent Ductus Arteriosus in Older Adults

When a PDA requires closure in older adults, the aortic end is often calcified and the ductus very short. A technique using CPB described by Goncalves-Estella and colleagues[G4] and later by O'Donovan and Beck[O1] is appropriate in this circumstance.

With the usual preparations (see Chapter 2), a median sternotomy is performed and the usual stay sutures and purse-string sutures placed. The aorta and pulmonary trunk are dissected apart. CPB is established with a single venous cannula, and cooling of the patient by the perfusate is begun. The head of the table is lowered to place the patient in a moderate Trendelenburg position. As the heart begins to slow from the cold perfusion, the ductus is obliterated by compressing the front wall of the LPA against it with the index finger. This is essential because otherwise ductal flow into the pulmonary artery will overdistend the pulmonary vascular bed and the right ventricle (this does not occur when the heart is ejecting adequately). When the nasopharyngeal temperature reaches 20°C to 22°C, the aorta is clamped and cold cardioplegic solution is infused into the aortic root or retrogradely into the coronary sinus (see "Technique of Retrograde Infusion" in Chapter 3). The perfusion temperature is stabilized at 20°C to 22°C, and flow is reduced to 0.5 $L \cdot min^{-1} \cdot m^{-2}$. The finger is removed, the distal pulmonary trunk is opened anteriorly and longitudinally, and the incision is continued into the LPA opposite the ductus. (If external pressure on the LPA does not control ductal flow during CPB cooling, perfusion is temporarily reduced to a low level, and the pulmonary artery incision is made such that the finger can be placed directly over the ostium of the ductus to control flow from it into the LPA. CPB flow rate is then increased until cooling is completed.)

The intracardiac sucker is positioned within the LPA beyond the ductus to aspirate blood entering it. The ductal orifice is closed by placing and tying one or more pledgeted

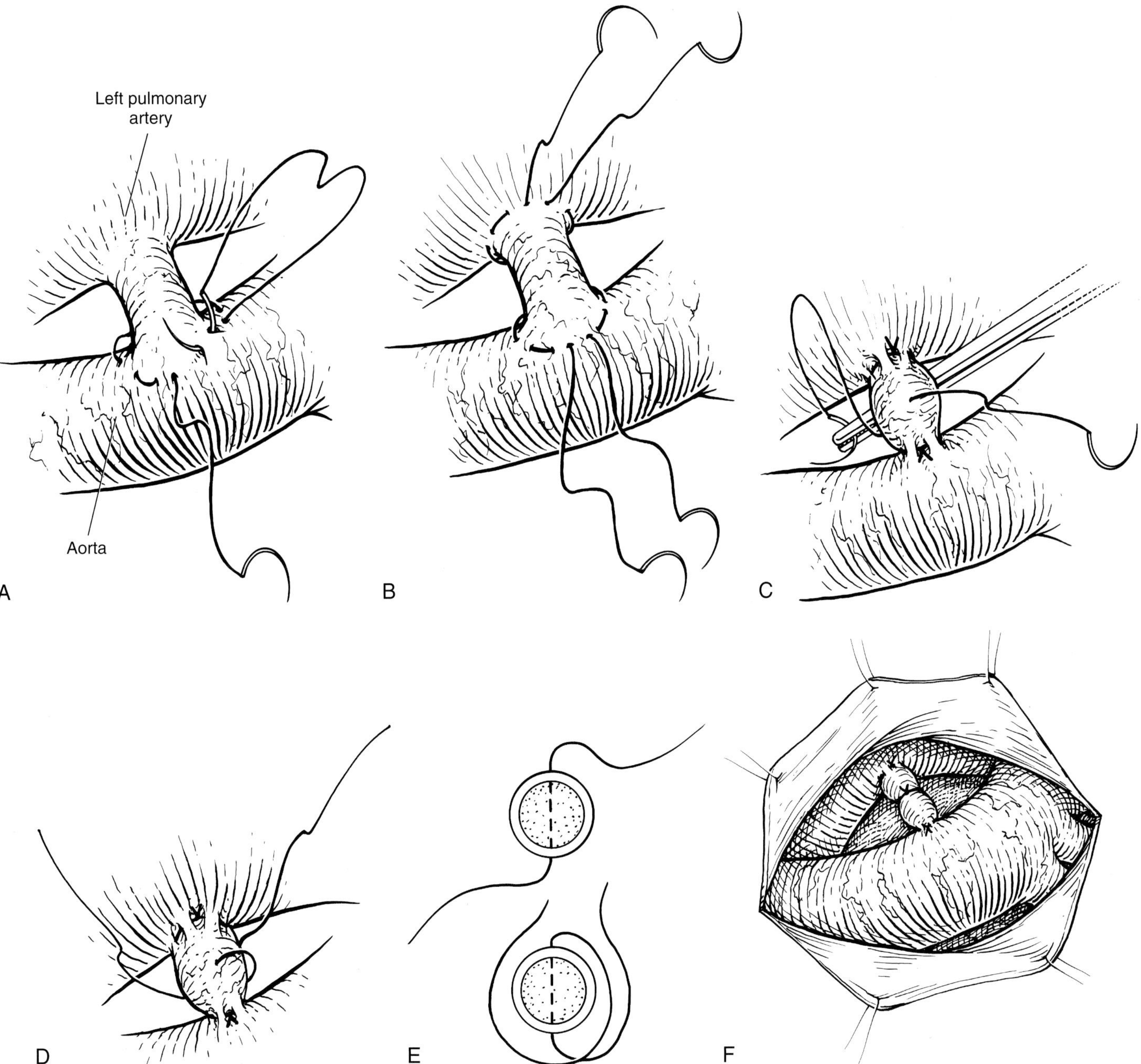

Figure 37-4 Closure of patent ductus arteriosus by ligation. **A,** Dissection has been completed as shown in Fig. 37-3. Adventitial purse-string suture of 5-0 or 6-0 polypropylene is placed around aortic end of ductus. **B,** Similar purse-string suture is placed around pulmonary end of ductus. **C,** The two purse-string sutures are snugly tied. Transfixion suture is placed through ductus. One end is passed beneath ductus. **D,** Other end of suture is passed beneath ductus in opposite direction, and the two ends are tied on anterior surface. **E,** Cross-sectional diagram showing scheme for passing ends of suture. **F,** Transfixion suture has been tied, leaving a space between it and other sutures.

mattress sutures of 3-0 or 4-0 polypropylene. This is usually readily accomplished because the pulmonary artery end of the ductus is rarely calcified, and the pulmonary artery tissues are strong enough to hold sutures well. If the orifice of the pulmonary artery end of the PDA is too large or immobile for this technique, an impervious patch of bovine pericardium, woven polyester, or polytetrafluorethylene can be used to close it, sewing the patch in place with continuous 4-0 or 5-0 polypropylene suture. Flows are then restored, the table leveled, and rewarming of the patient with the perfusate begun. Any leak from the ductus closure site is secured with additional sutures. The pulmonary arteriotomy is closed with a running stitch of fine polypropylene.

With strong suction on a venting catheter or needle that has been placed in the aortic root, the aortic clamp is released. The remainder of the operation is completed in the usual fashion (see "Completing Cardiopulmonary Bypass" in Section III of Chapter 2).

Closure of Patent Ductus Arteriosus in Premature Infants

Perioperative management and technique of operation are different when surgical closure of the ductus is indicated in the premature infant, most of whom weigh approximately 1000 g and some as little as 400 g. Precise management of ventilation, fluid administration, and body temperature, as well as a precise surgical technique, are essential for success.

Operation is usually performed in the neonatal intensive care unit. This simplifies the logistics and, when properly organized, can provide outcomes as good as those obtained in a conventional operating room.[C10,E4]

If the procedure is to be performed in the operating room, the infant is intubated in the neonatal nursery, and proper position of the tube is verified by a chest radiograph. The patient, covered by a plastic wrap blanket and cloth cap, is transported to the operating room in a prewarmed (37°C) transport isolette. The room is prewarmed to approximately 30°C, and the patient is placed on the right side on an infant operating table with overhead servocontrolled radiant warmers set at 37°C.

After preparation and draping, a left lateral incision of approximately 2.5 cm is made, cutting or reflecting the latissimus dorsi and posterior aspect of the serratus anterior. The chest is entered through the third or fourth interspace, and a small rib retractor is put into place. With a narrow malleable retractor, the lung is held forward by the first assistant. The ductus is usually large but is variable in position. It may course superiorly as well as anteriorly from the aorta and be immediately adjacent to the distal aortic arch. In this location it can be easily mistaken for the arch. It may course directly anteriorly and be well inferior to the arch.

The friable vascular tissue makes the usual complete dissection of the ductus inadvisable.[G15,K3,M7,T6] The mediastinal pleura is incised with fine scissors just superior to the aortic end of the ductus and then just inferior to it. The tissue plane is developed by gently spreading fine scissors. As the inferior tissue plane is developed, the back wall (or right side) of the ductus is seen; no attempt is made to pass an instrument around it. The ductus is temporarily and lightly occluded with a fine forceps, and a pulse oximeter on the foot confirms that it is the ductus, not aorta, and that the aortic arch is intact without interruption or coarctation. A medium-sized hemoclip on a holder is positioned well across the ductus at its aortic end; the tip of the clip must be *beyond* the ductus posteriorly. The adventitia of the aorta may be grasped and gently retracted toward the surgeon as the clip is placed. By closing the holder the ductus is closed.

A 12F catheter is brought out through a stab wound in the chest wall and placed on suction. Placing a chest tube is usually not necessary. The chest wall is closed with two pericostal sutures. The muscles are closed with a continuous fine absorbable suture (polyglycolic acid), and the closure is completed with a subcuticular stitch of fine absorbable sutures. When the procedure is performed in the operating room, the infant is transferred back to the neonatal intensive care unit in a prewarmed transfer isolette.

SPECIAL FEATURES OF POSTOPERATIVE CARE

Care after division or ligation of PDA is simple and follows the principles described in Chapter 5. The patient is usually extubated and the drainage catheter removed in the operating room or within a few hours of leaving it. When the transaxillary muscle-sparing technique is used, most patients can be discharged from the hospital within 24 hours.[C5,H4] When the operation is done with CPB, care is also simple and usual (see Chapter 5).

RESULTS

Early (Hospital) Death

Within 10 years of Gross and Hubbard's first successful case, hospital mortality for surgical closure of uncomplicated PDA had become very low. In 1951, Gross and Longino reported eight deaths (1.9%; CL 1%-3%) among their first 412 surgically treated cases.[G14] In 1955, Ash and Fischer reported no deaths (0%; CL 0%-6%) among 116 consecutive children (ages 4 months to 14 years) undergoing surgical closure.[A5] Other similar experiences reinforce the idea that the operation is safe and that hospital mortality approaches zero.[M6]

Incremental Risk Factors for Early Death

No risk factors for early death can be consistently identified. Operation in infancy or childhood, associated congenital anomalies, pulmonary hypertension, and mild or moderate increase of pulmonary vascular resistance do not increase the risk of hospital death, nor does the surgical technique used. However, by considering the entire span of time since Gross first successfully closed a PDA in 1938, certain situations can be presumed to increase risk.

When pulmonary vascular disease is severe and the shunt is bidirectional or dominantly right to left, risk is high; 5 of 14 such patients (36%; CL 21%-53%) died in the hospital in the early Mayo Clinic experience.[E5] Death was due to hemorrhage during operation (from the pulmonary artery suture line, because pulmonary artery pressure after closure was *higher* than systemic arterial pressure and the pulmonary artery was large and thin walled), or it occurred suddenly some days later without any demonstrable cause.[E5] However, no distinction with regard to reactivity of the pulmonary vascular bed was made in these patients. Thus, it is likely that with preoperative provocative testing, a subgroup of patients could be identified that would have lower operative risk.

When pulmonary vascular disease is mild or moderate, and thus when a large left-to-right shunt is present, there is no increased risk. Even in the early era, 16 among 271 patients undergoing repair of PDA at the Mayo Clinic had severe pulmonary hypertension but only mild or moderate pulmonary vascular disease and a large left-to-right shunt, and there were no (0%; CL 0%-11%) early or late deaths.[E5]

Older age minimally increases risk of surgical closure even in the absence of severe pulmonary vascular disease. This increase is principally from the technical problems posed by the friable and often calcified ductal wall in older patients, and the tendency of the long-standing volume overload of the left ventricle to predispose them to fatal arrhythmias. The mildly increased risk in the older age group is illustrated by the report of Black and Goldman in 1972, which described one death (2%; CL 0.2%-6%) in 53 adults (aged 14-55 years) undergoing surgical closure of a PDA. Death occurred at early reoperation for postoperative bleeding from a tear in the aorta.[B8] In recent years, the technical problems in older patients have been eased by use of an open technique (see Technique of Operation earlier in this chapter).

Time-Related Survival

Life expectancy is normal after surgical closure of an uncomplicated PDA in infancy or childhood. When moderate or severe pulmonary vascular disease has developed preoperatively, late deaths may result from its progression, as is the case in children with ventricular septal defect (see "Pulmonary Hypertension" under Results in Section I of Chapter 35).

When the operation is performed in adults with advanced chronic heart failure, premature late death is at times unavoidable. This is because the cardiomyopathy secondary to long-standing left ventricular volume overload is irreversible in some patients, in a way entirely analogous to the situation in patients with long-standing aortic valve regurgitation (see "Left Ventricular Structure and Function" under Results in Chapter 12).

Symptomatic and Functional Status

Disappearance of the signs and symptoms of heart failure is dramatic after surgical closure of a large PDA. Ash and Fischer recount that the marked hepatomegaly and splenomegaly in a 3-year-old girl with cardiac cachexia and advanced heart failure were no longer detectable 3 hours after surgical closure of the ductus, and cardiac size on chest radiography had returned to near normal within 4 months.[A5]

Physical Development

It has been presumed that when a large isolated PDA is closed in infancy, growth pattern becomes normal. However, growth retardation, particularly in regard to height, tends to persist, particularly when the operation is delayed beyond infancy or if the child has a rubella syndrome.[E7] The same may occur after repair of ventricular septal defect (see "Physical Development" under Results in Section I of Chapter 35).

Recurrence of Ductal Patency

Currently, prevalence of recurrent or persistent ductal patency approaches zero when division or appropriate ligation techniques are used.[L6,M6] In an earlier era, it did occur. In 1965, Jones reported 12 patients (20%; CL 14%-26%) with recurrent or persistent ductal patency out of 61 patients who had ductal ligation with heavy tape.[J5] Later, it became less common; Panagopoulos and colleagues reported only four cases (0.4%; CL 0.2%-0.8%) among 936 patients undergoing ductal closure, mostly by ligation.[P2] Trippestad and Efskind reported 20 among 639 traced cases (3.1%; CL 2.4%-4.0%).[T7]

False Aneurysm

False aneurysm is a rare complication of surgical ductal closure that usually occurs after ligation rather than division.[P3,P10,R7] Only rare cases of false aneurysm have been reported after ductal division, and these probably resulted from technical errors or infection.[C12,E3,H1,R5] Development of a false aneurysm is an indication for urgent reoperation.

Left Vocal Cord Paralysis

Transient and occasionally permanent left vocal cord paralysis resulting from manipulation or injury of the left recurrent laryngeal nerve occurs in 1% to 4% of patients following division or ligation of a PDA.[F2,M6] Prevalence is higher among infants with low birth weight.[B7,D2,F2,Z1]

Phrenic Nerve Paralysis

Phrenic nerve paralysis with elevation of the hemidiaphragm after PDA closure occurs in approximately 4% of patients.[F2] It usually occurs on the left side, usually in infants, and most frequently in preterm babies.[F2] It is not necessarily due to surgical damage to the phrenic nerve, because it may develop on the right side. It often regresses spontaneously but may persist for many months or indefinitely.

Chylothorax

Chylothorax is a rare complication of surgical ductal closure. Its management is discussed in Section II of Chapter 5.

INDICATIONS FOR OPERATION

Persistent PDA is an indication for closure, and the optimal age for operating is during the first year of life.[A5] Patients, either term or preterm, with *prolonged* PDA require closure in early life only when a large left-to-right shunt results in heart failure. In practice, this means that in term infants in the first month of life, PDA closure is indicated only when symptoms of heart failure are present. (For a discussion of the special situation in preterm infants, see "Patent Ductus Arteriosus in Preterm Infants" under Special Situations and Controversies later in this chapter.)

Beyond the first month of life, prophylactic closure of the PDA is indicated. In the absence of symptoms, operation may be delayed until about age 6 months. However, closure is indicated at any time before this when symptoms of heart failure or failure to thrive persist despite intense medical treatment. Older age is not a contraindication to closure of an isolated PDA in the absence of severe pulmonary vascular disease.

Severe pulmonary vascular disease is a contraindication to closure. The criteria of inoperability in this setting are the same as described for patients with ventricular septal defect (see Indications for Operation in Section I of Chapter 35). In the case of patients with PDA, the ductus may be temporarily occluded at operation; if pulmonary artery pressure does not decrease but remains severely elevated with no increase in aortic pressure, the shunt is *not* dominantly left to right. Closure of the ductus, therefore, will not reduce pulmonary artery pressure or left atrial pressure and therefore cannot trigger a favorable change in pulmonary vascular resistance. Repair is contraindicated in this situation. With preoperative provocative testing, abandoning closure in the operating room should be uncommon.

Until recently, indications for closure of PDA were indications for *operative* closure. This is probably still true in many institutions, but percutaneous closure must also be considered (see "Percutaneous [Catheter] Closure of Patent Ductus Arteriosus" under Special Situations and Controversies later in this chapter).

SPECIAL SITUATIONS AND CONTROVERSIES

Patent Ductus Arteriosus in Preterm Infants

Historical Note

In 1963, both Powell and De Cancq, independently, were apparently the first to close a PDA in a preterm infant by operation.[D3,P7] Subsequent improvement in the cardiovascular status of preterm infants after surgical closure of a PDA has been clearly demonstrated.[B3,J1]

Clinical Features and Diagnostic Criteria

The preterm infant with a PDA may have a continuous murmur, and under these circumstances diagnosis is made with confidence.[C8,E6] The shunt is considered large enough to be important if there is pulmonary plethora and cardiomegaly on the chest radiograph, if peripheral pulses are bounding, or if by echocardiography, the left atrial–aortic ratio is 1.5 or greater and Doppler color flow interrogation demonstrates a large left-to-right shunt.[J4]

A systolic murmur is less specific for PDA, but the diagnosis is made clinically if the murmur is associated with a hyperactive precordium, increased pulse pressure, or positive chest radiograph or echocardiogram. A few preterm infants have these positive clinical and laboratory findings of PDA without a murmur.[M8,T1]

Natural History

A high proportion of preterm infants have prolonged patency of the ductus arteriosus after birth. The frequency increases with decreasing gestational age and decreasing birth weight.[H7] Siassi and colleagues reported the presence of a PDA (based on presence of a long systolic murmur) in 77% of premature infants with a gestational age of 28 to 30 weeks, 44% with a gestational age of 31 to 33 weeks, and 21% with a gestational age of 34 to 36 weeks.[S3] Birth weights of less than 1000 g, 1000 to 1500 g, and 1500 to 2000 g were associated with a PDA prevalence of 83%, 47%, and 27%, respectively. Frequency of hemodynamically important PDA is less, however: approximately 40% when the birth weight is less than 1000 g and 10% when it is less than 1750 g.[E6,V2]

A PDA has the same hemodynamic effects in preterm infants as in term infants, as evidenced by collapsing pulses and radiographic evidence of increased pulmonary blood flow, left atrial enlargement, and cardiomegaly. Furthermore, experimental studies in preterm lambs have shown that the left-to-right shunt through the open ductus is associated with reduced effective systemic blood flow and organ hypoperfusion.[B4] This has led to the hypothesis that necrotizing enterocolitis in preterm infants may be associated with a large PDA, which is supported by results of a randomized trial of ductal closure in preterm babies and by other studies.[C3,V2]

A strong correlation exists between patency of the ductus arteriosus and idiopathic respiratory distress syndrome, although these may not be causally related.[E1,E2,T1] There is also an association between fluid administration and ductal patency; thus, PDA is less frequent in neonatal units that restrict fluids in preterm infants.[B5]

Technique of Operation

See Technique of Operation earlier in this chapter.

Special Features of Postoperative Care

Because surgical closure of a PDA is only one facet of care of a preterm infant, the patient is returned to the care of the neonatologist in the neonatal intensive care unit. The drainage catheter may be left until mechanical ventilation is no longer necessary, because pneumothorax occasionally develops in preterm infants maintained on a ventilator.

Early Results

Hospital mortality is approximately 10% to 20%.[H2,P1,P5,T8] It is not related to the interval between birth and operation, but, as in other circumstances in preterm infants, it is probably related to birth weight and gestational age. Death may be from continuing respiratory distress, intracranial hemorrhage, necrotizing enterocolitis, or a diffuse coagulopathy,[B10,P5] but it rarely occurs during the immediate perioperative period. In low-birth-weight preterm neonates, postoperative morbidity includes bronchopulmonary dysplasia, intraventricular hemorrhage, necrotizing enterocolitis, and retinopathy.[N1] There is no clear evidence that prevalence of intracranial hemorrhage is increased by surgical closure of the ductus.[S6] Whether ligation of the PDA is causally linked to these adverse outcomes remains to be determined.[N1]

Cardiac status usually improves immediately, and left atrial size is promptly reduced.[B10] At least one randomized study indicates overall benefit of early surgical closure of a PDA in preterm infants weighing less than 1500 g and requiring mechanical ventilation.[C11] Another randomized study of infants weighing 1000 g or less and requiring supplemental oxygen demonstrated reduction ($P = .001$) in necrotizing enterocolitis among those treated by early ligation.[C3]

Late Results

Among preterm infants requiring PDA closure, only half the hospital survivors are well 1 to 5 years later.[B10,D4] About one third have bronchopulmonary dysplasia on chest radiograph, with variable clinical findings. About one sixth have more severe complications, such as retrolental fibroplasia, blindness, and cerebral palsy.[B10,D4]

Indications for Operation

Recent publications have questioned the efficacy of PDA closure in preterm infants, whether by surgery or by pharmacologic therapy.[B6,N2] The analyses performed in these publications rely on review and meta-analysis of existing historical literature pertaining to management of PDA in premature infants. The retrospective nature of these analyses incorporates major assumptions and limits the veracity of the conclusions. The authors of these studies acknowledge that there currently are no randomized controlled prospective trials evaluating surgical closure, pharmacologic closure, and conservative medical management not aimed at closure, and that such studies are the only way to resolve this question definitively. Notwithstanding these opinions, the overwhelming consensus is that closure should be actively pursued in preterm infants with hemodynamically important PDA. Indications for operative closure of a PDA include respiratory distress (ventilator dependency and need for high FIO_2 in the absence of important shunt) and demonstration of a large PDA (collapsing pulses, left atrial enlargement by echocardiography, and a large $\dot{Q}p/\dot{Q}s$ by radionucleotide scanning). In many centers, closure is reserved for infants who do not respond to medical management, including a course of indomethacin or ibuprofen therapy, and for infants in whom pharmacologic therapy is contraindicated.[F7,H9,J3,O2,P4,V3] Failure of indomethacin treatment may approach 40% to 50%, particularly in low-birth-weight infants (<800 g).[P1,P5,T8] Surgical ligation should be considered the primary form of treatment in small preterm infants who have persistent cardiopulmonary compromise after pharmacologic therapy or an increased risk for development of complications from this therapy.[C3,G10,P5,J3]

Percutaneous (Catheter) Closure of Patent Ductus Arteriosus

Technical improvements and operator experience have made percutaneous closure of PDA an intervention of proven efficacy. Percutaneous closure is generally contraindicated in patients weighing less than 6 kg. Device closure was effective in 58 patients weighing 3.6 to 6.0 kg, but complication rates led these authors to conclude that surgical closure is first-line therapy.[A1] Two case reports document device closure in infants weighing 2.2 and 1.7 kg, but it is not recommended.[N3,P9] In earlier years, approximately 65% of patients had complete ablation of the shunt with this technique.[A4,R3] Currently, closure can be achieved in a high percentage of patients with umbrella or button coils or plugs.[B11,L4,L5,M4,R6,S2,S4,T2] Effective occlusion (no or trivial residual shunt) can be accomplished in up to 94% of patients.[F4,M1,R1,U1] Procedures are performed under local anesthesia and on an outpatient basis in many centers.[F3,M11,M13,P8,W1] Procedural mortality has been extremely low (1 of 1640 procedures [0.061%; CL 0.01%-0.21%] reviewed by Fortescue and colleagues).[F4] In this group of patients, embolization of the closure device occurred in 80 patients (4.9%; CL 4.3%-5.5%) and was successfully retrieved in 70. Aortic or LPA narrowing not requiring intervention occurred in 32 patients (2.0%; CL 1.6%-2.4%), significant hemolysis in 12 (0.73%; CL 0.52%-1.0%), and inguinal pseudoaneurysm or loss of pulse in 18 (1.1%; CL 0.83%-1.4%). Overall occurrence of minor complications was 8.8%.[F4] Procedural failure did not occur when PDA size was smaller than 1.5 mm. Infective endarteritis occurred in one patient, but follow-up to date is limited and variable in the reviewed studies. It is thus impossible to estimate the true risk of infective endarteritis with these techniques.[F4]

The ultimate role of outpatient closure of a PDA will be determined by its costs compared with those of operative closure, reproducibility of the results obtained, prevalence of complete and permanent closure, and occurrence of late complications resulting from a device residing in the ductus arteriosus.[F3,G6,G7,P1] Currently in patients with a PDA of large diameter or short length, surgical closure is advisable.

Thoracoscopic Closure of Patent Ductus Arteriosus

An alternative to percutaneous catheter closure of a PDA is thoracoscopic closure without thoracotomy. It is performed under general anesthesia using three or four incisions 3 to 7 mm in length in the left hemithorax.[L1,L2] The surgical field is viewed on a video screen. Once the ductus is dissected from the surrounding tissue, one or more clips are applied to close it. The technique has been used in neonates, children of all ages, and adults.[B12,C7,H10,L1] In the experience of Laborde and colleagues with 332 consecutive pediatric patients, mortality was zero (CL 0%-0.57%) and morbidity minimal.[L1] Three patients with persistent ductal patency required surgical closure. Subsequent series have confirmed the safety of the procedure, with no operative deaths.[D7,V1] When compared with open operation, more complications, particularly recurrent laryngeal nerve injury, occurred with the thoracoscopic technique.

REFERENCES

A

1. Abadir S, Boudjemline Y, Rey C, Petit J, Sassolas F, Acar P, et al. Significant persistent ductus arteriosus in infants less or equal to 6 kg: percutaneous closure or surgery? Arch Cardiovasc Dis 2009;102:533-540.
2. Abbott M. Atlas of congenital heart disease. New York: American Heart Association, 1936.
3. Acierno LJ. History of cardiology. New York: Parthenon, 1994.
4. Ali Khan MA, Mullins CE, Nihill MR, Yousef SA, Oufy SA, Abdullah M, et al. Percutaneous catheter closure of the ductus arteriosus in children and young adults. Am J Cardiol 1989;64:218.
5. Ash R, Fischer D. Manifestations and results of treatment of patent ductus arteriosus in infancy and childhood. An analysis of 138 cases. Pediatrics 1955;16:695.

B

1. Baden M, Kirks DR. Transient dilatation of the ductus arteriosus—the "ductus bump." J Pediatr 1974;84:858.
2. Balzer DT, Spray TL, McMullin D, Cottingham W, Canter CE. Endarteritis associated with a clinically silent patent ductus arteriosus. Am Heart J 1993;125:1192.
3. Baylen BG, Emmanouilides GC. Patent ductus arteriosus in the newborn. In Gregory GA, Thibeault DW, eds. Neonatal pulmonary care. Menlo Park, Calif: Addison-Wesley, 1979, p. 318.
4. Baylen BG, Ogata H, Ikegami M, Jacobs HC, Jobe AH, Emmanouilides GC. Left ventricular performance and regional blood flows before and after ductus arteriosus occlusion in premature lambs treated with surfactant. Circulation 1983;67:837.
5. Bell EF, Warburton D, Stonestreet BS, Oh W. Effect of fluid administration on the development of symptomatic patent ductus arteriosus and congestive heart failure in premature infants. N Engl J Med 1980;302:598.
6. Benitz WE. Treatment of persistent patent ductus arteriosus in preterm infants: time to accept the null hypothesis? J Perinatol 2010;30:241-252.
7. Benjamin JR, Smith PB, Cotten CM, Jaggers J, Goldstein RF, Malcolm WF. Long-term morbidities associated with vocal cord paralysis after surgical closure of a patent ductus arteriosus in extremely low birth weight infants. J Perinatol 2010;30:408-13.
8. Black LL, Goldman BS. Surgical treatment of the patent ductus arteriosus in the adult. Ann Surg 1972;175:290.
9. Blalock A. Operative closure of the patent ductus arteriosus. Surg Gynecol Obstet 1946;82:113.
10. Brandt B, Marvin WJ, Ehrenhaft JL, Heintz S, Doty DB. Ligation of patent ductus arteriosus in premature infants. Ann Thorac Surg 1981;32:167.
11. Bridges ND, Perry SB, Parness I, Keane JF, Lock JE. Transcatheter closure of a large patent ductus arteriosus with the clamshell septal umbrella. J Am Coll Cardiol 1991;18:1297.
12. Burke RP, Wernovsky G, van der Velde M, Hansen D, Castaneda AR. Video-assisted thoracoscopic surgery for congenital heart disease. J Thorac Cardiovasc Surg 1995;109:499.

C

1. Calder AL, Kirker JA, Neutze JM, Starling MB. Pathology of the ductus arteriosus treated with prostaglandins: comparisons with untreated cases. Pediatr Cardiol 1984;5:85.
2. Campbell M. Natural history of persistent ductus arteriosus. Br Heart J 1968;30:4.
3. Cassady G, Crouse DR, Kirklin JW, Strange MJ, Joiner CH, Godoy G, et al. A randomized controlled trial of very early prophylactic ligation of the ductus arteriosus in babies who weighed 1000 g or less at birth. N Engl J Med 1989;320:1511.
4. Cassels DE. The ductus arteriosus. Springfield, Ill: Charles C Thomas, 1973, p. 75.

5. Cetta F, Deleon SY, Roughneen PT, Graham LC, Lichtenberg RC, Bell TJ, et al. Cost-effectiveness of transaxillary muscle-sparing same-day operative closure of patent ductus arteriosus. Am J Cardiol 1997;79:1281.
6. Christie A. Normal closing time of the foramen ovale and the ductus arteriosus. Am J Dis Child 1930;40:323.
7. Chu JJ, Chang CH, Lin PJ, Liu HP, Tsai FC, Wu D, et al. Video-assisted thoracoscopic operation for interruption of patent ductus arteriosus in adults. Ann Thorac Surg 1997;63:175.
8. Clarkson PM, Orgill AA. Continuous murmurs in infants of low birth weight. J Pediatr 1974;84:208.
9. Clyman RI, Heymann MA. Pharmacology of the ductus arteriosus. Pediatr Clin North Am 1981;28:77.
10. Coster DD, Gorton ME, Grooters RK, Thieman KC, Schneider RF, Soltanzadeh H. Surgical closure of the patent ductus arteriosus in the neonatal intensive care unit. Ann Thorac Surg 1989;48:386.
11. Cotton RB, Stahlman MT, Bender HW, Graham TP, Catterton WZ, Kovar I. Randomized trial of early closure of symptomatic patent ductus arteriosus in small preterm infants. J Pediatr 1978;93:647.
12. Crafoord G. Discussion of paper by Gross RE. Complete division for the patent ductus arteriosus. J Thorac Surg 1947;16:314.
13. Cruickshank B, Marquis RM. Spontaneous aneurysms of the ductus arteriosus. Am J Med 1958;25:140.

D

1. Das JB, Chesterman JT. Aneurysms of the patent ductus arteriosus. Thorax 1956;11:295.
2. Davis JT, Baciewicz FA, Suriyapa S, Vauthy P, Polamreddy R, Barnett B. Vocal cord paralysis in premature infants undergoing ductal closure. Ann Thorac Surg 1988;46:214.
3. De Cancq HE Jr. Repair of patent ductus arteriosus in a 1417 g infant. Am J Dis Child 1963;106:402.
4. Dodge-Khatami A, Tschuppert S, Latal B, Rousson V, Doell C. Late morbidity during childhood and adolescence in previously premature neonates after patent ductus arteriosus closure. Pediatr Cardiol 2009;30:735-40.
5. DuBrow IW, Fisher E, Hastreiter A. Intermittent functional closure of patent ductus arteriosus in a ten-month old infant: hemodynamic documentation. Chest 1975;68:110.
6. d'Udekem Y, Rubay JE, Sluysmans T. A case of neonatal ductus arteriosus aneurysm. Cardiovasc Surg 1997;5:338.
7. Dutta S, Mihailovic A, Benson L, Kantor PF, Fitzgerald PG, Walton JM, et al. Thoracoscopic ligation versus coil occlusion for patent ductus arteriosus: a matched cohort study of outcomes and cost. Surg Endosc 2008;22:1643-8.

E

1. Edmunds LH Jr. Operation or indomethacin for the premature ductus. Ann Thorac Surg 1978;26:586.
2. Edmunds LH Jr, Gregory GA, Heymann MA, Kitterman JA, Rudolph AM, Tooley WH. Surgical closure of the ductus arteriosus in premature infants. Circulation 1973;48:856.
3. Egami J, Tada Y, Takagi A, Sato O, Idezuki Y. False aneurysm as a late complication of division of a patent ductus arteriosus. Ann Thorac Surg 1992;53:901.
4. Eggert LD, Jung AL, McGough EC, Ruttenberg HD. Surgical treatment of patent ductus arteriosus in preterm infants. Four-year experience with ligation in the newborn intensive care unit. Pediatr Cardiol 1982;2:15.
5. Ellis FH Jr, Kirklin JW, Callahan JA, Wood EH. Patent ductus arteriosus with pulmonary hypertension. J Thorac Surg 1956;31:268.
6. Ellison RC, Peckham GJ, Lang P, Talner NS, Lerer TJ, Lin L, et al. Evaluation of the preterm infant for patent ductus arteriosus. Pediatrics 1983;71:364.
7. Engle MA, Holswade GR, Goldbert HP, Glenn F. Present problems pertaining to patency of the ductus arteriosus. I. Persistence of growth retardation after successful surgery. Pediatrics 1958;21:70.

F

1. Falcone MW, Perloff JK, Roberts WC. Aneurysm of the nonpatent ductus arteriosus. Am J Cardiol 1972;29:422.
2. Fan LL, Campbell DN, Clarke DR, Washington RL, Fix EJ, White CW. Paralyzed left vocal cord associated with ligation of patent ductus arteriosus. J Thorac Cardiovasc Surg 1989;98:611.
3. Fedderly RT, Beekman RH 3rd, Mosca RS, Bove EL, Lloyd TR. Comparison of hospital charges for closure of patent ductus arteriosus by surgery and by transcatheter coil occlusion. Am J Cardiol 1996;77:776.
4. Fortescue EB, Lock JE, Galvin T, McElhinney DB. To close or not to close: the very small patent ductus arteriosus. Congenit Heart Dis 2010;5:354-65.
5. Franklin KJ. Ductus venosus (Arantii) and ductus arteriosus (Botalli). Bull Hist Med 1941;9:580.
6. French RK. The thorax in history. V. Discovery of the pulmonary transit. Thorax 1978;33:555.
7. Friedman WF, Hirschlau MJ, Printz MP, Pitlick PT, Kirkpatrick SE. Pharmacologic closure of patent ductus arteriosus in the premature infant. N Engl J Med 1976;295:526.
8. Fripp RR, Whitman V, Waldhausen JA, Boal DK. Ductus arteriosus aneurysm presenting as pulmonary artery obstruction: diagnosis and management. J Am Coll Cardiol 1985;6:234.

G

1. Gibson GA. Persistence of the arterial duct and its diagnosis. Edinb Med J 1900;8:1.
2. Gittenberger-de Groot AC. Persistent ductus arteriosus: most probably a primary congenital malformation. Br Heart J 1977;39:610.
3. Gittenberger-de Groot AC, Moulaert AJ, Harinck ME, Becker AE. Histopathology of the ductus arteriosus after prostaglandin E_1 administration in ductus dependent cardiac anomalies. Br Heart J 1978; 40:215.
4. Goncalves-Estella A, Perez-Villoria J, Gonzalez-Reoyo F, Gimenez-Mendez JP, Castro-Cels A, Castro-Llorens M. Closure of a complicated ductus arteriosus through the transpulmonary route using hypothermia. J Thorac Cardiovasc Surg 1975;69:698.
5. Graham EA. Aneurysm of the ductus arteriosus, with a consideration of its importance to the thoracic surgeon. Arch Surg 1940;41:324.
6. Gray DT, Fyler DC, Walker AM, Weinstein MC, Chalmers TC. Clinical outcomes and costs of transcatheter as compared with surgical closure of patent ductus arteriosus. The Patent Ductus Arteriosus Closure Comparative Study Group. N Engl J Med 1993;329:1517.
7. Gray DT, Weinstein MC. Decision and cost-utility analyses of surgical versus transcatheter closure of patent ductus arteriosus: should you let a smile be your umbrella? Med Decis Making 1998;18:187.
8. Graybial A, Strieder JW, Boyer NH. An attempt to obliterate the patent ductus arteriosus in a patient with subacute bacterial endocarditis. Am Heart J 1938;15:621.
9. Grollman JH Jr, Harris CH, Hamilton LC. Congenital diverticula of the aortic arch. N Engl J Med 1967;276:1178.
10. Grosfeld JL, Chaet M, Molinari F, Engle W, Engum SA, West KW, et al. Increased risk of necrotizing enterocolitis in premature infants with patent ductus arteriosus treated with indomethacin. Ann Surg 1996;224:350.
11. Gross RE. Complete division of the patent ductus arteriosus. J Thorac Surg 1947;16:314.
12. Gross RE. Complete surgical division of the patent ductus arteriosus. Surg Gynecol Obstet 1944;78:36.
13. Gross RE, Hubbard JP. Surgical ligation of a patent ductus arteriosus. Report of first successful case. JAMA 1939;112:729.
14. Gross RE, Longino LA. The patent ductus arteriosus. Observations from 412 surgically treated cases. Circulation 1951;3:125.
15. Gunning AJ. A simple, safe, surgical technique for closing the persistent ductus arteriosus in the preterm neonate. Ann R Coll Surg Engl 1983;65:214.

H

1. Hallman AL, Cooley DA. False aortic aneurysm following division and suture of a patent ductus arteriosus. Successful excision with hypothermia. J Cardiovasc Surg 1964;5:23.
2. Harting MT, Blakely ML, Cox CS Jr, Lantin-Hermoso R, Andrassy RJ, Lally KP. Acute hemodynamic decompensation following patent ductus arteriosus ligation in premature infants. J Invest Surg 2008;21:133-8.
3. Harvey W. The circulation of the blood. Franklin KJ, translator. Springfield, Ill: Charles C Thomas, 1958.
4. Hawkins JA, Minich LL, Tani LY, Sturtevant JE, Orsmond GS, McGough EC. Cost and efficacy of surgical ligation versus

transcatheter coil occlusion of patent ductus arteriosus. J Thorac Cardiovasc Surg 1996;112:1634.
5. Hay JD. Population and clinic studies of congenital heart disease in Liverpool. Br Med J 1966;2:661.
6. Heikkinen ES, Simila S, Laitinen J, Larmi T. Infantile aneurysm of the ductus arteriosus. Diagnosis, incidence, pathogenesis, and prognosis. Acta Paediatr Scand 1974;63:241.
7. Heymann MA. Patent ductus arteriosus. In Adams FH, Emmanouilides GC, eds. Heart disease in infants, children, and adolescents, 3rd ed. Baltimore: Williams & Wilkins, 1983.
8. Heymann MA, Rudolph AM. Control of the ductus arteriosus. Physiol Rev 1975;55:62.
9. Heymann MA, Rudolph AM, Silverman NH. Closure of the ductus arteriosus in premature infants by inhibition of prostaglandin synthesis. N Engl J Med 1976;295:530.
10. Hines MH, Bensky AS, Hammon JW Jr, Pennington G. Video-assisted thoracoscopic ligation of patent ductus arteriosus: safe and outpatient. Ann Thorac Surg 1998;66:853.
11. Houston AB, Gnanapragasam JP, Lim MK, Doig WB, Coleman EN. Doppler ultrasound and the silent ductus. Br Heart J 1991;65:97.

J

1. Jacob J, Gluck L, DiSessa T, Edwards D, Kulovich M, Kurlinski J, et al. The contribution of PDA in the neonate with severe RDS. J Pediatr 1980;96:79.
2. Jager BV, Wollenman OF Jr. An anatomical study of the closure of the ductus arteriosus. Am J Pathol 1942;18:595.
3. Jhaveri N, Moon-Grady A, Clyman RI. Early surgical ligation versus a conservative approach for management of patent ductus arteriosus that fails to close after indomethacin treatment. J Pediatr 2010;157:381-7.
4. Johnson GL, Breart GL, Gewitz MH, Brenner JI, Lang P, Dooley KJ, et al. Echocardiographic characteristics of premature infants with patent ductus arteriosus. Pediatrics 1983;72:846.
5. Jones JC. Twenty-five years' experience with the surgery of patent ductus arteriosus. J Thorac Cardiovasc Surg 1965;50:149.

K

1. Karwande SV, Rowles JR. Simplified muscle-sparing thoracotomy for patent ductus arteriosus ligation in neonates. Ann Thorac Surg 1992;54:164.
2. Keys A, Shapiro MJ. Patency of the ductus arteriosus in adults. Am Heart J 1943;25:158.
3. Kron IL, Mentzer RM Jr, Rheuban KS, Nolan SP. A simple, rapid technique for operative closure of patent ductus arteriosus in the premature infant. Ann Thorac Surg 1984;37:422.
4. Krovetz LJ, Warden HE. Patent ductus arteriosus. An analysis of 515 surgically proved cases. Dis Chest 1962;42:241.

L

1. Laborde F, Folliguet TA, Etienne PY, Carbognani D, Batisse A, Petrie J. Video-thoracoscopic surgical interruption of patent ductus arteriosus. Routine experience in 332 pediatric cases. Eur J Cardiothorac Surg 1997;11:1052.
2. Laborde F, Noirhomme P, Karam J, Batisse A, Bourel P, Saint Maurice O. A new video-assisted thoracoscopic surgical technique for interruption of patent ductus arteriosus in infants and children. J Thorac Cardiovasc Surg 1993;105:278.
3. Levine SA, Geremia AE. Clinical features of patent ductus arteriosus with special reference to cardiac murmurs. Am J Med Sci 1947; 213:385.
4. Lloyd TR, Fedderly R, Mendelsohn AM, Sandhu SK, Beekman RH 3rd. Transcatheter occlusion of patent ductus arteriosus with Gianturco coils. Circulation 1993;88:1412.
5. Lloyd TR, Rao PS, Beekman RH 3rd, Mendelsohn AM, Sideris EB. Atrial septal defect occlusion with the buttoned device (a multi-institutional U.S. trial). Am J Cardiol 1994;73:286.
6. Lucht U, Sondergaard T. Late results of operation for patent ductus arteriosus. Scand J Thorac Cardiovasc Surg 1971;5:223.

M

1. Magee AG, Stumper O, Burns JE, Godman MJ. Medium-term follow up of residual shunting and potential complications after transcatheter occlusion of the ductus arteriosus. Br Heart J 1994;71:63.
2. Majid AA. Closure of the patent ductus arteriosus with a Ligaclip through a minithoracotomy. Chest 1993;103:1512.
3. Mancini AJ. A study of the angle formed by the ductus arteriosus with the descending thoracic aorta. Anat Rec 1951;109:535.
4. Masura J, Walsh KP, Thanopoulous B, Chan C, Bass J, Goussous Y, et al. Catheter closure of moderate- to large-sized patent ductus arteriosus using the new Amplatzer duct occluder: immediate and short-term results. J Am Coll Cardiol 1998;31:878.
5. Matsushita T, Masuda S, Usui K, Yamada H. Spontaneous rupture of ductus arteriosus. Eur J Cardiothorac Surg 2009;36:396.
6. Mavroudis C, Backer CL, Gevitz M. Forty-six years of patent ductus arteriosus division at Children's Memorial Hospital of Chicago. Ann Surg 1994;220:402.
7. Mavroudis C, Cook LN, Fleischaker JW, Nagaraj HS, Shott RJ, Howe WR, et al. Management of patent ductus arteriosus in the premature infant: indomethacin versus ligation. Ann Thorac Surg 1983;36:561.
8. McGrath RL, McGuinness GA, Way GL, Wolfe RR, Nora JJ, Simmons MA. The silent ductus arteriosus. J Pediatr 1978;93:110.
9. McMurphy DM, Heymann MA, Rudolph AM, Melmon KL. Developmental change in constriction of the ductus arteriosus: response to oxygen and vasoactive substances in the isolated ductus arteriosus of the fetal lamb. Pediatr Res 1972;6:231.
10. Mitchell SC, Korones SB, Berendes HW. Congenital heart disease in 56,109 births. Incidence and natural history. Circulation 1971;43:323.
11. Mullins CE. Pediatric and congenital therapeutic cardiac catheterization. Circulation 1989;79:1153.
12. Munro JC. Surgery of the vascular system. Ligation of patent ductus arteriosus. Ann Surg 1907;46:335.
13. Musewe NN, Benson LN, Smallhorn JF, Freedom RM. Two-dimensional echocardiographic and color flow Doppler evaluation of ductal occlusion with the Rashkind prosthesis. Circulation 1989;80:1706.

N

1. Natarajan G, Chawla S, Aggarwal S. Short-term outcomes of patent ductus arteriosus ligation in preterm neonates: reason for concern? Am J Perinatol 2010;27:431-7.
2. Noori S. Patent ductus arteriosus in the preterm infant: to treat or not to treat? J Perinatol 2010;30:S31-S37.
3. Núñez FR, Álvarez AA, Trisac JL, Pardeiro CA. Percutaneous closure of patent ductus arteriosus in preterm infants. Rev Esp Cardiol 2010;63:740-41.

O

1. O'Donovan TG, Beck W. Closure of the complicated patent ductus arteriosus. Ann Thorac Surg 1978;25:463.
2. Ohlsson A, Walia R, Shah SS. Ibuprofen for the treatment of patent ductus arteriosus in preterm and/or low birth weight infants. Cochrane Database Syst Rev 2010:CD003481.

P

1. Palder SB, Schwartz MZ, Tyson KR, Marr CC. Association of closure of patent ductus arteriosus and development of necrotizing enterocolitis. J Pediatr Surg 1988;23:422.
2. Panagopoulos PH, Tatooles CJ, Aberdeen E, Waterston DJ, Bonham-Carter RE. Patent ductus arteriosus in infants and children: a review of 936 operations (1946-69). Thorax 1971;26: 1937.
3. Payne RF, Jordan SC. Postoperative aneurysms following ligation of the patent ductus arteriosus. Br J Radiol 1968;42:858.
4. Peckham GJ, Miettinen OS, Ellison RC, Kraybill EN, Gersony WM, Zierler S, et al. Clinical course to 1 year of age in premature infants with patent ductus arteriosus: results of a multicenter randomized trial of indomethacin. J Pediatr 1984;105:285.
5. Perez CA, Bustorff-Silva JM, Villasenor E, Fonkalsrud EW, Atkinson JB. Surgical ligation of patent ductus arteriosus in very low birth weight infants: is it safe? Am Surg 1998;64:1007.
6. Portsmann W, Wierny L, Warnke H, Gerstberger G, Romaniuk PA. Catheter closure of patent ductus arteriosus, 62 cases treated without thoracotomy. Radiol Clin North Am 1971;9:203.
7. Powell ML. Patent ductus arteriosus in premature infants. Med J Aust 1963;2:56.
8. Prieto LR, DeCamillo DM, Konrad DJ, Scalet-Longworth L, Latson LA. Comparison of cost and clinical outcome between

transcatheter coil occlusion and surgical closure of isolated patent ductus arteriosus. Pediatrics 1998;101:1020.
9. Prsa M, Ewert P. Transcatheter closure of a patent ductus arteriosus in a preterm infant with an Amplatzer vascular plug IV device. Catheter Cardiovasc Interv 2011;77:108-111.
10. Punsar S, Scheinin T, Tala P, Telivuo L. Postoperative aneurysm of the patent ductus arteriosus. Ann Chir Gynaecol (Fenn) 1962;51:385.

R

1. Rao PS, Kim SH, Choi JY, Rey C, Haddad J, Marcon F, et al. Follow-up results of transvenous occlusion of patent ductus arteriosus with the buttoned device. J Am Coll Cardiol 1999;33:820.
2. Rashkind WJ, Cuaso CC. Transcatheter closure of patent ductus arteriosus: successful use in a 3.5 kg infant. Pediatr Cardiol 1979;1:63.
3. Rashkind WJ, Mullins CE, Hellenbrand WE, Tait MA. Nonsurgical closure of patent ductus arteriosus: clinical application of the Rashkind PDA Occluder System. Circulation 1987;75:583.
4. Ravin A, Karley W. Apical diastolic murmur in patent ductus arteriosus. Ann Intern Med 1950;33:903.
5. Rosenkrantz JG, Kelminson LL, Paton BC, Vogel JH. False aneurysm after ligation of a patent ductus arteriosus. Ann Thorac Surg 1967;3:353.
6. Rosenthal E, Qureshi SA, Reidy J, Baker EJ, Tynan M. Evolving use of embolisation coils for occlusion of the arterial duct. Heart 1996;76:525.
7. Ross RJ, Feder FP, Spencer FC. Aneurysms of the previously ligated patent ductus arteriosus. Circulation 1961;23:350.
8. Rowe RD, Lowe JB. Auscultation in the diagnosis of persistent ductus arteriosus in infancy: a study of 50 patients. N Z Med J 1964;63:195.
9. Rudolph AM. The changes in the circulation after birth. Their importance in congenital heart disease. Circulation 1970;41:343.
10. Rudolph AM, Heymann HA, Spitznas U. Hemodynamic considerations in the development of narrowing of the aorta. Am J Cardiol 1972;30:514.

S

1. Santos MA, Moll JN, Drumond C, Araujo WB, Romano N, Reiss NB. Development of the ductus arteriosus in right ventricular outflow tract obstruction. Circulation 1980;62:818.
2. Schrader R, Hofstetter R, Fassbender D, Berger F, Bubmann WD, Ernst JM, et al. Transvenous closure of patent ductus arteriosus with Ivalon plugs. Multicenter experience with a new technique. Invest Radiol 1999;34:65.
3. Siassi B, Blanco C, Cabal LA, Coran AG. Incidence and clinical features of patent ductus arteriosus in low-birthweight infants: a prospective analysis of 150 consecutively born infants. Pediatrics 1976;57:347.
4. Sievert H, Niemoller E, Franz K, Kaltenbach M, Kober G, Rufenacht D, et al. Detachable balloon technique for transvenous closure of patent ductus arteriosus. J Interv Cardiol 1994;7:25.
5. Silver MM, Freedom RM, Silver MD, Olley PM. The morphology of the human newborn ductus arteriosus: a reappraisal of its structure and function with special reference to prostaglandin E_1 therapy. Hum Pathol 1981;12:1123.
6. Strange M, Myers G, Kirklin JK, Pacifico AD, Cassady G. Lack of effect of patent ductus arteriosus ligation on intraventricular hemorrhage in preterm infants. Clin Res 1983;31:913A.

T

1. Thibeault DW, Emmanouilides GC, Nelson RJ, Lachman RS, Rosengart RM, Oh W. Patent ductus arteriosus complicating the respiratory distress syndrome in preterm infants. J Pediatr 1975; 86:120.
2. Tometzki A, Chan K, De Giovanni J, Houston A, Martin R, Redel D, et al. Total UK multi-centre experience with a novel arterial occlusion device (Duct Occlud pfm). Heart 1996;76:520.
3. Touroff AS, Vesell H. Experiences in the surgical treatment of subacute *Streptococcus viridans* endarteritis complicating patent ductus arteriosus. J Thorac Surg 1940;10:59.
4. Touroff AS, Vesell H. Subacute *Streptococcus viridans* endarteritis complicating patent ductus arteriosus: recovery following surgical treatment. JAMA 1940;115:1270.
5. Tovar EA, Vana M Jr. VATS versus minithoracotomy for interruption of PDA in adults. Ann Thorac Surg 1997;64:1517.
6. Traugott RC, Will RJ, Schuchmann GF, Treasure RL. A simplified method of ligation of patent ductus arteriosus in premature infants. Ann Thorac Surg 1980;29:263.
7. Trippestad A, Efskind L. Patent ductus arteriosus. Surgical treatment of 686 patients. Scand J Thorac Cardiovasc Surg 1972;6:38.
8. Trus T, Winthrop AL, Pipe S, Shah J, Langer JC, Lau GY. Optimal management of patent ductus arteriosus in the neonate weighing less than 800 g. J Pediatr Surg 1993;28:1137.
9. Tutassaura H, Goldman B, Moes CA, Mustard WT. Spontaneous aneurysm of the ductus arteriosus in childhood. J Thorac Cardiovasc Surg 1969;57:180.

U

1. Uzun O, Dickinson D, Parsons J, Gibbs JL. Residual and recurrent shunts after implantation of Cook detachable duct occlusion coils. Heart 1998;79:220.

V

1. Vanamo K, Berg E, Kokki H, Tikanoja T. Video-assisted thoracoscopic versus open surgery for persistent ductus arteriosus. J Pediatr Surg 2006;41:1226-9.
2. van de Bor M, Verloove-Vanhorick SP, Brand R, Ruys JH. Patent ductus arteriosus in a cohort of 1338 preterm infants: a collaborative study. Paediatr Perinat Epidemiol 1988;2:328.
3. Vida VL, Lago P, Salvatori S, Boccuzzo G, Padalino MA, Milanesi O, et al. Is there an optimal timing for surgical ligation of patent ductus arteriosus in preterm infants? Ann Thorac Surg 2009;87: 1509-16.

W

1. Wessel DL, Keane JF, Parness I, Lock JE. Outpatient closure of the patent ductus arteriosus. Circulation 1988;77:1068.

Z

1. Zbar RI, Chen AH, Behrendt DM, Bell EF, Smith RJ. Incidence of vocal fold paralysis in infants undergoing ligation of patent ductus arteriosus. Ann Thorac Surg 1996;61:814.

38 Ventricular Septal Defect with Pulmonary Stenosis or Atresia

Section I Tetralogy of Fallot with Pulmonary Stenosis

DEFINITION

Tetralogy of Fallot (TF) is a congenital cardiac malformation characterized by underdevelopment of the right ventricular (RV) infundibulum, with anterior and leftward displacement of the infundibular (conal, outlet) septum and its parietal extension. Displacement (malalignment) of the infundibular septum is associated with RV outflow (pulmonary) stenosis (in extreme forms, atresia) and a large ventricular septal defect (VSD). Typically, the VSD is subaortic in position, but it may be beneath both the aorta and pulmonary trunk (juxta-arterial VSD) when the infundibular septum is absent. The RV and left ventricle (LV) are of equal thickness, and their systolic pressures are usually the same. The atrioventricular connection is concordant, and the aorta is biventricular in origin, overriding onto the RV. The amount of override varies widely. Importantly, there is fibrous continuity between the aortic and mitral valves (i.e., there is no subaortic infundibulum). This aorto-mitral fibrous continuity is the distinguishing morphologic characteristic separating TF from double outlet right ventricle with subaortic VSD (see Chapter 53).

This section considers only TF with pulmonary stenosis.

HISTORICAL NOTE

TF was first treated surgically by Blalock and Taussig in 1945, when they performed a palliative subclavian–pulmonary arterial shunt.[B16] Other types of systemic–pulmonary arterial shunts were introduced by Potts and colleagues in 1946,[P19] Waterston in 1962,[W4] Klinner in 1961,[K33,K34] Davidson in 1955,[D8] Laks and Castaneda in 1975,[L2] and de Leval and colleagues in 1981,[D11] among others. Palliation by direct relief of pulmonary stenosis with a closed technique was introduced by Sellors[S7] and Brock[B31,B32] in 1948.

TF was first successfully repaired by Lillehei and colleagues at the University of Minnesota in 1954 using controlled cross-circulation with another person serving as oxygenator.[L15] The first successful repair of TF using a pump-oxygenator was done by Kirklin and colleagues at the Mayo Clinic in 1955.[K26] Warden and Lillehei and colleagues introduced patch enlargement of the RV infundibulum in 1957,[W3] and Kirklin and colleagues reported using transanular patching in 1959.[K27] Use of an RV–pulmonary trunk conduit for TF with pulmonary atresia was reported by Kirklin and colleagues in 1965,[R3] and Ross and Somerville first reported use of a valved extracardiac conduit for this purpose in 1966.[R30] It was recognized very early that repairing TF in infants was associated with high mortality, and two-stage repair soon evolved. In 1969 at GLH, a policy of routine one-stage repair was adopted and later shown to provide good results.[B4,B5] However, a selective and more conservative approach with routine two-stage repair continued to be used by many surgeons.[A16,R20] Subsequently, a two-institution comparative study demonstrated one-stage repair to be equal or preferable to the two-stage approach.[K20] Prior to 1990, even those institutions practicing one-stage repair in neonates and infants generally only performed repair in the first 90 days of life in symptomatic patients, allowing asymptomatic patients to reach an older age or to develop symptoms before repair. Hanley and colleagues[P6] reported a policy of one-stage repair in early infancy in all patients with TF, regardless of symptomatic status. Symptomatic patients undergo repair at presentation, and asymptomatic patients electively at 6 to 8 weeks of life.

Thus, it has been almost 40 years since the first published reports of primary repair in neonates and infants, and more than 15 years since one-stage and two-stage repair have been compared with formal analysis. Nevertheless, current practice varies, both among individual surgeons and institutions, with one- and two-stage repair frequently practiced using varying protocols.

MORPHOLOGY

Developmental Considerations

TF with pulmonary stenosis encompasses a wide spectrum of morphologic subsets that vary primarily in details of RV outflow obstruction, VSD, and aortic overriding. All four major components of TF—RV outflow obstruction, VSD, overriding aorta, and RV hypertrophy—are linked embryologically. Van Praagh has advanced the concept of TF being the result of a "monology."[V2] The concept is that a small-volume subpulmonary infundibulum is the basic anomaly, resulting in pulmonary outflow tract obstruction (stenosis or atresia). There is a VSD because the small-volume infundibulum cannot fill the space above the trabecula septomarginalis (septal band; TSM) and the ventricular septum. The infundibular septum is malaligned anterosuperiorly above the RV (compared with normal) because of failure of normal expansile growth of the infundibulum. Failure of normal expansile growth of the infundibulum means that the infundibular outflow tract floor—the infundibular septum—fails to expand in a rightward, posterior, and inferior direction, thereby helping to close the interventricular foramen. Failure of this normal morphogenetic movement of the infundibular septum results in aortic overriding. Because the infundibular septum is abnormally anterosuperiorly malaligned above the RV, so too is the aortic valve, which is attached to what should be the LV outflow tract surface of the infundibular septum. RV hypertrophy is a secondary response to resulting RV afterload.[V1]

Thus, Van Praagh posits that embryologically, TF is a conotruncal malformation in which conotruncal septation is complete, but the infundibular septum is displaced. This anterior displacement is responsible for all of the morphologic characteristics of TF: crowding of the RV outflow tract and obstruction, overriding of the aorta, malalignment VSD, and RV hypertrophy.

Anderson, in contrast, argues that the "monology" concept is an oversimplification.[A14] His studies suggest two morphologic abnormalities that he considers pathognomonic for the lesion. (1) There is anterocephalad deviation of the outlet septum, but for obstruction of the RV outflow tract to occur, there must additionally be (2) an associated malformation of the septoparietal trabeculations, the muscular bars that reinforce the parietal wall of the RV. The squeeze produced between the malaligned outlet septum and the abnormally arranged septoparietal trabeculations identify the morphologic entity of tetralogy of Fallot.[A14]

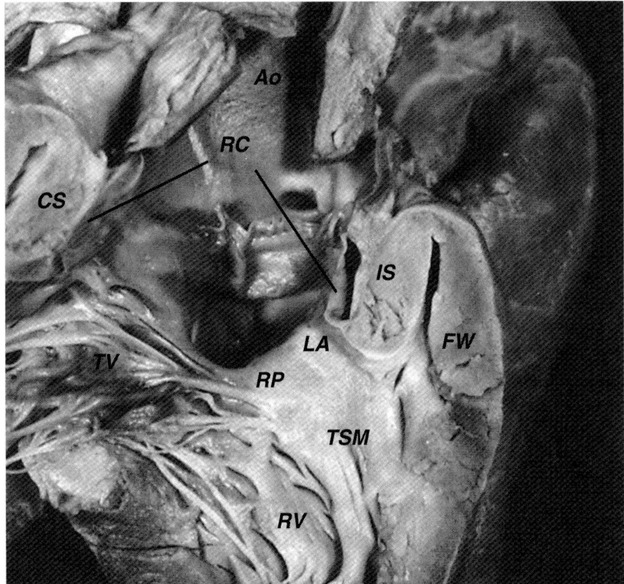

Figure 38-1 Autopsy specimen of tetralogy of Fallot with pulmonary stenosis, with right ventricle *(RV)* opened vertically and incision continued into overriding ascending aorta, dividing infundibular (outlet) septum and right aortic cusp transversely. Right aortic cusp clearly originates within the RV (overrides), its belly attaching to the infundibular septum and almost reaching its inferior edge. Septal end of infundibular septum is displaced anteriorly in front of the left anterior division of the trabecula septomarginalis (septal band; TSM). Right posterior division of TSM gives origin to tricuspid chordae (papillary muscle of the conus or medial papillary muscle). The gap between these two limbs of the TSM, which in a normal heart is occupied by the septal insertion of the infundibular septum, now forms inferior and anterior margins of ventricular septal defect, which is clearly related to this malalignment of the infundibular septum relative to the TSM. (In this and subsequent photographs of autopsied specimens, orientation is the traditional anatomic one. To view morphology as the surgeon does at operation, photograph needs to be rotated 90 degrees counterclockwise.) Key: *Ao,* Aorta; *FW,* anterior free wall; *IS,* infundibular septum; *LA,* left anterior division of trabecula septomarginalis; *RC,* right coronary cusp; *RP,* right posterior division of trabecula septomarginalis; *TSM,* trabecula septomarginalis; *TV,* tricuspid valve.

Right Ventricular Outflow Tract

Infundibulum

Infundibular stenosis associated with specific alterations in position of the infundibular septum is the hallmark of TF. Specifically, the septal (leftward) end of the infundibular septum is displaced anteriorly, inserting in front of the left anterior division of the TSM (septal band) (Fig. 38-1)[A12,V5] rather than between its two divisions, as in the normal heart (see Chapter 1, Fig. 1-5). In addition, the parietal (rightward) end of the infundibular septum is rotated anteriorly and passes anteriorly and inferiorly to reach the free wall of the RV (Fig. 38-2), so that the infundibular septum and its parietal extension may come to lie almost in a sagittal rather than the usual coronal (frontal) plane. Parietal and septal ends of the infundibular septum give rise to prominent muscle bands that attach to the right and left sides of the anterior RV free wall.[B12] The anterior free wall may show additional trabeculations or moderate thickening.

There is frequently a localized narrowing, the *os infundibulum*, which in 72% of cases lies in a transverse plane at the lower infundibular septal edge (see Fig. 38-2). This siting means that when the infundibular septum is well developed, there is a large infundibular chamber (or "third ventricle"; see Fig. 38-2), which in older patients occasionally becomes aneurysmal. In older patients, however, the os infundibulum is surrounded by fibrosis, which, when the chamber is small or absent, may extend into the RV–pulmonary trunk junction (pulmonary "anulus"). Less commonly (about 15% of cases), the major stenotic zone at the lower infundibular septal edge lies almost in a coronal plane, extending inferiorly from the lower infundibular septal edge. This occurs when hypertrophied muscle bands at the parietal end of the infundibular septum pass more inferiorly to join the free wall nearer to the RV apex, while on the septal (medial or leftward) aspect, there are not only inferiorly directed additional trabeculae, but also often an undue prominence and hypertrophy of TSM. Under these circumstances the inferior boundary of the os infundibulum may be formed by a prominent superiorly displaced moderator band.[A12] (When this type of low-lying infundibular stenosis is associated with a small or moderate-sized VSD, it is not termed TF; see Section V.) Both transverse and coronal plane stenoses are occasionally present.

When an *infundibular chamber* is present, its walls laterally and medially consist of numerous trabeculated spaces, some of which may form prominent blind recesses that do not lead directly to the valve "anulus," and occasionally an accessory opening is present. Endocardial fibrosis is not seen during the first 6 to 9 months of life and is seldom marked before age 2 years.[C23] Later, fibrosis seems to progress, which may lead to acquired infundibular atresia.

Generally, the infundibulum is somewhat longer, relative to total RV length, than it is in normal hearts.[B8,H29] When the infundibular septum is short (hypoplastic), infundibular stenosis reaches the pulmonary valve "anulus" without an intervening chamber. When the infundibular septum is absent, the VSD is juxta-arterial (doubly committed), extending superiorly to reach the pulmonary valve; infundibular stenosis is absent, and the posterior aspect of the RV outflow tract is formed by the VSD (Fig. 38-3).[N6] The pulmonary valve and sometimes its "anulus" are the main sites of the usually moderate stenosis in these hearts. However, once a VSD patch is in position, the hypertrophied RV walls and dextroposed aorta may combine with the patch to form severe subvalvar stenosis.

The infundibulum may be diffusely narrowed and hypoplastic. This is usually associated with severe cyanosis at birth or shortly thereafter. There is no localized os infundibulum (Fig. 38-4) nor increased trabeculations, nor important muscular hypertrophy. Nevertheless, stenosis is usually severe because narrowing occurs throughout the outflow tract (Fig. 38-5). Length of the stenosis in this morphologic variant is determined by length of the infundibular septum (see Fig. 38-4).

Pulmonary Valve

The pulmonary valve is stenotic to some degree in 75% of patients with TF. Approximately two thirds of stenotic valves are bicuspid (Table 38-1).[L9,N1] A three-cusp configuration occurs more commonly in nonstenotic valves. Even when nonstenotic, valve area is usually smaller than that of the

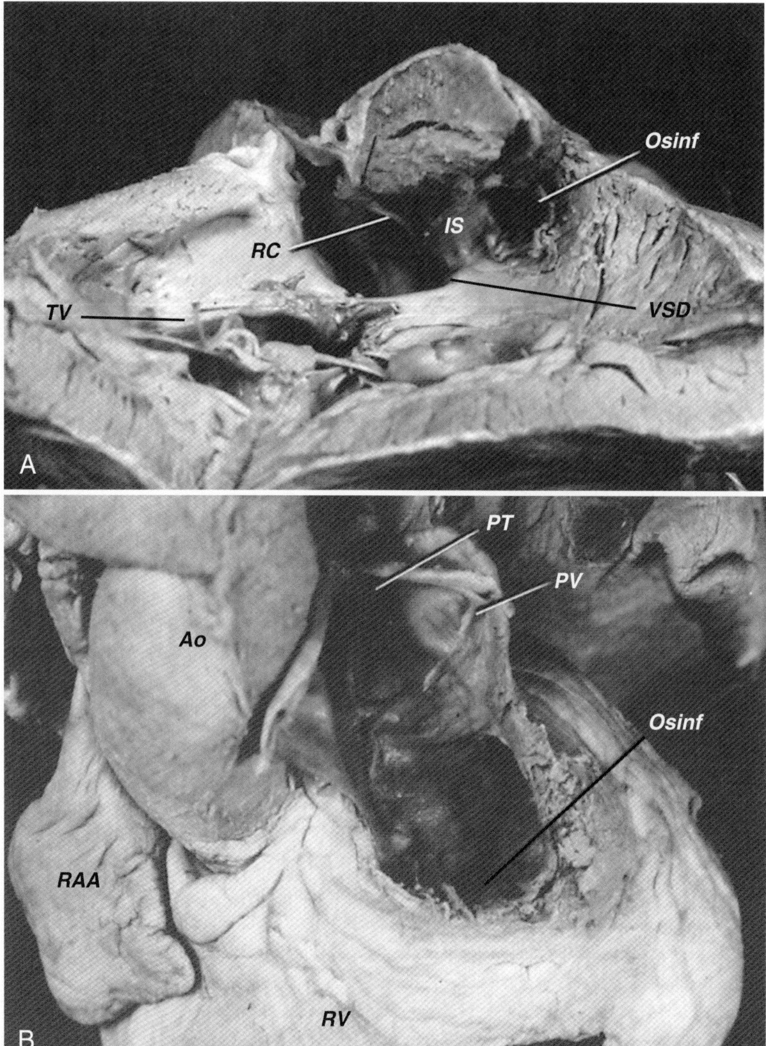

Figure 38-2 Autopsy specimen of tetralogy of Fallot with low-lying infundibular stenosis. Death occurred without surgical correction at age 3 years. **A,** Isolated infundibular stenosis viewed from below through opened right ventricle. **B,** Stenosis viewed from above after removing anterior wall of large infundibular chamber and opening front of pulmonary trunk. Stenosis is localized at lower border of infundibular septum (os infundibulum). Note that lateral (parietal) end of the septum is deviated anteriorly into almost a sagittal plane. Posterosuperior angle of ventricular septal defect is well seen *(arrow),* as is its proximity to right aortic cusp. Infundibular chamber is dilated and thin walled in association with the low, transversely placed infundibular stenosis. Pulmonary valve is tricuspid and not stenotic. Key: *Ao,* Aorta; *IS,* infundibular septum; *Osinf,* os infundibulum; *PT,* pulmonary trunk; *PV,* pulmonary valve; *RAA,* right atrial appendage; *RC,* right coronary cusp; *RV,* right ventricle; *TV,* tricuspid valve; *VSD,* ventricular septal defect.

aortic valve, which is the reverse of normal. The difference in size of these two valves is partly because the pulmonary valve is small and partly because the aortic valve is larger than normal.

Stenotic valve cusps are usually thickened, frequently severely so, a feature that increases the amount of obstruction at the valve level (Fig. 38-6). In approximately 10% of cases, cusps are replaced by sessile nubbins of fibromyxomatous tissue that offer little obstruction. Such vestigial valves are usually associated with a stenotic pulmonary "anulus." When the "anulus" is not severely narrowed and the valve is vestigial, severe pulmonary regurgitation results, a condition called *TF with absent pulmonary valve* (see Section III).

Pulmonary valve stenosis is usually caused by cusp tethering rather than by severe commissural fusion (see Table 38-1). The free edge of tethered cusps is considerably shorter than the diameter of the pulmonary trunk, so the valve cannot open adequately, and the pulmonary trunk is pulled inward at the point of commissural attachment. This produces a localized narrowing or corseting of the trunk at distal valve level. Thus, both the valve and trunk are tethered (see Fig. 38-6). In this situation the sinuses of Valsalva are frequently well formed, but entry into them between the cusp edge and pulmonary trunk wall is often also stenotic, resulting in slow filling of the sinuses with contrast medium on cineangiography. Cusps of a tethered valve may be fused for a short distance. Tethering is more common in a bicuspid valve, but can occur in a three-cusp valve.

Less commonly, the dominant morphology is thickened cusps associated with congenital commissural fusion, resulting in a concentric or eccentric stenotic orifice. An eccentric orifice can also result from a unicuspid configuration.

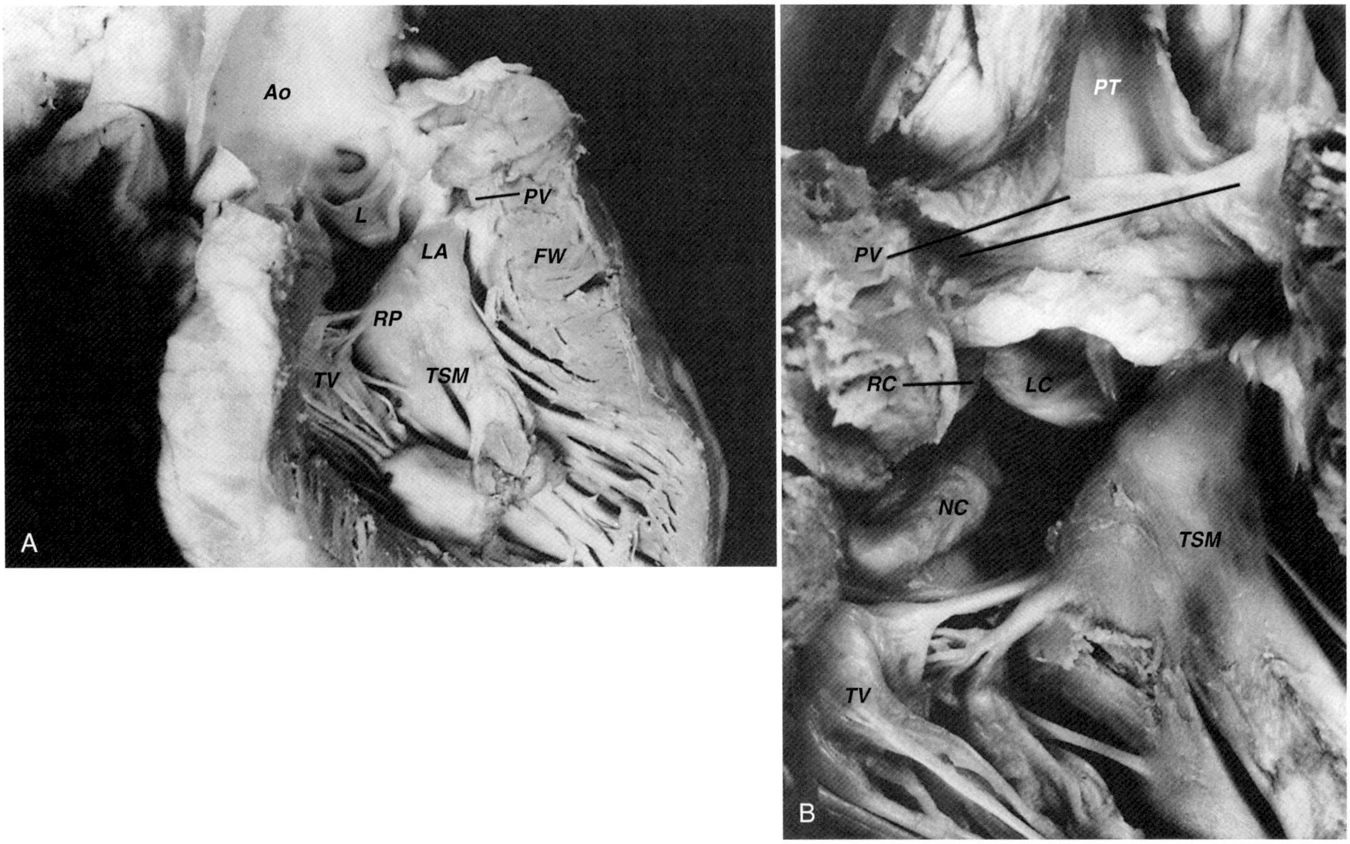

Figure 38-3 Autopsy specimen of tetralogy of Fallot with juxta-arterial ventricular septal defect (VSD). **A,** Viewed from opened right ventricle (RV) with incision carried across right cusp of aortic valve. **B,** Viewed after opening RV across pulmonary valve and trunk. Infundibular septum appears to be absent, and VSD is bounded superiorly by fused aortic and pulmonary valve "anuli." Trabecula septomarginalis (septal band) and RV free wall are severely hypertrophied. There is marked narrowing of pulmonary "anulus" and trunk and thickening and tethering of the valve cusps. Key: *Ao,* Aorta; *FW,* right ventricular free wall; *L,* left coronary cusp; *LA,* left anterior division at septal band; *LC,* left coronary aortic cusp; *NC,* noncoronary aortic cusp; *PT,* pulmonary trunk; *PV,* pulmonary valve; *RC,* right coronary aortic cusp; *RP,* right posterior division of septal band; *TSM,* trabecula septomarginalis (septal band); *TV,* tricuspid valve.

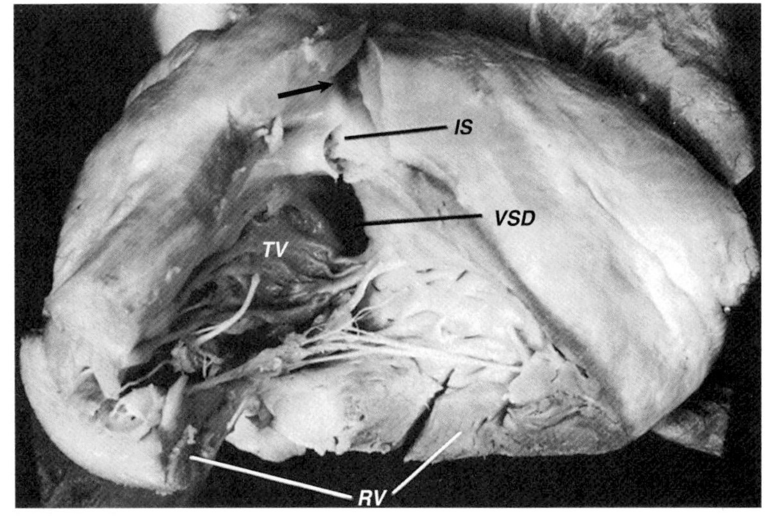

Figure 38-4 Autopsy specimen of tetralogy of Fallot with diffuse right ventricular *(RV)* outflow hypoplasia (same specimen as in Fig. 38-1). View is through opened RV. Stenotic infundibulum *(arrow)* is relatively short with a well-formed anteriorly displaced infundibular septum. There is no os infundibulum, but rather diffuse outflow tract narrowing without increased trabeculation or free wall thickening. Ventricular septal defect is conoventricular and perimembranous. Key: *IS,* Infundibular septum; *TV,* tricuspid valve; *VSD,* ventricular septal defect.

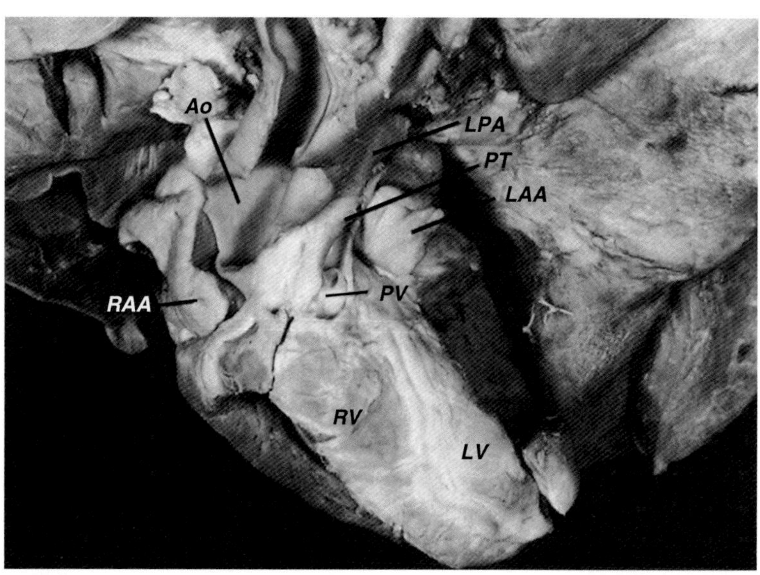

Figure 38-5 Specimen of tetralogy of Fallot with infundibular, valvar, and supravalvar pulmonary stenosis viewed from front. Aorta and pulmonary trunk have been opened. Pulmonary trunk is diffusely narrowed and continues directly into a left pulmonary artery of satisfactory size without any stenosis at its origin. Right pulmonary artery origin is not visible, passing at right angles directly beneath aorta. Key: *Ao,* Aorta; *LAA,* left atrial appendage; *LPA,* left pulmonary artery; *LV,* left ventricle; *PT,* pulmonary trunk; *PV,* pulmonary valve; *RAA,* right atrial appendage; *RV,* right ventricle.

Table 38-1 Pulmonary Valve Morphology in Tetralogy of Fallot[a]

Morphology	*n*	%
Valve Configuration		
Bicuspid	93	66
Three-cusp	21	15
Vestigial	14	10
Not recorded	13	9
Total	141	100
Valve Lesion		
Tethering alone	89	63
Commissural fusion alone	20	14
Tethering + fusion	8	6
Vestigial valve	14	10
Atretic valve (acquired)	2	1
Not recorded	8	6
Total	141	100

[a]Based on 141 patients undergoing repair (GLH experience, 1968-1978) of tetralogy of Fallot with pulmonary stenosis (excluding patients with subarterial ventricular septal defect, absent pulmonary valve, or congenital pulmonary atresia).

A fused stenotic pulmonary valve orifice may be beaded with tiny "vegetations" of fibrin. Progressive deposition of fibrin is presumably the mechanism of *acquired valvar atresia.*

Right Ventricular–Pulmonary Trunk Junction

The RV–pulmonary trunk junction is normally a muscular structure and, like the infundibulum, varies in diameter during the cardiac cycle. In TF, it is almost always smaller in diameter than the aortic "anulus" (the reverse of normal), and smaller than the normal junction. It is less likely to be stenotic when infundibular stenosis is low lying. The pulmonary "anulus" may become thick from fibrosis, which is usually an extension of endocardial thickening surrounding an intermediate- or high-level infundibular stenosis; in such cases, it is variably obstructive. It is small and obstructive when there is diffuse infundibular hypoplasia, resulting in diffuse RV outflow hypoplasia.

Pulmonary Trunk

Like the pulmonary valve and "anulus," the pulmonary trunk is nearly always smaller than normal, and smaller than the aorta. Reduction is most marked when there is diffuse RV outflow hypoplasia. Then, the pulmonary trunk is less than half the aortic diameter and is short (see Fig. 38-6), directed sharply posterior to its bifurcation. It is thus largely hidden from view at operation by the prominent aorta, which also displaces the origin of the trunk leftward and posteriorly.

When the pulmonary valve is markedly tethered, the pulmonary trunk is also tethered or corseted at its commissural attachments (see Fig. 38-6), and it may be very angulated or kinked at this point. This is the usual mechanism of supravalvar narrowing, and it is not associated with wall thickening. Rarely, however, there may be a discrete supravalvar narrowing beyond commissural level with diffuse wall thickening.

Pulmonary Trunk Bifurcation

The left pulmonary artery (LPA) is usually a direct continuation of the pulmonary trunk, with the right pulmonary artery (RPA) arising almost at right angles and close to it, but this pattern varies (Fig. 38-7). Uncommonly, the distal pulmonary trunk and origin of the RPA and LPA are moderately or severely narrowed *(bifurcation stenosis),* and in this situation the bifurcation may have a Y shape. A Y-shaped bifurcation is more common when the ductus arteriosus is absent (see "Aortic Arch and Ductus Arteriosus" later in this section).

Right and Left Pulmonary Arteries

Anomalies of the RPA and LPA are common in TF with pulmonary atresia (see Section II) but uncommon in TF with pulmonary stenosis, although any of the anomalies present in pulmonary atresia may occur in patients with

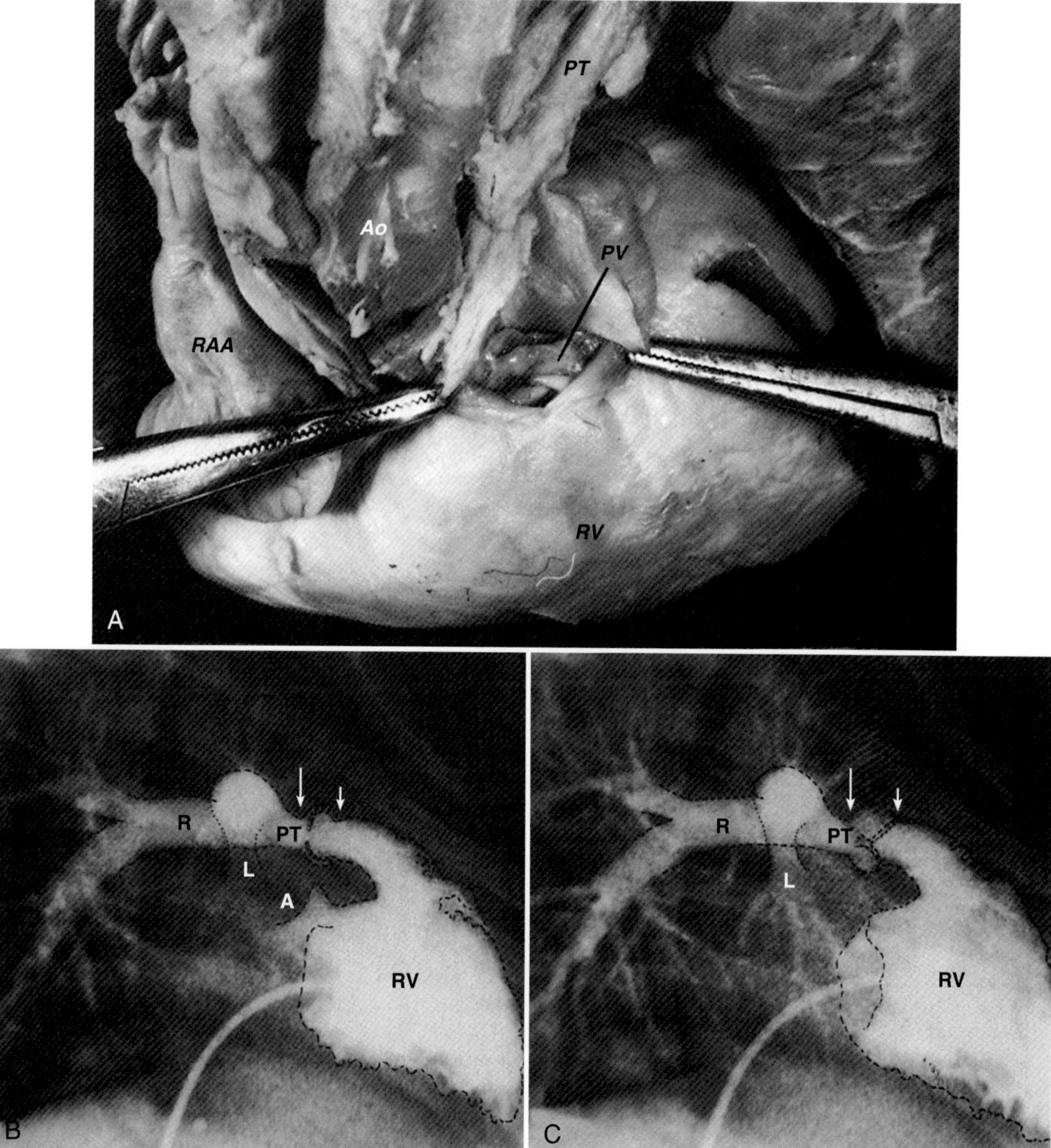

Figure 38-6 Specimen of tetralogy of Fallot showing thickened stenotic pulmonary valve *(PV)*, and right ventricular *(RV)* cineangiograms in the right anterior oblique projection showing same feature. **A,** Specimen showing stenotic PV viewed through opened pulmonary trunk *(PT)*. There are two thickened nonfused cusps, but PT wall is drawn inward where commissures attach (tethering). **B,** Early systolic frame. PV stenosis is due to valve tethering. Cusps are thickened and form a dome in systole from their attachments to pulmonary "anulus" *(small arrow)*. Supravalvar PT narrowing *(large arrow)* is localized to region between pulmonary sinuses and PT. **C,** Diastolic frame. Distal edges of thickened cusps remain approximated to narrowed PT wall, and the prominent sinuses may be slow to fill with contrast. Note shortness of PT. Key: *A,* Aortic valve; *Ao,* aorta; *L,* left pulmonary artery; *R,* right pulmonary artery; *RAA,* right atrial appendage. (From Calder and colleagues.[C2])

pulmonary stenosis (Table 38-2). Fellows and colleagues found pulmonary artery anomalies in 30% of infants having TF with pulmonary stenosis presenting in the first year of life.[F5] In particular, proximal LPA stenosis or hypoplasia, or both, can occur when certain configurations of the ductus arteriosus are present (see "Aortic Arch and Ductus Arteriosus" later in this section).

Distal Pulmonary Arteries and Veins

Pulmonary arteries and veins beyond the hilar positions are about normal in size in most patients.[H21,S10] Intraacinar arteries are smaller than normal, and their media are thinner.[J5] In addition, lung volume, alveolar size, and total alveolar number tend to be reduced.[H21,J5]

Dimensions of Right Ventricular Outflow Tract and Pulmonary Arteries

Hypoplasia of the RV outflow tract and pulmonary arteries in patients having TF with pulmonary stenosis is most marked centrally in the RV infundibulum and pulmonary trunk.[S10] On average, the RPA and LPA and their branches are not abnormally small. This does not deny the occasional existence of severe narrowing at the origin of the LPA or RPA (see Fig. 38-7). Elzenga and colleagues found juxtaductal proximal

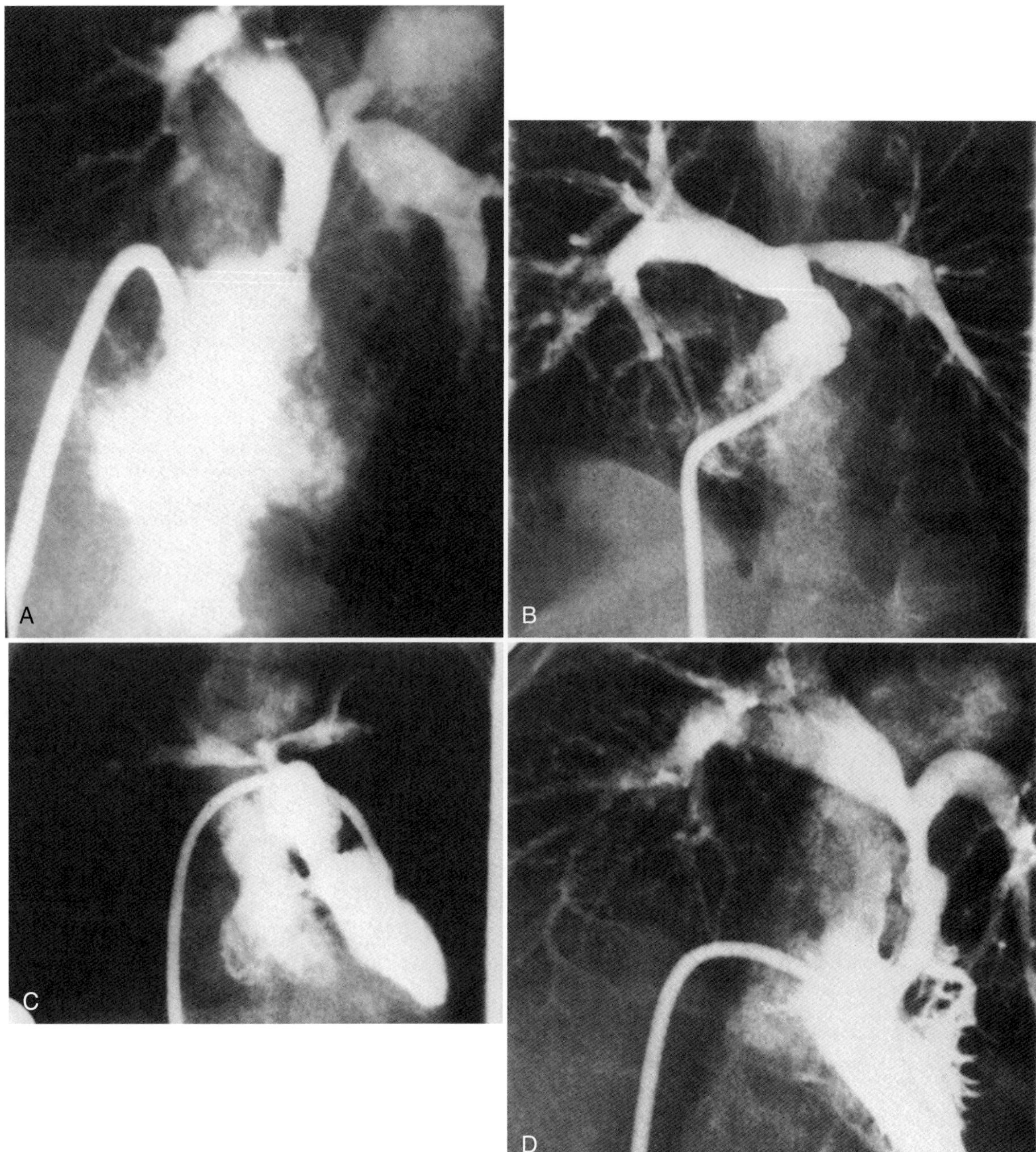

Figure 38-7 Cineangiograms after right ventricular injection showing stenoses at origins of pulmonary arteries in tetralogy of Fallot with pulmonary stenosis. **A,** Stenosis at origin of left pulmonary artery (LPA) in region of ductus arteriosus, which is closed at its aortic end. **B,** Stenosis at origin of LPA. This arrangement is unusual in that the LPA comes off at right angles. **C,** Bifurcation stenosis. Note that, as usual, the right pulmonary artery comes off at right angles to pulmonary trunk. **D,** Severe narrowing of distal pulmonary trunk. Note that first portion of LPA appears to be a continuation of pulmonary trunk.

stenoses of the LPA in 10% of patients having TF with pulmonary stenosis.[E9] There is great variability in these dimensions, however, making their careful pre-repair study important.

Convenient Morphologic Categories of Right Ventricular Outflow Obstruction

The nearly infinitely variable spectrum of RV outflow obstruction in TF can be conveniently categorized in a way that is surgically useful because it relates to difficulty in obtaining good relief of the pulmonary stenosis and therefore to surgical techniques and mortality (Box 38-1). This supplements earlier discussion of patterns of the infundibular portion of the obstruction. It might be inferred that transanular patching to relieve outflow tract obstruction would be more frequently required in those with "anulus" stenosis or diffuse hypoplasia, but a blanket rule is probably inappropriate.

Iatrogenic Pulmonary Arterial Problems

A transanular patch may later produce severe stenosis at the origin of the LPA or, less commonly, of the RPA.[F14]

Table 38-2 Major Associated Cardiac Anomalies in Patients Undergoing Repair of Tetralogy of Fallot[a]

	UAB, 1967 to 1982 (*n* = 713)		GLH, 1968 to 1978 (*n* = 205)		Total (*n* = 918)	
Anomaly	*n*	%	*n*	%	*n*	%
Multiple VSDs	20	2.8	2	1.0	22	2.4
Complete atrioventricular septal defect	20	2.8	0	0	20	2.2
Patent ductus arteriosus	29	4.1	8	3.9	37	4.0
Anomalous origin of LCA from pulmonary trunk	1	0.1	0	0	1	0.1
AP window	2	0.3	0	0	2	0.2
Subaortic stenosis	3	0.4	1	0.5	4	0.4
Moderate or severe aortic regurgitation	0	0	1	0.5	1	0.1
PAPVC	7	1.0	2	1.0	9	1.0
TAPVC	1	0.1	0	0	1	0.1
Unroofed coronary sinus	2	0.3	4	2.0	6	0.6
Straddling tricuspid valve	3	0.4	0	0	3	0.3
Small tricuspid valve anulus	2	0.3	0	0	2	0.2
Severe tricuspid regurgitation	2	0.3	1	0.5	3	0.3
Mitral stenosis	1	0.1	0	0	1	0.1
Dextrocardia	6	0.8	3	1.5	9	1.0
Situs ambiguous	2	0.3	0	0	2	0.2
Situs inversus totalis	2	0.3	3	1.5	5	0.5
Ebstein malformation	1	0.1	0	0	1	0.1
Underdeveloped RV	—	NT	3	1.5	3	0.3
RPA origin from ascending aorta	0	0	1	0.5	1	0.1
Pulmonary vascular disease	0	0	2	1.0	2	0.2
Endocarditis, RV outflow	0	0	2	1.0	3	0.2
TOTAL PATIENTS	87	12.2	26	13	113	12.3

[a]Categories are not mutually exclusive.
Key: *AP,* Aortopulmonary; *LCA,* left coronary artery; *NT,* not tabulated; *PAPVC,* partial anomalous pulmonary venous connection; *RV,* right ventricle; *RPA,* right pulmonary artery; *TAPVC,* total anomalous pulmonary venous connection; *VSD,* ventricular septal defect.

Box 38-1 Convenient Morphologic Categories of Right Ventricular Outflow Obstruction in Tetralogy of Fallot with Pulmonary Stenosis[a]

Isolated Infundibular Stenosis
This obstruction is encountered in a minority of cases. An infundibular chamber is usual when the level of stenosis is intermediate or low, but it may be absent when stenosis is high. When stenosis is at a low level, it is usually transversely oriented but may be in the coronal plane, and the infundibular chamber is usually large. Isolated infundibular stenosis may be at an intermediate level and transversely oriented. In this case, the infundibular septum is shorter than in the preceding type, and a moderate-sized or small chamber separates the stenotic zone from the pulmonary valve.

Infundibular Plus Valvar Stenosis
A combination of infundibular and valvar stenosis occurs in most cases. The valvar component may be due to an adequately sized "anulus" with leaflet obstruction, or to a hypoplastic "anulus." Low-level infundibular stenosis is less common than in isolated infundibular stenosis, but, again, when present it may be in either a transverse or coronal plane, or both. The pulmonary trunk may be diffusely small or tethered, but bifurcation stenosis is rare.

Diffuse Right Ventricular Outflow Hypoplasia
This morphologic subset is commonly seen in infants presenting with severe cyanosis. The pulmonary valve is usually bicuspid with thickened, tethered, stenotic cusps; the pulmonary "anulus" is small and obstructive; and the pulmonary trunk is half or less that of the aorta, often with associated tethering. The more severe the hypoplasia of the infundibulum and pulmonary trunk, the more severe is the narrowing of the first part of the right and left pulmonary arteries.

Dominant Valvar Stenosis
This obstruction is rare. The pulmonary "anulus" is frequently also stenotic, and when valve stenosis is produced by cusp tethering, the pulmonary trunk is also tethered. Infundibular stenosis is mild, but the infundibular septal deviation characteristic of tetralogy of Fallot is present. Examples of important valvar stenosis and a large ventricular septal defect without developmental anomalies of tetralogy of Fallot type in the infundibulum are uncommon (see Section V).

[a]These patterns of right ventricular infundibular obstruction are surgically useful, although they arbitrarily categorize what is in reality a continuous spectrum.

Important stenosis or kinking of an RPA or LPA may also be produced by an imprecise shunting operation (see "Technique of Shunting Operations" later in this section). The distal pulmonary artery may then become relatively hypoplastic because of poor pulmonary blood flow ($\dot{Q}p$).

Collateral Pulmonary Arterial Blood Flow

Patients virtually always have increased collateral pulmonary arterial blood flow, primarily from true bronchial arteries. Occasionally (less than 5% of patients), large aortopulmonary (AP) collateral arteries are present (see detailed discussion in "Alternative Sources of Pulmonary Blood Flow" in Section II).

Ventricular Septal Defect

In classic TF, the VSD is juxta-aortic and usually lies adjacent to or involves the membranous septum (conoventricular and perimembranous). It differs from the usual isolated VSD, however, in that it is associated with malalignment of the infundibular septum (see Fig. 38-2) and is virtually always large. Anterior displacement (malalignment) of the infundibular septum relative to the crest of the ventricular septum creates the VSD, rather than a deficiency of tissue. The infundibular septum may or may not be deficient or hypoplastic (see next paragraph), but deficiency of tissue is not necessary for the VSD to be present

The defect is more U-shaped than circular and is bounded superiorly and anteriorly by the free edge of the infundibular

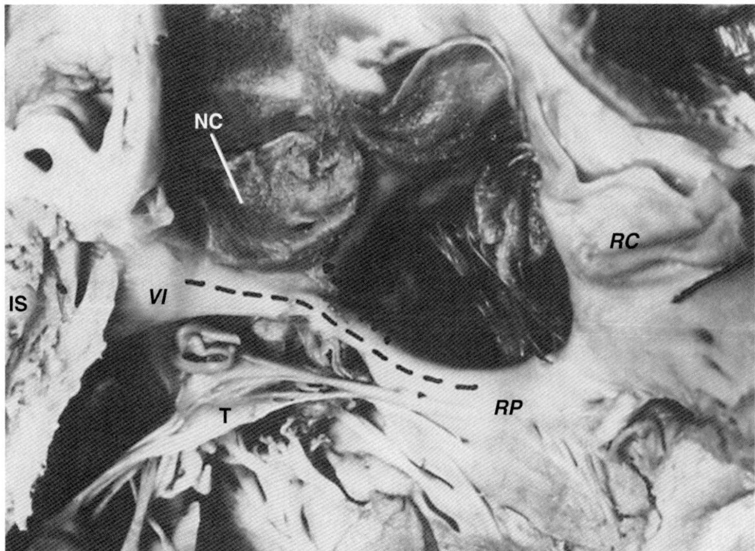

Figure 38-8 Specimen of tetralogy of Fallot demonstrating ventricular septal defect (VSD) and position of bundle of His. A narrow muscular bridge separates VSD from anterior tricuspid leaflet and tricuspid anulus. Right ventricle (RV) has been opened and the incision carried across infundibular septum and right coronary cusp *(RC)* out into the ascending aorta, as shown in Fig. 38-1. Narrow muscular bridge separating VSD from tricuspid valve is the continuity between right posterior division of trabecula septomarginalis and ventriculoinfundibular fold *(VI)*. VI joins the undersurface of the parietal end of infundibular septum. Sutures can be passed safely into this ridge along dashed line (or, alternatively, in base of tricuspid leaflet), but the margin for error is small because the course of the bundle of His *(dotted line)* is not far removed. Note marked RV overriding of RC. Key: *IS,* Infundibular septum; *NC,* noncoronary cusp; *RP,* right posterior division of trabecula septomarginalis (septal band); *RV,* right ventricle; *T,* anterior tricuspid leaflet.

septum (see Fig. 38-4). The septum may support part or most of the right aortic cusp, depending on the degree of aorta overriding the RV (see Fig. 38-1). Because of the anterior and leftward deviation of the parietal end (parietal extension) of the infundibular septum, the *posterosuperior* angle of the defect extends higher than that of the usual isolated conoventricular VSD (see Fig. 38-2, *A*) and can be more difficult to expose surgically, particularly if the parietal band is not fully mobilized (transected). When the infundibular septum is hypoplastic, the defect is larger and extends closer to the pulmonary valve; when the infundibular septum is absent, the VSD becomes juxtapulmonary (and juxta-arterial).

Posterosuperiorly, the VSD is bounded by muscle (the ventriculoinfundibular fold) adjacent to the rightward edge of the noncoronary aortic cusp (Fig. 38-8). This cusp may override considerably onto the RV (Fig. 38-9); then, the LV-aortic junction adjacent to the noncoronary cusp forms this boundary.

The *posterior* margin is variable. It is related to the base of the tricuspid anteroseptal leaflet commissure and to the right fibrous trigone (central fibrous body) at the nadir of the noncoronary aortic cusp. There is tricuspid-aortic-mitral fibrous continuity at this margin, and the membranous septum is absent—characteristics of a true perimembranous VSD. In some hearts the VSD extends inferiorly beneath the tricuspid septal leaflet more than usual, described as "inlet extension" of the VSD. When there is marked clockwise rotation of the overriding aortic root, the right trigone may form the posteroinferior angle of the defect, and the bundle of His (which perforates at this point) is exposed along the edge of the defect (Fig. 38-10). Occasionally the posterior margin may be formed by a remnant of fibrous tissue

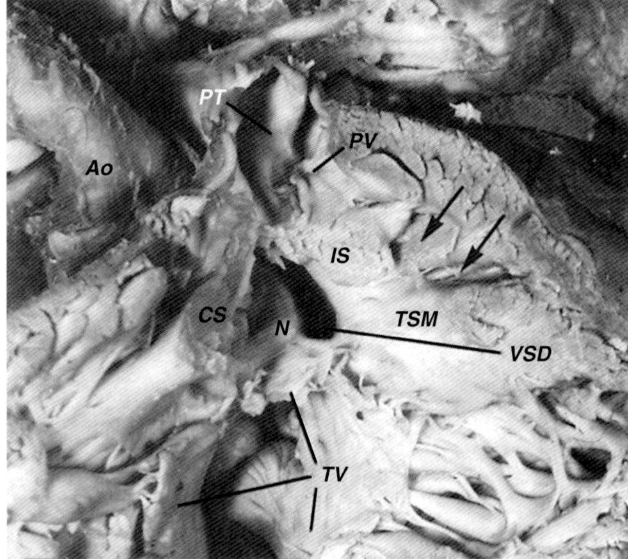

Figure 38-9 Specimen of tetralogy of Fallot with right ventricle and pulmonary trunk opened with an anterior incision and infundibular septum divided to expose ventricular septal defect. Accessory prominent muscular trabeculations are present in front of septal attachment of infundibular septum *(arrows)*, contributing to stenosis. Pulmonary valve is bicuspid and tethered, with mild cusp thickening. Marked overriding of aorta is visible, involving rightward margin of noncoronary cusp. Key: *Ao,* Aorta; *IS,* infundibular septum; *N,* noncoronary cusp; *PT,* pulmonary trunk; *PV,* pulmonary valve; *TSM,* trabecula septomarginalis; *TV,* tricuspid valve; *VSD,* ventricular septal defect.

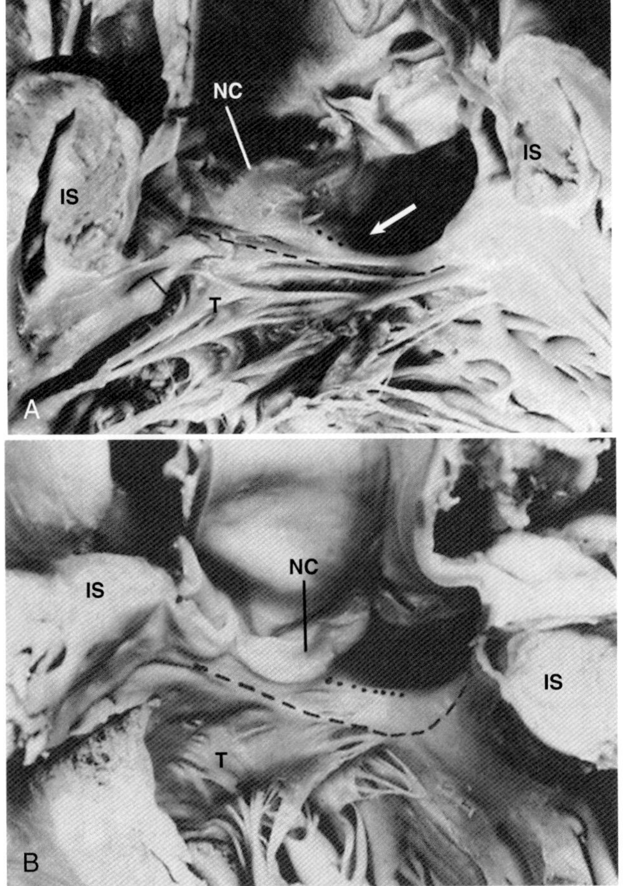

Figure 38-10 Two specimens of tetralogy of Fallot with perimembranous ventricular septal defect (VSD), opened as in Fig. 38-8. There is tricuspid-aortic-mitral fibrous continuity at the posterior margin (leftward in the photograph) of the VSD. **A,** Right fibrous trigone at nadir of noncoronary aortic cusp has been perforated by a pin passed from right atrial side at point of penetration of bundle of His; bundle extends from this point forward and slightly leftward along margin of VSD *(dotted line).* White arrow points to this area. VSD patch suture line must pass into base of septal tricuspid leaflet *(dashed line)* and not along lower VSD margin. **B,** Position of right fibrous trigone when there is important clockwise rotation of aortic root and right ventricular overriding of noncoronary and right aortic cusps. Bundle position is shown by dotted line and position of VSD suture line (passing into base of anterior tricuspid leaflet) by dashed line. Key: *IS,* Infundibular septum; *NC,* noncoronary cusp; *T,* tricuspid valve.

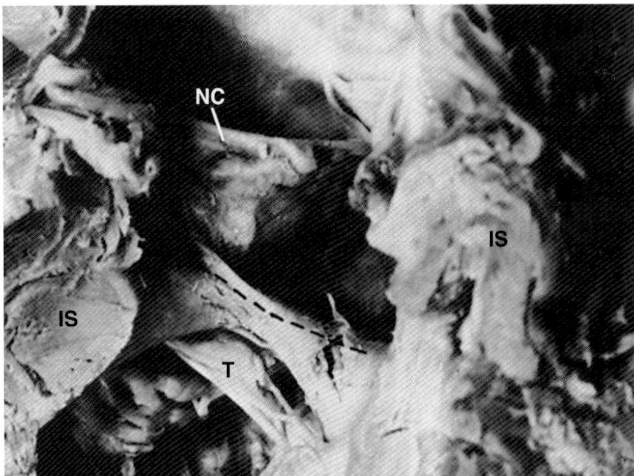

Figure 38-11 In this heart with tetralogy of Fallot, posterior muscular bridge is bulky and entirely hides right trigone that lies several millimeters caudal and leftward of margin of ventricular septal defect. His bundle will not be damaged by sutures passed into ridge along dashed line. Key: *IS,* Infundibular septum; *NC,* noncoronary cusp; *T,* tricuspid valve.

(membranous septum) projecting upward from the right trigone region. This tissue, also called the *membranous flap,* does not contain conduction tissue, and it can receive some of the sutures used to secure the VSD patch.[K41] Suzuki and colleagues found such a flap in about half of 158 TF hearts.[S32] Kurosawa and Imai[K40] found at least a remnant in all 68 of their surgical cases. In at least 20% of hearts, the posterior margin is formed by a muscular ridge of variable size that separates the right trigone from the base of the anterior tricuspid leaflet.[A9,B10,R10,S19] This ridge is formed by the right posterior division of the TSM as it becomes continuous with the ventriculoinfundibular fold (Fig. 38-11; see also Fig. 38-8). It displaces the right trigone and therefore the bundle of His away from the defect edge.

The *inferior* margin of the VSD is formed by the TSM as it cradles the VSD between its limbs. The papillary muscle of the conus (or corresponding chordae only) arises from the right posterior division of the TSM at the *anteroinferior* angle of the defect. Anomalous tricuspid chordal attachments to other margins of the defect are rare, in contrast to the situation in isolated perimembranous VSD.

The *anterior* margin of the VSD is formed by the leftward anterior division of the TSM as it becomes continuous with the inferior margin of the infundibular septum. When the TSM is poorly developed, the defect extends further anteriorly, and the VSD is described as having "anterior extension."

When the infundibular septum is absent, the VSD is juxta-arterial[N6] and is described as having "outlet extension." Posteriorly, this type of VSD is commonly separated from the tricuspid anulus by a 2- to 5-mm strip of muscle, but it may extend to the anulus. Aortic and pulmonary valve "anuli" are contiguous over about one third of their circumferences, being separated at this point by only a thin fibrous ridge where the infundibular septum would have been, if present (see Fig. 38-3). The two valves are often side by side, with the aorta more than usually dextroposed.[S19] TF with this type of VSD is morphologically similar to double outlet RV with a doubly committed (juxta-arterial) VSD (see Chapter 53), with the important distinction that in TF, fibrous continuity is maintained between the aortic valve and the central fibrous body, whereas in double outlet RV there is infundibular muscle beneath the aortic valve, and thus there is fibrous discontinuity between the aortic valve and central fibrous body.

In 3% to 15% of patients (see Table 38-2), one or more additional VSDs coexist with the typical juxta-aortic one (Fig. 38-12).[F5] Usually the additional VSD is muscular, and multiple muscular defects sometimes occur. It may also be in the inlet septum, either as an inlet septal VSD or a muscular defect (see "Inlet Septal Ventricular Septal Defect" under Morphology in Section I of Chapter 35).

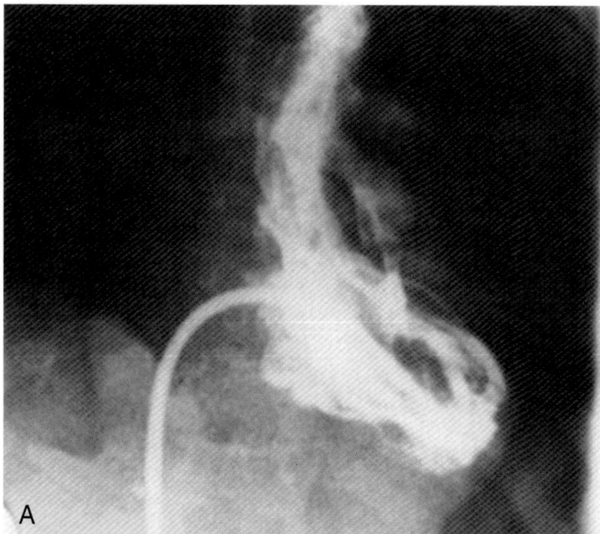

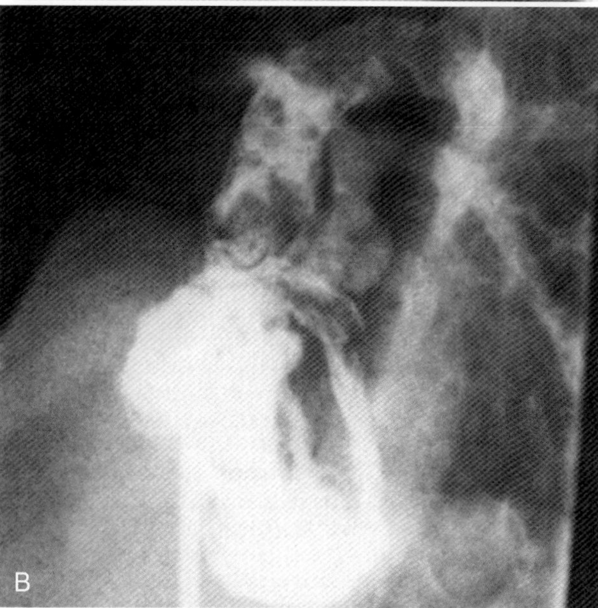

Figure 38-12 Cineangiograms of tetralogy of Fallot, pulmonary stenosis, and multiple ventricular septal defects (VSD). Note large trabecular VSD near apex as well as usual conoventricular VSD. **A,** Systolic frame. **B,** Diastolic frame.

Conduction System

The *sinus and atrioventricular nodes* are in their normal locations (see "Conduction System" in Chapter 1), and the bundle of His follows the same general course as in patients with isolated perimembranous VSDs (see "Location in Septum and Relationship to Conduction System" under Morphology in Section I of Chapter 35). Thus, the His bundle emerges through the right fibrous trigone at the base of the noncoronary cusp of the aortic valve and courses forward toward the papillary muscle of the conus along the inferior VSD margin or slightly to the left side of the defect edge.[F3,L8] In hearts showing marked clockwise rotation of the aortic root with RV overriding, the right trigone (and along with it the penetrating portion of the His bundle) is carried more rightward and superiorly and directly onto VSD margins (see Fig. 38-10).

By contrast, the bundle of His does not lie on the VSD margin when a muscle ridge is present (see Figs. 38-8 and 38-11),[D15] because the ridge projects superiorly above the right fibrous trigone; when the ridge is bulky, sutures can be safely placed into it.[B11]

Aorta

The aorta is biventricular in origin and more anteriorly placed than normal, often almost obscuring the smaller pulmonary trunk from view at operation. These changes are due to RV overriding, rotation, and enlargement of the aortic root. The proportion of aorta lying above the RV varies between 30% and 90%.[A12] Generally, about 50% of the aortic orifice is over the RV.

Aortic overriding is associated with a variable degree of clockwise rotation of the aortic root (as viewed from below). This rotation moves the base of the noncoronary cusp rightward and superiorly onto the posterosuperior margin of the VSD and away from the base of the anterior mitral leaflet so that in extreme cases, it may no longer be continuous with this structure. This cusp may then lie in part just beneath the extension of the infundibular septum. Rightward rotation of the left aortic cusp results in more of it becoming continuous with the anterior mitral leaflet. Simultaneously, the superiorly positioned right cusp moves to the left, and in extreme examples it may be just beneath the uppermost extension of the left anterior division of the trabecula septomarginalis at the anterosuperior VSD margin. An important point is that, despite the degree of aortic rotation, continuity of some portion of the aortic "anulus" and the anterior mitral leaflet is always maintained. As a result the VSD is always related to the aorta in TF. The VSD may *also* be related to the pulmonary valve when the infundibular septum is absent (see "Ventricular Septal Defect" in this section).

Degree of overriding and clockwise rotation of the aortic root relates to degree of underdevelopment of the RV outflow tract and to deviation (malalignment) of the infundibular septum. When these are minimal, as seen with isolated low-lying infundibular stenosis, the aorta is minimally affected; when there is diffuse RV outflow tract hypoplasia in association with a small, markedly deviated infundibular septum and posterior and leftward movement of the pulmonary trunk origin, the aorta is markedly rotated and dextroposed.

In patients with severe TF, the aortic root is larger than normal, even in infants. Occasionally in adults, it is greatly dilated. This may result in aortic valve regurgitation.

Aortic Arch and Ductus Arteriosus

The *ductus arteriosus* is absent in about 30% of patients born with TF. This does not mean a closed ductus (ligamentum arteriosum), but rather complete absence of any ductal structure. Absence of the ductus or ligamentum is about twice as common when there is a right, rather than left, aortic arch. The pulmonary artery bifurcation often takes on a Y-shaped configuration, also described as the "staghorn" or "seagull" configuration, in this setting. In the other 70% of patients in whom a ductal structure is present, it is patent at birth and closes over a normal time course unless pharmacologically maintained with PGE_1 for therapeutic reasons (cyanosis). The configuration of the ductus can vary from normal (an extension of the pulmonary trunk, creating an arch that somewhat parallels the aortic arch and inserts into the distal aortic isthmus) to abnormal, approximating the ductus orientation seen in pulmonary atresia (arising from the LPA and inserting more proximally into the aortic arch, without forming an arch). When the RV outflow tract obstruction is mild or moderate, the ductal configuration is more normal, reflecting ductal flow from the pulmonary trunk to aorta during fetal life, and more like that in pulmonary atresia when the RV outflow tract obstruction is severe, reflecting ductal flow from aorta to pulmonary trunk during fetal life. When the ductus originates from the LPA, the short proximal segment of LPA between the pulmonary trunk and ductus may be hypoplastic, and the LPA at the ductus insertion may become stenotic or even occluded when the ductus closes (so-called LPA coarctation). Rarely, there is physical discontinuity between the LPA and pulmonary trunk, with the isolated LPA arising from the ductus or ligamentum (Fig. 38-13).

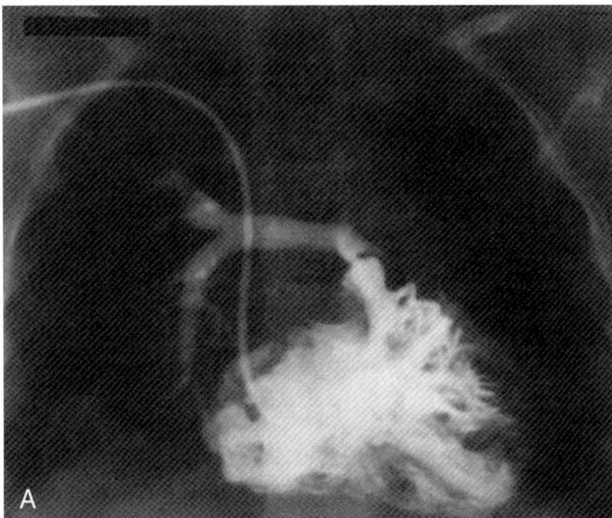

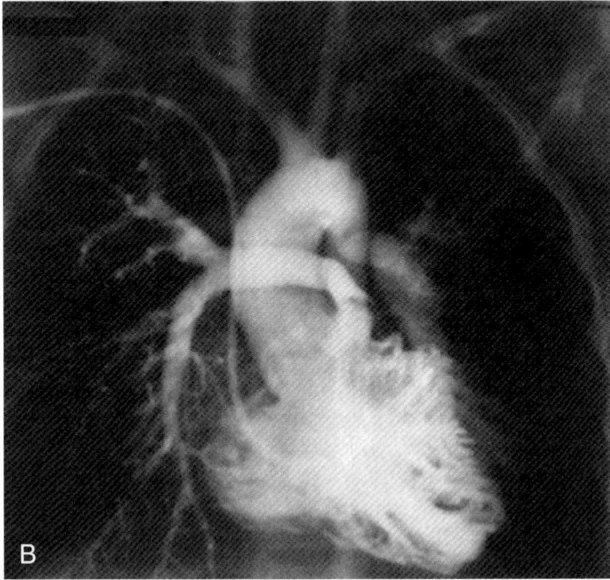

Figure 38-13 Cineangiogram of tetralogy of Fallot and absence of central portion of left pulmonary artery (LPA). **A,** Right ventricular injection shows lack of connection between pulmonary trunk and LPA. **B,** Later phase shows that hilar portion of LPA originates from ductus arteriosus.

A *left aortic arch* is present in about 75% of patients. In these, arch branching pattern is usually normal.

A *right aortic arch* is present in about 25% of patients. In 90% of these, there is mirror-image branching of the arch. Should a patent ductus arteriosus be present, it usually arises from the brachiocephalic or proximal left subclavian artery and joins the LPA.[S14] Rarely, there may be a right-sided ductus arteriosus to the RPA, usually arising from the upper descending thoracic aorta. In about 10% of patients, there is an aberrant left subclavian artery, analogous to the aberrant right subclavian artery of dysphagia lusoria in left aortic arch (see "Right Aortic Arch with Aberrant Left Subclavian Artery" in Section I of Chapter 51). In right aortic arch with aberrant left subclavian artery, the subclavian artery may arise directly from the descending aorta or from an aortic diverticulum. Thus, a ductus arteriosus may arise from the aortic diverticulum and pass to the left behind the esophagus to join the LPA.

Rarely, the left subclavian artery is sequestered or isolated from its aortic arch origin, but remains connected to the LPA by a patent ductus arteriosus. Often in these circumstances, there is vertebral steal, and on angiography the subclavian artery fills with contrast from the vertebral artery.

Right Ventricle

External dimensions of the sinus (inflow) portion of the RV are larger than normal due to hypertrophy, so the interventricular groove is displaced leftward and the LV lies more posteriorly than usual (clockwise rotation of ventricles). The RV sinus may be clearly separated from the infundibulum during systole by a transverse depression representing the site of maximal infundibular stenosis inferior to an infundibular chamber. RV wall thickness equals that of the LV and is therefore never excessive unless the large VSD is made restrictive by a fibrous flap valve on its right side (see Section IV). Normal trabeculations are, however, bulky and prominent. RV end-diastolic volume may be reduced and ejection fraction mildly depressed,[G24] typically in older children without TF repair, possibly the result of chronic hypoxia. Rarely (1.5% of cases), the sinus portion of the RV and tricuspid valve are underdeveloped (see Table 38-2).

Left Ventricle

The LV is usually normal in wall thickness[M3] but variable in volume. In patients with severe forms of TF with severe cyanosis, LV end-diastolic volume is normal or somewhat small,[L9,L10] but wall thickness remains normal. Uncommonly, the LV and mitral valve are truly hypoplastic,[G26] and rarely this may be so severe (end-diastolic volume < 30 mL $\cdot$ m^{-2}) as to contraindicate primary repair.[G26,N3]

The physiologic contributors to LV size are complex. The small pulmonary and thus left atrial blood flow tend to result in a small left atrium[M24,N1] and LV. However, the RV ejects blood into the LV as well as the aorta,[M24] and this tends to increase LV size. Mild or moderate degrees of LV hypoplasia may result from these physiologic factors, but true hypoplasia is of morphologic rather than functional origin.

LV systolic function is normal at birth but may become mildly reduced in older patients who have not undergone repair, particularly in severely cyanotic patients,[G25] presumably because of chronic hypoxia.

Table 38-3 Minor Associated Cardiac Anomalies in Patients Undergoing Repair of Tetralogy of Fallot with Pulmonary Stenosis or Atresia (*n* = 836)[a]

Anomaly	*n*	% of 836
Atrial septal defect	75	9
Persistent left superior vena cava	68	8
Anomalous origin of LAD from RCA	34	4
Aberrant origin of right subclavian artery	2	0.3
Absent right superior vena cava	1	0.2
Azygos extension of inferior vena cava	1	0.2
Congenital heart block	1	0.2
Juxtaposition of atrial appendages	1	0.2
Vascular ring	1	0.2

[a]UAB experience (1967 to July 1982).
Key: *LAD,* Left anterior descending coronary artery; *RCA,* right coronary artery.

Coronary Arteries

As in other cyanotic conditions, the coronary arteries become dilated and tortuous in children and adults. A large conal branch of the right coronary artery (RCA) usually courses obliquely across the free wall of the RV, and the presence of this vessel should be noted at the time of surgical repair.

The left anterior descending coronary artery (LAD) arises anomalously from the RCA in about 5% of patients (Table 38-3).[D1,F4,F5] The entire LAD may originate from the RCA and cross the anterior wall of the infundibulum a variable distance from the pulmonary valve, or only the distal part of the LAD may arise anomalously, in this case usually from the large conal branch of the RCA.

Rarely, the RCA originates from the left coronary artery, and equally uncommonly, there is anomalous origin of the left coronary artery from the pulmonary trunk (see Section II of Chapter 46).[A4]

Major Associated Cardiac Anomalies

Major associated cardiac anomalies are relatively uncommon (see Table 38-2). *Patent ductus arteriosus, multiple VSDs,* and *complete atrioventricular septal defect*[Z5] are most often seen.

Rarely, the RPA[K39] or LPA[M32] arises anomalously from the ascending aorta[K32] (see Chapter 45). This complicates the pathophysiology and repair, because the lung supplied by the pulmonary artery arising from the aorta usually has overcirculation, and the other usually has restricted flow due to the intracardiac anatomy.

Infrequently, *aortic valve regurgitation* coexists. This may be from typical cusp prolapse in TF with subarterial VSD (see Section II in Chapter 35).[M13] A bicuspid aortic valve occurs rarely in TF and may result in aortic regurgitation.[G19,V4] Occasionally, ill patients with TF in the second decade of life or older develop aortic regurgitation from endocarditis.[B7,C6] Massive dilatation of the aortic root from anuloaortic ectasia may result in aortic valve regurgitation,[C6] particularly in patients with large natural or surgically created systemic–pulmonary arterial shunts (see "Anastomotic" under Morphology in Chapter 26).

Minor Associated Cardiac Anomalies

Most infants undergoing repair of TF have a patent foramen ovale (PFO); when all ages are considered, a true atrial septal defect is found at operation in about 10%. Other minor associated cardiac anomalies are listed in Table 38-3.

CLINICAL FEATURES AND DIAGNOSTIC CRITERIA

Clinical Presentation

The hallmark clinical sign of TF is cyanosis. The severity of cyanosis and its variability depend on the specific morphology of the RV outflow tract. Infants with diffuse RV outflow hypoplasia, severe infundibular plus valvar plus anular stenosis, or severe infundibular plus valvar stenosis (see Box 38-1) are deeply cyanotic from birth and do not develop heart failure. They are breathless on feeding or other exertion. Hypoxic spells are rare, the cyanosis being constant and gradually worsening. It is seldom lessened by propranolol.

This situation contrasts with that in infants having dominant infundibular stenosis, in which onset of cyanosis is delayed and hypoxic (cyanotic) spells due to infundibular spasm may occur. These spells are often prevented or lessened in frequency by propranolol. Characteristically, they become less frequent with age, presumably because stenosis becomes fixed as a result of acquired endocardial fibrosis and thickening.

In up to 10% of patients who require surgical relief in infancy, presentation is initially as a large VSD with pulmonary plethora and sometimes heart failure at age 2 to 3 months, followed by gradually increasing cyanosis, frequently with cyanotic spells, at about age 6 months. In this group, stenosis is purely infundibular.

A minority of patients are acyanotic at rest and only mildly cyanotic during exercise because pulmonary stenosis is mild and right-to-left shunting minimal. In some the shunt is predominantly left to right. These individuals may remain acyanotic without spells and present at any age within the first or second decades of life with gradually increasing cyanosis and breathlessness as stenosis slowly increases in severity.

In patients with severe cyanosis and polycythemia, cerebral thrombosis may precipitate hemiplegia at any age (particularly in association with dehydration), or hemiplegia may follow paradoxical embolism or a brain abscess. The latter is heralded by fever, headache, and sometimes seizures. Massive hemoptysis may occur in older patients who are severely cyanotic, presumably from rupture of bronchial collateral vessels.

Cyanosis is always accompanied by effort dyspnea that is sometimes the dominant symptom, and as the child begins to walk (frequently much later than for a healthy child), cyanosis is often accompanied by squatting, which lessens its severity.[K28] There may be increased occurrence of respiratory infection, but not to the same extent as in patients with large isolated VSD; failure to thrive is also less striking.

Physical Examination

Cyanosis of variable degree is generally evident. Deeply cyanotic infants are often obese (in contrast to infants with isolated VSD). Severe symmetric clubbing of the fingers and toes is often present in children and adults, but not in infants.

Older patients may also have marked acne of the face and anterior chest. Jugular venous pressure is normal. The heart is not enlarged and is relatively quiet with an unimpressive RV lift. In those few patients with increased $\dot{Q}p$, the lift may be more marked than usual.

A precordial systolic thrill is rare. There is a moderate-intensity midsystolic pulmonary (ejection) murmur maximal in the second and third left intercostal spaces that becomes less prominent or even disappears when the stenosis is severe. When there is still a reasonable blood flow in the presence of moderate pulmonary stenosis, the systolic murmur is well heard posteriorly and in the axilla. In the presence of important cyanosis and low $\dot{Q}p$, the second heart sound is single, but in acyanotic patients it may be finely split with a low-intensity pulmonary component. Splitting is also present in moderately cyanotic patients with only a mildly reduced $\dot{Q}p$ when there are important pulmonary artery origin stenoses.

Signs of heart failure with venous pressure elevation and liver enlargement occur in patients with a systemic-to–pulmonary arterial shunt that is too large, or in a neonate on PGE_1 to maintain ductal patency. Heart failure may also appear in untreated severely cyanotic adults in the fourth or fifth decade of life, presumably secondary to myocardial fibrosis or in association with systemic hypertension or aortic regurgitation.

Laboratory Studies

Neonates or young infants who have severe TF with pulmonary stenosis usually present with marked reduction of arterial oxygen pressure ($Pa{O_2}$) and saturation ($Sa{O_2}$) and sometimes with metabolic acidosis. Polycythemia is rarely present, and, in fact, such infants are often anemic.

In older infants and children, red blood cell count and hematocrit are usually elevated, and degree of elevation is correlated with degree of arterial desaturation and thus with severity of the pulmonary stenosis. In older patients, hematocrit may reach 90%.

Most cyanotic patients have depressed platelet count and prolongation of most coagulation tests.

Chest Radiography

Chest radiographs in children usually show the typical boot-shaped heart of TF. In neonates and young infants the heart may be strikingly small, with an absent pulmonary artery segment along the left upper cardiac border and oligemic lung fields. In older patients, there may be a prominence of the left upper cardiac border caused by a large infundibular chamber. Large AP collaterals may alter the pulmonary blood flow pattern in one or both lungs. Plethora of one lung and oligemia of the other suggest anomalous origin of a pulmonary artery from the ascending aorta (see Chapter 45).

If there is a right aortic arch, posterior indentation of the shadow of the barium-filled esophagus results from an aberrant left or right subclavian artery.

Rib notching of the upper ipsilateral ribs may develop in the presence of a long-standing classic Blalock-Taussig (B-T) shunt, secondary to development of a rich collateral blood flow to the arm. This situation is rarely encountered in the current era because the classic B-T shunt is not commonly performed. Presumably, the same pathophysiology could develop after a modified B-T shunt if the subclavian artery were severely stenotic or occluded. Rarely, collaterals from the pleura to the lung may be sufficiently large, especially after poudrage or pleural stripping procedures, to result in bilateral rib notching in the lower half of the thorax. Patients in the second or third decade of life may show progressive kyphoscoliosis.

Electrocardiography

Electrocardiography (ECG) shows moderate RV hypertrophy consistent with RV pressure that is equal to but not greater than systematic pressure (in contrast to flap valve VSD; see Section IV). Occasionally, there is minimal RV hypertrophy, and in these circumstances RV underdevelopment should be suspected, although it may not be present. Left precordial leads are characterized by absent Q waves and low-voltage R waves. Occasionally the frontal plane vectorcardiographic pattern characteristic of atrioventricular septal defect is found in patients with typical TF.

Echocardiography

ECG is considered the definitive diagnostic procedure of choice in neonates and infants. The VSD, atrial septal status, aortic overriding, narrowing of the RV infundibulum, pulmonary valve, pulmonary trunk and bifurcation into the branch pulmonary arteries, and the ductus arteriosus, if present, can usually be seen with ECG (Fig. 38-14). Also, in experienced hands, two-dimensional (2D) echocardiography with Doppler color-flow interrogation has the same sensitivity and specificity for multiple VSDs in TF as does cineangiography. However, morphologic details of distal pulmonary artery branches as they approach the hilum may not be reliably visualized. Additional imaging is indicated when important abnormalities of the branch pulmonary arteries are identified, such as hypoplasia, discontinuity, or stenosis, and when abnormal arterial signals on Doppler interrogation are identified in the central and posterior mediastinum, suggestive of major AP collaterals.

Color Doppler imaging can also provide important physiologic information. Accurate estimates of the severity of obstruction across the RV outflow tract, as well as the site of obstruction (infundibular, valvar, supravalvar), can be obtained. Flow characteristics across the VSD and LV outflow tract can be used to confirm that pressures in the RV and LV are equal. Systolic function of the ventricles and competency of the inlet valves are also easily assessed, and flow patterns across the inlet valves in diastole can provide important information about ventricular diastolic function. In most cases the coronary artery pattern can be characterized, and anomalous patterns, such as the LAD arising from the RCA, can be identified.

Newer modalities of echocardiography, such as 3D echo, tissue Doppler, and strain rate imaging, hold further promise as noninvasive tools for improved morphologic and functional evaluation.[D2] Echocardiography can effectively diagnose TF in the fetus,[Y5] and can be helpful in planning early surgical intervention and in parental counseling.[H27]

In patients who have undergone operation for TF, whether palliative procedures or definitive repair, and in unoperated TF patients presenting well beyond infancy, echocardiography is an important part of the diagnostic workup; however, it is not definitive. Characterizing pulmonary vascular

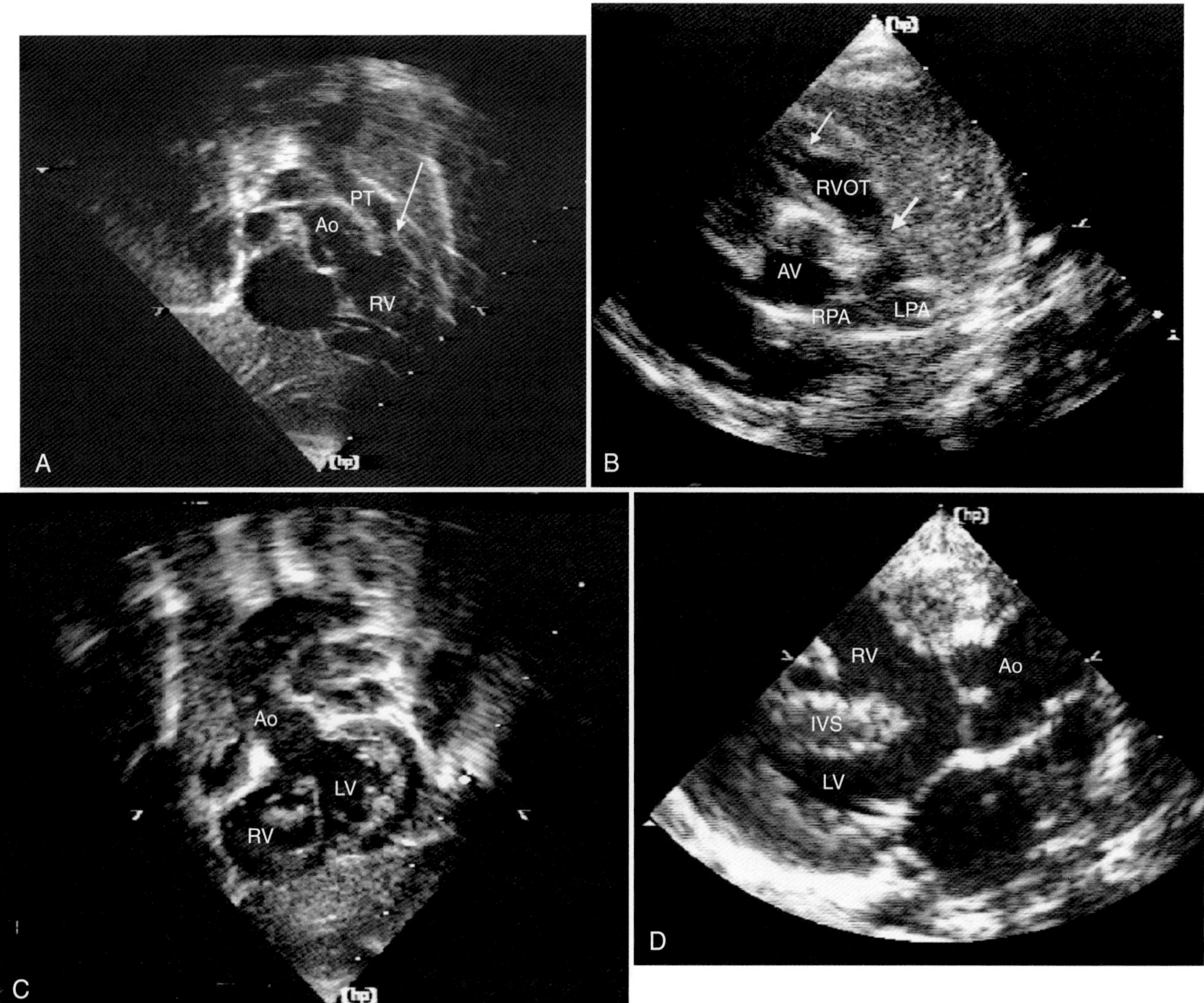

Figure 38-14 Echocardiograms of tetralogy of Fallot. **A,** Subxiphoid view. Narrowed right ventricular *(RV)* outflow tract due to infundibular hypertrophy *(arrow)* and anterior malalignment of infundibular septum. **B,** Parasternal short-axis view. Narrowed RV outflow tract due to infundibular hypertrophy *(thin arrow).* Pulmonary "anulus" and area distal to it are narrowed as well *(thick arrow).* **C,** Sagittal view from subxiphoid position. Overriding aorta is demonstrated. **D,** Parasternal long-axis view. Aorta is overriding interventricular septum and ventricular septal defect is imaged. Key: *Ao,* Aorta; *AV,* aortic valve; *IVS,* interventricular septum; *LPA,* left pulmonary artery; *LV,* left ventricle; *PT,* pulmonary trunk; *RA,* right atrium; *RPA,* right pulmonary artery; *RVOT,* right ventricular outflow tract.

resistance (Rp) and imaging the distal pulmonary arteries require cardiac catheterization.

Cardiac Catheterization and Angiography

Preoperative cardiac catheterization and angiography, although not routinely required when expertly interpreted echocardiography is available, precisely portray the hemodynamic state and morphology, particularly that of the distal pulmonary arteries. Peak pressure in the RV cavity (PRV) is similar to that in the left (PLV), and pulmonary artery pressure (PPA) is below normal. A systolic pressure gradient is demonstrable at infundibular and valvar levels when both zones are stenotic, but rarely at a more peripheral site. When proximal stenoses are severe, however, it may be impossible to enter the pulmonary trunk with a catheter.

There is right-to-left shunting at ventricular level and low $\dot{Q}p$, the severity of which reflect severity of stenosis. In acyanotic patients, there is minimal right-to-left shunting at rest or even a slight increase in $\dot{Q}p$, but in most patients, right-to-left shunting occurs on exercise. In severely cyanotic patients, PPA and Rp are not elevated preoperatively, even in the presence of important peripheral pulmonary artery stenosis or thrombosis, because of low $\dot{Q}p$. PPA may be elevated when there is a large $\dot{Q}p$ and an increase in Rp.

Biplane cineangiography demonstrates all the morphologic features of the malformation as well as morphology and dimensions of the RV–pulmonary trunk junction, pulmonary trunk, and RPA and LPA and their branches. Oblique[C2] and angled views[B2,S16] are used. Configuration of the RV sinus and infundibulum and degree and morphology of the RV outflow tract obstruction are studied. Morphology of the pulmonary valve and any tethering or narrowing of the pulmonary trunk at the level of the commissural attachments of the valve or beyond are noted. Bifurcation of the pulmonary trunk and origins of the LPA and RPA are studied with particular care because the surgeon cannot accurately assess presence or severity of stenoses in this area during operation. The

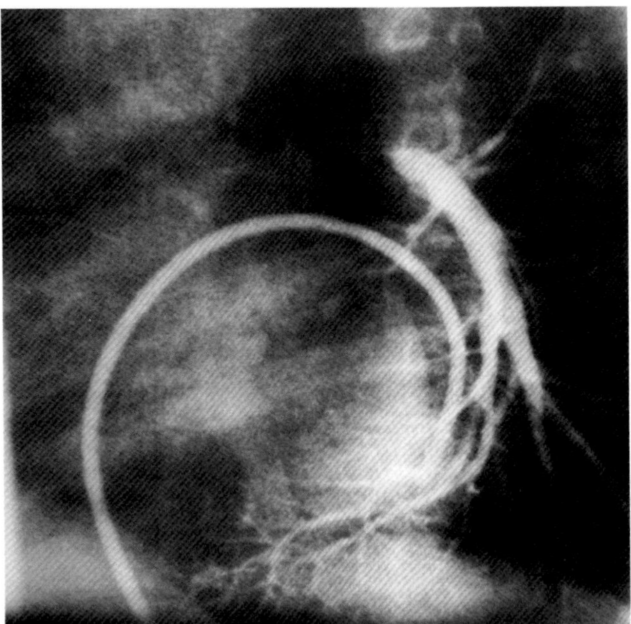

Figure 38-15 Pulmonary vein wedge injection in tetralogy of Fallot and absent central portion of left pulmonary artery demonstrating a left hilar pulmonary artery and its normal continuation. The artery was not visualized by right ventricular or aortic injection.

sitting-up position (cranially tilted frontal view) generally offers the best view, although oblique views also usually demonstrate origins of both pulmonary arteries. Presence, size, and morphology of various portions of the RPA and LPA are studied with care.

With proper profiling of the ventricular septum, the typical large VSD and overlying dextroposed aorta are identified (see Fig. 38-12). Additional VSDs, if present, are identified as well.

Coronary arterial anatomy can usually be seen following LV injection. Particular search is made for anomalous origin of the LAD from the RCA and for the rare but surgically important associated origin of the left coronary artery from the pulmonary trunk.

Follow-through frames are examined for evidence of large AP collateral arteries, and injection is made into the thoracic aorta[R11] and/or selectively into the collateral arteries[P1] if these are present. When the true LPA or RPA is not visualized following these injections, which must include late filming and sometimes also digital subtraction techniques, a *pulmonary vein wedge injection* is made to fill (retrogradely) the pulmonary arterial tree (Fig. 38-15).[F13,N9,S16,T1] When all techniques including this one fail to outline a central or hilar portion of a pulmonary artery, it can be safely assumed to be absent.

Any major associated cardiac anomalies are identified by the study. Previous palliative shunts or transanular patches are visualized, the former by selective injections if necessary. Any iatrogenic pulmonary arterial problems are defined in detail. Particular care is taken to visualize these to help the surgeon avoid misidentifying structures during repair.

Computed Tomography

Computed tomographic angiography (CTA) is used selectively in TF, both in neonates and infants, as a preoperative diagnostic test and in patients after palliative surgery or reparative surgery.[C15] It can define the branch and peripheral pulmonary arteries accurately and has replaced conventional angiography for many clinical indications (Fig. 38-16). The chief advantage is that it requires only peripheral intravenous access for contrast injection, thereby removing the risk of catheter-induced complications. Furthermore, CT images are 3D and amenable to image postprocessing (Fig. 38-17), whereas images from conventional angiography are projectional and overlapping vessels can be difficult to interpret. Conventional angiography has better spatial resolution, and

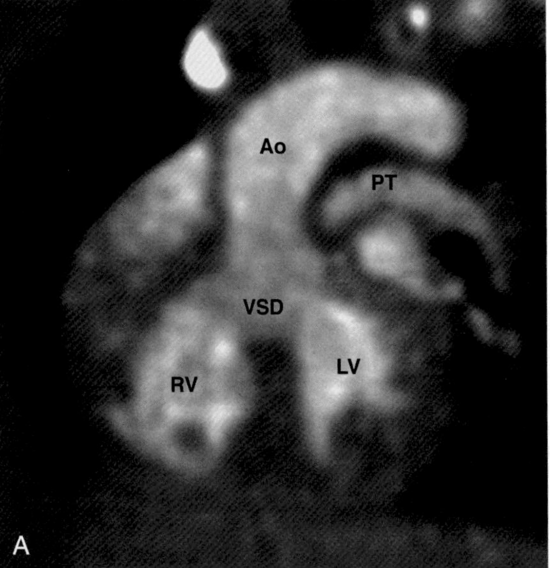

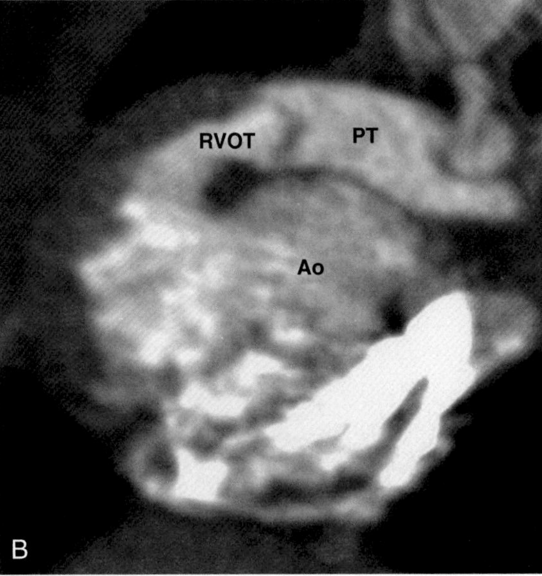

Figure 38-16 **A,** Short-axis computed tomographic angiography of a 2-week-old boy with tetralogy of Fallot shows aorta overriding ventricular septum. Right ventricle *(RV)* and left ventricle *(LV)* communicate through a malaligned ventricular septal defect *(VSD)*. Because the VSD is unrestrictive, RV pressure equalizes with LV pressure, promoting hypertrophy. **B,** Oblique image of the same 2-week-old boy shows a small pulmonary trunk compared with aorta. Both the RV outflow track and pulmonary valve are small. Therefore, the pulmonary stenosis found in a tetralogy of Fallot has supravalvar, valvar, and subvalvar components. Key: *Ao,* Aorta; *PT,* pulmonary trunk; *RVOT,* right ventricular outflow tract.

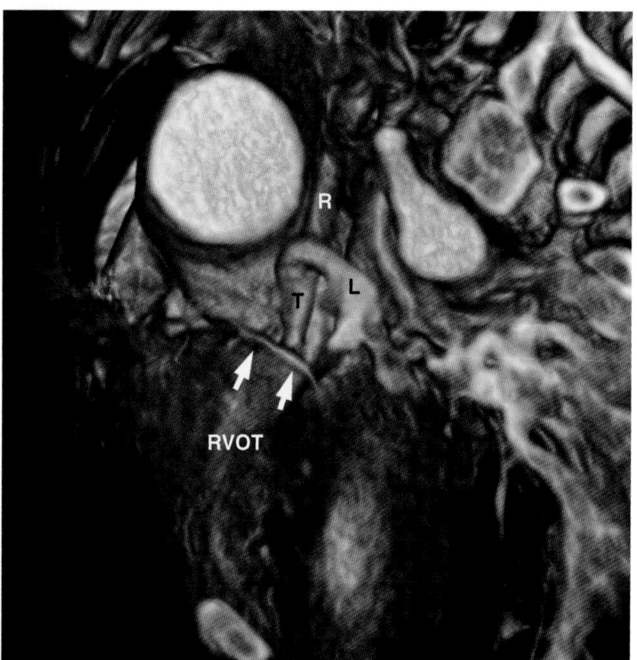

Figure 38-17 Volume-rendered computed tomographic angiography image of a 3-year-old girl with tetralogy of Fallot. Pulmonary trunk and right and left pulmonary arteries are small. Left anterior descending coronary artery abnormally arises from right coronary artery and cuts across *(arrows)* right ventricular outflow tract *(RVOT)*. Disruption of left anterior descending coronary artery during RVOT augmentation can cause left ventricular infarction. Key: *L,* Left; *R,* right; *T,* pulmonary trunk.

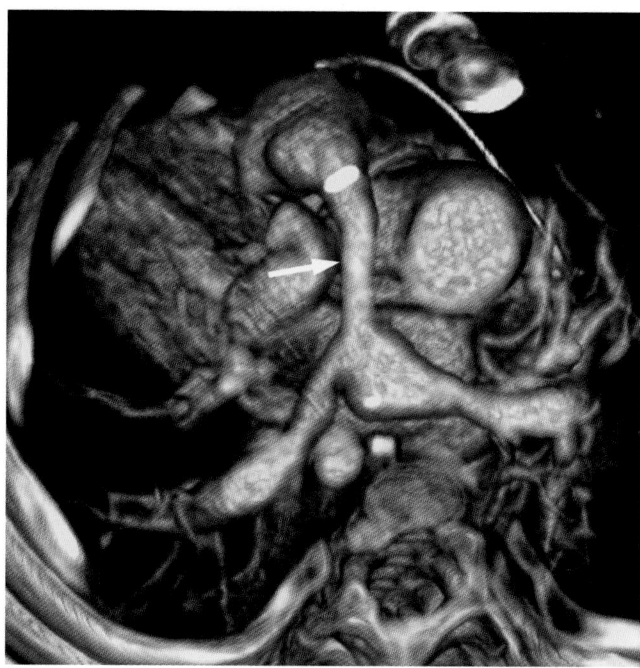

Figure 38-18 Volume-rendered computed tomographic angiography image of a 2-year-old boy who had a complete repair for tetralogy of Fallot with a right ventricle–to–pulmonary trunk conduit *(arrow)* and branch pulmonary artery reconstruction. Patient has outgrown original conduit and has proximal right pulmonary artery stenosis and requires pulmonary arterial reconstruction and conduit replacement.

selective branch injections may reveal flow dynamics in collateral branches better than CTA.

At the present time, when echocardiography is not sufficient to allay concerns about peripheral pulmonary artery abnormalities, CTA may be indicated to clarify the morphology. The decision to use conventional versus CTA is partly based on institutional expertise and preference; however, if hemodynamic information is required, or if major AP collaterals are suspected, catheterization is necessary.

In neonates and infants with suspected branch pulmonary artery abnormalities on echocardiography, in whom there is usually little concern about abnormal Rp, CTA is an excellent method for defining pulmonary artery stenoses and arborization abnormalities. In patients with systemic to pulmonary artery shunts, in whom concerns about Rp abnormalities are not present, CTA can define the morphologic details of the peripheral pulmonary arteries, systemic-pulmonary collateral vessels, and their pulmonary distributions. Cardiac-gated CTA can also reveal unanticipated coronary artery anomalies associated with TF (see Fig. 38-17). In postrepair TF patients with residual RV outflow tract abnormalities, CT can accurately characterize the morphology from the infundibulum to the peripheral pulmonary arteries and help detect native stenosis and conduit stenosis (Fig. 38-18) and aneurysm or pseudoaneurysm (Fig. 38-19).

Magnetic Resonance Imaging

Magnetic resonance imaging (MRI) is also used selectively in TF.[C15,S13] Generally speaking, CTA has higher spatial resolution than MRI, and therefore CT is preferred when finely detailed peripheral pulmonary vascular morphologic information is required. MRI can accurately define the anatomy of the RV outflow tract and branch pulmonary arteries (Figs. 38-20 and 38-21). MRI has the advantage that it does not use ionization radiation and is a good choice in larger patients and when repeated studies are anticipated.[G14] In neonates and infants, preoperative echocardiography is usually adequate and MRI is rarely indicated.

The major indication for MRI is in postrepair TF patients with chronic pulmonary regurgitation.[N12,O8] RV volume, pulmonary valve regurgitant fraction, coexisting pulmonary stenosis, and tricuspid valve regurgitant fraction can all be assessed quantitatively (Fig. 38-22). Serial examinations can accurately define trends in the values of these variables over time, and these trends can be helpful in determining the timing of reoperation. RV end-diastolic volume greater than 150 mL · m^{-2} in children has been identified as a threshold above which the RV is likely not to normalize its volume even after placement of a pulmonary valve prosthesis.[B35,D7]

When pacemakers or defibrillators are present, MRI is contraindicated. Under these conditions, CTA can be an excellent alternative.[G14]

NATURAL HISTORY

The natural history of patients having TF with pulmonary stenosis without major associated cardiac anomalies is variable[M15] and is determined primarily by severity of RV and pulmonary arterial outflow obstruction.[R37]

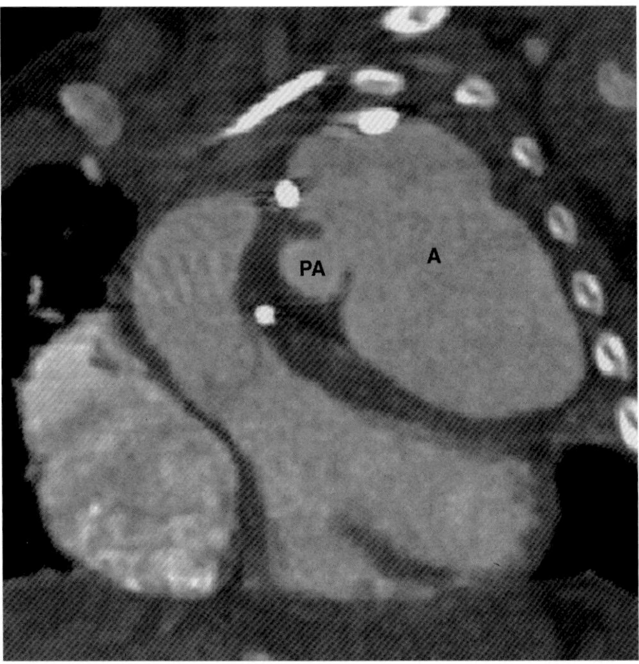

Figure 38-19 Computed tomographic angiography oblique image of a 2-year-old girl shows rupture of pulmonary conduit at its distal anastomosis, forming a large pseudoaneurysm. Key: *A,* Aneurysm; *PA,* pulmonary conduit.

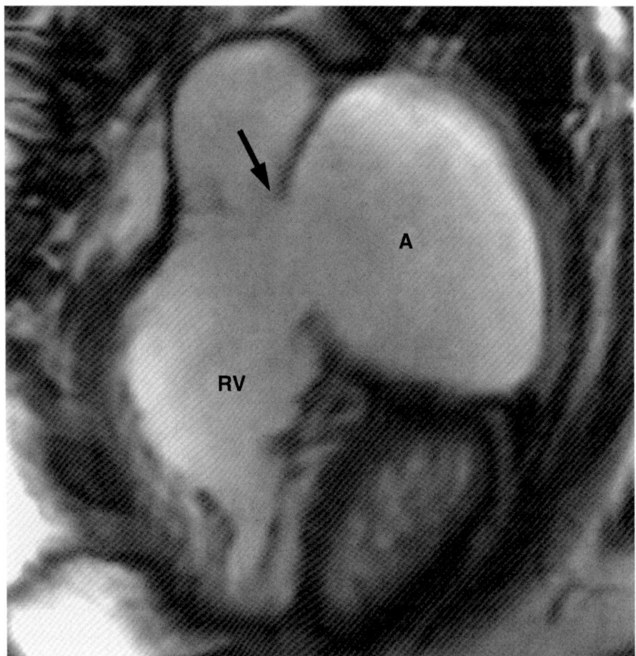

Figure 38-21 Bright-blood, steady-state free-precession magnetic resonance oblique image of a 6-year-old girl showing large rupture at outflow tract region of right ventricle that forms a pseudoaneurysm. Neck of aneurysm is below pulmonary valve *(arrow).* Key: *A,* Aneurysm; *RV,* right ventricle.

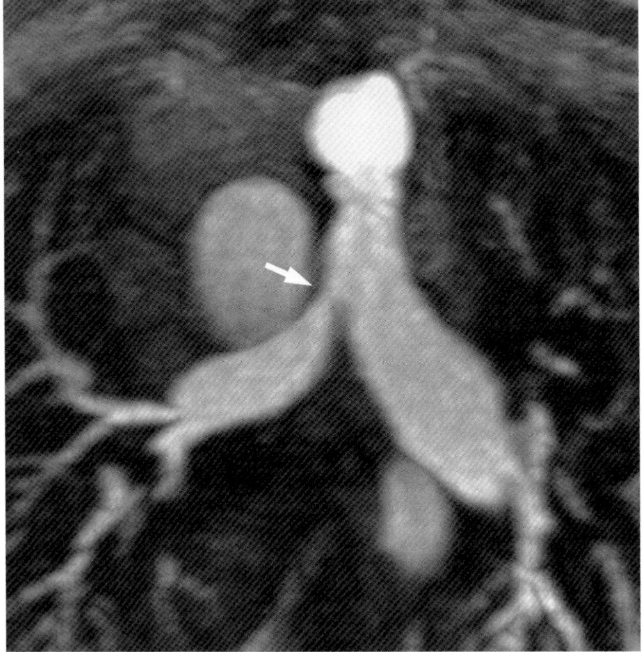

Figure 38-20 Axial image of central pulmonary arteries from contrast-enhanced magnetic resonance angiography of a 10-year-old boy who had a repaired tetralogy of Fallot showing a focal stenosis at origin of right pulmonary artery *(arrow).*

Symptoms and Survival

Twenty-five percent of surgically untreated infants die in the first year of life, but uncommonly in the first month (Fig. 38-23, *A* and *B*). These are the patients with the most severe obstruction to pulmonary blood flow. Forty percent are dead by age 3, 70% by age 10, and 95% by age 40. Instantaneous risk of death (hazard function) is greatest in the first year of life (Fig. 38-23, *C*). Risk then stays constant until about age 25, when it begins again to increase.

Hypoxic spells in the first few years of life are related to hyperactivity of the infundibulum. This and contraction of the infundibular septum and its parietal extension earlier in systole than in normal subjects[G23] produce variable and sometimes severe episodes of RV outflow tract obstruction and symptoms. Any sudden reduction of systemic vascular resistance also may precipitate a hypoxic spell.

About 25% of patients are acyanotic at birth and become cyanotic in the ensuing weeks, months, or years as pulmonary stenosis increases.[B21,G23] Progression of arterial desaturation, cyanosis, and polycythemia is variable and is furthered not only by increasing pulmonary stenosis but also by widespread tendency to thrombosis of the smaller pulmonary arteries, with progressive reduction in $\dot{Q}p$.[F6,R16] As part of this same tendency, death may result from cerebral thromboses or abscesses.

In those few patients surviving into the fourth and fifth decades of life, death is commonly from chronic heart failure due to secondary cardiomyopathy that results from RV pressure overload and chronic hypoxia and polycythemia.

Pulmonary Artery Thromboses

In severely cyanotic and polycythemic patients, diffuse pulmonary arterial thrombosis can occur. This is initially visible only microscopically,[F6] but rarely it progresses to occlusion of a lobar pulmonary artery or even an entire RPA or LPA. Usually, Rp is not importantly increased by this process, but rarely the thrombosis is so widespread and severe as to be a

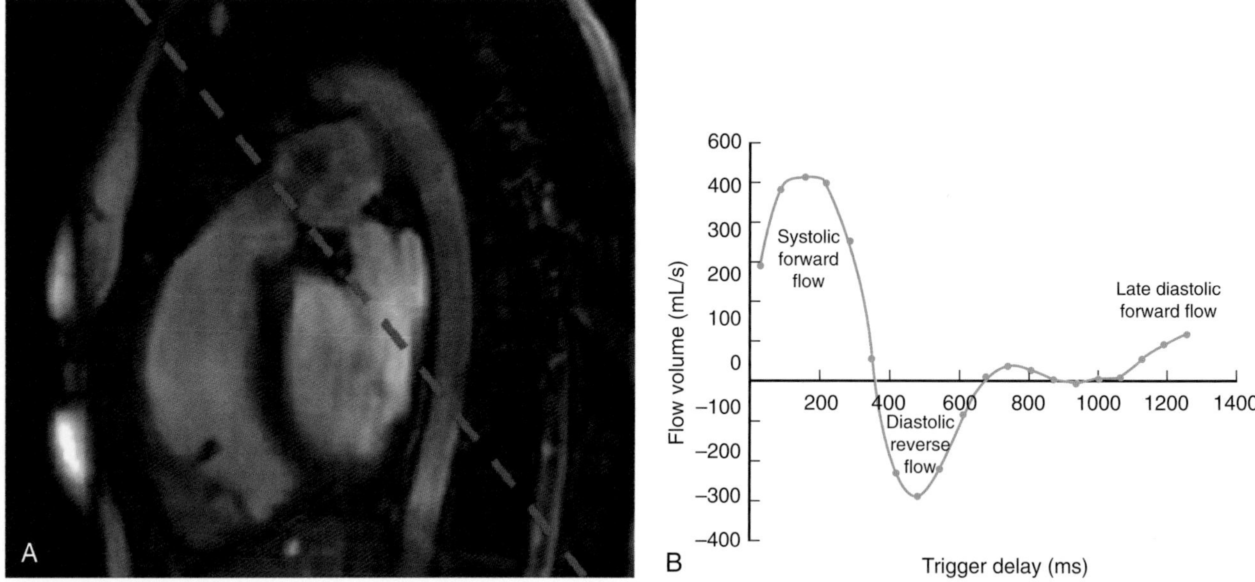

Figure 38-22 Right ventricular outflow tract cardiovascular magnetic resonance study of a patient with repaired tetralogy of Fallot with important late pulmonary regurgitation. **A,** Cine image. Red dotted line illustrates through-plane in which a non–breath-hold phase encoded velocity map was acquired. **B,** Flow curve obtained from same patient. Through integrating areas containing forward and reverse flow, a pulmonary regurgitation fraction of 34% was calculated. (From Shinebourne and colleagues.[S13])

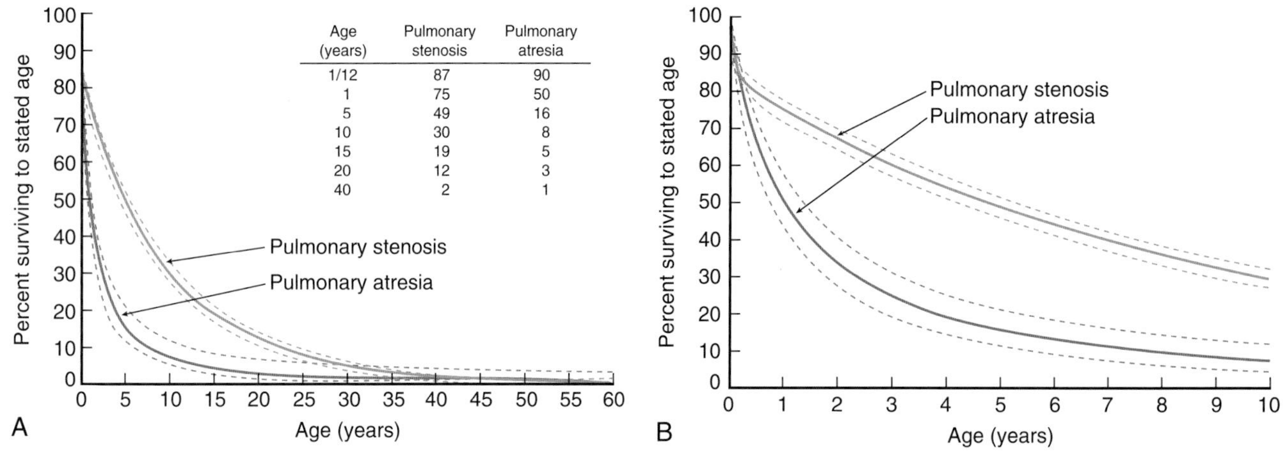

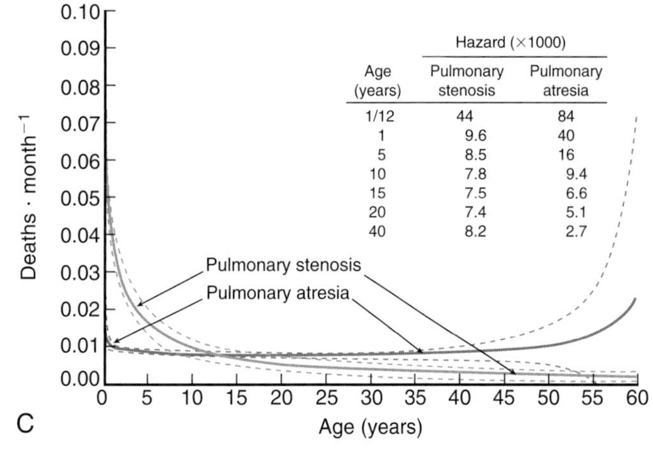

Age (years)	Pulmonary stenosis	Pulmonary atresia
1/12	87	90
1	75	50
5	49	16
10	30	8
15	19	5
20	12	3
40	2	1

Age (years)	Hazard (×1000) Pulmonary stenosis	Pulmonary atresia
1/12	44	84
1	9.6	40
5	8.5	16
10	7.8	9.4
15	7.5	6.6
20	7.4	5.1
40	8.2	2.7

Figure 38-23 Natural history of surgically untreated patients having tetralogy of Fallot with pulmonary stenosis or pulmonary atresia. **A,** Survival to age 60 years. Smooth lines represent survival of each group, and dashed lines enclose 70% confidence limits. **B,** Survival to age 10 years (expanded time scale). **C,** Hazard function according to age. (From Bertranou and colleagues.[B10])

cause of immediate and sometimes fatal pulmonary hypertension and RV failure following repair.

Pulmonary Vascular Disease

Pulmonary vascular disease rarely develops in surgically untreated patients. It may develop following too large a systemic to pulmonary arterial shunt (see "Interim Results after Classic Shunting Operations" later in this section). When a surgical shunt appears to be the cause, it is possible that preexistent pulmonary arterial thrombosis has compounded the problem.

Genetic History

Offspring of a parent who has TF are more likely to have the anomaly than offspring of parents without congenital heart disease. It is estimated that about 0.1% of live births have TF under the latter circumstances and about 1.5% under the former.[S2]

TECHNIQUE OF OPERATION

General Plan and Details of Repair Common to All Approaches

Surgical Evaluation

Outcome of repair of TF depends mainly on relief of pulmonary stenosis, whether infundibular, valvar, pulmonary arterial, or (as is usual) a combination of these. Therefore, the surgeon must come to the operating room with a clear mental image of the morphology as it has been displayed in the preoperative imaging studies, particularly as it relates to the RV and pulmonary arterial outflow obstruction.

After median sternotomy, external anatomy of the heart is studied, with particular attention to RV and pulmonary artery anatomy and configuration of coronary arteries crossing the RV. The preoperative imaging studies are mentally reviewed; these and observation of the heart determine the incision and details of repair.

Conceptual Approach to Surgery

The idealized goal of repair is to eliminate intracardiac shunting, reduce RV pressure and volume load to normal, and preserve normal myocardial function. This is accomplished by complete closure of the VSD (and atrial septal defect if present) and complete relief of the RV outflow tract obstruction while maintaining a competent pulmonary valve. This ideal is achieved in only a minority of patients, generally those with the most favorable RV outflow morphology, consisting of a normal or nearly normal pulmonary "anulus" and functioning pulmonary valve cusps (see discussion of variability of RV outflow tract morphology under Morphology in this section). In all other cases, the repair will fall short of ideal. Thus, in most cases, a number of important morphologically driven decisions must be made during repair, and these decisions will determine how closely the repair will approach the ideal. The decisions listed here (and discussed further in text that follows) often involve both technical and conceptual elements:

- Approaching the repair via transatrial or transventricular incisions
- Performing a transanular patch and determining width of the patch
- Preserving or sacrificing RCA branches
- Managing the RV outflow tract when an anomalous LAD is present
- Technically approaching abnormal pulmonary valve cusps, and preserving cusps when transanular patching is performed
- Managing atrial septal defects and PFOs
- Managing the tricuspid valve when septal leaflet function is compromised at VSD closure
- Dividing or resecting obstructing septal and parietal muscle bands in the RV outflow tract.

Approach

Surgical access to the VSD and RV outflow tract through a right atriotomy, supplemented by evaluating the pulmonary valve via a pulmonary arteriotomy in most cases, is advocated by some.[B13,E3,H31] This approach makes sense when a well-developed infundibulum is present; however, if there is diffuse hypoplasia of the RV outflow tract, and a full-length transanular patch is anticipated, this approach makes little sense. Additionally, if a small tricuspid valve is present, exposure through the right atrium may be difficult, especially in small infants, and more damage than good may result from traction on the myocardium and tricuspid valve. Nevertheless, initial approach through the pulmonary artery and right atrium is preferred in all situations by some.[K7,K39,K43,P13]

Transanular Patch The question of whether to use a transanular patch arises in many cases, and this decision is now known to have far-reaching implications for long-term outcome. Recent publications continue to emphasize the detrimental effects of large transanular incisions.[B22,M31,P4] A transanular patch creates obligatory pulmonary regurgitation, and when this is long-standing and severe, important RV dysfunction will inevitably occur (see Results later in this section). Degree of narrowing of the "anulus" can be expressed quantitatively by a *z* value—that is, the number of standard deviations (usually smaller) from normal. When the *z* value has been determined from echocardiography, corrected and transformed cineangiographic measurements, or MRI or CTA to be larger than −3, the surgeon's bias should be that a transanular patch is probably unnecessary (Fig. 38-24); when it is −3 or smaller, a patch is probably required. The surgeon's bias should also be that even with a transanular patch, when the *z* value of the "anulus" is less than −7 (<10% of cases), postrepair ratio of peak pressure in the RV to that in the LV ($P_{RV/LV}$) may be 1 or higher, even with a properly placed transanular patch (Fig. 38-25). It can be inferred from the findings outlined in Fig. 38-24 that the extremely small pulmonary valve "anulus" may in some cases be associated with diffuse hypoplasia of the distal pulmonary arteries. Thus, when a very small "anulus" is noted, preoperative evaluation of the distal pulmonary vasculature and Rp should be undertaken. If distal hypoplasia, elevated Rp, or both are observed, a reparative operation should avoided (at least temporarily) in favor of a shunt procedure. It must be emphasized that the *z* value is used only as a guideline. The pulmonary valve cusp configuration—number, thickness, and fusion—will influence the eventual gradient across the RV outflow tract after repair, and because of these variables, different gradients may result despite similar *z* values. Thus, the actual gradient should always be assessed after separation

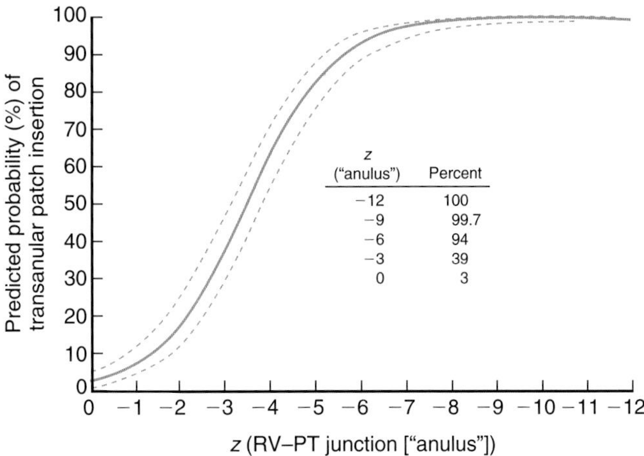

Figure 38-24 Probability of transanular patch insertion during repair of tetralogy of Fallot with pulmonary stenosis *(solid curve)*, according to dimension (*z* value) of right ventriculopulmonary trunk junction (pulmonary valve "anulus"). (See original paper for data and equation.) Dashed lines are 70% CLs. Key: *PT,* Pulmonary trunk; *RV,* right ventricular. (From Kirklin and colleagues.[K20])

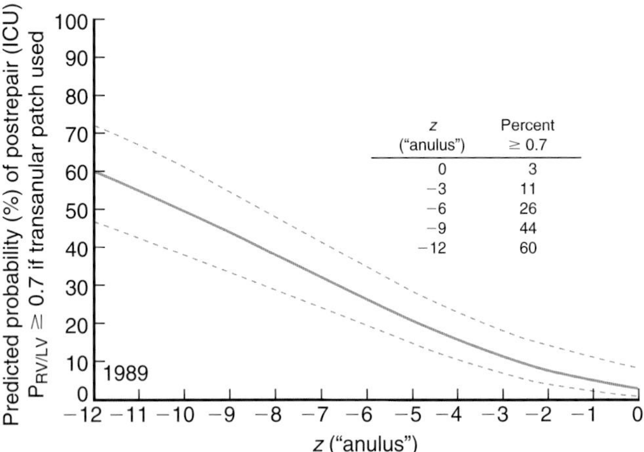

Figure 38-25 Probability of postrepair (ICU) $P_{RV/LV}$ being greater than 0.7 after a repair that includes insertion of a transanular patch, according to dimension (*z* value) of pulmonary "anulus" as determined on preoperative cineangiogram. (See original paper for data and equation.) Depiction as in Fig. 38-24. Key: $P_{RV/LV}$, Ratio of peak pressure in right ventricle to that in left ventricle. (From Kirklin and colleagues.[K20])

from cardiopulmonary bypass (CPB), at a minimum by intraoperative echocardiography, and preferably by direct pressure measurement.

Right Coronary Artery Branches As a general principle, visible-to-the-eye RV coronary artery branches should be preserved whenever possible. Occasionally visible branches must be transected to achieve acceptable RV outflow obstruction relief. Before transecting a branch, its course should be fully examined. Those that traverse the body of the RV, and even those smaller branches that supply muscle farther down on the RV infundibulum than the lower margin of the infundibular incision, should be preserved. When necessary, small transverse infundibular branches, with distal perfusion that stays above the lower margin of the infundibular incision, can be sacrificed.

Anomalous Left Anterior Descending Coronary Artery When an anomalous LAD arises from the RCA, modifying RV outflow tract management is often, but not always, necessary. Key factors are the exact course of the coronary artery and morphology of the infundibulum. In cases with a LAD that crosses high in the infundibulum near the valve anulus, and with low infundibular obstruction and a well-developed distal infundibular chamber, the obstruction can be addressed without endangering the coronary artery. On the other hand, when severe diffuse infundibular hypoplasia is present and the obstruction can be addressed only by placing a conduit from the RV to the pulmonary trunk, the RV-conduit anastomosis should be placed proximal to the coronary vessel. Occasionally the anomalous LAD is intramyocardial. This should be suspected when the left aortic sinus gives rise to an isolated circumflex coronary artery.

Pulmonary Valve The pulmonary valve cusps should be assessed carefully, especially when a transanular patch is necessary. There is a high likelihood of bicuspid valve when a transanular patch is needed (small anulus). Orientation of the two commissures may be directly anterior and posterior, directly left and right, or any position in between. With the exception of the direct lateral orientation, the transanular incision can be designed to cross the anulus precisely through the most anterior commissure, thereby preserving the function of both cusps. This maneuver minimizes the severity of pulmonary regurgitation that results from the transanular patching.

Atrial Septal Communications Managing the atrial septum can be essential to repair, particularly in neonates and infants. The combination of a transanular patch and high Rp can lead to postoperative RV failure. If the foramen ovale is patent under these conditions, it should be left patent. If the PFO has naturally closed, it can be reopened using a blunt instrument in most young infants. If a true atrial septal defect is present, it should be subtotally closed using a patch, leaving a small open flap that overlaps the edge of the limbus, to function like a PFO. The resulting cyanosis of atrial right to left shunting is well tolerated postoperatively, because chronic cyanosis is typically present preoperatively. In patients who do not receive a transanular patch, the atrial septum can typically be completely closed.

Tricuspid Valve Careful attention to the tricuspid valve during VSD closure is essential, particularly in small infants. Tethering of the septal leaflet and distortion of chordal structures during VSD closure is sometimes inevitable. Valve competency should be tested routinely after VSD closure. If regurgitation is present, tricuspid valve repair should be performed. Partial closure of the anterior septal leaflet commissure is effective in restoring tricuspid valve competency when septal leaflet tethering is present. A competent tricuspid valve is critical to achieving excellent outcome, especially if a transanular patch is used.

Right Ventricular Muscle Bundles Surgical myotomy or myectomy to manage obstructing septal, parietal, and free-wall muscle bundles in the infundibulum can have both short- and long-term implications for RV function. Despite its necessity, it remains one of the most destructive procedures in all of pediatric cardiac surgery. A minimalist approach is recommended in most cases. In neonates and infants, in whom fibrosis and excessive hypertrophy are not yet present, incision of obstructing septal and/or parietal bands without excision is all that is necessary. In many cases, if these muscle bundles are not obstructive, patching of the longitudinal infundibular incision is all that is needed to relieve infundibular obstruction. In older patients, when important fibrosis, hypertrophy, or both are present, simple incision may not relieve the obstruction, and excision may be required.

Preparations for Cardiopulmonary Bypass

Before establishing CPB, the ascending aorta is dissected free from the pulmonary trunk so that when the aortic clamp is in position, the pulmonary trunk and RPA are undistorted. Unless it is clear from preoperative imaging studies that the pulmonary trunk bifurcation and central and hilar portions of the LPA and RPA are free of stenoses or diffuse hypoplasia, these too are mobilized. On the left side, this is aided by cutting the pericardium down to the LPA, dissecting away and preserving the left phrenic nerve. The ligamentum (or ductus) arteriosum, if present, is dissected, ligated, and divided. Division of the ligamentum (or ductus) will prevent tethering of the proximal LPA, which can cause late kinking and obstruction, especially when a transanular patch is used at repair. On the right side the aorta is retracted anterior and to the left, and the RPA is dissected completely away from it out to the superior vena cava and beneath it if necessary.

Any surgically created shunts are at least partially dissected before establishing CPB (see later sections on repair after various shunts).

Technical Details of Repair

Immediately after CPB is established, all surgically created shunts are ligated or divided, and the ductus (if present) ligated and divided if this has not been accomplished prior to establishing CPB. Thereafter, once the heart is arrested, the right ventriculotomy or right atriotomy is made and the internal anatomy further visualized and conceptualized. The plan is to:

- Dissect and resect the infundibular stenosis (recalling that this may be at several levels).
- Visualize the pulmonary valve and open it if necessary.
- Estimate dimensions of the outflow tract, valve, and anulus with a Hegar dilator,[D18] and decide whether a transanular patch is needed.
- Repair the VSD.
- Evaluate the atrial septum and make a decision about closing any defects or leaving a PFO.
- Evaluate residual RV outflow tract obstruction following separation from CPB.

Repair is similar whether an RV or right atrial approach is chosen and is represented in Figs. 38-26 through 38-29, which should be studied in parallel with this text to obtain the most complete understanding of the pathologic anatomy and its repair.

Infundibular Dissection In patients presenting for surgery beyond early infancy, considerable RV infundibular muscle hypertrophy and fibrosis are typical, requiring a number of maneuvers during the infundibular dissection. The parietal extension of the infundibular septum is dissected away from the RV free wall and ventriculoinfundibular fold and is divided transversely 5 mm or so to the right of the attachment of the right coronary cusp of the aortic valve to the undersurface of the infundibular septum. This increases diameter of the infundibulum at its rightward end and improves exposure of the VSD from the RV approach. Any obstructive trabeculae along the left side of the outflow tract are also incised and partially removed. The aim is to increase the circumference of the infundibulum by enlarging each lateral recess in front of the infundibular septum. An obstruction at a low level (coronal plane) is relieved by dividing anomalous trabeculae above the moderator band while protecting adjacent papillary muscles; the moderator band is divided only when necessary to relieve the obstruction. When an os infundibulum is present at the level of the inferior edge of the infundibular septum, the *fibrous thickening* all around the ostial orifice is excised, as is any fibrous obstruction extending upstream toward the pulmonary valve. If the infundibular resection is performed using an RV infundibular incision, the

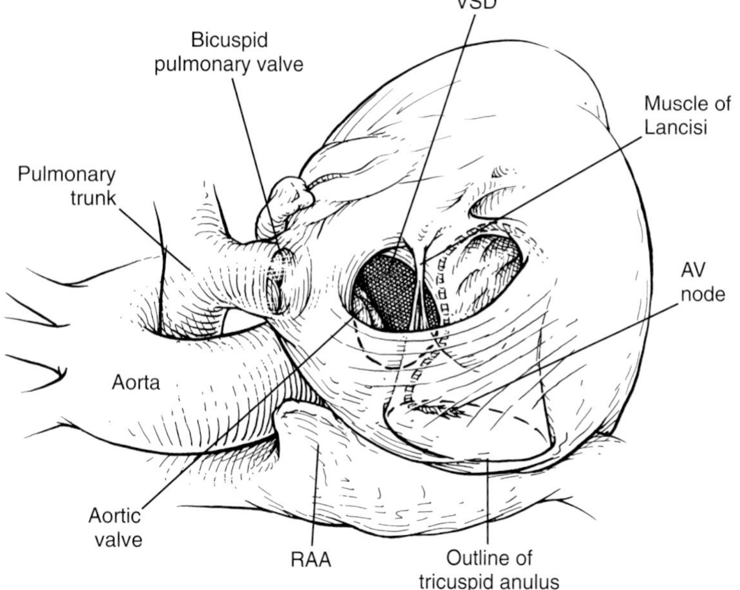

Figure 38-26 Anatomic substrate of repair of tetralogy of Fallot with pulmonary stenosis from right ventricular (RV) approach, shown as if RV free wall were in part translucent. Separation of pulmonary valve from aortic valve by infundibular septum is evident. Parietal extension arches to the right and over the RV outflow tract, blending in its termination with RV free wall. Posteriorly, ventricular septal defect *(VSD)* abuts tricuspid anulus. Ventriculoinfundibular fold borders VSD posterosuperiorly, but is unseen because it is overhung by the parietal extension. VSD comes into relationship anterosuperiorly and anteriorly with anteriorly displaced infundibular septum. This partially borders aorta as well in many patients, with an aortic cusp on its inferior surface. Anteroinferiorly, a valley-like area may be seen where infundibular septum merges with trabecula septomarginalis (septal band) that forms inferior border of VSD. Key: *AV,* Atrioventricular; *RAA,* right atrial appendage.

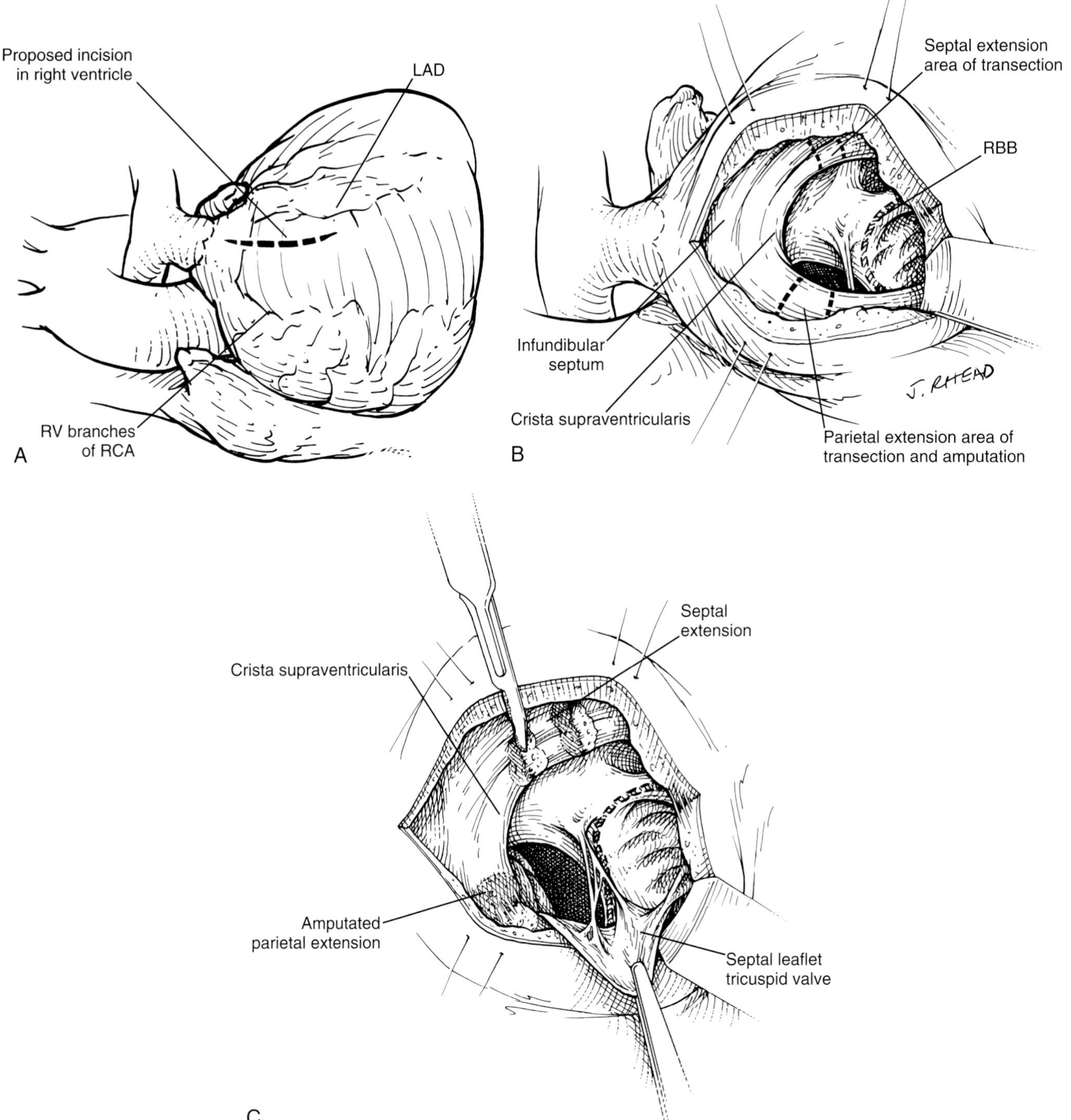

Figure 38-27 Repair of tetralogy of Fallot via right ventricular *(RV)* approach using vertical incision. **A,** Superiorly, incision stops short of pulmonary valve "anulus" and may vary according to presence and direction of a large conal branch of right coronary artery. **B,** RV incision is spread widely by retraction sutures. Parietal extension of infundibular septum is transected where it begins to fuse with RV free wall, dissected away from ventriculoinfundibular fold, and then amputated from infundibular septum. This uncovers the ventricular septal defect *(VSD)* and tricuspid valve. Ventriculoinfundibular fold remains unseen because it is overhung by the tricuspid valve anterior leaflet. **C,** Parietal extension has been mobilized (divided and partially amputated). Septal extension is likewise mobilized to maximize circumference of infundibular outflow tract.

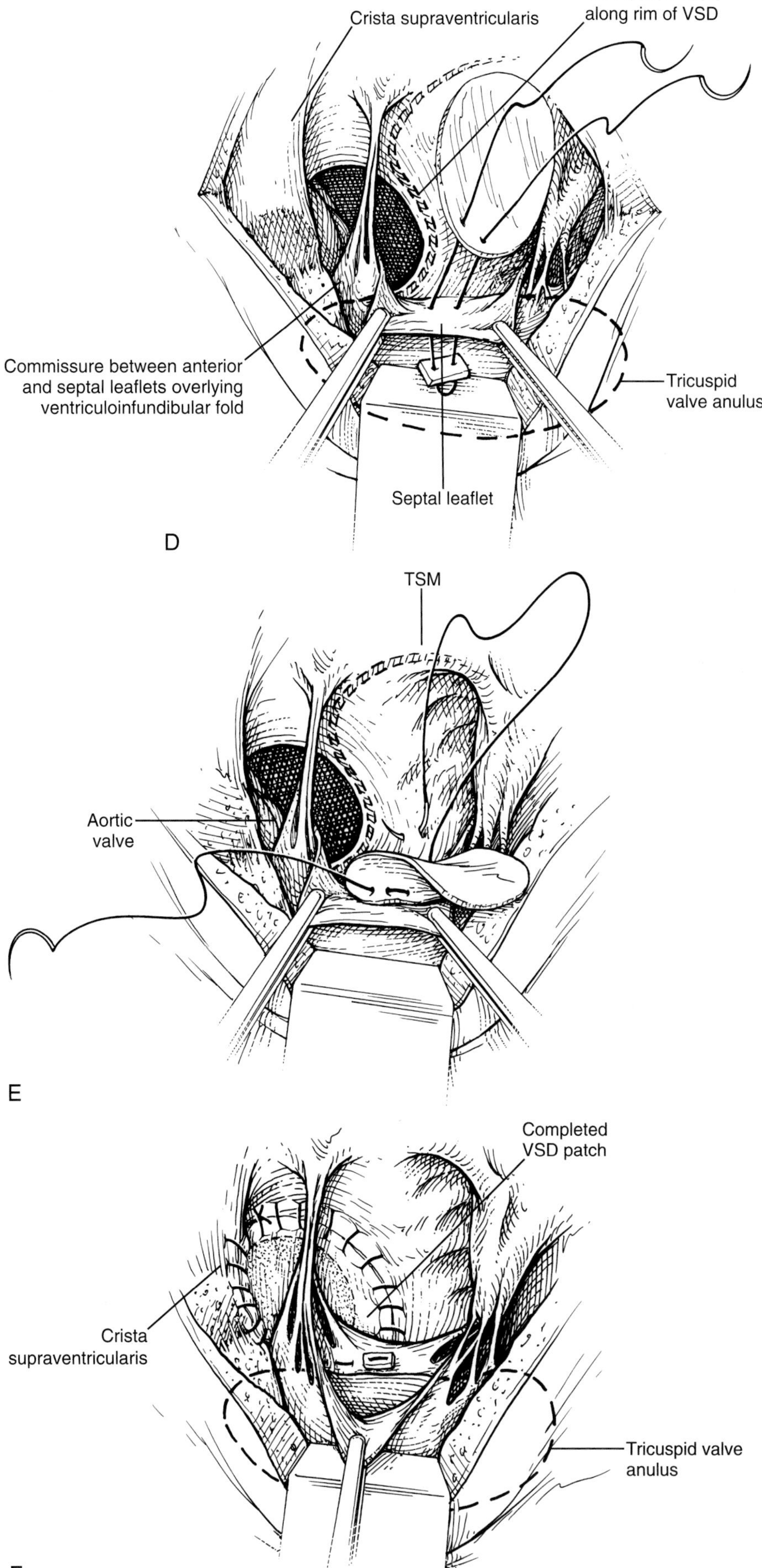

Figure 38-27, cont'd **D,** Pledgeted mattress suture is placed from right atrial side through base of commissural tissue between septal and posterior tricuspid leaflets and through patch. A few more stitches are taken, working posteriorly between base of septal leaflet and patch, followed by stitches through ventriculoinfundibular fold and patch. **E,** Suturing is continued onto parietal extension and infundibular septum, visualizing and staying close to aortic valve leaflets to avoid leaving a hole between muscular bands. Suture is then held. With other arm of suture, a few stitches are taken, working anteriorly between septal tricuspid leaflet and patch, weaving beneath any chordae crossing the VSD. When this has taken the suture line about 5 mm inferior to edge of the VSD, stitches are taken in septum, well back from VSD edge. **F,** Repair of VSD is completed. Note that suture line is away from bundle of His and its branches, except where it crosses the right bundle branch anteroinferiorly. Crista supraventricularis is pulled downward by the patch, which helps increase infundibular outflow circumference. Key: *LAD,* Left anterior descending coronary artery; *RBB,* right bundle branch; *RCA,* right coronary artery; *TSM,* trabecula septomarginalis.

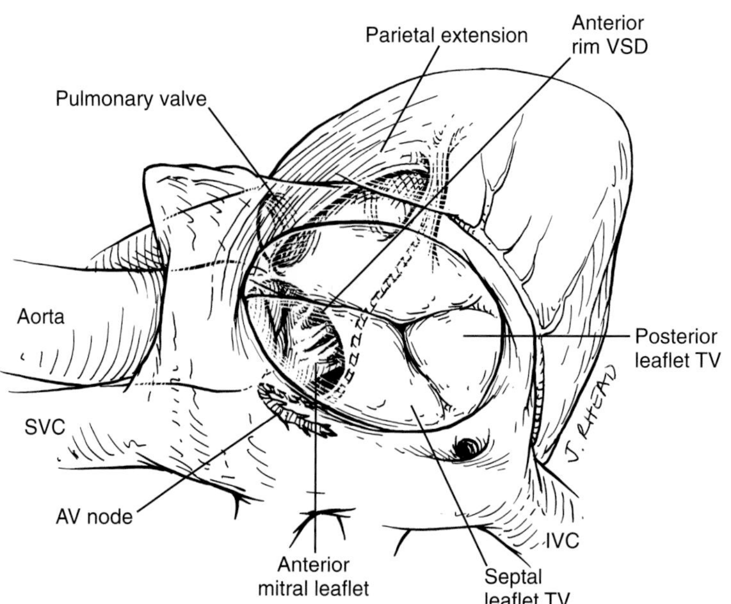

Figure 38-28 Anatomy of tetralogy of Fallot from perspective of right atrial approach, shown as if right atrial free wall and tricuspid valve were translucent. The striking difference from the right ventricular (RV) perspective (see Fig. 38-27) is apparent position of parietal extension. From right atrial perspective, the surgeon is looking beneath this, as parietal extension arches over the RV outflow tract. Ventriculoinfundibular fold is easily seen through tricuspid valve. Key: *AV,* Atrioventricular; *IVC,* inferior vena cava; *SVC,* superior vena cava; *TV,* tricuspid valve; *VSD,* ventricular septal defect.

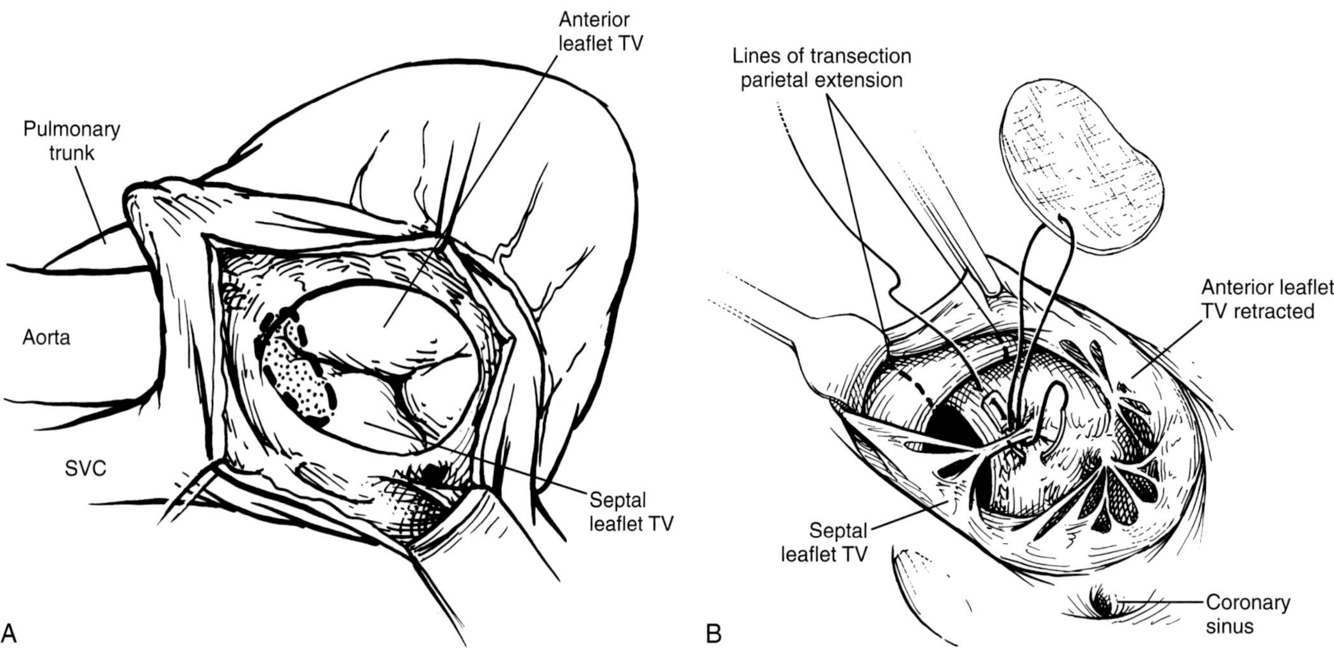

Figure 38-29 Repair of tetralogy of Fallot, right atrial approach. **A,** A high right atrial incision made close to the atrioventricular groove aids exposure. Ventricular septal defect (VSD) is located beneath anteroseptal commissure, indicated by dashed line. **B,** VSD is closed before amputating parietal extension. A pledgeted double-armed suture is begun at the anteroinferior aspect of VSD about 5 mm away from rim to avoid conduction fibers.

incision is closed with a patch of glutaraldehyde-treated autologous pericardium or other material (see "Decision and Technique for Transanular Patching" later in this section). Direct closure could narrow the outflow tract. When a transanular patch is needed, a glutaraldehyde-treated or untreated pericardial[H22] patch is inserted after extending the infundibular incision across the pulmonary "anulus."

This type of anatomic dissection is not possible in the presence of diffuse RV outflow hypoplasia and is often not possible when there is combined infundibular, valvar, and anular stenosis. These structures are all hypoplastic, a situation frequently encountered in patients who have become importantly symptomatic, as neonates or infants, and patch graft enlargement is often all that can be accomplished. In any event, particularly in infants, resection or even transection of RV muscle bundles that are not obstructive must be avoided[C8] because this unnecessarily impairs RV function.

Pulmonary Valvotomy If pulmonary valvotomy is needed, a vertical incision is made in the pulmonary trunk, taking care to avoid damaging the valve commissures (Fig. 38-30). The

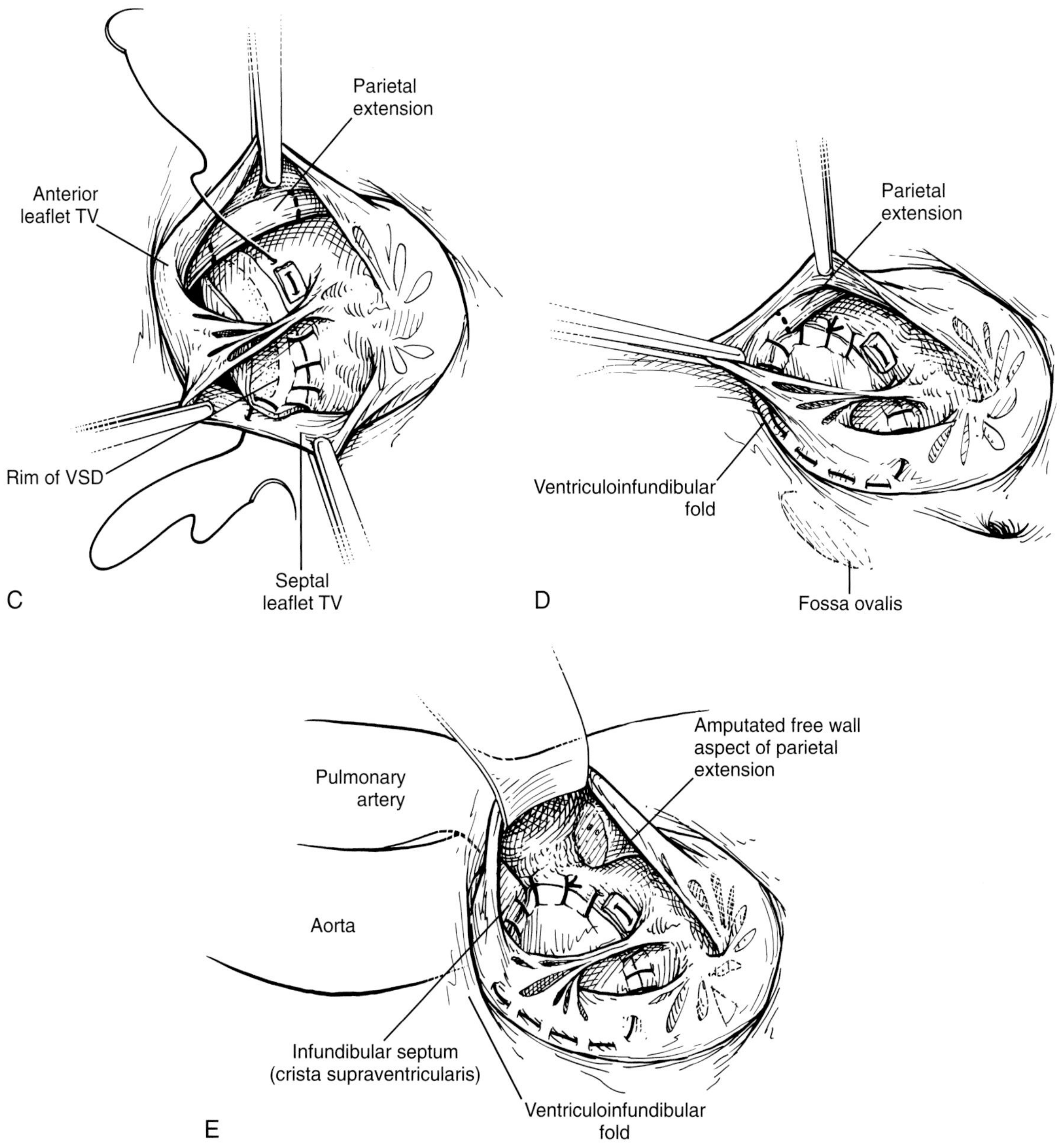

Figure 38-29, cont'd **C,** Suture line securing VSD patch is carried posteriorly to base of septal leaflet and then upward toward ventriculoinfundibular fold. **D,** Patch suture is completed, carrying second end of continuous suture anteriorly and superiorly at rim of VSD near base of aorta. This suture line thus marks the limit of infundibular resection at parietal extension. **E,** Parietal extension is transected at its origin from infundibular septum (staying outside VSD patch suture line). Remaining parietal muscle band is dissected up toward free wall and amputated. Exposure for accurate dissection is not as good as when using the RV approach. Key: *SVC,* Superior vena cava; *TV,* tricuspid valve; *VSD,* ventricular septal defect.

pulmonary arteriotomy is not made through a commissure between the cusps, because placing a patch in such an incision renders the valve regurgitant. Rarely can an adequate valvotomy be performed by simply dividing one or more sites of commissural fusion, because fusion is present in only 20% of stenotic valves and is almost always associated with important cusp thickening, particularly at the cusp free edge (see Morphology earlier in this section). After valvotomy, therefore, the surgeon may elect to excise the thickened cusp edge to relieve the stenosis, although some pulmonary valve regurgitation results. When there is cusp tethering only, the most common situation, the cusp edge may be cut from its attachment to the pulmonary artery wall over about 3 mm. This is done to one cusp at each commissure. Here, too, excising thickened cusp tissue may be required. Regurgitation from minor detachment of a cusp may be less than that from a transanular patch.[R25] If considerable cusp incision and detachment are required, regurgitation results; if there is also important residual narrowing, it is preferable to excise the cusps and place a transanular patch after completing the intraventricular part of the repair. If a transanular patch is not needed (see "Decision and Technique for Transanular Patching" later in this section), the pulmonary arteriotomy is closed, usually with a pericardial patch.

VSD Closure In children and adults, the VSD is closed with a filamentous polyester or polytetrafluoroethylene

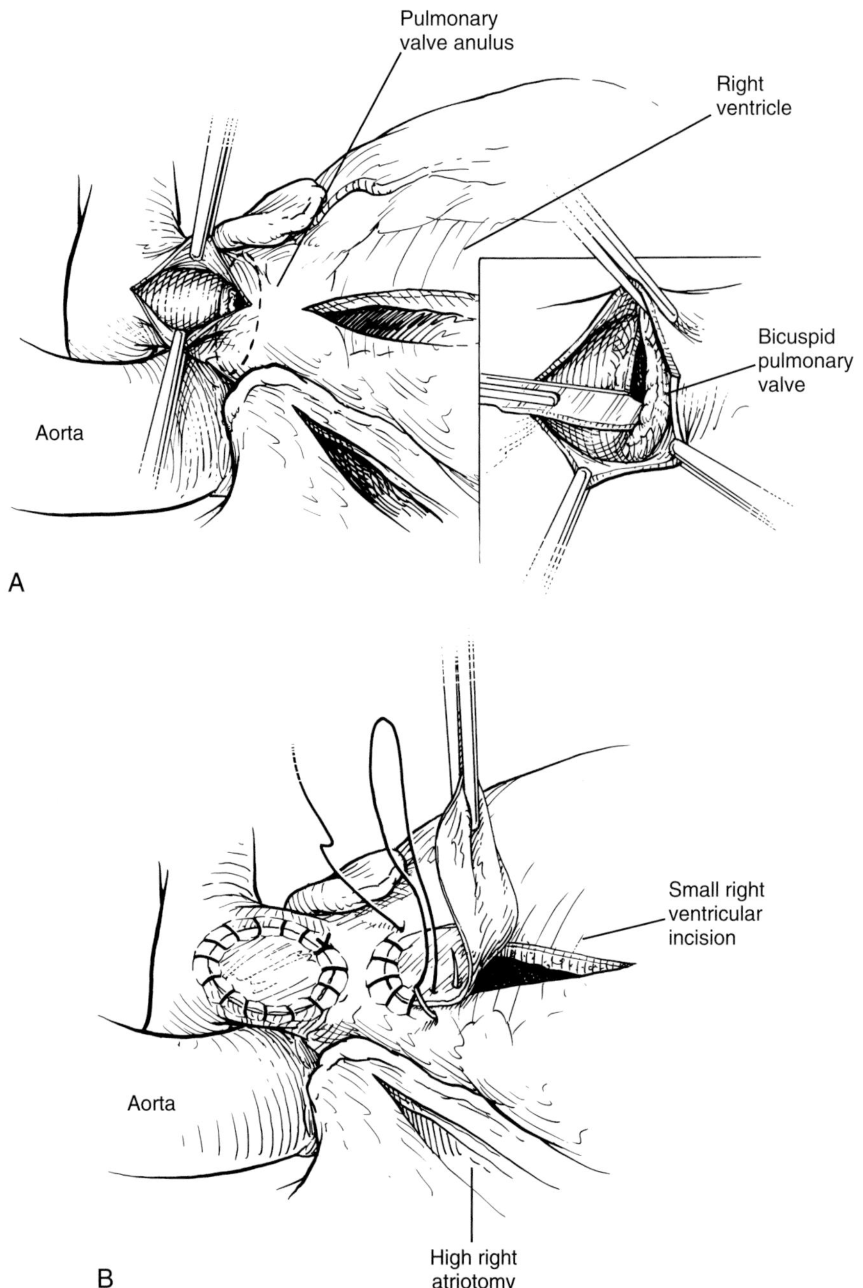

Figure 38-30 Repair of tetralogy of Fallot with separate infundibular and pulmonary arterial patches. **A,** Pulmonary trunk incision is shown extending to but not into pulmonary valve "anulus" *(dashed line).* Vertical ventriculotomy is also shown. *Inset,* Stenotic pulmonary valve seen through pulmonary arteriotomy. Fused commissures are incised with a knife to the pulmonary trunk wall. Fine tissue forceps steady the cusps on each side of commissure and provide even tension as incision is made. **B,** Unless pulmonary trunk is of normal width, which is uncommon, incision is closed with an oval pericardial or polytetrafluoroethylene patch. Patch is cut in the form shown, and its dimensions ensure that it is convex rather than flat.

(PTFE) patch; in neonates and infants, glutaraldehyde-treated pericardium works well. The patch is trimmed to be slightly larger than the VSD. Exposure may be obtained entirely with stay sutures; alternatively, the VSD is exposed through the right ventriculotomy by the assistant using two small curved retractors, one beneath both ends of the infundibular septum, which are pulled upward and apart. A third retractor is positioned in the lower margin of the ventriculotomy for gentle inferior traction. Sequencing of the suturing depends on whether the repair is from the right atrium or RV and is similar to that used for isolated VSD (see Figs. 38-26 through 38-29; see also Chapter 35 and Figs. 35-24 and 35-25). For example, through the RV it is usual to begin the continuous suture at the base of the tricuspid septal leaflet at the posterior-inferior aspect of the VSD. Via the right atrial approach, the suture is often begun anterior to the insertion of the medial papillary muscle (muscle of Lancisi).

Decision and Technique for Transanular Patching Preoperative imaging, usually by echocardiography and occasionally by cineangiography, is used to estimate the diameter of the pulmonary "anulus," and this information is used to assess the likelihood of whether a transanular patch will be

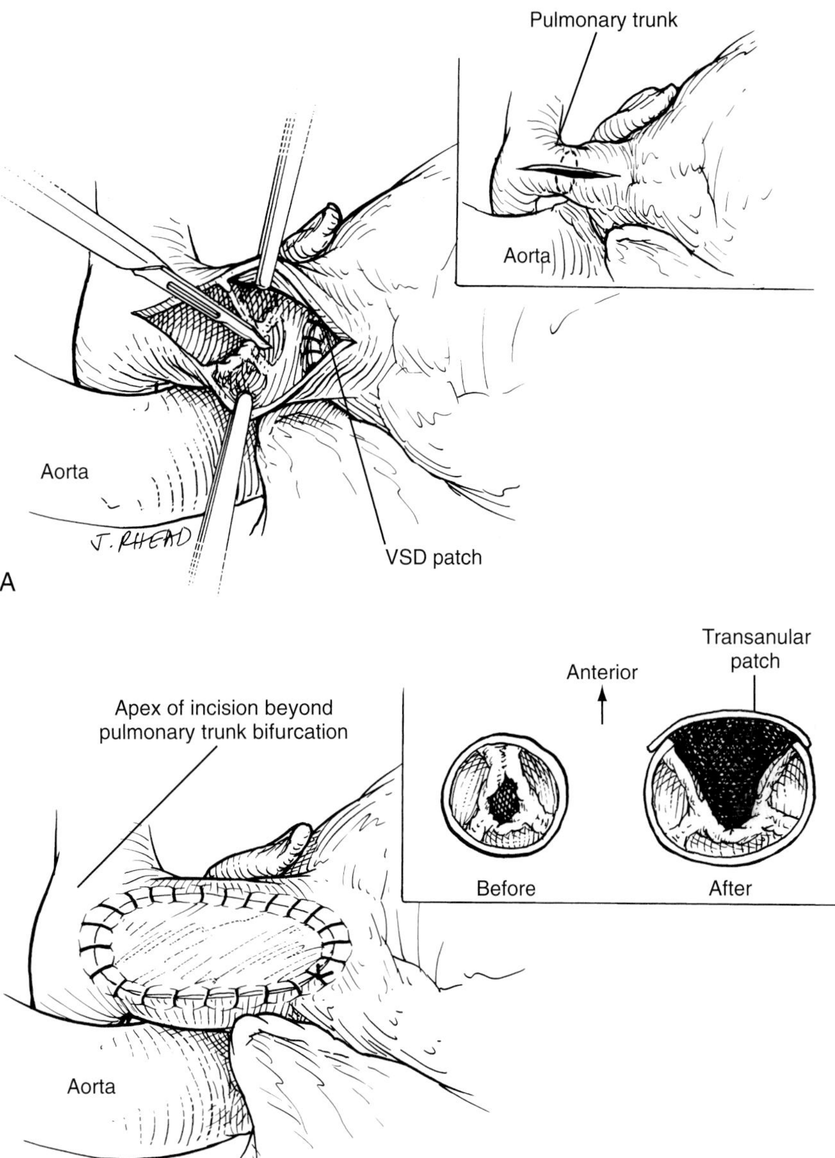

Figure 38-31 Use of transanular patch in repair of tetralogy of Fallot with pulmonary stenosis. **A,** Entire incision is made initially when a transanular patch is clearly indicated; otherwise, only a partial incision is made *(inset).* Note that incision extends beyond narrowest portion of pulmonary trunk, but only a short distance onto right ventricle. Pulmonary valve is excised completely and ventricular septal defect *(VSD)* repaired. **B,** A double-velour woven polyester (or polytetrafluoroethylene or pericardium) patch is trimmed to appropriate size and shape. When a polyester tube is used, it is elongated slightly by traction and cut to the correct length. It is then cut in half longitudinally and the ends trimmed. Note that distal end remains essentially square, with only corners trimmed off. When inserted, it forms a roof that is convex in all directions *(inset).*

necessary. In extreme cases (of both large and small "anuli"), this measurement can be highly predictive of whether or not a transanular patch will be needed. In many less extreme cases (z values between −2 and −4), intraoperative information will be used to decide when to place a transanular patch. The surgeon's bias regarding transanular patching is that it generally should not be necessary when the pulmonary "anulus" z value is larger than −3 as measured on the preoperative echocardiogram or cineangiogram. This is based on the high probability under these circumstances that the postrepair $P_{RV/LV}$ will be less than about 0.7,[K20] and on the anticipated increased need for insertion of a pulmonary valve very late postoperatively when a transanular patch has been placed.[K16] When the patient has TF with *subarterial* VSD, the "Asian" variant of TF, the surgeon's bias is that there is a three in four chance a transanular patch will be necessary.[V6]

Reassessment after closing the VSD is accomplished by estimating the diameter of the "anulus" with a Hegar dilator that passes snugly but not tightly through it. This provides one more precise estimate in borderline situations. This diameter is transformed to a z value as described in Chapter 1, Appendix Fig. 1D-1; generally this finding is similar to that obtained from the cineangiogram (but slightly smaller when the body surface area of the patient is less than 0.7 m^2 and slightly larger in patients with a body surface area greater than about 0.7 m^2).[B15] Generally, a transanular patch should not be placed when the z value is larger than −3. Otherwise, the incision is carried across the "anulus," the pulmonary valve excised, and the patch inserted (Fig. 38-31). If the situation is borderline, the lesser risk lies with inserting a transanular patch.

When a transanular patch is used, a major consideration is the distal extent of the incision in the pulmonary trunk, because this must be into an area of *distinctly greater diameter* than that of the "anulus," which is usually the narrowest area (Fig. 38-32). Otherwise, a transanular patch relieves only the small component of the high resistance produced by the length of the narrowing, and the gradient will persist

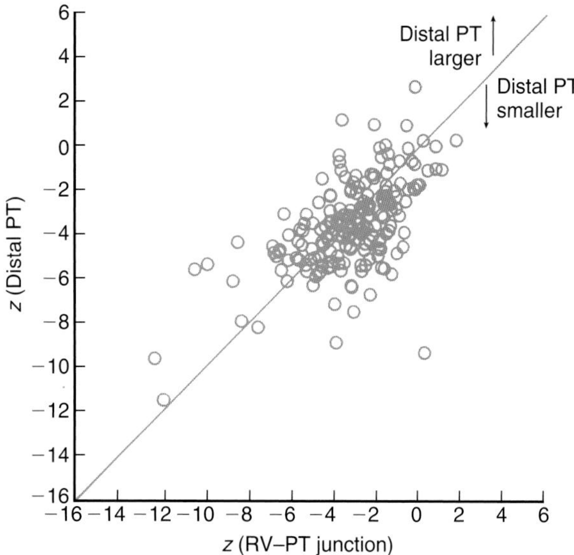

Figure 38-32 Scattergram illustrating relation between diameters of right ventricular–pulmonary trunk junction and those of distal portion of pulmonary trunk in patients having tetralogy of Fallot with pulmonary stenosis. In some patients with an anular *z* value of −4 or smaller, the distal pulmonary trunk is narrower than the "anulus." Key: *PT,* Pulmonary trunk; *RV,* right ventricle. (From Shimazaki and colleagues.[S10])

essentially unchanged and be at the junction of the patch and distal pulmonary trunk. In some patients the distal pulmonary trunk is narrower than the anulus; in these cases the incision is extended into the LPA, which usually continues in the same general direction as the pulmonary trunk and is usually proportionally larger than the distal pulmonary trunk. If the origin of the LPA is proportionally *no larger* than the distal pulmonary trunk, the incision and patch reconstruction should be carried into the midportion of the LPA, which is nearly always wider than the origin.[S10] Care must be taken to not damage the left phrenic nerve or left superior pulmonary vein. In neonates with a patent ductus, especially if they are on PGE_1, it is difficult to assess the proximal LPA, and patching that extends beyond the ductus onto the distal LPA should be performed.

The transanular patch may be of glutaraldehyde-treated or untreated autologous pericardium, processed bovine pericardium, or cut from a cylinder of preclotted double-velour woven polyester, collagen-impregnated knitted polyester, or PTFE. In neonates and young infants, autologous pericardium should be used exclusively. In older patients, collagen-impregnated polyester provides the benefit of precise sizing of the patch (an important consideration[F16,I4]), and when properly trimmed, its convexity is ensured, as is a relatively "square cut" of its distal end (see Fig. 38-31, *B*). Glutaraldehyde-treated pericardium has similar advantages. When a polyester tube is used, one is selected whose diameter corresponds to a *z* value of 0 to +2. Too large a transanular patch increases postoperative pulmonary regurgitation.[F16,I4,K42,O3,O4]

When the time comes for inserting the patch and the distal end of the incision is on the pulmonary trunk, the polyester tube is stretched *slightly* and cut to the length of the incision, cutting both ends squarely (see Fig. 38-31). The corrugated (crimped) nature of the tube provides sufficient length that it is convex longitudinally; the curve makes it a convex "roof" transversely. The tube is then cut longitudinally so that about three fifths of the circumference remains as the roof. Only the corners are trimmed at the distal end, leaving it very broad, while the proximal (RV) end is tapered. It is then sewn into place with a continuous 5-0 polypropylene suture (see Fig. 38-31, *B*).

When the incision has been carried onto the LPA, a slightly different technique is used, in the belief that the result is more apt to be geometrically correct. For this, a rectangular piece of pericardium is cut about 1.5 times wider than the apparent diameter of the LPA and about 1.5 times longer than the incision in the LPA. It is sewn into place with continuous 6-0 polypropylene sutures placed slightly farther apart in the patch than in the wall of the LPA. A polyester tube is used for the remainder of the reconstruction (Fig. 38-33). Alternatively, glutaraldehyde-treated pericardium can be used for both the transanular patch and the extension onto the LPA. Its length can be determined by measuring length of the incision from the RV to the pulmonary artery, and its maximum width is determined visually by holding the edges of the incision open at valve level and judging the size of the roof required to create a new pulmonary "anulus" whose diameter is no larger than three fourths the diameter of the ascending aorta. Alternatively, in infants, an 8-, 9-, or 10-mm Hegar dilator can be placed through the divided "anulus" and the width of the patch required to complete the roof over it measured. Both ends are cut almost transversely to create a blunt patch, particularly distally, and the patch is positioned using continuous 6-0 or 7-0 polypropylene sutures commencing at the distal end of the incision. The suture is placed using a running over-and-over technique, placing the first two or three throws along each side before pulling the pericardial patch into position as the suture is tightened. Suturing is continued down each side to anulus level, then the remainder of the right ventriculotomy is closed by incorporating the pericardial patch into it with continuous sutures. Deep bites of muscle are taken down each side and at the angle.

A monocusp may be attached to the pericardial roofing patch. The cusp diameter is fashioned somewhat larger than the planned roofed RV outflow. It is cut more or less circular and sutured to the patch when the latter suturing from distally reaches the valve "anulus."

Assessing Postrepair Right Ventricular Outflow Tract Obstruction

Measuring Postrepair (Operating Room [OR]) $P_{RV/LV}$ In older infants and beyond, the $P_{RV/LV}$ is helpful in assessing important residual RV outflow tract obstruction. After repair and separation from CPB, and preferably with the cannulae for CPB still in place, postrepair (OR) $P_{RV/LV}$ is obtained. The peripheral systemic systolic blood pressure can be used to estimate the P_{LV}. A polyvinyl catheter is placed through the right atrial wall and passed across the tricuspid valve into the RV to measure P_{RV}.

If a transanular patch has not been placed and postrepair (OR) $P_{RV/LV}$ is greater than 0.7, CPB should be reestablished and a transanular patch placed.

When a transanular patch has been placed and the ratio is greater than about 0.8, localizing the site of the gradient is vigorously pursued by pressure manometry or transesophageal echocardiography. If pressure gradient or localized obstruction is identified *between* the sinus portion of the RV

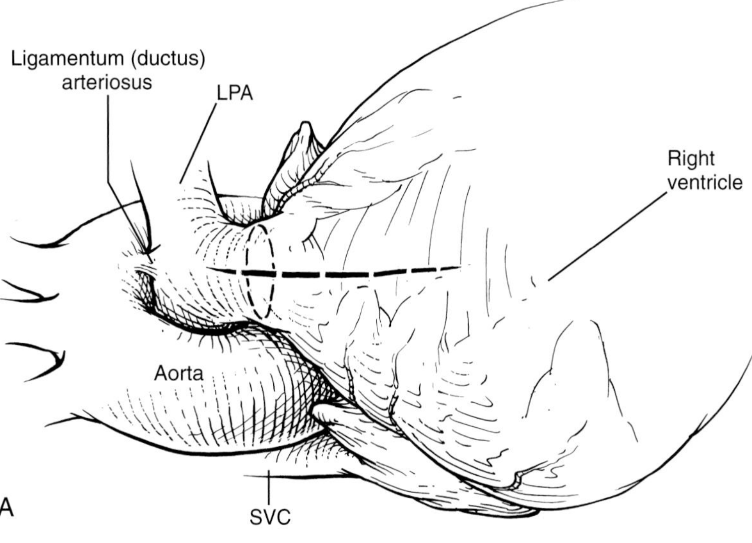

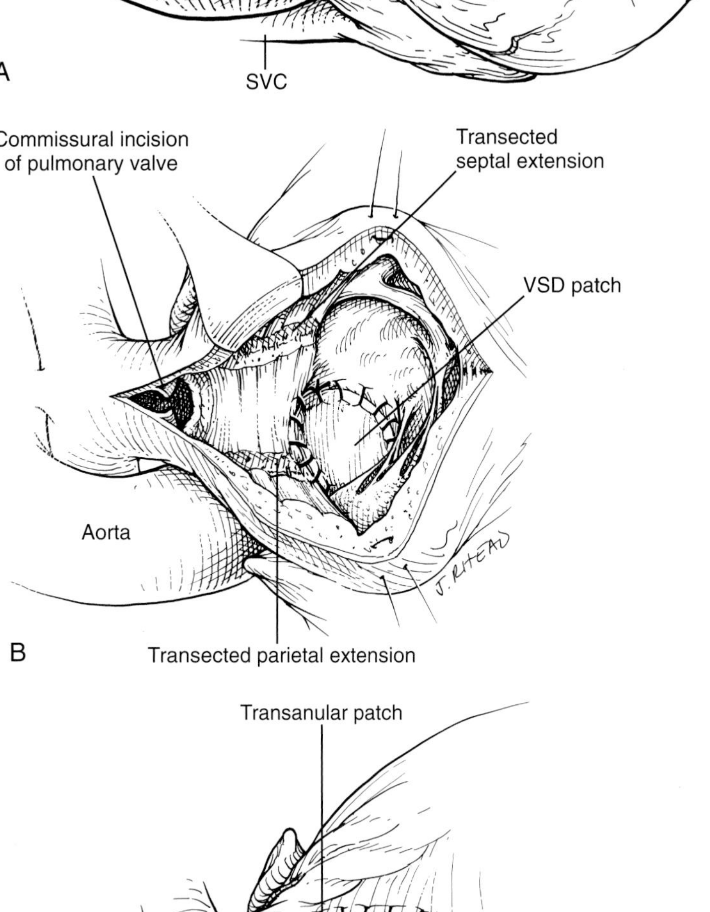

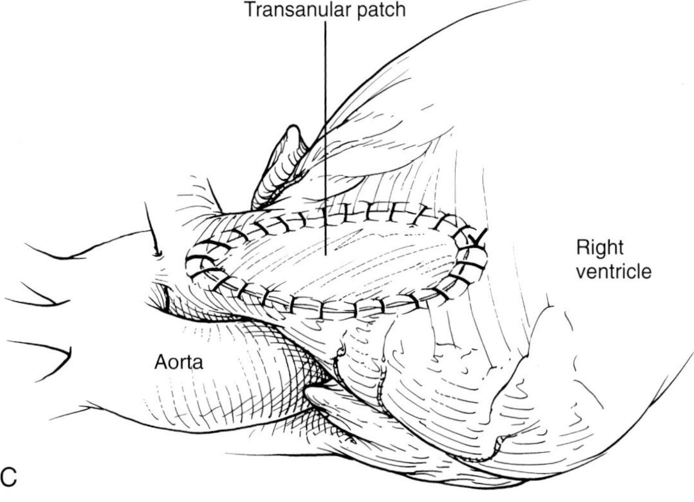

Figure 38-33 Repair of tetralogy of Fallot in neonates. **A,** A transanular right ventricular–pulmonary trunk incision is almost always used, keeping ventricular portion as cephalad as practicable. **B,** Pulmonary valve is incised fully to arterial wall and, if grossly distorted, resected fully. Parietal and septal extensions of the trabecula septomarginalis are incised at their origins from the infundibular septum, but resection of muscle is kept to a minimum. Ventricular septal defect *(VSD)* is closed as for the right ventricular approach (see Fig. 38-27). Often, pericardium is used for VSD patch. **C,** Transanular incision is closed with a polyester, polytetrafluoroethylene, or pericardial patch large enough to attain a mildly convex contour in all directions. Key: *LPA,* Left pulmonary artery; *SVC,* superior vena cava.

and distal end of the patch, CPB is reestablished and the situation corrected. If the operation has been properly performed (in which case the gradient is located at the distal end of the patch) and if the patch has been extended into a widened portion of the pulmonary trunk or LPA, little more can be done to relieve the obstruction.

If no correctable cause of the elevation of postrepair (OR) $P_{RV/LV}$ is found, and if the elevation is not extreme and the patient's condition is good, the patient should be sent to the intensive care unit (ICU) with continuous monitoring of RV pressure. There, over a few hours, postrepair (ICU) $P_{RV/LV}$ may fall to reasonable levels (see Special Features of Postoperative Care later in this section). If the patient's condition in the operating room is not good or if right atrial pressure is considerably elevated above left, then the situation is precarious, although uncommon, and requires action. CPB is reestablished, and a large hole is cut in the VSD patch, usually during a brief period of aortic clamping and through a right atriotomy.

Measuring Postrepair (OR) Right Ventricular Outflow Tract Pressure Gradient In neonates and young infants, compared with older patients, the $P_{RV/LV}$ is less helpful for assessing important residual RV outflow tract obstruction. There are several reasons for this. First, the data used to develop and interpret the ratio are from older patients, so the ratio thresholds predicting poor outcomes have not been validated in neonates. Second, and most important, the physiology in neonates and young infants is substantially different from that in older patients. Especially in the operating room post-CPB, systemic vascular resistance can be quite low, yielding systolic systemic arterial pressure (and thus the P_{LV}) as low as 50 mmHg. Also, Rp tends to be higher, so typically the P_{RV} may be as high as 40 to 45 mmHg without RV outflow tract obstruction. As a result, the $P_{RV/LV}$ may approach 1.0 without any residual RV outflow tract obstruction.

Nevertheless, assessment of residual obstruction, both when the pulmonary "anulus" is left intact and when a transanular patch is used, should be routinely performed. A polyvinyl catheter is placed in the RV as described in the previous section, to measure P_{RV}. Another catheter is placed in the pulmonary trunk and can be manipulated into the RPA and LPA, to obtain P_{PT}, P_{RPA}, and P_{LPA}. In a patient with an intact pulmonary valve "anulus," a gradient of 20 mmHg or more at the valve is an indication for revision with a transanular patch. In a patient with a transanular patch, a gradient of similar magnitude is an indication for revision at the specific site of the residual obstruction.

Management of Atrial Septum During repair, a PFO (present in about two thirds of patients[L9,R32]) should generally be closed in older infants and children. Rarely, a persistent atrial communication can be the source of paradoxical cerebral emboli late postoperatively.[L11] If a true atrial septal defect is not closed, there may be left-to-right shunting at atrial level. In neonates and infants, if a transanular patch is placed or if important pulmonary regurgitation is present, a PFO is left unclosed to allow decompression of any right atrial hypertension caused by acute RV failure.[C8,D16] Some arterial desaturation may be present in the first few postoperative days, but it then disappears as the RV remodels to accommodate the physiology of a high-volume, low-pressure circulation, as opposed to the preoperative physiology of a low-volume, high-pressure circulation. In fact, evidence of arterial desaturation is essentially proof that important RV failure is present.

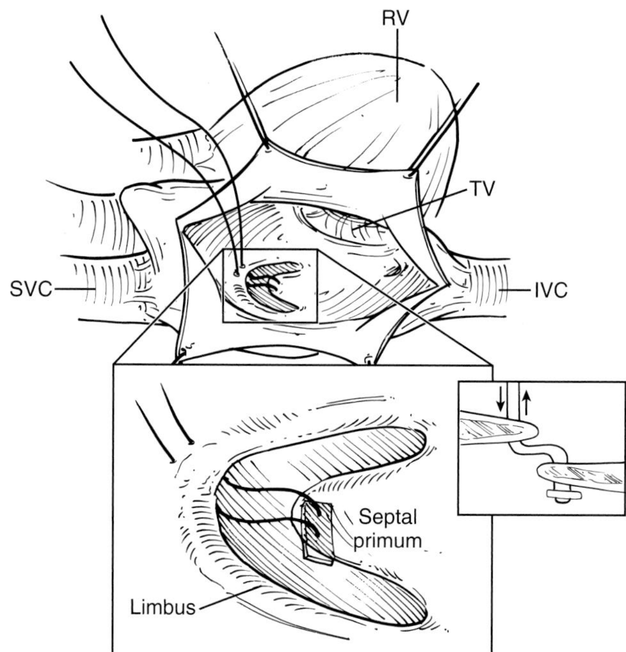

Figure 38-34 Technique of partial closure of patent foramen ovale (PFO) in patients undergoing infant tetralogy of Fallot repair. Using a standard right atriotomy, the limbus and free edge of the septum primum are identified. A single pledgeted mattress suture of 5-0 polypropylene is placed through edge of septum primum, with pledget positioned on left atrial surface of septum primum. Suture is then brought through limbus from left atrial side to right atrial side and is firmly tied. This reduces size of the PFO opening, but maintains its natural position and competence. Inset shows procedure from close up enface and profile perspectives. Key: *IVC,* Inferior vena cava; *RV,* right ventricle; *SVC,* superior vena cava; *TV,* tricuspid valve.

A PFO should be narrowed to a diameter of 3 to 4 mm. This is accomplished by suturing a portion of the free edge of the septum primum to the left side of the limbus (where it would naturally attach if spontaneous closure had occurred) using several 5-0 polypropylene mattress sutures (Fig. 38-34). This will preserve a functioning, but somewhat smaller, PFO. If the pulmonary valve is competent in neonates and infants after repair, important RV failure is unlikely, and the PFO can be closed at repair.

Repair of Uncomplicated Tetralogy of Fallot with Pulmonary Stenosis via Right Ventricle

After usual intraoperative preparations (see "Preparation for Cardiopulmonary Bypass" in Section III of Chapter 2), a median sternotomy is performed. Prompt control of major bleeding from collaterals is accomplished with electrocautery. The usual dissections are made (see "General Plan and Details of Repair Common to All Approaches" earlier in this section) and purse-string sutures and tapes placed. A polyester tube (see "Decision and Technique for Transanular Patching" earlier in this section) may be selected and pericardium may be removed and treated with glutaraldehyde.

CPB is established, and the patient's core temperature is cooled to 24° to 32°C using direct or indirect vena caval cannulation (see "Preparation for Cardiopulmonary Bypass in Section III of Chapter 2). The colder end of the spectrum should be considered in older, very cyanotic patients who may have developed substantial acquired systemic to pulmonary artery collaterals. Two venous cannulae are preferred; however, a single right atrial cannula can be used (see "One versus Two Venous Cannulae" under Special Situations and Controversies in Section III of Chapter 2). The cardioplegic catheter (or needle) is secured into the ascending aorta. An efficient system for venting the left heart is essential for precise repair of TF, because of the potential for high collateral flow return to the left atrium. The left atrial suction line may be inserted through the base of the right superior pulmonary vein through a purse-string suture and advanced across the mitral valve to vent the LV. The aorta is clamped and cold cardioplegic solution injected (see "Cold Cardioplegia, Controlled Aortic Root Reperfusion, and [When Needed] Warm Cardioplegic Induction" in Chapter 3). Efflux from the coronary sinus is aspirated and discarded or allowed to escape from the right atrium.

The RV is opened through a vertical (longitudinal) incision, sparing large conal and anterior branches of the RCA that cross the RV. If it is expected that the pulmonary valve will be adequate, the incision is made in the midportion of the RV infundibulum and extended nearly to, but not into, the pulmonary valve superiorly and just into the sinus portion of the RV (see Fig. 41-27, *A*).[K11] Two pledgeted stay sutures placed through each side of the incision are placed on traction for exposure (see Fig. 41-27, *B*). Alternatively, this can be achieved manually using a hand-held retractor.

Infundibular dissection is performed (see "General Plan and Details of Repair Common to All Approaches" earlier in this section and Figs. 38-26 and 38-27, *A* to *C*). The pulmonary valve is examined, and if it is stenotic, a valvotomy is performed through a pulmonary arteriotomy (see Fig. 38-30, *A*). Diameter of the valve anulus is estimated with Hegar dilators. If a transanular patch is considered necessary (see "Decision and Technique for Transanular Patching" earlier in this section), the infundibular incision is carried across the "anulus" before performing the infundibular dissection, paying attention to the position of the pulmonary valve commissures (see Fig. 38-31).

After the RV outflow tract is addressed, the VSD is closed using a patch (see Fig. 38-27, *D* to *F*). If the decision earlier in the operation has been not to use a transanular patch, measurements with Hegar dilators are repeated from the RV after VSD closure. If no further narrowing has resulted, the pulmonary arteriotomy and infundibular incision are closed with patches (see Fig. 38-30, *B*). Similarly, if a transanular incision has been used, it is closed with a patch of appropriate diameter (see "Decision and Technique for Transanular Patching" under Technical Details of Repair earlier in this section). The right atrium is opened and the atrial septum examined. If an atrial septal defect or PFO is present, it is managed as described in "Management of the Atrial Septum" under Technical Details of Repair earlier in this section). The right atriotomy is closed.

Rewarming and myocardial reperfusion (see Chapter 3) can be commenced at any point after VSD closure. Thus, by preference, the RV outflow tract patches can be placed and atrial septum addressed either with the aortic clamp in place or with rewarming and myocardial reperfusion initiated. Separation from CPB is performed in the usual way (see "Completing Cardiopulmonary Bypass" in Section III of Chapter 2).

Repair of Uncomplicated Tetralogy of Fallot with Pulmonary Stenosis via Right Atrium

This procedure is identical to repair through the RV up to the point that CPB is established. Aortic cannulation is standard. Bicaval venous cannulation is required. After commencing CPB, cooling is initiated. The left side is vented by placing a cannula through the right upper pulmonary vein across the mitral valve into the LV. Once the desired core temperature is achieved, the aorta is clamped and cardioplegia administered. The caval tapes are snugged, and a long right atriotomy is carried from the base of the appendage well inferiorly, a little anterior to the inferior vena cava cannula site. The right atrium, atrial septum, tricuspid valve, VSD, and RV outflow tract are examined (see Fig. 38-29, *A*).

With properly placed 6-0 polypropylene traction sutures on the septal and anterior leaflets of the tricuspid valve, edges of the VSD can usually be visualized,[1] although with more difficulty in TF than in isolated VSD because of the leftward and anterior displacement of the infundibular septum and its parietal extension.[K12] Alternatively, manual retraction by the surgical assistant using delicate instruments can achieve similar, or superior, exposure. The pathway from sinus to outflow portion of the RV is examined. The obstructive nature of the prominent parietal extension of the infundibular septum (see Figs. 38-28 and 38-29, *B*) is particularly well appreciated from this approach, and the infundibular chamber, if present, is easily visualized. The pulmonary valve can usually also be well seen. The VSD is repaired by sewing into place a patch (autologous glutaraldehyde pericardium or polyester velour) with continuous polypropylene (Fig. 38-29, *B* to *D*). It is closed before mobilizing and resecting the parietal band (as illustrated in Fig. 38-29). Often this allows better visualization of the borders of the VSD and, importantly, defines the limit of parietal extension to be resected (see Fig. 38-29, *B*). The VSD patch protects the aortic valve and crista during subsequent relief of outflow stenosis. Care should be taken not to cut or loosen the continuous patch suture anteriorly when resecting the parietal band. If needed, several interrupted sutures should be placed on this portion of the rim of the VSD patch.

RV outflow tract obstruction is addressed following VSD closure. The parietal extension is deeply incised 2 to 4 mm beyond its origin (toward the free wall) from the infundibular septum and 4 to 5 mm above the aortic cusps, which are visualized as the cut is made (see Fig. 38-29, *E*). The parietal extension is then dissected away from the ventriculoinfundibular fold (inner curvature of the RV) and from the anterior free wall of the RV and excised. The free wall of the RV is palpated occasionally from outside during this dissection to avoid perforating it. Any hypertrophied and obstructive trabeculae along the left side of the outflow tract are incised and removed together with the fibrous margins of the infundibulum. The infundibular chamber and areas just proximal to the pulmonary valve are examined to determine (in concert with the preoperative imaging studies) whether they need to be widened by an infundibular patch. Generally speaking, if this is the case, the atrial approach should not have been

[1]In about 5% of patients, aortic dextroposition is sufficiently severe that the cephalad (superior) borders of the VSD cannot be seen except with extreme traction on the tricuspid valve. In these cases, rather than using such strong traction, the right atrial approach is aborted and the RV approach used.

considered. This is because in TF, the VSD is always easier to expose and close through a ventriculotomy than through an atriotomy. Thus, if a ventriculotomy (infundibulotomy) is required because of a narrow infundibulum, the VSD should be closed through the infundibular incision. It makes little sense to close the VSD through the right atrium if an infundibular incision is required. The pulmonary valve is examined and the diameter of the "anulus" is estimated by passing a Hegar dilator antegrade across the RV outflow tract.

If a pulmonary valvotomy is needed, it is usually done through a vertical incision in the pulmonary trunk (see Fig. 38-30). After valvotomy, RV outflow diameter is again estimated by sizing the pulmonary valve orifice with Hegar dilators. The pulmonary arteriotomy is closed, usually with a pericardial patch. Management of an atrial septal defect or PFO and the remainder of the operation proceed as described for repair through the RV.

Repair of Tetralogy of Fallot in Infancy

A median sternotomy is performed and the heart exposed. A subtotal thymectomy is performed, paying careful attention to the phrenic nerve. If the echocardiogram or cineangiogram indicates that a transanular patch is required, and in borderline cases, the front of the pericardium is removed from where it joins the diaphragm to its most superior reflection from the aorta. This secures a piece of pericardium at least 6 cm long and 3 cm wide, tapering at both ends. The pericardium is stretched with its epicardial surface downward onto moist gauze or cardboard and is set aside for later use. Dissection of the pulmonary trunk, RPA, LPA, and ductus arteriosus or ligamentum arteriosum is easily and rapidly achieved.

CPB is established using aortic cannulation and, preferably, bicaval cannulation; however, single venous cannulation of the right atrium can be used. Standard continuous CPB with cooling to 28° to 32°C and cardioplegic cardiac arrest is preferred. The left heart is vented in standard fashion through the right upper pulmonary vein. Alternatively, hypothermic circulatory arrest can be used and is preferred by some. The ductus arteriosus, if present, is doubly ligated using two 5-0 polypropylene sutures and divided. The suture used to ligate the pulmonary artery end of the ductus should be placed precisely, at least 3 mm distal to the pulmonary artery origin of the ductus, to avoid constriction of the LPA branch or obstruction of the LPA lumen by extrusion of bulky ductal tissue. If a ligamentum is present, it should also be ligated and divided to avoid tethering of the LPA origin, which can cause late kinking and LPA obstruction, especially if pulmonary regurgitation and RV outflow tract dilatation develop. When imaging studies indicate that a transanular patch is not required and when dissection of the pulmonary trunk confirms that it is of adequate diameter, a vertical incision is made into the RV (see Fig. 38-27). The infundibular stenosis is completely relieved. This often involves simple transection of the parietal and septal extensions of the TSM, rather than resection (similar to that shown in Fig. 38-33, *B*). The pulmonary valve is examined from below and any stenosis relieved in the manner already described. The VSD is closed through the infundibular incision (similar to that shown in Fig. 38-27).

The tricuspid valve is retracted and the atrial septum exposed, looking retrograde from the RV into the right atrium. If a PFO is present, it is often possible to close or modify it from this approach; if not, the right atrium is opened and the PFO is managed through this approach. Or, if there is a more extensive atrial septal defect, the right atrium is opened and the defect closed using a pericardial patch with continuous polypropylene suture. If it has to be reduced in size, it is managed as described in Fig. 38-34. The right atrium is closed. The ventriculotomy is then closed with a narrow patch, also using a continuous suture.

When a transanular patch is indicated, the incision is carried across the "anulus" and out along the pulmonary trunk almost to the origin of the LPA, and a transanular pericardial patch is placed after VSD closure (see Fig. 38-33, *A*). Should there be LPA origin stenosis, the incision passes beyond this to reach the normal-diameter LPA (Fig. 38-35). If a transanular patch is used in neonates and young infants, the PFO should always be left open.

Repair of Tetralogy of Fallot with Stenosis at Origin of Left Pulmonary Artery

In this situation, there is usually sufficient hypoplasia of the pulmonary anulus and trunk that a transanular patch is also required (see Morphology earlier in this section). Repair is usually accomplished in exactly the manner described for situations in which the incision for placing a transanular patch must be extended onto the LPA (see "Decision and Technique for Transanular Patching" earlier in this section and see Fig. 38-35). In those uncommon instances in which a transanular patch is not needed, an incision is made across the stenosis in the origin of the LPA. A rectangular patch of pericardium is trimmed and sewn into place as described.

When there is virtual or total occlusion of the LPA origin, patch graft enlargement is not satisfactory. Instead, after locating the patent portion of the LPA beyond the zone of occlusion by dissecting along the chord of tissue that still connects it to the pulmonary trunk bifurcation, the patent LPA is opened longitudinally on its anterior surface for a short distance. The opened end is then sutured to the adjacent leftward edge of the pulmonary trunk with a running fine polypropylene suture to create a new posterior wall. The anterior wall is next created by a pericardial patch positioned as for reconstruction of a zone of stenosis (see earlier text). When the LPA is totally disconnected from the pulmonary trunk or is too small for this reconstruction, repair entails locating the LPA close to or adjacent to the lung hilum (usually by intrapleural dissection) and disconnecting it from any vessel, usually the ductus arteriosus, that supplies it. It is then usually possible to anastomose the LPA end to side to the leftward edge of the distal pulmonary trunk (mobilizing the trunk completely so that it will swing more easily to the left). If the LPA is narrowed proximally, however, a technique similar to that described earlier is employed.

Repair of Tetralogy of Fallot with Stenosis at Origin of Right Pulmonary Artery

This situation occurs uncommonly without associated LPA stenosis. In contrast to the LPA, the RPA is usually *not* an extension of the pulmonary trunk but comes off its side at a right angle. This makes the simple type of repair used for origin stenosis of the LPA less satisfactory, although it can be used when stenosis is not too severe.

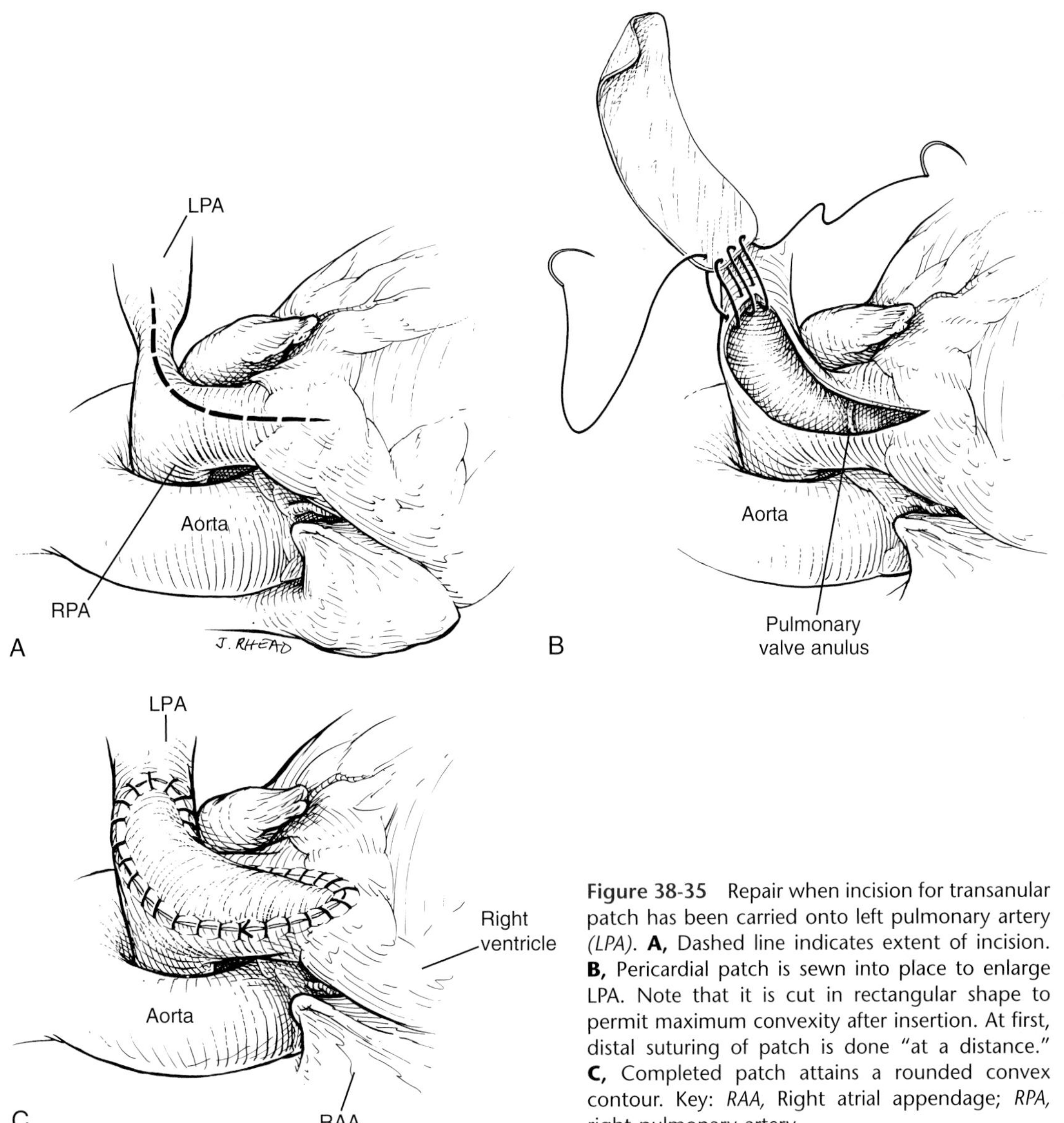

Figure 38-35 Repair when incision for transanular patch has been carried onto left pulmonary artery *(LPA)*. **A,** Dashed line indicates extent of incision. **B,** Pericardial patch is sewn into place to enlarge LPA. Note that it is cut in rectangular shape to permit maximum convexity after insertion. At first, distal suturing of patch is done "at a distance." **C,** Completed patch attains a rounded convex contour. Key: *RAA,* Right atrial appendage; *RPA,* right pulmonary artery.

Operation proceeds as usual until the VSD has been repaired. Then a small longitudinal incision is made in the pulmonary trunk to visualize the RPA orifice (Fig. 38-36, *A*). The origin of the RPA is excised from the pulmonary trunk. Lateral incisions are made to enlarge the orifice in the side of the pulmonary trunk (Fig. 38-36, *B*). The RPA is incised from its narrow orifice back into its wide portion. A rectangular piece of pericardium is trimmed and sewn to the RPA to make a markedly enlarged proximal RPA (Fig. 38-36, *C*). The proximal end of the reconstructed RPA is then sutured to the enlarged orifice in the side of the pulmonary trunk using continuous 6-0 or 7-0 polypropylene sutures, while taking care to avoid any purse-string effect (Fig. 38-36, *D*). Alternatively, the posterior edge of the opened RPA is sutured to the back wall of the opened pulmonary trunk; the rectangular piece of pericardium is then sewn to the remaining opening to widen it further.

Transection of the ascending aorta to improve exposure is rarely necessary.

Repair of Tetralogy of Fallot with Bifurcation Stenosis of Pulmonary Trunk

This condition requires appropriate reconstruction based on proper understanding of the morphology, although few papers discuss details of this repair.[L7] Both the LPA and RPA ostia are usually stenosed to a similar degree and over a short distance (<15 mm), and the distal pulmonary trunk is often similarly narrowed. The pulmonary trunk may be short, making the bifurcation proximal and more Y-shaped than usual.

In patients 5 years of age or older, the optimal procedure may be to replace the pulmonary valve, trunk, bifurcation, and proximal RPA and LPA with a pulmonary allograft (Fig. 38-37).[B36,C21] It is a less desirable operation in infants, however, because the allograft will almost certainly be outgrown and require earlier replacement than when used in older children. However, this procedure has the greatest probability of providing a good hemodynamic result in this complex situation.

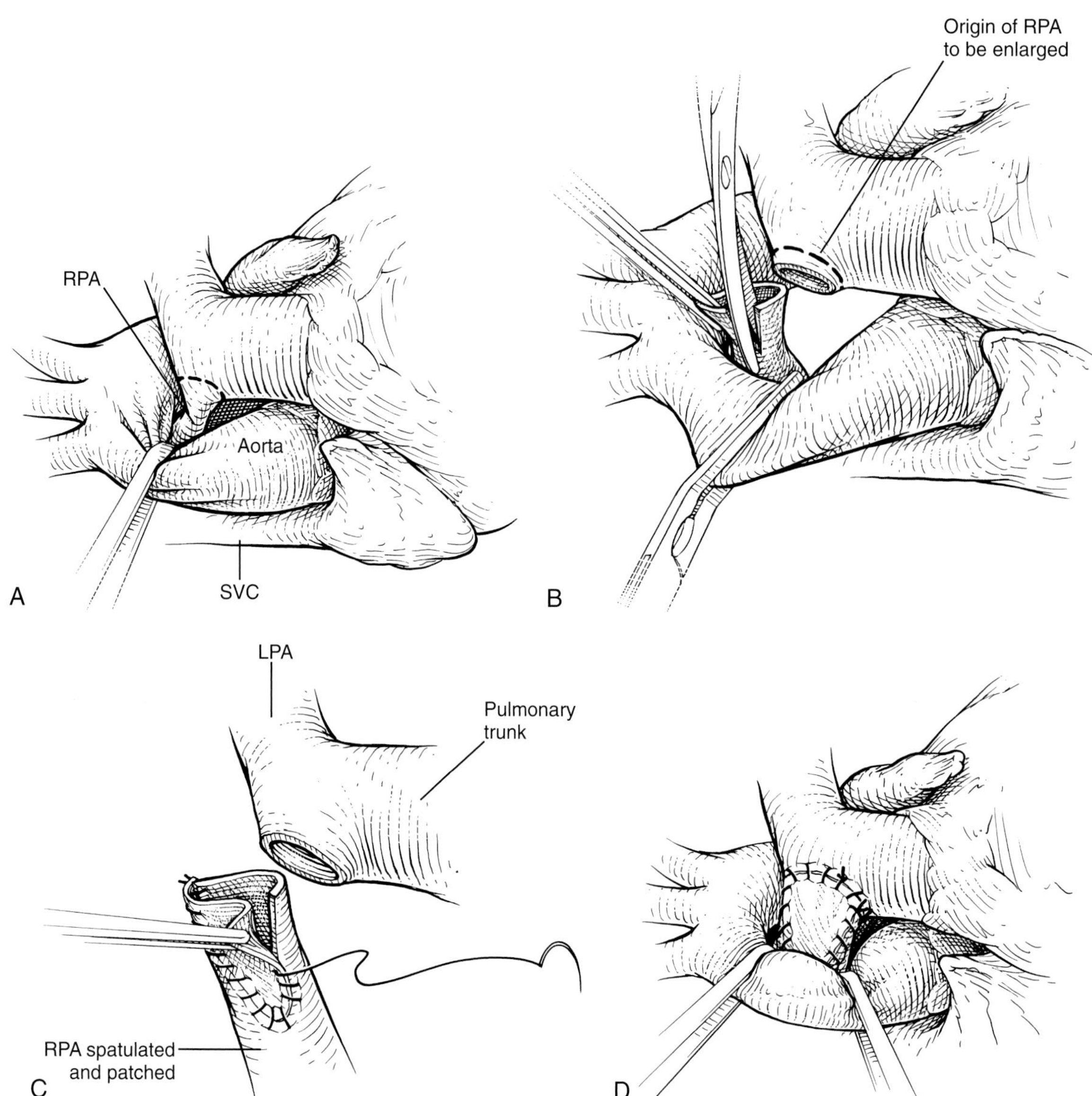

Figure 38-36 One type of repair of stenosis at origin of right pulmonary artery *(RPA)*. Initially, a small incision is made in pulmonary trunk through which stenotic orifice of RPA can be viewed from within. **A,** Ascending aorta has been mobilized to expose origin of RPA. Proposed incision for disconnecting RPA from pulmonary trunk is shown. **B,** RPA has been disconnected from pulmonary trunk. Resulting orifice in RPA can be enlarged as shown, but enlargement by *incision* is preferable. An incision is made down anterior aspect of RPA. **C,** RPA is enlarged with a pericardial patch. **D,** Enlarged RPA is reattached to enlarged aperture in pulmonary trunk. (At times, it may be easier to suture posterior wall of RPA to posterior aspect of pulmonary trunk orifice before making pericardial enlargement of RPA.) Key: *LPA,* Left pulmonary artery; *SVC,* superior vena cava.

Alternatively, and especially in infants, repair rather than replacement is indicated (Fig. 38-38). Complete mobilization of the aorta, pulmonary trunk, RPA, and LPA is required, preferably before CPB. The vertical ventriculotomy is carried across the anulus into the pulmonary trunk and extended to the bifurcation. A second incision is made on the anterior aspect of the branch pulmonary arteries, extending from the normal diameter of the distal LPA, across the stenotic region of the LPA, onto the RPA, and extending across the stenotic region of the RPA to the distal normal-diameter RPA. Thus, the two incisions described create a T shape. Autologous pericardial tissue or allograft pulmonary artery tissue is used to patch-augment the pulmonary trunk and branch pulmonary arteries. Two patches are used, the first to patch the branch pulmonary arteries (Fig. 38-38, *A*) and the second as the transanular patch, which extends distally to the first patch (Fig. 38-38, *B*).

Repair of Tetralogy of Fallot with Anomalous Origin of Left Anterior Descending Coronary Artery from Right Coronary Artery

In hearts in which there is a large coronary artery crossing the RV outflow tract close to the pulmonary "anulus" (usually an anomalously arising LAD from the RCA, but sometimes the entire left coronary artery coming from the RCA), relief of pulmonary stenosis must neither divide nor compromise flow through this vessel. Because such a vessel is occasionally

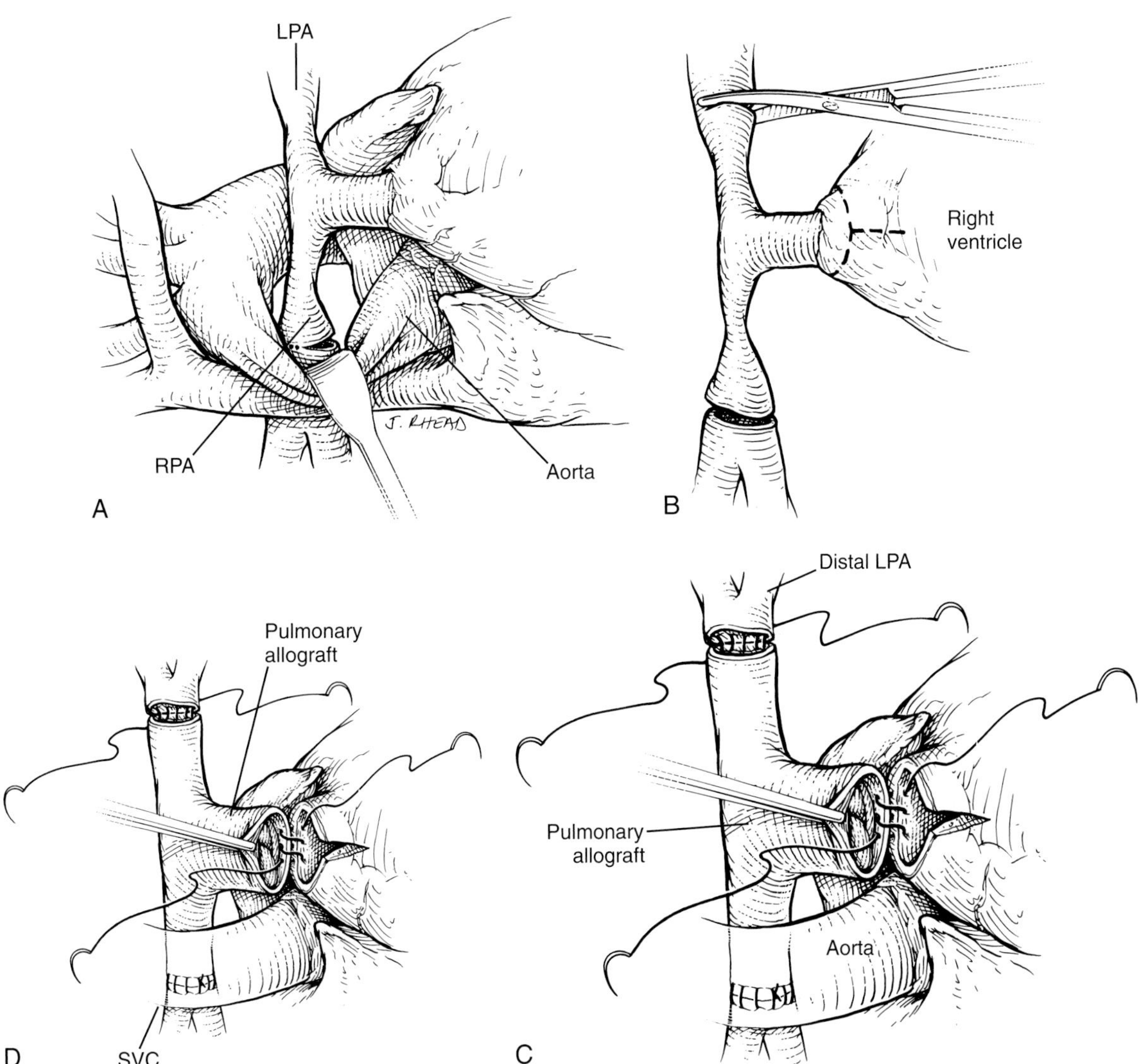

Figure 38-37 Repair of severe pulmonary trunk and bifurcation stenosis using a pulmonary valve allograft and its bifurcation. **A,** Dissection must be complete. For this, entire ascending aorta is completely freed from its posterior connections and from pulmonary trunk and its bifurcation. **B,** Superior vena cava is completely mobilized and right and left pulmonary arteries *(RPA and LPA)* dissected at least to the point where the first branch is visualized; that is, beyond the immediately prebranching level. **C,** Ascending aorta may be divided, but often the procedure can be performed without this step. Distal anastomoses are made first, taking care to transect the LPA and RPA beyond the narrow areas and to leave some redundancy in allograft bifurcation. **D,** Completion of the proximal anastomosis, often with a polyester (or pericardial) hood as shown. If transected, aorta is brought together end to end. Importantly, however, if aorta is enlarged and compresses the underlying allograft bifurcation or RPA, a short segment of polyester or polytetrafluoroethylene tube should be interposed between the two ends of the aorta. Key: *SVC,* Superior vena cava.

buried in muscle or fat and is not apparent on surface inspection at operation, preoperative imaging must be of sufficient quality to exclude this anomaly. When there is uncertainty, site of the usual course of the first part of the LAD is investigated during operation, and if the LAD is not there, it arises anomalously. When anomalous origin is present, technique of repair depends on morphology of the RV outflow obstruction, as usual. When the pulmonary "anulus" is of adequate diameter, either a vertical or transverse right ventriculotomy is made low in the outflow tract, well away from the coronary artery, and the infundibular stenosis is relieved from below. Alternatively, repair is accomplished via the right atrium. Any valvar stenosis is relieved via the pulmonary trunk.

When there is a small pulmonary "anulus" and proximal pulmonary trunk, a vertical ventriculotomy may be made after dissecting the anomalous artery from its bed in the RV wall over almost its entire length from its origin to near the interventricular groove. The incision is then carried beneath it and across the "anulus" into the pulmonary trunk. Infundibular stenosis is relieved in the usual fashion and a patch sufficiently large to relieve the stenosis positioned beneath the artery across the "anulus." If this is done, care is taken to avoid making the native pulmonary valve regurgitant by injudicious valvotomy. This technique can be used only when the RV outflow tract requires mild or moderate augmentation such that the width of the patch is not so great that the coronary artery will be distorted; severely hypoplastic RV outflow tracts should not be managed in this way. Alternatively, an allograft valved conduit can be used to augment the RV outflow tract, connecting the low infundibulum to the pulmonary trunk.

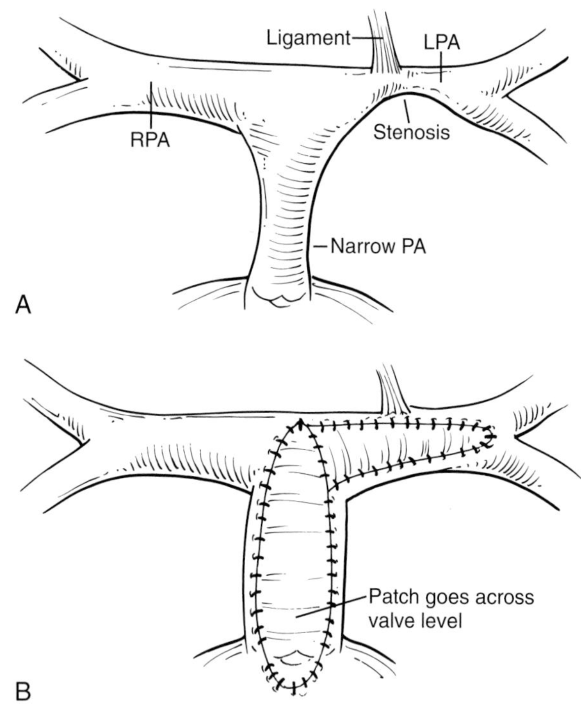

Figure 38-38 Repair of left pulmonary artery *(LPA)* stenosis in tetralogy of Fallot using two-patch technique. **A,** Typical right ventricular (RV) outflow tract hypoplasia and LPA stenosis present at ductus arteriosus or ligamentum arteriosum. **B,** Separate RV outflow tract patches and LPA patches are placed using a running monofilament suturing technique. This technique is useful when the angle of take-off of the LPA makes a single patch difficult to position correctly. Key: *PA,* Pulmonary artery; *RPA,* right pulmonary artery.

This technique may be used by choice, instead of the patch technique, when the infundibulum requires mild or moderate augmentation; it is the only option when marked augmentation is needed.

If the left coronary artery is damaged by the right ventriculotomy, the left internal thoracic artery can be taken down (see "Internal Thoracic Artery" under Technique of Operation in Chapter 7) and anastomosed to the distal left coronary artery. Alternatively, the coronary can be primarily repaired. This procedure can be life saving.

Repair of Tetralogy of Fallot after Blalock-Taussig Shunt or Polytetrafluoroethylene Interposition Shunt

Systemic-to–pulmonary artery shunts will have been created either through a thoracotomy (left or right) or a median sternotomy, and will consist of either a native systemic artery–pulmonary artery anastomosis (classic B-T shunt), or an interposition PTFE graft between the systemic and pulmonary artery. In the modern era, PTFE shunts are used much more commonly than classic B-T shunts, and a median sternotomy approach has commonly been used. However, variation in preferred shunt technique still exists, and older patients may be encountered with shunts placed using techniques rarely used today.

In many centers, median sternotomy has replaced lateral thoracotomy for primary systemic–pulmonary arterial shunts in neonates. Generally, a PTFE tube graft is used, connecting the brachiocephalic artery or brachiocephalic-subclavian junction to a pulmonary artery. In patients with a left aortic arch, the shunt is placed on the right side; with a right arch, it is on the left. At complete repair, access to the shunt is much better than that for all other types of shunts, with the graft positioned intrapericardially and centrally. Right-sided shunts are positioned medial to the superior vena cava and apposed to the lateral aspect of the ascending aorta, and on the left, just leftward of the ascending aorta. The shunt can be dissected prior to institution of CPB in most cases, the only exception being deeply cyanotic patients with a very small shunt. Interruption of the shunt is accomplished as CPB is initiated by placing appropriately sized hemostasis clips securely across the tube graft at the systemic and pulmonary ends. The graft is divided.

Median sternotomy in an older patient with TF and a *classic B-T shunt* is usually accompanied by profuse bleeding from arteries in front of and behind the sternum that have developed as part of the collateralization that follows subclavian artery ligation. While this bleeding is being controlled, rapid volume replacement should not be made with banked blood. This is because this low-calcium-content and low-pH blood passes directly across the VSD into the aorta and coronary arteries. If this cold, unmodified banked blood is infused rapidly, the heart may slow and even develop asystole. Warmed calcium-enriched blood may be used.

Left thoracotomy has often been used for shunt placement in neonates or small infants with a left aortic arch. Typically, a left PTFE tube graft has been used between the left subclavian artery and LPA. In part this was motivated by the ease with which it can be closed during repair. After sternotomy is performed, hemostasis secured, and sternal retractor inserted, and when the patient's condition is good, initial dissection is made. Because the graft lies deeply in the left chest, the approach is not beneath the thymus gland but over it, directly into the left pleural space. The few adhesions between the mediastinal pleura and lung are divided with the electrocautery. The PTFE tube graft is somewhat rigid and easily palpated. A small incision is made directly over it and carried down to it. At times a plane of dissection between the graft wall and surrounding tissue is easily established; if so, this dissection is carried out. Otherwise, the pericardium is opened and CPB established. The lungs are collapsed, and a plane of dissection is easily established around the graft. The shunt is clipped at each end and divided. Remainder of the operation is carried out as usual.

When a classic *right* B-T shunt is present in a patient with a left aortic arch, the pericardium is opened, and as the assistant elevates and retracts the ascending aorta to the left, the RPA is visualized coming from beneath the aorta. The superior vena cava is dissected off it and gently retracted rightward (in a few cases, exposure of the subclavian artery may be easier with the superior vena cava retracted to the left).[K30] Possible distortions of the RPA by the shunt are known from preoperative imaging studies, and these are kept in mind as dissection proceeds. Course of the right subclavian artery coming down to the RPA usually can be suspected from observation and palpation of a continuous thrill. The entire circumference of the subclavian artery may be freed along a short length by sharp dissection well superior to the anastomosis, and two heavy ligatures placed loosely around it. The artery is then temporarily occluded, and if vessel identification has been correct, the continuous thrill disappears, systolic and diastolic systemic arterial pressures increase, and pulse pressure narrows. If these things do not occur, the RPA has been misidentified as the subclavian artery or the shunt is small. The heart is cannulated, CPB is begun, ligatures around the subclavian artery are tied, and the operation proceeds as usual. An alternative preferred method is closure with hemostasis clips, in which case temporary ligatures are not placed.

When a classic *left* B-T shunt is present in a patient with a left or right aortic arch, the subclavian artery is approached from outside the pericardium. For this, the upper left pericardial stay sutures are placed on strong traction to the patient's right. Level of the LPA is noted before this maneuver; just cephalad (superior) to this level, the thymus gland and left phrenic nerve are dissected from the pericardium, sharply and over a limited area, because excessive dissection in this region can result in major bleeding that is difficult to control. A narrow retractor is slipped under the thymus, and the region of the subclavian artery is located by gentle palpation and sharp dissection beneath the thymus gland. The subclavian artery is dissected out as described for the right side, and the same tests are made for accuracy of identification. Operation then proceeds as described earlier.

If the left subclavian artery cannot be located by going over the thymus gland and phrenic nerve, an alternative method is used in patients with a right aortic arch. The brachiocephalic artery is identified beneath the brachiocephalic vein and traced distally to the point at which it bifurcates into left subclavian and left common carotid arteries. After identifying the left subclavian artery positively by the maneuvers described and by the fact that the anesthesiologist can feel the left common carotid (or left superficial temporal) pulse when the vessel is temporarily occluded, the operation proceeds as described.

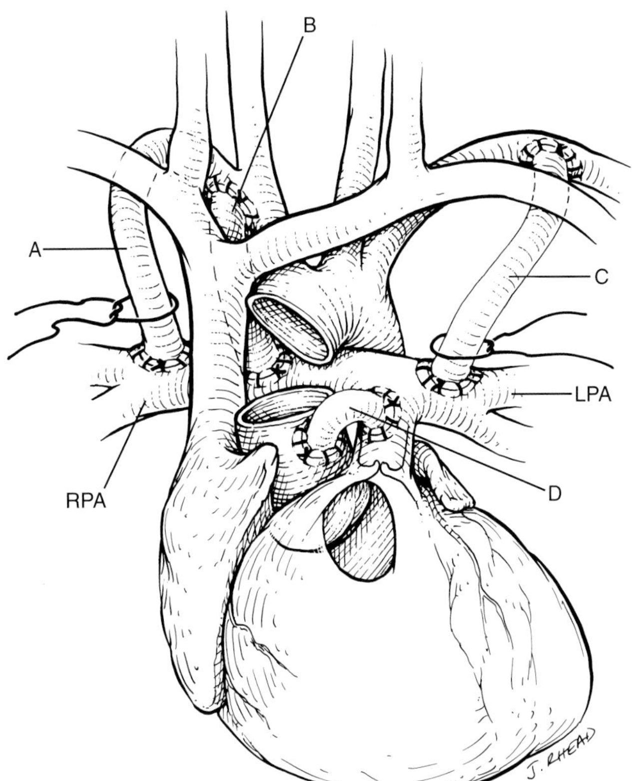

Figure 38-39 Composite diagram illustrating various positions of the usual systemic–pulmonary arterial shunts for augmenting pulmonary blood flow. *A,* Classic right Blalock-Taussig subclavian–pulmonary artery shunt with left (normal) aortic arch. *B,* Usual polytetrafluoroethylene (PTFE) interposition tube graft, shown between right pulmonary artery and brachiocephalic artery bifurcation. *C,* Left-sided PTFE interposition tube graft, shown between left pulmonary artery and left subclavian artery. *D,* Central shunt utilizing short PTFE tube between ascending aorta and pulmonary trunk. Key: *LPA,* Left pulmonary artery; *RPA,* right pulmonary artery.

Repair of Tetralogy of Fallot after Waterston and Potts Shunts

These shunts are of historical interest only; they are not used in current practice. In previous years, occasional older patients were seen for evaluation and repair who received the shunt many years before. Nearly all such patients have been repaired or have died; thus, it is rare to encounter such a patient currently. TF repair after Waterston[A8,E11,Y2] or Potts[G30,K25] shunt can be performed using well-described techniques, including those in editions 1 through 3 of this book.

Technique of Shunting Operations

Fig. 38-39 is a composite illustration of various positions used for systemic–pulmonary arterial shunts for augmenting pulmonary blood flow. General anesthesia with endotracheal intubation and controlled ventilation is used. Monitoring with an intraarterial catheter placed in an artery that will not serve as the systemic source of the shunt is established. Reliable intravenous access is obtained, either centrally or peripherally. Continuous pulse oxymetry is utilized. Details of each type of shunt follow.

Classic Right Blalock-Taussig Shunt

This is the original shunt described; however, it is typically not the first choice in modern practice. This is because it has the disadvantages of both sacrificing direct circulation to the right arm and delivering unpredictable flow to the pulmonary arteries. The artery can vary in size initially and can dilate over time. It may have some advantage in extremely small infants.

With the patient in left lateral decubitus position, a right lateral thoracic incision is made (Fig. 38-40, *A*, inset). The thorax is entered through either the top of the bed of the nonresected fourth rib or the third interspace. A rib spreader is positioned and gradually opened (see Fig. 38-40, *A*).

The first step in dissection is to securely identify the right superior pulmonary vein as it courses obliquely downward (medially and inferiorly) toward the heart to pierce the pericardium posterior to the phrenic nerve. The vein partially overlies the RPA; however, the RPA, in contrast to the vein, follows a straight course medially. With the lung retracted toward the surgeon, the periarterial sheath over the RPA is incised. Usually the superior branch of the RPA is first freed, in the process of which the main RPA (lying in a slightly different plane of dissection) can be easily overlooked. To find it, the superior surface of the right superior pulmonary vein is cleared, and it and the superior vena cava are elevated (Fig. 38-40, *A*). Dissection is carried centrally until the proximal RPA is identified as a single vessel, proximal to its first branch. With lateral traction on a loop of heavy suture placed around it, the RPA is dissected in the periarterial tissue plane

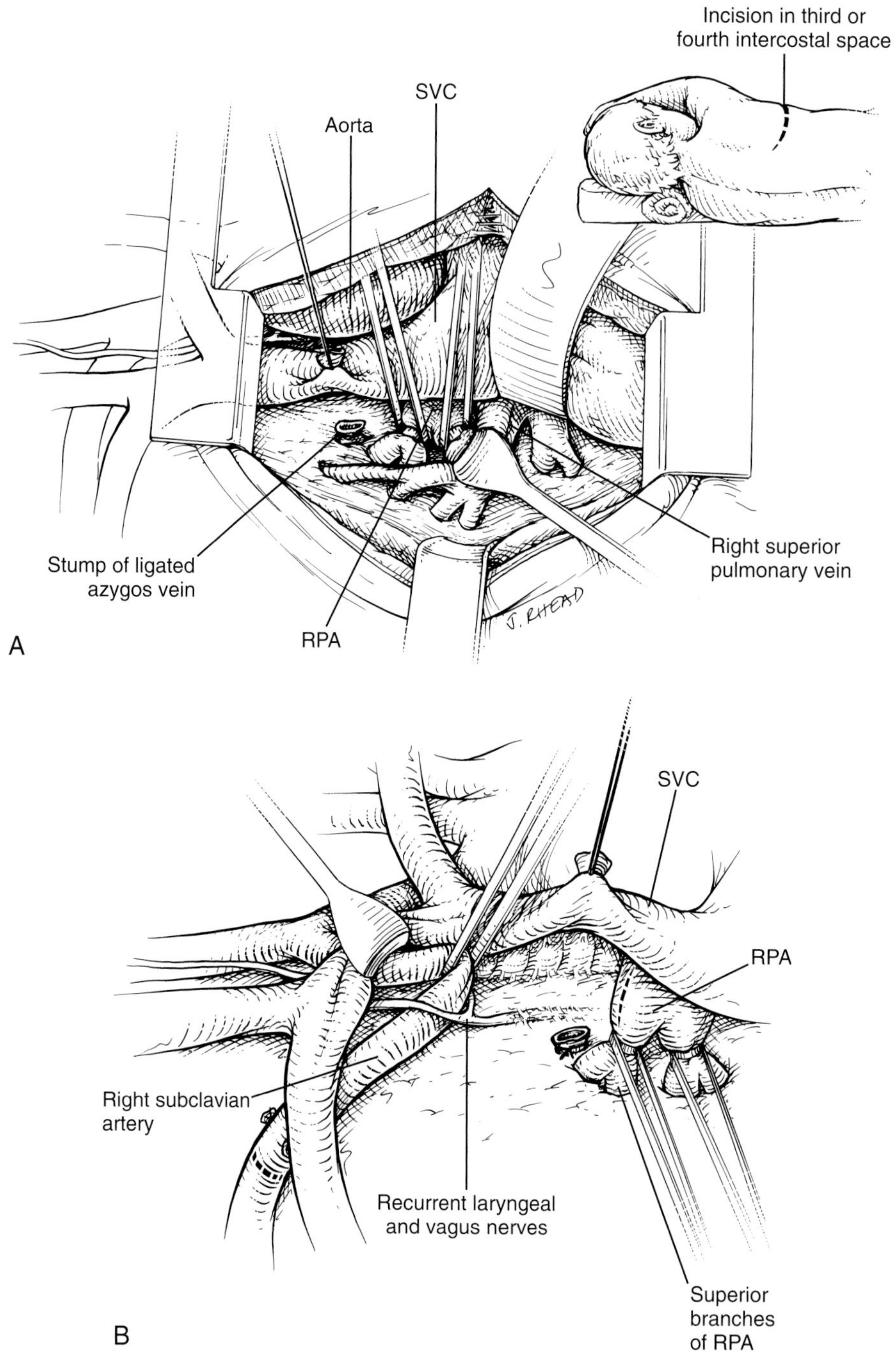

Figure 38-40 Classic right Blalock-Taussig shunt (left aortic arch). **A,** Right lateral thoracotomy is made in third or fourth intercostal space *(inset)*. Right pulmonary artery *(RPA)* and its branches are mobilized and azygos vein ligated and transected. **B,** Right subclavian artery is completely dissected, mobilized, and ligated just proximal or distal to its first branch. It is then divided as shown by dashed line and brought out from beneath the vagus nerve.

as far centrally as possible. The loop is then removed so that the RPA does not inadvertently become obstructed during the next phase of the operation.

The lung is packed off and retracted inferiorly. An incision is made in the mediastinal pleura over the azygos vein and carried superiorly to the top of the chest, parallel and posterior to the phrenic nerve. The azygos vein is divided between ligatures, and the soft tissue and right paratracheal lymph nodes are divided to provide a free pathway for the turned-down right subclavian artery. Any small veins overlying it are ligated and divided. Vagus and recurrent laryngeal nerves are identified, and the periarterial plane over the right subclavian artery is incised. By grasping only the adventitia of the often delicate subclavian artery, dissection is carried distally in the periarterial plane until the origins of internal thoracic and vertebral arteries are identified. These vessels are divided between ligatures, taking care that the proximal ligature is placed 1 to 2 mm away from the subclavian artery (Fig. 38-40, *B*). Anomalies in branching of the subclavian artery are frequent. The vagus nerve is gently retracted laterally, and

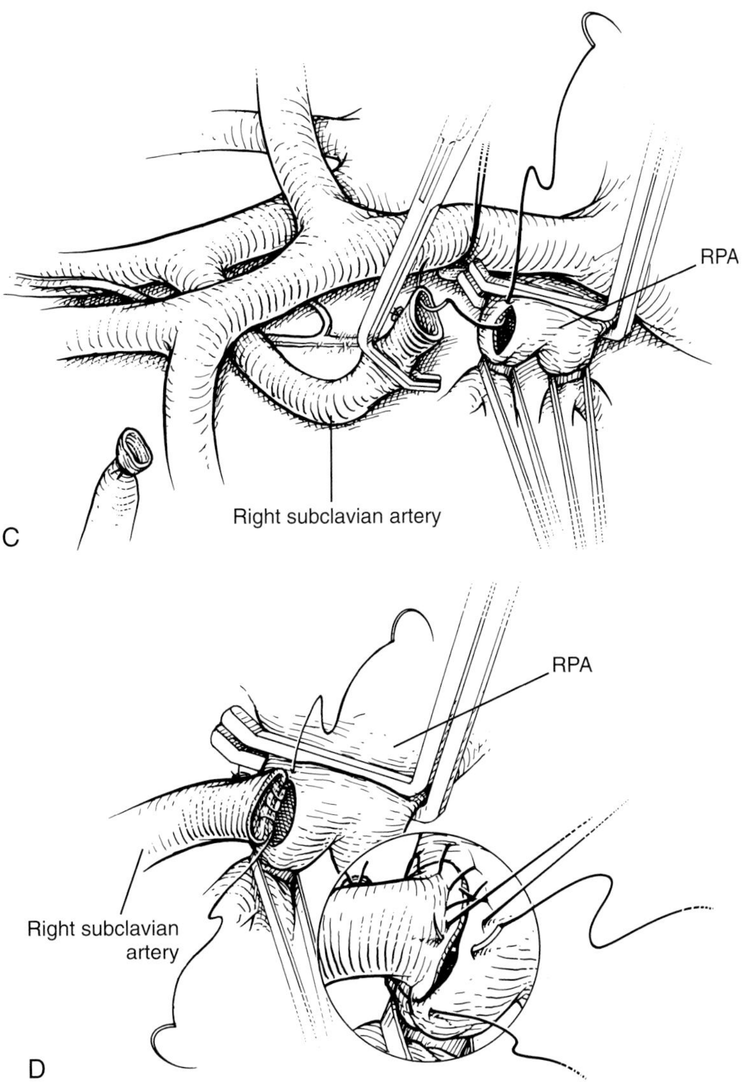

Figure 38-40, cont'd **C,** Subclavian artery has been divided and appropriate occluding devices placed on RPA. Incision in RPA is made on its very superior aspect. **D,** Anastomosis is made using interrupted or continuous 7-0 polypropylene sutures, starting posteriorly from within vessels. Inset shows completion of anastomosis. Key: *SVC,* Superior vena cava.

the periarterial plane over the subclavian artery medially is opened and dissected. The subclavian artery is divided between ligatures placed beyond the first two large branches, and a right-angled clamp is passed beneath the vagus nerve from its medial aspect superior to the recurrent laryngeal nerve (Fig. 38-40, *C*). The subclavian artery beyond the ligature is grasped with the clamp and pulled out from under the vagus nerve. Holding the artery *beyond* the ligature, dissection is carried centrally in the periarterial plane until the distal portion of the brachiocephalic artery and nearly the entire right common carotid artery are liberated. As dissection proceeds, a small artery is occasionally found arising from the origin of the subclavian from the brachiocephalic artery; this must be ligated and divided. The only thing limiting the turned-down length of the subclavian artery is the common carotid artery. Any obstructing bands in the paratracheal soft tissue are divided so that there is nothing in the pathway of the relocated right subclavian artery.

A light, straight arterial clamp with a handle long enough to allow easy holding by the first assistant is placed across the subclavian artery about 8 mm proximal to the point of final transection. The artery is cut squarely across, just proximal to its first branch. (Rarely the first branch comes off very proximally and the subclavian artery is unusually large beyond it. In such instances, the artery can be transected beyond this branch.) Double-looped elastic ligatures are placed around the upper branch and distal main RPA, snugged, and weighted laterally with heavy Kocher clamps. An appropriate-sized Baumgartner clamp is placed across the very proximal RPA, with the surgeon passing a right-angled clamp beneath the artery for lateral retraction as the first assistant tightens the clamp. A longitudinal incision is made *in the very superior surface* of the RPA (so that when the occluding devices are removed, there will be no torsion of the RPA).

Anastomosis is made with continuous or interrupted double-armed 7-0 polypropylene or polyester sutures, the continuous suture placed from within the respective arteries posteriorly (Fig. 38-40, *D*). The first assistant holds the two clamps such that the vessels are in perfect apposition and without tension during the anastomosis. Before placing the last few sutures, the lumina are examined and any tiny thrombi or debris irrigated away. After completing the anastomosis, in rather rapid succession the two doubly looped elastic ligatures are cut and removed, the clamp on the subclavian artery removed, and the proximal RPA clamp removed. Packing is placed lightly around the anastomosis, any unusual bleeding is controlled digitally, the lung is partially reexpanded, and 5 minutes are allowed to pass. During this time, a palpable continuous thrill should be present in the RPA. When the packs are removed, the field is usually dry. Rarely, an additional adventitial suture is needed.

A small chest catheter is brought out from the posterior gutter through about the seventh intercostal space and attached to gentle suction. The chest wall is closed and the lungs are well inflated before the ribs are brought together with absorbable suture. The wound is closed in layers with continuous fine polyglycolic acid sutures, and the skin approximated with a continuous subcuticular suture.

Interposition Shunt between Left Subclavian and Left Pulmonary Artery

This is a commonly performed procedure. It can be performed classically through a left thoracotomy or through a median sternotomy. The procedure performed through a thoracotomy is described.

Thoracotomy is as described for the classic B-T shunt, except on the left side. The LPA is identified and dissected out. The mediastinal pleura is opened over the left subclavian artery and contiguous portion of the aortic arch, and the periarterial sheath over these structures is opened. The subclavian artery is not mobilized.

The diameter of the graft is chosen based on the patient's weight and other factors. In normal-sized neonates or in the case of a very small LPA, a 3.5- or 4-mm PTFE tube graft is used, despite a possible small reduction in patency (see "Size" under Special Situations and Controversies, Systemic–Pulmonary Arterial Shunt, in Section II of Chapter 41 for discussion of criteria for selecting size of the PTFE tube graft).[M21] *Before* any occluding devices are placed, the proper length of the tube graft is determined. For this, the lung is partially inflated to bring the LPA into its usual position. When the anastomosis is completed, the graft should lie without tension and without redundancy (and thus potential kinking) between the proximal half of the subclavian artery and the superior surface of the LPA. The end of the graft that will be anastomosed to the subclavian artery is beveled (Fig. 38-41), the graft is placed in a temporary position, and the other end is cut square at the point that will make the length to the LPA correct.

A delicate side-biting clamp is placed deeply on the subclavian artery so that its handle lies inferiorly and the clamp occludes the artery both proximally and distally. A longitudinal incision is made in the excluded portion of the delicate subclavian artery, and an adventitial stay suture is placed on the anterior lip. The proximal anastomosis is made with a continuous 6-0 or 7-0 polypropylene suture. The clamp on the subclavian artery is not loosened or removed at this time (see variation in detail under "Systemic–Pulmonary Arterial Shunt" under Technique of Operation in Section II of Chapter 41). Elastic ligatures are looped twice around the upper branch and main LPA and snugged, and heavy Kocher clamps are placed on each for lateral traction. A C-shaped clamp is placed very proximally on the LPA, taking care not to compromise the ductus arteriosus. A longitudinal incision is made in the *superior* surface of the LPA, making this a little shorter than half the circumference of the PTFE tube graft. The distal anastomosis is made with continuous 6-0 or 7-0 polypropylene suture.

In quick succession, the doubly looped ligatures are cut and removed, the clamp on the subclavian artery is opened and carefully removed from the field, and the LPA clamp is opened and removed. A light pack is placed about each anastomosis, with light digital pressure if needed. A continuous thrill should be present in the LPA. Other evidences of patency include registration of an immediate increase in oxygen saturation (pulse oximeter) and an immediate increase in systolic and diastolic blood pressure when the shunt is briefly occluded with forceps. Five minutes are allowed to pass.

Remainder of the procedure is completed as described for the classic B-T shunt.

The interposition operation as an isolated procedure in patients with *left aortic arch* can be performed through a right thoracotomy. The PTFE tube graft is anastomosed proximally to the junction of the right subclavian and brachiocephalic arteries, which is in the cupola of the chest. This operation is more difficult than that on the left side. In comparison with the classic B-T anastomosis, the PTFE interposition shunt is a more reliable resistor and is easier to close later.

Right-Sided Interposition Shunt Through Median Sternotomy

The preferred systemic–pulmonary arterial shunt in neonates with left aortic arch is a right PTFE interposition shunt performed through a median sternotomy (Fig. 38-42, *A*). After sternotomy, most of the thymus gland is removed. The pericardium is opened in its superior portion and stay sutures applied. The posterior pericardium is opened over the RPA between the ascending aorta and superior vena cava. A small, fine side-biting (C-shaped) clamp is used to isolate the junction between the brachiocephalic and right subclavian arteries. A longitudinal incision is made, and the end of a beveled 3.5- or 4-mm PTFE tube is anastomosed to the incision (Fig. 38-42, *B*). A small, fine side-biting clamp is placed on the RPA as it is elevated with fine forceps; the clamp isolates the full width of the RPA. The other end of the PTFE tube graft is anastomosed to this opening (Fig. 38-42, *C*). Continuous 6-0 or 7-0 polypropylene on a cutting needle is used for both anastomoses. The clamps are removed sequentially, the RPA clamp first. After hemostasis is secured, the pericardium is loosely closed. The remainder of the sternotomy is closed in the usual manner. Although this technique has been used primarily in neonates, it is applicable to infants.

In patients with a right aortic arch, a left-sided PTFE interposition shunt from the left subclavian–brachiocephalic junction to the LPA is preferred. Details of the technique are the same as described for the right-sided shunt.

Classic Left Blalock-Taussig Shunt (in Patients with Right Aortic Arch)

Left thoracotomy incision and dissection of the LPA are as described in the preceding text. The left subclavian artery is dissected in the cupola of the chest, and maneuvers for freeing it, bringing it beneath the vagus nerve, and preparing it for anastomosis are those described for the right side (see Fig. 38-40). Occluding devices are placed, the anastomosis performed in the manner already described, and the operation

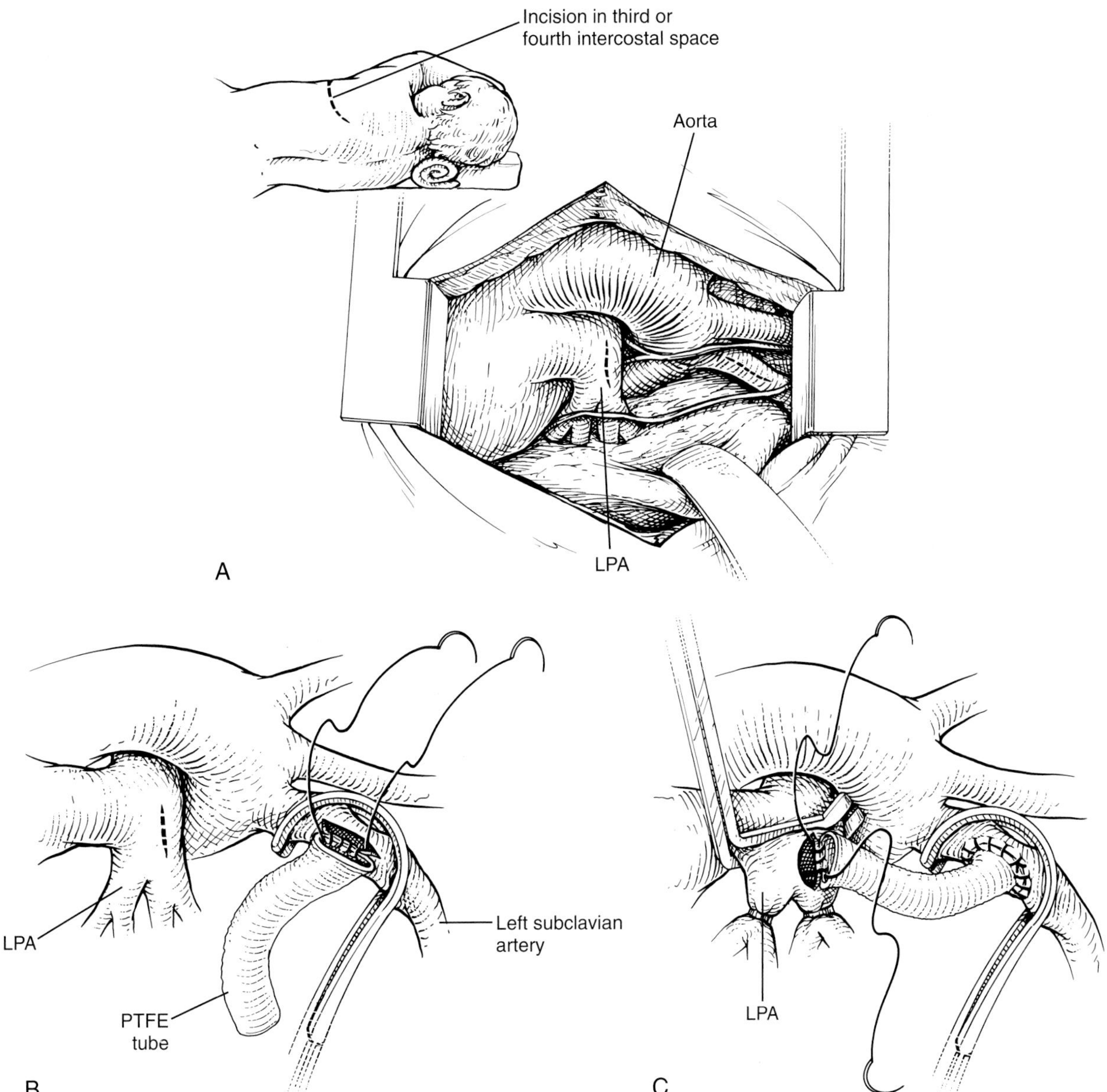

Figure 38-41 Left polytetrafluoroethylene (PTFE) interposition shunt (left aortic arch). **A,** Exposure and sites of incision *(dashed lines)* in pulmonary and subclavian arteries. **B,** PTFE graft has been trimmed for insertion. End-to-side anastomosis is made between graft and left subclavian artery. First portion of suture line is made by sewing from within, as shown. **C,** Distal anastomosis is made in a similar fashion. Direction of suturing (from medial to lateral) at both anastomoses minimizes possibility of tearing delicate subclavian or pulmonary artery. Note that clamp remains on subclavian artery until anastomosis is completed. Key: *LPA,* Left pulmonary artery; *PTFE,* polytetrafluoroethylene.

completed as described. This procedure has the same disadvantages as the right classic B-T shunt.

Right-Sided Interposition Shunt (in Patients with Right Aortic Arch)

This procedure in patients with right aortic arch proceeds exactly as the procedure on the left side in patients with left aortic arch (see Fig. 38-41).

SPECIAL FEATURES OF POSTOPERATIVE CARE

Repair

Management is by the general measures described in Chapter 5. Patients with TF have a particular tendency to increase their interstitial, pleural, and peritoneal fluids early postoperatively. Like other deeply cyanotic individuals, they probably have abnormal systemic and pulmonary capillary membranes, and this may make them particularly sensitive to the damaging effects of CPB (see "Response Variables" in Section II of Chapter 2). Therefore, particular care is taken lest loss of intravascular plasma to extravascular spaces produces undesirable hemoconcentration early postoperatively, and attention is given to the possible development of pleural and peritoneal fluid collections. If these develop, they should be aspirated.

Evaluation is complicated by the fact that in patients convalescing normally after repair of TF, with warm feet and good pedal pulses, arterial blood pressure tends to be as much as 10% lower than that in patients who are acyanotic

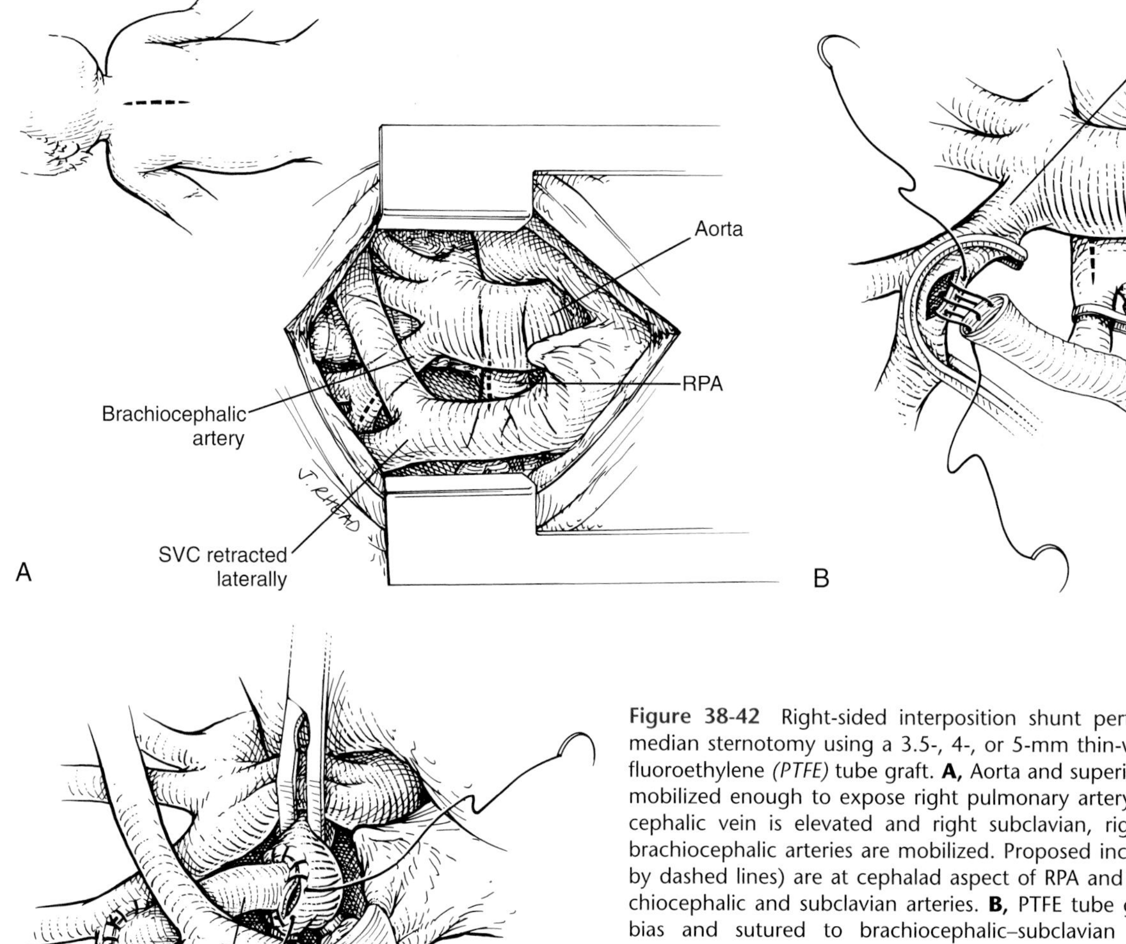

Figure 38-42 Right-sided interposition shunt performed through median sternotomy using a 3.5-, 4-, or 5-mm thin-walled polytetrafluoroethylene *(PTFE)* tube graft. **A,** Aorta and superior vena cava are mobilized enough to expose right pulmonary artery *(RPA)*. Brachiocephalic vein is elevated and right subclavian, right carotid, and brachiocephalic arteries are mobilized. Proposed incisions (indicated by dashed lines) are at cephalad aspect of RPA and junction of brachiocephalic and subclavian arteries. **B,** PTFE tube graft is cut on a bias and sutured to brachiocephalic–subclavian artery junction using continuous 6-0 or 7-0 polypropylene suture, beginning the anastomotic suture from within PTFE tube graft and systemic arteries. **C,** Shunt is completed after transecting PTFE tube graft squarely and using a suture technique similar to that for the systemic arterial anastomosis. Although not shown, subclavian artery clamp remains in place until RPA anastomosis is completed. Key: *SVC,* Superior vena cava.

preoperatively. Cardiac index is usually normal for this stage of convalescence, and tendency to hypotension is related to relatively low systemic vascular resistance.[T8] In the presence of other signs of normal convalescence, treatment of arterial blood pressure is not indicated.

The hemodynamic state is assessed continuously and management constantly reviewed to be certain of its appropriateness. Measurement of cardiac output is helpful, along with other determinants of adequacy of cardiovascular subsystem function (see "Cardiovascular Subsystem" in Section I of Chapter 5). An important right-to-left or left-to-right shunt must be identified, either by the indicator dilution method (see "Risk Factors for Low Cardiac Output" under Cardiovascular Subsystem in Section I of Chapter 5) or by 2D echocardiography with Doppler color flow interrogation. This is particularly important in neonates and infants, in whom the foramen ovale may have been left open for early postoperative decompression of the right atrium. Arterial desaturation is then the rule in the early hours after operation, and demonstrating right-to-left shunting at atrial level by echocardiography using color Doppler reassures that desaturation is not from pulmonary dysfunction (Fig. 38-43). Desaturation from right-to-left shunting usually decreases within 48 hours as RV function improves.

In the absence of shunting, values of left (PLA) and right (PRA) atrial pressures provide considerable insight into the relative function of the two ventricles. After repair of TF, these are usually similar, but one may be 2 to 4 mmHg higher than the other. Rarely, PLA is 5 to 10 mmHg higher than PRA. When this occurs, a residual left-to-right shunt at ventricular or great artery level must be sought and, if found, promptly closed by reoperation. Even relatively small postoperative residual left-to-right shunts may not be well tolerated in repaired TF patients. An important reason for this is that preoperative physiology in TF is that of a volume-underloaded heart, rather than the volume-overloaded preoperative physiology of lesions that tolerate postoperative small residual left-to-right shunts quite well, such as VSDs, atrioventricular septal defects, or truncus arteriosus. If no shunt is found, elevated PLA indicates LV hypoplasia or severe impairment of

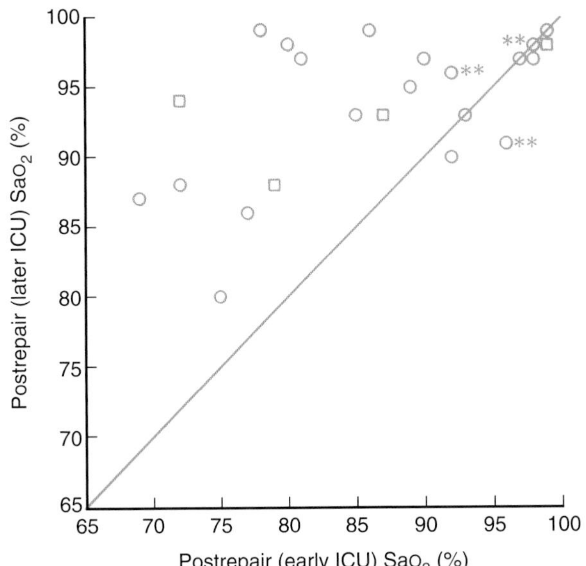

Figure 38-43 Relation of arterial oxygen saturation (Sa_{O_2}) on first arrival at intensive care unit after repair of tetralogy of Fallot *(horizontal axis)* to that present about 48 hours later *(vertical axis),* emphasizing arterial desaturation present early postoperatively when foramen ovale has been left open. Line of identity is shown. Squares represent patients who died postoperatively, and circles represent survivors. Patients identified by two asterisks had the foramen ovale closed. Key: *ICU,* Intensive care unit; *Sa_{O_2},* systemic arterial oxygen saturation. (From Di Donato and colleagues.[D16])

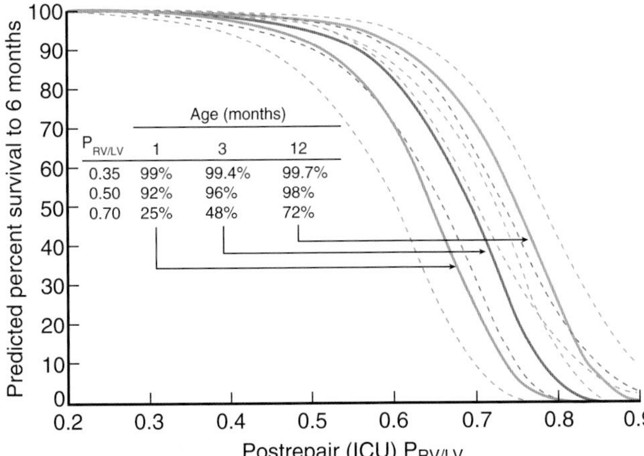

Figure 38-44 Effect of postrepair (ICU) $P_{RV/LV}$ on probability of early (6-month) survival after repair of tetralogy of Fallot. Additional effect of age at operation on this relation is also indicated. (See original paper for data and equations.) Key: *ICU,* Intensive care unit; *$P_{RV/LV}$,* ratio of peak pressure in right ventricle to that in left ventricle. (From Kirklin and colleagues.[K20])

LV systolic or diastolic function, and an inotropic agent and afterload reduction are indicated.

Rarely, PRA is 5 to 10 mmHg higher than PLA, indicating important volume or pressure overload of the RV or severe impairment of RV function. This situation is precarious and requires intense treatment, especially when postrepair $P_{RV/LV}$ is greater than about 0.7 (Fig. 38-44). If a transanular patch was not used, generally the patient should promptly be returned to the operating room and a patch placed. If a transanular patch is in place, as complete a repair as possible was obtained, and the patient's condition is reasonably good on only modest catecholamine support (e.g., 5 μg · kg^{-1} · min^{-1} of dopamine or dobutamine), then delay for a few hours is reasonable. If no improvement occurs, and particularly if postrepair $P_{RV/LV}$ is 0.8 or greater, risk of death approaches 50% and intervention is indicated. In neonates and young infants, the $P_{RV/LV}$ may not be as useful as in older patients. Anesthetized postoperative neonates may have low systemic vascular resistance and thus low systemic systolic blood pressure despite excellent cardiac output. In this setting, a relatively normal RV and pulmonary artery pressure may result in a $P_{RV/LV}$ as high as 0.8 or 0.9. Under these circumstances, the absolute P_{RV} should be carefully evaluated. Systolic P_{RV} over 50 mmHg should be investigated routinely, and that between 40 and 50 mmHg considered for investigation. Regardless of the patient's age, investigation, when indicated, is the same. A right ventriculogram and determination of site of the gradient by cardiac catheterization is performed. If an appreciable gradient is found in the RV or at the pulmonary "anulus," or a localized important uncorrected LPA or RPA origin or bifurcation stenosis is found, correction of these areas of residual stenosis at prompt reoperation is indicated.

However, if the original repair was complete, it is likely that none of these will be found. Instead, the gradient will be located at the distal transanular patch suture line. This circumstance is uncommon (1%-2% of patients), limited almost entirely to patients with severe hypoplasia of the "anulus" and pulmonary trunk. In that setting, and particularly without a distal widening (in the distal pulmonary trunk or LPA) into which the transanular patch can be extended, it may be impossible to make a geometrically proper patch.[K20,S10] If evaluation reveals that hypoplasia or discrete stenosis is present in the branch pulmonary arteries with normal distal pulmonary arterial development, then further patch augmentation of the pulmonary arteries is indicated. If the pulmonary artery hypoplasia is diffuse, a large perforation is made in the VSD, preventing the P_{RV} from becoming suprasystemic, and augmenting systemic output from right-to-left shunting across the VSD.

Particular attention is paid to the possible need for reoperation for bleeding. Preoperative polycythemia and depletion of many clotting factors, extensive collateral circulation, and damaging effects of CPB often combine to produce a considerable bleeding tendency. Intense treatment, particularly with platelet-rich plasma, is indicated. The usual criteria for reoperation are followed (see "Bleeding" in Section II of Chapter 5), and prompt reoperation is advised as soon as they are violated. This practice was one factor contributing to the considerable reduction in risk of operation in the early 1960s. Currently, with careful intraoperative hemostasis and definitive repair at a young age, reoperation for bleeding is rarely necessary.

After the patient leaves the ICU, body weight is followed closely because transient fluid retention is common, particularly when a transanular patch has been used. Pharmacologic management of right-sided heart failure is indicated.

Systemic–Pulmonary Arterial Shunting

In neonates and young infants, careful intraoperative and postoperative monitoring and control of Pa_{O_2}, pH, and buffer base are required (see "Neonates and Infants" in Section II of Chapter 5). The usual intense postoperative care and protocols are applied (see Chapter 5). An intraarterial catheter is used to monitor blood pressure, paying careful attention to the systolic/diastolic difference and absolute diastolic pressure. The patient is returned to the ICU ventilated through an endotracheal tube. A chest radiograph is obtained immediately. Ventilation is controlled postoperatively for at least several hours and up to a full day, until stable hemodynamics and confirmation of balanced systemic-pulmonary blood flow is assured. A combination of SaO_2, diastolic blood pressure and pulse pressure, and various signs that reflect systemic cardiac output are used to estimate the systemic-pulmonary blood flow balance. Assuming normal hematocrit and pulmonary gas exchange, an SaO_2 of about 80% usually reflects well-balanced systemic and pulmonary blood flow. Diastolic blood pressure ideally should be above 30 mmHg. Major diversions from these levels usually indicate an imbalance of systemic-pulmonary blood flow. A repeat chest radiograph should be performed to confirm that a pulmonary parenchymal process, and thus gas exchange, is not responsible. If this is ruled out, intravascular volume, pharmacologic (inotropes), and ventilator manipulation should be initiated to restabilize the balance of flow.

Maintaining an adequate cardiac output and blood pressure is an important factor in assuring shunt patency in the vulnerable period of the first 48 hours after surgery. Some centers use a heparin drip as an additional measure. Additionally, or alternatively, aspirin at 10 mg · kg^{-1} daily may be started and continued for the life of the shunt.

Infrequently, mild renal failure, and rarely, acute renal failure and anuria, develop after a simple shunting procedure. This is related to the renal pathology sometimes present in cyanotic patients with TF and to renal damage by radiopaque dye that may have been used for the cineangiogram a few hours or days before operation. Therefore, urine flow is carefully observed postoperatively.

A surgically created shunt *must* function. Therefore, auscultation is used to assess its patency during the entire postoperative hospitalization. If doubt develops concerning shunt function, immediate 2D echocardiography, cineangiographic study, or both are indicated. If it is poorly functioning, prompt reoperation is indicated. In older patients with large acquired systemic-to–pulmonary artery collaterals, a continuous murmur is present preoperatively, and therefore simple auscultation is not as useful early postoperatively. In this setting, if cyanosis has *not* improved, echocardiography and/or cineangiography is indicated.

RESULTS

Survival

Early (Hospital) Death

Although hospital mortality in a few series of heterogeneous groups of patients has been 1% or less,[A17,G33,P3,S20,S26,T2] in most series it varies between 2% and 5%[B9,C8,C12,G29,K6,K20,N2,R5,T10] (Fig. 38-45). TF repair in patients 90 days of age or younger at 32 centers participating in the Society of Thoracic Surgeons congenital heart database over a 3-year period from 2002 to 2005 was associated with a mortality of 6.1% (CL 3.6%-9.6%).[C28] In the same centers, mortality for shunt palliation was 8.3% (CL 5.4%-12%).[C28]

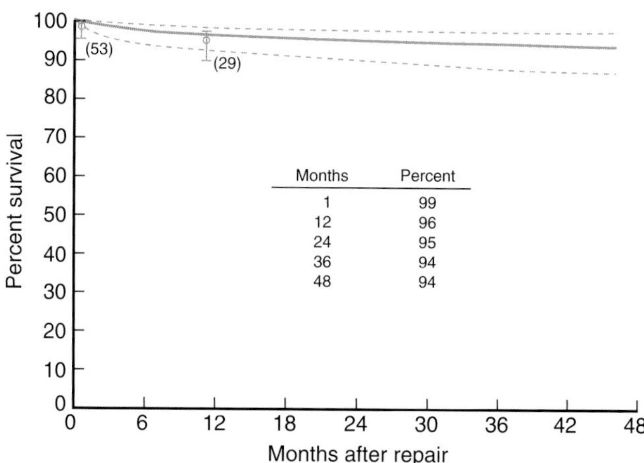

Figure 38-45 Survival after repair of tetralogy of Fallot in infancy. Circles represent two individual deaths. Vertical bars represent 70% confidence limits (CL). Solid line represents parametric survival estimates, and dashed lines enclose 70% CLs. (From Groh and colleagues.[G29])

Because the early rapidly declining phase of hazard does not flatten out until 3 to 6 months after operation (Fig. 38-46), hospital or 30-day mortality underestimates the risk of death early after repair.

Time-Related Survival and the Question of "Cure"

In considering survival after surgical repair, it must be recalled that deaths occurring *before* repair are not represented. Thus, an institution that delays repair until some specified age may have a few patients who, whether shunted or not, die before repair, whereas an institution that has a policy of one-stage repair in all symptomatic patients, no matter how young, may have an apparently higher mortality while actually saving more lives. Vobecky of Toronto's Hospital for Sick Children examined this issue in 270 TF patients younger than age 18 months.[V9] A few deaths occurred before palliation, between palliation and repair, and after repair (Table 38-4). Major noncardiac anomalies may preclude repair, and major associated malformations may increase operative risk at any age. At present, the data show nearly equal time-related survival for one-stage repair performed at any age and staged operation.

In one analysis, time-related survival after repair in heterogeneous groups of patients at 1 month and 1, 5, 10, and 20 years was about 94%, 92%, 91%, 90%, and 87%, respectively (Fig. 38-47).[K20] Patient-specific survivals and those of homogeneous groups of patients vary, with 10- and 20-year values as high as 97% in some circumstances (Fig. 38-48).[K7] In another analysis, overall time-related survival was 80% at 40 years.[H18] In that study, predicted 40-year survival for patients repaired in the latter part of the experience (operation performed in the year 1985) was 88%.

"Is the patient cured of TF?" This is a critical question that must be examined not only for the entire heterogeneous population of patients undergoing repair but also for specific patients, taking into account the strength and time-relatedness of their various risk factors. For operation to be curative, the hazard function for death after the early postoperative period (3-6 months) must be no greater than that for an age-sex-race–matched general population and have no late increase

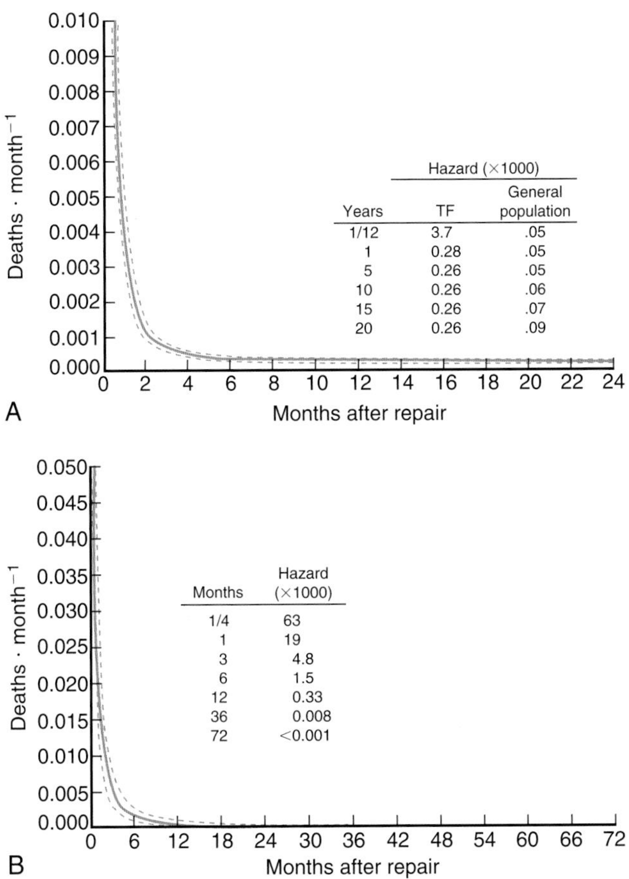

Figure 38-46 Hazard function for death after repair of tetralogy of Fallot *(TF)* with pulmonary stenosis from two different studies. In both, the rapidly declining early phase of hazard does not flatten appreciably until 3 to 6 months after repair. **A,** Hazard function from UAB study (1967 to May 1986; $n = 814$) with follow-up over 15 years. There is a constant phase of hazard extending for as long as patients were followed. **B,** Hazard function from combined Boston Children's Hospital–UAB study (September 1984 to 1989; $n = 176$), which has no late constant phase.[K20] Thus, the hazard function at 5 years, and presumably for a considerable period beyond, is the same as that of a matched general population (barely visible as dash-dot-dash line). (From Kirklin and colleagues.[K20])

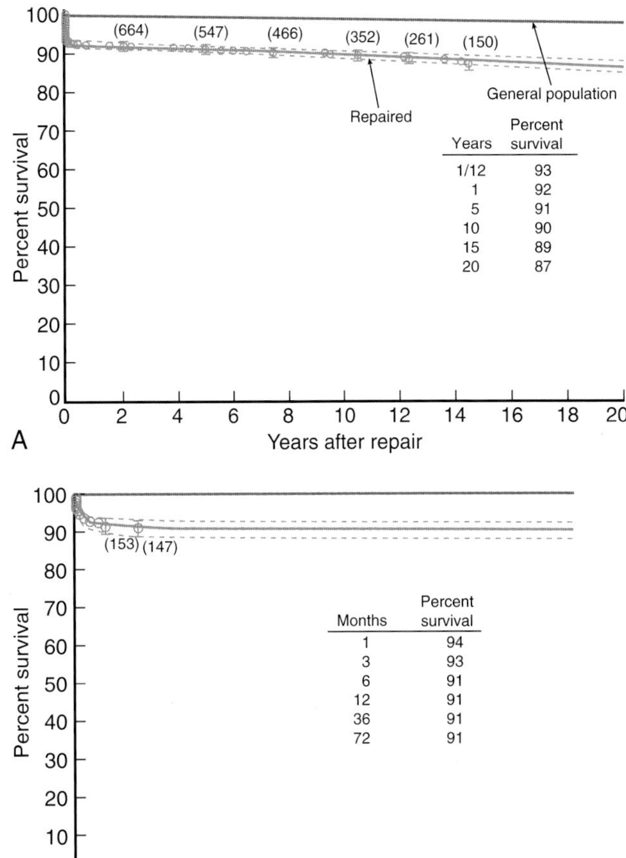

Figure 38-47 Survival after repair of tetralogy of Fallot with pulmonary stenosis in the two heterogeneous groups of patients whose hazard functions are depicted in Fig. 38-46. Each circle represents a death estimated by the Kaplan-Meier method. Vertical bars represent 70% confidence limits (CL) of these estimates. Solid line represents parametric estimate of survival, and dashed lines enclose its 70% CLs. Dash-dot-dash line represents survival of an age-sex-race–matched general population. **A,** Survival after repair in UAB study (1967 to May 1986; $n = 814$). **B,** Survival after repair in combined Boston Children's Hospital–UAB study (September 1984 to 1989; $n = 176$). (From Kirklin and colleagues.[K20])

Table 38-4 Time of Death of Infants with Isolated Tetralogy of Fallot ($n = 237$)

Timing of Death	No.	%
None	218	92
Before palliation	3	1.3
At palliation	2	0.8
Secondary palliation	1	0.4
After palliation/before repair	8	3.4
At repair	7	3.0
After repair	1	0.4
TOTAL DEATHS	22[a]	9.3

Data from Vobecky and colleagues.[V9]
[a]Fourteen deaths occurred before repair (5.9%; CL 4.3%-7.9%).

until that imposed by older age on the general population. Hazard function for death after repair in a heterogeneous group of patients has a constant hazard phase (as opposed to a rising phase) late postoperatively, as demonstrated in the analysis of early Mayo Clinic patients included in the study of Fuster and colleagues[F17] and subsequently reported by Murphy and colleagues.[M37] At 30 years, survival for patients who left the hospital alive was 86% compared with 96% in the general population ($P < .01$).

The 35-year follow-up of patients operated on by Lillehei and colleagues and the 30-year follow-up of patients operated on at Johns Hopkins Hospital are also consistent with presence of a low constant phase of hazard without a late rising phase.[H28,L14,L16]

Level of the constant hazard phase is about three times higher than that of a matched general population, but many patients had numerous risk factors. The hazard function for younger patients in the combined Boston Children's

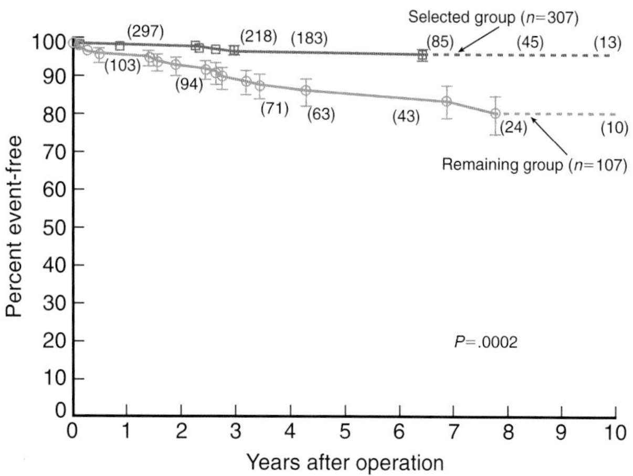

Figure 38-48 Freedom from premature late death, reoperation, arrhythmic symptoms, and heart failure among patients discharged from hospital alive after repair of tetralogy of Fallot with pulmonary stenosis. "Selected group" consisted of patients younger than age 20 years at repair, with no previous procedure or only a single Blalock-Taussig shunt, and a postrepair (OR) $P_{RV/LV}$ of 0.85 or less. (From Katz and colleagues.[K7])

Hospital–UAB data set, most of whom underwent primary (one-stage) repair, is behaving as if the constant hazard phase will be closer to that of a matched general population when they have been followed long enough for this to be identified. The Boston-UAB long-term data suggest that a late rise in the hazard function will not occur within the first 20 to 30 postoperative years (see Fig. 38-46).[C9,K20]

Thus, the inference is that time-related survival of most patients after repair of TF with pulmonary stenosis under proper circumstances is excellent, approaching that of the general population, but that the risk of death throughout life is slightly greater than that of the general population.

Modes of Death

Considering death with multiple subsystem failure to be basically death in subacute heart failure, only half the patients who died in hospital after repair in the combined Boston Children's Hospital–UAB study died this way. Pulmonary failure, hypermetabolic state, and catastrophic surgical or early postoperative events account for the remainder, a higher percentage than after most kinds of cardiac surgery in adults.[K20] Pathologic basis of the pulmonary failure has been described by Harms and colleagues,[H6] who found in their autopsy studies that extensive alveolar and interstitial edema and hemorrhage are characteristic of the lungs of patients dying early after repair of TF. This process is probably caused by the damaging effects of CPB (see Chapter 2),[H6,K18] to which severely cyanotic and polycythemic patients seem particularly sensitive. Thus, further improvement in results of repair may demand not only improved myocardial management but also lessening of the damaging effects of CPB and improved technical proficiency in the operating room and ICU when repair is being done in very small patients.

Incremental Risk Factors for Death

Incremental risk factors for death early and late after repair have been identified from a number of studies. A typical analysis from a single institution, identifying early hazard phase and late hazard phase risks, is shown in Table 38-5. There are a number of difficulties in definitively identifying risk factors for early death. These difficulties are that some variables were available for one analysis and not for another, that the risk factors may be different if procedural as well as patient characteristics are considered, and that some simultaneously determined "independent" risk factors are highly correlated and thus may be surrogates for one other (see "Variable Selection" in Section IV of Chapter 6). One of the most important difficulties is that in the current era, early mortality is so low that identifying risk factors for that phase is not possible.

Table 38-5 Incremental Risk Factors for Time-Related Death Following Corrective Repair of Tetralogy of Fallot ($n = 1181$)

Risk Factor for Death	Estimate	*P* value	Reliability (%)
Early hazard phase	−0.06	<0.001	99
Earlier date of corrective surgery (units = years)	−0.18	<0.001	92
Classic tetralogy of Fallot	−0.94	<0.001	75
Coexisting atrioventricular septal defect	+1.21	<0.001	98
Right aortic arch	+0.57	0.001	78
Previous central/Potts/Waterston shunt	+0.86	0.002	71
RV-PT conduit in classic tetralogy of Fallot	+1.05	0.03	—
Late hazard phase			
Coexisting atrioventricular septal defect	+2.01	<0.001	72
Branch pulmonary artery stenosis	+1.00	0.002	79
Double-outlet right ventricle variant	+1.47	0.001	66
Down syndrome	+1.33	<0.01	54

Data from Hickey and colleagues.[H18]
Reliability represents the percentage reliability of the *P* value as determined by percentage of bootstrap resamples for which the variable is included in the parametric model (inclusion threshold $P < .1$).
Key: *RV-PT,* Right ventricular-pulmonary trunk.

Young Age at Repair

Young age at repair[2] has been identified as a risk factor for death early after repair.[C19,C22,H2,P20,V8] There are, however, two important qualifications that accompany this observation. First, young age is not necessarily an immutable risk factor, because the age at which risk increases appreciably has been progressively reduced as experience and knowledge have grown. This improvement is illustrated by the UAB experience, in which risk of hospital death and predicted 20-year survival after repair in a 6-month-old infant improved considerably between 1967 and 1986 (Fig. 38-49). The

[2]Body surface area is a more statistically significant risk factor than young age in the majority of multivariable analyses, but most groups prefer to think in terms of age. Therefore, a regression analysis has been made of the relation of age to body surface area so that one can be used to estimate the other (see Appendix 38A).

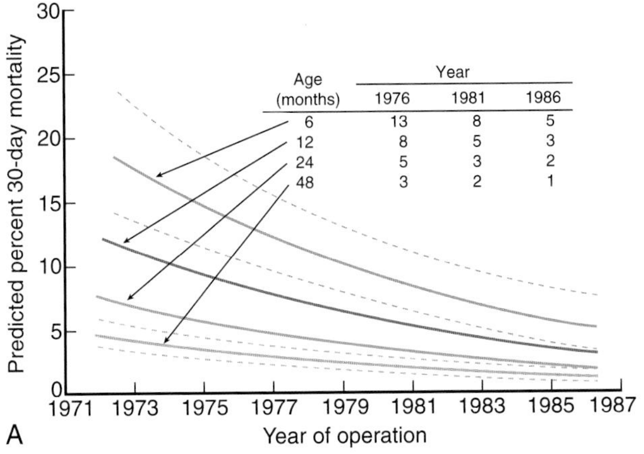

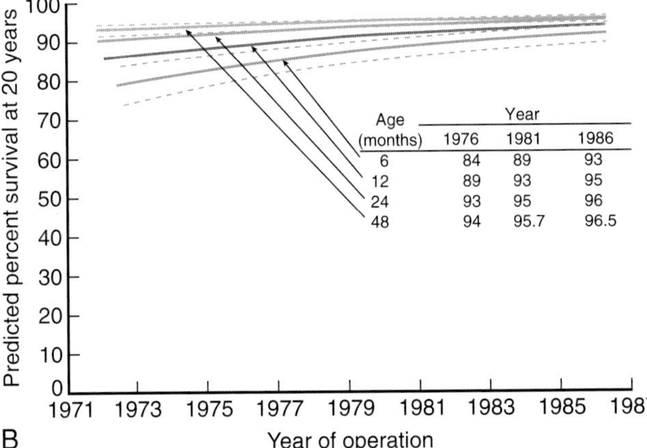

Figure 38-49 Nomograms illustrating decreasing strength across year of operation of the incremental risk of young age on early and late survival after repair of tetralogy of Fallot with pulmonary stenosis. (Nomogram is specific solution of multivariable risk factor equation from Kirklin and colleagues.[K16] Values entered for other variables in equation are in Appendix 38A). **A,** Predicted 30-day mortality. **B,** Predicted 20-year survival, including early deaths.

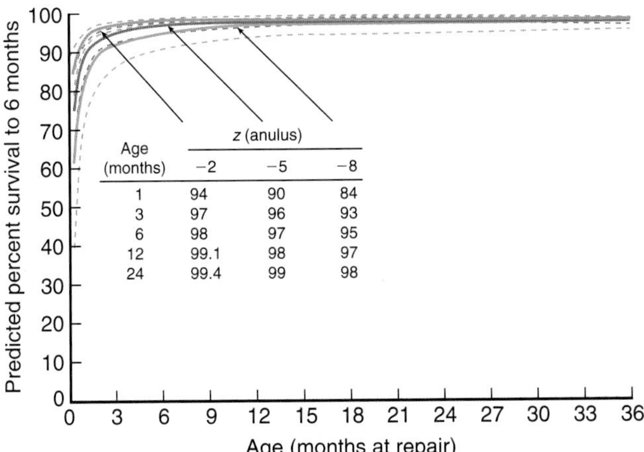

Figure 38-50 Nomogram illustrating incremental risk of young age and of dimension of pulmonary "anulus" on early survival after repair of tetralogy of Fallot with pulmonary stenosis in recent era. Note that effect of young age is stronger and more evident in patients with a very small "anulus" (*z* value of −8) than in the others, reflecting the usual incremental effect of one risk factor on another. (From Kirklin and colleagues.[K20])

incremental risk of young age in general is currently unapparent until age is younger than 3 months, and in some circumstances younger than 1 month (Fig. 38-50). Second, studies examining young age as a risk factor for early death have the inherent bias that only symptomatic patients were repaired in the neonatal period or early infancy. Because symptoms correlate with less favorable morphology of the RV outflow tract in patients with TF, it follows that patients who underwent repair at a very early age uniformly had less favorable morphology. Thus, there were no patients who underwent very early repair in these series with favorable morphology (asymptomatic). Even with multivariable analysis, it is difficult to overcome this bias.

Reduction of the age at which risk is increased is due in part to increasing technical expertise in intracardiac surgery and early postoperative care in the very young.[T10] Further improvements in these areas may completely neutralize the increased risk of young age. Control of the damaging effects of CPB (see Chapter 2) and improvement in the function of the heart early postoperatively, brought about by more effective intraoperative myocardial management, will assist in this effort.

Older Age at Repair

Older age has been identified as a risk factor for death early and late after repair (see Table 38-5). Its effect on survival late after repair is probably truly immutable (Fig. 38-51). This is because the bases of the incremental risk of older age lie in the adverse, and to a considerable extent irreversible, effect of long-standing RV hypertension, cyanosis, and polycythemia on cardiac structure and function,[B23] of cyanosis and polycythemia on renal function, and of volume overload on the LV of surgically created palliative shunts. For example, RV hypertrophy begins shortly after birth, continues as the child grows, and begins to be irreversible by age 4 years.[M7] It is in part to prevent these irreversible changes that repair is advisable early in life. A contraindication to early repair may be presence of an anomalous LAD from the RCA.[S20] Relative contraindications include complex pulmonary artery anatomy or very small pulmonary arteries. However, independent reports from Reddy, Stellin, Sousa-Uva, Starnes, and Groh and their colleagues[G29,R5,S20,S23,S26] document excellent results when early one-stage repair is applied routinely in neonates and infants.

Severity of Right Ventricle–Pulmonary Trunk Junction Hypoplasia

Severe hypoplasia of the RV–pulmonary trunk junction ("anulus") has been identified as a risk factor for death, at least early after repair (see Fig. 38-50). This may be related in part to the need for a ***transanular patch*** when the hypoplasia is severe, and to the correlation between severity of anular hypoplasia and ***postrepair*** $P_{RV/LV}$, even when a transanular patch is used and particularly when there is coexisting hypoplasia of the distal pulmonary trunk (see "Decision and Technique for Transanular Patching" earlier in this section). Thus, severity of anular hypoplasia, use of a transanular patch, and postrepair $P_{RV/LV}$ are all surrogates for one another in a complex manner that is difficult to quantify (Fig. 38-52).[K20]

Small Size of Right and Left Pulmonary Arteries

Important localized or diffuse hypoplasia of the RPA and LPA is uncommon in patients having TF with pulmonary

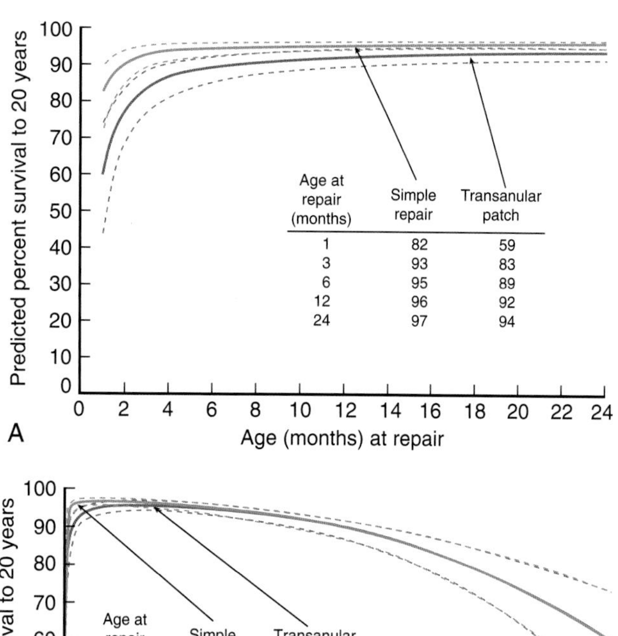

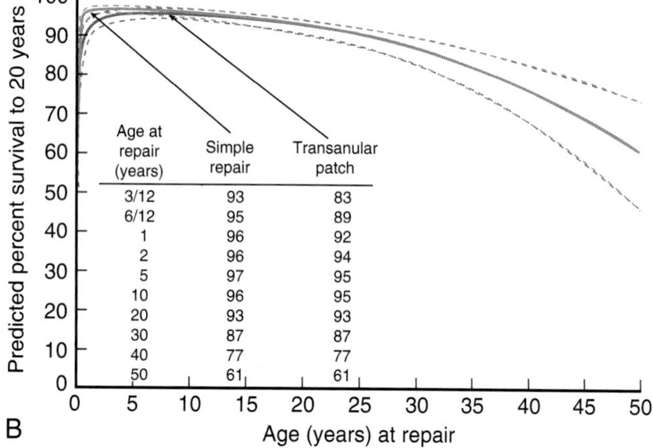

Figure 38-51 Nomograms illustrating incremental risk of older age at repair of tetralogy of Fallot with pulmonary stenosis in patients with and without a transanular patch. Note that adverse effects of older age on predicted, risk-adjusted survival begin at about age 5 to 7 years, but remain rather weak until after about age 20. Also noteworthy is lack of any adverse effect of transanular patching in older patients. (Nomograms are specific solutions of multivariable risk factor equation from original publication.[K16] Values entered for other variables in equation are in Appendix 38A.) **A,** Effect of young age (expanded horizontal axis). **B,** Effect of older age. (From Kirklin and colleagues.[K16])

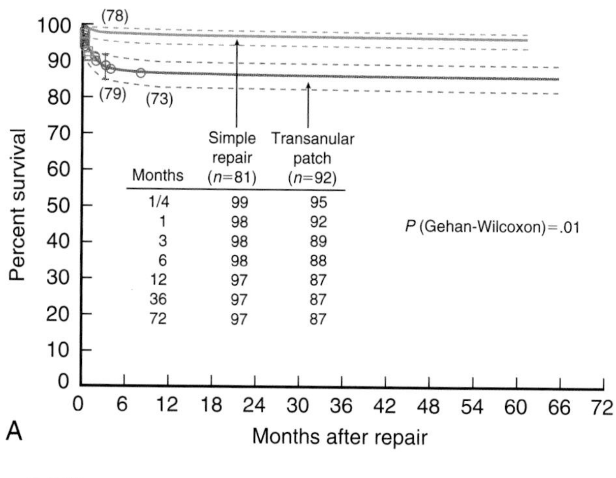

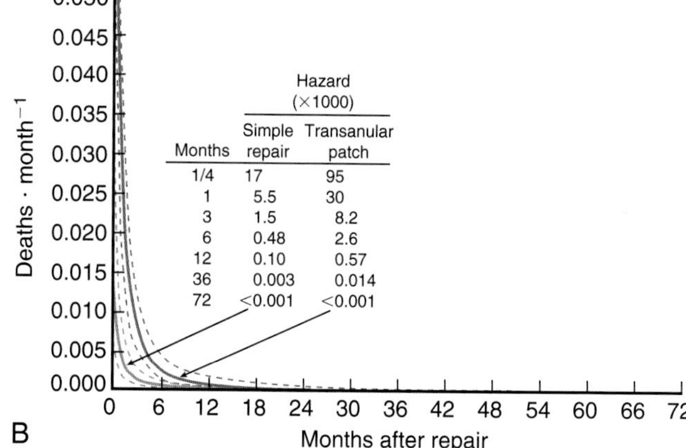

Figure 38-52 Survival after repair of tetralogy of Fallot with pulmonary stenosis with and without use of transanular patch. **A,** Survival. Depiction is as in Fig. 38-47. **B,** Hazard function. Depiction is as in Fig. 38-46. Note that the adverse effect of transanular patching on rate of death is no longer evident about 18 months after repair. (From Kirklin and colleagues.[K20])

stenosis.[S10] It is not surprising, then, that the diameters of these arteries have not been detected as correlates of postrepair $P_{RV/LV}$ nor as risk factors for premature death after repair.[G29,K20]

Transanular Patch

It remains arguable whether presence of a transanular patch is, per se, an incremental risk factor for premature death after repair of TF with pulmonary stenosis. Some studies find a higher mortality by univariable analysis among patients in whom a patch was used (see Fig. 38-52),[K35] whereas other studies do not.[H18]

In one analysis[K16] transanular patching was a risk factor for *early* death, but in another[K20] it was not. Even so, in the latter analysis survival through the early postoperative period (up to 6 months) was lower in patients receiving a transanular patch than in those in whom simple repair of TF had been performed (Fig. 38-52; see also Fig. 38-51).

Transanular patching was not a risk factor late postoperatively in earlier UAB[K16] and Mayo Clinic patients.[F17,M37] However, the increased chance of needing later reoperation and its attendant risk suggest that in a sufficiently large and well-matched comparison, use of a transanular patch may have a late increased risk (see "Reoperation and Other Reinterventions for Right Ventricular Outflow Problems" later in this section). Strength of the effect of transanular patching is weak when postrepair $P_{RV/LV}$ is low and more important when it is elevated. Apparently, the pulmonary regurgitation allowed by a transanular patch and the increase in RV volume are usually (unless postrepair $P_{RV/LV}$ is high) well tolerated acutely and chronically out to about 20 years by the previously hypertrophied RV.[M34] However, the natural history of patients with isolated congenital pulmonary valvar regurgitation[S21] suggests that by about 40 years after repair, RV dysfunction will have developed in some and could lead to premature death.

Postrepair $P_{RV/LV}$

Important residual pulmonary stenosis after repair, expressed as postrepair $P_{RV/LV}$, has been identified as a risk factor for premature death early and late after operation.[H15,K27,K31,K32,L18,R6,R36] This is true of postrepair (OR)

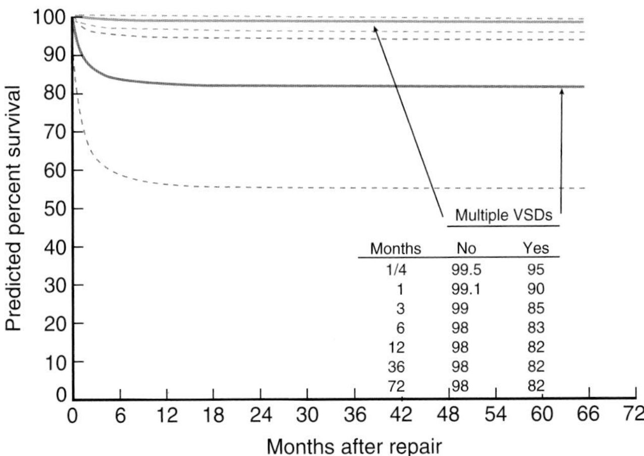

Figure 38-53 Nomogram illustrating adverse effect of multiple ventricular septal defects on survival early after repair of tetralogy of Fallot with pulmonary stenosis. Analysis is based on 176 patients undergoing repair at Boston Children's Hospital and UAB, 1985 to 1989. (Nomogram is specific solution of multivariable risk factor equation in original publication.[K20] Values entered for other variables in equation are in Appendix 38A.) Key: *VSD,* Ventricular septal defect. (From Kirklin and colleagues.[K20])

$P_{RV/LV}$, but the ratio as measured in the ICU about 24 hours after operation is a more powerful and precise predictor (see Fig. 38-44). The interaction of young age (or small patient size), small anulus, transanular patching, and postrepair $P_{RV/LV}$ is apparent from these same studies.[K16,K20] Although identified as a risk factor, postrepair $P_{RV/LV}$ is inversely correlated with size of the pulmonary valve "anulus" and of the distal pulmonary trunk.

Previous Palliative Operations

A single previously performed classic shunting operation is not a risk factor for death after repair, but more than one palliative operation has been shown to be.[K16] When a pulmonary artery has been importantly distorted by a shunting operation, an unusual occurrence under proper circumstances, risks of repair are increased.

Multiple Ventricular Septal Defects

Multiple VSDs are present in only 1% to 3% of patients having TF with pulmonary stenosis, but they have been identified as a strong risk factor for death in the early hazard phase, as evident in Fig. 38-53.[K20]

Coexisting Related Cardiac Anomalies

Coexisting *complete atrioventricular septal defect* complicates repair of TF with pulmonary stenosis, and a composite review of outcomes from 50 individual studies reported over a 40-year period imply higher surgical mortality than for simple TF (Table 38-6).[R15] Although mortality improved in the 1990s compared with prior years, it has not improved further and remains substantial. Nevertheless, mortality varied from study to study in this review, with some reports showing only a small incremental risk.[P2]

In one study, *Down syndrome,* rather than the atrioventricular septal defect itself, appeared to be the incremental risk factor (Table 38-7).[K20]

Historically, *large AP collateral arteries* were risk factors for death early after repair of TF with pulmonary stenosis. However, this may have been due to the greater frequency of important RPA and LPA hypoplasia in such patients, and of discontinuity between the pulmonary trunk and RPA or LPA.[K20] It is likely that early risk associated with AP collaterals has largely been neutralized, because current surgical mortality for patients with AP collateral arteries and TF *with pulmonary atresia* is now as low as 2%.[M6]

Table 38-6 Compilation of All Major Studies Reporting Surgical Mortality for Repair of Tetralogy of Fallot in Association with Complete Atrioventricular Septal Defect between 1965 and 2005

Year	Patients	Mortality (*n*)	Mortality (%)	CLs
1965-1990	106	21	20	16-25
1991-1998	120	13	11	7.9-15
1998-2005	120	12	10	7.2-14

Data from Ricci and colleagues.[R15]

Table 38-7 Confounding Effects of Down Syndrome and Coexisting Complete Atrioventricular Septal Defects on Non–Risk-Adjusted Survival in Patients with Tetralogy of Fallot

Category	*n*	Total Deaths after Entry: No.	%	CL (%)
No Down syndrome	177	13	7	5-10
No AV septal defect	173	13	8	5-10
AV septal defect	4	0	0	0-38
P (Fisher)			.7	
Down syndrome	19	9	47	34-62
No AV septal defect	10	2	20	7-41
AV septal defect	9	4	44	24-66
P (Fisher)			.3	
P (Normal vs. Down syndrome, χ^2)			.001	

Data from Kirklin and colleagues.[K20]
Key: *AV,* Atrioventricular; *CL,* 70% confidence limits.

Other Risk Factors

Although *high hematocrit* was frequently observed in an earlier era of delayed surgery, it is uncommon today; when seen, it may be a strong risk factor.[K1,R17]

Graham and colleagues proposed that small LV *end-diastolic volume* (<55% of normal for age) is an important risk factor for early death after repair.[G26] Nomoto and colleagues also reported that small LV volume is a risk factor, with a demonstrable increase in risk when preoperative LV end-diastolic volume is less than about 65% of normal.[N10] Oberhansli and Friedli reported similar findings.[O1]

Heart Block

Complete heart block is uncommon after repair. It occurred 7 of 814 patients (0.9%; CL 0.5%-1.3%) from 1967 to May 1986 at UAB, and in 0.6% (CL 0.1%-1.9%) of patients from September 1984 to 1989.[K16,K20] Right bundle branch block

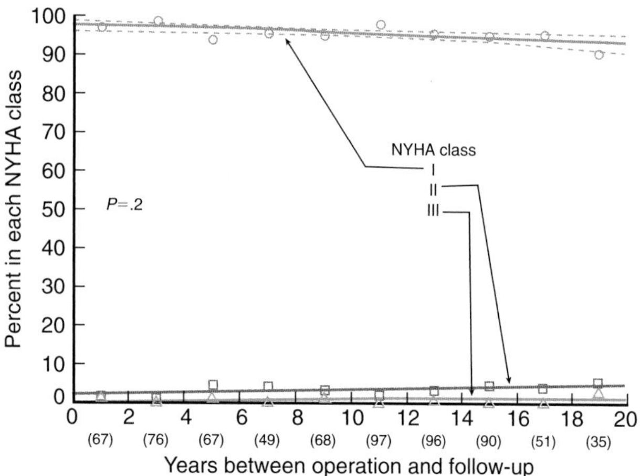

Figure 38-54 New York Heart Association (NYHA) functional class after repair of tetralogy of Fallot with pulmonary stenosis, according to interval between operation and last follow-up. Numbers in parentheses along horizontal axis represent number of patients available for functional class categorization at the odd-numbered interval below which number is positioned. Squares represent proportion of patients in functional class I at each interval; circles, those in class II; and triangles, those in class III. Solid line represents slope of solution of ordinal logistic (longitudinal) regression analysis, although the *P* value of .2 for the difference from zero slope indicates that change across time in the distribution of patients according to their NYHA functional class could be due to chance alone. (From Kirklin and colleagues.[K16])

and left anterior hemiblock[B19,R24,W12] occur in about the same frequency as after repair of isolated VSD (see "Conduction Disturbances" under Results in Chapter 35), and the combination is usually associated with a favorable course late postoperatively.[C1]

Junctional Ectopic Tachycardia

Junctional ectopic tachycardia occurs infrequently after repair of TF. Survival depends on aggressive treatment in the ICU with moderate core cooling and amiodarone (see "Atrial Arrhythmias" in Section I of Chapter 5).[W2] Thereafter, there is probably little risk of complete heart block. Repair by way of the right atrial–pulmonary artery approach may carry a higher risk of junctional ectopic tachycardia; however, there are no firm data to support this.

Functional Status

About 98% of patients are considered by themselves or their parents to be in New York Heart Association (NYHA) functional class I after repair.[K7,K20,P17,R27] Most importantly, this proportion has not declined over time, at least to 20 years (Fig. 38-54).

Some asymptomatic patients have reduced exercise capacity,[D12,W9] some have normal functioning capacity as judged by quantitative testing (Table 38-8), and some have the capacity of a trained athlete.[W9] Some patients with normal response to exercise testing have other abnormalities, such as limitation in chronotropic response to exercise.[P12]

Risk factors for impaired exercise tolerance have been identified, and these include older *age at repair*. Repair in the first 5 years of life results in a normal response to objective exercise testing.[J1,M36,P12] Patients averaging 12 years of age at operation have subnormal exercise capacity late postoperatively.[J1] *Residual RV hypertension*, expressed as PRV, $P_{RV/LV}$, or RV-to–pulmonary artery gradient, adversely affects functional status late after complete repair.[O2,P14,W9] Wessel and colleagues suggest that in the absence of other problems, PRV greater than 50 mmHg (corresponding roughly to $P_{RV/LV} > 0.7$) is likely to exert this effect (Table 38-9), although PRV greater than 70 mmHg may be a more realistic number (indeed, the relation is likely continuous but nonlinear).[W9] *Pulmonary valve regurgitation* after repair results in reduced exercise capacity regardless of RV systolic pressure.[D4,D12,M12,P14,R33,V7,W9] Consistent with this is the tendency of patients with transanular patches to have larger cardiothoracic ratios and RV volumes[E2] late postoperatively. In patients who have undergone repair without insertion of a valve for TF with absent pulmonary valve (Section III),

Table 38-8 Exercise Performance Under Standardized Conditions 1 or More Years after Repair of Tetralogy of Fallot[a]

Characteristic	10 Highest Performers[b]	10 Lowest Performers[c]	*P* (for Difference)
CT ratio	0.49	0.58	.001
PRV (mmHg)	39	76	.001
Age at repair (years)	5.83	10.7	.001
Pulmonary valve regurgitation (patients)	0/10	8/10	.0004
Previous Potts anastomosis (patients)	0/10	4/10	.04

Data from Wessel and colleagues.[W9]
[a]Mean values are given for continuous variables.
[b]Duration of exercise greater than 100% of normal for age.
[c]Duration of exercise 43% of normal for age.
Key: *CT*, Cardiothoracic; *PRV*, right ventricular pressure.

Table 38-9 Exercise Performance Under Standardized Conditions One or More Years after Repair of Tetralogy of Fallot, According to Right Ventricular Pressure and Presence of Pulmonary Regurgitation[a]

Right Ventricular Pressure Range and Regurgitation	Duration of Exercise (% of Normal Controls) Mean ± SD	*P* (for Difference)
PRV < 50 mmHg		
Pulmonary regurgitation: no	98 ± 20	
Pulmonary regurgitation: yes	75 ± 8.9	<.05
PRV > 50 mmHg		
Pulmonary regurgitation: no	88 ± 16	
Pulmonary regurgitation: yes	51 ± 30	<.02

Data from Wessel and colleagues.[W9]
Key: *PRV*, Right ventricular pressure; *SD*, standard deviation.
[a]Exclusive of patients with residual ventricular septal defects.

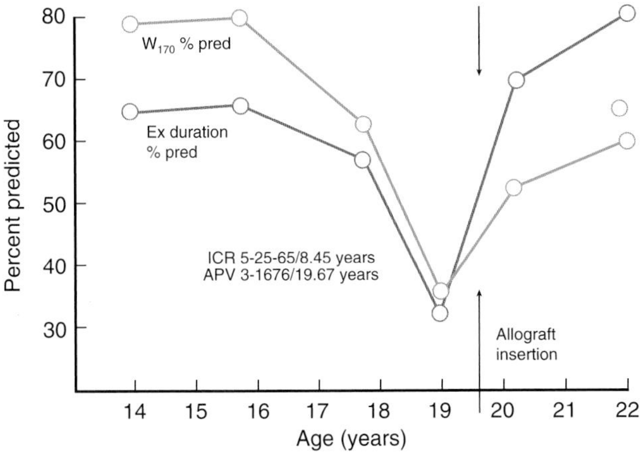

Figure 38-55 Results of serial exercise testing (work capacity above, exercise duration below, expressed as percentage of predicted value for age) after repair of tetralogy of Fallot with absent pulmonary valve. Intracardiac repair was performed without a valve in this patient at age 8.45 years, and exercise and work capacity steadily decreased. An allograft pulmonary valve was inserted when the patient was 19 years old, with subsequent improvement in performance. Key: *APV,* Allograft pulmonary valve; *Ex,* Exercise; *ICR,* intracardiac repair; *Pred,* predicted; *W,* work. (From Ilbawi and colleagues.[I5])

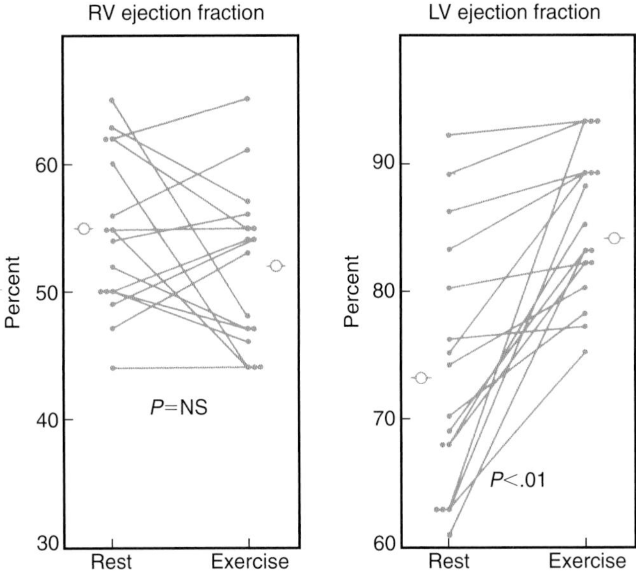

Figure 38-56 Right ventricular and left ventricular systolic function at rest and during exercise after repair of tetralogy of Fallot. Mean value for each set of data is indicated by open circle. Key: *LV,* Left ventricular; *NS,* not significant; *RV,* right ventricular. (From Reduto and colleagues.[R10])

subsequent insertion of a valve improves exercise capacity (Fig. 38-55).[I5] *Residual or recurrent VSDs* decrease exercise capacity.[W9,Z6] Furthermore, large residual or recurrent VSDs ($Qp/Qs > 2$) strongly predispose the patient to chronic heart failure late postoperatively.[R23]

Maximal oxygen uptake during exercise is only 30% to 40% of normal in patients corrected at an average age of 19.5 years.[B14] When repair is made at a still older age, the functional result is clearly worse than when it is performed in infancy or early childhood.[S28]

Right Ventricular Function

RV systolic and diastolic functions are variable late postoperatively and depend on preoperative status of the ventricle, extensiveness of the right ventriculotomy (if any) and muscular resection within the ventricle, care with which RV coronary arteries have been preserved, amount (if any) of postoperative RV systolic hypertension, and amount of pulmonary regurgitation. Relation of these to late RV systolic and diastolic function has not been well quantified, but general relations are evident.

Pulmonary regurgitation has its most evident effect on RV function. When a transanular patch has not been used and the pulmonary valve is competent, RV systolic function (ejection fraction) and end-diastolic volume may be normal late postoperatively.[B3,G24] However, even in this circumstance, RV ejection fraction may not increase normally with exercise (Fig. 38-56).[M27,R10] Global RV function (RV ejection fraction estimated by ventriculography) and contractile response to isoproterenol are better preserved after transatrial repair than after transventricular repair when measured in the early postoperative period; later clinical performance in the two groups is unknown.[M27] Also, in some patients with little or no pulmonary regurgitation, RV ejection fraction is depressed,[R8] no doubt related to other variables affecting it.

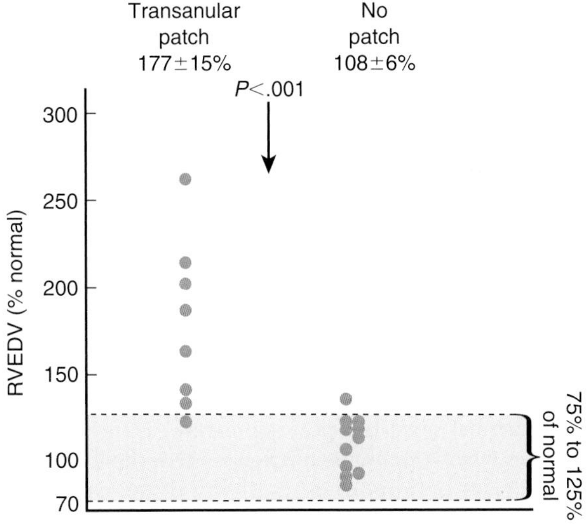

Figure 38-57 Right ventricular end-diastolic volume late after repair of tetralogy of Fallot. Patients are separated into those with and without a transanular patch. Stippled area represents normal values. Key: *RVEDV,* Right ventricular end-diastolic volume. (From Graham and colleagues.[G24])

When the pulmonary valve is regurgitant, RV systolic function and end-diastolic volume are less likely to be normal, and their abnormality correlates with amount of regurgitation.[R8] When a transanular patch has been used in the repair, ejection fraction is more likely to be low, and RV end-diastolic volume is increased, often severely so (Fig. 38-57).[B25,F16,G24] However, it has been suggested that increased RV wall thickness and consequently decreased ventricular compliance may limit volume expansion and RV enlargement. Reduced compliance may also protect against detrimental effects of pulmonary valve regurgitation.[G8] Decrease in ejection fraction is correlated with the increase in end-diastolic volume. Precise measurements of RV end-diastolic volume using MRI and CT imaging suggest that volume over 150 to 170 mL · m^{-2} will result in failure of the RV to remodel even after placement of a competent pulmonary valve.[B35,D7,G14,O8]

A resting systolic pressure up to 60 to 70 mmHg has little adverse effect on postrepair RV systolic and diastolic function. Higher systolic pressures produce dysfunction, but this is not well quantified.

Other potential determinants of postrepair RV function have not been correlated with it in a quantitative fashion.

Right Ventricular Aneurysms

RV aneurysms adversely affect RV function, but they are uncommon. True aneurysm is more common than false aneurysm and is presumably related to excessive thinning or devascularization of the RV free wall, or thinning and bulging of pericardium if it has been used as an infundibular or transanular patch.[S8] Most RV aneurysms develop within 6 months of operation, and true aneurysms stabilize and rarely progress. False aneurysm, in contrast, may progress rapidly and rupture.[R28]

Residual Right Ventricular Outflow Obstruction

Residual narrowing in the infundibulum at the RV–pulmonary trunk junction (with or without a transanular patch) or more distally can result in at least some residual RV outflow obstruction. Magnitude of obstruction is not evident at the end of operation, because both the gradient between the RV and distal pulmonary trunk and the postrepair $P_{RV/LV}$ are usually somewhat less late postoperatively than when measured in the operating room (Fig. 38-58). Dimensions of the RV–pulmonary junction enlarge proportionally to growth of the child after repair, whether or not a transanular patch was used (Fig. 38-59). However, disproportionate growth (i.e., "catch-up" growth) of the "anulus" does not occur without a transanular patch, and it cannot be expected that an "anulus" that is relatively small preoperatively and intraoperatively will become normal sized late postoperatively (Table 38-10). In some cases when a transanular patch is used, the junction will enlarge far out of proportion to growth of the child. This is caused by the same mechanism proposed for RV aneurysm formation: stretching and thinning of the patch, native tissue, or both.

Progression of originally unimportant residual RV outflow tract obstruction to important obstruction occurs uncommonly. Stiffening, thickening, and eventually even calcification of pulmonary valve cusps may occur and produce increasing RV hypertension, whether they are left in an intact "anulus" or beneath a transanular patch.[H11] Also, if mild to moderate infundibular obstruction is present immediately after surgery, progressive hypertrophy and fibrosis in the infundibulum may lead to an increase in obstruction. This usually becomes evident within a year of initial repair.

Important residual or recurrent RV outflow obstruction is an indication for reintervention if the obstruction is considered treatable. This is because of its adverse effect on RV function, particularly when considerable pulmonary regurgitation coexists.[I4]

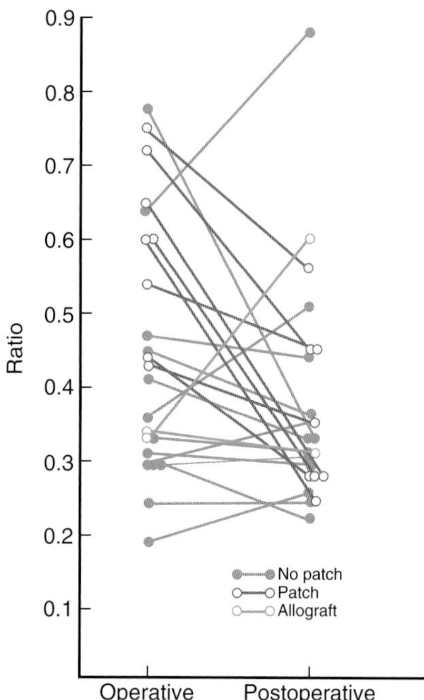

Figure 38-58 Right ventricular–to-aortic systolic pressure ratios (analogous to postrepair $P_{RV/LV}$) in the operating room after repair and at postoperative catheterization an average of 30 months later in 23 infants age 0.7 to 21 months at the time at operation. The child whose ratio increased to 0.87 had an inadequately relieved high-level infundibular and pulmonary "anulus" stenosis. Key: *Ratio,* Right ventricular to aortic peak pressure ratio. (From Calder and colleagues.[C2])

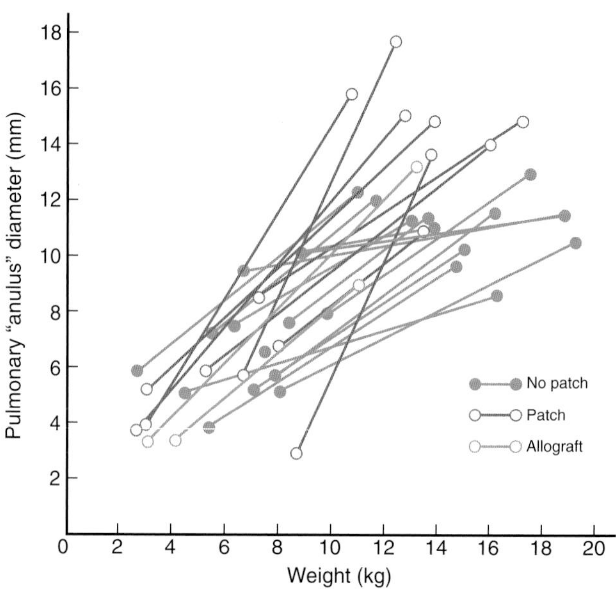

Figure 38-59 Diameter of right ventricular–pulmonary trunk junction ("anulus"), measured cineangiographically and corrected for magnification, in 23 infants age 0.7 to 21 months at repair. Leftward circle is immediately preoperative value, and rightward one is value obtained an average of 30 months later. (From Calder and colleagues.[C2])

Table 38-10 Change in Size of the Right Ventricular–Pulmonary Trunk Junction ("Anulus") after Repair of Tetralogy of Fallot[a]

	Pulmonary "Anulus"		
Type of Repair	***z* (Preop) Mean ± SD**	***z* (Late Postop) Mean ± SD**	***P* (for Difference)**
No transanular patch or allograft (*n* = 12)	−2.2 ± 1.5	−2.0 ± 1.2	.7
Transanular patch (*n* = 11)	−2.4 ± 1.8	1.1 ± 1.8	.004

Data from Calder and colleagues.[C2]
[a]Change over a 30-month period in 23 infants aged 0.7 to 21 months.
Key: *Postop,* Postoperative; *Preop,* preoperative; *SD,* standard deviation.

Table 38-11 Reasons for Reintervention after Repair of Tetralogy of Fallot with Pulmonary Stenosis[a]

Cause of Reintervention[b]	No.	% of 757
Persistent or recurrent RV outflow obstruction[c]	17	2
Pulmonary regurgitation	5	1
Residual or recurrent VSD	3	0.3
Large left-to-right shunt[d]	1	0.1
Valved conduit obstruction	2	0.2
Miscellaneous (four different categories)	4	1
TOTAL	32	4

[a]Based on follow-up and analysis of 757 hospital survivors (UAB experience, 1967 to May 1986).
[b]Reoperation: *n* = 31; balloon dilatation, *n* = 1.
[c]Obstruction was isolated and in the infundibulum in 4, at anulus in 1, at bifurcation of pulmonary trunk in 2, at origin of one or both pulmonary arteries in 2, and at multiple sites in 4. In one person each, it was associated with a small VSD, a right ventricular aneurysm, a small VSD and a right ventricular aneurysm, and severe tricuspid regurgitation.
[d]Through a recanalized classic Blalock-Taussig shunt and residual VSD.
Key: *RV,* Right ventricular; *VSD,* ventricular septal defect.

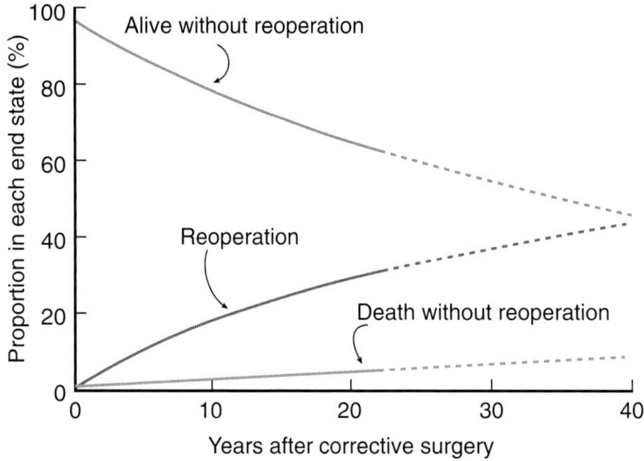

Figure 38-60 Time-related risk of reaching the mutually exclusive competing outcomes of (1) undergoing surgical reoperation, (2) death without reoperation, and (3) remaining alive without reoperation in a patient with tetralogy of Fallot and no associated cardiovascular anomalies or syndromes undergoing repair in year 1985. Lines represent parametric estimates. (From Hickey and colleagues.[H18])

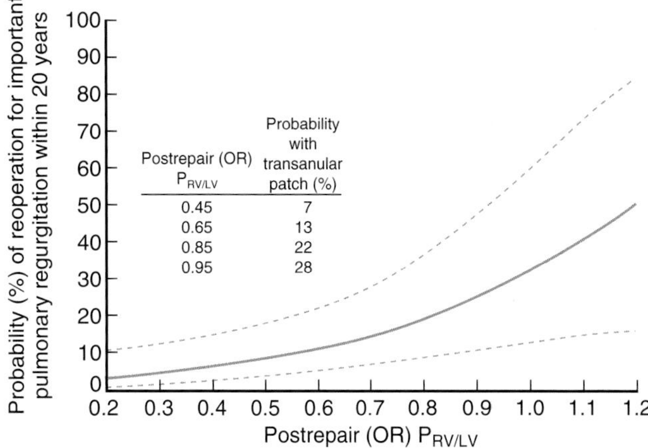

Figure 38-61 Nomogram illustrating effect of postrepair (OR) $P_{RV/LV}$ on probability of reoperation for pulmonary regurgitation within 20 years after repair of tetralogy of Fallot with pulmonary stenosis using a transanular patch. (Nomogram is specific solution of multivariable risk factor equation in original publication.) Key: *OR,* Operating room; $P_{RV/LV}$, ratio of peak pressure in right ventricle to that in left ventricle. (From Kirklin and colleagues.[K16])

Reoperation and Other Reinterventions for Right Ventricular Outflow Problems

Reoperations are infrequent in the first years after TF repair (Table 38-11), but by 30 years, half of all survivors require reoperation (Fig. 38-60).[H18] Risk of reoperation for RV outflow tract obstruction and pulmonary regurgitation both increase as time passes; however, the pattern is different. Most reoperations for obstruction occur early postoperatively, mostly in the first year, and then the rate slows but persists.[K16] The pattern of reoperation for pulmonary regurgitation varies depending on the study. In one study, the reoperation rate for pulmonary regurgitation was very low in the first years after repair and then increased substantially as time passed.[K36] In a report that covered operations performed between 1967 and 1986 that involved a transanular patch, Kirklin and colleagues reported freedom from reintervention for pulmonary regurgitation of 98% at 10 years and 88% at 20 years.[K16] In a recent (2009) study from Toronto, however, the hazard for pulmonary valve replacement was constant up to 4 decades after repair, at 0.8% per year.[H18] In an earlier (1997) study from Toronto, with follow-up extending to 36 years, only 1.2% of patients underwent reintervention for pulmonary regurgitation.[Y4] Furthermore, the study by Kirklin and colleagues identifies use of a transanular patch as a risk factor for subsequent pulmonary valve replacement, but the Toronto study does not. Although Kirklin and colleagues identify transanular patching as a risk factor, few patients in whom a transanular patch was inserted have undergone reoperation unless their postrepair (OR) $P_{RV/LV}$ was greater than about 0.7 (Fig. 38-61). Many of these differences and inconsistencies among studies probably reflect the subjective nature of the decision-making process related to the timing of reintervention for pulmonary regurgitation.

These classic studies notwithstanding, compelling data now exist showing that late serious problems arise in patients with isolated free pulmonary regurgitation; that is, pulmonary regurgitation without associated residual elevated RV pressure or residual left-to-right shunting. Free pulmonary regurgitation results in dilatation of the RV,[G15] RV dilatation correlates with prolonged QRS duration on ECG,[G7] and prolonged QRS duration is associated with sudden death.[G9] Reoperation as a marker of residual RV outflow tract problems in many analyses presents some difficulties and limitations. There are no accepted, standardized physiologic criteria for reoperation. This is of particular concern when the problem is pulmonary regurgitation. The long-term follow-up studies cited above show varying, but generally low, rates of reintervention for pulmonary regurgitation, even with follow-up of several decades or more. It must be kept in mind, however, that these studies used criteria for reintervention that are both more subjective and less strict than those used today. Also these studies rarely involve patients who originally underwent neonatal or even infant repair. They utilized presence of symptoms, onset of arrhythmias, and progressive tricuspid regurgitation as criteria for reintervention. More recently, a prolonged QRS complex of greater than 180 msec[G7,G9] and RV diastolic volume greater than 150 to 160 mL · m^{-2} have been added. Several studies using MRI indicate that enlarged RVs above about 150 to 170 mL · m^{-2} do not remodel to normal volume after a competent pulmonary valve is placed, although substantial volume reduction is observed.[B35,D7,G14,O8]

Inserting an allograft aortic or pulmonary valve, or a bioprosthetic valve, are the therapeutic options when intervention is required for pulmonary regurgitation, because they increase RV ejection fraction, decrease RV end-diastolic dimensions, and improve symptomatic status.[B26,F7] Survival after pulmonary valve replacement is excellent, with reports of 94% at 20 years.[H18] Percutaneous transcatheter pulmonary valve placement is an alternative in selected cases.[L22]

Reoperation for residual pulmonary stenosis is uncommon, with 95% of patients being free from it for at least 20 years (Fig. 38-62). Although rate of reoperation is highest early after repair, there is a constant phase of hazard as well, lasting as long as patients have been followed. The higher the postrepair (OR) $P_{RV/LV}$, the greater the probability of this type of reintervention, and the prevalence increases particularly steeply when the value is greater than about 0.7 (Fig. 38-63).

Early results for pulmonary valve replacement are good, even when additional procedures such as tricuspid valve repair or more complex RV outflow tract reconstruction are also performed. Thirty-day mortality of 2.6% (CL 1.2%-5.1%) has been reported, with 19% occurrence of postoperative arrhythmias, 13% respiratory complications, 13% renal complications, 13% reoperation during admission, and 3% myocardial infarction.[D21] Predictors of prolonged hospitalization include age greater than 45 years, number of previous sternotomies, and need for urgent operation.[D21]

Left Ventricular Function

LV systolic and diastolic function are variable late after operation. Risk factors for poor LV function include older age at repair, pre-repair status of LV (affected as it is by previous palliative operations), and residual or recurrent defects.

Patients undergoing repair during the first few years of life have normal or near-normal LV function not only at rest but also during stress.[B23,S31] Patients who are older at the time of

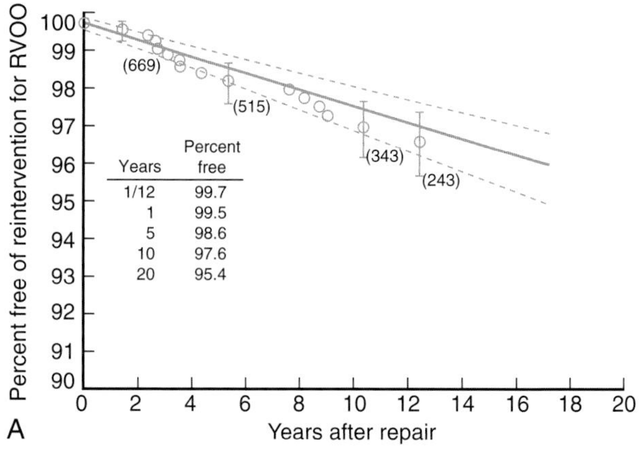

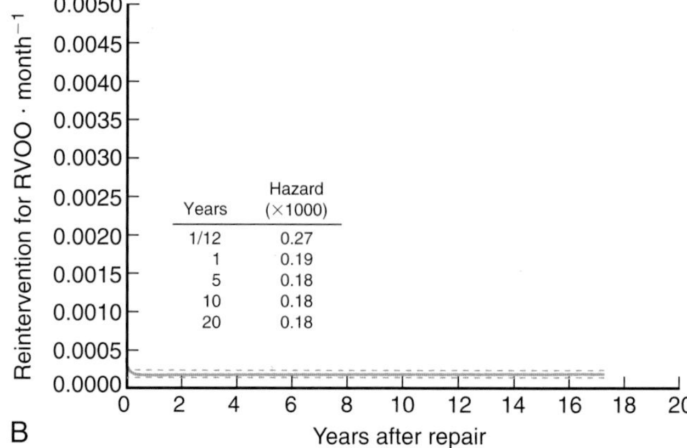

Figure 38-62 Reintervention for residual or recurrent right ventricular outflow obstruction after repair of tetralogy of Fallot with pulmonary stenosis (n = 793). (Based on the study of Kirklin and colleagues,[K16] exclusive of patients in whom a valved conduit was used in the repair [n = 21].) Depiction is as in Fig. 38-47. **A,** Time-related freedom from reintervention. Note greatly expanded vertical axis. **B,** Hazard function, which has a steeply declining early phase and a constant phase. Key: *RVOTO,* Right ventricular outflow tract obstruction.

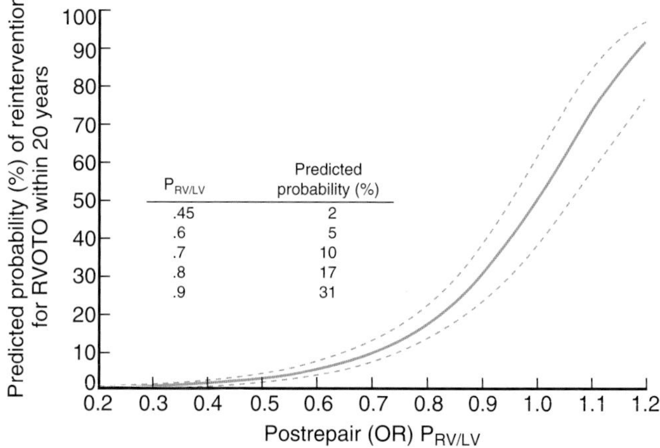

Figure 38-63 Nomogram illustrating relationship between postrepair (OR) $P_{RV/LV}$ and probability of reintervention for right ventricular outflow tract obstruction within 20 years. Analysis is based on 814 patients undergoing repair of tetralogy of Fallot and pulmonary stenosis at UAB from 1967 to May 1986. Key: *OR,* Operating room; $P_{RV/LV}$, ratio of peak pressure in right ventricle to that in left ventricle; *RVOTO,* right ventricular outflow tract obstruction. (Nomogram is specific solution of multivariable risk factor equation from Kirklin and colleagues.[K16])

repair[J2,O1] often have depressed LV ejection fraction at rest that intensifies during stress.[B23,J2] Less satisfactory function in patients undergoing repair at an older age may be due to myocardial damage from chronic preoperative hypoxia and to long-standing LV overload from systemic–pulmonary arterial shunts in most patients who are older at repair.[L5,R22] Other potential causes of LV dysfunction include intrinsic aortic root pathology. Aortic root dilatation and reduced aortic elasticity have been linked to aortic regurgitation, and aortic regurgitation to reduced LV function.[G31]

The age range at repair within which late postoperative LV function at rest and during exercise can be expected to be normal is not clearly defined. Some studies indicate that it extends to only age 2 to 3 years[B23,S31]; others suggest that it extends to as late as age 10 if shunting operations have not been necessary.[R10,R29]

Pulmonary Function

Patients with an optimal hemodynamic result from repair of TF in infancy or early childhood (closed VSD, PRV < 50 mmHg, and no pulmonary valve regurgitation) have normal lung volumes and capacities late postoperatively.[G10,W10] Conversely, patients with a less than optimal hemodynamic result and those operated on later in life have distinctly subnormal lung function. Postoperative pulmonary valve regurgitation has a particularly adverse effect on late postoperative lung volume and function.[W10]

Recurrent (Residual) Ventricular Septal Defects

Important recurrent or residual VSDs are uncommon, with reoperation being necessary in less than 1% of cases.[K1] Even small and hemodynamically unimportant leakage is infrequent.[B17] Routine left ventriculography done an average of 23 months postoperatively in 23 infants showed a tiny residual VSD in one (4%; CL 0.6%-14%).[C2] Others have reported small leakage in up to 10% of patients.[A5]

When important shunts are present, they are usually from inaccurate repair or dehiscence at the posteroinferior angle of the VSD.[C13]

Sudden Death and Important Arrhythmic Events

There has been much discussion about the possibility of sudden or arrhythmic death late after repair of TF with pulmonary stenosis,[G17,H5,Q1] but there is a lack of information about the circumstances under which this is likely to occur.

These events are more likely to occur in patients *not operated on in early life* and are unlikely when patients are repaired in the first few years of life.[D10,S29,T10] Thus, probability of sudden death or an important arrhythmic event (defined as a clearly arrhythmic death, intractable ventricular tachycardia, or insertion of a pacemaker for bradycardia developing late postoperatively) within 20 years of repair has occurred in less than 1% of patients who were younger than age 5 years at operation (Fig. 38-64).[K17] When the patient underwent repair in adult life, probability was 5% to 10%. Castaneda and colleagues found no sudden deaths and no important ventricular electrical instability in long-term follow-up of patients undergoing repair in infancy.[C8,C11,W1] Others have reported similar experiences with the relation between age and prevalence of sudden death late postoperatively.[K9,K37]

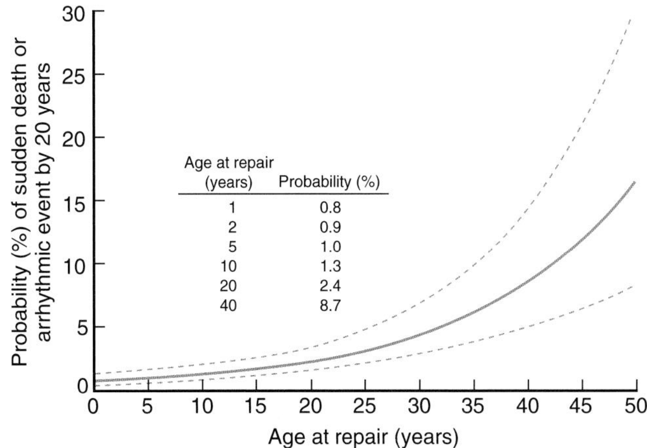

Figure 38-64 Nomogram illustrating relationship between age at repair and probability of sudden death or an important arrhythmic event within 20 years of repair of tetralogy of Fallot with pulmonary stenosis. (Multivariable equation is a specific solution of multivariable risk factor equation in original publication, as are values entered for other variables equation.) (From Kirklin and colleagues.[K17])

When *repairs are incomplete*, and particularly when this results in postoperative cardiomegaly, prevalence of ventricular arrhythmias and sudden death is higher.[W8] During long-term follow-up of the early Mayo Clinic patients, only 2% experienced sudden death; most had important cardiomegaly.[F17] Similar findings have been reported by others.[K10,W9]

When there is *important residual pulmonary stenosis*, prevalence of late postoperative arrhythmic events may be somewhat higher,[G4,G6] but the correlation is weak. Strong correlation has been demonstrated between *pulmonary regurgitation* and important ventricular arrhythmias late postoperatively.[Z2] Prolongation of the ECG QRS complex, which develops with the RV dilatation associated with pulmonary regurgitation, is associated with sudden death.[G7,G9]

Rarely, the *right ventriculotomy scar* may be arrhythmogenic. This should be considered as a possibility in patients with life-threatening ventricular arrhythmias only when cardiomegaly is absent and there is neither important pressure nor volume overload of the RV. Under these circumstances, electrophysiologic mapping is indicated. When the source of the arrhythmia can be localized to the right ventriculotomy scar, excising the scar and inserting a patch graft have been reported to be beneficial. Cryoablation techniques may also be effective in controlling arrhythmogenic foci localized to the ventriculotomy scar.

Infective Endocarditis

Infective endocarditis is rare after repair. No instances were observed with up to 10-year follow-up in two large studies.[K7,K20]

Interim Results after Classic Shunting Operations

Survival

Classic B-T and PTFE interposition shunts have a hospital mortality approaching zero and 1-month mortality of less than 1%.[A15,A18,B26,G34,I2,K21,K22,L3,S27,T12] Other types of shunting operations have a higher hospital mortality; however, they

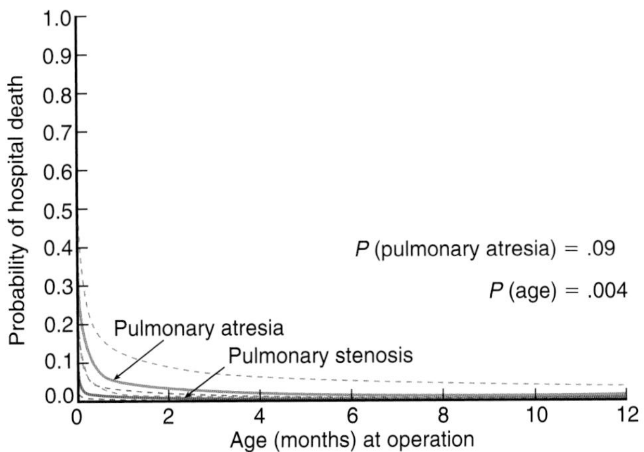

Figure 38-65 Nomogram illustrating effect of age on hospital mortality after repair of tetralogy of Fallot with pulmonary atresia versus pulmonary stenosis in patients with previous classic shunts. (Nomogram is specific solution of multivariable risk factor equation in original publication. Values entered for other variables are also given in original publication.) (From Kirklin and colleagues.[K22])

are rarely used in modern practice and are of historical interest only.[A18]

Probably the most important risk factor for early death after classic shunting procedures is *pulmonary arterial problems.*[K13] *Young age* adds an increment of risk to shunting operations, but a relatively small one (Fig. 38-65).

Interim Events

Early (<30 days) *nonfatal shunt closure* or narrowing occurs uncommonly (7%) in patients undergoing classic B-T or PTFE interposition shunt operations for TF.

Early and intermediate-term shunt closure or narrowing requiring reoperation occurs in 3% to 20% of heterogeneous groups of infants and children.[B26,D14,D20,K13,M21] Closure or important narrowing is considerably more common in neonates and young infants than in older patients (74% vs. 90% freedom at 2 years).[K13] However, closure may be less common in neonates and young infants when a PTFE interposition graft is used.[U1] Overall, shunt closure or narrowing results in unsatisfactory palliation within 3 years of shunting in about 40% of patients.[C4] This prevalence does not seem to differ among patients receiving a classic B-T shunt and those receiving a PTFE interposition graft.[C4] Use of aspirin seemingly does not increase long-term patency or reduce occurrence of localized shunt stenosis.[C14]

One manifestation of *reduced blood flow* in the arm on the side of a classic B-T shunt is that it becomes slightly shorter and smaller during the intermediate term after operation.[H7] Likewise, strength of the arm on the side of the shunt has been demonstrated to be less than normal, even though the patient is unaware of this.[Z3] When blood flow reduction is more severe than usual, gangrene of the hand can occur, although rarely.

Sudden death without explanation or autopsy, and nonfatal brain abscess each occur in about 1% of cases.[A16,K22] Improperly performed shunts of any kind result in a higher prevalence of unsatisfactory interim results, primarily because of iatrogenic pulmonary arterial problems.

Iatrogenic pulmonary arterial problems are reported to be uncommon after classic shunting or PTFE interposition shunting operations in early series.[B26,K22] However in the present era, because shunts are performed more frequently in patients with small pulmonary arteries, especially neonates, angiographic evidence of pulmonary artery distortion is fairly common late postoperatively and must be dealt with at the time of repair.[G18] From a historical perspective, these problems are much less frequent and less severe than those that were seen with obsolete shunts, such as Waterston and Potts shunts.[G11,N11,P5,R13,T3]

The key *beneficial interim results* of shunting procedures are increased $\dot{Q}p$, with consequent reduction in cyanosis and polycythemia, and improved functional capacity. NYHA functional class is usually I or II after shunting. SaO_2 at rest is usually 80% to 90%, but it always decreases with exercise, at times to as low as 50%.[H7,J3] These benefits are obtained at the expense of increased LV stroke volume, a stimulus to gradual development of LV dysfunction.

Another benefit of classic shunting procedures is the diffuse increase in size of the RPA and LPA.[G2,K19] The response of the valve and pulmonary "anulus" to shunting procedures is unpredictable. Some studies suggest that enlargement of the "anulus" can occur as a result of a shunting procedure,[A7,R20,V8] whereas others indicate that a stenotic valve can progress to atresia after shunting.[F1,M28]

Important pulmonary vascular obstructive disease does not occur with use of PTFE shunts if size of the shunt is chosen appropriately. Historically, vascular disease did develop after other shunts, such as a classic B-T, Waterston, or Potts shunt, but rarely before 5 years had passed.[H25,N8] Beyond this time, the proportion of patients who developed hypertensive pulmonary vascular disease increased with increasing shunt duration.[C24,D6,H3,R21,V10]

INDICATIONS FOR OPERATION

Diagnosis of TF is generally an indication for repair. Early repair is advisable because of the unfavorable natural history of the disease, particularly in the first year of life (see Fig. 38-23), advantages of repair before irreversible secondary myocardial and pulmonary changes occur, and low risks of repair in the current era. Yet the timing of repair remains controversial. When severe symptoms develop in the first 1 or 2 months of life, some favor one-stage repair, whereas others prefer an initial shunting operation followed within 12 months by repair.

When diagnosis is made in the neonatal period and the patient is, and remains, essentially asymptomatic or only mildly symptomatic, one-stage repair is typically deferred for a variable period. The ideal period of deferral, if any, is unclear and in current practice ranges from 2 to 24 months. A strong argument can be made that for institutions experienced in complex surgery in small infants, one-stage repair should be performed in the first 2 to 3 months.

Overall results with a two-stage protocol with an initial shunting operation for patients younger than about age 6 months and repair between age 6 and 24 months appear to be similar to those of one-stage repair, although such a protocol is not ideal.[K20] However, two-stage repair is probably prudent for institutions not well prepared for the intraoperative and early postoperative care required by neonates and small children undergoing intracardiac operations. It is also reasonable for surgeons who are not yet certain of their ability to achieve comparable results with one-stage repair in neonates and infants younger than about age 6 months.

When the LAD arises from the RCA, repair can be accomplished with usual techniques unless a "full-length" transanular patch is required. When a transanular patch is needed, there are two alternatives. One is to perform a systemic-to–pulmonary artery shunt in small symptomatic neonates and infants, deferring repair with a valved conduit for several years. The other is to perform a one-stage repair using a small valved conduit.

Multiplicity of VSDs in very young patients increases the risk of repair. Closure of apical muscular defects can often be accomplished percutaneously (see "Percutaneous Closure of Ventricular Septal Defects" under Special Situations and Controversies in Chapter 35). Thus, an initial shunting operation may be prudent, with subsequent percutaneous closure of muscular VSDs, followed by repair.

SPECIAL SITUATIONS AND CONTROVERSIES

Timing and Type of Initial Surgery

There remains wide variability in the initial surgical approach to TF.[F12,P6,T2,V1] It is becoming increasingly common to follow a protocol that involves only primary repair without use of palliative shunts; however, this approach is not universal[F12] and may not even be the most common. In an analysis of 196 patients undergoing surgery within the first 90 days of life from 32 centers participating in the Society of Thoracic Surgeons congenital heart database, 99 underwent primary repair and 97 shunt palliation.[C28]

Even when primary repair is used exclusively, there is variability in timing of repair. In patients with important symptoms, repair is performed immediately regardless of age.[K4,P6,R5,T2,V1] In asymptomatic patients, however, practices vary, ranging from elective repair as early as 8 to 12 weeks of age,[K4,P6] up to about 1 year of age.[V1]

Others prefer to perform a palliative shunt in symptomatic patients under a specific age, and primary repair above this age.[F12] The age threshold varies between 4 months and 1 year.

Currently, there is no conclusive evidence that any one of these protocols is superior.

Rationale for Use of Postrepair $P_{RV/LV}$

$P_{RV/LV}$ is easily measured in the operating room after repair, so when pulmonary artery pressure is known to be low, it is a convenient way of assessing adequacy of relief of pulmonary stenosis. It has the disadvantage of being difficult to measure late postoperatively, so in its place the ratio of peak PRV to peak radial, femoral, or aortic pressure is generally used. $P_{RV/LV}$ is neither better nor worse for assessing relief of pulmonary stenosis than is the theoretically more useful gradient between RV and pulmonary artery. Scanty data available concerning the relationship both of postrepair (OR) RV–pulmonary artery gradient to that of the next day or late postoperatively[G22,L4,S24] and of the gradient to late results are compatible with information and conclusions drawn from postrepair $P_{RV/LV}$.

Postrepair $P_{RV/LV}$ is related to pulmonary arteriolar resistance, size of the RPA and LPA,[M18] presence and severity of localized or segmental stenoses or incomplete distributions of the pulmonary arteries, and residual pulmonary trunk or RV outflow obstructions. It is also related to flow through the RV outflow tract, which may be increased postoperatively by residual left-to-right shunting across the VSD and by pulmonary valve regurgitation, or decreased by right-to-left flow through a PFO.

Postrepair $P_{RV/LV}$ should be interpreted with caution in neonates and small infants. Data correlating this ratio with medium and long-term outcome are based on patients repaired at an older age. Very young patients, especially those sedated and anesthetized perioperatively, may have low systemic vascular resistance and thus low systemic blood pressure. This may result in a $P_{RV/LV}$ that is high, above 0.7, even though the absolute RV systolic pressure is only 30 to 40 mmHg.

Initial Palliative Operations

In most institutions, a PTFE interposition shunt between the brachiocephalic or subclavian artery and pulmonary artery via a median sternotomy is preferred in all age groups. The PTFE shunt, introduced by Gazzaniga and colleagues in 1976,[G12,G13] is reliable even in young infants, with few late occlusions (see "Interim Results after Classic Shunting Operations" earlier in this section). This shunt has for the most part replaced the classic B-T shunt.

Although at one time the Waterston ascending aorta–RPA shunt was popular, most groups find it has higher mortality in infants,[A18,D3] a considerably higher proportion of iatrogenic RPA problems, and a relatively high prevalence of late pulmonary hypertension because of excessive $\dot{Q}p$.[G11] The same disadvantages pertain for the Potts descending aorta–LPA anastomosis.[D6] In addition, it is more difficult to perform than other shunts and more difficult to close later. These shunts are not performed in modern practice.

A central PTFE shunt between the ascending aorta and pulmonary trunk is another option. It has no proven advantage over a properly performed laterally placed PTFE interposition shunt; however, it will never result in branch pulmonary artery distortion. On the other hand, it may not allow as fine a regulation of pulmonary blood flow as the laterally placed interposition shunt.

Initial Palliation by β-Adrenergic Blockade

The possible advantage of β-adrenergic blockade with, for example, propranolol therapy for severe cyanosis and hypoxic spells in early infancy is that surgery may be deferred. Disadvantages are that propranolol does not always provide good palliation, and risk of repair may be higher in patients who are taking it.

Honey and colleagues showed in 1964 that β-adrenergic blockade usually alleviates paroxysmal hypoxic spells,[H26] and this has been confirmed by many others.[C27,K15,P18] When doses of about 2.5 $mg \cdot kg^{-1} \cdot day^{-1}$ of propranolol are used, relief of the hypoxic spells for at least 3 months occurs in 80% of patients.[G5] However, Garson and colleagues found this regimen to be more effective in patients older than 1 year, when it could be considered unnecessary, and less successful in infants age 6 months or less.[G5] However, their conclusion was that the drug was effective in very young patients if the dose was adequate (2-6 $mg \cdot kg^{-1} \cdot day^{-1}$ and serum propranolol levels about 100 $ng \cdot mL^{-1}$).

Initial Palliation by Balloon Valvotomy

Percutaneous balloon dilatation of the infundibulum and pulmonary valve, and percutaneous infundibular myectomy, have been reported to provide good relief of cyanosis and symptoms, with little risk, in some small patients.[B24,Q2,Q3,S21] However, the reports are anecdotal, and risks and effectiveness of the procedure in safely deferring repair remain to be clearly defined. Because repair can be performed safely at any age, these procedures are most applicable when extenuating circumstances increase surgical risk.

Monocusp Valves Beneath Transanular Patches

Many informal reports suggest that constructing monocusp valves, usually made of pericardium, beneath a transanular patch, or use of cusp-bearing allograft patches, are of value.[A1,F16,I6,M8,S15] They usually support the idea that these valves are competent in the early postrepair period but generally become regurgitant later. Over the long term, they do not appear to result in less pulmonary regurgitation than does a simple transanular patch.[G32,R12] Subsequent calcification of the cusp is potentially obstructive. Some enthusiastic formal reports have appeared,[P12] but evidence favoring their use is not persuasive.

Timing of Pulmonary Valve Replacement for Pulmonary Regurgitation Late after Repair

When this procedure should be performed to maximize effect and promote longevity of the RV remains unclear.[C18] Symptomatic deterioration of exercise ability, onset of clinical arrhythmia, or overt right heart failure from severe pulmonary regurgitation are unequivocal for pulmonary valve replacement. However, it is likely that these criteria represent a degree of hemodynamic deterioration that has progressed beyond the capacity for complete recovery ("reverse remodeling") after intervention. Therrien and colleagues[T7] showed that using these criteria, pulmonary valve replacement failed to provide for satisfactory RV reverse remodeling, with many patients suffering continued RV dilatation and low ejection fraction. Also, QRS duration stabilized (it continued to increase in a control group with similar follow-up duration), but failed to decrease to a normal level as one would have hoped. It can be argued that patients would benefit more if valve replacement were performed before onset of symptoms. However, this approach presents an additional problem. Currently, indications for pulmonary valve replacement in asymptomatic patients are being developed. Degree of RV dilatation, RV ejection fraction, and volume of pulmonary regurgitation can all be measured with precision using MRI, for example, but the need for and timing of pulmonary valve replacement late after TF on the basis of such measurements remain to be firmly established. For example, pulmonary regurgitant fraction and RV diastolic dimensions (as assessed by MRI) were not independently associated with impaired clinical status in long-term survivors of TF repair.[G15] However, numerous MRI studies show that recovery of RV function following pulmonary valve replacement was less likely if RV end-diastolic dimension exceeded 150 to 170 mL · m^{-2}.[B35,D7,O8] Similar arguments can be made for asymptomatic patients with prolonged QRS duration on ECG.

Percutaneous Pulmonary Valve Implantation

Percutaneous pulmonary valve implantation is a new option for patients with dysfunctional RV to pulmonary trunk conduits in selected TF patients who meet specific physiologic and anatomic criteria.[L22] The device can be used in cases of both RV outflow tract obstruction and pulmonary regurgitation. As of 2008, more than 500 percutaneous valves have been placed worldwide. In Lurz and Bonhoffer's experience with 230 of these cases followed for a mean of 28 months, freedom from reoperation was 93% at 10 months and 70% at 70 months.[L22] Currently, technology has not been modified to allow implantation in native outflow tracts.

Section II Tetralogy of Fallot with Pulmonary Atresia

DEFINITION

The definition of *tetralogy of Fallot with pulmonary stenosis* applies to TF with pulmonary atresia, except that in the latter there is no luminal continuity between the RV and pulmonary trunk (or both the RPA and LPA). Atresia is usually congenital but may be acquired.

HISTORICAL NOTE

As noted in Section I, Lillehei and colleagues first successfully repaired TF, and their original paper included a patient with pulmonary atresia.[L15] Rastelli and Kirklin reported the first use of an RV–pulmonary trunk extracardiac conduit to repair this anomaly in 1965.[R3] Ross and Somerville first reported use of a valved conduit for this purpose in 1966,[R30] as did Weldon and colleagues soon thereafter.[W7] Enlarging very hypoplastic pulmonary arteries by increasing pulmonary artery pressure and flow using a conduit connecting the RV to pulmonary arteries or by a systemic–pulmonary arterial shunt was reported by McGoon and colleagues and Kirklin and colleagues in 1977.[G16,K19]

The important role of large aortopulmonary (AP) collateral arteries in many patients having TF with pulmonary atresia appears to have been first addressed in a constructive manner by Macartney and colleagues.[M1] These investigators reported on the hemodynamic characteristics of these arteries in 1973[M1] and again in 1974.[M3] They introduced the concept of a multifocal blood supply to the pulmonary circulation through both the central pulmonary arteries and large AP collateral arteries.[M3] In 1980, Haworth and Macartney described in detail the large AP collateral arteries supplying blood to some pulmonary arterial segments by end-to-end anastomosis, and to others by end-to-side anastomosis.[H14] By then, the UAB group had described, in 1978, the adverse effect of incomplete distribution (arborization) of the pulmonary arteries on survival after repair of TF with pulmonary atresia.[A6] In 1981, Haworth, Macartney, and colleagues introduced the concept of unifocalization of pulmonary arterial supply as a first step to repair in patients with multifocal supply and large AP collateral arteries.[H15] Subsequently the surgical results of these procedures have accumulated (see

"Results after Staged Palliative Operations for Unifocalization" later in this section). Systematic one-stage complete repair in infancy, involving bilateral unifocalization and intracardiac repair via median sternotomy, was introduced by Reddy and Hanley in 1992 and reported in 1995.[R4] Percutaneous catheter dilatation of localized stenoses in the RPA and LPA was reported by Lock and colleagues in 1983,[L18] and closure of large AP collateral arteries using this technique was reported by Yamamoto and colleagues in 1979.[Y3]

MORPHOLOGY AND MORPHOGENESIS

Tetralogy of Fallot with Congenital Pulmonary Atresia

General morphology of the heart in TF with pulmonary atresia is similar to that in TF with pulmonary stenosis. The most important differences are that in TF with pulmonary atresia:

- No blood passes from RV to lungs; consequently, all pulmonary blood flow arises from the ductus arteriosus, collateral vessels, or fistulae.
- Pulmonary arterial anomalies are common.
- Large AP collateral arteries are common.

Right Ventricular Outflow Tract

Atresia, when congenital, may be in the infundibular area or at the RV–pulmonary trunk junction ("anulus").

Infundibular atresia is the most severe manifestation of RV outflow atresia in TF, occurring in about 70% of hearts.[A2] The RV infundibulum seems to be totally absent in such cases, or the infundibular septal elements may be present but nearly fused with the anterior RV free wall (Fig. 38-66). The VSD is usually large and extends nearly to the free wall of the RV anteriorly, as does the aortic valve. The RV in such hearts is usually massively hypertrophied.

When the *atresia is at the RV–pulmonary trunk junction*, the infundibulum is usually present, but the pathway is narrowed by marked hypertrophy of the infundibular structures (Fig. 38-67). Obstruction consists of a thick fibrous membrane (analog of the pulmonary valve) above the infundibulum. Length and width of the infundibulum is variable.

Pulmonary Trunk

The pulmonary trunk may be present and of reasonable size, but more commonly it is importantly hypoplastic (Fig. 38-68). Occasionally, it is represented by only a fibrous cord without a lumen. In about 5% of patients with duct-dependent pulmonary blood flow, it appears to be completely absent.[A13] In patients with collateral-dependent pulmonary blood flow, the pulmonary trunk as well as the central branch pulmonary arteries are absent in up to 23%.[M6]

No clear correlation has been developed between location and type of atresia and morphology of the pulmonary trunk.

An unusual variation of pulmonary trunk morphology has been recognized with increasing frequency recently, especially in patients with arborization abnormalities of the pulmonary artery branches. In this variant the pulmonary trunk arises from the proximal coronary artery system. Origins from the left main, right, and circumflex coronaries have all been identified.[A10] The true prevalence of this variant is not known, because most cases have been reported in isolation or in small groups[B20,K3,M22,W13,Y6]; however, when systematically sought in a population of patients with arborization abnormalities of the pulmonary artery branches, it has been found to occur in up to 10%.[A10]

Right and Left Pulmonary Arteries

Confluence of Right and Left Pulmonary Arteries About 20% to 30% of patients have nonconfluent RPAs and LPAs (discontinuity).[E5] This usually results from absence of the central portion of one or both of these arteries.[S11] Rarely, it is caused by atresia of at least the distal pulmonary trunk and origins of both pulmonary arteries. (Patients having TF with pulmonary stenosis rarely have discontinuity of the RPA and LPA.)

Confluent RPA and LPA may be associated with either a patent or atretic pulmonary trunk.

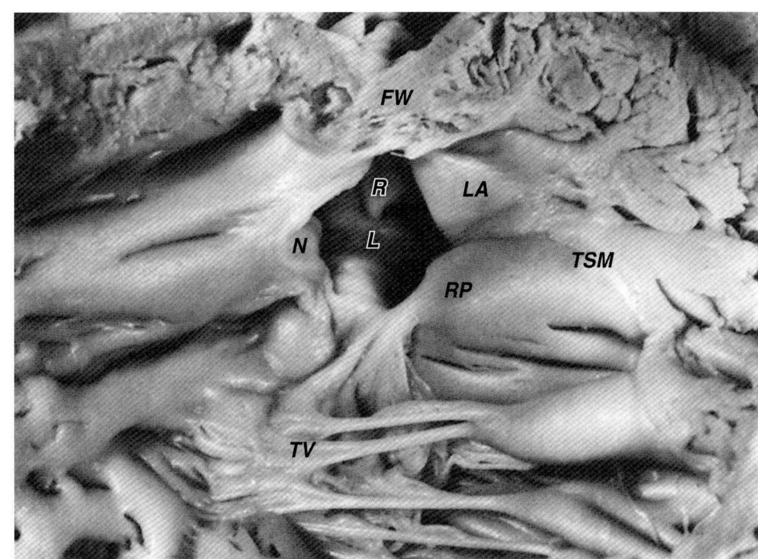

Figure 38-66 Specimen of tetralogy of Fallot with congenital infundibular atresia. Infundibular septum is small and divisions of trabecula septomarginalis prominent. Ventricular septal defect is perimembranous but extends anteriorly and superiorly almost to anterior free wall of ventricle. The danger of inadvertently cutting into the aortic root when making the right ventriculotomy is evident. There is marked overriding of noncoronary aortic cusp. Key: *FW,* Anterior free wall; *L,* left coronary cusp of aortic valve; *LA,* left anterior division of trabecula septomarginalis; *N,* noncoronary cusp of aortic valve; *R,* right coronary cusp of aortic valve; *RP,* right posterior division of trabecula septomarginalis; *TSM,* trabecula septomarginalis; *TV,* tricuspid valve.

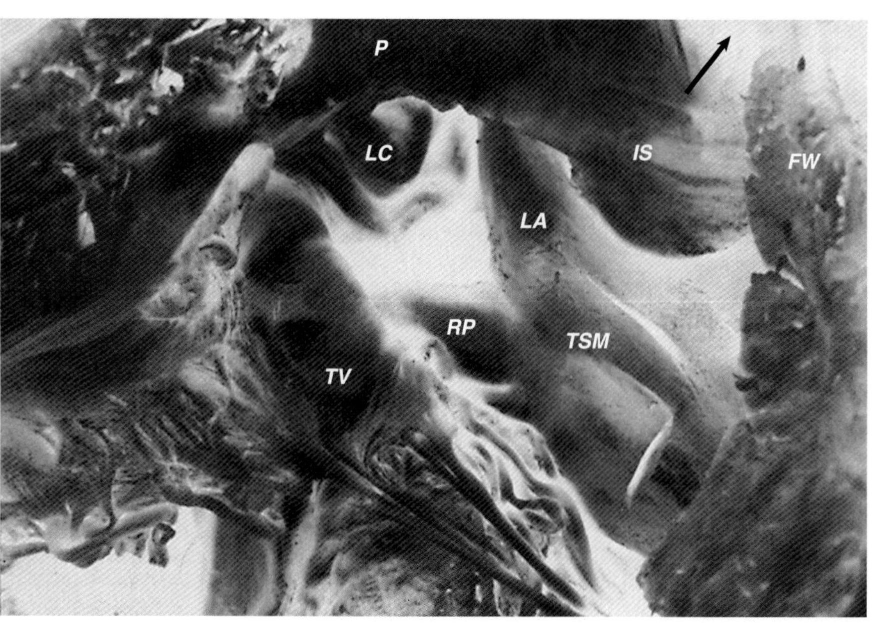

Figure 38-67 Autopsy specimen of tetralogy of Fallot with pulmonary atresia from a newborn. Anterior and leftward displacement of septal end of an unusually bulky infundibular septum is shown, inserting in front of left anterior division of trabecula septomarginalis rather than between its two divisions. Anterior and leftward deviation of parietal end of infundibular septum is also obvious, with the septum lying partway between a coronal and sagittal plane. There is a diminutive blind right ventricular outflow tract *(arrow)* in front of the infundibular septum. Key: *IS,* Infundibular septum; *FW,* anterior free wall; *LA,* left anterior division of trabecula septomarginalis; *LC,* left coronary cusp of aortic valve; *P,* parietal end of infundibular septum; *RP,* right posterior division of trabecula septomarginalis; *TSM,* trabecula septomarginalis; *TV,* tricuspid valve.

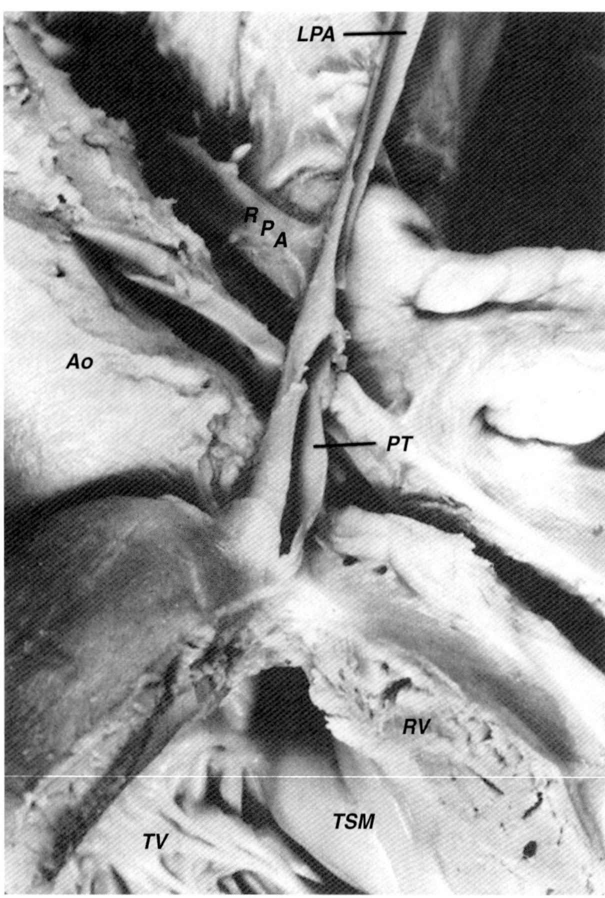

Figure 38-68 Autopsy specimen of tetralogy of Fallot with congenital pulmonary atresia (same specimen as Fig. 38-66). Proximally, the pulmonary trunk ends blindly; distally, it extends directly into small left pulmonary artery. By contrast, right pulmonary artery arises almost at right angles from pulmonary trunk. Key: *Ao,* Aorta; *LPA,* left pulmonary artery; *PT,* pulmonary trunk; *RPA,* right pulmonary artery; *RV,* opened right ventricular anterior wall; *TSM,* trabecula septomarginalis (septal band); *TV,* tricuspid valve.

Stenoses of Origins of Pulmonary Arteries Among patients with confluence of the RPA and LPA and normal distribution arborization of pulmonary arteries, about 10% have stenosis of the origin (central portion) of the RPA, and about 20% have stenosis of the LPA.[S11] The latter anomaly seems clearly related to extension onto the LPA of the process of ductal closure.[E8]

Distribution (Arborization) of Pulmonary Arteries An important feature of the morphology of TF with pulmonary atresia is frequent failure of the pulmonary arteries to distribute to all 20 pulmonary vascular segments.[A6,H14,S11] In this regard, patients with relatively normal caliber confluent central portions of the RPA and LPA are very different from those with either hypoplastic confluent branches or nonconfluent ones. Also, the presence or absence of a ductus arteriosus is an important factor determining arborization abnormalities. If a ductus arteriosus is present and the branch pulmonary arteries are confluent, arborization abnormalities and large AP collaterals are rarely if ever seen.[H14] If a ductus arteriosus is present and the branch pulmonary arteries are discontinuous, the branch pulmonary artery (usually the left) that receives flow from the ductus rarely if ever has arborization abnormalities, and that lung rarely if ever has large AP collaterals.[M6] In this setting, the opposite branch pulmonary artery (usually the right) is almost always hypoplastic and has arborization abnormalities or is completely absent, and the lung blood supply is solely from large AP collaterals.

In one series, distribution of the pulmonary arteries was complete to all 20 pulmonary arterial segments in slightly more than half (53%; CL 48%-58%)[S11] the patients with confluent RPA and LPA, and normal distribution was associated with relatively normal caliber of the confluent LPA and RPA (Table 38-12). In contrast, more than 80% of those with nonconfluent RPA and LPA or confluent but hypoplastic pulmonary arteries had incomplete distribution of one or both arteries, and in slightly more than one third of this group less than 10 pulmonary vascular segments were in continuity with a central or proximal extrapericardial portion

Table 38-12 Confluence or Nonconfluence of Central Pulmonary Arteries and Number of Pulmonary Artery Segments Centrally Connected in Patients with Tetralogy of Fallot with Pulmonary Atresia

No. of Pulmonary Artery Segments	Confluent (*n* = 132) No. of Patients	%		Nonconfluent[a] (*n* = 28) No. of Patients	%	
20	62	47		5	18	
19	8	6		2	7	
18	8	6		2	7	
17	13	10		0	0	
16	6	5		0	0	
15	8	6		0	0	
14	6	5		1	4	
13	6	5		0	0	
12	5	4		0	0	
11	4	3		0	0	
10	2	2		8	29	
9	2	4		1	4	
8	0	0		0	0	
7	0	0		2	7	
6	1	1		0	0	
5	0	0	4 (3%)	1	4	10 (36%)
4	1	1		0	0	
3	0	0		0	0	
2	0	0		0	0	
1	0	0		0	0	
0	0	0		6	21	
TOTAL	132	100		28	100	

Data from Shimazaki and colleagues.[S11]
[a]Absence of one or both central pulmonary arteries.

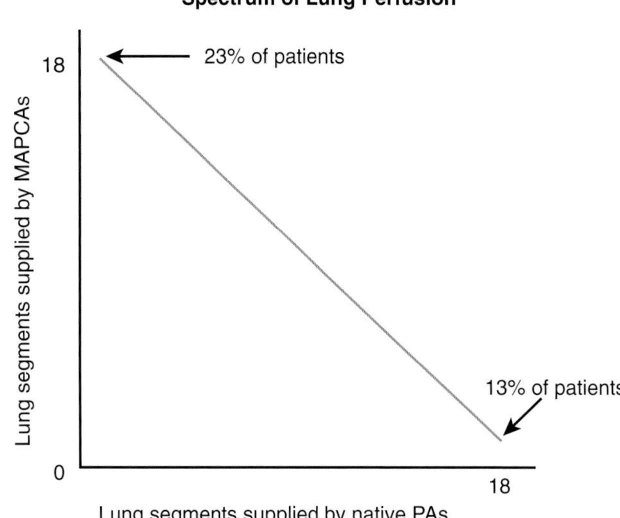

Figure 38-69 Spectrum of lung perfusion in pulmonary atresia with ventricular septal defect. This is a hypothetical relation between number of pulmonary segments perfused by native pulmonary arteries *(PAs)* and those perfused by major aortopulmonary collateral arteries *(MAPCAs)*.

of an ipsilateral pulmonary artery[S11] (see Table 38-12). Pulmonary arterial segments that are not connected to a central pulmonary artery usually receive large AP collateral arteries. As a general rule, there is an inverse correlation between the number of lung segments supplied by collaterals and those supplied by the native pulmonary arteries. Fig. 38-69 shows this relationship. In one large series of patients with pulmonary atresia and collateral-dependent pulmonary blood flow, 23% of all patients had no vascular distribution from native pulmonary arteries to the lungs, and 13% had complete vascular distribution from native pulmonary arteries to 18 lung segments (considered to be complete arborization in this study). The remaining 64% of patients had vascular distribution from both native pulmonary arteries and collaterals along the spectrum shown in Fig. 38-69.[M6] In contrast, most patients having TF with pulmonary stenosis have all 20 pulmonary arterial segments in continuity with a central or proximal extrapericardial portion of an ipsilateral pulmonary artery.

Stenoses of Pulmonary Arteries Stenoses of the pulmonary arteries beyond their origins are identified in only a small percentage of cases. However, when these small pulmonary arteries are subjected to increased pressure and flow after a palliative or corrective operation, they may enlarge in some areas and not in others.[F14,H15] Thus, localized areas of noncompliance in the pulmonary arterial walls may not present as stenoses until after a procedure that increases pulmonary blood flow.

Overall, stenoses are most common at the origin of the pulmonary artery on the side of the ductus arteriosus, when one is present. Such juxtaductal stenoses (pulmonary artery coarctations) were found in 65% of patients studied by Elzenga and colleagues.[E9]

Size of Pulmonary Arteries The immediately prebranching portion of the RPA and LPA varies widely, from normal caliber in some patients to extremely small in others—as low as McGoon ratios[P15] of about 0.5, which corresponds to a Nakata index[N4] of about 20 and a *z* value of about −10. These dimensions are particularly small in the subset with nonconfluence (discontinuity) of the RPA and LPA.[S11] In a subset of patients, intrapericardial pulmonary arteries are completely absent. In the series of 462 cases of TF with pulmonary atresia and large AP collaterals reported by Malhotra and Hanley, among the 77% of patients who had centrally confluent native pulmonary arteries, mean diameter of the branches was 2 mm.[M6] In general, patients with TF with pulmonary atresia have considerably smaller RPA and LPA than those with TF with pulmonary stenosis; in the latter group, these dimensions are similar to those in normal individuals.[B15,S10,S11]

Abnormal Hilar Branching Patterns Even when the pulmonary arteries distribute to all parts of the right and left lung, hilar branching patterns may be abnormal, particularly in patients with large AP collateral arteries.

Alternative Sources of Pulmonary Blood Flow

Large Aortopulmonary Collateral Arteries The most dramatic route of collateral flow is through large AP collateral

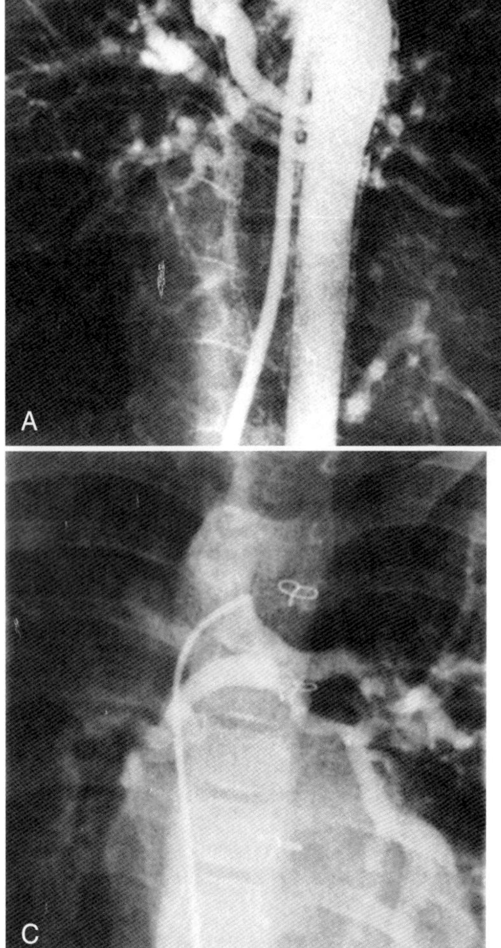

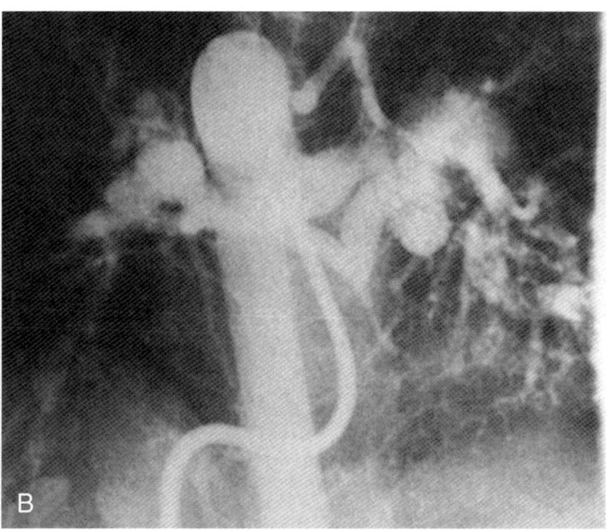

Figure 38-70 Large aortopulmonary (AP) collateral arteries in tetralogy of Fallot with pulmonary atresia. **A,** Two large AP collateral arteries come off right and anterior aspects of upper descending thoracic aorta and connect end to end with hilar arteries of right upper lobe. A smaller collateral artery supplies part of the lingula of left lower lobe. **B,** Large AP collateral artery passes to the left and joins end to side to hilar portion of left pulmonary artery (LPA) in a manifold. The Y-shaped distal pulmonary trunk and central LPA and right pulmonary artery (RPA) fill from this manifold. Another large AP collateral passes to the right above RPA. **C,** Branches of large AP collateral artery join end to end with hilar branches to left upper lobe, left lower lobe, and right lower lobe.

arteries, which are present in about 60% of patients having TF with pulmonary atresia (Fig. 38-70).[S11] In this context, "large" implies embryologic rather than acquired origin of the collaterals, the latter typically resulting in smaller, more numerous collateral vessels. Large collaterals occur rarely in TF with pulmonary stenosis. AP collateral arteries are large discrete arteries, typically from one to six in number but sometimes more, most commonly originating from the upper or mid-descending thoracic aorta.[R11] The most common origins after the mid-descending thoracic aorta are the aortic arch and the low thoracic aorta. Occasionally a collateral originates from the intraabdominal aorta. Regardless of origin, collaterals generally pursue a somewhat serpiginous course, occasionally passing through the esophageal wall, and most commonly terminate by joining an interlobar or intralobar pulmonary artery that arborizes normally within a pulmonary lobe or segment.[H14,M1]

AP collateral arteries arise from the aorta (or other source) either as elastic vessels with a wide lumen or as muscular arteries with stenotic areas.[H13] In either event, beyond their origins they resemble muscular systemic arteries. Areas of intimal proliferation (intimal pads) are frequent and result in stenoses. Extensive areas of these are prominent at branching points and at the junction of AP collateral arteries with pulmonary arteries. This process eventually results in stenoses in about 60% of collateral arteries.[H14,M20,M29] In most patients, stenoses are sufficient in number to prevent pulmonary overcirculation; when this is not the case, pulmonary overcirculation is present early in life, and pulmonary vascular disease develops in patients surviving past infancy.[H13,H16,T9] Even in the absence of clinical signs and symptoms of overcirculation, however, an unobstructed collateral may cause pulmonary vascular disease in the area of lung it supplies. Thus, both regional and localized overcirculation can occur.

Although stenoses in some cases are primarily related to structural abnormalities in the collateral vessel wall, in others they are acquired, the result of abnormal postnatal flow patterns. Severe stenoses have been documented angiographically in patients as young as age 3 to 4 months in vessels that showed normal caliber at neonatal angiography.[R6] Stenoses can evolve variably and unpredictably.

An AP collateral artery that joins end to end with an intrapulmonary artery changes in histologic appearance as it becomes a pulmonary artery and changes its positional relation to the bronchi. Thus, peripherally, its histologic appearance and position become typical for "true" pulmonary arteries.[H14] In this situation, the distal pulmonary arterial branches may be abnormally small[H14] and fewer in number than in normal individuals.

In about 50% of patients with large AP collateral arteries, the collateral enters end to side into a complex manifold in the hilum of the lung. This manifold usually includes the hilar portion of the pulmonary artery, and from this manifold interlobar and intralobar pulmonary arteries distribute distally, and central pulmonary arteries may fill retrogradely.[F2] The lung segments in this situation are said to have *dual supply* from the collateral and the true pulmonary artery. In other cases, the collateral distribution distally into the lung does not communicate with the central pulmonary artery system. In this situation, the involved lung segments are said to have *isolated supply* from the collateral only.

Less commonly, an AP collateral artery may connect end to side to a central pulmonary artery. Rarely, a single AP collateral artery on each side connects end to end with the hilar portion of the ipsilateral pulmonary artery.[J4,M3] It is this last form that gave origin to the erroneous appellation "truncus type IV."

AP collateral arteries are usually associated with abnormal branching patterns and incomplete distribution of the hilar portion of the pulmonary arteries. There may be associated single or multiple, localized or segmental, pulmonary arterial stenoses or diffuse hypoplasia.[H14,O6]

Paramediastinal Collateral Arteries These are no different from AP collaterals, with the exception that their systemic origin is from a vessel other than the aorta. A large right or left paramediastinal collateral artery occasionally arises from the right or left subclavian artery, most often on the side opposite that of the aortic arch. It may connect end to side to the right or left central or hilar pulmonary artery, or it may distribute end to end to the intrapulmonary arteries of the upper lobe. It may be difficult to distinguish such a collateral from an unusually positioned and tortuous patent ductus arteriosus if the collateral is the sole vascular supply to one lung.

Bronchial Collateral Arteries Systemic vessels that originate from the mid-descending thoracic aorta and follow the course of the trachea and major bronchi before communicating with the lung parenchyma are often designated as bronchial collateral arteries. These vessels are often adherent to the airways and give off numerous small branches that supply the walls of the airways. They tend to be thin walled and tortuous, but may be large and carry a large amount of collateral flow. Collaterals that fit this description can be found in some but not all patients with TF and pulmonary atresia. They may also occur in the same patients who have more typical AP collaterals.

Increased use of various collateral arteries in surgical reconstruction has stimulated their careful pathologic evaluation. The picture is complex. It is becoming increasingly clear that the distinction between bronchial collaterals and other AP collaterals, and between intraparenchymal and extraparenchymal vessels, is simplistic; rather, the course and structure of those vessels that carry these labels is highly variable and unpredictable. Thus, these distinct labels may not apply to many vessels.[H4] This observation corresponds with embryologic evidence that AP collateral artery formation occurs over extended periods during development.[D13]

Other Collaterals Small collateral channels may pass from coronary arteries to the bronchial arteries.[D1] Relatively large communications between the proximal right or left coronary artery and the central pulmonary artery confluence occur in up to 10% of cases.[A10] In rare cases a *fistula* between the RCA and pulmonary trunk may be the sole large collateral source of pulmonary blood flow.[K38] Even more rarely, an AP window may serve this function (see Chapter 44).[C10]

Acquired Collaterals These vessels are stimulated or promoted by several factors, primarily cyanosis and adhesions from previous surgery or procedures. They typically arise from intercostal, internal thoracic, and smaller mediastinal and diaphragmatic arteries and are almost always multiple (dozens or even hundreds), small, and tortuous. Thus, they are almost impossible to control or eliminate using either surgical techniques or interventional coil occlusion. This collateral circulation may be so well developed as to make even the most careful mobilization of the lung hazardous. Such situations are not encountered in infants who are not chronically cyanotic and who have not undergone previous surgical procedures.

Ductus Arteriosus

In the absence of AP collaterals, pulmonary circulation at birth is dependent on ductal flow to the site of pulmonary artery confluence. This represents about 40% of these patients. Ductus orientation and position are usually abnormal—a downwardly directed branch coming from beneath the left aortic arch.[C5] It is also longer and more tortuous than is otherwise the case (Fig. 38-71) and is often narrowed at its pulmonary end. In the setting of left aortic arch, a right-sided patent ductus arteriosus is rare. When present, it comes off the right subclavian or brachiocephalic artery, or if associated with an aberrant right subclavian artery, it may come from an aortic diverticulum and pass to the right behind the esophagus.

When the pulmonary arteries are confluent, presence of large (embryologic rather than acquired) AP collaterals almost always means that there will not be a ductus arteriosus. When the pulmonary arteries are not confluent, a ductus arteriosus may or may not be present (see "Distribution [Arborization] of Pulmonary Arteries" earlier in this section).

Morphogenesis

A feature that distinguishes patients having TF with pulmonary atresia from those with pulmonary stenosis is the association of pulmonary atresia with chromosome 22q11 deletion. The association is particularly high in those with pulmonary artery arborization abnormalities and large AP collaterals.[A11,C17,D17,H23,M10] This deletion is associated with clinical evidence of DiGeorge syndrome, or velocardiofacial syndrome, in approximately 90% of cases. In those cases, careful consideration must be given to the typical immunologic, calcium metabolism, and neurodevelopmental abnormalities that may be part of this syndrome.

Tetralogy of Fallot with Acquired Pulmonary Atresia

Pulmonary atresia may develop spontaneously after birth in patients born with TF with pulmonary stenosis, or may be stimulated by a palliative operation.[F1,N14] Acquired atresia is usually valvar, but may develop in the immediately subvalvar region or in the os infundibulum. This type of TF has the morphologic characteristics of TF with pulmonary stenosis.

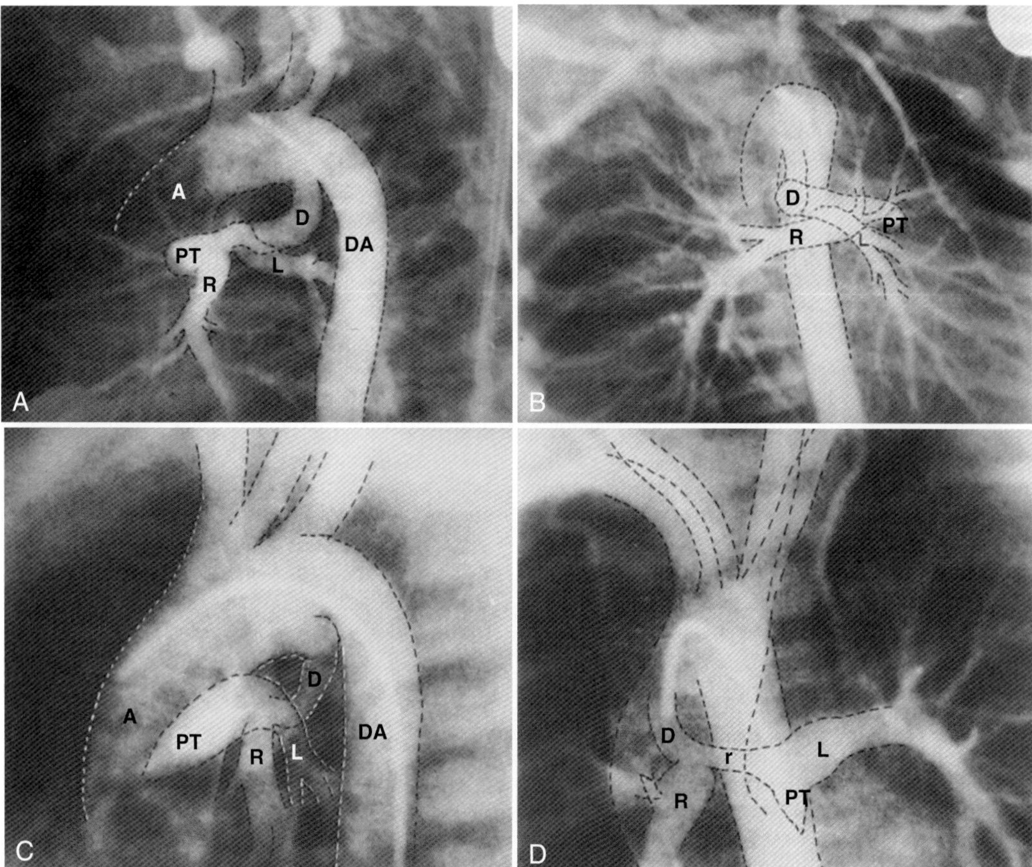

Figure 38-71 Arch aortography in tetralogy of Fallot (TF) with pulmonary atresia. Cineangiograms in **(A)** left anterior oblique (LAO) and **(B)** right anterior oblique projections show typical orientation of a left patent ductus arteriosus with left aortic arch. Ductus joins origin of left pulmonary artery (LPA). Contrast medium fills pulmonary trunk and right pulmonary artery (RPA) as well. LAO view shows normal (usual) brachiocephalic artery origins. Cineangiograms in lateral **(C)** and frontal **(D)** projections show typical orientation of patent ductus arteriosus when aortic arch is right sided. Here the right-sided ductus arises from distal arch to join the RPA. Contrast medium also fills the pulmonary trunk and LPA through narrowed proximal RPA. Key: *A,* Ascending aorta; *D,* patent ductus arteriosus; *DA,* descending aorta; *L,* left pulmonary artery; *PT,* pulmonary trunk; *R,* right pulmonary artery; *r,* proximal right pulmonary artery.

CLINICAL FEATURES AND DIAGNOSTIC CRITERIA

When the patient has TF with congenital pulmonary atresia and no AP or other large collateral arteries, cyanosis is usually evident during the first few days of life, becoming extreme as the ductus narrows and closes. This rapid progression is modified when there are large collaterals supplying the pulmonary bed, when the ductus stays open, or when an operation is performed.

Infants with pulmonary atresia and large AP collateral arteries present at birth with varying degrees of cyanosis. In approximately 80%, cyanosis is mild to moderate and hemodynamics are stable. In about 10%, presentation is with heart failure, which usually peaks at age 4 to 6 weeks as neonatal Rp decreases and Qp becomes large; cyanosis is mild. In about 10%, cyanosis is severe at birth, occasionally to the degree that hemodynamic instability develops. Regardless of presentation at birth, without intervention there is a general trend for cyanosis to worsen as collateral stenosis and pulmonary vascular disease develop. Both processes may occur in the same patient within different collateral areas.

Primary and secondary airway problems have been recognized with increasing frequency. The reasons are many, including upper airway extrinsic compression from a large aorta or collateral vessel[M17] to small airway hyperresponsiveness.[A2]

Children who first present at an older age are usually symptomatic, cyanotic, and polycythemic no matter what the source of collateral blood flow, because it has become inadequate by that time.

Physical examination discloses findings similar to those of patients who have TF with pulmonary stenosis. In pulmonary atresia, however, a systolic murmur is usually absent. There is frequently a continuous murmur from large AP collateral arteries, a patent ductus arteriosus, or a coronary–pulmonary artery fistula.[O7] The murmur is maximal over the site of the collateral at its point of stenosis and may therefore be heard to the left or right of the sternum or posteriorly.

Clinical presentation, examination, and special studies are similar to those described for TF with pulmonary stenosis, with some important distinctions.

Echocardiography

Echocardiography is diagnostic for all cases of TF with pulmonary atresia, but it is definitive only if confluent normal-caliber branch pulmonary arteries connected to a patent ductus arteriosus can be identified.

Catheterization and Angiography

Cardiac catheterization and angiography should be performed at birth in all patients with an echocardiographic diagnosis of TF with pulmonary atresia and non–duct-dependent pulmonary blood flow. The origin, course, and distribution of every collateral should be clearly identified. Characterization of the collateral blood supply to a given lung segment should be further assessed to determine whether the collateral vessel provides the sole blood supply or is part of dual or multiple sources of blood flow coming from other collaterals or from the central or "true" pulmonary arteries. Further assessment is performed to identify whether any of the sources of blood supply come from a ductus arteriosus or the coronary artery system. Central and peripheral stenoses are identified both external to and within the lung parenchyma. Finally, specific effort should be made to fully characterize the central true pulmonary arteries using collateral and pulmonary wedge injections. Only after this level of definition is achieved can an appropriate surgical management plan be formulated.

Although clinical status of the patient and specifics of the management plan may influence the need for repeat study at any time, in almost all cases, repeat cardiac catheterization and detailed angiography are required in a matter of months. The reason may be to reevaluate an infant at age 3 to 4 months immediately before a one-stage unifocalization and intracardiac repair, because collaterals can change dramatically in the first few months of life, or it may be to assess the results of a previous palliative procedure performed in the neonatal period. Clinical stability (i.e., a thriving infant with SaO_2 of 80% ± 5%) is not an indication to postpone cardiac catheterization. Such infants are likely to have important maldistribution of pulmonary blood flow despite their clinical stability, putting some lung segments at risk of developing pulmonary vascular disease due to overcirculation, and other segments at risk of being lost due to collateral occlusion.

In patients with ductus-dependent pulmonary blood flow with normally developed confluent pulmonary arteries, early repeat catheterization is typically not necessary, whether the initial neonatal procedure was one-stage repair or shunt placement. Although cardiac catheterization and standard angiography are absolute necessities in the workup of TF with pulmonary atresia and complex pulmonary arteries, newer imaging modalities such as 3D CTA or MRI currently provide an adjunctive role and may eventually take on increasing diagnostic importance in defining the complex morphology of abnormal pulmonary arteries and AP collaterals.[L6] Echocardiography is important in defining the intracardiac morphology, but has a subordinate role in the arterial assessment.[S17]

Computed Tomographic Angiography

This modality is being used increasingly in the neonatal period for TF with pulmonary atresia and large AP collaterals (Fig. 38-72). CTA in the neonatal period may prevent need for invasive catheterization if the CT demonstrates that a particular patient does not fall within one of several specific morphologic subgroups requiring neonatal surgery. The examples shown in Fig. 38-72 represent two specific subgroups that require neonatal surgery, according to the Stanford Management Protocol for TF with pulmonary atresia and aortopulmonary collaterals (Fig. 38-73). Because neonatal surgery is required in these subgroups, preoperative catheterization with detailed angiography of the collaterals is indicated. Catheterization can be deferred until the preoperative evaluation, typically at 3 to 4 months of life, in the majority (75%) of patients who make up the other morphologic subgroups.[M6] Thus, CT can serve as the definitive neonatal study in patients who will not require a neonatal operation. It should be emphasized that catheterization with angiography is strictly indicated if immediate surgery is anticipated.

NATURAL HISTORY

The natural history of patients with TF and congenital pulmonary atresia cannot be described simply, in part because of the great variability of morphology.[M26] This is reflected in the more complex hazard function for death compared with that for TF and pulmonary stenosis (see Fig. 38-23, C).[B10] It consists of a short-lasting early hazard phase, considerably more acute than for TF with pulmonary stenosis, that merges with a constant hazard phase (exponentially decreasing survival) that lasts to about age 50, followed by an increasing late hazard (with wide confidence limits). Unfortunately, morphologic characteristics of the anomaly corresponding to early death were not available to Bertranou and colleagues for their study of natural history, nor is it certain that reported groups of patients were an unselected sample of all patients born with this condition. This is particularly unfortunate in this condition, because it is likely that morphologic and physiologic characteristics influence survival.

Nevertheless, knowledge of the pathophysiology of the anomaly suggests that the shape of the natural history hazard function (see Fig. 38-23, *C*) may result from a mixture of different morphologic and physiologic subgroups that have been conveniently formed because of their surgical significance.

- *Confluent and normally distributing RPA and LPA and patent ductus arteriosus.* In this group, the only source of pulmonary blood flow is a patent ductus arteriosus, and the RPA and LPA are confluent, usually minimally hypoplastic, and distribute to all 20 pulmonary arterial segments.
- *Confluent, nonconfluent, or absent RPA and LPA with AP collaterals.*

The branch pulmonary arteries vary from confluent and almost normal size to confluent and severely hypoplastic, to nonconfluent, to completely absent. If they are not confluent, a ductus will connect to a normally arborizing (usually left) branch pulmonary artery, and the opposite branch pulmonary artery will be absent, with the lung solely supplied by AP collaterals. To add to the complexity, the degree of hypoplasia of the branch pulmonary arteries (as judged by their luminal diameter) does not necessarily correlate with the degree of arborization. Arborization of the pulmonary arteries, if present and confluent, may be to the majority of the lung segments or to a minority of lung segments. Segments not supplied by the pulmonary arteries are supplied by AP collaterals. There is an inverse relationship between the distribution of the pulmonary arteries and the distribution of the AP collaterals.

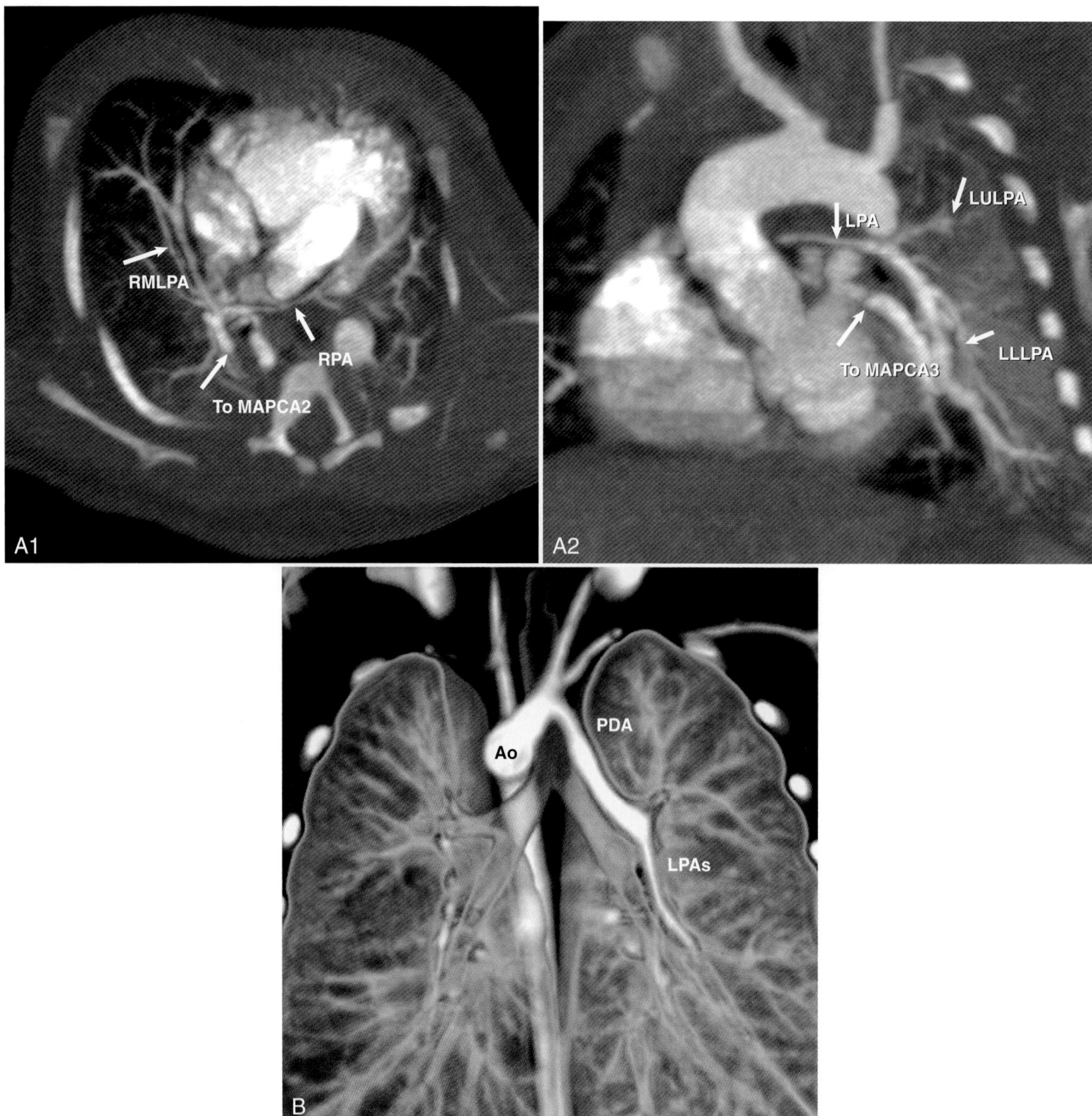

Figure 38-72 Computed tomographic angiography (CTA) of patients with pulmonary atresia with ventricular septal defect and large collateral arteries, illustrating the Stanford University management protocol. **A1** and **A2,** Two CTA images of a 1-week-old girl with very small centrally confluent native pulmonary arteries and large collaterals (MAPCAs). Images show a small right and left native right pulmonary arteries (RPA, LPA) and two major aortopulmonary collateral arteries (MAPCA2, MAPCA3) arising from the mid-thoracic descending aorta. Collaterals are connected peripherally to native pulmonary arteries. RML PA identifies right middle lobe branch of the RPA. LUL PA and LLL PA identify left upper and left lower branches of LPA. An additional very small collateral was present in this patient, but is not visualized in these images. According to the Stanford management protocol, this patient is identified as requiring neonatal surgery because of the normally arborizing and centrally confluent native pulmonary arteries, with all "dual-supply" collaterals. A neonatal preoperative cardiac catheterization with detailed angiography of the collaterals is required. **B,** Coronal cut of a volume-rendered image of airways and aorta in a 1-week old girl with large collaterals to right lung. There is a right-sided aortic arch. Peripheral LPA is connected to aorta through a patent ductus arteriosus originating from left brachiocephalic artery. According to the Stanford management protocol, this patient would require neonatal surgery because of the presence of the unilateral ductus. A preoperative neonatal catheterization would be required to define the details of the right lung collateral distribution. Key: *Ao,* Aortic arch; *LLL,* left lower lobe branch; *LPA,* left pulmonary artery; *LUL,* left upper lobe branch; *MAPCA,* major aortopulmonary collateral artery; *PA,* pulmonary artery; *PDA,* patent ductus arteriosus; *RML,* right middle lobe branch; *RPA,* right pulmonary artery.

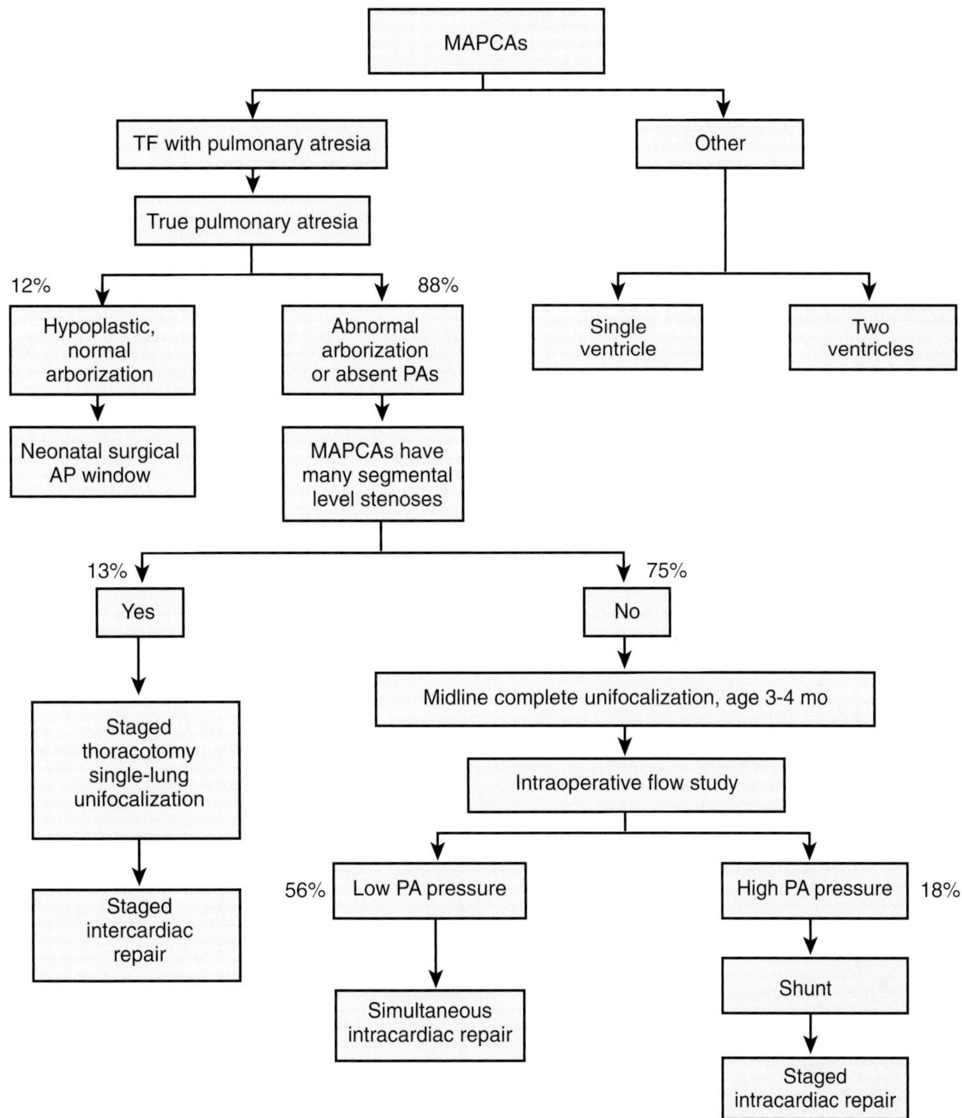

Figure 38-73 Treatment protocol for patients with tetralogy of Fallot and pulmonary atresia with major aortopulmonary collateral arteries. Key: *AP,* Aortopulmonary; *MAPCAs,* major aortopulmonary collateral arteries; *PA,* pulmonary artery; *TF,* tetralogy of Fallot.

There is a discrete separation between the first and second groups because of the normal pulmonary artery distribution, presence of a ductus arteriosus, and complete absence of collaterals in group one.

Natural History of Pathophysiologic Subgroups

Confluent and Normally Distributing Right and Left Pulmonary Arteries and Patent Ductus Arteriosus

About 40% of patients are in this category. This group is relatively homogeneous morphologically and physiologically. The ductus arteriosus appears to have its usual tendency to close, albeit probably more slowly than normal; without treatment, half of this group is probably dead of hypoxia by age 6 months and 90% by age 1 year.

Confluent, Nonconfluent, or Absent Right and Left Pulmonary Arteries with Aortopulmonary Collaterals

About 60% of patients are in this category. This group is extremely heterogeneous morphologically as well as physiologically. Cyanosis is always present, and symptoms may develop, depending on the number, size, and behavior of collateral vessels, but not as quickly nor as severely as in the group described in the preceding paragraph. Symptoms early in life are related either to severe cyanosis or to severe pulmonary overcirculation. Over time, a gradual increase in cyanosis is typical because of collateral stenosis with reduced pulmonary blood flow, Eisenmenger-like physiology in unobstructed collaterals, or both. Without interventional therapy, 10% of this group may die within the first few years of life, half by age 3 to 5 years, and 90% by age 10.

Pulmonary Arterial Disease

Patients with pulmonary atresia and AP collateral arteries probably differ from other patients with TF with respect to pulmonary arterial disease. The phrase *pulmonary arterial disease* rather than "pulmonary vascular disease" is used because of uncertainty regarding how much the increased pulmonary vascular resistance is due to hypoplasia and stenoses of the distal pulmonary arteries themselves and of the distal portions of the AP collateral arteries, versus how much is due to microvascular hypertensive pulmonary vascular disease.[R2] Without question, both mechanisms occur.

Pulmonary arterial disease tends to develop in those pulmonary arterial segments that are centrally connected. It progresses at a considerably accelerated rate, and perhaps even in fetal life or in the first few months after birth, in segments whose only or major source of pulmonary blood flow is large AP collateral arteries.[S12] Patients who survive without correction into the second and third decades of life often develop massive and sometimes fatal hemoptysis related to these large AP collaterals.[K8]

TECHNIQUE OF OPERATION

Repair of Tetralogy of Fallot with Acquired Pulmonary Atresia

Occasionally, and particularly in patients with pulmonary atresia that has developed after a shunting procedure, atresia is at the level of the infundibulum. The operation described for TF with pulmonary stenosis can then be done (see Technique of Operation in Section I), often without a transanular patch. When acquired atresia is at the pulmonary "anulus" and the pulmonary trunk is present (which it usually is), a transanular patch repair can be used, as described next under "Repair of Tetralogy of Fallot with Pulmonary Atresia and Confluent and Normally Distributing Right and Left Pulmonary Arteries and Patent Ductus Arteriosus." In about 90% of patients with TF and *acquired* pulmonary atresia, these straightforward repairs are feasible.

Repair of Tetralogy of Fallot with Pulmonary Atresia and Confluent and Normally Distributing Right and Left Pulmonary Arteries and Patent Ductus Arteriosus

This operation is generally performed in neonates and young infants in whom atresia is usually at the pulmonary "anulus," and the pulmonary trunk and confluence of the RPA and LPA are generally patent and of reasonable size. Occasionally, it is performed in older infants and in children who have been palliated by a shunting operation early in life. Operation proceeds much as described under Technique of Operation in Section I for TF with pulmonary stenosis with respect to CPB management, myocardial protection, and many technical details (see "Decision and Technique for Transanular Patching" and "Repair of Uncomplicated Tetralogy of Fallot with Pulmonary Stenosis via the Right Ventricle" under Technique of Operation for details of most aspects of the procedure except for those described in text that follows). There are, however, several important differences. The ductus arteriosus is always present and large and may be tortuous. It is dissected, and ligatures placed around it, prior to establishing CPB. It is then immediately ligated and divided as CPB is initiated (see "Closure of Associated Patent Ductus Arteriosus" under Technique of Operation in Section I of Chapter 35).

The VSD is always closed through a longitudinal incision in the RV infundibulum, never through the right atrial approach. The incision, RV muscle resection, and VSD closure are performed as described for TF with pulmonary stenosis under Technique of Operation in Section I.

There are several options for managing the RV-to-pulmonary trunk reconstruction. Preferably, a valved conduit is used to connect the RV to the pulmonary trunk. This is performed as described later in "Establishing Right Ventricle–to–Pulmonary Artery Continuity" under Repair of Tetralogy of Fallot with Pulmonary Atresia and Large Aortopulmonary Collaterals. Alternatively, it may be possible in some cases to make a single vertical incision in the RV infundibulum and extend it through the atresia to an appropriate point distally on the pulmonary trunk. This is appropriate when the atretic area is very short. Sufficient tissue must be present posteriorly at the site of the atresia so that growth of the area can proceed satisfactorily. The transanular patch must be appropriately contoured at the atretic area to accomplish satisfactory widening. The patch is roughly diamond shaped, with the widest portion applied to the atretic area. Great care is taken to avoid damage to the left anterior descending coronary artery (LAD) and right coronary artery by the patch suture line. Severe pulmonary regurgitation will be present immediately when this technique is used.

Management of the atrial septum will vary. If a valved conduit is used to reconstruct the RV outflow tract, closure of the atrial septal defect or PFO, if present, is performed. If a transanular patch is used, especially in neonates and young infants, a PFO is left open using the same criteria as given in "Managing the Atrial Septum" under Technique of Operation in Section I.

Repair of Tetralogy of Fallot with Pulmonary Atresia and Confluent, Nonconfluent, or Absent Right and Left Pulmonary Arteries and Aortopulmonary Collaterals

Vascular supply of blood to the lungs in this condition represents, arguably, the most variable and complex "lesion," both morphologically and physiologically, in congenital heart disease. As such, no single operative approach is applicable to all patients. That said, recent techniques have been developed, supported by midterm follow-up data, demonstrating that a majority of patients with TF with pulmonary atresia and large AP collaterals can be managed with one-stage repair in early infancy, involving left and right lung unifocalization, VSD closure, and RV outflow tract reconstruction.[L20,M16,M33,M38,M39,R4,R6,T4]

This approach can be applied to patients having relatively large confluent true pulmonary arteries, minor or moderate arborization abnormalities, severely hypoplastic confluent true pulmonary arteries with major arborization abnormalities and dominant collaterals, or completely absent intrapericardial true pulmonary arteries and collaterals only.

There are specific subpopulations, both morphologic and physiologic, in which the one-stage approach is contraindicated; these are discussed under "Alternatives to One-Stage Unifocalization and Intracardiac Repair" under Special Situations and Controversies later in this section. It should also be emphasized that individual surgeons selectively use one-stage repair based on morphologic details and their own experience.[C7,I8,M38,P11,P21,R7,R26,S3,W6]

One-Stage Unifocalization and Intracardiac Repair

In the text that follows, various components of the operation are described, including preliminary procedures leading up to it. These components include:

- Assessing intrapericardial true pulmonary artery system
- Identifying and assessing collateral system
- Managing sources of pulmonary blood flow on CPB
- Completing unifocalization
- Assessing adequacy of unifocalization
- Performing intracardiac repair
- Establishing RV-to–pulmonary arterial continuity
- Assessing complete repair

This procedure is typically performed in infants at approximately 3 to 4 months of age. Occasionally it is performed in neonates or in younger infants whose condition is unstable because of either profound cyanosis or severe pulmonary overcirculation, or in whom there are nonconfluent central pulmonary arteries and a ductus arteriosus providing blood flow to one of the lungs, with collateral supply to the contralateral lung.[R4]

Exposure is through median sternotomy. The skin incision is extended from the suprasternal notch to well below the xiphoid to provide adequate exposure for the extensive dissection that is necessary. If a thymus gland is present, it is subtotally removed, leaving a small remnant of thymic lobes above the brachiocephalic vein. The pericardium is opened anteriorly with a longitudinal incision; a piece of anterior pericardium may be removed and treated in glutaraldehyde for later use in the operation.

Assessing True Pulmonary Artery System The first task is to assess the intrapericardial true pulmonary artery system. Commonly there are confluent and very hypoplastic central pulmonary arteries with a small pulmonary trunk segment that ends blindly at the level of an atretic pulmonary valve (Fig. 38-74). The pulmonary trunk and branch pulmonary arteries are dissected over their entire course beginning centrally and moving to the periphery, clearly identifying major branches of the RPA and LPA as they enter the lung parenchyma.

Identifying and Assessing Collateral System The next task is to identify and assess the collateral system. This requires a clear mental image of it based on careful study of the preoperative angiograms. The technical maneuvers used in this part of the procedure are variable and depend on the number and positions of the large collateral arteries. This may take several hours to accomplish. Each large collateral artery is identified at its systemic source and dissected over its entire length to the point where it enters the lung parenchyma. The specific approach to each collateral depends on its point of origin. The most common site of origin is the upper descending aorta with the collaterals coursing anteriorly through the posterior mediastinum into the middle mediastinum and then into the lung hilum (see Fig. 38-74). It is best to approach these collaterals through direct mediastinal dissection rather than by entering the pleural space. With the ascending aorta retracted anteriorly and to the left and the superior vena cava retracted to the right (see Fig. 38-74), the posterior pericardial reflection is opened in the midline within the space bordered above by the tracheal bifurcation and below by the dome of the left atrium. If confluent central pulmonary arteries are present, it may be necessary to work around them as the posterior dissection proceeds. Once the posterior pericardium is opened and the soft tissue of the posterior mediastinum is entered, collateral vessels are easily identified. Further posterior dissection exposes the esophagus and descending aorta, allowing access to the origin of collaterals that arise from this aortic position (see Fig. 38-74).

Occasionally, large collateral arteries arise lower on the descending aorta or from the major head and neck vessels. Those arising from head and neck arteries can be accessed directly by dissecting the artery of origin and then exposing the collateral along its length until it enters lung parenchyma. Collaterals originating from the lower thoracic aorta and occasionally intraabdominally are best exposed by opening the appropriate pleural space anterior to the phrenic nerve and gently retracting the lung out of the pleural space to expose the descending aorta and collateral origin. These lower collaterals may enter the hilum of the lung directly or travel in the inferior pulmonary ligament before entering the lung parenchyma. It is not uncommon for collateral vessels to pass through the muscle of the esophagus before entering the lung tissue.

Managing Sources of Pulmonary Blood Flow on Cardiopulmonary Bypass Once the true pulmonary artery system and all collateral vessels have been identified and fully dissected, cannulation sutures are placed in preparation for CPB. Aortic and bicaval cannulation are standard (see Section III of Chapter 2). After full heparinization and aortic and bicaval venous cannulation, CPB is initiated. All collateral vessels (or remaining collaterals, if some are ligated prior to initiation of CPB) are rapidly ligated at their aortic or systemic vessel origin using appropriately sized permanent metal clips. Patients with TF generally have a large intracardiac return during repair because of acquired collateral flow to the pulmonary arteries; those with pulmonary atresia, and especially those with the large AP collateral arteries, may have a particularly large intracardiac return requiring special consideration. Thus, an important goal in patients who will be placed on CPB is to have control of as much pulmonary blood flow as possible. The surgeon should be aware of all sources of pulmonary flow. This is accomplished by detailed review of the preoperative cardiac catheterization and angiographic data. Possible sources include the ductus arteriosus, surgically created systemic–pulmonary arterial shunts, large AP collateral arteries, and acquired AP collaterals. Before commencing CPB, all sources should be surgically identified and dissected to the degree that instantaneous control can be achieved. This is most easily accomplished with the ductus or with surgically created shunts. Although more difficult, it is also necessary to dissect the origin of all large AP collaterals as described in the preceding text. Acquired collaterals, usually smaller in size but more numerous and diffuse, pose the greatest challenge. They usually arise from the internal thoracic artery, intercostal arteries, bronchial arteries, or other unnamed mediastinal vessels. If previous surgery has been performed, acquired collaterals may form at sites of pleural fusion. Some, and sometimes many, acquired collaterals can be coil occluded by an interventional cardiologist at preoperative catheterization. The surgeon should attempt to control remaining acquired collaterals during the operation before placing the patient on CPB (still, it is not unusual for intracardiac return to increase once CPB is established).

CPB is established with the perfusate at about 34°C and with ionized calcium at a normal level so that ventricular fibrillation does not occur before proper preparations are made for managing intracardiac return. After aortic and bicaval cannulation is accomplished, CPB is slowly established with the heart continuing to beat vigorously. A left

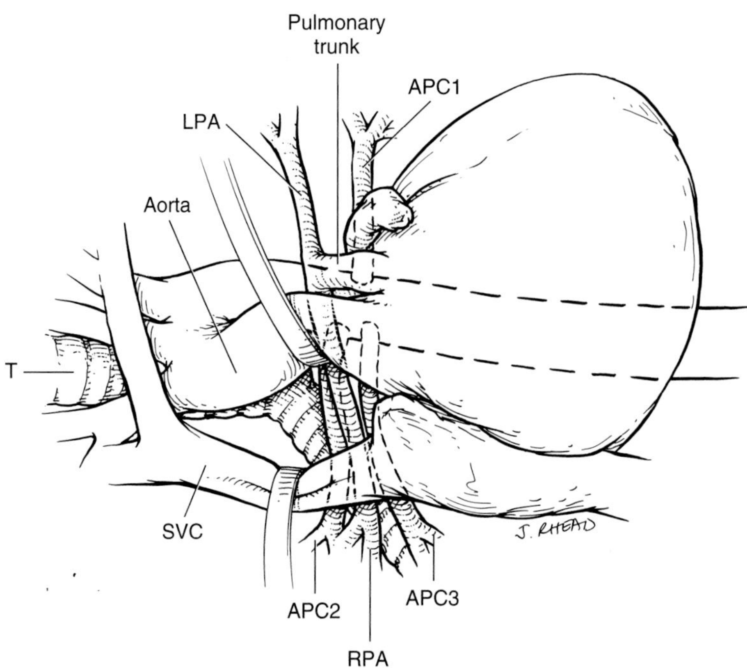

Figure 38-74 Anatomy of tetralogy of Fallot with pulmonary atresia, hypoplastic confluent central pulmonary arteries, and large aortopulmonary collateral arteries. This illustration provides a single example; however, it should be emphasized that extreme variability in number, origin, course, and size of large collateral arteries and true pulmonary arteries is found. Small pulmonary trunk extends to atretic pulmonary valve and is physically connected to the infundibulum. True pulmonary arteries are confluent and severely hypoplastic, and these central pulmonary arteries have limited distribution to the lungs. True left pulmonary artery *(LPA)* bifurcates to upper lobe and lingula only, and true right pulmonary artery *(RPA)* distributes to upper and middle lobes only. Three collateral vessels are present: one distributes to left lower lobe *(APC1)* and two distribute to right lung, one to right upper lobe *(APC2)* and one to right lower lobe *(APC3)*. Note that APC2 communicates with upper branch of true RPA, whereas APC1 and 3 have no proximal communication to true RPA and LPA. Thus, right upper lung field is said to have "dual-supply" blood flow from both collateral system (APC2) and true RPA, while left upper lung field has isolated blood supply from true LPA, and right lower lobe and left lower lobe have isolated blood supply, each from one collateral.

Prior to beginning cardiopulmonary bypass (CPB), true pulmonary arteries and all major collaterals are identified at their origin and dissected throughout their course until the vessels enter lung parenchyma. This often requires extensive dissection. Although collateral arteries may arise from many systemic arterial sites (see text for detailed description), the most common site of origin is the upper descending thoracic aorta, as illustrated. These collaterals are best identified, dissected, and rerouted for unifocalization by working through the central mediastinum as shown. Based on evaluation of preoperative angiograms, it may be beneficial to dissect and identify all major communications between collateral vessels and true pulmonary arteries.

As illustrated, ascending aorta is retracted anteriorly and to the left, either with a rigid retractor or a heavy stay suture placed into the adventitia. Superior vena cava *(SVC)* is mobilized completely, and commonly the azygos vein is ligated and divided. SVC is then retracted laterally to the right. This exposes the central mediastinum in the midline. If true central pulmonary arteries are present, these are fully dissected first so that they can be mobilized, allowing direct dissection into central mediastinum. To accomplish this, the pericardial reflection in the transverse sinus is opened in the midline, and space below tracheal bifurcation and above dome of left atrium is entered. Dissection transitions from central to posterior mediastinum, and upper thoracic descending aorta and esophagus are completely exposed. Collateral arteries are encountered in this dissection, and their origins from the upper thoracic aorta are easily identified. These collaterals are then dissected along their entire course until they enter lung parenchyma. It should be noted that collateral arteries commonly pass superficially through esophageal musculature; this must be recognized during the process of collateral dissection to avoid injuring the esophagus. Collaterals are commonly intertwined with secondary vagal nerve fibers, and it may be necessary to divide these to fully mobilize the collateral arteries. Once true pulmonary arteries and all collateral vessels have been fully identified and mobilized, preparation is made for CPB. Key: *Ao,* Aorta; *APC,* aortopulmonary collateral artery; *PT,* pulmonary trunk; *T,* trachea.

ventricular vent of appropriate size (10F for patients weighing 4.0 kg or less; 13F for patients weighing 4 to 10 kg; adult size for patients weighing more than 10 kg) is placed via a purse-string suture into the right upper pulmonary vein, and the vent tip is passed across the mitral valve into the LV. At this point, full CPB and vigorous venting are established, and immediately, all sources of pulmonary blood flow, previously identified and dissected at their systemic origin, are permanently closed using metal clips. If appropriate pre-CPB dissection has been accomplished, all major sources, including complex situations with up to eight large AP collaterals, can be controlled in 30 to 90 seconds. Commonly, especially in patients with baseline SaO_2 greater than 80%, a substantial portion of the multiple sources can be closed before initiation of CPB, with this process limited only by decrease in SaO_2. It is not unusual, particularly if the patient is in early infancy and has not undergone prior palliation, for these maneuvers to reduce intracardiac return to normal levels.

In older children who have been chronically cyanotic or palliated, acquired collateral vessels from the systemic to the pulmonary circulation have often developed. In these cases, control of the embryologic large AP collaterals may still leave substantial cardiac return through the acquired collaterals. Then, a larger LV vent and higher perfusion flow rates may be needed to account for the abnormally high runoff. Once CPB is established, perfusion temperature is gradually reduced, aiming for a core body temperature of 25°C.

In addition to these precautions against damage from large intracardiac return, cerebral perfusion can be further maintained at an adequate level by blood gas control despite rapid aortic runoff. Arterial P_{CO_2} is maintained at 45 mmHg or greater to maximize cerebral blood flow.

Completing Unifocalization The next task is to complete the unifocalization process. This again depends on number and positions of the collateral arteries and status of the central pulmonary artery system. Depending on number and complexity of collaterals, this aspect of the procedure may take several hours. It is performed without an aortic clamp so that the myocardium is well perfused in an empty beating state. Most collateral arteries can be connected directly to the central pulmonary artery system by working within the central mediastinal space previously dissected. Most commonly, long side-to-side anastomoses between the collaterals and true pulmonary arteries, extending from a midline position all the way to the periphery where the arteries enter the lung parenchyma, are performed using 7-0 absorbable monofilament suture (Fig. 38-75). Occasionally, collateral arteries arising from head and neck vessels or from much lower on the descending thoracic aorta can be connected in end-to-side fashion to the central system. Collateral arteries are usually connected to the superior-posterior, directly posterior, or inferior-posterior circumferential aspect of the central pulmonary artery system, leaving its anterior aspect untouched. Typically, collateral vessels that are candidates for unifocalization will not reach the true pulmonary artery easily if the collateral artery is rerouted over the hilum of the lung, and this technique is avoided.

Once all collateral vessels have been unifocalized, it is often beneficial to incise the remaining anterior aspect of the central true pulmonary arteries from left hilum to right hilum, and then patch them with a segment of cryopreserved allograft pulmonary artery. In this fashion, a completely unifocalized pulmonary artery system with newly reconstructed branch pulmonary arteries that are of normal or even supranormal diameter can be achieved, with no areas of circumferential pulmonary artery patch throughout the system.

With rare exceptions (i.e., small remote collaterals with single lung segment distribution or less), all isolated supply collaterals should be unifocalized because failure to do so will eliminate lung segments from the central pulmonary artery circulation after repair. In many cases, dual-supply collaterals (those that communicate with the true pulmonary arteries) should also be unifocalized. Even though a dual-supply collateral will distribute to the same distal vascular bed as that portion of the true pulmonary artery with which it communicates, the value of unifocalizing such a collateral is that it can be used to augment the diameter of the small true pulmonary artery. If the true pulmonary arteries are of adequate size, a dual-supply collateral need not be unifocalized and can be simply ligated at its origin.

If there is complete absence of true pulmonary arteries within the pericardium, collateral vessels from the right and left lungs can be easily connected to one another across the midline within the dissected central mediastinal space. Most frequently, on each side, all ipsilateral collateral vessels are first connected to one another with long side-to-side anastomoses, with the anastomoses beginning at the transected systemic end of the collaterals and extending to the lung parenchyma. Then the left side is connected to the right, achieving complete unifocalization and left-right confluence. Occasionally the older child or young adult will present as a good candidate for unifocalization. In this case more liberal use of circumferential synthetic material (no growth potential) is acceptable (Fig. 38-76). This should be avoided if possible in the growing infant and child.

Assessing Adequacy of Unifocalization Once unifocalization is complete, an assessment must be made regarding whether the pulmonary artery system will have adequately low resistance to allow intracardiac repair with subsequent low RV and pulmonary artery pressure. Following intracardiac repair, peak RV pressure should be less than 60% of peak systemic arterial pressure. Experienced surgeons can often predict this by size of the true pulmonary arteries and collateral arteries and adequacy of the unifocalization. In such cases, proceeding directly to intracardiac repair is indicated. In other circumstances, typically those in which neither the true pulmonary artery system nor the collateral system is sufficiently large to ensure low pulmonary arterial resistance, or in which unifocalization was difficult and a question remains regarding adequacy of anastomoses or positioning of the unifocalized vessels, it is most prudent to assess pulmonary arterial resistance objectively before deciding whether to move ahead with intracardiac repair.

Objective assessment can be made using an intraoperative blood flow study.[R7] The perfusionist primes a separate circuit, which draws blood from the venous reservoir and perfuses a cannula that is placed into the central portion of the newly unifocalized pulmonary artery system. Based on body surface area, controlled perfusion into the pulmonary artery circuit is then performed in incremental steps beginning at 20% of baseline indexed cardiac output and increasing in increments of 20% up to 100% indexed cardiac output. At each increment, after a steady state is achieved, pressure is measured using a small catheter placed into the pulmonary artery system and connected to a pressure transducer. During the assessment, careful attention is paid to the left atrial appendage. If the heart is not beating vigorously because of hypothermia or hypocalcemia, or if it is arrested with cardioplegia or is fibrillating, the left atrium and LV can be quickly overdistended by pulmonary venous return. To counter this, the LV vent is placed on vigorous suction and the vent pop-off valve is completely occluded. Even then, careful attention should be paid to the left atrial appendage to be sure that the vent system is not overwhelmed by pulmonary blood flow at higher incremental flows.

If mean P_{PA} remains less than 25 mmHg at full indexed cardiac output in a 3- to 4-month-old infant, intracardiac repair can proceed. These values have been shown to predict accurately that $P_{RV/LV}$ will be less than 0.5 following intracardiac repair in both controlled laboratory studies and in the clinical situation.[R7] In older children, a mean P_{PA} of 25 to 30 mmHg at full indexed cardiac output usually indicates ability to move ahead with intracardiac repair. If pressures increase to more than these threshold values at any incremental step in the pulmonary blood flow study, then the test is terminated and intracardiac repair is not performed. In this case, a central aorta to pulmonary artery shunt is performed from the left side of the ascending aorta to the central portion of the unifocalized pulmonary artery system using standard

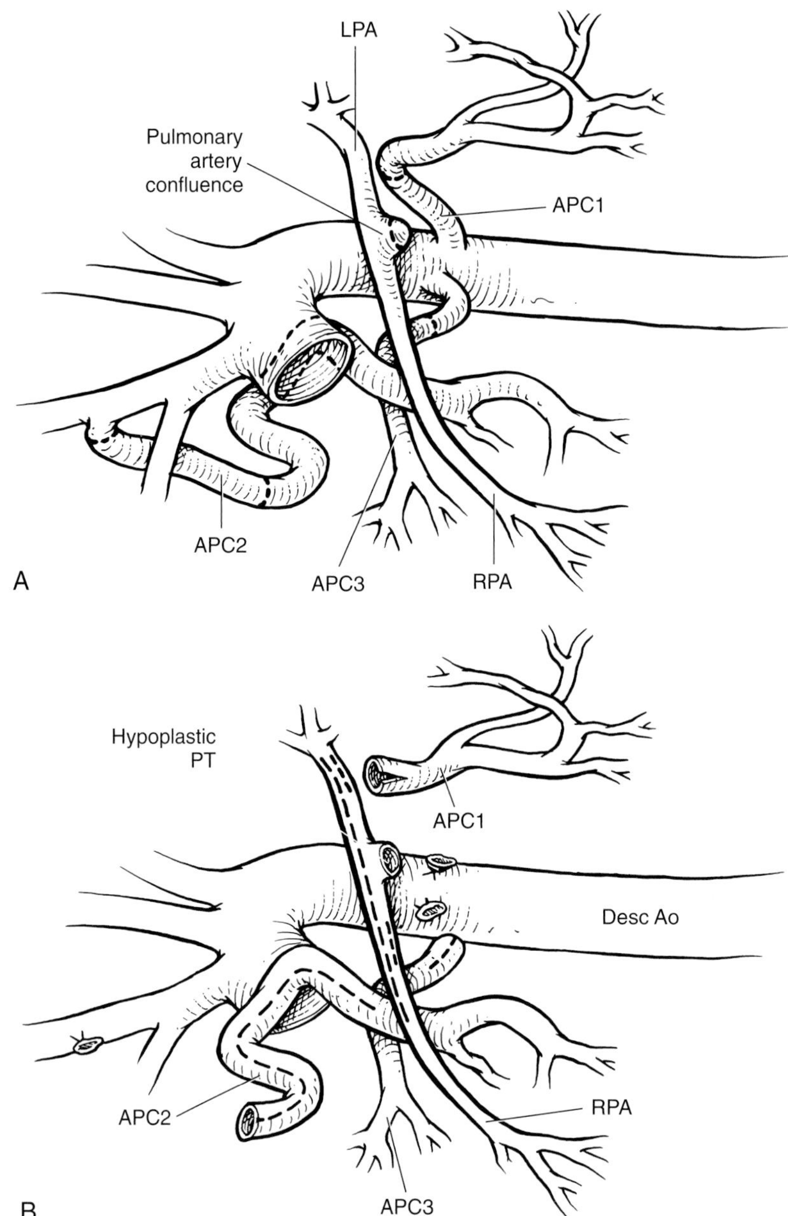

Figure 38-75 One-stage complete unifocalization and intracardiac repair via median sternotomy for tetralogy of Fallot with pulmonary atresia and large aortopulmonary collateral arteries. Median sternotomy preliminary dissection of true pulmonary arteries and collaterals, and cardiopulmonary bypass (CPB) details are described in the text, in Section III of Chapter 2, and in Fig. 38-74. Once CPB is established, previously dissected collateral vessels are immediately ligated at their systemic origin. This preserves entire length of each collateral so that this tissue can be used in the reconstruction that results in complete unifocalization. For clarity, heart, ascending aorta, and trachea have been eliminated in this figure. **A,** Hypoplastic centrally confluent true pulmonary arteries are present. Hypoplastic left pulmonary artery distributes to left upper lobe and hypoplastic right pulmonary artery *(RPA)* distributes to lateral aspect of right lower lobe. Three large collateral arteries are present. One arises from right carotid artery and takes a tortuous course *(dashed lines)* to provide blood flow to medial aspect of right lower lobe *(APC2)*. Two other collaterals arise from typical upper descending thoracic aortic position. One courses to right upper and middle lobes *(APC3)* and the second to left lower lobe *(APC1)*. The surgeon should be acutely aware, based on careful preoperative evaluation of the angiograms, of all stenotic areas within each collateral artery. Stenotic areas must be eliminated *(dashed lines on APC2)* if they are proximal within the collateral, or addressed surgically with either patching or some other form of augmentation if they are more distal. **B,** All three collateral arteries have been ligated and divided at their systemic origins. Hypoplastic pulmonary trunk has been transected just distal to atretic pulmonary valve. Unifocalization sites *(dashed lines)* have been chosen on the true pulmonary arteries in accordance with positions and lengths of collateral arteries to be unifocalized. In this case the two *short* dashed lines on the true pulmonary artery represent sites of implantation of the left and right mid-thoracic collateral vessels (APC1 and APC3). These incisions on the true pulmonary arteries are placed directly posterior. APC1 has been incised over part of its length to allow a side-to-side anastomosis within left hilum. Dashed line on APC3 identifies intended incision that will allow a side-to-side anastomosis with the true RPA. Tortuous APC2 has been mobilized, and the dashed line along its length indicates proposed incision that will allow performing an extensive side-to-side anastomosis onto the true pulmonary arteries beginning in the left hilum and extending all the way to the right hilum. The long incision on the true pulmonary artery, represented by the dashed line, is positioned on the superior-posterior aspect of the true pulmonary arteries.

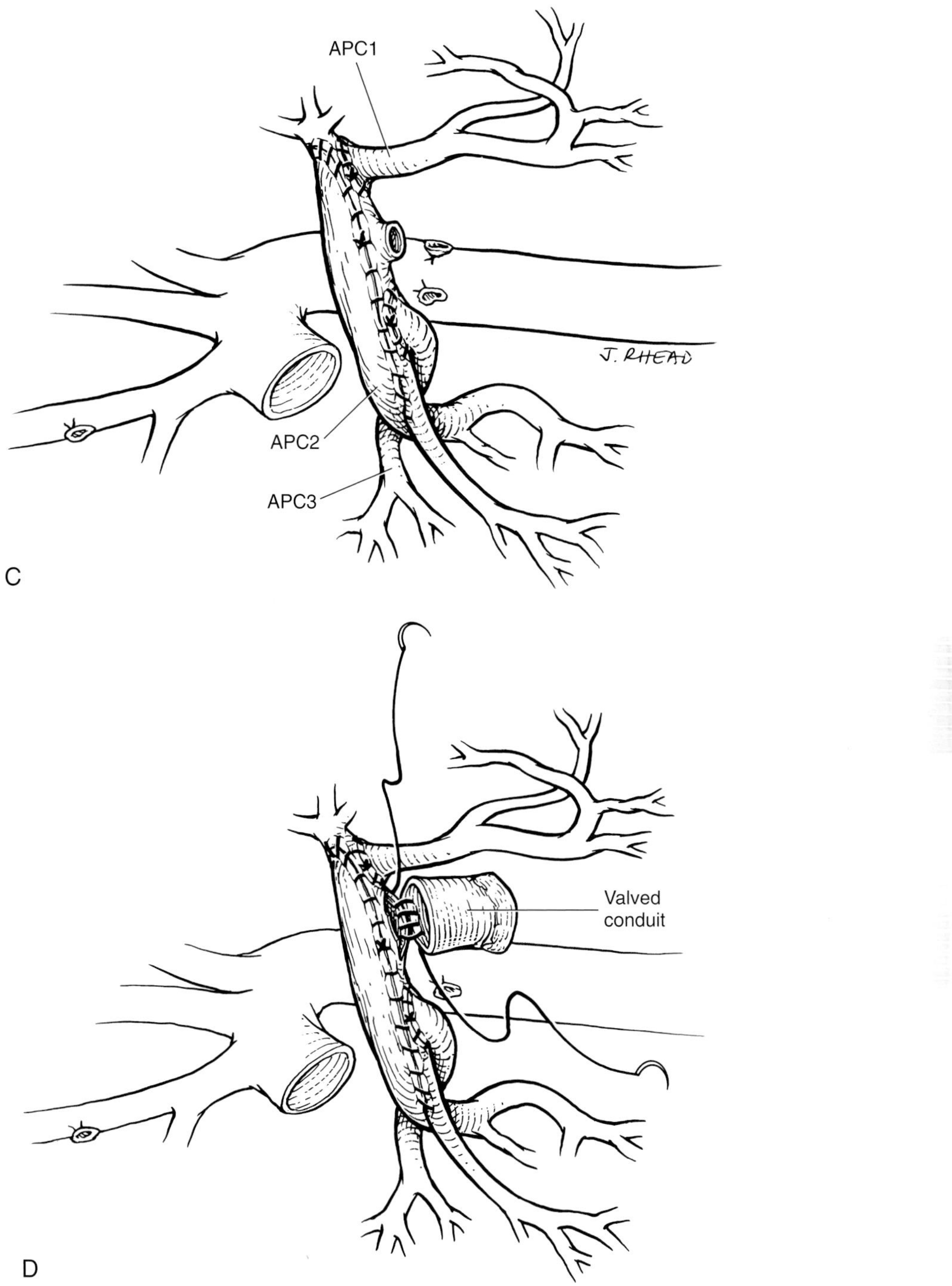

Figure 38-75, cont'd **C,** The three collateral vessels have been connected to the true pulmonary artery system as shown using running 7-0 absorbable monofilament sutures. Exquisite attention to detail and a three-dimensional vision of the result are required to avoid kinking, overstretching, and twisting of the delicate vessels. In this particular case, large tortuous collateral APC2 provides a large degree of "raw material" to augment the central pulmonary artery system adequately. In the absence of such abundant raw material, a less extensive anastomosis of the collateral to the true pulmonary artery would be performed, similar to the other two collateral anastomoses in this example, and the central pulmonary artery system would be augmented centrally from hilum to hilum with a patch of pulmonary arterial allograft tissue. At this point in the operation the decision is made whether to perform an intraoperative pulmonary blood flow study as an aid in designing the remainder of the operation. **D,** In this case operation is completed by ventricular septal defect (VSD) closure and right ventricular outflow tract conduit (see text for other options). The small opening at transected pulmonary trunk is enlarged to the left and right sides in order to perform distal anastomosis of valved allograft conduit into newly reconstructed central pulmonary artery system. This aspect of the procedure and remaining VSD closure and proximal conduit to right ventricular anastomosis is performed in standard fashion for tetralogy with pulmonary atresia without large aortopulmonary collateral arteries. Key: *APC,* Aortopulmonary collateral artery; *Desc Ao,* descending thoracic aorta; *PT,* pulmonary trunk.

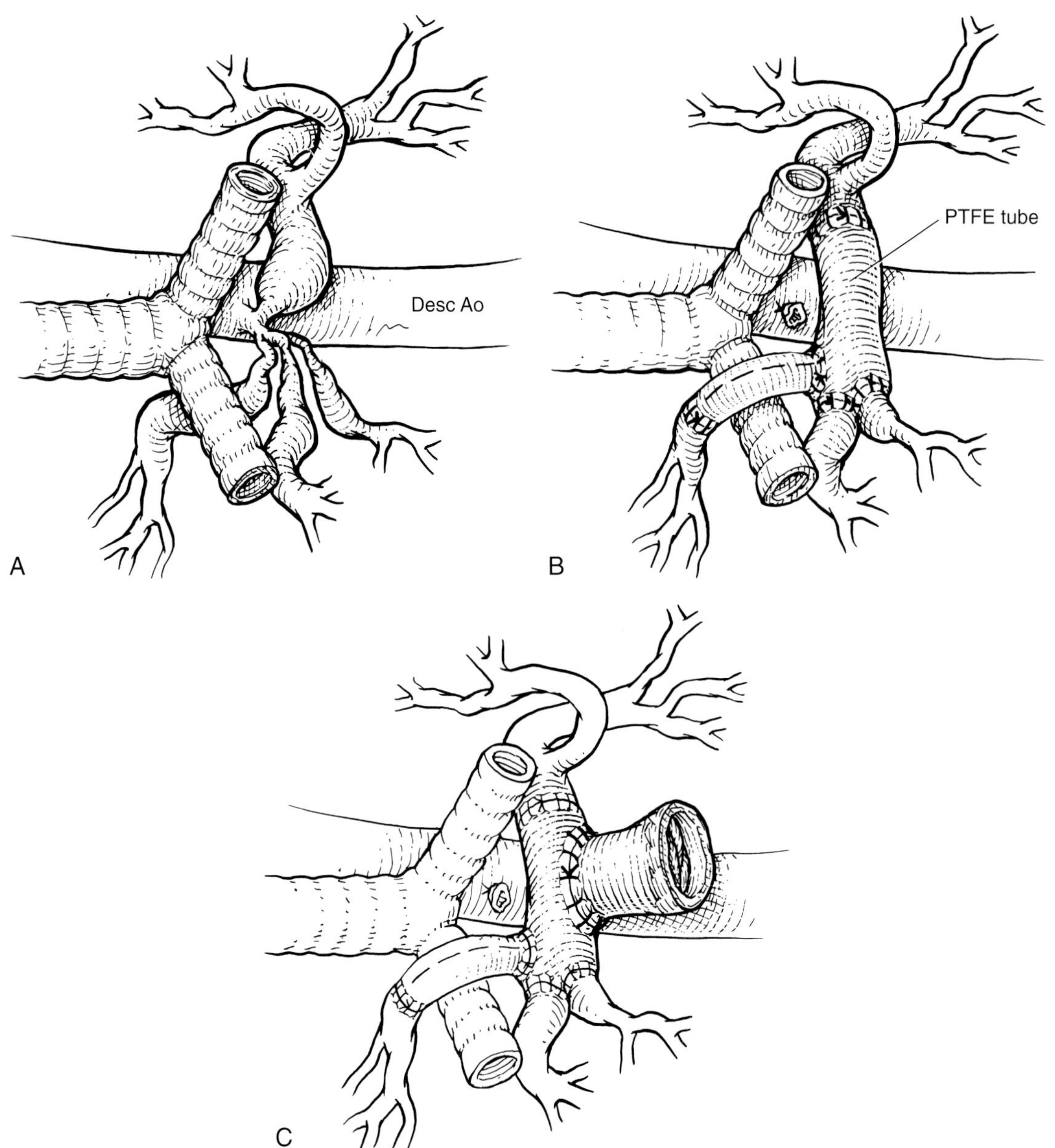

Figure 38-76 Alternative unifocalization repair of tetralogy of Fallot (TF) with pulmonary atresia and large aortopulmonary collateral arteries with absent true pulmonary arteries. In most cases when true pulmonary arteries are completely absent, central confluence between left- and right-sided collaterals is provided by creating direct continuity between collateral arteries from each side, working within the dissected space in central mediastinum, as described in Fig. 38-75. This is especially important in infants and young children, who require growth potential of living tissue. Occasionally a patient will present at an older age with stenotic but open collaterals with well-developed distal vasculature, as shown in this case. Under these conditions, native tissue-to-tissue anastomoses are not critical because growth potential is not required. For clarity, the heart and ascending aorta are eliminated from this figure. **A,** Four collateral vessels are shown arising from the upper mid-thoracic aorta. They have been exposed according to the dissection process described in the text and in Fig. 38-75. There is one large collateral vessel supplying the entire left lung; it is stenotic at its origin. Three separate collateral vessels, all stenotic at their origins and in their proximal segments, supply the right lung—one each to the right upper, right middle, and right lower lobes. **B,** All collaterals have been ligated and divided at their aortic origins. A polytetrafluoroethylene *(PTFE)* conduit of appropriate diameter is used to connect left and right sides. The large left-sided collateral is connected end to end to the PTFE tube graft, and the three right-sided collaterals are unifocalized either directly or with a separate smaller PTFE tube, after resecting proximal stenotic segments. **C,** Conduit placement and ventricular septal defect closure are performed as for typical TF with pulmonary atresia without large aortopulmonary collateral arteries. Key: *Desc Ao,* Descending thoracic aorta.

techniques for creating systemic–pulmonary arterial shunts (see "Techniques of Shunting Operations" in Section I). Size of the shunt is based on body size and on total pulmonary arterial resistance as assessed from the pulmonary blood flow study just completed. If resistance is particularly high, then a slightly larger shunt may be needed.

Intracardiac Repair If pulmonary arterial resistance is acceptable, intracardiac repair commences. The aorta is clamped and cardioplegic solution introduced into the aortic root in the usual manner (see "Cold Cardioplegia, Controlled Aortic Root Reperfusion, and [When Needed] Warm Cardioplegic Induction" in Chapter 3). After adequate cardiac arrest is achieved, superior and inferior caval tapes are tightened around the venous cannulae to isolate systemic venous return. A longitudinal incision is made in the infundibulum of the RV and the ventricular cavity is entered. Hypertrophied muscle is removed from the septal and parietal bands and infundibular free wall. This adequately exposes the VSD, which is then closed with either a glutaraldehyde-treated autologous pericardial patch or a woven polyester patch. Depending on the surgeon's preference, either a running nonabsorbable monofilament suture or interrupted pledgeted mattress sutures are used for attaching the patch to the borders of the VSD. All the same considerations are addressed in this situation as in VSD closure in more typical TF (see Technique of Operation in Section I).

A small right atriotomy is made and status of the atrial septum examined. If a competent but patent foramen ovale is present, it is usually left as is. A secundum atrial septal defect is typically closed either primarily or, if needed, with a pericardial or polyester patch attached with running nonabsorbable monofilament suture. If the atrial septum is intact, it is left in this state. If appropriate decisions have been made with respect to Rp, presence of a competent RV to pulmonary artery valved conduit usually allows for adequate RV function early postoperatively, minimizing the potential benefits of an open atrial septum (as described in the text that follows). The right atrial incision is then closed in standard fashion and the aortic clamp removed, allowing reperfusion of the myocardium.

At this point, RV-to–pulmonary artery reconstruction is undertaken. With adequate unifocalization and central pulmonary artery augmentation as described earlier, the conduit procedure is the same as used in the more straightforward case with duct-dependent TF, pulmonary atresia, and normally arborizing confluent central pulmonary arteries.

Establishing Right Ventricle-to–Pulmonary Artery Continuity Valved polyester conduits were used in the early era of this type of surgery; today, allograft conduits, either aortic valve with ascending aorta, or pulmonary valve with pulmonary trunk, with or without the bifurcation, are preferred. The allograft pulmonary valved conduit with its bifurcation is often the optimal replacement device.[B36,C21] When a bifurcated graft is not required, there is no secure evidence that the pulmonary or aortic valve allograft has an advantage over the other; however, the thinner wall of the pulmonary allograft may have more tendency to become aneurysmal if pulmonary artery pressure becomes importantly elevated.

During the early stages of the procedure, the allograft valved conduit is selected, thawed, and rinsed. In neonates and infants, depending on their size, a 10- to 18-mm-diameter valve can be used; in children older than age 5, a 22- to 25-mm-diameter valve can be used. These sizes should not be flow limiting.

Two somewhat different techniques of allograft insertion are used. In one (preferable), the proximal end of the allograft is sunk into the RV outflow tract and a piece of pericardium, allograft arterial wall, or polyester is used as a roof over the ventriculotomy (Fig. 38-77). The distal end of the allograft is attached to the newly reconstructed transverse central pulmonary artery system before making the proximal anastomosis of the allograft conduit directly onto the right ventriculotomy site. This method has the advantages of minimal use of foreign material on which a thick neointima may develop, and freedom from sternal compression. However, care must be taken that the allograft valve anulus retains its proper circular geometry and that the opening from RV into allograft is large.

In the second method, a woven polyester tube 2 to 5 mm larger than the diameter of the allograft valve anulus is sutured to the proximal end of the allograft. Before insertion, the proximal polyester end is cut in a severely beveled fashion so that it serves primarily as a roof on the ventriculotomy incision, with only a few millimeters of fully circular polyester conduit just proximal to the allograft. With care, the conduit can be kept completely away from the sternum. This technique has the advantage that the perfectly circular geometry of the allograft valve is well maintained and that with it all types of RV and pulmonary trunk morphology can be managed. It has the disadvantage of a very short 2- to 3-mm cylinder of polyester in the proximal end of the conduit.

There are situations in which one or the other method is mandated, depending on RV morphology and availability of the pulmonary trunk, but more often selection is one of preference.

Using either technique, the proximal end of the allograft is cut transversely about 5 mm below the nadir of the valve cusps, leaving the muscular remnant at least 4 mm thick (thicker than when the valve is used for aortic valve replacement). The conduit is not trimmed distally until the nature of the pulmonary artery confluence is established following completed unifocalization and central pulmonary artery augmentation and the distance between this and the right ventriculotomy is measured.

With the first method (see Fig. 38-77, *A*), a limited longitudinal incision is made in the superior RV wall where the pulmonary trunk would normally arise. Care is taken in extending the incision distally so that the anterior margin of the VSD and right coronary cusp of the aortic valve are not damaged. The RV opening is also enlarged proximally, and any thick trabeculations from the free wall, particularly inferiorly, are excised. The VSD is repaired in a fashion similar to that described for TF with pulmonary stenosis (see Fig. 38-27). The distal end of the allograft conduit is cut so that it is the correct shape and the conduit is the correct length. It must not be too long, or it may kink and possibly compress either branch of the pulmonary artery. The reconstructed or augmented pulmonary artery confluence is opened with an incision extending out along the RPA and LPA. The opening is made long enough to match exactly the diameter of the allograft. The distal anastomosis is made with continuous 5-0 or 6-0 polypropylene suture (Fig. 38-77, *B*). The proximal conduit anastomosis is made by commencing the suturing posteriorly where the allograft is apposed to the superior margin of the ventriculotomy and any remnant of infundibular septum. A 4-0 polypropylene suture is used, and often both the RV wall and superior edge of the VSD patch are picked up in the suture line to make it particularly secure posteriorly. The suture line is continued from the midline along both sides around about half the circumference of the conduit, and the sutures are held. A patch of pericardium, polyester, or allograft arterial wall is cut to an approximate semilunar shape and sutured into place to complete the anterior half of the anastomosis (Fig. 38-77, *C*). Its straight superior edge is anastomosed to the muscular portion of the graft as the first step, and its curved inferior edge is attached to the edges of the right ventriculotomy. Good bites of muscle are taken all around and care is used to avoid

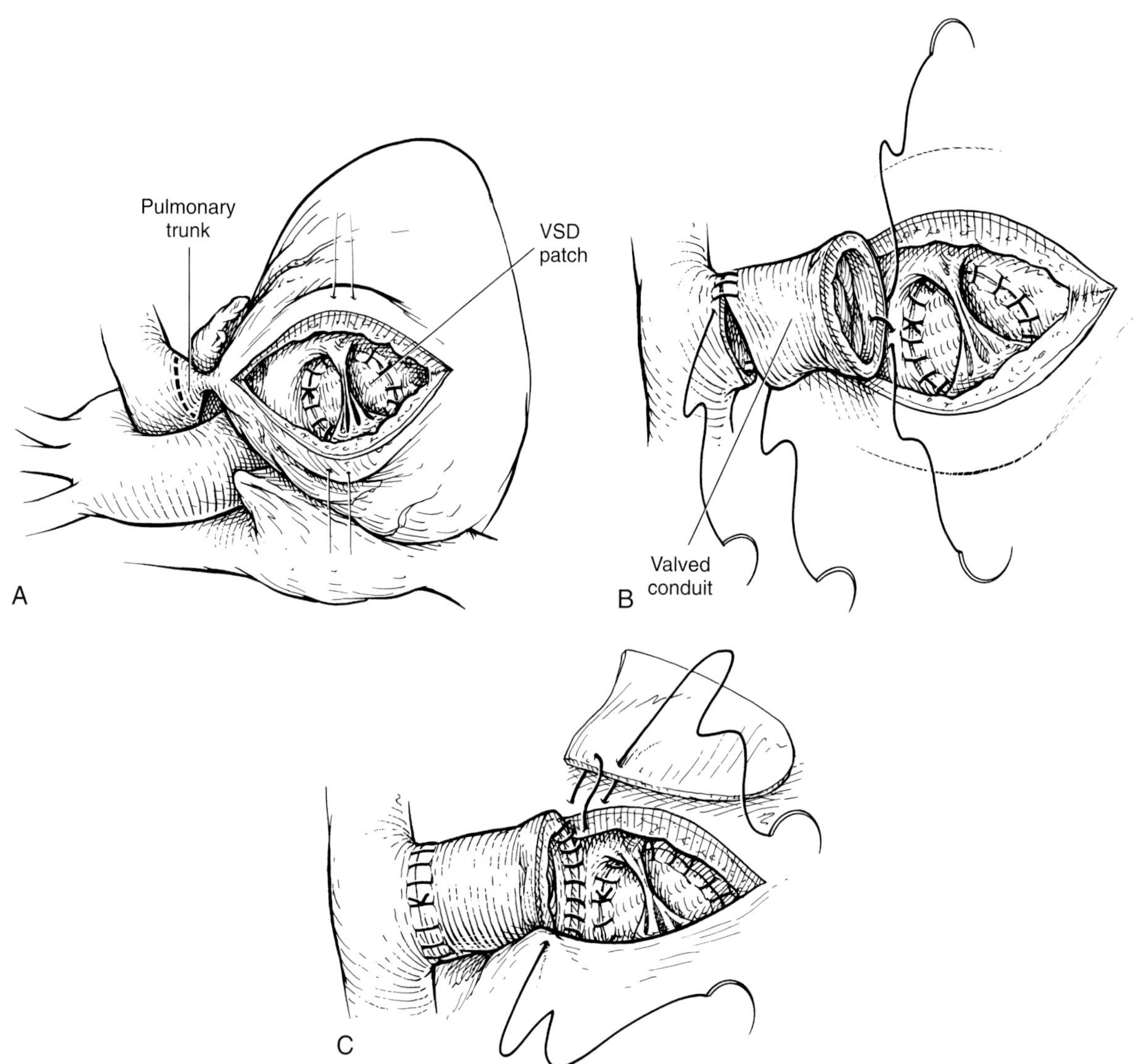

Figure 38-77 Right ventricular outflow tract conduit placement for tetralogy of Fallot (TF) with pulmonary atresia. Much of the surgical technique for repair of TF with pulmonary atresia is similar to that for TF with pulmonary stenosis (e.g., cardiopulmonary bypass [CPB], myocardial management, and intracardiac management of ventricular septal defect *[VSD]* and atrial septum). Management of these two malformations, however, deviates at several important points. Specific management of the pulmonary arteries depends on the form of pulmonary atresia. For duct-dependent atresia, ligation and division of ductus arteriosus is performed at commencement of CPB. For more complex forms of TF with pulmonary atresia and large aortopulmonary (AP) collateral arteries, complex reconstruction of the pulmonary vasculature is often required (see Figs. 38-74 to 38-76). Although in TF with pulmonary stenosis the VSD closure may be managed through a right atrial incision working through the tricuspid valve orifice, in TF with pulmonary atresia the VSD is always closed through an infundibular incision in the right ventricle (RV).

In the various parts of this figure (and in Fig. 38-78), pulmonary artery anatomy is that of normally arborizing, normal diameter, confluent branch pulmonary arteries with patent ductus arteriosus. However, RV outflow tract conduit placement is the same for more complex TF with pulmonary atresia in which the pulmonary artery system has been reconstructed through unifocalization. **A,** Ductus arteriosus has been ligated, taking care to avoid narrowing the left branch pulmonary artery. Dashed line on the distal pulmonary trunk shows site of transection in preparation for distal anastomosis of valved conduit to it. Opening in pulmonary trunk may need to be extended with incisions along left and right pulmonary arteries to accommodate circumference of the conduit. A longitudinal infundibular incision has been made and VSD closed with a patch and running suture technique. Note in this case that VSD has an inlet component. Hypertrophic muscle of the RV infundibulum and VSD closure are handled in a manner similar to that in TF with pulmonary stenosis. **B,** Ductus arteriosus has been divided. A pulmonary allograft valved conduit is shown with the distal anastomosis performed end to end, allograft to pulmonary trunk. A running suture technique using fine monofilament suture is used. Proximal aspect of conduit is then attached to RV. Conduit is placed into ventriculotomy with the suture line attaching its proximal end to the infundibular septum within the ventricular incision. Although not shown in this figure, commonly the proximal suture line incorporates the upper aspect of VSD patch, which is also attached to the anteriorly displaced edge of the infundibular septum. **C,** Posterior suture line of proximal conduit anastomosis is completed as it transitions onto free edge of infundibular incision. Proximal component of the reconstruction is completed using a roughly hemi-oval patch made of polyester, polytetrafluoroethylene, or glutaraldehyde-treated autologous pericardium. Straight edge of patch is sewn around remaining anterior aspect of proximal conduit, and curved edge is sewn around ventriculotomy site to complete the reconstruction. All sutures lines are running nonabsorbable monofilament suture.

damaging the valve cusps of the graft or the LAD. The conduit arises from the RV in nearly the same position as a normal pulmonary artery and passes superiorly and posteriorly directly to the pulmonary artery bifurcation. It is in little danger of being compressed by the sternum.

In the second method, a longitudinal incision is made in the downstream portion of the RV (Fig. 38-78, *A*). If a rudimentary infundibular septum and parietal extension are present, these are dissected away from the RV free wall. The VSD is repaired as described in "Ventricular Septal Defect Closure" under Technique of Operation for TF with pulmonary stenosis in Section I, and preparations are made for inserting the conduit. The conduit, once in position, should be directed toward the patient's left shoulder as it comes off the right ventriculotomy (it need not be oriented parallel to the ventriculotomy) and then curve gently back to the right to approach the pulmonary trunk with just a little redundancy and in an undistorted fashion. This is accomplished by cutting the distal end of the allograft exactly transversely (not obliquely). The proximal end of the conduit is cut obliquely so that the tubular part of the proximal polyester extension is only a few millimeters long and the rest is merely a hood (Fig. 38-78, *B*). The distal and proximal anastomoses are made using a running polypropylene suture (Fig. 38-78, *C*).

Completing the Procedure After reconstruction is completed, rewarming and separation from CPB is the same as for TF with pulmonary stenosis, as described in Section I (see also "Completing Cardiopulmonary Bypass" in Section III of Chapter 2).

Assessing Complete Repair Immediately after discontinuing CPB, postrepair (OR) $P_{RV/LV}$ is measured (see "Measuring Postrepair [OR] $P_{RV/LV}$" under Technique of Operation in Section I). A polyvinyl catheter is introduced into the right atrium and advanced into the RV. The level of postrepair (OR or ICU) $P_{RV/LV}$ that is acceptable in this situation is arguable. Thus, repair is left if the $P_{RV/LV}$ is less than about 0.7 and the patient is clinically stable. Although the probability of early death is low for a $P_{RV/LV}$ up to 0.9 (Fig. 38-79), important RV dysfunction occurs at midterm follow-up at these higher RV pressures. If the $P_{RV/LV}$ is greater than 0.7, or if cardiac output is compromised at levels between 0.5 and 0.7, the VSD patch is taken down and the conduit removed, and a central aortic-to–pulmonary artery shunt is placed. This situation, however, should be encountered rarely if the intraoperative blood flow study is used appropriately.

SPECIAL FEATURES OF POSTOPERATIVE CARE

Postoperative care is similar to that described for TF with pulmonary stenosis (see Section I). When the patient has come from the operating room with a complete repair, including closure of the VSD, and postrepair (ICU) $P_{RV/LV}$ (or some surrogate for it) is consistently less than about 0.7 and the patient is hemodynamically stable, further intervention is seldom needed. However, if the ratio approaches that level, there is a considerable probability of death (see Fig. 38-79), and either the cause of the residual obstruction must be removed or ameliorated or the VSD patch perforated. If the patient's original morphology was pulmonary atresia with confluent pulmonary arteries and a ductus arteriosus, the $P_{RV/LV}$ will rarely reach this value unless the RV-to–pulmonary trunk reconstruction (usually conduit) is technically inadequate, resulting in obstruction. Immediate revision of the conduit is indicated.

If the patient's original morphology involved AP collaterals that were unifocalized, the situation is more complex. Use of the intraoperative flow study will minimize the number of cases that result in an elevated $P_{RV/LV}$. However, should the situation arise, and the elevated pressure is proven not to be due to obstruction in the conduit but rather to elevated resistance in the pulmonary vascular bed, surgical revision is indicated. Cardiac catheterization should be performed to identify the precise cause of the elevated pressure. If surgically revisable obstruction is found in the reconstructed pulmonary arteries, revision aimed at relieving the obstruction is indicated. If there is no surgically correctable obstruction, the cause of the elevated pressure is elevated resistance in the pulmonary microvascular bed. In this case, if the $P_{RV/LV}$ is above 1.0, VSD perforation is performed; if the $P_{RV/LV}$ is between 0.7 and 1.0, VSD patch removal, conduit takedown, and placement of a systemic-to–pulmonary artery shunt is performed.

Occasionally, pulmonary hypertension is caused by reactivity in the microvascular bed rather than by proximal or fixed distal obstruction. This is more likely if the PPA and PRV had been low earlier postoperatively. Increased ventilatory support, sedation, and a trial of inhaled nitric oxide are typical maneuvers that are both diagnostic and therapeutic.

Postoperative airway difficulties are more common in TF with pulmonary atresia than in TF with pulmonary stenosis, especially if complex unifocalization was performed. *Large airway problems* caused by external compression by the aorta, unifocalized collaterals, or conduits can occur.[M17] Unmasking of subclinical, or exacerbation of clinically important, preoperative tracheobronchial malacia can also occur. Phrenic nerve injury is an important concern when extensive dissection has been performed. *Small airway reactivity* also appears to be more common than in TF with pulmonary stenosis, possibly related to an intrinsic predisposition,[M29] but also almost certainly related to direct trauma, autonomic nerve disruption, or airway blood supply disruption.[R4,S5] Careful and aggressive pulmonary toilet is an important component of treatment, both intraoperatively after CPB and in the ICU. Tracheobronchial suctioning and lavage, and even bronchoscopy, may be needed to keep airways free of both clear and bloody secretions.

A problem particular to certain unifocalization cases is lung reperfusion injury. This is most likely to occur in cases that preoperatively have severely underperfused segments of lung. The acute increase in flow and pressure into these vascular beds can result in important lung parenchymal edema, increased airway secretions, and pleural effusion. The process typically reaches a peak in severity 24 to 48 hours after surgery and resolves gradually over the following 3 to 5 days. The diagnosis is made by chest radiogram findings of pulmonary edema and consolidation, with evidence of intrapulmonary shunting (hypoxemia) in the appropriate clinical setting and with no evidence of infection. The treatment is largely expectant, with mechanical ventilator support until there is clinical evidence that the process has peaked and is resolving.

If the PLA is considerably higher than the PRA (see "Risk Factors for Low Cardiac Output" in Section I of Chapter 5), a left-to-right shunt may be present at some level. Unless

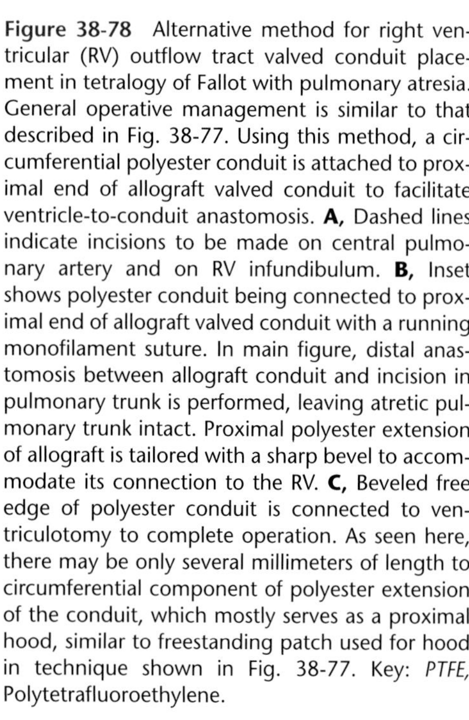

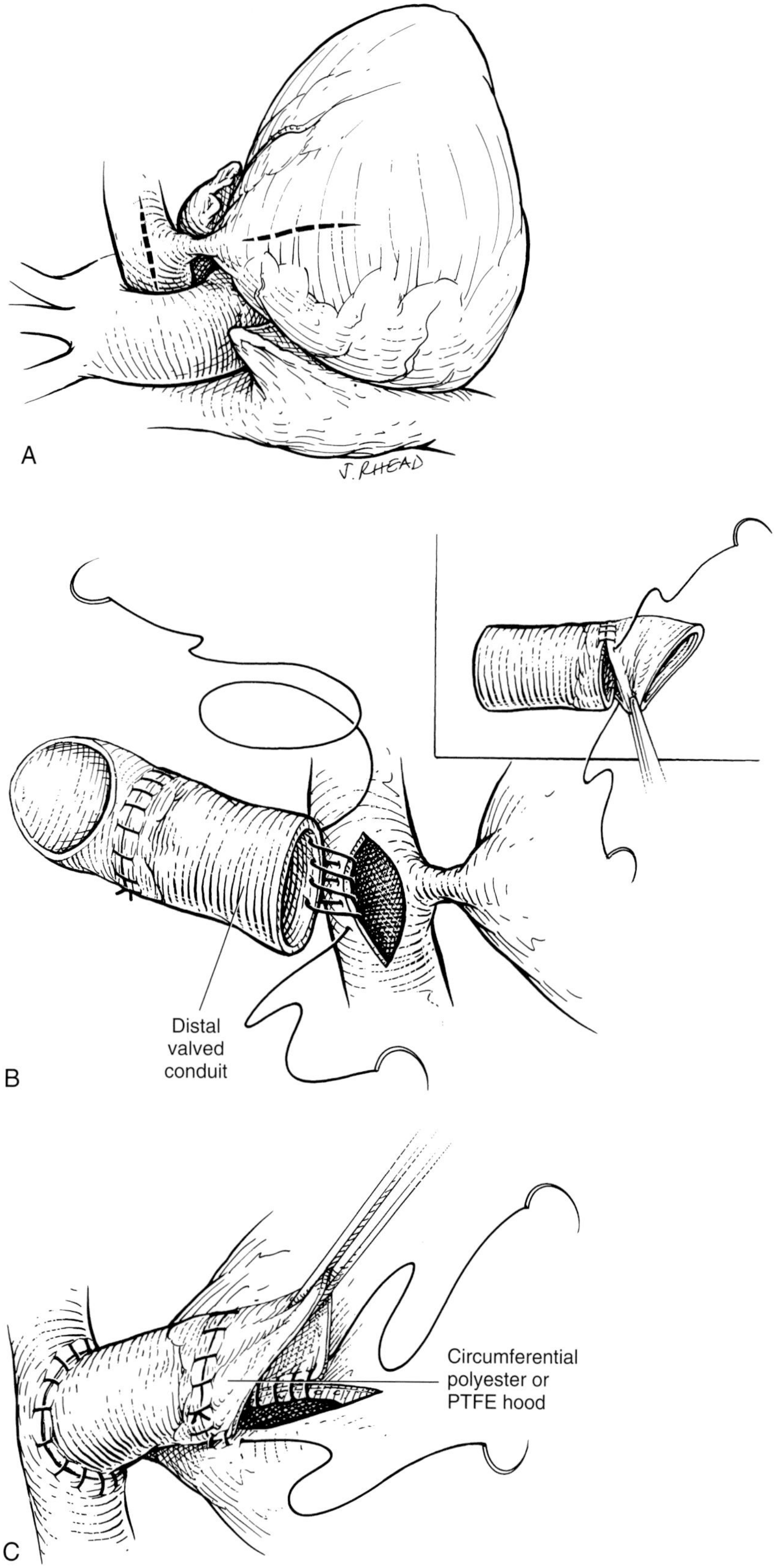

Figure 38-78 Alternative method for right ventricular (RV) outflow tract valved conduit placement in tetralogy of Fallot with pulmonary atresia. General operative management is similar to that described in Fig. 38-77. Using this method, a circumferential polyester conduit is attached to proximal end of allograft valved conduit to facilitate ventricle-to-conduit anastomosis. **A,** Dashed lines indicate incisions to be made on central pulmonary artery and on RV infundibulum. **B,** Inset shows polyester conduit being connected to proximal end of allograft valved conduit with a running monofilament suture. In main figure, distal anastomosis between allograft conduit and incision in pulmonary trunk is performed, leaving atretic pulmonary trunk intact. Proximal polyester extension of allograft is tailored with a sharp bevel to accommodate its connection to the RV. **C,** Beveled free edge of polyester conduit is connected to ventriculotomy to complete operation. As seen here, there may be only several millimeters of length to circumferential component of polyester extension of the conduit, which mostly serves as a proximal hood, similar to freestanding patch used for hood in technique shown in Fig. 38-77. Key: *PTFE,* Polytetrafluoroethylene.

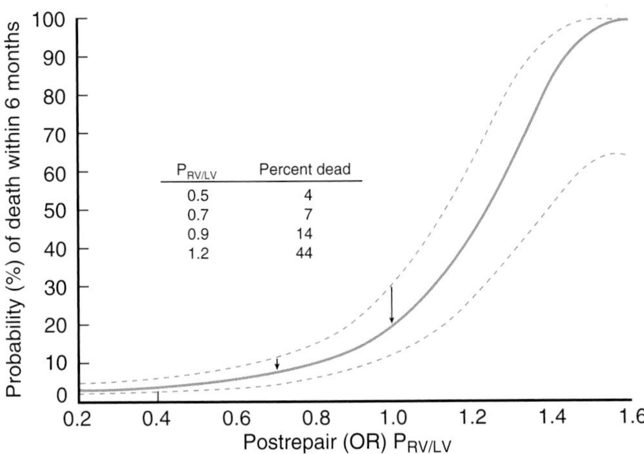

Figure 38-79 Nomogram illustrating relation between postrepair (OR) $P_{RV/LV}$ and death within 6 months of repair of tetralogy of Fallot with pulmonary atresia using a valved conduit. (Nomogram is specific solution of multivariable risk factor equation in original publication. Values entered for other variables are in original publication.) Key: $P_{RV/LV}$, Ratio of the peak pressure in right ventricle to that in left ventricle. (From Kirklin and colleagues.[K17])

the patient is convalescing well, an echocardiographic and cineangiographic search is made for sites of shunting that can be closed percutaneously or surgically.

RESULTS

After Repair

Early (Hospital) Death

Overall hospital mortality after repair in a heterogeneous population varies between less than 3% and up to 20%, depending on era, patient characteristics, and institution.

Most recent studies report hospital mortality of less than 5% for a heterogeneous population[H1] and less than 3% when patients undergoing extensive unifocalization procedures are excluded.[H20] When examining clinical series dealing only with complete repair involving unifocalization, hospital mortality historically has generally been less than 10%;[L7,M38,R6,T4] as experience with surgical management of this difficult group of patients has accumulated, the typical pattern of improved hospital mortality has emerged. Large series indicate that over the last 5 to 10 years, hospital mortality can be as low as 2%[B28,M6]; hospital mortality of less than 5% should be achievable.

Time-Related Survival

Overall time-related survival after repair, both for patients undergoing early repair without unifocalization and for those undergoing one-stage repair with unifocalization, has improved to the point that it is currently statistically indistinguishable from that of TF with pulmonary stenosis. Currently, 5-year survival for patients undergoing early repair without unifocalization (pulmonary atresia with confluent pulmonary arteries and ductus) is approximately 90%[H1,H24]; 2-year and 5-year survival for patients undergoing one-stage repair with unifocalization is 88% and 87%, respectively (Fig. 38-80) (for comparison, also see Fig. 38-47).[R6,M6]

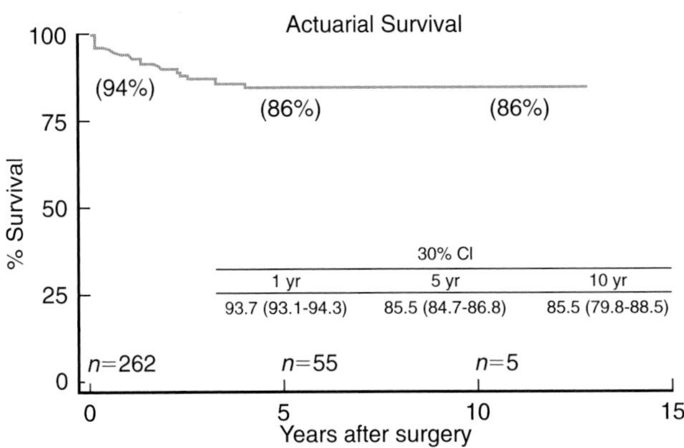

Figure 38-80 Survival in patients with pulmonary atresia, ventricular septal defect, and large systemic-to–pulmonary artery collaterals undergoing the surgical management protocol used by the Stanford group.[M6] Key: *CI,* Confidence interval.

Modes of Death

Most early postoperative deaths are attributable to acute cardiac failure, although some are due to acute or subacute pulmonary failure and a few to hypoxia or hemorrhage.[K24] In the large series of patients undergoing one-stage unifocalization and repair by Hanley and colleagues, acute hepatic failure was an important cause of death in the early years of the experience, accounting for much of the early 10% mortality; however, in the most recent decade, this cause has been virtually eliminated, with overall early mortality improving to approximately 2%.[M6] Most late postoperative deaths are due to chronic heart failure, although an appreciable number are sudden. These latter may be arrhythmic deaths. Unifocalized patients may experience fatal hemoptysis.

Incremental Risk Factors for Death

Variables relating to morphology of the pulmonary arterial circulation have traditionally been considered the strongest risk factors for death after repair, presumably accounting for most of the historical differences in outcome between these patients and those having TF with pulmonary stenosis. Available data for patients who do not require unifocalization, as well as for those who do, suggest that at least in the medium term, these variables can be and are being neutralized.[H20,R6]

Pulmonary Artery Abnormalities Size of central and proximal extracardiac right and left pulmonary arteries, congenitally nonconfluent right and left pulmonary arteries, and number of large AP collateral arteries have been identified as risk factors in early studies.[K24] With improvements in reconstructive techniques related to the central and branch pulmonary arteries, as well as unifocalization techniques, these factors have been completely neutralized.[M16,M39,R4,R6,R7,T4] It now seems clear that these previously identified pulmonary artery morphologic factors are surrogates for obstruction in the pulmonary artery system and elevated pulmonary vascular resistance (Rp). Carefully performed morphologic studies support this hypothesis. Shimizaki and colleagues found that late postrepair Rp was inversely related to number of pulmonary arterial segments connected (by nature) to an ipsilateral central pulmonary artery.[S12] Other studies and common experience indicate that the number of centrally connected pulmonary arterial segments is inversely related to the number of large AP collateral arteries.[S11] Thus, the incremental risk of the latter identified in early studies is probably a surrogate for that of increased Rp. Early and aggressive complete unifocalization of all collateral vessels and patch augmentation of centrally hypoplastic pulmonary arteries have eliminated the association between higher Rp and native pulmonary arterial arborization abnormalities.[R4,R6,R7]

Age (Size) Age older than about 5 to 8 years is a risk factor for death, primarily late after repair.[K17] The incremental risk of young age, once important, has largely been neutralized. This is evident in more recent experiences from institutions in which one-stage repair is typically performed in neonates and young infants.[D16,L20,R4,R6,T4]

Postrepair $P_{RV/LV}$ Higher postrepair $P_{RV/LV}$ is a risk factor for death after repair, probably an immutable one (see Fig. 38-79).[K17] This factor is the final common expression, which includes the influences of intrinsic Rp, degree of arborization of the pulmonary arteries (which includes completeness of unifocalization), size of the large pulmonary arteries, and precision with which any reconstruction or unifocalization has been accomplished.

Duration of Cardiopulmonary Bypass Duration of CPB was identified as a risk factor for death in early studies, particularly in the early period after repair.[K17,K24] Duration of CPB may carry risks related to CPB's intrinsic damaging effects, but it may also be a surrogate for technical complications during surgery. More recently, duration of CPB has not been associated with increased risk of early death in the large series of one-stage unifocalization and repair cases reported by Hanley and colleagues.[M6] Prolonged duration of CPB is a necessity in these patients in order to complete the unifocalization process, and thus does not represent difficulties or complications during surgery. Also, in more recent years, a reduction of the damaging effects of CPB has almost certainly been achieved.

Heart Block

Heart block is rare after repair, just as it is after repair of TF with pulmonary stenosis.

Functional Status

Most patients who survive repair have a good functional status (Table 38-13). Importantly, a tendency to declining functional status across time exists, but this may be attributable to chance alone (Fig. 38-81). Few objective studies of exercise performance have been reported.

Table 38-13 New York Heart Association Functional Class after Repair of Tetralogy of Fallot with Pulmonary Atresia

NYHA Class at Last Follow-up	*n*	% of 95
I	89	94
II	5	5
III	1	1
IV	0	0
Subtotal	95	100
Dead	39	
Alive, unknown class	5	
TOTAL	139	

Data from Kirklin and colleagues.[K24]

Pulmonary Artery Pressure and Resistance

As with other postoperative outcome events, information about PPA and Rp is limited. RV pressure can in no way substitute for PPA and Rp, because almost all patients have a pressure gradient between the RV and pulmonary arteries after repair. Shimazaki and colleagues found that 75% of patients had a gradient of at least 20 mmHg late after repair, and 10% had one of 60 mmHg.[S12] When patients undergoing repair in infancy or the neonatal period are considered, gradients progress inevitably over time, and at medium-term follow-up essentially all patients will have important gradients.

Early data suggested that about 50% of a heterogeneous group of patients will have elevated PPA and Rp late after repair, with elevated Rp correlating highly and inversely with extent of native pulmonary artery arborization.[S12] More recent data from patients undergoing surgical management plans that include early and complete correction of pulmonary artery arborization abnormalities demonstrate low PPA and Rp, both early and at medium-term follow-up and regardless of degree of original arborization,[R4,R6] indicating that this correlation is not immutable (Table 38-14). At midterm follow-up, $P_{RV/LV}$ was similar to the perioperative value, indicating that the unifocalized vascular bed grows over time.[M6]

Reintervention

Reoperations other than those on valved conduits and on peripheral pulmonary arteries in patients undergoing unifocalization are rare. Reintervention is infrequently needed to repair a residual or recurrent VSD or to close an overlooked large AP collateral artery (both in 3% of patients[K24]). Progressing dilatation of the aortic root and development of aortic valve regurgitation has required aortic valve replacement in 1% of patients.[K24] For patients undergoing early aggressive unifocalization, reoperation on the peripheral pulmonary

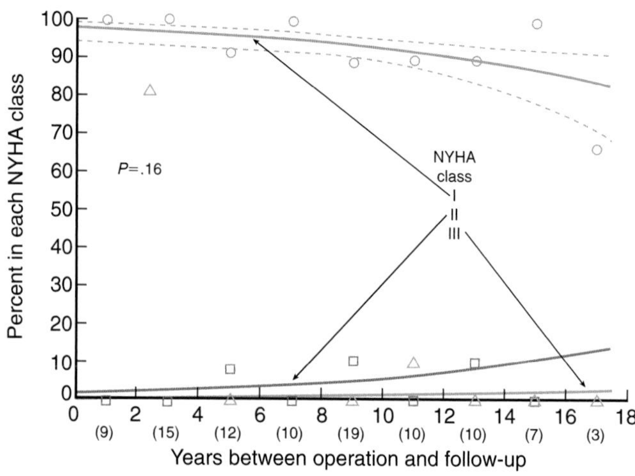

Figure 38-81 New York Heart Association *(NYHA)* functional class after repair of tetralogy of Fallot with pulmonary atresia, according to interval between operation and last follow-up. Details of presentation are similar to those of Fig. 38-54. *P* value of .16 for time trend in this ordinal logistic (longitudinal) regression analysis indicates that change across time in distribution of patients according to their NYHA functional class may be due to chance alone. (From Kirklin and colleagues.[K24])

Table 38-14 Perioperative Right-to–Left Ventricular Pressure Ratio in Patients Undergoing One-Stage Complete Unifocalization and Intracardiac Repair in Infancy[a]

Era	$P_{RV/LV}$ (Mean ± SD)
Total experience	0.41 ± 0.12
1992-1998	0.46 ± 0.14
1999-2005	0.37 ± 0.11

[a]The ratio improved when the periods between years 1992 through 1997 and 1998 through 2005 were compared.[M6]
Key: $P_{RV/LV}$, Ratio of right-to–left ventricular pressures.

arterial vasculature for persistent or recurrent obstruction is less than 15% at 5-year follow-up.[R6]

The most common reoperation is replacement of an obstructed xenograft or allograft valved conduit.[A3,B1,C20,I3,J6,M19,N13] Among a heterogeneous group of patients receiving these conduits for a variety of conditions, but most commonly for TF with pulmonary atresia, freedom from reoperation for conduit obstruction was 99%, 95%, 59%, and 11% at 3.5, 5, 10, and 15 years, respectively.[I4,K23,S4]

Among very young patients receiving 12-mm porcine valve xenografts in a polyester conduit, 3.5-, 5-, and 10-year freedom from replacement was 60%, 35%, and 9%, respectively, related in part to rapid growth of the patient.[B27] Time-related freedom from reoperation on allograft aortic and pulmonary valved conduits larger than about 21 mm is not yet known with a high degree of certainty. Currently, for properly preserved allograft aortic conduits, this appears to be about 95% at 5 years, falling to about 90% at 10 years and 60% at 20 years (Fig. 38-82, *A*).[K14,K23] The hazard function for reoperation has a steadily rising single phase (Fig. 38-82, *B*), suggesting that all such conduits may ultimately require replacement. Small patients require small allograft valved conduits, and the very small conduits required in neonates and infants clearly have a shorter reoperation-free interval than do larger conduits that can be used in children (Fig. 38-83). Despite these general trends, individual patient reoperation-free intervals can be quite variable, with some neonates having intervals up to a decade.

Prevalence and rate of reoperation for conduit obstruction are considerably greater when an allograft valved conduit is extended with a polyester cylinder than when it is not.[A9] It is not known whether this applies to proximal or distal extensions, or to both. A proximal polyester gusset in the RV does not seem to have this effect.[H12] Oversizing the conduit by too great a degree results in earlier reoperation.[A20]

Use of the valved bovine jugular vein conduit for RV to pulmonary artery reconstruction has received mixed reports. One individual institution report showed a high degree of midterm obstruction,[G20] whereas an eight-institution multi-institutional study,[B29] as well as individual institutional studies,[B33] showed midterm results that compare favorably with those of valved allografts.

After Palliative Operations for Increasing Pulmonary Blood Flow

Effect on Size of Pulmonary Arteries

Important enlargement of at least some portions of the pulmonary arteries can be obtained by increasing pulmonary

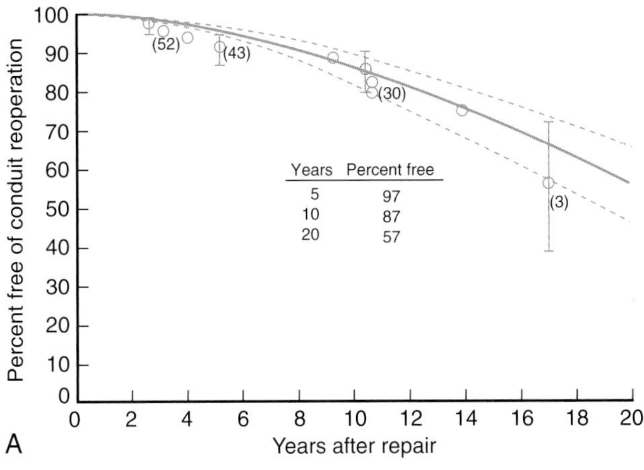

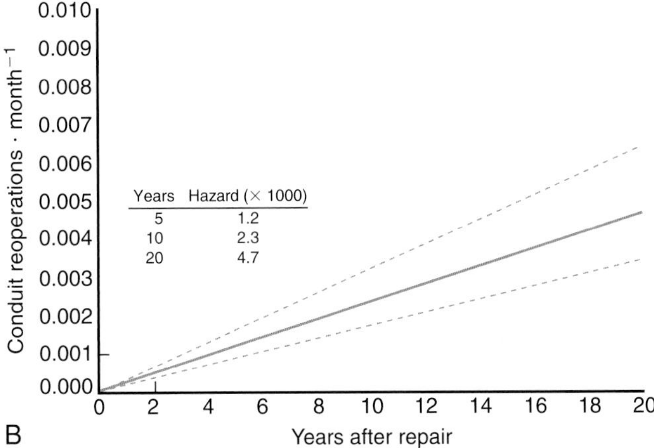

Figure 38-82 Freedom from conduit reoperation after placing an allograft valved conduit between ventricle and pulmonary trunk as part of cardiac repair. A polyester tube was used as a distal prolongation in a few patients, and this appeared to be disadvantageous. (Analysis is based on 58 patients operated on between 1966 and 1985. Data were supplied by D.N. Ross and J. Somerville.) **A,** Freedom from reoperation. Depiction is as in Fig. 38-47. **B,** Hazard function.

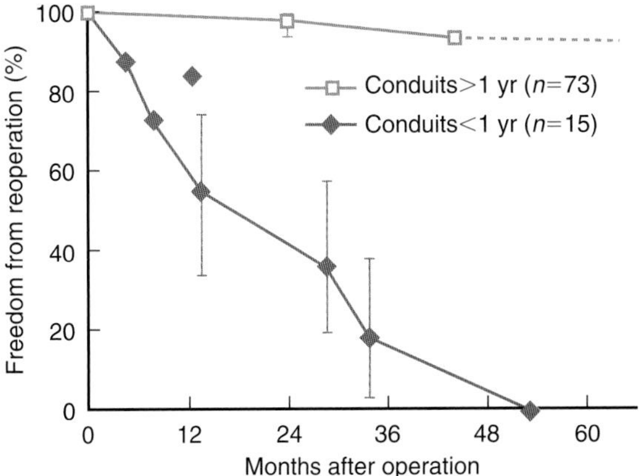

Figure 38-83 Freedom from reoperation for conduit obstruction according to age of patient (<age 1 year and >age 1 year) at time of insertion. Analysis includes patients in whom an allograft pulmonary or aortic valve conduit was used to construct right ventricular–pulmonary trunk continuity. (There was no difference in freedom between allograft pulmonary and allograft aortic valve conduits.) In patients younger than 1 year, the most common operation was repair of truncus arteriosus; in older patients, it was repair of tetralogy of Fallot with pulmonary atresia. Key: *yr,* Year. (From Hawkins and colleagues.[H12])

blood flow and pressure.[G16,K19] This observation has influenced a number of institutions to follow management plans in patients with small pulmonary arteries that include staging procedures to achieve increased flow and pressure into both the pulmonary arteries and collateral vessels. Various ways of achieving this have been described, including placing PTFE systemic–pulmonary arterial shunts, directly connecting central pulmonary arteries to the ascending aorta, placing RV–pulmonary trunk conduits or patches, and constructing shunts into individual or partially unifocalized collateral vessels.[M9,M23,P21,R26,S1,S3,W6] Although vessel growth clearly results from these procedures, it is difficult to document how frequently they lead to intracardiac repair with acceptable PRV and PPA. Reports suggest that approximately 20% of anastomoses performed in the palliative setting will occlude, and about half the patients undergoing staged palliative procedures will eventually undergo intracardiac repair. A substantial portion of these patients will have unacceptably high PPA.[I7,I8,M23,Y1]

Also well established is the fact that enlargement is not always diffuse, and there may remain areas of stenosis, presumably because pulmonary arterial walls are not uniformly compliant. Reasons for the noncompliance are not completely clear. Intrinsic abnormalities within the vessel wall and persistently abnormal blood flow patterns related to the palliative procedure may both play a role. These areas can be approached by percutaneous balloon dilatation or stenting, or by reoperation. An immediate favorable response can be achieved in more than 80% of cases; however, later stenosis and occlusion are common.[B34,E7,R9,R26,V11,Z4]

Likewise, the degree of enlargement that can be obtained in individual patients cannot be accurately predicted. However, it is correlated with the magnitude of increase in the Q̇p and PPA that can be brought about by the palliative procedure.[A11,G2] When the central pulmonary arteries are small, palliative RV–pulmonary trunk and systemic–pulmonary arterial shunts can provide maximal stimulus for pulmonary arterial enlargement. There is no reason to believe that this growth is any greater than that occurring in the pulmonary arteries and unifocalized collaterals following reparative surgery. Although there are no definitive data, there is a suggestion that focal areas of stenosis may be reduced in the setting of the normal pulmonary blood flow patterns that attend reparative, as opposed to palliative, operations.

Survival

Early mortality (1-month) for palliative operations, as reported in the mid-1980s, was 17%,[K22] with most of the deaths occurring in very small (young) infants with severe hypoplasia of the pulmonary arteries or other kinds of pulmonary arterial anomalies (Fig. 38-84). It is likely that mortality would be lower in a more contemporary series, considering recent improvements in perioperative care. Recent reports from institutions that emphasize palliative procedures for TF support this.[F12] Survival for at least 12 years has been good (75%) in patients receiving a systemic–pulmonary arterial shunt and no further procedures (see Fig. 38-84). These patients were deemed unsuitable for repair in the era of 1967 to 1983. There is no way, it seems, to compare in a risk-adjusted manner this survival with that had these same patients undergone one-stage repair or received no treatment. Most of the deaths occurred within the first 3 postoperative months.

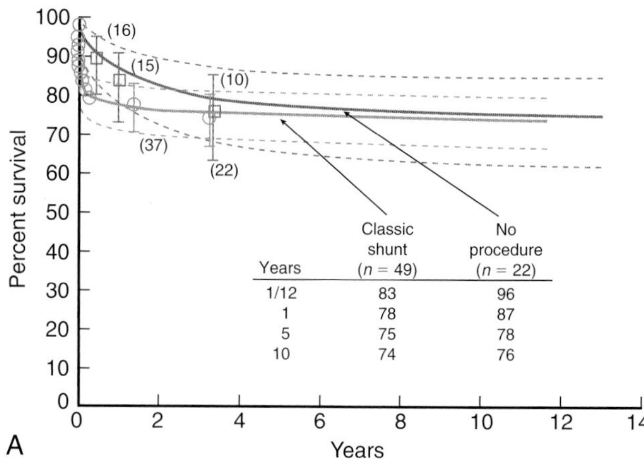

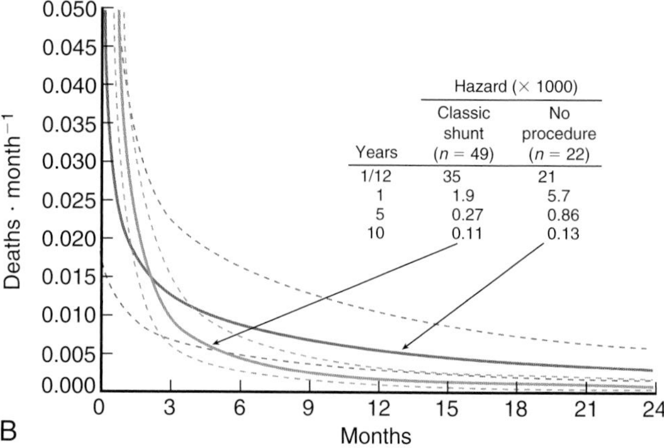

Figure 38-84 Time-related survival in patients having tetralogy of Fallot (TF) with pulmonary atresia who underwent no interventional therapy (*n* = 22) and who underwent only a systemic–pulmonary arterial shunt with no further intervention (*n* = 49). (Analysis is based on cross-sectional follow-up of 244 patients having TF with pulmonary atresia seen at UAB between 1967 and July 1983; follow-up was in mid-1986.) **A,** Survival. Depiction is as in Fig. 38-47. **B,** Hazard function for death.

Modes of Death

Death early after operation is usually due to acute cardiac failure, whereas late postoperatively it is usually from hypoxia.

Functional Status

There is little information on functional status; however, because all palliated patients have a completely mixed circulation, function is reduced in this population.

Results of No Interventional Therapy

Historical Perspective

Because there has been increasing recognition over the past 20 years that surgical or other interventional therapy is beneficial to patients with all forms of TF with pulmonary atresia, unselected patient cohorts receiving no intervention no longer exist.

Survival

Survival for at least 12 years in 22 patients receiving no interventional treatment was 75%, with most of the deaths occurring within a year of presentation (see Fig. 38-84). These were patients considered unsuitable for complete repair and too well oxygenated to require a systemic–pulmonary arterial shunt when they presented between 1967 and 1983. Most were older children who had fewer than 10 pulmonary arterial segments in continuity with central or hilar RPA or LPA. Again, there is no way to make a risk-adjusted comparison of their survival with that of patients who received interventional therapy. It is, however, almost a certainty that this patient group is highly selected and does not represent the newborn population with this malformation.

Modes of Death

Among the four patients who died within the follow-up period, one died of hypoxia and one of massive pulmonary hemorrhage. Mode of death was unknown in the other two.

Functional Status

Functional status of living patients was unknown, except in four. Two of these considered themselves to be fully active (NYHA class I), whereas one each was in NYHA classes II and III.

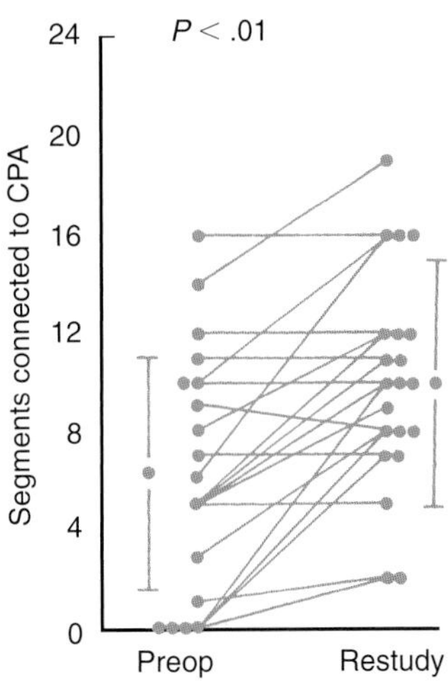

Figure 38-85 Number of pulmonary arterial segments connected centrally before and after unifocalization in 20 patients. $P < .01$ for difference in means (vertical bar represents one standard deviation). Key: *CPA,* Central pulmonary arteries; *Preop,* preoperative. (From Sullivan and colleagues.[S30])

After Staged Palliative Operations for Unifocalization

Results of unifocalization operations, performed as a preliminary step before complete repair in patients who have TF with pulmonary atresia and considerably incomplete distribution of the RPA and LPA, are not yet clear (see Special Situations and Controversies later in this section). Some reports refer only to a few patients; others contain information that is insufficient for assessing results. The best estimate based on available reports is that as many as half, but often less, actually undergo repair. Of those who do, a substantial percentage, even a majority, will have $P_{RV/LV}$ greater than 0.67.[I8,M23,P21,S3,W6,Y1]

One exemplary report from the Hospital for Sick Children at Great Ormond Street, London,[S30] states that among 26 infants and children undergoing staged unifocalization operations of various types through a lateral thoracotomy, most commonly with interposition of prosthetic tubes, 4 (15%; CL 8%-26%) died in hospital postoperatively. Eleven of 20 patients restudied had 10 or fewer pulmonary artery segments connected to central pulmonary arteries before the unifocalization procedure, whereas at restudy 9 were in this state (Fig. 38-85). Patency of the unifocalizing anastomoses varied between 5% and 100%, depending on the type of procedure. Seven (27%; CL 17%-39%) of the original group of 26 patients either underwent complete repair or were suitable for it.

A large experience has also been reported from the Mayo Clinic.[P21] Among 38 patients undergoing unifocalization, hospital mortality was 5% (CL 2%-12%), similar to that at Great Ormond Street. Sixty-one percent (CL 51%-70%) underwent complete repair, a higher prevalence than at Great Ormond Street; however, there is insufficient information to determine whether patient groups were comparable. Among the 23 patients undergoing complete repair, 21 (91%; CL 81%-97%) survived; these represent 55% (CL 46%-65%) of the original group, a higher prevalence than at Great Ormond Street. Of the 23 patients undergoing repair, 13% had postrepair (OR) $P_{RV/LV}$ greater than 0.85, and the mean value was 0.63.

Fifty-eight patients with TF and pulmonary atresia were reported from the Royal Children's Hospital in Melbourne, Australia, 34 of whom had unifocalization procedures. It is difficult to determine the outcome in these 34 separately from that of the entire group. However, among the 58 patients, 27 (47%; CL 39%-54%) either died after preliminary procedures or were ultimately considered unsuitable for repair. Results were good among the 30 patients who underwent repair, with one early death and three late deaths. In 2 of the 30 patients, late VSD patch fenestration was required because of $P_{RV/LV}$ greater than 1. Among 27 survivors who had undergone postoperative hemodynamic study, 5 (29%; CL 17%-45%) had postrepair $P_{RV/LV}$ of 0.7 to 0.9.[I8]

Thirty-four similar patients were reported from the Heart Institute of Japan at the Tokyo Women's Medical Colleges.[S3] Twenty-two had incomplete distribution of one or both pulmonary arteries. Among 16 of the 34 patients who underwent final repair, postrepair $P_{RV/LV}$ ranged between 0.36 and 1.00, with a mean of 0.71. In four other patients, a perforated VSD patch was used because severe elevation of postrepair $P_{RV/LV}$ was predicted if complete repair was done.

Clearly, some patients are correctable after a staged unifocalization operation and successfully undergo complete repair. For those whose repair is not successful, many factors may come into play, including natural attrition of healthy lung segments that occurs over time due to either vessel occlusion or pulmonary vascular obstructive disease, iatrogenic loss of lung segments directly related to palliative surgery, inability to create vascular continuity between lung segments due to scarring from prior palliative operations, and general cardiovascular complications related to chronic mixed circulation. Risk-adjusted, time-related probabilities of death and of importantly elevated postrepair $P_{RV/LV}$ are not yet available. As a general observation, however, the number of patients who achieve complete repair, *and in particular who achieve complete repair with a $P_{RV/LV}$ less than 0.5*, when the routine approach is initial palliation, appears to be substantially less than when the routine approach is early one-stage unifocalization and intracardiac repair.

INDICATIONS FOR OPERATION

Proper indications for operation, and their sequencing in the various subsets of patients who have TF with congenital pulmonary atresia, cannot be identified with certainty. This is not surprising, because the necessary patient-specific (risk-adjusted) comparisons of outcomes after no interventional treatment vs. the various types and combinations of procedures are not yet available. Therefore, indications can only be discussed in general terms for the major groups.

Confluent and Normally Distributing Right and Left Pulmonary Arteries and Patent Ductus Arteriosus

The highly unfavorable natural history of newborns in this subset, coupled with the fact that up to 95% survive complete repair in early life and 75% of those undergoing repair are alive and in good health for at least 10 years, indicates that complete repair as early in life as possible should be undertaken, almost always meaning neonatal repair. It must be emphasized, however, that equal outcomes appear to be achievable with neonatal shunting followed by later repair.

In those patients first seen after the neonatal period and usually living because of an AP anastomosis of some type, repair as soon as possible is likewise advisable.

Confluent, Nonconfluent, or Absent Pulmonary Arteries and Aortopulmonary Collaterals

Although the natural history is much more variable in this morphologic group, rarely do patients reach adult life in a healthy state if left untreated. Based on early surgical outcomes before 1990, it has been argued by some that surgical intervention is not indicated unless the individual is very symptomatic. More recent surgical results following both staged unifocalization and one-stage unifocalization and intracardiac repair demonstrate that repair with low PRV and PPA can be achieved in a high percentage of patients whether symptomatic or not. Although long-term outcome using these newer techniques is not yet known, the combination of low operative mortality and resultant low PRV suggests that outcomes over the long term are likely, in many cases, to be comparable with those achieved in the more favorable morphologic subset of patients with TF with pulmonary atresia and ductus-dependent, confluent, normally distributing pulmonary arteries. The most important principles in achieving results comparable with this more favorable group are incorporating blood supply from all lung segments into the central pulmonary artery system and achieving this in a timely manner such that the microvasculature in each lung segment remains undamaged.

SPECIAL SITUATIONS AND CONTROVERSIES

Alternatives to One-Stage Unifocalization and Intracardiac Repair

Situations may arise in the setting of large AP collaterals and true pulmonary artery arborization abnormalities in which one-stage unifocalization and intracardiac repair is not indicated. One of these is described earlier in which one-stage unifocalization through a midline sternotomy is accomplished, but Rp is proven to be elevated, intracardiac repair is aborted, and unifocalized pulmonary arteries are connected to the systemic circulation by a shunt. It has been demonstrated that approximately 80% to 90% of patients with large AP collaterals can achieve complete bilateral unifocalization through a midline sternotomy in one procedure in early infancy, and of these, approximately two thirds can undergo intracardiac repair at the same time. Of the one third of patients who undergo complete unifocalization, but in whom Rp is too high to permit immediate intracardiac repair, most achieve repair within 2 years.[R6]

There are various reasons why midline complete unifocalization is contraindicated in approximately 10% to 20% of patients with major AP collaterals. The most important is a lack of pulmonary vascular "raw materials." *Raw materials* are defined as the combination of true pulmonary arteries and major AP collaterals taken together. If both the true pulmonary artery system and AP collateral system are severely underdeveloped, an alternative approach should be considered. In the setting of poorly developed collaterals and absent true pulmonary arteries, a lateral thoracotomy with single lung unifocalization connected to an AP shunt may be the procedure of choice. This would be followed by a similar procedure on the contralateral lung at a future time. At a third procedure, a median sternotomy approach would be used to achieve vascular confluence between the left and right lungs, with later intracardiac repair and takedown of the previously placed shunts. Many techniques, using native tissue as well as prosthetic material, have been described to accomplish this type of reconstruction.[C7,I7,M23,P11,P21,R26,S3,Y1] In other situations the true central pulmonary arteries are present, confluent, but extremely hypoplastic in the mediastinum; however, they arborize to all or almost all of the lung segments, and communicate to the collateral system extensively within the lung parenchyma. In this situation, there are few if any isolated segments of lung that are supplied by only collateral flow. In this setting, creation in the neonatal or early infancy period of a central native tissue anastomosis between the ascending aorta and blind end of the pulmonary trunk can be performed to promote growth of the central system with communication to most lung segments. Following an interim period of central pulmonary artery growth, a second procedure with ligation of the dual-supply collateral sources at their systemic origin, and subsequent intracardiac repair and placement of an RV-to–pulmonary trunk conduit, can be accomplished.[I8,R24,W6]

It should be emphasized that there is wide variability among experienced surgeons in the approach to TF with pulmonary atresia and large AP collaterals. Experienced surgical teams may prefer one of the alternative surgical approaches described earlier as their procedure of choice.[P11,P21,R26,W6] One common approach is to perform an initial procedure that provides increased blood flow and pressure into the confluent hypoplastic central artery system whenever there exists confluent central pulmonary arteries. This can be accomplished through many techniques—for example, by creating the central systemic–pulmonary tissue-to-tissue connection described earlier.[R24,W6] Another approach is to create an RV-to–pulmonary trunk conduit using various tissue or synthetic prostheses, leaving the VSD open.[R26] A third approach is to create a prosthetic systemic–pulmonary arterial shunt to the pulmonary trunk or one of its branches.

There are several major concerns about all of these approaches when they are used unselectively as first-line management, especially when the central pulmonary arteries have limited arborization. First, they leave collateral flow untouched, allowing time for detrimental changes to occur in the lung vasculature supplied by collaterals, either in the form of overcirculation with development of pulmonary vascular obstructive changes or in the form of stenosis and occlusion leading to loss of lung segments. These negative effects inevitably lead to reduction in healthy lung cross-sectional area, increasing Rp. Another concern is that any surgical procedure is followed by scarring and adhesions, markedly reducing the surgeon's ability to manipulate, reroute, and unifocalize collaterals at subsequent operations. A final concern is that following any shunt or conduit procedure, no matter how small the shunt or conduit is, the flow and pressure transmitted into the distal vasculature of the true pulmonary arteries are likely to be pathologically elevated when there is a very limited distal bed in association with reduced arborization.

Regardless of the specific surgical approach, most programs with substantial experience with this lesion[M6,B28] believe that unifocalization of large collaterals is an important component of overall management; however, this view is not universally acknowledged.[B30]

Percutaneous Balloon Dilatation of Stenoses of Right and Left Pulmonary Arteries

Lock and colleagues first demonstrated the feasibility of this procedure.[L18,L19,R19] Intimal disruption with tearing of the media is one mechanism of dilatation, with the tears being subsequently filled in by scar tissue.[E4] In a multi-institutional study of a heterogeneous group of 156 patients, the largest subset of which had some form of pulmonary atresia, systolic pressure gradient across the stenosis was reduced only 10 to 14 mmHg, on average.[K2] A single-institution analysis of results in 135 patients indicated that about 60% of the procedures were satisfactory, defining this as a decrease of 20% or more of the peak pressure ratio between RV and aorta.[R31] Risk of death or other major complication was 1% to 3%. Patient age had no correlation with outcome. Effectiveness may be increased in the future by use of expandable stents.[M30,O5]

Effectiveness of balloon dilatation can also be assessed by its effect on normalizing the flow distribution in the lungs as measured by nuclear lung perfusion scan, even if PRV is not reduced. Following complete repair, normalization of homogeneous flow to the lungs can be promoted by balloon dilatation of lobar and segmental stenoses within the unifocalized pulmonary artery system.[R6]

Percutaneous Closure of Large Aortopulmonary Collateral Arteries

Yamamoto first demonstrated the feasibility of this procedure in 1979,[Y3] and Szarnicki and colleagues accomplished it by embolizing a Gianturco wire coil device in 1981.[S34] Subsequently, a number of studies have demonstrated the effectiveness and safety of percutaneous closure of large AP collateral arteries as long as proper precautions are taken. When wire coil uniformly coated with thrombogenic polyester strands is used, occlusion by thrombosis usually occurs within about 10 minutes.[F15] Other devices for promoting thrombosis have been used, including bucrylate adhesive[Z7] and detachable silicone balloons.[G28,T6] With wire coil and proper techniques, complete occlusion is achieved in about 70% of instances and subtotal occlusion in another 25%.[P13]

A large AP collateral artery should never be closed surgically or percutaneously when it connects end to end to distal pulmonary arteries, and thus is the sole or major source of blood flow to one or more pulmonary segments. Even when blood supply to a pulmonary segment occurs from dual sources, occlusion of the collateral source may not be indicated. For example, if upon review of detailed angiograms, it is determined that the collateral tissue can be used productively in surgical unifocalization, it should not be occluded prematurely. In this case, the collateral should be left open at catheterization and then ligated and divided during surgery, with its tissue used in the unifocalization and pulmonary artery augmentation process. When it is determined that tissue from a dual-supply collateral is not needed in surgical reconstruction and coil occlusion is being considered, it is prudent to occlude the vessel temporarily to be certain that its presence is not necessary for maintaining reasonable SaO_2.

Section III **Tetralogy of Fallot with Absent Pulmonary Valve**

DEFINITION

Tetralogy of Fallot with absent pulmonary valve is a subset of TF in which the pathologic and clinical states are determined largely by the vestigial, severely hypoplastic, nonfunctioning pulmonary valve cusps at the RV–pulmonary trunk junction.

HISTORICAL NOTE

The first apparent description was by Royer and Wilson in 1908.[R35] A second example was not reported until Kurtz and colleagues described their case in 1927.[K41]

MORPHOLOGY

The pulmonary valve cusps are myxomatous nubbins of valvar tissue at the RV–pulmonary trunk junction.[Z1] They are so severely hypoplastic that they are both nonfunctioning and only minimally stenotic. The pulmonary "anulus" is moderately narrow.[L1]

The VSD is large and similar to that in TF with pulmonary stenosis. The typical associated malalignment of the outlet septum contributes to infundibular narrowing. In addition, and perhaps related to the large flow, the RV outflow tract is often dilated and elongated.[Z6] The sinus portion of the RV is hypertrophied and its volume large.

The pulmonary trunk and central portions of the right pulmonary artery and left pulmonary artery are often aneurysmally dilated at birth.[S22] This dilatation may extend into the hilar portions of these arteries, particularly the right, which then produces tracheobronchial compression. This often results in either hyperexpansion from air trapping or collapse of lobes or even an entire lung.[L1]

Beyond their hilar portions, pulmonary arteries are usually of normal size. Rarely are distal branches hypoplastic or hilar branching pattern abnormal.[R28] However, segmental distribution of the RPA and LPA is abnormal. Instead of single segmental arteries, tufts of arteries entwine and compress the interpulmonary bronchi in some patients. This pathology, when present, may in part account for symptoms of severe pulmonary dysfunction seen in some neonates and young infants.[R1]

There is controversy regarding the histopathology of the dilated pulmonary arteries in this syndrome. Arensman and colleagues report a normal pulmonary arterial wall in five of six children, with one child having a reduction in the amount of elastic tissue.[A19] Osman and colleagues have reported similar findings,[O10] but histopathologic abnormalities have been reported by others.[M2,M25,O9,R1,R36] Whatever the histology, physiologic studies indicate a marked decrease in RPA compliance in sick small babies.[H19]

Cause of massive dilatation of the pulmonary arteries in utero is unclear, but when there is severe pulmonary regurgitation and a large VSD, absence of ductal flow between the pulmonary trunk and aorta seems to be essential to intrauterine survival.[Z6] Thus, a ductus arteriosus (or ligamentum) is almost always absent at autopsy[E10] unless the ductus connects to a pulmonary artery isolated from the pulmonary trunk. Thus, a likely cause of intrauterine dilatation of the pulmonary arteries is hemodynamic. The combination of a severely regurgitant valve in association with limited distal runoff from the pulmonary arteries from a combination of absence of a ductus and normally elevated intrauterine pulmonary vascular resistance (Rp) results in an exaggerated pulse pressure in the central pulmonary arteries.

There may be origin of the RPA or LPA from the ascending aorta,[C3] or a pulmonary artery (usually the left) may originate from a patent ductus arteriosus.[Z6] When a pulmonary artery arises from a ductus, it is not aneurysmally dilated, consistent with the hemodynamic explanation mentioned earlier.

CLINICAL FEATURES AND DIAGNOSTIC CRITERIA

TF with absent pulmonary valve generally results in both severe pulmonary regurgitation and a somewhat increased pulmonary blood flow ($\dot{Q}p$). Narrowing at the pulmonary "anulus" in combination with the large VSD results in low PPA and similar peak pressures in both ventricles.[L1] Part of the pressure gradient between the RV and pulmonary trunk is related to large $\dot{Q}p$ (the $\dot{Q}p/\dot{Q}s$ [ratio of $\dot{Q}p$ to systemic blood flow, $\dot{Q}s$] is generally 1.5 to 2.0); part is related to mild "anular" and infundibular narrowing.

When pulmonary regurgitation is severe, $\dot{Q}p$ increased, and pulmonary arteries dilated and compressing the tracheobronchial tree, presentation may be in early infancy, often in the first weeks of life, with heart failure and severe intractable tracheobronchitis and respiratory distress responding poorly to routine medical measures. In the most severe cases, presentation may be immediate at birth, with the neonate *in extremis* from an inability to breathe due to bronchial compression. Cyanosis is absent unless hypoxia develops from pulmonary complications. There is marked failure to thrive, and there may be low cardiac output, acidemia, and death.

In other cases, especially, but not always, when pulmonary regurgitation is less severe (in association with slightly more pulmonary stenosis, a near-normal $\dot{Q}p$, and less marked aneurysmal dilatation of the pulmonary arteries), presentation is later in life and less severe, usually confined to recurrent respiratory infections or mild heart failure. Notably, however, severity of the major morphologic and physiologic changes (size of the aneurysmal central pulmonary arteries and degree of pulmonary regurgitation) does not always predict severity of presentation. The important variable in critical neonatal presentation seems to be the inability of the airways to resist compression.

Physical Examination

Severely affected infants are in considerable respiratory distress, with tachypnea, subcostal retraction, and wheeze with rales and rhonchi audible throughout both lung fields. The heart is overactive and its rate rapid, pulse is of low volume, and there is obvious cardiomegaly, hepatomegaly, and raised venous pressure. There may be a precordial bulge. The infant is frail, cachectic, and febrile. On auscultation a to-and-fro murmur is audible along the left sternal edge, with the diastolic component often the more prominent. The second heart sound is single, and there may be an apical gallop.

Chest Radiography

Chest radiography is distinctive, showing from birth marked supracardiac mediastinal widening caused by aneurysmal dilatation of central and hilar pulmonary arteries, usually equal on both sides although sometimes asymmetric, with relatively oligemic lung fields. Segmental or lobar atelectasis is common, and sometimes an entire lung is collapsed. Aerated portions of the lung may be overinflated (Fig. 38-86). Atelectasis is

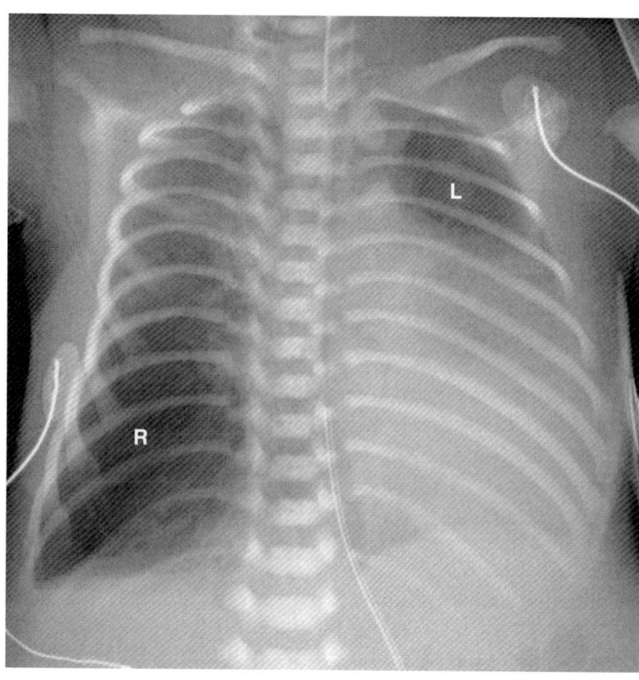

Figure 38-86 Chest radiograph of a newborn having tetralogy of Fallot with absent pulmonary valve. Heart is markedly enlarged. Hyperlucency is seen at the right lower lung *(R)* and left upper lung *(L)*, corresponding to areas of air trapping due to airway compressions by enlarged pulmonary arteries.

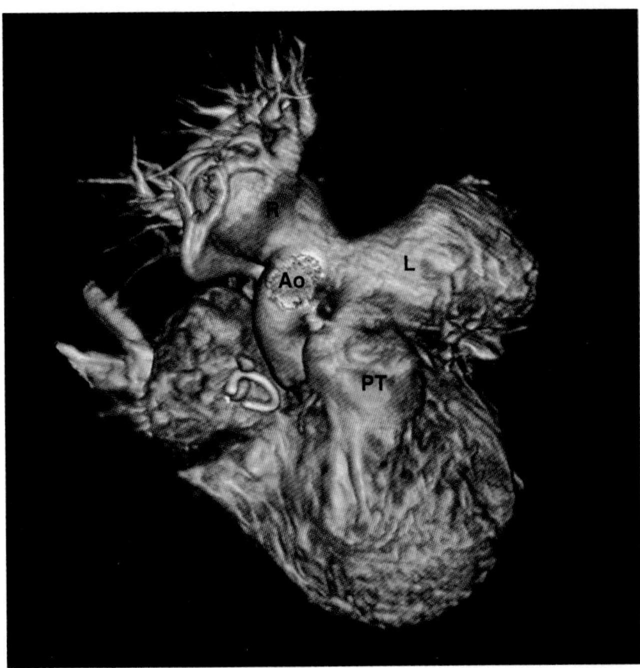

Figure 38-87 Volume rendering from a computed tomographic angiography image of a 5-year-old boy born with tetralogy of Fallot with absent pulmonary valve. The pulmonary trunk *(PT)*, right pulmonary artery *(R)*, and left pulmonary artery *(L)* are markedly enlarged compared with the aorta *(Ao)*.

associated with mediastinal shift, and in cases with partial or complete lung collapse, with acquired dextrocardia.[M25] In severe cases, there is considerable cardiomegaly. The left atrium may be pushed downward[M2] and the carina splayed with compression of lower trachea and both main bronchi.

Other Studies

The ECG is typical for patients with TF. In patients who are asymptomatic or mildly symptomatic and do not require neonatal surgery, 2D echocardiography is diagnostic and definitive. In unstable neonates and infants, further studies are indicated once the patient is resuscitated and stabilized. Currently, CTA provides the most information, characterizing the pulmonary artery and airway abnormalities and their interrelationships (Fig. 38-87). In some institutions cardiac catheterization is also performed, or is performed as an alternative to CT.

NATURAL HISTORY

TF with absent pulmonary valve is present in about 5% of patients born with a large VSD and pulmonary stenosis. A high percentage (perhaps 50%) die in the first year of life if untreated, and most in the first few months of life, from respiratory distress caused by the massively dilated RPA and LPA compressing the tracheobronchial tree.[A19,C3,D9,L1] Such critically ill infants also have heart failure associated with a left-to-right shunt, and the RV is markedly enlarged and systolic function reduced.[H19]

Patients who survive infancy, however, generally do well for 5 to 20 years, because RV outflow obstruction is only moderate and cyanosis mild or absent.[S9] They tend to become symptomatic ultimately and die of intractable RV failure as a result of its chronic pressure and volume overload.

TECHNIQUE OF OPERATION

When operation is delayed to age 3 to 5 years or older, the usual procedure is repair of the VSD and orthotopic insertion of an allograft aortic or pulmonary valve conduit (see "Establishing Right Ventricle–to–Pulmonary Artery Continuity" under Technique of Operation in Section II; see also Fig. 38-77). An end-to-end anastomosis is usually made between the distal end of the conduit and the divided pulmonary trunk. Usually no "roofing" of the right ventriculotomy is required, because the large infundibulum permits direct approximation.

In critically ill neonates and infants, a number of palliative operations have been used, but the corrective repair just described is preferred. In addition, however, elliptical strips of arterial wall are removed from the anterior and posterior aspects of the RPA, LPA, and pulmonary trunk bifurcation; the resultant defects are closed with a continuous suture before inserting the allograft valve cylinder.[G21,K5,S18,S25] This takes pressure off the underlying tracheobronchial tree. Waterston[W5] and Godart and colleagues[G21] report good results in infants using extensive pulmonary arterioplasty, closure of the VSD, infundibular resection, and placement of a transanular patch; a valved conduit is not used. Often the large pulmonary trunk can be transected, shortened, and moved ventrally and caudally to roof the infundibulum and relieve pressure from the tracheal bifurcation. Nevertheless, in unstable neonates and infants, it can be anticipated that residual airway problems will almost certainly persist following repair, even when aggressive reduction pulmonary arterioplasty is performed; therefore, normalizing the hemodynamics as much as possible by using a valved conduit is strongly recommended.

An alternative surgical approach for patients with airway compression involves translocating the pulmonary arteries anterior to the aorta[H30] in addition to VSD closure, conduit placement, and reduction pulmonary arterioplasty.

SPECIAL FEATURES OF POSTOPERATIVE CARE

When operation is performed electively in a patient age 3 to 5 years or older, care is the same as that usually given to patients after intracardiac surgery.

When operation has been performed urgently in neonates, infants, or young children, severe respiratory distress has usually been present and the patient receiving intensive treatment. This treatment (see Indications for Operation later in this section) is intensified in the postoperative period and then slowly withdrawn as the patient's condition improves.

RESULTS

Survival

Early (Hospital) Death

Historically, absent pulmonary valve syndrome has been associated with a high probability of hospital death after repair in young infants.[A19,I5,M14,P16] In the current era emphasizing pulmonary arterioplasty, Waterston and colleagues[W5] report 16%

mortality (CL 7%-29%) in infants, and Godart and colleagues[G21] 20% mortality (CL 6%-41%) in infants and 3.7% (CL 0.5%-12%) in children older than 1 year. Mortality in infants is related in part to their poor preoperative condition and severe respiratory problems. When operation is undertaken beyond the first year of life, respiratory problems have usually resolved or not been present, and hospital mortality is low.

Time-Related Survival

This, and the incremental risk factors for premature death, as well as other outcome events, are similar to those in other patients with TF whose repair includes insertion of an allograft valved conduit.

INDICATIONS FOR OPERATION

Help is urgently needed for small babies with this morphologic variant who present with severe respiratory distress. Some have unrelated congenital hypertrophic lobar emphysema, and a few have severe hypoplasia of the RPA and LPA; in either event, salvage may be impossible. In others an intense medical program is begun as soon as the condition is recognized. It includes managing the baby while continuously in a prone position on a hinged board placed in head-up position with maximal ventilator support.[A19] This allows the pulmonary arteries to fall forward and away from the bronchi, particularly the RPA.[A19] In the most severe cases, even this maneuver may be ineffective, and emergency sternotomy in the ICU may be required.[H17]

Most often, critically ill babies with this condition remain seriously ill even if ventilation is stabilized, and operation is required.

In patients with this morphology who require no special care in early life, repair is advised electively at 3 to 5 years of age.

Although various procedures have been recommended from time to time, that described under Technique of Operation is considered indicated. This is because alternative palliative procedures[B37,L17,O9] have not resulted in improved long-term outcomes.

Section IV **Tetralogy of Fallot with Flap Valve Ventricular Septal Defect**

DEFINITION

Tetralogy of Fallot with flap valve VSD is a subset of TF characterized by a thick fibrous flap hinged on the right side of a large VSD that narrows the interventricular communication and thereby limits right-to-left shunting.

MORPHOLOGY

The VSD is typical for TF. Its inferior margin either reaches the tricuspid anulus or is separated from it by a ridge of muscle (see "Ventricular Septal Defect" under Morphology in Section I). A fibrous flap is attached posteriorly to the aortic margin of the VSD, and its inferior margin may or may not be fused with the base and superior margin of the anterior tricuspid leaflet. Elsewhere, the flap is unattached, and it rarely plays any part in tricuspid valve function (Fig. 38-88). It can hinge freely toward the right, but its thickness and bulk prevent movement through the VSD into the LV. Therefore, in the presence of severe pulmonary stenosis and raised RV pressure, it virtually occludes the defect.[N7]

Pulmonary stenosis is typical of TF, but the infundibular component is made more evident by the severe degree of RV hypertrophy that involves chiefly the sinus portion of the ventricle because of high ventricular pressure. Thus, there may be a localized high-, intermediate-, or low-level infundibular stenosis, or the narrowing may be diffuse, and the valve may or may not be stenotic. Congenital pulmonary atresia is occasionally present and pulmonary artery branch origin stenosis may occur.

This subset of TF is one of a group of conditions in which there is an *accessory fibrous flap* or *pouch* or *excrescence* arising in the region of the atrioventricular valve apparatus and sometimes from the leaflets themselves.[C16,F8,I1] They have sometimes been called, usually erroneously, "aneurysms of the membranous septum."[P9] Such anomalies associated with the tricuspid valve may prolapse into the RV outflow tract and pulmonary valve and cause severe pulmonary stenosis,[C26,F9,P7] a phenomenon that may occur in the absence of a VSD.[E6] A mobile mass of fibrous tissue related to the tricuspid valve may prolapse through a VSD and produce LV outflow tract obstruction[M4,N5,S6]; this type of subaortic stenosis is easily corrected by operation.[M35] When transposition of the great arteries and VSD coexist, prolapse of accessory tricuspid valve tissue through the VSD results again in LV outflow tract obstruction, which is then subpulmonary (see Chapter 52).[H32,R18] In cases with congenitally corrected transposition of the great arteries (see Chapter 55), accessory valvar tissues of the right-sided, morphologically left atrioventricular valve may coexist; in this situation, the tendency is for the accessory tissue to prolapse in ball-valve fashion into the morphologically LV outflow tract, producing subpulmonary stenosis.[L12] This may occur with or without an associated VSD. Such prolapsing accessory tissue is uncommon, but appears to be more often associated with the systemic venous rather than the pulmonary venous (systemic) atrioventricular valve. Maclean and colleagues[M5] and Levy and colleagues[L12] each report such a case in which subaortic obstruction resulted. Such a phenomenon may rarely coexist with TF.[V3]

CLINICAL FEATURES AND DIAGNOSTIC CRITERIA

Right-to-left shunting through the restricted VSD may be large enough to produce important cyanosis; usually it is not, so when the atrial septum is also intact, the patient is acyanotic or only mildly cyanotic despite severe pulmonary stenosis. When pulmonary stenosis is severe, the virtually intact ventricular septum results in severe RV hypertrophy on ECG (in contrast to the moderate RV hypertrophy typical of TF), near-normal splitting of the second heart sound (because $\dot{Q}p$ and PPA are maintained at a near-normal level), and a prominent *a* wave in the jugular venous pulse. Presentation is similar to that of pulmonary stenosis with intact ventricular septum (see Chapter 37). These features and the larger cardiac silhouette on chest radiograph than in classic TF make the diagnosis likely. Echocardiography defines the

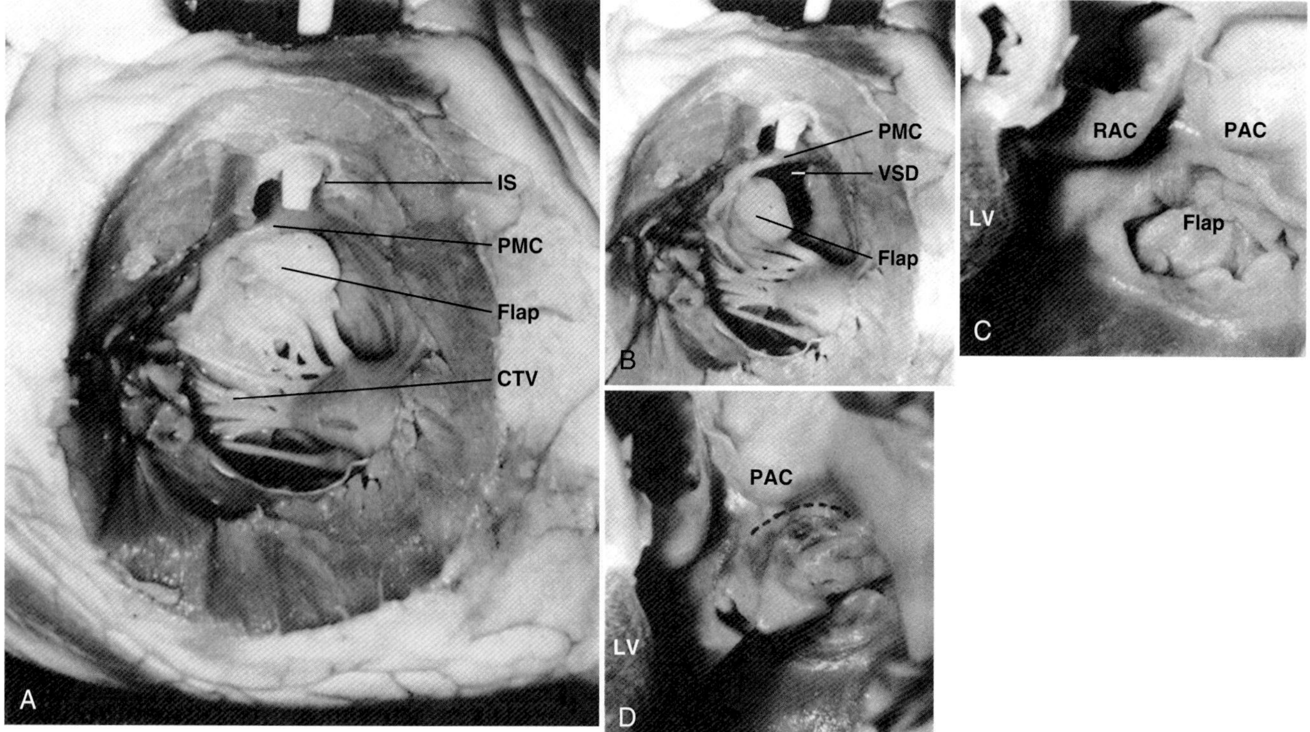

Figure 38-88 Tetralogy of Fallot with flap valve ventricular septal defect *(VSD)* and severe infundibular pulmonary stenosis. In this heart the pulmonary valve was normal and pulmonary trunk of near-normal size. **A** and **B,** Viewed from right ventricle (RV). Note extreme degree of RV hypertrophy and tight infundibular stenosis (probe). In this specimen the flap is continuous with anterior tricuspid leaflet. **B,** Flap has been moved rightward to expose large VSD. **C** and **D,** Viewed from left ventricle. Flap is hinged posteriorly *(dashed line)* beneath noncoronary aortic cusp and adjacent right cusp, where it becomes continuous with membranous septum. Key: *CTV,* Chordae of tricuspid valve; *IS,* infundibular septum; *LV,* left ventricle; *PAC,* posterior (noncoronary) aortic cusp; *PMC,* papillary muscle of conus (muscle of Lancisi); *RAC,* right aortic cusp.

intracardiac morphologic details and provides important information for estimating the degree of obstruction in the RV outflow tract and across the VSD. Cardiac catheterization is indicated only if there is a need to define pulmonary hemodynamics or morphology of the distal pulmonary arteries.

TECHNIQUE OF OPERATION

Intracardiac repair is similar to that for TF with pulmonary stenosis. However, severe RV hypertrophy makes relief of pulmonary stenosis more difficult and may also limit exposure of the VSD. Usually, wide excision of muscle is required. The fibrous flap is identified and excised unless it is atypical and part of the AV valve mechanism, which is rare. Then, its herniation into the VSD is simply reduced and the VSD repaired in the usual way. It may be necessary to attach the herniated portion to the tricuspid valve to prevent it from obstructing the RV outflow tract.

RESULTS

Hospital mortality after repair has, in the past, been relatively high.[F8] Four (24%; CL 12%-39%) of 17 patients in the GLH and UAB experiences died in hospital after repair (Table 38-15). One UAB death occurred in association with anomalous origin of the left main coronary artery from the pulmonary trunk and one GLH death in association with pulmonary atresia and a large fistulous communication between the left coronary artery and RV. Severe RV hypertrophy appears to be the primary incremental risk factor, and improved myocardial management may neutralize it. Late results in hospital survivors have been good.

INDICATIONS FOR OPERATION

Palliative shunting operations are inappropriate because they do not relieve the progressive RV pressure overload. Similarly, blind (or open) pulmonary valvotomy could result in excessive shunting from left to right through the VSD. One-stage repair is the proper treatment and is advisable when diagnosis is made.

Section V Double-Chamber Right Ventricle (Low-Lying Infundibular Pulmonary Stenosis with or without Ventricular Septal Defect)

DEFINITION

Low-lying infundibular pulmonary stenosis, so-called double-chamber RV, is a type of intraventricular stenosis that clearly separates the sinus (inflow) portion of the RV

Table 38-15 Hospital Mortality after Repair of Tetralogy with Flap Valve Ventricular Septal Defect (VSD) and Other Types of Pulmonary Stenosis and VSD

	UAB (1967 to July 1983)				GLH (1959 to 1983)			
		Hospital Deaths				Hospital Deaths		
Category	*n*	No.	%	CL (%)	*n*	No.	%	CL (%)
Tetralogy of Fallot with flap valve VSD	5	2	40	14-71	12	2	17	6-35
Low-lying infundibular PS[a]	48	1	2	0.3-7	45	2[b]	4	1-10
With VSD	41	1[c]	2	0.3-8	32	2	6	2-14
Without VSD	7	0	0	0-24	13	0	0	0-14
Other forms of infundibular PS[a]	22	0	0	0-8	—			
With VSD	17	0	0	0-11				
Without VSD	5	0	0	0-32				
Valvar PS with VSD	8	0	0	0-21	6	0	0	0-27
Valvar and infundibular PS (or atresia) with VSD	11	2	18	6-38	NA			

[a]In the GLH material, these two subsets are combined.
[b]Both deaths occurred in 1960, one in association with underdeveloped right ventricle.
[c]Operation in 1971; death with low cardiac output.
Key: *CL*, 70% Confidence limits; *NA*, not available; *PS*, pulmonary stenosis; *VSD*, ventricular septal defect.

from a typically, but not always, large and thin-walled infundibulum.[H10,L13] It is usually but not always associated with a small or moderate-sized and occasionally large VSD, which is usually juxtatricuspid in position, but it may have a narrow bar of muscle between it and the valve anulus. Also included in this section are similar cases with an intact ventricular septum, because they may be considered part of this overall spectrum. In many cases with intact ventricular septum, a VSD was present earlier in life, with spontaneous closure occurring because of the same process of hypertrophy and fibrosis that contributes to the RV obstruction.

Low-lying infundibular pulmonary stenosis may coexist with otherwise typical TF (see Section I).[L13] Low-lying infundibular pulmonary stenosis may also coexist with double outlet RV (see Chapter 53).[G3]

HISTORICAL NOTE

Like many cardiac anomalies, low-lying infundibular pulmonary stenosis was encountered by cardiac surgeons during the mid- and late 1950s, before the malformation was well recognized by morphologists as a discrete entity.[K29,S33,W11] However, case 1 in the 1933 report by Eakin and Abbott[E1] and cases 1 and 3 in the 1959 report by Blount and colleagues[B18] were examples of the entity, and Grant and colleagues clearly discussed this malformation in their 1961 publication.[G27] However, credit for the first description of the entity is generally given to Tsifutis and colleagues, who published their paper in the same year.[T11]

MORPHOLOGY

The important morphologic characteristics relate to the infundibulum, the ventricular septum, and the LV outflow tract. There can be substantial variation in all three areas.

The classic morphologic finding is the large thin-walled infundibular chamber, which gives rise to the appellation "two-chambered RV."[H10] The pulmonary valve and "anulus" are normal sized or large, as is the pulmonary trunk, and the right and left pulmonary arteries are virtually always large and free of stenoses or distributional anomalies. In some variations the infundibular chamber is not large. There is infundibular hypoplasia, and the anomalous muscle bundles arise from the infundibular septum a little more distally (downstream).

The stenosis is formed by accessory bulky muscle bundles concentrated at the junction of the sinus portion of the RV and infundibulum. In the most florid form, there is a bulky trabeculated muscular shelf lying almost in a coronal plane that separates a large, thin-walled infundibular chamber from a hypertrophied, thick-walled sinus portion containing the tricuspid valve apparatus and VSD. The shelf is often formed by medial and lateral anomalous muscle bundles that join the anterior free wall about halfway between ventricular apex and base.[B18] However, the shelf may be, in part, hypertrophied septoparietal bands.[R14] The stenotic ostium is usually centrally located, and in older patients it is surrounded by a bulky fibrous collar that further increases stenosis. There may be more than one ostium. This obstructing muscular diaphragm inserts so far inferiorly on the free wall that it lies nearly in a coronal plane, which predisposes the ventricular incision to be in the infundibular chamber. The muscular band on the right side usually seems to be the parietal extension of the infundibular septum.

The VSD is usually small or moderate in size, although it may be large or it may have closed, identified only by a fibrous dimple. It is usually perimembranous and juxtatricuspid and is overhung by thick tricuspid chordae, but it may have a bar of muscle at its posterior margin rather than abutting the tricuspid anulus. Importantly, the VSD, regardless of its size, does not demonstrate the characteristics of the VSD in the various forms of TF. Specifically, the infundibular septum is not anteriorly malaligned.

In about 5% of cases, important and otherwise typical subaortic stenosis (see Section II of Chapter 47) coexists with low-lying infundibular pulmonary stenosis.[R34] Why this relatively large proportion exists is unknown.[B6] A unifying theory, yet to be fully characterized, is the tendency for many of these patients to produce exuberant endocardial fibrosis that importantly contributes to the RV obstruction, closes or narrows the VSD, and extends across the VSD into the LV outflow tract, causing the subaortic stenosis (personal observation, Frank Hanley).

Other morphologic variations rarely exist. These include combined infundibular and valvar pulmonary stenosis with membranous or muscular VSD, or isolated valvar pulmonary stenosis with membranous or muscular VSD. It is likely that these cases represent coincidental occurrence of unrelated defects.

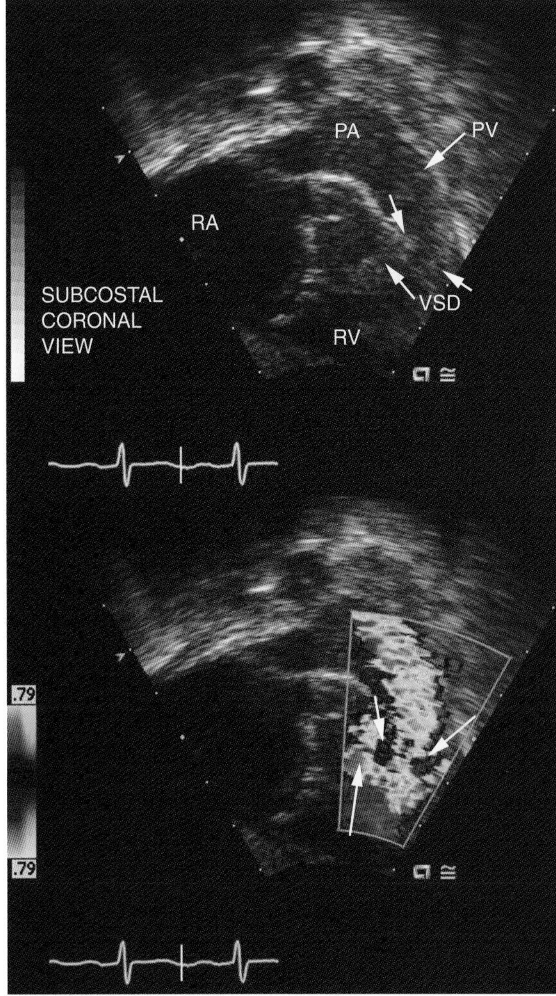

Figure 38-89 Subcostal coronal echocardiographic view in a patient with double-chambered right ventricle *(RV)*. Upper image is without color-flow Doppler. A ventricular septal defect *(VSD)* is present, positioned typically, proximal to the RV outflow tract obstruction. The muscular obstruction, shown between two unlabeled arrows, leads to a well-developed distal infundibular chamber, pulmonary valve *(PV)*, and pulmonary artery *(PA)*. Lower image is with color-flow Doppler. Paired arrows show muscular obstruction with narrowed flow signal. Single arrow shows flow through VSD. Key: *RA,* Right atrium.

CLINICAL FEATURES AND DIAGNOSTIC CRITERIA

Patients usually present with mild cyanosis in the midpart of the first decade of life, but they may present in the second decade or even in adult life. Increasingly, patients are diagnosed earlier in life, usually between 1 and 3 years of age, with clear evidence of mid-cavity RV obstruction. On examination the most striking feature is the loud systolic murmur, often grade 6 (heard with the stethoscope off the chest wall). Chest radiography is not specific, but the pulmonary trunk shadow along the upper left cardiac border is usually prominent.

Diagnosis is made by 2D echocardiography, which defines the typical mid-cavity RV obstruction, the VSD, if present, and the subaortic obstruction, if present (Figs. 38-89 and 38-90).

NATURAL HISTORY

Natural history can only be surmised. Because in some cases only a dimple remains in the perimembranous area at operation, the VSD presumably has a tendency to close spontaneously. Because few patients with this entity present in infancy, it is not surprising that the stenosis has been demonstrated to increase gradually in severity as the child grows.[C25,D5,F11,H8,H9] The progression can lead to complete infundibular atresia.[P10] Cyanosis is also presumed to be an acquired event. If a VSD is present, it will shunt left to right early in life before the RV obstruction progresses; no cyanosis will be present. If the VSD remains open and the RV obstruction progresses such that the VSD shunts right to left, cyanosis will develop.

TECHNIQUE OF OPERATION

Preparations for CPB, median sternotomy, and placement of stay sutures and purse-string sutures are as usual (see "Preparation for Cardiopulmonary Bypass" in Section III of Chapter 2). Examination of the heart may confirm presence of a characteristically large, thin-walled infundibular chamber, but this is not always evident externally. Usually a marginal branch of the right coronary artery courses over the underlying infundibular stenosis and should be preserved if the ventriculotomy approach to repair is used.

CPB is established, employing direct caval cannulation or caval cannulation via the right atrium (see Fig. 2-22 in Chapter 2). The left side is vented using a catheter placed through the right upper pulmonary vein. Mild hypothermia is typically used. The aortic root infusion catheter is inserted, the aorta clamped, and cold cardioplegia given (see "Cold Cardioplegia, Controlled Aortic Root Reperfusion, and [When Needed] Warm Cardioplegic Induction" in Chapter 3).

When the infundibulum is large and thin walled, repair can be through a transverse low infundibular incision or a right atrial incision.[F10,P8] With the infundibular incision the view is interesting and unique, because the interior of the smooth thin-walled infundibulum is exposed, and in its depth inferiorly is seen the ostium of the low-lying infundibular stenosis. A moment of carelessness could lead to misidentifying it as the VSD,[C23,L21] but further examination confirms it as the infundibulum because the tricuspid valve apparatus, lying entirely in the sinus portion of the RV, cannot be visualized.

Incision is made in the obstructing muscle mass anteriorly and to the left, which allows visualization of the interior of the sinus portion (proximal chamber) of the RV, tricuspid apparatus, and VSD. The part of the obstructing muscle mass that arches up and to the right from the infundibular septum (probably the parietal extension of the infundibular septum)

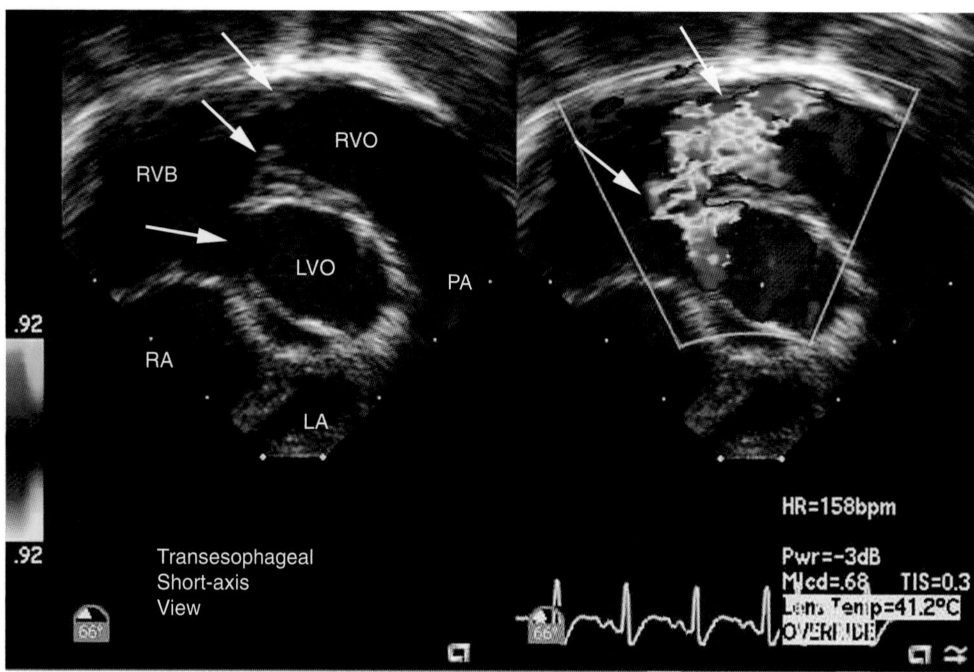

Figure 38-90 Transesophageal short-axis echocardiographic image of a patient with double-chambered right ventricle. Left image is without color-flow Doppler. Paired unlabeled arrows identify muscular obstruction. Single unlabeled arrow identifies ventricular septal defect, which is perimembranous. Right image shows color-flow Doppler pattern. Arrows identify ventricular septal defect flow and disturbed flow caused by muscular obstruction.

is dissected and largely resected. Before resecting the left side of the obstructive muscular collar, which is usually in part moderator band, location of the tricuspid papillary muscles is visualized, and they are protected as the left-sided heavy muscular band is dissected and largely amputated. There is then a wide exposure of the sinus portion of the RV and VSD. Although the VSD is typically small, it is repaired with a patch, just as for other VSDs in this area. If the VSD is small and overhung by thick chordae, a completely interrupted suture technique is preferable. The ventriculotomy is closed either primarily or with a narrow patch. The remainder of the procedure is completed as usual.

From the right atrial approach (Fig. 38-91, *A*), the obstructing muscle is located at its insertion anteriorly at the region of the moderator band. The anterior papillary muscle of the tricuspid valve is retracted. Relief of the muscular narrowing is accomplished much as for the atrial approach to classic TF, but exposure is easier because the obstruction is less anteriorly placed and more proximal in the RV. After muscle resection, the VSD, if present, is closed with a patch in a fashion similar to patch closure for isolated VSD by way of the right atrium (Fig. 38-91, *B*) (see Technique of Operation in Section I of Chapter 35). The right atriotomy is closed directly, and remainder of the procedure is completed as usual.

When the infundibular chamber is more hypoplastic, a vertical ventriculotomy and infundibular patching should probably be used routinely.

When associated subaortic obstruction is present, it should be addressed. If the patient has a large VSD, the fibrous tissue causing the obstruction in the LV outflow tract can often be visualized through the VSD and resected before closing the VSD. When the VSD is small or absent, the subaortic obstruction is addressed by way of an aortotomy, in a similar fashion to isolated subaortic membrane (see Chapter 47).

The morphology is so well suited to repair that usually no gradient is present after repair, nor are murmurs present postoperatively.

SPECIAL FEATURES OF POSTOPERATIVE CARE

Postoperative care is as usual (see Chapter 5).

RESULTS

Early (Hospital) Death

Hospital mortality after repair should approach zero.[G1,T5]

Time-Related Survival

Long-term results are excellent, with no late deaths and all patients asymptomatic.[G1,H6,T5] In the University of Michigan experience, among 20 patients followed for at least 20 years, 85% were in NYHA functional class I and only one (5%) had hemodynamically important impairment of cardiac function.[K43] Similarly, in the study by Telagh and colleagues,[T5] there was no functional or hemodynamic impairment at follow-up extending to 11 years.

INDICATIONS FOR OPERATION

Diagnosis of the malformation is an indication for elective repair.

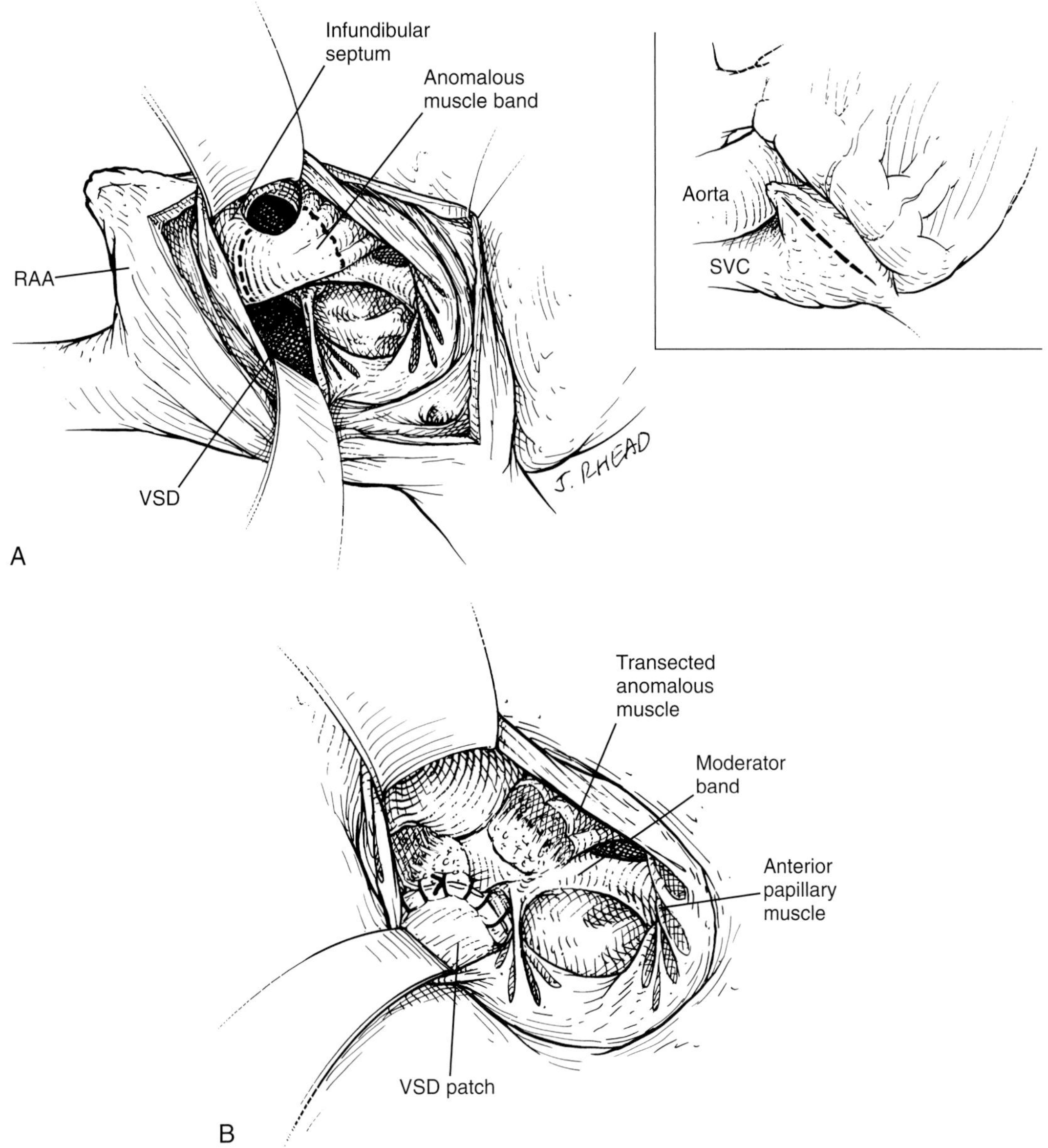

Figure 38-91 Low-lying infundibular pulmonary stenosis. **A,** *Inset* Usual high right atriotomy is made as for right atrial approach to repair tetralogy of Fallot (TF). Anomalous muscle band arises from moderator band and is downstream from ventricular septal defect *(VSD)*. Proposed incisions for resecting obstructing anomalous bands are shown *(dashed lines)*. **B,** After relief of the obstruction, VSD is closed in same manner as for TF. Key: *RAA,* Right atrial appendage; *SVC,* superior vena cava.

Section VI Other Forms of Infundibular or Valvar Pulmonary Stenosis and Ventricular Septal Defect

A few patients with infundibular pulmonary stenosis, with or without a VSD, do not meet the criteria for diagnosis of TF or low-lying infundibular stenosis. These are included in this section.

Some of these malformations may be similar in origin to low-lying infundibular pulmonary stenosis, except that there is infundibular hypoplasia and the anomalous muscle bundles arise from the infundibular septum a little more distally (downstream). Other examples in this subset probably represent instances in which the only discernible malformation at birth is a large VSD. With time, however, the parietal extension of the infundibular septum hypertrophies out of proportion to the rest of the right ventricle, and in some cases the VSD narrows or closes.[C25] Finally, occasionally valvar and infundibular stenosis may both coexist along with a VSD, in the absence of the typical morphology of TF.

Diagnosis, natural history, and techniques of repair are similar to those for low-lying infundibular pulmonary stenosis, except that a vertical ventriculotomy and infundibular patching should probably be used routinely. It is important to recognize the infundibular stenosis at time of repair of the VSD, because otherwise it can persist or worsen and reoperation may be required for relief.[D19,M11]

Indications for operation are the same as for low-lying infundibular pulmonary stenosis.

Surprisingly, isolated valvar pulmonary stenosis with VSD is only rarely reported in the literature. It does exist but is not common (and may well be underreported), and may merely represent chance coexistence of these two malformations. The combination is an indication for elective operation by the techniques described earlier.

38A Values of Variables Used in Nomograms

Values in Fig. 38-49

Specific values entered into the multivariable equation were hematocrit 50%, no more than one previous palliative operation, no Potts anastomosis, no previous direct approach to RV outlet obstruction, no multiple VSDs, no dextrocardia, no absence of unbranched hilar portion of one pulmonary artery, average prevalence of transanular patch placement (31%), and postrepair (OR) $P_{RV/LV}$ of 0.55. For age 6 months, 12 months, 24 months, and 48 months, body surface area was entered as 0.345 m^2, 0.4125 m^2, 0.5025 m^2, and 0.630 m^2, respectively.

Values in Fig. 38-51

Specific values entered into the multivariable equation were hematocrit 50%, no more than one previous palliative operation, no Potts anastomosis, no previous direct approach to RV outlet obstruction, no multiple VSDs, no dextrocardia, no absence of unbranched hilar portion of one pulmonary artery, date of operation 1988, and postrepair (OR) $P_{RV/LV}$ of 0.6.

Values in Fig. 38-53

Specific values entered into the multivariable equation were age 6 months at repair and postrepair (ICU) $P_{RV/LV}$ of 0.45.

38B Relation of Body Surface Area to Age

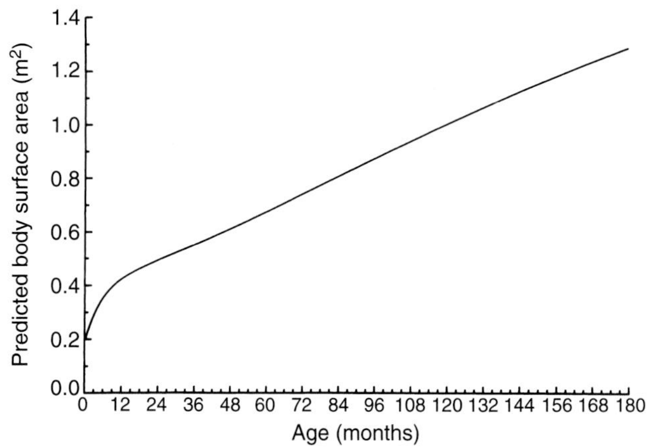

Figure 38B-1 Nomogram of equation relating body surface area to age in patients with tetralogy of Fallot. Equation is based on data from 1533 patients with tetralogy of Fallot and pulmonary stenosis or atresia (UAB experience). They ranged in age from 1 day to 57 years, and in body surface area from 0.12 to 2.3 m^2. The equation is as follows:

$$\mathrm{Ln(BSA)} = 4.504 + 27.82\, a^3 - 45.51 \cdot a^4 + 26.39 \cdot a^5 - 5.238 \cdot a^6$$

where $a = \mathrm{Ln}\,[\mathrm{Ln}(\text{age} + 9)]$, age is in months, *Ln* is the natural logarithm (double logarithmic transformation), and *Ln [BSA(m²)]* is the natural logarithm of body surface area.

REFERENCES

A

1. Abdulali SA, Silverton NP, Yakirevich VS, Ionescu MI. Right ventricular outflow tract reconstruction with a bovine pericardial monocusp patch. J Thorac Cardiovasc Surg 1985;89:764.
2. Ackerman MJ, Wylam ME, Feldt RH, Porter CJ, Dewald G, Scanlon PD, et al. Pulmonary atresia with ventricular septal defect and persistent airway hyperresponsiveness. J Thorac Cardiovasc Surg 2001;122:169.
3. Agarwal KC, Edwards WD, Feldt RH, Danielson GK, Puga FJ, McGoon DC. Pathogenesis of nonobstructive fibrous peels in right-sided porcine-valved extracardiac conduits. J Thorac Cardiovasc Surg 1982;83:584.
4. Akasaka T, Itoh K, Ohkawa Y, Nakayama S, Miyamoto H, Nishi T, et al. Surgical treatment of anomalous origin of the left coronary artery from the pulmonary artery associated with tetralogy of Fallot. Ann Thorac Surg 1981;31:469.
5. Albertal G, Swan HJ, Kirklin JW. Hemodynamic studies two weeks to six years after repair of tetralogy of Fallot. Circulation 1964;29:583.
6. Alfieri O, Blackstone EH, Kirklin JW, Pacifico AD, Bargeron LM Jr. Surgical treatment of tetralogy of Fallot with pulmonary atresia. J Thorac Cardiovasc Surg 1978;76:321.
7. Alfieri O, Blackstone EH, Parenzan L. Growth of the pulmonary anulus and pulmonary arteries after the Waterston anastomosis. J Thorac Cardiovasc Surg 1979;78:440.
8. Alfieri O, Locatelli G, Bianchi T, Vanini V, Parenzan L. Repair of tetralogy of Fallot after Waterston anastomosis. J Thorac Cardiovasc Surg 1979;77:826.
9. Almeida RS, Wyse RK, de Leval MR, Elliott MJ, Stark J. Long-term results of homograft valves in extracardiac conduits. Eur J Cardiothorac Surg 1989;3:488.
10. Amin Z, McElhinney DB, Reddy VM, Moore P, Hanley FL, Teitel DF. Coronary to pulmonary artery collaterals in patients with pulmonary atresia and ventricular septal defect. Ann Thorac Surg 2000;70:119.
11. Anaclerio S, Marino B, Carotti A, Digilio MC, Toscano A, Gitto P, et al. Pulmonary atresia with ventricular septal defect: prevalence of deletion 22q11 in the different anatomic patterns. Ital Heart J 2001;2:384.
12. Anderson RH, Allwork SP, Ho SY, Lenox CC, Zuberbuhler JR. Surgical anatomy of tetralogy of Fallot. J Thorac Cardiovasc Surg 1981;81:887.
13. Anderson RH, Devine WA, Del Nido P. The surgical anatomy of tetralogy of Fallot with pulmonary atresia rather than pulmonary stenosis. J Card Surg 1991;6:41.
14. Anderson RH, Jacobs ML. The anatomy of tetralogy of Fallot with pulmonary stenosis. Cardiol Young 2008;18:12-21.
15. Arciniegas E, Blackstone EH, Pacifico AD, Kirklin JW. Classic shunting operations as part of two-stage repair of tetralogy of Fallot. Ann Thorac Surg 1979;27:514.
16. Arciniegas E, Farooki ZQ, Hakimi M, Green EW. Results of two-stage surgical treatment of tetralogy of Fallot. J Thorac Cardiovasc Surg 1980;79:876.
17. Arciniegas E, Farooki ZQ, Hakimi M, Perry BL, Green EW. Early and late results of total correction of tetralogy of Fallot. J Thorac Cardiovasc Surg 1980;80:770.
18. Arciniegas E, Farooki ZQ, Hakimi M, Perry BL, Green EW. Classic shunting operations for congenital cyanotic heart defects. J Thorac Cardiovasc Surg 1982;84:88.
19. Arensman FW, Francis PD, Helmsworth JA, Benzing G 3rd, Schreiber JT, Schwartz DC, et al. Early medical and surgical intervention for tetralogy of Fallot with absence of pulmonic valve. J Thorac Cardiovasc Surg 1982;84:430.
20. Askovich B, Hawkins JA, Sower CT, Minich LL, Tani LY, Stoddard G, et al. Right ventricle-to-pulmonary artery conduit longevity: is it related to allograft size? Ann Thorac Surg 2007;84:907-911.

B

1. Bailey WW, Kirklin JW, Bargeron LM Jr, Pacifico AD, Kouchoukos NT. Late results with synthetic valved external conduits from venous ventricle to pulmonary arteries. Circulation 1977;56:II73.
2. Bargeron LM Jr, Elliott LP, Soto B, Bream PR, Curry GC. Axial cineangiography in congenital heart disease. Section I. Concept, technical and anatomic considerations. Circulation 1977;56:1075.
3. Barnard CN, Schrire V. The surgical treatment of the tetralogy of Fallot. Thorax 1961;16:346.
4. Barratt-Boyes BG, Neutze JM. Primary repair of tetralogy of Fallot in infancy using profound hypothermia with circulatory arrest and limited cardiopulmonary bypass: a comparison with conventional two-stage management. Ann Surg 1973;178:406.
5. Barratt-Boyes BG, Simpson M, Neutze JM. Intracardiac surgery in neonates and infants using deep hypothermia with surface cooling and limited cardiopulmonary bypass. Circulation 1971;43:I25.
6. Baumstark A, Fellows KE, Rosenthal A. Combined double chambered right ventricle and discrete subaortic stenosis. Circulation 1978;57:299.
7. Beach PM Jr, Bowman FO Jr, Kaiser GA, Malm JR. Total correction of tetralogy of Fallot in adolescents and adults. Circulation 1971;43:I37.
8. Becker AE, Connor M, Anderson RH. Tetralogy of Fallot: a morphometric and geometric study. Am J Cardiol 1975;35:402.
9. Bender HW Jr, Fisher RD, Conkle DM, Martin CE, Graham TP. Selective operative treatment for tetralogy of Fallot. Ann Surg 1976;183:685.
10. Bertranou EG, Blackstone EH, Hazelrig JB, Turner ME, Kirklin JW. Life expectancy without surgery in tetralogy of Fallot. Am J Cardiol 1978;42:458.
11. Bharati S, Lev M, Kirklin JW. Cardiac surgery and the conduction system, 2nd Ed. Mount Kisco, NY: Futura, 1992.
12. Bharati S, Paul MH, Idriss FS, Potkin RT, Lev M. The surgical anatomy of pulmonary atresia with ventricular septal defect: pseudotruncus. J Thorac Cardiovasc Surg 1975;69:713.
13. Binet JP, Hvass U, Bruniaux J, Langlois J, Planche C, Dreyfus G, et al. Complete correction of tetralogy of Fallot without opening the right ventricle. Arch Mal Coeur Vaiss 1980;73:1185.
14. Bjarke B. Oxygen uptake and cardiac output during submaximal and maximal exercise in adult subjects with totally corrected tetralogy of Fallot. Acta Med Scand 1975;197:177.
15. Blackstone EH, Kirklin JW, Bertranou EG, Labrosse CJ, Soto B, Bargeron LM Jr. Preoperative prediction from cineangiograms of postrepair right ventricular pressure in tetralogy of Fallot. J Thorac Cardiovasc Surg 1979;78:542.
16. Blalock A, Taussig HB. The surgical treatment of malformations of the heart in which there is pulmonary stenosis or pulmonary atresia. JAMA 1945;128:189.
17. Blondeau PH, Nottin R, d'Allaines C, Carpentier A, Soyer R, Bouchard F, et al. Communications interventricularies residuelles apres reparation complete de la tetralogie de Fallot. Coeur 1977;3:31.
18. Blount SG Jr, Vigoda PS, Swan H. Isolated infundibular stenosis. Am Heart J 1959;57:684.
19. Bocala RR, Guller B, Danielson GK, Feldt RH. Left anterior hemiblock and complete repair of tetralogy of Fallot (abstract). Pediatr Res 1974;8:347.
20. Bogers AJ, Rohmer J, Wolsky SA, Quaegebeur JM, Huysmans HA. Coronary artery fistula as source of pulmonary circulation in pulmonary atresia with ventricular septal defect. Thorac Cardiovasc Surg 1990;38:30.
21. Bonchek LI, Starr A, Sunderland CO, Menashe VD. Natural history of tetralogy of Fallot in infancy. Circulation 1973;48:392.
22. Boni L, Garcia E, Galletti L, Perez A, Herrera D, Ramos V, et al. Current strategies in tetralogy of Fallot repair: pulmonary valve sparing and evolution of right ventricle/left ventricle pressures ratio. Eur J Cardiothorac Surg 2009;35:885-90.
23. Borow KM, Green LH, Castaneda AR, Keane JF. Left ventricular function after repair of tetralogy of Fallot and its relationship to age at surgery. Circulation 1980;61:1150.
24. Boucek MM, Webster HE, Orsmond GS, Ruttenberg HD. Balloon pulmonary valvotomy: palliation for cyanotic heart disease. Am Heart J 1988;115:318.
25. Bove EL, Byrum CJ, Thomas FD, Kavey RE, Sondheimer HM, Blackman MS, et al. The influence of pulmonary insufficiency on ventricular function following repair of tetralogy of Fallot. Evaluation using radionuclide ventriculography. J Thorac Cardiovasc Surg 1983;85:691.
26. Bove EL, Kavey RE, Byrum CJ, Sondheimer HM, Blackman MS, Thomas FD. Improved right ventricular function following late pulmonary valve replacement for residual pulmonary insufficiency or stenosis. J Thorac Cardiovasc Surg 1985;90:50.
27. Boyce SW, Turley K, Yee ES, Verrier ED, Ebert PA. The fate of the 12 mm porcine valved conduit from the right ventricle to the

pulmonary artery. A ten-year experience. J Thorac Cardiovasc Surg 1988;95:201.
28. Brawn WJ, Jones T, Davies B, Barron D. How we manage patients with major aorta pulmonary collaterals. Semin Thorac Cardiovasc Surg Pediatr Card Surg Annu 2009:152-7.
29. Breymann T, Blanz U, Wojtalik MA, Daenen W, Hetzer R, Sarris G, et al. European Contegra multicentre study: 7-year results after 165 valved bovine jugular vein graft implantations. Thorac Cardiovasc Surg 2009;57:257-69.
30. Brizard CP, Liava'a M, d'Udekem Y. Pulmonary atresia, VSD and Mapcas: repair without unifocalization. Semin Thorac Cardiovasc Surg Pediatr Card Surg Annu 2009:139-44.
31. Brock RC. Pulmonary valvulotomy for relief of congenital pulmonary stenosis. Report of 3 cases. Br Med J 1948;1:1121.
32. Brock RC, Campbell M. Infundibular resection or dilatation for infundibular stenosis. Br Heart J 1950;12:403.
33. Brown JW, Ruzmetov M, Rodefeld MD, Vijay P, Darragh RK. Valved bovine jugular vein conduits for right ventricular outflow tract reconstruction in children: an attractive alternative to pulmonary homograft. Ann Thorac Surg 2006;82:909-16.
34. Brown SC, Eyskens B, Mertens L, Dumoulin M, Gewillig M. Percutaneous treatment of stenosed major aortopulmonary collaterals with balloon dilation and stenting: what can be achieved? Heart 1998;79:24.
35. Buechel ER, Dave HH, Kellenberger CJ, Dodge-Khatami A, Pretre R, Berger F, et al. Remodelling of the right ventricle after early pulmonary valve replacement in children with repaired tetralogy of Fallot: assessment by cardiovascular magnetic resonance. Eur Heart J 2005;26:2721-7.
36. Burczynski PL, McKay R, Arnold R, Mitchell DR, Sabino GP. Homograft replacement of the pulmonary artery bifurcation. J Thorac Cardiovasc Surg 1989;98:623.
37. Byrne JP, Hawkins JA, Battiste CE, Khoury GH. Palliative procedures in tetralogy of Fallot with absent pulmonary valve: a new approach. Ann Thorac Surg 1982;33:499.

C

1. Cairns JA, Dobell AR, Gibbons JE, Tessler I. Prognosis of right bundle branch block and left anterior hemiblock after intracardiac repair of tetralogy of Fallot. Am Heart J 1975;90:549.
2. Calder AL, Barratt-Boyes BG, Brandt PW, Neutze JM. Postoperative evaluation of patients with tetralogy of Fallot repaired in infancy. J Thorac Cardiovasc Surg 1979;77:704.
3. Calder AL, Brandt PW, Barratt-Boyes BG, Neutze JM. Variant of tetralogy of Fallot with absent pulmonary valve leaflets and origin of one pulmonary artery from the ascending aorta. Am J Cardiol 1980;46:106.
4. Calder AL, Chan NS, Clarkson PM, Kerr AR, Neutze JM. Progress of patients with pulmonary atresia after systemic to pulmonary arterial shunts. Ann Thorac Surg 1991;51:40l.
5. Calder AL, Kirker JA, Neutze JM, Starling MB. Pathology of the ductus arteriosus treated with prostaglandins. Comparison with untreated cases. Pediatr Cardiol 1984;5:85.
6. Capelli H, Ross D, Somerville J. Aortic regurgitation in tetrad of Fallot and pulmonary atresia. Am J Cardiol 1982;49:1979.
7. Carotti A, Di Donato RM, Squitieri C, Guccione P, Catena G. Total repair of pulmonary atresia with ventricular septal defect and major aortopulmonary collaterals: an integrated approach. J Thorac Cardiovasc Surg 1998;116:914.
8. Castaneda AR. Classical repair of tetralogy of Fallot: timing, technique, and results. Semin Thorac Cardiovasc Surg 1990;2:70.
9. Castaneda AR, Freed MD, Williams RG, Norwood WI. Repair of tetralogy of Fallot in infancy. Early and late results. J Thorac Cardiovasc Surg 1977;74:372.
10. Castaneda AR, Kirklin JW. Tetralogy of Fallot with aorticopulmonary window. Report of two surgical cases. J Thorac Cardiovasc Surg 1977;74:467.
11. Castaneda AR, Mayer J, Jonas R, Walsh EP, Lang P. Tetralogy of Fallot: repair in infancy. In: Crupi G, Parenzan L, Anderson RH, eds. Perspectives in pediatric cardiology, Vol. 2. Pediatric cardiac surgery, Part 1. New York: Futura Publishing, 1989.
12. Castaneda AR, Norwood WI. Fallot's tetralogy. In: Stark J, de Leval M, eds. Surgery for congenital heart defects. Orlando, Fla.: Grune & Stratton, 1983.
13. Castaneda AR, Sade RM, Lamberti J, Nicoloff DM. Reoperation for residual defects after repair of tetralogy of Fallot. Surgery 1974;76:1010.
14. Centazzo S, Montigny M, Davignon A, Chartrand C, Fournier A, Marchand T. Use of acetylsalicylic acid to improve patency of subclavian to pulmonary artery Gore-Tex shunts. Can J Cardiol 1993;9:243.
15. Chan FP. MR and CT imaging of the pediatric patient with structural heart disease. Semin Thorac Cardiovasc Surg Pediatr Card Surg Annu 2009:99-105.
16. Chesler E, Korns ME, Edwards JE. Anomalies of the tricuspid valve, including pouches, resembling aneurysms of the membranous ventricular septum. Am J Cardiol 1968;21:661.
17. Chessa M, Butera G, Bonhoeffer P, Iserin L, Kachaner J, Lyonnet S, et al. Relation of genotype 22qll deletion to phenotype of pulmonary vessels in tetralogy of Fallot and pulmonary atresia–ventricular septal defect. Heart 1998;79:186.
18. Cheung MM, Konstantinov IE, Redington AN. Late complications of repair of tetralogy of Fallot and indications for pulmonary valve replacement. Semin Thorac Cardiovasc Surg 2005;17:155-9.
19. Chiariello L, Meyer J, Wukasch DC, Hallman GL, Cooley DA. Intracardiac repair of tetralogy of Fallot. Five-year review of 403 patients. J Thorac Cardiovasc Surg 1975;70:529.
20. Ciaravella JM Jr, McGoon DC, Danielson GK, Wallace RB, Mair DD, Ilstrup DM. Experience with the extracardiac conduit. J Thorac Cardiovasc Surg 1979;78:920.
21. Clarke DR, Campbell DN, Pappas G. Pulmonary allograft conduit repair of tetralogy of Fallot. An alternative to transanular patch repair. J Thorac Cardiovasc Surg 1989;98:730.
22. Clayman JA, Ankeney JL, Liebman J. Results of complete repair of tetralogy of Fallot in 156 consecutive patients. Am J Surg 1975; 130:601.
23. Coates JR, McClenathan JE, Scott LW 3rd. The double-chambered right ventricle. A diagnostic and operative pitfall. Am J Cardiol 1964;14:561.
24. Cole RB, Muster AJ, Fixler DE, Paul MH. Long-term results of aortopulmonary anastomosis for tetralogy of Fallot. Circulation 1971;43:263.
25. Corone P, Doyon F, Gaudeau S, Guerin F, Vernant P, Ducam H, et al. Natural history of ventricular septal defect. A study involving 790 cases. Circulation 1977;55:908.
26. Cosio FG, Wang Y, Nicoloff DM. Membranous right ventricular outflow obstruction. Am J Cardiol 1973;32:1000.
27. Cumming GR, Carr W. Relief of dyspneic attacks in Fallot's tetralogy with propranolol. Lancet 1966;l:519.
28. Curzon CL, Milford-Beland S, Li JS, O'Brien SM, Jacobs JP, Jacobs ML, et al. Cardiac surgery in infants with low birth weight is associated with increased mortality: analysis of the Society of Thoracic Surgeons Congenital Heart Database. J Thorac Cardiovasc Surg 2008;135:546-51.

D

1. Dabizzi RP, Caprioli G, Aiazzi L, Castelli C, Baldrighi G, Parenzan L, et al. Distribution and anomalies of coronary arteries in tetralogy of Fallot. Circulation 1980;61:95.
2. Dadlani GH, John JB, Cohen MS. Echocardiography in tetralogy of Fallot. Cardiol Young 2008;18:22-8.
3. Daily PO, Stinson EB, Griepp RB, Shumway NE. Tetralogy of Fallot. Choice of surgical procedure. J Thorac Cardiovasc Surg 1978;75:338.
4. D'Allaines C, Sover R, Rioux C, Blondeau P, Cachera JP, Dubost C. Tetralogies de Fallot: Resultats a distance de la correction complete. Nouv Presse Med 1973;2:961.
5. Danilowicz D, Hoffman JI, Rudolph AM. Serial studies of pulmonary stenosis in infancy and childhood. Br Heart J 1975;37:808.
6. Daoud G, Kaplan S, Helmsworth JA. Tetralogy of Fallot and pulmonary hypertension. Am J Dis Child 1966;111:166.
7. Dave HH, Buechel ER, Dodge-Khatami A, Kadner A, Rousson V, Bauersfeld U, et al. Early insertion of a pulmonary valve for chronic regurgitation helps restoration of ventricular dimensions. Ann Thorac Surg 2005;80:1615-21.
8. Davidson JS. Anastomosis between the ascending aorta and the main pulmonary artery in the tetralogy of Fallot. Thorax 1955; 10:348.
9. D'Cruz I, Lendrum BL, Novak G. Congenital absence of the pulmonary valve. Am Heart J 1964;68:728.
10. Deanfield JE, Ho SY, Anderson RH, McKenna WJ, Allwork SP, Hallidie-Smith KA. Late sudden death after repair of tetralogy Fallot: a clinicopathologic study. Circulation 1983;67:626.

11. de Leval MR, McKay R, Jones M, Stark J, Macartney FJ. Modified Blalock-Taussig shunt. Use of subclavian artery orifice as flow regulator in prosthetic systemic–pulmonary artery shunts. J Thorac Cardiovasc Surg 1981;81:112.
12. Delisle G, Olley PM. Submaximal effort test in children with Fallot's tetralogy before and after surgical correction. Union Med Can 1974;103:886.
13. DeRuiter MC, Gittenbergerde Groot AC, Bogers AJ, Elzenga NJ. The restricted surgical relevance of morphologic criteria to classify systemic–pulmonary collateral arteries in pulmonary atresia with ventricular septal defect. J Thorac Cardiovasc Surg 1994;108:692.
14. Di Benedetto G, Tiraboschi R, Vanini V, Annecchino P, Aiazzi L, Caprioli C, et al. Systemic–pulmonary artery shunt using PTFE prosthesis (Gore-Tex). Early results and long-term follow-up on 105 consecutive cases. Thorac Cardiovasc Surg 1981;29:143.
15. Dickinson DF, Wilkinson JL, Smith A, Hamilton DI, Anderson RH. Variations in the morphology of the ventricular septal defect and disposition of the atrioventricular conduction tissues in tetralogy of Fallot. Thorac Cardiovasc Surg 1982;30:243.
16. Di Donato RM, Jonas RA, Lang P, Rome JJ, Mayer JE Jr, Castaneda AR. Neonatal repair of tetralogy of Fallot with and without pulmonary atresia. J Thorac Cardiovasc Surg 1991;101:126.
17. Digilio MC, Marino B, Grazioli S, Agostino D, Giannotti A, Dallapiccola B. Comparison of occurrence of genetic syndromes in ventricular septal defect with pulmonic stenosis (classic tetralogy of Fallot) versus ventricular septal defect with pulmonic atresia. Am J Cardiol 1996;77:1375.
18. Dobell AR, Charrette EP, Chughtai MS. Correction of tetralogy of Fallot in the young child. J Thorac Cardiovasc Surg 1968;55:70.
19. Dolara A, Dellocchio T, Diligenti LM, Manetti A, Vergassola R. Pulmonary infundibular stenosis developing after closure of ventricular septal defect. Acta Cardiol 1975;30:221.
20. Donahoo JS, Gardner TJ, Zahka K, Kidd BS. Systemic–pulmonary shunts in neonates and infants using microporous expanded polytetrafluoroethylene: immediate and late results. Ann Thorac Surg 1980;30:146.
21. Dos L, Dadashev A, Tanous D, Ferreira-Gonzalez IJ, Haberer K, Siu SC, et al. Pulmonary valve replacement in repaired tetralogy of Fallot: determinants of early postoperative adverse outcomes. J Thorac Cardiovasc Surg 2009;138:553-9.

E

1. Eakin WW, Abbott ME. Stenosis of the pulmonary conus at the lower bulbar orifice (conus a separate chamber) and closed interventricular septum with two illustrative cases. Presented at the Meeting of the American Association of Pathologists and Bacteriologists, Washington, DC, May 9, 1933.
2. Ebert PA. Second operations for pulmonary stenosis or insufficiency after repair of tetralogy of Fallot. Am J Cardiol 1982;50:637.
3. Edmunds LH Jr, Saxena NC, Friedman S, Rashkind WJ, Dodd PF. Transatrial resection of the obstructed right ventricular infundibulum. Circulation 1976;54:117.
4. Edwards BS, Lucas RV Jr, Lock JE, Edwards JE. Morphologic changes in the pulmonary arteries after percutaneous balloon angioplasty for pulmonary arterial stenosis. Circulation 1985;71:195.
5. Edwards JE, McGoon DC. Absence of anatomic origin from heart of pulmonary arterial supply. Circulation 1973;47:393.
6. Ehrenhaft JL, Theilen EO, Fisher J. Ectopic tricuspid leaflet producing symptoms of infundibular pulmonic stenosis. Ann Surg 1959;150:937.
7. El-Said HG, Clapp S, Fagan TE, Conwell J, Nihill MR. Stenting of stenosed aortopulmonary collaterals and shunts for palliation of pulmonary atresia/ventricular septal defect. Catheter Cardiovasc Interv 2000;49:430.
8. Elzenga NJ, Gittenbergerde Groot AC. The ductus arteriosus and stenoses of the pulmonary arteries in pulmonary atresia. Int J Cardiol 1986;11:195.
9. Elzenga NJ, von Suylen RJ, Frohn-Mulder I, Essed CE, Bos E, Quaegebeur JM. Juxtaductal pulmonary artery coarctation. An underestimated cause of branch pulmonary artery stenosis in patients with pulmonary atresia or stenosis and a ventricular septal defect. J Thorac Cardiovasc Surg 1990;100:416.
10. Emmanoulides GC, Thanopoulos B, Siassi B, Fishbein M. "Agenesis" of ductus arteriosus associated with the syndrome of tetralogy of Fallot and absent pulmonary valve. Am J Cardiol 1976;37:403.
11. Ergin MA, Griepp RB. Total correction of tetralogy of Fallot. How to deal with complicated ascending aorta–right pulmonary artery anastomosis. J Thorac Cardiovasc Surg 1979;77:469.

F

1. Fabricius J, Hansen PF, Lindeneg O. Pulmonary atresia developing after a shunt operation for Fallot's tetralogy. Br Heart J 1961;23:556.
2. Faller K, Haworth SG, Taylor JF, Macartney FJ. Duplicate sources of pulmonary blood supply in pulmonary atresia with ventricular septal defect. Br Heart J 1981;46:263.
3. Feldt RH, DuShane JW, Titus JL. The anatomy of the atrioventricular conduction system in ventricular septal defect and tetralogy of Fallot: correlations with the electrocardiogram and vectorcardiogram. Circulation 1966;34:774.
4. Fellows KE, Freed MK, Keane JF, Praagh R, Bernhard WF, Castaneda AC. Results of routine preoperative coronary angiography in tetralogy of Fallot. Circulation 1975;51:561.
5. Fellows KE, Smith J, Keane JF. Preoperative angiocardiography in infants with tetrad of Fallot. Review of 36 cases. Am J Cardiol 1981;47:1279.
6. Ferencz C. The pulmonary vascular bed in tetralogy of Fallot. I. Changes associated with pulmonary stenosis. Bull Johns Hopkins Hosp 1960;106:81.
7. Finck SJ, Puga FJ, Danielson GK. Pulmonary valve insertion during reoperation for tetralogy of Fallot. Ann Thorac Surg 1988;45:610.
8. Flanagan MF, Foran RB, Van Praagh R, Jonas R, Sanders SP. Tetralogy of Fallot with obstruction of the ventricular septal defect: spectrum of echocardiographic findings. J Am Coll Cardiol 1988;11:386.
9. Flege JB Jr, Vlad P, Ehrenhaft JL. Aneurysm of the triscuspid valve causing infundibular obstruction. Ann Thorac Surg 1967;3:446.
10. Ford DK, Bullaboy CA, Derkac WM, Hopkins RA, Jennings RB Jr, Johnson DH. Transatrial repair of double-chambered right ventricle. Ann Thorac Surg 1988;46:412.
11. Forster JW, Humphries JO. Right ventricular anomalous muscle bundle. Clinical and laboratory presentation and natural history. Circulation 1971;43:115.
12. Fraser CD Jr, McKenzie ED, Cooley DA. Tetralogy of Fallot: surgical management individualized to the patient. Ann Thorac Surg 2001;71:1556-63.
13. Freedom RM, Pongiglione G, Williams WG, Trusler GA, Moes CA, Rowe RD. Pulmonary vein wedge angiography: indications, results, and surgical correlates in 25 patients. Am J Cardiol 1983;51:936.
14. Freedom RM, Pongiglione G, Williams WG, Trusler GA, Rowe RD. Palliative right ventricular outflow tract construction for patients with pulmonary atresia, ventricular septal defect, and hypoplastic pulmonary arteries. J Thorac Cardiovasc Surg 1983;86:24.
15. Fuhrman BP, Bass JL, Castaneda-Zuniga W, Amplatz K, Lock JE. Coil embolization of congenital thoracic vascular anomalies in infants and children. Circulation 1984;70:285.
16. Furuse A, Mizuno A, Shindo G, Yamaguchi T, Saigusa M. Optimal size of outflow patch in total correction of tetralogy of Fallot. Jpn Heart J 1977;18:629.
17. Fuster V, McGoon DC, Kennedy MA, Ritter DG, Kirklin JW. Long-term evaluation (12 to 22 years) of open heart surgery for tetralogy of Fallot. Am J Cardiol 1980;46:635.

G

1. Galal O, Al-Halees Z, Solymar L, Hatle L, Mieles A, Darwish A, et al. Double-chambered right ventricle in 73 patients: spectrum of the disease and surgical results of transatrial repair. Can J Cardiol 2000;16:167-74.
2. Gale AW, Arciniegas E, Green EW, Blackstone EH, Kirklin JW. Growth of the pulmonary anulus and pulmonary arteries after the Blalock-Taussig shunt. J Thorac Cardiovasc Surg 1979;77:459.
3. Gallucci V, Scalia D, Thiene G, Mazzucco A, Valfre C. Double-chambered right ventricle: surgical experience and anatomical considerations. Thorac Cardiovasc Surg 1980;28:13.
4. Garson A Jr, Gillette PC, Gutgesell HP, McNamara DG. Stress-induced ventricular arrhythmia after repair of tetralogy of Fallot. Am J Cardiol 1980;46:1006.
5. Garson A Jr, Gillette PC, McNamara DG. Propranolol: the preferred palliation for tetralogy of Fallot. Am J Cardiol 1981; 47:1098.
6. Garson A Jr, Nihill MR, McNamara DG, Cooley DA. Status of the adult and adolescent after repair of tetralogy of Fallot. Circulation 1979;59:1232.

7. Gatzoulis MA, Balaji S, Webber SA, Siu SC, Hokanson JS, Poile C, et al. Risk factors for arrhythmia and sudden cardiac death late after repair of tetralogy of Fallot: a multicentre study. Lancet 2000;356:975-81.
8. Gatzoulis MA, Clark AL, Cullen S, Newman CG, Redington AN. Right ventricular diastolic function 15 to 35 years after repair of tetralogy of Fallot. Circulation 1995;91:1775.
9. Gatzoulis MA, Till JA, Somerville J, Redington AN. Mechanoelectrical interaction in tetralogy of Fallot. QRS prolongation relates to right ventricular size and predicts malignant ventricular arrhythmias and sudden death. Circulation 1995;92:231-7.
10. Gaultier C, Boule M, Thibert M, Leca F. Resting lung function in children after repair of tetralogy of Fallot. Chest 1986;89:561.
11. Gay WA Jr, Ebert PA. Aorta-to-right pulmonary artery anastomosis causing obstruction of the right pulmonary artery. Ann Thorac Surg 1973;16:402.
12. Gazzaniga AB, Elliott MP, Sperling DR, Dietrick WR, Eiseman JT, McRae DM, et al. Microporous expanded polytetrafluoroethylene arterial prosthesis for construction of aortopulmonary shunts. Experimental and clinical results. Ann Thorac Surg 1976;21:322.
13. Gazzaniga AB, Lamberti JJ, Siewers RD, Sperling DR, Dietrick WR, Arcilla RA, et al. Arterial prosthesis of microporous expanded polytetrafluoroethylene for construction of aortopulmonary shunts. J Thorac Cardiovasc Surg 1976;72:357.
14. Geva T. Indications and timing of pulmonary valve replacement after tetralogy of Fallot repair. Semin Thorac Cardiovasc Surg Pediatr Card Surg Annu 2006:11-22.
15. Geva T, Sandweiss BM, Gauvreau K, Lock JE, Powell AJ. Factors associated with impaired clinical status in long-term survivors of tetralogy of Fallot repair evaluated by magnetic resonance imaging. J Am Coll Cardiol 2004;43:1068-74.
16. Gill CC, Moodie DS, McGoon DC. Staged surgical management of pulmonary atresia with diminutive pulmonary arteries. J Thorac Cardiovasc Surg 1977;73:436.
17. Gillette PC, Yeoman MA, Mullins CE, McNamara DG. Sudden death after repair of tetralogy of Fallot. Electrocardiographic and electrophysiologic abnormalities. Circulation 1977; 56:566.
18. Gladman G, McCrindle BW, Williams WG, Freedom RM, Benson LN. The modified Blalock-Taussig shunt: clinical impact and morbidity in Fallot's tetralogy in the current era. J Thorac Cardiovasc Surg 1997;114:25.
19. Glancy DL, Morrow AG, Roberts W. Malformations of the aortic valve in patients with the tetralogy of Fallot. Am Heart J 1968;76:755.
20. Gober V, Berdat P, Pavlovic M, Pfammatter JP, Carrel TP. Adverse mid-term outcome following RVOT reconstruction using the Contegra valved bovine jugular vein. Ann Thorac Surg 2005; 79:625-31.
21. Godart F, Houyel L, Lacour-Gayet F, Serraf A, Sousa Uva M, Bruniaux J, et al. Absent pulmonary valve syndrome: surgical treatment and considerations. Ann Thorac Surg 1996;62:136.
22. Goor DA, Smolinksy A, Mohr R, Caspi J, Shem-Tov A. The drop of residual right ventricular pressure 24 hours after conservative infundibulectomy in repair of tetralogy of Fallot. J Thorac Cardiovasc Surg 1981;81:897.
23. Gotsman MS. Increasing obstruction to the outflow tract in Fallot's tetralogy. Br Heart J 1966;28:615.
24. Graham TP Jr, Cordell D, Atwood GF, Boucek RJ Jr, Boerth RC, Bender HW, et al. Right ventricular volume characteristics before and after palliative and reparative operation in tetralogy of Fallot. Circulation 1976;54:417.
25. Graham TP Jr, Erath HG Jr, Boucek RJ Jr, Boerth RC. Left ventricular function in cyanotic congenital heart disease. Am J Cardiol 1980;45:1231.
26. Graham TP Jr, Faulkner S, Bender H Jr, Wender CM. Hypoplasia of the left ventricle: rare cause of postoperative mortality in tetralogy of Fallot. Am J Cardiol 1977;40:454.
27. Grant RP, Downey FM, MacMahon H. The architecture of the right ventricular outflow tract in the normal human heart and in the presence of ventricular septal defects. Circulation 1961;24:223.
28. Grinnell VS, Mehringer CM, Hieshima GB, Stanley P, Lurie PR. Transaortic occlusion of collateral arteries to the lung by detachable valved balloons in a patient with tetralogy of Fallot. Circulation 1982;65:1276.
29. Groh MA, Meliones JN, Bove EL, Kirklin JW, Blackstone EH, Lupinetti FM, et al. Repair of tetralogy of Fallot in infancy: effect of pulmonary artery size on outcome. Circulation 1991;84:III206.
30. Gross RE, Bernhard WF, Litwin SB. Closure of Potts anastomoses in the total repair of tetralogy of Fallot. J Thorac Cardiovasc Surg 1969;57:72.
31. Grotenhuis HB, Ottenkamp J, de Bruijn L, Westenberg JJ, Vliegen HW, Kroft LJ, et al. Aortic elasticity and size are associated with aortic regurgitation and left ventricular dysfunction in tetralogy of Fallot after pulmonary valve replacement. Heart 2009;95:1931-6.
32. Gundry SR, Razzouk AJ, Boskind JF, Bansal R, Bailey LL. Fate of the pericardial monocusp pulmonary valve for right ventricular outflow tract reconstruction: early function, late failure without obstruction. J Thorac Cardiovasc Surg 1994;107:908.
33. Gustafson RA, Murray GF, Warden HE, Hill RC, Rozar GE Jr. Early primary repair of tetralogy of Fallot. Ann Thorac Surg 1988;45:235.
34. Guyton RA, Owens JE, Waumett JD, Dooley KJ, Hatcher CR Jr, Williams WH. The Blalock-Taussig shunt: low risk, effective palliation, and pulmonary artery growth. J Thorac Cardiovasc Surg 1983;85:917.

H

1. Hadjo A, Jimenez M, Baudet E, Roques X, Laborde N, Srour S, et al. Review of the long-term course of 52 patients with pulmonary atresia and ventricular septal defect. Anatomical and surgical considerations. Eur Heart J 1995;16:1668.
2. Hamilton DI, Di Eusanio G, Piccoli GP, Dickinson DF. Eight years experience with intracardiac repair of tetralogy of Fallot. Early and late results in 175 consecutive patients. Br Heart J 1981;46:144.
3. Hancock EW, Hultgren HN, March HW. Pulmonary hypertension after Blalock-Taussig anastomosis. Am Heart J 1964;67:817.
4. Hanley FL. MAPCAs, bronchials, monkeys, and men. Eur J Cardiothorac Surg 2006;29:643-4.
5. Harken AH, Horowitz LN, Josephson ME. Surgical correction of recurrent sustained ventricular tachycardia following complete repair of tetralogy of Fallot. J Thorac Cardiovasc Surg 1980;80:779.
6. Harms D, Hansen P, Fischer K, Bernhard A. Pathology of the "Fallot Lung." Virchows Arch Abt A Path Anat 1973;361:77.
7. Harris AM, Segel N, Bishop JM. Blalock-Taussig anastomosis for tetralogy of Fallot. A ten-to-fifteen year follow-up. Br Heart J 1964;26:266.
8. Hartmann AF Jr, Goldring D, Carlsson E. Development of right ventricular obstruction by aberrant muscular bands. Circulation 1964;30:679.
9. Hartmann AF Jr, Goldring D, Ferguson TB, Burford WH, Smith CH, Kissane JM, et al. The course of children with two chambered RV. J Thorac Cardiovasc Surg 1970;60:72.
10. Hartmann AF Jr, Tsifutis AA, Arvidsson H, Goldring D. The two-chambered right ventricle. Report of nine cases. Circulation 1962;26:279.
11. Hawe A, McGoon DC, Kincaid OW, Ritter DG. Fate of outflow tract in tetralogy of Fallot. Ann Thorac Surg 1972;13:137.
12. Hawkins JA, Bailey WW, Dillon T, Schwartz DC. Mid-term results with cryopreserved allograft valved conduits from the right ventricle to the pulmonary arteries. J Thorac Cardiovasc Surg 1992;104:910.
13. Haworth SG. Collateral arteries in pulmonary atresia with ventricular septal defect. A precarious blood supply. Br Heart J 1980;44:5.
14. Haworth SG, Macartney FJ. Growth and development of pulmonary circulation in pulmonary atresia with ventricular septal defect and major aortopulmonary collateral arteries. Br Heart J 1980;44:14.
15. Haworth SG, Rees PG, Taylor JF, Macartney FJ, de Leval M, Stark J. Pulmonary atresia with ventricular septal defect and major aortopulmonary collateral arteries: effect of systemic–pulmonary anastomosis. Br Heart J 1981;45:133.
16. Haworth SG, Reid L. Quantitative structural study of pulmonary circulation in the newborn with pulmonary atresia. Thorax 1977; 32:129.
17. Heinemann MK, Hanley FL. Preoperative management of neonatal tetralogy of Fallot with absent pulmonary valve syndrome. Ann Thorac Surg 1993;55:172-4.
18. Hickey EJ, Veldtman G, Bradley TJ, Gengsakul A, Manlhiot C, Williams WG, et al. Late risk of outcomes for adults with repaired tetralogy of Fallot from an inception cohort spanning four decades. Eur J Cardiothorac Surg 2009;35:156-64.

19. Hiraishi S, Bargeron LM, Isabel-Jones JB, Emmanouilides GC, Friedman WF, Jarmakani JM. Ventricular and pulmonary artery volumes in patients with absent pulmonary valve. Factors affecting the natural course. Circulation 1983;67:183.
20. Hirsch JC, Mosca RS, Bove EL. Complete repair of tetralogy of Fallot in the neonate: results in the modern era. Ann Surg 2000;232:508.
21. Hislop A, Reid L. Structural changes in the pulmonary arteries and veins in tetralogy of Fallot. Br Heart J 1973;35:1178.
22. Hjelms E, Pohlner P, Barratt-Boyes BG, Gavin JB. Study of autologous pericardial patch-grafts in the right ventricular outflow tracts in growing and adult dogs. J Thorac Cardiovasc Surg 1981;81:120.
23. Hofbeck M, Leipold G, Rauch A, Buheitel G, Singer H. Clinical relevance of monosomy 22q11.2 in children with pulmonary atresia and ventricular septal defect. Eur J Pediatr 1999;158:302.
24. Hofbeck M, Sunnegardh JT, Burrows PE, Moes CA, Lightfoot N, Williams WG, et al. Analysis of survival in patients with pulmonic valve atresia and ventricular septal defect. Am J Cardiol 1991; 67:737.
25. Hofschire PJ, Rosenquist GC, Ruckerman RN, Moller JH, Edwards JE. Pulmonary vascular disease complicating the Blalock-Taussig anastomosis. Circulation 1977;56:124.
26. Honey M, Chamberlain DA, Howard J. The effect of beta sympathetic blockade on arterial oxygen saturation in Fallot's tetralogy. Circulation 1964;30:501.
27. Hornberger LK, Sanders SP, Sahn DJ, Rice MJ, Spevak PJ, Benacerraf BR, et al. In utero pulmonary artery and aortic growth and potential for progression of pulmonary outflow tract obstruction in tetralogy of Fallot. J Am Coll Cardiol 1995;25:739-45.
28. Horneffer PJ, Zahka KG, Rowe SA, Manolio TA, Gott VL, Reitz BA, et al. Long-term results of total repair of tetralogy of Fallot in childhood. Ann Thorac Surg 1990;50:179.
29. Howell CE, Ho SY, Anderson RH, Elliott MJ. Variations within the fibrous skeleton and ventricular outflow tracts in tetralogy of Fallot. Ann Thorac Surg 1990;50:450.
30. Hraska V, Kantorova A, Kunovsky P, Haviar D. Intermediate results with correction of tetralogy of Fallot with absent pulmonary valve using a new approach. Eur J Cardiothorac Surg 2002; 21:711-5.
31. Hudapeth AS, Cordell AR, Johnston FR. Transatrial approach to total correction of tetralogy of Fallot. Circulation 1963;27:796.
32. Hu DC, Seward JB, Puga FJ, Fuster V, Tajik AJ. Total correction of tetralogy of Fallot at age 40 years and older: long-term follow-up. J Am Coll Cardiol 1985;5:40.

I

1. Idriss FS, Muster AJ, Paul MH, Backer CL, Mavroudis C. Ventricular septal defect with tricuspid pouch with and without transposition: anatomic and surgical considerations. J Thorac Cardiovasc Surg 1992;103:52.
2. Ilbawi MN, Grieco J, DeLeon SY, Idriss FS, Muster AJ, Berry TE, et al. Modified Blalock-Taussig shunt in newborn infants. J Thorac Cardiovasc Surg 1984;88:770.
3. Ilbawi MN, Idriss FS, DeLeon SY, Muster AJ, Berry TE, Paul MH. Long-term results of porcine valve insertion for pulmonary regurgitation following repair of tetralogy of Fallot. Ann Thorac Surg 1986;41:478.
4. Ilbawi MN, Idriss FS, DeLeon SY, Muster AJ, Gidding SS, Berry TE, et al. Factors that exaggerate the deleterious effects of pulmonary insufficiency on the right ventricle after tetralogy repair. Surgical implications. J Thorac Cardiovasc Surg 1987;93:36.
5. Ilbawi MN, Idriss FS, Muster AJ, Wessel HU, Paul MH, DeLeon SY. Tetralogy of Fallot with absent pulmonary valve. Should valve insertion be part of the intracardiac repair? J Thorac Cardiovasc Surg 1981;81:906.
6. Ionescu MI, Tandon AP, Macartney FJ. Long-term sequential hemodynamic evaluation of right ventricular outflow tract reconstruction using a valve mechanism. Ann Thorac Surg 1979; 27:426.
7. Ishizaka T, Yagihara T, Yamamoto F, Nichigaki K, Matsuki O, Uemura H, et al. Results and unifocalization for pulmonary atresia, ventricular septal defect and major aortopulmonary collateral arteries: patency of pulmonary vascular segments. Eur J Cardiothorac Surg 1996;10:331.
8. Iyer KS, Mee RB. Staged repair of pulmonary atresia with ventricular septal defect and major systemic to pulmonary artery collaterals. Ann Thorac Surg 1991;51:65.

J

1. James FW, Kaplan S, Schwartz DC, Chou TC, Sandker MJ, Naylor V. Response to exercise in patients after total surgical correction of tetralogy of Fallot. Circulation 1976;54:671.
2. Jarmakani JM, Graham TP Jr, Canent RV Jr, Jewett PH. Left heart function in children with tetralogy of Fallot before and after palliative or corrective surgery. Circulation 1972;46:478.
3. Jarmakani JM, Nakazawa M, Isabel-Jones J, Marks RA. Right ventricular function in children with tetralogy of Fallot before and after aortic to pulmonary shunt. Circulation 1976;53:555.
4. Jefferson K, Rees S, Somerville J. Systemic arterial supply to the lungs in pulmonary atresia and its relation to pulmonary artery development. Br Heart J 1972;34:418.
5. Johnson RJ, Haworth SG. Pulmonary vascular and alveolar development in tetralogy of Fallot: a recommendation for early correction. Thorax 1982;37:893.
6. Jonas RA, Freed MD, Mayer JE Jr, Castaneda AR. Long-term follow-up of synthetic right heart conduits. Circulation 1985; 72:II77.

K

1. Kahn DR. Discussion of paper by Dobell et al. J Thorac Cardiovasc Surg 1968;55:78.
2. Kan JS, Marvin WJ Jr, Bass JL, Muster AJ, Murphy J. Balloon angioplasty—branch pulmonary artery stenosis: Results from the Valvuloplasty and Angioplasty of Congenital Anomalies Registry. Am J Cardiol 1990;65:798.
3. Kaneko Y, Okabe H, Nagata N, Kobayashi J, Murakami A, Takamoto S. Pulmonary atresia, ventricular septal defect, and coronary-pulmonary artery fistula. Ann Thorac Surg 2001;71:355.
4. Kantorova A, Zbieranek K, Sauer H, Lilje C, Haun C, Hraska V. Primary early correction of tetralogy of Fallot irrespective of age. Cardiol Young 2008;18:153-7.
5. Karl TR, Musumeci F, de Leval M, Pincott JR, Taylor JF, Stark J. Surgical treatment of absent pulmonary valve syndrome. J Thorac Cardiovasc Surg 1986;91:590.
6. Karl TR, Sano S, Pornviliwan S, Mee RB. Tetralogy of Fallot: favorable outcome of nonneonatal transatrial, transpulmonary repair. Ann Thorac Surg 1992;54:903.
7. Katz NM, Blackstone EH, Kirklin JW, Pacifico AD, Bargeron LM Jr. Late survival and symptoms after repair of tetralogy of Fallot. Circulation 1982;65:403.
8. Kaufman SL, Kan JS, Mitchell SE, Flaherty JT, White RI Jr. Embolization of systemic to pulmonary artery collaterals in the management of hemoptysis in pulmonary atresia. Am J Cardiol 1986;58:1130.
9. Kavey RE, Blackman MS, Sondheimer HM. Incidence and severity of chronic ventricular dysrhythmias after repair of tetralogy of Fallot. Am Heart J 1982;103:342
10. Kavey RE, Thomas FD, Byrum CJ, Blackman MS, Sondheimer HM, Bove EL. Ventricular arrhythmias and biventricular dysfunction after repair of tetralogy of Fallot. J Am Coll Cardiol 1984; 4:126.
11. Kawashima Y, Kitamura S, Nakano S, Yagihara T. Corrective surgery for tetralogy of Fallot without or with minimal right ventriculotomy and with repair of the pulmonary valve. Circulation 1981;64:II147.
12. Kawashima Y, Mori T, Kitamura S, Hirose H, Nakano S, Yagihara T. Transpulmonary arterial, transright atrial repair of tetralogy of Fallot. J Jpn Surg Soc 1979;80:1259.
13. Kay PH, Capuani A, Franks R, Lincoln C. Experience with the modified Blalock-Taussig operation using polytetrafluoroethylene (Impra) grafts. Br Heart J 1983;49:359.
14. Kay PH, Ross DN. Fifteen years' experience with the aortic homograft: the conduit of choice for right ventricular outflow tract reconstruction. Ann Thorac Surg 1985;40:360.
15. Keck EW, Brode P. Beta-receptor blockade in Fallot's tetralogy. Dtsch Med Wochenschr 1970;95:766.
16. Kirklin JK, Kirklin JW, Blackstone EH, Milano A, Pacifico AD. Effect of transanular patching on outcome after repair of tetralogy of Fallot. Ann Thorac Surg 1989;48:783.
17. Kirklin JK, Kirklin JW, Blackstone EH, Pacifico AD, McConnell ME, Colvin EV, et al. Sudden death and arrhythmic events after repair of tetralogy of Fallot. In: Crupi G, Parenzan L, Anderson RH, eds. Perspectives in pediatric cardiology, Vol. 2. Pediatric cardiac surgery, Part 1. Mount Kisco, N.Y.: Futura, 1989, p. 204.

18. Kirklin JK, Westaby S, Chenoweth D, Blackstone EH, Kirklin JW, Pacifico AD. Complement and the damaging effects of cardiopulmonary bypass. J Thorac Cardiovasc Surg 1983;86:845.
19. Kirklin JW, Bargeron LM Jr, Pacifico AD. The enlargement of small pulmonary arteries by preliminary palliative operations. Circulation 1977;56:612.
20. Kirklin JW, Blackstone EH, Jonas RA, Shimazaki Y, Kirklin JK, Mayer JE Jr, et al. Morphologic and surgical determinants of outcome events after repair of tetralogy of Fallot and pulmonary stenosis: a two-institution study. J Thorac Cardiovasc Surg 1992;103:706.
21. Kirklin JW, Blackstone EH, Jonas RA, Shimazaki Y, Kirklin JK, Mayer JE Jr, et al. Morphologic and surgical determinants of outcome events after repair of tetralogy of Fallot and pulmonary stenosis. J Thorac Cardiovasc Surg 1992;103:706.
22. Kirklin JW, Blackstone EH, Kirklin JK, Pacifico AD, Aramendi J, Bargeron LM Jr. Surgical results and protocols in the spectrum of tetralogy of Fallot. Ann Surg 1983;198:251.
23. Kirklin JW, Blackstone EH, Maehara T, Pacifico AD, Kirklin JK, Pollock S, et al. Intermediate-term fate of cryopreserved allograft and xenograft valved conduits. Ann Thorac Surg 1987;44:598.
24. Kirklin JW, Blackstone EH, Shimazaki Y, Maehara T, Pacifico AD, Kirklin JK, et al. Survival, functional status, and reoperations after repair of tetralogy of Fallot with pulmonary atresia. J Thorac Cardiovasc Surg 1988;96:102.
25. Kirklin JW, Devloo RA. Hypothermic perfusion and circulatory arrest for surgical correction of tetralogy of Fallot with previously constructed Potts' anastomosis. Dis Chest 1961;39:87.
26. Kirklin JW, DuShane JW, Patrick RT, Donald DE, Hetzel PS, Harshbarger HC, et al. Intracardiac surgery with the aid of a mechanical pump-oxygenator system (Gibbon type): report of eight cases. Mayo Clin Proc 1955;30:201.
27. Kirklin JW, Ellis FH Jr, McGoon DC, DuShane JW, Swan HF. Surgical treatment for the tetralogy of Fallot by open intracardiac repair. J Thorac Surg 1959;37:22.
28. Kirklin JW, Karp RB. The tetralogy of Fallot. Philadelphia: WB Saunders, 1970.
29. Kirklin JW, Openshaw CR, Tompkins RG. Surgical treatment of infundibular stenosis with intact ventricular septum. Ann Surg 1953;137:228.
30. Kirklin JW, Payne WS. Surgical treatment for tetralogy of Fallot after previous anastomosis of systemic to pulmonary artery. Surg Gynecol Obstet 1960;110:707.
31. Kirklin JW, Payne WS, Theye RA, DuShuane JW. Factors affecting survival after open operation for tetralogy of Fallot. Ann Surg 1960;152:485.
32. Kirklin JW, Wallace RB, McGoon DC, DuShane JW. Early and late results after intracardiac repair of tetralogy of Fallot: 5-year review of 337 patients. Ann Surg 1965;162:578.
33. Klinner VW, Pasini M, Schaudig A. Anastomose zwischen systemund lungenarterie mit hilfe von kunststoffprothesen bei cyanotischen herzvitien. Thoraxchirurgie 1962;10:68.
34. Klinner W. Klinische und experimentelle untersuchungen zur operativen korrektur der Fallotschen tetralogie. Aus der Chirurgischen Klinik der Universitat Munchen, 1961.
35. Klinner W, Reichart B, Pfaller M, Hatz R. Late results after correction of tetralogy of Fallot necessitating outflow tract reconstruction. Comparison with results after correction without outflow tract patch. Thorac Cardiovasc Surg 1984;32:244.
36. Knott-Craig CJ, Elkins RC, Lane MM, Holz J, McCue C, Ward KE. A 26-year experience with surgical management of tetralogy of Fallot: risk analysis for mortality or late reintervention. Ann Thorac Surg 1998;66:506.
37. Kobayashi J, Hirose H, Nakano S, Matsuda H, Shirakura R, Kawashima Y. Ambulatory electrocardiographic study of the frequency and cause of ventricular arrhythmia after correction of tetralogy of Fallot. Am J Cardiol 1984;54:1310.
38. Krongrad E, Ritter DG, Hawe A, Kincaid OW, McGoon DC. Pulmonary atresia or severe stenosis and coronary artery-to-pulmonary artery fistula. Circulation 1972;46:1005.
39. Kuers PF, McGoon DC. Tetralogy of Fallot with aortic origin of right pulmonary artery. J Thorac Cardiovasc Surg 1973;65:327.
40. Kurosawa H, Imai Y. Surgical anatomy of the atrioventricular conduction bundle in tetralogy of Fallot. New findings relevant to the position of the sutures. J Thorac Cardiovasc Surg 1988;95:586.
41. Kurtz CM, Sprague HB, White PD. Congenital heart disease. Am Heart J 1927;3:77.
42. Kusuhara K, Miki S, Ueda Y, Ohkita Y, Tahata T, Komeda M, et al. Evaluation of corrective surgery for tetralogy of Fallot from late results by multivariate statistical analysis. Eur J Cardiothorac Surg 1988;2:124.
43. Kveselis D, Rosenthal A, Ferguson P, Behrendt D, Sloan H. Long-term prognosis after repair of double-chamber right ventricle with ventricular septal defect. Am J Cardiol 1984;54:1292.

L

1. Lakier JB, Stanger P, Heymann MA, Hoffman JI, Rudolph AM. Tetralogy of Fallot with absent pulmonary valve. Natural history and hemodynamic considerations. Circulation 1974;50:167.
2. Laks H, Castaneda AR. Subclavian arterioplasty for the ipsilateral Blalock-Taussig shunt. Ann Thorac Surg 1975;19:319.
3. Lamberti JJ, Carlisle J, Waldman JD, Lodge FA, Kirkpatrick SE, George L, et al. Systemic–pulmonary shunts in infants and children. J Thorac Cardiovasc Surg 1984;88:76.
4. Lang P, Chipman CW, Siden H, Williams RG, Norwood WI, Castaneda AR. Early assessment of hemodynamic status after repair of tetralogy of Fallot: a comparison of 24 hour (intensive care unit) and 1 year postoperative data in 98 patients. Am J Cardiol 1982;50:795.
5. Lange PE, Onnasch DG, Bernhard A, Heintzen PH. Left and right ventricular adaptation to right ventricular overload before and after surgical repair of tetralogy of Fallot. Am J Cardiol 1982;50:786.
6. Le Bret E, Mace L, Dervanian P, Folliguet T, Bourriez A, Zoghy J, et al. Images in cardiovascular medicine. Combined angiography and three-dimensional computed tomography for assessing systemic-to-pulmonary collaterals in pulmonary atresia with ventricular septal defect. Circulation 1998;98:2930.
7. Lecompte Y, Hazan E, Baillot F, Jarreau MM, Mathey J. La reparation chirurgicale de la voie pulmonaire dans la tetralogie de Fallot. Coeur 1977;3:739.
8. Lev M. The architecture of the conduction system in congenital heart disease. II. Tetralogy of Fallot. AMA Arch Pathol 1958; 67:572.
9. Lev M, Eckner FA. The pathologic anatomy of tetralogy of Fallot and its variations. Dis Chest 1964;45:251.
10. Lev M, Rimoldi HJ, Rowlatt DF. Quantitative anatomy of cyanotic tetralogy of Fallot. Circulation 1964;30:531.
11. Levine FH, Reis RL, Morrow AG. Incidence and significance of patent foramen ovale after correction of tetralogy of Fallot. Ann Thorac Surg 1972;13:464.
12. Levy MJ, Lillehei CW, Elliott LP, Carey LS, Adams P Jr, Edwards JE. Accessory valvular tissue causing subpulmonary stenosis in corrected transposition of great vessels. Circulation 1963;27:494.
13. Li MD, Coles JC, McDonald AC. Anomalous muscle bundle of the right ventricle. Its recognition and surgical treatment, Br Heart J 1978;40:1040.
14. Lillehei CW. Discussion of paper by Horneffer and colleagues. Ann Thorac Surg 1990;50:184.
15. Lillehei CW, Cohen M, Warden HE, Read RC, Aust JB, De Wall RA, et al. Direct vision intracardiac surgical correction of the tetralogy of Fallot, pentalogy of Fallot, and pulmonary atresia defects: report of first ten cases. Ann Surg 1955;142:418.
16. Lillehei CW, Varco RL, Cohen M, Warden HE, Gott VL, DeWall RA, et al. The first open heart corrections of tetralogy of Fallot. A 26-31 year follow-up of 106 patients. Ann Surg 1986;204:490.
17. Litwin SB, Rosenthal A, Fellows K. Surgical management of young infants with tetralogy of Fallot, absence of the pulmonary valve, and respiratory distress. J Thorac Cardiovasc Surg 1973;65:552.
18. Lock JE, Castaneda-Zuniga WR, Fuhrman BP, Bass JL. Balloon dilation angioplasty of hypoplastic and stenotic pulmonary arteries. Circulation 1983;67:962.
19. Lock JE, Niemi T, Einzig S, Amplatz K, Burke B, Bass JL. Transvenous angioplasty of experimental branch pulmonary artery stenosis in newborn lambs. Circulation 1981;64:886.
20. Lofland GK. The management of pulmonary atresia, ventricular septal defect, and multiple aorta pulmonary collateral arteries by definitive single stage repair in early infancy. Eur J Cardiothorac Surg 2000;18:480.
21. Lucas RV Jr, Varco RL, Lillehei CW, Adams P Jr, Anderson RC, Edwards JE. Anomalous muscle bundle of the right ventricle. Hemodynamic consequences and surgical considerations. Circulation 1962;25:443.

22. Lurz P, Gaudin R, Taylor AM, Bonhoeffer P. Percutaneous pulmonary valve implantation. Semin Thorac Cardiovasc Surg Pediatr Card Surg Annu 2009:112-7.

M

1. Macartney F, Deverall P, Scott O. Haemodynamic characteristics of systemic arterial blood supply to the lungs. Br Heart J 1973; 35:28.
2. Macartney FJ, Miller GA. Congenital absence of the pulmonary valve. Br Heart J 1970;32:483.
3. Macartney FJ, Scott O, Deverall PB. Haemodynamic and anatomical characteristics of pulmonary blood supply in pulmonary atresia with ventricular septal defect—including a case of persistent fifth aortic arch. Br Heart J 1974;36:1049.
4. Macedo ME, Sena Lino JA, Lima M, Salomao CS. Left ventricular outflow tract obstruction due to tricuspid valve prolapse through a high ventricular septal defect. Thorac Cardiovasc Surg 1983;31:110.
5. Maclean LD, Culligan JA, Kane DJ. Subaortic stenosis due to accessory tissue on the mitral valve. J Thorac Cardiovasc Surg 1963;45:382.
6. Malhotra SP, Hanley FL. Surgical management of pulmonary atresia with ventricular septal defect and major aortopulmonary collaterals: a protocol-based approach. Semin Thorac Cardiovasc Surg Pediatr Card Surg Annu 2009:145-51.
7. Manabe H. Recent advance in total correction of tetralogy of Fallot. Jpn Circ J 1984;48:1.
8. Marchand P. The use of a cusp-bearing homograft patch to the outflow tract and pulmonary artery in Fallot's tetralogy and pulmonary valvular stenosis. Thorax 1967;22:497.
9. Marelli AJ, Perloff JK, Child JS, Laks H. Pulmonary atresia with ventricular septal defect in adults. Circulation 1994;89:243.
10. Marino B, Digilio MC, Toscano A, Anaclerio S, Giannotti A, Feltri C, et al. Anatomic patterns of conotruncal defects associated with deletion 22q11. Genet Med 2001;3:45.
11. Maron BJ, Ferrans VJ, White RI Jr. Unusual evolution of acquired infundibular stenosis in patients with ventricular septal defect. Clinical and morphologic observations. Circulation 1973;48:1092.
12. Marx GR, Hicks RW, Allen HD, Goldberg SJ. Noninvasive assessment of hemodynamic responses to exercise in pulmonary regurgitation after operations to correct pulmonary outflow obstruction. Am J Cardiol 1988;61:595.
13. Matsuda H, Ihara K, Mori T, Kitamura S, Kawashima Y. Tetralogy of Fallot associated with aortic insufficiency. Ann Thorac Surg 1980;29:529.
14. McCaughan BC, Danielson GK, Driscoll DJ, McGoon DC. Tetralogy of Fallot with absent pulmonary valve. J Thorac Cardiovasc Surg 1985;89:280.
15. McCord MC, van Elk J, Blount G Jr. Tetralogy of Fallot clinical and hemodynamic spectrum of combined pulmonary stenosis and ventricular septal defects. Circulation 1957;16:736.
16. McElhinney DB, Reddy VM, Haley FL. Tetralogy of Fallot with major aortopulmonary collaterals: early total repair. Pediatr Cardiol 1998;19:289.
17. McElhinney DB, Reddy VM, Pian MS, Moore P, Hanley FL. Compression of the central airways by a dilated aorta in infants and children with congenital heart disease. Ann Thorac Surg 1999;67:1130.
18. McGoon DC, Baird DK, Davis GD. Surgical management of large bronchial collateral arteries with pulmonary stenosis or atresia. Circulation 1975;52:109.
19. McGoon DC, Danielson GK, Puga FJ, Ritter DG, Mair DD, Ilstrup DM. Late results after extracardiac conduit repair for congenital cardiac defects. Am J Cardiol 1982;49:1741.
20. McGoon MD, Fulton RE, Davis GD, Ritter DG, Neill CA, White RI Jr. Systemic collateral and pulmonary artery stenosis in patients with congenital pulmonary valve atresia and ventricular septal defect. Circulation 1977;56:473.
21. McKay R, de Leval MR, Rees P, Taylor JF, Macartney FJ, Stark J. Postoperative angiographic assessment of modified Blalock-Taussig shunts using expanded polytetrafluoroethylene (Gore-Tex). Ann Thorac Surg 1980;30:137.
22. McMahon CJ, Nihill MR. Origin of the main pulmonary artery from the left coronary artery in complex pulmonary atresia. Pediatr Cardiol 2001;22:347.
23. Metras D, Chetaille P, Kreitmann B, Fraisse A, Ghez O, Riberi A. Pulmonary atresia with ventricular septal defect, extremely hypoplastic pulmonary arteries, major aortopulmonary collaterals. Eur J Cardiothorac Surg 2001;20:590.
24. Miller GA, Kirklin JW, Rahimtoola SH, Swan HJ. Volume of the left ventricle in tetralogy of Fallot. Am J Cardiol 1965;16:488.
25. Miller RA, Lev M, Paul MH. Congenital absence of the pulmonary valve. The clinical syndrome of tetralogy of Fallot with pulmonary regurgitation. Circulation 1962;26:266.
26. Miller WW, Nadas AS, Bernhard WF, Gross RE. Congenital pulmonary atresia with ventricular septal defect. Review of the clinical course of fifty patients with assessment of the results of palliative surgery. Am J Cardiol 1968;21:673.
27. Miura T, Nakano S, Shimazaki Y, Kobayashi J, Hirose H, Sano T, et al. Evaluation of right ventricular function by regional wall motion analysis in patients after correction of tetralogy of Fallot. J Thorac Cardiovasc Surg 1992;104:917.
28. Mizuno A, Sato F, Hasegawa T, Tsuzuki M, Furuse A. Acquired obstruction of the right ventricular outflow tract in tetralogy of Fallot after Blalock-Taussig anastomosis. Report of two cases successfully treated with total correction. Jpn Heart J 1970;11:113.
29. Mocellin R, Krettek M, Sauer U, Buhlmeyer K. Pulmonary atresia with ventricular septal defect. Follow up and surgical results from 1963 to 1976 and diagnostic measures with special reference to large systemic-pulmonary collaterals. Z Kardiol 1977;66:382.
30. Moller JH, ed. Perspectives in pediatric cardiology: surgery of congenital heart disease, Vol. 6. Pediatric Cardiac Care Consortium 1984-1995, New York: Futura, 1998, p. 207.
31. Morales DL, Zafar F, Fraser CD Jr. Tetralogy of Fallot repair: the Right Ventricle Infundibulum Sparing (RVIS) strategy. Semin Thorac Cardiovasc Surg Pediatr Card Surg Annu 2009:54-8.
32. Morgan JR. Left pulmonary artery from ascending aorta in tetralogy of Fallot. Circulation 1972;45:653.
33. Moritz A, Marx M, Wollenek G, Domanig E, Wolner E. Complete repair of PA-VSD with diminutive or discontinuous pulmonary arteries by transverse thoracosternotomy. Ann Thorac Surg 1996; 61:646.
34. Mulla N, Simpson P, Sullivan NM, Paridon SM. Determinants of aerobic capacity during exercise following complete repair of tetralogy of Fallot with a transanular patch. Pediatr Cardiol 1997; 18:350.
35. Mullins CE, O'Laughlin MP, Vick GW 3rd, Mayer DC, Myers TJ, Kearney DL, et al. Implantation of balloon-expandable intravascular grafts by catheterization in pulmonary arteries and systemic veins. Circulation 1988;77:188.
36. Murphy JD, Freed MD, Keane JF, Norwood WI, Castaneda AR, Nadas AS. Hemodynamic results after intracardiac repair of tetralogy of Fallot by deep hypothermia and cardiopulmonary bypass. Circulation 1980;62:I168.
37. Murphy JG, Gersh BJ, Mair DD, Fuster V, McGoon MD, Ilstrup DM, et al. Long-term outcome in patients undergoing surgical repair of tetralogy of Fallot. N Engl J Med 1993;329:593.
38. Murthy KS, Krishnanaik S, Coelho R, Punnoose A, Arumugam SB, Cherian KM. Median sternotomy single stage complete unifocalization for pulmonary atresia, major aortopulmonary collateral arteries and VSD—early experience. Eur J Cardiothorac Surg 1999;16:21.
39. Murthy KS, Rao SG, Naik SK, Coelho R, Krishnan US, Cherian KM. Evolving surgical management for ventricular septal defect, pulmonary atresia, and major aortopulmonary collateral arteries. Ann Thorac Surg 1999;67:760.

N

1. Nagao GI, Daoud GI, McAdams AJ, Schwartz DC, Kaplan S. Cardiovascular anomalies associated with tetralogy of Fallot. Am J Cardiol 1967;20:206.
2. Naito Y. Study on total correction of tetralogy of Fallot: factors affecting operative mortality and surgical measures to improve operative results. Jpn J Assoc Thorac Surg 1972;20:131.
3. Naito Y, Fujita T, Yagihara T, Isobe F, Yamamoto F, Tanaka K, et al. Usefulness of left ventricular volume in assessing tetralogy of Fallot for total correction. Am J Cardiol 1985;56:356.
4. Nakata S, Imai Y, Takanashi Y, Kurosawa H, Tezuka K, Nakazawa M, et al. A new method for the quantitative standardization of cross sectional areas of the pulmonary arteries in congenital heart diseases with decreased pulmonary blood flow. J Thorac Cardiovasc Surg 1984;88:610.

5. Nanton MA, Belcourt CL, Gillis DA, Krause VW, Roy DL. Left ventricular outflow tract obstruction owing to accessory endocardial cushion tissue. J Thorac Cardiovasc Surg 1979;78:537.
6. Neirotti R, Galindez E, Kreutzer G, Rodriguez Coronel A, Pedrini M, et al. Tetralogy of Fallot with subpulmonary ventricular septal defect. Ann Thorac Surg 1978;25:51.
7. Neufeld HN, McGoon DC, DuShane JW, Edwards JE. Tetralogy of Fallot with anomalous tricuspid valve simulating pulmonary stenosis with intact septum. Circulation 1960;22:1083.
8. Newfeld EA, Waldman D, Paul MH, Muster AJ, Cole RB, Idriss F, et al. Pulmonary vascular disease after systemic–pulmonary arterial shunt operations. Am J Cardiol 1977;39:715.
9. Nihill MR, Mullins CE, McNamara DG. Visualization of the pulmonary arteries in pseudotruncus by pulmonary vein wedge angiography. Circulation 1978;58:140.
10. Nomoto S, Muraoka R, Yokota M, Aoshima M, Kyoku I, Nakano H. Left ventricular volume as a predictor of the postoperative hemodynamics and a criterion for total correction of the tetralogy of Fallot. J Thorac Cardiovasc Surg 1984;88:389.
11. Norberg WJ, Tadavarthy M, Knight L, Nicoloff DM, Moller JH. Late hemodynamic and angiographic findings after ascending aorta–pulmonary artery anastomosis. J Thorac Cardiovasc Surg 1978;76:345.
12. Norton KI, Tong C, Glass RB, Nielsen JC. Cardiac MR imaging assessment following tetralogy of Fallot repair. Radiographics 2006;26:197-211.
13. Norwood WI, Freed MD, Rocchini AP, Bernhard WF, Castaneda AR. Experience with valved conduits for repair of congenital cardiac lesions. Ann Thorac Surg 1977;24:223.
14. Norwood WI, Rosenthal A, Castaneda AR. Tetralogy of Fallot with acquired pulmonary atresia and hypoplasia of pulmonary arteries. Report of surgical management in infancy. J Thorac Cardiovasc Surg 1976;72:454.

O

1. Oberhansli I, Friedli B. Echocardiographic study of left and right ventricular dimension and left ventricular function in patients with tetralogy of Fallot, before and after surgery. Br Heart J 1979;41:40.
2. Oku H. Operative results and postoperative hemodynamic results in total correction of tetralogy of Fallot with special reference to patient's age and enlargement of right ventricular outflow tract. Nippon Geka Hokan 1976;45:87.
3. Oku H, Shirotani H, Yokoyama T, Yokota Y, Kawai J, Makino S, et al. Right ventricular outflow tract prosthesis in total correction of tetralogy of Fallot. Circulation 1980;62:604.
4. Oku H, Shirotani H, Yokoyama T, Yokota Y, Kawai J, Mori A, et al. Postoperative size of the right ventricular outflow tract and optimal age in complete repair of tetralogy of Fallot. Ann Thorac Surg 1978;25:322.
5. O'Laughlin MP, Perry SB, Lock JE, Mullins CE. Use of endovascular stents in congenital heart disease. Circulation 1991; 83:1923.
6. Olin CL, Ritter DG, McGoon DC, Wallace RB, Danielson GK. Pulmonary atresia: surgical considerations and results in 103 patients undergoing definitive repair. Circulation 1976;54:III35.
7. Ongley PA, Rahimtoola SH, Kincaid OW, Kirklin JW. Continuous murmurs in tetralogy of Fallot and pulmonary atresia with ventricular septal defect. Am J Cardiol 1966;18:821.
8. Oosterhof T, Mulder BJ, Vliegen HW, de Roos A. Cardiovascular magnetic resonance in the follow-up of patients with corrected tetralogy of Fallot: a review. Am Heart J 2006;151:265-72.
9. Opie JC, Sandor GG, Ashmore PG, Patterson MW. Successful palliation by pulmonary artery banding in absent pulmonary valve syndrome with aneurysmal pulmonary arteries. J Thorac Cardiovasc Surg 1983;85:125.
10. Osman MZ, Meng CC, Girdany BR. Congenital absence of the pulmonary valve. Report of eight cases with review of the literature. Am J Roentgenol Radium Ther Nucl Med 1969;106:58.

P

1. Pacifico AD, Kirklin JW, Bargeron LM Jr, Soto B. Surgical treatment of common arterial trunk with pseudotruncus arteriosus. Circulation 1974;50:II20.
2. Pacifico AD, Ricchi A, Bargeron LM Jr, Colvin EC, Kirklin JW, Kirklin JK. Corrective repair of complete atrioventricular canal defects and major associated cardiac anomalies. Ann Thorac Surg 1988;46:645.
3. Pacifico AD, Sand ME, Bargeron LM Jr, Colvin EC. Transatrial–transpulmonary repair of tetralogy of Fallot. J Thorac Cardiovasc Surg 1987;93:919.
4. Padalino MA, Vida VL, Stellin G. Transatrial–transpulmonary repair of tetralogy of Fallot. Semin Thorac Cardiovasc Surg Pediatr Card Surg Annu 2009:48-53.
5. Parenzan L, Alfieri O, Vanini V, Bianchi T, Villani M, Tiraboschi R, et al. Waterston anastomosis for initial palliation of tetralogy of Fallot. J Thorac Cardiovasc Surg 1981;82:176.
6. Parry AJ, McElhinney DB, Kung GC, Reddy VM, Brook MM, Hanley FL. Elective primary repair of acyanotic tetralogy of Fallot in early infancy: overall outcome and impact on the pulmonary valve. J Am Coll Cardiol 2000;36:2279-83.
7. Pate JW, Richardson RL Jr, Giles HH. Accessory tricuspid leaflet producing right ventricular outflow obstruction. N Engl J Med 1968;279:867.
8. Penkoske PA, Duncan N, Collins-Nakai RL. Surgical repair of double-chambered right ventricle with or without ventriculotomy. J Thorac Cardiovasc Surg 1987;93:385.
9. Perasalo O, Halonen PI, Pyorala K, Telivuo L. Aneurysm of the membranous ventricular septum causing obstruction of the right ventricular outflow tract in a case of ventricular septal defect. Acta Chir Scand 1961;283:123.
10. Perloff JK, Ronan JA Jr, de Leon AC Jr. Ventricular septal defect with the "two chambered right ventricle." Am J Cardiol 1965; 16:894.
11. Permut LC, Laks H, Aharon A. Surgical management of pulmonary atresia with ventricular septal defect and multiple aortopulmonary collaterals. Isr J Med Sci 1994;30:215.
12. Perrault H, Drblik SP, Montigny M, Davignon A, Lamarre A, Chartrand C, et al. Comparison of cardiovascular adjustments to exercise in adolescents 8 to 15 years of age after correction of tetralogy of Fallot, ventricular septal defect or atrial septal defect. Am J Cardiol 1989;64:213.
13. Perry SB, Radtke W, Fellows KE, Keane JF, Lock JE. Coil embolization to occlude aortopulmonary collateral vessels and shunts in patients with congenital heart disease. J Am Coll Cardiol 1989;13:100.
14. Piccoli GP, Dickinson DF, Musumeci F, Hamilton DI. A changing policy for the surgical treatment of tetralogy of Fallot: early and late results in 235 consecutive patients. Ann Thorac Surg 1982;33:365.
15. Piehler JM, Danielson GK, McGoon DC, Wallace RB, Fulton RE, Mair DD. Management of pulmonary atresia with ventricular septal defect and hypoplastic pulmonary arteries by right ventricular outflow construction. J Thorac Cardiovasc Surg 1980;80:552.
16. Pinsky WW, Nihill MR, Mullins CE, McNamara DG. Management of absent pulmonary valve syndrome. Am J Cardiol 1977; 39:311.
17. Poirier RA, McGoon DC, Danielson GK, Wallace RB, Ritter DG, Moodie DS, et al. Late results after repair of tetralogy of Fallot. J Thorac Cardiovasc Surg 1977;73:900.
18. Ponce FE, Williams LC, Webb HM, Riopel DA, Hohn AR. Propranolol palliation of tetralogy of Fallot: experience with long-term drug treatment in pediatric patients. Pediatrics 1973; 52:100.
19. Potts WJ, Smiths S, Gibson S. Anastomosis of the aorta to a pulmonary artery. JAMA 1946;132:627.
20. Puga FJ, DuShane JW, McGoon DC. Treatment of tetralogy of Fallot in children less than 4 years of age. J Thorac Cardiovasc Surg 1972;64:247.
21. Puga FJ, Leoni FE, Julsrud PR, Mair DD. Complete repair of pulmonary atresia, ventricular septal defect, and severe peripheral arborization abnormalities of the central pulmonary arteries. J Thorac Cardiovasc Surg 1989;98:1018.

Q

1. Quattlebaum TG, Varghese J, Neill CA, Donahoo JS. Sudden death among postoperative patients with tetralogy of Fallot. Circulation 1976;54:289.
2. Qureshi SA, Kirk CR, Lamb RK, Arnold R, Wilkinson JL. Balloon dilatation of the pulmonary valve in the first year of life in patients with tetralogy of Fallot: a preliminary study. Br Heart J 1988;60:232.
3. Qureshi SA, Parsons JM, Tynan M. Percutaneous transcatheter myectomy of subvalvar pulmonary stenosis in tetralogy of Fallot: a new palliative technique with an atherectomy catheter. Br Heart J 1990; 64:163.

R

1. Rabinovitch M, Grady S, David I, Van Praagh R, Sauer U, Buhlmeyer K, et al. Compression of intrapulmonary bronchi by abnormally branching pulmonary arteries associated with absent pulmonary valves. Am J Cardiol 1982;50:804.
2. Rabinovitch M, Herrera-deLeon V, Castaneda AR, Reid L. Growth and development of the pulmonary vascular bed in patients with tetralogy of Fallot with or without pulmonary atresia. Circulation 1981;64:1234.
3. Rastelli GC, Ongley PA, Davis GD, Kirklin JW. Surgical repair for pulmonary valve atresia with coronary-pulmonary artery fistula: report of case. Mayo Clin Proc 1965;40:521.
4. Reddy VM, Liddicoat JR, Hanley FL. Midline one-stage complete unifocalization and repair of pulmonary atresia with ventricular septal defect and major aortopulmonary collaterals. J Thorac Cardiovasc Surg 1995;109:832.
5. Reddy VM, Liddicoat JR, McElhinney DB, Brook MM, Stanger P, Hanley FL. Routine primary repair of tetralogy of Fallot in neonates and infants less than three months of age. Ann Thorac Surg 1995; 60:S592.
6. Reddy VM, McElhinney DB, Amin Z, Moore P, Parry AJ, Teitel DF, et al. Early and intermediate outcomes after repair of pulmonary atresia with ventricular septal defect and major aorto-pulmonary collateral arteries: experience with 85 patients. Circulation 2000;101:1826.
7. Reddy VM, Petrossian E, McElhinney DB, Moore P, Teitel DF, Hanley FL. One-stage complete unifocalization in infants: when should the ventricular septal defect be closed? J Thorac Cardiovasc Surg 1997;113:858.
8. Redington AN, Oldershaw PJ, Shinebourne EA, Rigby ML. A new technique for the assessment of pulmonary regurgitation and its application to the assessment of right ventricular function before and after repair of tetralogy of Fallot. Br Heart J 1988; 60:57.
9. Redington AN, Somerville J. Stenting of aortopulmonary collaterals in complex pulmonary atresia. Circulation 1996;94:2479.
10. Reduto LA, Berger HJ, Johnstone DE, Hellenbrand W, Wackers FJ, Whittemore R, et al. Radionuclide assessment of right and left ventricular exercise reserve after total correction of tetralogy of Fallot. Am J Cardiol 1980;45:1013.
11. Rees S, Somerville J. Aortography in Fallot's tetralogy and variants. Br Heart J 1969;31:146.
12. Regensburger D, Sievers HH, Lange PE, Heintzen PH, Bernhard A. Reconstruction of the right ventricular outflow tract in tetralogy of Fallot and pulmonary stenosis with a monocusp patch. Thorac Cardiovasc Surg 1981;29:345.
13. Reitman MJ, Galioto FM Jr, el-Said GM, Cooley DA, Hallman GL, McNamara DG. Ascending aorta to right pulmonary artery anastomosis. Immediate results in 123 patients and one month to six year follow-up in 74 patients. Circulation 1974;49:952.
14. Restivo A, Cameron AH, Anderson RH, Allwork SP. Divided right ventricle: a review of its anatomical varieties. Pediatr Cardiol 1984;5:197.
15. Ricci M, Tchervenkov CI, Jacobs JP, Anderson RH, Cohen G, Bove EL. Surgical correction for patients with tetralogy of Fallot and common atrioventricular junction. Cardiol Young 2008;18: 29-38.
16. Rich AR. A hitherto unrecognized tendency to the development of widespread pulmonary vascular obstruction in patients with congenital pulmonary stenosis (tetralogy of Fallot). Bull Johns Hopkins Hosp 1948;82:389.
17. Richardson JP, Clarke CP. Tetralogy of Fallot. Risk factors associated with complete repair. Br Heart J 1976;38:926.
18. Riemenschneider TA, Goldberg SJ, Ruttenberg HD, Gyepes MT. Subpulmonic obstruction in complete (d) transposition produced by redundant tricuspid tissue. Circulation 1969;39:603.
19. Ring JC, Bass JL, Marvin W, Fuhrman BP, Kulik TJ, Foker JE, et al. Management of congenital stenosis of a branch pulmonary artery with balloon dilation angioplasty. Report of 52 procedures. J Thorac Cardiovasc Surg 1985;90:35.
20. Rittenhouse EA, Mansfield PB, Hall DG, Herndon SP, Jones TK, Kawabori I, et al. Tetralogy of Fallot: selective staged management. J Thorac Cardiovasc Surg 1985;89:772.
21. Roberts WC, Friesinger GC, Cohen LS, Mason DT, Ross RS. Acquired pulmonic atresia. Total obstruction to right ventricular outflow after systemic to pulmonary arterial anastomoses for cyanotic congenital cardiac disease. Am J Cardiol 1969;24:335.
22. Rocchini AP, Keane JF, Freed MD, Castaneda AR, Nadas AS. Left ventricular function following attempted surgical repair of tetralogy of Fallot. Circulation 1978;57:798.
23. Rocchini AP, Rosenthal A, Freed M, Castaneda AR, Nadas AS. Chronic congestive heart failure after repair of tetralogy of Fallot. Circulation 1977;56:305.
24. Rodefeld MD, Reddy VM, Thompson LD, Suleman S, Moore PC, Teitel DF, et al. Surgical creation of aortopulmonary window in selected patients with pulmonary atresia with poorly developed aortopulmonary collaterals and hypoplastic pulmonary arteries. J Thorac Cardiovasc Surg 2002;123:1147.
25. Rohmer J, Van Der Mark F, Zijlstra WG. Pulmonary valve incompetence. II. Application of electromagnetic flow velocity catheters in children. Cardiovasc Res 1976;10:46.
26. Rome JJ, Mayer JE, Castaneda AR, Lock JE. Tetralogy of Fallot with pulmonary atresia. Rehabilitation of diminutive pulmonary arteries. Circulation 1993;88:1691.
27. Rosenthal A, Behrendt D, Sloan H, Ferguson P, Snedecor SM, Schork A. Long-term prognosis (15 to 26 years) after repair of tetralogy of Fallot. I. Survival and symptomatic status. Ann Thorac Surg 1984;38:151.
28. Rosenthal A, Gross RE, Pasternac A. Aneurysms of right ventricular outflow patches. J Thorac Cardiovasc Surg 1972;63:735.
29. Rosing DR, Borer JS, Kent KM, Maron BJ, Seides SF, Morrow AG, et al. Long-term hemodynamic and electrocardiographic assessment following operative repair of tetralogy of Fallot. Circulation 1978;58:I209.
30. Ross DN, Somerville J. Correction of pulmonary atresia with a homograft aortic valve. Lancet 1966;2:1446.
31. Rothman A, Perry SB, Keane JF, Lock JE. Early results and follow-up of balloon angioplasty for branch pulmonary artery stenoses. J Am Coll Cardiol 1990;15:1109.
32. Rowe RD, Vlad P, Keith JD. Experiences with 180 cases of tetralogy of Fallot in infants and children. Can Med Assoc J 1955;73:23.
33. Rowe SA, Zahka KG, Manolio TA, Horneffer PJ, Kidd L. Lung function and pulmonary regurgitation limit exercise capacity in postoperative tetralogy of Fallot. J Am Coll Cardiol 1991;17:461.
34. Rowland TW, Rosenthal A, Castaneda AR. Double-chamber right ventricle: experience with 17 cases. Am Heart J 1975;89:455.
35. Royer BF, Wilson JD. Incomplete heterotaxy with unusual heart malformations: case report. Arch Pediatr 1908;25:881.
36. Ruttenberg HD, Carey LS, Adams P, Edwards JE. Absence of the pulmonary valve in tetralogy of Fallot. Am J Roentgenol Radium Ther Nucl Med 1964;91:500.
37. Rygg IH, Olesen K, Boesen I. The life history of tetralogy of Fallot. Dan Med Bull 1971;18:25.

S

1. Sabri MR, Sholler G, Hawker R, Nunn G. Branch pulmonary artery growth after Blalock-Taussig shunts in tetralogy of Fallot and pulmonary atresia with ventricular septal defect: a retrospective, echocardiographic study. Pediatr Cardiol 1999;20:358.
2. Sanchez Cascos A. Genetics of Fallot's tetralogy. Br Heart J 1971;33: 899.
3. Sawatari K, Imai Y, Kurosawa H, Isomatsu Y, Momma K. Staged operation for pulmonary atresia and ventricular septal defect with major aortopulmonary collateral arteries. New technique for complete unifocalization. J Thorac Cardiovasc Surg 1989;98:738.
4. Schaff HV, DiDonato RM, Danielson GK, Puga FJ, Ritter DG, Edwards WD, et al. Reoperation for obstructed pulmonary ventricle–pulmonary artery conduits. J Thorac Cardiovasc Surg 1984;88:334.
5. Schulze-Neick I, Ho SY, Bush A, Rosenthal M, Franklin RC, Redington AN, Penny DJ. Severe airflow limitation after the unifocalization procedure: clinical and morphological correlates. Circulation 2000;102:III142.
6. Sellers RD, Lillehei CW, Edwards JE. Subaortic stenosis caused by anomalies of the atrioventricular valves. J Thorac Cardiovasc Surg 1964;48:289.
7. Sellors H. Surgery of pulmonary stenosis. A case in which the pulmonary valve was successfully divided. Lancet 1948;1:988.
8. Seybold-Epting W, Chiariello L, Hallman GL, Cooley DA. Aneurysm of pericardial right ventricular outflow tract patches. Ann Thorac Surg 1977;24:237.
9. Shimazaki Y, Blackstone EH, Kirklin JW. The natural history of isolated congenital pulmonary valve incompetence: surgical implications. Thorac Cardiovasc Surg 1984;32:257.

10. Shimazaki Y, Blackstone EH, Kirklin JW, Jonas RA, Mandell V, Colvin EV. The dimensions of the right ventricular outflow tract and pulmonary arteries in tetralogy of Fallot and pulmonary stenosis. J Thorac Cardiovasc Surg 1992;103:692.
11. Shimazaki Y, Maehara T, Blackstone EH, Kirklin JW, Bargeron LM Jr. The structure of the pulmonary circulation in tetralogy of Fallot with pulmonary atresia. J Thorac Cardiovasc Surg 1988; 95:1048.
12. Shimazaki Y, Tokuan Y, Lio M, Nakano S, Matsuda H, Blackstone EH, et al. Pulmonary artery pressure and resistance late after repair of tetralogy of Fallot with pulmonary atresia. J Thorac Cardiovasc Surg 1990;100:425.
13. Shinebourne EA, Babu-Narayan SV, Carvalho JS. Tetralogy of Fallot: from fetus to adult. Heart 2006;92:1353-9.
14. Shuford WH, Sybers RG. The aortic arch and its malformations with emphasis on the angiographic features. Springfield, Ill.: Charles C Thomas, 1974.
15. Sievers HH, Lange PE, Regensburger D, Yankah CA, Onnasch DG, Bursch J, et al. Short-term hemodynamic results after right ventricular outflow tract reconstruction using a cusp-bearing transanular patch. J Thorac Cardiovasc Surg 1983;86:777.
16. Singh SP, Rigby ML, Astley R. Demonstration of pulmonary arteries by contrast injection into pulmonary vein. Br Heart J 1978;40:55.
17. Smyllie JH, Sutherland GR, Keeton BR. The value of Doppler color flow mapping in determining pulmonary blood supply in infants with pulmonary atresia with ventricular septal defect. J Am Coll Cardiol 1989;14:1759.
18. Snir E, de Leval MR, Elliott MJ, Stark J. Current surgical technique to repair Fallot's tetralogy with absent pulmonary valve syndrome. Ann Thorac Surg 1991;51:979.
19. Soto B, Pacifico AD, Ceballos R, Bargeron LM Jr. Tetralogy of Fallot: an angiographic–pathologic correlative study. Circulation 1981;64:558.
20. Sousa-Uva M, Lacour-Gayet F, Komiya T, Serraf A, Bruniaux J, Touchot A, et al. Surgery for tetralogy of Fallot at less than six months of age. J Thorac Cardiovasc Surg 1994;107:1291.
21. Sreeram N, Saleem M, Jackson M, Peart I, McKay R, Arnold R, et al. Balloon pulmonary valvuloplasty for palliation of tetralogy of Fallot (abstract). J Am Coll Cardiol 1991;17:18A.
22. Stafford EG, Mair DD, McGoon DC, Danielson GK. Tetralogy of Fallot with absent pulmonary valve. Surgical considerations and results. Circulation 1973;48:III24.
23. Starnes VA, Luciani GB, Latter DA, Griffin ML. Current surgical management of tetralogy of Fallot. Ann Thorac Surg 1994; 58:211.
24. Starr A, Bonchek LI, Sunderland CO. Total correction of tetralogy of Fallot in infancy. J Thorac Cardiovasc Surg 1973;65:45.
25. Stellin G, Jonas RA, Goh TH, Brawn WJ, Venables AW, Mee RB. Surgical treatment of absent pulmonary valve syndrome in infants: relief of bronchial obstruction. Ann Thorac Surg 1983;36:468.
26. Stellin G, Milanesi O, Rubino M, Michielon G, Bianco R, Moreolo GS, et al. Repair of tetralogy of Fallot in the first six months of life; transatrial versus transventricular approach. Ann Thorac Surg 1995;60:S588.
27. Stephenson LW, Friedman S, Edmunds LH Jr. Staged surgical management of tetralogy of Fallot in infants. Circulation 1978; 58:837.
28. Strieder DJ, Aziz K, Zaver AG, Fellows KE. Exercise tolerance after repair of tetralogy of Fallot. Ann Thorac Surg 1975;19:397.
29. Sullivan ID, Presbitero P, Gooch VM, Aruta E, Deanfield JE. Is ventricular arrhythmia in repaired tetralogy of Fallot an effect of operation or a consequence of the course of the disease? A prospective study. Br Heart J 1987;58:40.
30. Sullivan ID, Wren C, Stark J, de Leval MR, Macartney FJ, Deanfield JE. Surgical unifocalization in pulmonary atresia and ventricular septal defect. A realistic goal? Circulation 1988;78:III5.
31. Sunderland CO, Rosenberg JA, Menashe VC, Lees MH, Bonchek LI, Starr A. Total correction of tetralogy of Fallot under two years of age. Postoperative hemodynamic evaluation (abstract). Circulation 1972;45:98.
32. Suzuki A, Ho SY, Anderson RH, Deanfield JE. Further morphologic studies on tetralogy of Fallot with particular emphasis on the prevalence and structure of the membranous flap. J Thorac Cardiovasc Surg 1990;99:528.
33. Swan H, Hederman WP, Vigoda PS, Blount SG Jr. The surgical treatment of isolated infundibular stenosis. J Thorac Cardiovasc Surg 1959;38:319.
34. Szarnicki R, Krebber HJ, Wack J. Wire coil embolization of systemic–pulmonary artery collaterals following surgical correction of pulmonary atresia. J Thorac Cardiovasc Surg 1981;81:124.

T

1. Takamiya M, Tauge I, Tadokoro M. Retrograde pulmonary arteriography: a new approach to opacification of pulmonary artery in pulmonary atresia, in Proceedings of the Thirteenth International Congress of Radiology, Madrid (abstract). International Congress Series No. 301. Amsterdam: Excerpta Medica, 1973, p. 233.
2. Tamesberger MI, Lechner E, Mair R, Hofer A, Sames-Dolzer E, Tulzer G. Early primary repair of tetralogy of Fallot in neonates and infants less than four months of age. Ann Thorac Surg 2008;86:1928-35.
3. Tay DJ, Engle MA, Ehlers KH, Levin AR. Early results and late developments of the Waterston anastomosis, Circulation 1974; 50:220.
4. Tchervenkov CI, Salasidis G, Cecere R, Beland MJ, Jutras L, Paquet M, et al. One-stage midline unifocalization and complete repair in infancy versus multiple-stage unifocalization followed by repair for complex heart disease with major aortopulmonary collaterals. J Thorac Cardiovasc Surg 1997;114:727.
5. Telagh R, Alexi-Meskishvili V, Hetzer R, Lange PE, Berger F, Abdul-Khaliq H. Initial clinical manifestations and mid- and long-term results after surgical repair of double-chambered right ventricle in children and adults. Cardiol Young 2008;18:268-74.
6. Terry PB, White RI Jr, Barth KH, Kaufman SL, Mitchell SE. Pulmonary arteriovenous malformations: physiologic observations and results of therapeutic balloon embolization. N Engl J Med 1983;308:1197.
7. Therrien J, Siu SC, Harris L, Dore A, Niwa K, Janousek J, et al. Impact of pulmonary valve replacement on arrhythmia propensity late after repair of tetralogy of Fallot. Circulation 2001;103: 2489-94.
8. Theye RA, Kirklin JW. Physiologic studies early after repair of tetralogy of Fallot. Circulation 1963;28:42.
9. Thiene G, Frescura C, Bini RM, Valente M, Gallucci V. Histology of pulmonary arterial supply in pulmonary atresia with ventricular septal defect. Circulation 1979;60:1066.
10. Touati GD, Vouhe PR, Amodeo A, Pouard P, Mauriat P, Leca F, et al. Primary repair of tetralogy of Fallot in infancy. J Thorac Cardiovasc Surg 1990;99:396.
11. Tsifutis AA, Hartmann AF Jr, Arvidsson H. Two-chambered right ventricle: report on seven patients. Circulation 1961;24:1058.
12. Tyson KR, Larrieu AJ, Kirchmer JT Jr. The Blalock-Taussig shunt in the first two years of life: a safe and effective procedure. Ann Thorac Surg 1978;26:38.

U

1. Ullom RL, Sade RM, Crawford FA Jr, Ross BA, Spinale F. The Blalock-Taussig shunt in infants: standard versus modified. Ann Thorac Surg 1987;44:539.

V

1. Van Arsdell GS, Maharaj GS, Tom J, Rao VK, Coles JG, Freedom RM, et al. What is the optimal age for repair of tetralogy of Fallot? Circulation 2000;102:III123-9.
2. Van Praagh R. The first Stella van Praagh memorial lecture: the history and anatomy of tetralogy of Fallot. Semin Thorac Cardiovasc Surg Pediatr Card Surg Annu 2009:19-38.
3. Van Praagh R, Corwin RD, Dahlquist EH Jr, Freedom RM, Mattioli L, Nebesar RA. Tetralogy of Fallot with severe left ventricular anomalous attachment of the mitral valve to the ventricular septum. Am J Cardiol 1970;26:93.
4. Van Praagh R, McNamara JJ. Anatomic types of ventricular septal defect with aortic insufficiency: diagnostic and surgical considerations. Am Heart J 1968;75:604.
5. Van Praagh R, Van Praagh S, Nebesar RA, Muster AJ, Sinha SN, Paul MH. Tetralogy of Fallot: underdevelopment of the pulmonary infundibulum and its sequelae. Am J Cardiol 1970;26:25.
6. Vargas FJ, Kreutzer GO, Pedrini M, Capelli H, Coronel AR. Tetralogy of Fallot with subarterial ventricular septal defect. Diagnostic and surgical considerations. J Thorac Cardiovasc Surg 1986;92:908.
7. Vetter HO, Reichart B, Seidel P, Kleinhans E, Bull U, Klinner W. Non-invasive assessment of right and left ventricular volumes 11 to 24 years after corrective surgery on patients with tetralogy of Fallot. Eur J Cardiothorac Surg 1990;4:24.

8. Villani M, Gamba A, Tiraboschi R, Crupi G, Parenzan L. Surgical treatment of tetralogy of Fallot. Recent experience using a prospective protocol. Thorac Cardiovasc Surg 1983;31:151.
9. Vobecky SJ, Williams WG, Trusler GA, Coles JG, Rebeyka IM, Smallhorn J, et al. Survival analysis of infants under age 18 months presenting with tetralogy of Fallot. Ann Thorac Surg 1993;56:944.
10. Von Bernuth G, Ritter DG, Frye RL, Weidman WH, Davis GD, McGoon DC. Evaluation of patients with tetralogy of Fallot and Potts anastomosis. Am J Cardiol 1971;27:259.
11. Vranicar M, Teitel DF, Moore P. Use of small stents for rehabilitation of hypoplastic pulmonary arteries in pulmonary atresia with ventricular septal defect. Catheter Cardiovasc Interv 2002;55:78.

W

1. Walsh EP, Rockenmacher S, Keane JF, Hougen TJ, Lock JE, Castaneda AR. Late results in patients with tetralogy of Fallot repaired during infancy. Circulation 1988;77:1062.
2. Walsh EP, Saul JP, Sholler GF, Triedman JK, Jonas RA, Mayer JE, et al. Evaluation of a staged treatment protocol for rapid automatic junctional tachycardia after operation for congenital heart disease. J Am Coll Cardiol 1997;29:1046.
3. Warden HE, DeWall RA, Cohen M, Varco RL, Lillehei CW. A surgical–pathologic classification for isolated ventricular septal defects and for those in Fallot's tetralogy based on observations made on 120 patients during repair under direct vision. J Thorac Surg 1957;33:21.
4. Waterston DJ. Treatment of Fallot's tetralogy in children under one year of age. Rozhl Chir 1962;41:181.
5. Watterson KG, Malm TK, Karl TR, Mee RB. Absent pulmonary valve syndrome: operation in infants with airway obstruction. Ann Thorac Surg 1992;54:1116.
6. Watterson KG, Wilkinson JL, Karl TR, Mee RB. Very small pulmonary arteries: central end-to-side shunt. Ann Thorac Surg 1991;52:1132.
7. Weldon CS, Rowe RD, Gott VL. Clinical experience with the use of aortic valve homografts for reconstruction of the pulmonary artery, pulmonary valve, and outflow portion of the right ventricle. Circulation 1968;37:II51.
8. Wessel HU, Bastanier CK, Paul MH, Berry TE, Cole RB, Muster AJ. Prognostic significance of arrhythmia in tetralogy of Fallot after intracardiac repair. Am J Cardiol 1980;46:843.
9. Wessel HU, Cunningham WJ, Paul MH, Bastanier CK, Muster AJ, Idriss FS. Exercise performance in tetralogy of Fallot after intracardiac repair. J Thorac Cardiovasc Surg 1980;80:582.
10. Wessel HU, Weiner MD, Paul MH, Bastanier CK. Lung function in tetralogy of Fallot after intracardiac repair. J Thorac Cardiovasc Surg 1981;82:616.
11. Williams GR, Richardson WR, Cayler GC, Campbell GC. Infundibular pulmonic stenosis with intact ventricular septum. Am Surg 1961;27:307.
12. Wolff GS, Rowland TW, Ellison RC. Surgically induced right bundle branch block with left anterior hemiblock. Circulation 1972;46:587.
13. Wu QY, Yang XB. Anomalous origin of the pulmonary artery from the right coronary artery. Ann Thorac Surg 2001;72:1396.

Y

1. Yagihara T, Yamamoto F, Nishigaki K, Matsuki O, Uemura H, Isizaka T, et al. Unifocalization for pulmonary atresia with ventricular septal defect and major aortopulmonary collateral arteries. J Thorac Cardiovasc Surg 1996;112:392.
2. Yamamoto N, Reul GJ, Kidd JN, Cooley DA, Hallman GL. A new approach to repair of pulmonary branch stenosis following ascending aorta–right pulmonary artery anastomosis. Ann Thorac Surg 1976;21:237.
3. Yamamoto S, Nozawa T, Aizawa T, Honda M, Mohri M. Transcatheter embolization of bronchial collateral arteries prior to intracardiac operation for tetralogy of Fallot. J Thorac Cardiovasc Surg 1979;78:739.
4. Yemets IM, Williams WG, Webb GD, Harrison DA, McLaughin PR, Trusler GA, et al. Pulmonary valve replacement late after repair of tetralogy of Fallot. Ann Thorac Surg 1997;64:526.
5. Yoo SJ, Lee YH, Kim ES, Ryu HM, Kim MY, Yang JH, et al. Tetralogy of Fallot in the fetus: findings at targeted sonography. Ultrasound Obstet Gynecol 1999;14:29-37.
6. Yoshigi M, Momma K, Imai Y. Coronary artery–pulmonary artery fistula in pulmonary atresia with ventricular septal defect. Heart Vessels 1995;10:163.

Z

1. Zach M, Beitzke A, Singer H, Hofler H, Schellmann B. The syndrome of absent pulmonary valve and ventricular septal defects—anatomical features and embryological implications. Basic Res Cardiol 1979;74:54.
2. Zahka KG, Horneffer PJ, Rowe SA, Neill CA, Manolio TA, Kidd L, et al. Long-term valvular function after total repair of tetralogy of Fallot. Relation to ventricular arrhythmias. Circulation 1988; 78:III14.
3. Zahka KG, Manolio TA, Rykiel MJ, Abel DL, Neill CA, Kidd L. Handgrip strength after the Blalock-Taussig shunt: 14 to 34 year follow-up. Clin Cardiol 1988;11:627.
4. Zahn EM, Lima VC, Benson LN, Freedom RM. Use of endovascular stents to increase pulmonary blood flow in pulmonary atresia with ventricular septal defect. Am J Cardiol 1992;70:411.
5. Zavanella C, Matsuda H, Subramanian S. Successful correction of a complete form of atrioventricular canal associated with tetralogy of Fallot. Case report. J Thorac Cardiovasc Surg 1977;74:195.
6. Zerbini EJ. The surgical treatment of the complex of Fallot: late results. J Thorac Cardiovasc Surg 1969;58:158.
7. Zuberbuhler JR, Dankner E, Zoltun R, Burkholder J, Bahnson HT. Tissue adhesive closure of aortic-pulmonary communications. Am Heart J 1974;88:41.

39 Pulmonary Stenosis and Intact Ventricular Septum

DEFINITION

Pulmonary stenosis and intact ventricular septum is a form of right ventricular outflow tract obstruction in which the stenosis can be valvar, infundibular, or both. Isolated infundibular stenosis is unusual. This chapter concerns primarily valvar pulmonary stenosis, with or without infundibular stenosis. When neonates present with the most severe form of this defect, the term *neonatal critical pulmonary stenosis* is used. When patients present beyond the neonatal period or in early infancy, the term *pulmonary stenosis* is used.

HISTORICAL NOTE

In 1913, as described by Dumont,[D7] Doyen first attempted to surgically relieve pulmonary stenosis in a 20-year-old woman who, in retrospect, is thought to have had infundibular obstruction. Thirty-five years later, in December 1948, Sellors performed a successful closed transventricular instrumental pulmonary valvotomy, closely following Doyen's technique.[S2] Brock performed three successful closed valvotomies in early 1948.[B5] These patients probably all had tetralogy of Fallot. Blalock and Kieffer applied this procedure to patients with pulmonary stenosis and intact ventricular septum soon thereafter, reporting 19 patients and two hospital deaths.[B4] Swan and colleagues surgically corrected pulmonary stenosis and intact ventricular septum by an open technique in about 1953, approaching the valve through a pulmonary arteriotomy during circulatory arrest, with the patient rendered moderately hypothermic by surface cooling.[S10] Other techniques evolved.[H5,L3,M12,S7]

Kirklin's experiences with closed valvotomy at Mayo Clinic led to an appreciation of the importance of acquired infundibular obstruction caused by hypertrophy[K5] and the need for a pump-oxygenator system that would allow relief by open operation.[K4] When cardiopulmonary bypass (CPB) became available in 1955, most surgeons began to use it to support patients during open valvotomy.

Surgical treatment of pulmonary stenosis was challenged in 1982 when Kan and colleagues reported successful percutaneous balloon valvuloplasty.[K1] This method of therapy is now applied to patients of all ages, and is, with the important exception of the morphologic variant called *pulmonary valvar dysplasia*,[K7] the initial procedure of choice.[C1,C3,L1,P1,Z1]

AGE CONSIDERATIONS

Symptoms, signs, and treatment of valvar pulmonary stenosis in the neonate presenting in severe distress during the first few days of life have long been recognized as different from those of patients presenting later in life. Interrelationships exist between neonatal valvar pulmonary stenosis and intact ventricular septum and pulmonary atresia and intact ventricular septum. Now that percutaneous techniques are used for therapy, different groups of physicians, as a rule, care for valvar pulmonary stenosis in patients presenting for treatment for the first time as adults and those presenting in early childhood. For all these reasons, this subject seems best approached according to age categories.

Section I Critical Valvar Pulmonary Stenosis in Neonates

MORPHOLOGY

Pulmonary Valve

The pulmonary valve is commonly a uniform fibrous cone with a circular, central, and stenotic orifice and two or three ridges on its pulmonary arterial side (Fig. 39-1). These ridges radiate from the central orifice to the periphery and outline two or three cusps that correspond to pulmonary sinuses of Valsalva, which are usually well formed. The valvar diaphragm is considerably thicker than normal cusp tissue, particularly around the ostium, but it is mobile.[G8] Thickening is produced by an increase in myxomatous tissue. Obstruction may be due to thickened, shortened, and rigid cusp tissue with little or no commissural fusion, known as *pulmonary valvar dysplasia*. This was described in 1969 by Koretzky, Edwards, and colleagues[K7] and further characterized by Stamm, Anderson, and colleagues.[S8] The right ventricular–pulmonary trunk junction *(anulus)* may be narrowed and the pulmonary trunk wall pulled inward or tethered at the site of commissural cusp attachment. The valve is often bicuspid. Although this condition may cause critical pulmonary stenosis in neonates, stenosis is typically moderate, a finding that is characteristic of Noonan syndrome.[N2,R9]

Pulmonary Arteries

Although it has been reported that in about 50% of neonates with critical pulmonary stenosis, right and left pulmonary arteries appear to be moderately or severely hypoplastic

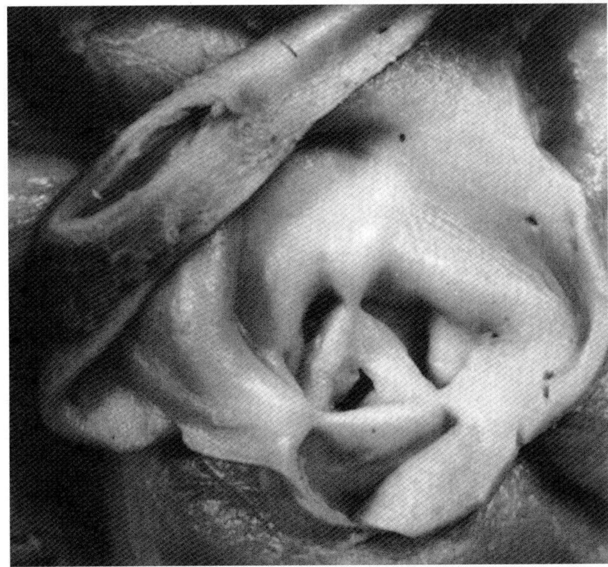

Figure 39-1 Specimen from a neonate with congenital valvar pulmonary stenosis and intact ventricular septum viewed through open, dilated pulmonary trunk. Fibrous cone with its central, very stenotic orifice; well-formed sinuses of Valsalva; and potential three-cusp valve structure are typical. Moderate right ventricular hypoplasia coexists (see Fig. 39-3).

Table 39-1 Critical Pulmonary Stenosis in Neonates: Relationship of Moderate or Severe Hypoplasia of Right and Left Pulmonary Arteries to Right Ventricular Cavity Size

		Moderate or Severe RPA and LPA Hypoplasia[b]	
RV Cavity Size[a]	*n*	No.	% of *n*
Enlarged (1-5)	3	0	0
Normal (0)	37	1	3
Mildly reduced (–1, –2)	30	0	0
Moderately reduced (–3)	11	1	9
Severely reduced (–4, –5)	3	1	33
Subtotal	84	3	4
Unknown	17	0	
TOTAL	101	3	

Data from Hanley and colleagues.[H2]
[a]Numbers in parentheses refer to grading of RV cavity size.
[b]Degree of hypoplasia of the pulmonary arteries was graded as 0 to –5. Hypoplasia was considered moderate or severe when graded –3, –4, or –5. Grading scheme was validated by comparison with actual measurements transformed to *z* values in patients for whom they were available.
Key: *LPA,* Left pulmonary artery; *RPA,* right pulmonary artery; *RV,* right ventricle.

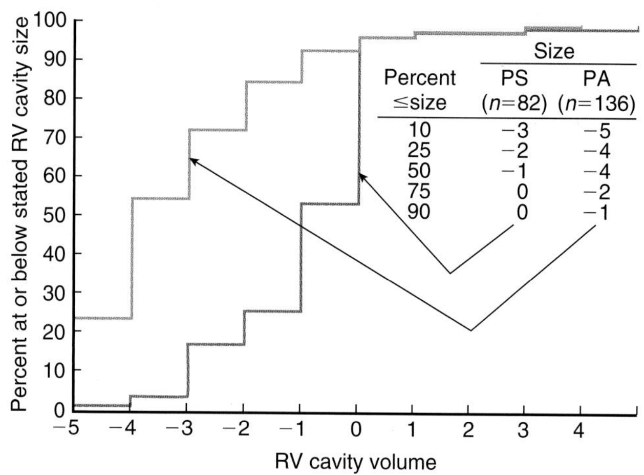

Figure 39-2 Cumulative frequency distribution of right ventricular (RV) cavity size in neonates with congenital pulmonary stenosis or atresia and intact ventricular septum (see Chapter 6 for details of construction). Zero represents normal RV cavity size, –5 represents severe RV hypoplasia, and +5 represents massive RV enlargement. The figure is based on data for 247 neonates. Only data for 82 patients with pulmonary stenosis and 136 with pulmonary atresia permitted an estimate of RV cavity size. Key: *PA,* Pulmonary atresia; *PS,* pulmonary stenosis; *RV,* right ventricular. (From Hanley and colleagues.[H2])

when imaged, this has not been confirmed by other studies[C2] (Table 39-1). As a rule, the appearance of pulmonary arterial hypoplasia is probably secondary to low pulmonary blood flow, because the pulmonary arteries are usually normal in size within a few years in those who survive interventional treatment.[C2]

Right Ventricle

Rarely, the right ventricular (RV) cavity is severely reduced in size. More commonly, mild or moderate reduction is present (Fig. 39-2). Reduction in cavity size relates in part to the amount of concentric RV hypertrophy produced by the RV outflow tract (RVOT) obstruction (Fig. 39-3).

Histologic appearance of the RV varies. Concentric RV hypertrophy is characterized by increased muscle cell size and diffuse fibrosis.[A1] The former is greater in the fibers near the endocardial surface; in some areas, muscle fibers can be seen to be disintegrating. Fibrosis is diffuse or patchy, but papillary muscles are the most severely affected. Fibrosis increases pari passu with hypertrophy and probably results from imbalance in the myocardial oxygen supply/demand ratio.[A1] Fibrosis of both endocardium and trabeculations is a marked feature when the RV is hypoplastic, contributing to poor compliance.

Neonates with critical pulmonary stenosis occasionally have severely enlarged RVs. This may represent coexisting important cardiomyopathy or (rarely) tricuspid valve disease. Prognosis is poor with or without valvotomy.

Tricuspid Valve

About 50% of neonates have normal tricuspid valve dimensions (within 2 standard deviations of the mean value for normal persons of the same size; see "Dimensions of Normal Cardiac and Great Artery Pathways" in Chapter 1). In the others, diameter is smaller than normal; in less than 10% the tricuspid valve is severely hypoplastic (Fig. 39-4). When it is markedly hypoplastic, it is apt to be grossly abnormal as well, with abnormal chordal attachments and fused cusps. Otherwise, the cusps and chordae usually are normal.

Right Ventricular Coronary Artery Fistulae

About 10% of neonates with critical pulmonary stenosis have RV sinusoids, but only 2% have RV coronary arterial fistulae. RV-dependent coronary circulation in such hearts is rare.

Right Atrium

The right atrium is usually large. There is generally at least a patent foramen ovale, and right-to-left shunting across it is a major contributor to arterial desaturation exhibited by many of these neonates.

Morphologic Correlates

RV cavity size and tricuspid valve dimension are not highly correlated in this condition, but mild to moderate hypoplasia is the rule in both locations.[H2] This is in contrast to pulmonary atresia and intact ventricular septum (see Morphology in Chapter 40), suggesting that reduction in RV cavity size in critical pulmonary stenosis is secondary to RV hypertrophy and thickening from outflow obstruction, rather than from genetic or developmentally induced hypoplasia. This is in harmony with the hypothesis that critical pulmonary stenosis develops relatively late in fetal life, in contrast to some types of pulmonary atresia.[T3]

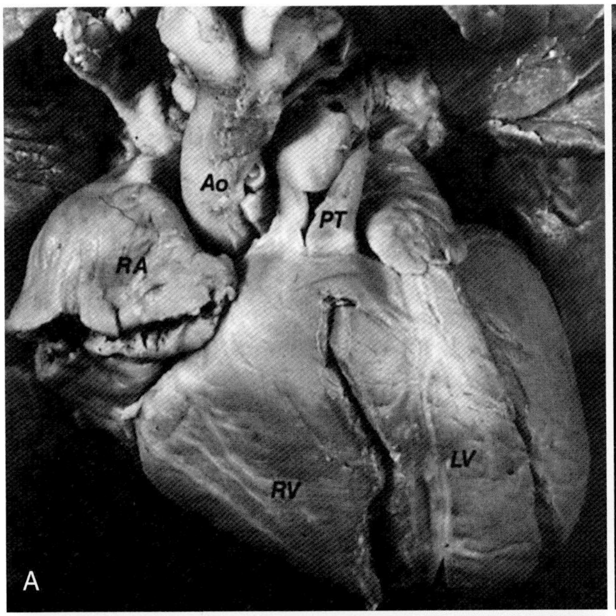

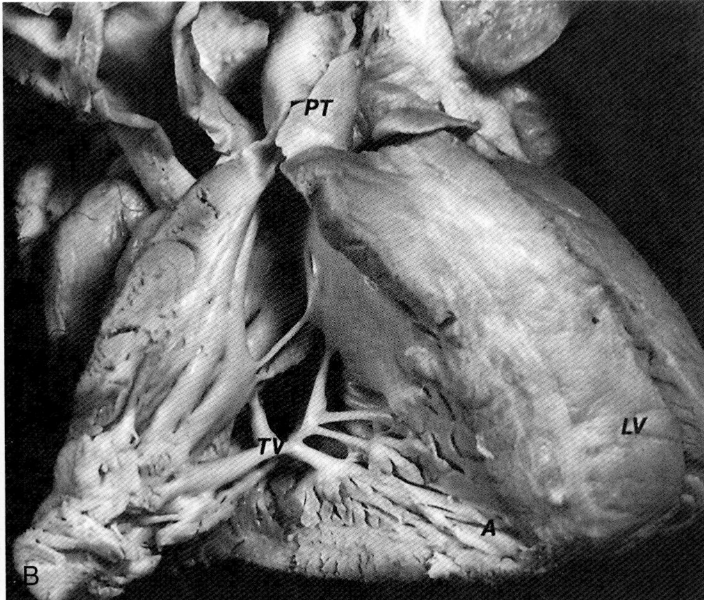

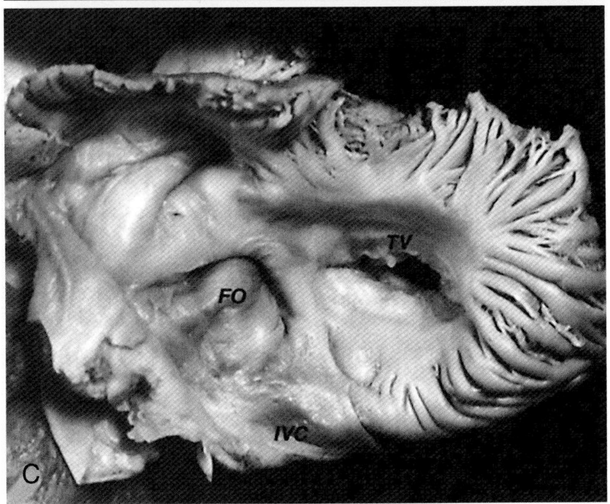

Figure 39-3 Specimen from a neonate with pulmonary stenosis and intact ventricular septum and moderate right ventricular (RV) hypoplasia. (Same specimen as in Fig. 39-1.) **A,** External dimensions of RV are moderately reduced, with displacement of left anterior descending coronary artery *(arrow)* toward the right. **B,** Opened RV shows almost complete obliteration of apical half of sinus portion of cavity by closely packed muscular trabeculations. These have had to be divided, along with the free wall, to display the potential cavity. Some dysplasia of tricuspid valve is apparent, with cusp thickening and shortening and abnormally attached and thickened sparse chordae. **C,** Somewhat stenotic tricuspid valve viewed from right atrial aspect. Its circumference was 32 mm, as was the mitral anular circumference. This heart is similar in some respects to those with pulmonary atresia and intact ventricular septum (see "Morphology" in Chapter 40). Key: *A,* Heavily trabeculated apical portion of cavity; *Ao,* aorta; *FO,* foramen ovale; *IVC,* inferior vena cava; *LV,* left ventricle; *PT,* pulmonary trunk; *RA,* right atrium; *RV,* right ventricle; *TV,* tricuspid valve.

Coexisting Cardiac Conditions

Coexisting cardiac conditions are uncommon. Ebstein malformation, which occurs in about 5% of patients with pulmonary atresia and intact ventricular septum, occurs in about 1% of those with critical pulmonary stenosis.[H2]

CLINICAL FEATURES AND DIAGNOSTIC CRITERIA

Neonates presenting with critical pulmonary stenosis and intact ventricular septum are usually critically ill, irritable, tachypneic, and severely hypoxic from right-to-left shunting at the atrial level. They usually present for treatment within a few days after birth and are generally of normal birth weight.[H2] When the atrial septum is intact, which is uncommon, cyanosis is absent.

Tachycardia and severity of heart failure often make auscultatory findings nondiagnostic. Physical findings of tricuspid regurgitation may be present. Chest radiograph usually shows a normal or somewhat enlarged heart. Pulmonary stenosis with hypoplastic RV is associated with less electrocardiographic (ECG) evidence of RV hypertrophy than expected.[F2] Diminished RV potentials are due to smallness of the RV cavity rather than to diminished muscle mass.[B6]

In a critically ill neonate with clear lung fields and a large cardiac silhouette, two-dimensional echocardiography provides near-certain diagnosis. The thick stenotic pulmonary valve is visualized, the RV cavity is seen, and size and cusp thickness of the tricuspid valve can be determined. Additionally, the pulmonary artery branch diameter can be accurately estimated, and color Doppler imaging can suggest presence of coronary artery anomalies such as RV-to–coronary artery fistulae.

Cardiac catheterization is indicated in essentially all cases for both diagnostic reasons (e.g., to define coronary artery anomalies) and therapy, because balloon pulmonary valvotomy is currently the treatment of choice. Cardiac catheterization usually shows peak RV pressure higher than that in the left ventricle (LV) or systemic arteries. Rarely, and in the presence of severe heart failure, peak RV pressure is less than that in the systemic circulation, despite severe valvar stenosis.

Cineangiography provides precise information regarding site of stenosis, size of RV cavity and infundibulum, presence or absence of tricuspid regurgitation, morphology of the pulmonary trunk and right and left pulmonary arteries, and presence or absence of RV-to–coronary artery fistulae (Fig. 39-5). The tricuspid valve is competent in about 10% of patients, and in the other 90% it is moderately or severely regurgitant (Hanley and colleagues and the Congenital Heart Surgeons Society: personal communication; 1992). Regurgitation, which is not well correlated with degree of RV hypertension (Fig. 39-6), is probably a manifestation of RV failure.

Currently, magnetic resonance and computed tomographic imaging are not routinely used in neonatal critical pulmonary stenosis, simply because these studies provide little added value to echocardiography and the mandatory cardiac catheterization. Recently, fetal echocardiography has been used to predict the postnatal fate of patients with critical

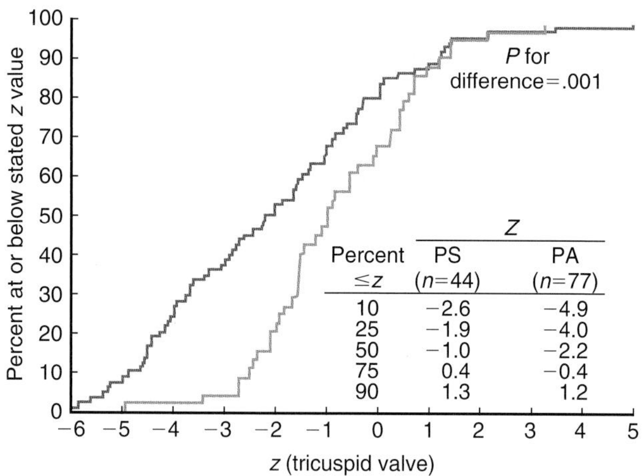

Figure 39-4 Cumulative frequency distribution of diameter of tricuspid valve, expressed as *z* value, in neonates with congenital pulmonary stenosis or atresia and intact ventricular septum. The *z* value of zero represents mean normal value, −2 represents 2 standard deviations (SD) below mean normal size, and +2 represents 2 SD above mean normal size. Figure is based on data for 247 neonates. Only data for 44 patients with pulmonary stenosis and 77 with pulmonary atresia permitted an estimate of tricuspid valve size. Key: *PA,* Pulmonary atresia; *PS,* pulmonary stenosis. (From Hanley and colleagues.[H2])

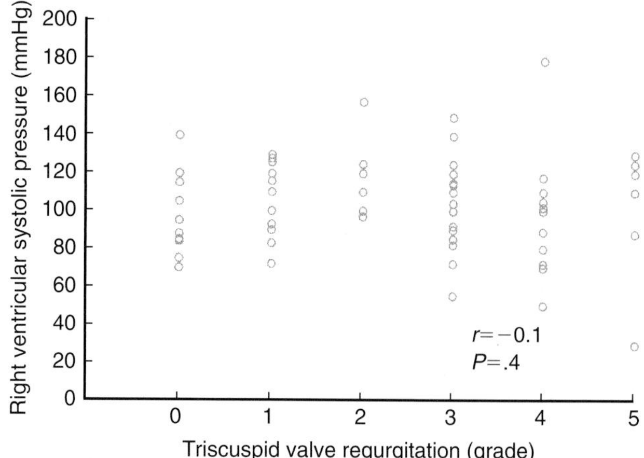

Figure 39-6 Scattergram illustrating lack of relationship between severity of tricuspid valve regurgitation and right ventricular peak pressure in neonates with critical pulmonary stenosis. (From Hanley and colleagues.[H2])

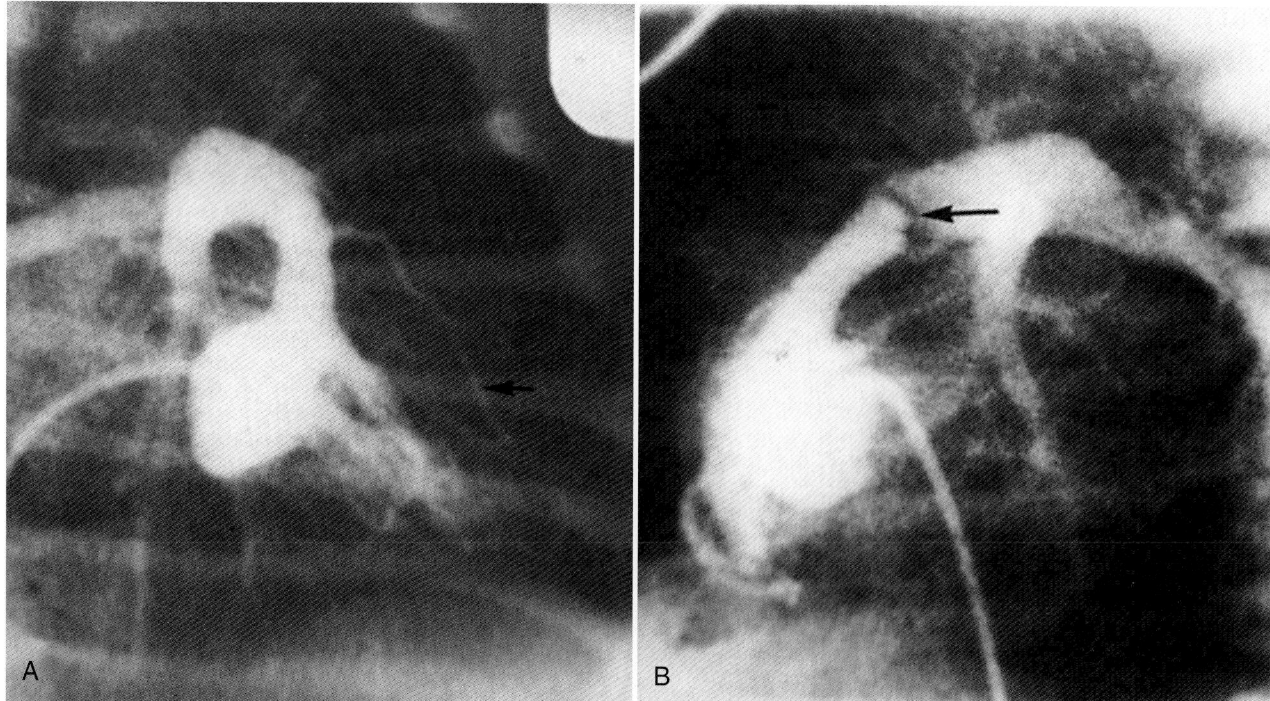

Figure 39-5 Cineangiogram of a neonate with extreme (pinhole) pulmonary stenosis and moderately severe right ventricular (RV) hypoplasia. **A,** Right anterior oblique view in diastole to show maximal degree of filling of apical half of sinus portion that is mainly occupied by thick muscular trabeculations. RV infundibulum, pulmonary trunk, and pulmonary artery branches are of good size. Left anterior descending coronary artery *(arrow)* is filling retrogradely from RV. There is no tricuspid regurgitation. **B,** Left anterior oblique view in systole demonstrates thickened domed pulmonary valve. A tiny central jet *(arrow)* is barely visible, but flow is sufficient to fill the pulmonary arteries well after several cardiac cycles.

pulmonary stenosis.[G3] The aim is to predict whether a two- or single-ventricle circulation will result following postnatal therapy. These techniques are more applicable to pulmonary atresia and intact ventricular septum but also have a role, albeit a lesser one, in pulmonary stenosis. Morphologic and physiologic characteristics identified at fetal echocardiographic interrogation can accurately predict the fate of the circulation following birth. These data can be used for planning postnatal therapy, parental counseling,[K2] and possibly prenatal intervention.[R10]

NATURAL HISTORY

Presentation is usually within the first 2 weeks, and mean age at operation in the series at Toronto Hospital for Sick Children was 3.9 days.[C2,M7] Most neonates in whom severe hypoxia develops, with or without heart failure, die without treatment, although some may live for a few months.[G5]

TECHNIQUE OF OPERATION

Percutaneous Balloon Valvotomy

The technique of percutaneous balloon valvotomy has been described in detail.[L1,P1,Z1] Briefly, a guidewire is introduced via the femoral vein across the pulmonary valve and maneuvered through the ductus arteriosus into the descending aorta. A wire-guided balloon 1.2 to 1.3 times the measured size of the anulus is placed across the pulmonary anulus. The balloon is inflated rapidly two or three times.[T1] Several case reports of fetal intervention for critical pulmonary stenosis using percutaneous balloon valvotomy have been reported, documenting technical success.[G1,T4] Efficacy of the procedure has not yet been documented.

Open Pulmonary Valvotomy Using Cardiopulmonary Bypass

When percutaneous balloon valvotomy has not been used or is unsuccessful, open pulmonary valvotomy using CPB is recommended.[H2] The surgical procedures of closed pulmonary valvotomy and open valvotomy with simple inflow stasis have also given good results; however, they are not currently recommended in most circumstances.[J2,M6] Operation may be performed using one or two venous cannulae and CPB with mild (32°C-34°C) or moderate (25°C-28°C) hypothermia as described in Chapter 2. A single venous cannula and mild hypothermia are chosen when a simple patent foramen ovale is present that will not be closed; two venous cannulae and moderate hypothermia are chosen when an atrial septal defect (ASD) will be closed.

Before establishing CPB, the ductus arteriosus is dissected and ligated immediately after initiating CPB. After establishing CPB and hypothermia, the aorta is clamped and cold cardioplegia administered (see "Cold Cardioplegia, Controlled Aortic Root Reperfusion, and [When Needed] Warm Cardioplegic Induction" in Chapter 3). Alternatively, operation may be done on the beating heart, without aortic clamping.

If two venous cannulae are used and an ASD is to be repaired, a small-caliber vent can be placed into the left side of the heart through a purse-string suture in the right pulmonary vein. Alternatively, the right atrium is opened through a small oblique incision, and a pump sump-sucker is placed across the foramen ovale and into the left atrium.

The pulmonary trunk is opened through a vertical incision, and fine stay sutures are placed on the edge of the incision for exposure. Two or three fused commissures can usually be seen, and these are opened with a knife, extending the incisions to the RV–pulmonary trunk junction. Because regurgitation is of less concern than residual narrowing, the incisions may be tailored to some extent to ensure that the valve has a wide opening. Portions of the valve are excised only when other methods fail to achieve a wide opening. Less commonly, the valve is dysplastic with three fully formed commissures and markedly thickened, even bulky, cusps. In this case, cusp debulking by partial resection of tissue is necessary to relieve obstruction. Rarely in neonates is there need to resect RV infundibular musculature. The pulmonary trunk is closed with one row of continuous 7-0 polypropylene suture. Usually, operation requires less than 15 minutes, and the aortic clamp, if used, is simply removed and de-airing accomplished. Remainder of the operation is completed in the usual manner (see "Completing Cardiopulmonary Bypass" in Section III of Chapter 2).

A patent foramen ovale, if present, is usually left open because the RV is very hypertrophied. The patient will benefit from allowing right-to-left atrial shunting until the RV remodels. If an ASD coexists, the decision is more complex because it is likely the patient will eventually develop significant left-to-right shunting through it once RV remodeling is complete. Judgment must be used in this setting. If there is concern that RV size and hypertrophy will result in perioperative RV failure, the ASD should be left open; it can be addressed at a later time once the RV has remodeled. If the RV is judged to be adequate, the ASD should be closed. Regardless of the initial decision, the physiology should be assessed carefully in the operating room following separation from CPB, and surgical readjustments (either opening or closing the ASD) made as necessary. Remainder of the operation is completed in the usual manner.

A concomitant systemic–pulmonary artery shunt may be added if PaO_2 is severely reduced (<30 mmHg) after discontinuing CPB. The neonate usually comes to the operating room well resuscitated by prostaglandin E_1 (PGE_1). However, in the rare circumstance in which this is not the case, methods employed for seriously ill adult patients will probably improve results (see "Cold Cardioplegia, Controlled Aortic Root Reperfusion, and [When Needed] Warm Cardioplegic Induction" in Chapter 3).

Consideration should be given to placing a fine polyvinyl catheter into the RV, inserted through the right atrium across the tricuspid valve. It is used perioperatively to monitor RV pressure and typically is removed 48 hours later in the intensive care unit (see Special Features of Postoperative Care later). Measurements in the operating room after repair are not as informative and cannot serve as a guide to concomitant infundibular resection (see Results).

Transesophageal echocardiography should be used routinely to assess the outflow tract after separation from CPB, paying particular attention to gradients at the valvar and infundibular level, degree of pulmonary and tricuspid valve regurgitation, RV function, and presence and degree of intraatrial shunting.

Transanular Patch

Although the likelihood of needing a transanular patch is greater when the RV cavity is small, the decision to place one at the initial surgical procedure is generally best made during operation.[H2] When surgery is performed as a secondary procedure, the decision is usually made preoperatively. Operation proceeds as described earlier for open pulmonary valvotomy. The interior of the RV infundibulum is inspected by looking through the pulmonary valve orifice. If it appears to be narrowed and if the diameter of the opened pulmonary valve (and thus presumably the "anulus") has a z value of −3 or less (see discussion of z value in "Standardization of Dimensions" under Dimensions of Normal Cardiac and Great Artery Pathways in Chapter 1), and particularly when the RV cavity is very small, a transanular patch is probably indicated.

Incision in the pulmonary trunk is carried across the anulus and down to the junction of the sinus and infundibular portions of the RV. The pulmonary valve cusps are excised. Conservative resection of hypertrophied muscular trabeculae in the infundibulum may be accomplished, but this is often impractical in neonates (see Fig. 38-11 in Chapter 38). An enlarging patch is fashioned from glutaraldehyde-treated or untreated autologous pericardium and sewn into place with continuous 6-0 or 7-0 polypropylene sutures (see "Decision and Technique for Transanular Patching" in Section I of Chapter 38). Remainder of the procedure, including placing the polyvinyl catheter, is as described in the preceding text. A systemic–pulmonary artery shunt is added only if PaO_2 is severely reduced after discontinuing CPB.

Systemic–Pulmonary Artery Shunt

If a systemic–pulmonary artery shunt is required as an isolated procedure (see Special Features of Postoperative Care later), a polytetrafluoroethylene (PTFE) interposition aortopulmonary shunt is made using a 3.5- or 4-mm tube via a median sternotomy. Whether shunting is an isolated procedure or concomitant to valvotomy or transanular patching, the PTFE tube is placed between the brachiocephalic trunk–right subclavian artery junction and the right pulmonary artery (see Technique of Operation in Section I of Chapter 38).

SPECIAL FEATURES OF POSTOPERATIVE CARE

Proper perioperative management of neonates is essential for success. Generally these deeply cyanotic and critically ill infants are started on PGE_1 intravenously in doses of 0.05 to 0.4 $\mu g \cdot kg^{-1} \cdot min^{-1}$ even before any studies are done; the resulting enlargement of the ductus arteriosus increases pulmonary blood flow and PaO_2 by the time of operation.[F6,N1,O3] PGE_1 is continued during percutaneous valvotomy and early thereafter until the RV has a chance to remodel.

Caution must be used lest pulmonary overcirculation develop in a neonate whose pulmonary valve has been widely opened. The infant is left intubated and ventilated. As PGE_1 is discontinued in the hours after the procedure, SaO_2 is monitored by pulse oximeter, or PaO_2 is measured frequently. If after 24 hours, PaO_2 remains well above 30 mmHg and the hemodynamic state is good, the neonate is gradually weaned from the ventilator and extubated. Even though some arterial desaturation persists, so long as PaO_2 stays above about 30 mmHg and the clinical condition remains good, the neonate is patiently followed in anticipation of continued improvement as the RV remodels and the pulmonary vascular resistance decreases. If PaO_2 falls to 30 mmHg or less, and if residual stenosis is mild or absent, a PTFE systemic–pulmonary artery shunt is performed. If important RVOT obstruction is present along with important hypoxia, a transanular patch as well as a systemic–pulmonary artery shunt is probably necessary.

If a primary surgical procedure is performed on the RVOT, the ductus has typically been ligated, and an appropriately sized systemic–pulmonary artery shunt may also have been placed. When a systemic–pulmonary artery shunt has been performed, the infant should be restudied at about age 6 to 12 months; plans should then be made for shunt closure by percutaneous or surgical means. In some surgical patients who do not receive a shunt at the time of the initial RVOT procedure, persistent cyanosis will occur, requiring return to surgery for placement of a shunt. Patients should be followed after hospital discharge until there is assurance that the RV–pulmonary artery peak pressure gradient is within acceptable limits. If it is not but can be remedied by further valvotomy, percutaneous techniques are generally recommended. In about 10% of patients, follow-up evaluation indicates important residual RV hypertension from "anular" or persistent infundibular narrowing; placing a transanular patch is then required to achieve the desired result.

RESULTS

Survival

Early (Hospital) Death

About 10% of heterogeneous groups of neonates die during initial hospitalization (Fig. 39-7). Risk-adjusted analysis indicates that early death occurs in only 6% of neonates treated by the surgical methods described in this chapter (Fig. 39-8). This very good result in critically ill patients is directly traceable to introduction of PGE_1, general improvement in neonatal cardiac surgery, and advent of percutaneous balloon valvotomy.[H2] Results of balloon valvotomy in neonates compare favorably with those of surgical valvotomy. Tabatabaei and colleagues were able to accomplish balloon dilatation in 35 of 37 neonates with critical valvar pulmonary stenosis (generally with suprasystemic RV pressure),[T1] with only 3 deaths (8%; CL 0%-16%). Others have reported similarly good survival.[F4,F5,T2,Z1]

Time-Related Survival

Survival for at least 4 years after birth in heterogeneous groups of treated neonates is about 80% (see Fig. 39-7). The rapidly declining appreciable early rate of death (hazard function) begins to flatten out considerably about 3 months after intervention. Risk-adjusted survival for at least 4 years can be presumed to be 94% (see Fig. 39-8), because death rarely occurred between 6 months and 4 years postoperatively in a large study.[H2] Gudausky and Beekman have reviewed mid- and long-term outcomes following balloon valvotomy in neonates, citing 6 studies since 1995 in addition to their own experience, totaling 221 patients.[G12] There were a total of 249 patients, with successful dilatation in 224 (90%). Follow-up ranged from 1 to 116 months. Twelve serious

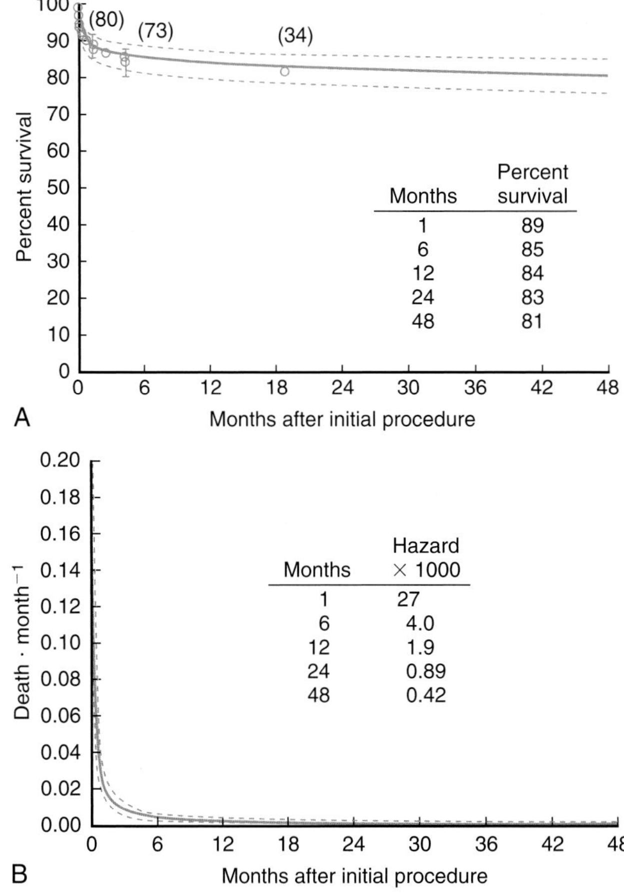

Figure 39-7 Death after first intervention in a heterogeneous group of 98 neonates with critical pulmonary stenosis. **A,** Survival. Each circle represents a death, and vertical bars represent 70% confidence limits of nonparametric estimates. Numbers in parentheses are number of patients traced after these estimates. Solid line represents a parametric estimate of survival enclosed within dashed 70% confidence bands. **B,** Hazard function *(solid line)* enclosed within 70% confidence bands *(dashed lines)*. (From Hanley and colleagues.[H2])

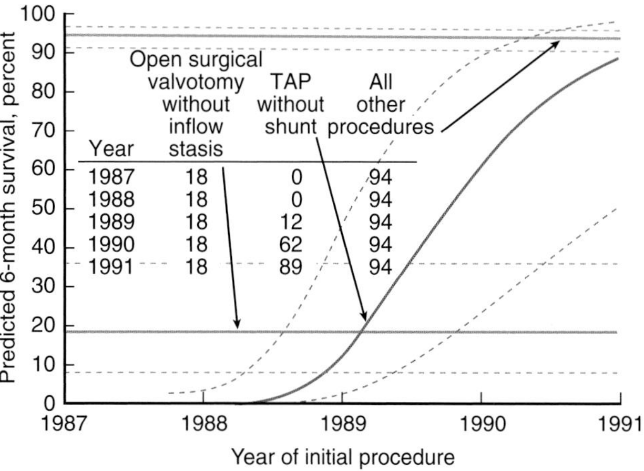

Figure 39-8 Risk-adjusted predicted percent survival for at least 6 months after initial intervention in neonates with critical pulmonary stenosis. "All other procedures" include percutaneous balloon valvotomy, closed surgical valvotomy, open surgical valvotomy with inflow stasis or cardiopulmonary bypass, and transanular patching (TAP) with concomitant systemic–pulmonary shunt. Solid lines represent a parametric estimate of survival enclosed within dashed 70% confidence bands. Dashed lines enclose the 70% confidence bands. The depiction is a specific solution of the multivariable equation in Table 39-2; –4 was entered for *z* value of tricuspid valve anulus, and grade 3 was entered for degree of tricuspid regurgitation. (From Hanley and colleagues.[H2])

Table 39-2 Incremental Risk Factors for Death at Any Time after Initial Accomplished Procedure[a]

Risk Factor		Single Hazard Phase *P* Value
Procedural		
	Open pulmonary valvotomy without inflow stasis	<.0001
	Transanular patching without a shunt[b]	
(Smaller)	+Dimension (*z* value) of RV-PT junction	.01
(Greater)	+Degree of tricuspid regurgitation	.0002
(Earlier)	+Date of procedure	.04

Data from Hanley and colleagues.[H2]
[a]Database consists of 101 neonates with critical pulmonary stenosis entered into a multiinstitutional study between January 1987 and 1991.[H2] Median age of entry was 3 days. Analysis was of 93 patients, excluding five with Ebstein anomaly, a large right ventricle, or both, and three (two are deceased) in which no procedure was performed.
[b]The three factors listed under transanular patching without a shunt are interaction terms; that is, they pertain only to patients in whom transanular patching without a shunt was performed, not to patients undergoing other types of procedure. Transanular patching without a shunt, when examined without interaction terms, had a low *P* value of .9.
Key: *PT,* Pulmonary trunk; *RV,* right ventricle.

complications resulted from the procedure, and 13 total deaths; 5 of the deaths were early and 8 were late.

Modes of Death

The mode of virtually all deaths is either hypoxia or acute cardiac failure.

Incremental Risk Factors for Premature Death

Although uncommon, RV enlargement of an appreciable degree is a highly lethal coexisting cardiac anomaly. This is probably a special situation in which there is a coexisting cardiomyopathy or tricuspid valve lesion (e.g., Ebstein malformation) already present in fetal life because of genetic or developmental factors. Aside from these rare cases, no general patient-specific risk factors for death are identifiable in neonates. This is unusual in patients with congenital heart disease.

For open pulmonary valvotomy *without* inflow stasis or CPB and for certain morphologic variants (see text that follows), transanular patching without a shunt is a risk factor, and these procedures should not be used[H2] (Table 39-2). Other procedures give good results, with few differences between them (Fig. 39-9). In neonates and young infants, transanular patching unaccompanied by a systemic–pulmonary artery shunt is an incremental risk factor when the pulmonary "anulus" is severely hypoplastic or when there is important tricuspid regurgitation. Patients in this situation usually have severe RV hypertrophy and reduced cavity size; without a shunt, they tend to have marked hypoxia from right-to-left shunting across a patent foramen ovale secondary to acute RV failure.

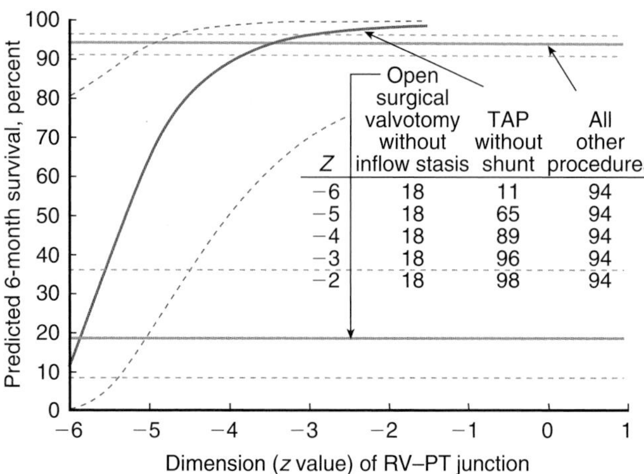

Figure 39-9 Risk-adjusted predicted percent survival for at least 6 months after first intervention in neonates with critical pulmonary stenosis. Depiction is similar to that in Figure 39-8. It indicates that in 1991 (value entered for date of operation), all procedures other than open pulmonary valvotomy without inflow stasis or cardiopulmonary bypass were followed by a 94% probability of survival for at least 6 months when the *z* value of right ventricle (RV)–pulmonary trunk (PT) junction ("anulus") was −4 or larger. When the anulus was severely hypoplastic, survival was not as good as after a transanular patch (TAP) without a shunt (see text). (Data from Hanley and colleagues.[H2])

Reintervention

About 75% of neonates successfully undergoing pulmonary valvotomy require no further procedure for at least 4 years.[H2] About 10% remain hypoxic and require a systemic–pulmonary artery shunt. In a few, repeat balloon valvotomy is needed. About 10% of those not initially receiving a transanular patch will need one at some point. Rarely (<2%), a two-ventricle system cannot be attained, and a superior cavopulmonary anastomosis or Fontan-type operation is ultimately required. Similarly, Rao reports occurrence of reintervention was 25% following initial balloon valvotomy.[R5]

Occasionally, closure of an ASD is required as the RV remodels and important left-to-right shunting develops in patients in whom the ASD was purposefully left open at the time of the neonatal procedure. The long-term implications of severe pulmonary regurgitation, primarily in those patients who received a transanular patch, remain unclear. In patients who fail to develop adequate SaO_2 (>85% at rest) and right atrial pressure (<12-15 mmHg at rest) with the atrial septum and any systemic–pulmonary artery shunt temporarily closed, a superior cavopulmonary anastomosis can be considered to reduce the workload of the RV, allowing closure of the ASD and systemic–pulmonary shunt. Occasionally, a Fontan-type operation is ultimately indicated.[G12]

Residual Right Ventricular Outflow Tract Obstruction

Limited information is available concerning residual gradients. In about 90%, any important residual gradient has disappeared or been overcome by repeat percutaneous valvotomy within 6 to 12 months of the initial procedure. Ultimately, the RV–pulmonary trunk gradient is usually about 20 mmHg.[M2,R1,R2,R6,R8,Z1] In unusual cases in which the gradient remains above about 50 mmHg, transanular patching is warranted. The mechanism by which percutaneous balloon valvotomy effects its good results is generally the ideal one of commissural splitting; tearing of pulmonary valve tissue is uncommon.[E4] The exception may be the dysplastic pulmonary valve, in which commissural fusion is not the dominant problem causing obstruction.[S8] Although Stamm, Anderson, and colleagues[S8] emphasize that balloon valvotomy is ineffective, based on morphologic characteristics of dysplastic valves, reports vary as to effectiveness of this procedure in this setting.[M1,M13,T5]

Morphologic and Functional Changes

Although some neonates initially have at least moderate reduction in RV cavity size, late after pulmonary valvotomy the RV cavity is normal or only mildly reduced in size in 90%. In only about 10% does an important degree of infundibular obstruction, cavity narrowing, or both persist.[C2] Following balloon valvotomy, pulmonary anulus and RV chamber size increase, cusp mobility improves, and cusp thickening resolves in the majority of cases studied by echocardiography 6 months to 8 years after intervention.[T1]

Whereas most patients have tricuspid regurgitation initially (in some cases, severe), more than 80% have no regurgitation late after valvotomy.[C2] However, in a few patients, moderate or severe regurgitation persists, and it is likely that the tricuspid valve is somewhat dysplastic in these patients. Pulmonary regurgitation following balloon valvotomy occurs with increasing frequency and severity over time in 41% to 88% of patients.[B3,G4] Need for surgical placement of a competent pulmonary valve prosthesis is unusual but reported.[B3]

INDICATIONS FOR OPERATION

Interventional treatment is indicated for all neonates. It may be accomplished by percutaneous balloon valvotomy or by open surgical valvotomy with CPB. Balloon valvotomy is the procedure of choice in most circumstances. An exception is when the patient has severe hypoplasia (*z* value of −4 or less) of the pulmonary "anulus" and severe reduction of RV cavity size; inserting a transanular patch and concomitantly constructing a systemic–pulmonary artery shunt are indicated as the initial procedure. When only a valvotomy has been performed, a subsequent systemic–pulmonary artery shunt, transanular patch, or both will be indicated in 10% to 20% of patients (see Special Features of Postoperative Care earlier). Surgical valvotomy is also the procedure of choice if expertise in percutaneous balloon valvotomy is lacking.

Section II **Pulmonary Stenosis in Infants, Children, and Adults**

MORPHOLOGY

Valvar pulmonary stenosis and intact ventricular septum in patients presenting after the neonatal period is a spectrum ranging from critical (pinhole) pulmonary stenosis, through severe pulmonary stenosis with a normal-sized or dilated RV, to moderate or mild valvar pulmonary stenosis that remains relatively stable throughout life.

Table 39-3 Morphologic Features of Pulmonary Stenosis with Intact Ventricular Septum in Infants, Children, and Adults[a]

	No.	% of Total Cases
Valve stenosis alone	82	59
Infundibular stenosis alone[b]	13	9
Valve + infundibular stenosis[c]	45	32
TOTAL	140	100
PT and/or branch PA origin stenosis	7	5
Hypoplastic right ventricle	19	14

[a]Based on 140 patients with pulmonary stenosis and intact ventricular septum undergoing repair at GLH, 1960 to 1979.
[b]This group is discussed in more detail in Section V of Chapter 38.
[c]Includes only patients receiving combined valvotomy and infundibular resection.
Key: *PA*, Pulmonary artery; *PT*, pulmonary trunk.

Pulmonary Valve

The pulmonary valve is usually better developed in infants and children with severe pulmonary stenosis than it is in neonates. Although the cusp tissue may have a myxomatous appearance and may be irregularly deformed and thickened, the two, three, or even four pulmonary valve cusps are relatively well formed with only partial commissural fusion.[G10,S3] In adults, the valve may become calcified, particularly when there has been preexisting infective endocarditis.[D5] In older patients, a variable amount of infundibular hypertrophy results in secondary infundibular stenosis. Occasionally, infundibular stenosis alone accounts for RV outflow tract obstruction (Table 39-3).

Pulmonary Arteries

Post-stenotic dilatation of the pulmonary trunk (see Fig. 39-5) is characteristic of this malformation and is present in about 70% of infants and children with this lesion.[F1,G6] The left pulmonary artery may be involved as well.

Right Ventricle

In older patients, in contrast to neonates, important hypoplasia of the RV is uncommon, although marked thickening of the ventricular wall is often seen. When this thickening involves the infundibular septum and free wall of the RV, severe subvalvar obstruction gradually develops.[K5] This has been anecdotally referred to as the "suicidal tendency" of the RV of patients with important pulmonary stenosis. In occasional cases, a low-lying and large moderator band or so-called anomalous muscle bands contribute to infundibular obstruction. In about 10% to 20% of patients, these are the only sites of obstruction, the valve being either normal or (rarely) bicuspid, but not stenotic (see Section V of Chapter 38).

Tricuspid Valve

In infants and children, the tricuspid valve is usually morphologically normal. However, mild regurgitation or, in the face of RV failure, moderate or severe regurgitation may develop.

Right Atrium

The right atrial wall is hypertrophied secondary to increased right atrial pressure. In about one fourth of infants and adults, the atrial septum is intact. However, in most the foramen ovale is patent, or there is a small ostium secundum ASD; right-to-left shunting results in cyanosis.[F2,K5] When a left-to-right shunt is present, there is usually a large ASD and only mild or moderate pulmonary stenosis.[R7]

Left Ventricle

Alterations in the LV (e.g., myocardial infarction, myocardial dysplasia, obstructive changes in the coronary arteries, abnormal media of the ascending aorta) have been shown occasionally to coexist with pulmonary stenosis and intact ventricular septum.[B2,S6] Muscular subaortic stenosis of the variety seen in hypertrophic obstructive cardiomyopathy may coexist. A combination of muscular subaortic and subpulmonary obstruction may be associated with abnormal facies and is a possible variant of Noonan syndrome.[N2] Important valvar pulmonary stenosis in infants and children can adversely affect LV function.[H3] This is largely the result of RV hypertension that displaces the septum toward the left and alters LV geometry.[S4] Cardiac output and LV function are adversely affected, but the abnormalities revert to normal after correction of the RV outflow obstruction.

Associated Anomalies

Pulmonary stenosis and intact ventricular septum occurs frequently in Noonan syndrome, which is characterized by small stature, hypertelorism, mild mental retardation, cardiac malformations (most commonly pulmonary stenosis), and at times ptosis, undescended testes, and skeletal malformations.[L5,N2] It is also associated with intrauterine rubella.

CLINICAL FEATURES AND DIAGNOSTIC CRITERIA

Symptoms

Infants may be symptomatic but usually have less severe symptoms than neonates. After the first year, patients often present because of a murmur only, produced by mild or moderate stenosis. In the second, third, and fourth decades, presentation may be with chronic RV failure. In all, 30% to 40% of patients are asymptomatic when first examined.[F1,K3] When symptoms occur, the earliest is often effort dyspnea, which results from inability to increase pulmonary (and thus systemic) blood flow with exercise because of the relatively fixed resistance of the pulmonary valve.[A3,F1]

Cyanosis appears when, in the presence of an interatrial communication, the RV becomes less compliant than the LV or its pressure becomes severely elevated. With a normally developed RV, this occurs only when its pressure is suprasystemic, and is associated with ECG evidence of considerable RV hypertrophy. When cyanosis is marked in older patients, polycythemia becomes severe, and all the complications associated with this condition can develop (see "Clinical Presentation" under Clinical Features and Diagnostic Criteria in Section I of Chapter 38).[M11] However, these patients rarely squat for symptomatic relief as do those with tetralogy of Fallot.[A3,F1]

Effort-related precordial pain is not uncommon and is presumably due to RV angina. Sudden death can occur in cyanotic and acyanotic children and in young adults.[M11,W3]

Patients in the second and third decades of life with severe and long-neglected pulmonary stenosis and intact ventricular septum show development of right heart failure with elevated jugular venous pressure, hepatomegaly, and ascites, which eventually leads to death.

Signs

Except in young infants with severe heart failure, a systolic murmur (best heard in the second left interspace) is present, often with a thrill. Peak intensity of the murmur occurs later in systole in those with severe rather than mild stenosis.[G2] The pulmonary component of the second sound may be normal, decreased, or inaudible, whereas the aortic component is usually obscured by the murmur. The tighter the pulmonary stenosis, the longer the RV ejection time and the greater the delay in pulmonary valve closure.[G2,V1]

In severe stenosis, an ejection click is absent because the dome of the pulmonary valve is pushed upward into the pulmonary trunk by the vigorous right atrial contraction before ventricular systole occurs. In some patients with mild stenosis, the abnormality of cusp movement may be insufficient to produce a click, although in other patients it may be prominent, the sound being magnified by a dilated pulmonary trunk.

The hypertrophied RV can often be appreciated as an RV heave palpable to the left of the sternum. The jugular venous "a" wave increases in amplitude as pulmonary stenosis increases in severity and is made more obvious by a noncompliant RV.[W3] In older children, diagnosis of associated RV hypoplasia is suspected when signs of pulmonary stenosis are combined with heart failure and cyanosis in the absence of severe RV hypertrophy on the ECG. Thus, in contrast to pulmonary stenosis with a normally developed RV, cyanosis may occur when its pressure is less than systemic and the ECG is unremarkable.[S1,W2]

Electrocardiography

Right atrial enlargement from moderate or severe pulmonary stenosis is reflected in prominent P waves in the ECG.[S5] When pulmonary stenosis is mild or moderate, the R-wave height in V_1 is less than 10 mm, or there is a pattern of incomplete right bundle branch block. When it is severe, the R or R′ in V_1 becomes greater than 10 mm and corresponding in its height to degree of RV hypertension.[E3]

Echocardiography

In children and adults, as well as neonates, two-dimensional echocardiography can provide near-certain diagnosis. The thickened, immobile, or domed pulmonary valve can be imaged, along with post-stenotic enlargement of the pulmonary trunk and RV thickening. Severity of stenosis can be estimated by Doppler evaluation of the flow across the pulmonary valve in systole, and this can be confirmed by similar evaluation of the velocity of flow in the tricuspid valve regurgitant jet, if present. Echocardiography can also be used to diagnose restrictive RV physiology by demonstrating forward flow across the pulmonary valve in late diastole. This physiology can be present in up to 42% of adults with moderate or severe stenosis and correlates with increased symptoms.[L2]

Cardiac Catheterization and Cineangiography

Techniques and findings are the same as those described in Section I.

NATURAL HISTORY

Pulmonary stenosis with intact ventricular septum accounts for about 10% of congenital heart disease and is thus a common malformation. Most surgical series show a predominance of females.

Patients Presenting in Infancy

Patients who survive the neonatal period to present later in infancy have a wide variation in degree of pulmonary valve narrowing. About 40% (CL 32%-47%) have mild obstruction, 47% (CL 39%-54%) moderate, and only 14% (CL 9%-20%) severe. However, these percentages probably underestimate the proportion of patients in this age group with severe obstruction. Nugent and colleagues found that 58% (CL 51%-64%) of an unselected group of infants presenting in the first 2 years (n = 81) with this entity had severe RV outflow obstruction.[N3] Even in early life, and probably more so as time passes, infundibular (muscular) narrowing adds to RV output resistance.

When RV outflow obstruction is severe in infants and young children, heart failure, cyanosis, or both are common (more so than in older patients who have developed the same degree of obstruction).[L4,N3] Prognosis of this group is poor. Levine and Blumenthal found that 56% of patients with heart failure died during follow-up.[L4]

Even when obstruction is moderate in this young age group, an important proportion have heart failure, with its same poor prognostic implication. It is probable that a degree of RV hypoplasia is often implicated in heart failure under these circumstances. According to Mody's study of 17 patients with moderate RV outflow tract obstruction in the first year, 53% (CL 38%-68%) experienced progression to a severe lesion in the next several years (average 4.5 years).[M8] Similar conclusions can be drawn from the data of Wennevold and Jacobsen and Danilowicz and colleagues.[D2,W1]

Even in asymptomatic infants with mild stenosis, Anand and Mehta reported rapid progression requiring intervention within 6 months in 15%.[A2] Experience of others, however, contradicts this, indicating that progression of mild pulmonary stenosis (gradient of <40 mmHg) in infants is rare and is similar to the natural history of mild pulmonary stenosis diagnosed in older children.[A4,D6]

Patients Presenting after Infancy

Patients with isolated pulmonary stenosis that produces mild RV outflow obstruction (peak pressure gradient between RV and pulmonary trunk ≤ 25 mmHg or RV peak pressure ≤ 50 mmHg) have a predicted probability of survival equal to that of an age-gender-ethnicity–matched general population.[H4] These patients rarely experience progression of pulmonary stenosis and therefore rarely require interventional therapy.[H4,M8,M9,M10] Recent studies by Rowland and colleagues and Gielen and colleagues corroborate earlier findings.[G7,R12]

Patients with moderately severe obstruction (peak pressure gradient between RV and pulmonary trunk > 25 mmHg but < 50 mmHg, or RV peak pressure > 50 mmHg but < 80 mmHg) sometimes experience progression in severity of their RV outflow obstruction. Without progression, as best as can be gleaned from currently available information, predicted probability of survival for at least 25 years is excellent.[H4]

Patients with severe pulmonary stenosis are susceptible to eventual development of chronic heart failure (and thus premature death), the tendency being greater the older the patient. Secondary changes in the severely stenotic valve probably make it more obstructive as time passes, with the outflow tract becoming more hypertrophied and stenotic and the RV becoming thicker, more fibrotic, less contractile, and less compliant.[H1] In women with severe pulmonary stenosis who are in New York Heart Association functional class I or II, pregnancy is not associated with an increase in fetal or maternal complications, in contrast to similar disease of the mitral or aortic valve.

Effect of Right Ventricular Hypoplasia

RV hypoplasia seems to affect natural history unfavorably. However, some patients with hypoplasia do not die in infancy but present later in life, usually with progressive cyanosis from a right-to-left shunt at atrial level. Left untreated, progressive right heart failure develops and causes death.

TECHNIQUE OF OPERATION

Comment

In infants, children, and adults, as in neonates, percutaneous balloon valvotomy is the treatment of choice for valvar pulmonary stenosis. If this is not successful, or is not indicated, open surgical valvotomy using CPB is performed. Balloon valvotomy is ineffective in most cases of dysplastic pulmonary valve, and when the valve anulus is hypoplastic (z value < −3). The surgical technique is that described in Section I. When transanular patching is necessary, the technique is also that described in Section I.

Open Operation during Cardiopulmonary Bypass

The general aspects of operation described in Section I are applicable to pulmonary valvotomy in infants and adults. After the pulmonary trunk is opened through a vertical incision, valvotomy is performed (Fig. 39-10). When edges of the cusps are bulky and obstructive, and particularly when the valve is bicuspid, partial or complete valvectomy may be necessary, because a taut bicuspid valve cannot open properly even after incision of the two fused commissures. RV, LV, and pulmonary artery pressures are measured at this point, but they are of little value in decision making (see Special Features of Postoperative Care later). A polyvinyl catheter is placed to measure RV pressure. It can be brought from the pulmonary artery out the low RV or alternatively, can be advanced forward from the right atrium through the tricuspid valve. Pressure measurements made the following morning may indicate the need for return to the operating room for relief of infundibular or anular stenosis.

When an infundibular resection is indicated (Fig. 39-11), a vertical infundibular incision is preferred. After resection, the incision is closed using an oval-shaped patch of PTFE or pericardium. In a few patients, a transanular patch is required because of a small pulmonary valve anulus. Patients requiring this often have dysplastic pulmonary valves. Cineangiogram or echocardiogram may suggest need for the transanular patch, but the final decision is usually made in the operating room. At the time of valvotomy through the pulmonary arteriotomy, the anulus is sized with Hegar dilators. If it is small (z value of −3 or less), the arteriotomy is carried across the anulus and down the infundibular free wall. If there is doubt about need for transanular patching, the pulmonary arteriotomy is left open and a vertical incision made in the infundibulum.

After muscle resection has been accomplished, the anulus is again sized by Hegar dilators passed through the valve from below. If it is too small, the two incisions are joined by cutting across the anulus, and a transanular patch is inserted (see "Decision and Technique for Transanular Patching" under Technique of Operation in Section I of Chapter 38). Deleon and colleagues have described a reconstructive operation for patients with dysplastic pulmonary valve with hypoplastic anulus that preserves valve function.[D4] However, the experience involves only two patients, and follow-up is limited.[D4]

In the occasional patient with stenosis of the pulmonary trunk or branches in whom these have not, or cannot, be treated adequately by balloon dilatation and stenting, the narrowed pulmonary branch is dissected to a point beyond the stenosis and an enlarging repair made (see Technique of Operation in Section I of Chapter 38). Preliminary dissection of these branches is best made during CPB cooling. These stenoses must be identified in detail at preoperative cardiac catheterization.

SPECIAL FEATURES OF POSTOPERATIVE CARE

Postoperative care is accomplished as described in Chapter 5. One special feature is that RV pressure should be assessed on the first postoperative day. This is accomplished by monitoring the RV pressure or withdrawal of the pulmonary artery pressure catheter that was placed at operation into the RV. These pressures are more reliable in predicting late results from operation than those taken in the operating room. However, if the patient's hemodynamic state is good, reoperation within a few days of the initial procedure is rarely necessary, even when RV pressure is high, because of the known tendency for infundibular hypertrophy to regress with time.

RESULTS

Survival

Early (Hospital) Death

Hospital mortality is essentially zero after percutaneous balloon valvotomy.[M1,M2,R1,R2] It is very low after surgical valvotomy as well and has been for many years.[D1,E1,M3,P2,R11] It approaches zero when patients with severe RV hypoplasia or advanced chronic heart failure are excluded.

Young age (down to 1 month) is not a risk factor. The few deaths that occur are associated either with severe

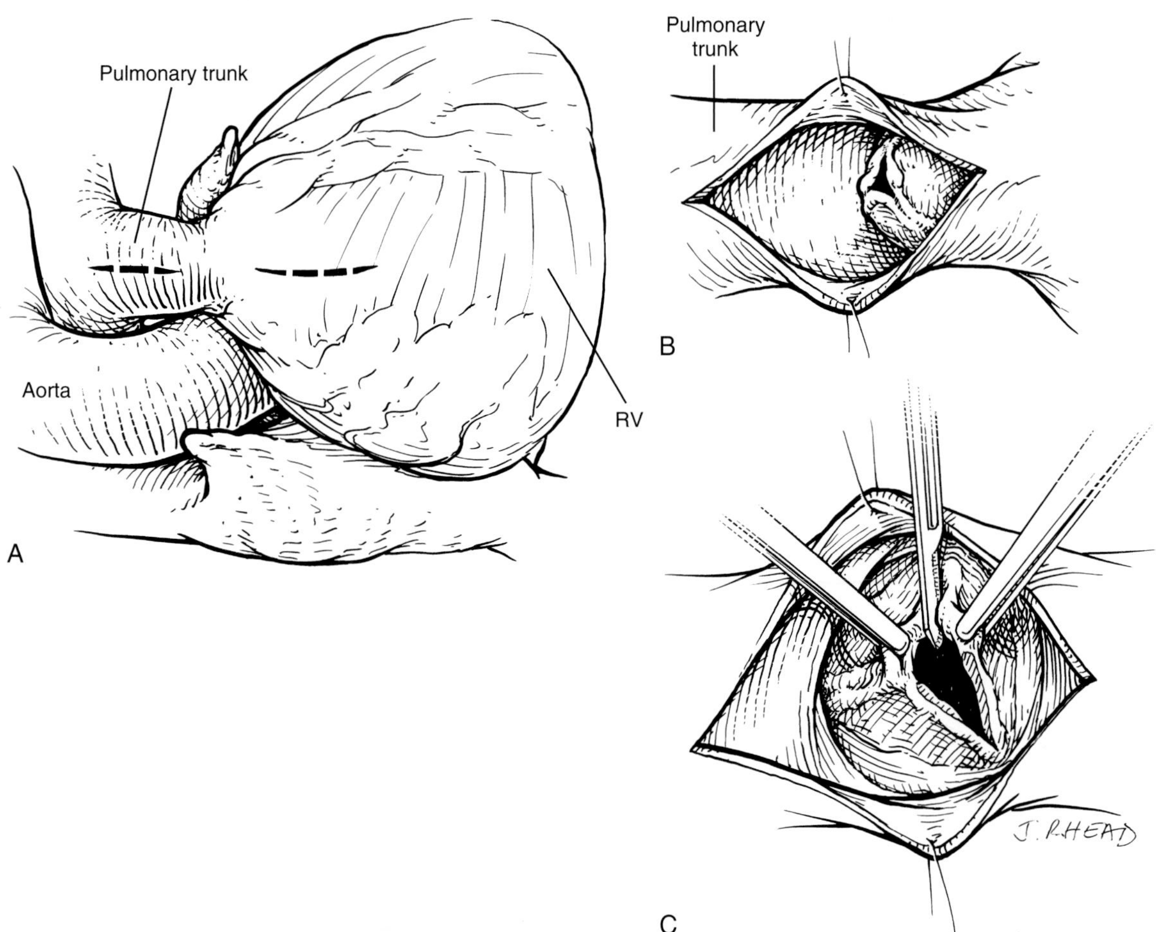

Figure 39-10 Pulmonary valvotomy through pulmonary trunk during cardiopulmonary bypass. **A,** Overview showing vertical incisions in pulmonary trunk and high right ventricle (RV). **B,** View of funnel-like stenosis of pulmonary valve. **C,** Commissures are incised sharply with a knife. As this is done, the surgeon and an assistant must carefully stabilize the cusp on either side to avoid inaccuracy in making the incision. If necessary, thickened valve tissue around the orifice may be resected, or a cusp may be partially detached. However, this is done only if the opening is otherwise unacceptable, because some degree of regurgitation results. When infundibular dissection and resection are also required, RV is opened through a vertical incision in the infundibulum. After performing the dissection and resection, vertical ventriculotomy is closed with a small oval patch of polytetrafluoroethylene or pericardium inserted with continuous polypropylene suture.

RV hypoplasia or, particularly in adults, advanced chronic heart failure.

Time-Related Survival

Long-term survival is the rule after surgical treatment. In the early Mayo Clinic experience, survival out to 25 years after hospital discharge was 91% in the overall group, but this was importantly affected by age at operation.[K6] Survival for at least 25 years after hospital discharge was 93% for those aged 0 to 4 years at operation, 100% for those aged 4 to 10 years at operation, 92% for those aged 11 to 20 years, and 71% for those older than 21 at operation.[K6] Although neonates were not represented in this experience, infants were, and this probably accounts for the effect of age in that era.

In a more recent longitudinal study of 51 patients, with follow-up ranging from 22 to 33 years (mean 25 years), late survival was 96%.[R11] Long-term survival is now available following balloon valvotomy. Fawzy and colleagues report 2- to 17-year follow-up (mean 10 years) in 90 patients, with no late deaths.[F3] All patients were older at the time of balloon intervention in this study, ranging from 15 to 54 years. Gupta and colleagues reported a single death in 166 patients,[G13] and Jarrar and colleagues report no late deaths in 62 patients[J1] during follow-up.

Hemodynamic Outcomes and Reintervention

Immediate relief of the gradient usually is obtained, and it is rare for adequate initial relief of obstruction to be temporary. On average, a peak RV pressure of 128 mmHg before valvotomy is reduced to 51 mmHg shortly after valvotomy.[K6] Completeness of relief of pulmonary stenosis can be determined only by late postoperative studies because of the usual, but not invariable, tendency for RV peak pressure to decrease over time after valvotomy.[E2,G11] This decline is believed to be due primarily to regression of RV hypertrophy and lessening of infundibular narrowing.[G9,K5,N3,R4] It is known, however, that adequate isolated pulmonary valvotomy does not invariably provide excellent relief of pulmonary stenosis, even in infants. Roos-Hesselink and colleagues report a low but definable incidence of restenosis.[R11] In 64 patients with follow-up ranging from 22 to 33 years, the reintervention rate was 15%. Two patients required reoperation for recurrent RVOT obstruction at 2 and 3 years after initial surgery, and

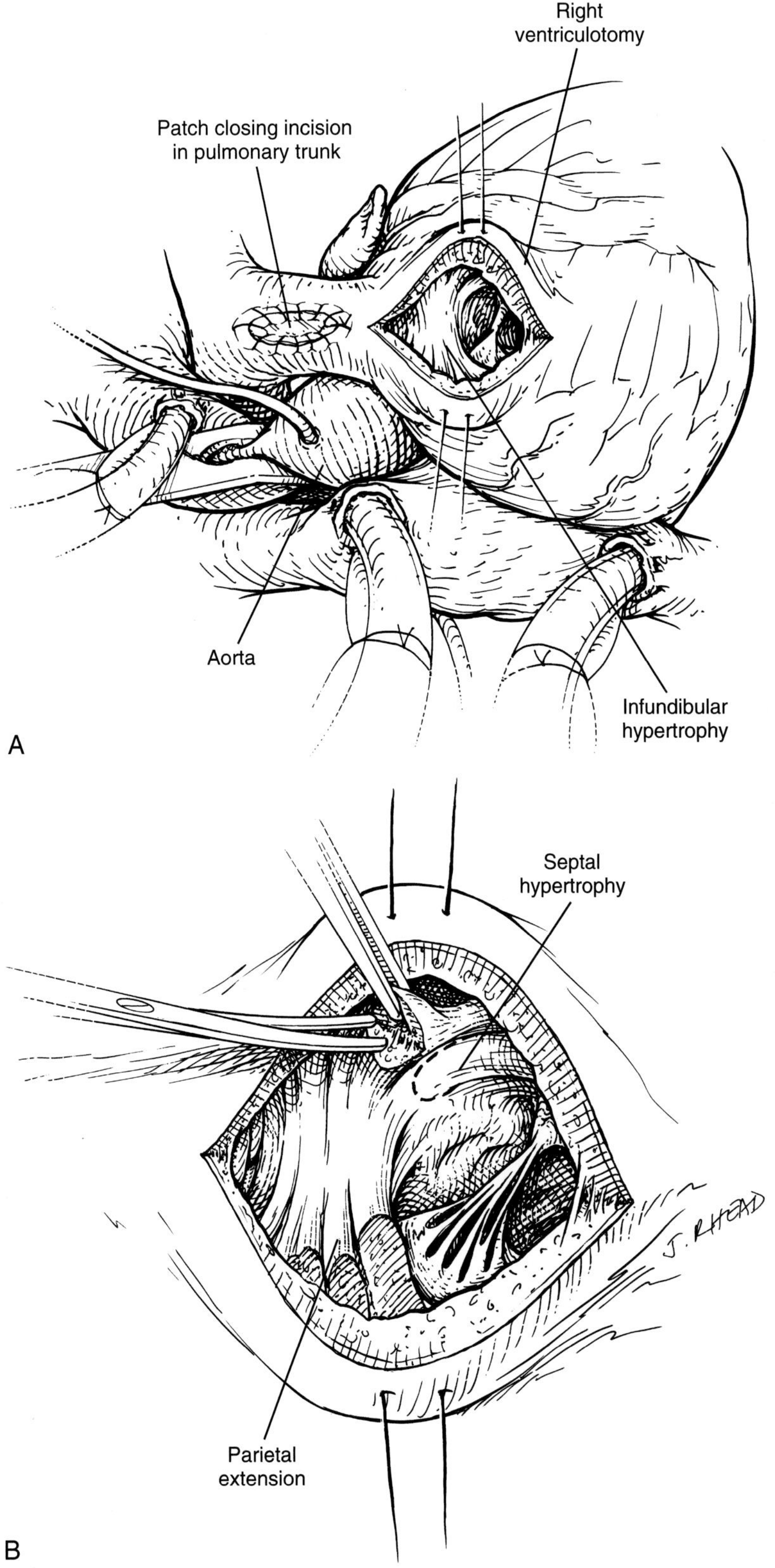

Figure 39-11 Infundibular resection for pulmonary stenosis with intact ventricular septum. In contrast to the situation in tetralogy of Fallot, this is a resection of muscle from the entire circumference of the severely hypertrophied outflow tract. **A,** Approach is through a vertical incision that will be closed with a polytetrafluoroethylene (PTFE), polyester, or pericardial patch as in tetralogy of Fallot. **B,** Working from below upward, muscle is cored out with a knife up to valve level. More muscle can be excised from recesses in front of either end of the infundibular septum than elsewhere. Excision is often also necessary from the walls (anterior, medial, and lateral) for a short distance below ventriculotomy.

Continued

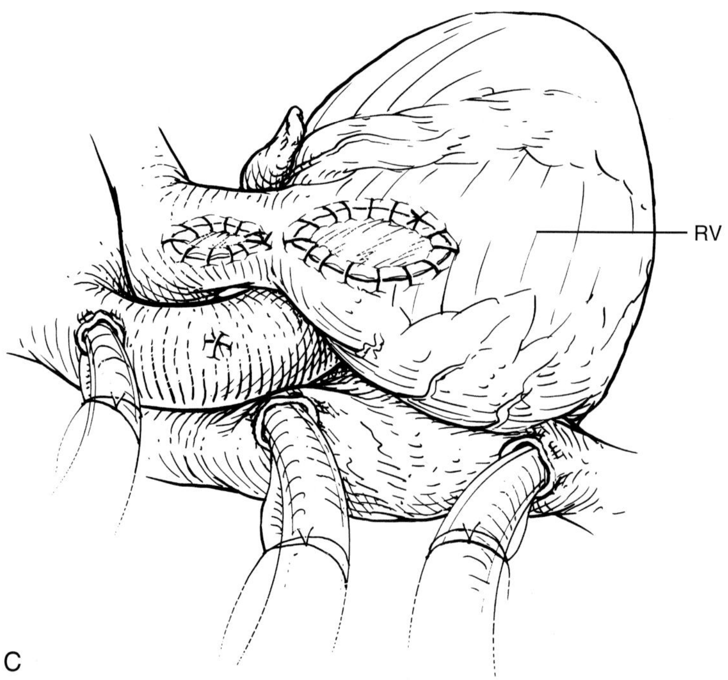

Figure 39-11, cont'd **C,** Both the pulmonary trunk incision and ventriculotomy are closed with small oval patches of PTFE, polyester, or pericardium. Key: *RV,* Right ventricle.

two required subsequent balloon dilatation at 16 and 18 years postoperatively. Additionally, six other patients required surgical reintervention, ranging from 16 to 24 years postoperatively, for severe pulmonary regurgitation. Five of these six had a transanular patch placed at initial operation. Moderate to severe pulmonary regurgitation was present at late follow-up in 37% of patients.

Earing and colleagues, on the other hand, reported more concerning long-term reintervention.[E1] In 53 patients with a mean follow-up of 33 years, reintervention for recurrent pulmonary stenosis was similarly low, but 21 patients (40%) required pulmonary valve replacement for severe regurgitation. This may reflect the extremely long follow-up, because other authors have recognized the progressive increase in symptomatic pulmonary regurgitation the longer the follow-up; however, equally important is that this cohort of patients underwent their original surgery in a different era. To this point, in this study, closed pulmonary valvotomy was importantly associated with need for late reoperation.

Hemodynamic results after percutaneous balloon valvotomy are similar to those just described (see Results in Section I). Fawzy and colleagues[F3] report a reduction in pulmonary valve gradient from 105 mmHg to 34 mmHg in their series of 90 patients (mean age 24 years). The infundibular gradient was large immediately following the procedure in 43 patients, all of whom underwent later recatheterization. The gradient decreased from 42 mmHg following the initial procedure to 13 mmHg at repeat study. Other reports document similar results.

Gudausky and Beekman[G12] summarize results from five large studies reported between 1994 and 2003. A total of 866 non-neonatal cases were included. Restenosis occurred in 20%, with 7% requiring repeat balloon valvotomy and 7% requiring surgery. Severe pulmonary insufficiency was present in 1%. Freedom from either surgical or balloon reintervention

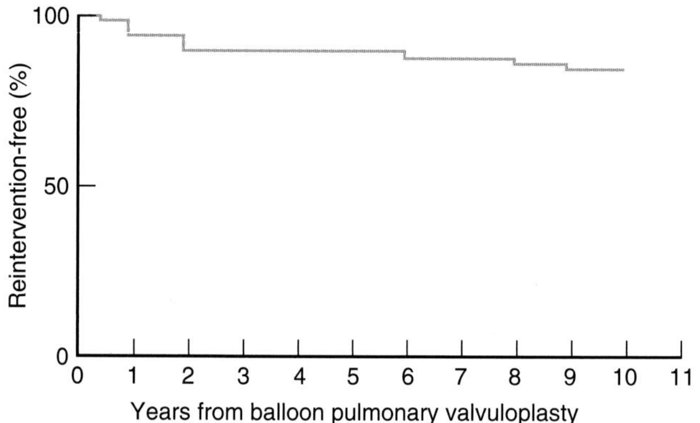

Figure 39-12 Actuarial reintervention-free rates after balloon dilatation of pulmonary valve. At 1, 2, 5, and 10 years, these were 94%, 89%, 88%, and 84%, respectively. (From Rao and colleagues.[R3])

at 5 and 10 years after intervention, reported by Rao and colleagues,[R3] was 88% and 84%, respectively (Fig. 39-12).

Comparison of Surgery and Balloon Valvotomy

Peterson and colleagues studied comparative outcomes between surgical and balloon valvotomy.[P2] Between 1969 and 2000, 62 patients underwent surgery, and 108 balloon valvotomy. Both techniques were effective, but there were differences at 10-year follow-up. Surgery reduced the gradient across the pulmonary valve more effectively than balloon valvotomy and had lower rates of restenosis and overall reintervention. Balloon valvotomy had a lower rate of moderate pulmonary regurgitation, which did not appear to influence reintervention rates in the two groups. Nevertheless, balloon valvotomy is today the procedure of choice because of its lower cost, shorter hospital stay, lower degree of invasiveness, and effectiveness. Based on the study of Earing and colleagues,[E1] it can be inferred that the reintervention rate in the surgery group studied by Peterson and colleagues[P2] will continue to rise with longer follow-up as symptoms from pulmonary regurgitation develop.

Cyanosis

Cyanosis may persist late postoperatively when the foramen ovale or ASD is not closed, even when stenosis has been relieved, as a result of impaired RV compliance.[D3,M5,O2] This can occur occasionally with a normally developed, severely hypertrophied RV, presumably secondary to diffuse fibrosis, but it is the rule in the hypoplastic RV. Data from Freed and colleagues suggest that the reversed atrial shunt may lessen as an infant or young child grows and as the RV increases in size, and later closure of the ASD thus may not be required.[F3] This favorable sequence cannot be expected in patients with hypoplastic RV, and it is well known that important hypoxia can occur from a right-to-left shunt through a small atrial communication.

Morphologic Changes

The sinus portion of the RV enlarges and becomes normal in size in most patients. The infundibulum enlarges in many patients, but as in tetralogy of Fallot (see Chapter 38), a narrow pulmonary anulus may fail to enlarge as the child grows. The apparent size of the pulmonary arteries increases, and in most patients they become normal sized. Tricuspid regurgitation, even when severe preoperatively, is usually absent or mild late postoperatively.

Functional Capacity

Most patients have an excellent late functional result. Stone and colleagues have shown that during exercise, children who have undergone pulmonary valvotomy have a normal relationship between cardiac output and oxygen consumption, no increase in RV end-diastolic pressure (preoperatively it increased), and less increase than preoperatively in RV peak systolic pressure.[S9]

The late result in patients with a hypoplastic RV is inferior to that in patients with a normally developed ventricle. Late mortality is higher, there may be a reversed shunt through an unclosed atrial communication, and there may be residual infundibular obstruction. There may also be persistent or recurrent right heart failure despite complete relief of stenosis. Although there are no techniques proven to be beneficial in managing the hypoplastic RV, a number of options are available in selected cases. Late heart failure may be prevented in this group, particularly in those who are young, by a complete valvotomy combined with enlargement of the RV cavity by excision of trabeculations. This may be particularly helpful if extensive endocardial fibrosis is present. In patients with persistent RV failure, volume unloading by creating a bidirectional superior cavopulmonary anastomosis may be beneficial.

INDICATIONS FOR OPERATION

When patients first show signs and symptoms at age 1 month or more, they are usually less critically ill than those presenting as neonates. Nonetheless, when diagnosis of severe stenosis is made, pulmonary valvotomy is advisable. As in critical pulmonary stenosis in neonates, percutaneous balloon valvotomy is usually the intervention indicated.[F4,O1,T1] Only in special circumstances is surgical intervention indicated. These include dysplastic valves, severely hypoplastic valves, severe infundibular stenosis, and associated intracardiac lesions requiring surgery.

Intervention is similarly advised in asymptomatic infants with severe stenosis. In those with moderate stenosis, intervention in infancy is debatable; it is not recommended when stenosis is mild. In older patients, management differs only in the group with moderate stenosis. In this subset, the older the age at diagnosis, the less likely there will be important progression and therefore less need for intervention.

In all patient groups beyond the neonatal period, a gradient across the pulmonary valve of 50 mmHg or greater is considered an indication for intervention. Presence and degree of RV hypoplasia are taken into account when deciding on intervention. Because of its effect in increasing cyanosis and heart failure, severe RV hypoplasia makes intervention more urgent in infants. In older children and adults presenting with this lesion, indications for intervention do not differ unless there is severe heart failure unresponsive to medical measures. Under these circumstances, risk of intervention is increased.

SPECIAL SITUATIONS AND CONTROVERSIES

Right Ventricular Hypoplasia in Children and Adults

When the RV is severely hypoplastic, symptoms and signs are substantially altered. Important symptoms are not necessarily present in infancy, but when they appear they tend to progress rapidly. Classically, there is a markedly prominent *a* wave and reversed (expiratory) splitting of the second heart sound.[W2] Pulmonary stenosis with hypoplastic RV is associated with less than the expected degree of RV hypertrophy, and in severe hypoplasia, LV forces are dominant despite severe stenosis.[E3] Diminished RV potentials are due to smallness of its cavity rather than to diminution in muscle mass.[B6] Balloon valvotomy may not be as effective in this group because of (1) frequent presence of organic infundibular obstruction, (2) necessity of closing the atrial communication to abolish the otherwise persistent right-to-left shunt, and (3) probable benefits of enlarging the RV cavity by excising muscle from its sinus portion.[W2] Taking all these factors into consideration, a surgical approach may be required. However, when severe heart failure is present, prognosis is still poor with any approach. In this setting, reducing volume load on the RV by performing a superior cavopulmonary anastomosis may be of benefit (see Special Situations and Controversies in Section III of Chapter 41).

Supravalvar Pulmonary Stenosis

The rarest form of pulmonary stenosis and intact ventricular septum is supravalvar pulmonary stenosis. It has been called *hourglass pulmonary stenosis*[M4] and is characterized by narrowing of the sinutubular junction, similar to that seen in supravalvar aortic stenosis. This lesion, like pulmonary valve dysplasia, does not respond to balloon dilatation[B1]; surgery is required. Various technical approaches have been described, all similar to those described for supravalvar aortic stenosis (see Section III of Chapter 47). The technique of repair can involve patching from the main pulmonary artery across the sinutubular junction into the sinus of Valsalva. Alternatively, repair using only native pulmonary artery tissue has been described.[B1]

REFERENCES

A

1. Allanby KD, Campbell M. Congenital pulmonary stenosis with closed ventricular septum. Guys Hosp Rep 1949;98:18.
2. Anand R, Mehta AV. Natural history of asymptomatic valvar pulmonary stenosis diagnosed in infancy. Clin Cardiol 1997;20:377.
3. Anderson IM, Nouri-Moghaddam S. Severe pulmonary stenosis in infancy and early childhood. Thorax 1969;24:312.
4. Ardura J, Gonzalez C, Andres J. Does mild pulmonary stenosis progress during childhood? A study of its natural course. Clin Cardiol 2004;27:519-22.

B

1. Bacha EA, Kalimi R, Starr JP, Quinones J, Koenig P. Autologous repair of supravalvar pulmonic stenosis. Ann Thorac Surg 2004; 77:734-6.
2. Becu L, Somerville J, Gallo A. "Isolated" pulmonary valve stenosis as part of more widespread cardiovascular disease. Br Heart J 1976;38:472.
3. Berman W Jr, Fripp RR, Raisher BD, Yabek SM. Significant pulmonary valve incompetence following oversize balloon pulmonary valveplasty in small infants: a long-term follow-up study. Catheter Cardiovasc Interv 1999;48:61-5.
4. Blalock A, Kieffer RF Jr. Valvulotomy for the relief of congenital valvular pulmonary stenosis with intact ventricular septum. Report of nineteen operations by the Brock method. Ann Surg 1950; 132:496.
5. Brock RC. Pulmonary valvulotomy for the relief of congenital pulmonary stenosis. Br Med J 1948;1:1121.
6. Brody DA. A theoretical analysis of intracavitary blood mass influence on the heart-lead relationship. Circ Res 1956;4:731.

C

1. Caspi J, Coles JG, Benson LN, Freedom RM, Burrows PE, Smallhorn JF, et al. Management of neonatal critical pulmonic stenosis in the balloon valvotomy era. Ann Thorac Surg 1990; 49:273.
2. Coles JG, Freedom RM, Olley PM, Coceani F, Williams WG, Trusler GA. Surgical management of critical pulmonary stenosis in the neonate. Ann Thorac Surg 1984;38:458.
3. Cooper R, Ritter S, Golinko R. Percutaneous balloon valvuloplasty (PBV): initial and long term results. J Am Coll Cardiol 1982;5:405.

D

1. Danielson GK, Exarhos ND, Weidman WH, McGoon DC. Pulmonic stenosis with intact ventricular septum. J Thorac Cardiovasc Surg 1971;61:228.
2. Danilowicz D, Hoffman JI, Rudolph AM. Serial studies of pulmonary stenosis in infancy and childhood. Br Heart J 1975;37:808.
3. De Castro CM, Nelson WP, Jones RC, Hall RJ, Hopeman AR, Jahnke EJ. Pulmonary stenosis: cyanosis, interatrial communication and inadequate right ventricular distensibility following pulmonary valvotomy. Am J Cardiol 1970;26:540.
4. Deleon SY, Dorotan J, Abdallah H, Kattash M, Hartz R. Annular and leaflet augmentation in Noonan's syndrome with dysplastic pulmonary valve. Pediatr Cardiol 2003;24:574-5.
5. Dinsmore RE, Sanders CA, Hawthorne JW, Austen WG. Calcification of the congenitally stenotic pulmonary valve. N Engl J Med 1966;275:99.
6. Drossner DM, Mahle WT. A management strategy for mild valvar pulmonary stenosis. Pediatr Cardiol 2008;29:649-52.
7. Dumont J. Chirurgie des malformations congenitales ou acquises du coeur. Presse Med 1913;21:860.

E

1. Earing MG, Connolly HM, Dearani JA, Ammash NM, Grogan M, Warnes CA. Long-term follow-up of patients after surgical treatment for isolated pulmonary valve stenosis. Mayo Clin Proc 2005;80:871-6.
2. Engle MA, Holswade GR, Goldberg HP, Lukas DS, Glenn F. Regression after open valvulotomy of infundibular stenosis accompanying severe valvular pulmonary stenosis. Circulation 1958; 17:862.
3. Engle MA, Ito T, Goldberg HP. The fate of the patient with pulmonic stenosis. Circulation 1964;30:554.
4. Ettedgui JA, Ho SY, Tynan M, Jones OD, Martin RP, Baker EJ, et al. The pathology of balloon pulmonary valvoplasty. Int J Cardiol 1987;16:285.

F

1. Fabricius J. Isolated pulmonary stenosis. Copenhagen: Munksgaard, 1959.
2. Farber S, Hubbard J. Fetal endomyocarditis—intrauterine infection as the cause of congenital cardiac anomalies. Am J Med Sci 1933;186:705.
3. Fawzy ME, Hassan W, Fadel BM, Sergani H, El Shaer F, El Widaa H, et al. Long-term results (up to 17 years) of pulmonary balloon valvuloplasty in adults and its effects on concomitant severe infundibular stenosis and tricuspid regurgitation. Am Heart J 2007; 153:433-8.
4. Fedderly RT, Beekman RH 3rd. Balloon valvuloplasty for pulmonary valve stenosis. J Interv Cardiol 1995;8:451.
5. Fedderly RT, Lloyd TR, Mendelsohn AM, Beekman RH. Determinants of successful balloon valvotomy in infants with critical pulmonary stenosis or membranous pulmonary atresia with intact ventricular septum. J Am Coll Cardiol 1995;25:460.
6. Freed MD, Heymann MA, Lewis AB, Roehl SL, Kensey RC. Prostaglandin E1 in infants with ductus arteriosus-dependent cyanotic congenital heart disease. Circulation 1981;64:899.

G

1. Galindo A, Gutierrez-Larraya F, Velasco JM, de la Fuente P. Pulmonary balloon valvuloplasty in a fetus with critical pulmonary stenosis/atresia with intact ventricular septum and heart failure. Fetal Diagn Ther 2006;21:100-4.
2. Gamboa R, Hugenholtz PG, Nadas AS. Accuracy of the phonocardiogram in assessing severity of aortic and pulmonic stenosis. Circulation 1964;30:35.
3. Gardiner HM, Belmar C, Tulzer G, Barlow A, Pasquini L, Carvalho JS, et al. Morphologic and functional predictors of eventual circulation in the fetus with pulmonary atresia or critical pulmonary stenosis with intact septum. J Am Coll Cardiol 2008;51:1299-308.
4. Garty Y, Veldtman G, Lee K, Benson L. Late outcomes after pulmonary valve balloon dilatation in neonates, infants and children. J Invasive Cardiol 2005;17:318-22.
5. Gersony WM, Bernhard WF, Nadas AS, Gross RE. Diagnosis and surgical treatment of infants with critical pulmonary outflow obstruction. Circulation 1967;35:765.
6. Gibson S, Clifton WM. Congenital heart disease. Am J Dis Child 1938;55:761.
7. Gielen H, Daniels O, van Lier H. Natural history of congenital pulmonary valvar stenosis: an echo and Doppler cardiographic study. Cardiol Young 1999;9:129.
8. Gikonyo BM, Lucas RV, Edwards JE. Anatomic features of congenital pulmonary valvar stenosis. Pediatr Cardiol 1987;8:109.
9. Gomez-Engler HE, Grunkemeier GL, Starr A. Critical pulmonary valve stenosis with intact ventricular septum. Thorac Cardiovasc Surg 1979;27:160.
10. Greene DG, Baldwin ED, Baldwin JS, Himmelstein A, Roh CE, Cournand A. Pure congenital pulmonary stenosis and idiopathic congenital dilatation of the pulmonary artery. Am J Med 1949;6: 24.
11. Griffith BP, Hardesty RL, Siewers RD, Lerberg DB, Ferson PF, Bahnson HT. Pulmonary valvulotomy alone for pulmonary stenosis: results in children with and without muscular infundibular hypertrophy. J Thorac Cardiovasc Surg 1982;83:577.
12. Gudausky TM, Beekman RH 3rd. Current options, and long-term results for interventional treatment of pulmonary valvar stenosis. Cardiol Young 2006;16:418-27.
13. Gupta D, Saxena A, Kothari SS, Juneja R. Factors influencing late course of residual valvular and infundibular gradients following pulmonary valve balloon dilatation. Int J Cardiol 2001;79:143-9.

H

1. Hameed AB, Goodwin TM, Elkayam U. Effect of pulmonary stenosis on pregnancy outcomes–a case-control study. Am Heart J 2007;5:852-4.
2. Hanley FL, Sade RM, Freedom RM, Blackstone EH, Kirklin JW. Outcomes in critically ill neonates with pulmonary stenosis and intact ventricular septum: a multiinstitutional study. Congenital Heart Surgeons Society. J Am Coll Cardiol 1993;22:183.
3. Harinck E, Becker AE, Groot AC, Oppenheimer-Dekker A, Versprille A. The left ventricle in congenital isolated pulmonary valve stenosis. Br Heart J 1977;39:429.
4. Hayes CJ, Gersony WM, Driscoll DJ, Keane JF, Kidd L, O'Fallon WM, et al. The second natural history study of congenital heart defects: results of treatment of patients with pulmonary valvar stenosis. Circulation 1993;87:I28.
5. Himmelstein A, Jameson AG, Fishman AP, Humphreys GH 2nd. Closed transventricular valvulotomy for pulmonic stenosis. Description of a new valvulotome and results based on pressures during operation. Surgery 1957;42:121.

J

1. Jarrar M, Betbout F, Farhat MB, Maatouk F, Gamra H, Addad F, et al. Long-term invasive and noninvasive results of percutaneous balloon pulmonary valvuloplasty in children, adolescents, and adults. Am Heart J 1999;138:950-4.
2. Jonas RA, Castaneda AR, Norwood WI, Freed MD. Pulmonary valvotomy under normothermic caval inflow occlusion. Aust N Z J Surg 1985;55:39.

K

1. Kan JS, White RI Jr, Mitchell SE, Gardner TJ. Percutaneous balloon valvuloplasty: a new method for treating congenital pulmonary valve stenosis. N Engl J Med 1982;307:540.
2. Kawazu Y, Inamura N, Kayatani F. Prediction of therapeutic strategy and outcome for antenatally diagnosed pulmonary atresia/stenosis with intact ventricular septum. Circ J 2008;72:1471-5.
3. Keith JD, Rowe RD, Vlad P. Heart disease in infancy and childhood. New York: Macmillan, 1967.
4. Kirklin JW. Open-heart surgery at the Mayo Clinic. The 25th Anniversary. Mayo Clin Proc 1980;55:339.
5. Kirklin JW, Connolly DC, Ellis FE Jr, Burchell HB, Edwards JE, Wood EH. Problems in the diagnosis and surgical treatment of pulmonic stenosis with intact ventricular septum. Circulation 1953; 8:849.
6. Kopecky SL, Gersh BJ, McGoon MD, Mair DD, Porter CJ, Ilstrup DM, et al. Long-term outcome of patients undergoing surgical repair of isolated pulmonary valve stenosis: follow-up at 20 to 30 years. Circulation 1988;78:1150.
7. Koretzky ED, Moller JH, Korns ME, Schwartz CJ, Edwards JE. Congenital pulmonary stenosis resulting from dysplasia of valve. Circulation 1969;40:43.

L

1. Lababidi Z, Wu JR. Percutaneous balloon pulmonary valvuloplasty. Am J Cardiol 1983;52:560.
2. Lam Y, Kaya M, Goktekin O, Gatzoulis M, Li W, Henein M. Restrictive right ventricular physiology: its presence and symptomatic contribution in patiens with pulmonary valvular stenosis. J Am Coll Cardiol 2007;15:1491.
3. Leca-Chetochine F, Thibert M, Neveux JY, Louville Y, Fiemeyer A, Mathey J. Anatomical aspects and surgical treatment of pulmonary stenoses and atresias with intact interventricular septum in the newborn and the infant under 6 months. Arch Mal Coeur Vaiss 1976;69:639.
4. Levine OR, Blumenthal S. Pulmonic stenosis. Circulation 1965;32:III33.
5. Linde LM, Turner SW, Sparkes RS. Pulmonary valvular dysplasia: a cardiofacial syndrome. Br Heart J 1973;35:301.

M

1. Marantz PM, Huhta JC, Mullins CE, Murphy DJ, Nihill MR, Ludomirsky A, et al. Results of balloon valvuloplasty in typical and dysplastic pulmonary valve stenosis: Doppler echocardiographic follow-up. J Am Coll Cardiol 1988;12:476.
2. McCrindle BW, Kan JS. Long-term results after balloon pulmonary valvuloplasty. Circulation 1991;83:1915.
3. McGoon DC, Kirklin FW. Pulmonic stenosis with intact ventricular septum. Treatment utilizing extracorporeal circulation. Circulation 1958;17:180.
4. Milo S, Fiegel A, Shem-Tov A, Neufeld HN, Goor DA. Hour-glass deformity of the pulmonary valve: a third type of pulmonary valve stenosis. Br Heart J 1988;60:128-33.
5. Mirowski M, Shah KD, Neill CA, Taussig HB. Long-term (10 to 13 years) follow-up study after transventricular pulmonary valvotomy for pulmonary stenosis with intact ventricular septum. Circulation 1963;28:906.
6. Mistrot J, Neal W, Lyons G, Moller J, Lucas R, Castaneda A, et al. Pulmonary valvulotomy under inflow stasis for isolated pulmonary stenosis. Ann Thorac Surg 1976;21:30.
7. Mitchell SC, Korones SB, Berendes HW. Congenital heart disease in 56,109 births. Incidence and natural history. Circulation 1971; 43:323.
8. Mody MR. The natural history of uncomplicated valvular pulmonic stenosis. Am Heart J 1975;90:317.
9. Moller JH, Adams P Jr. The natural history of pulmonary valvular stenosis. Am J Cardiol 1965;16:654.
10. Moller I, Wennevold A, Lyngborg KE. The natural history of pulmonary stenosis. Cardiology 1973;58:193.
11. Moss AJ, Adams FH, Emmanouilides GC, eds. Heart disease in infants, children, and adolescents, 2nd Ed. Baltimore: Williams & Wilkins, 1977, p. 226.
12. Murphy DA, Murphy RD, Gibbons JE, Dobell RC. Surgical treatment of pulmonary atresia with intact intraventricular septum. J Thorac Cardiovasc Surg 1971;62:213.
13. Musewe NN, Robertson MA, Benson LN, Smallhorn JF, Burrows PE, Freedom RM, et al. The dysplastic pulmonary valve: echocardiographic features and results of balloon dilatation. Br Heart J 1987;57:364.

N

1. Neutze JM, Starling MB, Elliott RB, Barratt-Boyes BG. Palliation of cyanotic congenital heart disease in infancy with E-type prostaglandins. Circulation 1977;55:238.
2. Noonan JA, Ehmke DA. Associated noncardiac malformations in children with congenital heart disease. J Pediatr 1963;63:468.
3. Nugent EW, Freedom RM, Nora JJ, Ellison RC, Rowe RD, Nadas AS. Clinical course in pulmonary stenosis. Circulation 1977;56:I38.

O

1. O'Connor BK, Beekman RH, Lindauer A, Rocchini A. Intermediate-term outcome after pulmonary balloon valvuloplasty: comparison with a matched surgical control group. J Am Coll Cardiol 1992; 20:169.
2. Oakley CM, Braimbridge MV, Bentall HH, Cleland WP. Reversed interatrial shunt following complete relief of pulmonary valve stenosis. Br Heart J 1964;26:662.
3. Olley PH, Coceani F, Bodach E. E-type prostaglandins: a new emergency O2 therapy for certain cyanotic congenital heart malformations. Circulation 1976;53:728.

P

1. Pepine CJ, Gessner IH, Feldman RL. Percutaneous balloon valvuloplasty for pulmonic valve stenosis in the adult. Am J Cardiol 1982;50:1442.
2. Peterson C, Schilthuis JJ, Dodge-Khatami A, Hitchcock JF, Meijboom EJ, Bennink GB. Comparative long-term results of surgery versus balloon valvuloplasty for pulmonary valve stenosis in infants and children. Ann Thorac Surg 2003;76:1078-82.

R

1. Rao PS. Balloon dilatation in infants and children with dysplastic pulmonary valves: short-term and intermediate-term results. Am Heart J 1988;116:1168.
2. Rao PS, Fawzy ME, Solymar L, Mardini MK. Long-term results of balloon pulmonary valvuloplasty of valvar pulmonic stenosis. Am Heart J 1988;115:1291.
3. Rao PS, Galal O, Patnana M, Buck SH, Wilson AD. Results of three to 10 year follow up of balloon dilatation of the pulmonary valve. Heart 1998;80:591.
4. Rao PS, Liebman J, Borkat G. Right ventricular growth in a case of pulmonic stenosis with intact ventricular septum and hypoplastic right ventricle. Circulation 1976;53:389.

5. Rao PS. Percutaneous balloon pulmonary valvuloplasty: state of the art. Catheter Cardiovasc Interv 2007;69:747-63.
6. Rey C, Marache P, Francart C, Dupuis C. Percutaneous transluminal balloon valvuloplasty of congenital pulmonary valve stenosis, with a special report on infants and neonates. J Am Coll Cardiol 1988;11:815.
7. Roberts WC, Shemin RJ, Kent KM. Frequency and direction of interatrial shunting in valvular pulmonic stenosis with intact ventricular septum and without left ventricular inflow or outflow obstruction. Am Heart J 1980;99:142.
8. Robertson M, Benson LN, Smallhorn JS, Musewe N, Freedom RM, Moes CA, et al. The morphology of the right ventricular outflow tract after percutaneous pulmonary valvotomy: long term follow up. Br Heart J 1987;58:239.
9. Rodriquez-Fernandez HZ, Char F, Kelly D, Rowe RD. The dysplastic pulmonic valve and the Noonan's syndrome (abstract). Circulation 1972;45/46:II98.
10. Roman KS, Fouron JC, Nii M, Smallhorn JF, Chaturvedi R, Jaeggi ET. Determinants of outcome in fetal pulmonary valve stenosis or atresia with intact ventricular septum. Am J Cardiol 2007;99: 699-703.
11. Roos-Hesselink JW, Meijboom FJ, Spitaels SE, vanDomburg RT, vanRijen EH, Utens EM, et al. Long-term outcome after surgery for pulmonary stenosis (a longitudinal study of 22-33 years). Eur Heart J 2006;27:482-8.
12. Rowland DG, Hammill WW, Allen HD, Gutgesell HP. Natural course of isolated pulmonary valve stenosis in infants and children utilizing Doppler echocardiography. Am J Cardiol 1997;79:344.

S

1. Schieken RM, Friedman S, Pierce WS. Severe congenital pulmonary stenosis with pulmonary valvular dysplasia syndrome. Ann Thorac Surg 1973;15:570.
2. Sellors TH. The surgery of pulmonary stenosis. Lancet 1948;1:988.
3. Selzer A, Carnes WH, Noble CA Jr, Higgins WH Jr, Holmes RO. The syndrome of pulmonary stenosis with patent foramen ovale. Am J Med 1949;6:3.
4. Sholler GF, Colan SD, Sanders SP. Effect of isolated right ventricular outflow obstruction on left ventricular function in infants. Am J Cardiol 1988;62:778.
5. Silverman BK, Nadas AS, Wittenborg MH, Goodale WT, Gross RE. Pulmonary stenosis with intact ventricular septum. Am J Med 1956;20:53.
6. Somerville J, Becu L. Proceedings: "Isolated" pulmonary valve stenosis: a possible misnomer. Br Heart J 1976;38:316.
7. Srinivasan V, Konyer A, Broda JJ, Subramanian S. Critical pulmonary stenosis in infants less than three months of age: a reappraisal of closed transventricular pulmonary valvotomy. Ann Thorac Surg 1982;34:46.
8. Stamm C, Anderson RH, Ho SY. Clinical anatomy of the normal pulmonary root compared with that in isolated pulmonary valvular stenosis. J Am Coll Cardiol 1998;31:1420-5.
9. Stone FM, Bessinger FB Jr, Lucas RV Jr, Moller JH. Pre- and postoperative rest and exercise hemodynamics in children with pulmonary stenosis. Circulation 1974;49:1102.
10. Swan H, Zeavin L, Blount SG Jr, Virtue RW. Surgery by direct vision in the open heart during hypothermia. JAMA 1953;153:1081.

T

1. Tabatabaei H, Boutin C, Nykanen DG, Freedom RM, Benson LN. Morphologic and hemodynamic consequences after percutaneous balloon valvotomy for neonatal pulmonary stenosis: medium-term follow-up. J Am Coll Cardiol 1996;27:473.
2. Talsma M, Witsenburg M, Rohmer J, Hess J. Determinants for outcome of balloon valvuloplasty for severe pulmonary stenosis in neonates and infants up to six months of age. Am J Cardiol 1993;71:1246.
3. Todros T, Presbitero P, Gaglioti P, Demarie D. Pulmonary stenosis with intact ventricular septum: documentation of development of the lesion echocardiographically during fetal life. Int J Cardiol 1988;19:355.
4. Tulzer G, Arzt W, Franklin RC, Loughna PV, Mair R, Gardiner HM. Fetal pulmonary valvuloplasty for critical pulmonary stenosis or atresia with intact septum. Lancet 2002;360:1567-8.
5. Tynan M, Baker EJ, Rohmer J, Jones OD, Reidy JF, Joseph MC, et al. Percutaneous balloon pulmonary valvuloplasty. Br Heart J 1985;53:520.

V

1. Vogelpoel L, Schrire V. Auscultatory and phonocardiographic assessment of pulmonary stenosis with intact ventricular septum. Circulation 1960;22:55.

W

1. Wennevold A, Jacobsen JR. Natural history of valvular pulmonary stenosis in children below the age of two years. Eur J Cardiol 1978;8:371.
2. Williams JC, Barratt-Boyes BG, Lowe JB. Underdeveloped right ventricle and pulmonary stenosis. Am J Cardiol 1963;11:458.
3. Wood P. Pulmonary stenosis with normal aortic root. In Disease of the heart and circulation, 2nd Ed. Philadelphia: JB Lippincott, 1956, p. 408.

Z

1. Zeevi B, Keane JF, Fellows KE, Lock JE. Balloon dilation of critical pulmonary stenosis in the first week of life. J Am Coll Cardiol 1988;11:821.

40 Pulmonary Atresia and Intact Ventricular Septum

DEFINITION

Pulmonary atresia and intact ventricular septum is a congenital malformation in which the pulmonary valve is atretic and no ventricular septal defect exists. It coexists with variable degrees of right ventricular (RV) and tricuspid valve hypoplasia, and variable degrees of coronary artery abnormalities. This chapter discusses this malformation in the setting of atrioventricular and ventriculoarterial concordant connections.

HISTORICAL NOTE

In 1839, Peacock collected records of seven patients with pulmonary atresia and intact ventricular septum and gave credit to John Hunter for reporting the first case in 1783.[P4] Hunter described a premature male who died 13 days after birth. The RV had "scarcely any cavity," and the tricuspid valve was "especially small." Coronary sinusoids and RV–coronary artery fistulae were recognized by Grant in 1926 and later by others.[G10,K1,L2,S10,W4] RV-dependent coronary circulation began to be recognized at least in 1975 by Essed and colleagues and more recently by others.[B7,C1,E6,G7]

In 1955, Greenwold and colleagues at Mayo Clinic described two types of RV in this malformation: (1) small and (2) normal-sized or large.[G11,G12] Subsequently, the idea evolved that values for RV cavity size and tricuspid valve dimensions, as well as morphologic details, comprised a spectrum embracing virtually all values between the extremes.[G4,Z2] Greenwold and colleagues also suggested that pulmonary valvotomy was appropriate treatment when the RV was near normal in size.[G11,G12] In 1961, Davignon and colleagues at Mayo Clinic suggested that a systemic–pulmonary artery shunt be performed when the RV was small.[D4] Reports of successful surgery from the University of Minnesota, Mayo Clinic, and Henry Ford Hospital appeared in 1961.[B3,D4,Z1] The combination of a systemic–pulmonary artery shunt with an RV outflow operation was described by Bowman and colleagues in 1971 and by Trusler and colleagues in 1976.[B8,T2] In 1993, Hanley and colleagues introduced the concept that optimal outcomes are best achieved when neonatal and subsequent surgical management are specifically tailored to the variable morphology of this malformation.[H1]

MORPHOLOGY

Hearts with pulmonary atresia and intact ventricular septum include a spectrum extending from mild concomitant abnormalities of the RV and tricuspid valve to the most severe. Whether the entity of pulmonary stenosis and intact ventricular septum, particularly critical pulmonary stenosis in neonates, is part of this spectrum can be debated (see Section I of Chapter 39). Evidence supporting the continuum of these two entities is that at least some hearts at adjoining ends of the spectra have similar RV and tricuspid valvar abnormalities. It has been hypothesized that the later the narrowing of the pulmonary valve develops in fetal life, including progression to atresia, the more fully and normally developed are the tricuspid valve, RV cavity, and RV myocardium. Conversely, the earlier these developments occur in fetal life, the more likely that these structures will be hypoplastic and abnormal.[A2,K3,T1] This hypothesis is also consistent with the concept that there is a continuity of the spectra of pulmonary atresia with intact ventricular septum and pulmonary stenosis with intact ventricular septum.

Pulmonary Valve

The nature of the structure at the junction of the RV and pulmonary trunk is arguable. Van Praagh and colleagues imply that fibrous components are pulmonary valve remnants.[V1] Others point out that in many cases, there is only poorly structured imperforate fibrous tissue overlying muscular atresia.[A5,E1,Z2] In any event, commissural ridges may be prominent and converge to meet in the center of the "valve," an appearance similar to that in pulmonary valve stenosis.[Z2] In some patients, commissural ridges are present only in the periphery, the center being a smooth fibrous membrane.[B9] In the combined U.K.-Ireland multicenter study of 183 patients, 75% had membranous atresia and 25% muscular atresia.[D1] Of greater importance is the nature of the structures immediately below the RV–pulmonary trunk junction (see "Right Ventricle" and "Tricuspid Valve" in text that follows).

Table 40-1 Right Ventricular Cavity Size in Pulmonary Atresia and Intact Ventricular Septum[a]

RV Cavity Size[b]	n	% of 136
Normal (0)	5	4
Mildly reduced (−1, −2)	28	21
Moderately reduced (−3)	25	18
Severely reduced (−4, −5)	78[c]	57
Subtotal	136	100
Unknown	27	
TOTAL	163[d]	

Data from Hanley and colleagues.[H1]
[a]Based on data from 171 neonates with pulmonary atresia and intact ventricular septum in the Congenital Heart Surgeons Society study. Size of pulmonary arteries was known in 84.
[b]Cavity size was graded (0, normal to −5, severe hypoplasia) based on echocardiographic and cineangiographic findings.
[c]Five of six patients with moderate or severe hypoplasia of right and left pulmonary arteries on cineangiography had severely reduced right ventricular cavity size (information available for 84 of 136 patients).
[d]In addition, eight patients had enlarged right ventricular cavities, and one (12%) of these had moderately hypoplastic pulmonary arteries.
Key: *RV*, Right ventricle.

Pulmonary Arteries

The pulmonary trunk is usually nearly normal in size, but uncommonly is severely hypoplastic.[C3,C9,E1,E5,Z2] Rarely, the pulmonary trunk is represented only by a fibrous cord.[V1]

Right and left pulmonary arteries are usually normal in diameter or slightly hypoplastic.[E3,V1] Uncommonly, they are moderately or severely hypoplastic, usually in patients with severely reduced RV cavity size (Table 40-1). Rarely, there are major arborization abnormalities of the native pulmonary arteries in association with large aortopulmonary collaterals. Four such patients have been encountered by F.L. Hanley and colleagues (personal communication, February 2012).

Right Ventricle

Size of the RV cavity is variable. In about 5% of patients, it is enlarged (see Chapter 38, Fig. 38-2 and Chapter 39, Table 39-1). Ebstein malformation and severe tricuspid regurgitation may coexist with the latter.[A7,B8,C10,F8,M8,V3,Z2] Many individuals with this combination die in fetal life.[A2] Rarely, the RV wall may be very thin (*Uhl anomaly* or *parchment right ventricle*[C10]) and the cavity nontrabeculated adjacent to the tricuspid valve and heavily trabeculated in its apical half.

Much more frequently, cavity size is reduced, severely so in about 60% of patients. This appears to be the result of massive wall hypertrophy extending into the ventricular cavity. Often, this completely obliterates the infundibular cavity, and the atresia can be termed *muscular* in such cases.[B14] At times, the apical-trabecular cavity is completely obliterated; in the most extreme cases, both portions are obliterated. Although these cavities are obliterated, the respective portions of the RV are not absent. Cavity obliteration can be localized by echocardiography as well as by anatomic studies.[M5] Cavity obliteration has been further characterized in the U.K.-Ireland multicenter study.[D1] All three components of the RV (inlet, trabecular, and infundibular) were present in all cases, but with different degrees of cavity obliteration from muscular ingrowth. A "unipartite" ventricle due

Table 40-2 Prevalence of Coronary Artery Abnormalities in Pulmonary Stenosis and Atresia and Intact Ventricular Septum[a]

	PS		PA	
Category	**No.**	**% of 86**	**No.**	**% of 145**
Coronary sinusoids—present:	9	10	72	50
Without RV-cor fistulae	7	8	8	5
With RV-cor fistulae	2	2	64	45
Without RV dependence	2	2	52	36
With RV dependence[b]	0	0	12	9
Subtotal	86		145	
Unknown	15		26	
TOTAL	101		171	

Data from Hanley and colleagues.[H1]
[a]Based on data from 274 patients (two with unknown type of right ventricular outflow obstruction) in the Congenital Heart Surgeons Society study.
[b]In this study, it was not possible to place each patient in the spectrum of right ventricular dependency (see text). The phrase "with RV dependence" describes patients in whom dependence was judged to be so extreme that decompression of the right ventricle would be fatal.
Key: *Cor,* Coronary; *PA,* pulmonary atresia; *PS,* pulmonary stenosis; *RV,* right ventricular.

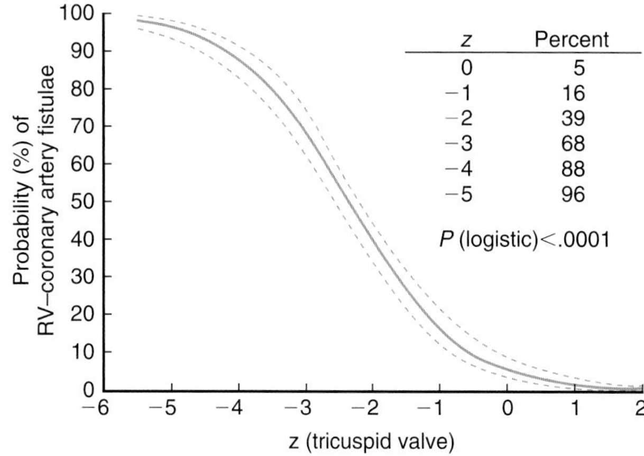

Figure 40-1 Nomogram of a regression equation (univariable) expressing the relation between dimensions of the tricuspid valve expressed as *z* value (see "Dimensions of Normal Cardiac and Great Artery Pathways" in Chapter 1) and probability of the presence of right ventricular–coronary artery fistulae in pulmonary atresia with intact ventricular septum. Key: *RV,* Right ventricle. (From Hanley and colleagues.[H1])

to muscular obliteration of the infundibular and trabecular components was present in 8%. A "bipartite" ventricle due to muscular obliteration of the trabecular component alone was present in 34%. There were no cases of muscular obliteration of the infundibulum alone. A "tripartite" ventricle was present in the remaining 58%.

There is associated diffuse fibrosis of the hypertrophied muscle and, especially when the RV cavity is small, a modest degree of RV endocardial fibroelastosis.[C8,E3,P3,Z2] Bulkley and colleagues found typical myocardial fiber disarray in 69% of the RV free wall and in 73% of the ventricular septum in this condition.[B13] The potential for impaired left ventricular (LV) as well as RV dysfunction is evident.

Right Ventricular–Coronary Artery Fistulae

Coronary sinusoids, or dilated portions of the coronary microcirculation, can be detected by cineangiography in about half of patients[C1,C9] (Table 40-2). In some cases, fistulous connections between the RV cavity and these sinusoids form multiple small communications into branches of left or right coronary arteries.[E3,G10,L2,W4] Occasionally they converge into a single large vessel that empties into the left anterior descending or right coronary artery. In many cases, the fistulae are minor. In the multicenter U.K.-Ireland study, 58% of patients had completely normal coronary circulation, 15% had minor filling of the coronary arteries with RV injection at catheterization, and about 25% had major fistulae, with about one third of these having no coronary connection to the aorta.[D1]

Prevalence of RV–coronary arterial fistulae is inversely related to dimensions of the tricuspid valve (and hence of the RV cavity) (Fig. 40-1) and amount of tricuspid regurgitation. It is also directly related to RV systolic pressure.[F4,H1,P2] However, the milieu for development of fistulae may be a consequence of genetically or developmentally induced myocardial abnormalities. Immunohistochemical studies demonstrate abnormal density and orientation of capillaries and myocyte disarray in the presence of fistulae.[O4]

Desaturated RV blood, although vital in the presence of proximal coronary obstructions, compromises myocardial oxygen supply in regions to which it is distributed by these fistulae. This may account in part for the myocardial abnormalities described later in this chapter.[E3,O3,V1] Complexity of oxygen delivery to the myocardium is evidenced by the fact that the left anterior descending artery (or any coronary artery) may fill through these fistulae from the RV in systole, and from the aorta in the normal manner during diastole.[F5] There results a spectrum of percentages of LV myocardium dependent on the RV for coronary perfusion, albeit desaturated; the percentage depends on location and severity of proximal coronary artery stenoses as well as on the fistulae. At some critical point, sufficient myocardium is in jeopardy of developing such severe ischemia when RV hypertension is relieved that RV decompression becomes contraindicated as a surgical option. In an analysis by Giglia and colleagues of 16 patients with coronary angiography and subsequent RV surgical decompression, 7 of 7 (100%; CL 77%-100%) with no coronary stenosis survived, 4 of 6 (67%; CL 39%-88%) with stenosis in one major coronary survived, and 0 of 3 (0%; CL 0%-46%) with stenosis in two major coronaries survived.[G6]

When less severe coronary abnormalities are present in association with fistulae, regional LV wall motion abnormalities are commonly identifiable before RV decompression, and they increase after decompression; however, severe global LV dysfunction is unusual.[G2]

In about 10% of patients (20% of those with RV–coronary fistulae), coronary circulation or some critical part of it is derived entirely or nearly so from the RV in the manner described, defining *RV-dependent coronary circulation.*[G7] This may occur because of development of arterial obstructions in the left main or right coronary arteries, or both, or in the proximal portion of the left anterior descending artery (R.M. Freedom, personal communication, 1991). No correlates of RV dependence are known beyond those for RV–coronary artery fistulae.[H1] Proximal coronary arterial occlusions etiologic to the dependence may develop in fetal life; some develop or progress after birth.[G7]

RV-dependent coronary circulation is a major consideration in planning therapy (see Indications for Operation later in this chapter). The difficulty is in deciding how much myocardium at risk is considered too much, triggering the management decision to avoid decompressing the hypertensive RV. To address this difficulty, Calder and colleagues identified coronary abnormalities in 116 patients.[C2] They determined that presence of coronary fistulae alone did not correlate with mortality. The presence and extent of coronary interruptions, and the amount of LV myocardium that was RV dependent (determined with a 15-point scoring system), did correlate with mortality.

The problem, however, is even more complex than solely determining the amount of myocardium at risk, because even a small amount of extremely ischemic myocardium may be the source of a life-threatening dysrhythmia. Recently, LV coronary abnormalities unrelated to the presence of fistulae, sinusoids, or coronary interruptions have been discovered. Hwang and colleagues showed that patients with pulmonary atresia with intact ventricular septum, regardless of the presence of fistulae, have decreased density of intramyocardial arterioles relative to normal and hypertrophied hearts.[H8]

Tricuspid Valve

The tricuspid valve is usually abnormal in this malformation.[A5,B14,F4] Occasionally the abnormality is simply small size, but usually the leaflets are thickened and the chordae are abnormal in number and attachment. Local agenesis and incomplete leaflet separation occur. The importance of these abnormalities has been emphasized by Davignon and colleagues and by Paul and Lev.[D4,P3]

In about 10% of neonates, *z* value of the tricuspid valve is less than −5, and in 50% it is −2.2 or less (Fig. 40-2). (See Appendix Fig. 40A-1 for a nomogram for estimating the *z* value of the tricuspid valve.) Dimensions of the tricuspid valve are well correlated with those of the RV cavity, in contrast to dimensions in neonates with critical pulmonary stenosis, in whom they are not correlated.[B14,E3,E5,F4,Z2]

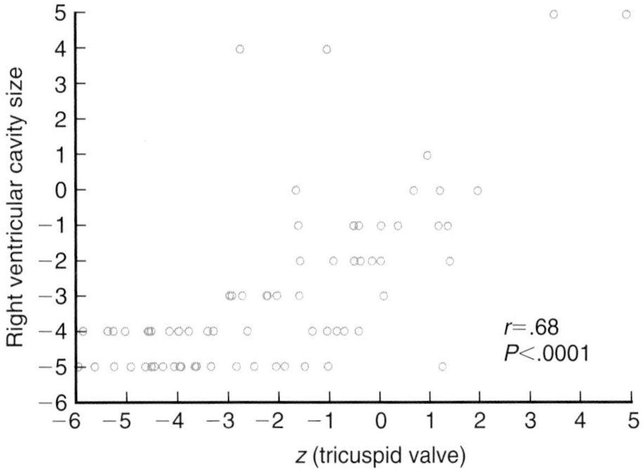

Figure 40-2 Relationship between diameter of the tricuspid valve (by echocardiography), expressed as *z* value, and size of the right ventricular cavity (grade estimated subjectively from echocardiographic and cineangiographic studies) in patients with pulmonary atresia and intact ventricular septum (n = 71). (From Hanley and colleagues.[H1])

In uncommon cases in which dimensions of the tricuspid valve are large, its leaflets usually show features of Ebstein malformation, with enlargement of the anterior leaflet and downward displacement onto the ventricle of the origin of a dysplastic septal leaflet. The posterior leaflet may or may not be abnormal.[B4] These valves are usually severely regurgitant.[B2] Another pathologic lesion of the tricuspid valve has been recognized in patients with dilated RV and severe tricuspid regurgitation—that of unguarded tricuspid orifice, in which the inferior (mural) leaflet is absent rather than displaced.[A6]

Right Atrium

The right atrium is enlarged, and it is more enlarged when there is severe tricuspid regurgitation. An interatrial communication is present in all cases, usually a patent foramen ovale of adequate size.[E1] However, shortly after birth the foramen becomes restrictive in some patients. The eustachian valve is frequently prominent.

Left-Sided Chambers

The left atrium is usually hypertrophied and somewhat enlarged, and the mitral orifice is usually larger than normal. The LV shows some hypertrophy and endocardial fibroelastosis.[C8] A convex bulging of the interventricular septum into the LV cavity has been noted, with some speculating that this might produce subaortic obstruction.[Z2] Clinical and postmortem studies have demonstrated evidence of LV myocardial ischemia in virtually all patients[F10,H3]; perhaps related to this, LV compliance is depressed in many.[S9]

Aorta

The aorta usually has adult morphology without isthmic narrowing and is usually left sided.[M8]

Ductus Arteriosus

The ductus arteriosus is patent at birth but has the usual tendency to close. Orientation of the ductus is typical for pulmonary atresia of all forms, with an obtuse proximal and acute distal angle at its aortic attachment. Usually the bronchial arteries are normal, and important aortopulmonary collateral arteries absent.[E1]

Coexisting Cardiac Anomalies

Other than Ebstein malformation, coexisting cardiac anomalies are uncommon.[B11]

CLINICAL FEATURES AND DIAGNOSTIC CRITERIA

Symptoms and Signs

Fetal distress is usually not evident except in those with a large RV. Delivery is typically uncomplicated and at term.[E5] The babies are generally well developed (Fig. 40-3) and are likely initially to appear healthy except for cyanosis.[B3,B11] Cyanosis is usually obvious on the first day and becomes rapidly more severe as the ductus closes and there is respiratory distress and progressing metabolic acidosis.[D8,G8] In the New England series, 81% of babies presented during the first week

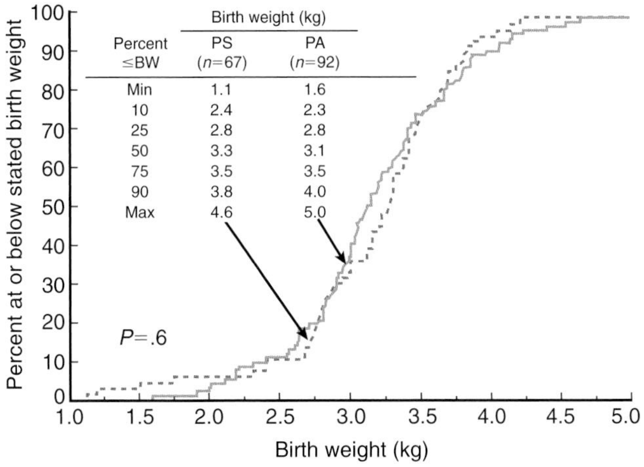

Figure 40-3 Cumulative frequency distribution of birth weight of neonates with pulmonary atresia or stenosis with intact ventricular septum. Key: *BW,* Birth weight; *Max,* maximum; *Min,* minimum; *PA,* pulmonary atresia; *PS,* pulmonary stenosis. (From Hanley and colleagues.[H1])

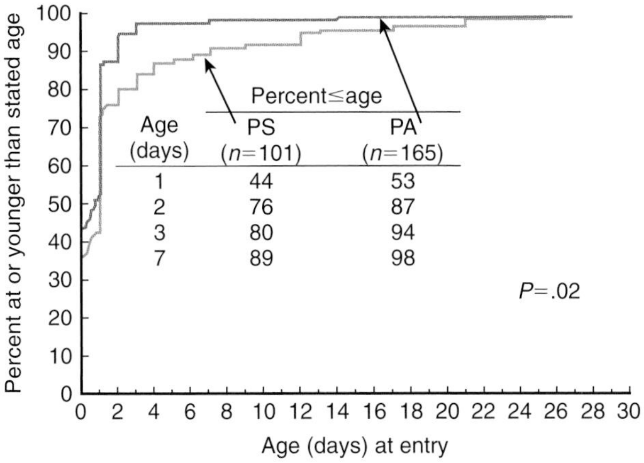

Figure 40-4 Cumulative frequency distribution of age at entry into the hospital of an inception cohort of neonates with pulmonary atresia or stenosis and intact ventricular septum. Key: *PA,* Pulmonary atresia; *PS,* pulmonary stenosis. (From Hanley and colleagues.[H1])

of life; in a more recent study, 94% presented in the first 3 days[B11] (Fig. 40-4).

Absence of an RV impulse in a cyanotic infant with a palpable LV should arouse suspicion of pulmonary atresia and intact ventricular septum, tricuspid atresia, Ebstein malformation, or critical pulmonary stenosis with hypoplastic RV.[B5,P5] Typically, no murmur or a systolic murmur of tricuspid regurgitation is heard, sometimes with a thrill.[B3,B5,E1] Despite presence of a patent ductus arteriosus, a continuous murmur is seldom heard.[C3,E1] The second heart sound is single.[P5]

Classic findings on chest radiography include clear lung fields with diminished (or normal) vascular markings and a flat or concave pulmonary trunk segment. Heart size is variable and may be large, even when the RV cavity is small.

Electrocardiography

P waves can be normal at birth, but evidence of right atrial enlargement develops quickly, and within a few weeks, prominent right atrial P waves are uniformly present.[B3,C8,P5,S5] Mean

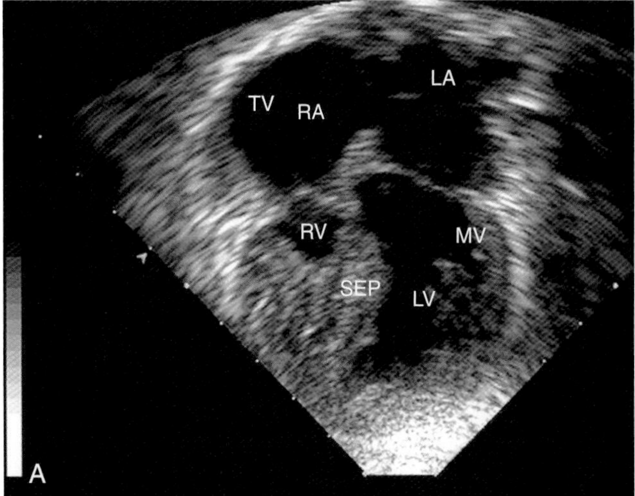

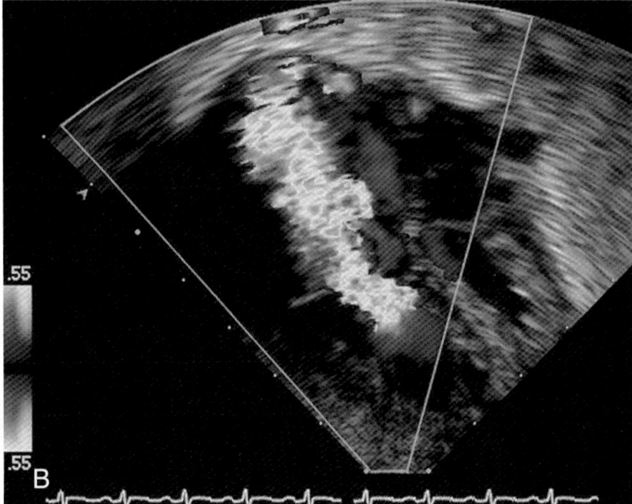

Figure 40-5 Intracardiac findings in pulmonary atresia and intact ventricular septum. **A,** Apical four-chamber view revealing hypoplastic and massively hypertrophied right ventricular (RV) cavity. Note ventricular septum bulging into left ventricle (LV), indicating severe RV hypertension. Tricuspid valve (TV) anulus is small, about 50% of the diameter of the mitral valve (MV) anulus. A large atrial septal defect is present. **B,** Apical four-chamber view with color Doppler in systole, showing severe tricuspid valve regurgitation. Right atrium (RA) is markedly enlarged. Key: *LA,* Left atrium; *SEP,* ventricular septum.

QRS axis in the frontal plane is usually normal or shows a rightward deviation, and the RV hypertrophy pattern usually present in the neonate is absent.[C8,G1,M3,S7] However, electrocardiographic evidence of RV hypertrophy may be present even though the RV cavity is small, precluding its use to predict RV cavity size.

Echocardiography

Two-dimensional echocardiography is diagnostic (Fig. 40-5). Also, dimensions of the tricuspid valve, RV cavity size, and nature of the outflow obstruction (membranous or muscular) can be determined with confidence. Of importance is the fact that RV–coronary artery fistulae can be identified accurately by two-dimensional echocardiography with pulsed Doppler color flow ultrasound imaging[S2,V2] (Fig. 40-6). However,

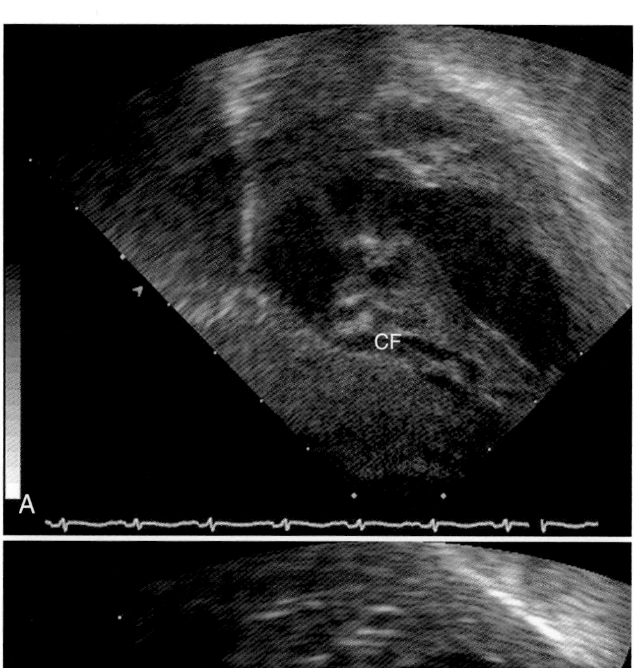

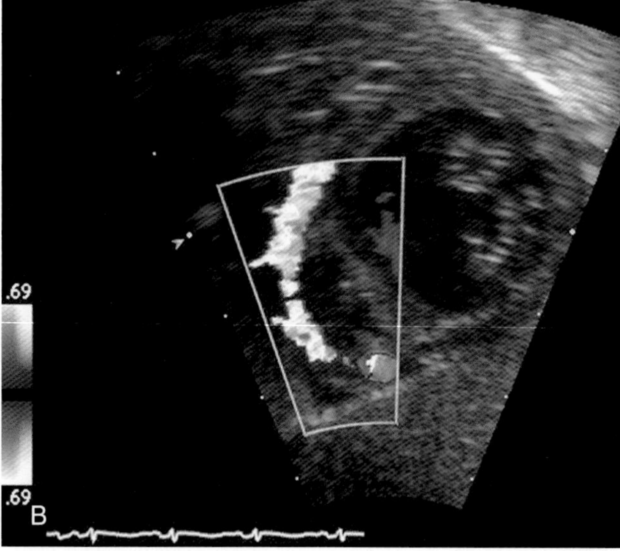

Figure 40-6 Echocardiographic identification of right ventricular (RV)–coronary artery fistulae. **A,** Subcostal coronal view showing miniscule hypertrophied RV chamber with large coronary fistula (CF). **B,** Subcostal sagittal view with color Doppler showing flow in RV–coronary artery fistula.

echocardiographic evaluation is limited: fistula size, extent of fistula formation, and presence of proximal coronary arterial stenosis cannot as yet be accurately delineated.

Tricuspid valve *z* value can be highly predictive of RV-dependent coronary circulation, indicating need for further angiographic evaluation.[S4] Fetal echocardiography can identify the anomaly with reasonable accuracy,[M1] but this does not appear to affect postnatal outcome favorably.[D2] Nevertheless, the morphology determined at fetal echocardiographic evaluation can be used to predict postnatal outcome and thus can be employed as an important prenatal counseling tool.[S1]

Cardiac Catheterization and Cineangiography

When pulmonary atresia with intact ventricular septum is diagnosed by echocardiography, cardiac catheterization and angiography are indicated to search for coronary arterial stenoses, coronary sinusoids, and RV-coronary fistulae. If these are present, extent of LV myocardial dependence on the RV must be established.

Right atrial mean pressure is usually higher than left, and a prominent *a* wave can be seen on the pressure tracing.[C3,C8] RV peak pressure is usually higher than or equal to systemic pressure, although it may be less in association with severe tricuspid regurgitation and a thin-walled RV.[C3,D8,G4,J2,S7] Systemic arterial saturation is low, but varies according to flow through the patent ductus arteriosus. Size and configuration of the RV cavity can be displayed by RV angiography (Fig. 40-7). In Ebstein anomaly with severe tricuspid regurgitation presenting in the neonatal period in association with high pulmonary vascular resistance, RV systole may fail to open a normal pulmonary valve; high-quality angiography will prevent the mistaken diagnosis of pulmonary atresia.[N3]

Quantitative cineangiographic studies indicate reduced RV function in essentially all cases. LV function and end-diastolic volume are also abnormal unless a normal LV mass is present.[S6]

Cardiac Magnetic Resonance Imaging and Computed Tomography Angiography

These imaging modalities are not typically used during the neonatal period. They may, however, be useful in evaluating older patients. Evaluation of cavity size and degree of musculature of the RV can be accurately determined using cardiac magnetic resonance (CMR) imaging (Fig. 40-8). Delayed-enhancement CMR can be used to determine the status of the myocardium as well (Fig. 40-9). Volume-rendered computed tomography (CT) angiography imaging can also accurately define abnormal coronary connections (Fig. 40-10).

NATURAL HISTORY

Pulmonary atresia and intact ventricular septum is an uncommon malformation, occurring in 1% to 1.5% of individuals born with congenital heart disease.[F6,M10] It was present in 3% of critically ill infants with congenital heart disease in the New England series.[B11] It is highly lethal, with about 50% of individuals dying within 2 weeks of birth and about 85% by age 6 months (Fig. 40-11). Death is caused by severe hypoxia and metabolic acidosis and usually coincides with spontaneous closure of the ductus arteriosus. Rarely, patients survive into young adult life. McArthur and colleagues describe a 21-year-old whose pulmonary blood flow came from a right coronary–pulmonary arterial fistula, and Robicsek and colleagues describe another patient of similar age who survived because of a congenital aortopulmonary window.[M6,R3]

TECHNIQUE OF OPERATION

Overview

No single neonatal operation is standard for pulmonary atresia with intact ventricular septum; rather, several surgical procedures, either in isolation or in combination, are indicated based on the details of the morphology in each case[H1] (see Indications for Operation later in this chapter for a description of the best initial operation for each morphologic variant). The initial operation most commonly indicated for

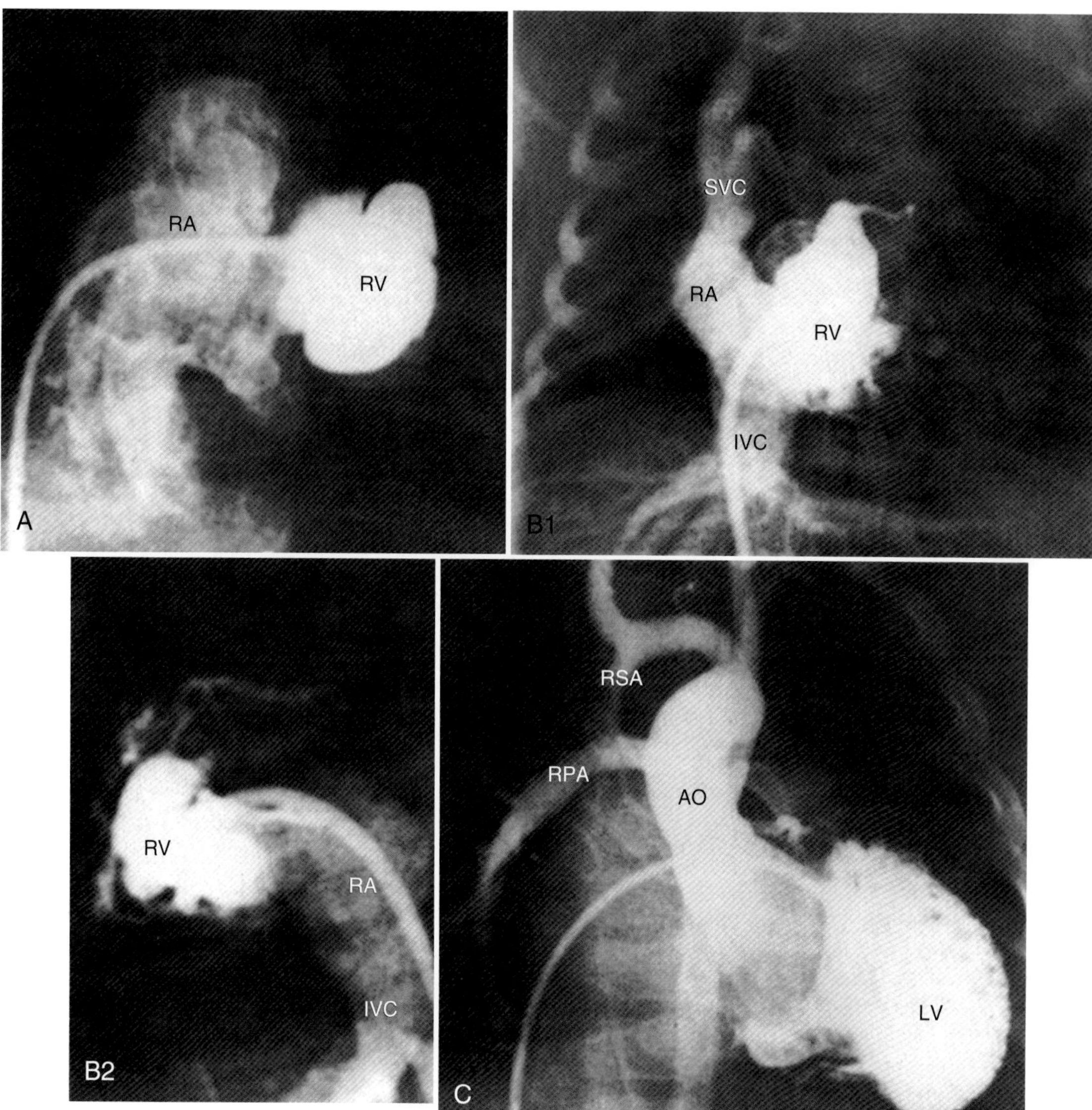

Figure 40-7 Cineangiograms in neonates with pulmonary atresia and intact ventricular septum. **A,** Right ventriculogram, frontal view. Small right ventricle (RV) has smooth borders, infundibular cavity is obliterated, and tricuspid valve shows severe regurgitation. **B,** Right ventriculogram from another patient in *(B1)* frontal and *(B2)* lateral views. The RV is very small, but its walls are trabeculated. Sinusoid channels are connected with coronary circulation. **C,** Left ventriculogram in frontal view in another patient. The left ventricle (LV) has its usual appearance and supports the aorta. A right Blalock-Taussig shunt has been made. Key: *AO,* Aorta; *IVC,* inferior vena cava; *RA,* right atrium; *RPA,* right pulmonary artery; *RSA,* right subclavian artery; *SVC,* superior vena cava.

this entity is concomitant transanular patching, systemic–pulmonary artery shunting, and ductal ligation. The next most common procedure is an isolated systemic-to–pulmonary artery shunt and ductal ligation.

For all of the procedures described, postnatal preoperative management is similar. Following birth, an arterial pressure monitoring catheter is placed, preferably into the left radial artery. (A right radial artery catheter should be avoided because of the possibility that a systemic-to–pulmonary artery shunt originating from the right subclavian artery will be part of the surgical procedure.) A reliable intravenous line is placed into either the femoral or umbilical vein. In general, deep intravenous lines into the upper body, such as into the subclavian or jugular veins, should be avoided to minimize thrombosis in the upper body venous system, because many patients will ultimately require a bidirectional cavopulmonary shunt as part of their overall surgical management. A prostaglandin E_1 (PGE_1) infusion is started as soon as possible to maintain ductal patency and is continued until after the surgical procedure.[C4,C7,E4,F3,H4,N2,O2] The full dose is $0.1\ mg \cdot kg^{-1} \cdot min^{-1}$; when the ductus is confirmed to be open, the dose often can be reduced.

Endotracheal intubation and mechanical ventilation are usually necessary, either as part of general resuscitative measures, or as a result of inhibition of intrinsic ventilatory drive due to PGE_1. A low inspired oxygen fraction and controlled hypercarbia are used to counter the tendency for overcirculation through the ductus arteriosus. Low-dose inotropic support with dopamine or milrinone may be needed to support the systemic circulation.

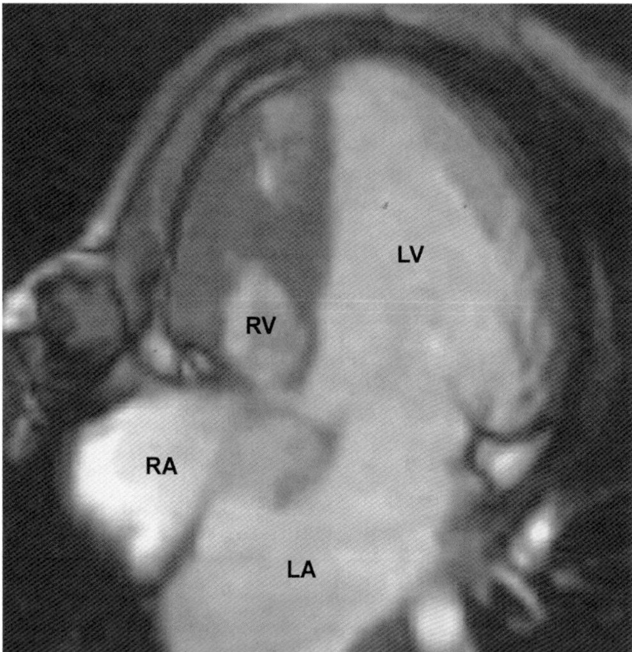

Figure 40-8 Four-chamber view from a bright-blood, steady-state free precession cardiac magnetic resonance imaging scan of a 15-year-old boy with pulmonary atresia with intact ventricular septum. The right atrium (RA) is aligned with the small and dysplastic right ventricle (RV). The tricuspid valve is small. Central venous return flows through an atrial septal defect (not shown) and mixes with pulmonary venous return in the left atrium (LA) before entering the left ventricle (LV).

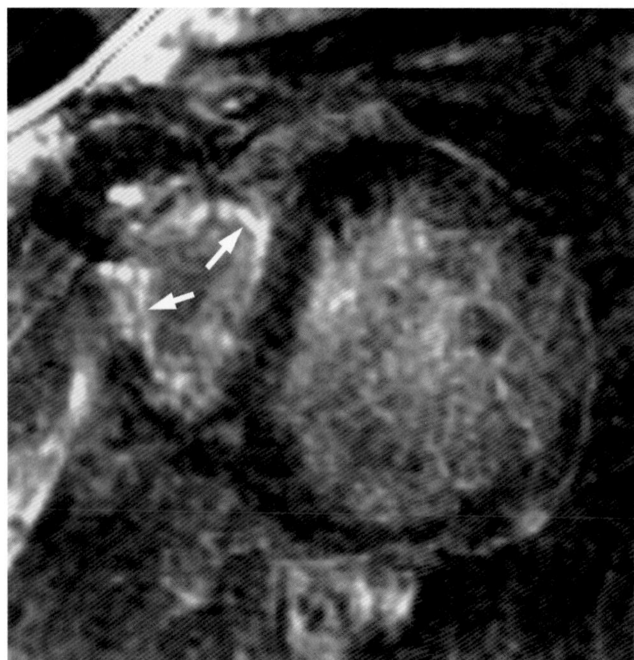

Figure 40-9 Mid–short axis view of the ventricles from a delayed-enhancement cardiac magnetic resonance imaging scan of a 10-year-old boy with pulmonary atresia with intact ventricular septum showing endocardial delayed enhancement *(arrows)*. This is the result of endocardial infarction and fibrosis secondary to suprasystemic right ventricular pressure, which impedes endocardial coronary flow.

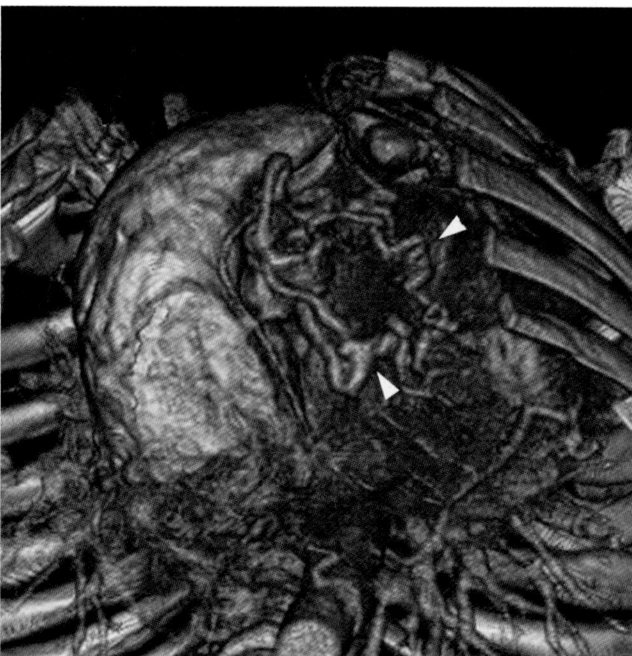

Figure 40-10 Volume-rendered computed tomography angiogram of right ventricular inferior wall in a 10-year-old boy with pulmonary atresia with intact ventricular septum. A number of coronary fistulae arise from the right coronary artery and terminate in right ventricular sinusoidal spaces *(arrowheads)*.

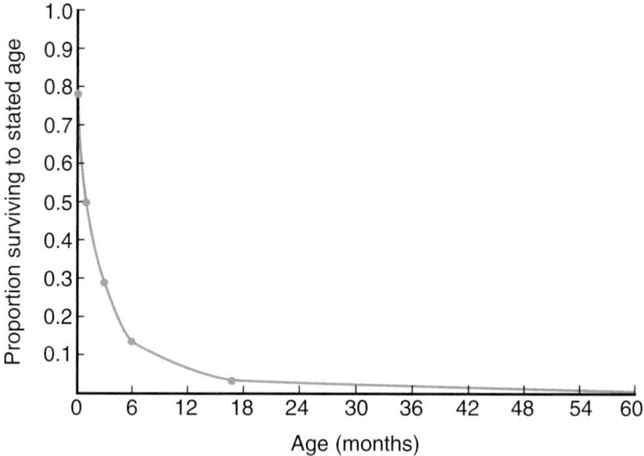

Figure 40-11 Freehand estimate of survival of surgically untreated patients with pulmonary atresia and intact ventricular septum based on reports in the literature.[B11,D4,D8,D9,F6,F7,L5,M8,M10,M13,S11,W3]

Concomitant Placement of Transanular Patch and Systemic–Pulmonary Artery Shunt

A median sternotomy is made through an incision that is carried a little farther into the neck than usual to provide better exposure of the brachiocephalic trunk and subclavian arteries. After the pericardium is opened and stay sutures applied, the right pulmonary artery between the aorta and superior vena cava is dissected.

A 3.5-mm expanded polytetrafluoroethylene (PTFE) tube (3.0 mm if the neonate is smaller than about 2.5 kg) is cut to proper length. Without giving heparin at this time, a fine

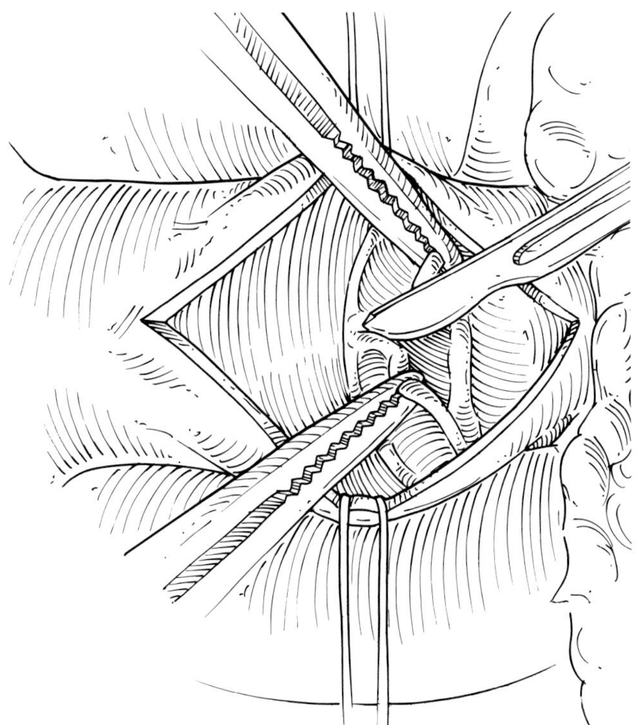

Figure 40-12 Technique of surgical pulmonary valvotomy for pulmonary atresia with intact ventricular septum. Median sternotomy is used. Cardiopulmonary bypass (CPB) with single venous cannulation, at normothermic or mild hypothermic temperature, is initiated. The ductus arteriosus is ligated (not shown). Aortic clamping is not performed. After CPB is established, the valve is exposed through a longitudinal incision in the pulmonary trunk. Fused commissures of the valve are identified. Using a knife with a #15 blade, the commissures are incised precisely along the fusion point between leaflets, beginning centrally and moving to the anulus. Arteriotomy is closed either primarily or with a narrow glutaraldehyde-treated autologous pericardial patch, using 7-0 polypropylene running suture.

side-biting clamp is placed to exclude the brachiocephalic trunk–subclavian artery junction, and an incision is made in the anterolateral aspect of the arterial wall. An end-to-side anastomosis is made between one end of the expanded PTFE graft and the artery, using 7-0 polypropylene suture. A clamp is placed as far medially on the right pulmonary artery as possible, and another as far laterally as possible but medial to the superior vena cava, and the pulmonary artery is opened longitudinally between them. Alternatively, a single fine side-biting (C) clamp is used. Great care is taken to ensure the clamp does not interfere with ductal flow to the left pulmonary artery or cause coronary artery compression at the aortic origin. The distal end of the expanded PTFE tube is anastomosed to this opening. Clamps are removed.

The ductus arteriosus is dissected and ligated. The pulmonary trunk is dissected minimally. A piece of pericardium is removed, treated with glutaraldehyde, and cut to proper dimensions (see "Decision and Technique for Transanular Patching" under Technique of Operation in Section I of Chapter 38). The usual aortic cannula is employed, and a single venous cannula is positioned (see "One Versus Two Venous Cannulae" under Special Situations and Controversies in Section III of Chapter 2).

Cardiopulmonary bypass (CPB) is established, with the perfusate warm and normocalcemic. The neonate's temperature is maintained at approximately 34°C during CPB. The surgically created shunt is temporarily occluded by placing a vascular clamp on the PTFE tube. The operation may be done with the heart beating, or cold cardioplegia and controlled reperfusion may be used (see "Cold Cardioplegia, Controlled Aortic Root Reperfusion, and [When Needed] Warm Cardioplegic Induction" in Chapter 3).

A longitudinal incision is made in the pulmonary trunk, and the cartilaginous valve plate is incised. The incision is carried proximally onto the RV, taking care to find and stay in the cavity of the infundibulum and to extend it to the sinus portion and distally along the pulmonary trunk, stopping just before the bifurcation. The patch, preferably made from glutaraldehyde-treated autologous pericardium, is sewn into place with 7-0 polypropylene continuous suture. The suture line does not include the full thickness of the incised RV wall, but rather incorporates the epicardium and about 30% of the outer thickness of the RV wall. The foramen ovale must not be closed.

The aortic clamp is released (or controlled reperfusion accomplished), and preparations are made for discontinuing CPB. The vascular clamp is removed from the PTFE tube, and when normothermia is regained, CPB is discontinued and the remainder of the operation completed as usual.

Other Initial Operations

Other initial operations are indicated based on specific morphology. These include isolated placement of a systemic to pulmonary artery shunt and ductal ligation; isolated placement of a transanular patch and ductal ligation using CPB; pulmonary valvotomy, placement of a systemic-to–pulmonary artery shunt, and ductal ligation using CPB; and isolated pulmonary valvotomy and ductal ligation using CPB (Fig. 40-12).

SPECIAL FEATURES OF POSTOPERATIVE CARE

Postoperative care is the same as described under "Special Features of Postoperative Care" in Chapter 39 for critical pulmonary stenosis in neonates. As in the case with pulmonary stenosis, need for an additional surgical procedure is continually assessed.

RESULTS

Survival

Early (Hospital) Death

Overall hospital mortality of a heterogeneous group of neonates with pulmonary atresia and intact ventricular septum, virtually all of whom have had one or more procedures, has been about 20%.[H1] However, the hazard function for death does not level off appreciably until 3 to 6 months (Fig. 40-13). This plus the wide variability of morphology and of procedures makes the unadjusted figure of little value. More recent studies that have followed, in general, the guidelines described under Indications for Operation (see later) show improved early survival. In one study,[J1] there was 1 hospital death among 47 patients (2.1%; CL 0.4%-6.8%), and in another,[H5] 5 early deaths among 44 patients (11%; CL

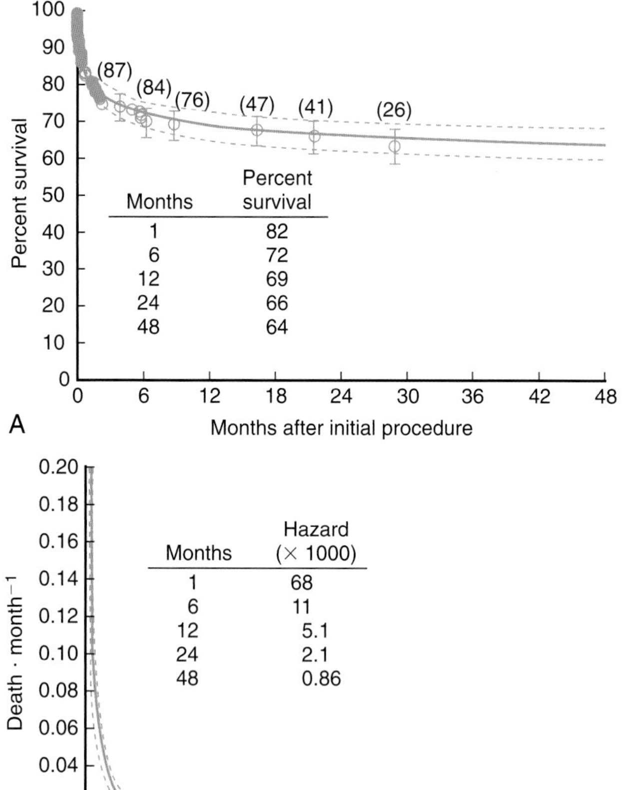

Figure 40-13 Survival after initial procedure (performed, on average, at age 3 days) of neonates with pulmonary atresia and intact ventricular septum (n = 171). Circles represent individual deaths, and vertical bars represent 70% confidence limits of nonparametric estimates. Solid line represents parametrically determined continuous point estimates, and dashed lines enclose 70% confidence limits. Excluded were patients having abnormally large right ventricles with or without Ebstein malformation (n = 13, of whom 11 died) and those having had no procedure (n = 8, among whom 7 died; 3 are among the 13 just mentioned). Depiction is of 153 patients. **A,** Survival. **B,** Hazard function. (From Hanley and colleagues.[H1])

6.7%-18%). A 40-year single-institution study of 210 patients also documents that survival has improved over time.[D10]

Time-Related Survival

Only about 60% of a heterogeneous group of neonates with pulmonary atresia and intact ventricular septum were alive 1 year after entrance into the hospital for treatment, as were 60% at 2 years and 58% at 4 years.[H1] The hazard function for death remains high but declining for the first 3 months, but after about 36 months it is only a little higher than that of an age-sex-race–matched general population. Patients with an abnormally large RV, with or without Ebstein malformation, have a particularly poor outlook regardless of treatment; about 85% die within the first year.[H1,H5] Excluding this small group of patients, 1-month, 1-year, and 4-year survival has been somewhat better than in the heterogeneous group (see Fig. 40-13). Some recent single-institution reports suggest slightly better long-term outcome.[H5,O1,R6,Y1]

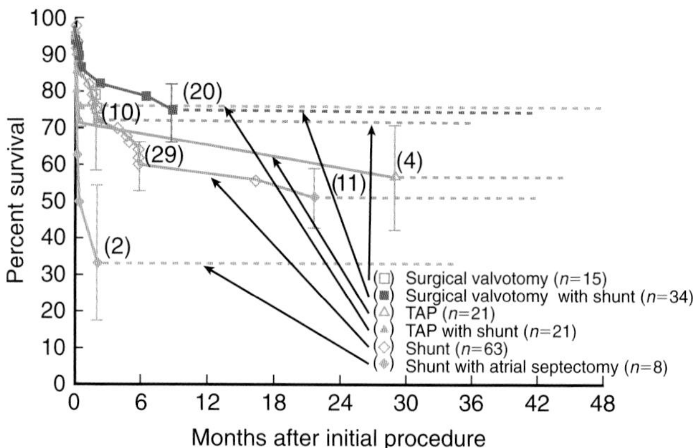

Figure 40-14 Survival after various initial procedures in a heterogeneous group of patients with pulmonary atresia and intact ventricular septum. In addition, eight patients (seven of whom died) underwent no procedure, and one underwent an unknown procedure. No patient had an initial percutaneous procedure. In general, patients who received a pulmonary-systemic shunt (with or without atrial septectomy) had the smallest tricuspid valves (z value ≤ -3). Key: *TAP,* Transanular patching. (From Hanley and colleagues.[H1])

Table 40-3 Incremental Risk Factors for Death in Pulmonary Atresia and Intact Ventricular Septum[a]

Risk Factor	Single Hazard Phase *P*[b]
Patient	
(Lower) Birth weight	<.0001
RV-dependent circulation	.03
(Smaller) Dimension (z value) of tricuspid valve overall	.03
If valvotomy or transanular patching performed with a shunt	.001
Procedural	
(Earlier) Date of shunt alone	.002

Data from Hanley and colleagues.[H1]
[a]Based on 171 neonates with pulmonary atresia in the Congenital Heart Surgeons Society study (1987-1991). Excluded were patients with Ebstein malformation or right ventricular cavity size greater than normal (n = 13, 11 of whom died) and those having no procedure (8, among whom 7 died; 3 are among the 13 just mentioned), leaving 153 neonates who actually underwent a procedure. Time zero was time of first intervention.
[b]Coefficients, their standard deviation, and other details of the multivariable equation resulting from the analysis are in cited article.[H1]
Key: *RV,* Right ventricle.

Modes of Death

The most common modes of death are acute heart failure and hypoxia.

Incremental Risk Factors for Premature Death

Survival after different initial procedures has varied widely (Fig. 40-14), but prevalence of small tricuspid valves and RV cavities has varied among the procedure groups. A more reliable understanding of the patient-specific and procedural risk factors for death is obtained by multivariable analysis (Table 40-3); validation of the analysis is shown in Appendix Fig. 40B-1.

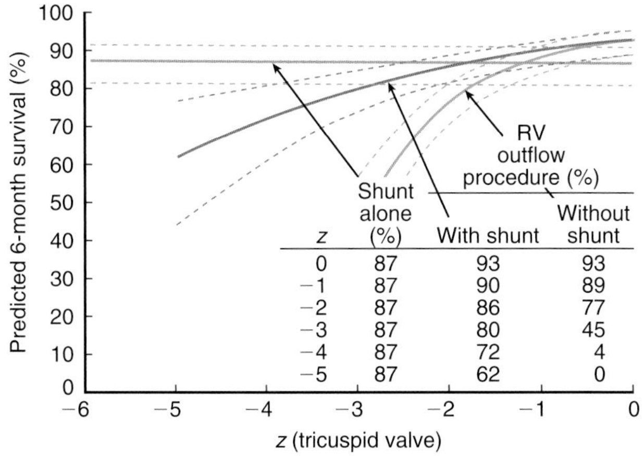

Figure 40-15 Nomogram of a specific solution of a multivariable equation illustrating effects of dimension of tricuspid valve (expressed as *z* value) and type of initial procedure on survival in neonates with pulmonary atresia and intact ventricular septum (see Table 40-3). Values for other variables entered into equation are birth weight 3.1 kg, right ventricular (RV)-dependent circulation, number, and in the case of a shunt operation, date of operation 1991. This nomogram is a rational basis for therapy. (From Hanley and colleagues.[H1])

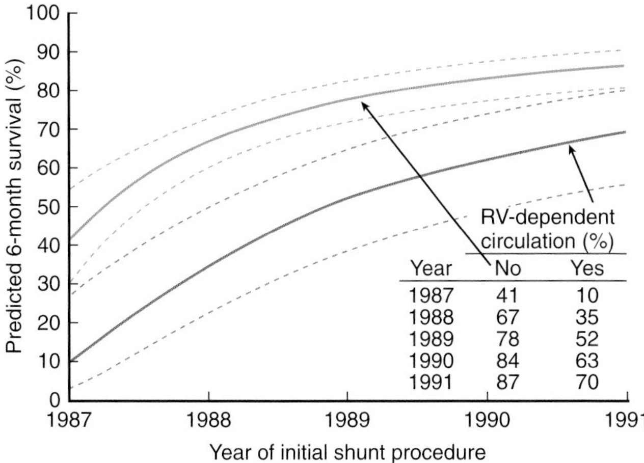

Figure 40-16 Nomogram of a specific solution of multivariable equation (see Table 40-3) demonstrating improvement in survival after an initial shunt procedure that has occurred across time, and effect of a right ventricular (RV)-dependent circulation. Value entered for birth weight is 3.1 kg. (From Hanley and colleagues.[H1])

Dimensions of Tricuspid Valve

Small size (*z* value of diameter) of the tricuspid valve is a strong risk factor for death (Fig. 40-15). An exception is the case of neonates in whom the initial procedure is a systemic–pulmonary artery shunt alone. When that procedure is used, survival is unrelated to dimension of the tricuspid valve (see Fig. 40-15). Survival after shunting appears to have improved recently, probably related to increased experience with making systemic–pulmonary artery shunts in neonates (Fig. 40-16). The recent two-center study by Fenton and colleagues is relevant to this discussion.[F2] They assessed survival among 35 patients who underwent a shunt-alone initial procedure. Although they did not measure tricuspid valve diameter, they evaluated RV cavity size, which is known to correlate with tricuspid valve size. Early mortality was low and unrelated to RV size. Interestingly, however, they demonstrated that interim mortality (defined as occurring after successful neonatal surgery but before the second-stage operation) was substantial: 15%. Furthermore, when they evaluated only patients with very small RV cavities, interim mortality was 24%.

Right Ventricular–Dependent Coronary Circulation

An RV-dependent coronary circulation is a powerful risk factor for death.[C2,C9,H5] In a study among 12 such patients, only 4 (CL 18%-52%) survived 1 or more years.[H1] There is evidence, however, that even this powerful risk factor has recently been neutralized to some extent (see Fig. 40-16). In a 2006 study focusing only on patients with RV-dependent coronary circulation, overall mortality was 19%.[G13] All patients were managed as neonates with a systemic-to–pulmonary artery shunt only; all deaths occurred within 3 months of the procedure. Notably, all three patients with no coronary-to-aorta connection died. All surviving patients have gone on to a bidirectional cavopulmonary connection or Fontan without further mortality. In another recent study, 2 of 5 patients (CL 14%-71%) with RV-dependent coronary circulation died.[H5]

The severity of coronary abnormalities and fistulae affect more than survival; they are also associated with reduced LV function at late follow-up.[D10]

Systemic–Pulmonary Artery Shunt

In the past, systemic–pulmonary artery shunting alone has been associated with lower overall survival than when other procedures were used (see Fig. 40-14). More recently, survival with a shunt alone has improved strikingly (see Fig. 40-16). This is the only procedure associated with reasonable survival in patients with very small tricuspid valves.

Birth Weight

As in nearly all types of congenital heart disease requiring treatment early in life, low birth weight is an important risk factor for death.[L4]

Interim Interventions after Initial Procedure

This section discusses further interim interventions performed before the definitive intervention leading to a separated two-ventricle system or a single-ventricle Fontan system. Patients whose initial procedure is a transanular patch and a systemic–pulmonary artery shunt generally do not require further interim procedures. This is an important advantage of this operation as the initial procedure. With it, the opportunity for maximal RV (and tricuspid valve) growth exists during the critical early weeks and months of life when myocardial hyperplasia is possible.

Among patients whose initial procedure is pulmonary valvotomy or placement of a transanular patch without a concomitant systemic–pulmonary artery shunt, about half require a systemic-pulmonary shunt within a few weeks (Fig. 40-17). The smaller the dimensions of the tricuspid valve, the greater the probability that a subsequent systemic–pulmonary artery shunt will be needed ($P = .04$) (Fig. 40-18).

Patients whose initial procedure is a pulmonary valvotomy with or without a concomitant shunt often subsequently require placement of a transanular patch (Fig. 40-19). No correlates with subsequent placement of such a patch have been identified. This suggests that a transanular patch should

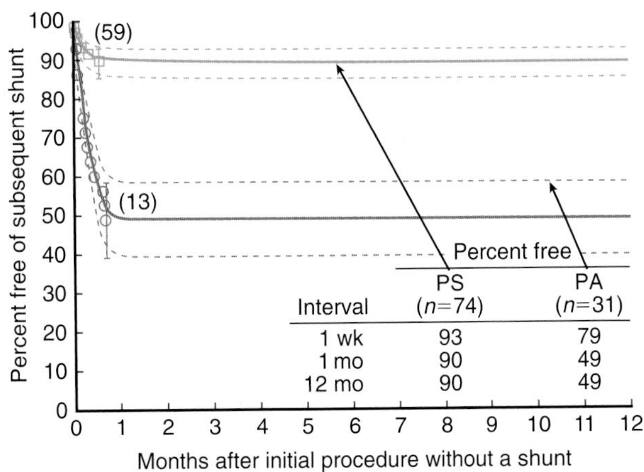

Figure 40-17 Freedom from a subsequent shunt operation in neonates with pulmonary stenosis or atresia and intact ventricular septum undergoing an initial valvotomy (balloon or surgical) or insertion of a transanular patch without a concomitant shunt (n = 105). (Format is as in Fig. 40-13.) Patients with Ebstein malformation or with a right ventricular cavity size greater than normal, or both, were not included in this analysis. Key: *PA,* Pulmonary atresia; *PS,* pulmonary stenosis. (From Hanley and colleagues.[H1])

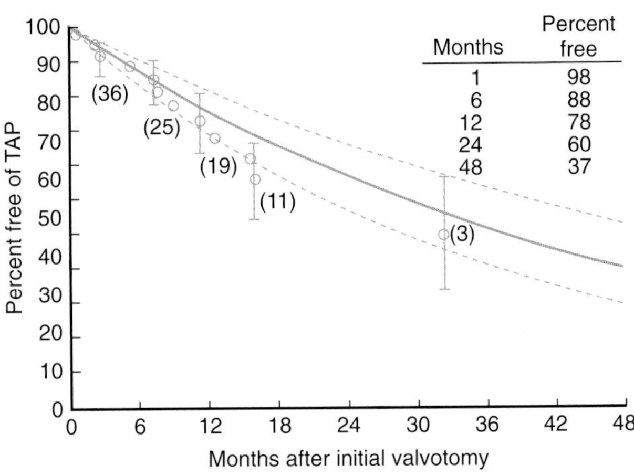

Figure 40-19 Freedom from a transanular patch (TAP) in neonates with pulmonary atresia and intact ventricular septum undergoing an initial pulmonary valvotomy with or without a concomitant shunt operation (n = 46). (Format is as in Fig. 40-13.) Patients with Ebstein malformation, right ventricular cavity size greater than normal, or both were not included in this analysis. Multivariable analysis identified no risk factors for this event. (From Hanley and colleagues.[H1])

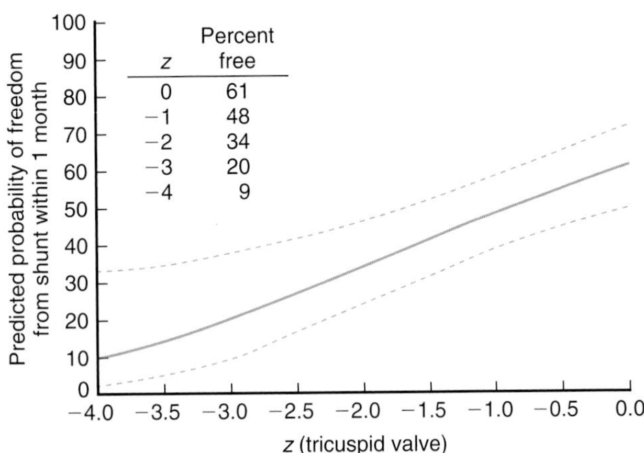

Figure 40-18 Nomogram of a specific solution of a multivariable equation illustrating the relationship between dimensions of the tricuspid valve (expressed as z value) and probability of being free of a subsequent shunt operation after initial pulmonary valvotomy or placement of a transanular patch without a concomitant shunt. (From Hanley and colleagues[H1]; see citation for coefficients and their standard deviation.)

be incorporated into the initial procedure whenever there is doubt about adequacy of the pathway through the infundibular portion of the RV.

Patients who initially have only a systemic–pulmonary artery shunt should be a select group characterized by marked hypoplasia of the tricuspid valve and RV, or RV-dependent coronary artery circulation (see Indications for Operation later). The goal is survival to age 3 to 6 months, when a bidirectional superior cavopulmonary shunt can be performed, eventually followed by a Fontan operation (see Indications for Operation in Chapter 41). About 85% of patients who receive an initial systemic–pulmonary artery shunt only appear to be able to achieve the goal of a Fontan operation.[H1]

Definitive Procedures

It is not possible at present to know the prevalence of achieving (at some time) a separated two-ventricle repair. It appears to be about 60% to 70% in patients with a tricuspid valve z value of −2 or greater, and less than 10% in those with very small z values.[H1]

Theoretically, in all patients in whom a separated two-ventricle repair cannot be accomplished, a single-ventricle Fontan system should eventually be achievable. The limiting factor in this group is survival to the time of a Fontan operation. Thus, the problem is analogous to that in patients with hypoplastic left heart physiology. Results of the Fontan operation in patients with pulmonary atresia and intact ventricular septum appear to be the same as in patients with other congenital cardiac anomalies.[M2,N1] Patients with severe coronary abnormalities may, however, be at increased late risk.[P6]

A more difficult question is whether all patients not able to achieve a two-ventricle repair *should* eventually undergo a Fontan, or whether an alternative procedure should serve as the definitive operation in selected patients. For example, certain patients with tricuspid valve z values that are moderately small may best be served by a definitive operation consisting of a bidirectional superior cavopulmonary shunt combined with closure of the atrial septal defect and a procedure creating unobstructed RV to pulmonary artery flow, the so-called one-and-a-half ventricle repair[B4,C5,G3,K2,M12,M15] (see Special Situations and Controversies). In patients in whom the tricuspid valve and RV are functional, procedures may occasionally be necessary to correct tricuspid valve regurgitation.[R1]

Other Outcomes

Myocardial perfusion has been shown to be abnormal at mid- to late follow-up.[E2] The abnormalities are not restricted to patients with identified coronary fistulae, but include patients with apparently normal coronary arteries. Exercise capacity is reduced in all patients with pulmonary atresia with intact ventricular septum, regardless of the definitive procedure.[N4,S3] Late follow-up also demonstrates progressive right atrial dilatation, indicating abnormalities of the RV and tricuspid valve, and a tendency to develop arrhythmias.[M9]

INDICATIONS FOR OPERATION

Presence of the malformation is generally an indication for operation because of its high lethality. As soon as the diagnosis is suspected, the neonate is resuscitated and stabilized, as described under Technique of Operation. Once the diagnosis is established and the baby is stabilized and in good condition, operation is undertaken, but in view of the favorable effect of PGE_1, it is not done as an emergency.

Selection of the initial intervention is based in large part on the estimated probability that a separated two-ventricle system will ultimately be possible.[B6,C6,D5] Indications given in this section are based on the work of de Leval and colleagues and on the findings of the Congenital Heart Surgeons Society study[D5,H1] (see Table 40-3 and Figs. 40-15 to 40-19). These two studies are entirely consistent with each other, as are those of other recent studies.[A1,A4,B6,C6,C9]

The inference from all available information is that the best guide to the type of initial operation is size of the tricuspid valve. A z value equal to or less than −4 (and by implication a very small RV chamber) makes probability of death after placement of a transanular patch with a concomitant shunt greater than after a systemic–pulmonary artery shunt alone (see Fig. 40-15). Furthermore, an achieved separated two-ventricle system has been extremely uncommon when the original z value of the tricuspid valve has been less than −3.[H1] (This line of reasoning could be altered were it to be shown that growth of the hypoplastic tricuspid valve could be made disproportionally greater than that of the body as a whole.) Thus, in patients with pulmonary atresia and a z value of the tricuspid valve equal to or less than −4, an initial systemic–pulmonary artery shunt is indicated.

At age 3 to 6 months, a bidirectional superior cavopulmonary shunt is performed, followed by a Fontan operation (see Indications for Operation in Chapter 41). So long as a total cavopulmonary type of connection is used for the Fontan procedure, nothing need be done to the tricuspid valve. Any evident RV–coronary artery fistula should be closed, unless there is RV-dependent coronary circulation. When the z value of the tricuspid valve is greater than −4, the inference is that risk of death will be no greater (see Fig. 40-15), and probability of a separated two-ventricle system greater, when a transanular patch is placed (or, in special circumstances, a pulmonary valvotomy performed) and a concomitant shunt is placed rather than a systemic–pulmonary artery shunt alone.

Ideally, some objective method of determining need for a transanular patch should be available, but the decision must rest on the subjectively evaluated "adequacy" of the infundibular cavity, the "anulus," and the pulmonary valve tissue itself. In the absence of any clear evidence of a substantial advantage of valvotomy in this setting, and because about 40% of those in whom a valvotomy has been done have required a subsequent transanular patch, a transanular patch should be used whenever doubt arises.[H1]

When an RV outflow operation is being performed as described, need for a concomitant systemic–pulmonary artery shunt is moderately related to RV cavity size and thus to dimension of the tricuspid valve (see Fig. 40-18). As a general guide, a concomitant systemic–pulmonary artery shunt should be performed, especially when the z value of the tricuspid valve is less than about −2 (indicating a small RV cavity).

When the initial procedure has been done under the hypothesis that a separated two-ventricle system will be possible, testing of that hypothesis should begin 6 to 12 months after the initial procedure. The shunt is temporarily occluded, ideally percutaneously. If arterial oxygen saturation remains high, the shunt is permanently closed by percutaneous or surgical techniques (for percutaneous technique, see "Percutaneous Closure of Large Aortopulmonary Collateral Arteries" under Special Situations and Controversies in Section II of Chapter 38). The atrial septal defect is temporarily occluded, again ideally by percutaneous techniques. If right atrial pressure remains below 12 to 15 mmHg, cardiac output is adequate, and oxygen saturation of blood in the right atrium is maintained (any decrease in cardiac output is compensated for by rise in arterial oxygen saturation), the defect should be closed permanently by a surgical or percutaneous technique (see "Closure of Atrial Septal Defects by Percutaneous Techniques" under Special Situations and Controversies in Chapter 30).[B1]

When the patient does not tolerate shunt closure, a separated two-ventricle system may not be possible, and consideration should be given to beginning the process leading to a Fontan operation or some other definitive procedure, such as the "one-and-a-half ventricle" repair as discussed earlier under "Definitive Procedures." When closure of the atrial septal defect is not well tolerated, a prolonged period of procrastination may be wise if the patient's clinical state is good.

Neonates with RV-dependent coronary circulation represent a special problem (see "Right Ventricular–Coronary Artery Fistulae" earlier under Morphology). When after detailed study, a considerable portion of the LV myocardium is judged to be in jeopardy of developing severe ischemia, decompression or thrombolytic exclusion of the RV is contraindicated.[C9] The recent study by Calder[C2] provides quantitative information on the amount of LV myocardium at risk of ischemia and how it relates to outcome. These patients may be treated the same as other patients with severely hypoplastic tricuspid valves and RVs, so long as the type of Fontan operation allows fully saturated blood to enter the RV. In time, cardiac transplantation may prove the optimal treatment for this small subset of patients.

SPECIAL SITUATIONS AND CONTROVERSIES

Percutaneous Valvotomy

It has been recognized for some time that percutaneous techniques could become the initial procedure for neonates in whom the pathway through the infundibulum is reasonably wide and the atresia "membranous." In 1991, this was achieved successfully by laser valvotomy followed by balloon dilatation.[P1] Other reports have followed, with mixed outcome.[B12,F1,G5,G9,O4,R4,W2]

Shinebourne and colleagues recommend percutaneous valvotomy in all cases of membranous atresia with an RV and tricuspid valve that have the potential for a biventricular repair. Even in this favorable subgroup, 60% will remain duct dependent and require a systemic-to-pulmonary artery shunt.[S8] Similarly, Humpl and colleagues attempted percutaneous valvotomy in a highly selected subgroup.[H7] Of 30 patients, the valve could not be perforated in 3 (10%; CL 4.6%-19%), 14 required a shunt (47%; CL 36%-57%), and 4 (13%; CL 7.1%-23%) required RV outflow surgery. Thus, more than two thirds of the group required surgical intervention. In the study by Hirata and colleagues, only 2 of 17 patients (12%; CL 4.2%-25%) undergoing percutaneous valvotomy did not require an additional neonatal surgical procedure involving either a shunt or the RV outflow tract.[H5] Similar outcomes were observed by McLean and Pearl.[M7]

In the U.K.-Ireland multicenter study, neonates undergoing percutaneous valvotomy had an increased risk of reintervention to increase pulmonary blood flow relative to those undergoing initial surgery.[D3] Thus, this method has the same limitations as surgical valvotomy or transanular patching without a concomitant shunt—particularly the potential delay of weeks or months in maximizing the stimulus to RV growth—and is associated with a higher likelihood of reintervention than these initial surgical procedures (see "Interim Interventions after Initial Procedure" earlier under Results).

Formalin Infiltration of Ductus Arteriosus

In 1975, Rudolph and colleagues introduced formalin infiltration of the wall of the ductus via a left thoracotomy as a means of maintaining patency and avoiding need for an artificial shunt.[R5] In carefully selected patients with favorable anatomy, this technique may provide outcome similar to that of surgical intervention.[A3] Others have observed ductal closure within a few weeks or months of the procedures, and its use is not currently recommended.[D6,D7,M14]

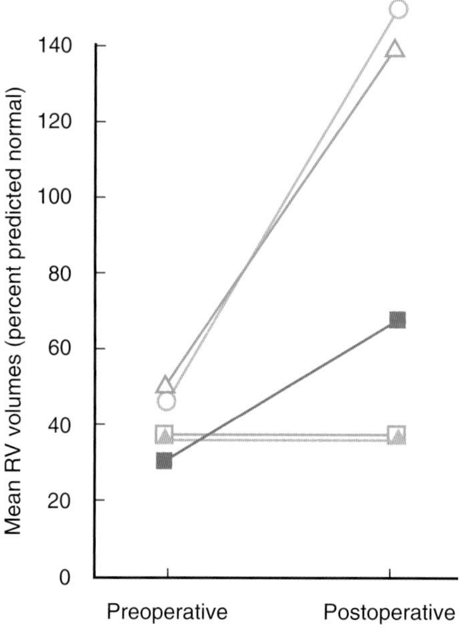

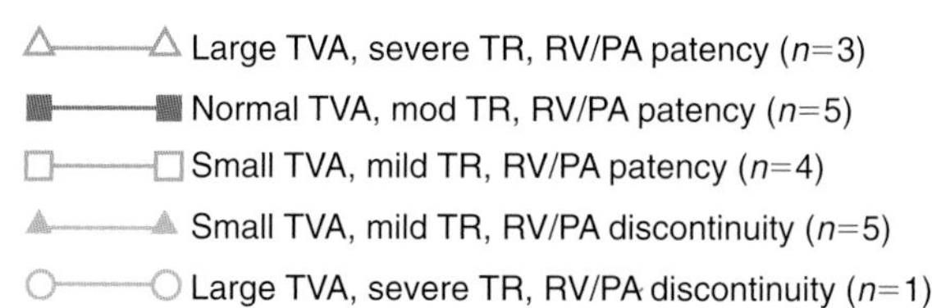

Figure 40-20 Change in right ventricular (RV) end-diastolic volume after palliative operations for pulmonary atresia and intact ventricular septum. Mean RV end-diastolic volumes are expressed as percentage of expected volume both before operation and at time of last assessment. Key: *PA,* Pulmonary artery; *TR,* tricuspid regurgitation; *TVA,* tricuspid valve anulus. (From Patel and colleagues.[P2])

Right Ventricle–to-Aorta Conduit

Use of an RV-to-aorta conduit for patients with RV-dependent coronary circulation has been used by several groups to limit myocardial ischemia.[F9,L1] Although outcomes have been good, the extremely limited use of this procedure prevents adequate assessment of its effectiveness.

Tricuspid Valve Closure in the Presence of Right Ventricular–Coronary Fistulae

Several groups advocate closing the tricuspid valve orifice in the setting of RV-coronary fistulae without major coronary abnormalities.[W1,W5] Limited experience prevents adequate analysis of this procedure.

Tricuspid Valve Growth

The tricuspid valve and RV cavity tend under some circumstances to increase in size as the patient grows.[G9,L5,M4,M13,S11] However, there is little evidence that *disproportionate* enlargement occurs as growth of the child proceeds, no matter what the surgical procedure. The only evidence for disproportionate growth comes from a recent study by Huang and colleagues of 40 patients undergoing initial neonatal surgical pulmonary valvotomy and shunt.[H6] They showed that on average, there was no change in tricuspid valve z value over time; however, on an individual patient basis, 32% showed tricuspid valve enlargement of at least +2 z values at follow-up.

There is evidence that the RV cavity increases in size, but this may result from iatrogenic pulmonary or tricuspid regurgitation or both (Fig. 40-20). The tricuspid valve appears to grow *proportionally* with the child when there is forward flow across the tricuspid and pulmonary valves, but not otherwise[D6,H2,L3] (Fig. 40-21). With growth of the RV, right ventricular–coronary artery fistulae may disappear.[P2] However, important abnormalities of RV compliance usually remain.[G9] Thus, there is at present no basis for determining treatment on anything other than z value of the tricuspid valve before initial therapy.

Bidirectional Cavopulmonary Shunt in Right Ventricular–Dependent Coronary Circulation

It is widely acknowledged that the blood entering the RV (and thus perfusing the coronary circulation) following a total cavopulmonary connection type of Fontan in patients with RV-dependent coronary circulation will be fully or almost fully saturated. Miyaji and colleagues recently have shown that the blood entering the RV after a superior cavopulmonary shunt ("bidirectional Glenn") is also more saturated than that under conditions of a systemic-to-pulmonary shunt.[M11] This raises the question of whether there is value

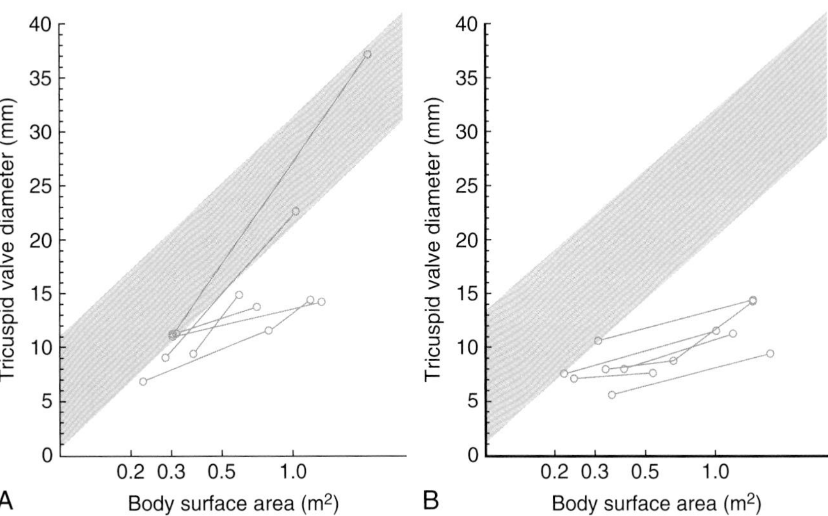

Figure 40-21 Tricuspid valve diameter related to body surface area (BSA, logarithmic scale) during growth of infants surviving an initial operation for pulmonary atresia and intact ventricular septum. Shaded area indicates 2 standard deviations around mean normal value. **A,** Patients in whom a pathway from right ventricle (RV) to pulmonary artery was created. **B,** Patients without RV-to–pulmonary artery continuity. (From de Leval and colleagues.[D6])

in performing an early superior cavopulmonary shunt in patients with RV-dependent coronary circulation.

Right Ventricular Sinus Myectomy

Because it is well accepted that the RV in this malformation is intrinsically tripartite and only becomes bipartite or unipartite from muscular ingrowth and cavity obliteration, it is logical to infer that removal of the excess muscle may have therapeutic value in selected cases. Bryant and colleagues studied this in 16 patients.[B10] They concluded that the procedure leads to an immediate increase in RV volume and is associated with achievement of a biventricular repair in 87% of selected patients. Of concern, they also noted that tricuspid valve growth in relation to somatic growth was minimal, potentially limiting long-term success of this procedure.

Assessment of Functional Benefit of Biventricular Versus Univentricular Definitive Procedures

Evidence supporting the generally held view that a biventricular repair is superior to a Fontan is limited at best. Redington and colleagues showed that a biventricular repair in patients with this malformation had restrictive RV physiology, with antegrade flow across the pulmonary valve during atrial contraction.[R2] This implies limited functional capacity. Exercise capacity was assessed by Sanghavi and colleagues and found to be similar in patients with biventricular repair and Fontan.[S3] Patients in both groups had subnormal peak $\dot{V}O_2$, with increasing impairment associated with increasing age. Based on these findings, it is not surprising that Numata and colleagues were unable to demonstrate a benefit in exercise capacity of the so-called one-and-a-half ventricle repair over the Fontan.[N4]

40A *z* Value of Tricuspid Valve

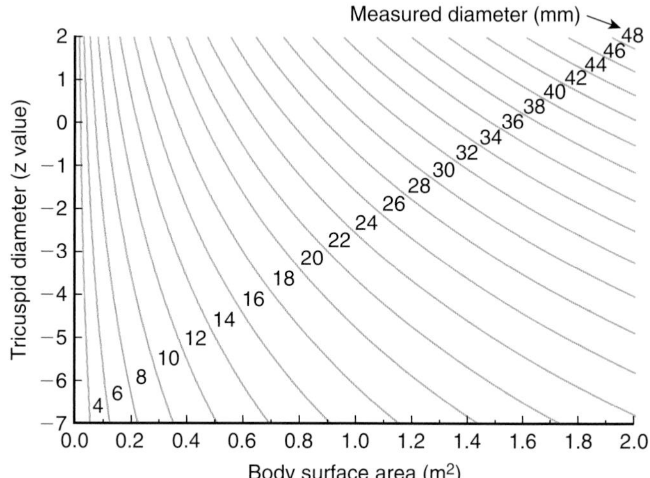

Figure 40A-1 Nomogram for conversion of diameter of tricuspid valve (obtained by echocardiography) to *z* value. Nomogram assumes a circular shape of tricuspid valve, which is usually the case in patients with pulmonary atresia and intact ventricular septum. (For a description of *z* value and its method of determination, see "Dimensions of Normal Cardiac and Great Artery Pathways" in Chapter 1.)

40B Validation of Multivariable Analysis

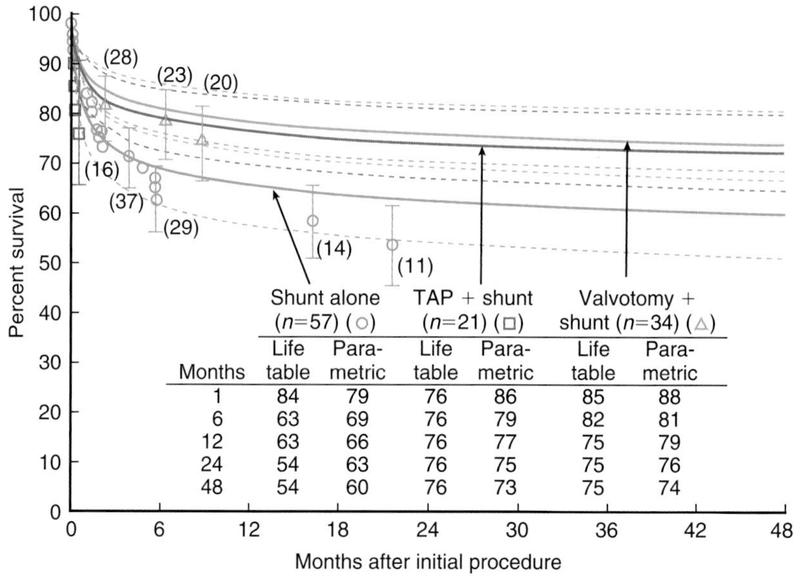

	Shunt alone (*n*=57) (○)		TAP + shunt (*n*=21) (□)		Valvotomy + shunt (*n*=34) (△)	
Months	Life table	Parametric	Life table	Parametric	Life table	Parametric
1	84	79	76	86	85	88
6	63	69	76	79	82	81
12	63	66	76	77	75	79
24	54	63	76	75	75	76
48	54	60	76	73	75	74

Figure 40B-1 Validation of multivariable risk factor equation (see Table 40-3) for death after initial procedure in patients with pulmonary atresia and intact ventricular septum. Patients with Ebstein malformation, right ventricular cavity size greater than normal, or both were not included in this analysis. Symbols represent nonparametric survival estimates, and vertical bars represent confidence limits for each of the three major treatment groups. Solid lines indicate parametrically estimated survival, and dashed lines enclose their 70% confidence limits, which are obtained by averaging parametric estimates for each patient within each group (see "Parametric Hazard Function Regression" in Section IV of Chapter 6). Note close correspondence of average parametric estimate to nonparametric estimate. (From Hanley and colleagues.[H1])

REFERENCES

A

1. Alboliras ET, Julsrud PR, Danielson GK, Puga FJ, Schaff HV, McGoon DC, et al. Definitive operation for pulmonary atresia with intact ventricular septum. J Thorac Cardiovasc Surg 1987;93:454.
2. Allan LD, Crawford DC, Tynan MJ. Pulmonary atresia in prenatal life. J Am Coll Cardiol 1986;8:1131.
3. Alwi M, Geetha K, Bilkis AA, Lim MK, Hasri S, Haifa AL, et al. Pulmonary atresia with intact ventricular septum percutaneous radiofrequency-assisted valvotomy and balloon dilation versus surgical valvotomy and Blalock Taussig shunt. J Am Coll Cardiol 2000;35:468.
4. Amodeo A, Keeton BR, Sutherland GR, Monro JL. Pulmonary atresia with intact ventricular septum: is neonatal repair advisable? Eur J Cardiothorac Surg 1991;5:17.
5. Anderson RH, Anderson C, Zuberbuhler JR. Further morphologic studies on hearts with pulmonary atresia and intact ventricular septum. Cardiol Young 1991;1:105.
6. Anderson RH, Silverman NH, Zuberbuhler JR. Congenitally unguarded tricuspid orifice: its differentiation from Ebstein's malformation in association with pulmonary atresia and intact ventricular septum. Pediatr Cardiol 1990;11:86.
7. Azcarate AO, Gonzalez LF, Alarcon AV. Atresia pulmonar con tabique interventricular integro. Arch Inst Cardiol Mex 1974;44:388.

B

1. Bass JL, Fuhrman BP, Lock JE. Balloon occlusion of atrial septal defect to assess right ventricular capability in hypoplastic right heart syndrome. Circulation 1983;68:1081.
2. Becker AE, Becker MJ, Edwards JE. Pathologic spectrum of dysplasia of the tricuspid valve. Arch Pathol 1971;91:161.
3. Benton JW Jr, Elliott LP, Adams P Jr, Anderson RC, Hong CY, Lester RG. Pulmonary atresia and stenosis with intact ventricular septum. Am J Dis Child 1962;104:83.
4. Bharati S, McAllister HA Jr, Chiemmongkoltip P, Lev M. Congenital pulmonary atresia with tricuspid insufficiency: morphologic study. Am J Cardiol 1977;40:70.
5. Bialostozky D, Attie F, Lupi E, Contreras R, Espino Vela J. Pulmonary atresia with intact intraventricular septum. I. Arch Inst Cardiol Mex 1974;44:195.
6. Billingsley AM, Laks H, Boyce SW, George B, Santulli T, Williams RG. Definitive repair in patients with pulmonary atresia and intact ventricular septum. J Thorac Cardiovasc Surg 1989;97:746.
7. Blackman MS, Schneider B, Sondheimer HM. Absent proximal left main coronary artery in association with pulmonary atresia. Br Heart J 1981;46:449.
8. Bowman FO Jr, Malm JR, Hayes CJ, Gersony WM, Ellis K. Pulmonary atresia with intact ventricular septum. J Thorac Cardiovasc Surg 1971;61:85.
9. Braunlin EA, Formanek AG, Moller JH, Edwards JE. Angiopathological appearances of pulmonary valve in pulmonary atresia with intact ventricular septum. Interpretation of nature of right ventricle from pulmonary angiography. Br Heart J 1982;47:281.
10. Bryant R 3rd, Nowicki ER, Mee RB, Rajeswaran J, Duncan BW, Rosenthal GL, et al. Success and limitations of right ventricular sinus myectomy for pulmonary atresia with intact ventricular septum. J Thorac Cardiovasc Surg 2008;136:735-42.
11. Buckley LP, Dooley KJ, Fyler DC. Pulmonary atresia and intact ventricular septum in New England (abstract). Am J Cardiol 1976;37:124.
12. Buheitel G, Hofbeck M, Singer H. Balloon dilatation of the pulmonary valve within the first 40 days of life in critical valvular pulmonary stenosis, Fallot's tetralogy and following surgical or interventional high-frequency opening of pulmonary atresia. Z Kardiol 1995;84:64.
13. Bulkley BH, D'Amico B, Taylor AL. Extensive myocardial fiber disarray in aortic and pulmonary atresia. Relevance to hypertrophic cardiomyopathy. Circulation 1983;67:191.
14. Bull C, de Leval MR, Mercanti C, Macartney FJ, Anderson RH. Pulmonary atresia and intact ventricular septum: a revised classification. Circulation 1982;66:266.

C

1. Calder AL, Co EE, Sage MD. Coronary arterial abnormalities in pulmonary atresia with intact ventricular septum. Am J Cardiol 1987;59:436.
2. Calder AL, Peebles CR, Occleshaw CJ. The prevalence of coronary arterial abnormalities in pulmonary atresia with intact ventricular septum and their influence on surgical results. Cardiol Young 2007;17:387-96.
3. Celermajer JM, Bowdler JD, Gengos DC, Cohen DH, Stuckey DS. Pulmonary valve fusion with intact ventricular septum. Am Heart J 1968;76:452.
4. Christensen NC, Fabricus J. Medical manipulation of the ductus arteriosus. Lancet 1975;2:406.
5. Clapp SK, Tantengco MV, Walters HL 3rd, Lobdell KW, Hakimi M. Bidirectional cavopulmonary anastomosis with intracardiac repair. Ann Thorac Surg 1997;63:746.
6. Cobanoglu A, Metzdorff MT, Pinson CW, Grunkemeier GL, Sunderland CO, Starr A. Valvotomy for pulmonary atresia with intact ventricular septum. A disciplined approach to achieve a functioning right ventricle. J Thorac Cardiovasc Surg 1985;89:482.
7. Coceani F, Olley PM. The response of the ductus arteriosus to prostaglandins. Can J Physiol Pharmacol 1973;51:220.
8. Cole RB, Muster AJ, Lev M, Paul MH. Pulmonary atresia with intact ventricular septum. Am J Cardiol 1968;21:23.
9. Coles JG, Freedom RM, Lightfoot NE, Dasmahapatra HK, Williams WG, Trusler GA, et al. Long-term results in neonates with pulmonary atresia and intact ventricular septum. Ann Thorac Surg 1989;47:213.
10. Cote M, Davignon A, Fouron JC. Congenital hypoplasia of right ventricular myocardium (Uhl's anomaly) associated with pulmonary atresia in a newborn. Am J Cardiol 1973;31:658.

D

1. Daubeney PE, Delany DJ, Anderson RH, Sandor GG, Slavik Z, Keeton BR, et al. Pulmonary atresia with intact ventricular septum: range of morphology in a population-based study. J Am Coll Cardiol 2002;39:1670-9.
2. Daubeney PE, Sharland GK, Cook AC, Keeton BR, Anderson RH, Webber SA. Pulmonary atresia with intact ventricular septum: impact of fetal echocardiography on incidence at birth and postnatal outcome. Circulation 1998;98:562.
3. Daubeney PE, Wang D, Delany DJ, Keeton BR, Anderson RH, Slavik Z, et al. Pulmonary atresia with intact ventricular septum: predictors of early and medium-term outcome in a population-based study. J Thorac Cardiovasc Surg 2005;130:1071.
4. Davignon AL, Greenwold WE, DuShane JW, Edwards JE. Congenital pulmonary atresia with intact ventricular septum—clinicopathologic correlation of two anatomic types. Am Heart J 1961;62:591.
5. de Leval M, Bull C, Hopkins R, Rees P, Deanfield J, Taylor JF, et al. Decision making in the definitive repair of the heart with a small right ventricle. Circulation 1985;72:II52.
6. de Leval M, Bull C, Stark J, Anderson RH, Taylor JF, Macartney FJ. Pulmonary atresia and intact ventricular septum: surgical management based on a revised classification. Circulation 1982;66:272.
7. Deanfield JE, Rees PG, Bull CM, de Leval M, Stark J, Macartney FJ, et al. Formalin infiltration of ductus arteriosus in cyanotic congenital heart disease. Br Heart J 1981;45:573.
8. Dhanavaravibul S, Nora JJ, McNamara DG. Pulmonary valvular atresia with intact ventricular septum: problems in diagnosis and results of treatment. J Pediatr 1970;77:1010.
9. Dobell AR, Grignon A. Early and late results in pulmonary atresia. Ann Thorac Surg 1977;24:264.
10. Dyamenahalli U, McCrindle BW, McDonald C, Trivedi KR, Smallhorn JF, Benson LN, et al. Pulmonary atresia with intact ventricular septum: management of, and outcomes for, a cohort of 210 consecutive patients. Cardiol Young 2004;14:299-308.

E

1. Edwards JE, Carey LS, Neufeld HN, Lester RG. Pulmonary atresia with intact ventricular septum. In Congenital heart disease. Philadelphia: WB Saunders, 1965, p. 576.
2. Ekman-Joelsson BM, Berggren H, Boll AB, Sixt R, Sunnegardh J. Abnormalities in myocardial perfusion after surgical correction of pulmonary atresia with intact ventricular septum. Cardiol Young 2008;18:89-95.
3. Elliott LP, Adams P Jr, Edwards JE. Pulmonary atresia with intact ventricular septum. Br Heart J 1963;25:489.

4. Elliott RB, Starling MB, Neutze JM. Medical manipulation of the ductus arteriosus. Lancet 1975;1:140.
5. Ellis K, Casarella WJ, Hayes CJ, Gersony WM, Bowman FO Jr, Malm JR. Pulmonary atresia with intact ventricular septum. Am J Roentgenol Radium Ther Nucl Med 1972;116:501.
6. Essed CE, Klein HW, Krediet P, Vorst EJ. Coronary and endocardial fibroelastosis of the ventricles in the hypoplastic left and right heart syndromes. Virchows Arch A Pathol Anat Histol 1975;368:87.

F

1. Fedderly RT, Lloyd TR, Mendelsohn AM, Beekman RH. Determinants of successful balloon valvotomy in infants with critical pulmonary stenosis or membranous pulmonary atresia with intact ventricular septum. J Am Coll Cardiol 1995;25:460.
2. Fenton KN, Pigula FA, Gandhi SK, Russo L, Duncan KF. Interim mortality in pulmonary atresia with intact ventricular septum. Ann Thorac Surg 2004;78:1994-8.
3. Freed MD, Heymann MA, Lewis AB, Roehl SL, Kensey RC. Prostaglandin E1 infants with ductus arteriosus-dependent congenital heart disease. Circulation 1981;64:899.
4. Freedom RM, Dische MR, Rowe RD. The tricuspid valve in pulmonary atresia and intact ventricular septum. Arch Pathol Lab Med 1978;102:28.
5. Freedom RM, Harrington DP. Contributions of intramyocardial sinusoids in pulmonary atresia and intact ventricular septum to a right-sided circular shunt. Br Heart J 1974;36:1061.
6. Freedom RM, Keith JD. Pulmonary atresia with normal aortic root. In Keith JD, Rowe RD, Vlad P, eds. Heart disease in infancy and childhood. 3rd Ed. New York: Macmillan, 1978, p. 506.
7. Freedom RM, White RI Jr, Ho CS, Gingell RL, Hawker RE, Rowe RD. Evaluation of patients with pulmonary atresia and intact ventricular septum by double catheter technique. Pediatr Cardiol 1974; 33:892.
8. Freedom RM, Wilson G, Trusler GA, Williams WG, Rowe RD. Pulmonary atresia and intact ventricular septum. Scand J Thorac Cardiovasc Surg 1983;17:1.
9. Freeman JE, DeLeon SY, Lai S, Fisher EA, Ow EP, Pifarre R. Right ventricle-to-aorta conduit in pulmonary atresia with intact ventricular septum and coronary sinusoids. Ann Thorac Surg 1993;56:1393.
10. Fyfe DA, Edwards WD, Driscoll DJ. Myocardial ischemia in patients with pulmonary atresia and intact ventricular septum. J Am Coll Cardiol 1986;8:402.

G

1. Gamboa R, Gersony WM, Nadas AS. The electrocardiogram in tricuspid atresia and pulmonary atresia with intact ventricular septum. Circulation 1966;34:24.
2. Gentles TL, Colan SD, Giglia TM, Mandell VS, Mayer JE, Sanders SP. Right ventricular decompression and left ventricular function in pulmonary atresia with intact ventricular septum: the influence of less extensive coronary anomalies. Circulation 1993; 88:II183.
3. Gentles TL, Keane JF, Jonas RA, Marx GE, Mayer JE Jr. Surgical alternatives to the Fontan procedure incorporating a hypoplastic right ventricle. Circulation 1994;90:II1.
4. Gersony WM, Bernhard WF, Nadas AS, Gross RE. Diagnosis and surgical treatment of infants with critical pulmonary outflow obstruction. Circulation 1967;35:765.
5. Gibbs JL, Blackburn ME, Uzun O, Dickinson DF, Parsons JM, Chatrath RR. Laser valvotomy with balloon valvoplasty for pulmonary atresia with intact ventricular septum: five years' experience. Heart 1997;77:225.
6. Giglia TM, Mandell VS, Connor AR, Mayer JE Jr, Lock JE. Diagnosis and management of right ventricle-dependent coronary circulation in pulmonary atresia with intact ventricular septum. Circulation 1992;86:1516.
7. Gittenberger-de Groot AC, Sauer U, Bindl L, Babic R, Essed CE, Buhlmeyer K. Competition of coronary arteries and ventriculo-coronary arterial communications in pulmonary atresia with intact ventricular septum. Int J Cardiol 1988;18:243.
8. Gootman NL, Scarpelli EM, Rudolph AM. Metabolic acidosis in children with severe cyanotic congenital heart disease. Pediatrics 1963;31:251.
9. Graham TP Jr, Bender HW, Atwood GF, Page DL, Sell CG. Increase in right ventricular volume following valvulotomy for pulmonary atresia or stenosis with intact ventricular septum. Circulation 1974;50:II69.
10. Grant RT. An unusual anomaly of the coronary vessels in the malformed heart of a child. Heart 1926;13:273.
11. Greenwold WE. A clinico-pathologic study of congenital tricuspid atresia and of pulmonary stenosis or pulmonary atresia with intact ventricular septum (thesis). University of Minnesota, November 1955.
12. Greenwold WE, DuShane JW, Burchell HB, Bruwer A, Edwards JE. Congenital pulmonary atresia with intact ventricular septum: two anatomic types (abstract). Circulation 1956;14:945.
13. Guleserian KJ, Armsby LB, Thiagarajan RR, del Nido PJ, Mayer JE Jr. Natural history of pulmonary atresia with intact ventricular septum and right-ventricle-dependent coronary circulation managed by the single-ventricle approach. Ann Thorac Surg 2006;81: 2250-8.

H

1. Hanley FL, Sade RM, Blackstone EH, Kirklin JW, Freedom RM, Nanda NC. Outcomes in neonatal pulmonary atresia with intact ventricular septum. A multiinstitutional study. J Thorac Cardiovasc Surg 1993;105:406.
2. Hanseus K, Bjorkhem G, Lundstrom NR, Laurin S. Cross-sectional echocardiographic measurements of right ventricular size and growth in patients with pulmonary atresia and intact ventricular septum. Pediatr Cardiol 1991;12:135.
3. Hausdorf G, Gravinghoff L, Keck EW. Effects of persisting myocardial sinusoids on left ventricular performance in pulmonary atresia with intact ventricular septum. Eur Heart J 1987;8:291.
4. Heymann MA, Rudolph AM. Ductus arteriosus dilatation by prostaglandin E_1 in infants with pulmonary atresia. Pediatrics 1977; 59:325.
5. Hirata Y, Chen JM, Quaegebeur JM, Hellenbrand WE, Mosca RS. Pulmonary atresia with intact ventricular septum: limitations of catheter-based intervention. Ann Thorac Surg 2007;84:574-80.
6. Huang SC, Ishino K, Kasahara S, Yoshizumi K, Kotani Y, Sano S. The potential of disproportionate growth of tricuspid valve after decompression of the right ventricle in patients with pulmonary atresia and intact ventricular septa. J Thorac Cardiovasc Surg 2009;138:1160-6.
7. Humpl T, Soderberg B, McCrindle BW, Nykanen DG, Freedom RM, Williams WG, et al. Percutaneous balloon valvotomy in pulmonary atresia with intact ventricular septum: impact on patient care. Circulation 2003;108:826-32.
8. Hwang MS, Taylor GP, Freedom RM. Decreased left ventricular coronary artery density in pulmonary atresia and intact ventricular septum. Cardiology 2008;109:10-4.

J

1. Jahangiri M, Zurakowski D, Bichell D, Mayer JE, del Nido PJ, Jonas RA. Improved results with selective management in pulmonary atresia with intact ventricular septum. J Thorac Cardiovasc Surg 1999;118:1046.
2. Jimenez MQ, Sarachaga IH, Granados FM, Martul EV, Fanjul IT, Dieguez CG, et al. Atresia pulmonar con tabique interventricular integro. Arch Inst Cardiol Mex 1976;46:182.

K

1. Kauffman SL, Anderson DH. Persistent venous valves, maldevelopment of the right heart, and coronary artery–ventricular communications. Am Heart J 1963;66:664.
2. Kreutzer C, Mayorquim RC, Kreutzer GO, Conejeros W, Roman MI, Vazquez H, et al. Experience with one and a half ventricle repair. J Thorac Cardiovasc Surg 1999;117:662.
3. Kutsche LM, Van Mierop LH. Pulmonary atresia with and without ventricular septal defect: a different etiology and pathogenesis for the atresia in the 2 types? Am J Cardiol 1983;51;932.

L

1. Laks H, Gates RN, Grant PW, Drant S, Allada V, Harake B. Aortic to right ventricular shunt for pulmonary atresia and intact ventricular septum. Ann Thorac Surg 1995;59:342.
2. Lauer RM, Fink HP, Petry EL, Dunn MI, Diehl AM. Angiographic demonstration of intramyocardial sinusoids in pulmonary-valve atresia with intact ventricular septum and hypoplastic right ventricle. N Engl J Med 1964;271:68.

3. Lewis AB, Wells W, Lindesmith GG. Evaluation and surgical treatment of pulmonary atresia and intact ventricular septum in infancy. Circulation 1983;67:1318.
4. Lightfoot NE, Coles JG, Dasmahapatra HK, Williams WG, Chin K, Trusler GA, et al. Analysis of survival in patients with pulmonary atresia and intact ventricular septum treated surgically. Int J Cardiol 1989;24:159.
5. Luckstead EF, Mattioli L, Crosby IK, Reed WA, Diehl AM. Two-stage palliative surgical approach for pulmonary atresia with intact ventricular septum (Type I). Am J Cardiol 1972;29:490.

M

1. Maeno YV, Boutin C, Hornberger LK, McCrindle BW, Cavalle-Garrido T, Gladman G, et al. Prenatal diagnosis of right ventricular outflow tract obstruction with intact ventricular septum, and detection of ventriculocoronary connections. Heart 1999;81: 661.
2. Mair DD, Julsrud PR, Puga FJ, Danielson GK. The Fontan procedure for pulmonary atresia with intact ventricular septum: operative and late results. J Am Coll Cardiol 1997;29:1359.
3. Mangiardi JL, Sullivan JJ, Bifulco E, Lukash L. Congenital tricuspid stenosis with pulmonary atresia. Am J Cardiol 1963;11:726.
4. Mansfield PB, Hall DG, Rittenhouse EA, Sauvage LR, Herndon PS, Stamm SJ. Surgical treatment of pulmonary atresia with right ventricular hypoplasia and intact septum. Mod Prob Pediatr 1983; 22:167.
5. Marino B, Franceschini E, Ballerini L, Marcelletti C, Thiene G. Anatomical-echocardiographic correlations in pulmonary atresia with intact ventricular septum. Use of subcostal cross-sectional views. Int J Cardiol 1986;11:103.
6. McArthur JD, Munsi SC, Sukumar IP, Cherian G. Pulmonary valve atresia with intact ventricular septum. Circulation 1971;44: 740.
7. McLean KM, Pearl JM. Pulmonary atresia with intact ventricular septum: initial management. Ann Thorac Surg 2006;82: 2214-20.
8. Miller GA, Restifo M, Shinebourne EA, Paneth M, Joseph MC, Lennox SC, et al. Pulmonary atresia with intact ventricular septum and critical pulmonary stenosis presenting in first month of life. Br Heart J 1973;35:9.
9. Mishima A, Asano M, Sasaki S, Yamamoto S, Saito T, Ukai T, et al. Long-term outcome for right heart function after biventricular repair of pulmonary atresia and intact ventricular septum. Jpn J Thorac Cardiovasc Surg 2000;48:145-52.
10. Mitchell SC, Korones SB, Berendes HW. Congenital heart disease in 56,109 births. Circulation 1971;43:323.
11. Miyaji K, Murakami A, Takasaki T, Ohara K, Takamoto S, Yoshimura H. Does a bidirectional Glenn shunt improve the oxygenation of right ventricle-dependent coronary circulation in pulmonary atresia with intact ventricular septum? J Thorac Cardiovasc Surg 2005;130:1050-3.
12. Miyaji K, Shimada M, Sekiguchi A, Ishizawa A, Isoda T, Tsunemoto M. Pulmonary atresia with intact ventricular septum: long-term results of "one and a half ventricular repair." Ann Thorac Surg 1995;60:1762.
13. Moller JH, Girod D, Amplatz K, Varco RL. Pulmonary valvotomy in pulmonary atresia with hypoplastic right ventricle. Surgery 1970; 68:630.
14. Moulton AL, Bowman FO Jr, Edie RN, Hayes CJ, Ellis K, Gersony WM. Pulmonary atresia with intact ventricular septum. Sixteen-year experience. J Thorac Cardiovasc Surg 1979;78:527.
15. Muster AJ, Zales VR, Ilbawi MN, Backer CL, Duffy CE, Mavroudis C. Biventricular repair of hypoplastic right ventricle assisted by pulsatile bidirectional cavopulmonary anastomosis. J Thorac Cardiovasc Surg 1993;105:112.

N

1. Najm HK, Williams WG, Coles JG, Rebeyka IM, Freedom RM. Pulmonary atresia with intact ventricular septum: results of the Fontan procedure. Ann Thorac Surg 1997;63:669.
2. Neutze JM, Starling MB, Elliott RB, Barratt-Boyes BG. Palliation of cyanotic congenital heart disease in infancy with E-type prostaglandins. Circulation 1977;55:238.
3. Newfeld EA, Cole RB, Paul MH. Ebstein's malformation of the tricuspid valve in the neonate. Functional or anatomic pulmonary outflow tract obstruction. Am J Cardiol 1967;19:727.
4. Numata S, Uemura H, Yagihara T, Kagisaki K, Takahashi M, Ohuchi H. Long-term functional results of the one and one half ventricular repair for the spectrum of patients with pulmonary atresia/stenosis with intact ventricular septum. Eur J Cardiothorac Surg 2003;24:516-20.

O

1. Odim J, Laks H, Plunkett MD, Tung TC. Successful management of patients with pulmonary atresia with intact ventricular septum using a three tier grading system for right ventricular hypoplasia. Ann Thorac Surg 2006;81:678-84.
2. Olley PM, Coceani F, Bodach E. E-type prostaglandins. A new emergency therapy for certain cyanotic congenital heart malformations. Circulation 1976;53:728.
3. Oosthoek PW, Moorman AF, Sauer U, Gittenberger-de Groot AC. Capillary distribution in the ventricles of hearts with pulmonary atresia and intact ventricular septum. Circulation 1995;91:1790.
4. Ovaert C, Qureshi SA, Rosenthal E, Baker EJ, Tynan M. Growth of the right ventricle after successful transcatheter pulmonary valvotomy in neonates and infants with pulmonary atresia and intact ventricular septum. J Thorac Cardiovasc Surg 1998;115:1055.

P

1. Parsons JM, Rees MR, Gibbs JL. Percutaneous laser valvotomy with balloon dilatation of the pulmonary valve as primary treatment for pulmonary atresia. Br Heart J 1991;66:36.
2. Patel RG, Freedom RM, Moes CA, Bloom KR, Olley PM, Williams WG, et al. Right ventricular volume determinations in 18 patients with pulmonary atresia and intact ventricular septum. Analysis of factors influencing right ventricular growth. Circulation 1980; 61:428.
3. Paul MH, Lev M. Tricuspid stenosis with pulmonary atresia. Circulation 1960;22:198.
4. Peacock TB. Malformation of the heart: atresia of the orifice of the pulmonary artery. Trans Pathol Soc Lond 1869;20:61.
5. Perloff JK. Pulmonary atresia with intact ventricular septum. In Perloff JK, ed. The clinical recognition of congenital heart disease. Philadelphia: WB Saunders, 1978, p. 604.
6. Powell AJ, Mayer JE, Lang P, Lock JE. Outcome in infants with pulmonary atresia, intact ventricular septum, and right ventricle-dependent coronary circulation. Am J Cardiol 2000;86:1272.

R

1. Reddy VM, McElhinney DB, Brook MM, Silverman NH, Stanger P, Hanley FL. Repair of congenital tricuspid valve abnormalities with artificial chordae tendineae. Ann Thorac Surg 1998;66:172.
2. Redington AN, Penny D, Rigby ML, Hayes A. Antegrade diastolic pulmonary arterial flow as a marker of right ventricular restriction after complete repair of pulmonary atresia with intact septum and critical pulmonary valvar stenosis. Cardiol Young 1992;2:382-6.
3. Robicsek F, Bostoen H, Sanger PW. Atresia of the pulmonary valve with normal pulmonary artery and intact ventricular septum in a 21-year-old woman. Angiology 1966;17:896.
4. Rosenthal E, Qureshi SA, Kakadekar AP, Anjos R, Baker EJ, Tynan M. Technique of percutaneous laser-assisted valve dilatation for valvar atresia in congenital heart disease. Br Heart J 1993;69: 556.
5. Rudolph AM, Heymann MA, Fishman N, Lakier JB. Formalin infiltration of the ductus arteriosus. A method for palliation of infants with selected congenital cardiac lesions. N Engl J Med 1975;292:1263.
6. Rychik J, Levy H, Gaynor JW, DeCampli WM, Spray TL. Outcome after operations for pulmonary atresia with intact ventricular septum. J Thorac Cardiovasc Surg 1998;116:924.

S

1. Salvin JW, McElhinney DB, Colan SD, Gauvreau K, del Nido PJ, Jenkins KJ, et al. Fetal tricuspid valve size and growth as predictors of outcome in pulmonary atresia with intact ventricular septum. Pediatrics 2006;118:e415-20.
2. Sanders SP, Parness IA, Colan SD. Recognition of abnormal connections of coronary arteries with the use of Doppler color flow mapping. J Am Coll Cardiol 1989;13:922.

3. Sanghavi DM, Flanagan M, Powell AJ, Curran T, Picard S, Rhodes J. Determinants of exercise function following univentricular versus biventricular repair for pulmonary atresia/intact ventricular septum. Am J Cardiol 2006;97:1638-43.
4. Satou GM, Perry SB, Gauvreau K, Geva T. Echocardiographic predictors of coronary artery pathology in pulmonary atresia with intact ventricular septum. Am J Cardiol 2000;85:1319.
5. Schrire V, Sutin GJ, Barnard CN. Organic and functional pulmonary atresia with intact ventricular septum. Am J Cardiol 1961;8:100.
6. Scognamiglio R, Daliento L, Razzolini R, Boffa GM, Pellegrino PA, Chioin R, et al. Pulmonary atresia with intact ventricular septum: a quantitative cineventriculographic study of the right and left ventricular function. Pediatr Cardiol 1986;7:183.
7. Shams A, Fowler RS, Trusler GA, Keith JD, Mustard WT. Pulmonary atresia with intact ventricular septum. Report of 50 cases. Pediatrics 1971;47:370.
8. Shinebourne EA, Rigby ML, Carvalho JS. Pulmonary atresia with intact ventricular septum: from fetus to adult: congenital heart disease. Heart 2008;94:1350-7.
9. Sideris EB, Olley PM, Spooner E, Farina M, Foster E, Trusler G, et al. Left ventricular function and compliance in pulmonary atresia with intact ventricular septum. J Thorac Cardiovasc Surg 1982; 84:192.
10. Sissman NJ, Abrams HL. Bidirectional shunting in a coronary artery-right ventricular fistula associated with pulmonary atresia and an intact ventricular septum. Circulation 1965;32:582.
11. Subramanian S. Surgical treatment of complex cyanotic anomalies in infants: pulmonary atresia with intact ventricular septum. In Davila JC, ed. Second Henry Ford Hospital International Symposium on Cardiac Surgery. E. Norwalk, Conn.: Appleton & Lange, 1977, p. 316.

T

1. Todros T, Presbitero P, Gaglioti P, Demarie D. Pulmonary stenosis with intact ventricular septum: documentation of development of the lesion echocardiographically during fetal life. Int J Cardiol 1988;19:355.
2. Trusler GA, Yamamoto N, Williams WG, Izukawa T, Rowe RD, Mustard WT. Surgical treatment of pulmonary atresia with intact ventricular septum. Br Heart J 1976;38:957.

V

1. Van Praagh R, Ando M, Van Praagh S, Senno A, Hougen TJ, Novak G, et al. Pulmonary atresia: anatomic considerations. In Kidd BS, Rowe RD, eds. The child with congenital heart disease after surgery. Mount Kisco, N.Y.: Futura, 1976, p. 103.
2. Velvis H, Schmidt KG, Silverman NH, Turley K. Diagnosis of coronary artery fistula by two-dimensional echocardiography, pulsed Doppler ultrasound and color flow imaging. J Am Coll Cardiol 1989;14:968.
3. Vlad P. Pulmonary atresia with intact ventricular septum. In Barratt-Boyes BG, Neutze JM, Harris EA, eds. Heart disease in infancy. Baltimore: Williams & Wilkins, 1973, p. 245.

W

1. Waldman JD, Karp RB, Lamberti JJ, Sand ME, Ruschhaupt DG, Agarwala B. Tricuspid valve closure in pulmonary atresia and important RV-to-coronary artery connections. Ann Thorac Surg 1995; 59:933.
2. Wang JK, Wu MH, Chang CI, Chen YS, Lue HC. Outcomes of transcatheter valvotomy in patients with pulmonary atresia and intact ventricular septum. Am J Cardiol 1999;84:1055.
3. Weisz D, Gootman N, Silbert D, Voleti C, Wisoff BG. Pulmonary atresia with intact ventricular septum. N Y State J Med 1977;77: 2068.
4. Williams RR, Kent GB Jr, Edwards JE. Anomalous cardiac blood vessel communicating with the right ventricle. Arch Pathol 1951; 52:480.
5. Williams WG, Burrows P, Freedom RM, Trusler GA, Coles JG, Moes CA, et al. Thromboexclusion of the right ventricle in children with pulmonary atresia and intact ventricular septum. J Thorac Cardiovasc Surg 1991;101:222.

Y

1. Yoshimura N, Yamaguchi M, Ohashi H, Oshima Y, Oka S, Yoshida M, et al. Pulmonary atresia with intact ventricular septum: strategy based on right ventricular morphology. J Thorac Cardiovasc Surg 2003;126:1417-26.

Z

1. Ziegler RF, Taber RE. Diagnostic criteria and successful surgery in an operable form of complete pulmonary valve atresia. Circulation 1962;26:807.
2. Zuberbuhler JR, Anderson RH. Morphological variations in pulmonary atresia with intact ventricular septum. Br Heart J 1979; 41:281.

41 Tricuspid Atresia and Single-Ventricle Physiology

Section I Tricuspid Atresia and Single-Ventricle Physiology

DEFINITION

Tricuspid Atresia

Tricuspid atresia is a congenital cardiac malformation in which the right atrium, in the setting of ventricular D-loop, fails to open into a ventricle through an atrioventricular (AV) valve. Thus, there is univentricular AV connection consisting of a left-sided mitral valve between morphologically left atrium and left ventricle (LV). Atrial situs is almost invariably solitus (normal) in association with ventricular D-loop, and the right ventricle (RV) is hypoplastic. A ventricular septal defect (VSD) usually is present. Ventriculoarterial connection may be concordant or discordant (transposed great arteries). Rarely, tricuspid atresia occurs in situs inversus with ventricular L-loop (mirror-image pattern).

Patients with atrial situs solitus and ventricular L-loop in which the left-sided left atrium is separated from a left-sided hypoplastic morphologically RV by an atretic left-sided (tricuspid) AV valve are excluded from this discussion; they are considered in Chapter 56.

Single-Ventricle Physiology

Single-ventricle physiology is present when there is impossibility or inadvisability of surgically reconstructing a functional two-ventricle heart with separated in-series pulmonary and systemic circulations. The spectrum of surgical management of single-ventricle physiology is generally similar for tricuspid atresia, other types of univentricular AV connection (see Chapter 56), and other anomalies without two adequate ventricles (see "Fontan versus Intracardiac Repair for Complex Morphology" later in this section) and is based on the Fontan operation. All such anomalies have in common the limitation of single-ventricle physiology, regardless of their specific morphology. Therefore, the Fontan operation and all its modifications and applications, as well as the spectrum of pre-Fontan palliative operations, are discussed fully in this chapter.

HISTORICAL NOTE

In 1906, Kuhne apparently recognized the entity of congenital tricuspid atresia and described its two basic morphologic subsets: hearts with concordant ventriculoarterial connection and hearts with discordant connection.[K31] In 1949, Edwards and Burchell further emphasized these two subsets and added presence or absence of pulmonary stenosis as another categorizing feature.[E1] Tandon and Edwards added further descriptive features in 1974.[T2] The clinical features of tricuspid atresia were described by Bellet and colleagues in 1933 and by Taussig and by Brown in 1936.[B9,B31,T6] Controversy arose early and continues as to whether tricuspid atresia should be considered a subset of single ventricle (see Historical Note in Chapter 56).[R3] From a surgical point of view, it is best considered as such, but tradition and its prevalence support presenting it as a separate entity.

Systemic–pulmonary arterial shunts developed in 1945 by Blalock and Taussig and later by Potts and by Waterston (see Historical Note in Section I of Chapter 38) were soon applied to cyanotic patients with tricuspid atresia. In 1958, Glenn specifically applied the superior vena cava–to–right pulmonary artery anastomosis to patients with tricuspid atresia.[G20] The basis for the classic Glenn shunt was experimental studies reported by Carlon and colleagues in 1951, by Glenn and colleagues, and by Robicsek and colleagues, showing that systemic venous pressure was adequate to drive pulmonary blood flow.[C6,G21,N9,P4,R15] In Moscow, Bakuljev and Kolesnikov independently developed these same concepts.[B1] In 1966, Haller and colleagues demonstrated experimentally the possibility of performing a bidirectional superior cavopulmonary anastomosis.[H4] This was applied clinically by Azzolina and colleagues in 1974, and in 1985, Hopkins and colleagues further refined the procedure with an end-to-side anastomosis of superior vena cava (SVC) to undivided right pulmonary artery (RPA).[A23,H14] Abrams and colleagues applied this idea in the form of a side-to-side anastomosis of SVC to undivided RPA.[A1,S1] In 1984, Kawashima and colleagues added a further improvisation in patients with either one or two SVCs, and azygos or hemiazygos continuation of the inferior vena cava (IVC) into an SVC, with only splanchnic and coronary venous blood draining into the right atrium.[K10] They divided the SVC (both, if there were two), closed its cardiac end, and anastomosed the SVC end to side to the pulmonary artery after closing the pulmonary trunk. This *total cavopulmonary shunt* was an incompleted Fontan operation in which only splanchnic and coronary venous blood drained directly to the systemic arterial circulation.[D11,J10,J11,P19]

Successful repair of tricuspid atresia with separation of right and left circulations was accomplished in 1968 by Fontan and colleagues and was reported in 1971.[F11,F16] This was preceded by experimental studies in 1943 by Starr and colleagues, demonstrating that destroying a dog's RV did not result in systemic venous hypertension[S34]; in 1949 by Rodbard and Wagner, demonstrating that the RV could be bypassed[R16]; and in 1954 by Warden, DeWall, and Varco, demonstrating the feasibility of bypassing the RV with a right atrial–pulmonary artery anastomosis.[W3] Based on these experiments, Hurwitt and colleagues reported an unsuccessful attempt to correct tricuspid atresia by a right atrial–to–pulmonary artery anastomosis in 1955.[H21] Fontan's procedure involved constructing a cavopulmonary (Glenn) anastomosis with, in the first patient, a direct anastomosis between right atrial appendage and proximal end of the divided RPA. In the subsequent two patients, one of whom had discordant ventriculoarterial connection, an aortic allograft valved conduit was placed between right atrium and RPA. In all three patients, an allograft valve was inserted into the IVC ostium, foramen ovale closed, and pulmonary trunk ligated or divided. In 1973, Kreutzer and colleagues reported a modification of Fontan's operation in which the patient's pulmonary trunk with its intact pulmonary valve was excised from the RV and anastomosed to the right atrial appendage after closing the VSD and atrial septal defect (ASD). A Glenn procedure was not performed, and no IVC valve was used.[K28]

Other early reports of successful repairs were those of Ross and Somerville and of Stanford and colleagues.[R22,S32] Fontan subsequently modified the operation that he and Baudet had originally performed[F12,F13]; many others have as well.[B18,B21,D22,H9,N4] Bjork described direct anastomosis between right atrial appendage and RV outflow tract in patients with a normal pulmonary valve, using a roof of pericardium to avoid a synthetic tube graft.[B18] Direct right atrial–pulmonary artery connection, used by Fontan in his first case, has been modified and widely used.[D22,G2,G3,K29]

The extracardiac conduit Fontan modification, in which the IVC is disconnected from the right atrium and connected by a prosthetic tube to the RPA outside the heart, has become popular. A bidirectional superior cavopulmonary connection completes the procedure. This was first described by Humes for use only in special cases of complex venous anatomy.[H20] It was subsequently modified for use as the procedure of choice for all Fontan candidates by Marcelletti and colleagues and further modified as a closed heart, partial bypass, or off-bypass procedure by Petrossian and colleagues.[M9,P13]

Choussat and Fontan and colleagues formalized a set of risk factors ("ten commandments") for the Fontan operation in 1979.[C21] In 1988, Laks and colleagues introduced the concept of deliberately making the separation between caval and pulmonary venous pathways incomplete, and then adjusting or closing the communication early postoperatively by percutaneous manipulation of a snare.[B16,L3,L6] Bridges and colleagues modified this approach by closing the residual aperture using catheter techniques late postoperatively.[B29]

Although the Fontan operation was introduced as a treatment for tricuspid atresia, it was soon realized that it was applicable to many other forms of univentricular AV connection. In 1976, Yacoub reported its use for single ventricle,[Y1] and by 1980, for many other anomalies with one severely hypoplastic ventricle.[M10] The Fontan operation has subsequently been used to treat a group of patients who have two adequate ventricles and AV valves but who are judged by some surgeons to have intracardiac morphology too complex for biventricular repair.[R24]

MORPHOLOGY AND MORPHOGENESIS

In tricuspid atresia, there is no direct connection between right atrium and RV, but the left atrium connects through the mitral valve to the LV. Atresia is usually muscular (75% of cases), meaning the AV connection is absent; it may be membranous with an imperforate AV connection.[A17,S4] In the *muscular type*, presence of a tiny dimple in the right atrial floor may or may not represent the atretic valve. The dimple has been said to lie above the LV or ventricular septum in most cases and may then transilluminate from the LV.[A17,B15,R11,R20,W6] In such instances, it may represent a remnant of membranous AV septum.[A18]

The *membranous type* has three variants. In one, a fibrous diaphragm blocks the AV orifice, and remnants of the valvar apparatus are occasionally found beneath the membrane in the RV. This has been called *tricuspid atresia with imperforate valve membrane*.[A16,S4] It is often associated with left-sided juxtaposition of atrial appendages and discordant ventriculoarterial connection.[D17] Overall, juxtaposed atrial appendages are found in 11% of patients with tricuspid atresia.[T7] In a second, there is classic Ebstein anomaly (see Chapter 42) that is imperforate because of completely fused leaflets that are also fused to the wall of a small RV[A17,R4,W6] (Fig. 41-1). In a third and rarer variant, there is an AV septal defect in which the right-sided valve is imperforate and blocks the opening between right atrium and RV (Fig. 41-2). An autopsy series, focused on left-sided structures in tricuspid atresia, identified a high prevalence of mitral valve and LV abnormalities, including cleft mitral valve, muscularized subvalvar apparatus, and abnormal muscle bundles.[O13]

There are two major morphologic subsets of tricuspid atresia:

- Origins of great arteries are normal (concordant ventriculoarterial connection; 60% to 70% of cases).
- Origins of great arteries are transposed (discordant ventriculoarterial connection; about 30% to 40% of cases).[A20,E1,S25]

Rarely, the ventriculoarterial connection is double outlet right ventricle (DORV) or double outlet left ventricle (DOLV) or single outlet with truncus arteriosus.[A17] Other rare variants exist, and it has been estimated that only about 80% of patients diagnosed as having tricuspid atresia actually have the typical two morphologies.[A16,F17]

Tricuspid Atresia and Concordant Ventriculoarterial Connection (Normally Related Great Arteries)

This form of tricuspid atresia was referred to as *type 1* by Edwards and Burchell and by Vlad.[E1,V10] Atria are usually in situs solitus. The right atrium and its appendage are enlarged and thick walled, and an interatrial communication is present, usually through a fossa ovalis ASD (Fig. 41-3). The valve of the fossa ovalis may be redundant and bulge into the left atrium and contain multiple fenestrations. The ASD is generally large; by hemodynamic studies, Dick and colleagues found that only 4% of patients had a restrictive ASD.[D16] Uncommonly, the defect is an ostium primum ASD in association with a cleft left AV valve, and rarely there is a common atrium (see Morphology in Chapter 34).

The eustachian valve is often prominent, and in about 5% of cases it extends superiorly to form a veil or partition across the right atrium, so-called cor triatriatum dexter (see Morphology in Chapter 32).[B15,T13] At operation, this may be confusing to the unprepared surgeon.

The left atrium is morphologically normal but enlarged from obligatory shunting of systemic venous blood across the ASD. The mitral valve is usually larger than normal, as is the LV, because both systemic and pulmonary venous return pass through them. The LV is also hypertrophied and its

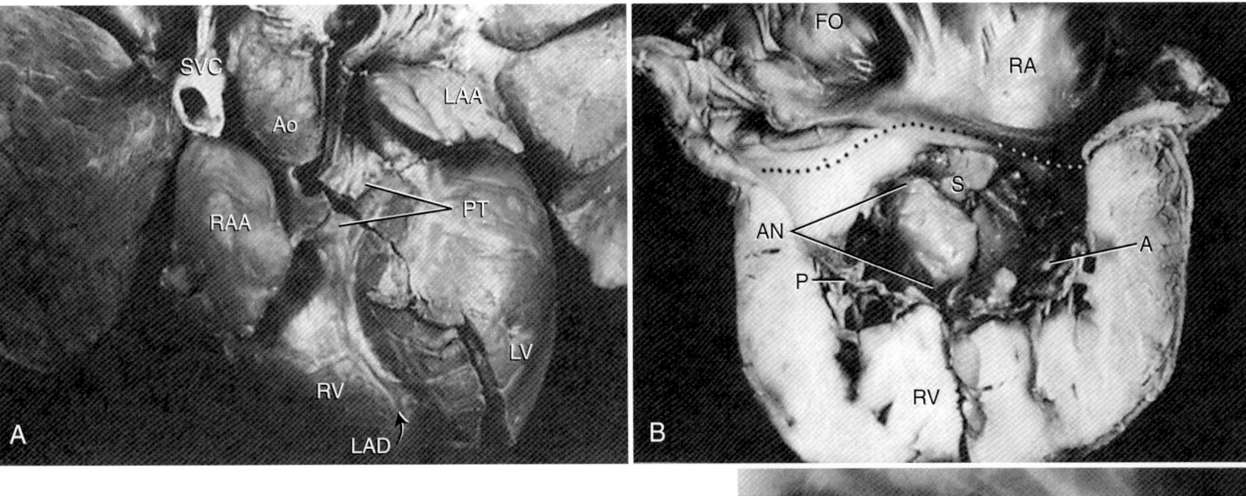

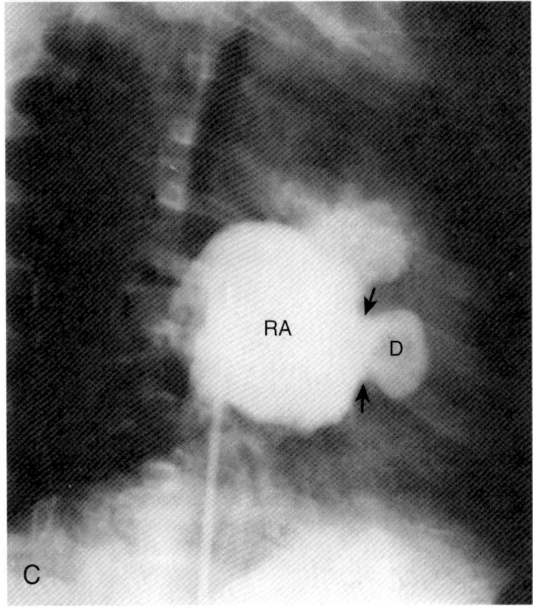

Figure 41-1 Specimen and cineangiogram of tricuspid atresia coexisting with Ebstein malformation. **A,** Exterior view of heart shows displaced left anterior descending coronary artery *(LAD)* and small right ventricle *(RV)* to its right. Cordlike pulmonary trunk remnant wraps around proximal aorta where it arises from left ventricle *(LV)*. **B,** Interior of RV and right atrium *(RA)*. Septal and posterior leaflets are downwardly displaced from tricuspid anulus *(dotted line)*. All three leaflets are loosely adherent to RV wall and join to form an imperforate membrane. Aneurysmal bulge of septal leaflet covers a potential ventricular septal defect. The blind RV is markedly hypertrophied. **C,** Cineangiogram frame from a similar patient in right anterior oblique projection shows site of tricuspid anulus *(arrow)* and blind diverticulum formed by fused leaflets. Key: *A,* Anterior leaflet; *AN,* aneurysm, septal leaflet; *Ao,* aorta; *D,* diverticulum; *FO,* fossa ovalis; *LAA,* left atrial appendage; *P,* posterior tricuspid leaflet; *PT,* pulmonary trunk; *RAA,* right atrial appendage; *S,* septal tricuspid leaflet; *SVC,* superior vena cava.

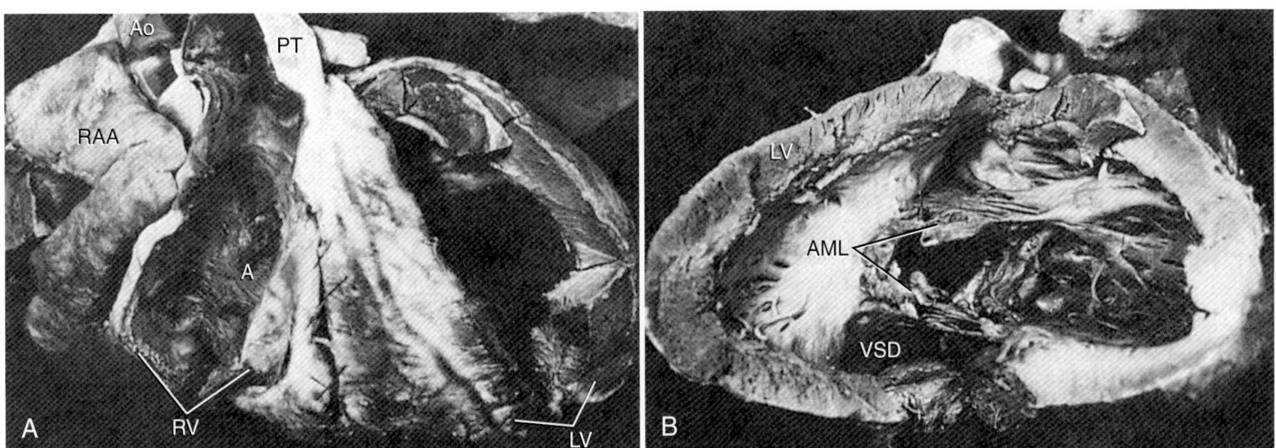

Figure 41-2 Specimen of tricuspid atresia with an atrioventicular (AV) septal defect. **A,** Frontal view with thin-walled, small right ventricle *(RV)* and pulmonary trunk *(PT)* open. Rightward portions of AV valve are fused to form an imperforate fibrous membrane. Note large, thick-walled left ventricle *(LV)*. Pulmonary valve is normal. Ventricular septal defect *(VSD)* is not visible in this view. **B,** View of opened LV to show typical scooped-out ventricular septal crest and superior and inferior leaflets of left side of AV valve. VSD is adjacent to inferior leaflet. Key: *A,* Imperforate membrane; *AML,* left AV valve leaflets; *Ao,* aorta; *RAA,* right atrial appendage.

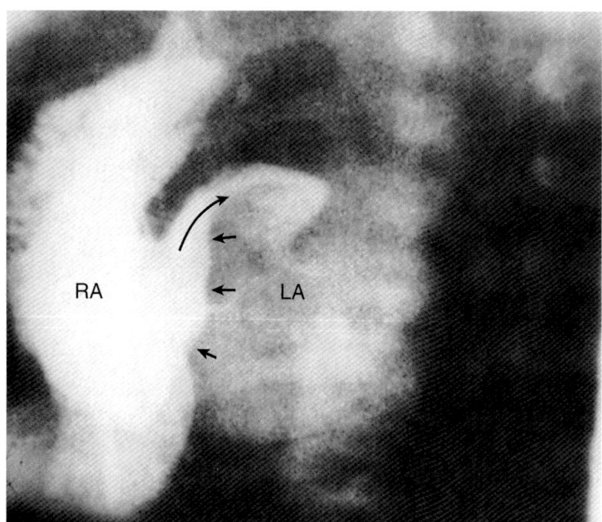

Figure 41-3 Cineangiogram frame in tilted left anterior oblique projection in tricuspid atresia that shows right-to-left atrial shunt through a stretched patent foramen ovale *(large arrow)*. Valve of fossa ovalis is outlined by small arrows. There is no right ventricular filling. Key: *LA,* Left atrium; *RA,* right atrium.

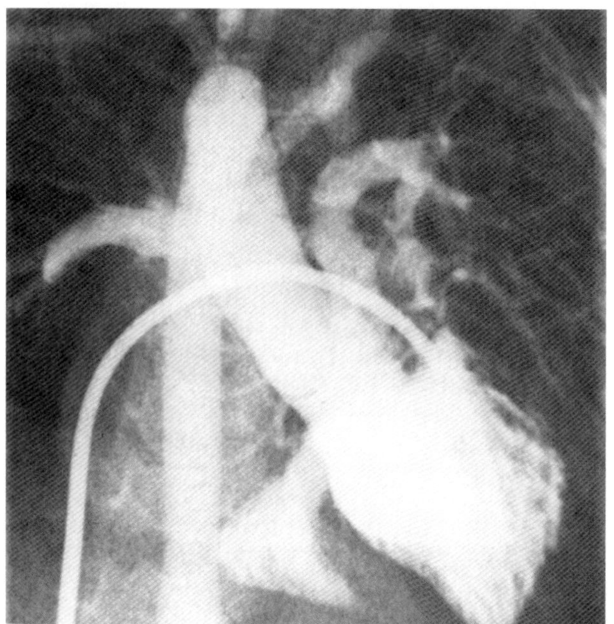

Figure 41-4 Cineangiogram of tricuspid atresia and concordant ventriculoarterial connection in four-chamber view. Injection is into left ventricle, which is mildly enlarged. Severely hypoplastic sinus portion of right ventricle is evident, as is the infundibular outlet portion. Pulmonary valve "anulus" and pulmonary arteries are slightly small but not restrictive. Bifurcation of pulmonary trunk is normal, as is usually the case.

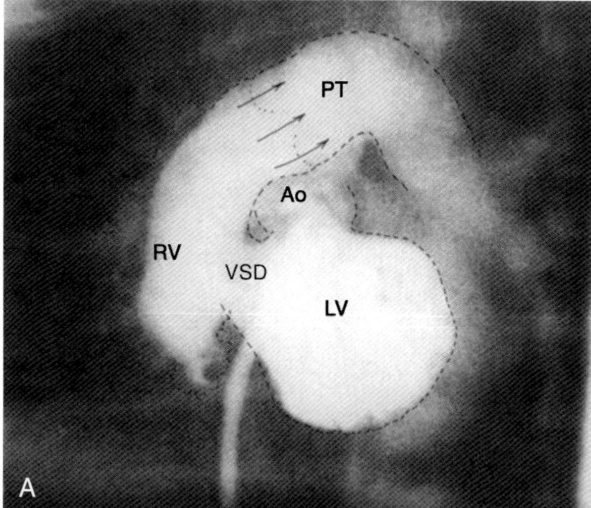

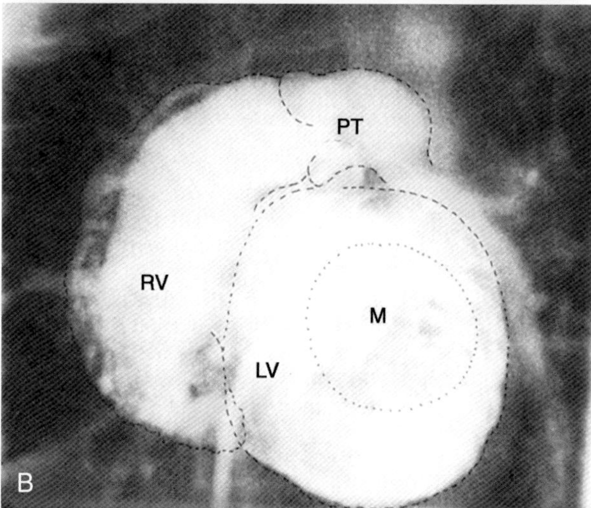

Figure 41-5 Cineangiogram in left anterior oblique projection of tricuspid atresia and a reasonably large right ventricle *(RV)*. **A,** Systolic frame shows a large ventricular septal defect *(VSD)* entering RV and a wide channel to pulmonary trunk *(PT)*. **B,** Enlargement of both right and left ventricles in diastole and large mitral valve orifice. Key: *Ao,* Aorta; *LV,* left ventricle; *M,* mitral orifice.

trabeculations typically fine, although anomalous muscle bands near the posterior papillary muscle are occasionally present.

The normally positioned RV is highly abnormal and typically similar to the small RV of double inlet left ventricle (DILV; see Morphology in Chapter 56).[D6] In most hearts it consists of a distal tubular smooth-walled portion with a thin free wall and a smaller proximal trabeculated portion into which a VSD usually opens (Fig. 41-4). The VSD varies in size and position and is sometimes multiple. In general, the larger the VSD, the larger the RV. The VSD usually lies below the infundibular (conal) septum, and from the LV side is separated from the noncoronary aortic cusp by infundibular muscle. When the VSD is large, it may extend inferiorly to the membranous septum, or it may be entirely muscular, lower in the septum, and sometimes slit-like. The VSD and trabeculated portion of the RV into which it opens are frequently separated from the smooth-walled distal portion by a narrow opening that looks like an os infundibulum (see "Infundibulum" under Morphology in Section I of Chapter 38). Like other VSDs, it frequently narrows spontaneously and is therefore often small and may close completely. In some hearts, the RV is large and has a true sinus portion (Fig. 41-5).

In 85% to 95% of patients, pulmonary blood flow is obstructed.[S25] Obstruction most commonly occurs at the os infundibulum, or it may occur at the VSD or throughout the entire infundibulum (Fig. 41-6). The pulmonary valve is bicuspid in about 20% of cases, but usually it and the "anulus,"

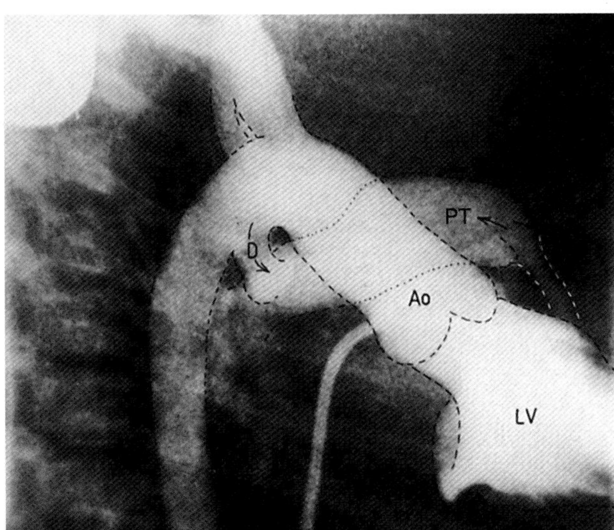

Figure 41-6 Cineangiogram in right anterior oblique projection in tricuspid atresia with severe infundibular pulmonary stenosis beneath a normal, although small, pulmonary valve. There is also a patent ductus arteriosus. Key: *Ao,* Aorta; *D,* patent ductus arteriosus; *LV,* left ventricle; *PT,* pulmonary trunk.

although a little smaller than normal, are not obstructive (diameter usually within 1 standard deviation of normal). The pulmonary trunk and branch pulmonary arteries are usually a little small, but only uncommonly (about 5% of patients) are they severely hypoplastic and restrictive to flow.[B15,C33]

In about 10% of cases in this subset, the pulmonary valve is atretic. Under these circumstances, trunk and branch pulmonary arteries are usually small, and pulmonary blood flow ($\dot{Q}p$) is via a patent ductus arteriosus or aortopulmonary collateral artery. The RV is usually extremely small, represented only by a minuscule endothelium-lined slit that is often inapparent on gross examination.[B15] The same is usually true when a VSD is absent. However, an RV chamber may be found in tricuspid atresia without a VSD.[F17,M12,M44]

Absent pulmonary valve is rarely described with type 1 tricuspid atresia. In a report documenting three newly described cases, it was noted that only 24 previous cases had been described.[L22] A number of associated lesions that are atypical for the more usual forms of tricuspid atresia are commonly found when there is absent pulmonary valve, including absence of a VSD, RV myocardial dysplasia, and abnormalities or even absence of the right coronary artery.

Some 5% to 15% of cases have no infundibular or pulmonary stenosis and normal or increased $\dot{Q}p$.[S25] The VSD is larger than usual. Coronary arteries are normally distributed, and the system is usually right dominant. The well-formed anterior descending coronary artery is displaced rightward by the large LV. The conduction system is basically normal but is affected by abnormalities present. Thus, the AV node is in its usual position in the AV septum between coronary sinus and dimple of atretic tricuspid valve.[B13,D18] It penetrates the abnormally formed central fibrous body to the left side of the ventricular septum and becomes the branching bundle in the lower confines of the pars membranacea.[B14,G26] Here it gives off most of the posterior radiation of the left bundle branch. Bifurcation of the bundle and formation of the right bundle branch occur at the posteroinferior angle of the VSD on the LV side. The right bundle branch proceeds here on the LV side and then intramyocardially along the inferior

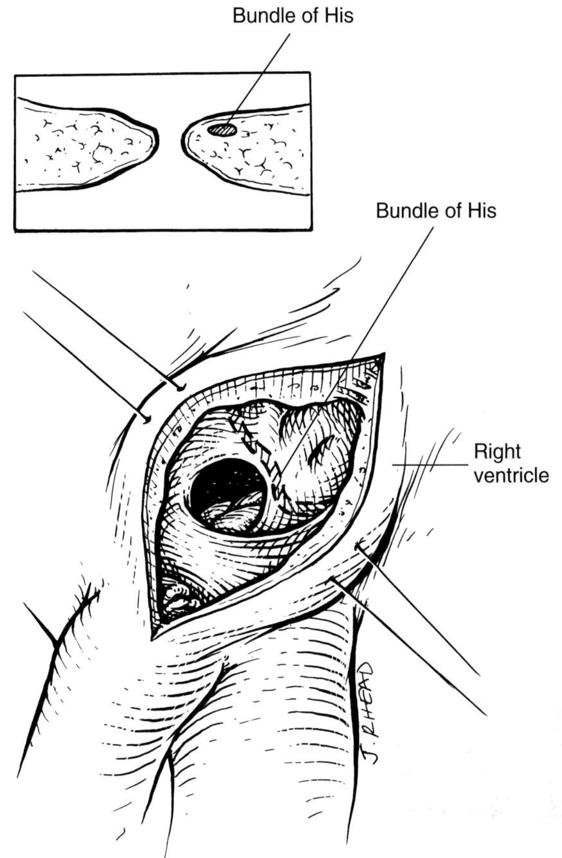

Figure 41-7 Conduction system in tricuspid atresia and concordant ventriculoarterial connection. Perspective is through a longitudinal incision in incomplete right ventricular chamber just below pulmonary valve. Ventricular septal defect is visible, with aortic valve also visible through it. Dashed line shows course of bundle of His, and inset shows protection of bundle from the surgeon by thickness of ventricular septum. (From Bharati and colleagues.[B14])

(caudal) border of the VSD. Then it emerges on the RV side and proceeds along the hypoplastic trabecula septomarginalis (septal band) (Fig. 41-7).

Major associated anomalies in this subset of tricuspid atresia are uncommon, but a persistent left SVC entering the coronary sinus occurs in about 15% of cases. Partially unroofed coronary sinus with coronary sinus–left atrial communication (see Morphology in Chapter 33) occurs in 1% to 5% of patients. This is important for the atriopulmonary type of Fontan repair, when high right atrial pressure will produce an important right-to-left shunt through it, even though a shunt was not apparent preoperatively.

Tricuspid Atresia and Discordant Ventriculoarterial Connection (Transposed Great Arteries)

In this tricuspid atresia subset (called *type 2* by Edwards and Burchell[E1]), the aorta arises from the RV, and the pulmonary trunk from the LV (Fig. 41-8). Generally, the aorta is anterior and to the right of the pulmonary trunk (D-malposition) in the position characteristic of transposition of the great arteries (see Morphology in Chapter 52), but uncommonly there is L-malposition.[T2,T3]

Atrial anatomy is generally similar to that described in the preceding text. However, left juxtaposition of the atrial

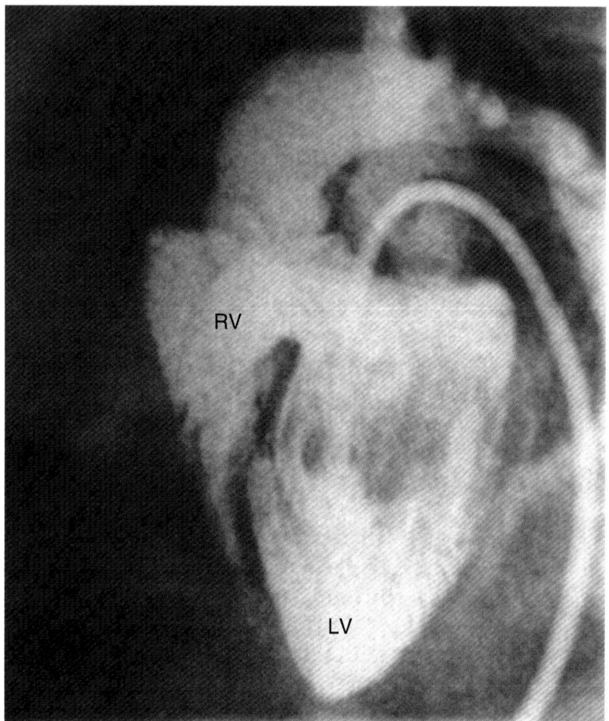

Figure 41-8 Tricuspid atresia and discordant ventriculoarterial connection. Injection is into left ventricle (LV) in this long axis view; aorta is seen to arise from right ventricle (RV), which is usually larger than when aorta arises from LV. Single ventricular septal defect is large and subaortic in position. There is moderate subpulmonary stenosis (poorly seen in this view) in LV outflow tract, and LV is typically larger than normal.

appendages occurs in about 10%, and in about half, the ASD is small.[B15,W6]

The RV is larger and thicker walled than usual. It tends to be a single smooth-walled cavity without a proximal trabeculated portion and is, in actuality, a subaortic outlet chamber. The VSD is usually subaortic in position. Commonly it is small, or becomes small, and then represents important subaortic stenosis. In one series, aortic or subaortic stenosis was present in 40%.[S25] The VSD, however, may be large and unobstructive.

The LV is normal although enlarged. Pulmonary valve and anulus are usually normal or as large as the pulmonary trunk. Thus, $\dot{Q}p$ is usually large. Subpulmonary stenosis in the LV occurs in about 20% to 30% of cases, and occasionally pulmonary atresia is present. These conditions result in low $\dot{Q}p$ and hypoxia.

Coronary arteries usually arise from the posterior aortic sinuses of Valsalva, those facing the pulmonary trunk, as in transposition of the great arteries (see "Coronary Arteries" under Morphology in Chapter 52). Associated cardiac anomalies usually involve the aortic arch. Obstruction coexists in about 25% to 35% of cases, with coarctation occurring more frequently than interrupted aortic arch.

Other Aspects of Single-Ventricle Physiology

Wolff-Parkinson-White syndrome is associated with tricuspid atresia.[H1] The morphology that results in single-ventricle physiology has other systemic effects. For example, levels of natriuretic peptides (both atrial natriuretic peptide and B-type natriuretic peptide) are abnormal; furthermore, they are distinctively abnormal compared with other forms of heart disease, including congenital defects with biventricular physiology.[S40]

CLINICAL FEATURES AND DIAGNOSTIC CRITERIA

Symptoms and Signs

Tricuspid Atresia and Concordant Ventriculoarterial Connection

Patients in this subset of tricuspid atresia are usually cyanotic from birth because of limited $\dot{Q}p$ from RV outflow obstruction. Dick and colleagues reported that in 50% of patients, congenital heart disease is recognized on the first day of life.[D16] Cyanosis is severe, progressive, and often accompanied by hypoxic spells characterized by increased cyanosis, dyspnea, and occasionally syncope. These spells may occur in the first 6 months and are a grave prognostic sign. In patients with increasing obstruction to pulmonary blood flow from progressive infundibular stenosis or VSD closure, cyanosis becomes rapidly more severe, and those who were previously acyanotic may become cyanotic in a matter of a few months. Clubbing of the fingers is common in children who survive beyond the first 2 years, but it may occasionally develop as early as 3 or 4 months. Squatting is uncommon, but dyspnea is often apparent with crying or feeding.

Most patients have loud, harsh, ejection systolic murmurs that are loudest over the lower left sternal border; these may be associated with an apical mid-diastolic rumble from large mitral valve flow. In cases of progressive obstruction to pulmonary flow, murmurs decrease or disappear. A continuous ductus arteriosus murmur may also be heard in patients with pulmonary atresia and occasionally in infants with pulmonary stenosis.

A minority of patients have no obstruction to pulmonary blood flow and a nonrestrictive VSD. These patients may present in infancy with signs and symptoms of excessive pulmonary blood flow, or they may have more or less normal $\dot{Q}p$ and only mild cyanosis. In the latter, physical findings, chest radiograph, and electrocardiogram (ECG) are similar to those of other patients with normal origin of the great arteries.

Tricuspid Atresia and Discordant Ventriculoarterial Connection

Patients in this subset of tricuspid atresia often present in early life with symptoms and signs of excessive pulmonary blood flow (see "Clinical Findings" under Clinical Features and Diagnostic Criteria in Section I of Chapter 35). Usually an apical mid-diastolic rumble is heard, and there is fixed splitting of the second heart sound at the base. However, moderate subvalvar pulmonary stenosis occasionally results in either mildly increased or normal $\dot{Q}p$. Such patients usually present after the neonatal period and sometimes after infancy, with mild cyanosis and few if any symptoms. Physical findings are similar to those in patients with tricuspid atresia and concordant ventriculoarterial connection. If aortic coarctation or interrupted aortic arch is present, the neonate presents with a duct-dependent systemic circulation and pulmonary overcirculation.

Chest Radiography

Chest radiography is usually characteristic of reduced $\dot{Q}p$ and RV hypoplasia in typical pulmonary undercirculated patients with tricuspid atresia and *concordant ventriculoarterial connection*. Pulmonary vascular markings are reduced and hilar shadows diminutive. The left apical heart border may be rounded, forming a high, arched contour. The vascular pedicle is narrow, and the left border in the area of the pulmonary trunk is usually concave. Radiographic appearance of the heart may resemble that of tetralogy of Fallot or occasionally appear normal.

Chest radiography in patients with tricuspid atresia and *discordant ventriculoarterial connection* usually shows pulmonary plethora and cardiomegaly, and the narrow supracardiac waist and LV contour make it resemble simple transposition.

Electrocardiography

The ECG in the subset with *concordant ventriculoarterial connection* demonstrates left axis deviation (0° to −90°) in about 90% of patients, LV hypertrophy in virtually all, and abnormalities of the P wave,[D16,O8] which is frequently tall (>2.5 mV) and notched.

The ECG may show left axis deviation in the subgroup with *discordant ventriculoarterial connection,* but a normal QRS axis between 0 and +90 degrees is present in more than half of patients.

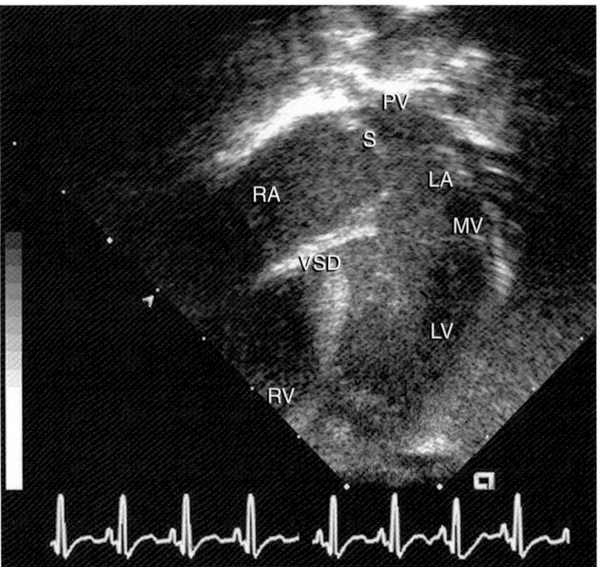

Figure 41-9 Four-chamber echocardiogram view of tricuspid atresia and concordant ventriculoarterial connection. Note restrictive ventricular septal defect *(VSD)* and hypoplastic right ventricular *(RV)* chamber. There is platelike tricuspid atresia present, with an atrial septal *(S)* defect and bowing of atrial septum from right to left. Pulmonary veins *(PV)* can be seen draining to back of left atrium. Left atrium *(LA)*, mitral valve *(MV)*, and left ventricle *(LV)* are of normal size. Key: *RA,* Right atrium.

Two-Dimensional Echocardiography

Echocardiography with color flow Doppler interrogation confirms the clinical impression of tricuspid atresia and usually provides definitive diagnosis (Fig. 41-9). Position of the great arteries and size and position of the diminutive RV and large LV can be determined (Fig. 41-10). In discordant ventriculoarterial connection, size of VSD relative to aortic "anulus" must be determined because this importantly affects the surgical procedure chosen. The aortic arch is examined for obstruction. RV size is determined because in this setting, it is functionally a subaortic outlet chamber. LV contractility is assessed. Flow across the atrial septum is assessed, which is unobstructed in most but not all cases.

Cardiac Catheterization and Cineangiography

Cardiac catheterization and cineangiography are not routinely performed. Indications for catheterization include inadequate echocardiographic evaluation, suspicion of inadequate or abnormal pulmonary arteries, concerns about pulmonary vascular resistance (Rp), and need for catheter-based intervention (e.g., restrictive atrial septum).

Computed Tomography and Magnetic Resonance Imaging

Computed tomography (CT) and magnetic resonance imaging (MRI) are rarely indicated in the newborn period. They can, however, be of great value at subsequent stages to assess valve abnormalities, complex subaortic obstruction, arch obstruction, ventricular mass, ventricular function, peripheral and central vascular dynamics, and abnormal venous and arterial connections associated with chronic single-ventricle physiology.[R12]

NATURAL HISTORY

Tricuspid atresia occurs more commonly than any other type of univentricular AV connection and accounts for 1% to 3% of congenital heart disease. The early natural history is determined primarily by presence and severity of obstruction to pulmonary blood flow and later by LV cardiomyopathy that develops in response to volume overload (see "Cardiomyopathy" later in this section).

Tricuspid Atresia and Concordant Ventriculoarterial Connection

Patients in this subset usually have important RV outflow obstruction and are cyanotic at birth. In most, the VSD narrows rapidly (in common with the general tendency of muscular VSDs to close spontaneously [see "Spontaneous Closure" under Natural History in Section I of Chapter 35]), $\dot{Q}p$ diminishes still further, cyanosis worsens, and hypoxia increases, causing the death of 90% of surgically untreated patients by age 1 year[C4,R1] (Fig. 41-11).

When these patients have a normal or increased $\dot{Q}p$, natural history is more favorable than in any other subset (see Fig. 41-11). Some die in early infancy of heart failure secondary to large $\dot{Q}p$, but spontaneous VSD narrowing and progression of infundibular narrowing usually produce a more balanced flow and better hemodynamic state within a few months of birth. Mild cyanosis and mild to moderate exercise intolerance persist at a plateau level for several years. Spontaneous narrowing of most VSDs continues, however, and

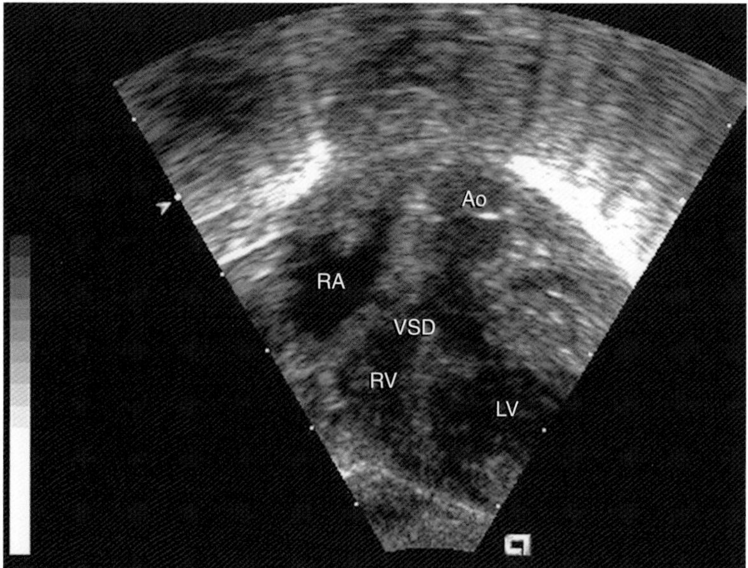

Figure 41-10 Subcostal echocardiogram view of tricuspid atresia and concordant ventriculoarterial connection, demonstrating ventriculoarterial connection. Right atrium *(RA)*, right ventricle *(RV)*, left ventricle *(LV)*, and ascending aorta *(Ao)* are shown. Aorta is aligned with LV without obstruction. Ventricular septal defect *(VSD)* is small and restrictive, and RV cavity is hypoplastic.

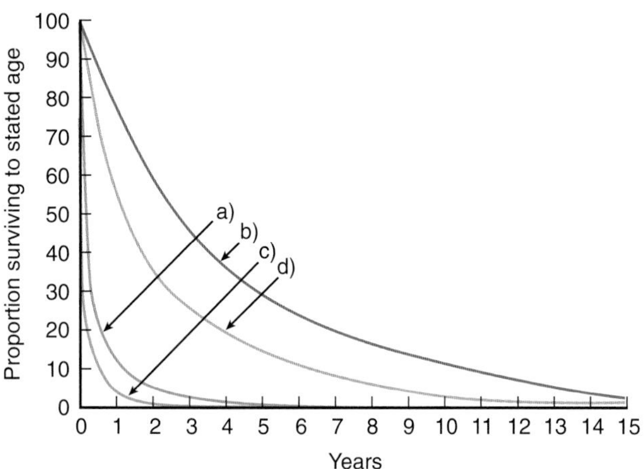

Figure 41-11 Free-hand representation of life expectancy of surgically untreated patients with tricuspid atresia. *a)*, Patients with concordant ventriculoarterial connection and reduced pulmonary blood flow at birth. *b)*, Patients with concordant ventriculoarterial connection and normal or increased pulmonary blood flow at birth. *c)*, Patients with discordant ventriculoarterial connection (transposition) and increased pulmonary blood flow at birth. *d)*, Patients with discordant ventriculoarterial connection and decreased or normal pulmonary blood flow at birth. (Data in part from Vlad[V10] and Dick and colleagues.[D16])

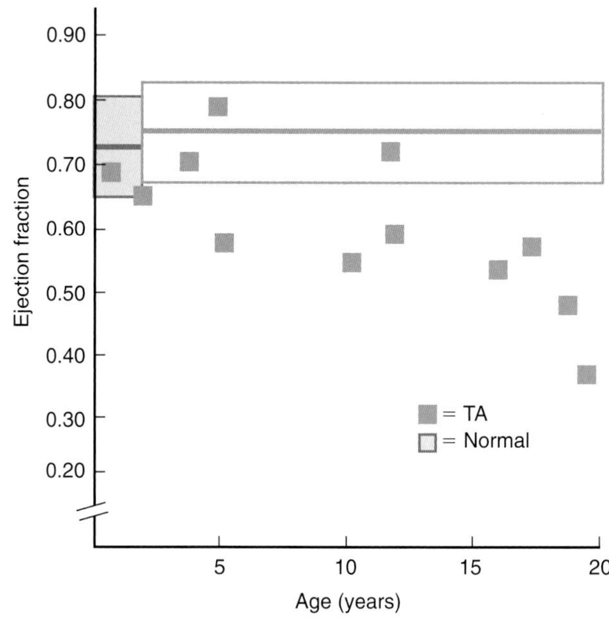

Figure 41-12 Left ventricular ejection fraction in patients with tricuspid atresia *(TA)* and surgically created systemic–pulmonary arterial shunts *(solid squares)* compared with normal subjects *(shaded area)*. Note that it becomes progressively more depressed as patients age. (From LaCorte and colleagues.[L1])

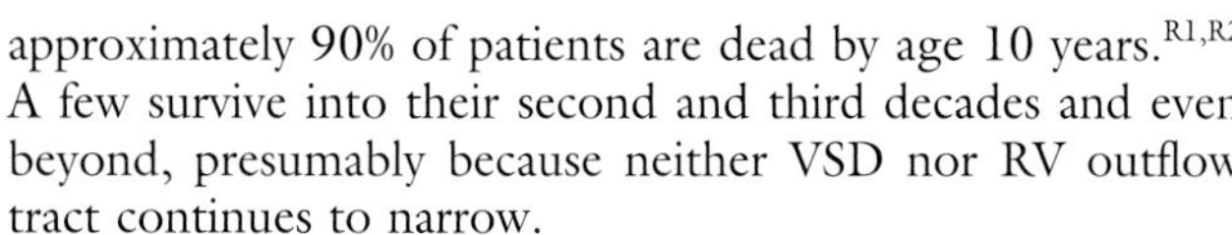

approximately 90% of patients are dead by age 10 years.[R1,R2] A few survive into their second and third decades and even beyond, presumably because neither VSD nor RV outflow tract continues to narrow.

In patients who survive into the second decade and longer, chronic LV volume overload usually produces a secondary LV cardiomyopathy and reduced systolic function (Fig. 41-12), and mitral regurgitation may develop. These factors produce a lower LV output and consequently increasing cyanosis and heart failure.

Tricuspid Atresia and Discordant Ventriculoarterial Connection

Surgically untreated patients in this subset usually have markedly increased $\dot{Q}p$, because the LV ejects directly and without restriction into the pulmonary trunk. Any tendency to VSD closure worsens the pulmonary plethora and, by producing subaortic stenosis, reduces systemic blood flow ($\dot{Q}s$). This unfavorable situation results in death of most babies by age 1 year (see Fig. 41-11). If there is coexisting important aortic

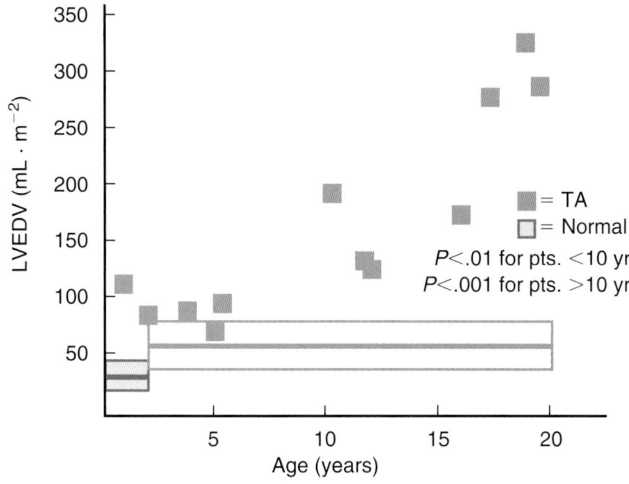

Figure 41-13 Left ventricular end-diastolic volume *(LVEDV)* in patients with tricuspid atresia *(TA)* and systemic–pulmonary arterial shunts. Presentation is as in Fig. 41-12. Note progressive increase with time in LV size. Key: *pts.,* Patients; *yr,* years. (From LaCorte and colleagues.[L1])

coarctation or interruption, natural history is heavily influenced by duct-dependent systemic perfusion. The majority of such infants suffer circulatory collapse and death in the first weeks of life within hours or days of ductal closure.

A few patients have mild or moderate LV (subpulmonary) outflow narrowing at birth and decreased $\dot{Q}p$. Progression of VSD narrowing (and RV outflow obstruction) is slower in this subset, so approximately 50% of patients survive to about age 2 years (see Fig. 41-11). Hypoxia worsens with time, however, and about 90% of surgically untreated subjects are dead by age 6 or 7 years.

Cardiomyopathy

The volume-overloaded LV, receiving both pulmonary and systemic venous return in patients with tricuspid atresia, plays an important role in natural history. Surgically untreated infants with diminished $\dot{Q}p$ have depressed LV systolic function (reduced ejection fraction) and end-diastolic volume larger than normal.[L1,N7] Reduced ejection fraction at this young age may be related to hypoxia. In patients who live beyond about age 5 years, ejection fraction becomes progressively more depressed (see Fig. 41-12) and LV volume progressively larger[L1] (Fig. 41-13). This is related to progression of LV cardiomyopathy secondary to chronic volume overload.[N7] In some patients, this leads to gradual development of mitral regurgitation in the second, third, and fourth decades. Recent evidence suggests the cardiomyopathy is due to a combination of volume overload and ischemia, with the ischemia partially due to an inadequately developed capillary network within the LV.[B17]

TECHNIQUE OF OPERATION

General Plan for Surgical Management of Single-Ventricle Physiology

The Fontan operation is considered the surgical end point for patients whose cardiac anomalies do not allow a two-ventricle circulation. The original Fontan operation was performed exclusively in patients with tricuspid atresia, but it is now applied to all forms of univentricular AV connection (see Chapters 40, 49, and 56), as well as to a number of other conditions in which complete two-ventricle circulations cannot easily be achieved (see Chapter 58). Soon after the original operative description, Fontan himself modified the procedure; it therefore seems unnecessary to term each subsequent modification a "modified Fontan." All forms of Fontan operation aim to divert systemic (with or without coronary) venous return to the pulmonary arterial circulation (either directly or by pathways through the heart), leaving one ventricle to provide essentially all energy driving blood flow in an in-series circulation. Each of the various techniques of achieving this separated pulmonary and systemic in-series circulation has advantages and disadvantages. Widely used techniques are described in sections that follow, and techniques that may be useful in specific cases are described under Special Situations and Controversies in Section IV.

Staged Palliation

Most patients with tricuspid atresia and those with other forms of univentricular AV connection (single-ventricle physiology) require preliminary surgical palliation before the Fontan operation. This usually involves:

- *First-stage palliation* in the neonatal period (see Section II)
- Commonly, *second-stage palliation* at some point between 3 months and 1 year to create a superior cavopulmonary connection in order to remove or reduce volume load on the single ventricle (see Section III)
- *Third-stage palliation,* the Fontan procedure, is then performed, typically between ages 1 and 5 years, depending on a number of factors (see Section IV)

Physiology and presentation, technique of operation, special features of postoperative care, results, indications for operation, and special situations and controversies of each palliative stage are discussed in separate sections that follow.

Specific Techniques of Operation

Morphologic variations of tricuspid atresia encompass most of the physiologic circumstances encountered when managing all other forms of single-ventricle physiology; therefore, specific discussion of the surgical management of tricuspid atresia presents an excellent opportunity to outline most techniques for managing all forms of single-ventricle physiology, from birth to Fontan completion. Several unique exceptions exist and are discussed in Chapters 49 and 58.

RESULTS

Results of first-stage palliation are presented in Section II, those of second-stage palliation in Section III, and those of third-stage palliation (Fontan operation) in Section IV.

Overall outcome for single-ventricle patients followed from early infancy was assessed in 405 patients by Lee and colleagues.[L15] These patients had the entire spectrum of single-ventricle morphology, but included only 14 with hypoplastic left heart physiology; thus, this relatively high-risk lesion did not have a major influence on overall results. Tricuspid atresia, double inlet ventricle, DORV, and unbalanced

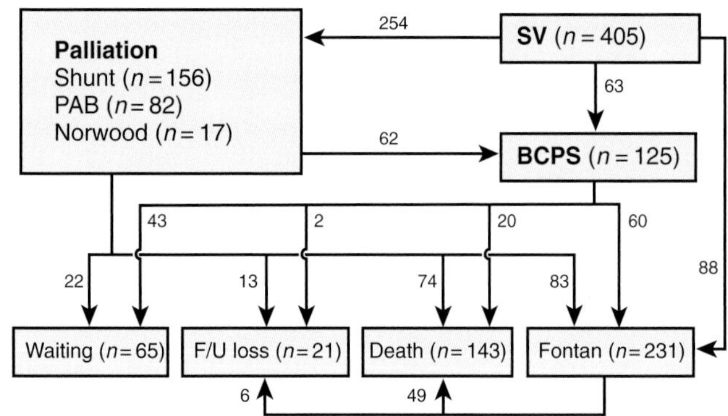

Figure 41-14 Surgical management and current status of 405 single-ventricle patients. Key: *BCPS,* Bidirectional superior cavopulmonary shunt; *F/U loss,* lost to follow-up; *PAB,* pulmonary artery band; *SV,* single ventricle; *waiting,* waiting for Fontan. (From Lee and colleagues.[L15])

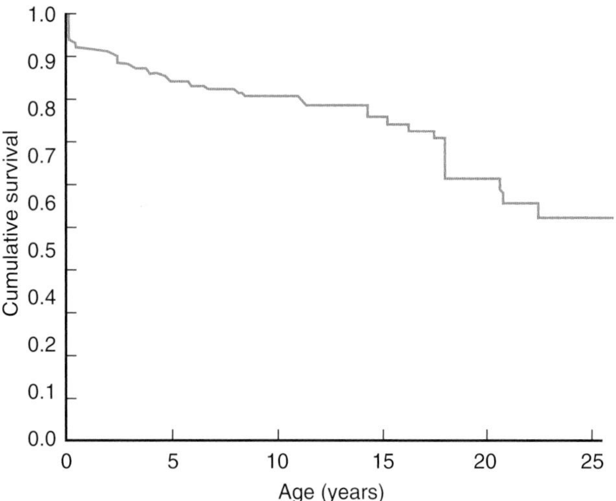

Figure 41-15 Kaplan-Meier survival from birth of 140 patients with transposed great arteries and either double inlet left ventricle or tricuspid atresia. (From Lan and Lakes.[L9])

AV septal defect accounted for 379 of the 405 cases. Patients were managed with a variety of surgical procedures (Fig. 41-14), but the goal was to achieve a Fontan circulation. Survival was thus influenced by operative mortality at each operation, interstage mortality, and mortality following the Fontan operation. The study showed a 10-year survival of 60%. Lan and colleagues examined 140 cases of DILV or tricuspid atresia with discordant ventriculoarterial connection and reported survival of 80% at 10 years[L9] (Fig. 41-15).

INDICATIONS FOR OPERATION

Patients in whom only one ventricle has an AV connection and is of sufficient size and power to provide energy for generating in-series pulmonary and systemic blood flows are considered for the Fontan operation. In most of these patients, the heart has a univentricular AV connection (see "Atrioventricular Connection" under Morphology in Chapter 56), one subset of which is tricuspid atresia. The Fontan operation may also be indicated for a few patients with concordant or discordant AV connections in whom one ventricle is too small or dysplastic, or both, to provide sufficient energy for generating adequate blood flow in a two-ventricle circulation (see Chapters 40, 49, and 58).[A7] Also, there are some cases in which two adequately sized and functioning ventricles exist in association with adequate inlet valves, but they cannot be septated because of complex relationships among the ventricles, great arteries, and VSDs. Such patients may best be treated with a Fontan procedure (see Chapter 53).[R24]

Some data suggest that a hypoplastic RV of less than 30% normal size does not contribute to the circulation, indicating that the Fontan operation should be performed if this threshold value is met.[I4]

SPECIAL SITUATIONS AND CONTROVERSIES

Moderately Hypoplastic Ventricle

If the RV is hypoplastic but greater than 30% normal size, then it may be of benefit to incorporate it into the right-sided circulation with a functioning inlet and outlet valve and a superior cavopulmonary anastomosis.[H5,M49] This procedure has been called the *one-and-a-half ventricle repair.*

Although definite proof of its efficacy is lacking, the one-and-a-half ventricle repair, used both to avoid the Fontan operation and to unload the normally developed but failing RV, has gained fairly wide acceptance as a useful procedure in both settings.[C23,K27,M38,M49,R9,V1]

Fontan versus Intracardiac Repair for Complex Morphology

Under certain morphologic circumstances, biventricular repair, although theoretically possible, may not be advisable, and consideration should be given to performing the Fontan operation. These circumstances include but are not limited to:

- Unbalanced AV septal defect
- Moderate right heart hypoplasia
- Moderate left heart hypoplasia
- DORV with uncommitted VSD
- Tricuspid atresia with VSD and moderately developed RV
- Pulmonary atresia with intact ventricular septum with moderate RV hypoplasia or dysfunction
- Ebstein anomaly with moderate RV hypoplasia or dysfunction
- Marked straddling of one AV valve, with AV and ventriculoarterial discordant connections, in association with VSD and pulmonary atresia or stenosis

In these anomalies, there may be two reasons to question a standard biventricular repair:

- Concern about ability of the hypoplastic ventricle or AV valve to function adequately
- Overall complexity of the procedure required to achieve a standard biventricular repair

Occasionally, both ventricles and inlet valves are of normal size and morphology is not particularly complex, but one ventricle demonstrates marked dysfunction (e.g., tetralogy of Fallot with markedly reduced RV function). In these circumstances, biventricular repair, Fontan operation, superior cavopulmonary anastomosis with intracardiac repair (one-and-a-half ventricle repair) and transplantation[G1] are theoretically possible. No clear criteria exist in these complex clinical settings for deciding among the options.[D8] Furthermore, there are no compelling data to suggest that long-term functional status of patients with one type of reconstruction is superior to the alternatives (e.g., one-and-a-half ventricle repair vs. Fontan).[H5] One single-institution study suggests that based on short-term and midterm survival, the Fontan is superior to complex intracardiac reconstructions.[D12] Other centers, however, do not agree with the findings.

Classic Glenn Operation

The classic Glenn operation (SVC-RPA anastomosis) is rarely performed in the current era. Most were performed as definitive operations prior to development, or at least wide acceptance, of the Fontan operation.

Early mortality for the procedure has been low, generally about 5%, when performed in infants older than about age 6 months and in children. In some respects it facilitates a later Fontan operation, because half the operation has been performed, similar to the situation following bidirectional superior cavopulmonary anastomosis. Interruption of the RPA, a necessary step in the classic Glenn operation, is in general disadvantageous from a technical standpoint.

Long-term results of the classic Glenn anastomosis in patients not suitable for complete repair are generally satisfactory.[E2] About 85% survive at least 10 years after creation of the shunt, which usually remains patent for at least that length of time.[B5,C8,C21,M17,T14] Kopf and colleagues report only 50% are still functional 20 years postoperatively, with 10- and 20-year survivals of 84% and 66%, respectively.[K25]

When symptoms recur, they may be caused by shunt closure, but also by rising hematocrit (with consequent decrease in right lung pulmonary blood flow), decreasing left lung pulmonary blood flow due to progressive narrowing of the VSD or pulmonary valve or subvalvar area, or by increasing flow through venovenous collaterals developing from the upper body to the lower body around the ligated SVC.[B5,B19,C8,L5]

The operation is followed in many patients by redistribution of pulmonary blood flow in the right lung.[B19,L5] Using ventilation/perfusion lung scans, Cloutier and colleagues demonstrated a decreased ratio of upper lobe–to–lower lobe pulmonary blood flow.[C26] Presumably as a more advanced manifestation of the same underlying process, right-sided pulmonary arteriovenous fistulae form late after the Glenn procedure, generally confined to the right lower lobe.[C1,C26,M17,M29,V2] In Kopf and colleagues' 30-year follow-up study, pulmonary arteriovenous fistulae developed in the right lung of 33% of patients.[K25] They found that a longer interval between operation and observation increased the probability of these fistulae being present. Right-to-left shunting and cyanosis usually develop with sufficient severity to warrant therapeutic fistula embolization in about one third of those afflicted.[K25] If fistulae are multiple and diffuse, embolization may not be an option.

Alternative Definitive Operations Other Than the Fontan

In most centers, the Fontan operation is considered the definitive operation for patients with single-ventricle physiology. Some patients will not meet physiologic criteria for the Fontan, most commonly because of elevated Rp or elevated ventricular end-diastolic pressure. For these patients, the definitive operation may be the superior cavopulmonary anastomosis, commonly with an additional source of pulmonary blood flow.[C3] In a minority of centers, the bidirectional superior cavopulmonary anastomosis with an additional source of pulmonary blood flow is considered the preferred definitive operation for patients with single-ventricle physiology.[Y3] There are no data comparing long-term outcomes after this procedure with those after the Fontan.

Section II First-Stage Neonatal Palliation of Single-Ventricle Physiology

The purpose of neonatal surgical intervention for tricuspid atresia and all forms of single-ventricle physiology is to balance systemic and pulmonary blood flow ($\dot{Q}p/\dot{Q}s$), provide unobstructed mixing at the atrial level, and ensure unobstructed systemic cardiac output.

CONCORDANT VENTRICULOARTERIAL CONNECTION

Clinical Features and Diagnostic Criteria

Inadequate Pulmonary Blood Flow

Because in this subset, the patient most commonly presents with reduced $\dot{Q}p$, or with duct-dependent $\dot{Q}p$ resulting from obstruction at or below the pulmonary valve, neonatal surgical palliation is required. This is achieved by some form of *systemic–pulmonary arterial shunt* designed to increase $\dot{Q}p$.

Excessive Pulmonary Blood Flow

Occasionally, there is little or no obstruction at or below the pulmonary valve, and the patient presents with excessive $\dot{Q}p$; surgical palliation to reduce it is required. This is achieved with a *pulmonary trunk band*. On occasion, neonates present with either well-balanced or moderately increased $\dot{Q}p$ across the right ventricular (RV) outflow tract. If $\dot{Q}p$ is truly well balanced, neonatal surgical palliation may be avoided. Such patients need careful monitoring, because resistance across the VSD, hypoplastic RV, and pulmonary valve can change rapidly in the first few weeks of life. Some will require a systemic–pulmonary arterial shunt if blood flow to the lungs decreases over time; others will remain with relatively well-balanced $\dot{Q}p/\dot{Q}s$ and may not require surgery until their superior cavopulmonary connection.

When there is little or no resistance across the VSD and RV outflow tract, however, markedly increased $\dot{Q}p$ gradually develops. This usually is not a problem in the first week of life when resistance in the pulmonary microvascular bed remains somewhat elevated, but such patients eventually require a pulmonary trunk band to establish appropriate balance between $\dot{Q}p$ and $\dot{Q}s$. Careful consideration should be given to timing of banding in such patients, even if diagnosis is made in the first few days of life. It is beneficial to delay placing the band until $\dot{Q}p$ increases somewhat, in concert with the normal postnatal decrease in pulmonary resistance (Rp) (see "Timing of Pulmonary Trunk Banding" under Indications for Operation later in this section).

Technique of Operation

Preoperative Management

Before undertaking any surgical procedure, overall cardiopulmonary stability should be ensured. These neonates are typically stable and come to the operating room breathing spontaneously and on little pharmacologic support other than, in some cases, prostaglandin E_1 (PGE_1) infusion to maintain ductal patency. However, if they present in an uncompensated state, either with overcirculation of the pulmonary circuit or with undercirculation and profound cyanosis, it is prudent to resuscitate them aggressively before operation. This may include use of PGE_1, inotropic agents, diuretics, mechanical ventilation with appropriate manipulations, nutritional support, and treatment of sepsis. Following stabilization, a period of observation is usually beneficial to allow recovery of systemic end-organ damage before surgical intervention. However, circumstances may require urgent operation despite inadequate resuscitation. For example, a previously undiagnosed and stable infant may present at several weeks of life with a recently closed ductus, resulting in ongoing critical cyanosis.

Systemic–Pulmonary Arterial Shunt

After anesthesia induction, an indwelling arterial catheter is placed, preferably in the left radial artery. Reliable intravenous access is achieved, preferably via peripheral extremity vein; subclavian and internal jugular veins should be specifically avoided because they tend to develop deep venous thrombosis that can importantly complicate subsequent management at the time of superior cavopulmonary shunt (see Section III). It is similarly important to avoid femoral vein cannulation, because most patients with univentricular AV connection require multiple cardiac catheterization evaluations, preferably via the femoral vein.

The preferred incision for performing a systemic–pulmonary arterial shunt is median sternotomy. This incision has multiple advantages over traditional lateral thoracotomy:

- Both lungs can be completely ventilated throughout the procedure. This can be especially important in unstable infants.
- The shunt can be placed more centrally on the left or right branch pulmonary artery, thereby reducing prevalence of right or left upper lobe pulmonary artery branch stenosis.
- Maximal flexibility is achieved.
- If the ductus arteriosus is to be ligated during the shunt procedure, it can be accomplished effectively.
- If central pulmonary artery stenosis at the site of ductus insertion is present or suspected, pulmonary arterioplasty can be performed.
- If the patient becomes unstable during the procedure and requires cardiopulmonary bypass (CPB), there is access for cannulation.
- Occurrence of musculoskeletal deformities induced by a lateral incision, such as scoliosis, is eliminated.

The single disadvantage of median sternotomy is risk of hemorrhage from inadvertent cardiotomy on repeat sternotomy at subsequent procedures. This can be minimized by leaving intact the anterior aspect of the pericardial sack overlying the ventricular mass at the first procedure.

Median sternotomy is performed (see "Incision" in Section III of Chapter 2). The typically large thymus gland is mobilized or partially removed, and only the upper pericardial reflection over the great arteries is opened, leaving intact the portion overlying the ventricular mass. Sites on both systemic and pulmonary circuits are chosen for placing the shunt (see "Systemic–Pulmonary Arterial Shunt" under Special Situations and Controversies later in this section). Usually a modified Blalock-Taussig shunt is performed (Fig. 41-16) using an expanded polytetrafluoroethylene (PTFE) vascular graft of specified internal diameter, placed between the brachiocephalic–right subclavian artery junction, and central portion of the RPA (see "Systemic–Pulmonary Arterial Shunt" under Special Situations and Controversies later in this section). Systemic and pulmonary arterial sites are prepared using sharp dissection. The patient is heparinized ($3\ mg \cdot kg^{-1}$ intravenously). An appropriately sized partial occlusion vascular clamp is used to isolate the brachiocephalic–right subclavian arterial segment, which is incised over a length appropriate to create an orifice that matches the expanded PTFE graft.

Focus on detail is necessary to create a functional and reliable shunt. Attention is given to the *angle of takeoff* of the brachiocephalic artery origin and brachiocephalic-subclavian arterial junction. The expanded PTFE graft is tailored with a bevel to maximize laminar flow at the arterial graft anastomosis. Anastomosis is then performed with running 7-0 nonabsorbable monofilament suture.

After the anastomosis is completed, the partial occlusion clamp on the arterial segment is removed and replaced with a small clamp occluding the graft. This allows the arterial segment to assume its natural position, thereby permitting the surgeon to judge exactly the *length of the graft* in preparation for its anastomosis to the RPA. Attention to detail is necessary because a graft tailored to an inappropriate length may kink or distort the involved arteries. Typically, no bevel is necessary at the graft-RPA connection, and end-to-side anastomosis is performed at a 90-degree angle. After trimming the graft to an appropriate length, a partial occlusion clamp is placed on the central portion of the RPA that lies to the right of the ascending aorta and left of the SVC; it should not involve the right upper pulmonary artery. An incision of appropriate length is made in the sequestered segment of RPA, and anastomosis proceeds using a technique similar to that of the previous anastomosis. Before completing it, heparinized saline may be infused into the graft and pulmonary artery segments to flush remnants of blood that may have accumulated. The clamp is then removed from the RPA. Before removing the clamp on the shunt, the ductus arteriosus (if present) is exposed, and a heavy silk ligature with a snare is placed around it. The clamp is then removed from the shunt, and the snare on the ductus is gently tightened to occlude it.

A period of hemodynamic adjustment then ensues. The surgeon should pay careful attention to change in systemic arterial oxygen saturation (SaO_2) as indicated by pulse oximetry and by change in hemodynamics as indicated by heart rate and systolic, diastolic, and mean blood pressures. New

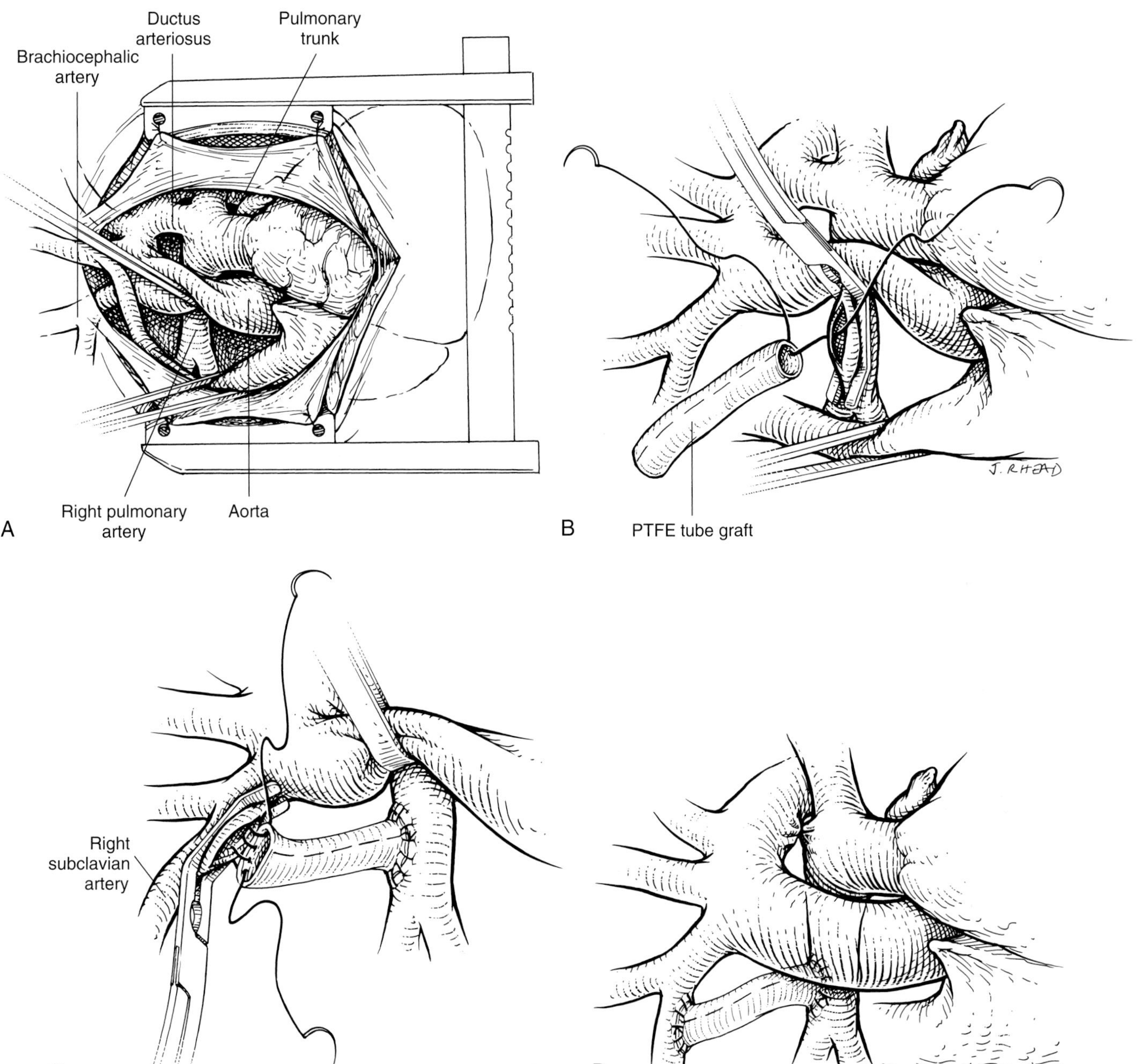

Figure 41-16 Right modified Blalock-Taussig shunt through median sternotomy. Although either anastomosis can be performed first, here the graft–right pulmonary artery (RPA) anastomosis is performed first, followed by the graft–subclavian artery anastomosis. (See text for description of procedure in opposite order.) **A,** After median sternotomy, thymus gland is subtotally resected and pericardium opened along its upper aspect. Aorta is retracted to left side, and superior vena cava to right side, exposing RPA. Brachiocephalic artery and its bifurcation into right subclavian and carotid arteries are dissected cephalad to brachiocephalic vein. **B,** Side-biting vascular clamp is placed on RPA in such a way that clamp itself holds aorta to patient's left. Care is taken that incision in superior aspect of RPA does not encroach on its bifurcation into upper and lower branches, but is kept as central as possible. An appropriately sized polytetrafluoroethylene *(PTFE)* tube graft is then connected to RPA incision, using a continuous suture technique and 7-0 nonabsorbable monofilament suture (see text for a more detailed discussion of factors involved in determining choice of shunt size). Posterior aspect of anastomosis is performed first, followed by anterior aspect. **C,** After the graft to pulmonary artery anastomosis is completed, a side-biting vascular clamp is placed on exposed right subclavian artery or right subclavian–brachiocephalic artery junction. Sequestered segment of artery is incised over an appropriate length to match circumference of PTFE tube graft. Graft is tailored to an appropriate length and beveled to avoid kinking or distorting subclavian and right pulmonary arteries. Anastomosis is performed using a technique similar to that described for graft-to–pulmonary artery anastomosis **(B)**. **D,** Shunt is shown with anastomoses completed and aorta and superior vena cava in their normal positions. Additionally, ductus arteriosus has been ligated with a 5-0 polypropylene suture following blunt circumferential dissection with a small right-angled clamp.

steady-state values for these variables are judged against baseline conditions, which may vary among infants. In general, SaO_2 between 75% and 85% is considered acceptable. SaO_2 below this range should raise concerns about a technical problem with the shunt, an inadequately sized shunt, or unsuspected distal pulmonary artery problems. SaO_2 above this range should raise concern that the shunt is too large. This latter concern is heightened if systemic arterial diastolic blood pressure is less than 25 to 30 mmHg.

Once stability has been achieved, the snare is removed from the ductus, and it is permanently ligated. PGE_1 infusion is stopped. Mediastinal drainage and closing the median sternotomy are as usual (see "Completing Operation" in Section III of Chapter 2).

Pulmonary Trunk Banding

Pulmonary trunk banding is usually performed via median sternotomy, lateral thoracotomy, or anterior parasternal incision. Median sternotomy is preferred for the same reasons described in the preceding text for placing a systemic–pulmonary arterial shunt; patient preparation is also similar. If the surgeon prefers a lateral thoracotomy or anterior parasternal incision, it is performed on the left side. In other patients with univentricular AV connection with conotruncal abnormalities that result in position of the pulmonary trunk to the right of the aortic root, a right lateral incision is chosen.

Preferred median sternotomy is performed as described in Chapter 2, and the thymus gland is mobilized or partially removed. The pericardium is opened only at its superior border over the great arteries, with care taken to leave it intact over the ventricular mass. The tissue plane between ascending aorta and pulmonary trunk is developed over a limited area halfway between the sinutubular junction of the pulmonary trunk and origin of the RPA (Fig. 41-17, *A*).

Aggressive dissection in this area is discouraged because it increases the chances of migration of the band over time. Once circumferential access to the pulmonary trunk is achieved, the band is placed around it. Choice of band material may vary; however, material that prevents important fibrosis and calcification and has a low risk of erosion into the pulmonary trunk should be chosen. Width of band material should be broad (at least 2.5 mm) to minimize erosion. Preferred choice of band is a 3-mm-wide strip fashioned from a relatively thick (0.3 to 0.4 mm) silicone rubber sheet. This material incites minimal reaction in surrounding tissues.

After placing the band around the pulmonary trunk (Fig. 41-17, *B*), its free ends are secured together to create a circumferential ring (Fig. 41-17, *C*). Formulas can be used to estimate the appropriate circumferential length, but individual physiologic variability usually dictates adjustments be made. Free ends of the band are initially secured together at a point that allows only minimal circumferential narrowing of the pulmonary trunk. Following this initial placement, two sutures are placed at points 180 degrees opposite each other on the circumference of the band, attaching the band to the adventitia of the proximal portion of the pulmonary trunk (see Fig. 41-17, *C*). These sutures prevent pressure-driven distal band migration on the pulmonary trunk. Migration is common if the band is not secured.

Once the band is positioned, but before it has been adjusted to its final circumference, it is prudent to temporarily place a catheter into the distal pulmonary trunk to measure pressure distal to the band. Difference in systemic arterial and

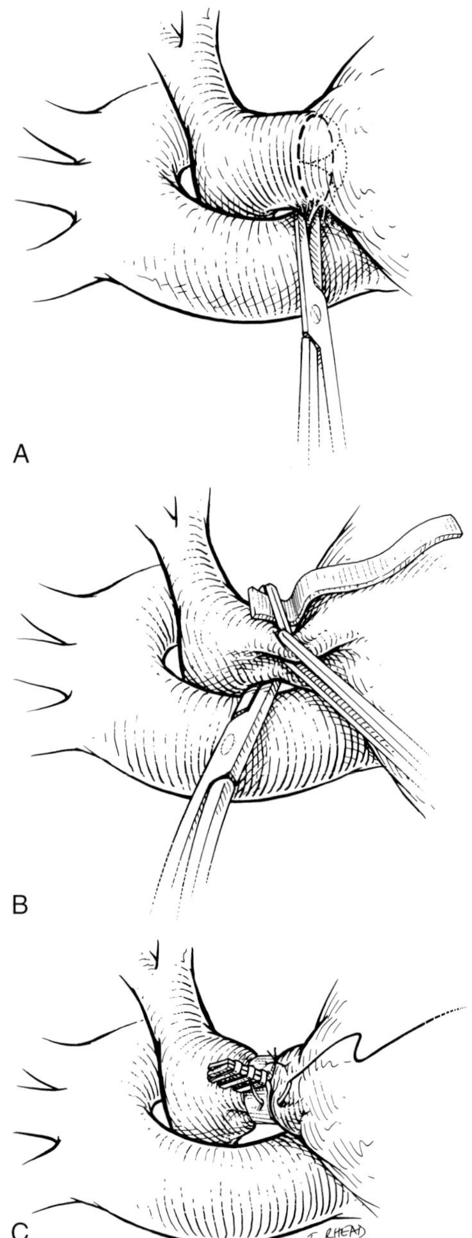

Figure 41-17 Pulmonary trunk (PT) band placement in neonate or young infant. **A,** Anatomy of PT and aorta is shown in tricuspid atresia and normally related great arteries, exposed through the preferred standard median sternotomy. It should be noted that tops of pulmonary valve commissures *(dotted lines)* are within millimeters of origin of right pulmonary artery. Circumferential dissection around PT is purposefully limited to minimize potential for distal band migration. Opening between PT and aorta is only large enough to just allow passage of band. **B,** After circumferential dissection, PT is stabilized and manipulated with forceps while a right-angled clamp is placed around it. A segment of band material (3-mm-wide strip of reinforced silicone rubber sheeting is preferred) is positioned around PT as shown. Care is taken to place band just distal to sinutubular junction but also proximal to origin of right pulmonary artery. **C,** Band is appropriately positioned circumferentially. Ends of band are overlapped anteriorly, and medium-sized metal clips are placed to secure them. Successively lower clips are placed to adjust band tightness. Once band is appropriately tightened (see text for details), two separate 5-0 monofilament nonabsorbable sutures are placed at left and right lateral aspects of PT, attaching band to PT adventitia. This is performed to further minimize potential for distal band migration.

distal pulmonary artery pressure provides an accurate assessment of band gradient. The surgeon then gradually reduces band circumference, evaluating both band gradient and SaO_2 as end points. Both vary depending on physiologic circumstances; however, a typical band gradient in a neonate will be in the range of 40 to 70 mmHg, and SaO_2 should range between 75% and 85%. Band circumference is adjusted by placing metal clips in the vicinity where the two free ends of the band were initially secured together (see Fig. 41-17, *C*). These clips are placed sequentially, with each subsequent clip placed just below the most recently placed one, gradually approaching the physiologic end points just described. Appropriately adjusting $\dot{Q}p$ with a pulmonary trunk band can be somewhat difficult. This is because pulmonary blood flow occurs only in systole, and the band is a two-dimensional resistor with little length. As a result, small changes in band circumference result in marked resistance changes and, therefore, marked $\dot{Q}p$ changes. Because flow across the band occurs only in systole, $\dot{Q}p$ varies with changes in systemic arterial pressure. It is therefore critical that the anesthesiologist create circumstances during band adjustment such that systemic blood pressure approximates that expected in the awake infant. This can usually be achieved by appropriate choice of anesthetic and volume management.

Once the band is appropriately adjusted, an indwelling right atrial catheter and atrial and ventricular pacing wires are placed as described earlier in this section for the systemic–pulmonary arterial shunt. Mediastinal drainage and median sternotomy closure are as described in "Completing Operation" in Section III of Chapter 2.

Special Features of Postoperative Care

Systemic–Pulmonary Arterial Shunting Procedures

After completing the procedure, it is not necessary to reverse the heparin with protamine; instead, the heparin is allowed to metabolize slowly. Beginning on the first postoperative night, aspirin is given rectally (1 mg · kg^{-1} · day^{-1}) to prevent thrombus formation in the shunt.

Some degree of hemodynamic instability and modest metabolic acidosis are common in the first few postoperative hours. It is prudent to support the patient over the first postoperative day with mechanical ventilation and close observation. Occasionally, low-dose inotropic support is indicated.

Pulmonary Trunk Banding

As Rp gradually decreases after placement of a pulmonary trunk band, it is occasionally necessary to reoperate to tighten the band further. Need for readjusting it can be minimized by appropriately timing the initial banding (see "Timing of Pulmonary Trunk Banding" under Indications for Operation later in this section).

Results

Systemic–Pulmonary Arterial Shunting Procedures

Early mortality for patients with tricuspid atresia and other types of univentricular communications and reduced $\dot{Q}p$ is low (Tables 41-1 and 41-2) and similar to that for shunts performed for palliation of tetralogy of Fallot (see "Interim Results after Classic Shunting Operations" in Section I of Chapter 38). As expected, early mortality from multi-institution reports is somewhat higher than in the single-institution reports cited in these tables. A three-institution report revealed 3 early deaths in 23 cases (13%; CL 6%-24%).[W1] Under most circumstances, pulmonary artery distortion by the shunt is uncommon.[C33]

In patients who cannot subsequently have a Fontan operation, palliation has been good, and 5-year survival without definitive operation is about 90%.[C33] Intermediate time-related survival, including mortality of subsequent interventions, is about 85% at 10 years when the shunt is initially performed after the first few months of life[M40,S35,T1,V9] (Fig. 41-18). However, substantially worse survival was reported by Franklin and colleagues for a patient group in which many required operation early in life; this may be more representative[F18,F19] (Fig. 41-19). Risk of dying is highest in the first few months following the shunt procedure (Fig. 41-20). Then, after 5 to 10 years, many patients begin to deteriorate. This is related to cyanosis, which is due to relative narrowing of the Blalock-Taussig shunt commensurate with patient growth, as well as to LV cardiomyopathy secondary

Table 41-1 Hospital Mortality after Surgical Procedures for Tricuspid Atresia

		Hospital Deaths			
Operation	***n***	**No.**	**%**	**CL (%)**	
Systemic–pulmonary artery shunting	69	5	7	4-12	
Blalock-Taussig	31	2	6	2-15	} 3/44, 7%; CL 3%-13%
PTFE interposition	13	1	8	1-24	
Others	25	2	8	3-18	
Glenn operation	11	2	18	6-38	
Revisions of shunts	8	2	25	9-50	
Open palliative procedures	7	1	14	2-41	
Pulmonary trunk banding	6	0	0	0-27	
Coarctation repair and pulmonary trunk banding	1	0	0	0-86	
Miscellaneous other palliative procedures	6	1	17	2-46	
TOTAL	108	11	10	7-14	

Data from Cleveland and colleagues.[C25]
Key: *CL*, 70% confidence limits; *PTFE*, polytetrafluoroethylene.

Table 41-2 Hospital Mortality after Initial and Subsequent Palliative Operations for Single Ventricle

		Hospital Deaths			
Operation	***n***	**No.**	**%**	**CL (%)**	
Systemic–pulmonary artery shunting	73	6	8	5-13	
Blalock-Taussig	41	1	2	0.3-8	1/55, 2%; CL 0.2%-6% (Blalock-Taussig and PTFE interposition)
PTFE interposition	14	0	0	0-13	
Other shunts	18	5	28	16-43	
Pulmonary trunk banding	4	0	0	0-38	
Atrial septectomy	9	0	0	0-19	
Repair only of associated cardiac anomaly	7	2	29	10-55	
Combined closed palliative procedures	9	0	0	0-19	
Others[a]	9	2	22	8-45	
TOTAL	111	10	9	6-13	

Data from Stefanelli and colleagues.[S35]
[a]Seven exploratory cardiotomies, including or not including pulmonary valvotomy or a valved extracardiac conduit (seven cases, one hospital death), and two revisions of previous procedures (one hospital death).
Key: *CL,* 70% confidence limits; *PTFE,* polytetrafluoroethylene.

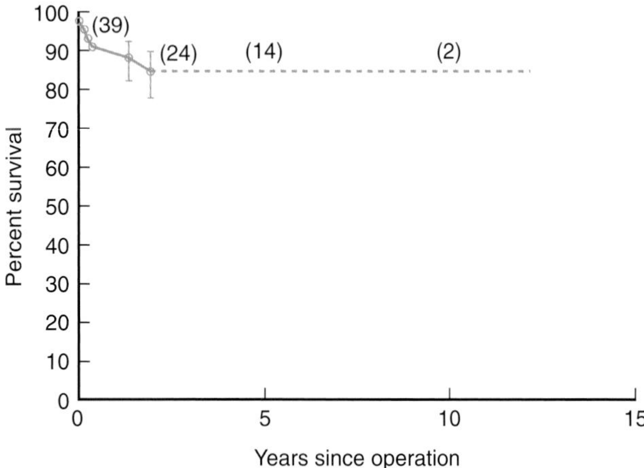

Figure 41-18 Survival, including hospital deaths, after a classic shunting operation done as the primary operation for single ventricle. Patients were not censored at the time of a subsequent procedure. Each circle represents a death. Vertical bars represent 70% confidence limits, and numbers in parentheses represent patients remaining at risk. Dashed line indicates traced patients without an event. (From Stefanelli and colleagues.[S35])

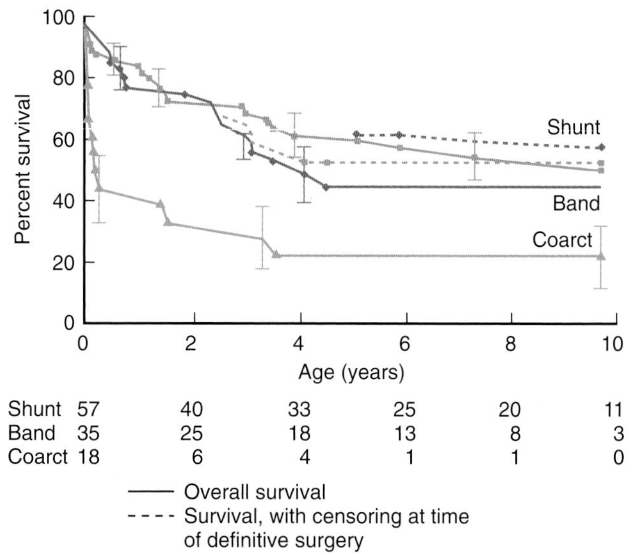

Figure 41-19 Survival of patients with double inlet ventricle after an initial systemic–pulmonary arterial shunt, pulmonary trunk banding, or repair of coarctation (or interrupted aortic arch) plus pulmonary trunk banding in early life. Vertical bars represent 70% confidence limits; numbers are patients at risk. Key: *Band,* Pulmonary trunk banding; *Coarct,* coarctation or interrupted aortic arch; *Shunt,* systemic–pulmonary arterial shunt. (From Franklin and colleagues.[F19])

to chronic volume overload, which worsens with time (see "Cardiomyopathy" under Natural History in Section I).

Pulmonary Trunk Banding

Early mortality after pulmonary trunk banding has been reported to be substantial—25% to 35%.[H15,L13,V3] This high mortality likely reflects that this information spans many years and thus includes many patients receiving bands in the 1970s, when mortality in general was high for complex cases. It may also reflect difficulty of achieving physiologic balance of $\dot{Q}p$ and $\dot{Q}s$ compared with a systemic–pulmonary arterial shunt. In the current era, mortality of less than 5% should be expected (see Tables 41-1 and 41-2). Low mortality (no early deaths in 10 cases) (0%; CL 0%-17%) in the current era is confirmed even in multi-institutional reports.[W1]

Outcome following pulmonary trunk banding, like systemic–pulmonary arterial shunting, is somewhat influenced by intracardiac anatomy. For example, with tricuspid atresia or DILV and discordant ventriculoarterial connection, the tendency for subaortic stenosis to develop or progress is a frequent and unfavorable sequel to the banding procedure (see "Physiology and Presentation" under Discordant Ventriculoarterial Connection later in this section).[F20,F22,F25,K3,P7,S29] Subaortic stenosis not only increases risk of death before definitive repair but also after the Fontan operation; this is due to the resulting increase in main ventricular chamber muscle mass and corresponding decrease in ventricular compliance.[S12]

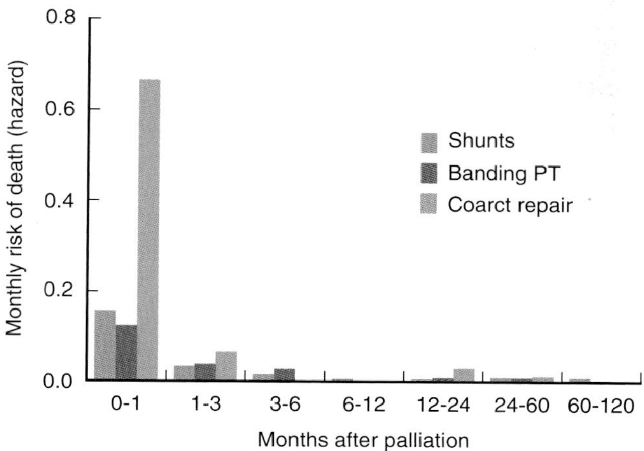

Figure 41-20 Histogram of hazard function (death · mo^{-1}) after palliative procedure indicated and before definitive surgery. Key: *Coarct,* Coarctation; *PT,* pulmonary trunk; *Shunts,* systemic–pulmonary arterial shunts. (From Franklin and colleagues.[F19])

Indications for Operation

Systemic–Pulmonary Arterial Shunt

Presence of severe cyanosis (SaO_2 < 70%-75%) early in life or of duct dependency are indications for performing a systemic–pulmonary arterial shunt. Causes for cyanosis other than restrictive Q̇p (e.g., reversible lung disease, anemia, obstructive pulmonary venous connection) must be ruled out.

The shunt does not facilitate later decision making about a Fontan operation, and it somewhat complicates its later performance.

Pulmonary Trunk Banding

When Q̇p is large enough to produce serious heart failure early in life, the pulmonary trunk should probably be banded. If increased Q̇p is insufficient to produce important heart failure in the early weeks of life, banding is not performed.

Timing of Pulmonary Trunk Banding If a pulmonary trunk band is placed too early following birth when distal Rp is still high, the surgeon will be limited by the patient's cyanosis when attempting to tighten the band to an appropriate level. As Rp gradually decreases after placing such a band, it is commonly necessary to reoperate to tighten the band further. Need for readjusting the band can be minimized by appropriately timing the initial banding. The ideal time varies based on individual physiologic characteristics, but the procedure is usually best performed in the second, third, or fourth week of life. In the physiologic setting of low distal Rp and relatively high Q̇p, the situation is optimal for placing the band with an appropriate tightness that ensures long-term balance between Q̇p and Q̇s.

DISCORDANT VENTRICULOARTERIAL CONNECTION

Clinical Features and Diagnostic Criteria

In this subset, neonates typically present a different set of physiologic considerations from those with concordant ventriculoarterial connection. Because the pulmonary valve is in fibrous continuity with the mitral valve and arises directly from the LV, obstruction to pulmonary blood flow is unusual and unrestrictive Q̇p the rule. The aorta arises from the hypoplastic RV, and as a result, the LV must eject through the VSD (bulboventricular foramen) and underdeveloped RV into the aorta. If the outflow tract from LV to aorta and the aortic arch are well developed, the patient can be managed effectively in a fashion similar to that described for tricuspid atresia and concordant ventriculoarterial connection with excessive Q̇p using a pulmonary trunk band as described in the preceding text.

Tricuspid atresia and discordant ventriculoarterial connection, however, commonly manifests with important obstruction in the systemic circulation.[L2] Obstruction typically occurs at two levels: subaortic and aortic arch. *Subaortic obstruction* is due to a combination of restrictive VSD and muscular obstruction in the underdeveloped incomplete RV. *Arch obstruction* may be due to discrete aortic coarctation alone, a diffusely hypoplastic arch in combination with discrete coarctation, or interrupted aortic arch. Many patients with DILV have physiology similar to that just described (see Clinical Features and Diagnostic Criteria in Chapter 56).

Patients in whom subaortic stenosis becomes evident shortly after birth typically have a small or moderate-sized VSD[M18] and often coexisting hypoplasia of the aortic arch with associated aortic coarctation or interrupted aortic arch.[F24] Any type of coexisting aortic arch obstruction increases by sevenfold the probability that severe subaortic stenosis will be present.[K3] Narrowing may be accelerated by maneuvers that reduce volume load on the heart, such as pulmonary trunk banding or takedown of a systemic–pulmonary arterial shunt at the time of a bidirectional superior cavopulmonary shunt or Fontan procedure. Some studies suggest that subaortic stenosis will ultimately develop in up to 80% of such patients who undergo pulmonary banding early in life.[F20,F23,K3]

Even when the VSD is large at the time of a Fontan operation, it may narrow thereafter and subaortic stenosis may appear.[R5] Narrowing may occur immediately at the time of the Fontan operation if important volume unloading occurs, either by removing a pulmonary artery band with pulmonary trunk occlusion or by removing a systemic–pulmonary arterial shunt. However, if the patient is undergoing three-stage palliation, it is more likely for the volume load to be dramatically reduced at the time of second-stage bidirectional superior cavopulmonary shunt, and subaortic stenosis is more likely to develop at that time.

In summary, subaortic stenosis is a potential problem in patients in whom the aorta arises above an incomplete ventricle (or outlet chamber). Probability of its appearance is increased by smallness of the VSD (bulboventricular foramen), coexisting aortic arch obstruction, and maneuvers that reduce ventricular volume load. Even in the absence of associated factors, it may still develop. Subaortic stenosis is least likely to occur when the aortic valve is large, the VSD is large, and no arch obstruction is present.

Technique of Operation

Preoperative Management

Neonates with this morphology have the potential to be acutely ill in a manner similar to those with hypoplastic left heart physiology; therefore, preoperative stabilization should be similar to that for patients with hypoplastic left heart physiology (see Box 49-1 under "Definition," and

"Preoperative Management" in Chapter 49). Even when the VSD is large at birth, it may spontaneously narrow, and subaortic obstruction then becomes apparent.

Pulmonary Trunk Banding and Aortic Arch Reconstruction

This technique is described for tricuspid atresia and discordant ventriculoarterial connection with aortic arch obstruction, but is applicable to any patient with univentricular AV connection, aortic arch obstruction, and excessive $\dot{Q}p$ (Fig. 41-21). The patient is positioned in right lateral decubitus position, and a standard left posterolateral thoracotomy is made through the fourth intercostal space (see "Alternative Primary Incisions" under Incisions in Section III of Chapter 2). Description of the arch repair is similar to that for isolated coarctation in the neonate (see Technique of Operation in Section I of Chapter 48 for details).

Following arch reconstruction, a longitudinal incision in the pericardium is made 1 cm anterior to the left phrenic nerve. Depending on extent of the thymus gland, modest mobilization of its left lobe may be necessary. Once the pericardium is opened, the pulmonary trunk is identified in the transposed position, posterior and to the left of the ascending aorta. (In patients with DILV and L-transposition, the pulmonary trunk is posterior and to the right.) The plane between adjacent walls of ascending aorta and pulmonary trunk are carefully dissected, gaining circumferential access around the pulmonary trunk midway between its sinutubular junction and origin of the RPA. The RPA origin is particularly difficult to visualize through a left thoracotomy incision; however, it must be carefully located before positioning the band. Following this, details related to placing and adjusting the band are similar to those described previously (see "Pulmonary Trunk Banding" under Technique of Operation earlier in this section) for placing a pulmonary artery band through a median sternotomy (see Fig. 41-17).

Proximal Pulmonary Trunk to Aortic Connection with Arch Repair

This technique is described for tricuspid atresia and discordant ventriculoarterial connection with subaortic and arch obstruction, but is applicable to all forms of univentricular AV connection with subaortic and arch obstruction[V4] (Fig. 41-22). After anesthesia induction, placing indwelling peripheral arterial and venous catheters, and supine positioning, a median sternotomy is performed (see "Preparation for Cardiopulmonary Bypass" in Section III of Chapter 2). The thymus gland is subtotally removed and the pericardium opened anteriorly over the heart. The plane between pulmonary trunk and ascending aorta is carefully dissected and the entire aortic arch mobilized, including the first 1 to 2 cm of each arch vessel. The central pulmonary artery, ductus arteriosus, and descending aorta to the level of the first pair of intercostal arteries are also mobilized. The patient is then prepared for CPB. If the aortic arch is hypoplastic but not preocclusive (>2-3 mm in diameter), adequate perfusion on CPB can be achieved by cannulating the aortic system alone using a 6F or 8F aortic cannula.[M27] If the ascending aorta is of adequate size, it can be cannulated directly (as shown in Fig. 41-22), or alternatively, if it is hypoplastic, the base of the brachiocephalic artery can be cannulated. The arterial cannula (or cannulae) is secured in place with standard purse-string sutures and snares. If the aortic arch is interrupted, or is in continuity but with preocclusive narrowing at the isthmus and coarctation, dual arterial cannulation of the proximal pulmonary trunk and the aortic system is performed. (This variation is not shown in Fig. 41-22, but see Technique of Operation in Chapter 48 for a detailed description of cannulation technique and CPB management when the arch is interrupted.) Temporary occlusion of branch pulmonary arteries is achieved either with snares or vascular clamps if perfusion is performed through the pulmonary trunk and ductus arteriosus to the descending thoracic aorta.

Venous cannulation is through a purse string in the right atrial appendage. After cannulation, CPB is instituted and preferably carried out using continuous antegrade cerebral perfusion (see Fig. 41-22). Alternatively, some surgeons prefer to use circulatory arrest (see "Technique in Neonates, Infants, and Children" in Section IV of Chapter 2). These CPB management techniques are also discussed in detail in the description of the Norwood procedure for hypoplastic left heart physiology (see "Norwood Procedure Using Continuous Perfusion" under Technique of Operation in Chapter 49). In particular, the techniques described in Chapter 49 for performing continuous antegrade cerebral perfusion are widely applicable to all forms of neonatal arch obstruction with associated hypoplastic arch and ascending aorta. Once the target perfusion temperature is reached, antegrade cerebral perfusion established, and cardiac arrest induced with cardioplegia, the obstructed aortic arch is addressed, as described in Fig. 41-22.

If the aortic arch is in continuity but hypoplastic, the aortic isthmus is ligated with a 5-0 polypropylene suture, and ductus and coarctation tissue distal to it are removed (see Fig. 41-22, *A*). A small vascular clamp can be placed across the descending aorta at the level of the first set of intercostal vessels to stabilize the aorta and deliver it into the anterior mediastinum. A longitudinal incision is made in the posterior aspect of the upper ascending aorta and proximal aortic arch (see Fig. 41-22, *A*), and the descending aorta is anastomosed to this incision with a running 7-0 monofilament absorbable suture, thereby repairing the arch obstruction (Fig. 41-22, *B*). In the case of true aortic arch interruption, the isthmus ligature is not necessary, and arch repair otherwise proceeds as described.

With the arch obstruction addressed, antegrade cerebral perfusion is terminated and full-body bypass is again established (see "Norwood Procedure Using Continuous Perfusion" under Technique of Operation in Chapter 49). Attention is turned to the proximal pulmonary trunk–to-aortic anastomosis. This can be accomplished in several ways, one of which is described in detail in Fig. 41-22, *B*. Although unusual in neonates with tricuspid atresia, if preoperative evaluation suggests that potential or real obstruction exists at the atrial septum, the right atrium is opened during continuous bypass, and the septum primum is removed to create an unobstructed atrial communication. During this maneuver, the single venous cannula in the right atrium must be temporarily clamped, and cardiotomy suction devices used within the two vena caval orifices to provide exposure for the atrial septal resection. The right atriotomy is then closed with a running 6-0 polypropylene monofilament suture. Venous drainage via the right atrial cannula is then reestablished and rewarming begun.

An appropriately sized expanded PTFE tube graft is then used to create a modified Blalock-Taussig shunt (see Fig.

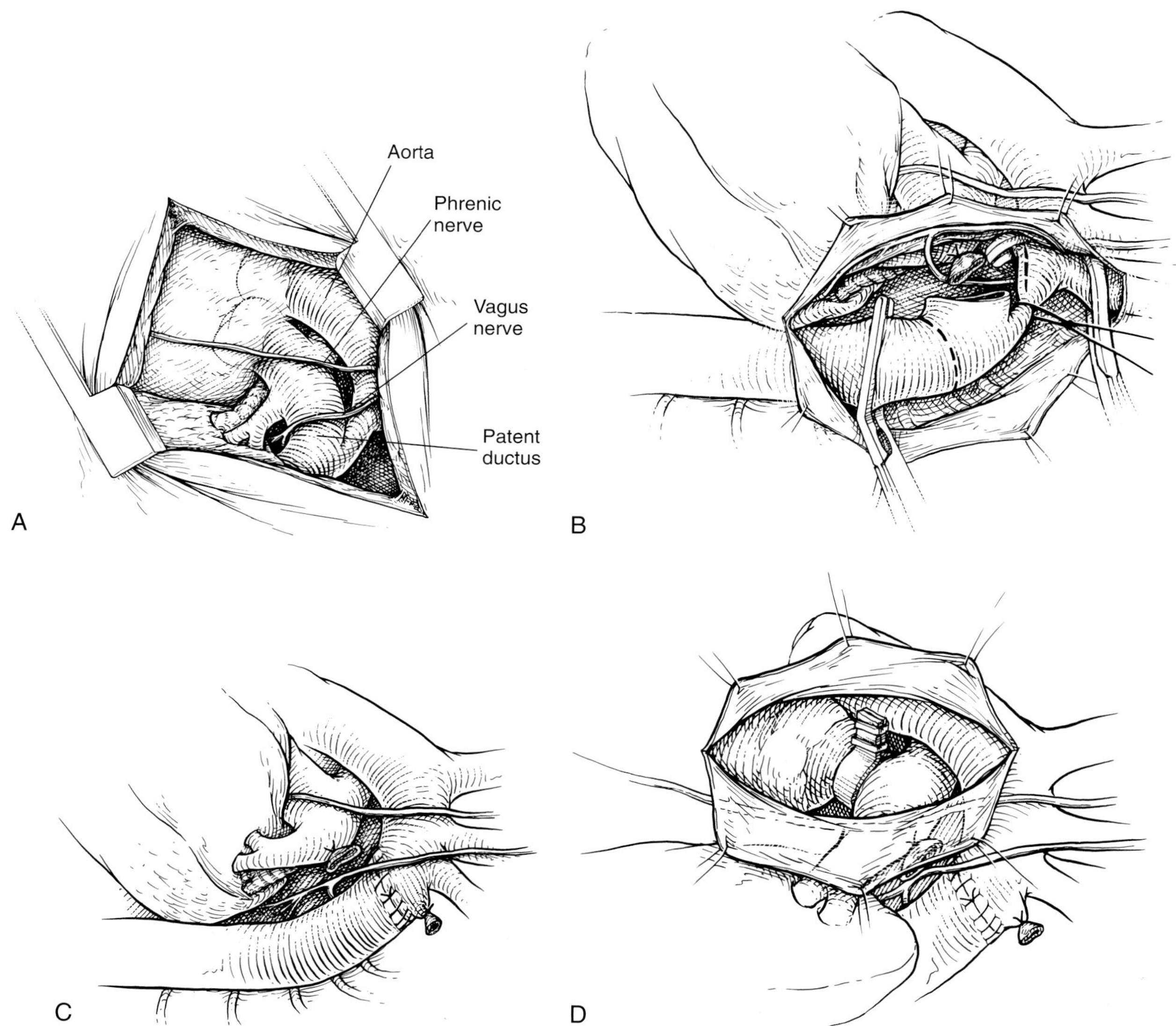

Figure 41-21 Repair of hypoplastic aortic arch and pulmonary trunk band placement via left thoracotomy. **A,** Standard left posterolateral thoracotomy is performed through fourth intercostal space, and ribs are retracted. Adventitia overlying distal aortic arch and left pulmonary artery is shown. Positions of phrenic and vagus nerves are indicated. Large ductus arteriosus is noted, along with severe hypoplasia of aortic isthmus and moderate hypoplasia of distal aortic arch. Great arteries are in transposed position, with aorta anterior and pulmonary trunk posterior. Left lung has been deflated and retracted in an inferior direction. **B,** Adventitia overlying distal aortic arch is opened and retracted with sutures. Aortic arch obstruction is managed in standard fashion for neonatal aortic coarctation (see Section I of Chapter 48 for full discussion of technical and management issues related to aortic arch obstruction in the neonate). After appropriate dissection of aorta and ductus, vascular clamps are placed, and ductus arteriosus is ligated and divided, as is hypoplastic aortic isthmus. All remaining ductal tissue is removed from descending aorta, and a longitudinal incision is made on undersurface of aortic arch *(dashed lines)*. Descending aorta is connected end to side to undersurface of aortic arch between left subclavian and brachiocephalic arteries. **C,** Repaired arch with ligated and divided hypoplastic aortic isthmus and ligated and divided ductus arteriosus. **D,** Inferiorly retracted lung is now repositioned with more direct posterior retraction to better expose proximal intrapericardial great arteries. Incision in pericardial sack is made anterior and parallel to phrenic nerve to expose proximal pulmonary trunk in preparation for placing pulmonary trunk band. Pulmonary trunk is carefully dissected in limited fashion just above tops of pulmonary valve commissures and below origin of right pulmonary artery (see Fig. 41-17). Identification of right pulmonary artery origin may be difficult from the left thoracotomy perspective. Using a small right-angled clamp, circumferential dissection is achieved and a 3-mm-diameter band, taken from a sheet of reinforced silicone rubber, is placed around proximal pulmonary trunk. Band is then tightened and secured to prevent migration, as described in Fig. 41-17.

41-22, *B*). Details of the shunt procedure are similar to those described earlier in this section for isolated neonatal systemic–pulmonary arterial shunt.

Principles of rewarming and separation from bypass are those described in "Completing Cardiopulmonary Bypass" in Section III of Chapter 2. Following separation from CPB, management considerations with regard to pharmacology, physiology, and sternal wound (immediate or delayed sternal closure) are the same as described in the management of hypoplastic left heart physiology following the Norwood procedure (see "Special Features of Postoperative Care" in Chapter 49).

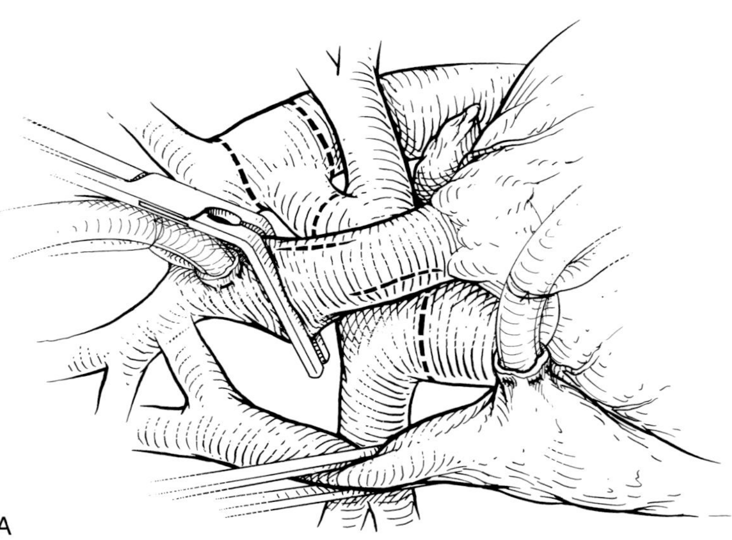

Figure 41-22 Construction of proximal pulmonary trunk to aortic anastomosis (Damus-Kaye-Stansel operation), using continuous cardiopulmonary bypass (CPB), for complex systemic outflow tract obstruction. **A,** Surgical exposure is through median sternotomy, with subtotal resection of thymus gland. Pericardium is opened widely with a longitudinal incision. Great arteries are transposed with a hypoplastic ascending aorta and aortic arch, aortic coarctation, and large ductus arteriosus. Pulmonary trunk is dilated. Great arteries and their branches are dissected in a fashion similar to that performed for interrupted aortic arch (see Technique of Operation in Section II of Chapter 48). Systemic arterial and right atrial cannulation sites for CPB are positioned so that procedure can be performed using continuous CPB. In this illustration, the systemic arterial cannula is placed within the aorta at base of brachiocephalic artery (see text for other sites of cannulation). Dashed lines indicate areas of transection or incision required to create proximal pulmonary trunk–to-aortic anastomosis and repair hypoplastic aortic arch. Standard, moderately hypothermic CPB is established, as are cardiac arrest and cardioplegic myocardial protection. In cases with aortic continuity, as shown, ductus arteriosus is ligated at its pulmonary artery end as bypass is begun. Once target core temperature is achieved on CPB, aorta is clamped as shown and cardioplegia delivered to myocardium. As aortic clamp is placed, systemic perfusion flow is reduced to 30 mL $\cdot$ min^{-1} $\cdot$ kg^{-1} to reflect reduced distribution of flow, which is limited to upper body. Aortic clamp is adjusted to a more superior and oblique position such that perfusion to brachiocephalic and left carotid arteries is unobstructed, and left posterolateral aspect of upper ascending aorta is easily accessible to perform arch reconstruction (see Technique of Operation in Section II of Chapter 48). Operation proceeds by first addressing aortic arch, and then by creating proximal pulmonary trunk–to-aortic anastomosis. All ductal tissue is removed from descending aorta and isthmus, as shown by dashed lines. Left posterolateral aspect of upper ascending aorta is incised along dashed line shown, and descending aorta is connected to ascending aorta end to side, using 7-0 monofilament absorbable suture and a continuous suturing technique. After arch reconstruction is completed, attention is turned to proximal pulmonary trunk–to-aortic reconstruction. Dashed lines on distal pulmonary trunk and on right lateral aspect of proximal ascending aorta represent incisions required to create this anastomosis.

Modified Norwood Anastomosis

The Norwood anastomosis used in this setting is a slight modification of the procedure used in first-stage repair of patients with classic hypoplastic left heart physiology. It combines the Damus-Kaye-Stansel anastomosis with extensive augmentation (enlargement) of the hypoplastic aortic arch and upper descending thoracic aorta (see Chapter 49).[C12,R25] It is important to emphasize that the augmentation patch used is of a slightly different shape from that described for the typical patient with hypoplastic left heart physiology. This is necessary because with either tricuspid atresia and discordant ventriculoarterial connection, or with double inlet ventricle with L-loop and discordant ventriculoarterial connection, orientation of the great arteries is different from that in patients with normally related great arteries (i.e., found in aortic atresia and other classic forms of hypoplastic left heart physiology).

Muscular Resection to Relieve Subaortic Obstruction

This technique is described for patients with tricuspid atresia and discordant ventriculoarterial connection with subaortic obstruction at the bulboventricular foramen (VSD) or incomplete RV, but is applicable to all patients with univentricular AV connection in whom the aorta arises from an incomplete ventricle. Other lesions that result in a similar problem include DILV with discordant ventriculoarterial connection, and mitral atresia with concordant ventriculoarterial connection (see Chapter 56).

Patient preparation, median sternotomy, and cardiac exposure are similar to that described in the preceding text. In the unusual case that there has been no previous surgery, upon opening the pericardium, it is immediately noticed that aorta and diminutive RV are anterior. More commonly, previous surgery (including previous median sternotomy) has been performed. Caution should be exercised upon repeat median sternotomy, because the anterior aorta may be in close proximity to the posterior sternal table. The patient is prepared for CPB by placing purse strings in the ascending aorta just below the brachiocephalic artery origin and in SVC and IVC. Aortic and bicaval cannulation is then performed in standard fashion, the patient is placed on CPB, and moderate hypothermia is achieved. The aorta is clamped, and cardioplegia is administered through the aortic root (see "Single-Dose Cold Cardioplegia in Neonates and Infants" in Chapter 3).

The VSD is best approached through an incision in the incomplete ventricle (outlet chamber) just below the aortic

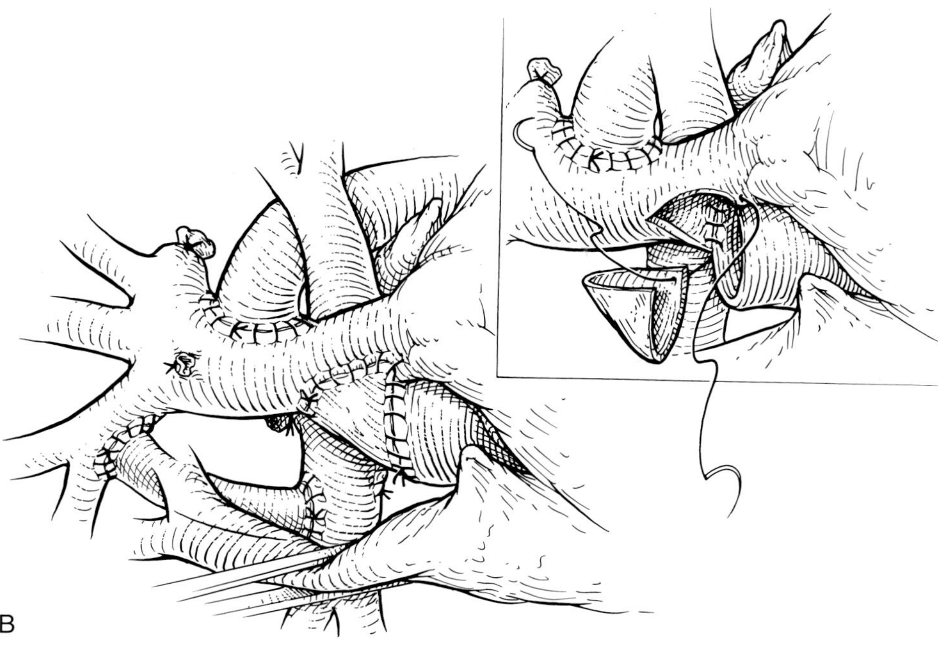

Figure 41-22, cont'd **B,** Pulmonary trunk is transected between sinutubular junction and origin of right pulmonary artery. Opening in distal pulmonary trunk is closed with either a patch or a primary transverse closure using continuous suture technique. Proximal ascending aorta is incised longitudinally on its right lateral aspect beginning just above sinutubular junction and extending to superiorly placed aortic clamp. Proximal end of right lateral aortic incision is extended posteriorly in a circumferential direction at a 90-degree angle from original longitudinal incision to create a posterior aortic flap *(inset)*. Base of this flap is then connected to adjacent posteromedial circumference of transected pulmonary trunk. The anterior-anterolateral component of the aorta-to–pulmonary trunk connection is completed using a patch of pulmonary artery allograft tissue or glutaraldehyde-treated autologous pericardium. To complete the procedure, an appropriately sized expanded polytetrafluoroethylene tube graft is used to create a systemic–pulmonary arterial shunt from brachiocephalic–subclavian artery junction to proximal right pulmonary artery (see "Systemic–Pulmonary Arterial Shunt" under Technique of Operation in Section II). Completed reconstruction is shown.

valve (Fig. 41-23, *A*). This incision is later closed by an enlarging patch.[C17] Alternatively, the VSD may be approached through the aorta; however, this exposure may be limited because the aortic valve and aorta are typically hypoplastic.[N5,S28] Some have considered the risk of surgically induced heart block to be high in this procedure, but risk is substantially reduced using currently available knowledge about the location of the conduction tissue. When the VSD is observed through an incision in the outlet chamber (morphologic RV), the relationship of the conduction system to the VSD is the same as with any conoventricular VSD, with the conduction tissue at the posterior inferior rim of the defect. This is true whether the underlying morphology is tricuspid atresia and discordant ventriculoarterial connection, or double inlet single LV and discordant AV and ventriculoarterial connections.[C17] Confusion regarding this issue has arisen because the conduction system *appears* to be positioned on the "anterior" rim of the VSD when viewed from the perspective of the main ventricular chamber of either tricuspid atresia and discordant ventriculoarterial connection or DILV and discordant AV and ventriculoarterial connections. This confusion is the result of difficulty in conceptualizing the spatial arrangement of the two ventricular chambers and ventricular septum with this exposure, which involves an atrial incision, substantial rotation of the heart, and visualization of the VSD through an AV (typically mitral) valve.

The preferred approach is a vertical incision made in the outlet chamber free wall directly in line with the course of the ascending aorta (see Fig. 41-23, *A*). This incision should be made only after all major coronary artery branches are identified, because the incision should not cut across any of these. Once the outlet chamber has been entered, the VSD is identified and a full-thickness wedge of septum is removed from the anterior and anterior apical aspects of the rim of the defect (Fig. 41-23, *B*).

Obstructing muscle bundles within the outlet chamber are excised. The outlet chamber is enlarged by closing the ventriculotomy with an enlarging patch, typically of polyester or glutaraldehyde-treated pericardium, using running monofilament suture (Fig. 41-23, *C*). The process of separation from bypass and chest closure is standard.

Special Features of Postoperative Care

These are detailed under Special Features of Postoperative Care in Chapter 49.

Results

Pulmonary Trunk Banding and Aortic Arch Reconstruction

In early-era reports, both early and intermediate-term survival have been unfavorable in patients with single-ventricle physiology following initial coarctation repair, with or without pulmonary trunk banding (see Fig. 41-19) (see "Results of Repair of Coarctation in Patients with Other Major

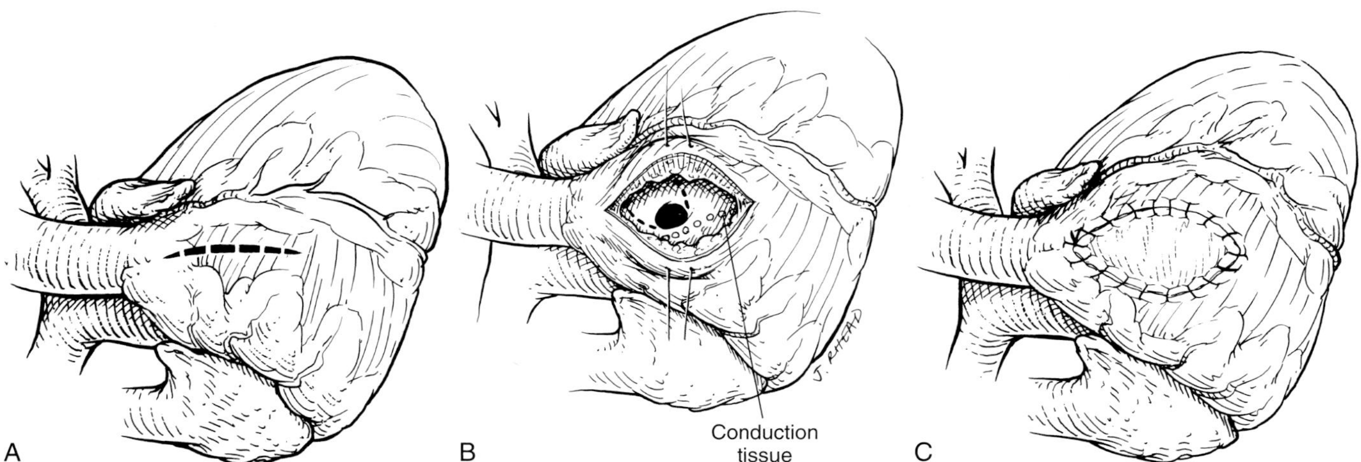

Figure 41-23 Direct relief of subaortic obstruction in univentricular hearts with transposed great arteries. **A,** Median sternotomy exposure and standard cardiopulmonary bypass technique using moderate hypothermia and cardioplegic myocardial protection are utilized. Longitudinal incision in subaortic area of incomplete right ventricular (RV) chamber is used to expose subaortic obstruction. **B,** Internal anatomy of incomplete and hypoplastic RV chamber is shown. Dashed lines show incisions used to resect muscle that result in enlarging the ventricular septal defect (VSD). Wedge of full-thickness septal muscle between these two incisions is removed, taking care to avoid injury to adjacent aortic valve and underlying atrioventricular valve. Position of wedge resection is also designed to avoid conduction tissue positioned along posteroinferior rim of VSD, represented by open circles. **C,** Incision in free wall of incomplete RV is closed with a patch designed to augment subaortic chamber. Patch material can be polyester, glutaraldehyde-treated autologous pericardium, or polytetrafluoroethylene. Care is taken to avoid injury or obstruction to major coronary branches running along free wall of incomplete RV during incision closure.

Coexisting Intracardiac Anomalies" in Section I of Chapter 48). Risk of death early after the procedure has been particularly high (see Fig. 41-20). This may be due to associated instability that accompanies single-ventricle physiology. Although these data are for patients with DILV with arch obstruction, it is likely that similar outcomes pertain to patients with tricuspid atresia and discordant ventriculoarterial connection with aortic arch obstruction. More recent reports show better early and midterm outcomes. Odim and colleagues reported no early mortality (0%; CL 0%-12%) and an 87% survival at mean follow-up of 68 months in 15 patients undergoing aortic arch reconstruction and pulmonary trunk banding.[O5]

Proximal Pulmonary Trunk to Aortic Connection with Arch Repair

This procedure carries a substantial early mortality (≈35%).[R25] Although limited data are available for evaluating it, certain insights can be gained by comparing the Damus-Kaye-Stansel and shunt procedure with the Norwood procedure, because there are important parallels between them (see "First-Stage Reconstruction [Norwood Procedure]" under Results in Chapter 49). Regurgitation of the original aortic or pulmonary valve, either immediate or delayed (perhaps due to distortion of the great arteries), and hemodynamic instability relating to a pulmonary circulation arising from a systemic–pulmonary arterial shunt all can be problems if the Damus-Kaye-Stansel procedure is used in this setting. Despite high early mortality, intermediate-term results in hospital survivors appear to be good.[C8,L21,P7]

Modified Norwood Anastomosis

Early mortality ranges from 0% to 35%.[B24,R25] Reports with better outcomes tend to be from more recent series.[B24] It should be expected that outcomes from the modified Norwood procedure will be somewhat better in this morphologic population compared with patients with aortic atresia and other forms of hypoplastic left heart physiology because of fewer morphologic risk factors.

Muscular Resection to Relieve Subaortic Obstruction

Knowledge of results of this operation is incomplete because of the great heterogeneity of patients receiving it, relatively small experience with it, and lack of complete and long-term follow-up.[A15,C17,G13,R23,S28] Hospital mortality of 11% (CL 1%-33%) has been reported by Cheung and colleagues among 9 patients.[C17] The death occurred in a patient operated on in the first year of life at the time of VSD enlargement. One patient required repeat surgical enlargement. Deaths after hospital dismissal were related to subsequent procedures. More recently, Cerillo and colleagues reported no early mortality after 6 resections (0%; CL 0%-27%).[C9]

Indications for Operation

When designing the appropriate operative procedure, the *status of the aortic arch* must be assessed. If the ascending aorta and arch are widely patent, associated subaortic obstruction is less likely. If obstruction is identified at the aortic arch, the subaortic region must be carefully evaluated because obstruction at this level is commonly present. Accurately evaluating the subaortic region may be difficult in the preoperative setting of a patent ductus arteriosus, because the LV ejects only part of the systemic cardiac output (upper-body component) across the VSD to the aortic valve; the remainder (lower-body output) is delivered from the LV directly across the pulmonary valve and ductus arteriosus to the thoracic aorta. As a result, absence of a gradient (determined either by echocardiography or cardiac catheterization) between LV and aorta is an unreliable gauge of future outflow tract adequacy once the aortic arch is repaired and the ductus arteriosus removed. Under these circumstances, the entire systemic cardiac output must cross the VSD and subaortic region. Because physiologic variables are unreliable, one must rely on morphologic details of the sizes of the VSD, subaortic region, and aortic valve itself in judging adequacy of the LV-to-aortic outflow tract. Echocardiographic characterization of VSD size has been suggested as a predictor of long-term adequacy of the LV outflow tract.[M18]

However, if obstruction is documented preoperatively in this setting, then the systemic LV outflow tract will be clearly inadequate. If so, the operative procedure entails repair of the obstructed aortic arch, creating a proximal pulmonary trunk–to-aortic anastomosis (Damus-Kaye-Stansel procedure) and a systemic–pulmonary arterial shunt. This combination essentially achieves the same result as that achieved by aortic arch reconstruction in the Norwood procedure for hypoplastic left heart physiology (see Indications for Operation in Chapter 49). The Damus-Kaye-Stansel procedure with aortic arch reconstruction, or modifications of Norwood aortic arch reconstruction that some surgeons prefer, can be applied to other forms of univentricular AV connection in the setting of aortic arch and subaortic obstruction, most commonly DILV with discordant ventriculoarterial connection and mitral atresia with VSD and concordant ventriculoarterial connection (see Indications for Operation in Chapter 56).[B26,V4]

For a detailed description of aortic arch reconstruction in hypoplastic left heart physiology, see the description of the Norwood operation under Technique of Operation in Chapter 49. Most forms of aortic arch obstruction in combination with subaortic obstruction occur in the setting of ventriculoarterial discordant connection. Orientation of the great vessels, therefore, is quite different from that in typical hypoplastic left heart physiology. As a result, the Norwood type aortic arch reconstruction is somewhat modified.

SPECIAL SITUATIONS AND CONTROVERSIES

Concordant Ventriculoarterial Connection

Systemic–Pulmonary Arterial Shunt

Site Systemic–pulmonary arterial shunts can be placed at sites on the systemic and pulmonary arterial systems other than that described previously in this chapter. These alternative sites may be chosen for practical reasons relating to individual anatomy or simply surgeon preference. Anatomic variations that may determine site of the shunt include situs inversus, atrial isomerism, right-sided aortic arch, and abnormal arch branching patterns. In patients with small central pulmonary arteries, it may be wise to site the pulmonary arterial anastomosis on the pulmonary trunk segment, if one is present, to avoid distorting or occluding either left or right pulmonary arteries. Regardless of site, the systemic–pulmonary arterial connection is performed using a specific length and diameter of extended PTFE tube graft (see text that follows).

Size Diameter of the expanded PTFE graft is the most important determinant of resistance within a systemic–pulmonary arterial connection and therefore is the prime regulator of $\dot{Q}p$. Other factors, such as graft length and site of origin on the systemic circulation, also influence resistance but to a lesser degree (Poiseuille resistance relationships). Once the appropriate diameter is chosen for the graft, these other factors can be used in individual patients to help further regulate pulmonary blood flow to create the ideal balance between $\dot{Q}p$ and $\dot{Q}s$. A 3.5-kg infant is typically well served using a 3.5-mm-diameter graft connected to the brachiocephalic–right subclavian arterial junction. A larger infant, or one who has particularly small pulmonary arteries or manifests physiology indicative of elevated Rp, might best be served by a similar 3.5-mm tube graft connected directly to the brachiocephalic artery or even ascending aorta. With these adjustments, resistance in the artery giving rise to the tube graft is reduced, and therefore overall resistance across the connection is less, compared with a graft constructed with a more distal (smaller diameter) systemic connection. On the other hand, a smaller infant or one who manifests physiology indicative of very low Rp preoperatively may best be served by a 3.5-mm-diameter graft connected entirely to the right subclavian artery. In this case, the subclavian artery contributes additional resistance to that of the tube graft. A 3-mm-diameter tube graft may be considered in particularly small infants, such as those with a body weight 2.5 to 3 kg or less (see "Type" in text that follows).

Type Technique of Operation in this section describes the preferred modified Blalock-Taussig shunt using an expanded PTFE tube graft. Systemic–pulmonary arterial shunts using direct arterial tissue-to-tissue connection, such as end-to-side connection of the subclavian artery to the RPA (classic Blalock-Taussig shunt),[T2] direct ascending aorta–to-RPA connection (Waterston shunt), descending aorta–to–left pulmonary artery connection (Potts shunt), and central ascending aortic–to–pulmonary trunk connection, are rarely if ever used in the setting of normally developed branch pulmonary arteries. These connections all have disadvantages of unreliable regulation of $\dot{Q}p$ or high prevalence of pulmonary artery distortion.

There is no foolproof formula for choosing optimal shunt diameter and connection to create perfectly balanced $\dot{Q}p$. Careful evaluation of patient size, pulmonary arterial anatomy, and physiologic behavior of the pulmonary vasculature preoperatively, and the surgeon's own experience, all are considerations when choosing size, site, and type of shunt that will best serve an individual patient. A surgeon who typically uses precise and accurate surgical technique will achieve a 3.5-mm orifice at systemic and pulmonary artery anastomoses when a 3.5-mm tube graft is used; one who typically uses less precise and accurate technique will likely create anastomoses at both sites that are smaller than the 3.5-mm tube graft. In this case, a surgeon may come to realize over time that a larger-diameter graft provides the appropriate degree of pulmonary flow.

Aspirin Use Although the use of aspirin following shunt placement is widely practiced, until recently there has been little documented evidence of its efficacy. The recent multicenter study by Li and colleagues[L20] shows that risk of thrombosis and death are both lower when aspirin is used. The study involved a wide range of morphologic lesions, and aspirin daily dosage varied, with 80% of patients receiving 20 to 40 mg $\cdot$ day^{-1}. The efficacy of aspirin did not vary with dosage.

Left Pulmonary Artery Stenosis

Occasionally, infants with this subset of tricuspid atresia have either hypoplasia or a discrete stenosis in the proximal left pulmonary artery in the region of the ductus arteriosus. This lesion will almost certainly become rapidly progressive once PGE_1 infusion is stopped. It is usually prudent to address it at the initial shunt procedure. Individual judgment is required regarding the method of relieving the stenosis. A patch can

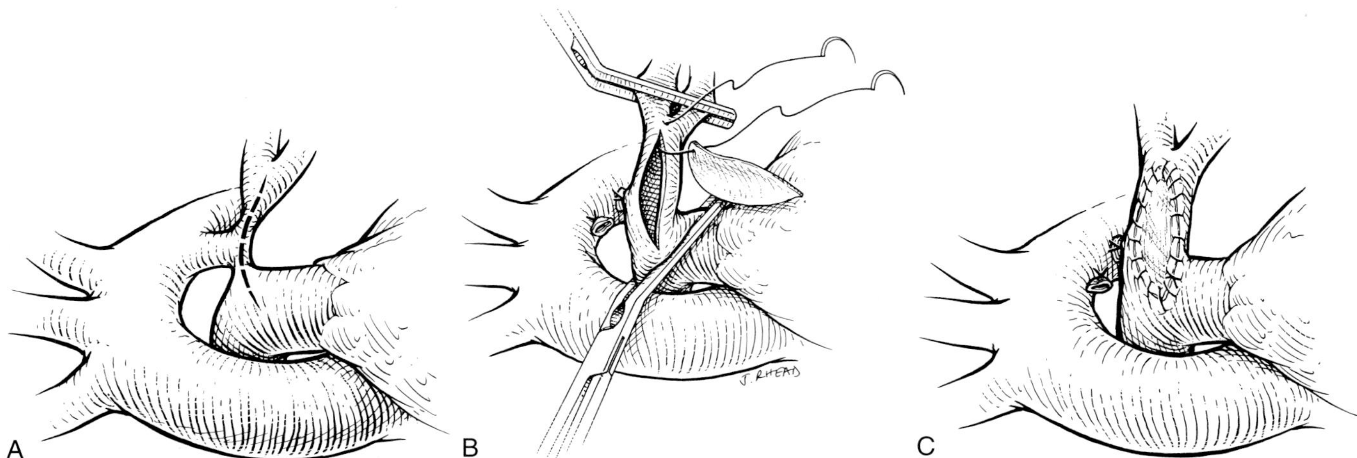

Figure 41-24 Repair of periductal left pulmonary artery (LPA) stenosis in neonate. **A,** Exposure of pulmonary trunk and LPA is shown through a median sternotomy. Ductus arteriosus insertion at site of LPA stenosis is evident. Dashed line represents incision that will be made for patch repair of hypoplastic segment. **B,** After blunt circumferential dissection of ductus arteriosus, 5-0 polypropylene suture ligatures are placed on aortic and pulmonary artery ends of ductus, and it is ligated and divided. Typically, a right modified Blalock-Taussig shunt has already been performed to ensure pulmonary blood flow to right lung while LPA reconstruction is performed (see Fig. 41-16 and further discussion in text). Two vascular clamps isolate LPA. Care is taken to avoid injury to left phrenic nerve. Central clamp is placed at junction of LPA with pulmonary trunk, providing enough tissue sequestered between the two clamps such that entire stenosis can be addressed. LPA is opened with a longitudinal incision across stenotic area and extending well beyond stenosis on each side. This may require incising onto pulmonary trunk. An appropriately fashioned patch of expanded polytetrafluoroethylene is then used to augment LPA. Diameter of patch at maximal area of stenosis should be determined such that luminal area at stenotic point is 40% to 50% larger than normal LPA diameter. Patch is sewn into place beginning distally and moving centrally with a running 7-0 monofilament nonabsorbable suture. **C,** Completed repair is shown, with a widely patent LPA lumen and undistorted lobar pulmonary artery branches.

be placed across the segment of concern (Fig. 41-24), or the segment can be excised and the distal left pulmonary artery reattached to the side of the pulmonary trunk. Either technique can be performed without using CPB, allowing the shunt to perfuse the right lung only during left pulmonary artery reconstruction. Occasionally with more complex central pulmonary artery stenosis, CPB support is necessary to achieve satisfactory reconstruction.

Discordant Ventriculoarterial Connection

Aortic Arch Obstruction without Apparent Subaortic Obstruction

When this subset of tricuspid atresia exists with important aortic arch obstruction but without evidence of clear subaortic obstruction, surgical management in the neonatal period is controversial.[F21] Some surgeons prefer to act on the established observation that presence of aortic arch hypoplasia increases the likelihood of subaortic obstruction, and in all such cases they perform a proximal pulmonary trunk–to-aortic connection (Damus-Kaye-Stansel anastomosis[B26,D3,K11,R25,S33]) with arch reconstruction, or a modified Norwood.[B24,J5] This approach has the advantage of removing uncertainty related to adequacy of LV systemic outflow. Its disadvantages are magnitude and risk of the procedure, which usually involves a prolonged period of CPB, myocardial ischemia, and in many hands, cerebral ischemia. This risk is warranted if subaortic obstruction exists; it may not be warranted if in fact the equivocal subaortic region is adequate.

Thus, some surgeons prefer to make an individual evaluation of the subaortic region. If its morphologic characteristics suggest the LV-to-aortic outflow tract will be adequate, an isolated arch repair and pulmonary trunk band is performed.[K1,M36,O5,R17] The advantage of this approach is that CPB and organ ischemia are avoided, and complexity of the procedure minimized. Acute morbidity and mortality with this operation are clearly lower than with the former approach. The disadvantage, however, is that the subaortic region remains a concern. Therefore, careful and frequent evaluation of the subaortic region, beginning in the immediate postoperative period, must be undertaken.

Mild subaortic obstruction for a short period may not negatively affect function of the single ventricle. Recent evidence suggests that patients with subaortic gradients up to 40 mmHg for up to about a 6-month duration, who initially underwent pulmonary artery banding and only later DKS procedures, did not have negative effects on ventricular function or reduced candidacy for later Fontan.[C14]

Assessment of the subaortic area must be ongoing over the course of the patient's life. If LV-to-aortic outflow obstruction develops, the patient must undergo one of several subsequent procedures to relieve it. If subaortic obstruction occurs in the first several months following aortic arch repair and pulmonary trunk banding, the most appropriate procedure is a proximal aortic–to–pulmonary trunk connection (Damus-Kaye-Stansel anastomosis) and systemic–pulmonary artery shunt. Before this procedure is done, the banded pulmonary trunk must be assessed carefully to confirm that no damage to the pulmonary valve has occurred from the band. Distortion or damage to the pulmonary valve resulting from the banding procedure may increase the chances of important neoaortic regurgitation following the proximal pulmonary trunk–to-aortic connection. When careful attention is given to technical details, competence of the native pulmonary valve can usually be preserved.[D1,F6] If the pulmonary valve is regurgitant, the only remaining surgical alternative is to incise and excise the obstructing subaortic muscle at the level of the VSD and hypoplastic RV chamber. Such a procedure, however, carries an important risk of morbidity in the small infant or neonate with respect to ventricular function and conduction integrity.

If subaortic obstruction develops later in infancy following neonatal arch reconstruction and pulmonary trunk banding, proximal aortic to pulmonary trunk connection (Damus-Kaye-Stansel anastomosis) can be performed at the time of superior cavopulmonary connection, obviating need for a systemic–pulmonary artery shunt. Again, careful evaluation of the adequacy of the pulmonary valve must be undertaken, and the alternative of a subaortic muscle resection must be given consideration.

If subaortic obstruction develops in a patient who previously received arch reconstruction and pulmonary trunk banding as a neonate, and who has subsequently undergone either a superior cavopulmonary shunt or a Fontan procedure, risk/benefit analysis of each of the two procedures that can be used to relieve the obstruction is substantially altered. Forward flow across the pulmonary valve is eliminated or markedly reduced at the time of the superior cavopulmonary shunt and must be eliminated at the time of the Fontan. If subaortic obstruction develops subsequently, long-standing lack of flow across the pulmonary valve, with stasis of the valve cusps, increases concern about its long-term function in the systemic circulation. Muscle resection to enlarge the VSD and subaortic region, although never without morbidity, becomes a more attractive option under these circumstances. In the larger patient, accurate resection at the level of the VSD may relieve obstruction with less risk of injuring the conduction system or major coronary branches in the septum.

Arterial Switch Operation

The technique used for neonates with simple transposition of the great arteries (see "Arterial Switch Operation" under Technique of Operation in Chapter 52) has been described in a limited number of patients with subaortic obstruction complicating the various forms of univentricular AV connection described in this chapter.[F26,F27] This technique has one major disadvantage and as a result is not commonly used. Although the arterial switch itself relieves subaortic obstruction completely, restriction at the VSD and outlet chamber regulates $\dot{Q}p$. Obstruction can be quite variable and, as a result, regulation of $\dot{Q}p$ can be unpredictable, resulting in patient instability or need for further procedures to stabilize or rebalance $\dot{Q}p$.

A single report is the basis for assessing risk of the procedure in this setting.[K3] From this experience, 5 of 6 (83%; CL 54%-98%) critically ill neonates were hospital survivors of the arterial switch procedure (accompanied by aortic arch repair and atrial septectomy), and 4 of the 6 (67%; CL 38%-88%) were still awaiting definitive Fontan operation at the time of the report. No late follow-up of this experience is available.

Other Palliative Operations

Early mortality after palliative procedures discussed in the text that follows should be low. Procedures should not interfere with, and indeed should facilitate, later Fontan operation, and they should provide good long-term palliation for patients in whom the completed Fontan operation is not possible.

Atrial Septectomy

Atrial septectomy, usually performed for patients with mitral atresia, can be performed with low mortality either as an isolated procedure or combined with pulmonary trunk banding or a systemic–pulmonary arterial shunt procedure (see Table 41-2). This success, however, is not universal. Shore and colleagues report a high mortality (23%; CL 10%-41%).[S22]

Hybrid Palliation

The hybrid procedure, initially designed as a neonatal alternative to the Norwood operation for patients with aortic atresia and other forms of hypoplastic left heart physiology (see Chapter 49), has occasionally been applied to other single-ventricle patients with systemic outflow obstruction and unobstructed pulmonary blood flow.[C2]

Other Operations in Neonatal Period

Other operations are indicated for specific physiologic circumstances. These primarily include anomalous pulmonary venous connection and occasionally AV valve regurgitation. Outcomes after surgical management of single-ventricle patients with associated anomalous pulmonary venous connection, especially when obstructed, are poor. Sinzobahamvya and colleagues report 1-year actuarial survival of 31%.[S24] Lodge and colleagues report 1-year survival of 53%, but when transplantation is included, midterm survival without need for transplant is about 25%.[L24]

Section III **Second-Stage Palliation**

CLINICAL FEATURES AND DIAGNOSTIC CRITERIA

The second stage of the three-stage management plan for patients with tricuspid atresia and other forms of single-ventricle physiology has three purposes:

- Eliminate inefficiencies of the completely mixed circulation as early in life as possible
- Correct or eliminate existing morphologic abnormalities before Fontan operation
- Allow for ventricular remodeling in response to the acute reduction in volume load[W4]

Eliminating physiologic inefficiencies of the completely mixed circulation is accomplished by partially separating pulmonary and systemic venous circuits. By directing desaturated SVC blood exclusively into the pulmonary arteries, using a superior cavopulmonary shunt or hemi-Fontan connection, efficiency of gas exchange is improved such that the systemic–pulmonary arterial connection (via either a systemic–pulmonary arterial shunt or pulmonary trunk band) can be eliminated or markedly reduced. This results in dramatic reduction in workload of the single ventricle to a level that approaches that in an intact normal circulation.[A11,J6] The new physiology has important positive implications for improved functional status and long-term preservation of the myocardium.[M2,M16,S10] This is an important consideration because failure of the myocardium is one of the most important causes of long-term morbidity and mortality in single-ventricle patients, both with and without Fontan physiology (see "Cardiomyopathy" under Natural History in Section I).[F15,P2] Reduction in ventricular work is accomplished without compromising gas exchange or SaO_2, which typically remains above 80%. Additionally, diastolic shunt runoff is eliminated, increasing aortic diastolic pressure and improving coronary perfusion.

Considering the beneficial effects of the physiology associated with the superior cavopulmonary shunt compared with that of a completely mixed circulation, it seems prudent to perform the cavopulmonary shunt as soon as it is safe to do so. The major deterrent to performing it in the neonate is elevated pulmonary resistance (Rp) following birth. In theory, the superior cavopulmonary shunt should be possible within 4 to 8 weeks after birth when Rp has decreased to normal. Based on these concepts, there has been a general trend toward performing the superior cavopulmonary shunt in early infancy.[B23,C13,R6,S26] This experience has shown that it can be performed at age 8 to 10 weeks, with morbidity similar to that seen in infants age 6 months and older. However, the experience of one of the authors (Hanley FL: personal communication, 2002) has shown that the procedure is associated with increased morbidity when performed between age 4 and 6 weeks.[R7] This experience shows that the morbidity is not related to persistent elevation in Rp, because pressure in the cavopulmonary system is not elevated. Rather, it is related to unacceptable cyanosis. It thus appears that factors other than elevated Rp, such as poor ventilation/perfusion matching or exaggerated responses in the lung to CPB, may play important roles in determining the lower age limit for safely performing the superior cavopulmonary shunt.

The second purpose for performing the second-stage operation is to correct or eliminate any existing morphologic abnormalities before the Fontan procedure is performed. The second-stage procedure is preventive in this regard. Early removal of the synthetic systemic–pulmonary arterial shunt and creation of a tissue-to-tissue cavopulmonary connection prevent branch pulmonary artery distortion and eliminate any possibility of developing pulmonary vascular obstructive disease. Additionally, the second-stage operation provides the opportunity to correct other malformations such as branch pulmonary artery hypoplasia or stenosis, arch obstruction, subaortic obstruction, AV valve regurgitation, restrictive atrial septum, or anomalous pulmonary venous connection. Careful early attention to these issues preserves and maximizes overall cardiopulmonary function and markedly simplifies the technical procedure at the Fontan operation.

The third purpose of the second-stage operation is to allow for ventricular remodeling, which necessarily occurs with acute reduction in volume loading, to happen prior to the Fontan. Acute volume reduction results in temporary relative ventricular hypertrophy, lower ejection fraction, and diastolic filling abnormalities.[G27,W4] These changes resolve over time. Thus, ventricular mass and function will return toward normal well before the Fontan operation if a second-stage procedure is performed. The acute ventricular changes associated with volume reduction are better tolerated under conditions of the superior cavopulmonary shunt physiology than under conditions of Fontan physiology.

TECHNIQUE OF OPERATION

Preoperative Management

Prior to proceeding with second-stage palliation, assessment with echocardiography, and usually cardiac catheterization, is performed. Echocardiography primarily evaluates existing intracardiac morphologic abnormalities and identifies new or evolving ones, such as AV valve regurgitation or ventricular outlet obstruction. Cardiac catheterization primarily is used to evaluate morphology of pulmonary artery branches and measure Rp, a critically important value in determining the advisability of creating a cavopulmonary shunt (see Indications for Operation later in this section). At catheterization, pulmonary artery pressure can accurately be estimated by measuring pulmonary venous wedge pressure, thus simplifying the procedure.[G25] Recently, some have argued that routine catheterization is not necessary and should be performed only when noninvasive evaluation by echocardiography, computed tomography angiography (CTA), or cardiac MRI suggests that abnormalities of ventricular end-diastolic pressure and Rp are likely to be present.[B30,F5,F9,M31,P16,R19]

Bidirectional Superior Cavopulmonary Shunt

This palliative operation diverts SVC blood from either one or bilateral superior venae cavae to the pulmonary arteries, with preservation of continuity between right and left pulmonary arteries. Usually, patients will have undergone previous palliative procedures involving either a systemic–pulmonary arterial shunt or a pulmonary trunk band. Operation is typically performed through a median sternotomy with or without CPB.

Using Cardiopulmonary Bypass

When CPB is used, the ascending aorta and SVC at the brachiocephalic–jugular vein junction are cannulated, and a calcium-supplemented blood prime is used with either mild or no hypothermia (Fig. 41-25, *A*). After partial bypass is initiated, the heart is allowed to remain beating, and all sources of systemic-to-pulmonary blood flow are controlled. If the decision is made to remove all extra sources of pulmonary blood flow permanently, it can be done at this point. If a systemic–pulmonary arterial shunt is present, it is ligated either with heavy suture material or metal clips and always divided (see Fig. 41-25, *A*). If a pulmonary trunk band is present or any forward flow exits from heart to pulmonary arteries, the pulmonary trunk is transected between vascular clamps, and proximal and distal ends are oversewn with running monofilament suture. Care should be taken to avoid creating a blind pouch when the proximal pulmonary trunk is transected, because this pouch may serve as a nidus for thrombus formation, with the potential for systemic embolization. If the decision is made to keep an extra source of pulmonary blood flow, the systemic–pulmonary arterial shunt is temporarily controlled with vascular clamps, whereas a pulmonary trunk band need not be addressed at this time in the procedure.

Vascular clamps are placed across the SVC at the cavoatrial junction and close to the venous cannulation site. The SVC is transected as it crosses the RPA. The azygos vein is ligated to avoid late decompression of superior cavopulmonary shunt flow into the lower body. The SVC stump attached to the right atrium is oversewn with a running monofilament suture. An appropriately sized partial occlusion vascular clamp is then placed on the cephalad aspect of the RPA, and it is incised over an appropriate length to accommodate the circumference of the transected SVC. If a systemic–pulmonary arterial shunt has been previously placed into the RPA, all shunt material is completely removed from it before creating the anastomosis between SVC and RPA (Fig. 41-25, *B*). An end-to-side anastomosis of SVC to RPA is performed using 7-0 absorbable monofilament suture. The patient is then separated from CPB, and cannulae are removed (Fig. 41-25, *C*). Atrial pressure is monitored with an indwelling catheter, and pulmonary artery pressure is measured before chest closure.

If the patient has a preexisting systemic–pulmonary arterial shunt and the decision is made to allow the shunt to remain patent as an extra source of pulmonary blood flow, it is usually necessary to reduce shunt flow substantially (Fig. 41-25, *E*). It can be reduced by placing either sutures or

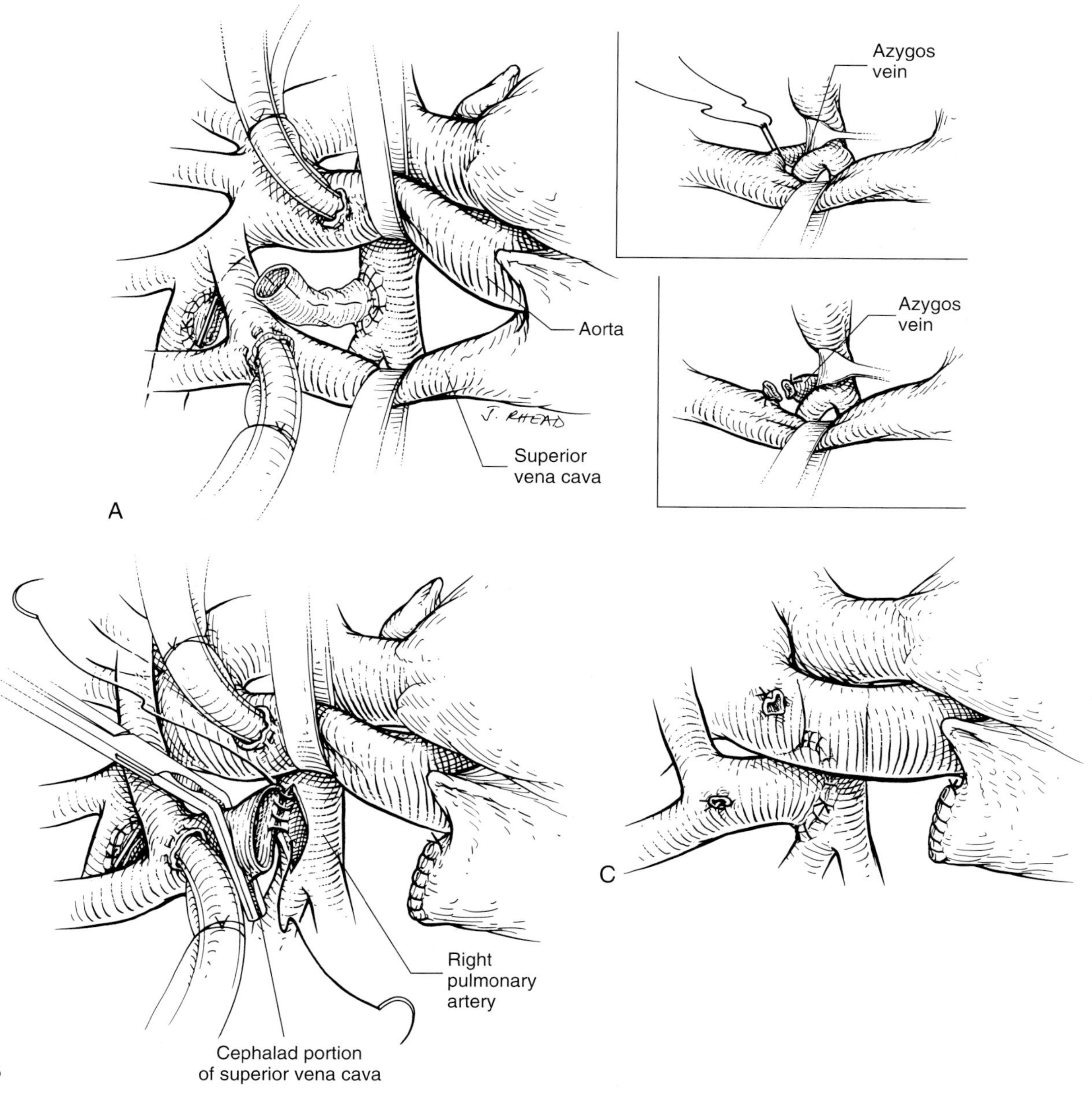

Figure 41-25 Creation of right-sided bidirectional superior cavopulmonary shunt. **A,** Surgical exposure is through a standard median sternotomy as shown. Procedure can be performed on partial cardiopulmonary bypass (CPB), as shown here, by cannulating ascending aorta and cephalad portion of superior vena cava (SVC). At institution of CPB, the dissected and exposed previously placed right subclavian artery–to–pulmonary artery shunt is immediately ligated at its proximal origin and divided. As shown in the two insets, azygos vein is doubly ligated and divided. **B,** SVC has been divided between clamps and cardiac end oversewn with a continuous monofilament suture. Old polytetrafluoroethylene shunt is completely removed from right pulmonary artery (RPA), and RPA opening is enlarged to accommodate diameter of SVC. Cephalad portion of SVC is then connected to RPA end to side using absorbable fine monofilament continuous suture. Posterior aspect of anastomosis is completed first, as shown, followed by anterior component. SVC clamp is then removed, and patient is separated from CPB in standard fashion. **C,** Completed procedure.

Continued

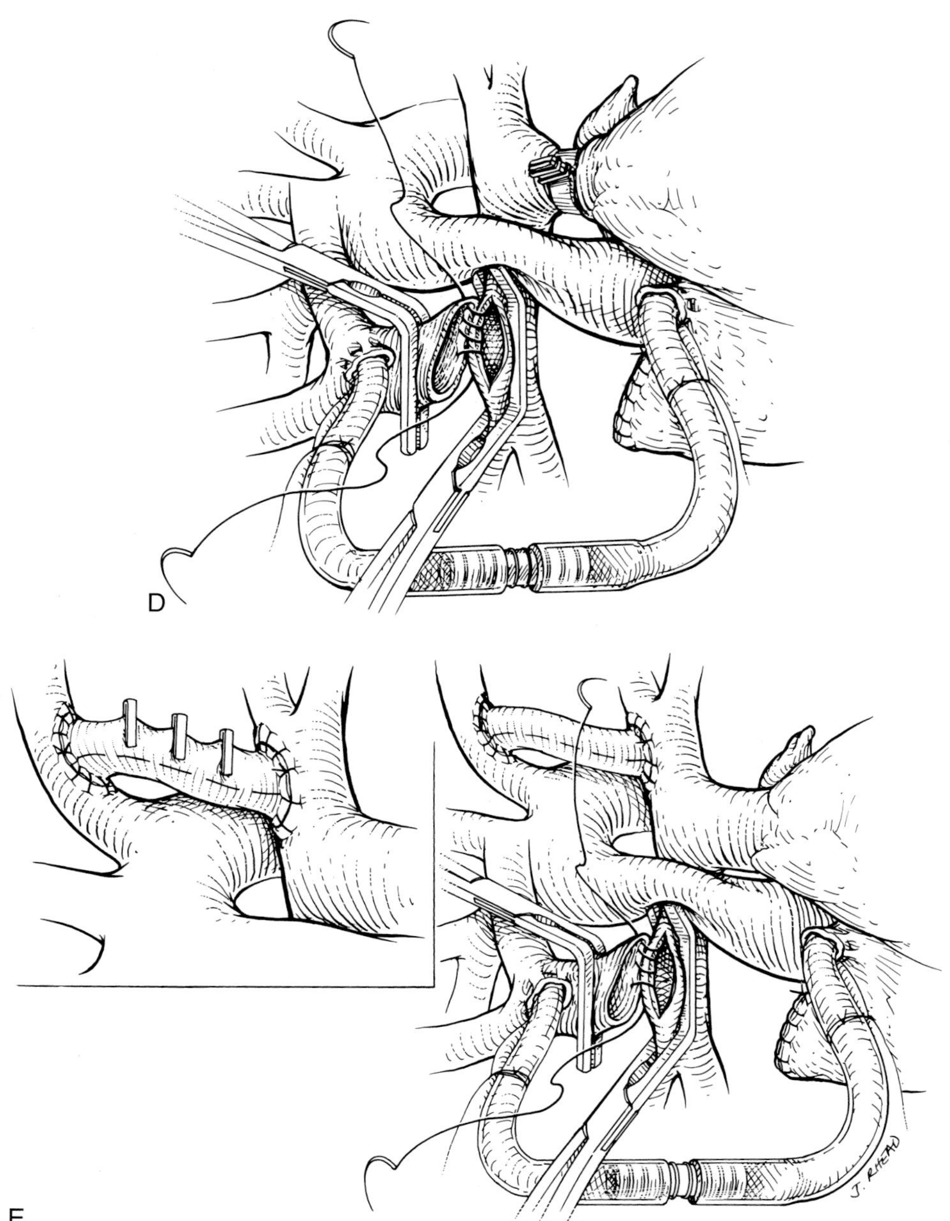

Figure 41-25, cont'd **D,** Illustration of one of many conditions that allow this shunt to be performed without CPB. Exposure is through median sternotomy. Previously placed pulmonary trunk band is shown. After mobilizing SVC and RPA, two appropriately sized right-angled venous cannulae are inserted into SVC at brachiocephalic–jugular vein junction and into right atrial appendage. They are carefully de-aired and connected together following full heparinization to provide continuous SVC-to–right atrial flow while creating the SVC-to-RPA anastomosis. After cannulae are secured and flow established through them, vascular clamps are placed on SVC just inferior to upper cannula and at SVC–right atrial junction. SVC is transected as it crosses over RPA. Transected cardiac end of SVC is oversewn with a continuous monofilament suture. A partial occlusion clamp is placed on superior aspect of RPA, taking care not to disrupt forward flow through pulmonary trunk band site to left pulmonary artery, and an incision is made in sequestered portion of RPA to accommodate circumference of SVC. SVC is connected end to side to RPA using a fine absorbable monofilament suture with continuous technique. Upon completion of anastomosis, SVC and RPA clamps are removed, and caval and right atrial cannulae are clamped and removed, establishing bidirectional superior cavopulmonary shunt–to–pulmonary artery flow. Based on patient's hemodynamic response, pulmonary trunk band is further tightened, or pulmonary trunk is completely occluded (see text for full discussion of factors involved in this decision). **E,** Similar to **D**, except that existing pulmonary blood source is through a left modified Blalock-Taussig shunt rather than from forward flow across banded pulmonary trunk. Reconstruction proceeds exactly as in **D**, except that at completion of procedure, after physiologic assessment of patient has been made, shunt is modified appropriately or eliminated using medium-sized metal clips (see text for full discussion of factors involved in shunt management at time of bidirectional superior cavopulmonary shunt). As shown in inset, shunt diameter is narrowed using several metal clips.

metal clips along the length of the shunt to partially reduce its internal diameter. Shunt flow can be reduced in a quantitative fashion by carefully observing changes in hemodynamics as shunt diameter is narrowed, and by adhering to the following process. Preoperative catheterization data are reviewed, and thus the surgeon has a good idea of amount of flow through the shunt under baseline preoperative conditions. After the bidirectional superior cavopulmonary shunt is completed and the patient removed from CPB and in a hemodynamic steady-state, the change in systemic diastolic blood pressure that occurs when the temporarily occluded shunt is opened is observed. This maneuver can be repeated several times to get a reliable measurement. The shunt can then be permanently narrowed to achieve a diastolic blood pressure at a level between the two values observed when the shunt was completely open and when it was occluded. This provides a semiquantitative estimate of reduction in shunt flow. Additional information that can be used to adjust the extra source of flow is absolute pressure within the SVC and pulmonary arteries following the bidirectional superior cavopulmonary shunt. As a general rule, mean pulmonary arterial pressures should be less than 15 mmHg, and pulse pressure in the pulmonary artery should be less than 5 mmHg.

If the preexisting source of pulmonary blood flow was through a pulmonary trunk band or stenotic pulmonary valve and it is decided to leave this as an extra source of flow, it is usually necessary to adjust the band or further narrow the pulmonary trunk after creating the bidirectional cavopulmonary anastomosis. Changes in systemic diastolic blood pressure are insensitive indicators of changes in flow across a pulmonary trunk band; measuring distal mean pulmonary artery pressure and pulsatility responses with the band site open and with it temporarily occluded is the best way to adjust flow across the pulmonary valve or pulmonary trunk band. The standard method for placing and adjusting a pulmonary trunk band is used (see Fig. 41-21, *D*).

Without Using Cardiopulmonary Bypass

When CPB is not used, it is prudent to decompress the upper-body venous system while creating the cavopulmonary anastomosis if a single SVC is present. Before placing venous cannulae, the patient is fully heparinized (3 mg · kg^{-1}). Two venous cannulae are placed, one in the SVC and the other in the right atrial appendage, de-aired, and connected together (Fig. 41-25, *D*).

If bilateral SVCs are present, decompression is usually not needed. If the preexisting source of pulmonary blood flow is either a right- or left-sided systemic–pulmonary arterial shunt, the operation proceeds by creating the first cavopulmonary anastomosis on the side opposite the preexisting source of pulmonary blood flow. Once this anastomosis is completed, it can serve as an adequate source of pulmonary blood flow while the systemic–pulmonary arterial shunt is removed in preparation for creating the second cavopulmonary connection on the side where the shunt existed.

Hemi-Fontan Operation

The hemi-Fontan operation is physiologically similar to a bidirectional superior cavopulmonary shunt, but important differences exist. The hemi-Fontan requires hypothermic CPB and cardiac arrest because it is an open cardiac procedure, technical details of the operation are more complex, and potential for sinoatrial node injury is increased.[D23] Some surgeons prefer the hemi-Fontan operation because it is believed that this procedure makes a subsequent lateral tunnel Fontan simpler to perform.[D23,J6] Others who use the lateral tunnel Fontan prefer the bidirectional superior cavopulmonary shunt. If the subsequent Fontan operation will be an extracardiac conduit Fontan, the hemi-Fontan operation provides no advantage.

The hemi-Fontan operation consists of diverting SVC flow to the pulmonary arteries by creating a right atrial–to-RPA anastomosis. After CPB, hypothermia, and cardiac arrest are achieved in standard fashion, an incision in the roof of the right atrium is spiraled onto the back of the SVC (Fig. 41-26, *A*). A complementary incision is made on the caudad aspect of the RPA, and the two structures are sewn together to complete the anastomosis (Fig. 41-26, *B-C*). A right atrial free-wall incision is made, and a pulmonary allograft patch is placed inside the superior aspect of the right atrium, partitioning the inferior vena caval, coronary sinus, and pulmonary venous flow from the hemi-Fontan anastomosis (Fig. 41-26, *D*). A large atrial septal opening is created if necessary, and any central pulmonary artery abnormalities may be corrected at the same procedure. Managing preexisting sources of pulmonary blood flow is similar to that described in the preceding text for the bidirectional superior cavopulmonary shunt. Upon completion of the Fontan operation, if a lateral tunnel Fontan is to be used, the intraatrial patch is removed, and the lateral tunnel baffle can be easily placed while working solely within the right atrium.

The hemi-Fontan operation can be simplified by performing a standard bidirectional superior cavopulmonary shunt and connecting the cardiac stump of the transected SVC into the caudad surface of the RPA. The procedure is completed within the right atrium by placing a patch over the right atrial–SVC orifice.[S22] Although this modification simplifies the surgical anastomosis, it also requires hypothermic CPB and cardiac arrest, because it is an open cardiac procedure. At the time of the Fontan operation, the intraatrial patch is removed.

SPECIAL FEATURES OF POSTOPERATIVE CARE

In general, care is routine. Hemodynamics are typically stable. The patient should be positioned with the head elevated 30 degrees because of the elevated SVC pressure. Aggressive pulmonary toilet is particularly important because important desaturation can occur with this physiology if gas exchange is not efficient. The hematocrit should be maintained at 45% at least. Duration of mechanical ventilation should be minimized; however, while the patient is mechanically ventilated, care should be taken to keep Pa_{CO_2} at approximately 45 mmHg.

RESULTS

Bidirectional Superior Cavopulmonary Shunt

Hospital mortality is about 5% to 10%.[B23,C13,L8,M1,M16,R6] However, this may partly reflect additional risk from concomitant procedures. Early palliation has generally been excellent, with Sa_{O_2} averaging 85%.[B28,L8,M25] Midterm results can be estimated from only limited data, because currently

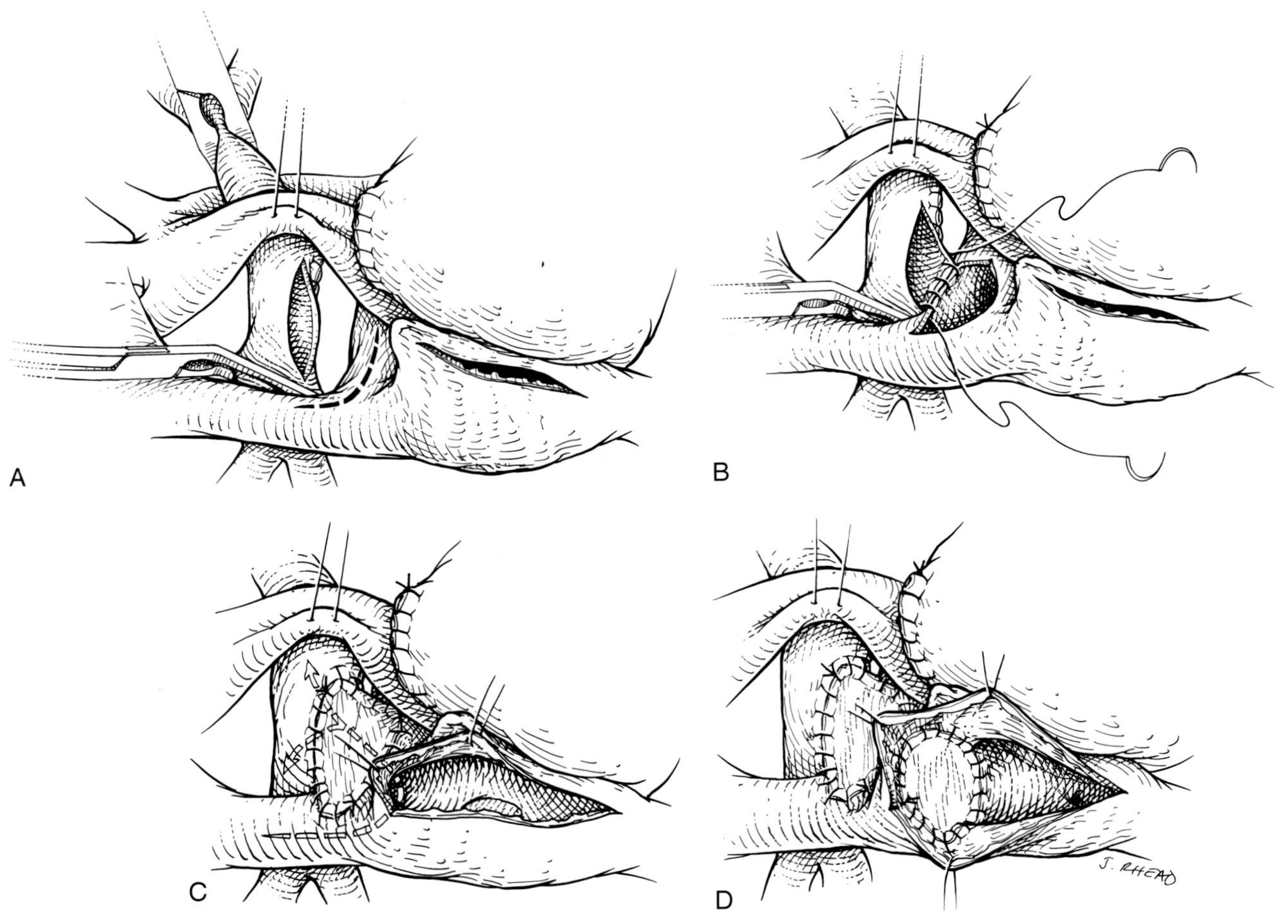

Figure 41-26 Hemi-Fontan operation. **A,** Full-flow cardiopulmonary bypass (CPB), hypothermia, and cardiac arrest with cardioplegia are required for this procedure. Pulmonary trunk has been divided and proximal portion oversewn with a running monofilament suture. Opening in transected distal pulmonary trunk is also oversewn. Branch pulmonary arteries are controlled with vascular clamps or snares. Incision is made on inferior surface of right pulmonary artery (RPA) where it lies adjacent to superior vena cava (SVC) and dome of right atrial chamber. Dome of right atrium and undersurface of SVC are opened by a spiral incision along dashed line as shown. **B,** Posterior row of anastomosis between right atrium and RPA is made using running monofilament absorbable suture. **C,** Anterior portion (roof) of anastomosis is completed by incorporating a patch of pulmonary allograft, as shown here. This creates a wide pathway that will conduct SVC blood to pulmonary arteries along dashed line illustrated. Separate incision in free wall of right atrium is made. **D,** Another patch of pulmonary allograft tissue is used to close orifice of SVC in right atrium. This effectively isolates the SVC-to–pulmonary artery pathway, allowing inferior vena caval, pulmonary venous, and coronary sinus blood to pass directly to systemic circulation. Right atrial incision is then closed.

most patients receiving a bidirectional Glenn procedure go on to a Fontan operation. Available reports suggest 1-year survival of about 90% and 5-year survival of more than 80%.[A8,H8,P17] Risk factors for death include elevated pulmonary artery pressure, total anomalous pulmonary venous connection, heterotaxy, RV morphology, AV valve regurgitation, and very young age.[A8,R6,S5,S23] Age between 2 and 6 months and bidirectional superior cavopulmonary shunt as a second-stage operation in appropriately selected patients are not risk factors for death.[C13,P14,R6]

Risk factors for prolonged intensive care and hospital stays include length of CPB, RV morphology, elevated central venous pressure, elevated transpulmonary gradient, and low weight for age at the time of the procedure.[A13,K22]

The operation facilitates, more so than the classic Glenn operation, a subsequent completed Fontan operation, because the RPA has not been divided. In patients not suitable for the completed Fontan operation, long-term palliation, although not known, will probably be similar to that achieved by the classic Glenn operation (see "Classic Glenn Operation" under Special Situations and Controversies in Section I).

Hemi-Fontan Operation

Early mortality for the hemi-Fontan operation is in the range of 5% to 10%.[D23,J6] The operation considerably facilitates the subsequent procedure of conversion to the lateral tunnel form of completed Fontan procedure, but does not facilitate conversion to the extracardiac conduit form. There is evidence that the hemi-Fontan compromises sinus node function at least temporarily.[C28]

INDICATIONS FOR OPERATION

Second-Stage Palliation

Although there is no absolute indication for the bidirectional superior cavopulmonary shunt or hemi-Fontan as the second stage of a three-stage plan to completion Fontan, it is widely believed that the second-stage procedure is beneficial and therefore indicated in most patients with single-ventricle physiology[M15,S3,S10] (see "General Plan for Surgical Management of Single-Ventricle Physiology" in Section I). The procedure should be performed between age 3 and 6 months to achieve maximum benefit. The bidirectional superior cavopulmonary shunt and hemi-Fontan achieve the same physiologic result; however, morbidity of the two procedures may be different (see "Hemi-Fontan Operation" under Technique of Operation in this section). If an extracardiac conduit Fontan is contemplated, the bidirectional superior cavopulmonary shunt is the clear choice for the second-stage procedure, whereas if a lateral tunnel Fontan is contemplated, the hemi-Fontan may produce certain technical advantages.

Generally accepted contraindications to the procedure are:

- Age younger than 6 weeks
- Mean pulmonary artery pressure greater than 30 mmHg regardless of Rp
- Rp greater than 4 units · m^2
- Pulmonary venous obstruction

These must be eliminated or corrected, sometimes with interim surgical or interventional procedures, before proceeding with the superior cavopulmonary shunt or hemi-Fontan. A recent study suggests that patients with baseline (room air) Rp as high as 6 units · m^2 can successfully undergo a superior cavopulmonary anastomosis if the Rp falls to less than 3.5 units · m^2 in 100% oxygen, albeit with increased risk of death.[H22] Inhaled nitric oxide may be beneficial in such high-risk cases.[A3]

Bidirectional Superior Cavopulmonary Shunt as Primary Procedure

Patients who are not dependent on the ductus arteriosus for pulmonary blood flow, who maintain SaO_2 greater than 70% to 75%, and who do not have excessive $\dot{Q}p$ with pulmonary hypertension (mean pulmonary artery pressure > 25 mmHg) or failure to thrive may be considered for a primary bidirectional superior cavopulmonary shunt at about age 8 weeks.

SPECIAL SITUATIONS AND CONTROVERSIES

Three-Stage Palliation Plan

The three-stage surgical plan is neither mandatory nor universally practiced. Some centers selectively choose patients for the Fontan procedure following neonatal (first-stage) palliation only, whereas others routinely follow the three-stage plan. Currently, however, it is most commonly held that advantages of the second-stage bidirectional superior cavopulmonary shunt outweigh its disadvantages.[M25,P17] Its main advantages are described at the beginning of this section. Additionally, evidence suggests that other complex measures of ventricular mechanics improve following the second-stage procedure.[T4,T5] Disadvantages cited by some include acute surgical risks of an additional procedure, inadequate pulmonary artery growth under conditions of low $\dot{Q}p$, development of aortopulmonary collateral vessels in response to low $\dot{Q}p$ and cyanosis, development of abnormal venovenous channels, and formation of intrapulmonary arteriovenous malformations[B12,G8,I1,M32,S30] Important controversy exists regarding the clinical relevance of many of these disadvantages. It is generally believed, however, that the mortality risk (which is low) associated with the bidirectional superior cavopulmonary shunt is outweighed by its benefits, pulmonary artery size (diameter) may not correlate with Fontan outcome, and pulmonary artery growth may continue relatively normally following the shunt. Also, it is recognized that both acquired aortopulmonary collaterals and intrapulmonary arteriovenous malformations usually form gradually and in a small fraction of patients.[F14,R8] As a result, interventional catheterization or an early Fontan procedure, when necessary, can eliminate or minimize these developments in most patients.[B20]

Retaining Additional Source of Pulmonary Blood Flow

Another important management issue at the time of the second-stage procedure is whether to retain an additional source of pulmonary blood flow along with the bidirectional superior cavopulmonary shunt.[F29] Proponents of this practice argue that a controlled extra source of flow can provide a "normal" ($\dot{Q}p/\dot{Q}s$ of 1) or close to normal amount of flow to the lungs, promoting normal pulmonary artery growth and possibly providing necessary humoral or hemodynamic factors (flow and pulsation) to eliminate or reduce the tendency for developing aortopulmonary collaterals and intrapulmonary arteriovenous malformations, with few or no ill effects.[B10,C7,Y6] Opponents make two points:

- Even if the extra flow causes pulmonary artery growth and reduces collateral formation, there is no clinical benefit in terms of eventual Fontan candidacy or outcome.[C24,G23,S6]
- Evidence exists that morbidity is increased and that an extra source of flow continues to place an increased, albeit limited, volume load on the single ventricle.[L7,M5]

Although the controversy is unresolved, a middle ground with appropriate patient selection and operative management might well maximize overall outcome. For example, patients with RV morphology, reduced ventricular function, or a common or regurgitant AV valve might best be managed without an extra source of pulmonary blood flow, based on careful risk/benefit analysis. On the other hand, patients with normal ventricular function, especially those with LV morphology or two ventricles, normally formed and competent AV valves, small pulmonary arteries, or certain forms of heterotaxy syndrome (that predispose to forming intrapulmonary AV malformations) might benefit from a carefully constructed extra source of pulmonary blood flow that augments $\dot{Q}p/\dot{Q}s$ by an accurately determined additional 0.3 to 0.5.

Use of Cardiopulmonary Bypass

It has been shown that the superior cavopulmonary anastomosis can be created safely without the use of CPB.[H23,L23] The decision regarding use of CPB is based on several practical considerations. Avoiding CPB is an option if an existing source of pulmonary blood flow can be maintained while the bidirectional superior cavopulmonary shunt is being constructed,[L8] such as when the original source of pulmonary blood flow is a pulmonary artery band, central shunt, or shunt placed on the opposite side of the proposed bidirectional superior cavopulmonary shunt, or when bilateral superior venae cavae are present. When one of these exists, surgeon preference determines whether to use CPB or to avoid it. Even when these conditions do not exist, techniques have been devised to avoid bypass (see Fig. 41-25, *D-E*).[M48]

The only situation in which CPB is absolutely necessary is when there is a single source of preexisting pulmonary blood flow through a systemic–pulmonary arterial shunt that is positioned such that the shunt must be completely removed to perform the bidirectional superior cavopulmonary shunt. This situation is commonly present when the SVC is unilateral and on the right side and the patient has received a previous right-sided modified Blalock-Taussig shunt.

Section IV Third-Stage Palliation (Fontan Operation)

CLINICAL FEATURES AND DIAGNOSTIC CRITERIA

In typical three-stage surgical palliation for patients with tricuspid atresia, as well as for other forms of single-ventricle physiology, the patient presents for the Fontan procedure having already undergone a bidirectional superior cavopulmonary shunt or a hemi-Fontan procedure. At the Fontan operation, all IVC blood flow is directed into the pulmonary circulation, leaving only pulmonary venous blood and coronary sinus blood to return to the common atrial chamber and single ventricle. Thus, this operation achieves almost complete separation of systemic and pulmonary circulations. Some centers routinely create a separate communication between systemic and pulmonary venous circulations (adjustable ASD, or fenestrated Fontan). In certain circumstances, this may provide a hemodynamic benefit, although it is achieved at the expense of increased mixing of desaturated blood with pulmonary venous return, thereby reducing SaO_2.

At the time of the Fontan operation, other morphologic and hemodynamic issues may also require attention. If any systemic–pulmonary arterial connections exist, either natural or surgically created, every effort must be made to eliminate them, either at operation or by the interventional cardiologist at the time of preoperative cardiac catheterization. Additionally, other issues such as distortion or hypoplasia of branch pulmonary arteries, AV valve regurgitation, obstruction at any level in the systemic circulation, and abnormal systemic venoatrial connections should be addressed at the time of the Fontan.

In some cases, patients have not previously undergone typical first-stage neonatal palliation and second-stage bidirectional superior cavopulmonary shunt. Sometimes only one or the other of these procedures has been performed, and occasionally no previous surgical intervention has been required. If a bidirectional superior cavopulmonary shunt has not been performed, it is performed at the Fontan operation along with the IVC-to–pulmonary artery connection.

Preoperative Evaluation

Standard preoperative evaluation involves cardiac catheterization and echocardiography.[N1] Echocardiography is performed primarily to evaluate ventricular function and define details of intracardiac anatomy and physiology such as AV valve morphology and function. Cardiac catheterization is performed for two reasons:

- As a *diagnostic study* to evaluate morphology and hemodynamics that cannot be directly assessed by echocardiography. These include morphology of the distal pulmonary arterial system, which is assessed by angiography, and hemodynamic variables, including atrial filling pressure, ventricular end-diastolic pressure, pulmonary artery pressure, $\dot{Q}p$, $\dot{Q}s$, and systemic vascular resistance (Rs) and pulmonary vascular resistance (Rp). These data are used to select appropriate patients to undergo the Fontan operation and provide details for designing the operation. The specific physiologic data used to select patients for the Fontan operation are discussed under Indications for Operation later in this section.
- To determine whether any *cardiologic intervention* will be needed before surgery. Potential interventional procedures include closing systemic–pulmonary arterial shunts, systemic–pulmonary artery collateral vessels, and systemic venoatrial connections, as well as balloon dilatation or stenting of peripheral pulmonary arteries or aortic coarctation.

Recently, some have argued that routine catheterization is unnecessary; in their view, catheterization should be performed only when noninvasive evaluation by echocardiography, CT, angiography, and cardiac MRI suggest that abnormalities of end-diastolic pressure and pulmonary vascular resistance are likely to be present.[F5,F9,P16,R19] Currently, this approach is taken by only a small minority of programs that manage Fontan patients. (The approach is taken somewhat more frequently during preoperative evaluation prior to the superior cavopulmonary anastomosis.) An important argument for preoperative catheterization is that acquired aortopulmonary collaterals develop in essentially all patients with single-ventricle physiology and present a potential volume load on the single ventricle. These can be coil occluded at the time of catheterization. Although there is universal acknowledgment of the development of these collaterals, opinions differ regarding their clinical significance.[B22,K2,M28,S38]

In patients with prior atriopulmonary Fontan and atrial dysrhythmias, formal electrophysiologic evaluation is performed preoperatively.

TECHNIQUE OF OPERATION

Fontan connection can be achieved in a number of ways. Currently, the two most frequently used methods are the *extracardiac conduit* and *lateral tunnel total cavopulmonary connections*. The Society of Thoracic Surgeons (STS) Congenital Heart Database indicates that as of 2009, about two thirds of Fontans are of the extracardiac conduit type.[J8] In their classic forms, both include a bidirectional superior cavopulmonary shunt or hemi-Fontan. The *atriopulmonary* connection, formerly the most frequently performed Fontan variant, is no longer considered a first-line option because of its related complications.

Other recently described techniques for creating the IVC-to–pulmonary artery connection are options.[G27,H24,O6,V5] They include the extracardiac lateral tunnel technique,[L17] extracardiac pericardial tube technique,[G27,K7,P3,W13,Y2] and direct IVC-to–pulmonary trunk connection. The latter is applicable only in a limited number of patients who have morphology favorable for a direct tissue-to-tissue connection. These procedures are not yet widely embraced.

Experimental evidence using computational fluid dynamics suggests that a Y-graft extracardiac conduit demonstrates better flow characteristics, during both rest and exercise, than a single tube either with or without an offset between IVC and SVC connections.[M13] This design has not been tested clinically, and concerns about thrombosis in the smaller-diameter limbs of the graft remain a concern at present.

Extracardiac Conduit Fontan Operation

Preparations for operation and median sternotomy are generally as described under "Incision" in Section III of Chapter 2. Operative technique is described for the patient with tricuspid atresia who has previously undergone neonatal palliation and subsequent second-stage palliation with a bidirectional cavopulmonary shunt. However, the general operative plan can be applied to all patients with single-ventricle physiology who have undergone similar neonatal and second-stage palliation. Details of the procedure require modifications appropriate to morphology, such as atrial isomerism, situs inversus, interrupted IVC, and distortions in pulmonary artery, systemic venous, or pulmonary venous systems. Techniques applicable to these morphologic variations are discussed in other chapters.

It is particularly important for the skin overlying the femoral vessels to be prepped into the surgical field. This is prudent for the usual reasons relating to reoperative sternotomy, but also because in some patients, especially those weighing more than 20 kg, peripheral venous cannulation may simplify the surgical procedure (see "Cardiopulmonary Bypass Established by Peripheral Cannulation" in Section III of Chapter 2).

After median sternotomy, complete dissection of the previously created superior cavopulmonary shunt and pulmonary artery system out to the hilum bilaterally is performed, including the pulmonary artery segment under the ascending aorta (Fig. 41-27, *A*). It is important to mobilize any adhesions around right-sided pulmonary veins as they enter the left atrium. The RPA is mobilized beyond the origin of the right upper lobe pulmonary artery such that it and lower-lobe pulmonary arteries are clearly identified circumferentially (see Fig. 41-27, *A*). A standard arterial purse string is placed in the ascending aorta and, in patients weighing less than 20 kg, a purse string is placed in the IVC at the reflection of the diaphragm.

If the intrathoracic segment of the IVC is relatively short, it may be necessary to take down the diaphragmatic reflection onto the IVC to place the purse string as low as possible. For patients weighing more than 20 kg, the option of cannulating the femoral vein for venous drainage of the IVC system is a reasonable option. The patient is then fully heparinized (3 mg · kg^{-1}). Usually the upper anastomosis of the Fontan connection can be performed before instituting CPB.

A segment of central pulmonary trunk and RPA proximal to the previously placed bidirectional superior cavopulmonary shunt is isolated in preparation for the upper anastomosis. This is accomplished without interrupting flow from the SVC to right lung by placing a vascular clamp obliquely across the peripheral RPA close to the bidirectional superior cavopulmonary shunt anastomosis, such that a long segment of the inferior (caudal) aspect of the pulmonary trunk and RPA is isolated. The left pulmonary artery is clamped on the left side of the ascending aorta (Fig. 41-27, *B*). This completely isolates the central pulmonary artery system. In some cases, it may be necessary to disconnect the pulmonary trunk from the heart if this has not been done previously. The inferior (caudal) surface of the central pulmonary trunk and RPA is then opened, beginning in the periphery at approximately the level of the previously placed bidirectional superior cavopulmonary shunt and extending it centrally to the pulmonary trunk beneath the ascending aorta.

A PTFE tube graft is then selected to create the extracardiac conduit. The tube graft should be at least 2 cm in diameter and larger if possible, to accommodate growth to adulthood. Placing large conduits in small children may create IVC–conduit diameter mismatch, raising concerns about flow disruption and thrombosis. A 2-cm graft generally fits nicely in children who weigh 15 kg or more, although there can be wide variation in IVC diameter for the same body surface area.[A9] Akio and colleagues have reported a series of extracardiac conduits in patients weighing less than 10 kg without an increase in morbidity (see "Timing of Fontan Operation" under Indications for Operation later in this section).[I3] In patients who weigh more than 20 kg, a 22- or even 24-mm PTFE tube graft can easily be accommodated. Itatani and colleagues argue that smaller-diameter conduits (16 to 18 mm) provided superior flow characteristics when studied 1 year postoperatively in 3-year-old patients[I8]; however, there are concerns that these conduits may be of inadequate size as these children grow.

Before creating the proximal anastomosis, the PTFE graft is beveled such that the free edge of the graft matches the length of the extensive incision in the right and central pulmonary arteries. In this way, the proximal anastomosis can also be used to patch-augment any central pulmonary artery distortion or hypoplasia. Occasionally the proximal anastomosis must be extended across the central pulmonary artery to the left pulmonary artery if there is proximal left pulmonary artery stenosis. This can easily be accomplished, because the left pulmonary artery is controlled by a vascular clamp at the left hilum. The anastomosis itself is performed with running 5-0 or 6-0 monofilament suture (Fig. 41-27, *C*). SaO_2 is well maintained with ongoing SVC flow into the right lung only.

On rare occasions, the appropriate length of pulmonary artery cannot be sequestered without causing either hemodynamic instability or inadequate oxygenation, and CPB must be instituted to create the proximal anastomosis of the conduit to the RPA. When this is necessary, a separate purse string is placed in the SVC, and normothermic CPB is initiated after cannulating the ascending aorta, SVC, and IVC in standard fashion. A calcium-supplemented blood prime allows the heart to remain beating throughout the procedure.

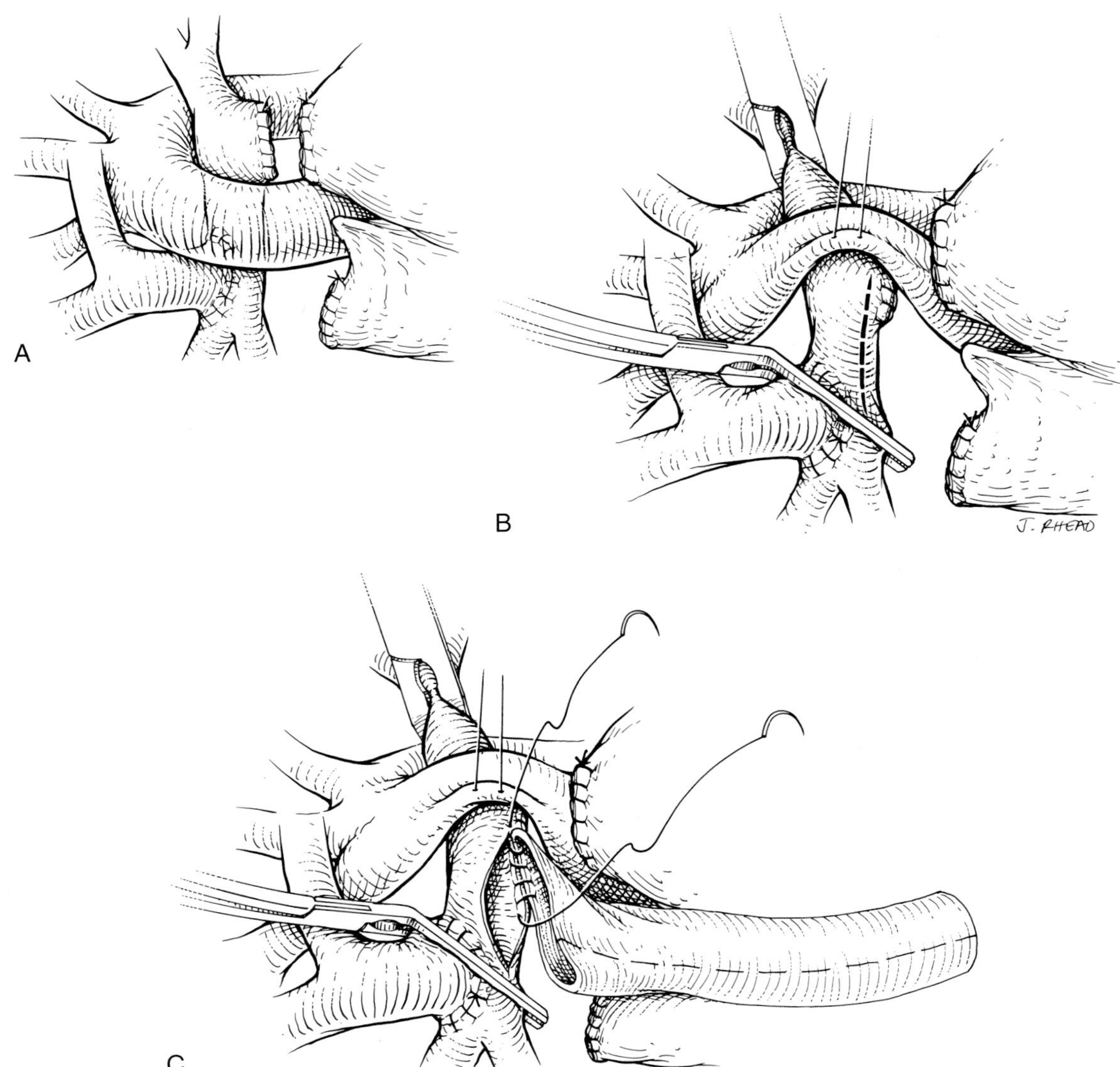

Figure 41-27 Extracardiac conduit Fontan operation. **A,** Exposure is through standard median sternotomy. Most often this a reoperative median sternotomy, because most patients will have undergone several previous procedures. Typically, a bidirectional superior cavopulmonary shunt has been previously performed, as shown here. In this case, there is no additional source of pulmonary blood flow. Once sternum is opened, adhesions are dissected in order to completely mobilize previous superior vena cava (SVC)-to–right pulmonary artery (RPA) anastomosis. Pulmonary artery system is dissected from right upper and lower arterial branch junction to pulmonary trunk, working from right to left under ascending aorta. Occasionally, proximal left pulmonary artery (LPA) is dissected as well, working on left side of ascending aorta. Goal of this dissection is to mobilize an extensive length of RPA and pulmonary trunk for proximal Fontan anastomosis. **B,** Patient is heparinized, and central portion of pulmonary artery is isolated by placing two vascular clamps, one obliquely across RPA close to previously constructed bidirectional superior cavopulmonary shunt, and the other on the central or LPA as far to the left as possible. In this depiction, LPA is controlled on left side of ascending aorta. Inferior surface of right and central pulmonary artery is incised *(dashed line)* over an appropriate length to accept the circumference of a sharply beveled 20-mm-diameter expanded polytetrafluoroethylene (PTFE) tube graft. Care is taken that clamp adjacent to previously placed superior cavopulmonary anastomosis does not obstruct SVC flow to RPA, which is required for systemic oxygenation. **C,** Anastomosis between graft and pulmonary artery is performed using nonabsorbable fine monofilament suture and a continuous technique, beginning with posterior aspect and finishing with anterior aspect of anastomosis.

Assuming that CPB is not used, after the proximal anastomosis is completed, the graft and pulmonary arteries are de-aired, a vascular clamp is placed across the PTFE graft, and the branch pulmonary artery clamps are completely removed (Fig. 41-27, *D*). This reestablishes bidirectional superior cavopulmonary flow.

The ascending aorta and IVC are cannulated and connected to a centrifugal pump at approximately 50 mL · kg · min^{-1} without an oxygenator, to achieve pump-assisted IVC decompression. Two large vascular clamps are placed across the IVC, one at the cavoatrial junction and the other just at the level of IVC cannulation (Fig. 41-27, *E-F*). If the femoral vein is used for lower body venous cannulation instead of the IVC, the clamp on the IVC is placed at the level of the diaphragm. The IVC is then transected and the cardiac stump oversewn with a running 3-0 polypropylene suture. The PTFE graft is then tailored to the appropriate length and anastomosed end to end to the IVC at the diaphragm with

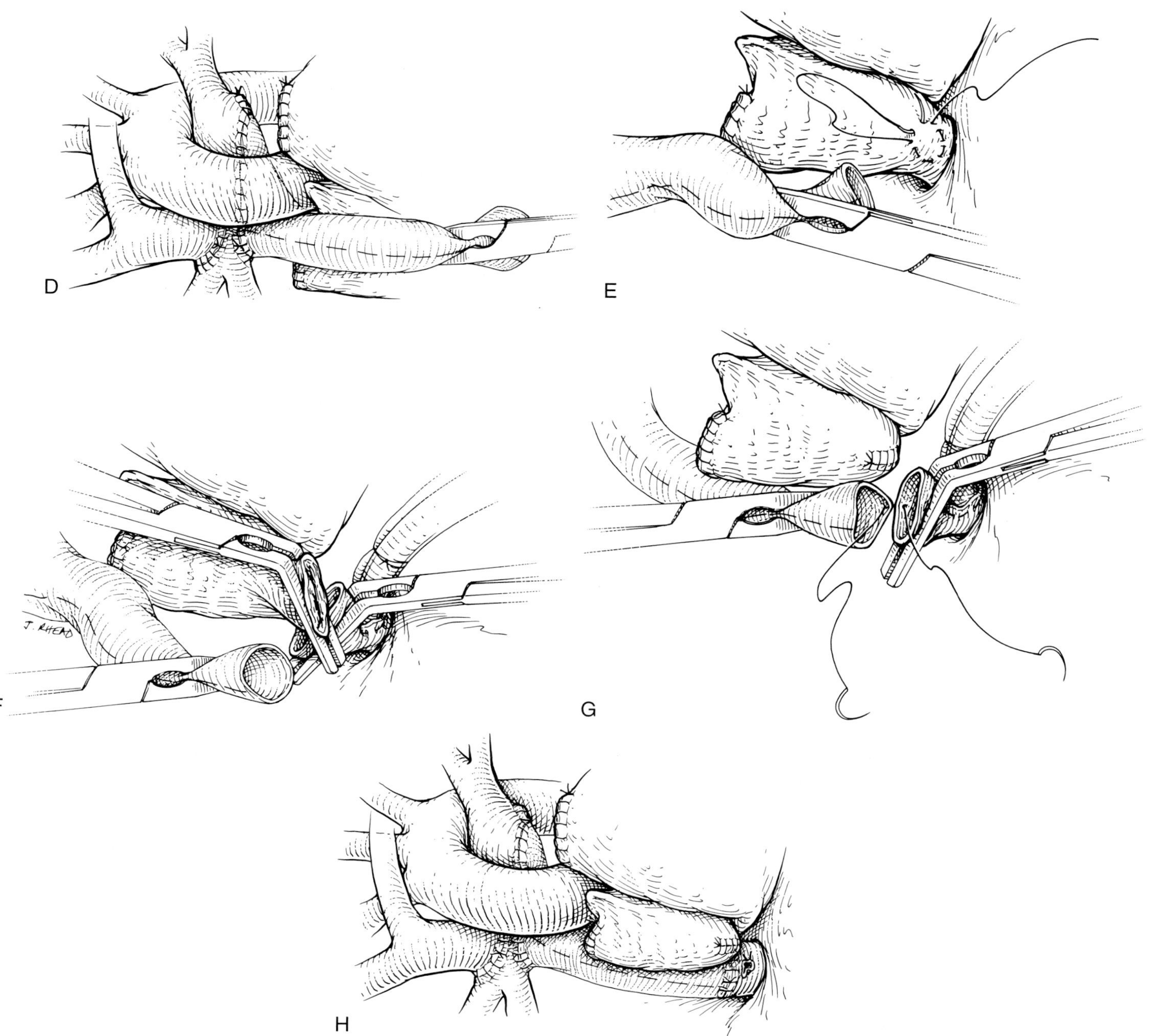

Figure 41-27, cont'd **D,** Proximal anastomosis is completed, and pulmonary artery vascular clamps have been removed. These are replaced with a single clamp on midportion of tube graft. This allows reestablishing bidirectional SVC-to–pulmonary artery flow. **E,** Inferior vena cava (IVC) is examined, and PTFE graft is tailored to appropriate length for end-to-end graft to IVC. An IVC purse string is placed at its diaphragmatic reflection. During graft to IVC anastomosis, interruption of caval flow is necessary. During this period, IVC blood can be rerouted into either right atrium or ascending aorta in several ways as described in text. **F,** Once IVC decompression is accomplished, two large vascular clamps are placed on it, one at the atriocaval junction and the other just cephalad to venous cannula. IVC is transected between clamps. **G,** IVC remnant on right atrium is oversewn with a nonabsorbable heavy monofilament continuous suture technique. PTFE tube is connected end to end to diaphragmatic component of IVC using a nonabsorbable fine monofilament suture and a continuous technique as shown, with anastomosis beginning at posterior aspect of circumference of IVC. **H,** Completed extracardiac conduit Fontan with previously placed bidirectional superior cavopulmonary shunt.

a running 5-0 polypropylene suture (Fig. 41-27, *G*). This anastomosis can typically be performed in about 10 minutes.

Alternative extracorporeal circulation techniques can be used to construct the IVC-to–PTFE conduit anastomosis. One of these eliminates use of the pump described in previous text. Purse strings are placed on the right atrial appendage and IVC, and both are cannulated with large venous cannulae, which are then connected together to provide passive IVC decompression to the right atrium while the IVC is clamped and transected and the PTFE graft–to-IVC anastomosis performed. This technique is currently used by the authors as well as others.[P12,U1,Y4] Another technique involves simply clamping the IVC (which completely interrupts IVC flow) while the PTFE-to-IVC anastomosis is performed.[S20]

Following completion of the anastomosis, the patient is decannulated as needed (Fig. 41-27, *H*). Pressure-monitoring catheters are placed in the common atrium and IVC at the cannulation site to measure Fontan pathway and left-sided filling pressures and calculate transpulmonary gradient. These catheters are removed as soon as hemodynamic stability is ensured. Temporary atrial and ventricular pacing wires are placed along with appropriately positioned drainage tubes in the pleural and pericardial spaces, and the sternotomy is closed in standard fashion.

Extracardiac Conduit Fontan Operation with Deliberately Incomplete Atrial Partitioning

Incomplete atrial partitioning with the extracardiac conduit Fontan is usually unnecessary, particularly when the procedure is performed without CPB or with minimal CPB.[P12] (The reasons for this are detailed in "Fontan Operation with Deliberately Incomplete Atrial Partitioning" under Indications for Operation later in this section.) In essence, in creating a complete extracardiac conduit Fontan, the damaging effects of both CPB and myocardial ischemia are avoided, attenuating the transient hemodynamic disturbances that have made incomplete atrial partitioning necessary to ensure superior outcomes.

If hemodynamics following the Fontan procedure requires a communication between the Fontan conduit and atrium, this can be assessed after completing the Fontan as described; the connection can be accomplished without CPB. With the patient still heparinized, side-biting clamps are placed on the free wall of the right atrium and adjacent conduit, and a connection is made between these structures in one of two ways. First, a carefully controlled punch incision of predetermined diameter can be made in the conduit to regulate size of the fenestration. A second larger incision can be made in the sequestered segment of atrial wall, and free edges of the atrial incision can then be sewn widely around the punch hole in the conduit to create a fenestration. Second, small incisions can be made in both conduit and right atrial free wall, and a PTFE tube graft of approximately 8-mm diameter can be sewn between the two structures to create a tunnel-like communication. One of the authors (FLH) has used both of these techniques since 1992.[P12] Either communication can be regulated with a large snare if the surgeon prefers. The tube graft fenestration can also be closed using interventional catheterization.[B25]

Lateral Tunnel Fontan Operation

Preparation for operation and median sternotomy incision are generally those described in "Preparation for Cardiopulmonary Bypass" in Section III of Chapter 2. After anesthesia induction, a short double-lumen catheter is inserted percutaneously into the right internal jugular vein and advanced centrally (see subsequent text about early removal). In small patients, it may extend too far, interfering with SVC cannulation or with a total cavopulmonary connection; in that case the surgeon cuts off excess length. Inserting a polyvinyl catheter through the right superior pulmonary vein into the left atrium to measure ventricular loading is particularly important.

Risk of thrombosis around catheters in caval veins and their branches is increased in patients undergoing a Fontan operation (or bidirectional superior cavopulmonary shunt); therefore, any inserted for operation should be removed early postoperatively as soon as hemodynamic stability is achieved.

Aortic cannulation and cardioplegia purse-string sutures are placed as usual, as are those for direct SVC and IVC cannulation (see "Preparation for Cardiopulmonary Bypass" in Section III of Chapter 2, and Fig. 41-23). However, particular attention is paid to placing the SVC purse string as far cephalad as possible so that it does not interfere with a bicaval-pulmonary connection if chosen. Also, an elliptical shape of the purse string, with the long access of the ellipse oriented longitudinally, is particularly important so that tying it down later only minimally narrows the SVC. Purse string and cannulation may be on the brachiocephalic vein. Any previously made systemic–pulmonary arterial anastomosis is dissected (see "Repair of Tetralogy of Fallot after Blalock-Taussig or Polytetrafluoroethylene Interposition Shunt" under Technique of Operation in Section I of Chapter 38) and closed immediately after start of CPB.

CPB is established, systemic hypothermia achieved, aorta clamped, and cold cardioplegic infusion given. Perfusate temperature is rapidly lowered on CPB by taking the heat exchanger water bath to 4°C. Body temperature is stabilized, usually at 25°C, before administering cardioplegia. The technique of controlled myocardial reperfusion can be used after repair is completed (see "Cold Cardioplegia, Controlled Aortic Root Reperfusion, and [When Needed] Warm Cardioplegic Induction" in Chapter 3).

Although practiced in only a small minority of programs, some surgeons perform the operation using hypothermic circulatory arrest, in which case the body temperature is brought to 15°C to 18°C. During cooling, a left atrial vent may be inserted through the base of the right superior pulmonary vein, or the field may be freed of blood by a pump-oxygenator sump-sucker placed across the foramen ovale after the right atrium is opened.

The pulmonary trunk is completely dissected away from the ascending aorta, and right and left pulmonary arteries are mobilized out to their first branch. This is usually begun before CPB is established, but is completed after establishing CPB and closing any systemic–pulmonary arterial shunts (Fig. 41-28, *A*). To prevent serious bleeding after CPB, meticulous hemostasis must be obtained with electrocautery as dissection is being accomplished.

The right atrium is opened through an oblique incision placed a little more anteriorly than usual (to preserve more posterior right atrial wall to serve as part of the intraatrial tunnel that will be created), and the pump-oxygenator sump-sucker is placed across the foramen ovale into the left atrium (see Fig. 41-28, *A*).

The pulmonary trunk is transected as close to the valve as convenient, and the proximal end is closed with two rows of continuous 4-0 polypropylene sutures (Fig. 41-28, *B*). During dissection, division, and closure of the pulmonary trunk, care is taken not to disturb the left coronary artery. It is tempting to leave the distal end of the pulmonary trunk open for later anastomosis to the cardiac end of the transected SVC, but this anastomosis can rarely be performed without tension and angulation of the trunk and first part of the left pulmonary artery. Therefore, the distal end of the pulmonary trunk is usually closed with two rows of continuous 6-0

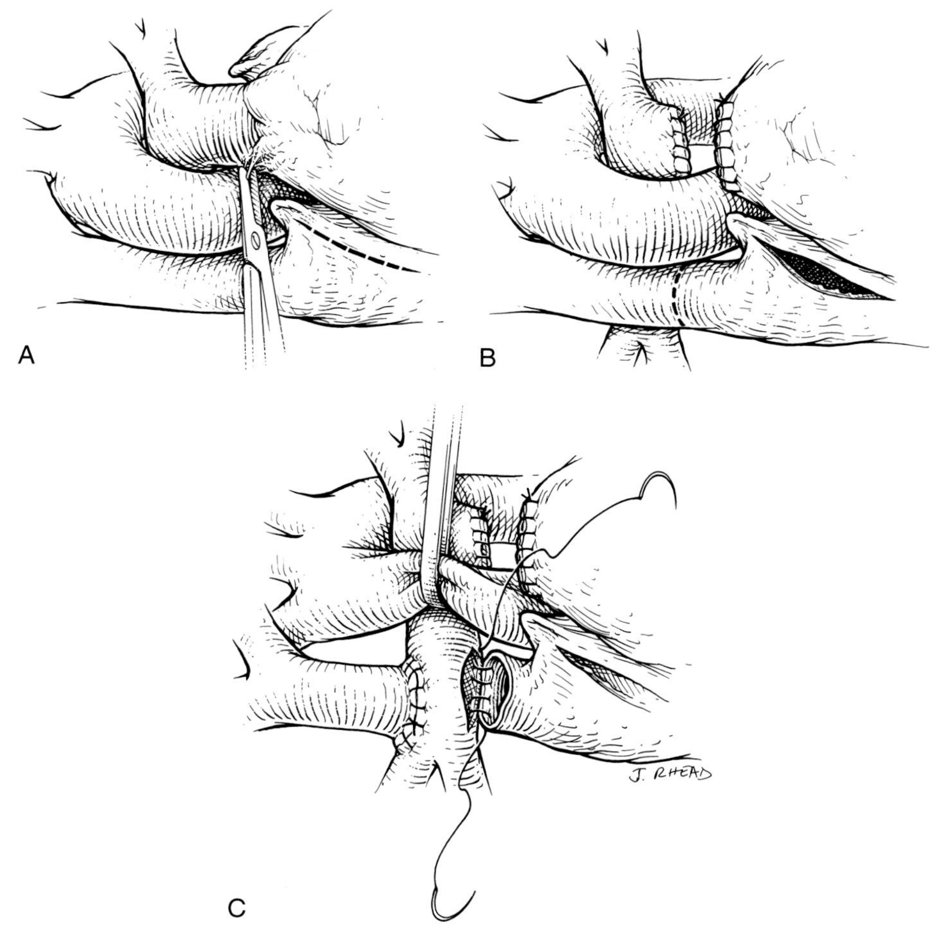

Figure 41-28 Lateral tunnel Fontan operation. Operation is shown for tricuspid atresia and normally related great arteries with well-developed main and branch pulmonary arteries. **A,** Exposure is through a standard median sternotomy, and standard cardiopulmonary bypass (CPB) with moderate hypothermia and cardioplegia is used. In this case, a bidirectional superior cavopulmonary shunt has not yet been performed. Dashed line indicates incision to be made in right atrial appendage. Operation proceeds by separating pulmonary trunk from aorta using sharp dissection. **B,** Right and left pulmonary arteries are dissected to their first branches in a manner similar to that used for arterial switch operation. After separating ascending aorta and pulmonary trunk, superior vena cava (SVC) is mobilized and azygos vein identified. CPB is then instituted with aortic cannulation and separate high SVC and inferior vena cava (IVC) cannulae. If any systemic–pulmonary arterial connections exist, these are also taken down immediately upon institution of CPB. Pulmonary trunk is transected at level of pulmonary valve, and each end is oversewn with a continuous monofilament suture. Dashed line on SVC shows point of eventual transection required to completed Fontan procedure. Somewhat anteriorly placed incision on right atrial free wall is also shown. Entry into right atrium provides access to left side of heart, allowing a pump sump-sucker to be placed across foramen ovale to decompress it. **C,** Anastomosis between cephalad portion of divided SVC and an incision in the superior surface of right pulmonary artery (RPA) is performed as shown, using a continuous 7-0 monofilament absorbable suture. This is performed exactly as shown in technique used for bidirectional superior cavopulmonary shunt (see Fig. 41-22). Cardiac end of divided SVC is connected to incision in inferior aspect of RPA as shown, using a continuous 7-0 monofilament absorbable suture.

Continued

polypropylene sutures placed as a whip stitch (see Fig. 41-28, *B*). However, if the distal pulmonary trunk segment has little length (which may be the case when a pulmonary trunk band has previously been placed too far distally), a patch of pericardium or allograft pulmonary artery is used for closure to maintain a wide pathway between right and left pulmonary arteries.

Success requires that the central unbranched hilar portions of right and left pulmonary arteries be enlarged if they are small. This can be accomplished by making a long incision in the midportion of the anterior wall of the left and right pulmonary arteries extending to the area of origin of the first branch on both sides. Inserting a widening patch-graft is accomplished with continuous 6-0 polypropylene sutures.[N8] If available, a pulmonary arterial allograft serves best as the patch-graft material. Otherwise, aortic allograft or autologous pericardium, untreated or treated with glutaraldehyde, may be used. Incision for anastomosis to the right atrium or cavae is then best made in the native pulmonary arterial wall rather than in the patch. This procedure can neutralize the incremental risk of small central right and left pulmonary arteries only if the branching portions of these arteries are of reasonable size.

If a previous bidirectional superior cavopulmonary shunt has not been performed, the SVC is transected at the point where it crosses the RPA; the transection is usually

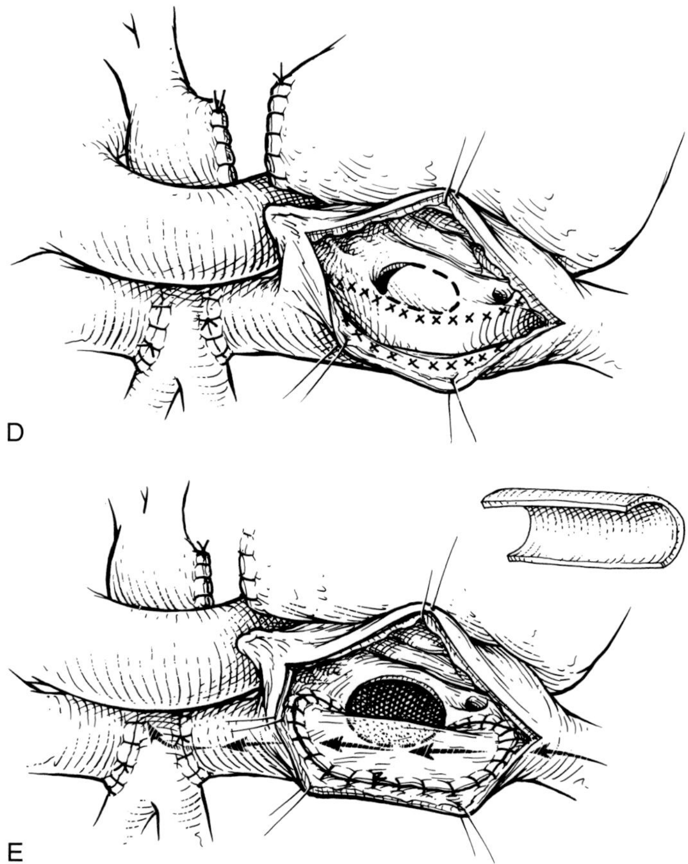

Figure 41-28, cont'd **D,** Internal aspect of right atrium is then examined. Floor of fossa ovalis *(dashed lines)* is excised to make a large intraatrial communication, leaving posterior and superior portions of limbus intact and taking care not to injure area of atrioventricular node. Preparation is then made for the intraatrial lateral tunnel baffle that will be fashioned from a tube of polytetrafluoroethylene (PTFE). Line of x's shows proposed suture line of synthetic baffle, extending around both cavoatrial orifices. Coronary sinus is allowed to drain into new pulmonary venous atrium. **E,** Convex PTFE baffle has been cut to size such that it will make up approximately half the circumference of proposed intraatrial tunnel. It is sewn into place with a continuous 5-0 polypropylene suture. Other half of circumference of tunnel is made up of posterolateral aspect of atrial septum and right atrial free wall to provide growth potential of tunnel. Right atrium is closed. See text for techniques applicable to other previous palliative procedures.

just proximal to the azygos vein, which is divided between ligatures to help mobilize the cephalic end of the SVC. A longitudinal incision is made along the superior surface of the RPA, and the cephalic end of the SVC is anastomosed to this opening (Fig. 41-28, *B-C*). A longitudinal incision is made along the inferior surface of the RPA, a little more medially placed than the previous incision, and anastomosis made between the central end of the divided SVC and this opening (see Fig. 41-28, *C*). In most cases the sinus node artery can be seen and avoided.

A tunnel within the right atrium is required to conduct IVC and hepatic venous blood to the cardiac end of the SVC; generally, some heavy atrial trabeculations must be excised to clear that pathway. The ASD may need to be enlarged, particularly if the right AV valve will be the main pathway for pulmonary venous blood to reach the systemic ventricle (Fig. 41-28, *D*). A patch cut from a PTFE tube is selected, trimmed, and sewn into place. The suture line is started between the coronary sinus and IVC orifices and continued cephalad along the atrial septum as near the ASD as possible until the leftward edge of the SVC is reached. With the other arm of the suture, the suture line is carried over the IVC orifice, along the inside of the right atrial wall, and then over the SVC (Fig. 41-28, *D-E*).

The coronary sinus, as with the extracardiac conduit Fontan, now drains into the low-pressure left atrium; this arrangement is physiologically preferred, in contrast to an atriopulmonary Fontan, in which the coronary sinus drains to the high-pressure systemic venous circuit. Ilbawi and colleagues have shown that coronary sinus pressure greater than 15 mmHg depresses systemic ventricular output, although Ward and colleagues' and Eicken and colleagues' data appear to disprove this.[E3,I5,W2]

Collateral blood flow to the pulmonary circulation is often large in patients undergoing the Fontan operation, and particular care must be taken to avoid overdistention of the left atrium (and pulmonary veins) and systemic ventricle during final stages of repair. This can be accomplished by suction on the vent placed across the foramen ovale into the left atrium and by free drainage of blood from the pulmonary arteries into the right atrium through the anastomoses. The vent can be conveniently introduced through the right atrial appendage. In any event, as the right atrium is being closed, necessitating removal of the pump sump-sucker, care must be used to prevent undue elevation of left atrial and ventricular pressure until cardiac action has returned. Toward this end, the caval tapes may be released before the atrium is closed, and suction on the caval cannulae can help decompress the pulmonary arteries and thereby the left atrium. After the heart is closed, aortic root reperfusion is established and de-airing begun. The remainder of operation is completed in the usual manner (see "Completing Operation" in Section III of Chapter 2).

At times, it may be more convenient to use a right atrial flap as the inner part of the wall of the tunnel.[P19] Depending on the anatomic situation in the individual patient, this atrial inner wall may be made from either anterior or posterior portions of right atrial wall.

Some prefer not to use the orifice of the cardiac end of the transected SVC to make the anastomosis to the RPA, but rather to close the central end and use a separate incision in the superior aspect of the right atrium for the anastomosis. A roof for the anastomosis is then made with allograft pulmonary arterial wall or pericardium. The intraatrial baffle is constructed so that it conducts IVC blood to the new opening.

When possible, as the repair is being completed, provision is made for measuring pressure in the pulmonary artery, venae cavae, and left atrium. Sites of insertion of fine polyvinyl catheters depend on the specific procedure used. Two right atrial and two RV myocardial electrodes are placed at the end of operation.

Provision for adequate drainage of the pericardium is particularly important. While the patient is still on CPB, a large window is made between the pericardial and right pleural spaces by excising a large piece of pericardium anterior to the phrenic nerve. A window is made between the pericardial and left pleural spaces by tilting the heart up anteriorly and making a large incision in the posterior pericardium well behind the phrenic nerve from within the pericardium. One posteriorly placed and one anteriorly placed drainage tube is brought out from each pleural space.

Lateral Tunnel Fontan Operation with Deliberately Incomplete Atrial Partitioning

Under some circumstances (see Indications for Operation later in this section), incomplete atrial partitioning is considered advantageous in performing the Fontan operation.[G13] This has been accomplished in two ways in the setting of the lateral tunnel procedure.

Laks and colleagues leave a small defect in the suture line that attaches the PTFE to the atrium. They place one pledgeted polypropylene mattress suture through the edge of the PTFE at the site of the defect, bring the suture outside the heart through the posterior atrial wall, and pass the ends through another pledget and secure them on a snugger (a section of an 8F pediatric suction catheter)[L3,L4,P6] (Fig. 41-29, *A*). The end of the suture is left beneath the closure of the linea alba (Fig. 41-29, *B*). Pushing the snugger down makes

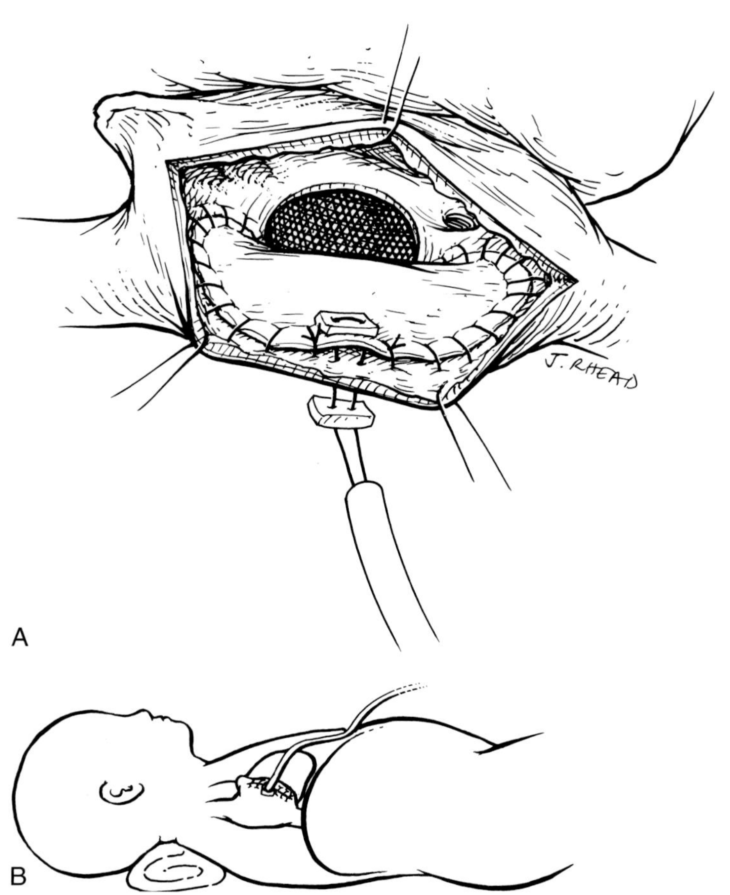

Figure 41-29 Lateral tunnel Fontan operation with deliberately incomplete atrial partitioning using "adjustable atrial septal defect." **A,** After intraatrial polytetrafluoroethylene (PTFE) lateral tunnel baffle is placed, a small (approximately 6 mm) aperture is left in midportion of baffle suture line where baffle is attached to right atrial free wall, as shown. This aperture is controlled by a mattress suture using heavy 2-0 polypropylene suture with felt pledgets placed on both sides, connected to a snare. Length of snare is tailored to reach subxyphoid area prior to closure of right atrium. Snare is tested to demonstrate effectiveness of mechanism for opening and closing the aperture. Right atrium is then closed and patient separated from cardiopulmonary bypass in standard fashion. Prior to closing sternal incision, hemodynamics are assessed and aperture adjusted to maximize early hemodynamics. **B,** Prior to closing sternum, snare length is carefully determined to reach the subcutaneous position in subxyphoid region. Snare is secured at determined level of aperture patency that results in ideal early hemodynamics by placing multiple large metal clips at subcutaneous end of snare. This allows easy access to snare either early or late postoperatively for further aperture adjustment. Metal clips serve not only to stabilize snare but also as a convenient radiologic and tactile landmark, should early or late aperture adjustment be necessary.

the interatrial communication smaller. The residual aperture is adjusted to an appropriate size before closing the chest. In the intensive care unit (ICU), the aperture is made larger, smaller, or nonexistent by simply removing a few sutures from the skin and linea alba closure, removing clips holding the snugger in position, and repositioning and securing the snugger.

An alternative is a fixed fenestration in the lateral tunnel PTFE baffle. At operation, after the tunnel is placed in the atrium, a hole is made in it equidistant from the two suture lines and somewhat inferior to the center of the tunnel. The hole is made with a 4-mm aortic punch for patients weighing less than about 12 kg, with a 5-mm punch for those weighing about 12 to 30 kg, and with a 6-mm punch for larger patients.[K24] Postoperatively, the patient is evaluated continuously for the possibility and proper time, if at all, for closure of the interatrial communication (see Special Features of Postoperative Care later in this section). When the time is appropriate, the patient is taken to the cardiac catheterization laboratory, where the communication is temporarily closed by a percutaneously inserted balloon; if the hemodynamic state remains good, the communication is closed permanently with a percutaneously inserted occlusion device.[R16] Otherwise, the communication is left open and closure is reconsidered later.

SPECIAL FEATURES OF POSTOPERATIVE CARE

Care usually given after intracardiac operations is appropriate (see Section IV of Chapter 5). However, some aspects of care are of particular importance.

Monitoring

The patient leaves the operating room with catheters in the IVC and left atrium as well as the usual arterial catheter. Not only are these devices useful in general management of patients after a complete or partial (bidirectional superior cavopulmonary shunt, hemi-Fontan, or fenestrated) Fontan operation, they also provide information critical to making rational decisions for patients who are not convalescing normally. Catheters in caval veins are removed as soon as possible.

General Measures

The patient is nursed in semi-Fowler's position, and positive end-expiratory pressure is not used.[W11] Because of the adverse effect of positive intrathoracic pressure on $\dot{Q}p$, inspiratory ventilation pressures are kept as low as possible, and spontaneous breathing is encouraged as early as possible.[P8,R10] Extubation is usually accomplished within 2 to 48 hours of operation. Stay in the ICU is usually 48 to 72 hours, rather than the usual 24 hours, because cardiac physiology is not fully normalized.

There is more than the usual tendency for fluid to leave the intravascular compartment and pass into the interstitial space and into the pleural, pericardial, and peritoneal cavities. The cause is multifactorial and includes increase in microvascular permeability resulting from CPB (if used), and at least mild increase in right atrial and caval pressures.[A10,F14,S27] Because of this tendency for transcapillary fluid loss, 5% albumin or stable plasma protein solution may be necessary to maintain adequate ventricular loading.

Every effort is made to keep body cavities free of fluid and atrial and caval pressures low. Pleural effusions drain through the tubes placed at operation, and the wide opening made between the pericardial space and both pleural spaces prevents pericardial tamponade. On occasion, a peritoneal catheter may have to be inserted in the ICU to drain rapidly developing ascites.

Occasionally, serous drainage may insidiously become chylous, perhaps because the leaking microvascular pores gradually enlarge with time with passage of macromolecules, such that ultimately chylomicrons can pass.[S27] In any event, when the fluid becomes chylous, ligation of the thoracic duct rarely is useful, and surgical attempts to promote pleural symphysis often fail. Adequate tube drainage, high caloric intake, fluid restriction, and aggressive use of diuretics are the mainstays of treatment (see "Chylothorax" in Section II of Chapter 5). In cases of persistent chylous effusion, more aggressive measures can be effective in eliminating it. These include nothing by mouth (NPO) status, with all nutrition provided parenterally, and administration of synthetic somatostatin analogs such as octreotide.[C10,C11]

Careful follow-up is required for at least 3 to 6 weeks. The tendency to fluid retention, hepatomegaly, and ascites may persist for most of this time, making sodium and fluid restriction and diuretic therapy necessary. Also, fluid retention and even chylous accumulations may appear to be mild during hospitalization, but with increased activity after hospital dismissal, larger accumulations of fluid or chyle may develop in body cavities. This may be recognized only when pulmonary or cardiac dysfunction appears to develop rather suddenly. If this occurs, immediate hospitalization and intensive treatment are necessary; these late accumulations can be rapidly fatal if untreated.

Preventing Atrial Thrombosis

Although atrial or Fontan pathway thrombosis is uncommon (see "Thromboembolic Complications" under Results later in this section), it is a serious complication warranting special consideration. It appears reasonable to believe that this is more apt to occur in patients with elevated Fontan pathway pressures or in those who are slow to recover because of chronic effusions or some other complication. Thus, patients in these categories are placed on warfarin therapy beginning about 3 days postoperatively and continuing for 6 to 12 weeks. Thereafter, lifelong therapy with aspirin ($80\ mg \cdot day^{-1}$) is advisable. It should be noted that for the atriopulmonary Fontan, Fontan pathway thrombosis is atrial thrombosis; for the lateral tunnel Fontan, atrial thrombosis may be in the Fontan pathway or in the systemic side of the atrium; and for the extracardiac conduit Fontan, the atrium is completely excluded from the Fontan pathway and is not at risk for thrombosis.

Should acute thrombosis occur early postoperatively, particularly if it causes obstruction or is associated with pulmonary embolization, immediate surgical exploration, or in some cases thrombolytic therapy, is indicated.[D2]

Strategic Importance of Fontan Pathway Pressure

Patients often have a Fontan pathway pressure of 16 mmHg or less a few hours after entering the ICU, and they generally convalesce well. When pressure is higher than this, and particularly when it progressively increases—often as a result of a need to augment blood volume to maintain cardiac output—a potentially lethal situation may be developing, and a thoughtful and prompt analysis is indicated.[K18] When a fenestrated Fontan operation has been performed, the warning sign may be severe arterial desaturation rather than elevation of Fontan pathway pressure. Narrowing the fenestration may simply substitute elevation of pressure for arterial desaturation; therefore, treatment strategies for these two developments are similar.

Treatment strategy for these patients first considers left atrial pressure (PLA). If it is elevated to within a few mmHg of Fontan pathway pressure and if it too rises as the hours pass, main chamber ventricular dysfunction or AV valve dysfunction (regurgitation or stenosis) is probably etiologic to the poor hemodynamic state. PLA greater than 10 mmHg is not well tolerated, because this results in unacceptably high Fontan pathway pressure, even in the face of a normal Rp and transpulmonary pressure gradient. Two-dimensional echocardiographic examination in the ICU is indicated. If ventricular dysfunction is present, an increase in inotropic support may improve the hemodynamics. If new-onset AV valve regurgitation is present, reoperation and valve repair should be considered. If these efforts are unsuccessful or are not feasible, the only option is mechanical ventricular support in preparation for transplantation (see Chapter 21).

If Fontan pathway pressure remains 12 mmHg or more higher than PLA, and pulmonary arterial pressure is similarly elevated, then pulmonary vascular disease, pulmonary arteriolar spasm, or small size of pulmonary arteries may be responsible. The patient is hyperventilated to an arterial $Pa\text{CO}_2$ of 25 to 30 mmHg, arterial $Pa\text{O}_2$ is maximized (short of having an $F\text{IO}_2$ of 1.0), and inhaled nitric oxide is initiated in a dose of 20 to 40 ppm.[G5] If these do not soon bring about improvement, it must be concluded that the problem is pulmonary vascular disease or small pulmonary arteries, and not pulmonary arteriolar spasm. Modification or takedown of the Fontan operation must be considered. Improved knowledge of stress-related metabolic and hormonal changes, and of inflammatory responses to surgery, may provide additional modes of therapy.[H12,M4] Aprotinin has been associated with reduced Fontan pathway pressure.[T15]

If Fontan pathway pressure is high and left atrial and pulmonary artery pressures are not, then an obstruction exists in the newly created pathways. If Fontan pathway pressure is greater than 16 mmHg or if pressure increases as the hours pass, serious consideration must be given to reoperation for obstruction of the pathway. Echocardiographic or angiographic study may be desirable before the final decision is made.

Takedown or Modification of Fontan Operation

Under certain circumstances, and usually within 12 hours of operation, the hemodynamic state of the patient may be sufficiently poor that probability of survival seems low, and modification or takedown of the Fontan operation is advisable as an emergency procedure.[D9]

When a completed Fontan operation has been performed, takedown should be done as soon as circumstances requiring it are identified. These are a poor hemodynamic state and presence of an elevated pulmonary arterial pressure (greater than 18 mmHg) and elevated PLA (>10 mmHg) with a relatively normal transpulmonary pressure gradient. In the case of a lateral tunnel Fontan, after CPB and cardioplegia are established, the right atrium is opened and the patch placed to form the intraatrial tunnel is removed, resulting in a wide open interatrial communication. The cardiac end of the SVC is closed by a patch placed from within the right atrium. Essentially, this is conversion of a completed Fontan operation to a hemi-Fontan.[D23] The extracardiac conduit Fontan can be taken down simply by removing the conduit from the undersurface of the pulmonary artery and connecting it to the side of the right atrium. This procedure is performed using normothermic, beating-heart CPB with aortic and IVC cannulation. A large partial-occlusion vascular clamp is used to sequester the portion of the right atrial wall that will receive the IVC conduit.

When a poor hemodynamic state exists in the setting of elevated pulmonary artery pressure and low PLA—that is, an elevated transpulmonary pressure gradient—establishing a fenestration if one is not present or enlarging an existing fenestration or adjustable ASD may be beneficial. Following a complete lateral tunnel Fontan, this requires return to CPB, opening the right atrium, and creating an appropriately sized hole in the PTFE patch. If a complete extracardiac conduit Fontan exists, the communication can be performed without return to CPB by placing an 8-mm-diameter PTFE tube graft between the extracardiac conduit and right atrial appendage using partial occlusion vascular clamps to isolate segments of the conduit and the right atrium (see "Extracardiac Conduit Fontan with Deliberately Incomplete Atrial Positioning" under Technique of Operation earlier in this section). If an incompleted Fontan with an adjustable ASD had been performed originally, then opening the skin and fascia overlying the controlling snare around the ASD is performed and ASD size adjusted. If these maneuvers fail to improve the hemodynamic state, Fontan takedown is undertaken.

Fontan Operation with Deliberately Incomplete Atrial Partitioning

It has been hypothesized that some failures and deaths after a completed Fontan operation are due to temporary pulmonary vascular or parenchymal dysfunction (presumably related to the damaging effects of CPB) and to temporary myocardial dysfunction (presumably related to inadequate myocardial management).[B29] This hypothesis is supported by the finding of increased ventricular wall thickness (myocardial edema) and decreased ventricular compliance and volume immediately after the Fontan operation, with regression of these responses to surgery over the several weeks or months thereafter.[G14]

Thus, in the early postoperative period, when $Sa\text{O}_2$ increases to 85% or greater and Fontan pathway pressure decreases to 15 mmHg or less, closure of the aperture by snugging down the suture controlling the adjustable ASD or by a percutaneously placed device may be considered.[P15] A valuable indicator that the incompleted Fontan operation can be made complete is cessation in formation of pleural effusions.[B29] With closure of the residual aperture, $Sa\text{O}_2$ should approach 100%, but Fontan pathway and PLA responses can be variable. Fontan pathway pressure may increase to greater than 15 mmHg, PLA may decrease to less than 7 to 8 mmHg, and the cardiac index may fall, evidence that the aperture should be reopened. When Fontan pathway pressure remains at or less than 15 mmHg, and PLA remains sufficiently high that cardiac output remains good, the residual aperture can be permanently closed.

Although this general plan has often been successful, at times morbidity is increased by closing the residual aperture. In the early postoperative period, timing of atrial communication closure remains controversial. Delayed closure several months after the Fontan operation is practiced at many centers, and this strategy may be more prudent than one that attempts to close the communication in the postoperative period. In essence, there is little reason to close the communication early unless SaO_2 decreases to unacceptable levels (<75%) in association with low pressure (<15 mmHg) in the pulmonary arteries, indicating that the communication is too large. Regardless of timing of closure, assessing hemodynamic consequences of closure should be made by temporarily closing the communication first. In some cases, hemodynamic response will suggest that the communication be left open permanently. Fenestration closure may benefit patients at midterm follow-up[G22]; however, others argue that patients are better off with the fenestration left open.[O9]

RESULTS

Completed Fontan Operation

A considerable body of knowledge is available about early and late results after completed Fontan operation.[G12] Effects of temporary or permanent partial Fontan operations, of lateral tunnel and extracardiac conduit variations, and of minimal use or avoidance of CPB have been documented at early but not late follow-up.

Survival

Early (Hospital) Death Thirty-day or hospital mortality has improved over the past decade and currently is 0% to 4%,[C22,H6,H16,J2,M30,M34,P12,S7] substantially better than earlier reports of about 20% in heterogeneous groups of patients.[A19,D26,F14,F15,K20,M23] Improvement in survival is documented both in series that report Fontan operations performed exclusively in more recent calendar years and in series that cover a wider range of calendar years in which improved survival is documented for more recent calendar years.[B6,B20,C27,D5,I2,J1,L12,M22,M23,M50,P13,S36] Equal results have been achieved with extracardiac conduit and lateral tunnel techniques, and with the entire spectrum of CPB management techniques, from off-pump series to series using hypothermic circulatory arrest.[J2,K32,M34,P12]

Time-Related Survival Overall, in heterogeneous groups of patients undergoing completed Fontan operation in the time period from approximately 1970 to 1985, 5-, 10-, and 15-year survivals, including early mortality, were about 70%, 65%, and 50%, respectively[D7,D14,F14,T1,W12] (Fig. 41-30, *A*). The hazard function for such patients had three phases (Fig. 41-30, *B*), and in none was it similar to that of the general population. In a series of 216 tricuspid atresia patients undergoing the Fontan over a 25-year period at the Mayo Clinic, overall survival was 79%.[M6] Outcomes improved substantially within each decade of this experience, with 56/59 patients alive from the final decade. Long-term follow-up is becoming available for more recent patients who have undergone a bidirectional superior cavopulmonary shunt (bidirectional Glenn or hemi-Fontan) followed by a lateral tunnel or

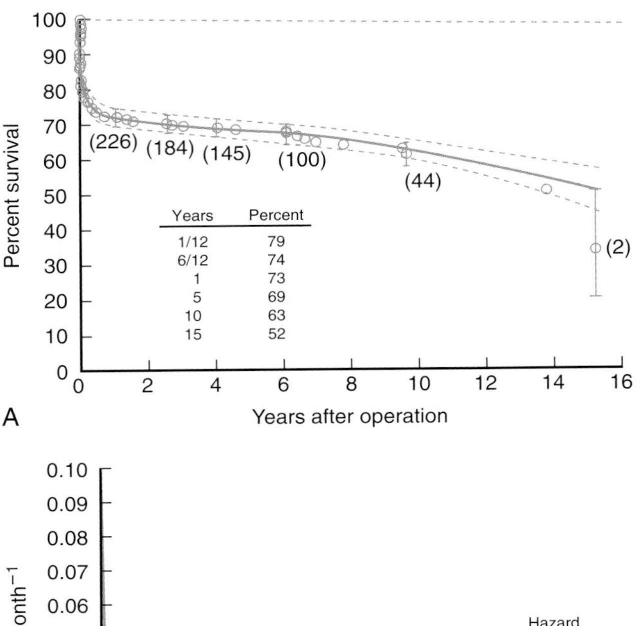

Years	Percent
1/12	79
6/12	74
1	73
5	69
10	63
15	52

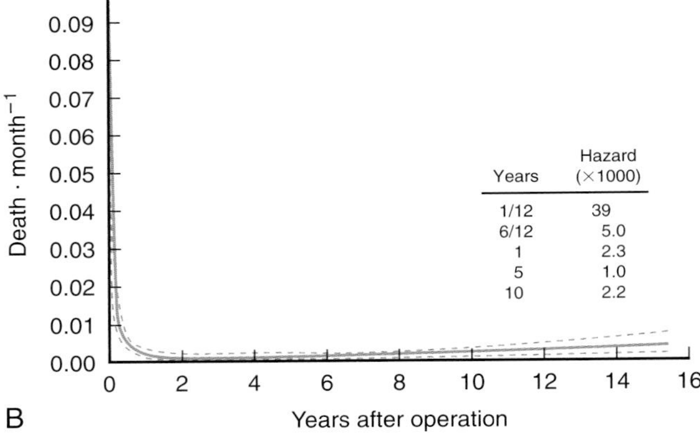

Years	Hazard (×1000)
1/12	39
6/12	5.0
1	2.3
5	1.0
10	2.2

Figure 41-30 Survival after Fontan operation in a heterogeneous group of patients (n = 334; deaths = 110). **A,** Survival. Solid lines are parametric estimates, and dashed lines enclose their 70% confidence limits (CL). Each circle represents a death and is positioned according to Kaplan-Meier estimator; vertical bars are 70% CLs of nonparametric estimates, and numbers in parentheses are patients remaining at risk. Dash-dot-dash line represents survival of an age-sex-race–matched general population. **B,** Hazard function for death. Note gradually rising late phase of hazard, becoming evident about 8 years after operation. (From Fontan and colleagues.[F14])

extracardiac conduit total cavopulmonary Fontan. Midterm survival is markedly improved, with 1- to 5-year survival approaching and exceeding 90%.[A12,K19,H16,L8] Petrossian and colleagues report 10-year actuarial freedom from Fontan failure of any kind, including death, takedown, or transplantation, at 90%[P12] (Fig. 41-31). Others report similar outcomes.[G16,H13,T16]

Survival after a "Perfect" Fontan Operation Because many deaths after the Fontan operation have been due to circumstances that can be avoided in the present era, the persistent and rising hazard function for death (see Fig. 41-30, *B*) could be a result of now avoidable circumstances. However, analysis of survival under circumstances that can be considered ideal indicates that the late, slow-rising phase of hazard is still present (Fig. 41-32, *A*). Under ideal circumstances, 15-year survival is predicted to be 73% (Fig. 41-32, *B*), a prediction supported by the experience of others.[D26] A recent analysis revisiting the idea of the perfect Fontan shows that in the modern era, using an extracardiac conduit for the Fontan, outcomes equal to that predicted by Fontan and

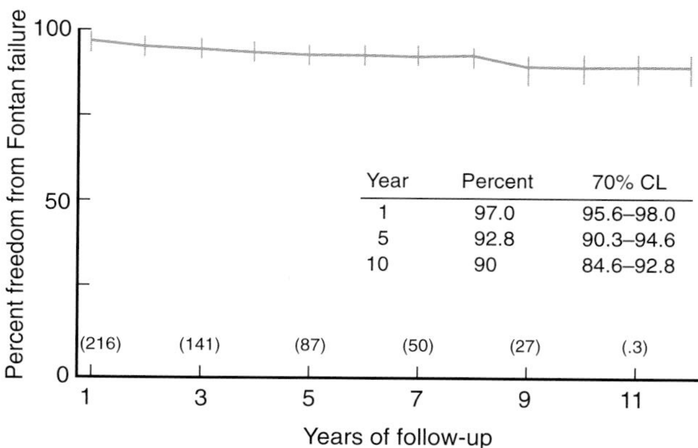

Figure 41-31 Freedom from Fontan failure, including death, takedown, and transplantation, after 216 extracardiac conduit Fontan procedures. Vertical bars are 70% confidence limits. (From Petrossian and colleagues.[P12])

colleagues' original "perfect Fontan" equations can be achieved routinely in all patients.[K17] Other recent series document 10-year survival superior to that achieved with the classic "perfect Fontan" (see Fig. 41-31). These data simply reflect the gradual improvement in outcome that has occurred over the last 2 decades.

Declining survival late postoperatively and rising late hazard for death under good circumstances are different from those after repair of tetralogy of Fallot (see "Time-Related Survival and the Question of 'Cure'" under Results in Section I of Chapter 38), as is the gradually declining functional capability after the Fontan operation (Fig. 41-33). These suggest that the Fontan operation should be considered an excellent palliative operation but not a curative one. The fact that no risk factors (other than older age at operation) have been identified for the late phase of hazard suggests that this is related to the circulatory state after the Fontan operation. This state may predispose to subtle morphologic and functional changes in the pulmonary circulation similar to those that occur after the bidirectional superior cavopulmonary shunt.[C1,M17,M29] Also, there may be gradual deterioration of structure and function of the congenitally abnormal ventricular chamber. The latter could be contributed to by high coronary sinus pressure, unless it has been diverted into the left atrium.[I5] Also, additional congenital cardiac and myocardial anomalies are common in the univentricular hearts of patients who undergo the Fontan operation, and these may gradually impair cardiac function as time passes. It remains to be seen whether the proposed advantages of the extracardiac-conduit Fontan procedure—which removes the atrium from the Fontan circuit, avoiding right atrial foreign material and suture, eliminating myocardial ischemia at operation, and removing the coronary sinus from the Fontan circuit—will result in improved laminar flow, reduced dysrhythmias, preserved ventricular function, and reduced thrombotic and obstructive complications, thereby reducing the slope of the late hazard phase.

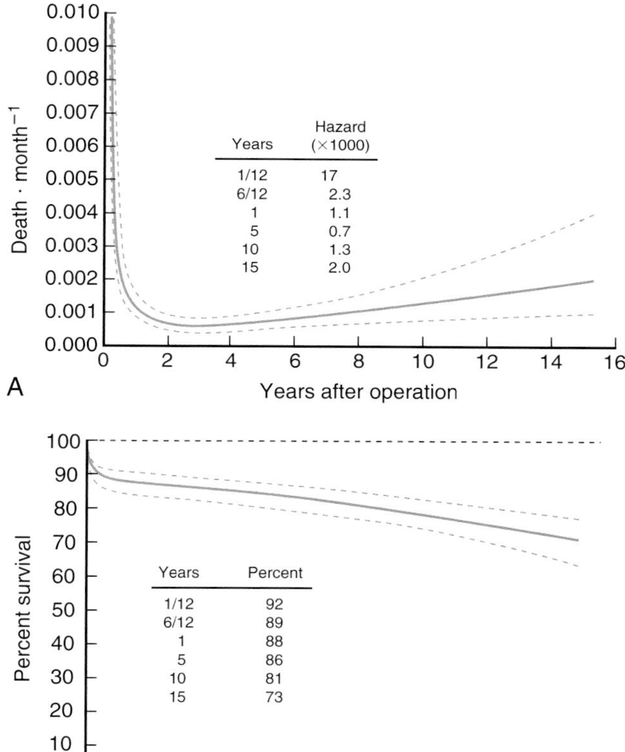

Figure 41-32 Survival after a "perfect" Fontan operation. Solid lines are parametric estimates enclosed between 70% confidence limits. Dash-dot-dash line represents estimates for a matched general population. **A,** Nomogram of predicted hazard function for death. Equation for nomogram is based on multivariable risk factor equation (see Table 41-4), entering optimal values within the realm of realism for each risk factor. Details are described in the publication.[F14] Note that greatly expanded vertical axis makes hazard function appear to be higher than that of Fig. 41-30, *B*; in fact, it is lower. **B,** Corresponding predicted survival. (From Fontan and colleagues.[F15])

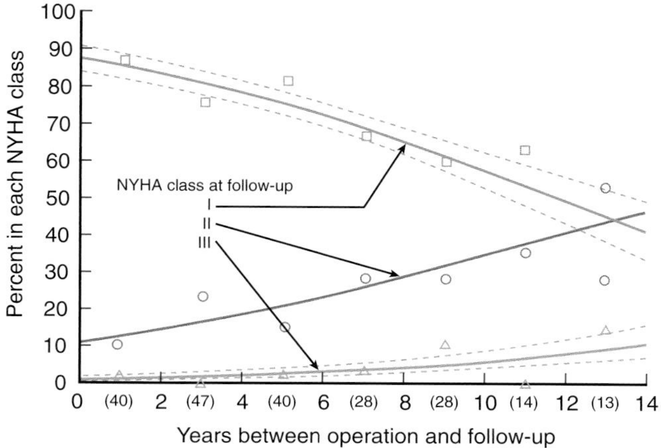

Figure 41-33 Time-related New York Heart Association (NYHA) functional class of patients after Fontan operation. Parentheses enclose number of patients followed up within intervals. Squares, circles, and triangles represent actual percentages; solid lines are parametrically determined percentages, with dashed lines enclosing 70% confidence limits around the percentages for NYHA classes I and III (see "Longitudinal Outcomes" in Section IV of Chapter 6). (From Fontan and colleagues.[F15])

Table 41-3 Modes of Death, Both Early and Intermediate Term, after Fontan Operation

Mode of Death	*n*	% of 110
Cardiac failure	80	73
Acute	50[a]	45
Subacute	23	21
Chronic	7	6
Acute pulmonary failure	1	1
Persistent fluid accumulation	11	10
Neurologic dysfunction	9	8
Sudden	4	4
Hemorrhage	2	2
Arrhythmic death	2	2
TOTAL	110	100

Data from Fontan and colleagues.[F15]
[a]Three occurred perioperatively after late reoperation for Fontan operation, and two occurred after late reoperation for Fontan pathway obstruction.

Table 41-4 Incremental Risk Factors for Death or Takedown after Fontan Operation

Risk Factor[a]		Hazard Phase	
		Early[a]	Late
	Patient		
(Younger)	Age	•	
(Older)	Age	•	•
	Morphologic:		
	Left AV valve atresia	•	
(Greater)	Main chamber hypertrophy	•	
(Smaller)	Dimensions of pulmonary arteries	•	
(Higher)	Pulmonary artery pressure	•	
	Procedure		
	Nonuse of cardioplegia	•	
(Longer)	Global myocardial ischemic time with cardioplegia	•	
	RA-PA (rather than RV) anastomosis	•	
	RA-to-PT valved conduit	•	
	Direct RA-to-PT anastomosis with linear RA incision	•	

Data from Fontan and colleagues.[F14]
[a]Shaping parameters and coefficients are in original publication.[F14]
Key: *AV,* Atrioventricular; *PT,* pulmonary trunk; *RA,* right atrium, *RV,* right ventricle.

Modes of Death

For patients undergoing the Fontan operation in the 1970s and 1980s, acute cardiac failure early postoperatively was the most common mode of death. Chronic cardiac failure, which first appears several years before death, and sudden death are the most common modes late postoperatively.

Assigning a mode of death after a Fontan operation is difficult because of frequent occurrence of fluid retention, which may have obvious hemodynamic causes (e.g., myocardial failure, elevated Rp, Fontan pathway obstruction) or may occur in the absence of any specific hemodynamic abnormality other than the existence of the Fontan itself. This fluid retention often appears primarily as persistent accumulations of pleural fluid or, less often, of ascitic or pericardial fluid. This tendency has been shown to be considerably less when a bidirectional superior cavopulmonary shunt has preceded the Fontan procedure.[Z2] In any event, in only about 10% of patients who die does persistent fluid accumulation in pericardial, pleural, or peritoneal spaces without hemodynamic insufficiency appear to be the mode of death (Table 41-3).

Incremental Risk Factors for Death

Acute Ventricular Decompression An important potential risk factor still remains to be investigated: namely, sudden "decompression" of the ventricular chamber by the Fontan operation. Decompression at the time of Fontan can be avoided by surgical staging, as described in this chapter, using one of two techniques: bidirectional superior cavopulmonary shunt or a hemi-Fontan operation.[W4] In this case, decompression is achieved at the time of second-stage palliation (see Section III), not at the time of the Fontan operation. It has not been shown definitely that avoiding ventricular decompression at the time of the Fontan improves outcome.

Deterioration The incremental risk factor for a late rising phase of hazard for death may be the post-Fontan state. It may result from:

- Long-standing nonpulsatile pulmonary artery flow generated by the systemic venous pressure
- Abnormality of the dominant ventricle per se

The latter may be an immutable congenital anomaly or may be acquired during postnatal life, either from the abnormal hemodynamic state existing before Fontan repair or from myocardial ischemia at previous operations. (A similar late-rising phase of hazard occurs in patients with discordant AV connection undergoing a two-ventricle repair.)

Younger Age at Operation In older studies, younger age at time of the Fontan operation was a risk factor for death (or complete takedown of a Fontan operation) early after operation[B6,D26,F14,K20] (Table 41-4). The nature of the relationship was such that risk of death (or takedown) early postoperatively began to increase as age of operation approached 3 years, and then increased more steeply as age was reduced to younger than 2 years[B6,F14,M23] (Fig. 41-34). Good results can be obtained from performing the Fontan operation in infants and children younger than 2 years, yet the probability of surviving has been documented to be less than in older patients.[M23,M24,W5] It should be emphasized, however, that this documentation is now 15 to 20 years old.

Certainly, mortality of 55% for patients younger than 4 years[M24] in older reports is no longer the case.[M23,M50,S37] The incremental risk of young age may have been neutralized by staged, fenestrated, incompleted Fontan operations, and by avoiding use of CPB, although this is not yet fully documented.[K4,M50]

Older Age at Operation Older age at operation is not a risk factor for death early postoperatively.[H20] Burkhart and colleagues[B33] report an 8.3% operative mortality, Ovroutski and colleagues[O14] and Veldtman and colleagues[V7] 13%, and Fujii and colleagues[F30] 4%, when operation is performed in

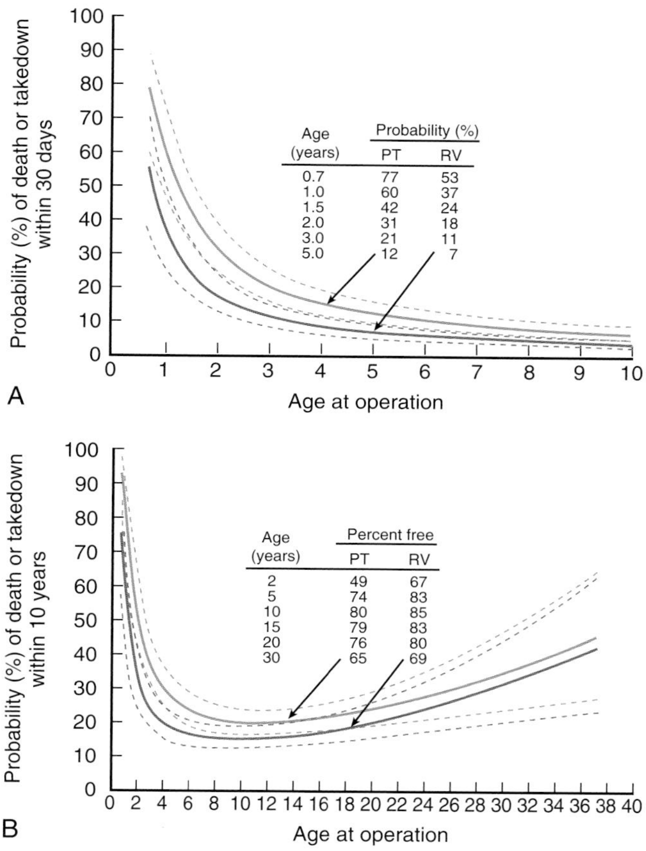

Figure 41-34 Illustration of incremental risk of younger and older age on outcome (death or takedown of repair) after Fontan operation. Illustration is a nomogram of a specific solution of a multivariable risk factor equation.[F15] **A,** Effect of young age on risk of death (or takedown) early (within 30 days) after operation. **B,** Effect of older age on late (10 years) outcome. Key: *PT,* Right atrial–to–pulmonary trunk anastomosis; *RV,* right atrium–to–right ventricle connection. (From Fontan and colleagues.[F14])

selected adults. It slightly increased risk of death late after the Fontan operation (Fig. 41-34, *B*) in one study,[F15] but this was not found by others.[D26,M46,V7]

Cardiac Morphology Cardiac morphology has been reported to be importantly related to outcome after the Fontan operation; specifically, tricuspid atresia has been found to have more favorable outcomes than other anomalies, and all anomalies with the morphologic LV as the main chamber have been reported to have more favorable outcomes than those with a right or indeterminate main ventricle.[B6,B8,D26,M19,R24,W8] There are exceptions; three studies found no influence of ventricular morphology on outcome.[H1,H16,T16]

A related morphologic feature that has also been identified as a risk factor is left AV valve atresia[M23] (see Table 41-4). This may not be a morphologic risk factor per se, but rather a morphologic arrangement that until recently resulted in use of a complex baffle for partitioning the atria. Such baffles often resulted in some obstruction of the pulmonary venous pathway to the right or a common AV valve, and this probably was the true risk factor.[M23] Various forms of total cavopulmonary connection, including the extracardiac conduit and lateral tunnel Fontan techniques (see Figs. 41-27 and 41-28), have overcome this problem, and left AV valve atresia may not be a risk factor in the future.

Small Size of Central Right and Left Pulmonary Arteries Small size of central right and left pulmonary arteries has been identified by some as a risk factor for death (or takedown) early after the Fontan operation,[F14] although others have not found this to be so.[A2] As is often the case, the controversy may relate to differing patient populations, patient data, and surgical techniques. In nearly all studies, only the prebranching pulmonary artery dimensions have been studied. If small size is limited to prebranching portions of right and left pulmonary arteries and if these portions are enlarged by patch-grafting at Fontan repair, one may expect to find little relationship between small size and outcome, as was the case in the study of Bridges and colleagues.[B27] Failure to perform surgical enlargement may leave small pulmonary artery size as a risk factor. Thus, according to the combined University of Bordeaux–UAB experience, when the prebranching portions of the right and left pulmonary arteries are small (McGoon ratio less than about 1.5 [see Figs. 1F-1, 1F-2, and 1F-3 in Chapter 1], a z value of less than about −3.5, or a cross-sectional area index [Nakata index] of less than about 160 $mm^2 \cdot m^{-2}$), risk of early death is increased[F14] (Fig. 41-35). Nakata and colleagues suggested, as a more restrictive guideline for considering patients at high risk, an index of less than 250 $mm^2 \cdot m^{-2}$.[N2] However, rarely was augmentation of the central pulmonary arteries performed in these patients.

By contrast, the Mayo Clinic group has suggested that size of right and left pulmonary arteries measured in the operating room is not related to outcome, even when augmentation is not done. However, the patients on whom they made measurements were selected based on *not* having small pulmonary arteries, so inferences about small size are not possible from their data. There are few studies relating size of pulmonary arteries measured *after enlargement* to outcome.

If pulmonary arterial narrowing extends into more distal portions of right and left pulmonary arteries, their small sizes may be a risk factor for death. Pulmonary artery "distortion" was found to be a powerful risk factor for death, but such distortion has been uncommonly found.[M7,M23,M35]

Elevated Pulmonary Artery Pressure and Pulmonary Vascular Resistance Elevated mean pulmonary artery pressure (PPA) and Rp have been known to increase risk of the Fontan operation since Choussat and colleagues' classic paper[C21]; this has been confirmed in subsequent studies.[B6,B29,D26,F14,K20,M23] Risk is particularly elevated when PPA is greater than 15 to 20 mmHg, unless the elevation is explained by a large $\dot{Q}p$ or important AV valve regurgitation. Rp would be expected to predict outcome more precisely, but in many patients it is difficult to measure determinants of this value, and the value is not highly sensitive to presence of multiple peripheral thrombi.[J12] Nonetheless, with Rp greater than 2 to 4 units · m^2, probability of good outcome is less.[B8]

Advanced Main Chamber Ventricular Hypertrophy Advanced main chamber ventricular hypertrophy and increased muscle mass is an important risk factor for death[D26,F14,K16,M50,S12] (see Table 41-4). Early survival (out to 6 months) after a Fontan operation in a 5-year-old child with favorable features and mild LV hypertrophy is estimated to be 99%, but it is 78% when moderately severe LV hypertrophy

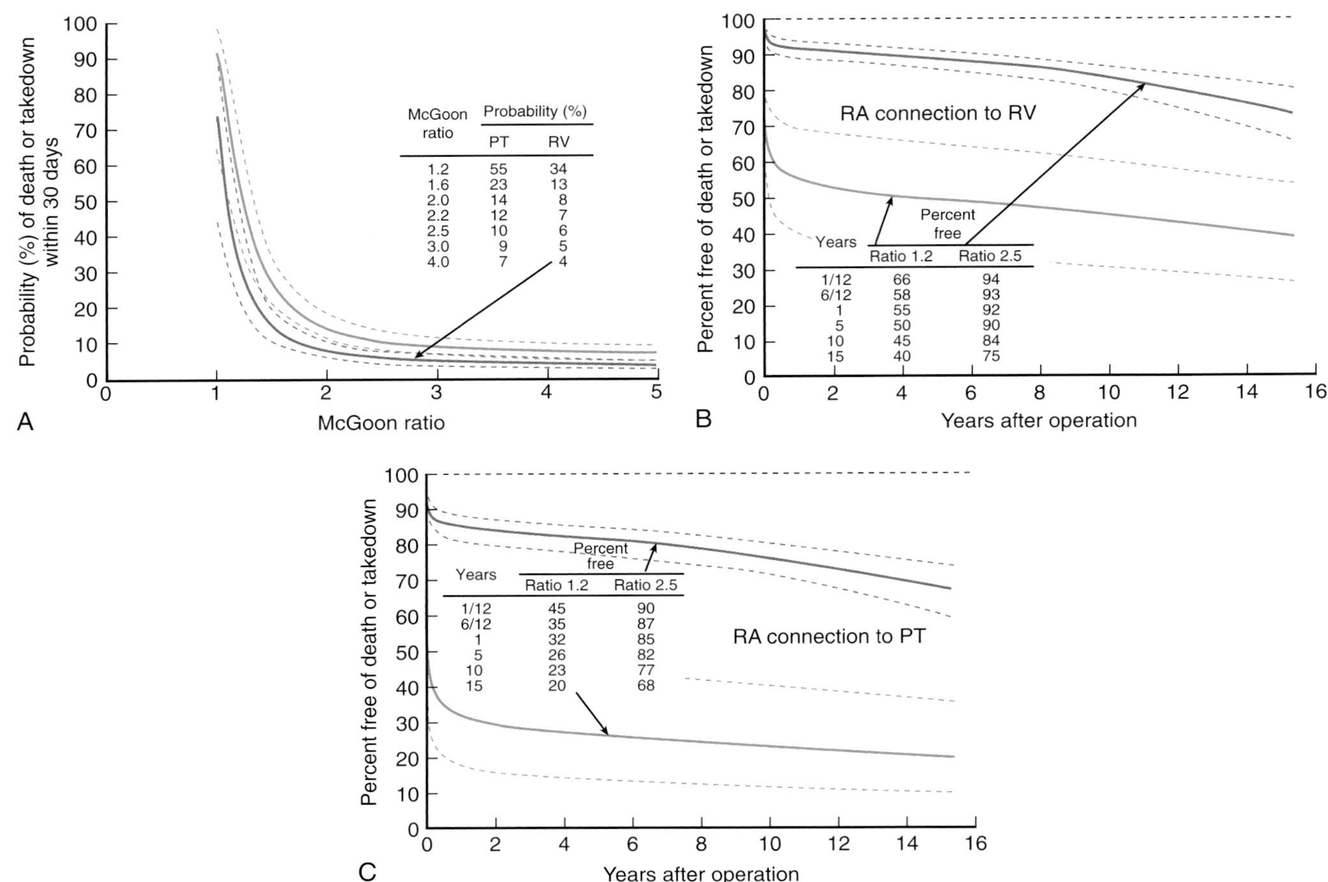

Figure 41-35 Nomogram of solutions of multivariable equation (see Table 41-4) illustrating effect of small size of central pulmonary arteries on outcome after Fontan operation when augmentation of central right and left pulmonary arteries is not performed. (See original paper for details of specific solution of multivariable equation.[F14]) **A,** Probability of death or takedown within 30 days of operation, according to sum of diameters of prebranching portions of right and left pulmonary arteries, expressed as McGoon ratio (see "Dimensions of the Pulmonary Arteries" and Appendix 1F in Chapter 1). **B,** Percent free of death or takedown out to 16 years postoperatively when a *right atrial–to–right ventricular connection* is made, according to whether pulmonary arteries are small (McGoon ratio of 1.2) or large (ratio of 2.5). **C,** Percent free of death or takedown out to 16 years postoperatively when a *right atrial–to–pulmonary arterial connection* is made, according to size of pulmonary arteries. Key: *PT,* Right atrium–to–pulmonary trunk anastomosis **(A)** and pulmonary trunk **(B, C)**; *RA,* right atrium; *RV,* right atrium–to–right ventricle connection **(A)** and right ventricle **(B, C)**. (From Fontan and colleagues.[F14])

is present.[K16] This risk factor adversely affects ventricular compliance (diastolic function) and, when advanced, systolic function as well.[S12] These observations have led to the widely held current practice of aggressive surgical relief of ventricular outflow obstruction in the staging of patients with single-ventricle physiology (see Section III). Although not advisable, relief of ventricular outflow obstruction can be performed simultaneously with the Fontan.[H11]

Atrial Isomerism Atrial isomerism (see Chapter 58), with its usually concurrent asplenia or polysplenia, has been identified as a risk factor for death.[B6,B8,D26,K20] This risk factor may relate in large part to abnormal systemic venous connections to the heart, and these may be neutralized by modifications of surgical technique (see "Persistent Left Superior Vena Cava with Hemiazygos Extension of Interior Vena Cava" under Special Situations and Controversies later in this section). Recent techniques may have neutralized the risk of heterotaxy. Early mortality in 21 patients undergoing operation from 1995 to 2004 was only 9.5% (2 deaths; CL 3.3%-21%), and 10-year survival of a larger cohort of 142 patients from the same series was 57%.[B7] In other studies, recent experience defines the risk of early mortality at 0% to 13%.[A25,M37,S31] Risk may also relate to dysfunction of the common AV valve, which is often present.

Functional Status

Many patients consider themselves fully active after the Fontan operation; it was previously reported that 94% of patients are in New York Heart Association (NYHA) functional class I or II.[F13] Now that intermediate-term follow-up information is available out to at least 20 years, it is known that NYHA functional class gradually deteriorates.[F15,G11] Nearly 90% of patients are in NYHA functional class I at 1 year after operation, but this is true in only about 56% of patients at 10 years (see Fig. 41-33). This information supports the inference that the Fontan operation is a palliative procedure, with increasing disability developing in some patients by 10 years and in an increasing percentage thereafter. In patients with lateral tunnel or extracardiac conduit connections, exercise capacity is also well below normal, and daily activity limitations are related to older age, further supporting this inference.[M47,R13,Y5]

Other variables may affect functional status. In a large multicenter study, the extracardiac conduit Fontan was noted to have better functional status than the lateral tunnel Fontan as measured by oxygen consumption during exercise testing.[A14] In the same study, LV morphology also was associated with better functional status than either RV or indeterminate ventricular morphology. In a large multicenter evaluation, the presence of heterotaxy did not affect functional status.[A22] The study by Shiraishi and colleagues suggests that in patients undergoing an extracardiac conduit Fontan, earlier age at completion of the procedure results in better long-term hemodynamics and exercise capacity.[S21] In contrast, the study by Napoleone and colleagues found no differences based on age at which the Fontan was performed.[P1] Whether the RV is incorporated into the Fontan circuit or not, pharmacologic afterload reduction does not improve exercise tolerance.[K26,W7] Others have documented subnormal performance on objective exercise testing in patients who claim unrestricted activity with complete absence of symptoms. Nevertheless, subnormal performance represents a considerable improvement over preoperative status.[A19,D24,D25,K23,N6] Exercise capacity is severely restricted in Fontan patients at moderately high altitudes.[D5]

Somatic growth does not improve after the Fontan operation if the patient had previously undergone a bidirectional superior cavopulmonary shunt, mainly because catch-up growth has already occurred (somatic growth does improve after the bidirectional superior cavopulmonary shunt, demonstrating catch-up growth that was lost during the volume overloaded previous state).[V11]

Hemodynamic Status

Notwithstanding good functional status in most patients for at least several years after the Fontan operation, objectively studied hemodynamic state is usually subnormal.[A6,A19,B4,C19,F10,H7,K23,P2] Peterson and colleagues, studying 16 patients (5 of whom had a valve used in the Fontan repair) with average follow-up of 25 months, found that resting and exercise cardiac indexes were not different from those of healthy children.[P10] The mechanism used by the patients to achieve high cardiac outputs during exercise was an increase in heart rate. However, ventricular ejection fraction was low, 0.45 ± 0.11 at rest and 0.51 ± 0.13 at peak exercise, and ventricular end-diastolic volumes were considerably greater than those of healthy children. Findings by Shachar and colleagues were similar, indicating reduced ejection fraction and increased left ventricular end-diastolic volume at rest and exercise.[S14]

An important aspect of the hemodynamic state after the Fontan operation is increase in Fontan pathway pressure during exercise.[L4,S14] Its elevation can lead to reflux into caval and hepatic veins during atrial systole.[D20] Observant patients occasionally note that garments become tight around the waist during exercise, presumably because of increased Fontan pathway pressure and hepatic swelling. $\dot{Q}p$ is biphasic after the atriopulmonary Fontan operation, from both right atrial relaxation and contraction as well as left atrial emptying into the main ventricular chamber.[D20,H2,L4,M39]

Not surprisingly, the respiratory cycle strongly affects $\dot{Q}p$ after certain types of Fontan operations, and perhaps after all types.[R10] $\dot{Q}p$ is increased with normal inspiration and is considerably augmented during strenuous inspiration. It is nearly stopped during the Valsalva maneuver.

Ventricular morphology influences hemodynamics. The presence of LV morphology results in better ejection fraction, AV valve function, and semilunar valve function compared with right or indeterminate ventricular morphology.[A14]

De Leval and colleagues have studied flow characteristics of the total cavopulmonary connection, finding that laminar flow is maintained to a greater extent when SVC and IVC pulmonary artery connections are offset, avoiding direct collision of the two bloodstreams, and when 90-degree angled configurations of the cavopulmonary connections are avoided.[D10] Experimental studies have shown that the extracardiac conduit connection provides superior hemodynamics when compared with either the atriopulmonary or lateral tunnel connection[L10]; clinical studies have not been performed. Using three-dimensional phased-contrast MRI in the clinical setting, altered flow patterns in the pulmonary arteries were found equally in atriopulmonary and lateral tunnel Fontans.[M43] Extracardiac conduit Fontans were not evaluated.

Cardiac Rhythm

Importance of sinus rhythm postoperatively remains arguable, primarily because of uncertainty about hemodynamic events after the Fontan operation. There is little doubt that sinus rhythm enhances performance of the main ventricular chamber, because of "atrial kick." Dynamics of flow from cavae to pulmonary arteries are less firmly established. Acute animal experiments of Matsuda and colleagues and of Shemin and colleagues indicate that loss of sinus rhythm does not alter flow through an atriopulmonary conduit regardless of whether it contains a valve.[M20,S18] However, using Doppler techniques, Bull and colleagues showed that in patients with an atriopulmonary connection, pulmonary flow accelerates during atrial systole.[B32] This was also observed by Ishikawa and colleagues using low-pressure contrast injection into the pulmonary artery.[I7]

Although sinus rhythm may not have a demonstrable direct effect on flow from right atrium to pulmonary arteries, it may influence this flow indirectly by permitting a lower PLA than otherwise would be the case. Also, because sinus rhythm seems to provide at least some pulsatility in the pulmonary arterial circulation, it may be advantageous in minimizing late changes in the pulmonary circulation. Loss of sinus rhythm and other supraventricular dysrhythmias, especially atrial flutter, are common after the atriopulmonary Fontan and increase with longer follow-up.[P5,P9] Freedom from supraventricular tachydysrhythmias at 20 years after the atriopulmonary-type Fontan can be as low as 46%. Electrophysiologic ablation procedures are initially successful, but recurrence is common.[W9]

The lateral tunnel Fontan is also associated with a high prevalence of loss of sinus rhythm in some studies.[C30,K5,K8,M8] In contrast, one study finds a greater loss of sinus rhythm in extracardiac conduit than in lateral tunnel Fontans; however, the follow-up period was almost twice as long in the extracardiac conduit group, putting the validity of this comparison into question.[D19] Experimental work in animal models suggests that the foreign body and suture line inherent in the lateral tunnel and hemi-Fontan techniques can induce supraventricular rhythm disturbance.[B2,G6] Early and midterm follow-up studies indicate that loss of sinus rhythm and other supraventricular dysrhythmias are markedly reduced following the extracardiac conduit Fontan compared historically with lateral tunnel and atriopulmonary Fontan operations.[P12,P13] It should be emphasized, however, that randomized and long-term follow-up studies are not available.

Loss of sinus rhythm and occurrence of supraventricular dysrhythmias may have complex etiologies and likely are not exclusively the result of the type of Fontan connection.[F8] Influence of previous operations, such as atrial septectomy or AV valve repair or replacement, myocardial ischemia from prior insults both intraoperatively and perioperatively, type of superior cavopulmonary connection (bidirectional superior cavopulmonary shunt vs. hemi-Fontan), and prior hemodynamic circumstances (chronic volume loads or obstructions) are all likely to affect atrial rythym.[M8]

Sudden death has occurred in some patients late after operation (see Table 41-3). Multiform premature ventricular contractions appear to be present late postoperatively in about one third of patients and asymptomatic bradycardia in about 20%.[C16] These findings suggest that disturbances of cardiac rhythm may cause some late failures of the Fontan operation. Many of the factors mentioned in the previous paragraph may influence ventricular rhythm as well.

Complete heart block is rare after the Fontan operation.[G3]

Abnormalities of Pulmonary Circulation

Decrease in upper-to–lower lobe pulmonary blood flow perfusion ratio was observed by Cloutier and colleagues in most patients after the Fontan operation, similar to that seen in those who had undergone the classic Glenn operation[C26] (see "Classic Glenn Operation" under Special Situations and Controversies in Section I). To date, however, pulmonary arteriovenous fistulas have been observed uncommonly after the Fontan operation.[M41,P18]

A longer interval between operation and time of observation clearly increases prevalence of pulmonary arteriovenous fistulas after a classic Glenn operation.[K25] Thus, long follow-up is required to document the impression that this complication is uncommon.

Nevertheless, it is becoming increasingly clear that pulmonary arteriovenous fistulas are much less likely to form following Fontan completion. There is increasing anecdotal evidence that fistulas that form after a bidirectional superior cavopulmonary shunt regress following the Fontan. Pathophysiology of these fistulas remains elusive, and various etiologic factors have been suggested, including reduced $\dot{Q}p$, nonpulsatile flow, cyanosis, and lack of splanchnic venous blood in the pulmonary circulation. Using contrast echocardiography, a sensitive method for identifying pulmonary arteriovenous fistulae, it has been shown that patients with single-ventricle physiology at any stage in their surgical reconstruction—that is, at the stage with completely mixed circulation with a systemic–pulmonary arterial shunt or at the stage with a bidirectional superior cavopulmonary shunt—were more likely to show evidence of fistulae than patients with separated circulations.[B12] Echocardiographic evidence of fistulae, however, did not necessarily predict clinical cyanosis.

Protein-Losing Enteropathy

An important complication of the Fontan operation is protein-losing enteropathy. It is characterized by depressed serum albumin concentration with no obvious cause.[H10] It may be suggested by late postoperative onset of generalized edema and pleural or peritoneal fluid accumulations. Patients may or may not have diarrhea. α_1-Antitrypsin clearance is abnormally high, and because of low serum protein, total serum calcium is abnormally low. Special studies show excessive loss of serum proteins from the gastrointestinal tract; endoscopic investigations show prominent lymph vessels in the jejunal mucosa. This *gastrointestinal protein loss* occurs before clinical evidence of protein-losing enteropathy.[T10]

About 13% of patients develop evidence of protein-losing enteropathy by 10 years, and interval between operation and its appearance ranges widely, from 1 month to 16 years.[F2,M33] Protein-losing enteropathy is associated with death, with near 50% mortality 5 years after diagnosis.

Protein-losing enteropathy is not limited to patients who have undergone the Fontan operation. It has been reported in almost all situations in which there is chronically elevated central venous pressure, including heart failure, chronic constrictive pericarditis, and atrial switch operations for transposition of the great arteries.[D4,M39,W10] It has also been observed in patients who have undergone SVC-RPA anastomosis and in patients with isolated SVC obstruction after an atrial switch operation.[G19,H10] Presumably, the combination of increased lymph production from increased IVC pressure and impaired lymph drainage from increased SVC pressure contribute to this complication. Other potential influences are an elevated systemic inflammatory state and changes in mesenteric vascular resistance.[O11]

It may be relieved by reoperations that result in a lower right atrial pressure, such as when bidirectional superior cavopulmonary shunt or Fontan revisions are used to relieve systemic venous pathway obstruction. However, there is considerable early mortality after reoperation.

Correcting other hemodynamic abnormalities when right atrial pressure is low has resulted in regression.[V8] Creating a late fenestration has been reported to result in resolution of protein-losing enteropathy in three of five cases.[R26,V12] Nonsurgical therapy, including use of steroids and heparin, has been associated with its resolution.[K12,Z1] Resolution has been reported after pacemaker placement in two patients with sinus node dysfunction,[C29] and in two patients following diaphragm placation for phrenic nerve palsy.[L19] In a multicenter study, transplantation was found to effectively reverse protein-losing enteropathy.[B11]

Thromboembolic Complications

The cumulative occurrence of thrombotic complications ranges from 3% to 16%, and of embolic complications from 3% to 19%, according to a recent literature review.[J3] However, essentially all the primary reports reviewed involved patients predominantly receiving their operation prior to the modern era. Most of the studies indicate that these complications occur either early, within the first year after the Fontan, or late, beyond 10 years after surgery. Massive thrombi may form in the right atrium, particularly in atriopulmonary Fontan connections. Thus, in about half of the few cases reported, thrombi developed within a few weeks of operation; in the other half, they became evident a number of years later.[D21,P20] Although infrequent, occurring early or over the intermediate term in about 10% of patients, this complication is of importance[C32] because a large thrombus or a piece of it may migrate from the right atrium and occlude the Fontan anastomosis or fill the RV or pulmonary arteries with sufficient thrombi to be fatal. Recently, a high prevalence of thrombus has been documented in the Fontan pathway when this complication was sought by routine echocardiography in asymptomatic patients, and embolic complications have been reported as high as 29%.[B3,R21]

Presumably, slower-than-normal flow through the cavae and presence of foreign material predispose patients to thrombus formation and subsequent embolization. However, acquired abnormalities of the clotting system may be involved. In a study of this specific problem, the most common and most pronounced of these was a presumably acquired deficiency of protein C.[C32] Additional deficiencies in proteins and factor VII have been identified, which may relate in part to chronic impairment of liver function.[J7,O4] The extracardiac conduit and lateral tunnel Fontan techniques currently favored by most centers may reduce thrombotic complications by maintaining laminar flow and reducing stasis. At midterm follow-up, the risk of thrombosis is almost nonexistent in a large series of extracardiac conduit Fontans.[P12]

Neurologic Complications

Neurodevelopmental outcome is reported to be generally within the normal range.[U2] Thromboembolic cerebrovascular events have been reported, but their true prevalence is not known. Association of these events with ligated pulmonary artery segments and with fenestrations have been cited.[O10,Q1] Intracerebral venous thrombosis has been reported. Overall prevalence of stroke ranges from 3% to 9% over a 15-year period.[D27]

Desaturation after Fontan

Early and late systemic desaturation can occur from various systemic venous channels connecting to the pulmonary veins, coronary sinus, or left-sided atrial structures that may become manifest immediately or develop over time.[F4,G8,S39] Evaluation with cardiac catheterization is indicated to distinguish these entities from lung disease or intrapulmonary arteriovenous malformations, and to define specific morphology of the venous connections. Surgical or interventional closure of the connection is indicated.

Reoperation

Takedown Reoperation for takedown of the Fontan operation has been necessary in a few patients in whom death has seemed otherwise inevitable. In earlier eras, risk of takedown (with substitution of a systemic–pulmonary arterial shunt) has been high, with 3 of 7 patients dying after the procedure in the combined University of Bordeaux–UAB experience (43%; CL 20%-68%).[F14] Most of these patients were seriously ill when takedown was performed.

Mayer and colleagues also reported a high mortality (100%; CL 79%-100%) among 8 patients treated in this manner, but 2 survived and did well after takedown to a bidirectional superior cavopulmonary shunt (0%; CL 0%-61%).[M23] With this latter type of takedown, results in the future may be better (see "Takedown or Modification of Fontan Operation" earlier under Technique of Operation).

Reoperation for Pathway Obstruction Reoperation for pathway obstruction has been the most common type of reoperation after the Fontan operation, and freedom from it has not been as high as desirable[G18] (Fig. 41-36). Furthermore, in this group of patients, instantaneous risk of requiring reoperation for pathway obstruction increased throughout follow-up, suggesting that with certain

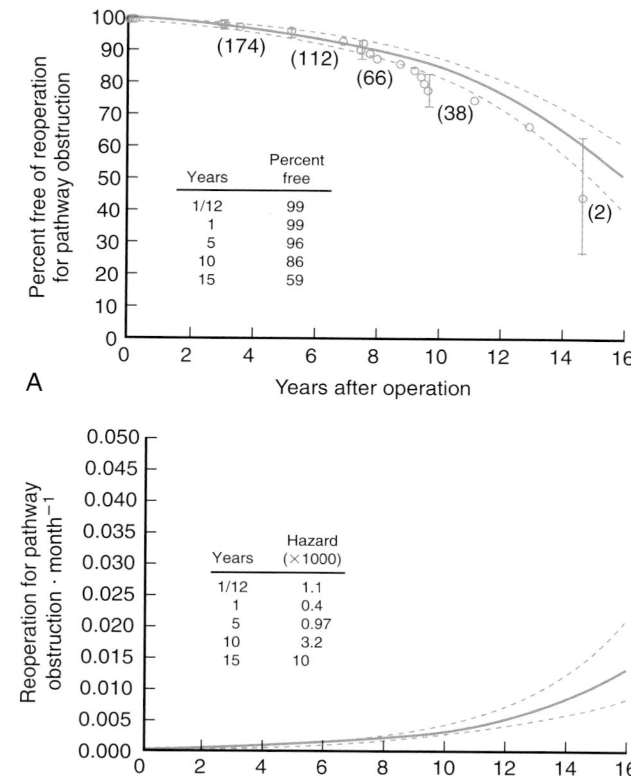

Figure 41-36 Reoperation for pathway obstruction after Fontan operation in a heterogeneous group of patients. Depiction is as in Fig. 41-30, *A*. **A,** Time-related freedom from reoperation. **B,** Hazard function. Note its gradual rise. (From Fernandez and colleagues.[F3])

techniques of creating these pathways (see text that follows), nearly all patients will at some time require surgical revision of the pathway.[F3] Hospital mortality after reoperation has been high: 5 of 21 patients (24%; CL 14%-37%) in the University of Bordeaux–UAB experience.[F14] However, among hospital survivors, late survival and functional status have been as satisfactory as after the original Fontan operation.

Need for reoperation for pathway obstruction has varied considerably, depending on the type of Fontan operation. Direct nonvalved connections between right atrium and either RV or pulmonary trunk have had a low prevalence of reoperations for pathway obstruction (Table 41-5), specifically, 4 instances among 200 patients (2%; CL 1%-3.6%). By contrast, 17 of 134 patients (13%; CL 9.6%-16%) receiving conduit connections, either valved or nonvalved, underwent reoperations for pathway obstruction.[F3] Pathway obstruction has not been evident following the extracardiac conduit and lateral tunnel Fontans, but follow-up has been shorter than for older procedures.[L14,O2,P12]

Other Reoperations In about 5% of patients undergoing the atriopulmonary Fontan operation for double inlet ventricle, closure of the right-sided AV valve dehisced and required reoperation.[F3] Likewise, re-repair of the ASD has been required in about 2% of patients. Cardiac transplantation was required late postoperatively in four patients in the combined University of Bordeaux–UAB experience for progressive myocardial failure.[F14] This final form of treatment may be required with increasing frequency in the future.

Table 41-5 Site and Type of Distal Right Atrial Connection in Fontan Operation and Prevalence of Reoperation for Pathway Obstruction

		Reoperation for Pathway Obstruction		
Site and Type of Distal RA Connection	*n*	**No.**	**%**	**CL (%)**
Right ventricle	114	14	12	9-16
Conduit	69	12	17	13-23
Valved	20	2	10	3-22
Xenograft	1	0	0	0-85
Allograft	19	2	11	4-23
Nonvalved	49	10	20	14-28
Direct	45	2	4	1-10
Simple	32	2	6	2-14
Roofed	13	0	0	0-14
Pulmonary artery	220	7	3	2-5
Conduit	65	5	8	4-13
Valved	63	5	8	4-13
Xenograft	11	1	9	1-28
Allograft	52	4	8	4-14
Nonvalved	2	0	0	0-61
Direct	155	2	1.3	0.4-3
Simple	118	2	2	0.6-4
Roofed	37	0	0	0-5
TOTAL	334	21	6	5-8

Data from Fernandez and colleagues.[F3]
Key: *RA,* Right atrial.

As the extracardiac conduit and lateral tunnel Fontan procedures have come into favor, they are being used with increasing frequency to revise atriopulmonary and AV Fontan connections. Indications include obstruction in the systemic venous Fontan pathway, thrombus formation in the right atrium, right pulmonary vein compression, and atrial dysrhythmias.[K30,M11,M26] Use of the maze procedure, its modifications (see "Maze III Procedure" and "Modified Maze Procedures" under Results in Section IV of Chapter 16), or intraoperative cryoablation may be indicated in a substantial portion of these patients.[M21] These Fontan revisions have achieved substantial improvement in almost all patients. Operative mortality is about 10%.[M11] It has been suggested from experimental studies that simply performing a bidirectional superior cavopulmonary shunt in patients with an atriopulmonary Fontan and dilated right atrial chamber and impaired hemodynamics may be beneficial, although there are no clinical data to support this.[L11]

Fontan Operation with Deliberately Incomplete Atrial Partitioning

A number of operations have evolved that, despite their name, are *not* a Fontan operation. They have in common partial diversion of systemic venous blood to the pulmonary arteries and thus, an *incomplete* separation of pulmonary and systemic circulations. Some are intended as preliminary procedures to a Fontan operation, whereas others, such as the permanently "fenestrated Fontan," replace the Fontan operation. Results of these operations have to be considered separately from those of a completed Fontan operation, although it is not yet known whether they are different.

The Fontan operation with deliberately incomplete atrial partitioning (fenestrated Fontan, Fontan with adjustable ASD) is difficult to evaluate because of the small number of patients in whom it has been performed and absence of risk-adjusted comparisons with other approaches. Early mortality has been 0% to 5%.[B29,J1,K24,L3,L6,L7,M23,S36] Early closure of the residual aperture has been possible in at least 50% of patients, but this proportion, as well as the early and late results, varies according to characteristics of the patients being operated on and policies of the responsible physicians.[B29] Both techniques, the method of Laks and colleagues[L3] and that of percutaneous catheter closure,[R18] are well controlled and achieve secondary closure of the residual aperture (when this is elected) with low risk and good success. Late results of the specific subgroup of patients receiving permanently fenestrated Fontan operation have not yet been determined.

INDICATIONS FOR OPERATION

Fontan Operation

Most patients will have previously undergone palliative operations as newborns and again later in infancy, although a small group will have undergone one or no previous procedures. The Fontan procedure is rarely performed before age 1 year and typically not before age 18 to 24 months. Certain physiologic and morphologic criteria must be met for the Fontan to succeed. Currently, there are no clear indications for specifically performing either the extracardiac conduit Fontan or the lateral tunnel Fontan, although there is general consensus that these forms of total cavopulmonary Fontan are preferred over variations that include the right atrium.[C20,C31,M34,P12] Despite lack of established superiority of one or the other of these, important differences between the two operations exist.[M9,P13] These differences may ultimately be found to be important factors influencing outcome (see "Extracardiac Conduit versus Lateral Tunnel Fontan" in Special Situations and Controversies).

Many criteria, classically expounded by Choussat, Fontan, and colleagues, for performing a completed Fontan operation are arguable.[C21] However, Rp greater than about 4 units · m^2 seems a clear contraindication. Pathologic data from lung biopsy have not aided in making this decision.[G10] When Rp is 2 to 4 units · m^2, a bidirectional superior cavopulmonary shunt (or a hemi-Fontan procedure[K21]) or a fenestrated Fontan operation rather than a completed Fontan operation may be indicated (see Section III). If subsequent evaluation confirms adequacy of the pulmonary vascular bed, the preliminary procedure can be converted to a total cavopulmonary connection. Evaluation of $\dot{Q}p$ and Rp should be performed shortly before the intended Fontan procedure, because they can be affected over time by factors such as chronic pulmonary microemboli.[O7]

When branches of right and left pulmonary arteries are small, a Fontan operation will probably not succeed, although it can be argued that this should be the case only if they are small enough to cause elevation in Rp.[S13] For these cases, only a systemic–pulmonary arterial shunt is feasible. Small size of central portions of right and left pulmonary arteries is not a contraindication to repair, but enlargement of these arteries should probably be combined with a bidirectional superior cavopulmonary shunt or hemi-Fontan operation, which can later be converted to a completed Fontan operation.

The same strategy can be used when ventricular function is impaired. In general, ventricular end-diastolic pressure of greater than 10 to 12 mmHg (in absence of a large $\dot{Q}$ or important AV valvar regurgitation) or an ejection fraction of less than 45% raise questions as to the suitability of the patient for a Fontan repair and suggest a preliminary procedure of the type described.

Poorly planned, multiple, uncoordinated palliative operations deny many patients the opportunity for a successful Fontan operation.[M35,S35,T1] Therefore, the entire therapeutic plan must be in hand before the first procedure is performed (see Section I).

Timing of Fontan Operation

Because the tube graft for an extracardiac conduit Fontan operation should be 2 cm in diameter or larger (this is the diameter of the average adult IVC), it is reasonable to delay the Fontan procedure in patients with single-ventricle physiology who have previously undergone a bidirectional superior cavopulmonary shunt until they weigh 15 kg or more, assuming other physiologic or morphologic developments do not require earlier intervention. A 2-cm-diameter graft can be placed in children who are somewhat smaller (weighing 11 to 12 kg), but this is not ideal, because of the size mismatch between graft and vessels. Conditions that might require earlier performance of the Fontan include development of intrapulmonary arteriovenous malformations and acquired aortopulmonary collaterals. Additionally, patients who are symptomatic and cyanotic under conditions of bidirectional superior cavopulmonary shunt physiology may also be candidates for earlier Fontan. Recent studies suggest that the extracardiac conduit can be performed earlier, using 16- and 18-mm-diameter grafts, with excellent results; however, long-term follow-up is not available.[I8] The lateral tunnel Fontan can be performed earlier without concern that the child will outgrow the tunnel, because the tunnel has growth potential. Some institutions routinely perform the lateral tunnel Fontan at about 2 years of age.[J2,M34]

Fontan Operation with Deliberately Incomplete Atrial Partitioning

Incomplete atrial partitioning with the extracardiac conduit Fontan is usually not necessary to achieve excellent outcomes.[P12,T10] There are several reasons for this. The operation can be accomplished without inducing hypothermia or CPB, resulting in no inflammatory response. The aorta is not clamped, so there is no myocardial ischemia. As a result, systolic and diastolic ventricular function are not compromised even temporarily. Rp is minimally affected in the perioperative period, because the circulation is not exposed to an extracorporeal circuit. Therefore, the transient elevation of cardiac filling pressures and Rp that are usually encountered when hypothermia, CPB, and myocardial ischemia are used are markedly attenuated. Nevertheless, according to the STS database, currently 75% of all Fontans are fenestrated.[J8] Because two thirds of all Fontans are extracardiac conduits, this indicates that many extracardiac conduit Fontans are also being fenestrated. It is not clear from the STS report whether it is primarily the extracardiac conduits performed using CPB that are receiving a fenestration, or whether particular institutions and surgeons are using the fenestration independent of CPB management.

The lateral tunnel Fontan requires full CPB, hypothermia, and aortic clamping with administration of cardioplegia, and thus patients undergoing this procedure typically have perioperative perturbations in ventricular filling pressure and Rp. Most[J2,M34] institutions that routinely perform the lateral tunnel Fontan use incomplete atrial partitioning, but some never do.[H17]

The argument remains whether a fenestrated Fontan operation should be done as a routine procedure or only in high-risk situations. In any event, use of some form of incomplete atrial partitioning seems advantageous in high-risk patients, especially when CPB is used to perform the procedure.

SPECIAL SITUATIONS AND CONTROVERSIES

Definitive Palliation Other Than Fontan Operation

Although the predominant view is that the Fontan is the best available definitive palliation for patients with single-ventricle physiology, few or no definitive data support this view. Some studies suggest that final palliation in the form of superior cavopulmonary shunt or aortopulmonary shunt provide long-term palliation that compares favorably with the Fontan.[G7]

Conversion of Atriopulmonary Fontan to Cavopulmonary Fontan Operation

Increasingly, patients who have previously undergone Fontan surgery with atriopulmonary connections of various kinds present with complications specifically related to them, including giant right atrium, right atrial thrombosis, compression of right pulmonary veins, atrial dysrhythmias, and obstruction at the atriopulmonary connection. They may present for Fontan revision, but only if ventricular function and Rp are adequate to sustain the Fontan circulation once the complications described previously are surgically addressed (if ventricular function is compromised and it is not due to a surgically correctable hemodynamic cause, or if the Rp is elevated, the only option is transplantation[H18]). The Fontan conversion operation entails removing the atriopulmonary connection and creating either an extracardiac conduit IVC-to–pulmonary artery connection or a lateral tunnel inferior cavopulmonary connection. Additionally, atrial reduction plasty, thrombus removal, and atrial dysrhythmia surgery, such as a formal maze procedure or one of its modifications (see "Interruption of Macro-reentrant Circuits" in Section IV of Chapter 16), may also be performed.[A4,K30,M11,M26]

Another reason for Fontan conversion is to remove coronary sinus drainage from the high-pressure systemic venous compartment and place it in the low-pressure pulmonary venous compartment. It has been argued that elevated coronary sinus pressure reduces coronary perfusion pressure, which in theory may reduce coronary flow reserve; however, recent data suggest that the site of the coronary sinus drainage does not influence coronary flow reserve.[E3]

Giardini and colleagues[G17] have documented that peak oxygen uptake improved and heart failure symptoms resolved when studied 6 months after conversion. Most conversions have been performed using the extracardiac conduit[A4,G17,K15,M26,S17]; however, Morales and colleagues[M42] provide evidence that lateral tunnel and extracardiac conduit revisions have equal outcomes.

In appropriately chosen candidates, early mortality is 0% to 5%.[A4,G17,K15,M26,M42,S17] Outcomes will be optimized if appropriate preoperative medical management of the failing Fontan is undertaken.[G15]

Routine Use of Fontan Operation with Deliberately Incomplete Atrial Partitioning

Some institutions routinely fenestrate,[J2,M34] and others rarely or never do.[H17,P12] The advantages of fenestrating are reported to be improved perioperative hemodynamics, lower early mortality, and reduced pleural effusions. The need for routine fenestration has been supported[A5] and has been questioned.[H6,O1,P12]

Improvement in perioperative hemodynamics does occur in selected cases—specifically in those that have a systemic inflammatory response or temporary myocardial dysfunction as a result of the operation. These perturbations are more likely to occur when CPB is used and when cardiac arrest is used during CPB. Thus, fenestration is likely to be beneficial when the Fontan is performed using CPB, and of little or no benefit in most cases when CPB is not used.

The evidence that fenestration improves early mortality and reduces duration of effusions is not convincing. Table 41-6 shows that the majority of studies examining the effects of fenestration on effusions indicate that absence of a fenestration is not a risk factor for effusions, and Table 41-7 shows no difference in duration of effusions based on whether a fenestration is performed. Table 41-8 lists all studies examining the association between fenestration (or not) and early death. Four of the eight studies, and importantly the four most recent ones, show no association. Table 41-9 lists early mortality in studies that routinely use a fenestration, and in those that do not. Results are similar.

Table 41-6 Single-Institution Studies Examining "Absence of Fenestration" as a Risk Factor for Effusions: Multivariable Analysis

		Risk of Effusions	
Study	**Year**	**Yes**	**No**
Airan et al.[A5]	2000	•	
Gaynor et al.[G9]	2002	•	
Lemler et al.[L18]	2002	•	
Fedderly et al.[F1]	2001		•
Atik et al.[A21]	2002		•
McGuirk et al.[M30]	2003		•
Gupta et al.[G28]	2004		•
Schreiber et al.[S8]	2006		•
Meyer et al.[M34]	2006		•
Hosein et al.[H16]	2007		•
Mascio et al.[M14]	2009		•

Extracardiac Conduit versus Lateral Tunnel Fontan Operation

When usual morphologic variants are being considered, there remains considerable difference of opinion as to the best way to construct the Fontan physiology. Currently, extracardiac conduit or lateral tunnel cavopulmonary variants are preferred by most surgeons, largely because of the many long-term complications associated with the atriopulmonary connection. These complications include atrial dysrhythmia, loss of sinus node function, giant right atrium, atrial thrombus formation, compression of right pulmonary veins, and loss of laminar flow (see Clinical Features and Diagnostic Criteria earlier in this section). Any form of total cavopulmonary connection will address many of these complications, but controversy exists as to whether the lateral tunnel or the extracardiac conduit is better. According to the STS database, two thirds of all recent Fontans are extracardiac conduits, and one third are lateral tunnels.[J8] Some surgeons perform both operations, having specific indications for each, but most surgeons perform predominantly one or the other in the belief that they are choosing the operation that provides the least overall morbidity.

No definitive data support the superiority of either the lateral tunnel or extracardiac conduit Fontan. There are distinct differences between these two techniques, and it is a matter of speculation as to how these differences translate into patient benefit. The lateral tunnel procedure provides reasonable laminar flow and has the advantage of growth potential; however, it is an open cardiac procedure requiring CPB, hypothermia, and myocardial ischemia, which may have both immediate postoperative effects and long-term implications. The procedure also requires substantial manipulation of tissue in the region of the sinoatrial node and sinoatrial nodal artery, and atrial suture and foreign body load exposed to the systemic circulation is substantial. As a result, there are concerns regarding maintaining sinus rhythm and avoiding atrial dysrhythmias. The extracardiac conduit provides hemodynamics that most closely approximate laminar flow.[L10] It can be performed as a closed cardiac procedure without hypothermia, myocardial ischemia, or CPB, reducing the risks related to CPB, as well as the CPB-related systemic inflammatory response[K9] and the transient physiologic perturbations that increase the need for fenestration.[P12] Minimal or no manipulation of the right atrium is typical, and suture and foreign body load in the right atrium is eliminated, removing stimuli for dysrhythmia and systemic thromboembolic phenomena.[P12,P13] The sinoatrial node and sinoatrial nodal artery regions are completely avoided. It can be argued, therefore, that the immediate postoperative and long-term ventricular mechanics, sinus node function, and atrial rhythm status are maximized. The extracardiac conduit, however, does not have growth potential and in general is performed in slightly older children to allow for a full-sized conduit. This delay until Fontan completion, and concern regarding long-term obstructive problems, have been cited as theoretical disadvantages.

Although there are no randomized trials comparing the two procedures, there exists a substantial body of data evaluating a wide spectrum of outcomes for each. Mahnke and colleagues noted a greater occurrence of cerebrovascular accidents in lateral tunnel than in extracardiac conduit Fontans, but follow-up was shorter in the latter group.[M3] Azakie,[A24]

Table 41-7 Single-Institution Studies Examining Duration of Effusions, Categorized by Use of Fenestration or Not

Fenestration			No Fenestration		
Study	Year	Chest Tube Drainage (median days)	Study	Year	Chest Tube Drainage (median days)
Azakie et al.[A24]	2001	8	Hsu et al.[H17]	1997	5
Kumar et al.[K32]	2003	9	Gupta et al.[G28]	2004	10
Woods et al.[W13]	2003	7	Petrossian et al.[P12]	2006	8
Meyer et al.[M34]	2006	2	Schreiber et al.[S7]	2007	4
Hosein et al.[H16]	2007	8	Hosein et al.[H16]	2007	8
			Harada et al.[H6]	2009	11

Table 41-8 Single-Institution Studies Examining "Absence of Fenestration" as a Risk Factor for Death: Multivariable Analysis

		Risk of Death	
Study	Year	Yes	No
Jacobs & Norwood[J2]	1994	•	
Gentles et al.[G11]	1997	•	
Airan et al.[A5]	2000	•	
Gaynor et al.[G9]	2002	•	
Schreiber et al.[S9]	2004		•
Meyer et al.[M34]	2006		•
Hosein et al.[H16]	2007		•
Kim et al.[K14]	2008		•

Nurnberg,[N10] Lee,[L16] and Robbers-Visser[R14] and their colleagues all identified the lateral tunnel as an independent risk factor for both early and midterm atrial dysrhythmias, but Hakacova and colleagues did not.[H3] Fiore and colleagues showed that there was no difference in outcomes for the two operations with respect to early or late mortality, dysrhythmias, thromboembolic events, neurologic complications, or readmissions for effusions; however, they noted that the extracardiac conduit required fewer fenestrations but used a greater amount of resources.[F7] In contrast, Kumar and colleagues examined multiple outcome measures both early and midterm and found no differences between the groups, including resource utilization.[K32] None of these studies note an increased thrombosis risk for extracardiac conduit Fontans, and Petrossian and colleagues have documented a close to zero occurrence of thrombosis both early and up to 10 years after the extracardiac conduit operation.[P12]

Midterm follow-up of a large series of extracardiac conduit Fontan procedures indicates that performing the Fontan procedure at 3 to 4 years of age does not result in development of significant complications such as pulmonary arteriovenous malformations or acquired systemic to pulmonary artery collaterals.[P12] It is also well documented that the extracardiac conduit operation can be performed without aortic clamping and even without CPB, whereas the lateral tunnel operation requires both.[P12,S20] Longer length of hospital stay has been linked to a greater need for perioperative fluid administration, which is secondarily linked to use of CPB.[S2] Avoiding CPB and reducing its length are associated with reduced effusions, providing indirect evidence supporting the advantages of the extracardiac conduit technique.[S19] There is no evidence to support the contention that the extracardiac conduit develops stenosis over time. Follow-up of up to 10 years reveals that the extracardiac conduit does not develop obstruction as the child grows,[P12] and formal measurement of the conduit by angiography at midterm follow-up indicates the conduit diameter shows little or no change from the diameter at insertion.[L14,O2] In the Pediatric Heart Network multicenter study that retrospectively examined outcomes for the Fontan in 546 patients, the lateral tunnel Fontan was shown to have lower exercise performance than the extracardiac conduit Fontan.[A14]

Transplantation Following Fontan Operation

Patients with Fontan physiology may become candidates for transplantation for several reasons. One is that a critically important physiologic variable becomes abnormal, and as a result, the circulation can no longer be sustained. There are two such variables: ventricular function and Rp. If ventricular function decreases to the point that end-diastolic filling pressure becomes elevated, or if Rp becomes elevated, the Fontan circulation will fail, and transplantation is the only therapeutic option. Another reason is that intractable complications of the Fontan circulation develop, despite preserved ventricular function and low Rp. These complications include protein-losing enteropathy and plastic bronchitis. Patients who present for transplantation with preserved ventricular function and Fontan-related complications may have a particularly high mortality,[G24] implying that earlier transplantation may be necessary when these intractable complications develop. Protein-losing enteropathy will reverse after successful transplantation.[B11,G4] Some studies report that survival after transplantation in Fontan patients is similar to that of patients undergoing transplantation for other causes, with 1-year survival of 72% and 5-year survival of 68%,[C15,J9] whereas others report much higher early and late mortality.[P11] In a multicenter study assessing 98 patients, survival after transplantation in Fontan patients was slightly less than in other children with congenital heart disease and in those without congenital heart disease.[B11]

Hepatic Function in Fontan Patients

Hepatic dysfunction is universally recognized following the Fontan operation. Liver abnormalities correlate with older age and with time since the Fontan operation. Some studies correlate elevated systemic venous pressure and poor cardiac

Table 41-9 Single-Institution Studies Examining Early Mortality, Categorized by Use of Fenestration or Not

Fenestration						No Fenestration					
Study	Year	*n*	No.	%	CL (%)	Study	Year	*n*	No.	%	CL (%)
Jacobs & Norwood[J2]	1994	112	5	4.5	2.5-7.5	Jacobs & Norwood[J2]	1994	88	11	12	8.8-17
Woods et al.[W13]	2003	54	3	5	2.5-11	Hsu et al.[H17]	1997	61	3	4.9	2.2-9.6
Meyer et al.[M34]	2006	144	2	1.4	0.5-3.3	Tokunaga et al.[T11]	2002	99	0	0	0-1.9
Petrossian	2006	49	0	0	0-3.8	Petrossian et al.[P12]	2006	236	4	1.7	0.9-3.1
Jacobs et al.[J2]	2008	100	0	0	0-1.9	Schreiber et al.[S7]	2007	132	2	1.5	0.5-3.5
						Ocello et al.[O1]	2007	100	6	6.0	3.6-9.5
						Harada et al.[H6]	2009	72	0	0	0-2.6

function with liver abnormalities,[C5,F28,K13] and others do not.[N3] Liver abnormalities include fibrosis and cirrhosis, with their attendant consequences, and synthetic dysfunction, which particularly affects the coagulation system.[N3,O3,O4,T12]

Use of Long-Term Anticoagulation

It is well recognized that the Fontan population is at high risk for thrombotic complications, second only to the nonbiological prosthetic valve population. Thus, anticoagulation therapy is an important consideration in this population. There are currently no prospective studies examining the efficacy of long-term anticoagulation following the Fontan operation; however, one study that recognized pulmonary emboli in 17% of Fontan patients also found that this complication did not occur if patients were on warfarin therapy.[V6] Another study showed no benefit for the use of warfarin.[M3] Nevertheless, practices vary widely. Some advocate no routine therapy but use varying pharmacologic regimens including aspirin, warfarin, or heparin for patients with risk factors for thrombosis.[C18,K6] Others recommend aspirin routinely but no additional therapy.[J4] Still others recommend warfarin therapy, citing their experience that this approach reduces thrombosis when compared with no therapy or aspirin therapy.[S11]

Type of Operation for Tricuspid Atresia

When the cardiac malformation is tricuspid atresia and concordant ventriculoarterial connection, most patients will undergo either an extracardiac conduit or lateral tunnel Fontan; however, there is a possibility that the RV can become sufficiently functional to provide some benefit to the pulmonary circulation.[B32,G29] Therefore, consideration can be given to performing an initial nonvalved right atrial–RV connection, generally at age 3 to 5 years. The RV enlarges considerably after this procedure, at least in some patients. If the ventricle becomes 30% or greater of normal size, the secondary insertion at age 8 to 10 years of an allograft valved conduit between right atrium and RV should provide a reasonably effective two-ventricle system. However, risk of conduit compression by the sternum must be overcome for this to be a generally useful alternative.

Bowman and colleagues were the first to demonstrate progressive RV enlargement when a valved right AV conduit was used.[B21] Pumping action of the enlarged ventricle can contribute to Qp and reduction of Fontan pathway pressure.[B32,G29,O12] Moreover, pulmonary artery systolic and pulse pressures can increase almost to normal. Fontan and colleagues also reported data from standardized exercise testing supporting the idea that an allograft valve in the connection between right atrium and RV provides a better late functional result than does a nonvalved connection.[F13] Del Torso and colleagues also noted less abnormality in both ejection fraction and hemodynamic response to exercise in patients with an AV connection than in those with an atriopulmonary connection.[D13] Magnitude of the hemodynamic advantages of a valved connection between right atrium and RV seem sufficient to affect functional status and survival late postoperatively,[F14] but this remains to be proven.

Valved Fontan Pathway

Studies suggest that a valve does not function when the RV is totally excluded, as in the Kreutzer modification of the Fontan procedure, even though the valve remains structurally perfect.[I7] Bull and colleagues also showed echocardiographically that the valve in a valved allograft conduit between right atrium and pulmonary artery closed momentarily or not at all.[B32] In similar circumstances, Sharratt and colleagues demonstrated delayed opening and slow closing of the conduit valve, suggesting that its presence in the pulmonary circuit may not contribute much to the hemodynamic state.[S16] Finally, in acute animal experiments, Shemin and colleagues showed that flow through a right atrial–to–pulmonary artery conduit was similar whether a valve was present or not.[S18]

Persistent Left Superior Vena Cava with Hemiazygos Extension of Inferior Vena Cava

As a part of the complex cardiac anatomy that usually coexists with atrial isomerism (see Morphology in Chapter 58) and sometimes in the absence of atrial isomerism, a persistent left SVC receiving IVC return via the hemiazygos vein may drain into the upper left corner of the left or common atrium. When the hepatic veins attach to the atrium well to the right, a slightly modified form of lateral tunnel total cavopulmonary connection can be used in which the left SVC is disconnected from the left atrium, the atrial opening oversewn, and the end of the left SVC anastomosed end to side to an incision in the left pulmonary artery. Occasionally, the left SVC lies virtually parallel to the left pulmonary artery, and then a side-to-side anastomosis without caval division permits a better fit of the two structures. In this case, the left SVC-atrial junction should be closed securely with a ligature and several pledgeted mattress transfixion sutures. The right-sided SVC is managed as usual in this variant of the lateral tunnel total cavopulmonary connection, but the intraatrial tunnel brings only hepatic vein blood (not IVC blood) to the anastomosis of the cardiac end of the SVC to the RPA. Alternatively, the extracardiac conduit technique can be used, with the conduit connecting the hepatic venous confluence to the pulmonary artery system.[H19]

In some hearts with these complex venous drainages, the hepatic veins enter a common atrium in the midline or to the left of it. This, and sometimes position of orifices of pulmonary veins, can make connection of hepatic veins to the cardiac end of the SVC possible only by a long and circuitous tunnel if the lateral tunnel technique is being considered. The extracardiac conduit Fontan does not present this limitation under these morphologic circumstances and can be used effectively. The conduit can be routed to either the left or right of the cardiac mass to reach the pulmonary arterial system.

The total cavopulmonary shunt of Kawashima, which permanently leaves hepatic venous blood draining to the pulmonary venous atrium, has also been suggested as an option under these circumstances.[K10] After this operation, resting SaO_2 has been between 87% and 92% but decreases with exercise.[K10] There is also the important concern of pulmonary arteriovenous malformations, which develop frequently following this procedure. As a result, the Kawashima variant is no longer recommended as a long-term solution.

Preoperative Cardiac Catheterization

Some have suggested that the Fontan operation can be performed without cardiac catheterization,[F5,F9,P16] but this approach is not widely accepted. Other studies suggest that catheterization should be performed using actual measurement of oxygen uptake rather than relying on predicted oxygen uptake in calculating cardiac output and pulmonary vascular resistance, because predicted values underestimate Rp.[S15]

Several other studies indicate that pulmonary artery pressure can be accurately estimated by measuring pulmonary venous wedge pressure in single-ventricle patients, thus obviating the need to directly measure pulmonary artery pressure.[M45,T8]

REFERENCES

A

1. Abrams LD. Side-to-side cavopulmonary anastomosis for the palliation of "primitive ventricle." Br Heart J 1977;39:926.
2. Adachi I, Yagihara T, Kagisaki K, Hagino I, Ishizaka T, Kobayashi J, et al. Preoperative small pulmonary artery did not affect the midterm results of Fontan operation. Eur J Cardiothorac Surg 2007;32:156-62.
3. Agarwal HS, Churchwell KB, Doyle TP, Christian KG, Drinkwater DC Jr, Byrne DW, et al. Inhaled nitric oxide use in bidirectional Glenn anastomosis for elevated Glenn pressures. Ann Thorac Surg 2006;81:1429-34.
4. Agnoletti G, Borghi A, Vignati G, Crupi GC. Fontan conversion to total cavopulmonary connection and arrhythmia ablation: clinical and functional results. Heart 2003;89:193-8.
5. Airan B, Sharma R, Choudhary SK, Mohanty SR, Bhan A, Chowdhari UK, et al. Univentricular repair: is routine fenestration justified? Ann Thorac Surg 2000;69:1900-6.
6. Akagi T, Benson LN, Green M, DeSouza M, Harder JR, Gilday DL, et al. Ventricular function during supine bicycle exercise in univentricular connection with absent right atrioventricular connection. Am J Cardiol 1991;67:1273.
7. Alboliras ET, Julsrud PR, Danielson GK, Puga FJ, Schaff HV, McGoon DC, et al. Definitive operation for pulmonary atresia with intact ventricular septum. Results in twenty patients. J Thorac Cardiovasc Surg 1987;93:454.
8. Alejos JC, Williams RG, Jarmakani JM, Galindo AJ, Isabel-Jones JB, Drinkwater D, et al. Factors influencing survival in patients undergoing the bidirectional Glenn anastomosis. Am J Cardiol 1995;75:1048.
9. Alexi-Meskishvili V, Ovroutski S, Ewert P, Dahnert I, Berger F, Lange PE, et al. Optimal conduit size for extracardiac Fontan operation. Eur J Cardiothorac Surg 2000;18:690-5.
10. Allen SJ, Laine GA, Drake RE, Gabel JC. Superior vena caval pressure elevation causes pleural effusion formation in sheep. Am J Physiol 1988;255:H492.
11. Allgood NL, Alejos J, Drinkwater DC, Laks H, Williams RG. Effectiveness of the bidirectional Glenn shunt procedure for volume unloading in the single ventricle patient. Am J Cardiol 1994; 74:834.
12. Amodeo A, Galletti L, Marianeschi S, Picardo S, Giannico S, DiRenzi P, et al. Extracardiac Fontan operation for complex cardiac anomalies: seven years experience. J Thorac Cardiovasc Surg 1997;114:1020.
13. Anderson JB, Beekman RH 3rd, Border WL, Kalkwarf HJ, Khoury PR, Uzark K, et al. Lower weight-for-age z score adversely affects hospital length of stay after the bidirectional Glenn procedure in 100 infants with a single ventricle. J Thorac Cardiovasc Surg 2009;138:397-404.
14. Anderson PA, Sleeper LA, Mahony L, Colan SD, Atz AM, Breitbart RE, et al. Contemporary outcomes after the Fontan procedure: a Pediatric Heart Network multicenter study. J Am Coll Cardiol 2008;52:85-98.
15. Anderson RH, Penkoske PA, Zuberbuhler JR. Variable morphology of ventricular septal defect in double inlet left ventricle. Am J Cardiol 1985;55:1560.
16. Anderson RH, Rigby ML. The morphologic heterogeneity of "tricuspid atresia" (editorial). Int J Cardiol 1987;16:67.
17. Anderson RH, Wilkins JL, Gerlis LM, Smith A, Becker AE. Atresia of the right atrioventricular orifice. Br Heart J 1977;39:414.
18. Ando M, Satami G, Takao A. Atresia of tricuspid or mitral orifice: anatomic spectrum and morphogenetic hypothesis. In Van Praagh R, Takao A, eds. Etiology and morphogenesis of congenital heart disease. Mount Kisco, NY: Futura, 1980, p. 421.
19. Annecchino FP, Brunelli F, Borghi A, Abbruzzese P, Merlo M, Parenzan L. Fontan repair for tricuspid atresia: experience with 50 consecutive patients. Ann Thorac Surg 1988;45:430.
20. Annecchino FP, Fontan F, Chauve A, Quaegebeur J. Palliative reconstruction of the right ventricular outflow tract in tricuspid atresia: a report of 5 patients. Ann Thorac Surg 1980;29:317.
21. Atik E, Ikari NM, Martins TC, Barbero-Marcial M. Fontan operation and the cavopulmonary technique: immediate and late results according to the presence of atrial fenestration. Arq Bras Cardiol 2002;78:162-6.
22. Atz AM, Cohen MS, Sleeper LA, McCrindle BW, Lu M, Prakash A, et al. Functional state of patients with heterotaxy syndrome following the Fontan operation. Cardiol Young 2007;17 Suppl 2:44-53.
23. Azzolina G, Eufrate S, Pensa P. Tricuspid atresia: experience in surgical management with a modified cavopulmonary anastomosis. Thorax 1972;27:111.
24. Azakie A, McCrindle BW, Van Arsdell G, Benson LN, Coles J, Hamilton R, et al. Extracardiac conduit versus lateral tunnel cavopulmonary connections at a single institution: impact on outcomes. J Thorac Cardiovasc Surg 2001;122:1219-28.
25. Azakie A, Merklinger SL, Williams WG, Van Arsdell GS, Coles JG, Adatia I. Improving outcomes of the Fontan operation in children with atrial isomerism and heterotaxy syndromes. Ann Thorac Surg 2001;72:1636-40.

B

1. Bakulev AN, Kolesnikov SA. Anastomosis of superior vena cava and pulmonary artery in the surgical treatment of certain congenital defects of the heart. J Thorac Cardiovasc Surg 1959;37:693.
2. Balaji S, Case CL, Sade RM, Gillette PC. Arrhythmias and electrocardiographic changes after the hemi-Fontan procedure. Am J Cardiol 1994;73:828.

3. Balling G, Vogt M, Kaemmerer H, Eicken A, Meisner H, Hess J. Intracardiac thrombus formation after the Fontan operation. J Thorac Cardiovasc Surg 2000;119:745.
4. Barber G, Di Sessa T, Child JS, Perloff JK, Laks H, George BL, et al. Hemodynamic responses to isolated increments in heart rate by atrial pacing after a Fontan procedure. Am Heart J 1988;115:837.
5. Bargeron LM Jr, Karp RB, Barcia A, Kirklin JW, Hunt D, Deverall PB. Late deterioration of patients after superior vena cava to right pulmonary artery anastomosis. Am J Cardiol 1972;30:211.
6. Bartmus DA, Driscoll DJ, Offord KP, Humes RA, Mair DD, Schaff HV, et al. The modified Fontan operation for children less than 4 years old. J Am Coll Cardiol 1990;15:429.
7. Bartz PJ, Driscoll DJ, Dearani JA, Puga FJ, Danielson GK, O'Leary PW, et al. Early and late results of the modified Fontan operation for heterotaxy syndrome: 30 years of experience in 142 patients. J Am Coll Cardiol 2006;48:2301-5.
8. Behrendt DM, Rosenthal A. Cardiovascular status after repair by Fontan procedure. Ann Thorac Surg 1980;29:322.
9. Bellet S, Stewart HL. Congenital heart disease, atresia of tricuspid orifice. Am J Dis Child 1933;45:1247.
10. Berdat PA, Belli E, Lacour-Gayet F, Planche C, Serraf A. Additional pulmonary blood flow has no adverse effect on outcome after TCPC. J Thorac Cardiovasc Surg 2004;52:280-6.
11. Bernstein D, Naftel D, Chin C, Addonizio LJ, Gamberg P, Blume ED, et al. Outcome of listing for cardiac transplantation for failed Fontan: a multi-institutional study. Circulation 2006;114:273-80.
12. Bernstein HS, Brook MM, Silverman NH, Bristow J. Development of pulmonary arteriovenous fistulae in children after cavopulmonary shunt. Circulation 1995;92:II309.
13. Bharati S, Lev M. The conduction system in tricuspid atresia with and without regular (D-) transposition. Circulation 1977;56:423.
14. Bharati S, Lev M, Kirklin JW. Cardiac surgery and the conduction system. 2nd Ed. Mount Kisco, NY: Futura, 1992.
15. Bharati S, McAllister HA Jr, Tatooles CJ, Miller RA, Weinberg M Jr, Bucheleres HG, et al. Anatomic variations in underdeveloped right ventricle related to tricuspid atresia and stenosis. J Thorac Cardiovasc Surg 1976;72:383.
16. Billingsley AM, Laks H, Boyce SW, George B, Santulli T, Williams RG. Definitive repair in patients with pulmonary atresia and intact ventricular septum. J Thorac Cardiovasc Surg 1989;97:746.
17. Binotto MA, Higuchi Mde L, Aiello VD. Left ventricular remodeling in hearts with tricuspid atresia: morphologic observations and possible basis for ventricular dysfunction after surgery. J Thorac Cardiovasc Surg 2003;126:1026-32.
18. Bjork VO, Olin CL, Bjarke BB, Thoren CA. Right atrial–right ventricular anastomosis for correction of tricuspid atresia. J Thorac Cardiovasc Surg 1979;77:452.
19. Boruchow IB, Swenson EW, Elliott LP, Bartley TD, Wheat MW Jr, Schiebler GL. Study of the mechanisms of shunt failure after superior vena cava–right pulmonary artery anastomosis. J Thorac Cardiovasc Surg 1970;60:531.
20. Bove EL. Current status of staged reconstruction for hypoplastic left heart syndrome. Pediatr Cardiol 1998;19:308.
21. Bowman FO, Malm JR, Hayes CJ, Gersony WM. Physiological approach to surgery for tricuspid atresia. Circulation 1978;58:I83.
22. Bradley SM. Management of aortopulmonary collateral arteries in Fontan patients: routine occlusion is not warranted. Semin Thorac Cardiovasc Surg Pediatr Card Surg Annu 2002;5:55-67.
23. Bradley SM, Mosca RS, Hennein HA, Crowley DC, Kulik TJ, Bove EL. Bidirectional superior cavopulmonary connection in young infants. Circulation 1996;94:II5.
24. Bradley SM, Simsic JM, Atz AM, Dorman BH. The infant with single ventricle and excessive pulmonary blood flow: results of a strategy of pulmonary artery division and shunt. Ann Thorac Surg 2002;74:805-10.
25. Bradley TJ, Human DG, Culham JA, Duncan WJ, Patterson MW, LeBlanc JG, et al. Clipped tube fenestration after extracardiac Fontan allows for simple transcatheter coil occlusion. Ann Thorac Surg 2003;76:1923-8.
26. Brawn WJ, Sethia B, Jagtap R, Stumper OF, Wright JG, DeGiovanni JV, et al. Univentricular heart with systemic outflow obstruction: palliation by primary Damus procedure. Ann Thorac Surg 1995;59:1441.
27. Bridges ND, Farrell PE Jr, Pigott JD 3rd, Norwood WI, Chin AJ. Pulmonary artery index: a nonpredictor of operative survival in patients undergoing modified Fontan repair. Circulation 1989;80:I216.
28. Bridges ND, Jonas RA, Mayer JE, Flanagan MF, Keane JF, Castaneda AR. Bidirectional cavopulmonary anastomosis as interim palliation for high risk Fontan candidates. Circulation 1990;82:IV170.
29. Bridges ND, Lock JE, Castaneda AR. Baffle fenestration with subsequent transcatheter closure, modification of the Fontan operation for patients at increased risk. Circulation 1990;82:1681.
30. Brown DW, Gauvreau K, Powell AJ, Lang P, Colan SD, Del Nido PJ, et al. Cardiac magnetic resonance versus routine cardiac catheterization before bidirectional Glenn anastomosis in infants with functional single ventricle: a prospective randomized trial. Circulation 2007;116:2718-25.
31. Brown JW. Congenital tricuspid atresia. Arch Dis Child 1936;11:275.
32. Bull C, de Leval MR, Stark J, Taylor JF, Macartney FJ. Use of a subpulmonary ventricular chamber in the Fontan circulation. J Thorac Cardiovasc Surg 1983;85:21.
33. Burkhart HM, Dearani JA, Mair DD, Warnes CA, Rowland CC, Schaff HV, et al. The modified Fontan procedure: early and late results in 132 adult patients. J Thorac Cardiovasc Surg 2003;125:1252-9.

C

1. Calabrese CT, Carrington CB, Harley RA Jr, Rojas RH, Glenn WW. The long-term functional and morphological changes in the pulmonary circulation following cava-pulmonary artery shunt. J Surg Res 1968;8:593.
2. Caldarone CA, Benson L, Holtby H, Li J, Redington AN, Van Arsdell GS. Initial experience with hybrid palliation for neonates with single-ventricle physiology. Ann Thorac Surg 2007;84:1294-300.
3. Calvaruso DF, Rubino A, Ocello S, Salviato N, Guardi D, Petruccelli DF, et al. Bidirectional Glenn and antegrade pulmonary blood flow: temporary or definitive palliation? Ann Thorac Surg 2008;85:1389-96.
4. Campbell M. Tricuspid atresia and its prognosis with and without surgical treatment. Br Heart J 1961;23:699.
5. Camposilvan S, Milanesi O, Stellin G, Pettenazzo A, Zancan L, D'Antiga L. Liver and cardiac function in the long term after Fontan operation. Ann Thorac Surg 2008;86:177-82.
6. Carlon CA, Mondini PG, de Marchi R. Surgical treatment of some cardiovascular diseases. J Int Coll Surg 1951;16:1.
7. Caspi J, Pettitt TW, Ferguson TB Jr, Stopa AR, Sandhu SK. Effects of controlled antegrade pulmonary blood flow on cardiac function after bidirectional cavopulmonary anastomosis. Ann Thorac Surg 2003;76:1917-22.
8. Ceithaml EL, Puga FJ, Danielson GK, McGoon DC, Ritter DG. Results of the Damus-Stansel-Kaye procedure for transposition of the great arteries and for double-outlet right ventricle with subpulmonary ventricular septal defect. Ann Thorac Surg 1984;38:433.
9. Cerillo AG, Murzi B, Giusti S, Crucean A, Redaelli S, Vanini V. Pulmonary artery banding and ventricular septal defect enlargement in patients with univentricular atrioventricular connection and the aorta originating from an incomplete ventricle. Eur J Cardiothorac Surg 2002;22:192-9.
10. Chan EH, Russell JL, Williams WG, Van Arsdell GS, Coles JG, McCrindle BW. Postoperative chylothorax after cardiothoracic surgery in children. Ann Thorac Surg 2005;80:1864-70.
11. Chan SY, Lau W, Wong WH, Cheng LC, Chau AK, Cheung YF. Chylothorax in children after congenital heart surgery. Ann Thorac Surg 2006;82:1650-6.
12. Chang AC, Farrell PE Jr, Murdison KA, Baffa JM, Barber G, Norwood WI, et al. Hypoplastic left heart syndrome: hemodynamic and angiographic assessment after initial reconstructive surgery and relevance to modified Fontan procedure. J Am Coll Cardiol 1991;17:1143.
13. Chang AC, Hanley FL, Wermovsky G, Rosenfeld HM, Wessel DL, Jonas RA, et al. Early bidirectional cavopulmonary shunt in young infants: postoperative course and early results. Circulation 1993;88:149.
14. Chang YH, Kim WH, Lee JY, Kim SJ, Lee C, Hwang SW, et al. Pulmonary artery banding before the Damus-Kaye-Stansel procedure. Pediatr Cardiol 2006;27:594-9.
15. Chen JM, Davies RR, Mital SR, Mercando ML, Addonizio LJ, Pinney SP, et al. Trends and outcomes in transplantation for complex congenital heart disease: 1984 to 2004. Ann Thorac Surg 2004;78:1352-61.

16. Chen SC, Nouri S, Pennington DG. Dysrhythmias after the modified Fontan procedure. Pediatr Cardiol 1988;9:215.
17. Cheung HC, Lincoln C, Anderson RH, Ho SY, Shinebourne EA, Pallides S, et al. Options for surgical repair in hearts with univentricular atrioventricular connection and subaortic stenosis. J Thorac Cardiovasc Surg 1990;100:672.
18. Cheung YF, Chay GW, Chiu CS, Cheng LC. Long-term anticoagulation therapy and thromboembolic complications after the Fontan procedure. Int J Cardiol 2005;102:509-13.
19. Chin AJ, Franklin WH, Andrews BA, Norwood WI Jr. Changes in ventricular geometry early after Fontan operation. Ann Thorac Surg 1993;56:1359.
20. Chopra PS, Rao P. Corrective surgery for tricuspid atresia: which modification of Fontan-Kreutzer procedure should be used? A review. Am Heart J 1992;123:758.
21. Choussat A, Fontan I, Besse P, Vallot F, Chauve A, Bricand H. Selection criteria for Fontan's procedure. In Anderson RH, Shinebourne EA, eds. Pediatric cardiology. 1977. Edinburgh: Churchill Livingstone, 1978.
22. Chowdhury UK, Airan B, Kothari SS, Talwar S, Saxena A, Singh R, et al. Specific issues after extracardiac Fontan operation: ventricular function, growth potential, arrhythmia, and thromboembolism. Ann Thorac Surg 2005;80:665-72.
23. Clapp SK, Tantengco MV, Walters HL 3rd, Lobdell KW, Hakimi M. Bidirectional cavopulmonary anastomosis with intracardiac repair. Ann Thorac Surg 1997;63:746.
24. Cleuziou J, Schreiber C, Cornelsen JK, Horer J, Eicken A, Lange R. Bidirectional cavopulmonary connection without additional pulmonary blood flow in patients below the age of 6 months. Eur J Cardiothorac Surg 2008;34:556-62.
25. Cleveland DC, Kirklin JK, Naftel DC, Kirklin JW, Blackstone EH, Pacifico AD, et al. Surgical treatment of tricuspid atresia. Ann Thorac Surg 1984;38:447.
26. Cloutier A, Ash JM, Smallhorn JF, Williams WG, Trusler GA, Rowe RD, et al. Abnormal distribution of pulmonary blood flow after the Glenn shunt or Fontan procedure: risk of development of arteriovenous fistulae. Circulation 1985;72:471.
27. Cochrane AD, Brizard CP, Penny DJ, Johansson S, Comas JV, Malm T, et al. Management of the univentricular connection: are we improving? Eur J Cardiothorac Surg 1997;12:107.
28. Cohen MI, Bridges ND, Gaynor JW, Hoffman TM, Wernovsky G, Vetter VL, et al. Modifications to the cavopulmonary anastomosis do not eliminate early sinus node dysfunction. J Thorac Cardiovasc Surg 2000;120:891-900.
29. Cohen MI, Rhodes LA, Wernovsky G, Gaynor JW, Spray TL, Rychik J. Atrial pacing: an alternative treatment for protein-losing enteropathy after the Fontan operation. J Thorac Cardiovasc Surg 2001;121:582-3.
30. Cohen MI, Wernovsky G, Vetter VL, Wieand TS, Gaynor JW, Jacobs ML. Sinus node function after a systematically staged Fontan procedure. Circulation 1998;98:II352.
31. Coles JG, Leung M, Kielmanowicz S, Freedom RM, Benson LN, Rabinovitch M, et al. Repair of tricuspid atresia: utility of right ventricular incorporation. Ann Thorac Surg 1988;45:384.
32. Cromme-Dijkhuis AH, Henkens CM, Bijleveld CM, Hillege HL, Bom VJ, van der Meer J. Coagulation factor abnormalities as possible thrombotic risk factors after Fontan operations. Lancet 1990;336:1087.
33. Crupi G, Alfieri O, Locatelli G, Villani M, Parenzan L. Results of systemic-to-pulmonary artery anastomosis for tricuspid atresia with reduced pulmonary blood flow. Thorax 1979;34:290.

D

1. Daenen W, Eyskens B, Meyns B, Gewillig M. Neonatal pulmonary artery banding does not compromise the short-term function of a Damus-Kaye-Stansel connection. Eur J Cardiothorac Surg 2000;17:655-7.
2. Dajee H, Deutsch LS, Benson LN, Perloff JK, Laks H. Thrombolytic therapy for superior vena caval thrombosis following superior vena cava–pulmonary artery anastomosis. Ann Thorac Surg 1984;38:637.
3. Damus PS, Thomson NB Jr, McLoughlin TG. Arterial repair without coronary relocation for complete transposition of the great vessels with ventricular septal defect. Report of a case. J Thorac Cardiovasc Surg 1982;83:316.
4. Davidson JD, Waldmann TA, Goodman DS, Gordon RS. Protein-losing enteropathy in congestive heart failure. Lancet 1961;1:899.
5. Day RW, Orsmond GS, Sturtevant JE, Hawkins JA, Doty DB, McGough E. Early and intermediate results of the Fontan procedure at moderately high altitude. Ann Thorac Surg 1994;57:170.
6. Deanfield JE, Tommasini G, Anderson RH, Macartney FJ. Tricuspid atresia: analysis of coronary artery distribution and ventricular morphology. Br Heart J 1982;48:485.
7. de Brux JL, Zannini L, Binet JP, Neveux JY, Langlois J, Hazan E, et al. Tricuspid atresia. Results of treatment in 115 children. J Thorac Cardiovasc Surg 1983;85:440.
8. DeLeon SY, Ilbawi MN, Idriss FS, Backer CL, Ohtake S, Zales VR, et al. Direct tricuspid closure versus atrial partitioning in Fontan operation for complex lesions. Ann Thorac Surg 1989;47:761.
9. DeLeon SY, Ilbawi MN, Idriss FS, Muster AJ, Gidding SS, Berry TE, et al. Fontan type operation for complex lesions. Surgical considerations to improve survival. J Thorac Cardiovasc Surg 1986;92:1029.
10. de Leval MR, Dubini G, Migliavacca F, Jalali H, Camporini G, Redington A, et al. Use of computational fluid dynamics in the design of surgical procedures: application to the study of competitive flows in cavo-pulmonary connections. J Thorac Cardiovasc Surg 1996;111:502.
11. de Leval MR, Kilner P, Gewillig M, Bull C. Total cavopulmonary connection: a logical alternative to atriopulmonary connection for complex Fontan operations. J Thorac Cardiovasc Surg 1988;96:682.
12. Delius RE, Rademecker MA, de Leval MR, Elliott MJ, Stark J. Is a high-risk biventricular repair always preferable to conversion to a single ventricle repair? J Thorac Cardiovasc Surg 1996;112:1561.
13. del Torso S, Kelly MJ, Kalff V, Venables AW. Radionuclide assessment of ventricular contraction at rest and during exercise following the Fontan procedure for either tricuspid atresia or single ventricle. Am J Cardiol 1985;55:1127.
14. de Vivie ER, Ruschewski W, Koveker G, Risch D, Weber H, Beuren AJ. Fontan procedure—indication and clinical results. Thorac Cardiovasc Surg 1981;29:348.
15. di Carlo D, Williams WG, Freedom RM, Trusler GA, Rowe RD. The role of cava-pulmonary (Glenn) anastomosis in the palliative treatment of congenital heart disease. J Thorac Cardiovasc Surg 1982;83:437.
16. Dick M, Fyler DC, Nadas AS. Tricuspid atresia. Clinical course in 101 patients. Am J Cardiol 1975;36:327.
17. Dickinson DF, Wilkinson JL, Smith A, Anderson RH. Atresia of the right atrioventricular orifice with atrioventricular concordance. Br Heart J 1979;42:9.
18. Dickinson DF, Wilkinson JL, Smith A, Becker AE, Anderson RH. Atrioventricular conduction tissues in univentricular hearts of left ventricular type with absent right atrioventricular connection ("tricuspid atresia"). Br Heart J 1979;42:1.
19. Dilawar M, Bradley SM, Saul JP, Stroud MR, Balaji S. Sinus node dysfunction after intraatrial lateral tunnel and extracardiac conduit Fontan procedures. Pediatr Cardiol 2003;24:284-8.
20. DiSessa TG, Child JS, Perloff JK, Wu L, Williams RG, Laks H, et al. Systemic venous and pulmonary arterial flow patterns after Fontan's procedure for tricuspid atresia or single ventricle. Circulation 1984;70:898.
21. Dobell AR, Trusler GA, Smallhorn JF, Williams WG. Atrial thrombi after the Fontan operation. Ann Thorac Surg 1986;42:664.
22. Doty DB, Marvin WJ Jr, Lauer RM. Modified Fontan procedure. Methods to achieve direct anastomosis of right atrium to pulmonary artery. J Thorac Cardiovasc Surg 1981;81:470.
23. Douville EC, Sade RM, Fyfe DA. Hemi-Fontan operation in surgery for single ventricle: a preliminary report. Ann Thorac Surg 1991;51:893.
24. Driscoll DJ, Danielson GK, Puga FJ, Schaff HV, Heise CT, Staats BA. Exercise tolerance and cardiorespiratory response to exercise after the Fontan operation for tricuspid atresia or functional single ventricle. J Am Coll Cardiol 1986;7:1087.
25. Driscoll DJ, Feldt RH, Mottram CD, Puga FJ, Schaff HV, Danielson GK. Cardiorespiratory response to exercise after definitive repair of univentricular atrioventricular connection. Int J Cardiol 1987;17:73.
26. Driscoll DJ, Offord KP, Feldt RH, Schaff HV, Puga FJ, Danielson GK. Five- to fifteen-year follow-up after Fontan operation. Circulation 1992;85:469.
27. du Plessis AJ, Chang AC, Wessel DL, Lock JE, Wernovsky G, Newburger JW, et al. Cerebrovascular accidents following the Fontan operation. Pediatr Neurol 1995;12:230.

E

1. Edwards JE, Burchell HB. Congenital tricuspid atresia: a classification. Med Clin North Am 1949;1177.
2. Edwards WS, Bargeron LM Jr. The superiority of the Glenn operation for tricuspid atresia in infancy and childhood. J Thorac Cardiovasc Surg 1968;55:60.
3. Eicken A, Sebening W, Genz T, Kaemmerer H, Lange R, Busch R, et al. Site of coronary sinus drainage does not significantly affect coronary flow reserve in patients long term after Fontan operation. Pediatr Cardiol 2006;27:102-9.

F

1. Fedderly RT, Whitstone BN, Frisbee SJ, Tweddell JS, Litwin SB. Factors related to pleural effusions after Fontan procedure in the era of fenestration. Circulation 2001;104:I148-51.
2. Feldt RH, Driscoll DJ, Offord KP, Cha RH, Perrault J, Schaff HV, et al. Protein-losing enteropathy after the Fontan operation. J Thorac Cardiovasc Surg 1996;112:672.
3. Fernandez G, Costa F, Fontan F, Naftel DC, Blackstone EH, Kirklin JW. Prevalence of reoperation for pathway obstruction after Fontan operation. Ann Thorac Surg 1989;48:654.
4. Fernandez-Martorell P, Sklansky MS, Lucas VW, Kashani IA, Cocalis MW, Jamieson SW, et al. Accessory hepatic vein to pulmonary venous atrium as a cause of cyanosis after the Fontan operation. Am J Cardiol 1996;77:1386.
5. Festa P, Ait Ali L, Bernabei M, De Marchi D. The role of magnetic resonance imaging in the evaluation of the functionally single ventricle before and after conversion to the Fontan circulation. Cardiol Young 2005;15 Suppl 3:51-6.
6. Fiore AC, Rodefeld M, Vijay P, Turrentine M, Seithel C, Ruzmetov M, et al. Subaortic obstruction in univentricular heart: results using the double barrel Damus-Kaye Stansel operation. Eur J Cardiothorac Surg 2009;35:141-6.
7. Fiore AC, Turrentine M, Rodefeld M, Vijay P, Schwartz TL, Virgo KS, et al. Fontan operation: a comparison of lateral tunnel with extracardiac conduit. Ann Thorac Surg 2007;83:622-30.
8. Fishberger SB, Wernovsky G, Gentles TL, Gauvreau K, Burnett J, Mayer JE Jr, et al. Factors that influence the development of atrial flutter after the Fontan procedure. J Thorac Cardiovasc Surg 1997;113:80.
9. Fogel MA. Is routine cardiac catheterization necessary in the management of patients with single ventricles across staged Fontan reconstruction? No! Pediatr Cardiol 2005;26:154-8.
10. Fogel MA, Weinberg PM, Chin AJ, Fellows KE, Hoffman EA. Late ventricular geometry and performance changes of functional single ventricle throughout staged Fontan reconstruction assessed by magnetic resonance imaging. J Am Coll Cardiol 1996;28:212.
11. Fontan F, Baudet E. Surgical repair of tricuspid atresia. Thorax 1971;26:240.
12. Fontan F, Choussat A, Brom AG, Chauve A, Deville C, Castro-Cels A. Repair of tricuspid atresia—surgical considerations and results. In Anderson RH, Shinebourne EA, eds. Pediatric cardiology. 1977. Edinburgh: Churchill Livingstone, 1978.
13. Fontan F, Deville C, Quaegebeur J, Ottenkamp J, Sourdille N, Choussat A, et al. Repair of tricuspid atresia in 100 patients. J Thorac Cardiovasc Surg 1983;85:647.
14. Fontan F, Fernandez G, Costa F, Naftel DC, Tritto F, Blackstone EH, et al. The size of the pulmonary arteries and the results of the Fontan operation. J Thorac Cardiovasc Surg 1989;98:711.
15. Fontan F, Kirklin JW, Fernandez G, Costa F, Naftel DC, Tritto F, et al. Outcome after a "perfect" Fontan operation. Circulation 1990;81:1520.
16. Fontan F, Mounicot FB, Baudet E, Simonneau J, Gordo J, Gouffrant JM. "Correction" de l'atresie tricuspidienne. Rapport de deux cas "corriges" par l'utilisation d'une technique chirurgicale nouvelle. Ann Chir Thorac Cardiovasc 1971;10:39.
17. Forrest P, Bini RM, Wilkinson JL, Arnold R, Wright JG, McKay R, et al. Congenital absence of the pulmonic valve and tricuspid valve atresia with intact ventricular septum. Am J Cardiol 1987; 59:482.
18. Franklin RC, Spiegelhalter DJ, Anderson RH, Macartney FJ, Rossi Filho RI, Rigby ML, et al. Double-inlet ventricle presenting in infancy. II. Results of palliative operations. J Thorac Cardiovasc Surg 1991;101:917.
19. Franklin RC, Spiegelhalter DJ, Rossi Filho RI, Macartney FJ, Anderson RH, Deanfield JE, et al. Double-inlet ventricle presenting in infancy. III. Outcome and potential for definitive repair. J Thorac Cardiovasc Surg 1991;101:924.
20. Franklin RC, Sullivan ID, Anderson RH, Shinebourne EA, Deanfield JE. Is banding of the pulmonary trunk obsolete for infants with tricuspid atresia and double inlet ventricle with a discordant ventriculoarterial connection? Role of aortic arch obstruction and subaortic stenosis. J Am Coll Cardiol 1990;16:1455.
21. Fraser CD Jr. Management of systemic outlet obstruction in patients undergoing single ventricle palliation. Semin Thorac Cardiovasc Surg Pediatr Card Surg Annu 2009:70-5.
22. Freed MD, Rosenthal A, Plauth WH Jr, Nadas AS. Development of subaortic stenosis after pulmonary banding. Circulation 1973; 48:III7.
23. Freedom RM, Benson LN, Smallhorn JF, Williams WG, Trusler GA, Rowe RD. Subaortic stenosis, the univentricular heart and banding of the pulmonary artery: an analysis of the courses of 43 patients with univentricular heart palliated by pulmonary artery banding. Circulation 1986;73:758.
24. Freedom RM, Dische MR, Rowe RD. Pathologic anatomy of subaortic stenosis and atresia in the first year of life. Am J Cardiol 1977;39:1035.
25. Freedom RM, Sondheimer H, Sische R, Rowe RD. Development of "subaortic stenosis" after pulmonary arterial banding for common ventricle. Am J Cardiol 1977;39:78.
26. Freedom RM, Trusler GA. Arterial switch for palliation of subaortic stenosis in single ventricle and transposition: no mean feat! Ann Thorac Surg 1991;52:415.
27. Freedom RM, Williams WG, Fowler RS, Trusler GA, Rowe RD. Tricuspid atresia, transposition of the great arteries, and banded pulmonary artery. Repair by arterial switch, coronary artery reimplantation, and right atrioventricular valved conduit. J Thorac Cardiovasc Surg 1980;80:621.
28. Friedrich-Rust M, Koch C, Rentzsch A, Sarrazin C, Schwarz P, Herrmann E, et al. Noninvasive assessment of liver fibrosis in patients with Fontan circulation using transient elastography and biochemical fibrosis markers. J Thorac Cardiovasc Surg 2008; 135:560-7.
29. Frommelt MA, Frommelt PC, Berger S, Pelech AN, Lewis DA, Tweddell JS, et al. Does an additional source of pulmonary blood flow alter outcome after a bidirectional cavopulmonary shunt? Circulation 1995;92:II240.
30. Fujii Y, Sano S, Kotani Y, Yoshizumi K, Kasahara S, Ishino K, et al. Midterm to long-term outcome of total cavopulmonary connection in high-risk adult candidates. Ann Thorac Surg 2009;87:562-70.

G

1. Gajarski RJ, Towbin JA, Garson A Jr. Fontan palliation versus heart transplantation: a comparison of charges. Am Heart J 1996;131:1169.
2. Gale AW, Danielson GK, McGoon DC, Mair DD. Modified Fontan operation for univentricular heart and complicated congenital lesions. J Thorac Cardiovasc Surg 1979;78:831.
3. Gale AW, Danielson GK, McGoon DC, Wallace RB, Mair DD. Fontan procedure for tricuspid atresia. Circulation 1980;62:91.
4. Gamba A, Merlo M, Fiocchi R, Terzi A, Mammana C, Sebastiani R, et al. Heart transplantation in patients with previous Fontan operations. J Thorac Cardiovasc Surg 2004;127:555-62.
5. Gamillscheg A, Zobel G, Urlesberger B, Berger J, Dacar D, Stein JI, et al. Inhaled nitric oxide in patients with critical pulmonary perfusion after Fontan-type procedures and bidirectional Glenn anastomosis. J Thorac Cardiovasc Surg 1997;113:435.
6. Gandhi SK, Bromberg BI, Rodefeld MD, Schuessler RB, Boineau JP, Cox JL, et al. Lateral tunnel suture line variation reduces atrial flutter after the modified Fontan operation. Ann Thorac Surg 1996;61:1299.
7. Gatzoulis MA, Munk MD, Williams WG, Webb GD. Definitive palliation with cavopulmonary or aortopulmonary shunts for adults with single ventricle physiology. Heart 2000;83:51-7.
8. Gatzoulis MA, Shinebourne EA, Redington AN, Rigby ML, Ho SY, Shore DF. Increasing cyanosis early after cavopulmonary connection caused by abnormal systemic venous channels. Br Heart J 1995;73:182.
9. Gaynor JW, Bridges ND, Cohen MI, Mahle WT, Decampli WM, Steven JM, et al. Predictors of outcome after the Fontan operation: is hypoplastic left heart syndrome still a risk factor? J Thorac Cardiovasc Surg 2002;123:237-45.

10. Geggel RL, Mayer JE Jr, Fried R, Helgason H, Cook EF, Reid LM. Role of lung biopsy in patients undergoing a modified Fontan procedure. J Thorac Cardiovasc Surg 1990;99:451.
11. Gentles TL, Gauvreau K, Mayer JE Jr, Fishberger SB, Burnett J, Colan SD, et al. Functional outcome after the Fontan operation: factors influencing late morbidity. J Thorac Cardiovasc Surg 1997;114:392.
12. Gentles TL, Mayer JE Jr, Gauvreau K, Newburger JW, Lock JE, Kupferschmid JP, et al. Fontan operation in five hundred consecutive patients: factors influencing early and late outcome. J Thorac Cardiovasc Surg 1997;114:376-91.
13. Geva T, Ott DA, Ludomirsky A, Argyle SJ, O'Laughlin MP. Tricuspid atresia associated with aortopulmonary window: controlling pulmonary blood flow with a fenestrated patch. Am Heart J 1992;123:260.
14. Gewillig MH, Lundstrom UR, Deanfield JE, Bull C, Franklin RC, Graham TP Jr, et al. Impact of Fontan operation on left ventricular size and contractility in tricuspid atresia. Circulation 1990;81:118.
15. Ghanayem NS, Berger S, Tweddell JS. Medical management of the failing Fontan. Pediatr Cardiol 2007;28:465-71.
16. Giannico S, Hammad F, Amodeo A, Michielon G, Drago F, Turchetta A, et al. Clinical outcome of 193 extracardiac Fontan patients: the first 15 years. J Am Coll Cardiol 2006;47:2065-73.
17. Giardini A, Pace Napoleone C, Specchia S, Donti A, Formigari R, Oppido G, et al. Conversion of atriopulmonary Fontan to extracardiac total cavopulmonary connection improves cardiopulmonary function. Int J Cardiol 2006;113:341-4.
18. Girod DA, Fontan F, Deville C, Ottenkamp J, Choussat A. Long-term results after the Fontan operation for tricuspid atresia. Circulation 1987;75:605.
19. Gleason WA Jr, Roodman ST, Laks H. Protein-losing enteropathy and intestinal lymphangiectasia after superior vena cava–right pulmonary artery (Glenn) shunt. J Thorac Cardiovasc Surg 1979;77:843.
20. Glenn WW. Circulatory bypass of the right side of the heart. IV. Shunt between superior vena cava and distal right pulmonary artery—report of clinical application. N Engl J Med 1958;259:117.
21. Glenn WW, Patino JF. Circulatory bypass of the right heart. I. Preliminary observations on the direct delivery of vena caval blood into the pulmonary arterial circulation. Azygous vein-pulmonary artery shunt. Yale J Biol Med 1954;27:147.
22. Goff DA, Blume ED, Gauvreau K, Mayer JE, Lock JE, Jenkins KJ. Clinical outcome of fenestrated Fontan patients after closure: the first 10 years. Circulation 2000;102:2094-9.
23. Gray RG, Altmann K, Mosca RS, Prakash A, Williams IA, Quaegebeur JM, et al. Persistent antegrade pulmonary blood flow post-Glenn does not alter early post-Fontan outcomes in single-ventricle patients. Ann Thorac Surg 2007;84:888-93.
24. Griffiths ER, Kaza AK, Wyler von Ballmoos MC, Loyola H, Valente AM, Blume ED, et al. Evaluating failing Fontans for heart transplantation: predictors of death. Ann Thorac Surg 2009;88:558-64.
25. Gruenstein DH, Spicer RL, Shim D, Beekman RH 3rd. Pulmonary venous wedge pressure provides an accurate assessment of pulmonary artery pressure in children with a bidirectional Glenn shunt. J Interv Cardiol 2003;16:367-70.
26. Guller B, DuShane JW, Titus JL. The atrioventricular conduction system in two cases of tricuspid atresia. Circulation 1969;40:217.
27. Gundry SR, Razzouk AJ, del Rio MJ, Shirali G, Bailey LL. The optimal Fontan connection: a growing extracardiac lateral tunnel with pedicled pericardium. J Thorac Cardiovasc Surg 1997;114: 552.
28. Gupta A, Daggett C, Behera S, Ferraro M, Wells W, Starnes V. Risk factors for persistent pleural effusions after the extracardiac Fontan procedure. J Thorac Cardiovasc Surg 2004;127:1664-9.
29. Gussenhoven WJ, The HK, Schippers L, Bos E, Roelandt J, Ligtvoet C. Growth and function of the right ventricular outflow tract after Fontan's procedure for tricuspid atresia: a two-dimensional echocardiographic study. Thorac Cardiovasc Surg 1986;34:236.

H

1. Hager A, Zrenner B, Brodherr-Heberlein S, Steinbauer-Rosenthal I, Schreieck J, Hess J. Congenital and surgically acquired Wolff-Parkinson-White syndrome in patients with tricuspid atresia. J Thorac Cardiovasc Surg 2005;130:48-53.
2. Hagler DJ, Seward JB, Tajik AJ, Ritter DG. Functional assessment of the Fontan operation: combined M-mode, two-dimensional and Doppler echocardiographic studies. J Am Coll Cardiol 1984; 4:756.
3. Hakacova N, Lakomy M, Kovacikova L. Arrhythmias after Fontan operation: comparison of lateral tunnel and extracardiac conduit. J Electrocardiol 2008;41:173-7.
4. Haller JA Jr, Adkins JC, Worthington M, Rauenhorst J. Experimental studies on permanent bypass of the right heart. Surgery 1966;59:1128.
5. Hanley FL. The one and a half ventricle repair—we can do it, but should we do it? J Thorac Cardiovasc Surg 1999;117:659.
6. Harada Y, Uchita S, Sakamoto T, Kimura M, Umezu K, Takigiku K, et al. Do we need fenestration when performing two-staged total cavopulmonary connection using an extracardiac conduit? Interact Cardiovasc Thorac Surg 2009;9:50-4.
7. Harrison DA, Liu P, Walters JE, Goodman JM, Siu SC, Webb GD, et al. Cardiopulmonary function in adult patients late after Fontan repair. J Am Coll Cardiol 1995;26:1016.
8. Hawkins JA, Shaddy RE, Day RW, Sturtevant JE, Orsmond GS, McGough EC. Mid-term results after bidirectional cavopulmonary shunts. Ann Thorac Surg 1993;56:833.
9. Henry JN, Devloo RA, Ritter DG, Mair DD, Davis GD, Danielson GK. Tricuspid atresia. Successful surgical "correction" in two patients using porcine xenograft valves. Mayo Clin Proc 1974; 49:803.
10. Hess J, Kruizinga K, Bijleveld CM, Hardjowijono R, Eygelaar A. Protein-losing enteropathy after Fontan operation. J Thorac Cardiovasc Surg 1984;88:606.
11. Hiramatsu T, Imai Y, Kurosawa H, Takanashi Y, Aoki M, Shinoka T, et al. Midterm results of surgical treatment of systemic ventricular outflow obstruction in Fontan patients. Ann Thorac Surg 2002;73:855-61.
12. Hiramatsu T, Imai Y, Takanashi Y, Seo K, Terada M, Nakazawa M. Hemodynamic effects of human atrial natriuretic peptide after modified Fontan procedure. Ann Thorac Surg 1998;65:761.
13. Hirsch JC, Goldberg C, Bove EL, Salehian S, Lee T, Ohye RG, et al. Fontan operation in the current era: a 15-year single institution experience. Ann Surg 2008;248:402-10.
14. Hopkins RA, Armstrong BE, Serwer GA, Peterson RJ, Oldham HN Jr. Physiological rationale for a bidirectional cavopulmonary shunt. A versatile complement to the Fontan principle. J Thorac Cardiovasc Surg 1985;90:391.
15. Horowitz MD, Culpepper WS 3rd, Williams LC 3rd, Sundgaard-Riise K, Ochsner JL. Pulmonary artery banding: analysis of a 25-year experience. Ann Thorac Surg 1989;48:444.
16. Hosein RB, Clarke AJ, McGuirk SP, Griselli M, Stumper O, De Giovanni JV, et al. Factors influencing early and late outcome following the Fontan procedure in the current era. The "Two Commandments"? Eur J Cardiothorac Surg 2007;31:344-53.
17. Hsu DT, Quaegebeur JM, Ing FF, Selber EJ, Lamour JM, Gersony WM. Outcome after the single-stage, nonfenestrated Fontan procedure. Circulation 1997;96:II335-40.
18. Huddleston CB. The failing Fontan: options for surgical therapy. Pediatr Cardiol 2007;28:472-6.
19. Humes RA, Feldt RH, Porter CJ, Julsrud PR, Puga FJ, Danielson GK. The modified Fontan operation for asplenia and polysplenia syndromes. J Thorac Cardiovasc Surg 1988;96:212.
20. Humes RA, Mair DD, Porter CB, Puga FJ, Schaff HV, Danielson GK. Results of the modified Fontan operation in adults. Am J Cardiol 1988;61:602.
21. Hurwitt ES, Young D, Escher DJ. The rationale of anastomosis of the right auricular appendage to the pulmonary artery in the treatment of tricuspid atresia. J Thorac Surg 1955;30:503.
22. Hussain A, Arfi AM, Hussamuddin M, Haneef AA, Jamjoom A, Al-Ata J, et al. Comparative outcome of bidirectional Glenn shunt in patients with pulmonary vascular resistance > or = 3.5 woods units versus < 3.5 woods units. Am J Cardiol 2008;102: 907-12.
23. Hussain ST, Bhan A, Sapra S, Juneja R, Das S, Sharma S. The bidirectional cavopulmonary (Glenn) shunt without cardiopulmonary bypass: is it a safe option? Interact Cardiovasc Thorac Surg 2007;6:77-82.
24. Hvass U, Pansard Y, Bohm G, Depoix JP, Enguerrand D, Worms AM. Bicaval pulmonary connection in tricuspid atresia using an extracardiac tube of autologous pediculated pericardium to bridge inferior vena cava. Eur J Cardiothorac Surg 1992,6:49.

I

1. Ichikawa H, Yagihara T, Kishimoto H, Isobe F, Yamamoto F, Nishigaki K, et al. Extent of aortopulmonary collateral blood flow as a risk factor for Fontan operation. Ann Thorac Surg 1995;59:433.
2. Iemura J, Oku H, Saga T, Kitayama H, Matumoto T. Total extracardiac right heart bypass using a polytetrafluoroethylene graft. J Card Surg 1997;12:32.
3. Ikai A, Fujimoto Y, Hirose K, Ota N, Tosaka Y, Nakata T, et al. Feasibility of the extracardiac conduit Fontan procedure in patients weighing less than 10 kilograms. J Thorac Cardiovasc Surg 2008; 135:1145-52.
4. Ilbawi MN, Idriss FS, DeLeon SY, Kucich VA, Muster AJ, Paul MH, et al. When should the hypoplastic right ventricle be used in a Fontan operation? An experimental and clinical correlation. Ann Thorac Surg 1989;47:533.
5. Ilbawi MN, Idriss FS, Muster AJ, DeLeon SY, Berry TE, Duffy CE, et al. Effects of elevated coronary sinus pressure on left ventricular function after the Fontan operation. J Thorac Cardiovasc Surg 1986;92:231.
6. Imai Y, Kurosawa H, Fujiwara T, Fukuchi S, Matsuo K, Kawada M, et al. Palliative repair of aortic atresia associated with tricuspid atresia and transposition of the great arteries. Ann Thorac Surg 1991;51:646.
7. Ishikawa T, Neutze JM, Brandt PW, Barratt-Boyes BG. Hemodynamics following the Kreutzer procedure for tricuspid atresia in patients under 2 years of age. J Thorac Cardiovasc Surg 1984;88:373.
8. Itatani K, Miyaji K, Tomoyasu T, Nakahata Y, Ohara K, Takamoto S, et al. Optimal conduit size of the extracardiac Fontan operation based on energy loss and flow stagnation. Ann Thorac Surg 2009;88:565-73.

J

1. Jacobs ML, Norwood WI Jr. Fontan operation: influence of modifications on morbidity and mortality. Ann Thorac Surg 1994; 58:945-52.
2. Jacobs ML, Pelletier GJ, Pourmoghadam KK, Mesia CI, Madan N, Stern H, et al. Protocols associated with no mortality in 100 consecutive Fontan procedures. Eur J Cardiothorac Surg 2008;33: 626-32.
3. Jacobs ML, Pourmoghadam KK. Thromboembolism and the role of anticoagulation in the Fontan patient. Pediatr Cardiol 2007; 28:457-64.
4. Jacobs ML, Pourmoghadam KK, Geary EM, Reyes AT, Madan N, McGrath LB, et al. Fontan's operation: is aspirin enough? Is Coumadin too much? Ann Thorac Surg 2002;73:64-8.
5. Jacobs ML, Rychik J, Murphy JD, Nicolson SC, Steven JM, Norwood WI. Results of Norwood's operation for lesions other than hypoplastic left heart syndrome. J Thorac Cardiovasc Surg 1995;110:1555.
6. Jacobs ML, Rychik J, Rome JJ, Apostolopoulou S, Pizarro C, Murphy JD, et al. Early reduction of the volume work of the single ventricle: the hemi-Fontan operation. Ann Thorac Surg 1996; 62:456.
7. Jahangiri M, Shore D, Kakkar V, Lincoln C, Shinebourne E. Coagulation factor abnormalities after the Fontan procedure and its modifications. J Thorac Cardiovasc Surg 1997;113:989.
8. Jaquiss RD, Imamura M. Single ventricle physiology: surgical options, indications and outcomes. Curr Opin Cardiol 2009; 24:113-8.
9. Jayakumar KA, Addonizio LJ, Kichuk-Chrisant MR, Galantowicz ME, Lamour JM, Quaegebeur JM, et al. Cardiac transplantation after the Fontan or Glenn procedure. J Am Coll Cardiol 2004; 44:2065-72.
10. Jonas RA, Castaneda AR. Modified Fontan procedure: atrial baffle and systemic venous to pulmonary artery anastomotic techniques. J Card Surg 1988;3:91.
11. Jonas RA, Mayer JE, Castaneda AR. Invited letter concerning: total cavopulmonary connection. J Thorac Cardiovasc Surg 1988;96:830.
12. Juaneda E, Haworth SG. Pulmonary vascular structure in patients dying after a Fontan procedure. The lung as a risk factor. Br Heart J 1984;52:575.

K

1. Kajihara N, Asou T, Takeda Y, Kosaka Y, Nagafuchi H, Oyama R, et al. Staged surgical approach in neonates with a functionally single ventricle and arch obstruction: pulmonary artery banding and aortic arch reconstruction before placement of a bidirectional cavopulmonary shunt in infants. Pediatr Cardiol 2010;31:33-9.
2. Kanter KR, Vincent RN. Management of aortopulmonary collateral arteries in Fontan patients: occlusion improves clinical outcome. Semin Thorac Cardiovasc Surg Pediatr Card Surg Annu 2002; 5:48-54.
3. Karl TR, Watterson KG, Sano S, Mee RB. Operations for subaortic stenosis in univentricular hearts. Ann Thorac Surg 1991;52:420.
4. Kaulitz R, Ziemer G, Luhmer I, Paul T, Kallfelz HC. Total cavopulmonary anastomosis in patients less than three years of age. Ann Thorac Surg 1995;60:S563.
5. Kaulitz R, Ziemer G, Paul T, Peuster M, Bertram H, Hausdorf G. Fontan-type procedures: residual lesions and late interventions. Ann Thorac Surg 2002;74:778-85.
6. Kaulitz R, Ziemer G, Rauch R, Girisch M, Bertram H, Wessel A, et al. Prophylaxis of thromboembolic complications after the Fontan operation (total cavopulmonary anastomosis). J Thorac Cardiovasc Surg 2005;129:569-75.
7. Kavarana MN, Pagni S, Recto MR, Sobczyk WL, Yeh T Jr, Mitchell M, et al. Seven-year clinical experience with the extracardiac pedicled pericardial Fontan operation. Ann Thorac Surg 2005;80:37-43.
8. Kavey RE, Gaum WE, Byrum CJ, Smith FC, Kveselis DA. Loss of sinus rhythm after total cavopulmonary connection. Circulation 1995;92:II304.
9. Kawahira Y, Uemura H, Yagihara T. Impact of the off-pump Fontan procedure on complement activation and cytokine generation. Ann Thorac Surg 2006;81:685-9.
10. Kawashima Y, Kitamura S, Matsuda H, Shimazaki Y, Nakano S, Hirose H. Total cavopulmonary shunt operation in complex cardiac anomalies. J Thorac Cardiovasc Surg 1984;87:74.
11. Kaye MP. Anatomic correction of transposition of great arteries. Mayo Clin Proc 1975;50:638.
12. Kelly AM, Feldt RH, Driscoll DJ, Danielson GK. Use of heparin in the treatment of protein-losing enteropathy after Fontan operation for complex congenital heart disease. Mayo Clinic Proc 1998;73:777.
13. Kiesewetter CH, Sheron N, Vettukattill JJ, Hacking N, Stedman B, Millward-Sadler H, et al. Hepatic changes in the failing Fontan circulation. Heart 2007;93:579-84.
14. Kim SJ, Kim WH, Lim HG, Lee JY. Outcome of 200 patients after an extracardiac Fontan procedure. J Thorac Cardiovasc Surg 2008;136:108-16.
15. Kim WH, Lim HG, Lee JR, Rho JR, Bae EJ, Noh CI, et al. Fontan conversion with arrhythmia surgery. Eur J Cardiothorac Surg 2005;27:250-7.
16. Kirklin JK, Blackstone EH, Kirklin JW, Pacifico AD, Bargeron LM Jr. The Fontan operation: ventricular hypertrophy, age, and date of operation as risk factors. J Thorac Cardiovasc Surg 1986; 92:1049.
17. Kirklin JK, Brown RN, Bryant AS, Naftel DC, Colvin EV, Pearce FB, et al. Is the "perfect Fontan" operation routinely achievable in the modern era? Cardiol Young 2008;18:328-36.
18. Kirklin JW, Fernandez G, Fontan F, Naftel DC, Ebner A, Blackstone EH. Therapeutic use of right atrial pressures early after the Fontan operation. Eur J Cardiothorac Surg 1990;4:2.
19. Knight W, Mee RB. A cure for pulmonary arteriovenous fistulas. Ann Thorac Surg 1995;59:999.
20. Knott-Craig CJ, Danielson GK, Schaff HV, Puga FJ, Weaver AL, Driscoll DD. The modified Fontan operation: an analysis of risk factors for early postoperative death or takedown in 702 consecutive patients from one institution. J Thorac Cardiovasc Surg 1995; 109:1237.
21. Knott-Craig CJ, Fryar-Dragg T, Overholt ED, Razook JD, Ward KE, Elkins RC. Modified hemi-Fontan operation: an alternative definitive palliation for high-risk patients. Ann Thorac Surg 1995;60:S554.
22. Kogon BE, Plattner C, Leong T, Simsic J, Kirshbom PM, Kanter KR. The bidirectional Glenn operation: a risk factor analysis for morbidity and mortality. J Thorac Cardiovasc Surg 2008;136: 1237-42.
23. Kondoh C, Hiroe M, Nakanishi T, Nakazawa M, Nakae S, Imai Y, et al. Left ventricular characteristics during exercise in patients after Fontan's operation for tricuspid atresia. Heart Vessels 1988;4:34.
24. Kopf GS, Kleinman CS, Hijazi ZM, Fahey JT, Dewar ML, Hellenbrand WE. Fenestrated Fontan operation with delayed

transcatheter closure of atrial septal defect: improved results in high-risk patients. J Thorac Cardiovasc Surg 1992;103:1039.
25. Kopf GS, Laks H, Stansel HC, Hellenbrand WE, Kleinman CS, Talner NS. Thirty-year follow-up of superior vena cava–pulmonary artery (Glenn) shunts. J Thorac Cardiovasc Surg 1990;100:662.
26. Kouatli AA, Garcia JA, Zellers TM, Weinstein EM, Mahony L. Enalapril does not enhance exercise capacity in patients after Fontan procedure. Circulation 1997;96:1507.
27. Kreutzer C, Mayorquim RC, Kreutzer GO, Conejeros W, Roman MI, Vazquez H, et al. Experience with one and a half ventricle repair. J Thorac Cardiovasc Surg 1999;117:662.
28. Kreutzer G, Galindez E, Bono H, de Palma C, Laura JP. An operation for the correction of tricuspid atresia. J Thorac Cardiovasc Surg 1973;66:613.
29. Kreutzer GO, Vargas FJ, Schlichter AJ, Laura JP, Suarez JC, Coronel AR, et al. Atriopulmonary anastomosis. J Thorac Cardiovasc Surg 1982;83:427.
30. Kreutzer J, Keane JF, Lock JE, Walsh EP, Jonas RA, Castaneda AR, et al. Conversion of modified Fontan procedure to lateral atrial tunnel cavopulmonary anastomosis. J Thorac Cardiovasc Surg 1996; 111:1169.
31. Kuhne M. Uber zwei Falle kongenitaler atresie des ostium venosum dextrum. Jahrb Kinderheildd Physi Erziehung 1906;63:235.
32. Kumar SP, Rubinstein CS, Simsic JM, Taylor AB, Saul JP, Bradley SM. Lateral tunnel versus extracardiac conduit Fontan procedure: a concurrent comparison. Ann Thorac Surg 2003;76:1389-97.

L

1. La Corte MA, Dick M, Scheer G, La Farge CG, Fyler DC. Left ventricular function in tricuspid atresia. Angiographic analysis in 28 patients. Circulation 1975;52:996.
2. Lacour-Gayet F, Serraf A, Fermont L, Bruniaux J, Rey C, Touchot A, et al. Early palliation of univentricular hearts with subaortic stenosis and ventriculoarterial discordance. J Thorac Cardiovasc Surg 1992; 104:1238.
3. Laks H, Haas GS, Pearl MJ, Sadeghi AM, George B, Santuli TV, et al. The use of an adjustable intraatrial communication in patients undergoing the Fontan and other definitive heart procedures (abstract). Circulation 1988;78:357.
4. Laks H, Milliken JC, Perloff JK, Hellenbrand WE, George BL, Chin A, et al. Experience with the Fontan procedure. J Thorac Cardiovasc Surg 1984;88:939.
5. Laks H, Mudd JG, Standeven JW, Fagan L, Willman VL. Long term effect of the superior vena cava–pulmonary artery anastomosis on pulmonary blood flow. J Thorac Cardiovasc Surg 1977;74:253.
6. Laks H, Pearl J, Wu A, Haas G, George B. Experience with the Fontan procedure including use of an adjustable intraatrial communication. In Crupi G, Parenzan L, Anderson RH, eds. Perspectives in pediatric cardiac surgery. Pt. 2. Mount Kisco, NY: Futura, 1989, p. 205.
7. Lamberti JJ, Mainwaring RD, Spicer RL, Uzark KC, Moore FJ. Factors influencing perioperative morbidity during palliation of the univentricular heart. Ann Thorac Surg 1995;60:550.
8. Lamberti JJ, Spicer RL, Waldman JD, Grehl TM, Thompson D, George L, et al. The bidirectional cavopulmonary shunt. J Thorac Cardiovasc Surg 1990;100:22.
9. Lan YT, Chang RK, Laks H. Outcome of patients with double-inlet left ventricle or tricuspid atresia with transposed great arteries. J Am Coll Cardiol 2004;43:113-9.
10. Lardo AC, Webber SA, Friehs I, del Nido PJ, Cape EG. Fluid dynamic comparison of intraatrial and extracardiac total cavopulmonary connections. J Thorac Cardiovasc Surg 1999;117:697.
11. Lardo AC, Webber SA, Iyengar A, del Nido PJ, Friehs I, Cape EG. Bidirectional superior cavopulmonary anastomosis improves mechanical efficiency in dilated atriopulmonary connections. J Thorac Cardiovasc Surg 1999;118:681.
12. Laschinger JC, Redmond JM, Cameron DE, Kans JS, Ringel RE. Intermediate results of the extracardiac Fontan procedure. Ann Thorac Surg 1996;62:1261.
13. LeBlanc JG, Ashmore PG, Pineda E, Sandor GG, Patterson MW, Tipple M. Pulmonary artery banding: results and current indications in pediatric cardiac surgery. Ann Thorac Surg 1987;44:628.
14. Lee C, Lee CH, Hwang SW, Lim HG, Kim SJ, Lee JY, et al. Midterm follow-up of the status of Gore-Tex graft after extracardiac conduit Fontan procedure. Eur J Cardiothorac Surg 2007; 31:1008-12.
15. Lee JR, Choi JS, Kang CH, Bae EJ, Kim YJ, Rho JR. Surgical results of patients with a functional single ventricle. Eur J Cardiothorac Surg 2003;24:716-22.
16. Lee JR, Kwak J, Kim KC, Min SK, Kim WH, Kim YJ, et al. Comparison of lateral tunnel and extracardiac conduit Fontan procedure. Interact Cardiovasc Thorac Surg 2007;6:328-30.
17. Lemler MS, Ramaciotti C, Stromberg D, Scott WA, Leonard SR. The extracardiac lateral tunnel Fontan, constructed with bovine pericardium: comparison with the extracardiac conduit Fontan. Am Heart J 2006;151:928-33.
18. Lemler MS, Scott WA, Leonard SR, Stromberg D, Ramaciotti C. Fenestration improves clinical outcome of the Fontan procedure: a prospective, randomized study. Circulation 2002;105:207-12.
19. Lemmer J, Stiller B, Heise G, Hubler M, Alexi-Meskishvili V, Weng Y, et al. Postoperative phrenic nerve palsy: early clinical implications and management. Intensive Care Med 2006;32:1227-33.
20. Li JS, Yow E, Berezny KY, Rhodes JF, Bokesch PM, Charpie JR, et al. Clinical outcomes of palliative surgery including a systemic-to-pulmonary artery shunt in infants with cyanotic congenital heart disease: does aspirin make a difference? Circulation 2007;116: 293-7.
21. Lin AE, Laks H, Barber G, Chin AJ, Williams RG. Subaortic obstruction in complex congenital heart disease: management by proximal pulmonary artery to ascending aorta end to side anastomosis. J Am Coll Cardiol 1986;7:617.
22. Litovsky S, Choy M, Park J, Parrish M, Waters B, Nagashima M, et al. Absent pulmonary valve with tricuspid atresia or severe tricuspid stenosis: report of three cases and review of the literature. Pediatr Dev Pathol 2000;3:353-66.
23. Liu J, Lu Y, Chen H, Shi Z, Su Z, Ding W. Bidirectional Glenn procedure without cardiopulmonary bypass. Ann Thorac Surg 2004;77:1349-52.
24. Lodge AJ, Rychik J, Nicolson SC, Ittenbach RF, Spray TL, Gaynor JW. Improving outcomes in functional single ventricle and total anomalous pulmonary venous connection. Ann Thorac Surg 2004;78:1688-95.

M

1. MacIver RH, Stewart RD, Backer CL, Mavroudis C. Results with continuous cardiopulmonary bypass for the bidirectional cavopulmonary anastomosis. Cardiol Young 2008;18:147-52.
2. Mahle WT, Wernovsky G, Bridges ND, Linton AB, Paridon SM. Impact of early ventricular unloading on exercise performance in preadolescents with single ventricle Fontan physiology. J Am Coll Cardiol 1999;34:1637-43.
3. Mahnke CB, Boyle GJ, Janosky JE, Siewers RD, Pigula FA. Anticoagulation and incidence of late cerebrovascular accidents following the Fontan procedure. Pediatr Cardiol 2005;26:56-61.
4. Mainwaring RD, Lamberti JJ, Hugli TE. Complement activation and cytokine generation after modified Fontan procedure. Ann Thorac Surg 1998;65:1715.
5. Mainwaring RD, Lamberti JJ, Uzark K, Spicer RL. Bidirectional Glenn: is accessory pulmonary blood flow good or bad? Circulation 1995;92:II294.
6. Mair DD, Puga FJ, Danielson GK. The Fontan procedure for tricuspid atresia: early and late results of a 25-year experience with 216 patients. J Am Coll Cardiol 2001;37:933-9.
7. Malcic I, Sauer U, Stern H, Kellerer M, Kuhlein B, Locher D, et al. The influence of pulmonary artery banding on outcome after the Fontan operation. J Thorac Cardiovasc Surg 1992;104:743.
8. Manning PB, Mayer JE, Wernovsky G, Fishberger SB, Walsh EP. Staged operation to Fontan increases the incidence of sinoatrial node dysfunction. J Thorac Cardiovasc Surg 1996;111:833.
9. Marcelletti C, Corno A, Giannico S, Marino B. Inferior vena cava-pulmonary artery extracardiac conduit. J Thorac Cardiovasc Surg 1990;100:228.
10. Marcelletti C, Mazzera E, Olthof H, Sebel PS, Duren DR, Losekoot TG, et al. Fontan's operation: an expanded horizon. J Thorac Cardiovasc Surg 1980;80:764.
11. Marcelletti CF, Hanley FL, Mavroudis C, McElhinney DB, Abella RF, Marianeschi SM, et al. Revision of previous Fontan connections to total extracardiac cavopulmonary anastomosis: a multicenter experience. J Thorac Cardiovasc Surg 2000;119:340.
12. Marin-Garcia J, Roca J, Blieden LC, Lucas RV, Edwards JE. Congenital absence of the pulmonary valve associated with tricuspid atresia and intact ventricular septum. Chest 1973;64:658.

13. Marsden AL, Bernstein AJ, Reddy VM, Shadden SC, Spilker RL, Chan FP, et al. Evaluation of a novel Y-shaped extracardiac Fontan baffle using computational fluid dynamics. J Thorac Cardiovasc Surg 2009;137:394-403.
14. Mascio CE, Wayment M, Colaizy TT, Mahoney LT, Burkhart HM. The modified Fontan procedure and prolonged pleural effusions. Am Surg 2009;75:175-7.
15. Masuda M, Kado H, Shiokawa Y, Fukae K, Suzuki M, Murakami E, et al. Clinical results of the staged Fontan procedure in high-risk patients. Ann Thorac Surg 1998;65:1721.
16. Masuda H, Kawamura K, Tohda K, Shozawa T, Sageshima M, Honma M. Endocardium of the left ventricle in volume-loaded canine heart. Acta Pathol Jpn 1989;39:111.
17. Mathur M, Glenn WW. Long-term evaluation of cava-pulmonary artery anastomosis. Surgery 1973;74:899.
18. Matitiau A, Geva T, Colan SD, Sluysmans T, Parness IA, Spevak PJ, et al. Bulboventricular foramen size in infants with double-inlet left ventricle or tricuspid atresia with transposed great arteries: influence on initial palliative operation and rate of growth. J Am Coll Cardiol 1992;19:142.
19. Matsuda H, Kawashima Y, Kishimoto H, Hirose H, Nakano S, Kato H, et al. Problems in the modified Fontan operation for univentricular heart of the right ventricular type. Circulation 1987;76:III45.
20. Matsuda H, Kawashima Y, Takano H, Miyamoto K, Mori T. Experimental evaluation of atrial function in right atrium-pulmonary artery conduit operation for tricuspid atresia. J Thorac Cardiovasc Surg 1981;81:762.
21. Mavroudis C, Backer CL, Deal BJ, Johnsrude CL. Fontan conversion to cavopulmonary connection and arrhythmia circuit cryoablation. J Thorac Cardiovasc Surg 1998;115:547.
22. Mavroudis C, Zaies VR, Backer CL, Muster AJ, Latson LA. Fenestrated Fontan with delayed catheter closure. Circulation 1992;86:II85.
23. Mayer JE Jr, Bridges ND, Lock JE, Hanley FL, Jonas RA, Castaneda AR. Factors associated with marked reduction in mortality for Fontan operations in patients with single ventricle. J Thorac Cardiovasc Surg 1992;103:444.
24. Mayer JE Jr, Helgason H, Jonas RA, Lang P, Vargas FJ, Cook N, et al. Extending the limits for modified Fontan procedures. J Thorac Cardiovasc Surg 1986;92:1021.
25. Mazzera E, Corno A, Picardo S, Di Donato R, Marino B, Costa D, et al. Bidirectional cavopulmonary shunts: clinical applications as staged or definitive palliation. Ann Thorac Surg 1989;47:415.
26. McElhinney DB, Reddy VM, Moore P, Hanley FL. Revision of previous Fontan connections to extracardiac or intraatrial conduit cavopulmonary anastomosis. Ann Thorac Surg 1996;62:1276.
27. McElhinney DB, Reddy VM, Silverman NH, Hanley FL. Modified Damus-Kaye-Stansel procedure for single ventricle, subaortic stenosis, and arch obstruction in neonates and infants: midterm results and techniques for avoiding circulatory arrest. J Thorac Cardiovasc Surg 1997;114:718-26.
28. McElhinney DB, Reddy VM, Tworetzky W, Petrossian E, Hanley FL, Moore P. Incidence and implications of systemic to pulmonary collaterals after bidirectional cavopulmonary anastomosis. Ann Thorac Surg 2000;69:1222-8.
29. McFaul RC, Tajik AJ, Mair DD, Danielson GK, Seward JB. Development of pulmonary arteriovenous shunt after superior vena cava–right pulmonary artery (Glenn) anastomosis. Circulation 1977;55:212.
30. McGuirk SP, Winlaw DS, Langley SM, Stumper OF, de Giovanni JV, Wright JG, et al. The impact of ventricular morphology on midterm outcome following completion total cavopulmonary connection. Eur J Cardiothorac Surg 2003;24:37-46.
31. McMahon CJ, Eidem BW, Bezold LI, Vargo T, Neish SR, Bricker JT, et al. Is cardiac catheterization a prerequisite in all patients undergoing bidirectional cavopulmonary anastomosis? J Am Soc Echocardiogr 2003;16:1068-72.
32. Mendelsohn AM, Bove EL, Lupinetti FM, Crowley DC, Lloyd TR, Beekman RH 3rd. Central pulmonary artery growth patterns after the bidirectional Glenn procedure. J Thorac Cardiovasc Surg 1994;107:1284.
33. Mertens L, Hagler DJ, Sauer U, Somerville J, Gewillig M. Protein-losing enteropathy after the Fontan operation: an international multi-center study. J Thorac Cardiovasc Surg 1998;115:1063.
34. Meyer DB, Zamora G, Wernovsky G, Ittenbach RF, Gallagher PR, Tabbutt S, et al. Outcomes of the Fontan procedure using cardiopulmonary bypass with aortic cross-clamping. Ann Thorac Surg 2006;82:1611-20.
35. Mietus-Snyder M, Lang P, Mayer JE, Jones RA, Castaneda AR, Lock JE. Childhood systemic–pulmonary shunts: subsequent suitability for Fontan operation. Circulation 1987;76:III39.
36. Miura T, Kishimoto H, Kawata H, Hata M, Hoashi T, Nakajima T. Management of univentricular heart with systemic ventricular outflow obstruction by pulmonary artery banding and Damus-Kaye-Stansel operation. Ann Thorac Surg 2004;77:23-8.
37. Miyaji K. [Fontan procedure for asplenia syndrome]. Kyobu Geka 2003;56:304-7.
38. Miyaji K, Shimada M, Sekiguchi A, Ishizawa A, Isoda T, Tsunemoto M. Pulmonary atresia with intact ventricular septum: long-term results of "one and a half ventricular repair." Ann Thorac Surg 1995;60:1762.
39. Moodie DS, Feldt RH, Wallace RB. Transient protein-losing enteropathy secondary to elevated caval pressures and caval obstruction after the Mustard procedure. J Thorac Cardiovasc Surg 1976;72:379.
40. Moodie DS, Ritter DG, Tajik AH, McGoon DC, Danielson GK, O'Fallon WM. Long-term follow-up after palliative operation for univentricular heart. Am J Cardiol 1984;53:1648.
41. Moore JW, Kirby WC, Madden WA, Gaither NS. Development of pulmonary arteriovenous malformations after modified Fontan operations. J Thorac Cardiovasc Surg 1989;98:1045.
42. Morales DL, Dibardino DJ, Braud BE, Fenrich AL, Heinle JS, Vaughn WK, et al. Salvaging the failing Fontan: lateral tunnel versus extracardiac conduit. Ann Thorac Surg 2005;80:1445-52.
43. Morgan VL, Graham TP Jr, Roselli RJ, Lorenz CH. Alterations in pulmonary artery flow patterns and shear stress determined with three-dimensional phase-contrast magnetic resonance imaging in Fontan patients. J Thorac Cardiovasc Surg 1998;116:294.
44. Mori K, Ando M, Satomi G, Nakazawa M, Momma K, Takao A. Imperforate tricuspid valve with dysplasia of the right ventricular myocardium, pulmonary valve, and coronary artery. Pediatr Cardiol 1992;13:24.
45. Mori Y, Nakanishi T, Ishii T, Imai Y, Nakazawa M. Relation of pulmonary venous wedge pressures to pulmonary artery pressures in patients with single ventricle physiology. Am J Cardiol 2003; 91:772-4.
46. Mott AR, Feltes TF, McKenzie ED, Andropoulos DB, Bezold LI, Fenrich AL, et al. Improved early results with the Fontan operation in adults with functional single ventricle. Ann Thorac Surg 2004; 77:1334-40.
47. Muller J, Christov F, Schreiber C, Hess J, Hager A. Exercise capacity, quality of life, and daily activity in the long-term follow-up of patients with univentricular heart and total cavopulmonary connection. Eur Heart J 2009;30:2915-20.
48. Murthy KS, Coelho R, Naik SK, Punnoose A, Thomas W, Cherian KM. Novel techniques of bidirectional Glen shunt without cardiopulmonary bypass. Ann Thorac Surg 1999;67:1771.
49. Muster AJ, Zales VR, Ilbawi MN, Backer CL, Duffy CE, Mavroudis C. Biventricular repair of hypoplastic right ventricle assisted by pulsatile bidirectional cavopulmonary anastomosis. J Thorac Cardiovasc Surg 1993;105:112.
50. Myers JL, Waldhausen JA, Weber HS, Arenas JD, Cyran SE, Gleason MM, et al. A reconsideration of risk factors for the Fontan operation. Ann Surg 1990;211:738.

N

1. Nakanishi T. Cardiac catheterization is necessary before bidirectional Glenn and Fontan procedures in single ventricle physiology. Pediatr Cardiol 2005;26:159-61.
2. Nakata S, Imai Y, Takanashi Y, Kurosawa H, Tezuka K, Nakazawa M, et al. A new method for the quantitative standardization of cross-sectional areas of the pulmonary arteries in congenital heart diseases with decreased pulmonary blood flow. J Thorac Cardiovasc Surg 1984;88:610.
3. Narkewicz MR, Sondheimer HM, Ziegler JW, Otanni Y, Lorts A, Shaffer EM, et al. Hepatic dysfunction following the Fontan procedure. J Pediatr Gastroenterol Nutr 2003;36:352-7.
4. Neveux JY, Dreyfus G, Leca F, Marchand M, Bex JP. Modified technique for correction of tricuspid atresia. J Thorac Cardiovasc Surg 1981;82:457.
5. Newfeld EA, Nikaidoh H. Surgical management of subaortic stenosis in patients with single ventricle and transposition of the great vessels. Circulation 1987;76:III29.

6. Nir A, Driscoll DJ, Mottram CD, Offord KP, Puga FJ, Schaff HV, et al. Cardiorespiratory response to exercise after the Fontan operation: a serial study. J Am Coll Cardiol 1993;22:216.
7. Nishioka K, Kamiya T, Ueda T, Hayashidera T, Mori C, Konishi Y, et al. Left ventricle volume characteristics in children with tricuspid atresia before and after surgery. Am J Cardiol 1981; 47:1105.
8. Norwood WI, Pigott JD. Hypoplastic left-sided heart syndrome. In Grillo HC, Austen WG, Wilkins EW, Mathisen DJ, Vlahakes GJ, eds. Current therapy in cardiothoracic surgery. Toronto: B.C. Decker, 1989, p. 473.
9. Nuland SB, Glenn WW, Guilfoil PH. Circulatory bypass of the right heart. III. Some observations on long-term survivors. Surgery 1958;43:184.
10. Nurnberg JH, Ovroutski S, Alexi-Meskishvili V, Ewert P, Hetzer R, Lange PE. New onset arrhythmias after the extracardiac conduit Fontan operation compared with the intraatrial lateral tunnel procedure: early and midterm results. Ann Thorac Surg 2004; 78:1979-88.

O

1. Ocello S, Salviato N, Marcelletti CF. Results of 100 consecutive extracardiac conduit Fontan operations. Pediatr Cardiol 2007;28: 433-7.
2. Ochiai Y, Imoto Y, Sakamoto M, Kajiwara T, Sese A, Watanabe M, et al. Mid-term follow-up of the status of Gore-Tex graft after extracardiac conduit Fontan procedure. Eur J Cardiothorac Surg 2009;36:63-8.
3. Odegard KC, McGowan FX Jr, DiNardo JA, Castro RA, Zurakowski D, Connor CM, et al. Coagulation abnormalities in patients with single-ventricle physiology precede the Fontan procedure. J Thorac Cardiovasc Surg 2002;123:459-65.
4. Odegard KC, McGowan FX Jr, Zurakowski D, Dinardo JA, Castro RA, del Nido PJ, et al. Procoagulant and anticoagulant factor abnormalities following the Fontan procedure: increased factor VIII may predispose to thrombosis. J Thorac Cardiovasc Surg 2003;125:1260-7.
5. Odim JN, Laks H, Drinkwater DC Jr, George BL, Yun J, Salem M, et al. Staged surgical approach to neonates with aortic obstruction and single-ventricle physiology. Ann Thorac Surg 1999;68:962-8.
6. Okabe H, Nagata N, Kaneko Y, Kobayashi J, Kanemoto S, Takaoka T. Extracardiac cavopulmonary connection of Fontan procedure with autologous pedicled pericardium without cardiopulmonary bypass. J Thorac Cardiovasc Surg 1998;116:1073.
7. Olson TM, Driscoll DJ, Edwards WD, Puga FJ, Danielson GK. Pulmonary microthrombi. J Thorac Cardiovasc Surg 1993;106:739.
8. O'Neill CA. Left axis deviation in tricuspid atresia and single ventricle. Circulation 1955;12:612.
9. Ono M, Boethig D, Goerler H, Lange M, Westhoff-Bleck M, Breymann T. Clinical outcome of patients 20 years after Fontan operation—effect of fenestration on late morbidity. Eur J Cardiothorac Surg 2006;30:923-9.
10. Oski JA, Canter CE, Spray TL, Kan JS, Cameron DE, Murphy AM. Embolic stroke after ligation of the pulmonary artery in patients with functional single ventricle. Am Heart J 1996;132:836.
11. Ostrow AM, Freeze H, Rychik J. Protein-losing enteropathy after Fontan operation: investigations into possible pathophysiologic mechanisms. Ann Thorac Surg 2006;82:695-700.
12. Ottenkamp J, Rohmer J, Quaegebeur JM, Brom AG, Fontan F. Nine years' experience of physiological correction of tricuspid atresia: long-term results and current surgical approach. Thorax 1982;37:718.
13. Ottenkamp J, Wenink AC. Anomalies of the mitral valve and of the left ventricular architecture in tricuspid valve atresia. Am J Cardiol 1989;63:880.
14. Ovroutski S, Alexi-Meskishvili V, Ewert P, Nurnberg JH, Hetzer R, Lange PE. Early and medium-term results after modified Fontan operation in adults. Eur J Cardiothorac Surg 2003;23:311-6.

P

1. Pace Napoleone C, Oppido G, Angeli E, Giardini A, Resciniti E, Gargiulo G. Results of the modified Fontan procedure are not related to age at operation. Eur J Cardiothorac Surg 2010; 37:645-50.
2. Parikh SR, Hurwitz RA, Caldwell RL, Girod DA. Ventricular function in the single ventricle before and after Fontan surgery. Am J Cardiol 1991;67:1390.
3. Park HK, Youn YN, Yang HS, Yoo BW, Choi JY, Park YH. Results of an extracardiac pericardial-flap lateral tunnel Fontan operation. Eur J Cardiothorac Surg 2008;34:563-9.
4. Patino JF, Glenn WW, Guilfoil PH, Hume M, Fenn J. Circulatory bypass of the right heart. II. Further observations on vena caval pulmonary artery shunts. Surg Forum 1956;6:189.
5. Paul T, Ziemer G, Luhmer L, Bertram H, Hecker H, Kallfelz HC. Early and late atrial dysrhythmias after modified Fontan operation. Pediatr Med Chir 1998;20:9.
6. Pearl JM, Laks H. Current status of the modified Fontan procedure. In Yacoub M, Pepper J, eds. Annual of cardiac surgery. Philadelphia: Current Science, Ltd., 1991, p. 64.
7. Penkoske PA, Freedom RM, Williams WG, Trusler GA, Rowe RD. Surgical palliation of subaortic stenosis in the univentricular heart. J Thorac Cardiovasc Surg 1984;87:767.
8. Penny DJ, Hayek Z, Redington AN. The effect of positive and negative extrathoracic pressure ventilation on pulmonary blood flow after the total cavopulmonary shunt procedure. Int J Cardiol 1991; 30:128.
9. Peters NS, Somerville J. Arrhythmias after the Fontan procedure. Br Heart J 1992,68:199.
10. Peterson RJ, Franch RH, Fajman WA, Jennings JG, Jones RH. Noninvasive determination of exercise cardiac function following Fontan operation. J Thorac Cardiovasc Surg 1984;88:263.
11. Petko M, Myung RJ, Wernovsky G, Cohen MI, Rychik J, Nicolson SC, et al. Surgical reinterventions following the Fontan procedure. Eur J Cardiothorac Surg 2003;24:255-9.
12. Petrossian E, Reddy VM, Collins KK, Culbertson CB, MacDonald MJ, Lamberti JJ, et al. The extracardiac conduit Fontan operation using minimal approach extracorporeal circulation: early and midterm outcomes. J Thorac Cardiovasc Surg 2006;132: 1054-63.
13. Petrossian E, Reddy VM, McElhinney DB, Akkersdijk GP, Moore P, Parry AJ, et al. Early results of the extracardiac conduit Fontan operation. J Thorac Cardiovasc Surg 1999;117:688.
14. Petrucci O, Khoury PR, Manning PB, Eghtesady P. Outcomes of the bidirectional Glenn procedure in patients less than 3 months of age. J Thorac Cardiovasc Surg 2010;139:562-8.
15. Pihkala J, Yazaki S, Mehta R, Lee KJ, Chaturvedi R, McCrindle BW, et al. Feasibility and clinical impact of transcatheter closure of interatrial communications after a fenestrated Fontan procedure: medium-term outcomes. Catheter Cardiovasc Interv 2007;69: 1007-14.
16. Prakash A, Khan MA, Hardy R, Torres AJ, Chen JM, Gersony WM. A new diagnostic algorithm for assessment of patients with single ventricle before a Fontan operation. J Thorac Cardiovasc Surg 2009;138:917-23.
17. Pridjian AK, Mendelsohn AM, Lupinetti FM, Beekman RH 3rd, Dick M 2nd, Serwer G, et al. Usefulness of the bidirectional Glenn procedure as staged reconstruction for the functional single ventricle. Am J Cardiol 1993;71:959.
18. Puga FJ. The modified Fontan operation. J Thorac Cardiovasc Surg 1989;98:150.
19. Puga FJ, Chiavarelli M, Hagler DJ. Modifications of the Fontan operation applicable to patients with left atrioventricular valve atresia or single atrioventricular valve. Circulation 1987;76:III53.
20. Putnam JB Jr, Lemmer JH Jr, Rocchini AP, Bove EL. Embolectomy for acute pulmonary artery occlusion following Fontan procedure. Ann Thorac Surg 1988;45:335.

Q

1. Quinones JA, Deleon SY, Bell TJ, Cetta F, Moffa SM, Freeman JE, et al. Fenestrated Fontan procedure: evolution of technique and occurrence of paradoxical embolism. Pediatr Cardiol 1997; 18:218.

R

1. Rao PS. Natural history of the ventricular septal defects in tricuspid atresia and its surgical implications. Br Heart J 1977;39:276.
2. Rao PS. Further observations on the spontaneous closure of physiologically advantageous ventricular septal defects in tricuspid atresia: surgical implications. Ann Thorac Surg 1983;35:121.

3. Rao PS. Is the term "tricuspid atresia" appropriate? Am J Cardiol 1990;66:1251.
4. Rao PS, Jue KL, Isabel-Jones J, Ruttenberg HD. Ebstein's malformation of the tricuspid valve with atresia. Differentiation from isolated tricuspid atresia. Am J Cardiol 1973;32:1004.
5. Razzouk AJ, Freedom RM, Cohen AJ, Williams WG, Trusler GA, Coles JG, et al. The recognition, identification of morphologic substrate, and treatment of subaortic stenosis after a Fontan operation. An analysis of twelve patients. J Thorac Cardiovasc Surg 1992;104:938.
6. Reddy VM, Liddicoat JR, Hanley FL. Primary bidirectional superior cavopulmonary shunt in infants between 1 and 4 months of age. Ann Thorac Surg 1995;59:1120.
7. Reddy VM, McElhinney DB, Moore P, Haas GS, Hanley FL. Outcomes after bidirectional cavopulmonary shunt in infants less than 6 months old. J Am Coll Cardiol 1997;29:1365.
8. Reddy VM, McElhinney DB, Moore P, Petrossian E, Hanley FL. Pulmonary artery growth after bidirectional cavopulmonary shunt: is there a cause for concern? J Thorac Cardiovasc Surg 1996; 112:1180.
9. Reddy VM, McElhinney DB, Silverman NH, Marianeschi SM, Hanley FL. Partial biventricular repair for complex congenital heart defects: an intermediate option for complicated anatomy or functionally borderline right heart complex. J Thorac Cardiovasc Surg 1998;116:21.
10. Redington AN, Penny D, Shinebourne EA. Pulmonary blood flow after total cavopulmonary shunt. Br Heart J 1991;65:213.
11. Rigby ML, Gibson DG, Joseph MC, Lincoln JC, Shinebourne EA, Shore DF, et al. Recognition of imperforate atrioventricular valves by two-dimensional echocardiography. Br Heart J 1982;47:329.
12. Robbers-Visser D, Jan Ten Harkel D, Kapusta L, Strengers JL, Dalinghaus M, Meijboom FJ, et al. Usefulness of cardiac magnetic resonance imaging combined with low-dose dobutamine stress to detect an abnormal ventricular stress response in children and young adults after Fontan operation at young age. Am J Cardiol 2008;101:1657-62.
13. Robbers-Visser D, Kapusta L, van Osch-Gevers L, Strengers JL, Boersma E, de Rijke YB, et al. Clinical outcome 5 to 18 years after the Fontan operation performed on children younger than 5 years. J Thorac Cardiovasc Surg 2009;138:89-95.
14. Robbers-Visser D, Miedema M, Nijveld A, Boersma E, Bogers AJ, Haas F, et al. Results of staged total cavopulmonary connection for functionally univentricular hearts; comparison of intra-atrial lateral tunnel and extracardiac conduit. Eur J Cardiothorac Surg 2010; 37:934-41.
15. Robicsek F, Temesvari A, Kadar RL. A new method for the treatment of congenital heart disease associated with impaired pulmonary circulation. Acta Med Scand 1956;154:151.
16. Rodbard S, Wagner D. Bypassing the right ventricle. Proc Soc Exp Biol Mod 1949;71:69.
17. Rodefeld MD, Ruzmetov M, Schamberger MS, Girod DA, Turrentine MW, Brown JW. Staged surgical repair of functional single ventricle in infants with unobstructed pulmonary blood flow. Eur J Cardiothorac Surg 2005;27:949-55.
18. Rome JJ, Keane JF, Perry SB, Spevak PJ, Lock JE. Double-umbrella closure of atrial defects. Circulation 1990;82:751.
19. Ro PS, Rychik J, Cohen MS, Mahle WT, Rome JJ. Diagnostic assessment before Fontan operation in patients with bidirectional cavopulmonary anastomosis: are noninvasive methods sufficient? J Am Coll Cardiol 2004;44:184-7.
20. Rosenquist GC, Levy RJ, Rowe RD. Right atrial-left ventricular relationships in tricuspid atresia: position of the presumed site of the atretic valve as determined by transillumination. Am Heart J 1970;80:493.
21. Rosenthal DN, Friedman AH, Kleinman CS, Kopf GS, Rosenfeld LE, Hellenbrand WE. Thromboembolic complications after Fontan operations. Circulation 1995;92:I1287.
22. Ross DN, Somerville J. Surgical correction of tricuspid atresia. Lancet 1973;1:845.
23. Rothman A, Lang P, Lock JE, Jonas RA, Mayer JE, Castaneda AR. Surgical management of subaortic obstruction in single left ventricle and tricuspid atresia. J Am Coll Cardiol 1987;10:421.
24. Russo P, Danielson GK, Puga FJ, McGoon DC, Humes R. Modified Fontan procedure for biventricular hearts with complex forms of double-outlet right ventricle. Circulation 1988;78:III20.
25. Rychik J, Murdison KA, Chin AJ, Norwood WI. Surgical management of severe aortic outflow obstruction in lesions other than the hypoplastic left heart syndrome: use of a pulmonary artery to aorta anastomosis. J Am Coll Cardiol 1995;59:1120.
26. Rychik J, Rome JJ, Jacobs ML. Late surgical fenestration for complications after the Fontan operation. Circulation 1997;96:33.

S

1. Salmon AP, Sethia B, Silove ED, Goh D, Mitchell I, Alton H, et al. Cavopulmonary anastomosis as long-term palliation for patients with tricuspid atresia. Eur J Cardiothorac Surg 1989; 3:494.
2. Salvin JW, Scheurer MA, Laussen PC, Mayer JE, Jr., Del Nido PJ, Pigula FA, et al. Factors associated with prolonged recovery after the Fontan operation. Circulation 2008;118:S171-6.
3. Sandor GG, Patterson MW, LeBlanc JG. Systolic and diastolic function in tricuspid valve atresia before the Fontan operation. Am J Cardiol 1994;73:292.
4. Scalia D, Russo P, Anderson RH, Macartney FJ, Hegerty AS, Ho SY, et al. The surgical anatomy of hearts with no direct communication between the right atrium and the ventricular mass—so-called tricuspid atresia. J Thorac Cardiovasc Surg 1984;87:743.
5. Scheurer MA, Hill EG, Vasuki N, Maurer S, Graham EM, Bandisode V, et al. Survival after bidirectional cavopulmonary anastomosis: analysis of preoperative risk factors. J Thorac Cardiovasc Surg 2007;134:82-9.
6. Schreiber C, Cleuziou J, Cornelsen JK, Horer J, Eicken A, Lange R. Bidirectional cavopulmonary connection without additional pulmonary blood flow as an ideal staging for functional univentricular hearts. Eur J Cardiothorac Surg 2008;34:550-5.
7. Schreiber C, Horer J, Vogt M, Cleuziou J, Prodan Z, Lange R. Nonfenestrated extracardiac total cavopulmonary connection in 132 consecutive patients. Ann Thorac Surg 2007;84:894-9.
8. Schreiber C, Kostolny M, Horer J, Cleuziou J, Holper K, Tassani-Prell P, et al. Can we do without routine fenestration in extracardiac total cavopulmonary connections? Report on 84 consecutive patients. Cardiol Young 2006;16:54-60.
9. Schreiber C, Kostolny M, Weipert J, Holper K, Vogt M, Hager A, et al. What was the impact of the introduction of extracardiac completion for a single center performing total cavopulmonary connections? Cardiol Young 2004;14:140-7.
10. Schwartz SM, Gordon D, Mosca RS, Bove EL, Heidelberger KP, Kulik TJ. Collagen content in normal, pressure, and pressure-volume overloaded developing human hearts. Am J Cardiol 1996; 77:734.
11. Seipelt RG, Franke A, Vazquez-Jimenez JF, Hanrath P, von Bernuth G, Messmer BJ, et al. Thromboembolic complications after Fontan procedures: comparison of different therapeutic approaches. Ann Thorac Surg 2002;74:556-62.
12. Seliem M, Muster AJ, Paul MH, Benson DW Jr. Relation between preoperative left ventricular muscle mass and outcome of the Fontan procedure in patients with tricuspid atresia. J Am Coll Cardiol 1989;14:750.
13. Senzaki H, Isoda T, Ishizawa A, Hishi T. Reconsideration of criteria for the Fontan operation. Influence of pulmonary artery size on postoperative hemodynamics of the Fontan operation. Circulation 1994;89:266.
14. Shachar GB, Fuhrman BP, Wang Y, Lucas RV Jr, Lock JE. Rest and exercise hemodynamics after the Fontan procedure. Circulation 1982;65:1043.
15. Shanahan CL, Wilson NJ, Gentles TL, Skinner JR. The influence of measured versus assumed uptake of oxygen in assessing pulmonary vascular resistance in patients with a bidirectional Glenn anastomosis. Cardiol Young 2003;13:137-42.
16. Sharratt GP, Johnson AM, Monro JL. Persistence and effects of sinus rhythm after Fontan procedure for tricuspid atresia. Br Heart J 1979;42:78.
17. Sheikh AM, Tang AT, Roman K, Baig K, Mehta R, Morgan J, et al. The failing Fontan circulation: successful conversion of atriopulmonary connections. J Thorac Cardiovasc Surg 2004; 128:60-6.
18. Shemin RJ, Merrill WH, Pfeifer JS, Conkle DM, Morrow AG. Evaluation of right atrial–pulmonary artery conduits for tricuspid atresia. J Thorac Cardiovasc Surg 1979;77:685.
19. Shikata F, Yagihara T, Kagisaki K, Hagino I, Shiraishi S, Kobayashi J, et al. Does the off-pump Fontan procedure ameliorate the volume and duration of pleural and peritoneal effusions? Eur J Cardiothorac Surg 2008;34:570-5.

20. Shiraishi S, Uemura H, Kagisaki K, Koh M, Yagihara T, Kitamura S. The off-pump Fontan procedure by simply cross-clamping the inferior caval vein. Ann Thorac Surg 2005;79:2083-8.
21. Shiraishi S, Yagihara T, Kagisaki K, Hagino I, Ohuchi H, Kobayashi J, et al. Impact of age at Fontan completion on postoperative hemodynamics and long-term aerobic exercise capacity in patients with dominant left ventricle. Ann Thorac Surg 2009;87:555-61.
22. Shore D, Jones O, Rigby ML, Anderson RH, Lincoln C. Atresia of left atrioventricular connection. Br Heart J 1982;47:35.
23. Silvilairat S, Pongprot Y, Sittiwangkul R, Woragidpoonpol S, Chuaratanaphong S, Nawarawong W. Factors influencing survival in patients after bidirectional Glenn shunt. Asian Cardiovasc Thorac Ann 2008;16:381-6.
24. Sinzobahamvya N, Arenz C, Reckers J, Photiadis J, Murin P, Schindler E, et al. Poor outcome for patients with totally anomalous pulmonary venous connection and functionally single ventricle. Cardiol Young 2009;19:594-600.
25. Sittiwangkul R, Azakie A, Van Arsdell GS, Williams WG, McCrindle BW. Outcomes of tricuspid atresia in the Fontan era. Ann Thorac Surg 2004;77:889-94.
26. Slavik Z, Lamb RK, Webber SA, Devlin AM, Keeton BR, Monro JL, et al. Bidirectional superior cavopulmonary anastomosis: how young is too young? Heart 1996;75:78.
27. Smith EE, Naftel DC, Blackstone EH, Kirklin JW. Microvascular permeability after cardiopulmonary bypass: an experimental study. J Thorac Cardiovasc Surg 1987;94:225.
28. Smolinsky A, Castaneda AR, Van Praagh R. Infundibular septal resection: surgical anatomy of the superior approach. J Thorac Cardiovasc Surg 1988;95:486.
29. Somerville J, Becu L, Ross D. Common ventricle with acquired subaortic obstruction. Am J Cardiol 1974;34:206.
30. Srivastava D, Preminger T, Lock JE, Mandell V, Keane JF, Mayer JE Jr, et al. Hepatic venous blood and the development of pulmonary arteriovenous malformations in congenital heart disease. Circulation 1995;92:1217.
31. Stamm C, Friehs I, Duebener LF, Zurakowski D, Mayer JE Jr, Jonas RA, et al. Improving results of the modified Fontan operation in patients with heterotaxy syndrome. Ann Thorac Surg 2002; 74:1967-78.
32. Stanford W, Armstrong RG, Cline RE, King TD. Right atrium pulmonary artery allograft for correction of tricuspid atresia. J Thorac Cardiovasc Surg 1973;66:105.
33. Stansel HC Jr. A new operation for d-loop transposition of the great vessels. Ann Thorac Surg 1975;19:565.
34. Starr I, Jeffers WA, Meade RH. The absence of conspicuous increments of venous pressure after severe damage to the right ventricle of the dog, with a discussion of the relation between clinical congestive failure and heart disease. Am Heart J 1943;26: 291.
35. Stefanelli G, Kirklin JW, Naftel DC, Blackstone EH, Pacifico AD, Kirklin JK, et al. Early and intermediate-term (10-year) results of surgery for univentricular atrioventricular connection ("single ventricle"). Am J Cardiol 1984;54:811.
36. Stein DG, Laks H, Drinkwater DC, Permut LC, Louie HW, Pearl JM, et al. Results of total cavopulmonary connection in the treatment of patients with a functional single ventricle. J Thorac Cardiovasc Surg 1991;102:280.
37. Stellin G, Mazzucco A, Bortolotti U, del Torso S, Faggian G, Fracasso A, et al. Tricuspid atresia versus other complex lesions. J Thorac Cardiovasc Surg 1988;96:204.
38. Stern HJ. The argument for aggressive coiling of aortopulmonary collaterals in single ventricle patients. Catheter Cardiovasc Interv 2009;74:897-900.
39. Strumper O, Wright JG, Sadiq M, DeGiovanni JV. Late systemic desaturation after total cavopulmonary shunt operations. Br Heart J 1995;74:282.
40. Sun LS, Dominguez C, Mallavaram NA, Quaegebeur JM. Dysfunction of atrial and B-type natriuretic peptides in congenital univentricular defects. J Thorac Cardiovasc Surg 2005;129:1104-10.

T

1. Tam CK, Lightfoot NE, Finlay CD, Coles J, Williams WG, Trusler GA, et al. Course of tricuspid atresia in the Fontan era. Am J Cardiol 1989;63:589.
2. Tandon R, Edwards JE. Tricuspid atresia. A re-evaluation and classification. J Thorac Cardiovasc Surg 1974;67:530.
3. Tandon R, Marin-Garcia J, Moller JM, Edwards JE. Tricuspid atresia with l-transposition. Am Heart J 1974;88:417.
4. Tanoue Y, Sese A, Imoto Y, Joh K. Ventricular mechanics in the bidirectional glenn procedure and total cavopulmonary connection. Ann Thorac Surg 2003;76:562-6.
5. Tanoue Y, Sese A, Ueno Y, Joh K, Hijii T. Bidirectional Glenn procedure improves the mechanical efficiency of a total cavopulmonary connection in high-risk Fontan candidates. Circulation 2001;103:2176-80.
6. Taussig HB. The clinical and pathological findings in congenital malformation of the heart due to defective development of the right ventricle associated with tricuspid atresia or hypoplasia. Bull Johns Hopkins Hosp 1936;59:435.
7. Thoele DG, Ursell PC, Ho SY, Smith A, Bowman FO, Gersony WM, et al. Atrial morphologic features in tricuspid atresia. J Thorac Cardiovasc Surg 1991;102:606.
8. Thompson J, Moore P, Teitel DF. Pulmonary venous wedge pressures accurately predict pulmonary arterial pressures in children with single ventricle physiology. Pediatr Cardiol 2003; 24:531-7.
9. Thompson LD, Petrossian E, McElhinney DB, Abrikosova NA, Moore P, Reddy VM, et al. Is it necessary to routinely fenestrate an extracardiac Fontan? J Am Coll Cardiol 1999;34:539-44.
10. Thorne SA, Hooper J, Kemp M, Somerville J. Gastro-intestinal protein loss in late survivors of Fontan surgery and other congenital heart disease. Eur Heart J 1998;19:514.
11. Tokunaga S, Kado H, Imoto Y, Masuda M, Shiokawa Y, Fukae K, et al. Total cavopulmonary connection with an extracardiac conduit: experience with 100 patients. Ann Thorac Surg 2002;73:76-80.
12. Tomita H, Yamada O, Ohuchi H, Ono Y, Arakaki Y, Yagihara T, et al. Coagulation profile, hepatic function, and hemodynamics following Fontan-type operations. Cardiol Young 2001;11:62-6.
13. Trento A, Zuberbuhler JR, Anderson RH, Park SC, Siewers RD. Divided right atrium (prominence of the eustachian and thebesian valves). J Thorac Cardiovasc Surg 1988;96:457.
14. Trusler GA, Williams WG. Long-term results of shunt procedures for tricuspid atresia. Ann Thorac Surg 1980;29:312.
15. Tweddell JS, Berger S, Frommelt PC, Pelech AN, Lewis DA, Fedderly RT, et al. Aprotinin improves outcome of single-ventricle palliation. Ann Thorac Surg 1996;62:1329.
16. Tweddell JS, Nersesian M, Mussatto KA, Nugent M, Simpson P, Mitchell ME, et al. Fontan palliation in the modern era: factors impacting mortality and morbidity. Ann Thorac Surg 2009; 88:1291-9.

U

1. Uemura H, Yagihara T, Yamashita K, Ishizaka T, Yoshizumi K, Kawahira Y. Establishment of total cavopulmonary connection without use of cardiopulmonary bypass. Eur J Cardiothorac Surg 1998;13:504.
2. Uzark K, Lincoln A, Lamberti JJ, Mainwaring RD, Spicer RL, Moore JW. Neurodevelopmental outcomes in children with Fontan repair of functional single ventricle. Pediatrics 1998;101:630.

V

1. Van Arsdell GS, Williams WG, Maser CM, Streitenberger KS, Rebeyka IM, Coles JG, et al. Superior vena cava to pulmonary artery anastomosis: an adjunct to biventricular repair. J Thorac Cardiovasc Surg 1996;112:1143.
2. Van Den Bogaert-Van Heesvelde AM, Derom F, Kunnen M, Van Egmond H, Devloo-Blancquaert A. Surgery for arteriovenous fistulas and dilated vessels in the right lung after the Glenn procedure. J Thorac Cardiovasc Surg 1978;76:195.
3. Van Nooten G, Deuvaert FE, De Paepe J, Primo G. Pulmonary artery banding. Experience with 69 patients. J Cardiovasc Surg 1989;30:334.
4. van Son JA, Reddy VM, Haas GS, Hanley FL. Modified surgical techniques for relief of aortic obstruction in [S,L,L] hearts with rudimentary right ventricle and restrictive bulboventricular foramen. J Thorac Cardiovasc Surg 1995;110:909.
5. van Son JA, Reddy M, Hanley FL. Extracardiac modification of the Fontan operation without use of prosthetic material. J Thorac Cardiovasc Surg 1995;110:1766.
6. Varma C, Warr MR, Hendler AL, Paul NS, Webb GD, Therrien J. Prevalence of "silent" pulmonary emboli in adults after the Fontan operation. J Am Coll Cardiol 2003;41:2252-8.

7. Veldtman GR, Nishimoto A, Siu S, Freeman M, Fredriksen PM, Gatzoulis MA, et al. The Fontan procedure in adults. Heart 2001;86:330-5.
8. Ventriglia F, Mundo L, Bosco G, Colloridi V. Regression of post-Fontan protein-losing enteropathy. After surgical correction of hemodynamic faults other than high right atrial pressure. Tex Heart Inst J 1996;23:233.
9. Villani M, Crupi G, Locatelli G, Tiraboschi R, Vanini V, Parenzan L. Experience in palliative treatment of univentricular heart including tricuspid atresia. Herz 1979;4:256.
10. Vlad P. Tricuspid atresia. In Keith JD, Rowe RD, Vlad P, eds. Heart disease in infancy and childhood. 3rd Ed. New York: Macmillan, 1978, p. 518.
11. Vogt KN, Manlhiot C, Van Arsdell G, Russell JL, Mital S, McCrindle BW. Somatic growth in children with single ventricle physiology impact of physiologic state. J Am Coll Cardiol 2007; 50:1876-83.
12. Vyas H, Driscoll DJ, Cabalka AK, Cetta F, Hagler DJ. Results of transcatheter Fontan fenestration to treat protein losing enteropathy. Catheter Cardiovasc Interv 2007;69:584-9.

W

1. Wald RM, Tham EB, McCrindle BW, Goff DA, McAuliffe FM, Golding F, et al. Outcome after prenatal diagnosis of tricuspid atresia: a multicenter experience. Am Heart J 2007;153:772-8.
2. Ward KE, Fisher DJ, Michael L. Elevated coronary sinus pressure does not alter myocardial blood flow or left ventricular contractile function in mature sheep. J Thorac Cardiovasc Surg 1988;95: 511.
3. Warden HE, De Wall RA, Varco RL. Use of the right auricle as a pump for the pulmonary circuit. Surg Forum 1954;5:16.
4. Watanabe M, Aoki M, Fujiwara T. Transition of ventricular function and energy efficiency after a primary or staged Fontan procedure. Gen Thorac Cardiovasc Surg 2008;56:498-504.
5. Weber HS, Gleason MM, Myers JL, Waldhausen JA, Cyran SE, Baylen BG. The Fontan operation in infants less than 2 years of age. J Am Coll Cardiol 1992;19:828.
6. Weinberg PM. Anatomy of tricuspid atresia and its relevance to current forms of surgical therapy. Ann Thorac Surg 1980;29:306.
7. Weipert J, Koch W, Haehnel JC, Meisner H. Exercise capacity and mid-term survival in patients with tricuspid atresia and complex congenital cardiac malformations after modified Fontan operation. Eur J Cardiothorac Surg 1997;12:574.
8. Weipert J, Meisner H, Haehnel C, Paek SU, Sebening F. Surgical evaluation of the modified Fontan procedure. Herz 1992; 17:246.
9. Weipert J, Noebauer C, Schreiber C, Kostolny M, Zrenner B, Wacker A, et al. Occurrence and management of atrial arrhythmia after long-term Fontan circulation. J Thorac Cardiovasc Surg 2004;127:457-64.
10. Wilkinson P, Pinto B, Senior JR. Reversible protein-losing enteropathy with intestinal lymphangiectasia secondary to chronic constrictive pericarditis. N Engl J Med 1965;273:1178.
11. Williams DB, Kiernan PD, Metke MP, Marsh HM, Danielson GK. Hemodynamic response to positive end-expiratory pressure following right atrium–pulmonary artery bypass (Fontan procedure). J Thorac Cardiovasc Surg 1984;87:856.
12. Williams WG, Rubis L, Fowler RS, Rao MK, Trusler GA, Mustard WT. Tricuspid atresia: results of treatment in 160 children. Am J Cardiol 1976;38:235.
13. Woods RK, Dyamenahalli U, Duncan BW, Rosenthal GL, Lupinetti FM. Comparison of extracardiac Fontan techniques: pedicled pericardial tunnel versus conduit reconstruction. J Thorac Cardiovasc Surg 2003;125:465-71.

Y

1. Yacoub MH, Radley-Smith R. Use of a valved conduit from right atrium to pulmonary artery for "correction" of a single ventricle. Circulation 1976;54:III63.
2. Yalcinbas YK, Erek E, Salihoglu E, Sarioglu A, Sarioglu T. Early results of extracardiac Fontan procedure with autologous pericardial tube conduit. Thorac Cardiovasc Surg 2005;53:37-40.
3. Yamada K, Roques X, Elia N, Laborde MN, Jimenez M, Choussat A, et al. The short- and mid-term results of bidirectional cavopulmonary shunt with additional source of pulmonary blood flow as definitive palliation for the functional single ventricular heart. Eur J Cardiothorac Surg 2000;18:683-9.
4. Yetman AT, Drummond-Webb J, Fiser WP, Schmitz ML, Imamura M, Ullah S, et al. The extracardiac Fontan procedure without cardiopulmonary bypass: technique and intermediate-term results. Ann Thorac Surg 2002;74:S1416-21.
5. Yin Z, Wang C, Zhu H, Zhang R, Wang H, Li X. Exercise tolerance in extracardiac total cavopulmonary connection. Asian Cardiovasc Thorac Ann 2009;17:39-45.
6. Yoshida M, Yamaguchi M, Yoshimura N, Murakami H, Matsuhisa H, Okita Y. Appropriate additional pulmonary blood flow at the bidirectional Glenn procedure is useful for completion of total cavopulmonary connection. Ann Thorac Surg 2005;80:976-81.

Z

1. Zellers TM, Brown K. Protein-losing enteropathy after the modified Fontan operation: oral prednisone treatment with biopsy and laboratory proved improvement. Pediatr Cardiol 1996;17:115.
2. Zellers TM, Driscoll DJ, Humes RA, Feldt RH, Puga FJ, Danielson GK. Glenn shunt: effect on pleural drainage after modified Fontan operation. J Thorac Cardiovasc Surg 1989;98:725.

42 Ebstein Anomaly

DEFINITION

Ebstein anomaly is a congenital defect of the tricuspid valve in which origins of the septal or posterior leaflets or both are displaced downward into the right ventricle, and the leaflets are variably deformed. Characteristically, the anterior leaflet is enlarged and "sail-like." There is a wide spectrum of severity; in the mildest asymptomatic forms, the valve may appear normal at first sight, and classification as Ebstein anomaly may be debatable.[S7]

This chapter discusses Ebstein anomaly in hearts with atrioventricular concordant connection and without other major cardiac anomalies. Ebstein-type tricuspid atresia and Ebstein anomaly associated with pulmonary atresia and with atrioventricular discordant connection are discussed elsewhere (see Chapters 40, 41, and 55). Details of Wolff-Parkinson-White syndrome, which is occasionally associated with Ebstein anomaly, are presented in Chapter 16.

HISTORICAL NOTE

Wilhelm Ebstein's scholarly description of the tricuspid valve abnormality bearing his name was published in 1866.[E1] His report describes a single autopsy specimen and includes a hypothesis of pathophysiology based on correlation of the morphology with clinical notes on the deeply cyanosed patient supplied by a colleague (Ebstein did not apparently

Table 42-1 Autopsy Findings in 16 Hearts with Ebstein Anomaly[a]

	Leaflet Origin				Leaflet Size		
Tricuspid Leaflet	**Totally Absent**	**Normal**	**Displaced**	**Adherent**	**Normal**	**Small**	**Elongated**
Septal	1	0	10	8[b]	2	11[c]	1
Posterior	1	3	5	7	1	1	12
Anterior	0	14	1	0	0	0	15[d]

Data from GLH group.
[a]Dilatation of the functional ventricle was present in 15, of the atrialized chamber in 4, and of the tricuspid anulus in 12. There was an atrial communication in all specimens (small probe-patent foramen ovale in 2, an enlarged foramen ovale in 7, and fossa ovalis atrial septal defect in 7).
[b]In two hearts, the whole cusp was adherent.
[c]In three hearts, up to half the leaflet was missing.
[d]In three hearts, the elongation was slight.

see the patient, Joseph Prescher, alive).[A7,S4] According to the historical review by Mann and Lie, the second case was not described until 20 years later, and the first description in the English literature was by MacCallum in 1900.[M4] The eponym *Ebstein's disease* was first suggested by Arnstein in 1927 and was used by Yater and Shapiro in their 1937 review article that reported the sixteenth case and the first to be examined by both radiography and electrocardiography.[A8,Y1] These investigators commented that "it would appear impossible to make the diagnosis during life." In 1950, Engle and colleagues as well as Reynolds suggested that the disease was associated with a clinical syndrome that should make diagnosis possible.[E3,R6] In 1951, Van Lingen and colleagues and Soloff and colleagues made the diagnosis during life using cardiac catheterization and angiography, respectively.[S17,V3] In 1955, Lev and colleagues described a patient with coexisting Wolff-Parkinson-White (WPW) syndrome and provided histologic details of the course of the conducting tissue in this anomaly.[L2]

Palliative surgery was attempted unsuccessfully using a Blalock-Taussig shunt in 1950.[E2] A superior vena cava–to–right pulmonary artery anastomosis (Glenn procedure[G6]) was used successfully by Gasul and colleagues in 1959 and subsequently by McCredie and colleagues and Scott and colleagues.[G1,G2,M9,S6] Barnard and Schrire were the first to report the use of prosthetic valve replacement in 1962, followed by Cartwright and colleagues and Lillehei and colleagues.[B3,C4,L4] Hardy and colleagues reported the first successful valvuloplasty in 1964 based on the concepts of Hunter and Lillehei.[H1,H5] A similar technique was used by Bahnson in 1965.[B1]

MORPHOLOGY AND MORPHOGENESIS

Tricuspid Valve

Both the origin of the tricuspid valve from the atrioventricular (AV) ring and its chordal attachments within the right ventricle (RV) are malpositioned, and the leaflets are malformed.[A4,A6,B4,L3,S5,Z1] The leaflets are either enlarged or reduced in size and are frequently dysplastic (thickened and distorted). These deformities vary widely in severity (Table 42-1). In the mildest forms, the valve is functionally near normal[P3]; in the fully developed syndrome, function is severely compromised. Displacement of the origin of the leaflets from the AV ring is reasonably constant. The septal leaflet appears always to be affected, the posterior leaflet nearly always, and the anterior leaflet seldom (Fig. 42-1). As noted by Anderson and colleagues, when both the septal and posterior leaflets are displaced,[A6] the point of maximum displacement is usually at the commissure between them. Thus, the functional tricuspid anulus is rotated apically and anteriorly (Fig. 42-2). In the few cases in which the anterior leaflet is displaced, the commissural area between it and the septal leaflet, attached to the right trigone at the point of penetration of the bundle of His, remains in normal position[L2] (see Fig. 42-1). In many patients, the apparent displacement is due to adherence of the base of the leaflet to the RV wall (see Table 42-1 and Fig. 42-1). Adherence of leaflet tissue to the underlying myocardium is thought to represent a failure of delamination during development.[K1] This failure effectively moves the hinge points of the septal and posterior leaflets (the functional anulus) into the ventricular cavity. When adherence is incomplete, there is a potential or obvious pocket beneath the leaflet.

The septal or posterior leaflet may be partially absent, in which case the belly of the leaflet is small or absent (see Fig. 42-1). The posterior leaflet is more often elongated than reduced in size (see Table 42-1), due in part to lack of a commissure between the posterior and anterior cusps. This was the case in 8 of 15 hearts examined at autopsy at GLH. The septal–posterior leaflet commissure may also occasionally be absent. Leaflet enlargement and elongation are characteristic of the anterior leaflet, which has been described as sail-like. The leaflet is usually diffusely thickened or ridged and occasionally consists partly of muscle. All the leaflets are frequently dysplastic, and isolated accessory leaflets may occur.[L3]

Distal leaflet attachments are variable and usually abnormal. Displaced and dysplastic posterior and septal leaflets frequently have multiple short chordae connecting to multiple small papillary muscles (see Fig. 42-1). The sail-like anterior leaflet may also have multiple short chordae arising around most of its free edge, binding it relatively closely to the septum and occasionally to the free wall, or the leaflet edge may be directly adherent to the anterior papillary muscle and moderator band or the posterior edge of the septal band.[Z1] Presence of a free anterior leaflet is an important morphologic detail, because it greatly increases the likelihood of a successful repair. Leaflet fenestrations are common, with the opening typically guarded by a single papillary muscle, which gives rise to chords that attach to the periphery of the fenestration.

If the entire free margin of the leaflets is adherent and imperforate, one variety of tricuspid atresia is produced (see Chapter 41).[R3,Z1] When the adherence is partial, the large

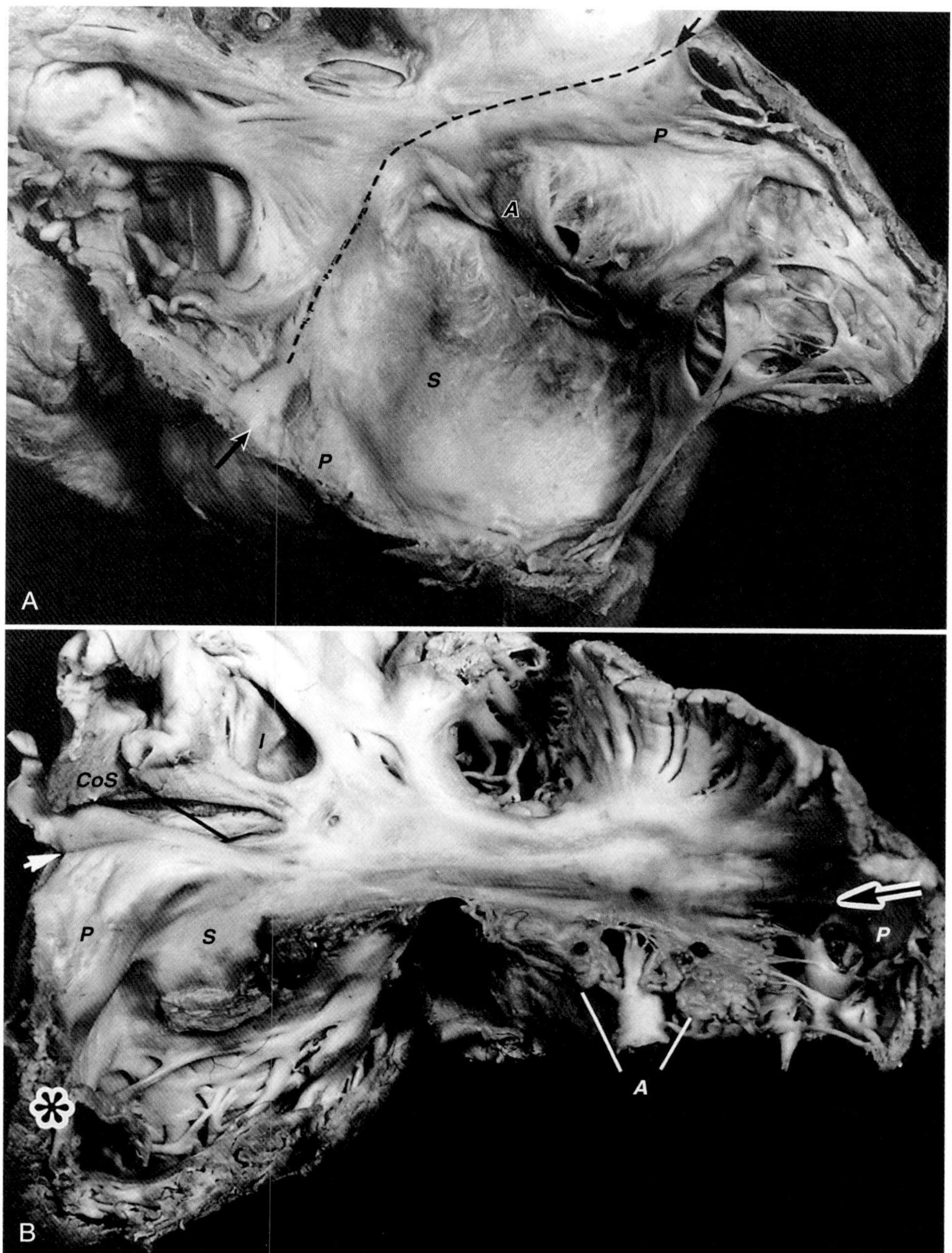

Figure 42-1 Autopsy specimens of Ebstein anomaly with varying degrees of tricuspid valve deformity. Right atrium and right ventricle have been opened. **A,** Site of true atrioventricular ring is marked by dashed line between arrows. All three leaflets are enlarged and elongated (anterior leaflet is poorly displayed). Septal leaflet is completely adherent to ventricular septal surface and has abnormal distal chordal attachments, as does posterior leaflet. Note normal leaflet origin at right trigone (anteroseptal commissure). **B,** Septal leaflet origin is displaced well downward into ventricle, and leaflet tissue is diminutive and dysplastic. Posterior leaflet is adherent from the ring to point marked with large asterisk. Anterior leaflet origin is normal, its belly is mildly elongated and cleft, and there are multiple short chordal attachments.

Continued

anterior leaflet produces a variable degree of stenosis between the portion of ventricle proximal to it (atrialized ventricle) and that distal to it (functional or ventricularized ventricle), because blood can pass only between openings that remain between the leaflet margin and ventricular wall (or through the commissures when these are present) (Fig. 42-3). Stiffness of the anterior leaflet contributes to stenosis.

Although important stenosis is uncommon, most Ebstein valves are regurgitant, often severely so (Fig. 42-4). This is contributed to by marked dilatation of the true tricuspid anulus and the RV, as by well as by morphologic abnormalities of the tricuspid valve.

The functional tricuspid orifice is determined by the hinge points of the valve leaflets, which rotate around the aortic root. The resultant functional valve orifice resides at the junction of the inlet and apical trabecular portions of the RV. We emphasize Anderson's focus on this rotational understanding of Ebstein anomaly to differentiate it from

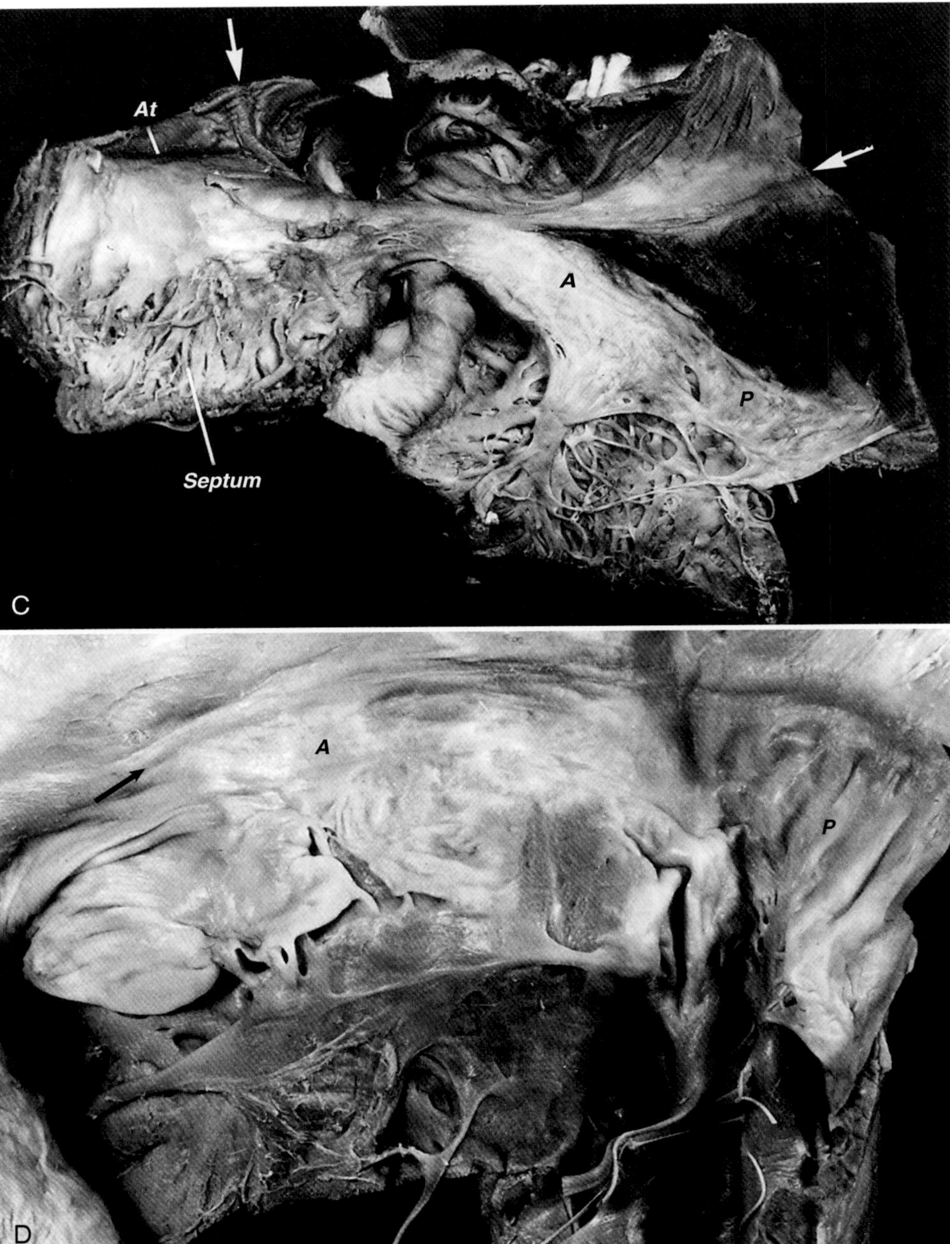

Figure 42-1, cont'd **C,** Septal leaflet is absent except for a strand of fibrous tissue. Anterior leaflet origin is downwardly displaced (except at right trigone), as is the posterior leaflet origin. Darkened, bruised portion of ventricular wall is thinned, atrialized ventricle. **D,** Elongated anterior and posterior leaflets originating normally from ring *(arrow)* but with poor commissural development. Central part of distal anterior leaflet edge is completely fused to a broad muscle group on the right ventricular free wall; adjacent to this are thickened, short chordae. Septal leaflet is not visible. Key: *A,* Anterior tricuspid valve leaflet; *At,* atrialized ventricle; *CoS,* coronary sinus; *P,* posterior tricuspid valve leaflet; *S,* septal tricuspid valve leaflet.

tricuspid valve dysplasia, which is often mistaken for Ebstein anomaly.[B8,V4]

Right Ventricle

Rotational displacement of the valve divides the RV into proximal *(atrialized)* and distal *(ventricularized)* portions. The proximal portion lies between the true tricuspid anulus and the valve attachment and comprises a variable portion of the posterior and inferior (diaphragmatic) aspects of the ventricular cavity (see Figs. 42-3 and 42-4). The right coronary artery denotes location of the true tricuspid anulus.

The proximal portion is atrialized in about one fourth of hearts in which the posterior and septal leaflets are severely displaced (Fig. 42-5). This atrialized portion of ventricular wall is dilated. Uncommonly, it is so thin as to seem aneurysmal, in which case it is largely fibrous tissue, and the endocardium is smooth. When very thin, it moves paradoxically during ventricular systole and may also expand during atrial systole. Its electrical potentials are ventricular, but its

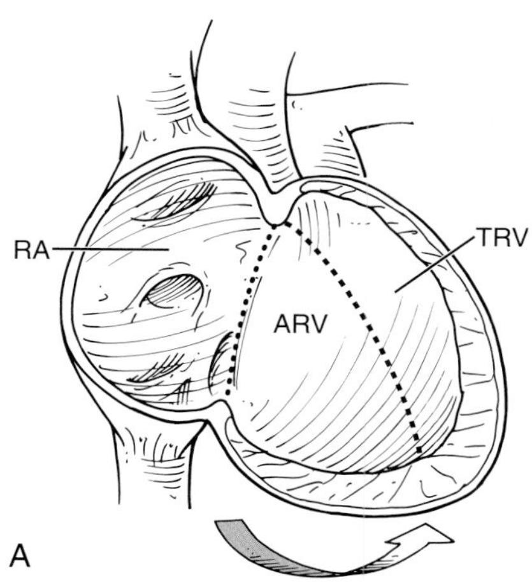

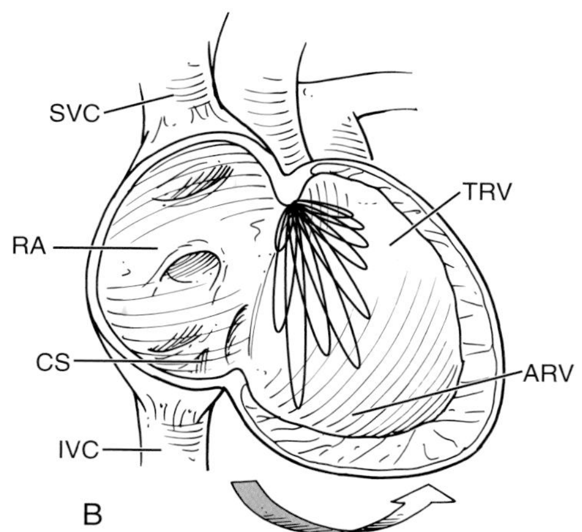

Figure 42-2 Functional tricuspid valve anulus in Ebstein anomaly. **A,** Normal proximal tricuspid attachments at atrioventricular junction *(circular dotted line)* and direction of hinge line *(square dotted line)*. Displacement of valve orifice is rotational *(flat arrow)*. **B,** Location of functional orifice of the abnormal valve *(black ovals)* as observed in the series of hearts examined by Schreiber and colleagues.[S5] Key: *ARV,* Atrialized right ventricle; *CS,* coronary sinus; *IVC,* inferior vena cava; *RA,* right atrium; *SVC,* superior vena cava; *TRV,* true right ventricle.

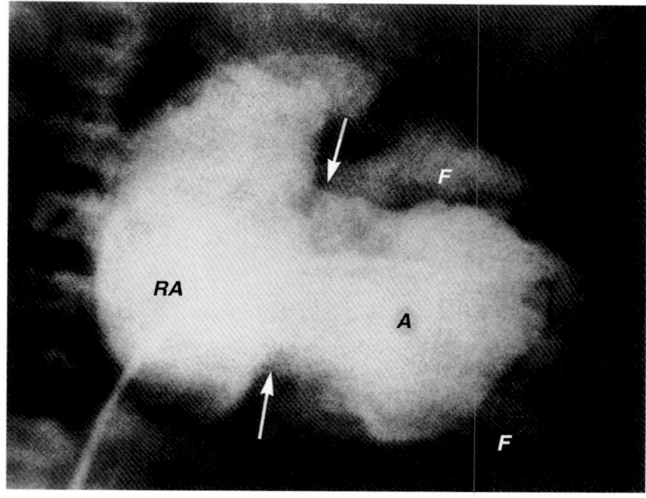

Figure 42-3 Cineangiogram in right anterior oblique projection of Ebstein anomaly. Injection is into a large atrialized right ventricle, demonstrating dome formed by the fused leaflets. Free reflux is present into right atrium *(RA)* through atrioventricular ring *(arrows)*. Relatively small functional (ventricularized) ventricle is poorly outlined because displaced valve is stenotic (virtual tricuspid atresia). Key: *A,* Atrialized portion of right ventricle; *F,* functional portion of right ventricle.

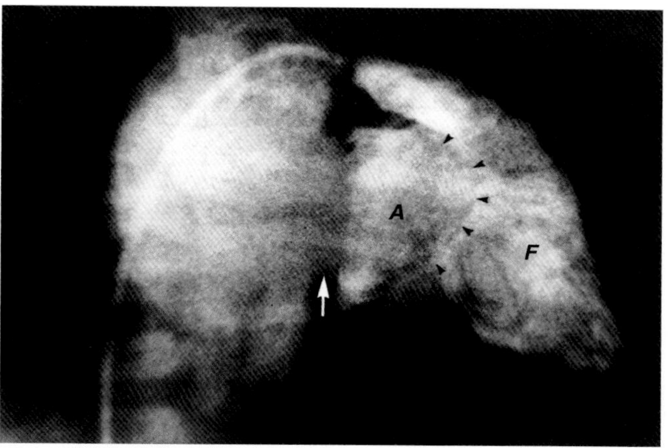

Figure 42-4 Cineangiogram in right anterior oblique projection of neonate with pulmonary atresia and Ebstein anomaly. Injection was into right ventricle, but catheter has recoiled into right atrium. Curved margin *(black arrowheads)* represents a dome formed by abnormally tethered distal edge of tricuspid leaflets. This margin separates atrialized ventricle from functional ventricle. There is severe tricuspid regurgitation. Normally positioned atrioventricular ring is readily identified *(white arrow)*. Key: *A,* Atrialized portion of right ventricle; *F,* functional portion of right ventricle.

pressure pulse has an atrial contour. More commonly, the wall of the atrialized portion is thicker than this and contains variable amounts of muscle.

The functional ventricularized portion of the RV lies distal (downstream) to the displaced valve and is therefore smaller than the normal RV. However, this feature is modified by RV dilatation, which is an almost constant finding. The functional portion consists of the infundibulum (conus), trabeculated apex, and that portion of the ventricle beneath the large anterior cusp (anterolateral recess)[A4] (Figs. 42-6 and 42-7).

Ebstein anomaly is more than a valve abnormality, in that the RV has an underlying myopathy. The dilated functional ventricle is usually thinner walled than normal and contains fewer muscle fibers. Anderson and Lie suggested there may be a congenital paucity of myocardial cells in the RV, such that dilatation of both portions of the ventricle is part of the developmental anomaly rather than entirely its hemodynamic consequence.[A5]

In 1988, Carpentier proposed a *classification system* based on size of the functional RV and adequacy of the anterior leaflet for repair[A9,C3]:

- Type A: volume of true RV is adequate.
- Type B: a large atrialized component of RV is present, and anterior leaflet of tricuspid valve moves freely.

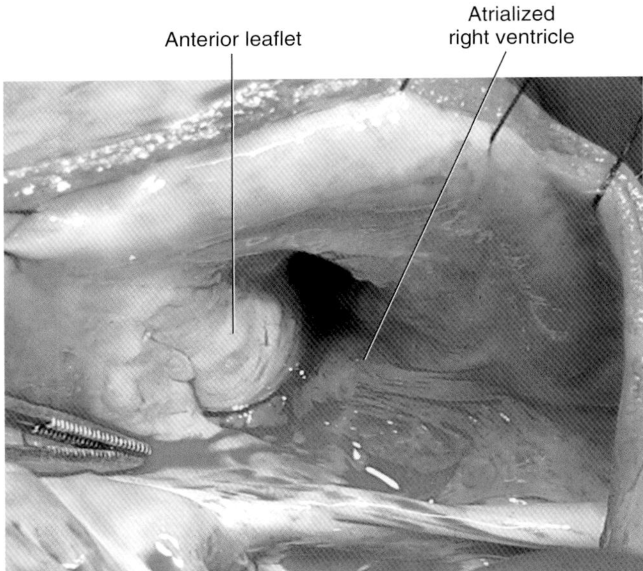

Figure 42-5 Morphology of Ebstein anomaly. This image at operation shows typical Ebstein anomaly. Septal and posterior leaflets are displaced below tricuspid anulus and are fused to endocardium of right ventricle, producing an atrialized portion. Anterior leaflet of tricuspid valve is enlarged and sail-like.

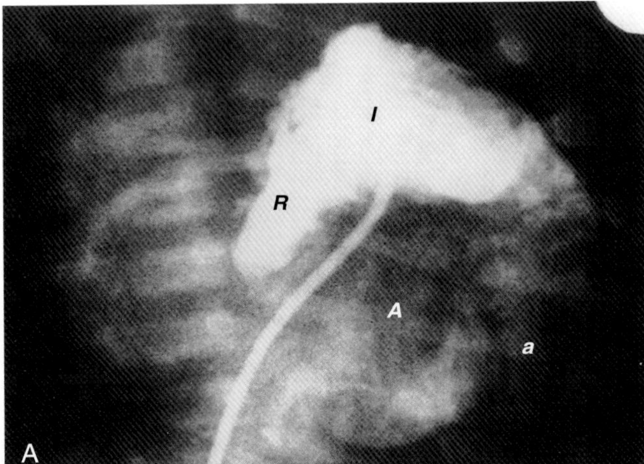

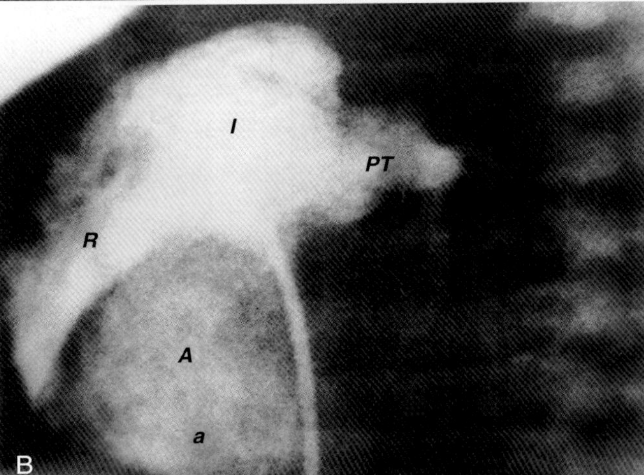

Figure 42-6 Right anterior oblique **(A)** and left anterior oblique **(B)** cineangiogram frames of Ebstein anomaly. Injection was into outflow portion of the functional (ventricularized) right ventricle, which also extends around the anterior and rightward free-wall aspects of the atrialized portion to form the anterolateral recess. Apical portion of functional ventricle fills poorly and is superimposed on atrialized portion in left anterior oblique view. Key: *a,* Apical portion of functional right ventricle; *A,* atrialized portion of right ventricle; *I,* outflow portion of the functional right ventricle; *PT,* pulmonary trunk; *R,* anterolateral recess.

- Type C: movement of anterior leaflet is severely restricted and may cause obstruction of RV outflow tract.
- Type D: RV is nearly completely atrialized, except for a small infundibular component.

Right Atrium

The right atrium is enormously dilated in advanced cases. There is usually an interatrial communication (60% of autopsy specimens, 42% at catheterization, and 21 of 22 surgical cases in Watson's collective review), most commonly a patent foramen ovale, although an atrial septal defect (ASD) of any type may be present.[W1] Interatrial communication was present in 94% of patients at operation in the series reported by Danielson and colleagues.[D4] Rarely, an ostium primum AV septal defect coexists.

The bundle of His and AV node lie in their usual locations, although the right bundle and node may be compressed by thickened endocardium (a possible explanation of the frequent right bundle branch block pattern in the electrocardiogram).[B7,H3,L2,L3] WPW syndrome is present in about 14% of persons with Ebstein anomaly.[D4,T5]

Left Ventricle

Monibi and colleagues and Ng and colleagues report that abnormal left ventricular contraction and contour and mitral valve prolapse are frequently present.[M13,N5] Marked dilatation of the RV produces leftward septal shift and compression and posterior displacement of the left ventricle. Daliento and colleagues studied nine autopsied hearts and found the ventricular septum normal in six and thin in three, which could account for the exaggerated leftward diastolic movement observed by angiography in 24 of 26 patients.[D1] Severe leftward displacement produced a "banana" appearance of the left ventricle. Regional left ventricular wall motion abnormality was observed in 67% of patients. In a Mayo Clinic experience of over 500 surgical patients with Ebstein anomaly, 9% had moderate or severe LV dysfunction.[B14] When mitral valve prolapse is present, the valve is frequently nodular and thickened.[C1,D1,L2,R8] A Mayo Clinic study of 106 patients identified left ventricular abnormalities in 39%, of whom 18% had left ventricular dysplasia resembling noncompaction.[A10]

Lungs

In severe Ebstein anomaly associated with fetal and neonatal distress or death, both lungs are usually hypoplastic but otherwise normal. The hypoplasia is secondary to gross cardiomegaly from severe tricuspid regurgitation.[L1]

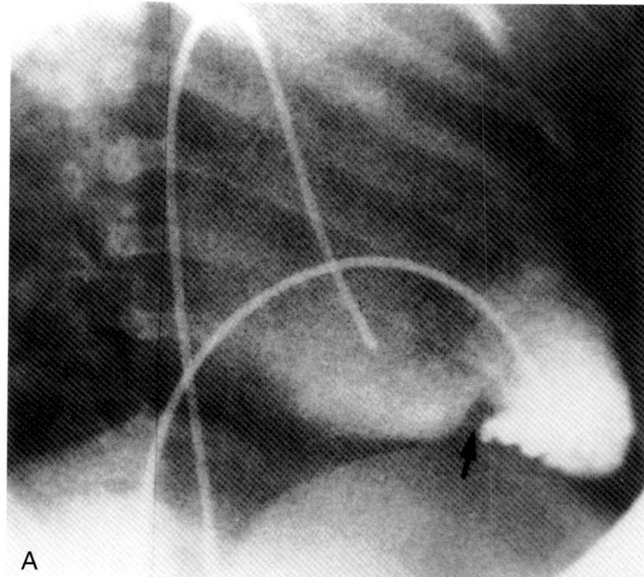

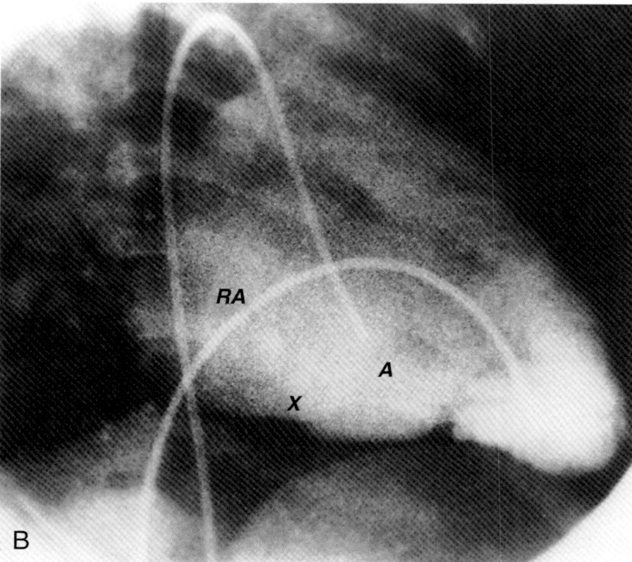

Figure 42-7 Right anterior oblique cineangiographic frames of Ebstein anomaly. Injection was into right ventricular apex. **A,** Early frame showing reflux through displaced leaflets into atrialized ventricle. Deep notch *(arrow)* represents attachment of a dysplastic posterior leaflet to inferior wall. **B,** Later frame showing more extensive filling of atrialized ventricle and right atrium *(RA)*. X marks position of true atrioventricular ring. Key: *A,* Atrialized right ventricle.

Associated Anomalies

An ASD is present in 80% to 95% of patients with Ebstein anomaly.[B13,D4] *Pulmonary atresia* or *stenosis* may be present in up to one third of autopsied hearts (see Chapters 39 and 40).[B4] Others include ventricular septal defect, tetralogy of Fallot, patent ductus arteriosus, transposition of the great arteries, coarctation of the aorta, and congenital mitral stenosis.[B4,K11,L3,W1]

In *congenitally corrected transposition* with atrial situs solitus, the tricuspid valve lies within a left-sided, systemic, morphologically right ventricle. Although 30% of these left-sided valves are regurgitant, this is frequently due to Ebstein anomaly.[A3,A6] This Ebstein anomaly differs from the usual right-sided form in that dilatation of the AV ring and separation of the morphologic RV into atrialized and ventricularized portions are uncommon. The anterior leaflet is also less prominent and may be cleft (see Chapter 55).

CLINICAL FEATURES AND DIAGNOSTIC CRITERIA

Mechanisms Underlying Clinical Presentation and Natural History

Three primary pathophysiologic features predominate in patients with Ebstein anomaly:

- RV abnormalities
- Tricuspid valve abnormalities
- Accessory conduction pathways (WPW syndrome)

Their severity determines secondary pathophysiologic features, clinical presentation, and natural history.

Right Ventricular Abnormalities

Severity of RV abnormality is partly related to the extent to which the number of muscle fibers in the ventricular wall is reduced.[A5] Nearly all patients have at least mild RV cavity enlargement and wall thinning. In the most severe cases, the RV cavity is greatly enlarged and free wall extremely thin.[R7] The ventricular septum is often abnormal as well, with leftward bulging and consequent reduction in cavity size of the left ventricle, impairing left ventricular function.[B6,D1] In the most advanced examples, the RV free wall is paper thin, a condition referred to as *Uhl disease.*

Extensiveness of the atrialized portion of the RV, which exhibits systolic expansion rather than contraction, importantly affects RV performance. RV dysfunction, along with tricuspid valve regurgitation, is responsible for right atrial enlargement and its wall thickening, which are at times extreme.

In aggregate, these abnormalities of RV structure and function underlie the variable cardiomegaly exhibited by patients with Ebstein anomaly: hepatomegaly, ascites, and fluid retention that may be advanced; cyanosis that is occasionally extreme, resulting from right-to-left shunting across a patent foramen ovale or ASD; and paroxysms of supraventricular and occasionally ventricular tachyarrhythmias that can cause advanced disability and sometimes sudden death.

Tricuspid Valve Abnormalities

Tricuspid regurgitation, usually present to some degree, exacerbates the abnormalities of RV structure and function. Degree of regurgitation is determined by the valve's morphologic anomalies. Those valves in which the anterior leaflet is tightly tethered and adherent to the underlying RV free wall and septum and, to a lesser extent, those in which the posterior leaflet is displaced and immobilized, are more likely to be regurgitant.[R7]

Pulmonary hypoplasia, a feature that contributes to neonatal death, is correlated with the degree of tricuspid regurgitation, occurring in association with severe regurgitation and gross cardiomegaly. If these features are corrected, the lungs presumably grow normally.[L1]

Wolff-Parkinson-White Syndrome

Arrhythmic features of WPW syndrome, present in about 14% of patients, may dominate the clinical picture in patients whose tricuspid valve and RV anomalies are mild (see Section III in Chapter 16).

Associated Anomalies

In general, coexisting cardiac anomalies have little impact on the clinical features and course of patients with Ebstein anomaly. Exceptions are congenital pulmonary stenosis or atresia; when these coexist with Ebstein anomaly, death in utero or soon after birth is common. A patent foramen ovale or ASD, present in many patients, is necessary for right-to-left shunting and for the occasional paradoxical embolus or cerebral abscess that develops, but otherwise usually plays little role in the etiology of signs and symptoms. However, in the uncommon circumstance of only mild RV and tricuspid abnormalities, important left-to-right shunting may occur across an ASD.

Symptoms and Signs

Breathlessness in association with cyanosis, severe cardiomegaly, and often heart failure may appear during the first week of life. However, many patients have milder symptoms and do not present until later in life. Nonetheless, objective exercise testing shows that their functional capacity is less than normal.[B2] Oxygen saturation at rest is a major predictor of exercise tolerance.[M1] Mild dyspnea and fatigue may become evident in childhood or early adult life, or more severe symptoms and signs of various types may develop. If heart failure develops, the patient becomes severely limited by breathlessness and fatigue.

Cyanosis is a common sign of Ebstein anomaly, occurring in more than half of patients and severe in about one third.[K11] It may appear at birth, but in most patients onset is in infancy or early childhood.

Palpitations caused by various types of arrhythmia are also common.[B9] Severe arrhythmic symptoms are frequent in patients of all ages and may be disabling. WPW syndrome is the best known type of arrhythmia, but less specific types of supraventricular tachycardias are more common. Numerous electrophysiologic abnormalities have been identified, which no doubt account for the frequent occurrence and persistence of arrhythmic symptoms even after operation.[H3,K2] Symptoms are more severe when there are important associated cardiac anomalies.

A malar flush, similar to the so-called mitral facies, was noted by Ebstein's colleague and occurs in about one third of patients.[S3] It is unrelated to cyanosis or polycythemia or to cardiac output.[K11]

The left anterior chest is often prominent in association with marked cardiomegaly, and there may be a systolic thrill along the left sternal edge originating from the tricuspid valve. Characteristically, the precordium and apex remain quiet despite marked cardiomegaly. Jugular venous pressure is generally unremarkable and rarely suggests tricuspid regurgitation or stenosis, even though free tricuspid regurgitation is revealed by imaging studies.[W4] This is related to the large size and compliance of both the right atrium and atrialized RV, as well as the low RV and pulmonary artery pressure. Congestive hepatosplenomegaly is commonly observed and may lead to hepatic fibrosis.[D10]

On auscultation the most constant finding is wide splitting of the first sound with accentuation of the delayed component caused by closing (or termination of motion[C8,F1]) of the large anterior tricuspid leaflet. Delayed tricuspid valve closure is probably mechanical rather than related to right bundle branch block, although Crews and colleagues considered it correlated with the latter.[C8,G5] The large anterior leaflet is also responsible for an opening snap in diastole, and there may be an atrial fourth sound. The pulmonary component of the second sound is delayed and soft (in relation to the right bundle branch block) or absent when pulmonary artery pressure is low. A pansystolic murmur maximal at the lower left sternal edge is due to tricuspid regurgitation and is heard in about one third of patients. Finally, there is usually a diastolic murmur, often low pitched and sometimes scratchy in quality, commencing with the opening snap and sometimes augmented by the fourth sound. The diastolic murmur is presumably due to movement of blood across the malformed tricuspid orifice.

Chest Radiography

In classic Ebstein anomaly, the chest radiograph shows marked cardiomegaly with a rounded or boxlike cardiac contour beneath a narrow pedicle (Fig. 42-8). In the posteroanterior view the whole of the silhouette is then formed by the right atrium and RV, and because of their minimal excursion and the normal or oligemic lung fields, the silhouette has a peculiarly sharp edge. However, as with other features of the disease, there is wide variation in heart size.[S3] In a few cases, it remains normal; in most, it is only moderately enlarged.[K11]

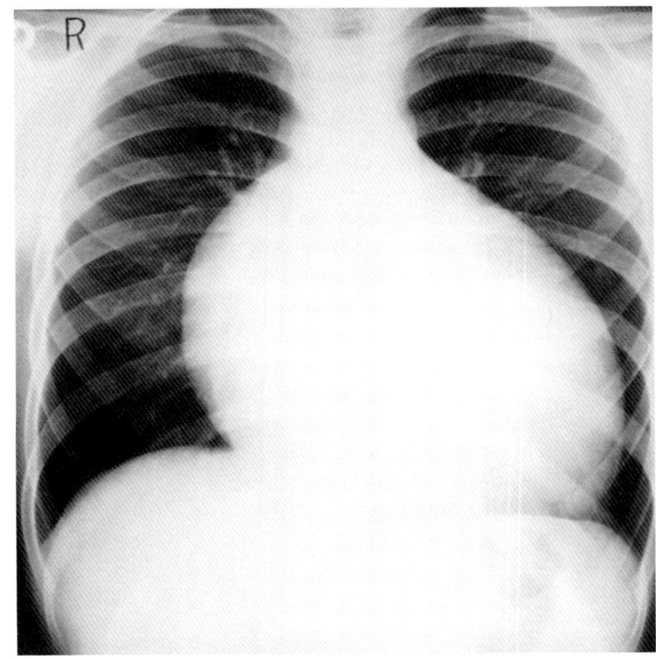

Figure 42-8 Chest radiograph of a 12-year-old girl with classic Ebstein anomaly.

Electrocardiography

A right bundle branch pattern together with a relatively low-amplitude R wave in right-sided chest leads and right atrial hypertrophy are characteristic of the anomaly. According to Kumar and colleagues, height of the P wave varies inversely with arterial oxygen saturation ($r = .82$, $P < .001$).[K11] In addition, the taller the P wave, the shorter the survival time ($P < .001$). RV hypertrophy does not occur in uncomplicated Ebstein anomaly, and inverted T waves in leads V_1 to V_4 are fairly common. Using intraluminal electrode catheters, Kastor and colleagues demonstrated prolonged intra–right atrial and infranodal conduction in patients with a large right atrium and well-defined atrialized ventricle.[K2]

In approximately 14% of patients, the electrocardiogram shows type B (right-sided) WPW syndrome. In any cyanotic patient with this type of preexcitation, Ebstein anomaly should be considered. Supraventricular arrhythmias occur in more than half of patients, and they may be paroxysmal and recurrent. Paroxysmal atrial tachycardia, atrial fibrillation, and nodal rhythm can all occur, as can first-degree heart block. Serious ventricular arrhythmias resulting from RV dilatation may also occur.[D10]

Echocardiography

Two-dimensional echocardiography has become definitive for diagnosis and anatomic evaluation of Ebstein anomaly[B6,M2,M6,N6,S13] (Fig. 42-9). It is possible to identify Ebstein anomaly by the characteristic degree of displacement of the septal leaflet of the tricuspid valve (>8 mm · m^{-2}) and the presence of an elongated, redundant anterior tricuspid valve leaflet.[A2,S10] The feasibility of tricuspid repair rather than replacement can be determined with this method of imaging.[S13] A right-to-left atrial shunt and tricuspid regurgitation can be demonstrated using Doppler color flow interrogation.

Historically, M-mode echocardiography usually demonstrated delayed tricuspid valve closure and displacement of the tricuspid valve to the left. According to Giuliani and colleagues, the greater the delay in tricuspid valve closure, the more severe the disease.[G5] Wide excursion of the anterior leaflet, a decreased E-F slope, increased RV dimensions, and paradoxical septal motion can also be demonstrated.

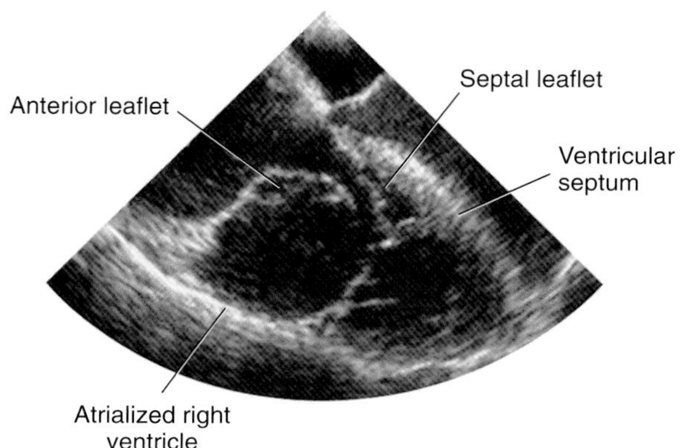

Figure 42-9 Two-dimensional echocardiogram of Ebstein anomaly. There is characteristic displacement of hinge point of septal leaflet below natural tricuspid anulus and adherence to septal wall. Anterior leaflet is elongated.

Cardiac Catheterization and Cineangiography

Currently, cardiac catheterization and cineangiography are required only when specific hemodynamic details need to be identified,[S13] or in patients about aged 40, when the coronary tree should be examined.

In the past, cardiac catheterization showed that the mean right atrial pressure is often modestly elevated, and the pressure pulse may have either a dominant *a* or *v* wave. These correlate poorly with degree of tricuspid regurgitation or stenosis. An additional *s* wave preceding the *v* wave and interrupting the *c* wave is said to indicate tricuspid regurgitation.[G5,K11,S3] The right atrial waveform is also recorded in the atrialized portion of the RV so that the tricuspid valve is noted to be displaced well toward the left of the spine. An *electrode catheter* may define the position and size of the atrialized RV chamber.[M9,Y3] RV systolic pressure is normal or low, and RV end-diastolic pressure is frequently elevated, more so when there is the syndrome of chronic heart failure. It is uncommon to record an important gradient across the tricuspid valve, although Takayasu and colleagues noted this in 8 of 26 cases and considered that stenosis could still be important in its absence.[K11,T1]

When there is an interatrial communication, the shunt through it is usually right to left in association with systemic arterial desaturation and a reduced pulmonary blood flow ($\dot{Q}p$). The right-to-left shunt can be quantified by indicator dilution. The shunt may occasionally be left to right, and the resultant increase in $\dot{Q}p$ may be associated with heart failure.[M8] Direction of shunting is no doubt influenced by RV compliance.

In the newborn with Ebstein anomaly, a functional pulmonary outflow obstruction can occur.[N4] Thus, a normal pulmonary valve may fail to open following a right-sided injection of contrast media because of the combination of massive tricuspid regurgitation, poor RV contraction, and a high neonatal pulmonary vascular resistance with or without a large shunt at ductal level. High-quality imaging is therefore necessary to distinguish this situation from true pulmonary atresia.

Cineangiography (see Figs. 42-3 to 42-7) is usually diagnostic as long as there is important displacement and dysplasia of the septal or posterior leaflets.[D13] In the right anterior oblique projection, the conjoined posterior and anterior leaflets, and therefore the distal limit of the atrialized ventricle, can frequently be identified. Contrast media trapped beneath the posterior leaflet can indicate the degree of its adherence to, and level of its origin from, the diaphragmatic border of the RV, which may be notched at this point.[S17] The site of the true anulus is also visible more proximally. An injection into the functional RV enables tricuspid regurgitation to be assessed together with size and behavior of the functional ventricle. Angiography in left anterior oblique projection also permits visualization of the right-to-left shunt at atrial level, and any ventricular septal defects can be localized by left ventriculography.

NATURAL HISTORY

Ebstein anomaly is uncommon, with a prevalence of 0.5% and occurring in less than 1% of subjects with congenital heart disease.[K3] The incidence is equal in both sexes. Familial Ebstein anomaly has been reported rarely.[E2,G8,S16] It occurs

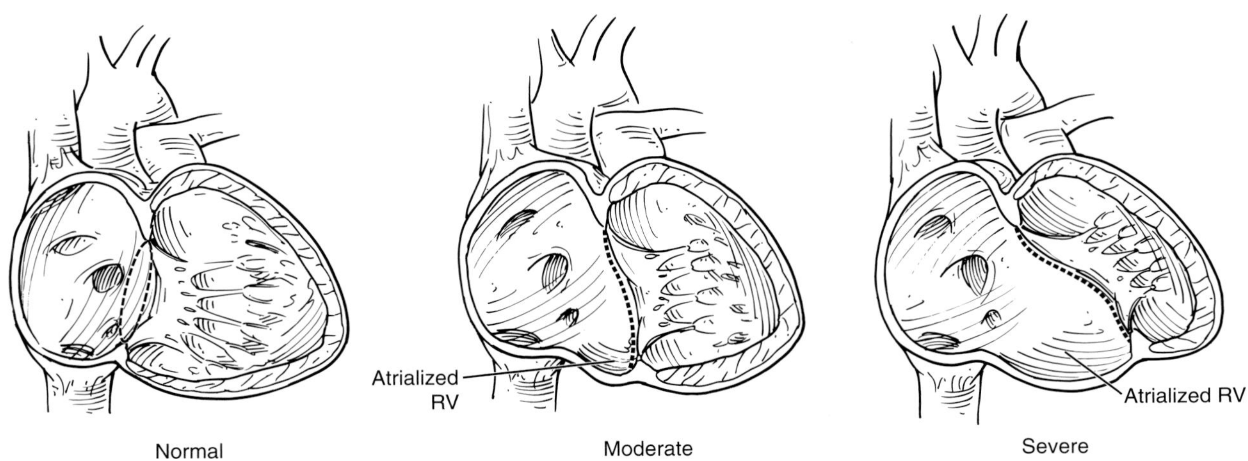

Figure 42-10 Changes in tricuspid anular dimension with progression of rotational tricuspid valve displacement from normal *(left panel)* to moderate *(middle panel)* to severe *(right panel)*. Dotted line indicates functional tricuspid placement with increasing severity of Ebstein anomaly. (From Malhotra and colleagues.[M3])

with more frequency in babies of mothers who are on lithium medication during pregnancy.[L5,R1]

The natural history is determined primarily by the three primary pathophysiologic features described in Clinical Features and Diagnostic Criteria earlier in this chapter. Extent and severity of these relate to age at presentation; thus, age at presentation tends to correlate with prognosis. The presentation takes two general forms: symptomatic neonatal and infant presentation, and presentation in older children and adults.

Table 42-2 Celermajer Scale for Neonatal Ebstein Anomaly

Grade	Ratio (RA+ARV): (RV+LA+LV)	Risk of Death (%)
1	<0.5	0
2	0.5 to 0.99	10
3	1 to 1.49	44 to 100
4	≥1.50	100

Data from Celermajer and colleagues.[C6]
Key: *ARV*, Atrialized right ventricle; *LA*, left atrium; *LV*, left ventricle; *RA*, right atrium; *RV*, right ventricle.

Presentation during First Week of Life

Ebstein anomaly is a recognized cause of death in utero.[G4,H4,L1] When severe tricuspid regurgitation accompanies Ebstein anomaly at birth, the elevated newborn pulmonary vascular resistance worsens it. $\dot{Q}p$ may be ductal dependent. The resultant severe hypoxemia (right-to-left shunting through an ASD), coupled with marked right-sided heart failure, may also be accompanied by low cardiac output if the ASD is restrictive. This is because maintenance of normal cardiac output requires shunting at the atrial level through a nonrestrictive ASD. Low cardiac output may also result from abnormal ventricular interactions caused by paradoxical septal bowing and flattening of the left ventricle. The hypoxemia may be aggravated by pulmonary dysfunction secondary to lung compression by marked cardiomegaly. Although lung hypoplasia has been suggested,[C6,L1] pathologic studies indicate that the lungs are rarely hypoplastic in surviving newborns, but are instead compressed by the enlarged heart.[T2]

Celermajer and colleagues from Great Ormond Street identified neonates with good and poor outcomes based on a score (Celermajer Score or Great Ormond Street Ratio)[A9,C5] derived from echocardiographic measurements of the right atrium, RV, left atrium, and left ventricle.[C6] The score is calculated from a four-chamber echocardiographic view in which the combined area of the anatomic right atrium plus atrialized RV is divided by the sum of the areas of the functional (nonatrialized) RV, left atrium, and left ventricle (Table 42-2). The outlook is generally dismal for patients with Celermajer grades 3 or 4[C6,Y2] (severe Ebstein anomaly; Fig. 42-10). Importantly, patients with Ebstein anomaly who survive after presentation early in life have a good chance of long-term survival.[G3]

Many studies have probably underestimated the incidence and severity of this entity in neonates. The review by Vacca and colleagues of 108 clinical or autopsy cases reported between 1866 and 1957 recorded only two patients younger than 1 month.[V1] In Watson's collective review of 505 cases, only 35 (7%) were younger than 1 year (half were younger than 1 month).[W1] In Bialostozky and colleagues' review of 65 patients, neonates were not included.[B9] In a Mayo Clinic series, only 10 of 67 patients were diagnosed in infancy.[G5] In a Boston Children's Hospital series, 12 of their 55 patients (22%) were seen during the first week of life, and 34 (64%) were younger than 2 years.[K11] Eleven of the 34 died early. These series must have been in some way selective and therefore are not useful in assessing natural history. In contrast, Schiebler and colleagues' earlier study from the Mayo Clinic found that 12 of 23 patients presented during the neonatal period, and of these, 5 died.[S3] Roberson and Silverman reported that among 16 consecutive patients diagnosed in utero or presenting during the first 3 days of life, 7 died before age 3 months; all had severe RV and tricuspid morphologic abnormalities.[R7] In the 40-institution administrative registry of the Pediatric Health Information System (PHIS), of 464 neonates diagnosed with Ebstein anomaly from January 2003 to January 2008, 415 with complete data, mortality during initial hospitalization among 257 (62%) managed medically was 22% (56/257; CL 19%-25%).[G7]

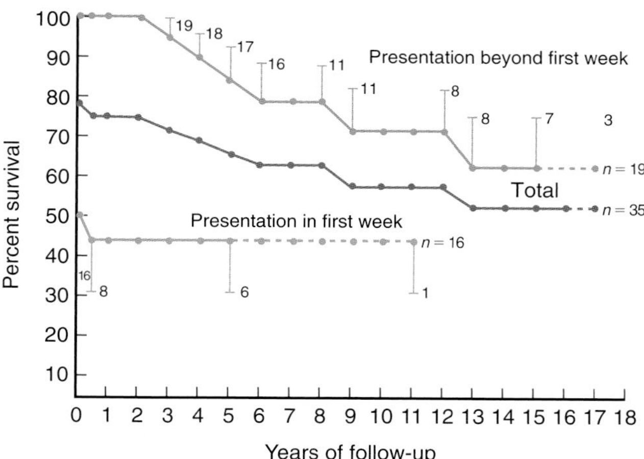

Figure 42-11 Survival of patients with Ebstein anomaly, total and stratified according to age at presentation. Numbers of patients at risk are noted. *P* value for difference between the two stratified curves is .01. (From GLH group.)

Presentation in Infancy

Presentation in infancy is associated with less risk of death and milder symptoms than occur with neonatal presentation (Fig. 42-11), although some studies suggest an increased mortality until presentation is beyond about 6 months.[G5,K11,W1] Beyond this age, Watson's series indicates a prognosis similar to that of older children.[W1] He states that "whereas 72% of those under 1 year were in heart failure, 71% of the children and adolescents had little or no disability."

Presentation in Childhood and Adult Life

Patients presenting after infancy often have mild symptoms. Prognosis is generally good, consistent with less severe RV and tricuspid valve pathophysiology.[S11] Patients presenting in adult life are often acyanotic and have a normal-sized heart.[G4] However, even these patients, who report few symptoms, have clearly definable abnormalities. Without preexcitation, nearly half have episodic supraventricular tachyarrhythmias, although these usually produce few symptoms.[S18] Exercise tolerance measured by objective testing is often reduced.[B2,D15,M1,S2] The degree of tricuspid regurgitation does not correlate with symptoms, but as time passes, left ventricular dysfunction often appears as symptoms develop.[S2]

Death in this group of patients is often due to paroxysmal embolization or paradoxical supraventricular tachycardia, with heart failure appearing either much later or not at all. An atrial level communication increases the risk of paradoxical embolism, brain abscess, and sudden death.

Modes of Death

Heart failure is the mode of death in somewhat less than half of patients who die of causes related to their heart disease after the neonatal period.[K11,W1] Sudden death, presumably caused for the most part by arrhythmias other than those associated with WPW, occurs in about 60% (CL 43%-77%) of these patients.[G3,G4,W1] Sudden death correlates with marked cardiomegaly, rather than with New York Heart Association (NYHA) status.[G3] Cerebral abscess and paradoxical emboli account for most of the remaining deaths, particularly in patients older than about 50 years.[G4,M7] Infective endocarditis is rare.

TECHNIQUE OF OPERATION

Repair of Tricuspid Valve and Atrial Septal Defect Closure

The usual preparations are made for operation, anesthetic management (see Chapter 4), and cardiopulmonary bypass (CPB) (see Chapter 2). Before commencing CPB, the atrialized portion of the RV is assessed, noting particularly whether it moves paradoxically.

CPB is established using two venous cannulae, and the patient's body temperature is lowered to about 25°C. The aorta is occluded and tourniquets secured around the venae cavae and cannulae. Cold cardioplegia may be administered directly into the aortic root or into the coronary sinus after the atrium is opened (see "Technique of Retrograde Infusion" in Chapter 3). The right atrium is incised parallel to the AV groove. A sump-sucker is placed across the atrial septum into the left atrium.

The atrial septum and tricuspid valve are examined (Fig. 42-12). The anterior leaflet of the tricuspid valve is studied with particular care, because successful repair of a regurgitant tricuspid valve relies on it. The anterior leaflet is rarely displaced into the RV, but if it is, the tricuspid valve may require replacement (see "Replacement of Tricuspid Valve" in text that follows). However, if the displacement is limited to that portion near the commissure, repair may be possible. Extreme thickening of the anterior leaflet, and particularly the dense attachment of its free edge to the underlying RV endocardium, makes successful repair unlikely and therefore contraindicates it.[D4]

Tricuspid valve repair with ASD closure is the preferred operation.[K5] Most repairs are designed to convert the tricuspid valve into a monoleaflet valve using the anterior leaflet to establish valve competence. The most important features that predict successful repair are a mobile, free leading edge of the anterior leaflet and attachment of more than 50% of it at the anatomic tricuspid anulus. A variety of maneuvers have been used to mobilize and extend this leading edge, with or without plication of the atrialized portion of the RV.

The method devised by Danielson and colleagues is the best tested.[D2,D5,D6,M2,T3] It plicates the atrialized portion of the ventricle, narrows the tricuspid orifice in a selective manner, and results in a monoleaflet valve that is usually competent or nearly so. A modification of the Danielson method in which the tricuspid valve anulus is remodeled by an anuloplasty ring is shown in Fig. 42-13.[D14] Dearani and colleagues have also recommended moving the anterior leaflet closer to the ventricular septum by displacing the major papillary muscles supporting the anterior leaflet to a position closer to the septum. This is accomplished by placing pledgeted mattress sutures from the papillary muscle to the ventricular septum[A9,D12] (Fig. 42-14).

An alternative is the Carpentier repair, in which the anterior leaflet is mobilized and detached from the anulus. The atrialized ventricle is plicated vertically, at right angles to the direction used by Danielson[C3] (Fig. 42-15). The anterior leaflet is advanced and reattached to the true anulus. This

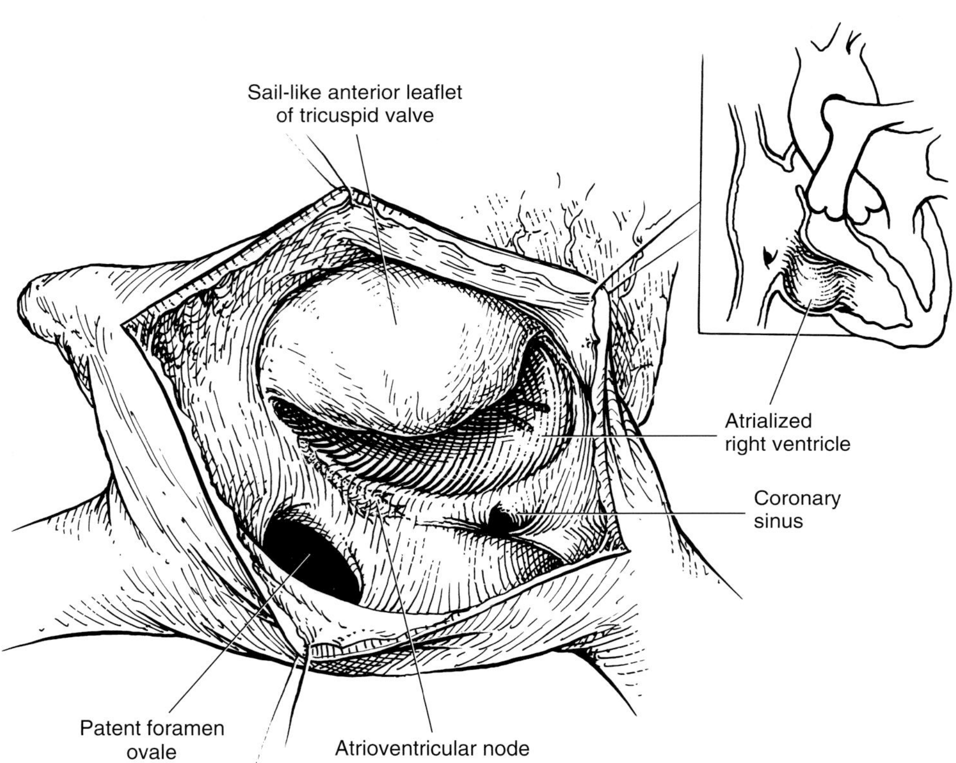

Figure 42-12 Morphology of interior of right atrium in Ebstein anomaly at operation. Septal and posterior leaflets of tricuspid valve are adhered to septum and right ventricular (RV) wall. Downward displacement of tricuspid valve divides RV into a proximal atrialized portion and a distal ventricularized portion. Anterior leaflet is enlarged and elongated, described as sail-like. There is a foramen ovale type of atrial septal defect. Coronary sinus, atrioventricular node, and bundle of His are in their usual locations.

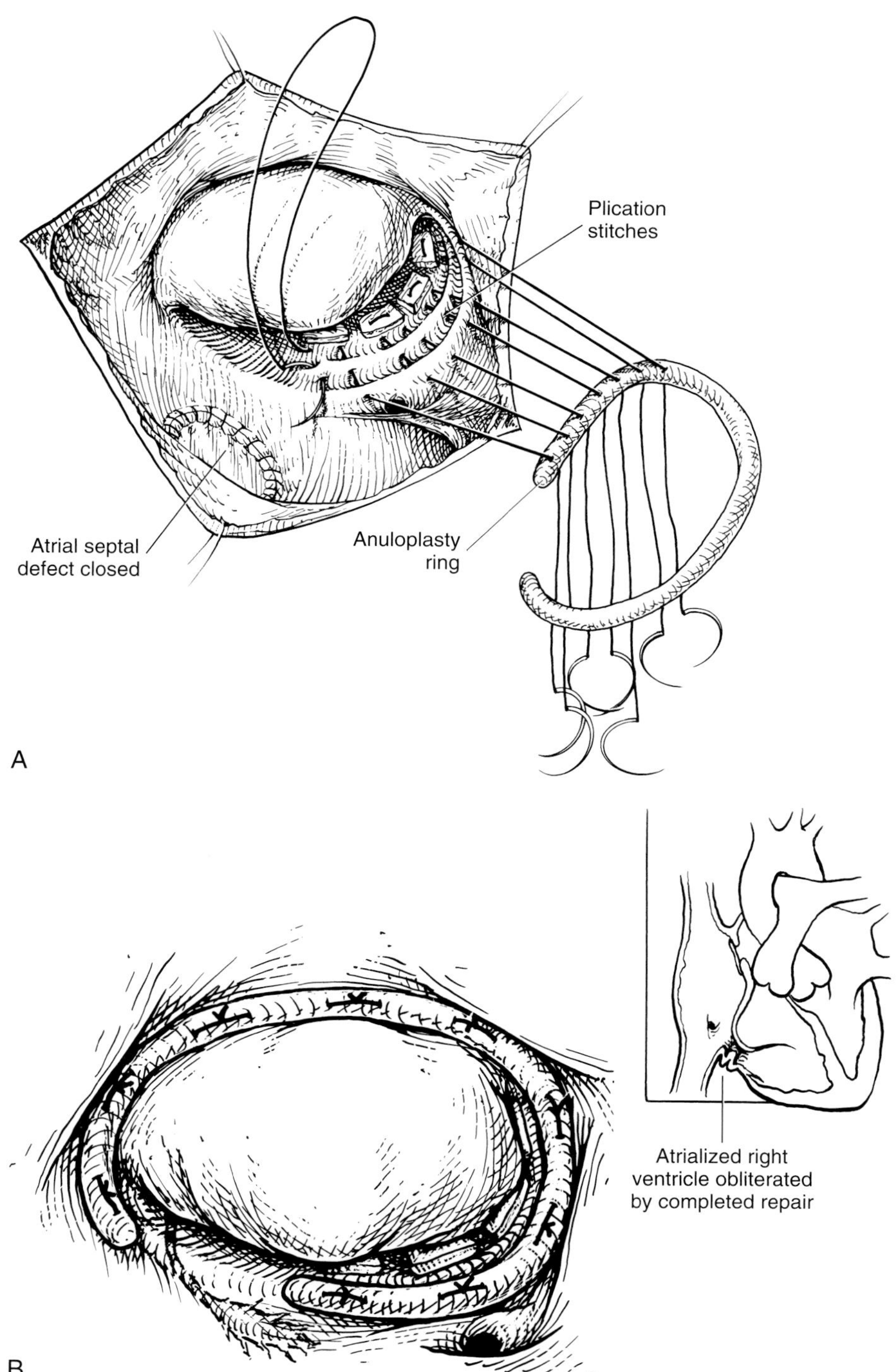

Figure 42-13 Repair of regurgitant tricuspid valve in Ebstein anomaly using a modification of the Danielson method.[D5,D6,D14] **A,** A series of pledget-reinforced mattress sutures are placed at base of the septal and posterior leaflets of tricuspid valve. Stitches are continued to plicate atrialized portion of right ventricle (RV) up to the natural location of the valve anulus. Stitches are passed through a Carpentier anuloplasty ring. Atrial septal defect is closed by pericardial patch. **B,** Plication sutures are tied over anuloplasty ring to remodel the anulus and obliterate atrialized portion of the RV to complete the repair. Large anterior leaflet occludes the atrioventricular orifice.

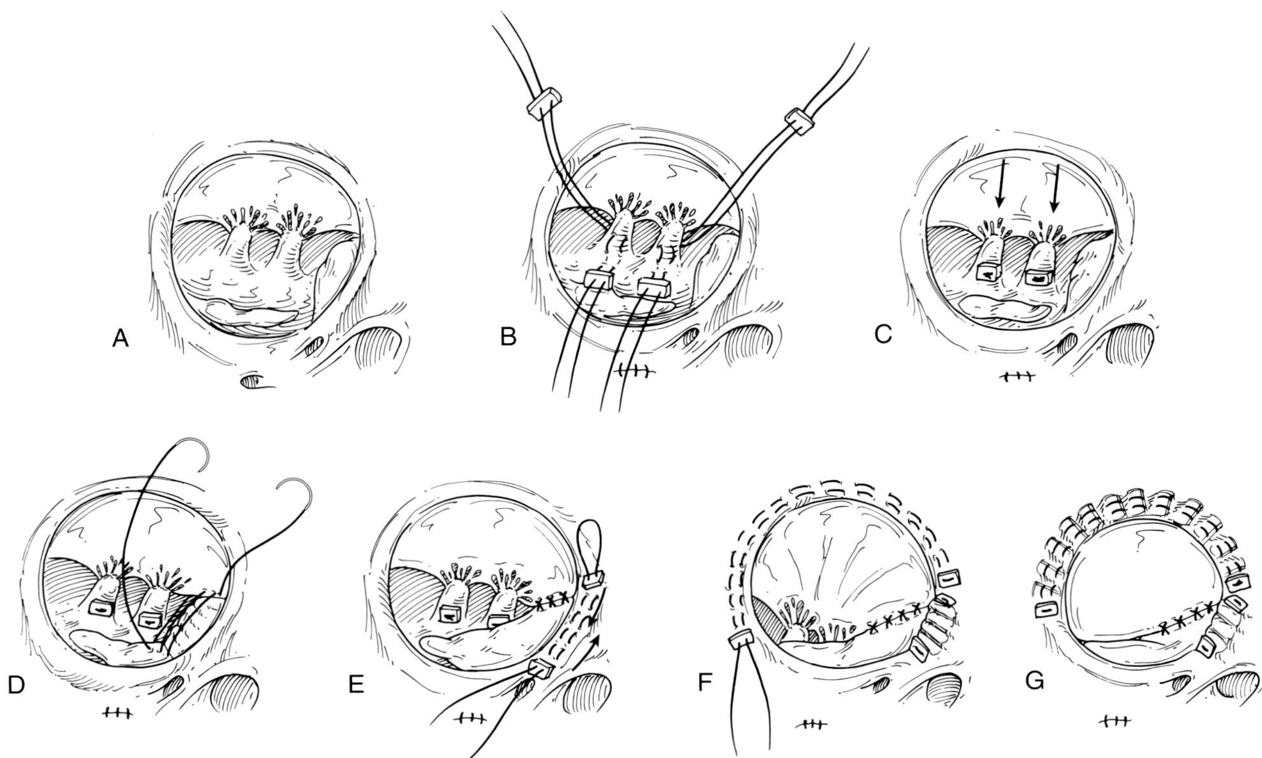

Figure 42-14 Diagram of modified Mayo Clinic method of tricuspid valve repair technique used for Ebstein anomaly. **A,** Two papillary muscles arise from free wall of right ventricle, with short chordal attachments to leading edge of anterior leaflet. Septal leaflet is diminutive and only a ridge of tissue. Posterior leaflet is not well formed and is adherent to underlying endocardium. A small patent foramen ovale is present. **B-C,** Base of each papillary muscle is moved toward ventricular septum at the appropriate level with horizontal mattress sutures backed with felt pledgets. Patent foramen ovale is closed by direct suture. **D,** Posterior angle of tricuspid orifice is closed by bringing right side of anterior leaflet down to the septum and plicating the nonfunctional posterior leaflet in the process. **E,** A posterior anuloplasty is performed to narrow diameter of tricuspid anulus; the coronary sinus marks posterior and leftward extent of anuloplasty. **F,** An anterior purse-string anuloplasty is performed to further narrow tricuspid anulus. This anuloplasty stitch is tied down over a 25-mm valve sizer in an adult to prevent tricuspid stenosis. **G,** Completed repair that allows anterior leaflet to function as a monoleaflet valve. (From Dearani and colleagues. Used with permission of Mayo Foundation for Medical Education and Research.)

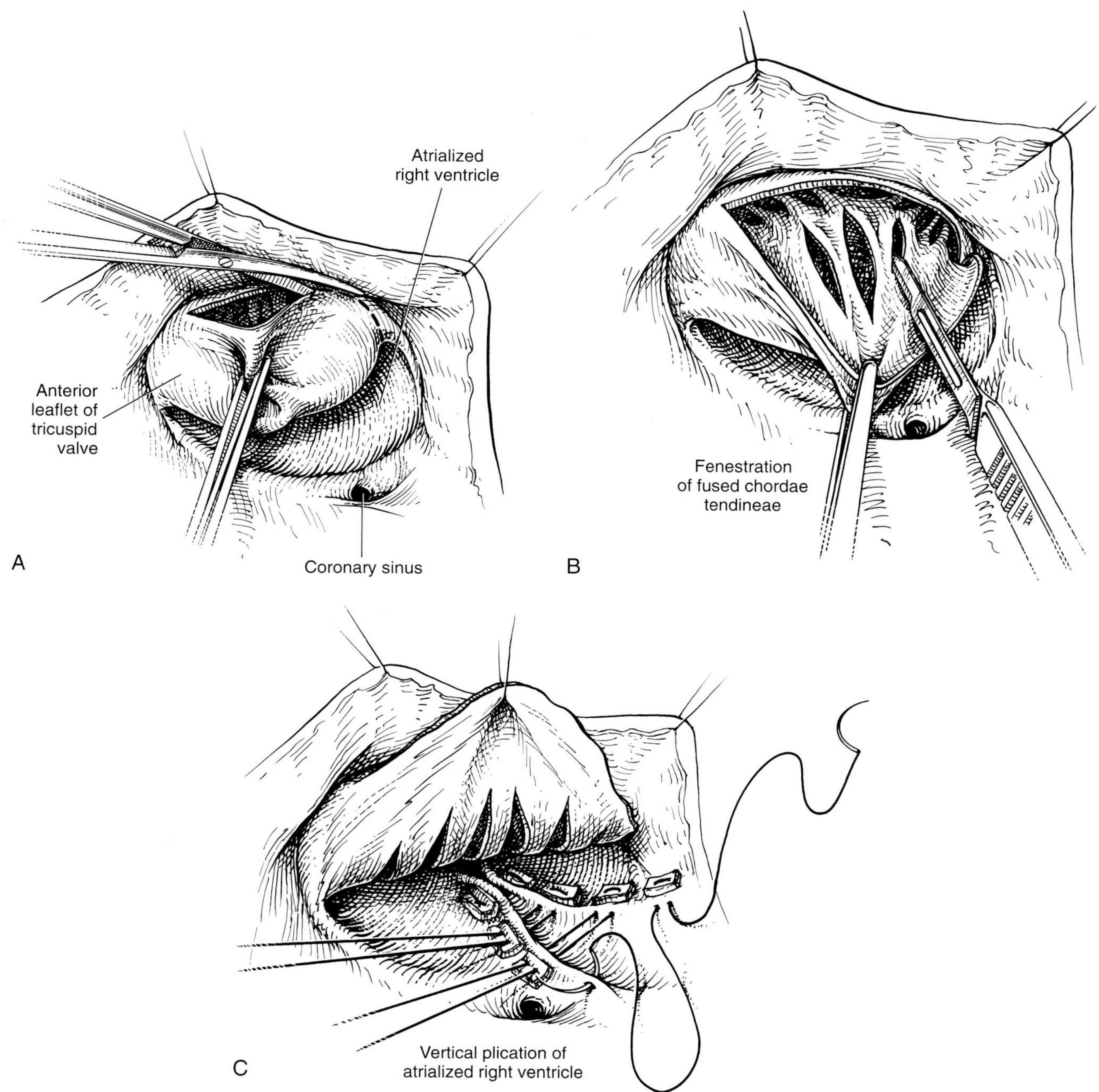

Figure 42-15 Repair of regurgitant tricuspid valve in Ebstein anomaly using the Carpentier method.[C3] **A,** Three fourths of the enlarged anterior leaflet and as much as possible of the posterior leaflet are detached from the anulus. Incision is continued to the point at which valve begins to be displaced on ventricular wall at atrialized portion of right ventricle (RV). **B,** Detached leaflet is everted to expose support mechanism. There is usually chordal fusion, which may be marked in some cases. Fenestrations are made in the support mechanism to lengthen chordae and relieve obstruction below leaflets. **C,** Unique aspect of repair is placing pledget-reinforced plication stitches in atrialized portion of RV to create a vertical plication. Plication stitches are continued from base of leaflet attachment to ventricle to true anulus. Anulus is narrowed by this technique. A few stitches are placed in floor of right atrium. Plication stitches may be woven across atrialized portion for better obliteration of this portion of ventricle.

Continued

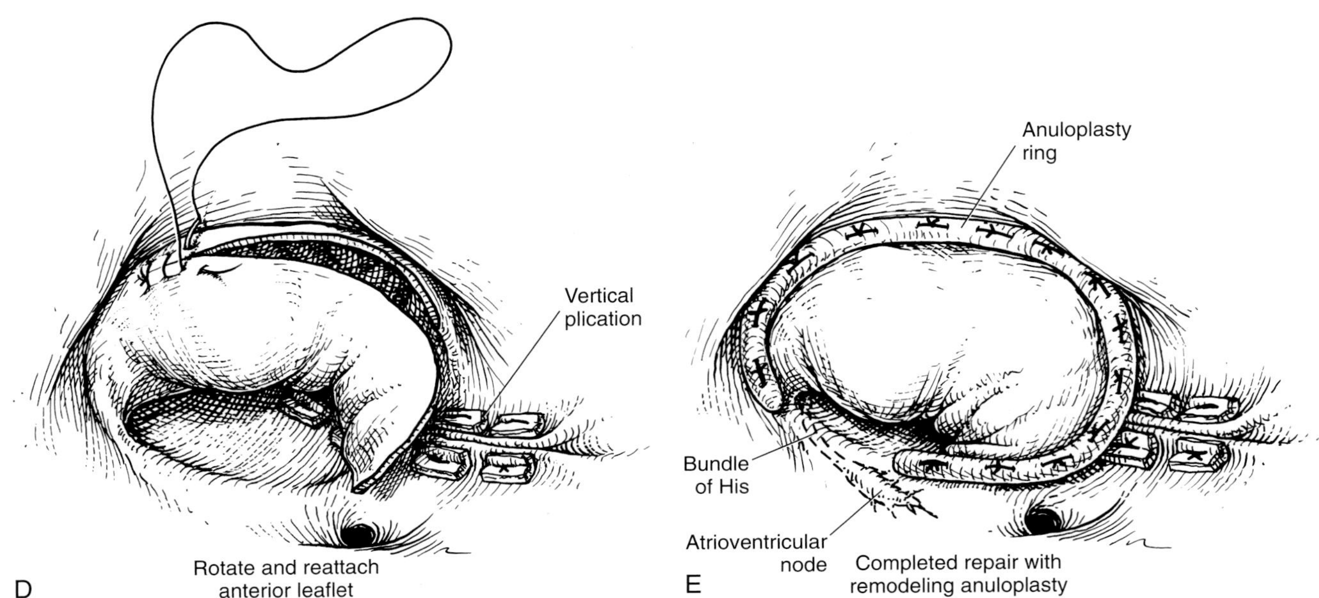

Figure 42-15, cont'd **D,** Detached portion of tricuspid leaflet is rotated clockwise to cover tricuspid orifice beyond plication and as far toward septum as it will reach comfortably. Leaflet is reattached to anulus by continuous suture. **E,** Repair is supported by a Carpentier anuloplasty ring, which also remodels shape of anulus. It is attached to tricuspid anulus by a series of mattress sutures placed at perimeter of anulus. These stitches are most easily placed before anterior leaflet is reattached. A gap in the anuloplasty ring protects conduction system from injury.

repair may result in more normal size and shape of the RV than does the Danielson technique.

A further extension of the Carpentier repair has been proposed by da Silva and colleagues[D7] and termed the *cone procedure* (Fig. 42-16). The anterior and posterior leaflets are detached from the anulus as a single unit, mobilized from their anomalous attachments in the RV, and rotated in a clockwise fashion to be sutured to the septal border of the anterior leaflet. The rotated leaflets are reattached to the true anatomic anulus. When possible, the septal leaflet is detached and incorporated into the repair. The anatomic anulus is plicated with two sutures at its true anular level. This repair does not incorporate an anuloplasty ring. da Silva and colleagues incorporate a longitudinal plication of the atrialized portion, but the value of this maneuver is controversial (see "Indications for Plication of Atrialized Ventricle" under Special Situations and Controversies). da Silva and colleagues recommend closing the foramen ovale in a valved fashion (see Fig. 42-16).

The technique described by Ullman and Sebening[U1] also involves mobilizing and reattaching the septal, anterior, and posterior leaflets to allow anterior leaflet coaptation with the septal leaflet at the anatomic anular level without exclusion of the atrialized ventricle. The anuloplasty technique pioneered by Sebening involves narrowing the tricuspid valve orifice with a pledgeted mattress suture placed from the center of the anatomic anulus of the anterior leaflet to the native anulus on the opposite side, creating a double orifice valve. The posterior anulus can be closed with additional pledgeted sutures or left open, as needed to produce a competent valve. Variations of this technique have been reported by Hetzer[K10,N1] and by Hanley's group,[M3] who recommend the "play it where it lies" approach (Fig. 42-17) in which no attempt is made to reattach the septal or posterior leaflet at the level of the anatomic anulus.

Others have used autologous or bovine pericardium to augment the anterior leaflet[O1] or septal leaflet[B10] (Fig. 42-18) to increase the area of leaflet coaptation. Midterm follow-up on a small number of patients has indicated good valve function.

Use of a *bidirectional cavopulmonary shunt* as an adjunctive procedure to create a one-and-a-half ventricle repair is an important surgical option to consider in valve reconstruction procedures.[M3,Q2] A protocolized approach to application of a one-and-a-half ventricle strategy (see Special Situations and Controversies) may increase the frequency of successful valve repair with aggressive anuloplasty techniques that may create some degree of tricuspid valve stenosis in order to eliminate regurgitation.[M3]

Replacement of Tricuspid Valve

In about 20% to 30% of patients, immobility or morphology of the tricuspid valve prevents repair and valve replacement is required.[D4] For this, the leaflet tissue is excised (Fig. 42-19, *A*), leaving a more generous portion of the base of the anterior and septal leaflets where they attach to the membranous septum and right trigone at the point of penetration of the bundle of His. The general suture technique for inserting the valve prosthesis is described in Chapters 11 and 14. When the septal and posterior leaflets are displaced into the RV, or the septal leaflet is absent, sutures may be passed through the usual location of the tricuspid ring. Alternatively, the suture line in this area can be placed well posterior to the AV node area and coronary sinus, as described by Barnard and Schrire.[B3] The replacement valve is usually a large mechanical prosthesis (Fig. 42-19, *B*) or stent-mounted xenograft. A pulmonary allograft mounted in a short polyester sleeve has been used.[M11] A mitral allograft could also be considered.[A1,R2]

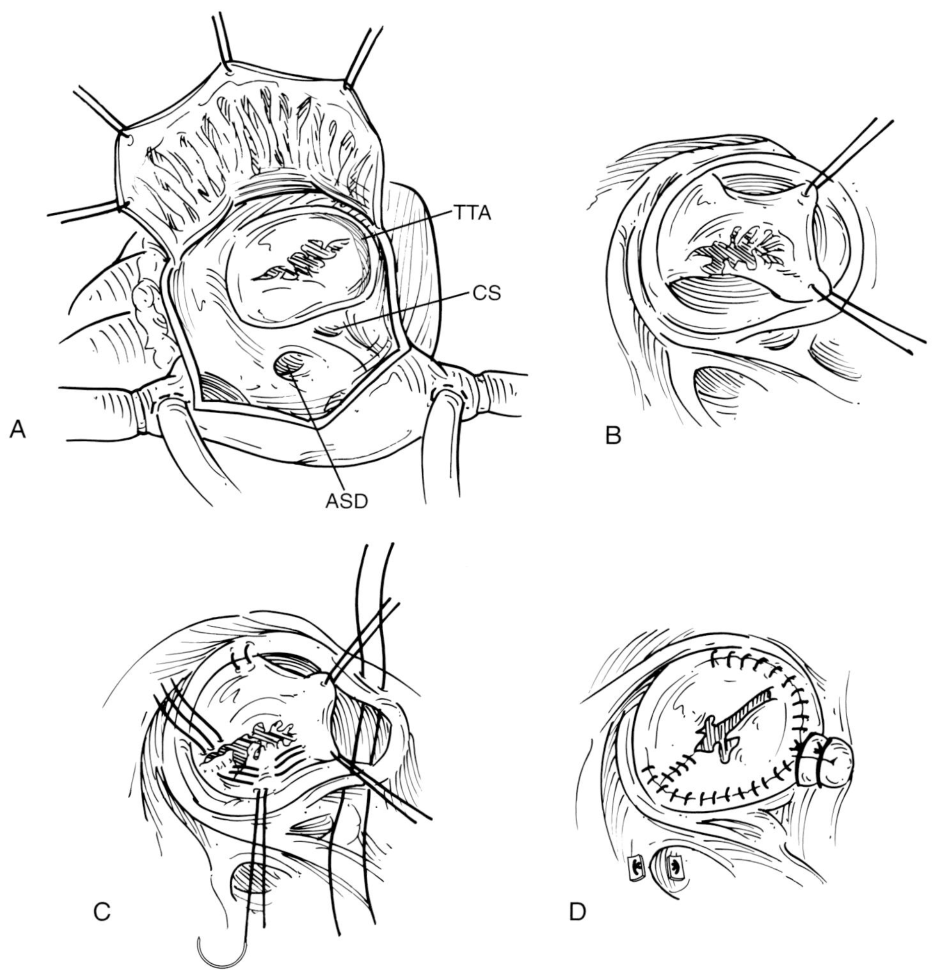

Figure 42-16 Operative steps for Ebstein anomaly repair with cone procedure. **A,** Opened right atrium showing displacement of tricuspid valve. **B,** Detached part of anterior and posterior leaflet forming a single piece. **C,** Clockwise rotation of posterior leaflet edge to be sutured to anterior leaflet septal edge and plication of true tricuspid anulus *(TTA)*. **D,** Completed valve attachment to true tricuspid anulus and valved closure of atrial septal defect *(ASD)*. Key: *CS*, Coronary sinus. (From da Silva and colleagues.[D7])

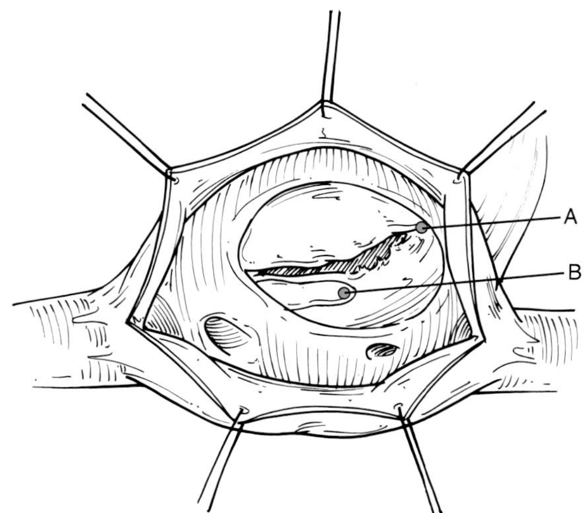

Figure 42-17 "Play it where it lies" approach to repair of Ebstein anomaly. Operation involves limited plication of tricuspid valve. Points *A* and *B* are approximated with one or two mattress sutures at the level of the native valve, not to the level of the true tricuspid anulus. This results in approximating apical aspects of septal and anterior leaflets, effectively creating a bicuspid valve. (From Malhotra and colleagues.[M3])

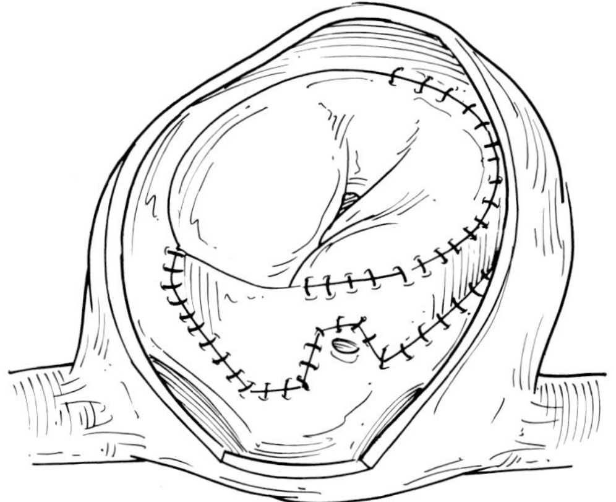

Figure 42-18 Leaflet augmentation procedure for Ebstein anomaly. Patch of polytetrafluoroethylene is tailored to form a new septal anulus, attached to the atrium remote from the area of the atrioventricular node. Accommodation for coronary sinus is made by placing a notch in the patch. Tailored patch in place, defining a new septal anulus and an armature, onto which leaflet advancement is performed, attached at the plane of the reconstructed anulus. All suture material is remote from the atrioventricular node and bundle of His. (From Bichell and colleagues.[B10])

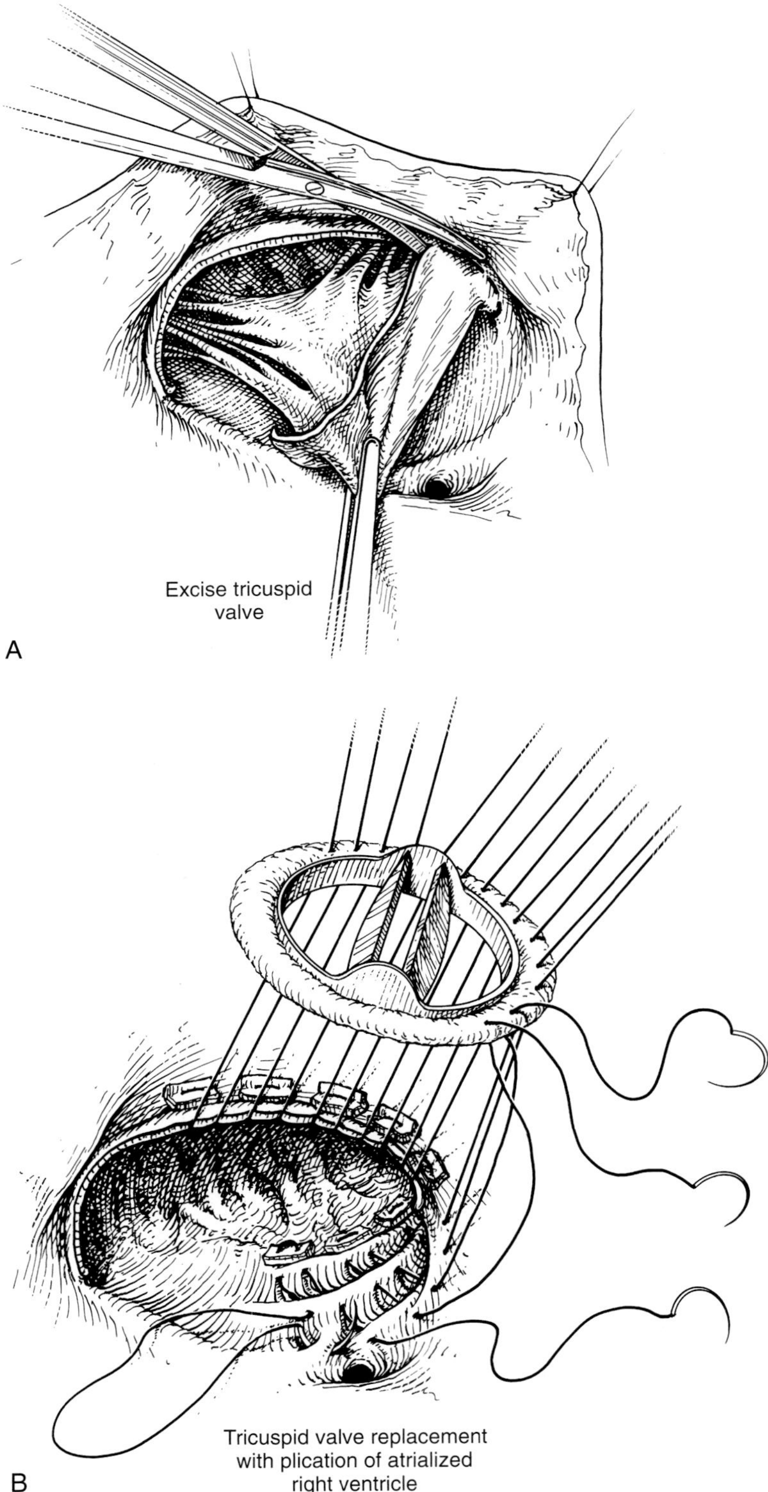

Figure 42-19 Replacement of tricuspid valve in Ebstein anomaly. **A,** Valve is excised. **B,** Valve is replaced with a mechanical prosthesis or stent-mounted xenograft. Device is attached to anulus by pledget-reinforced mattress sutures. Atrialized portion of the right ventricle may be plicated by sutures used to attach the prosthesis. (From Doty and colleagues.[D14])

When the atrialized ventricle is thin walled and fibrous and moves paradoxically, it is plicated by passing sutures used to position the valve first through tissue that forms the margin of the atrialized ventricle (corresponding to attachment of the displaced septal and posterior leaflets) and then through the true tricuspid ring. The valve is seated and sutures tied and cut. If the atrialized ventricle has been plicated, this portion may be further obliterated by a running polypropylene suture placed from outside the heart, taking care not to compromise the arterial supply of the remainder of the RV

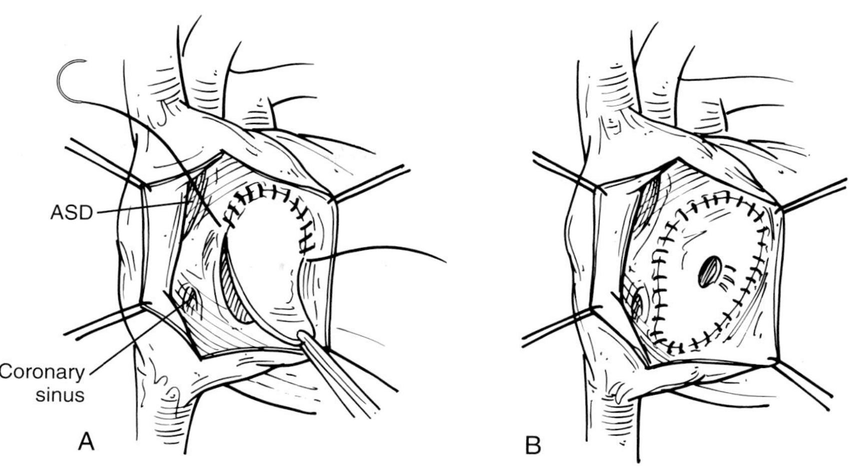

Figure 42-20 Fenestrated patch closure of tricuspid valve in Starnes procedure. **A,** Glutaraldehyde-fixed autologous pericardial patch is sewn at anatomic level of tricuspid valve anulus. **B,** A 4-mm coronary punch is used to create a fenestration in the patch. Coronary sinus remains on right atrial side of patch. Key: *ASD,* Atrial septal defect. (From Reemtsen and colleagues.[R4])

by occluding large coronary arteries. Plication is probably unnecessary in most cases when valve replacement is performed.[W2]

The interatrial communication is closed. In many instances, the septal tissue is stretched and the fossa ovalis tissue thinned. A patch must then be used (pericardium is ideal); it is positioned without tension using a continuous 4-0 polypropylene suture (see Fig. 42-13, *A*). Direct suture is avoided unless the tissues are strong and the defect small, which is uncommon. The left atrium is deliberately not emptied of blood, and the patch suture line is completed at the highest point (superiorly) to avoid air entrapment on the left side of the septum.

The right atriotomy is closed. When the atrium is very large, its size may be reduced by excising an ellipse from the lateral wall. The procedure is completed in the usual fashion, including placement of atrial and ventricular pacing wires and left and right atrial pressure catheters (see Chapter 2).

Simple Atrial Septal Defect Closure

Simple ASD closure may be done as described for closure in conjunction with valve replacement. However, this procedure is rarely indicated in patients with Ebstein anomaly.

Ventricular Exclusion in Critically Ill Neonates (Starnes Operation)

The Starnes operation is designed to abolish the detrimental tricuspid regurgitation by patch closing the tricuspid valve, creating a widely opened and nonrestrictive ASD, and establishing controlled pulmonary blood flow through a systemic-to–pulmonary artery shunt. A single ventricle palliation strategy is then pursued.[S18]

CPB is established. Bicaval cannulation may be used (see "Venous Cannulation" in Section III of Chapter 2) and the operation performed during hypothermic CPB. Alternatively, a single venous cannula may be used and the intraatrial portion of the operation performed during hypothermic circulatory arrest. Cold cardioplegia is used (see "Cold Cardioplegia, Controlled Aortic Root Reperfusion, and [When Needed] Warm Cardioplegic Induction" in Chapter 3). The right atrium is opened obliquely. The ASD is enlarged by excising all remnants of the septum primum (floor of the fossa ovalis). The tricuspid valve is closed by sewing into place an appropriately sized pericardial patch, sewn at the anatomic level of the tricuspid anulus. The coronary sinus is maintained on the atrial side of the patch. The patch is fenestrated with a 4-mm punch (Fig. 42-20). The right atrium is reduced in size by removing a segment of the right atrial free wall, and then is closed. If this portion of the procedure is done during hypothermic circulatory arrest, CPB is reestablished. If pulmonary regurgitation is present, the proximal main pulmonary trunk is closed.

A systemic-pulmonary shunt is created. Starnes and colleagues prefer a central shunt of 4-mm polytetrafluoroethylene (PTFE) tube interposed between the ascending aorta and pulmonary trunk.[S18] Alternatively, a 3.5- or 4-mm PTFE tube may be interposed between the brachiocephalic–right carotid artery junction and the medial aspect of the right pulmonary artery (see "Reconstructive Surgery" in Chapter 49), or between the right lateral aspect of the ascending aorta and anterior aspect of the right pulmonary artery. After rewarming has been accomplished, the remainder of the operation is completed in the usual manner (see "Completing Cardiopulmonary Bypass" in Section III of Chapter 2). The sternum is generally left open and the skin closed with a patch of bovine pericardium. The sternum can usually be closed in the intensive care unit 48 to 72 hours later.

Treatment of Arrhythmias

Dearani and colleagues at the Mayo Clinic[A9] recommend routine electrophysiologic evaluation in children and adults undergoing Ebstein repair. If arrhythmic substrate is identified (e.g., WPW syndrome is present), and there is a history of life-threatening paroxysmal arrhythmia, the accessory conduction pathways are divided at the same operation, after proper electrophysiologic study[M12,S8] (see Technique of Intervention in Section III of Chapter 16). This is generally done before valve repair or replacement. Alternatively, these pathways may be obliterated preoperatively in the electrophysiology laboratory.[O2]

Supraventricular arrhythmia such as atrial flutter and fibrillation may occur paroxysmally or chronically as the right atrium enlarges. A right-sided maze procedure may be done at the time of operation.[S19,T4]

Table 42-3 Hospital Mortality According to Management Strategy Among 415 Neonates with Ebstein Anomaly

		Hospital Mortality		
Strategy	***n***	**No.**	**%**	**CL (%)**
Medical management	257	56	22	19-25
Percutaneous procedure	29	2	6.9	2.4-16
Percutaneous procedure and surgery	11	7	64	44-81
Systemic-to-pulmonary shunt	63	17	27	21-34
Tricuspid valve repair	16	5	31	18-47
Single-ventricle palliation	36	13	36	27-46
Transplantation	3	0	0	0-47
TOTAL	415	98	24	21-26

Modified from Pediatric Health Information System, 2003-2008.[G7]

SPECIAL FEATURES OF POSTOPERATIVE CARE

Postoperative care is as usual after repair or replacement of the tricuspid valve for Ebstein anomaly (see Chapter 5). Convalescence is generally rapid and normal.

Critically ill neonates undergoing the Starnes operation, however, require the type of care accorded all neonates in whom pulmonary blood flow originates exclusively from the systemic circulation (see "General Care of Neonates and Infants" in Chapter 5). Additionally, pulmonary artery vasodilatation is encouraged by nitric oxide administration (see Chapter 5). Lowering pulmonary vascular resistance decreases the tendency to RV distention (see Special Situations and Controversies). Further operations and procedures follow the Fontan pathway strategies (see Indications for Operation and Special Situations and Controversies in Section IV of Chapter 41).

RESULTS AFTER REPAIR

Survival

Mortality after Surgery in the Neonatal Period

Historically, hospital mortality has been high (>50%) for critically ill neonates who undergo emergency or urgent operation. However, with current techniques of intensive neonatal medical management and surgical and percutaneous therapy as needed, survival has importantly improved. Thus, in the 40-institution report of the PHIS, overall hospital mortality of neonates initially managed by percutaneous procedures with or without surgery was 22% (9/40; CL 15%-31%), for those managed by systemic-to–pulmonary shunting 27%, for those undergoing tricuspid valve repair 31%, and for those receiving a transplant 0%[G7] (Table 42-3). Notably, half the neonates were medically managed, and 15% were managed by placement of a systemic-to–pulmonary system shunt, 9.6% by a percutaneous procedure, 8.7% by single ventricle palliation, and 3.9% by tricuspid valve repair.

Among 16 neonates undergoing surgical intervention between 1992 and 2005, Starnes and colleagues reported a hospital mortality of 31% with a variety of surgical procedures (Reemtsan 2006). The best survival occurred in the 10 patients (80% hospital survival; CL 59%-93%) who underwent patch fenestration as part of a RV exclusion procedure (Starnes operation). No late deaths were reported, all had undergone a subsequent bidirectional Glenn, and three had a completed Fontan.

Knott-Craig and colleagues[K8] have pursued tricuspid valve repair and two-ventricle physiology, creating a competent monoleaflet valve based on the anterior leaflet, partially closing the ASD, and performing a reduction atrioplasty. Hospital survival among neonates exceeded 65%, but mortality was 55% (6/11; CL 35%-73%) among patients with anatomic pulmonary atresia.

An experience with surgical intervention in 24 neonates with Ebstein anomaly reported by Shinkawa and colleagues[S14] supports a policy of shunt only in the presence of refractory cyanosis without severe tricuspid regurgitation. In the presence of severe regurgitation and refractory heart failure, RV exclusion provided possibly superior hospital (73%, 8/11; CL 53%-87%) and late survival (63%) compared with tricuspid valve repair (25%, 1/4; CL 4.0%-62% for hospital and late survival).

Early (Hospital) Death in Children and Adults

Thirty-day mortality in the Mayo Clinic series of 539 patients (1972-2006) was 6.1% (33 deaths; CL 5.0%-7.4%), but 2.7% after 2001, which is representative of what can be accomplished in these often ill patients.[B14] Augustin and colleagues reported two hospital deaths among 60 patients (3.3%; CL 1.1%-7.7%) (1974-1995).[A11] These results are improved over those obtained in an earlier era. A multicenter study from the European Congenital Heart Surgeons Association reported a hospital mortality of 8.3% (CL 5.4%-12%) among 96 patients undergoing tricuspid valve repair or replacement between 1992 and 2005.[S1] In patients operated on from September 1993 to September 2008, Malhotra and colleagues report no early (0%; CL 0%-3.3%) or late mortality in a group of 57 non-neonatal patients (median age 8 years, range 7 months to 40 years), among whom 95% had valve repairs and 54% had concomitant cavopulmonary shunts.[M3] Using near routine excision of atrialized RV, detachment and repair of the tricuspid valve leaflets, and anulus plication, Wu and colleagues[W6] reported no early mortality (0%; CL 0%-2.3%) among 83 patients operated on between 1997 and 2006.[B12,K6,M10,P1,R9,W6,S7,S9] Among 52 children aged 5 months to 12 years undergoing repair of Ebstein anomaly at the Mayo Clinic between 1974 and 2003, early mortality was 5.8% (3/52; CL 2.6%-11%), with no deaths since 1984 (0/31; CL 0%-5.9%).[B11] da Silva and colleagues reported a 2.5% hospital mortality (1/40; CL 0.4%-8.2%) among 40 patients undergoing the cone procedure between 1993 and 2005.[D7]

Mode of death is usually acute cardiac failure, probably related to preoperative RV enlargement and dysfunction. Improved methods of myocardial management, increasing prevalence and success of tricuspid valve repair rather than replacement, and possibly selective use of bidirectional cavopulmonary shunts have contributed to reduced early mortality.

Time-Related Survival

The seriousness of Ebstein anomaly is well demonstrated in a long-term follow-up study of a heterogeneous group of patients without major associated cardiac anomalies, 18 of whom (n = 48) underwent 22 operations.[G3] Median survival for the overall group was 47 years. Survival was similar in patients who presented during the first 3 days of life but survived to 6 months of age, and those who presented after 3 months of age. All four patients in whom permanent atrial fibrillation developed died within 5 years.

Late deaths are uncommon after tricuspid valve repair (or replacement) and ASD closure, with about 80% of patients surviving long term.[B5,D5,W2] In the Mayo Clinic cohort of 539 patients, 10- and 20-year survival was 85% and 71%, respectively, with no important difference in late survival between patients undergoing valve repair vs. replacement.[B14] Among 52 children undergoing repair, 15-year survival was 90%.[B11] Deaths are often sudden and attributable to rhythm disturbances. Although it seems that late survival and freedom from reoperation would be better after successful valve repair than replacement, the Mayo Clinic analysis indicates no difference in late reoperation-free survival between patients receiving tricuspid valve repair vs. replacement among patients 12 years of age or older.[B11] However, among patients under age 12, reoperation-free survival is superior for those undergoing valve repair.[B14]

Preoperative risk factors for late mortality include higher hematocrit (worse cyanosis), severe mitral valve regurgitation, prior cardiac operations, and moderate to severe reduction in RV systolic function.[B14] Left ventricular dysfunction is also a risk factor for early and late mortality, despite the finding of improved left ventricular systolic function in most such patients following Ebstein anomaly repair.[B14]

Right Ventricular Function

Little is known about the long-term fate of RV function after *neonatal surgery* for Ebstein anomaly. However, Reemtsen and colleagues compared echocardiographic findings at 6 to 204 months (median 30 months) with those immediately prior to the Starnes procedure performed in the neonatal period. The Great Ormond Street ratio (see Table 42-2) and RV size decreased prior to the bidirectional Glenn, indicating RV regression.[R5] Left ventricular septal impingement on left ventricular cavity dimensions decreased an average of 38%, with normalization of left ventricular morphology and systolic function. These findings have important implications in predicting favorable outcomes after the Fontan operation if a single-ventricle strategy is selected in the neonatal period.

Functional Status

Most patients (about 85%) achieve good functional status (NYHA class I or II) and improved performance during objective exercise testing postoperatively, although many are severely limited preoperatively.[B14,D3,D15,S12,S15] Residual symptoms, when present, are usually related to troublesome, non-WPW supraventricular arrhythmias.[W2] Failure to plicate the atrialized portion of the RV has not been shown to decrease the probability of a good functional result.[S9] The effect of a bidirectional cavopulmonary shunt on late functional status has been incompletely studied, but favorable midterm functional status has been reported.[K4,M3]

Tricuspid Valve Function after Repair and Freedom from Reoperation

Although many reports indicate absent or mild tricuspid regurgitation early and midterm after repair,[A11,C3,D3,Q1] concerns remain about the important occurrence of late tricuspid valve replacement. Several areas of controversy relate to the optimal methods to prevent late, progressive tricuspid regurgitation. The Danielson and Carpentier techniques (see Technique of Operation) rely on creating essentially a monoleaflet valve that coapts against the RV septum in the area of the septal leaflet. This area has been observed as the site of recurrent tricuspid regurgitation,[D7] which theoretically may be obviated by direct leaflet coaptation in the septal area, as is achieved with the cone procedure (see Technique of Operation).

da Silva and colleagues reported no reoperations for tricuspid valve replacement, but one for re-repair and a 9% occurrence of moderately severe early tricuspid regurgitation among 40 patients who underwent the cone procedure.[D7] Freedom from further tricuspid regurgitation has been maintained in the intermediate term.[D8,D9] Whether this technique and repair principles provide an important improvement in late valve function will require further long-term studies.

Postrepair Rhythm Disturbances

Complete heart block is uncommon after repair, despite the distorted morphology in the region of the bundle of His.

WPW has mostly been cured by concomitant sectioning of the accessory pathways (see Chapter 16), which can be accomplished without increasing operative risk.[M12,S8] However, episodic non-WPW supraventricular tachycardia continues late postoperatively in about 20% of patients.[C3,W2] Uncommonly, even after successful surgical relief of WPW syndrome, late sudden death occurs. The substrate for atrial arrhythmias is enhanced by the large right atrium, RV dysfunction, and tricuspid regurgitation that frequently accompany Ebstein anomaly late after operation. Stulak and colleagues at the Mayo Clinic[S19] reported greater than 90% freedom from late recurrence of atrial fibrillation or flutter with a right-sided maze procedure plus isthmus ablation. An ongoing area of controversy relates to the possible benefit of a prophylactic right-sided maze procedure at the time of Ebstein anomaly repair.[V2]

RESULTS OF OTHER PROCEDURES

Repair of Atrial Septal Defect Alone

The risk associated with simple ASD closure is low in properly selected patients. In the combined UAB-GLH experience, nine patients with either left-to-right or right-to-left shunts and competent but abnormal tricuspid valves underwent simple ASD closure, with no hospital deaths (CL 0%-19%; Table 42-4). It is surprising that closure of the ASD was well tolerated in the face of preoperative right-to-left shunting, but this was also the experience at the Mayo Clinic and has been the case in pulmonary stenosis with intact ventricular septum (see Chapter 39).[W5]

When a left-to-right shunt is present preoperatively, late results are good (see Table 42-4). Thus, in the combined UAB-GLH experience, three patients in this category were hospital survivors; two had excellent long-term results, and one had WPW syndrome with episodic arrhythmias.

If the indication is appropriate, late results of simple ASD closure are also good in patients with right-to-left shunting preoperatively and important cyanosis. At late postoperative

Table 42-4 Late Results of Atrial Septal Defect Closure without Tricuspid Valve Repair or Replacement[a]

Age at Operation (Years)	Shunt	Preop NYHA Class	Length of Follow-Up (Years)	Postop NYHA Class	Comments
0.2	L → R	IV	6	I	Moderate-sized VSD also closed
8	L → R	II	3.2	I	Kent bundle cut; pulmonary valvotomy performed; SV tachycardia PO
11	L → R	II	18	II	WPW, with episodic dysrhythmia PO
13	R → L	III	10	I	Episodic SV tachycardia PO
14	0	I	4	I	Operation for suspected RA myxoma
17	R → L[b]	I	3	I	Operation for peripheral embolism; episodic SV tachycardia PO
20	R → L	II	14	II	Episodic severe dysrhythmia PO
26	L → R	III	6	II	Kent bundles cut; severe dysrhythmias PO
32	R → L	IV	3		Late death at operation for TVR
40	R → L	III	12	II	Episodic severe SV tachycardia PO
59	L → R	II	1	I	

Data from combined UAB-GLH experience.
[a]ASD repair alone was performed in eight; ASD and VSD repair in one; ASD repair and pulmonary valvotomy in one; ASD repair in patient with suspected myxoma in one. One patient with ASD repair and tricuspid valvotomy, not included in this table, died 2 weeks after hospital discharge.
[b]Bidirectional, but dominantly R → L.
Key: *ASD,* Atrial septal defect; *L → R,* left to right; *NYHA,* New York Heart Association; *postop/PO,* postoperative; *preop,* preoperative; *R → L,* right to left; *RA,* right atrial; *SV,* supraventricular; *TVR,* tricuspid valve replacement; *VSD,* ventricular septal defect; *WPW,* Wolff-Parkinson-White syndrome.

follow-up, four of five such patients in the UAB-GLH experience were alive and acyanotic, but all had episodic arrhythmias, severe in three cases. Two patients considered themselves functionally normal (NYHA class I), whereas two were in NYHA class II (see Table 42-4). One patient had an initially good result, and then cyanosis and severe disability recurred. Three years after his initial operation, he died after reoperation for reclosure of the septal defect and tricuspid valve replacement.

Tricuspid Valvotomy

The rare occurrence of tricuspid stenosis invites tricuspid valvotomy, but severe regurgitation may result.[P1] If the Carpentier technique of fenestration to restore or substitute for interchordal spaces is not satisfactory, valve replacement is indicated.[C3]

Pulmonary Valvotomy

Pulmonary valvotomy can have low hospital mortality in patients with Ebstein anomaly when indications are appropriate. This procedure may be life saving in neonates, because it decreases the degree of tricuspid regurgitation.

INDICATIONS FOR OPERATION

Neonates presenting in extremis, usually in the first week of life, are immediately intubated and begun on prostaglandin E_1, appropriate catecholamine support, aggressive treatment of metabolic acidosis, and other intensive therapy (see Special Situations and Controversies). Once stabilized, a Starnes procedure is performed, particularly if the patient has a Celermajer grade of 3 or 4 (see Special Situations and Controversies). If the patient's condition does not stabilize, operation is performed at an exceptionally high risk. Extracorporeal membrane oxygenation (ECMO) should be considered in such circumstances, either before or following emergency operation.

In the absence of severe cyanosis or symptoms of heart failure, medical management is advisable. Surgical intervention should be considered with the development of heart failure symptoms, worsening cyanosis, progressive increase in heart size, reduction in ventricular systolic function, or the appearance of atrial or ventricular tachyarrhythmias.[A9] The presence of severe tricuspid regurgitation and moderate cyanosis secondary to right-to-left shunting through the ASD should prompt earlier surgical intervention. Severe limitations and severe hypoxia are not contraindications to repair, although increased hospital mortality in patients in functional NYHA class IV argues strongly in favor of advising operation before disability is this advanced. The correlation between sudden death and cardiomegaly argues for operation when the cardiothoracic ratio reaches 0.60 or greater, regardless of symptoms.[G3]

Among patients under about 12 to 14 years of age, valve repair is greatly preferable to replacement. In older teenagers and adults, tricuspid valve replacement is a suitable option if repair appears unlikely to succeed.

Simple repair of the ASD is indicated when there is a large left-to-right shunt ($\dot{Q}p/\dot{Q}s > 2$), with or without symptoms of heart failure, and little or no tricuspid regurgitation. Simple repair of the ASD, *without* repair (or replacement if needed) of the tricuspid valve, is otherwise rarely advisable.

In patients with WPW syndrome that is producing life-threatening arrhythmia, the accessory conduction pathways should be divided or ablated, and the valve defect should be treated concomitantly on its merits.[S7] Atrial communications should be closed at the time of accessory pathways division. Other arrhythmias are not an indication for operation, because their occurrence is not altered by correction of the valve defect. However, they are undoubtedly less well tolerated in the presence of severe tricuspid regurgitation, cardiomegaly, and cyanosis, and can then be an added indication for operation on the valve.

SPECIAL SITUATIONS AND CONTROVERSIES

Morphology

Confusion as to morphologic classification has arisen in some infants who have pulmonary atresia and minor downward displacement (or adherence) of the septal tricuspid leaflet origin (see Chapter 40).[B8] When this is the only Ebstein-like leaflet abnormality present, the defect is not classified or treated as Ebstein anomaly. In a number of infants with pulmonary atresia, however, the tricuspid valve shows additional typical and often florid features of Ebstein anomaly in association with severe regurgitation. Such patients form one variety of complex Ebstein anomaly.

Management of Critically Ill Neonates with Ebstein Anomaly

When neonates with Ebstein anomaly present with severe cyanosis, prostaglandin infusion is initiated to maintain or restore ductal patency. Urgent echocardiographic evaluation is performed to establish the diagnosis and evaluate the RV outflow tract. If antegrade flow through the pulmonary valve is absent, the pulmonary atresia may be functional (elevated pulmonary vascular resistance coupled with severe tricuspid regurgitation and RV dysfunction) or anatomic.[J1] A trial of inhaled nitric oxide is warranted to lower pulmonary vascular resistance and promote antegrade flow through the pulmonary valve if it is patent.[J1] If nitric oxide is helpful in bridging a marginal patient through the neonatal period, the addition of oral sildenafil may be useful.[P2] Other standard measures for critical ill neonates with Ebstein anomaly include placement of umbilical arterial and venous catheters and mechanical ventilation with the minimum effective airway pressure and tidal volumes of 10 to 15 $mL \cdot kg^{-1}$ to recruit areas of atelectasis.[K7,K9] If the RV outflow tract is functional, a trial of prostaglandin weaning is indicated. If SaO_2 is maintained at 70% or greater without heart failure, surgical intervention may not be necessary.

If prostaglandin weaning is not successful, two situations may occur. If the circulation is stable without evidence of heart failure and the only problem is unacceptable cyanosis, a systemic-to–pulmonary shunt may be the only necessary procedure. However, if heart failure and circulatory compromise persist, the tricuspid valve itself must be addressed, either through the Starnes procedure or valve reconstruction (see Technique of Operation).

In planning for continued medical therapy vs. the likelihood of needing surgical intervention, calculation of the Celermajer score[C6] is useful in predicting risk of death (see Table 42-2).

Type of Prosthesis for Tricuspid Valve Replacement

A stent-mounted glutaraldehyde-preserved porcine bioprosthesis or bovine pericardial bioprosthesis may be considered optimal in most patients with Ebstein anomaly, but both are subject to the usual problems of a bioprosthesis.[W3] Mechanical prostheses may also be used to achieve long-term durability, but anticoagulant therapy is required.[C7] An analysis of the Mayo Clinic experience identified use of a bioprosthetic valve (vs. mechanical prosthetic valve) as an independent predictor of long-term survival.[B15,N2] An allograft, either a stent-mounted pulmonary or aortic valve, or a directly attached mitral allograft supported by an anuloplasty ring, could also be considered.[A1,M11]

Indications for Plication (or Resection) of Atrialized Ventricle

Indications for plication of an atrialized ventricle at the time of tricuspid valve replacement are controversial. Potential *advantages* of plication (or resection) include (1) reducing the size of the nonfunctional RV, potentially increasing transit of blood by improved systolic function; (2) improving left ventricular function by alleviating left ventricular compression and septal bowing; (3) moving the anterior leaflet closer to the septum by elevating the papillary muscles; and (4) providing more space for lung expansion, especially in neonates. The major potential disadvantage relates to possible distortion of or injury to the right coronary artery and its branches, which could worsen RV function and contribute to ventricular arrhythmias.[B14] Some suggest that omitting routine plication compromises RV function postoperatively[H2,T6]; others believe that plication is indicated only when the atrialized portion of the RV is very thin walled and aneurysmal (probably about 10% to 15% of cases).[K6,N3,P1] Plication may be considered unnecessary in even these cases, because good function has resulted without it.[C2,C8,W2]

Plication of the atrialized ventricle is performed routinely in some methods of tricuspid valve repair, for which it is an integral part of the anuloplasty portion of the repair. However, several reported techniques emphasize the need for only partial plication near the functional anulus[M3] as part of the anuloplasty procedure, without need to plicate the remainder of the atrialized portion.

Excision or Plication of Right Atrial Wall

Excision or plication of the right atrial wall was suggested by Timmis and colleagues, who considered it important "to promote atrial emptying and lessen the likelihood of clot formation" when a mechanical prosthesis was used.[T6] Danielson and colleagues incorporate excision of the right atrial wall in their repair.[D6,M10] The simplicity of this maneuver during valve replacement or repair makes it an attractive step when the right atrium is markedly enlarged.

Role of Bidirectional Cavopulmonary Shunt and One-and-a-Half Ventricle Repair

The vast majority of patients with Ebstein anomaly can undergo successful biventricular repair. However, creating a "one-and-a-half" ventricle repair can be an effective strategy if reducing the tricuspid anulus to a z value of less than −2 (or about 2.5 cm in the adult) is necessary to eliminate important tricuspid regurgitation in an infant or child with normal pulmonary vascular resistance. In this instance, functional tricuspid stenosis is managed by constructing a bidirectional cavopulmonary shunt with division of the superior vena cava at its junction with the right atrium (see Chapter 41).[M3] This strategy may also be useful when the RV is severely dysfunctional,[Q2] as long as the left atrial and pulmonary artery pressures are low. By reducing the RV stroke volume required to maintain effective cardiac output, RV work requirement is reduced and preload of the left ventricle optimized.[M3] Furthermore, the adverse effect on left ventricular function by a massively enlarged RV can be ameliorated.[D12] Bidirectional cavopulmonary shunt may also reduce residual tricuspid regurgitation.[M5] Dearani and colleagues have recommended the following criteria for constructing a bidirectional cavopulmonary shunt: left ventricular end-diastolic pressure less than 15 mmHg, transpulmonary gradient less than 10 mmHg, and mean pulmonary artery pressure less than 18 to 20 mmHg.[D12] Malhotra and colleagues[M3] recommend performing a bidirectional cavopulmonary shunt if, at the end of the repair, right atrial pressure is more than 1.5 times left atrial pressure.

The potential disadvantages of this approach include possible facial suffusion secondary to elevated jugular venous pressure and pulsations in the head and neck veins, development of collateral veins and pulmonary arteriovenous fistulas, and compromise of access for pacemaker leads.

Malhotra and colleagues[M3] reported an experience of valve repair in 54 of 57 patients with Ebstein anomaly, of whom 55% received a bidirectional cavopulmonary shunt (half of these in adults). Freedom from subsequent valve replacement was 92% at 4 years, with 95% of patients in NYHA class I. Van Arsdell and colleagues reported 90% 10-year survival following one-and-a-half ventricle repair.[V2]

Indications for Single-Ventricle Pathway

The potential advantages of RV exclusion (Starnes procedure) for severely ill neonates with Ebstein anomaly are discussed under "Survival" in Results after Repair. Such patients, if they survive the initial neonatal procedure, have a high likelihood of survival through the bidirectional Glenn stage.

A particularly high-risk morphologic subset of Ebstein anomaly is hearts with the combination of severe tricuspid regurgitation and anatomic pulmonary atresia.[K8,R4] Symptomatic infants and children with this combination are likely best treated with a single-ventricle strategy. Polimenakos and colleagues have also applied this strategy successfully in an adult Ebstein patient with severe RV dysfunction, tricuspid regurgitation, and RV outflow obstruction.[P4]

REFERENCES

A

1. Acar C, Tolan M, Berrebi A, Gaer J, Gouzeo R, Marchix T, et al. Homograft replacement of the mitral valve: graft selection, technique of implantation, and results in forty-three patients. J Thorac Cardiovasc Surg 1996;111:367.
2. Ammash NM, Warnes CA, Connolly HM, Danielson GK, Seward JB. Mimics of Ebstein's anomaly. Am Heart J 1997;134:508.
3. Anderson KR, Danielson GK, McGoon DC, Lie JT. Ebstein's anomaly of the left-sided tricuspid valve. Pathological anatomy of the valvular malformation. Circulation 1977;58:1.
4. Anderson KR, Lie JT. Pathologic anatomy of Ebstein's anomaly of the heart revisited. Am J Cardiol 1978;71:739.
5. Anderson KR, Lie JT. The right ventricular myocardium in Ebstein's anomaly. A morphometric histopathologic study. Mayo Clin Proc 1979;54:181.
6. Anderson KR, Zuberbuhler JR, Anderson RH, Becker AE, Lie JT. Morphologic spectrum of Ebstein's anomaly of the heart. A review. Mayo Clin Proc 1979;54:174.
7. Anderson RH. The triangle of Koch in the setting of Ebstein's malformation. Rev Esp Cardiol 2010;63:633-4.
8. Arnstein A. Eine Seltene Missbildung der Trikuspikalklappe ("Ebsteinische Krankheit"). Virchows Arch [A] 1927;266:274.
9. Attenhofer Jost CH, Connolly HM, Dearani JA, Edwards WD, Danielson GK. Ebstein's anomaly. Circulation 2007;115:277-85.
10. Attenhofer Jost CH, Connolly HM, O'Leary PW, Warnes CA, Tajik AJ, Seward JB. Left heart lesions in patients with Ebstein anomaly. Mayo Clin Proc 2005;80:361-8.
11. Augustin N, Schmidt-Habelmann P, Wottke M, Meisner H, Sebening F. Results after surgical repair of Ebstein's anomaly. Ann Thorac Surg 1997;63:1650.

B

1. Bahnson HT, Bauersfeld SR, Smith JR. Pathological anatomy and surgical correction of Ebstein's anomaly. Circulation 1965;31:3.
2. Barber G, Danielson GK, Heise CT, Driscoll DJ. Cardiorespiratory response to exercise in Ebstein's anomaly. Am J Cardiol 1985; 56:509.
3. Barnard CN, Schrire Y. Surgical correction of Ebstein's malformation with a prosthetic tricuspid valve. Surgery 1963;54:302.
4. Becker AE, Becker MJ, Edwards JE. Pathologic spectrum of dysplasia of the tricuspid valve: features in common with Ebstein's malformation. Arch Pathol 1971;91:167.
5. Behl PR, Blesovsky A. Ebstein's anomaly: sixteen years' experience with valve replacement without plication of the right ventricle. Thorax 1984;39:8.
6. Benson LN, Child JS, Schwaiger M, Perloff JK, Schelbert HR. Left ventricular geometry and function in adults with Ebstein's anomaly of the tricuspid valve. Circulation 1987;75:353.
7. Bharati S, Lev M, Kirklin JW. Cardiac surgery and the conduction system, 2nd Ed. Mount Kisco, N.Y.: Futura, 1992.
8. Bharucha T, Anderson RH, Lim ZS, Vettukattil JJ. Multiplanar review of three-dimensional echocardiography gives new insights into the morphology of Ebstein's malformation. Cardiol Young 2010;20:49-53.
9. Bialostozky D, Horwitz S, Espino-Vela J. Ebstein's malformation of the tricuspid valve. A review of 65 cases. Am J Cardiol 1972; 29:826.
10. Bichell DP, Mora BN, Mathewson JW, Kirkpatrick SK, Tyner JJ, McLees-Palinkas T. Modified technique for the surgical treatment of severe tricuspid valve deformity in Ebstein's anomaly. Ann Thorac Surg 2007;83:678-80.
11. Boston US, Dearani JA, O'Leary PW, Driscoll DJ, Danielson GK. Tricuspid valve repair for Ebstein's anomaly in young children: a 30-year experience. Ann Thorac Surg 2006;81:690-6.
12. Bove EL, Kirsh MM. Valve replacement for Ebstein's anomaly of the tricuspid valve. J Thorac Cardiovasc Surg 1979;78:229.
13. Brickner ME, Hillis LD, Lange RA. Congenital heart disease in adults. Second of two parts. N Engl J Med 2000;342:334-42.
14. Brown ML, Dearani JA, Danielson GK, Cetta F, Connolly HM, Warnes CA, et al. Functional status after operation for Ebstein anomaly: the Mayo Clinic experience. J Am Coll Cardiol 2008; 52:460-6.
15. Brown ML, Dearani JA, Danielson GK, Cetta F, Connolly HM, Warnes CA, et al. Comparison of the outcome of porcine bioprosthetic versus mechanical prosthetic replacement of the tricuspid valve in the Ebstein anomaly. Am J Cardiol 2009;103:555-61.

C

1. Cabin HS, Roberts WC. Ebstein's anomaly of the tricuspid valve and prolapse of the mitral valve. Am Heart J 1981;101:177.
2. Caralps JM, Aris A, Bonnin JO, Solanes H, Torner M. Ebstein's anomaly: surgical treatment with tricuspid replacement without right ventricular plication. Ann Thorac Surg 1981;31:277.
3. Carpentier A, Chauvaud S, Mace L, Relland J, Mihaileanu S, Marino JP, et al. A new reconstructive operation for Ebstein's anomaly of the tricuspid valve. J Thorac Cardiovasc Surg 1988; 96:92.
4. Cartwright RS, Smeloff EA, Cayler GG, Fong W, Huntley AC, Blake JR, et al. Total correction of Ebstein's anomaly by means of tricuspid replacement. J Thorac Cardiovasc Surg 1964;47:755.
5. Celermajer DS, Bull C, Till JA, Cullen S, Vassillikos VP, Sullivan ID, et al. Ebstein's anomaly: presentation and outcome from fetus to adult. J Am Coll Cardiol 1994;23:170-6.
6. Celermajer DS, Cullen S, Sullivan ID, Spiegelhalter DJ, Wyse RK, Deanfield JE. Outcome in neonates with Ebstein's anomaly. J Am Coll Cardiol 1992;19:1041-6.

7. Charles RG, Barnard CN, Beck W. Tricuspid valve replacement for Ebstein's anomaly: a 19-year review of the first case. Br Heart J 1981;46:578.
8. Crews TL, Pridie RB, Benham R, Leatham A. Auscultatory and phonocardiographic findings in Ebstein's anomaly. Correlation of first heart sound with ultrasonic records of tricuspid valve movement. Br Heart J 1972;34:681.

D

1. Daliento L, Angelini A, Ho SY, Frescura C, Turrini P, Baratella MC, et al. Angiographic and morphologic features of the left ventricle in Ebstein malformation. Am J Cardiol 1997;80:1051.
2. Danielson GK. Ebstein's anomaly: editorial comments and personal observations. Ann Thorac Surg 1982;34:396.
3. Danielson GK. Discussion of Carpentier A, Chauvaud S, Mace L, Relland J, Mihaileanu S, Marino JT, Abry B, Guibourt P. A new reconstructive operation for Ebstein's anomaly of the tricuspid valve. J Thorac Cardiovasc Surg 1988;96:92.
4. Danielson GK, Driscoll DJ, Mair DD, Warnes CA, Oliver WC Jr. Operative treatment of Ebstein's anomaly. J Thorac Cardiovasc Surg 1992;104:1195.
5. Danielson GK, Fuster V. Surgical repair of Ebstein's anomaly. Ann Surg 1982;196:499.
6. Danielson GK, Maloney JD, Devloo RA. Surgical repair of Ebstein's anomaly. Mayo Clin Proc 1979;54:185.
7. da Silva JP, Baumgratz JF, da Fonseca L, Franchi SM, Lopes LM, Tavares GM, et al. The cone reconstruction of the tricuspid valve in Ebstein's anomaly. The operation: early and midterm results. J Thorac Cardiovasc Surg 2007;133:215-23.
8. da Silva JP, da Fonseca L. Ebstein's anomaly of the tricuspid valve: the cone repair. Semin Thorac Cardiovasc Surg Pediatr Card Surg Annu 2012 (in press).
9. da Silva JP, da Fonseca da Silva L, Moreira LF, Lopes LM, Franchi SM, Lianza AC, et al. Cone reconstruction in Ebstein's anomaly repair: early and long-term results. Arq Bras Cardiol 2011; 97:199-208.
10. Dearani JA, Danielson GK. Congenital heart surgery nomenclature and database project: Ebstein's anomaly and tricuspid valve disease. Ann Thorac Surg 2000;69:S106.
11. Dearani JA, Danielson GK. Ebstein's anomaly. In: Sellke FW, del Nido PJ, Swanson SJ, eds. Sabiston & Spencer: Surgery of the chest. 7th ed. Philadelphia: Elsevier Saunders, 2005:2223-35.
12. Dearani JA, O'Leary PW, Danielson GK. Surgical treatment of Ebstein's malformation: state of the art in 2006. Cardiol Young 2006;16:S12-20.
13. Deutsch V, Wexler L, Blieden LC, Yahini JH, Neufeld HN. Ebstein's anomaly of tricuspid valve: critical review of roentgenological features and additional angiographic signs. Am J Roentgenol Radium Ther Nucl Med 1975;125:395.
14. Doty DB. Cardiac surgery: operative technique. St. Louis: Mosby-Year Book, 1997, p. 96.
15. Driscoll DJ, Mottram CD, Danielson GK. Spectrum of exercise intolerance in 45 patients with Ebstein's anomaly and observations on exercise tolerance in 11 patients after surgical repair. J Am Coll Cardiol 1988;11:831.

E

1. Ebstein W. Ueber einen sehr seltenen Fall von Insufficient der valvula tricuspidalis, bedingt durch eine angedorene hochgradige missbildung derselben. Arch Anat Physiol 1866;328.
2. Emanuel R, O'Brien K, Ng R. Ebstein's anomaly: genetic study of 26 families. Br Heart J 1976;38:5.
3. Engle MA, Payne TP, Bruins C, Taussig HB. Ebstein's anomaly of the tricuspid valve. Report of 3 cases and analysis of clinical syndrome. Circulation 1950;1:1246.

F

1. Fontana ME, Wooley CF. Sail sound in Ebstein's anomaly of the tricuspid valve. Circulation 1972;46:155.

G

1. Gasul BM, Weinberg MJ, Lendrum BL, Fell EH. Indications for and evaluation of surgical therapy in congenital heart disease. Prog Cardiovasc Dis 1960;3:763.
2. Gasul BM, Weinberg M Jr, Luan LL, Fell EH, Bicoff J, Steiger Z. Superior vena cava–right main pulmonary artery anastomosis. JAMA 1959;171:1979.
3. Gentles TL, Calder AL, Clarkson PM, Neutze JM. Predictors of long-term survival with Ebstein's anomaly of the tricuspid valve. Am J Cardiol 1992;69:377.
4. Genton E, Blount SG Jr. The spectrum of Ebstein's anomaly. Am Heart J 1967;73:395.
5. Giuliani ER, Fuster V, Brandenberg RO, Mair DD. Ebstein's anomaly: the clinical features and natural history of the tricuspid valve. Mayo Clin Proc 1979;54:163.
6. Glenn WL. Circulatory bypass of the right side of the heart: shunt between superior vena cava and right pulmonary artery. Report of clinical application. N Engl J Med 1958;259:117.
7. Goldberg SP, Jones RC, Boston US, Haddad LM, Wetzel GT, Chin TK, et al. Current trends in the management of neonates with Ebstein's anomaly. World J Pediat Congen Heart Surg 2011; 2:554-7.
8. Gueron M, Hirsch M, Stern J, Cohen W, Levy MJ. Familial Ebstein's anomaly with emphasis on the surgical treatment. Am J Cardiol 1966;18:105.

H

1. Hardy KL, May IA, Webster CA, Kimball KG. Ebstein's anomaly: a functional concept and successful definitive repair. J Thorac Cardiovasc Surg 1964;48:927.
2. Hardy KL, Roe BB. Ebstein's anomaly: further experience with definitive repair. J Thorac Cardiovasc Surg 1969;58:553.
4. Hornberger LK, Sahn DJ, Kleinman CS, Copel JA, Reed KL. Tricuspid valve disease with significant tricuspid insufficiency in the fetus: diagnosis and outcome. J Am Coll Cardiol 1991;17:167.
3. Ho SY, Goltz D, McCarthy K, Cook AC, Connell MG, Smith A, et al. The atrioventricular junctions in Ebstein malformation. Heart 2000;83:444-9.
5. Hunter SW, Lillehei CW. Ebstein's malformation of the tricuspid valve with suggestions of a new form of surgical therapy. Dis Chest 1958;33:297.

J

1. Jaquiss RD, Imamura M. Management of Ebstein's anomaly and pure tricuspid insufficiency in the neonate. Semin Thorac Cardiovasc Surg 2007;19:258-63.

K

1. Kanani M, Moorman AF, Cook AC, Webb S, Brown NA, Lamers WH, et al. Development of the atrioventricular valves: clinicomorphological correlations. Ann Thorac Surg 2005;79:1797-804.
2. Kastor JA, Goldreyer BN, Josephson ME, Perloff JK, Scharf DL, Manchester JH, et al. Electrophysiologic characteristics of Ebstein's anomaly of the tricuspid valve. Circulation 1975;52:987.
3. Keith JD, Rowe RD, Vlad P. Heart disease in infants and children. New York: Macmillan Company, 1958.
4. Kim S, Al-Radi O, Friedberg M, et al. Superior vena cava to pulmonary artery anastomosis as an adjunct to biventricular repair: 38-year follow-up. Ann Thorac Surg 2009;87:1475-83.
5. Kirklin JK. Christiaan Barnard's contribution to the surgical treatment of Ebstein's malformation. 1963. Ann Thorac Surg 1991; 51:147.
6. Kitamura S, Johnson JL, Redington JV, Mendez A, Zubiate P, Kay JH. Surgery for Ebstein's anomaly. Ann Thorac Surg 1971;11:320.
7. Knott-Craig CJ, Goldberg SP. Management of neonatal Ebstein's anomaly. Semin Thorac Cardiovasc Surg Pediatr Card Surg Annu 2007:112-6.
8. Knott-Craig CJ, Goldberg SP, Overholt ED, Colvin EV, Kirklin JK. Repair of neonates and young infants with Ebstein's anomaly and related disorders. Ann Thorac Surg 2007;84:587-93.
9. Knott-Craig CJ, Overholt ED, Ward KE, Ringewald JM, Baker SS, Razook JD. Repair of Ebstein's anomaly in the symptomatic neonate: an evolution of technique with 7-year follow-up. Ann Thorac Surg 2002;73:1786-93.
10. Komoda T, Komoda S, Nagdyman N, Berger F, Hetzer R. Combination of a Hetzer operation and a Sebening stitch for Ebstein's anomaly. Gen Thorac Cardiovasc Surg 2007;55:355-9.
11. Kumar AJ, Fyler DC, Miettinen OS, Nadas AS. Ebstein's anomaly. Clinical profile and natural history. Am J Cardiol 1971;28:84.

L

1. Lang D, Oberhoffer R, Cook A, Sharland G, Allan L, Fagg N, et al. Pathologic spectrum of malformations of the tricuspid valve in prenatal and neonatal life. J Am Coll Cardiol 1991;17:1161.
2. Lev M, Gibson S, Millar RA. Ebstein's disease with Wolff-Parkinson-White syndrome: report of a case with histopathologic study of possible conduction pathways. Am Heart J 1955;49:724.
3. Lev M, Liberthson RR, Joseph RH, Seten CE, Eckner FA, Kunske RD, et al. The pathologic anatomy of Ebstein's disease. Arch Pathol 1970;90:334.
4. Lillehei CW, Kalke BR, Carlson RG. Evolution of corrective surgery for Ebstein's anomaly. Circulation 1967;35:I111.
5. Long WA, Willis PW 4th. Maternal lithium and neonatal Ebstein's anomaly: evaluation with cross-sectional echocardiography. Am J Perinatol 1984;1:182-4.

M

1. MacLellan-Tobert SG, Driscoll DJ, Mottram CD, Mahoney DW, Wollan PC, Danielson GK. Exercise tolerance in patients with Ebstein's anomaly. J Am Coll Cardiol 1997;29:1615.
2. Mair DD, Seward JB, Driscoll DJ, Danielson GK. Surgical repair of Ebstein's anomaly: selection of patients and early and late operative results. Circulation 1985;72:II70.
3. Malhotra SP, Petrossian E, Reddy VM, Qiu M, Maeda K, Suleman S, et al. Selective right ventricular unloading and novel technical concepts in Ebstein's anomaly. Ann Thorac Surg 2009;88:1975-81.
4. Mann RJ, Lie JT. The life story of Wilhelm Ebstein (1836-1912) and his almost overlooked description of a congenital heart disease. Mayo Clin Proc 1979;54:197.
5. Marianeschi SM, McElhinney DB, Reddy VM, Silverman NH, Hanley FL. Alternative approach to the repair of Ebstein's malformation: intracardiac repair with ventricular unloading. Ann Thorac Surg 1998;66:1546-50.
6. Marino JP, Mihaileanu S, El Asmar B, Chauvaud S, Mace L, Relland J, et al. Echocardiography and color-flow mapping evaluation of a new reconstructive surgical technique for Ebstein's anomaly. Circulation 1989;80:I197.
7. Mathews JL, Pennington WS, Isobe JH, Gaskin TA, Dumas JH, Kahn DR. Paradoxical embolization with Ebstein's anomaly. Arch Surg 1983;118:1101.
8. Mayer FE, Nadas AS, Ongley PA. Ebstein's anomaly. Presentation of 10 cases. Circulation 1957;16:1057.
9. McCredie RM, Oakley C, Mahoney EB, Yu PN. Ebstein's disease: diagnosis by electrode catheter and treatment by partial bypass of the right side of the heart. N Engl J Med 1962;267:174.
10. McFaul RC, Davis Z, Giuliani ER, Ritter DG, Danielson GK. Ebstein's malformation. Surgical experience at the Mayo Clinic. J Thorac Cardiovasc Surg 1976;72:910.
11. McKay R, Sono J, Arnold RM. Tricuspid valve replacement using an unstented pulmonary homograft. Ann Thorac Surg 1988;46:58.
12. Misaki T, Watanabe G, Iwa T, Watanabe Y, Mukai K, Takahasi M, et al. Surgical treatment of patients with Wolff-Parkinson-White syndrome and associated Ebstein's anomaly. J Thorac Cardiovasc Surg 1995;110:1702.
13. Monibi AA, Neches WH, Lenox CC, Park SC, Mathews RA, Zuberbuhler JR. Left ventricular anomalies associated with Ebstein's malformation of the tricuspid valve. Circulation 1978;57:303.

N

1. Nagdyman N, Ewert P, Komoda T, Alexi-Meskisvili V, Weng Y, Berger F, et al. Modified repair in patients with Ebstein's anomaly. J Heart Valve Dis 2010;19:364-70.
2. Najafi H, Hunter JA, Dye WS, Javid H, Julian OC. Ebstein's malformation of the tricuspid valve. Ann Thorac Surg 1967;4:334.
3. Nawa S, Kioka Y, Sano S, Shirakawa K, Ozaki K, Beika M, et al. Surgical correction of Ebstein's anomaly by tricuspid valve replacement and its late problems. J Cardiovasc Surg (Torino) 1984;25:142.
4. Newfeld EA, Cole RB, Paul MH. Ebstein's malformation of the tricuspid valve in the neonate. Functional and anatomic pulmonary outflow tract obstruction. Am J Cardiol 1967;19:727.
5. Ng R, Somerville J, Ross D. Ebstein's anomaly: late results of surgical correction. Eur J Cardiol 1979;9:39.
6. Nihoyannopoulos P, McKenna WJ, Smith G, Foale R. Echocardiographic assessment of the right ventricle in Ebstein's anomaly: relation to clinical outcome. J Am Coll Cardiol 1986;8:627.

O

1. Ogus NT, Indelen C, Yildirim T, Selimoglu O, Basaran M. Pericardial patch augmentation of both anterior and septal leaflets in Ebstein's anomaly. Ann Thorac Surg 2007;83:676-8.
2. Okishige K, Azegami K, Goseki Y, Ohira H, Sasano T, Yamashita K, et al. Radiofrequency ablation of tachyarrhythmias in patients with Ebstein's anomaly. Int J Cardiol 1997;60:171.

P

1. Peterffy A, Bjork VO. Surgical treatment of Ebstein's anomaly. Early and late results in 7 consecutive cases. Scand J Thorac Cardiovasc Surg 1979;13:1.
2. Pham P, Hoyer A, Shaughnessy R, Law YM. A novel approach incorporating sildenafil in the management of symptomatic neonates with Ebstein''s anomaly. Pediatr Cardiol 2006;27:614-7.
3. Pocock WA, Tucker RB, Barlow JB. Mild Ebstein's anomaly. Br Heart J 1969;31:327.
4. Polimenakos AC, Reemtsen BL, Wells WJ, Starnes VA. Right ventricular exclusion procedure with total cavopulmonary connection: an alternative operative approach in adults with severe Ebstein anomaly. J Thorac Cardiovasc Surg 2008;135:1182-3.

Q

1. Quaegebeur JM, Sreeram N, Fraser AG, Bogers AJ, Stumper OF, Hess J, et al. Surgery for Ebstein's anomaly: the clinical and echocardiographic evaluation of a new technique. J Am Coll Cardiol 1991;17:722.
2. Quinonez LG, Dearani JA, Puga FJ, O'Leary PW, Driscoll DJ, Connolly HM, et al. Results of the 1.5-ventricle repair for Ebstein anomaly and the failing right ventricle. J Thorac Cardiovasc Surg 2007;133:1303-10.

R

1. Radford DJ, Graff RF, Neilson GH. Diagnosis and natural history of Ebstein's anomaly. Br Heart J 1985;54:517-22.
2. Ramsheyi A, D'Attellis N, Le Lostec Z, Fegueux S, Acar C. Partial mitral homograft for tricuspid valve repair. Ann Thorac Surg 1997;64:1486.
3. Rao PS, Jue KL, Isabel-Jones J, Ruttenberg HD. Ebstein's malformation of the tricuspid valve with atresia differentiation from isolated tricuspid atresia. Am J Cardiol 1973;32:1004.
4. Reemtsen BL, Fagan BT, Wells WJ, Starnes VA. Current surgical therapy for Ebstein anomaly in neonates. J Thorac Cardiovasc Surg 2006;132:1285-90.
5. Reemtsen BL, Polimenakos AC, Fagan BT, Wells WJ, Starnes VA. Fate of the right ventricle after fenestrated right ventricular exclusion for severe neonatal Ebstein anomaly. J Thorac Cardiovasc Surg 2007;134:1406-12.
6. Reynolds G. Ebstein's disease. A case diagnosed clinically. Guys Hosp Rep 1950;99:276.
7. Roberson DA, Silverman NH. Ebstein's anomaly: echocardiographic and clinical features in the fetus and neonate. J Am Coll Cardiol 1989;14:1300.
8. Roberts WC, Glancy DL, Seningen RP, Maron BJ, Epstein SE. Prolapse of the mitral valve is described in two patients with Ebstein's anomaly of the tricuspid valve. Am J Cardiol 1976;38:377.
9. Ross D, Somerville J. Surgical correction of Ebstein's anomaly. Lancet 1970;2:280.

S

1. Sarris GE, Giannopoulos NM, Tsoutsinos AJ, Chatzis AK, Kirvassilis G, Brawn WJ, et al. Results of surgery for Ebstein anomaly: a multicenter study from the European Congenital Heart Surgeons Association. J Thorac Cardiovasc Surg 2006;132:50-7.
2. Saxena A, Fong LV, Tristam M, Ackery DM, Keeton BR. Late noninvasive evaluation of cardiac performance in mildly symptomatic older patients with Ebstein's anomaly of tricuspid valve. J Am Coll Cardiol 1991;17:182.
3. Schiebler GL, Adams P Jr, Anderson RC, Amplatz K, Lester RG Clinical study of 23 cases of Ebstein's anomaly of the tricuspid valve. Circulation 1959;19:165.
4. Schiebler GL, Gravenstein JS, Van Mierop LH. Ebstein's anomaly of the tricuspid valve. Translation of original description with comments. Am J Cardiol 1968;22:867.

5. Schreiber C, Cook A, Ho SY, Augustin N, Anderson RH. Morphologic spectrum of Ebstein's malformation: revisitation relative to surgical repair. J Thorac Cardiovasc Surg 1999;117:148.
6. Scott LP 3rd, Dempsey JJ, Timmis HH, McClenathan JE. Surgical approach to Ebstein's disease. Circulation 1963;27:574.
7. Sealy WC. The cause of the hemodynamic disturbances in Ebstein's anomaly based on observations at operation. Ann Thorac Surg 1979;27:536.
8. Sealy WC, Gallagher JJ, Pritchett EL, Wallace AG. Surgical treatment of tachyarrhythmias in patients with both an Ebstein's anomaly and a Kent bundle. J Thorac Cardiovasc Surg 1978;75:847.
9. Senoo Y, Ohishi K, Nawa S, Teramoto S, Sunada T. Total correction of Ebstein's anomaly by replacement with a biological aortic valve without plication of the atrialized ventricle. J Thorac Cardiovasc Surg 1976;72:243.
10. Seward JB. Ebstein's anomaly: ultrasound imaging and hemodynamic evaluation. Echocardiography 1993;10:641.
11. Seward JB, Tajik AJ, Feist DJ, Smith HC. Ebstein's anomaly in an 85-year-old man. Mayo Clin Proc 1979;54:193.
12. Shigenobu M, Mendez MA, Zubiate P, Kay JH. Thirteen years' experience with Kay-Shiley disc valve for tricuspid replacement in Ebstein's anomaly. Ann Thorac Surg 1980;29:423.
13. Shina A, Seward JB, Edwards WD, Hagler DJ, Tajik AJ. Two-dimensional echocardiographic spectrum of Ebstein's anomaly: detailed anatomic assessment. J Am Coll Cardiol 1984;3:356.
14. Shinkawa T, Polimenakos AC, Gomez-Fifer CA, Charpie JR, Hirsch JC, Devaney EJ, et al. Management and long-term outcome of neonatal Ebstein anomaly. J Thorac Cardiovasc Surg 2010;139:354-8.
15. Silver MA, Cohen SR, McIntosh CL, Cannon RO 3rd, Roberts WC. Late (5 to 132 months) clinical and hemodynamic results after either tricuspid valve replacement or anuloplasty for Ebstein's anomaly of the tricuspid valve. Am J Cardiol 1984;54:627.
16. Simcha A, Bonham-Carter RE. Ebstein's anomaly. Clinical study of 32 patients in childhood. Br Heart J 1971;33:46.
17. Soloff LA, Stauffer HM, Zatuchni J. Ebstein's disease: report of the first case diagnosed during life. Am J Med Sci 1951; 222:554.
18. Starnes VA, Pitlick PT, Bernstein D, Griffin ML, Choy M, Shumway NE. Ebstein's anomaly appearing in the neonate. A new surgical approach. J Thorac Cardiovasc Surg 1991;101:1082.
19. Stulak JM, Dearani JA, Puga FJ, Zehr KJ, Schaff HV, Danielson GK. Right-sided Maze procedure for atrial tachyarrhythmias in congenital heart disease. Ann Thorac Surg 2006;81:1780-5.

T

1. Takayasu S, Obunai Y, Konno S. Clinical classification of Ebstein's anomaly. Am Heart J 1978;95:154.
2. Tanaka T, Yamaki S, Ohno T, Ozawa A, Kakizawa H, Iinuma K. The histology of the lung in neonates with tricuspid valve disease and gross cardiomegaly due to severe regurgitation. Pediatr Cardiol 1998;19:133-8.
3. Theodoro DA, Danielson GK, Kiziltan HT, Driscoll DJ, Mair DD, Warnes CA, et al. Surgical management of Ebstein's anomaly: a 25-year experience. Circulation 1997;96:507.
4. Theodoro DA, Danielson GK, Porter CJ, Warnes CA. Right-sided Maze procedure for right atrial arrhythmias in congenital heart disease. Ann Thorac Surg 1998;65:149.
5. Theodoro DA, Danielson GK, Warnes CA, Porter CJ. Ebstein's anomaly with associated Wolff-Parkinson-White syndrome: operative treatment. Circulation 1996;94:120.
6. Timmis HH, Hardy JD, Watson DG. The surgical management of Ebstein's anomaly. The combined use of tricuspid valve replacement, atrioventricular plication and atrioplasty. J Thorac Cardiovasc Surg 1967;53:385.

U

1. Ullmann MV, Born S, Sebening C, Gorenflo M, Ulmer HE, Hagl S. Ventricularization of the atrialized chamber: a concept of Ebstein's anomaly repair. Ann Thorac Surg 2004;78:918-25.

V

1. Vacca JB, Bussman DW, Mudd JG. Ebstein's anomaly. Complete review of 108 cases. Am J Cardiol 1958;1:210.
2. Van Arsdell G. Can we modify late functional outcome in Ebstein anomaly by altering surgical strategy? (editorial comment). J Am Coll Cardiol 2008;52:467-9.
3. Van Lingen B, McGregor M, Kaye J, Meyer MJ, Jacobs HD, Braudo JL, et al. Clinical and cardiac catheterization. Findings compatible with Ebstein's anomaly of the tricuspid valve. A report of 2 cases. Am Heart J 1952;43:77.
4. Vettukattil JJ, Bharucha T, Anderson RH. Defining Ebstein's malformation using three-dimensional echocardiography. Interact Cardiovasc Thorac Surg 2007;6:685-90.

W

1. Watson H. Natural history of Ebstein's anomaly of the tricuspid valve in childhood and adolescence: an international cooperative study of 505 cases. Br Heart J 1974;36:417.
2. Westaby S, Karp RB, Kirklin JW, Waldo AL, Blackstone EH. Surgical treatment in Ebstein's malformation. Ann Thorac Surg 1982; 34:388.
3. Williams JB, Karp RB, Kirklin JW, Kouchoukos NT, Pacifico AD, Zorn GL Jr, et al. Considerations in selection and management of patients undergoing valve replacement with glutaraldehyde-fixed porcine bioprostheses. Ann Thorac Surg 1980;30:247.
4. Wood P. Diseases of the heart and circulation, 2nd Ed. London: Eyre and Spottiswoode, 1968, p. 412.
5. Wright JL, Burchell HB, Kirklin JW, Wood EH. Congenital displacement of the tricuspid valve (Ebstein's malformation). Report of a case with closure of the associated foramen ovale for correction of the right to left shunt. Proc Mayo Clin 1954;29:278.
6. Wu Q, Huang Z, Pan G, Wang L, Li L, Xue H. Early and midterm results in anatomic repair of Ebstein anomaly. J Thorac Cardiovasc Surg 2007;134:1438-42.

Y

1. Yater WM, Shapiro MJ. Congenital displacement of a tricuspid valve (Ebstein's disease): review and report of a case with electrocardiographic abnormalities and detailed histological study of the conduction system. Ann Intern Med 1937;11:1043.
2. Yetman AT, Freedom RM, McCrindle BW. Outcome in cyanotic neonates with Ebstein's anomaly. Am J Cardiol 1998;81:749-54.
3. Yim BJ, Yu PN. Value of an electrode catheter in diagnosis of Ebstein's disease. Circulation 1958;17:543.

Z

1. Zuberbuhler JR, Allwork SP, Anderson RH. The spectrum of Ebstein's anomaly of the tricuspid valve. J Thorac Cardiovasc Surg 1979;77:202.

43 Truncus Arteriosus

DEFINITION

Truncus arteriosus (persistent truncus arteriosus, truncus arteriosus communis, common aorticopulmonary trunk) is a congenital cardiovascular malformation in which one great artery arising from the base of the heart by way of a single semilunar (truncal) valve gives origin to the coronary, systemic, and one or two pulmonary arteries proximal to the origin of the brachiocephalic branches. It is one of several diagnoses within the phylum of common ventriculoatrial junction (see http://www.ipccc.net/). A ventricular septal defect (VSD) is almost always present beneath the truncal valve.

This definition excludes those hearts in which there are no true pulmonary arteries and in which the lungs are supplied only by large aortopulmonary arteries (Collett and Edwards type IV[C7]), characteristic of tetralogy of Fallot and pulmonary atresia with absence of the pulmonary trunk and the central and hilar portions of the right and left pulmonary arteries (see "Morphology" under Tetralogy of Fallot with Pulmonary Atresia in Section II of Chapter 38). Excluded also from discussion in this chapter are hearts with a common arterial trunk but an intact ventricular septum.[A2] Whether hearts in which there is a VSD but no interventricular communication during diastole (because the semilunar cusps close against the crest of the ventricular septum) should be considered to have an intact septum is controversial.[A5,C2,D6,V2]

HISTORICAL NOTE

The first well-documented case of truncus arteriosus was reported by Wilson in 1798,[W4] and existence of the entity was confirmed by accurate clinical and autopsy reports of a 6-month-old infant by Buchanan in 1864.[B11] In the early literature, there was frequent confusion with a single arterial trunk and, although Vievordt clarified this aspect in 1898 (quoted by Victoria and colleagues[V3]), confusion existed as late as 1930 when Shapiro[S5] distinguished it from hearts with aortic and pulmonary atresia. Lev and Saphir proposed the basic morphologic criteria defining the anomaly in 1942,[L5] and in 1949 Collett and Edwards[C7] reviewed previously published cases and proposed a classification. An alternative classification was suggested by the Van Praaghs in 1965.[V2]

Surgical treatment was initially confined to banding of one or both pulmonary arteries.[A9,H6,S9] Intracardiac repair was first successfully accomplished in 1962 at the University of Michigan using a nonvalved polytetrafluoroethylene (PTFE) conduit; the patient was alive and well 11 years later.[B3] Experimental work using ascending aortic allografts including the aortic valve was reported from Japan by Arai and colleagues in 1965[A8] and by Rastelli and colleagues at the Mayo Clinic in 1967.[R2,S4] Before this, in 1966, Ross and Somerville had successfully used an ascending aortic allograft in reconstructing tetralogy of Fallot with pulmonary atresia.[R3]

McGoon and colleagues were the first to successfully repair truncus arteriosus using an ascending aortic allograft and valve conduit (cylinder) in September 1967.[M5,W1] Weldon and Cameron reported a successful repair in 1967.[W2] Binet used a xenograft valve incorporated within a polyester cylinder in 1971 (see discussion of paper by Moore and colleagues[M13]), and Bowman and colleagues reported use of a glutaraldehyde-treated porcine aortic valve in a polyester cylinder in 1973.[B8]

The first successful conduit repair in infancy was carried out in a 6-week-old infant by Barratt-Boyes in 1971, as reported by Girinath.[G3]

MORPHOGENESIS AND MORPHOLOGY

Morphogenesis

Deletion of chromosome 22q11 is present in a substantial number of patients with conotruncal abnormalities. About one third of subjects with truncus arteriosus have been found to have 22q11 deletion,[G4,M12] and many of these have additional characteristic features of DiGeorge syndrome, velocardiofacial syndrome, or conotruncal face syndrome. As such, their natural history and also their course following operation may be complicated by hypocalcemia, palatal abnormalities, learning disability, and other noncardiac problems.

Morphology

Truncus arteriosus is classified based on origins of the pulmonary arteries from the truncal artery (Collett and Edwards[C7]) and also on degree of development of the ascending aorta and ductus arteriosus in cases with a single pulmonary artery (Van Praagh and Van Praagh[V2]).

Truncal Artery

The arterial trunk (truncal artery) is larger than a normal aorta and is the only vessel arising from the base of the heart. It originates in part from both ventricles, but usually is more over the right than left ventricle.[B5,C8,T2] In an autopsy series of 56 cases, the trunk was equally balanced over both ventricles in 50%. In the remainder, it was either exclusively or predominantly over the right ventricle in 40% and over the left ventricle in 10%.[A1] In the unbalanced cases, the VSD was much more likely to be smaller (both shallower and narrower). From the truncal artery arise the coronary arteries and one or both pulmonary arteries.

Table 43-1 Site of Origin of Pulmonary Arteries in Truncus Arteriosus ($n = 202$)[a]

Site	No.	%
Single pulmonary trunk (I)[b]	140	69
Separate left and right pulmonary artery orifices close together (II)	41	20
Separate orifices at lateral aspects of truncus (III)	14	7
Common pulmonary orifice without a common trunk	4	2
Other arrangement	3	1.5

Data from Williams and colleagues.[W3]
[a]148 patients underwent repair.
[b]I, II, and III refer to approximate type of Collett and Edwards.

Pulmonary Arteries

The pulmonary arteries usually originate just downstream from the truncal valve on the left posterolateral aspect of the truncus artery, although their origin may lie truly laterally, truly posteriorly,[A6] or (rarely) anterolaterally (Table 43-1).[W3] There is frequently a single orifice leading into a short pulmonary trunk (type I of Collett and Edwards), which then divides into left and right pulmonary arteries that follow a normal course (Figs. 43-1 and 43-2). Alternatively and less commonly, the orifice is double, the left and right branches arising separately side by side (Fig. 43-3) or occasionally with the orifice of the left pulmonary artery superior (anterior) to the right rather than to the left of it (type II of Collett and Edwards). Types I and II merge into each other and are best considered together. They comprise the majority of cases[B5,C1,C7,C8] (89% of the Toronto surgical series).[W3]

Rarely, ostia of left and right pulmonary arteries may be widely separated and arise from opposite lateral walls of the truncal artery at either the same or different levels above the valve (type III of Collett and Edwards). This arrangement poses special problems for repair.[S11]

Occasionally, only one pulmonary artery originates from the truncal artery. The arterial vascular supply to the opposite lung arises either from a patent ductus arteriosus as a complete branch pulmonary artery or from large aortopulmonary collateral arteries, as in tetralogy of Fallot with pulmonary atresia.[M8,V1] When the left pulmonary artery is the one that does not originate from the truncus (or is absent), the right often continues to arise from the left posterolateral surface of the proximal truncal artery.[C1,V2] The term *hemitruncus* has been used to describe the condition of the common arterial trunk giving rise to only one branch pulmonary artery,[G7] but the term is more commonly used to describe the slightly more common "origin of right (or left) pulmonary artery from the aorta." In the latter, of course, there are two separate semilunar valves (see Chapter 45).

Stenosis of the origin of one or both branch pulmonary arteries is more frequent than absence of the origin; it is probably underestimated in autopsy compared with cineangiographic studies. It was noted in five clinical cases (10%) in one series.[C1]

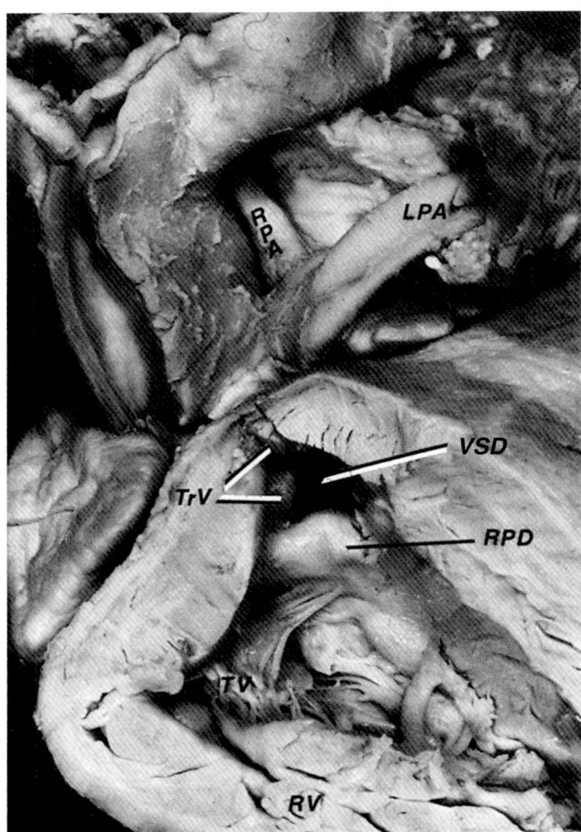

Figure 43-1 Autopsy specimen from 12-day-old neonate with type I truncus arteriosus. A distinct short pulmonary trunk arises from the left lateral aspect of truncal artery. Right ventricle (RV) has been opened, revealing its thick wall. Ventricular septal defect (VSD) lies immediately beneath truncal valve. Note that defect's lower margin is separated from the tricuspid valve (TV) by a prominent right posterior division of the septal band (trabecula septomarginalis). Infundibular septum is absent. Key: *LPA,* Left pulmonary artery; *RPA,* right pulmonary artery; *RPD,* right posterior division of septal band; *TrV,* truncal valve.

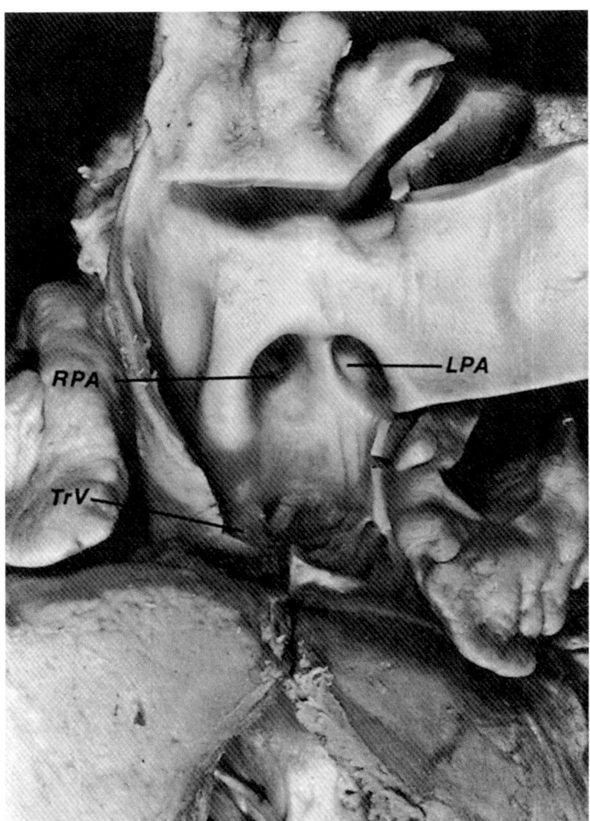

Figure 43-3 Autopsy specimen from a 4-week-old infant with type II truncus arteriosus. Proximal carina between left and right pulmonary arteries is well seen lying flush with posterolateral wall of widely opened truncal artery. Truncal valve (TrV) is quadricuspid with moderately abnormal leaflets, which clinically were considered to be both stenotic and regurgitant. Key: *LPA,* Left pulmonary artery; *RPA,* right pulmonary artery.

Figure 43-2 Autopsy specimen from 6-week-old infant with type I truncus arteriosus viewed from opened right ventricle and truncal artery. Truncal valve has three cusps of normal appearance. Orifice of pulmonary trunk arises from truncal artery close to the commissure between right and left cusps of truncal valve. There is lack of continuity between the right posterior division of septal band (trabecula septomarginalis) and ventriculoinfundibular fold, allowing tricuspid–truncal valve fibrous continuity at posteroinferior margin of ventricular septal defect (VSD). Bundle of His therefore lies along this edge of VSD. Key: *L,* Left cusp of truncal valve; *LAD,* left anterior division of septal band; *PA,* pulmonary artery; *R,* right cusp of truncal valve; *RPD,* right posterior division of septal band; *S,* septal band; *TV,* tricuspid valve, *VIF,* ventriculoinfundibular fold.

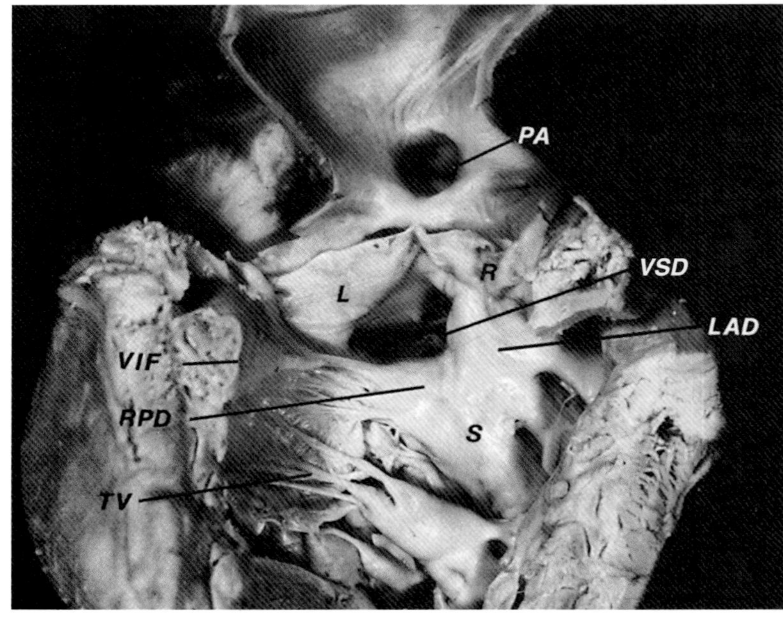

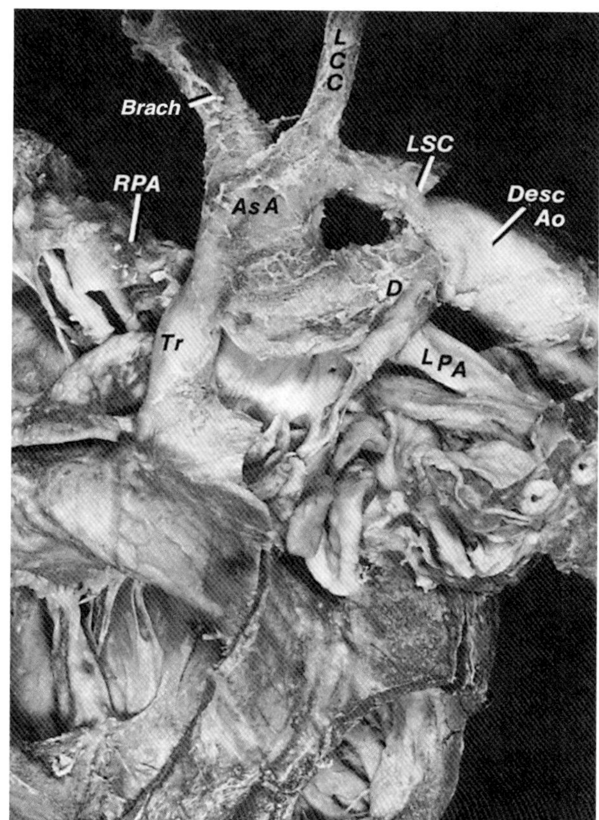

Figure 43-4 Autopsy specimen from 7-day-old neonate with truncus arteriosus (Van Praagh type 4). A large patent ductus arteriosus is similar in diameter to the descending aorta. There is also severe coarctation of the aorta consisting of a short, nearly atretic segment and a hypoplastic arch between left common carotid (LCC) and left subclavian (LSC) arteries. Truncal artery (opened anteriorly) is wider than usual with this arrangement. Origins of left and right pulmonary arteries (not visible in photograph) are widely separated. Key: *AsA,* Ascending aorta; *Brach,* brachiocephalic artery; *D,* patent ductus arteriosus; *Desc Ao,* descending aorta; *LPA,* left pulmonary artery; *RPA,* right pulmonary artery; *Tr,* truncal artery.

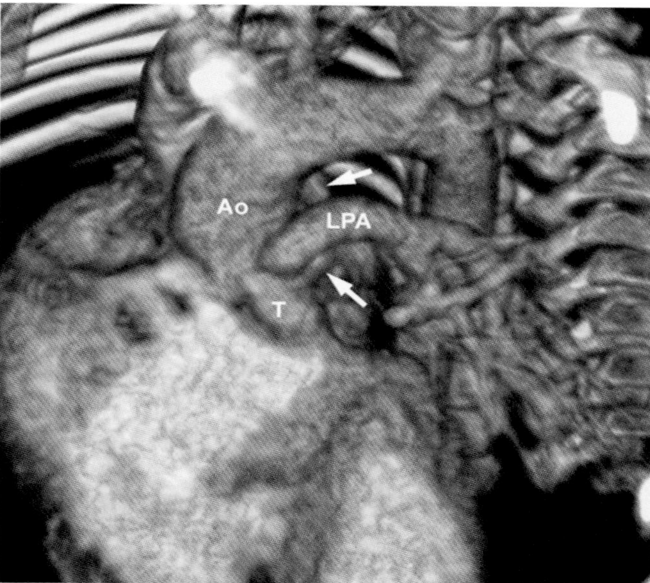

Figure 43-5 A volume-rendered image from a computed tomography angiogram of a 2-week-old neonate with truncus arteriosus, type II of Collette and Edwards. It shows that left and right branch pulmonary arteries *(arrow)* arise separately from the truncus arteriosus. Aorta is normal in appearance. Key: *Ao,* Aorta; *LPA,* left pulmonary artery; *T,* truncus.

Ascending Aorta and Ductus Arteriosus

In truncus arteriosus, there is reciprocal development between ascending and transverse aortic arches (arising from fourth aortic arch) and ductus arteriosus (arising from sixth aortic arch).[V2] Thus, in the majority of cases the ascending aorta is a direct continuation of the truncus artery and of about the same diameter (see Fig. 43-1), whereas the ductus arteriosus is usually entirely absent. Rarely a ductus is present with a well-developed arch.[M9]

By contrast, when the ductus arteriosus is present, the transverse arch is usually absent (interrupted aortic arch) and the ascending aorta is underdeveloped. The ductus is a direct continuation of the truncus artery, arching leftward to join the descending aorta (Fig. 43-4). In this situation, left and right pulmonary artery branches usually arise separately from superior and inferior (leftward and rightward) walls of the truncal artery (type III of Collett and Edwards). The ascending aorta now arises from the superior rightward aspect of the truncus artery as the relatively smaller branch. Usually the transverse aorta is interrupted beyond the origin of the left common carotid artery (type B interrupted aortic arch; see "Types" under Morphology in Section II of Chapter 48), or there is severe coarctation including tubular hypoplasia of the aortic isthmus and arch[T3] (see Fig. 43-4). This arrangement (Van Praagh type A4) was present in 12% of the cases of Van Praagh and colleagues and 14% (28 of 303) of the Toronto surgical series.[C1,W3]

Coronary Arteries

Orifices of the coronary arteries have a variable relationship to the sinuses of Valsalva above the truncal cusps (Fig. 43-5). A minority (≈20%) arise centrally (more or less normally) within the sinuses; about 80% (whether the usual two or a single orifice) are at the margin of the sinus or at the upper margin of a commissure.[S13] In at least a third of cases, one coronary orifice (usually the left) is displaced cephalad above the sinutubular ridge and must be differentiated from the pulmonary artery orifices at the time of repair. In about two thirds of cases, the left coronary artery arises from the left posterior aspect of the truncal artery, and the right coronary artery from the right anterior aspect in a position similar to normal.[A3,C6] Deviations from this pattern occur in the remainder of cases and include a single ostium (found in 18% of hearts reported by de la Cruz and colleagues[D4]), closely approximated right and left ostia, and small, slitlike, or stenotic and kinked proximal left coronary artery.[A3,B5,C8,L4,S6,V2]

Rarely, a coronary artery may arise from a pulmonary artery rather than the truncal artery; Daskalopoulos and colleagues report the circumflex artery's origin from the right pulmonary artery in a patient in whom pulmonary artery banding was not tolerated.[D2] The proximal part of the left anterior descending coronary artery is frequently displaced to the left of the interventricular sulcus and does not reach it until about halfway down the front of the heart. It tends to be small. Larger-than-normal diagonal branches from the

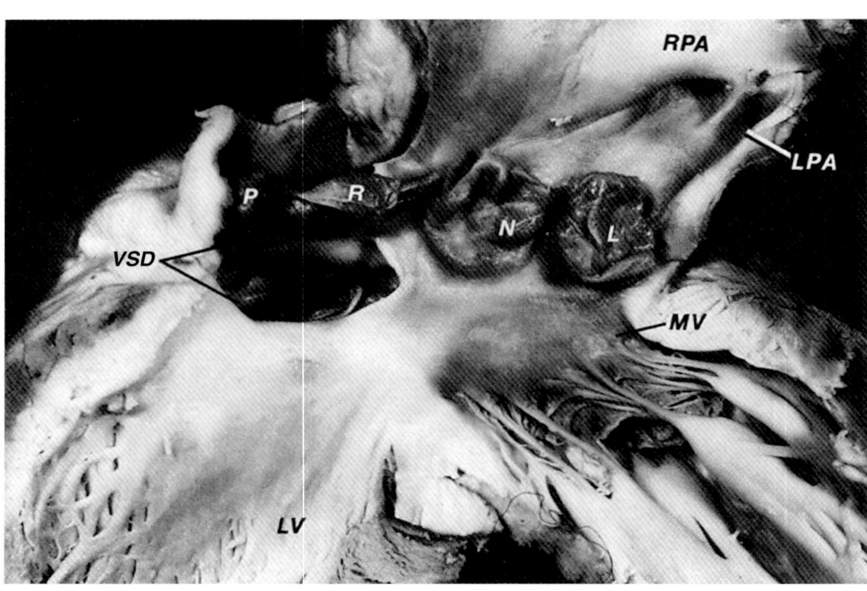

Figure 43-6 Autopsy specimen from a 3-day-old neonate with type II truncus arteriosus, in which the truncal artery and left ventricle (LV) have been opened to demonstrate fibrous continuity between anterior leaflet of the mitral valve (MV) and noncoronary (N) and left coronary (L) truncal valve cusps, as in the normal heart. Truncal valve is quadricuspid, with ventricular septal defect (VSD) lying directly beneath its right and pulmonary cusps. Key: *LPA,* left pulmonary artery; *P,* pulmonary truncal cusp; *R,* right truncal cusp; *RPA,* right pulmonary artery.

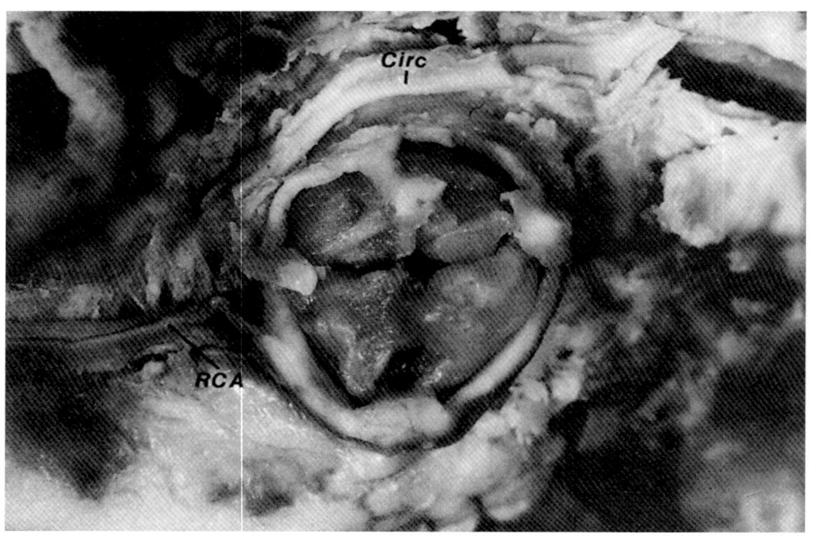

Figure 43-7 Autopsy specimen from 3-week-old neonate with truncus arteriosus showing a severely abnormal truncal valve viewed from above. The four cusps are thickened, nodular, myxomatous, and stiff. Clinically, the valve was considered stenotic. Key: *Circ,* Circumflex coronary artery; *RCA,* right coronary artery.

right coronary artery cross the anterior right ventricle inferior to conal branches, contributing to the blood supply of the upper interventricular septum and occasionally part of the left ventricle.[A3,B5] Damage to these vessels during surgical repair can seriously compromise the myocardium.[A3]

Semilunar Valve

The single truncal valve is posterior and inferior in position, similar to the normal aortic valve, although it points more anteriorly.[C1] There is fibrous continuity between its posterior cusps and the anterior mitral leaflet, as in the normal heart[C1] (Fig. 43-6). It has three cusps in half to two thirds of cases, and four cusps in most of the remainder.[S13] Rarely the valve is bicuspid. Not infrequently a raphe is present and partially divides a cusp into two, but it is doubtful whether there are ever more than four well-formed cusps.[V2] There may be variations in length and width of individual cusps, but in most patients who survive infancy, the cusps are well formed (see Figs. 43-2 and 43-6). However, in all cases, details of the structure of the truncal valve are different from those of the normal aortic valve.[S13]

In autopsy material, obvious severe myxomatous thickening of the cusps is present in a third of cases and is much more common in those dying as neonates (Fig. 43-7). Less severe myxomatous changes are present in two thirds of older infants (Fig. 43-8), and microscopic increase in thickness of the distal portions of the cusps is apparent in many more.[B2] Severe myxomatous changes often are associated with severe truncal valve regurgitation, and their frequency in autopsy specimens from neonates and young infants corresponds to the high prevalence of truncal valve regurgitation in neonates and young infants who develop severe heart failure or die. These morphologic changes are also reminiscent of those seen in congenital valvar aortic stenosis in the neonate (see "Morphology" in Section I of Chapter 47) and may make the valve stenotic.[B12,G2,L3,P3] Rarely, stenosis is contributed to

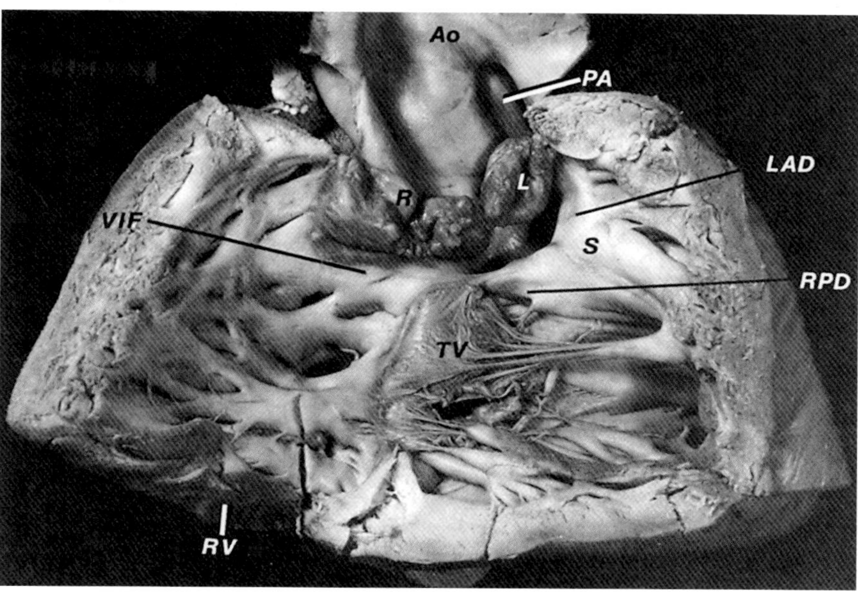

Figure 43-8 Autopsy specimen from 3-week-old neonate with type I truncus arteriosus. Truncal artery and right ventricle (RV) have been opened. Tricuspid truncal valve has severely abnormal cusps. A diminutive muscular ridge separates truncal and tricuspid valves at postero-inferior margin of ventricular septal defect. Key: *Ao,* Aorta (in fact, truncal artery beyond takeoff of pulmonary arteries); *L,* left truncal cusp; *LAD,* left anterior division of septal band; *PA,* pulmonary artery; *PT,* pulmonary trunk origin; *R,* right truncal cusp; *RPD,* right posterior division of septal band; *S,* septal band (trabecula septomarginalis); *TV,* tricuspid valve; *VIF,* ventriculoinfundibular fold.

by commissural fusion.[B2] A redundant truncal valve leaflet may obstruct the pulmonary trunk ostium during ventricular ejection when the ostium is proximally placed.[C1]

Ventricular Septal Defect

The VSD is high, anterior, usually large, and juxtatruncal in position. It is typically stated that the truncal valve forms its superior margin (see Figs. 43-2 and 43-6). Consistent with this observation is the fact that the infundibular septum is absent in truncus arteriosus, so there is no infundibular structure to form the superior margin of the VSD, leaving the superior margin to be formed by the valve itself. Another way to characterize the VSD is to describe it as *U shaped*—that is, with no superior margin. This perspective can be best appreciated if one examines a specimen with the truncal valve leaflets opened to the position they occupy during systole. Inferiorly and anteriorly, the VSD is bounded by the two divisions of the septal band (trabecula septomarginalis [TSM]) and posteriorly by the free wall muscle band that separates the semilunar from the tricuspid valve (the ventriculoinfundibular fold) (see Fig. 43-2).

Usually the junction of the right posterior division of the TSM and ventriculoinfundibular fold forms a muscle bridge that separates the defect from the tricuspid valve and right trigone (see Fig. 43-1) and therefore from the bundle of His.[B5,C4,C8,V2] Occasionally, this muscle bridge is absent (see Fig. 43-2) or poorly formed (see Fig. 43-8); the lower margin of the defect then approaches the tricuspid anulus, or the VSD becomes juxtatricuspid in position, in which case the His bundle is at risk of damage during repair.[B4] In these hearts, there may be fibrous truncal-tricuspid-mitral valve continuity. Part of the membranous ventricular septum may still be present at the posteroinferior margin of the VSD.

Right Ventricle

The infundibular (conal) septum is absent from the right ventricular outflow tract.[C8,V2] Contrariwise, it has been asserted that the infundibular septum can be recognized fused to the distal anterior (free) right ventricular wall; rarely, there is a persistent blind right ventricular outflow pouch in front of it.[V2] The right ventricle is nearly always hypertrophied and enlarged.

Left Ventricle

In contrast to the right ventricular outflow tract, the left ventricular outflow tract is relatively normal in hearts with truncus arteriosus (see Fig. 43-6), and flow from this chamber into the truncal artery is restricted only in the unusual situation when the truncal artery originates mainly from the right ventricle and the VSD is small. A pressure gradient demonstrable on catheter withdrawal from left ventricle to aorta in such rare instances will lie at the VSD level rather than at the truncal valve. Although a moderate-sized VSD is not restrictive before surgical repair, it may prove so afterward and thus may need to be enlarged at operation (see Technique of Operation later).

Associated Anomalies

The most common associated cardiac and noncardiac anomalies are shown in Tables 43-2 and 43-3. About 10% to 20% of patients with truncus arteriosus have coexisting interrupted aortic arch or coarctation with patency of the ductus arteriosus.[S1] Truncus arteriosus is rarely associated with atrioventricular discordant connection, situs inversus, asplenia or polysplenia, or dextrocardia. Double inlet ventricle is also rare,[V2] although mitral stenosis or atresia with left ventricular hypoplasia occurs.

Frequent total absence of the ductus arteriosus has already been mentioned together with association of a widely patent ductus arteriosus in patients in whom there is also aortic arch interruption or, less often, aortic coarctation or atresia. When hearts with aortic arch interruption are excluded, right aortic arch is as common in truncus arteriosus as in tetralogy of Fallot (25%-35%).[C1,V2] Anomalous aortic branch origins occur frequently, usually of the subclavian arteries (10%). A persistent left superior vena cava drains to the coronary sinus in about 10% of patients, and occasionally there is partial anomalous pulmonary venous connection. Patent foramen ovale is

Table 43-2 Associated Congenital Anomalies in Truncus Arteriosus Communis Patients

Anomaly	No. of Patients	Percent
Cardiac		
VSD	29	100
Truncal valve, regurgitation (mild/moderate)	15 (9/5)	51.7
Truncal valve, stenosis (mild/moderate)	8 (6/2)	27.6
Secundum ASD/PFO	11	37.9
Right aortic arch	7	24.1
Coronary anomalies	4	13.8
Persistent LSVC	3	10.3
IAA:	2	6.9
Type A	1	
Type B	1	
PDA	2[a]	6.9
Noncardiac		
DiGeorge syndrome	9	31
Hypocalcemia	3	10.3
von Willebrand disease	2	6.9
Hypothyroidism	1	3.1
Esophageal atresia + tracheoesophageal fistula	1	3.1
Anovestibular fistula	1	3.1
Other	4	13.8

Adapted from Kalavrouziotis and colleagues.[K1]
[a]The two patients with IAA are excluded.
ASD, Atrial septal defect; *IAA,* interrupted aortic arch; *LSVC,* left superior vena cava; *PDA,* patent ductus arteriosus; *PFO,* patent foramen ovale; *VSD,* ventricular septal defect.

Table 43-3 Associated Congenital Cardiovascular Anomalies

Anomaly	Patients	
	Number	Percentage
Major		
Truncal stenosis/regurgitation (severe)	7	12
IAA	6	10
Non-confluent pulmonary arteries	4	7
TAPVR	1	2
Minor		
Secundum ASD/PFO	15	25
Other (right aortic arch, coarctation, anomalous systemic-venous connection, DiGeorge syndrome	13	22
Other than three truncal leaflets	15	25
Coronary anomaly	6	10

From Brown and colleagues.[B10]
Key: *ASD,* Atrial septal defect; *IAA,* interrupted aortic arch; *PFO,* patent foramen ovale; *TAPVR,* total anomalous pulmonary venous return.

common, and atrial septal defect of moderate or large size is found in about 10% of patients. Mitral valve anomalies of various types are present with similar frequency. Other rare lesions include atrioventricular septal defect, double aortic arch,[C7] and according to Bharati and colleagues,[B5] tricuspid stenosis and (rarely) atresia.

Extracardiac congenital defects are not uncommon and may occasionally contribute to death. DiGeorge syndrome (thymic and parathyroid aplasia or hypoplasia) is known to be associated with truncus arteriosus.[F2]

CLINICAL FEATURES AND DIAGNOSTIC CRITERIA

Symptoms

Presenting symptoms are almost always tachypnea, tachycardia, irritability, and unwillingness to take either breast or bottle feedings during the early weeks of life, all manifestations of heart failure.[A4] Rarely, respiratory distress is aggravated by compression of the left upper lobe bronchus between an anteriorly placed left pulmonary artery and the posterior aortic arch.[C1,H1] Even more rarely, an aneurysmal truncal artery associated with interrupted aortic arch may severely compress the right main bronchus and produce total right lung collapse. Mild cyanosis accompanies these symptoms in about one third of cases but rarely is the presenting feature. By contrast, in those infants who survive for longer periods, recurrent respiratory infections, dyspnea, and failure to thrive are usually present, and cyanosis is more apparent secondary to rising pulmonary vascular resistance. Older children may occasionally present with increasing cyanosis (Eisenmenger syndrome) and fail to give a history of heart failure in infancy.

Physical Examination

On examination, signs of heart failure are accompanied by a jerky to collapsing arterial pulse produced by rapid runoff from the truncal artery into the pulmonary arteries. The heart is overactive, and a prominent left parasternal systolic murmur and often thrill are appreciated. There is frequently an ejection click coinciding with full opening of the truncal valve,[A10] and an apical gallop rhythm may be present, although it is surprisingly rare in neonates. An aortic early diastolic murmur (from truncal valve regurgitation) is highly suggestive of truncus arteriosus, particularly when it is accompanied by pulmonary plethora on chest radiograph and right aortic arch. The second heart sound is usually single but split in about one third of cases. A continuous murmur is noted occasionally and is most often due to stenosis at the origin of one or both pulmonary arteries. Important truncal valve stenosis is a confusing feature and usually results in diminished peripheral pulses accompanied by a harsh ejection systolic murmur and thrill, maximal in the right upper intercostal spaces.[B12,L2]

Chest Radiography

Chest radiography shows marked cardiomegaly as well as plethoric lung fields in neonates and infants. The pulmonary trunk segment is deficient (as in transposition), but a high origin or arching of the left pulmonary artery may be evident in older children as a "comma" sign on the left upper mediastinal border.[C1] A solitary right pulmonary artery arising from the left side of the truncus artery may give a similar appearance. The hemithorax may be smaller and vascularity less on the side of the "absent" branch pulmonary artery (when this lung is supplied by bronchial collaterals or by a relatively small patent ductus arteriosus). In truncus arteriosus with aortic arch interruption, the descending aorta is often prominent in the chest radiograph.[C1] In those few infants who survive without treatment, pulmonary plethora subsides, as does cardiomegaly, from increasing pulmonary vascular disease.

Electrocardiography

Electrocardiography (ECG) usually shows combined ventricular hypertrophy and a normal or slightly rightward axis, although left ventricular hypertrophy is usually dominant in the tracing (occasionally it is absent).[C1] P pulmonale can occur.[V3]

Echocardiography

Two-dimensional echocardiography can be diagnostic and is usually definitive, with infrequent occurrence of only minor errors[T7] (Fig. 43-9). It demonstrates a single vessel overriding the ventricular septum and reveals abnormalities in the truncal valve cusps.[A10,H2,P3] In addition, origins of pulmonary arteries can be predicted with some accuracy, and presence of major associated abnormalities, particularly interrupted aortic arch, can be determined.

Cardiac Catheterization and Angiography

Cardiac catheterization and angiography may still be performed in the occasional neonate or young infant to define the pulmonary arteries, and hemodynamic state when there is an atypical physiologic presentation, such as severe cyanosis, or when there is suspicion on echocardiography that the pulmonary artery morphology is complex (e.g., unilateral aortopulmonary collaterals). Magnetic resonance imaging (MRI) and computed tomography (CT) compete with traditional angiography when structural details and some physiologic details require definition (see "Computed Tomography Angiography and Magnetic Resonance Imaging" later). There is an absolute indication for catheterization in patients who present after 6 months of life to define the status of the pulmonary microvasculature.

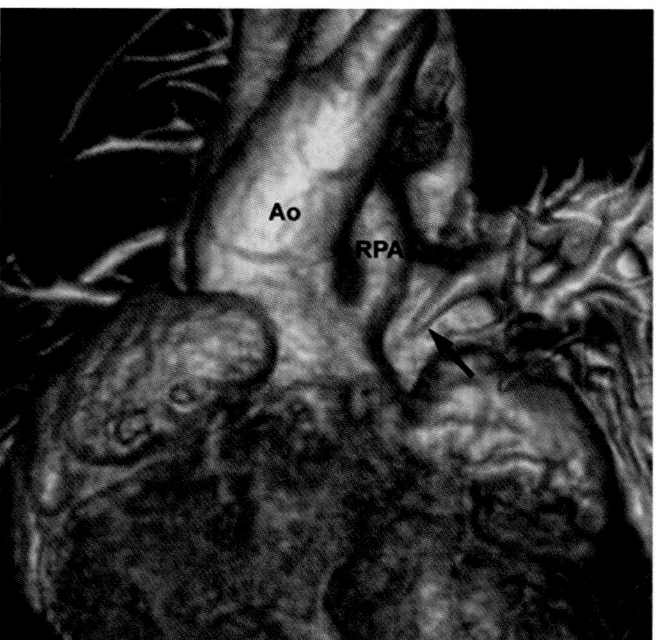

Figure 43-9 A volume-rendered image from a computed tomography angiogram of a 1-year old with complex truncus in which the right pulmonary artery (RPA) branch, but not the left *(arrow)*, arises from truncal root, coursing to the right lung posterior to ascending aorta (Ao). Left pulmonary artery has an atretic proximal component. Left lung is supplied by aortopulmonary collateral arteries.

In neonates and young infants with typical physiology, there is left-to-right shunting at the ventricular level with a high pulmonary-to-systemic blood flow ratio ($\dot{Q}p/\dot{Q}s$) and systemic pressures in the right ventricle and pulmonary artery. The high pulmonary blood flow keeps aortic oxygen saturation at 85% or more.[M2] Pulmonary vascular resistance is mildly raised (2-4 units · m^2). Atypical physiology may occur. Rarely, when the VSD is restrictive and the truncal origin is mainly from the right ventricle, left ventricular pressure may exceed that in the right. When there is truncal valve stenosis, there is a withdrawal gradient across it. The site of stenosis may be difficult to identify preoperatively. Pulmonary artery pressure is often slightly below systemic pressure, but it is importantly reduced when there is stenosis at the origin of one or the other artery.

The progressive rise in pulmonary vascular resistance that occurs in virtually all children who survive infancy is associated with a fall in $\dot{Q}p$ and therefore in arterial oxygen saturation. Arterial oxygen saturations less than 80% are usually an indication that pulmonary vascular resistance is beyond the operable range.[M2]

Cineangiography with contrast injections into both ventricles and ascending aorta demonstrates the exact site of origin of the pulmonary arteries and differentiates this lesion from patent ductus arteriosus. Special views are required to demonstrate the origin of right and left pulmonary artery branches to assess any proximal stenosis. Should one pulmonary artery fail to outline after routine contrast injections, the origin and distribution of the blood supply to the other lung must be identified. This is usually possible by injections into the upper descending thoracic aorta and its branches, defining either a ductus or large collaterals. In addition, a pulmonary vein wedge injection can be used to retrogradely fill true pulmonary arteries that fill either inadequately or not at all from an aortic injection.

These studies also provide information on alignment of the truncal artery and truncal valve with the two ventricles, truncal valve cusp thickening, and truncal valve stenosis or regurgitation. A bicuspid or quadricuspid valve may show doming in systole without stenosis being present. Site of the VSD is demonstrated, as are the two ventricles.

Computed Tomography Angiography and Magnetic Resonance Imaging

CT angiography (CTA) and MRI are not routinely indicated, but these imaging modalities may be indicated in specific circumstances in both neonates and older children. CTA provides excellent spatial resolution (Fig. 43-10). When echocardiography suggests complex pulmonary artery problems such as stenosis or discontinuity, but there is no concern about pulmonary vascular resistance, CTA can

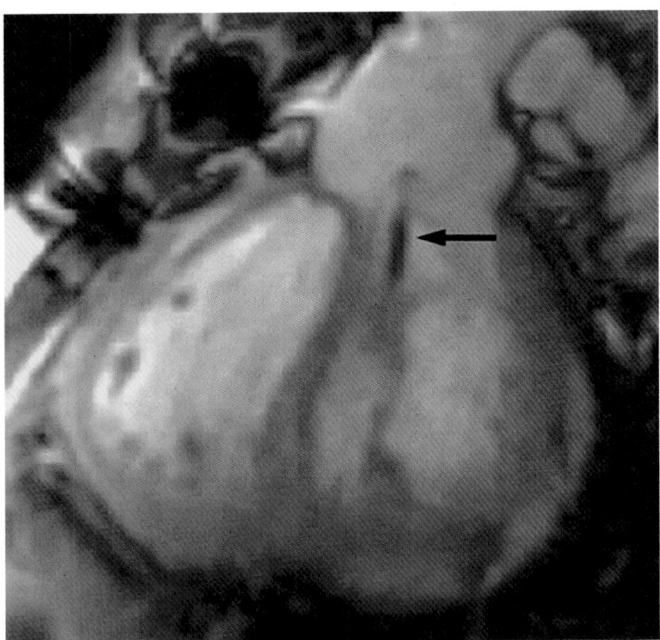

Figure 43-10 Bright-blood, steady-state free precession magnetic resonance imaging scan longitudinal to aortic valve in a 10 year old with repaired truncus arteriosus. Aortic regurgitation jet *(arrow)* is seen beneath truncal valve. Regurgitant fraction can be calculated.

define the morphologic details, and cardiac catheterization can be avoided (Fig. 43-11). MRI can quantify the regurgitant fraction of an abnormal truncal valve, providing objective data for longitudinal follow-up and decision making (Fig. 43-12).

NATURAL HISTORY

Truncus arteriosus is rare, occurring in 2.8% of cases of congenital heart disease in the cardiac registry report by Calder and colleagues[C1] and in 1.7% of the autopsy series of Tandon and colleagues.[T1] The natural history of patients with truncus arteriosus is unfavorable. No series follow a cohort of patients from birth, so exact data are not available. However, several studies when taken in aggregate provide an accurate estimate of survival without surgical treatment. Marcelletti and colleagues report on 23 cases prior to the era of intervention.[M3] Ten patients presented in the neonatal or infancy period (Table 43-4). Additional reports of autopsy cases by Calder and the Van Praaghs,[C1,V2] Collett, Edwards, and colleagues,[C7,F1] and Bharati, Lev, and colleagues[B5] imply similar mortality to the Marcelletti report. In two reports, the median age of death was 5 weeks,[C1,F1] and in another, two thirds were dead before reaching age 6 months.[C7] Similar statistics are available from the review of 357 cases by Fontana and Edwards.[F1] Bharati and colleagues report a

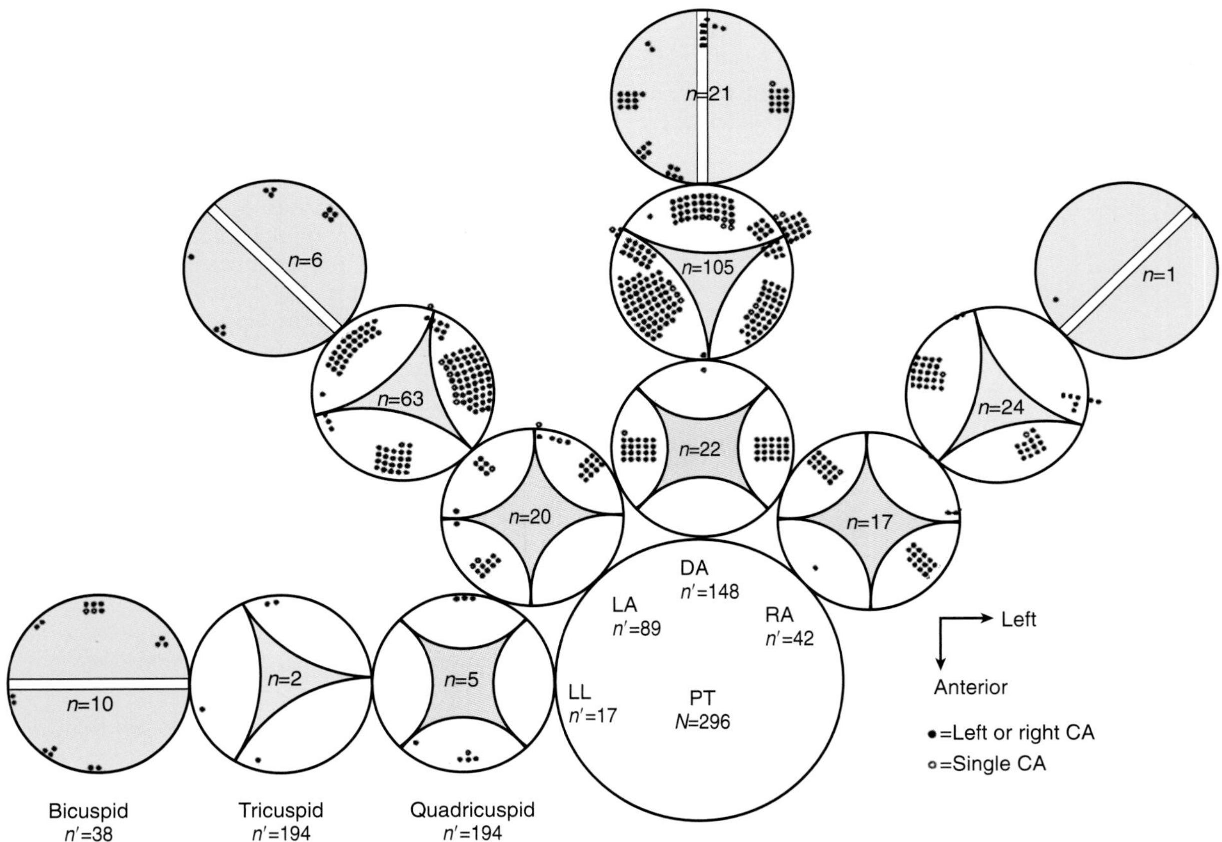

Figure 43-11 Position and rotation of trunk and coronary artery ostial positional variations in 296 cases of truncus arteriosus. For orientation, large circle represents position of a pulmonary root if it had formed. Trunk rotation places it in the left lateral (LL), left anterior (LA), direct anterior (DA), or right anterior (RA) position relative to the imaginary pulmonary root. Commissural positions for bicuspid, tricuspid, and quadricuspid valves are shown for each rotational position. Left and right coronary ostial *(closed dots)* and single coronary ostial *(open dots)* positions are shown relative to commissures. Key: *CA,* Coronary artery; *PT,* pulmonary trunk.

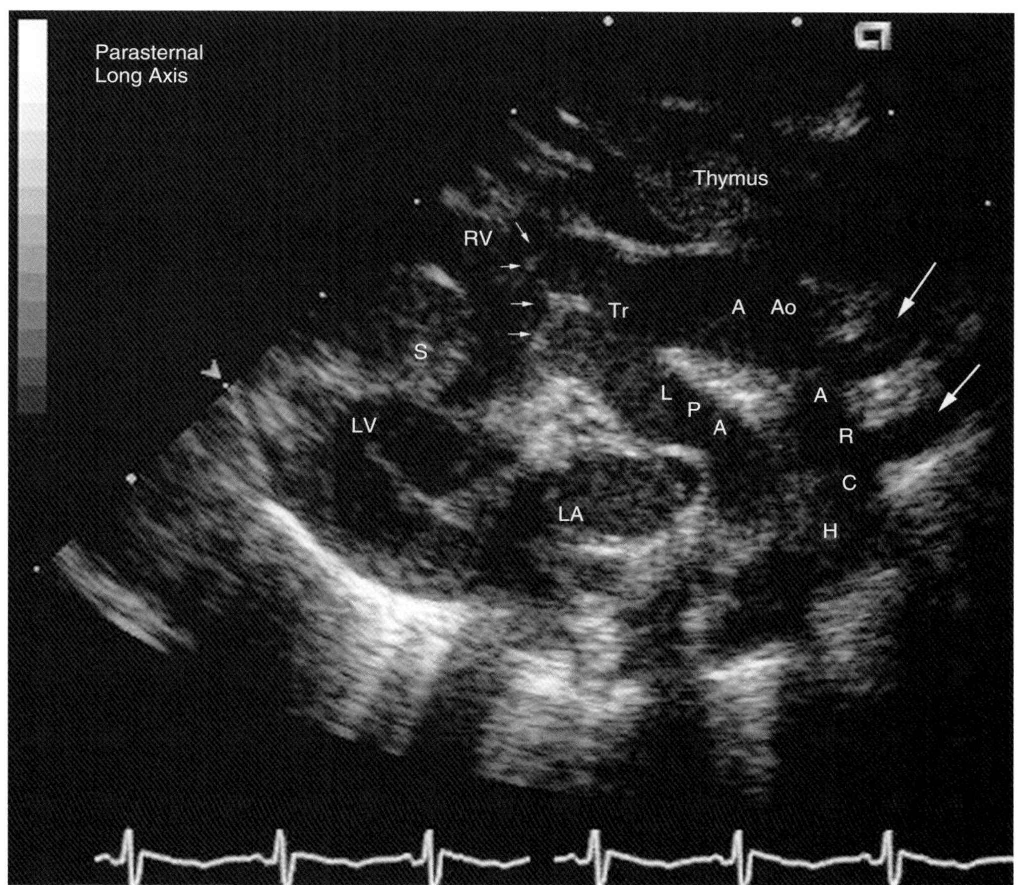

Figure 43-12 Parasternal long-axis echocardiographic view showing important morphologic characteristics of truncus arteriosus. Small arrows show thickened truncal valve overriding crest of intraventricular septum (s), with the ventricular septal defect evident above septal crest and below truncal valve. Left pulmonary artery (LPA) is seen exiting from left and posterior aspect of common trunk (TR). Large arrows identify arch branches. Coronary arteries are not well visualized in this view. Right pulmonary artery is out of the plane of this view. Key: *A Ao,* Ascending aorta; *ARCH,* aortic arch; *LA,* left atrium; *LV,* left ventricle; *RV,* right ventricle.

Table 43-4 Natural History of Truncus Arteriosus for Patients Presenting before Age 1 Year

							Death	
Case	Sex, Age at Diagnosis	Symptoms	Systemic O_2 Sat., %	Systemic Arterial Pressure, mm Hg	Rp, U m^2	Associated Defects	Time after 1st Exam	Cause
1	F, 8 days	HF, C	89	—	*	—	10 days	HF†
2	F, 2 mo	HF	90	85	*	—	Few days	HF†
3	F, 2 mo	HF	—	—	*	—	Few days	HF†
4	F, 3 mo	HF	—	—	*	—	Few days	HF†
5	F, 5 mo	HF	80	80	*	Mild TVR	1 1⁄12 yr	HF
6	F, 6 mo	HF	82	84	*	—	8½ yr	HF
7	F, 6 mo	HF	92	73	1.4	PDA, ASD	2 mo	Ventricular† & tachyarrhythmias
8	M, 8 mo	HF	90	—	*	—	Few days	HF†
9	F, 1 yr	HF, C	86	80	*	PDA, tricuspid regurg., LPA absent	1 mo	HF
10	M, 1 yr	Asymp.	91	88	7.0	—	12 yr	ARI

Adapted from Marcelletti and colleagues.[M3]
*Where no value is given, the pulmonary artery pressure was unknown.
†Autopsy performed at Mayo Clinic; specimen available.
Key: *ARI,* Acute respiratory infection; *ASD,* atrial septal defect; *Asymp.,* asymptomatic; *C,* cyanosis; *HF,* heart failure; *LPA,* left pulmonary artery; *PDA,* patent ductus arteriosus; *Rp,* pulmonary resistance; *Sat.,* saturation; *TVR,* truncal valve regurgitation.

mean age of death of 6 months in 177 cases.[B5] Other isolated case reports[C3,H8] confirm that some subjects, perhaps 10%, survive into adolescence or young adult life, but usually with severe pulmonary vascular disease.

Based on all these reports, about 50% of those born with this condition survive beyond the first month of life, 30% beyond 3 months, 15% beyond 6 months, and 10% beyond 1 year. There is little further mortality beyond this age until pulmonary vascular disease becomes severe and death occurs with Eisenmenger syndrome in about the third decade of life. Death in infancy is invariably due to heart failure, and when it occurs in the neonatal period, severe truncal valve regurgitation and large left-to-right shunt play contributing roles. The situation may be compounded by severe respiratory infection, as in other malformations with large left-to-right shunts in early life.

Longer-term survivors may occasionally succumb from infective endocarditis or cerebral abscess,[C7] but most eventually die from consequences of severe pulmonary vascular disease (see "Pulmonary Vascular Disease" under Natural History in Section I of Chapter 35). When pulmonary vascular disease develops during the first year of life or later (and it typically develops more rapidly than in patients with isolated VSD[M3]), the patient has a good chance of surviving at least into the teens, as is usually the case with Eisenmenger syndrome. Thus 7 of 10 Mayo Clinic patients with pulmonary vascular resistance greater than 8 units · m^2 at diagnosis before 1 year of age were alive (without treatment) 1 to 15 years (average 8.3 years) later.[M3]

Rather remarkably, a few patients survive infancy and early childhood without developing severe pulmonary vascular disease despite large left-to-right shunts.[J2] These patients probably represent less than half of those surviving beyond 1 year of age and less than 5% of all those born with truncus arteriosus.

Survival is adversely affected by severe truncal valve regurgitation,[E1] as noted earlier, or by truncal valve stenosis.[G1] Even in older patients, truncal valve regurgitation is present in 60% to 70% of cases.[H3] Regurgitation may be predominantly into the right ventricle. Survival is also adversely affected by coexisting interrupted aortic arch or coarctation.[V2] Survival is also less favorable when there are other associated severe lesions such as left ventricular hypoplasia and a small or atretic mitral valve, complete atrioventricular septal defect, or serious extracardiac anomalies.

Survival is favorably affected by pulmonary stenosis (narrowing at the origins of the pulmonary trunk or right or left pulmonary arteries). Four of the first 28 (14%) truncus patients repaired beyond infancy at the Mayo Clinic had naturally occurring pulmonary artery stenosis.[M6]

TECHNIQUE OF OPERATION

Repair by whatever technique chosen is usually performed during mildly to moderately hypothermic cardiopulmonary bypass (CPB) using a distally placed aortic cannula, one right atrial or two vena caval cannulae, and a left-sided vent placed through the right upper pulmonary vein. Although there is no technical reason to use deep hypothermia with either low-flow CPB or circulatory arrest, some surgeons prefer it. The branch pulmonary arteries are exposed and temporarily occluded with either nontraumatic microvascular clips or snares immediately after CPB is established.

Ideally, myocardial management is accomplished with cold blood cardioplegia using antegrade cardioplegia infused directly into the truncal root (also while the branch pulmonary arteries are occluded). When moderate or severe truncal regurgitation is present, the patient is cooled on CPB to the target temperature (or until ventricular fibrillation occurs spontaneously), the truncal root is clamped and opened, and cardioplegia is delivered directly into the coronary ostia (see "Methods of Myocardial Management during Cardiac Surgery" in Chapter 3). However, surgeon preference and morphologic findings may dictate other combinations.

Repair with Allograft Aortic or Pulmonary Valved Conduit

Following primary median sternotomy, a piece of pericardium may be taken and laid aside in a moist sponge. The proper-sized allograft aortic or pulmonary valved conduit (10-12 mm for a neonate, 12-14 mm for an infant) is selected, and its processing for insertion is begun (see Appendix 12A in Chapter 12 and Technique of Repair in Section II of Chapter 38).

Left and right pulmonary arteries are dissected in preparation for immediate temporary occlusion at the institution of CPB, as described earlier. The usual purse-string sutures are placed (see "Preparation for Cardiopulmonary Bypass" in Section III of Chapter 2), positioning the one for aortic cannulation as far downstream as possible so that the aortic clamp (placed proximal, or upstream, to the cannula) will be as far distal as possible on the ascending aorta.

Once CPB has been established and the pulmonary arteries controlled, cooling to the target core temperature is accomplished. The aorta is clamped and cardioplegia delivered. Snares on the pulmonary arteries are released, and repair is begun. The pulmonary trunk origin is detached from the truncal artery (Fig. 43-13, *A-B*); in truncus type II, an appropriate ellipse of truncal wall is included in the excision. The incision for detachment is begun on the left side, typically only several millimeters distal to the sinutubular junction of the truncal valve. The incision is initially made only large enough so that the interior of the truncal artery and valve, ostia of the coronary arteries, and orifices of right and left pulmonary arteries can be directly visualized. High origin of the left coronary artery should be distinguished from a pulmonary artery orifice. Detachment is then completed while viewing all these structures from within. The resulting orifice in the truncal root is closed with two rows of continuous 4-0 or 5-0 polypropylene sutures, using the second row to bring adventitia over the first row. This is done carefully to avoid distorting the coronary arteries or the truncal valve; a patch is often used for closure if direct repair risks distortion.

Alternatively, in some cases of truncus type I, the main pulmonary trunk may have enough length before it bifurcates into the two pulmonary branches such that it can be controlled directly rather than controlling the two branch pulmonary arteries individually. When this is possible, a vascular clamp can be placed across the base of the pulmonary trunk flush against the truncal root immediately upon the institution of CPB. When this is possible, the pulmonary trunk can then be separated from the truncal root, and the truncal root sutured at the clamp while the core cooling is taking

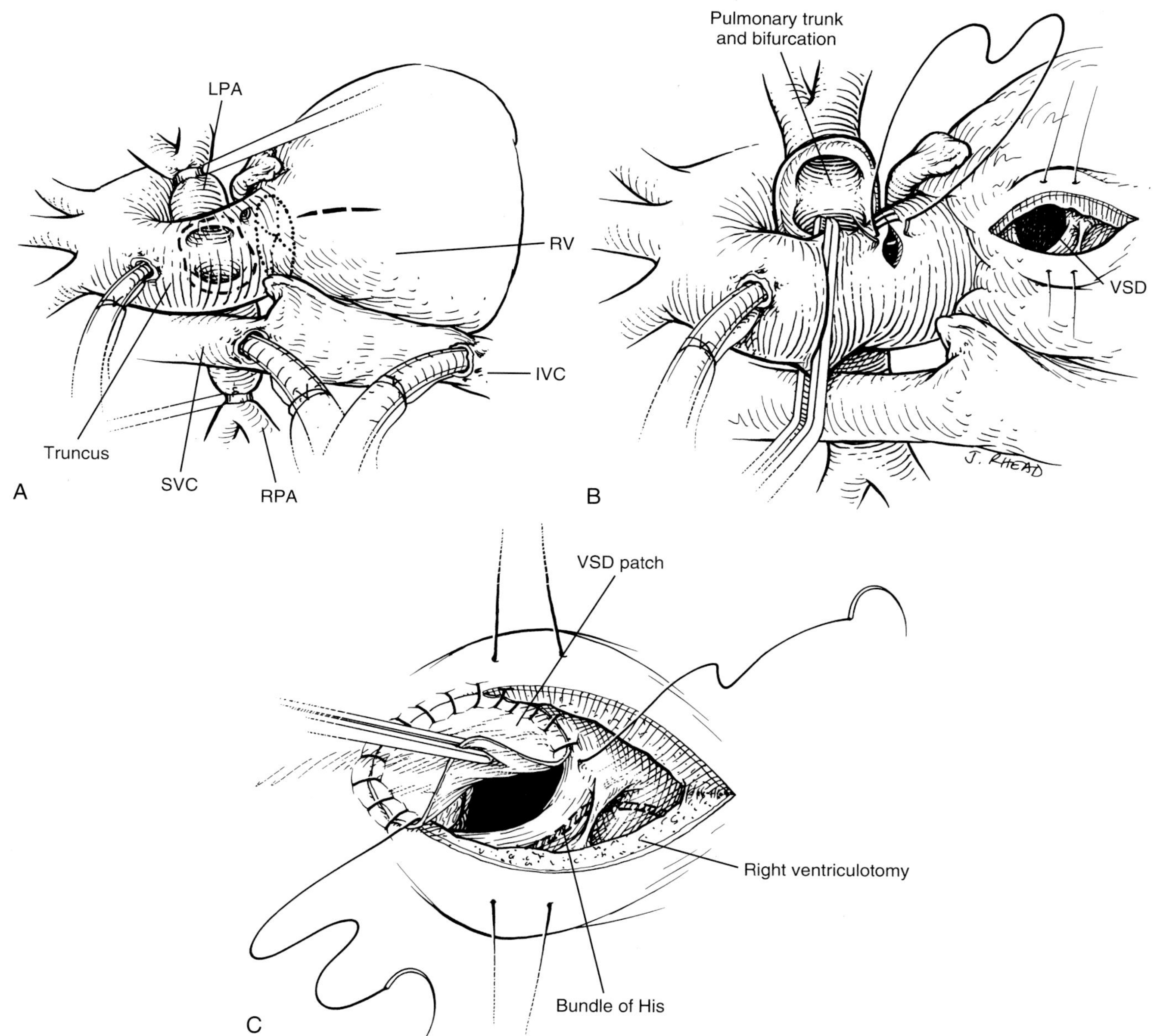

Figure 43-13 Repair of truncus arteriosus I, II with allograft valve cylinder. **A,** After establishing cardiopulmonary bypass and clamping the aorta, pulmonary arteries are temporarily occluded while cardioplegic solution is infused, and incision for separation of pulmonary trunk from truncus artery is begun. After looking through the incision and determining the precise origin of coronary and pulmonary arteries, excision of pulmonary trunk is completed. Dashed line represents proposed vertical right ventriculotomy. **B,** Pulmonary trunk has been cut away from truncal artery, and suture line in the latter is near completion. Distal end of pulmonary trunk is prepared for conduit. Longitudinal ventriculotomy has been made. Ventricular septal defect (VSD) illustrated is typical, with a band of muscle (see Fig. 43-1) separating it from tricuspid anulus. **C,** VSD is closed by suturing patch to edges of VSD, the atrioventricular node and bundle of His being away from this edge. Key: *IVC,* Inferior vena cava; *LPA,* left pulmonary artery; *RPA,* right pulmonary artery; *RV,* right ventricle; *SVC,* superior vena cava.

Continued

place prior to aortic clamping and cardioplegia. Thus, the subsequent period of aortic clamping can be substantially shortened.

When the pulmonary trunk or separately arising (but closely related) left and right pulmonary arteries arise from the posterior aspect of the truncal artery, they are excised as part of a large button of truncal wall. The opening into the truncus is closed with a patch. The distal end of the allograft valve cylinder is then anastomosed to the large button. Similarly, when widely separated right and left pulmonary arteries come off the lateral truncal walls at the same level above the truncal valve, they are excised along with a strip of posterior truncal wall or with the entire circumference of that part of the truncal artery. Excised origins of the pulmonary arteries and adjacent aortic wall are converted into a tube, to which the distal end of the allograft valve cylinder is anastomosed.[G6,S11] The transected truncal root is reconstituted by end-to-end anastomosis. Complete mobilization of the distal portion of the ascending aorta, arch, and brachiocephalic arteries should nearly always

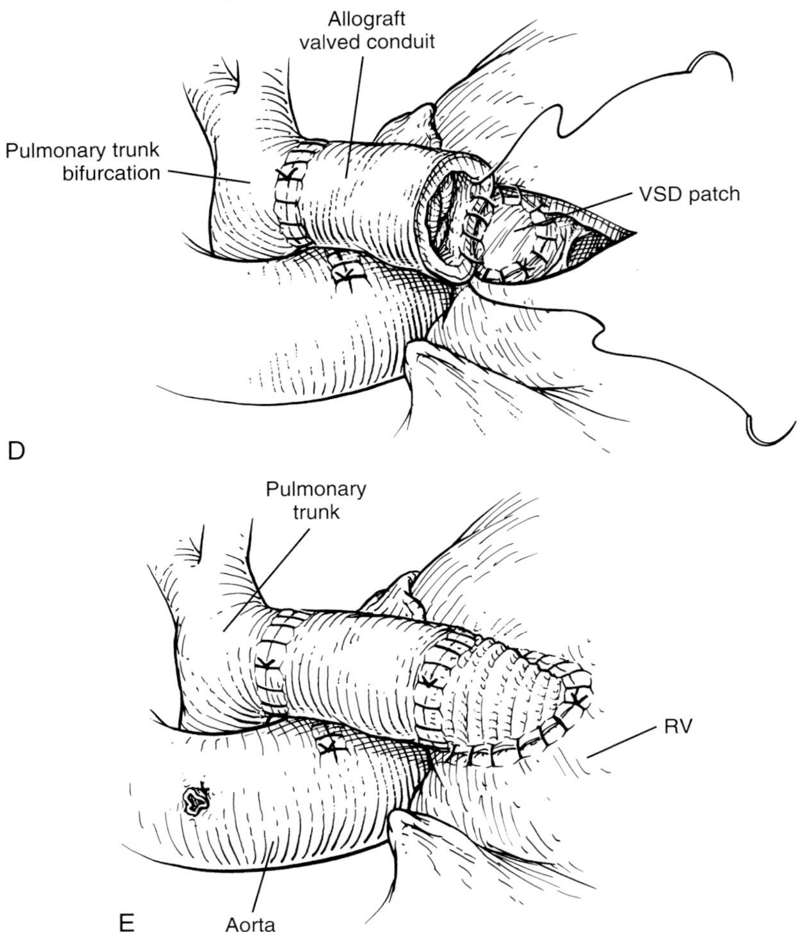

Figure 43-13, cont'd D, Allograft valved conduit has been anastomosed distally to pulmonary trunk. Posterior half of proximal anastomosis has been made. A small pericardial, polytetrafluroethylene, or polyester patch is trimmed and sutured into place to fill defect between allograft and right ventricular wall. Note that posterior proximal suture line incorporates upper portion of VSD patch suture line for additional purchase. **E,** Repair is completed using a triangular hood of pericardium or synthetic material.

allow direct anastomosis.[L1] The alternative of interposing a short segment of polyester graft is undesirable.[G6]

When widely spaced left and right pulmonary arteries arise from the lateral truncal wall at different levels above the truncal valve, pulmonary arteries are removed separately from the truncal root, each with a segment of surrounding truncal tissue. The branch pulmonary arteries are sewn together behind the truncal root to create continuity, using the extra truncal tissue to create a short tunnel that will be used to accept the distal aspect of the right ventricle to pulmonary conduit. The two separate defects in the truncal root are repaired with patches. A longitudinal right ventriculotomy is made just proximal to the truncal valve, essentially parallel to and to the right of the left anterior coronary artery; stay sutures may be placed for exposure. Alternatively, the opening may be enlarged to an oval shape by excising muscle from the anterior wall, leaving adequate tissue along the right and left sides so that neither the left anterior descending nor right coronary arteries will be compromised during subsequent suturing.

The VSD is repaired through the right ventriculotomy as described for tetralogy of Fallot (see "Repair of Uncomplicated Tetralogy of Fallot with Pulmonary Stenosis via Right Ventricle" under Technique of Operation in Section I of Chapter 38). However, in most cases of truncus arteriosus, there is a rim of muscle between the VSD and tricuspid anulus (ventriculoinfundibular fold; see Morphology earlier); this facilitates repair of the VSD, because sutures may be placed in this muscular rim posteroinferiorly without producing heart block or tethering the septal leaflet of the tricuspid valve (Fig. 43-13, *C*). If the VSD extends far posteriorly and is juxtatricuspid as well as juxtatruncal, the appropriate suture technique must be used (away from the rim of the VSD) (see Technique of Operation in Section I of Chapters 35 and 38).[B4] As in repair of tetralogy of Fallot with pulmonary atresia (see Section II of Chapter 38), the superior sutures may pass into the anterior right ventricular wall where it forms the distal margin of the circular VSD opening. If the lower margin of the VSD lies so close to the truncal valve that the left ventricular outflow tract would be narrowed following patch closure, the VSD is enlarged by excising a wedge of muscle from its anteroinferior margin. The defect is then closed with a polyester, PTFE, or pericardial patch in a manner similar to that used in repair of double-outlet right ventricle (see Fig. 53-13 in Chapter 53).

While the heart is still under cardioplegic arrest, the atrial septum is addressed if necessary. In most circumstances when a valved right ventricular outflow tract conduit is used, both secundum atrial septal defects and patent foramen ovales should be closed. If two caval cannulae are used for CPB, the cavae are snared at this point. If a single right atrial cannula is used, it is positioned into the inferior vena cava at this point. A right atriotomy is made. In the case of a single right atrial cannula, a cardiotomy suction device is positioned into the superior vena cava orifice. The atrial defect is then closed either primarily or with an autologous pericardial patch, as appropriate, using a continuous 5-0 or 6-0 polypropylene suture. The atriotomy incision is then closed.

Before placing the right ventricular outflow tract conduit, the aortic clamp is removed and core rewarming started. The allograft valve cylinder is then trimmed to an appropriate length. A conduit that is too long tends to kink the pulmonary trunk bifurcation or the back wall of the conduit itself. Either an aortic or pulmonary allograft valved conduit can be used; however, pulmonary is preferred in those requiring augmentation of the native pulmonary trunk bifurcation or stenotic pulmonary artery orifice.[H5]

If there is narrowing at the origins of the right or left pulmonary artery, the offending artery is opened longitudinally across the stenosis, and a tongue of allograft is left on the distal end of the conduit, widening this point. The distal conduit–to–pulmonary artery end-to-end anastomosis is constructed with continuous 6-0 or 7-0 polypropylene. The proximal end of the conduit may be anastomosed directly to the right ventriculotomy (Fig. 43-13, *D*). The posterior portion of the conduit suture line may also pick up adjacent edges of the VSD patch and right ventricular wall. A hood of pericardial or allograft arterial wall patch is usually needed to complete the anterior portion of the proximal attachment of the allograft to the ventriculotomy (Fig. 43-13, *E*). To avoid conduit valve compression or distortion and valvar regurgitation, the valve should be placed distal to its usual anatomic position, away from the back of the closed sternum. As this anastomosis is being made, rewarming is accomplished, and the remainder of the operation is completed in the usual manner (see "Completing Cardiopulmonary Bypass" in Section III of Chapter 2).

In neonates with typical preoperative physiology and in whom a post-CPB transesophageal echocardiogram shows normal left ventricular and right ventricular function, a right atrial volume and pressure monitoring polyvinyl catheter should be placed if one has not been placed preoperatively by the anesthesiology team. Pulmonary artery and left atrial catheters are not needed.

In older patients in whom pulmonary hypertensive episodes can be expected with a high likelihood, in patients with atypical preoperative physiology, and in those with reduced ventricular function by echocardiography post-CPB, a very important step is placing fine polyvinyl catheters in the left atrium, right atrium, and pulmonary artery by way of the right ventricle so that postoperative care may be rational, with particular regard for paroxysmal pulmonary hypertensive crisis. As for other repairs using right ventricular–to–pulmonary artery conduits, conduit reoperation may be expected in the future. Therefore, some form of pericardial closure should be considered, usually using PTFE pericardial membrane to protect the anteriorly placed conduit from injury during resternotomy.

Repair of Truncus I, II with Autologous Tissue for Right Ventricular Outflow Tract

Preliminary steps in the operation are the same as those already described, and mildly or moderately hypothermic CPB is established in a similar fashion. The snares previously placed around left and right pulmonary arteries are snugged down, cooling of the patient is begun, the aorta is clamped and cold cardioplegia given, the left side of the heart is vented via the right upper pulmonary vein, and the snares are removed.

A longitudinal incision is made into the anterosuperior aspect of the left pulmonary artery and extended inferiorly into the truncal root toward the left sinus of Valsalva (Fig. 43-14, *A*). The interior of the truncal root is inspected through the incision, and orifices of left and right pulmonary arteries, coronary ostia (particularly that of the left coronary artery), and truncal valve cusps are identified. A woven polyester, PTFE, or pericardial patch (with or without immersion in glutaraldehyde) is then sewn into place to partition the truncal root into aortic and pulmonary trunks (Fig. 43-14, *B*).

A vertical incision is made into the right ventricle, extending it nearly to the truncal wall over the left-sided sinus of Valsalva. The VSD is repaired. The posterior wall of the right ventricular–pulmonary trunk pathway is created by suturing the inferior flap of the initial left pulmonary artery/truncal root incision to the superior aspect of the right ventricular borders of the ventriculotomy (Fig. 43-14, *C*). The anterior wall is created by suturing into place a patch of autologous or bovine pericardium or synthetic material (Fig. 43-14, *D*). Barbero-Marcial, the innovator of this method, uses a bovine pericardial patch, to the undersurface of which has been attached a bovine pericardial monocuspid valve.[B1] The remainder of operation is completed in the usual manner.

When the pulmonary trunk or separate but closely related left and right pulmonary arteries arise from the posterior aspect of the truncal artery, excision is as described in the previous section. A modification of the technique may then be necessary because of the distance between the opening into the pulmonary arteries and right ventriculotomy.[B1] In this modification, the left atrial appendage is interposed to create the posterior wall of the right ventricular–pulmonary arterial pathway (Fig. 43-15).

Repair of Truncus with Single Branch Pulmonary Artery Arising from Truncal Root

Morphology of this lesion is highly variable, and experience with each type is limited.[M8] If the lung that does not have an arterial connection to the truncal root is supplied by a true branch pulmonary artery connected to a ductus arteriosus, single-stage neonatal repair is recommended. The technique of creating pulmonary artery continuity is similar to that described previously for widely separated branch pulmonary arteries that arise at different levels above the truncal valve. Care must be taken to eliminate the ductal tissue from the anastomosis.

If the lung that does not have an arterial connection to the truncal root is supplied by aortopulmonary collaterals, several options are available. If the collaterals are few and

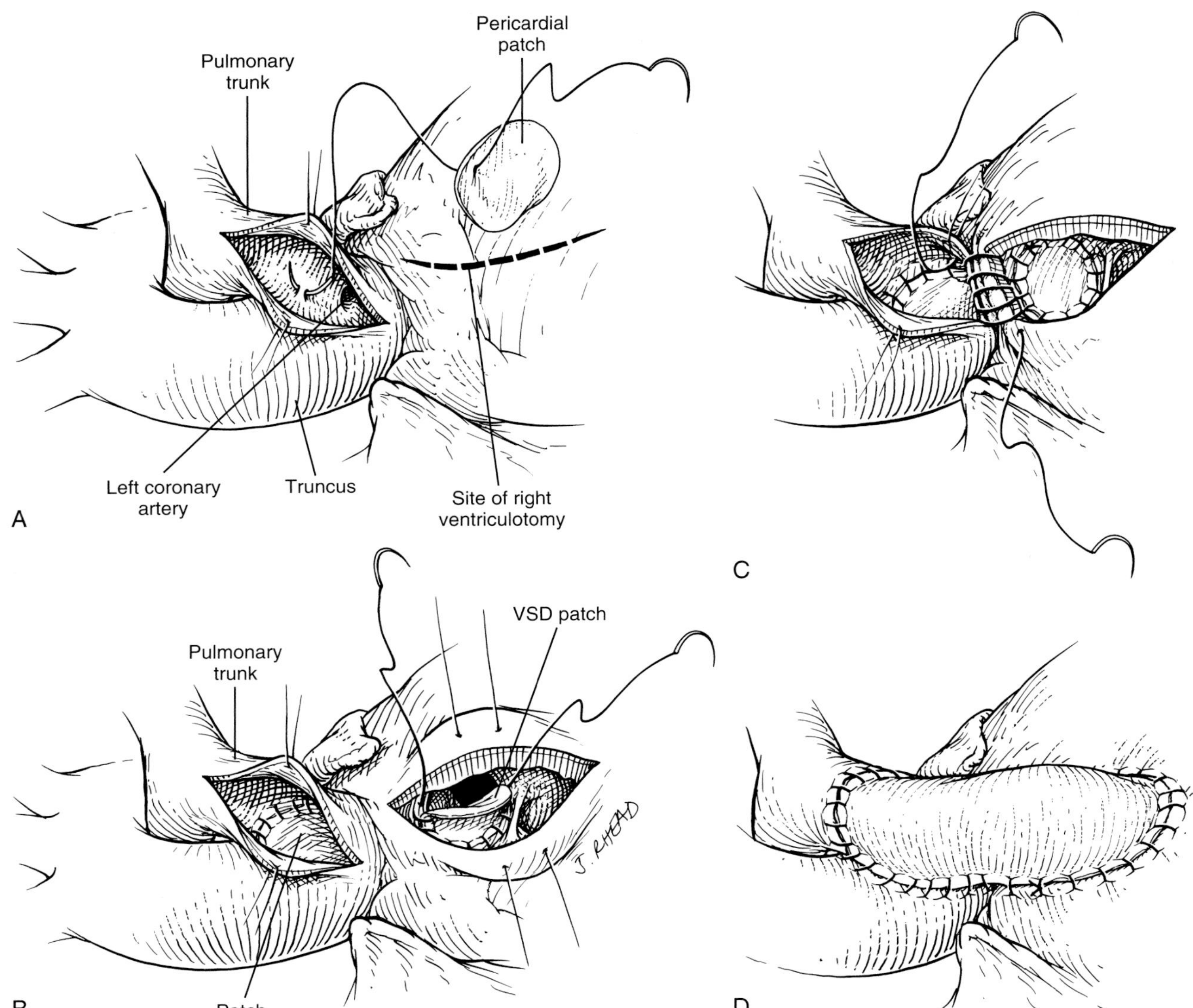

Figure 43-14 Repair of truncus arteriosus I, II with autologous tissue (Barbero-Marcial and colleagues[B1]). **A,** Incision is made into pulmonary trunk and adjacent portion of truncal artery. Proposed right ventriculotomy *(dashed line)* begins just beneath left side of sinuses of Valsalva and extends downward and slightly leftward, avoiding (inasmuch as possible) large diagonal branches of right coronary artery. Usually the incision opens widely after stay sutures are placed, but if it does not, some free right ventricular wall may be excised. **B,** Patch is placed to separate completely neoaorta from neopulmonary trunk. Illustration shows that the patch is placed clearly on the pulmonary trunk side of cusps of neoaortic valve and coronary ostia (i.e., anteriorly). After separating neopulmonary artery from truncus (now neoaorta) the ventricular septal defect (VSD) is closed with a patch. **C,** Inferior aspect of original "truncal" incision is attached to upper portion of right ventriculotomy using fine polypropylene suture. **D,** A roof is placed on the opening with essentially the same technique and materials used for inserting a transanular patch in repair of tetralogy of Fallot (see "Decision and Technique for Transanular Patching" under Technique of Operation in Section I of Chapter 38). NOTE: Barbero-Marcial places a monocusp valve in the outflow patch that closes against the posterior suture line between pulmonary trunk and right ventricle.

large, unifocalization and complete repair in one stage is preferred. The technique of unifocalization is similar to that described for single-stage unifocalization using a median sternotomy (see Chapter 38). The unifocalized lung arterial supply is then made continuous with the "normal" pulmonary artery from the opposite lung, and intracardiac repair is accomplished. If the collaterals are multiple and complex, an initial thoracotomy is performed to unifocalize the arterial supply and create a vascular hilar confluence in the affected lung. The unifocalized vessel is then connected to a systemic-to–pulmonary artery shunt.

At a second-stage procedure through a median sternotomy—which can be performed days to weeks later—vascular continuity of the two lungs is created and intracardiac repair performed. After taking down the previously created shunt and removing the pulmonary artery from the truncal root, the right and left pulmonary arteries are made confluent with each other behind the truncal artery, either by direct anastomosis or with interposition of an autologous pericardial tube. After the VSD has been repaired, a valved conduit is interposed between the confluent pulmonary and right ventriculotomy.

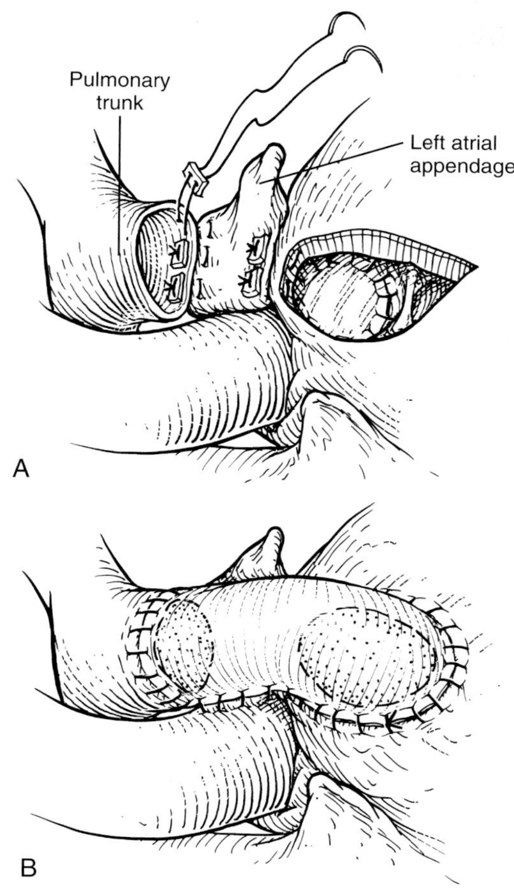

Figure 43-15 Barbero-Marcial's modification of autologous tissue method for use when opening into pulmonary arteries is far removed from right ventriculotomy.[B1] **A,** Creation of posterior wall of right ventricular–pulmonary arterial pathway by interposing left atrial appendage. Pulmonary arteries have previously been disconnected from aorta in some manner, often with end-to-end anastomosis for reconstruction of pulmonary arteries. **B,** Completed pathway, using a pericardial or synthetic patch for roof.

Repair of Truncus Arteriosus with Interrupted Arch

One-stage repair from the anterior approach is the preferred procedure.[D3,D7,F3,G5,S1,S2,S3] We recommend using extracorporeal circulatory management without circulatory arrest. After standard exposure through a median sternotomy, the thymus gland is subtotally resected and the pericardium opened. The great vessels are dissected above the brachiocephalic vein into the base of the neck, providing full exposure of the brachiocephalic artery. A purse-string suture is placed in the midportion of the brachiocephalic artery in preparation for arterial cannulation (Fig. 43-16, *A-B*). Purse-string sutures are placed in the superior and inferior venae cavae for venous cannulation and in the right upper pulmonary vein in preparation for left-sided venting. Depending on patient size, either a 6F or 8F arterial cannula is used to perfuse the systemic circulation through the brachiocephalic artery. Bicaval cannulation with appropriately sized right-angled venous cannulae is also performed.

Once CPB is initiated, the two branch pulmonary arteries are temporarily occluded with either snares or vascular clamps, allowing perfusion of the lower body through the ductus arteriosus. After a core body temperature of 25°C is achieved, the ductus arteriosus is ligated and divided just distal to the left branch pulmonary artery origin, and perfusion flow is reduced to 30 to 40 $mL \cdot kg^{-1} \cdot min^{-1}$, effectively establishing antegrade selective cerebral perfusion. The aorta is clamped and cardioplegia introduced into the aortic root. Caval snares are tightened to provide occlusive venous return, and a vent is placed through the right upper pulmonary vein purse string, across the mitral valve, and into the left ventricle.

The distal ductus arteriosus and proximal descending aorta are dissected to the second set of intercostal vessels, and a curved vascular clamp is placed on the descending aorta to prevent backbleeding. All ductal tissue is resected from the descending aorta. The aortic clamp is then adjusted by moving it superiorly to allow arterial perfusion to the brachiocephalic and left carotid arteries while leaving the ascending aorta available for aortic arch reconstruction. This is achieved by placing the aortic clamp in a slightly oblique position as shown in Fig. 43-16, *C*.

Arch reconstruction as shown in Fig. 43-16, *C* and *D* is performed, using the left subclavian artery to establish arch continuity. The pulmonary trunk confluence is removed from the side of the common trunk in standard fashion. The ascending aorta is then incised from the opening in the truncal root that resulted from removing the pulmonary arteries, up to the arch. The ascending aorta, arch, and proximal descending aorta are augmented with a patch similar in length and shape to the patch used in stage-one reconstruction for patients with hypoplastic left heart physiology (see Chapter 49).

Alternatively, a direct descending-to-ascending aortic anastomosis can be performed. In this case, an appropriately sized incision is made in the left posterolateral aspect of the ascending aorta to accommodate the diameter of the descending aorta. A primary end-to-side anastomosis of the descending aorta to the ascending aorta is done (Fig. 43-16, *F*) using a nonabsorbable monofilament suture.

Once the arch repair is completed, the aortic clamp is repositioned at the mid–ascending aorta, reestablishing total body perfusion, and perfusion flow rate is increased appropriately. Additional doses of cardioplegia are given through the aortic root as appropriate every 20 to 25 minutes.

The cardiac portion of the repair is performed in standard fashion through a right ventricular infundibular incision, with patch closure of the VSD, assessment of the atrial septum with maintenance of a competent foramen ovale, and placement of a right ventricle–to–pulmonary trunk valved allograft conduit (Fig. 43-16, *E*). Rewarming and separation from CPB are performed in standard fashion (see "Completing Cardiopulmonary Bypass" in Section III of Chapter 2).

An alternative approach is to use hypothermic circulatory arrest. The aortic cannula is placed distally into the ascending aorta, and a single venous cannula is placed into the right atrium at its junction with the inferior vena cava. Two periods of hypothermic circulatory arrest are used: to reconstruct the aortic arch and again to close the VSD (although the second period of arrest is not uniformly necessary).

Using either technique just described, it is imperative to achieve adequate resection of ductal tissue so that later anastomotic stenosis in the arch does not occur. When primary descending-to-ascending aortic anastomosis is used, the connection is made as distally on the arch as possible to prevent compression of the left bronchus.

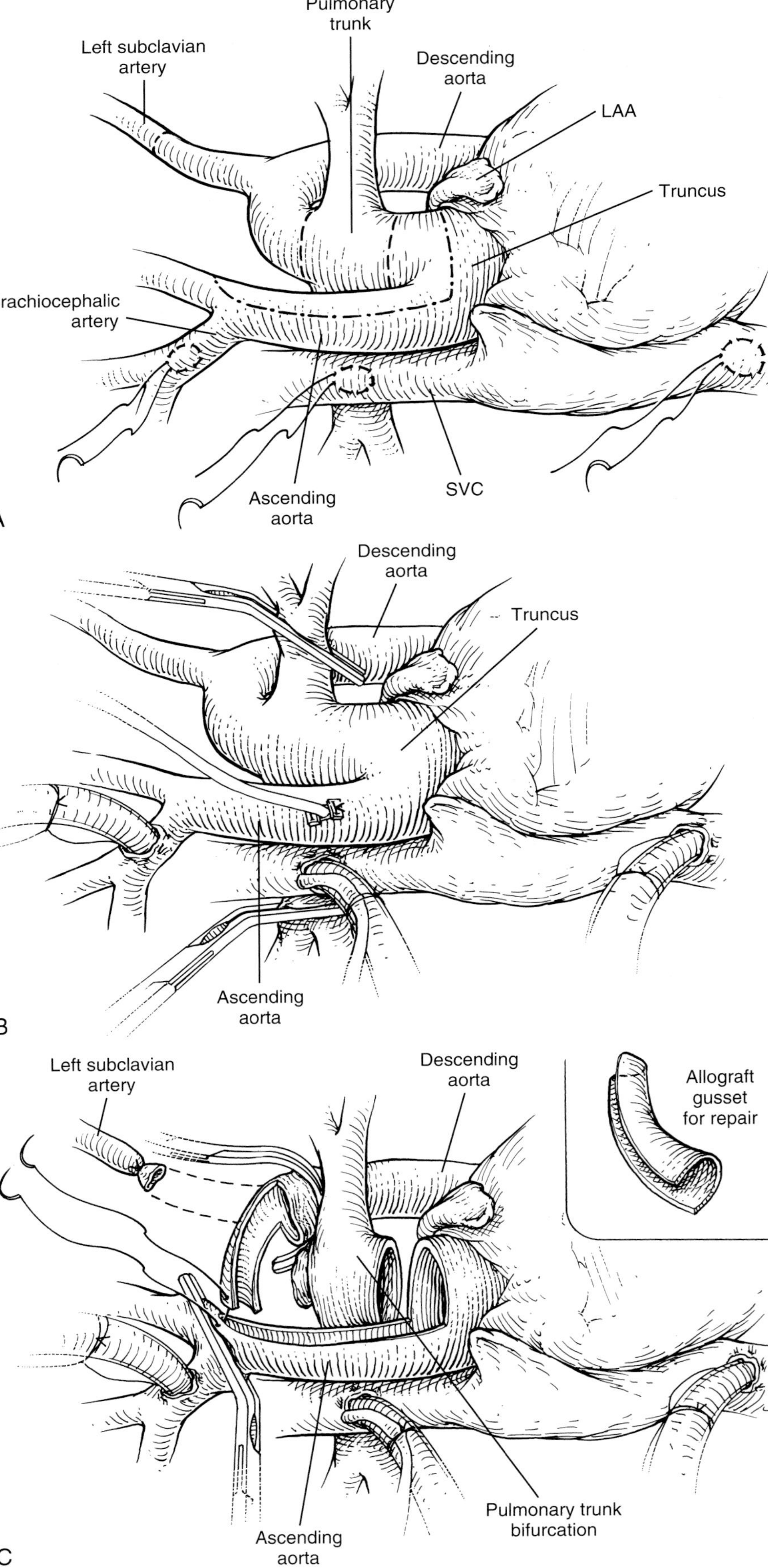

Figure 43-16 Repair of truncus arteriosus with interrupted aortic arch. **A,** The malformation characteristically has a vertically oriented ascending aorta originating from a broad truncus. Proposed incisions to isolate the pulmonary artery branches and bifurcation are indicated by dashed line. Incision to open ascending aorta is indicated by dot-dashed line. **B,** Two venous cannulae are positioned, and arterial return is via brachiocephalic artery, which has been fully mobilized to accommodate anticipated leftward displacement of ascending aorta. Pulmonary artery branches are temporarily occluded while delivering cold cardioplegia. **C,** Diminutive aortic arch and descending aorta are thoroughly mobilized and all ductal tissue resected (see Technique of Operation in Section II of Chapter 48). Transection of left subclavian artery enhances mobilizing the ascending aorta, which has been opened in preparation for augmentation. Augmentation is by a segment of cryopreserved pulmonary allograft fashioned by confluence of donor pulmonary trunk and left pulmonary artery (LPA) to produce a curvilinear gusset, and amplified by spatulation of proximal left subclavian artery. Key: *LAA,* Left atrial appendage; *SVC,* superior vena cava.

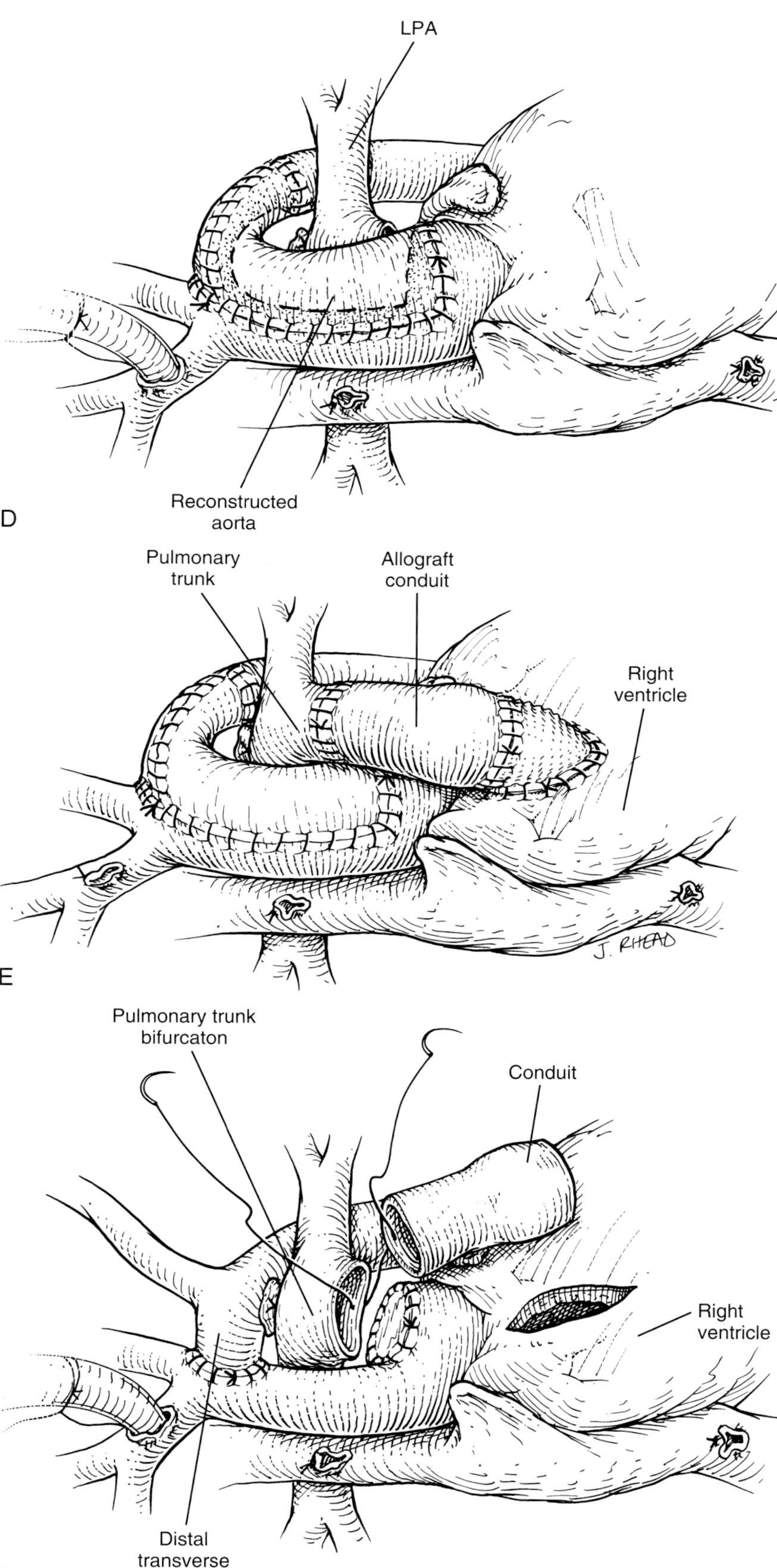

Figure 43-16, cont'd **D,** Descending aorta has been attached to ascending aorta and neoaorta augmented by the allograft gusset. **E,** Operation is completed as usual for truncus arteriosus by closing ventricular septal defect through a right ventriculotomy and connecting the isolated pulmonary trunk to the right ventricle using a valved allograft conduit. **F,** Alternative traditional repair. Ascending and descending aortae are fully mobilized. All ductal tissue is resected. Pulmonary trunk is isolated from truncus arteriosus and the latter closed with a small patch. Descending aorta is anastomosed directly to low ascending aorta. After closure of ventricular septal defect, right ventricle is connected to pulmonary trunk with a valved conduit.

If bronchial compression is still of concern, alternative arch reconstructive techniques, such as that shown in Fig. 43-16, *A* to *E* or the technique described by McKay and colleagues,[M7] can be used. The McKay technique involves placing the distal aortic segment beneath (posterior to) the pulmonary arteries and anastomosing it to the defect left in the truncal artery by excision of the pulmonary trunk.[M7] The ascending aortic valved allograft from the right ventricle to pulmonary trunk is placed anterior to the reconstructed aortic pathway.

Other techniques are described for bringing the pulmonary arteries anterior to the aorta.[P2] It has also been reported that success has been achieved by leaving the ductus arteriosus open to serve as a permanent pathway to the descending aorta and performing the usual operation for truncus arteriosus.[D3,G5,M2] However, in most patients who are under consideration for surgery in the neonatal period, the ductus is not a reliable long-term pathway, because it will narrow and close.

SPECIAL FEATURES OF POSTOPERATIVE CARE

Neonates and infants who have undergone repair of truncus arteriosus require the same standard intensive care required for all patients undergoing complex cardiac repair. If repair is undertaken after 12 weeks of age, a right ventricular or pulmonary artery pressure catheter is required because these patients are particularly susceptible to pulmonary hypertensive crises, the prevention and management of which are described under "General Care of Neonates and Infants" in Section IV of Chapter 5.

RESULTS

Survival

Early (Hospital) Death

Non–risk-adjusted hospital mortality of 17% (CL 12%-24%) was reported by Hanley and colleagues[H4] in 63 neonates and infants operated on between 1986 and 1991. Patients included those with interrupted aortic arch, severe coronary anomalies, and severe truncal valve regurgitation. In patients without these risk factors, there was no early mortality. Similarly, hospital mortality of 11% (CL 7%-17%) was reported in 46 neonates and infants operated on during the same period by Bove and colleagues.[B7] Kalavrouziotis and colleagues[K1] reported a 3.4% early mortality in 29 patients operated on between 1993 and 2005, and Thompson and colleagues[T4] reported a 5% mortality in 65 consecutive neonates operated on between 1992 and 1999. These studies are representative of what can be accomplished in the current era in institutions properly experienced to perform this type of surgery in neonates and young infants.

With the exception of the 1984 study by Ebert and colleagues[E2] that reported a mortality of 11%, most earlier studies reported much higher early mortality.[D7,M11] No deaths (0%; CL 0%-24%) were reported by Sano and colleagues[S1] among 7 neonates and infants undergoing repair of truncus arteriosus and interrupted aortic arch,[S1] and Tlaskal and colleagues[T5] reported 1 death (12%) in 8 patients. In marked contrast to these single-institution studies, the multiinstitutional Congenital Heart Surgeons Society report of 50 patients with truncus arteriosus with interrupted aortic arch operated on from 1987 to 1997 showed an early mortality of about 50%.[K2]

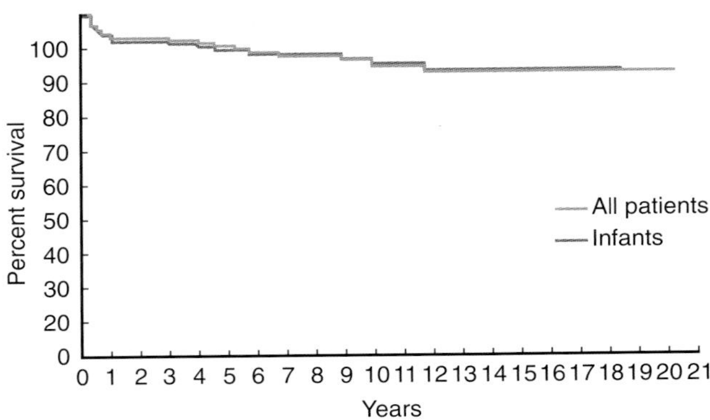

At risk:
All patients 165 137 128 121 114 110 104 101 93 83 70 61 44 39 24 16 7 6 3 1 1
Infants 133 110 103 98 92 88 83 81 74 68 57 52 35 30 18 11 4 3 1

Figure 43-17 Survival among hospital survivors of complete truncus repair. Survival curves are shown for all patients and for infants (patients under age 1 year at repair). Number of patients remaining at risk is shown beneath graph. (From Rajasinghe and colleagues.[R1])

The single-institution reports by Miyamoto and colleagues[M10] and Sinzobahamvya and colleagues[S8] also showed an early mortality of about 50% in patients undergoing operation from 1987 to 2007.

Time-Related Survival

For patients undergoing repair of truncus arteriosus during the first year of life, 10-year and 20-year survival is about the same as operative (30-day) and hospital survival, because few patients die after hospital discharge.[B9,B10,D7,M14,P1,R1,W3] A representative report is that by Rajasinghe and colleagues (Fig. 43-17). Among 165 patients surviving initial repair, there were 23 late deaths (median follow-up 10.5 years), 10 related to reoperation.[R1]

Modes of Death

Most deaths occur early after operation, and the mode is usually acute cardiac failure.

Incremental Risk Factors for Premature Death after Repair

Hanley and colleagues[H4] performed a multivariable analysis of 63 patients; interrupted aortic arch, severe truncal valve regurgitation, severe coronary artery abnormalities, and age older than 100 days at operation were identified as risk factors for early death. The multivariable analysis by Brown and colleagues[B10] indicated that earlier year of operation and coexisting interrupted aortic arch were risk factors. More recent studies, not surprisingly, suggest that morphologic factors such as interrupted aortic arch and truncal valve regurgitation may no longer be risks.[J1,T4] Thompson and colleagues,[T4] however, show that some of these previously identified risk factors continue to be of clinical concern but fall just short of reaching statistical significance as risk factors (Table 43-5). Other variables have not been clearly identified as risk factors, but they have not been rigorously studied. They are discussed briefly in the text that follows.

Table 43-5 Results of Cox Regression Analysis for Factors Associated with Poorer Survival Over Time

Independent Variable	Odds Ratio[a,b]	*P* Value
Demographic Variables		
Age ≤1 week	4.2 (0.7-15)	.12
Weight ≤2.5 kg	10.2 (1.7-61)	.01
Female sex	1.0 (0.2-6.2)	.98
Associated Anomalies		
Moderate or severe truncal valve regurgitation	4.6 (0.8-27)	.09
Interruption of aortic arch	5.2 (0.9-31)	.07
Coronary artery anomalies	1.0 (0.1-8.0)	.99
Nonconfluent pulmonary arteries	0.1 (0.0-8300)	.72
Surgical Variables[c]		
Duration of cardiopulmonary bypass	0.98 (0.96-1.0)	.16
Duration of cardioplegic arrest	0.99 (0.96-1.0)	.13
Truncal valve procedure (repair or replacement)	4.4 (0.9-22)	.07
Truncal valve replacement	11.0 (1.8-66)	.009

From Thompson and colleagues.[T4]
[a]Numbers in parentheses are 95% confidence intervals.
[b]An odds ratio >1 indicates shorter freedom from reintervention.
[c]Repair of interrupted aortic arch is not listed, because all patients with an interrupted arch underwent concurrent repair, and the odds ratio and *P* value were identical.

Age at Repair

Young age has been neutralized in institutions properly prepared for neonatal cardiac surgery, where risk after neonatal repair has been reduced to about 10%.[B7,H4] In fact, many recent series involve only neonates.[T4] Older age at may be a risk factor for premature death after repair, both early and late. However, age is probably a surrogate for severity of pulmonary vascular disease[H4] (see later).

Low Birth Weight

Low birth weight has been identified as a risk factor for early death in two single-institution studies, one of 65 consecutive neonatal repairs and the other of 61 patients younger than 6 months of age at repair.[D1,T4]

Type of Truncus Arteriosus

Types I and II truncus arteriosus are so similar that no difference in risk of death after operation has been identified.[T6] Relatively few patients with truncus arteriosus type III have undergone repair, but increased complexity of operation is expected to increase risk of death to some extent.

Size of Ventricular Septal Defect

Closure of relatively small VSDs may result in some degree of left ventricular outflow obstruction; surgical enlargement of such defects risks interference with septal coronary arteries. Thus, small size of the VSD may be a risk factor.

Predominance of Origin of the Truncal Artery

The more the truncal artery lies over the right ventricle, the greater the probability that VSD closure will narrow the left ventricular outflow tract (particularly when the VSD is small and has not been surgically enlarged), potentially increasing the risk of death early after operation. Possibly this risk factor and that of small VSD size can be neutralized by appropriate VSD enlargement and proper contouring of the VSD patch.

Small Size of Right and Left Pulmonary Arteries

Small branch pulmonary arteries may present risk, especially if proximal obstruction is not addressed at surgical reconstruction.

Truncal Valve Abnormalities

Narrowing of the truncal valve may be difficult to identify and evaluate because flow through it, comprising both systemic and pulmonary flow, is large. Preoperative evaluation typically indicates obstruction across the truncal valve because of the high flow; however, true stenosis is rare and has not been specifically identified as a risk factor. Severe truncal valve regurgitation itself is a well-identified risk factor for death after repair.[E2,H4] This is probably related to both its unfavorable effect postoperatively and its interference with myocardial management intraoperatively.[D5] Treatment of truncal valve regurgitation, either by valvuloplasty or by using an allograft valve conduit placed by the "mini" root-replacement technique (see "Allograft Aortic Valve Cylinder" under Technique of Operation in Chapter 12) is the most important modification of the operation for neutralizing incremental risk of truncal regurgitation (see Appendix 6C in Chapter 6).[B7]

Truncus with Only One Branch Pulmonary Artery Connected to the Truncal Root

Neonates and infants undergoing repair of truncus with only one branch pulmonary artery connected to the truncal root undergo a complex single- or two-stage operation, increasing risk. Nonetheless, repair has been accomplished in 10 infants by Mee, with a 20% (CL 7%-41%) hospital mortality and no post-discharge deaths in a follow-up of nearly 5 years.[M8]

In patients who do not undergo repair during the first 6 months of life, pulmonary vascular disease develops rapidly in the lung supplied from the truncus arteriosus, increasing both early and late risks of repair.[M1]

Major Associated Cardiac Anomalies

Major associated cardiac anomalies increase overall risks. Repair of truncus arteriosus and interrupted arch has been associated with risk of early death in up to 50% of patients,[B10,H4] but more recent studies bring this association into question.[J1]

Pulmonary Vascular Disease

Irreversible pulmonary vascular disease is rarely an issue when repair is performed during the first 3 months of life. The likelihood of postoperative pulmonary hypertensive episodes, however, increases in infants who are repaired after the first 3 weeks of age.[H4] These episodes are a manifestation of a damaged pulmonary vasculature, but the vasculature can remodel and become normal when hemodynamics are normalized with early repair. Progressive damage to the pulmonary vasculature may play an important role in the increased risk of death observed in patients operated on later than 3 months of age.[H4]

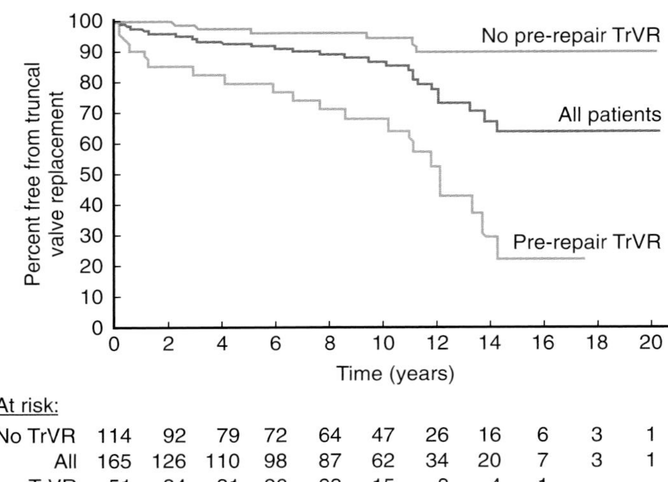

At risk:

	0	2	4	6	8	10	12	14	16	18	20
No TrVR	114	92	79	72	64	47	26	16	6	3	1
All	165	126	110	98	87	62	34	20	7	3	1
TrVR	51	34	31	26	23	15	8	4	1		

Figure 43-18 Freedom from truncal valve replacement in all patients and in patients with and without truncal valve regurgitation (TrVR) before complete truncus repair. Number of patients remaining at risk is shown beneath graph. (From Rajasinghe and colleagues.[R1])

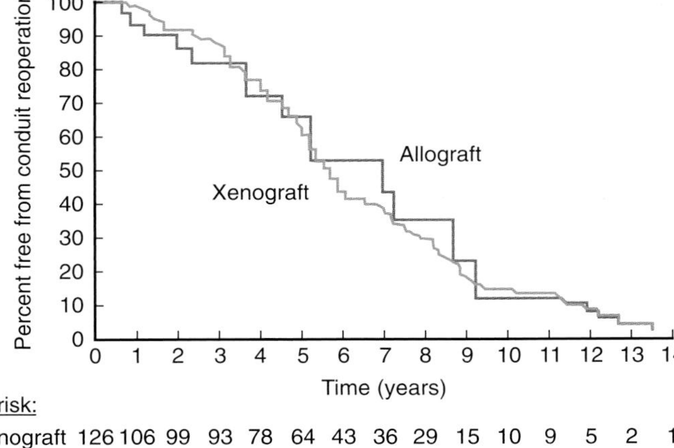

At risk:

	0	1	2	3	4	5	6	7	8	9	10	11	12	13	14
Xenograft	126	106	99	93	78	64	43	36	29	15	10	9	5	2	1
Allograft	39	29	22	18	13	10	7	5	3	2	1	1			

Figure 43-19 Freedom from conduit reoperation according to type of right ventricle–pulmonary trunk conduit used at initial truncus repair. Solid line represents estimates for xenografts and dashed line for allografts. Number of patients remaining at risk is shown beneath graph. (From Rajasinghe and colleagues.[R1])

Progressing Truncal Valve Regurgitation

Rajasinghe and colleagues show that pre-repair truncal valve regurgitation portends only a 20% freedom from eventual truncal valve replacement, and also that a few valves with no pre-repair truncal regurgitation will have to be replaced (Fig. 43-18).[M4,R1] Henaine and colleagues showed the same associations.[H7] Most patients have mild regurgitation 1 to 2 years after repair, and occasionally moderate regurgitation is observed at that time. Mortality for truncal valve replacement can be high when performed in children early after initial truncus repair, but mortality for late truncal valve replacement is low.[M4]

Conduit Replacement

Conduit replacement or revision is almost inevitable (Fig. 43-19). Mean time to conduit replacement was 5.5 years in the study by Rajasinghe and colleagues.[R1] The only factor associated with shorter time to replacement is smaller conduit size at initial repair.[R1] Type of conduit (aortic allograft, pulmonary allograft, or xenograft) does not seem to affect the interval between initial repair and need for reoperation.[C5,R1] Avoidance of a conduit and use of the direct right ventricle–to–pulmonary artery connection at the initial operation may reduce the need for reoperation on the right ventricular outflow tract,[D1] but the need for catheter-based intervention for obstruction is higher using the direct connection. Thus, the requirement for intervention of any kind (surgical and catheter-based combined) is the same for both conduit and direct connection techniques.[C5] In the series by Honjo and colleagues, freedom from intervention for right ventricular outflow tract obstruction was only 50% at 5 years.[H10] The jugular venous valved conduit has been evaluated in a prospective multicentered study and appears to be equivalent to allograft conduits in most respects.[H9] Time to conduit replacement was similar, and both right ventricular outflow tract gradient and valve regurgitation showed similar progression in the two conduit types. Progression of stenosis after catheter intervention for stenosis was significantly slower in the jugular vein conduit.

INDICATIONS FOR OPERATION

Diagnosis of truncus arteriosus is an indication for repair. Because about 50% of surgically untreated patients die during the first month of life, repair should be recommended as early as possible, rather than deferring it to some predetermined age.[A7,B6,B7,S12] This is true whether or not important cardiac anomalies coexist. In children older than 6 months at presentation, operation may be complicated, or even contraindicated, by presence of important elevation of pulmonary vascular resistance. Cardiac catheterization with assessment of pulmonary vascular resistance will determine operability. Criteria for inoperability are the same as for patients with VSD (see Indications for Operation in Section I of Chapter 35).

SPECIAL SITUATIONS AND CONTROVERSIES

Importance of a Valve in Repair

An unsettled matter is the importance of a right ventricular outflow valve. Several groups have reported success with use of valveless conduits.[B3,S7,S10] Although there are no randomized trials comparing the valveless direct connection technique and the valved conduit technique, two studies that use both techniques retrospectively evaluated outcomes.[C5,D1] Fewer total reinterventions were needed in the direct connection patients in one study[D1] but not in the other.[C5] Early mortality did not differ in one study.[C5] In the other,[D1] it was significantly higher in the direct connection group (22% vs. 8%) by univariable analysis; however, multivariable analysis did not confirm the univariable finding. The study authors believe that the validity of the multivariable analysis may be questionable because of the small number of patients and events. To further confuse matters, biases may exist in these retrospective studies that make inferences difficult. For example, in the study by Danton and colleagues,[D1] neonates and young infants (patients not likely to have pulmonary hypertension) predominantly received the valveless direct connection, and older patients (with higher risk for pulmonary hypertension) received valved conduits. These biases may affect timing and prevalence of right ventricular outflow tract reintervention and mortality.

REFERENCES

A

1. Adachi I, Seale A, Uemura H, McCarthy KP, Kimberley P, Ho SY. Morphologic spectrum of truncal valvar origin relative to the ventricular septum: correlation with the size of ventricular septal defect. J Thorac Cardiovasc Surg 2009;138:1283-9.
2. Alves PM, Ferrari AH. Common arterial trunk arising exclusively from the right ventricle with hypoplastic left ventricle and intact ventricular septum. Int J Cardiol 1987;16:99.
3. Anderson KR, McGoon DC, Lie JT. Surgical significance of the coronary arterial anatomy in truncus arteriosus communis. Am J Cardiol 1978;41:76.
4. Anderson RC, Obata W, Lillehei CW. Truncus arteriosus. Clinical study of 14 cases. Circulation 1957;26:586.
5. Anderson RH, Thiene G. Categorization and description of hearts with a common arterial trunk. Eur J Cardiothorac Surg 1989; 3:481.
6. Angelini P, Verdugo AL, Illera JP, Leachman RD. Truncus arteriosus communis. Unusual case associated with transposition. Circulation 1977;56:1107.
7. Appelbaum A, Bargeron LM Jr, Pacifico AD, Kirklin JW. Surgical treatment of truncus arteriosus with emphasis on infants and small children. J Thorac Cardiovasc Surg 1976;71:436.
8. Arai T, Tsuzuki Y, Nazi M, Kurashize K, Kayanazi H, Nishida H. Experimental study on bypass between the right and left ventricle and aorta by means of homograft with valve. Bull Heart Inst Jpn 1965;9:49.
9. Armer RM, De Oliveira PF, Lurie PR. True truncus arteriosus: review of 17 cases and report of surgery in 7 patients (abstract). Circulation 1961;24:878.
10. Assad-Morell JL, Seward JB, Tajik AJ, Hagler DJ, Giuliani ER, Ritter DG. Echo-phonocardiographic and contrast studies in conditions associated systemic arterial trunk over-riding the ventricular septum. Truncus arteriosus, tetralogy of Fallot and pulmonary atresia with ventricular septal defect. Circulation 1976;53:663.

B

1. Barbero-Marcial M, Riso A, Atik E, Jatene A. A technique for correction of truncus arteriosus types I and II without extracardiac conduits. J Thorac Cardiovasc Surg 1990;99:364.
2. Becker AE, Becker MJ, Edwards JE. Pathology of the semilunar valve in persistent truncus arteriosus. J Thorac Cardiovasc Surg 1971;62:16.
3. Behrendt DM, Kirsh MM, Stern A, Sigmann J, Perry B, Sloan H. The surgical therapy for pulmonary artery–right ventricular discontinuity. Ann Thorac Surg 1974;18:122.
4. Bharati S, Karp R, Lev M. The conduction system in truncus arteriosus and its surgical significance: a study of five cases. J Thorac Cardiovasc Surg 1992;104:954.
5. Bharati S, McAllister HA Jr, Rosenquist GC, Miller RA, Tatooles CJ, Lev M. The surgical anatomy of truncus arteriosus communis. J Thorac Cardiovasc Surg 1974;67:501.
6. Bove EL, Beekman RH, Snider AR, Callow LB, Underhill DJ, Rocchini AP, et al. Repair of truncus arteriosus in the neonate and young infant. Ann Thorac Surg 1989;47:499.
7. Bove EL, Lupinetti FM, Pridjian AK, Beekman RH 3rd, Callow LB, Snider AR, et al. Results of a policy of primary repair of truncus arteriosus in the neonate. J Thorac Cardiovasc Surg 1993;105:1057.
8. Bowman FO Jr, Hancock WD, Malm JR. A valve-containing dacron prosthesis: its use in restoring pulmonary artery-right ventricular continuity. Arch Surg 1973;107:724.
9. Brawley RK, Gardner TJ, Donahoo JS, Neill CA, Rowe RD, Gott VL. Late results after right ventricular outflow tract reconstruction with aortic root homografts. J Thorac Cardiovasc Surg 1972;64:314.
10. Brown JW, Ruzmetov M, Okada Y, Vijay P, Turrentine MW. Truncus arteriosus repair: outcomes, risk factors, reoperation and management. Eur J Cardiothorac Surg 2001;20:221-7.
11. Buchanan A. Malformation of the heart. Undivided truncus arteriosus. Heart otherwise double. Trans Pathol Soc Lond 1864;15:89.
12. Burnell RH, McEnery G, Miller GA. Truncal valve stenosis. Br Heart J 1971;33:423.

C

1. Calder L, Van Praagh R, Van Praagh S, Sears WP, Corwin R, Levy A, et al. Truncus arteriosus communis. Clinical angiocardiographic and pathologic findings in 100 patients. Am Heart J 1976;92:23.
2. Carr I, Bharati S, Kusnoor VS, Lev M. Truncus arteriosus communis with intact ventricular septum. Br Heart J 1979;42:97.
3. Carr FB, Goodale RH, Rockwell AE. Persistent truncus arteriosus in a managed 36 years. Arch Pathol 1935;19:833.
4. Ceballos R, Soto B, Kirklin JW, Bargeron LM Jr. Truncus arteriosus. An anatomical-angiographic study. Br Heart J 1983;49:589.
5. Chen JM, Glickstein JS, Davies RR, Mercando ML, Hellenbrand WE, Mosca RS, et al. The effect of repair technique on postoperative right-sided obstruction in patients with truncus arteriosus. J Thorac Cardiovasc Surg 2005;129:559-68.
6. Chiu IS, Wu SJ, Chen MR, Chen SJ, Wang JK. Anatomic relationship of the coronary orifice and truncal valve in truncus arteriosus and their surgical implication. J Thorac Cardiovasc Surg 2002;123:350-2.
7. Collett RW, Edwards JE. Persistent truncus arteriosus: a classification according to anatomic types. Surg Clin North Am 1949; 29:1245.
8. Crupi G, Macartney FJ, Anderson RH. Persistent truncus arteriosus. A study of 66 autopsy cases with special reference to definition and morphogenesis. Am J Cardiol 1977;40:569.

D

1. Danton MH, Barron DJ, Stumper O, Wright JG, De Giovannni J, Silove ED, et al. Repair of truncus arteriosus: a considered approach to right ventricular outflow tract reconstruction. Eur J Cardiothorac Surg 2001;20:95-104.
2. Daskalopoulos DA, Edwards WD, Driscoll DJ, Schaff HV, Danielson GK. Fatal pulmonary artery banding in truncus arteriosus with anomalous origin of circumflex coronary artery from right pulmonary artery. Am J Cardiol 1983;52:1363.
3. Davis JT, Ehrlich R, Blakemore WS, Lev M, Bharati S. Truncus arteriosus with interrupted aortic arch: report of a successful surgical repair. Ann Thorac Surg 1985;39:82.
4. de la Cruz MV, Cayre R, Angelini P, Noriega-Ramos N, Sadowinski S. Coronary arteries in truncus arteriosus. Am J Cardiol 1990; 66:1482.
5. de Leval MR, McGoon DC, Wallace RB, Danielson GK, Mair DD. Management of truncal valvular regurgitation. Ann Surg 1974; 180:427.
6. Deely WJ, Hagstrom JW, Engle MA. Truncus insufficiency. Common truncus arteriosus with regurgitant truncal valve: report of 4 cases. Am Heart J 1963;65:542.
7. Di Donato RM, Fyfe DA, Puga FJ, Danielson GK, Ritter DG, Edwards WD, et al. Fifteen-year experience with surgical repair of truncus arteriosus. J Thorac Cardiovasc Surg 1985;89:414.

E

1. Ebert PA. Truncus arteriosus. In Parenzan L, Crupi G, Graham G, eds. Congenital heart disease in the first 3 months of life. Bologna, Italy: Patron Editore, 1981.
2. Ebert PA, Turley K, Stanger P, Hoffman JI, Heymann MA, Rudolph AM. Surgical treatment of truncus arteriosus in the first six months of life. Ann Surg 1984;200:451.

F

1. Fontana RS, Edwards JE. A review of 357 cases studied pathologically. In Fontana RS, ed. Congenital cardiac disease. Philadelphia: WB Saunders, 1962, p. 95.
2. Freedom RM, Rosen FS, Nadas AS. Congenital cardiovascular disease and anomalies of the third and fourth pharyngeal pouch. Circulation 1972;46:165.
3. Fujiwara K, Yokota Y, Okamoto F, Kiyota Y, Sugawara E, Iemura J, et al. Successful surgical repair of truncus arteriosus with

interrupted aortic arch in infancy by an anterior approach. Ann Thorac Surg 1988;45:441.

G

1. Gelband H, Van Meter S, Gersony WM. Truncal valve abnormalities in infants with persistent truncus arteriosus. A clinicopathologic study. Circulation 1972;45:397.
2. Gerlis LM, Wilson N, Dickinson DF, Scott O. Valvar stenosis in truncus arteriosus. Br Heart J 1984;52:440.
3. Girinath MR. Case presentation: truncus arteriosus: repair with homograft reconstruction in infancy. In Barratt-Boyes BG, Neutze JM, Harris EA, eds. Heart disease in infancy. Diagnosis and surgical treatment. Edinburgh: Churchill Livingstone, 1973, p. 234.
4. Goldmuntz E, Clark BJ, Mitchell LE, Jawad AF, Cuneo BF, Reed L, et al. Frequency of 22q11 deletions in patients with conotruncal defects. J Am Coll Cardiol 1998;32:492.
5. Gomes MM, McGoon DC. Truncus arteriosus with interruption of the aortic arch: report of a case successfully repaired. Mayo Clin Proc 1971;46:40.
6. Griepp RB, Stinson EB, Shumway NE. Surgical correction of types II and III truncus arteriosus. J Thorac Cardiovasc Surg 1977;73:345.
7. Guadalupi P, Spadoni I, Vanini V. Repair of hemitruncus with autologous arterial ring and valved bioconduit. Ann Thorac Surg 2000;70:1708-10.

H

1. Habbema L, Losekoot TG, Becker AE. Respiratory distress due to bronchial compression in persistent truncus arteriosus. Chest 1980;77:230.
2. Hagler DJ, Tajik AJ, Seward JB, Mair DD, Ritter DG. Wide-angle two-dimensional echocardiographic profiles of conotruncal abnormalities. Mayo Clin Proc 1980;55:73.
3. Hallermann FJ, Kincaid OW, Tsakiris AG, Ritter DG, Titus JL. Persistent truncus arteriosus: a radiographic and angiocardiographic study. Am J Roentgenol Radium Ther Nucl Med 1969;107:827.
4. Hanley FL, Heinemann MK, Jonas RA, Mayer JE Jr, Cook NR, Wessel DL, et al. Repair of truncus arteriosus in the neonate. J Thorac Cardiovasc Surg 1993;105:1047.
5. Hawkins JA, Bailey WW, Dillon T, Schwartz DC. Midterm results with cryopreserved allograft valved conduits from the right ventricle to the pulmonary arteries. J Thorac Cardiovasc Surg 1992;104:910.
6. Heilbrunn A, Kittle CF, Diehl AM. Pulmonary arterial banding in the treatment of truncus arteriosus. Circulation 1964;29:102.
7. Henaine R, Azarnoush K, Belli E, Capderou A, Roussin R, Planche C, et al. Fate of the truncal valve in truncus arteriosus. Ann Thorac Surg 2008;85:172-8.
8. Hicken P, Evans D, Heath D. Persistent truncus arteriosus with survival to the age of 38 years. Br Heart J 1966;28:284.
9. Hickey EJ, McCrindle BW, Blackstone EH, Yeh T Jr, Pigula F, Clarke D, et al. Jugular venous valved conduit (Contegra) matches allograft performance in infant truncus arteriosus repair. Eur J Cardiothorac Surg 2008;33:890-8.
10. Honjo O, Kotani Y, Akagi T, Osaki S, Kawada M, Ishino K, et al. Right ventricular outflow tract reconstruction in patients with persistent truncus arteriosus: a 15-year experience in a single Japanese center. Circ J 2007;71:1776-80.

J

1. Jahangiri M, Zurakowski D, Mayer JE, del Nido PJ, Jonas RA. Repair of the truncal valve and associated interrupted arch in neonates with truncus arteriosus. J Thorac Cardiovasc Surg 2000; 119:508-14.
2. Juaneda E, Haworth SG. Pulmonary vascular disease in children with truncus arteriosus. Am J Cardiol 1984;54:1314.

K

1. Kalavrouziotis G, Purohit M, Ciotti G, Corno AF, Pozzi M. Truncus arteriosus communis: early and midterm results of early primary repair. Ann Thorac Surg 2006;82:2200-6.
2. Konstantinov IE, Karamlou T, Blackstone EH, Mosca RS, Lofland GK, Caldarone CA, et al. Truncus arteriosus associated with interrupted aortic arch in 50 neonates: a Congenital Heart Surgeons Society study. Ann Thorac Surg 2006;81:214-22.

L

1. Lacour-Gayet F, Serraf A, Komiya T, Sousa-Uva M, Bruniaux J, Touchot A, et al. Truncus arteriosus repair: influence of techniques of right ventricular outflow tract reconstruction. J Thorac Cardiovasc Surg 1996;111:849.
2. Ledbetter MK, Tandon R, Titus JL, Edwards JE. Stenotic semilunar valve in persistent truncus arteriosus. Chest 1976;69:182.
3. Lee MH, Bellon EM, Liebman J, Perrin EV. Truncal valve stenosis. Am Heart J 1973;85:397.
4. Lenox CC, Debich DE, Zuberbuhler JR. The role of coronary artery abnormalities in the prognosis of truncus arteriosus. J Thorac Cardiovasc Surg 1992;104:1728.
5. Lev M, Saphir O. Truncus arteriosus communis persistens. J Pediatr 1943;20:74.

M

1. Mair DD, Ritter DG, Danielson GK, Wallace RB, McGoon DC. Truncus arteriosus with unilateral absence of a pulmonary artery. Criteria for operability and surgical results. Circulation 1977;55:641.
2. Mair DD, Ritter DG, Davis GD, Wallace RB, Danielson GK, McGoon DC. Selection of patients with truncus arteriosus for surgical correction: anatomic and hemodynamic considerations. Circulation 1974;49:144.
3. Marcelletti C, McGoon DC, Mair DD. The natural history of truncus arteriosus. Circulation 1976;54:108.
4. McElhinney DB, Reddy VM, Rajasinghe HA, Mora BN, Silverman NH, Hanley FL. Trends in the management of truncal valve insufficiency. Ann Thorac Surg 1998;65:517-24.
5. McGoon DC, Rastelli GC, Ongley PA. An operation for the correction of truncus arteriosus. JAMA 1968;205:69.
6. McGoon DC, Rastelli GC, Wallace RB. Discontinuity between right ventricle and pulmonary artery: surgical treatment. Ann Surg 1970;172:680.
7. McKay R, Miyamoto S, Peart I, Battistessa SA, Wren C, Cunliffe M, et al. Truncus arteriosus with interrupted aortic arch: successful correction in a neonate. Ann Thorac Surg 1989;48:587.
8. Mee RB. Surgical repair of hemitruncus: principles and techniques. J Card Surg 1987;2:247.
9. Mello DM, McElhinney DB, Parry AJ, Silverman NH, Hanley FL. Truncus arteriosus with patent ductus arteriosus and normal aortic arch. Ann Thorac Surg 1997;64:1808-10.
10. Miyamoto T, Sinzobahamvya N, Kumpikaite D, Asfour B, Photiadis J, Brecher AM, et al. Repair of truncus arteriosus and aortic arch interruption: outcome analysis. Ann Thorac Surg 2005;79:2077-82.
11. Moller JH, ed. Perspectives in pediatric cardiology, Vol. 6. Surgery of congenital heart disease: Pediatric Cardiac Care Consortium 1984-1995, Armonk, New York: Futura Publishing Co. Inc.
12. Momma K, Ando M, Matsuoka R. Truncus arteriosus communis associated with chromosome 22q11 deletion. J Am Coll Cardiol 1997;30:1067.
13. Moore CH, Martelli V, Ross DN. Reconstruction of right ventricular outflow tract with a valved conduit in 75 cases of congenital heart disease. J Thorac Cardiovasc Surg 1976;71:11.
14. Moseley PW, Ochsner JL, Mills NL, Chapman J. Management of an infected Hancock prosthesis after repair of truncus arteriosus. J Thorac Cardiovasc Surg 1977;73:306.

P

1. Parenzan L, Alfieri O. Surgical repair of persistent truncus arteriosus in infancy. In Anderson RH, Shinebourne EA, eds. Pediatric cardiology, 1977, Edinburgh: Churchill Livingstone, p. 551.
2. Park CS, Jhang WK, Ko JK, Kim YH, Yun TJ. Lecompte operation: is it still a viable option for truncus arteriosus? J Thorac Cardiovasc Surg 2008;136:1384-6.
3. Patel RG, Freedom RM, Bloom KR, Rowe RD. Truncal or aortic valve stenosis in functionally single arterial trunk. A clinical hemodynamic and pathologic study of six cases. Am J Cardiol 1978; 42:800.

R

1. Rajasinghe HA, McElhinney DB, Reddy VM, Mora BN, Hanley FL. Long-term follow-up of truncus arteriosus repaired in infancy: a twenty-year experience. J Thorac Cardiovasc Surg 1997;113:869.

2. Rastelli GC, Titus JL, McGoon DC. Homograft of ascending aorta and aortic valve as a right ventricular outflow. Arch Surg 1967; 95:698.
3. Ross DN, Somerville J. Correction of pulmonary atresia with a homograft aortic valve. Lancet 1966;2:1446.

S

1. Sano S, Brawn WJ, Mee RB. Repair of truncus arteriosus and interrupted aortic arch. J Card Surg 1990;5:157.
2. Schumacher G, Schreiber R, Meisner H, Lorenz HP, Sebening F, Buhlmeyer K. Interrupted aortic arch: natural history and operative results. Pediatr Cardiol 1986;7:89.
3. Scott WA, Rocchini AP, Bove EL, Behrendt DM, Beekman RH, Dick M 2nd, et al. Repair of interrupted aortic arch in infancy. J Thorac Cardiovasc Surg 1988;96:564.
4. Seki S, Rastelli GC, McGoon DC, Titus JL. Replacement of the pulmonary artery with a pulmonary arterial homograft. J Thorac Cardiovasc Surg 1970;60:853.
5. Shapiro PF. Truncus solitarius pulmonalis. A rare type of congenital cardiac anomaly. Arch Pathol 1930;10:671.
6. Shrivastava S, Edwards JE. Coronary arterial origin in persistent truncus arteriosus. Circulation 1977;55:551.
7. Singh A, de Leval M, Stark J. Total correction of type I truncus arteriosus in a 6-month-old infant. Br Heart J 1975;37:1314.
8. Sinzobahamvya N, Boscheinen M, Blaschczok HC, Kallenberg R, Photiadis J, Haun C, et al. Survival and reintervention after neonatal repair of truncus arteriosus with valved conduit. Eur J Cardiothorac Surg 2008;34:732-7.
9. Smith GW, Thompson WM Jr, Dammann JF Jr, Muller WH Jr. Use of the pulmonary artery banding procedure in treating type II truncus arteriosus. Circulation 1964;29:I108.
10. Spicer RL, Behrendt D, Crowley DC, Dick M, Rocchini AP, Uzark K, et al. Repair of truncus arteriosus in neonates with the use of a valveless conduit. Circulation 1984;70:I26.
11. Stark J, Gandhi D, de Leval M, Macartney F, Taylor JF. Surgical treatment of persistent truncus arteriosus in the first year of life. Br Heart J 1978;40:1280.
12. Sullivan H, Sulayman R, Replogle R, Arcilla RA. Surgical correction of truncus arteriosus in infancy. Am J Cardiol 1976;38:113.
13. Suzuki A, Ho SY, Anderson RH, Deanfield JE. Coronary arterial and sinusal anatomy in hearts with a common arterial trunk. Ann Thorac Surg 1989;48:792.

T

1. Tandon R, Hanck AJ, Nadas AS. Persistent truncus arteriosus: a clinical, hemodynamic and autopsy study of 19 cases. Circulation 1963;28:1050.
2. Thiene G, Bortolotti U, Gallucci V, Terribile V, Pellegrino PA. Anatomical study of truncus arteriosus communis with embryological and surgical considerations. Br Heart J 1976;38:1109.
3. Thiene G, Cucchini F, Pellegrino PA. Truncus arteriosus communis associated with underdevelopment of the aortic arch. Br Heart J 1975;37:1268.
4. Thompson LD, McElhinney DB, Reddy M, Petrossian E, Silverman NH, Hanley FL. Neonatal repair of truncus arteriosus: continuing improvement in outcomes. Ann Thorac Surg 2001; 72:391-5.
5. Tlaskal T, Hucin B, Kucera V, Vojtovic P, Gebauer R, Chaloupecky V, et al. Repair of persistent truncus arteriosus with interrupted aortic arch. Eur J Cardiothorac Surg 2005;28:736-41.
6. Trowitzsch E, Sluysmans T, Parness IA, Spevak PJ, Colan SD, Mayer JE, et al. Anatomy and surgical outcome in infants with truncus arteriosus (abstract). J Am Coll Cardiol 1991;17:110a.
7. Tworetzky W, McElhinney DB, Brook MM, Reddy VM, Hanley FL, Silverman NH. Echocardiographic diagnosis alone for the complete repair of major congenital heart defects. J Am Coll Cardiol 1999;33:228-33.

V

1. van der Horst RL, Gotsman MS. Type 3c truncus arteriosus. Case report with clinical and surgical implications. Br Heart J 1974; 36:1046.
2. Van Praagh R, Van Praagh S. The anatomy of common aorticopulmonary trunk (truncus arteriosus communis) and its embryonic implications. A study of 57 necropsy cases. Am J Cardiol 1965; 16:406.
3. Victoria BE, Krovetz LJ, Elliott LP, Van Mierop LH, Bartley TD, Gessner IH, et al. Persistent truncus arteriosus in infancy. Am Heart J 1969;77:13.

W

1. Wallace RB, Rastelli GC, Ongley PA, Titus JL, McGoon DC. Complete repair of truncus arteriosus defects. J Thorac Cardiovasc Surg 1969;57:95.
2. Weldon CS, Cameron JL. Correction of persistent truncus arteriosus. J Cardiovasc Surg 1968;9:463.
3. Williams JM, de Leeuw M, Black MD, Freedom RM, Williams WG, McCrindle BW. Factors associated with outcomes of persistent truncus arteriosus. J Am Coll Cardiol 1999;34:545.
4. Wilson J. A description of a very unusual malformation of the human heart. Philos Trans R Soc Lond [Biol] 1798;18:346.

44 Aortopulmonary Window

DEFINITION

Aortopulmonary window (APW) is a round, oval, or sometimes spiral opening between the ascending aorta and pulmonary trunk, occurring as a congenital anomaly in hearts with separate aortic and pulmonary valves. This malformation has also been termed *aortic septal defect; aortopulmonary fistula, fenestration, or septal defect;* and *aorticopulmonary window, fistula, fenestration, or septal defect.*[R1]

HISTORICAL NOTE

The first report of an APW was by Elliotson in 1830, and in the American literature by Cotton about 70 years later.[C6,E1] The first reported correct clinical diagnoses are attributed to Dodds and Hoyle in 1949 and to Gasul and colleagues in 1951.[D5,G2]

In 1952, Gross reported successful ligation of an APW using a closed technique.[G3] Scott and Sabiston in 1953 and Fletcher and colleagues in 1954 reported successful division of an APW by a closed technique.[F2,S3] The operation was difficult and hazardous, however.

The advent of open operation with cardiopulmonary bypass (CPB) in 1954 to 1955 made it easier to correct this malformation. Division of the connection between aorta and pulmonary trunk was used in early cases at the Mayo Clinic. In 1957, Cooley and colleagues reported three successful repairs using this method.[C5] Bjork advised closure of the defect by the simple method of patching it from within the pulmonary trunk (Bjork VO: 1964, personal communication). This was later also suggested by Putnam and Gross.[P2] In 1968, Wright and colleagues reported the transaortic approach to intraluminal closure by direct suture.[W1] A year later, Deverall and colleagues reported use of a transaortic approach, but with polyester patch closure.[D2]

Johansson and colleagues described a "sandwich"-type closure in 1978.[J3] Schmid and colleagues closed APW without CPB, using a felt strip technique.[S2] Richardson and colleagues used a contoured polyester patch, and Kitagawa and colleagues rerouted the pulmonary trunk for distal APW defects.[K2,R1] Messmer closed the defect using a pulmonary trunk flap and closed the pulmonary trunk with a pericardial patch.[M3] Di Bella and Gladstone used only a pulmonary trunk flap to close the defect.[D3] Kawata and colleagues closed an APW using a vascular clip in an infant weighing 758 g.[K1]

MORPHOLOGY

An APW is usually a large defect between the aorta and pulmonary trunk, although in about 10% of patients the defect is small. The pulmonary arteries are normally related to the pulmonary trunk. As the term *window* implies, there is little or no length to the communication in most patients. It is nearly always a single orifice, although it may be fenestrated.

Several classifications have been proposed to describe the location of the anomalous "window" on the ascending aorta and its relationship to the branch pulmonary arteries. Mori and colleagues proposed the terms *proximal, distal,* and *total* to describe the location within the ascending aorta[M4]; Richardson and colleagues used the term *type I* to describe proximal defects and *type II* to indicate defects in the distal ascending aorta.[R1] Ho and colleagues added the term *intermediate* to describe defects with upper and lower edges suitable for percutaneous closure.[H2] Jacobs and colleagues[J1] from the Society of Thoracic Surgeons' Congenital Heart Surgery Database Committee recommended the terms *type I–proximal defect, type II–distal defect, type III–total defect,* and *intermediate defect* (Fig. 44-1).

Proximal (type I) APWs are located in the proximal ascending aorta (see Fig. 44-1). The window is in the left lateral wall of the ascending aorta, usually close to the orifice of the left coronary artery, and in the contiguous right wall of the pulmonary trunk inferior to the origin of the right pulmonary artery.[N1] It is not surprising, therefore, that occasionally the right coronary artery, and rarely the left, may be transposed onto the pulmonary trunk close to the edge of the defect.[B4,B7,D6,D7,L2] This must always be considered in the surgical treatment of APW.[K4] When viewed from within the pulmonary trunk, the APW can be confused with the orifice of the right pulmonary artery. The proximal type occurs in about 90% of APW cases.[B6,F3,T4]

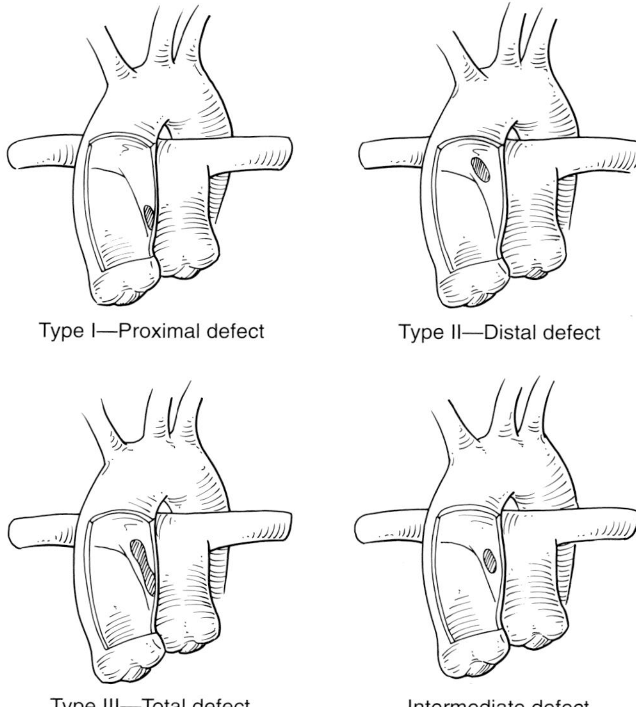

Figure 44-1 Classification scheme recommended by Society of Thoracic Surgeons' Congenital Heart Surgery Database Committee for aortopulmonary window. Type I is a proximal defect located just above sinus of Valsalva, a few millimeters above semilunar valve. Proximal defects have little inferior rim separating defect from semilunar valves. Type II is a distal defect located in uppermost portion of ascending aorta. It corresponds to Richardson type II lesion, where defect overlies a portion of right pulmonary artery. Distal defects are noted to have a well-formed inferior rim but little superior rim. Type III is a total defect involving majority of ascending aorta. Type IV is the intermediate defect; these have adequate superior and inferior rims and are the group most suitable for possible device closure.

Rarely, the opening between the aorta and the origin of the right pulmonary artery from the pulmonary trunk is more downstream in the ascending aorta (*distal* or *type II APW*).[D6,M2,M4,R1] The orifice may lie between the aorta and right pulmonary artery; such defects have a spiral opening.[B2,D6,K4]

In rare instances, the APW may involve nearly the entire ascending aorta (*total* or *type III*).

When the communication is such that the right pulmonary artery takes its origin from the ascending aorta and is not related to the pulmonary trunk, the defect is called *anomalous origin of the right pulmonary artery from the ascending aorta* (see Chapter 45).

Because of the association between APW (particularly distally located ones) and anomalous origin of the right pulmonary artery from the ascending aorta, the APW may open between the right pulmonary artery and aorta.[D6,M4] The right pulmonary artery may straddle the APW ("unroofing" of the right pulmonary artery) or may originate completely from the aorta while maintaining continuity with the left pulmonary artery by way of the APW.[B2] Finally, the two conditions may simply coexist.[G4]

APW is accompanied by other cardiac anomalies in about 50% of cases,[K3,K4] of which interrupted aortic arch (IAA) (about 90% of which are type A and the rest type B) is the most frequently observed major associated lesion[D4,K4] (although this combination is rare among all patients with congenital heart disease). Other major associated lesions include ventricular septal defect (VSD), tetralogy of Fallot, transposition of the great arteries (Vannini V: personal communication, 1980), anomalous origin of a coronary artery, aortic isthmic hypoplasia, and subaortic stenosis.[C1,C3,D7,F1,T1,T2]

Rarely, there is a complex syndrome of the APW, usually in the downstream portion of the ascending aorta, with aortic origin of the right pulmonary artery, intact ventricular septum, patent ductus arteriosus, and interrupted aortic arch or severe coarctation (Berry syndrome).[A1,B2,C2,D1,T1] This is a particularly lethal combination; most affected infants die shortly after birth.

From 5% to 10% of patients with the malformation have less severe associated cardiac anomalies such as right aortic arch (7%), ostium secundum atrial septal defects, or patent ductus arteriosus.[B4,C4,D2,F1]

The rarity of IAA with APW is such that among 472 neonatal patients with IAA reported in a Congenital Heart Surgeon's Society study, 20 (4%) had IAA with APW[K3] (Fig. 44-2).

CLINICAL FEATURES AND DIAGNOSTIC CRITERIA

In infants with isolated APW, symptoms and signs of heart failure usually develop early in life, and their presentation is similar to that of infants with a large VSD. These infants are generally small, underdeveloped, and tachypneic, and they tend to have repeated respiratory infections.[T3]

On examination, the left precordium is prominent because of marked cardiomegaly. The second heart sound at the base is usually accentuated. The murmur is usually only systolic and of variable intensity.[D2,M5,N1] In about 15% of patients, it is continuous because the APW is smaller and pulmonary hypertension less than usual.[M5,N1] When the left-to-right shunt through the defect is large, there are peripheral signs of rapid aortic runoff (e.g., jerky or collapsing peripheral pulses), but these signs are not evident when heart failure is marked or pulmonary vascular resistance is severely elevated.

Chest radiograph and electrocardiogram (ECG) findings are similar to those of infants and young children with VSD or large patent ductus arteriosus, giving evidence of left and right ventricular enlargement and large pulmonary blood flow.[B4] Left atrial enlargement (a result of large pulmonary blood flow) is usually prominent.

Differential diagnoses before special study include large patent ductus arteriosus (see Chapter 37), truncus arteriosus (see Chapter 43), and, in patients beyond the infant age group, VSD with aortic regurgitation (see Section II of Chapter 35) and ruptured sinus of Valsalva aneurysm (see Chapter 36).

Since the early 1990s, diagnosis has relied exclusively on two-dimensional (2D) echocardiography.[M1,P1,S1,T4] Nevertheless, other imaging techniques are useful. Garver and colleagues correlated echocardiography, angiography, and magnetic resonance imaging (MRI) to achieve accurate diagnosis in APW.[G1] Prior to the advent of 2D echocardiography,

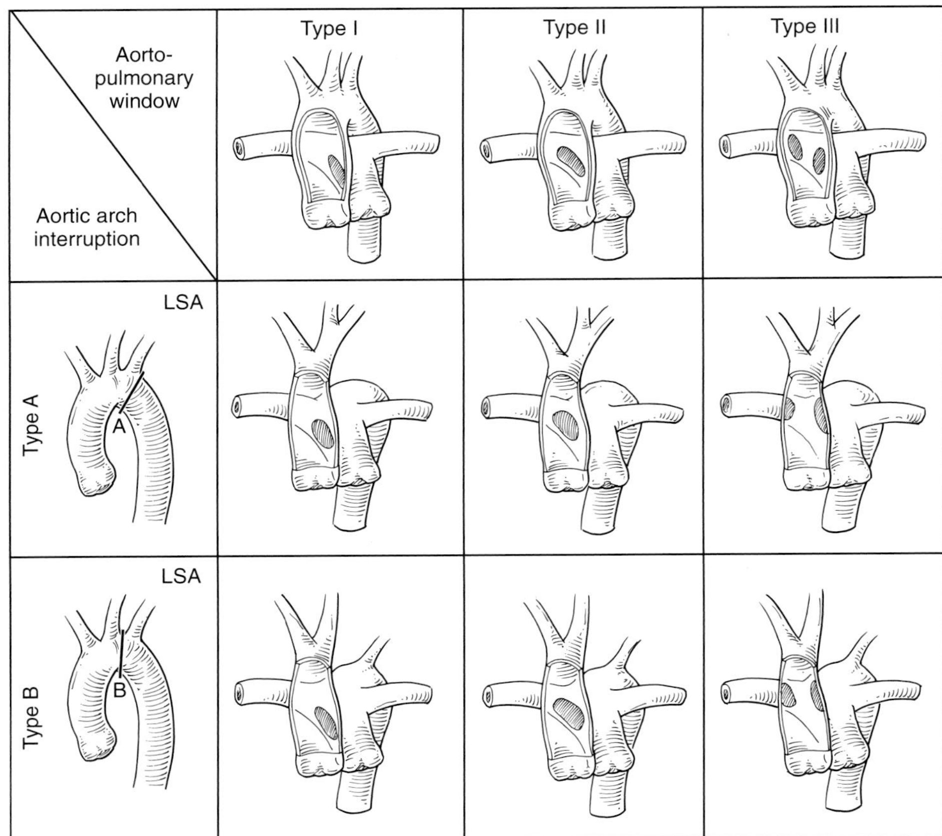

Figure 44-2 Morphologic subtypes of aortopulmonary window in interrupted aortic arch. Key: *LSA,* Left subclavian artery.

cardiac catheterization and cineangiography were used to provide the definitive diagnosis and identify associated cardiac anomalies. Cardiac catheterization shows blood oxygen saturation in the pulmonary artery is elevated over that in the right ventricle and right atrium in most cases. Occasionally, oxygen saturation in the right ventricle is increased over that in the right atrium, which may suggest VSD or truncus arteriosus until cineangiography shows this to be from pulmonary valve regurgitation associated with APW. Ascending aortic angiography shows rapid filling of the pulmonary trunk through the APW, as well as separate aortic and pulmonary valves. Because location of the APW varies and coronary arteries may arise from the pulmonary trunk, visualization of all anomalies must be accurate.

NATURAL HISTORY

APW is a rare malformation, occurring in about 0.2% of cases of congenital heart disease.[B1,H1,R2] There is no known tendency for APWs to close spontaneously. The natural history of infants with large APWs is at least as unfavorable as that of infants with persistently large VSD (see Natural History in Section I of Chapter 35). In the absence of surgical correction, mortality in the first year of life has been estimated at 40%.[T4] In fact, patients with large APWs are rarely seen in childhood or adult life, and those who survive beyond early life have important pulmonary vascular disease.[M2] This natural history is, therefore, similar to that of surgically untreated older patients with large VSD.

TECHNIQUE OF OPERATION

Because APW often coexists with other important cardiac anomalies, the basic technique of repair must be modified and adapted to the individual situation. However, every effort should be made to accomplish a one-stage repair. A special combination is APW and anomalous origin of the right pulmonary artery from the ascending aorta, in which the APW may be left open anatomically but functionally closed by connecting it to the orifice of the right pulmonary artery by one of several techniques.[D4,G4,K2,R1] The discussion that follows pertains specifically to *isolated APWs.*

Diagnosis can usually be verified at operation from outside the heart. The first portion of the aorta and pulmonary trunk form a large confluence that suggests truncus arteriosus. However, separate semilunar valve "anuli" can usually be verified by finding a dimple between the two great arteries where they arise from the heart. Even in young infants, the left ventricle is enlarged, usually about grade 3 on a scale of 0 to 6, as are the left atrium and right ventricle. In older children, ventricular enlargement and hypertrophy are severe.

The operation may be done with CPB (see Section III of Chapter 2) unless the infant weighs less than about 2.5 kg, in which case hypothermic circulatory arrest may be used (see Section IV of Chapter 2). Particular care must be taken in selecting the site for aortic cannulation, which must be as far downstream as possible. Also, before establishing CPB, a limited dissection is made between the aorta and pulmonary trunk, downstream from the APW but proximal to the aortic

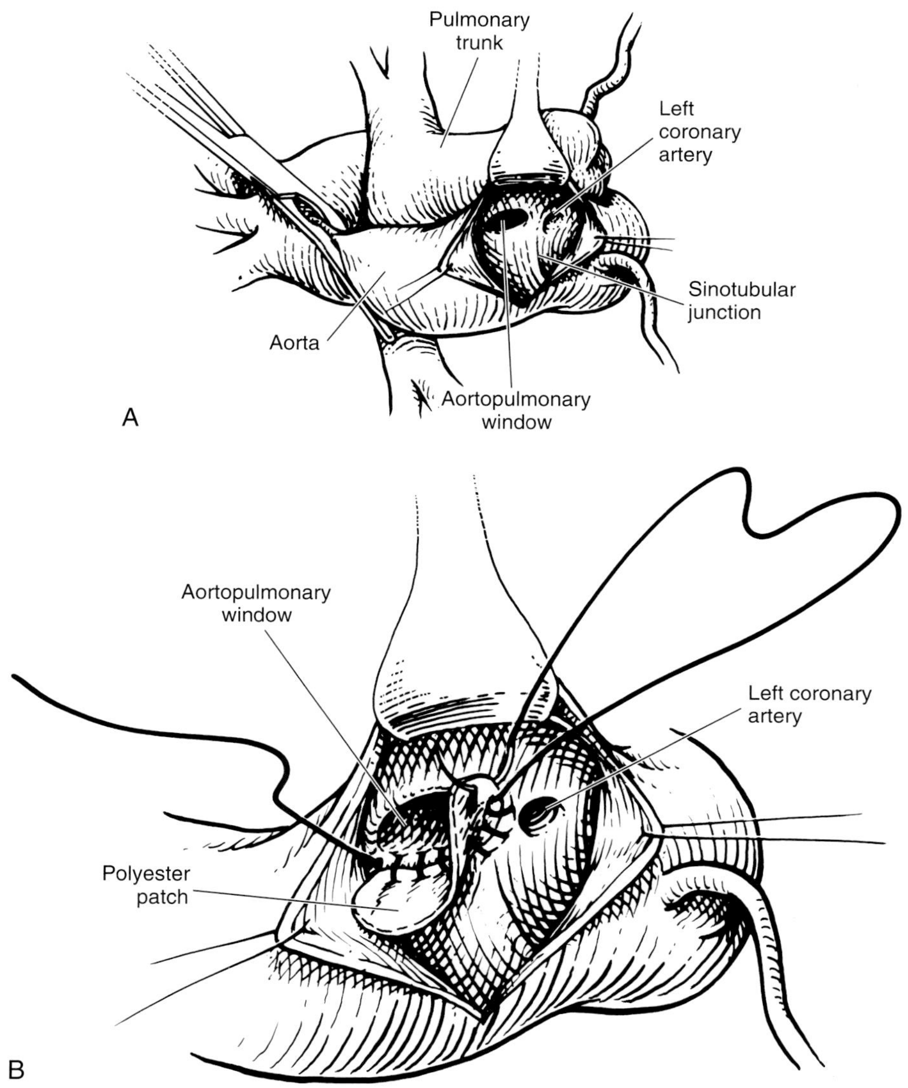

Figure 44-3 Repair of type I aortopulmonary window (APW). **A,** Operation is performed on cardiopulmonary bypass with aorta occluded. APW is exposed through a transverse aortotomy. It is located just above sinutubular junction. Origin of left coronary artery is identified because it may have a close relationship with inferior margin of APW. **B,** APW is closed with a polyester, polytetrafluoroethylene, or pericardial patch to create a partition between aorta and pulmonary trunk. Left coronary artery is protected from inclusion in suture line.

cannulation site. Care is taken to identify and protect the right pulmonary artery during this dissection and while placing the aortic clamp. A single venous cannula may be used, or the cavae may be cannulated directly. The right atrium is opened and a pump-oxygenator sump sucker placed across the foramen ovale into the left atrium.

As soon as CPB has been initiated and core cooling begun, a side-biting clamp (e.g., small Cooley clamp) is placed across the window from the pulmonary trunk side to occlude the window; alternatively, separate tourniquets may be placed on left and right pulmonary arteries. The aortic occlusion clamp is positioned exactly at the place provided by the prior dissection. Cold cardioplegic solution is injected into the ascending aorta or retrogradely via the coronary sinus (see "Methods of Myocardial Management during Cardiac Surgery" in Chapter 3).

Repair can be done through either the aorta or pulmonary trunk, and even the older technique of complete division has given good results.[P2] However, an initial approach through the aorta is generally recommended to facilitate clear identification of the aortic valve and right and left coronary orifices in relation to the defect. The aorta is opened transversely at the level of the APW (Fig. 44-3, *A*). Both coronary arteries must be identified. If one is anomalously positioned in the pulmonary trunk, the patch for closure of the window must be positioned so that both coronary ostia are on the aortic side of the patch. Small or moderate-sized APWs may be closed by direct suture, using one or two rows of continuous 4-0 polypropylene sutures. A large window is closed with a polyester, polytetrafluoroethylene (PTFE), or pericardial patch sewn into place with continuous 4-0 or 5-0 polypropylene sutures[C3,R1] (Fig. 44-3, *B*). The aortotomy incision is then closed with one row of continuous polypropylene sutures. The remainder of the operation, including the de-airing procedure, is carried out as usual (see "De-airing the Heart" in Section III of Chapter 2).

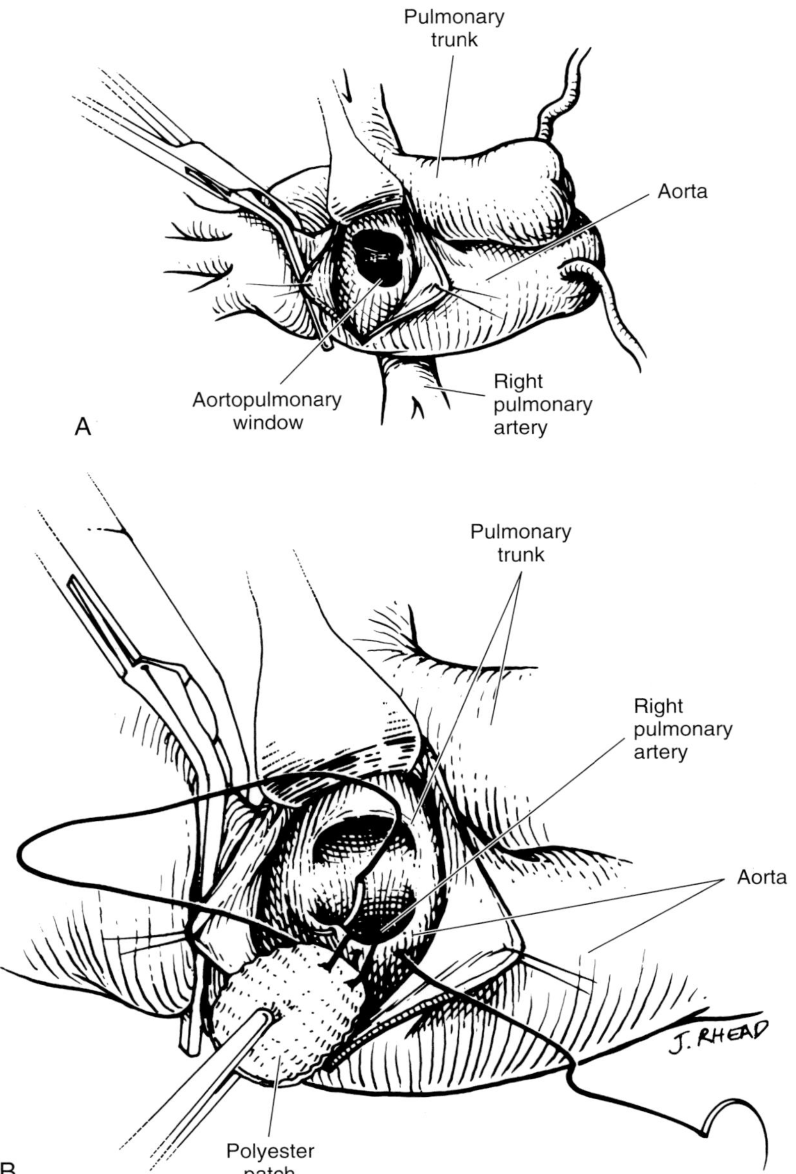

Figure 44-4 Repair of type II aortopulmonary window (APW). **A,** Operation is performed on cardiopulmonary bypass. Aortic perfusion cannula is placed in aortic arch to allow occlusion of aorta near origin of brachiocephalic artery. APW is exposed through a transverse aortotomy. It is located on posterior aspect of aorta and involves the pulmonary trunk at origin of right pulmonary artery. **B,** Partition between aorta and pulmonary trunk is created using a polyester patch. There must be some contour to the patch to avoid stenosis of proximal right pulmonary artery. Edge of aorta at right side of window must be identified and the patch attached to aortic edge to prevent communication of aorta with right pulmonary artery.

If the APW involves the front wall of the proximal right pulmonary artery (type II), approach is made through a vertical or transverse aortotomy (Fig. 44-4, *A*) and the defect closed with a patch that extends out along the right pulmonary artery[R1] (Fig. 44-4, *B*).

Alternatively, a vertical incision may be made in the anterior wall of the APW itself, more or less transecting its anterior half.[J3] After carefully identifying orifices of the right pulmonary artery and left coronary artery, the patch for closure is sutured to the posterior, superior, and inferior walls of the window. The incision into the window is then closed by incorporating the front edge of the patch, with each stitch passing through the aortic wall, the patch, and the pulmonary trunk wall. This technique allows visualization of the left coronary ostium and orifice of the right pulmonary artery and provides a secure partitioning of the ascending aorta from the pulmonary trunk. Unless there is aneurysmal thinning around the window, this technique seems useful.

A modification of this technique is required when the right coronary artery arises from the pulmonary trunk just to the left of the anterior wall of the APW. Then the anterior incision into the window curves to the left into the pulmonary trunk to create a flap of anterior pulmonary trunk wall that includes the origin of the right coronary artery.[A2,L2] The flap should be large enough to cover the entire window. It is sewn into position over the window with a continuous polypropylene stitch. Repair is completed by closing the defect in the pulmonary trunk with a pericardial patch.

Rarely, the right coronary artery arises from the anterior aspect of the pulmonary trunk at some distance from the APW. In that situation, the right coronary artery can be taken as a button from the pulmonary trunk, mobilized, and reimplanted into the aorta at a site distinct from the APW, which is closed with a separate patch.[L1] Similar methods (flap reconstruction or reimplantation) can be used to repair APW with an anomalous origin of the left coronary artery from the posterior wall of the pulmonary trunk.[B5,L1]

SPECIAL FEATURES OF POSTOPERATIVE CARE

Postoperative care is as usual (see Chapter 5). The hemodynamic state is generally excellent because the left ventricle is large, no ventriculotomy has been made, and duration of myocardial ischemia is less than 1 hour. When repair has been performed in a neonate or infant, care appropriate to this age group is used (see Section IV, Chapter 5).

RESULTS

Early (Hospital) Death

Hospital mortality is low after repair of APW unless unusual circumstances are present; no deaths occurred among 18 patients undergoing primary repair at UAB and the University of California at San Francisco (Table 44-1), and one death occurred among 11 infants reported by Tiraboschi and colleagues.[T3] Even with coexisting major anomalies or low birth weight, risk of total repair may also be low.[C1,C3,D4,K1,K3,M1]

Time-Related Survival

Time-related survival is excellent when the operation is performed in infancy. McElhinney and colleagues followed patients for up to 25 years after operation.[M1] Eighteen patients with Richardson type I or II were operated on at age 6 months or less. Eleven were categorized as complex because of presence of associated severe anomalies, most commonly interrupted aortic arch. One patient died 4 months after operation from unspecified respiratory complications. There were no other late deaths. Tkebuchava and colleagues reported similar long-term results.[T4] Ten patients with types I and II defects were operated on, 77% with associated anomalies. One patient with associated interrupted aortic arch died. There were no late deaths among patients followed up to 22 years. In the Congenital Heart Surgeons' Society analysis of 19 patients who underwent surgical repair of IAA and APW, 1- and 10-year survival was 91% and 84%, respectively.[K3]

In those rare circumstances in which repair of a large APW is done in older children, the late result may be compromised by pulmonary vascular disease. The probability of "surgical cure" depends on age at operation and level of pulmonary vascular resistance at the time of operation (see Chapter 35).

Table 44-1 Hospital Mortality after Primary Repair of Aortopulmonary Window

Age (Months) ≤	<	UAB[a] n	UCSF[b] n	Hospital Deaths No.	%	CL
	3	2	3	0	0	
3	6	5	5	0	0	
6	12	1	0	0	0	
12	24	1	0	0	0	
24	48	1	0	0	0	
48		0	0	—	—	
Total		10	8	0	0	0%-17%

[a]1967 to July 1, 1983.
[b]1972 to 1996.[M1]
Key: *CL,* 70% confidence limits; *UCSF,* University of California at San Francisco.

Reinterventions

Although reported cases are too few for meaningful analysis, simple ligation appears to increase the likelihood of incomplete closure or pulmonary artery distortion severe enough to require reintervention, either with catheter techniques or reoperation.[B3,J2,T4] In one study, transpulmonary repair was also associated with a greater chance of reintervention.[J1]

In the setting of IAA with APW, reinterventions are much more likely. In the Congenital Heart Surgeons' Society multi-institutional analysis, by 5 years after repair, 51% of patients required arch reintervention (2 of whom had bronchial compression), 6% pulmonary artery reintervention, and 43% were alive without further intervention. Arch reinterventions were more likely in patients with type B IAA.[K3] Thus, in IAA with APW, long-term survival is excellent, but late sequelae related to the arch repair of IAA are likely.

INDICATIONS FOR OPERATION

Symptomatic infants with APW should be operated on promptly when the diagnosis is made. Elective repair is advised before age 3 months.

Older children should be operated on unless high pulmonary vascular resistance renders them inoperable. The criteria of operability described for patients with VSD are applicable to those with large APWs (see Indications for Operation in Section I of Chapter 35).

ALTERNATIVE PROCEDURES AND CONTROVERSIES

Transcatheter Closure of Aortopulmonary Window

Stamato and colleagues reported successful closure of an APW using a modified double umbrella occluder system delivered via a catheter.[S4] Tulloh and Rigby also used a Rashkind double umbrella device for closure of a small APW estimated to be 3 mm in diameter.[T5] Jureidini and colleagues deployed a 12-mm buttoned device in a 3.7-mm diameter APW in a 27-year-old patient.[J4] Experience to date is limited, and success using this approach requires secure positioning of the device to occlude the orifice of the APW without impinging on the ostium of the left coronary artery.

REFERENCES

A

1. Abbruzzese PA, Merlo M, Chiappa E, Bianco R, Ferrero F, Cappone CM. Berry syndrome, a complex aortopulmonary malformation: one-stage repair in a neonate. Ann Thorac Surg 1997;64:1167.

2. Aydin H, Ozisik K, Surer S, Bolat A, Koc M, Kutsal A. Translocation of anomalous right coronary artery to aortic side of the aortopulmonary window: a different approach for a rare combination. J Card Surg 2009;24:567-9.

B

1. Bagtharia R, Freedom RM, Yoo SJ. Aortopulmonary window. In: Freedom RM, Yoo SJ, Mikailian H, Williams WG, eds. The natural and modified history of congenital heart disease. Malden, Mass.: Wiley-Blackwell, 2004:237-40.
2. Berry TE, Bharati S, Muster AJ, Idriss FS, Santucci B, Lev M, et al. Distal aortopulmonary septal defect, aortic origin of the right pulmonary artery, intact ventricular septum, patent ductus arteriosus and hypoplasia of the aortic isthmus: a newly recognized syndrome. Am J Cardiol 1982;49:108.
3. Bhan A, Gupta M, Abraham S, Sharma R, Kothari SS, Juneja R. Surgical experience of aortopulmonary window repair in infants. Interact Cardiovasc Thorac Surg 2007;6:200-3.
4. Blieden LC, Moller JH. Aorticopulmonary septal defect. An experience with 17 patients. Br Heart J 1974;36:630.
5. Bourlon F, Kreitmann P, Jourdan J, Grinneiser D, Schmitt R, Dor V. Anomalous origin of left coronary artery with aortopulmonary window—a case report with surgical correction and delayed control. Thorac Cardiovasc Surg 1981;29:91-2.
6. Brook MM, Heymann MA. Aortopulmonary window. In: Allen HD, Gutgesell HP, Clark EB, Driscott DJ, eds. Moss and Adams' heart disease in infants, children and adolescents. Philadelphia: Lippincott William and Wilkins 2001:670-4.
7. Burroughs JT, Schumutzer KJ, Linder F, Neuhans G. Anomalous origin of the right coronary artery with aorticopulmonary window and ventricular septal defect. J Cardiovasc Surg 1968;3:142.

C

1. Castaneda AR, Kirklin JW. Tetralogy of Fallot with aorticopulmonary window. Report of two surgical cases. J Thorac Cardiovasc Surg 1977;74:467.
2. Chiemmongkoltip P, Moulder PV, Cassels DE. Interruption of the aortic arch with aorticopulmonary septal defect and intact ventricular septum in a teenage girl. Chest 1971;60:324.
3. Clarke CP, Richardson JP. The management of aortopulmonary window. Advantages of transaortic closure with a Dacron patch. J Thorac Cardiovasc Surg 1976;72:48.
4. Coleman EN, Barclay RS, Reid JM, Stevenson JG. Congenital aortopulmonary fistula combined with persistent ductus arteriosus. Br Heart J 1967;29:571.
5. Cooley DA, McNamara DG, Latson JR. Aorticopulmonary septal defect: diagnosis and surgical treatment. Surgery 1957;42:101.
6. Cotton AC. Report of a case of anuria. Arch Pediatr 1899;16: 774.

D

1. Davies MJ, Dyamenahalli U, Leanage RR, Firmin RK. Total one-stage repair of aortopulmonary window and interrupted aortic arch in a neonate. Pediatr Cardiol 1996;17:122.
2. Deverall PB, Lincoln JC, Aberdeen E, Bonham-Carter RE, Waterston DJ. Aortopulmonary window. J Thorac Cardiovasc Surg 1969;57:479.
3. Di Bella I, Gladstone DJ. Surgical management of aortopulmonary window. Ann Thorac Surg 1998;65:768.
4. Ding WX, Su ZK, Cao DF, Jonas RA. One-stage repair of absence of the aortopulmonary septum and interrupted aortic arch. Ann Thorac Surg 1990;49:664.
5. Dodds JH, Hoyle C. Congenital aortic septal defect. Br Heart J 1949;11:390.
6. Doty DB, Richardson JV, Falkovsky GE, Gordonova MI, Burakovsky VI. Aortopulmonary septal defect: hemodynamics, angiography, and operation. Ann Thorac Surg 1981;32:244.
7. D'Souza VJ, Chen MY. Anomalous origin of coronary artery in association with aorticopulmonary window. Pediatr Cardiol 1996; 17:316.

E

1. Elliotson J. Case of malformation of the pulmonary artery and aorta. Lancet 1830;1:247.

F

1. Faulkner SL, Oldham RR, Atwood GF, Graham TP Jr. Aortopulmonary window, ventricular septal defect, and membranous pulmonary atresia with a diagnosis of truncus arteriosus. Chest 1974;65:351.
2. Fletcher G, DuShane JW, Kirklin JW, Wood EH. Aorticopulmonary septal defect. Report of a case with surgical division along with successful resuscitation from ventricular fibrillation. Mayo Clin Proc 1954;29:285.
3. Freitas I, Parames F, Rebelo M, Martins JD, Pinto MF, Kaku S. Aortopulmonary window. Experience of eleven cases. Rev Port Cardiol 2008;27:1597-603.

G

1. Garver KA, Hernandez RJ, Vermilion RP, Goble MM. Images in cardiovascular medicine. Correlative imaging of aortopulmonary window: demonstration with echocardiography, angiography, and MRI. Circulation 1997;96:1036.
2. Gasul BM, Fell EH, Casas R. The diagnosis of aortic septal defect by retrograde aortography: report of a case. Circulation 1951;4:251.
3. Gross RE. Surgical closure of an aortic septal defect. Circulation 1952;5:858.
4. Gula G, Chew C, Radley-Smith R, Yacoub M. Anomalous origin of the right pulmonary artery from the ascending aorta associated with aortopulmonary window. Thorax 1978;33:265.

H

1. Hew CC, Bacha EA, Zurakowski D, del Nido PJ Jr, Jonas RA. Optimal surgical approach for repair of aortopulmonary window. Cardiol Young 2001;11:385-90.
2. Ho SY, Gerlis LM, Anderson C, Devine WA, Smith A. The morphology of aortopulmonary window with regard to classification and morphogenesis. Cardiol Young 1994;4:146-55.

J

1. Jacobs JP, Quintessenza JA, Gaynor JW, Burke RP, Mavroudis C. Congenital heart surgery nomenclature and database project: aortopulmonary window. Ann Thorac Surg 2000;69:S44-9.
2. Jansen C, Hruda J, Rammeloo L, Ottenkamp J, Hazekamp MG. Surgical repair of aortopulmonary window: thirty-seven years of experience. Pediatr Cardiol 2006;27:552-6.
3. Johansson L, Michaelsson M, Westerholm CJ, Abeg T. Aortopulmonary window: a new operative approach. Ann Thorac Surg 1978;25:564.
4. Jureidini SB, Spadaro JJ, Rao PS. Successful transcatheter closure with the buttoned device of aortopulmonary window in an adult. Am J Cardiol 1998;81:371.

K

1. Kawata H, Kishimoto H, Ueno T, Nakajima T, Inamura N, Nakada T. Repair of aortopulmonary window in an infant with extremely low birth weight. Ann Thorac Surg 1996;62:1843.
2. Kitagawa T, Katoh I, Taki H, Wakisaka Y, Egawa Y, Takahashi Y, et al. New operative method for distal aortopulmonary septal defect. Ann Thorac Surg 1991;51:680.
3. Konstantinov IE, Karamlou T, Williams WG, Quaegebeur JM, del Nido PJ, Spray TL, et al. Surgical management of aortopulmonary window associated with interrupted aortic arch: a Congenital Heart Surgeons Society study. J Thorac Cardiovasc Surg 2006; 131:1136-41.
4. Kutsche LM, Van Mierop LH. Anatomy and pathogenesis of aorticopulmonary septal defects. Am J Cardiol 1987;59:443-7.

L

1. Leobon B, Le Bret E, Roussin R, Kortas C, Ly M, Sigal-Cinqualbre A, et al. Technical options for the treatment of anomalous origins of right or left coronary arteries associated with aortopulmonary windows. J Thorac Cardiovasc Surg 2009;138:777-8.
2. Luisi SV, Ashraf MH, Gula G, Radley-Smith R, Yacoub M. Anomalous origin of the right coronary artery with aortopulmonary window: functional and surgical considerations. Thorax 1980;35:446.

M

1. McElhinney DB, Reddy VM, Tworetzky W, Silverman NH, Hanley FL. Early and late results after repair of aortopulmonary septal defect and associated anomalies in infants <6 months of age. Am J Cardiol 1998;81:195.

2. Meisner H, Schmidt-Habelmann P, Sebenning F, Klinner W. Surgical correction of aortopulmonary septal defects. A review of the literature and report of eight cases. Dis Chest 1968;53:750.
3. Messmer BJ. Pulmonary artery flap for closure of aortopulmonary window. Ann Thorac Surg 1994;57:498.
4. Mori K, Ando M, Takao A, Ishikawa S, Imai Y. Distal type of aortopulmonary window. Report of 4 cases. Br Heart J 1978;40:681.
5. Morrow AG, Greenfield LJ, Braunwald E. Congenital aorto-pulmonary septal defect. Clinical and hemodynamic findings, surgical technique, and results of operative correction. Circulation 1962;25:463.

N

1. Neufeld HN, Lester RG, Adams P Jr, Anderson RC, Lillehei CW, Edwards JE. Aorticopulmonary septal defect. Am J Cardiol 1962; 9:12.

P

1. Pieroni DR, Gingell RL, Roland JM, Chung CY, Broda JJ, Subramanian S. Two-dimensional echocardiographic recognition and surgical management of aortopulmonary septal defect in the premature infant. Thorac Cardiovasc Surg 1982;30:180.
2. Putnam TC, Gross RE. Surgical management of aortopulmonary fenestration. Surgery 1966;59:727.

R

1. Richardson JV, Doty DB, Rossi NP, Ehrenhaft JL. The spectrum of anomalies of aortopulmonary septation. J Thorac Cardiovasc Surg 1979;78:21.
2. Rowe RD. Aortopulmonary septal defect. In Keith JD, Rowe RD, Vlad P, eds. Heart disease in infancy and childhood, 3rd Ed. New York: Macmillan, 1978.

S

1. Satomi G, Nokamura K, Imai Y, Takao A. Two-dimensional echo-cardiographic diagnosis of aorticopulmonary window. Br Heart J 1980;43:351.
2. Schmid FX, Hake U, Iversen S, Schranz D, Oelert H. Surgical closure of aortopulmonary window without cardiopulmonary bypass. Pediatr Cardiol 1989;10:166.
3. Scott HW Jr, Sabiston DC Jr. Surgical treatment for congenital aorticopulmonary fistula. Experimental and clinical aspects. J Thorac Surg 1953;25:26.
4. Stamato T, Benson LN, Smallhorn JF, Freedom RM. Transcatheter closure of an aortopulmonary window with a modified double umbrella occluder system. Cathet Cardiovasc Diagn 1995;35:165.

T

1. Tabak C, Moskowitz W, Wagner H, Weinberg P, Edmunds LH Jr. Aortopulmonary window and aortic isthmic hypoplasia. Operative management in newborn infants. J Thorac Cardiovasc Surg 1983; 86:273.
2. Tandon R, DaSilva CL, Moller JH, Edwards JE. Aorticopulmonary septal defect coexisting with ventricular septal defect. Circulation 1974;50:188.
3. Tiraboschi R, Salomone G, Crupi G, Manasse E, Salim A, Carminati M, et al. Aortopulmonary window in the first year of life: report on 11 surgical cases. Ann Thorac Surg 1988;46:438.
4. Tkebuchava T, von Segesser LK, Vogt PR, Bauersfeld U, Jenni R, Künzli A, et al. Congenital aortopulumonary window: diagnosis, surgical technique and long-term results. Eur J Cardiothorac Surg 1997;11:293-7.
5. Tulloh RM, Rigby ML. Transcatheter umbrella closure of aortopul-monary window: case report. Heart 1997;77:479.

W

1. Wright JS, Freeman R, Johnston JB. Aortopulmonary fenestration. A technique of surgical management. J Thorac Cardiovasc Surg 1968;55:280.

45 Origin of the Right or Left Pulmonary Artery from the Ascending Aorta

DEFINITION

Anomalous origin of a pulmonary artery from the ascending aorta is a condition in which the right pulmonary artery (RPA) or rarely, the left pulmonary artery (LPA), arises from the ascending aorta in the presence of separate aortic and pulmonary valves and without interposition of ductal tissue. This condition is sometimes referred to as *hemitruncus*. *Hemitruncus* is also used to describe a subset of truncus arteriosus (see Chapter 43). Rarely, both right and left pulmonary arteries arise from the ascending aorta in the presence of two separate semilunar valves.

Origins of one or both pulmonary arteries from the transverse aortic arch via a ductus arteriosus or collateral arteries and from the descending thoracic aorta via collateral arteries are not discussed; these conditions are most commonly part of tetralogy of Fallot, but they can occur in the presence of other intracardiac defects or even with normal intracardiac morphology (see Chapter 38). When both the RPA and LPA or only one pulmonary artery arise from the ascending aorta with a common semilunar valve, the condition is a subset of truncus arteriosus (see Chapter 43).

HISTORICAL NOTE

The first description of this entity was by Fraentzel, who in 1868 reported the case of a 25-year-old woman dying in heart failure, with the RPA arising from the ascending aorta and an aortopulmonary window.[F3] In 1914, Doering reported aortic origin of the RPA in an infant dying at age 8 months whose only associated anomaly was a patent ductus arteriosus.[D2] Bopp, in 1949, gave a detailed report of this condition[B5]; since then, and with development of cardiac catheterization and angiography, other cases have been reported.

In 1957, Caro and colleagues corrected the malformation by disconnecting the RPA from the ascending aorta and connecting it with an interposition graft to the pulmonary trunk.[C3] The patient, a 23-year-old man, died a short time after operation. The first successful repair, which was in a 12-month-old infant, was reported in 1961 by Armer and colleagues.[A1] They interposed a graft between the pulmonary trunk and distal end of the divided RPA and closed a coexisting patent ductus arteriosus. In 1967, Kirkpatrick and colleagues reported the first successful cases of retroaortic direct anastomosis of the divided RPA to the pulmonary trunk.[K6] The first report of successful surgical treatment of aortic origin of the LPA, in a 6-week-old infant, was by Herbert and colleagues in 1973.[H1]

MORPHOGENESIS AND MORPHOLOGY

Morphogenesis

Anomalous origin of the RPA from the ascending aorta is related to development of the aortopulmonary septum by fusion of the right and left conotruncal ridges. As such, this defect has developmental morphogenesis similar to aortopulmonary window (see Chapter 44). Severe unequal partitioning of the aortopulmonary trunk by conotruncal ridges results in more dorsal development of the aorta. In this situation, the right sixth aortic arch originates solely from the ascending aorta and is not related to the pulmonary trunk. The result of severe conotruncal ridge malalignment is anomalous origin of the RPA from the ascending aorta, which has been classified by Richardson and colleagues as *aortopulmonary septal defect type III*.[R2]

Morphology

Anomalous Origin of Right Pulmonary Artery

The RPA usually arises from the right or posterior aspect of the ascending aorta (Fig. 45-1) in this condition, but occasionally it arises from the leftward posterior aspect.[C2] Its origin is usually within 1 to 3 cm of the aortic valve.[B4,G1,K3,W1,W2] Uncommonly, it arises from the distal portion of the ascending aorta just proximal to the origin of the brachiocephalic

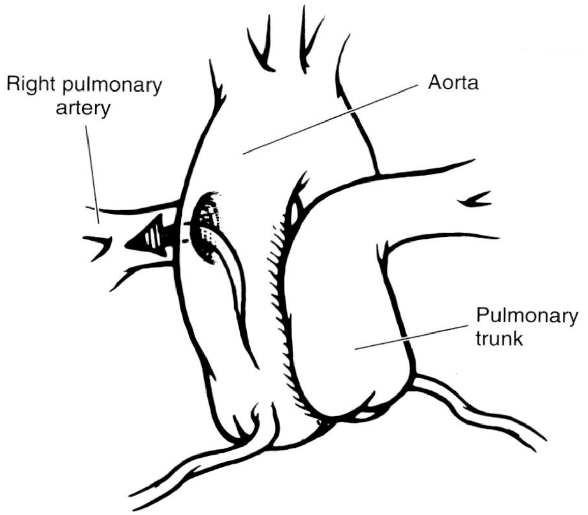

Figure 45-1 Origin of right pulmonary artery (RPA) from ascending aorta, also referred to as *aortopulmonary septal defect type III* (see Chapter 44).[R2] RPA takes its origin from right lateral aspect of ascending aorta. There is a large blood flow shunt from aorta to RPA.

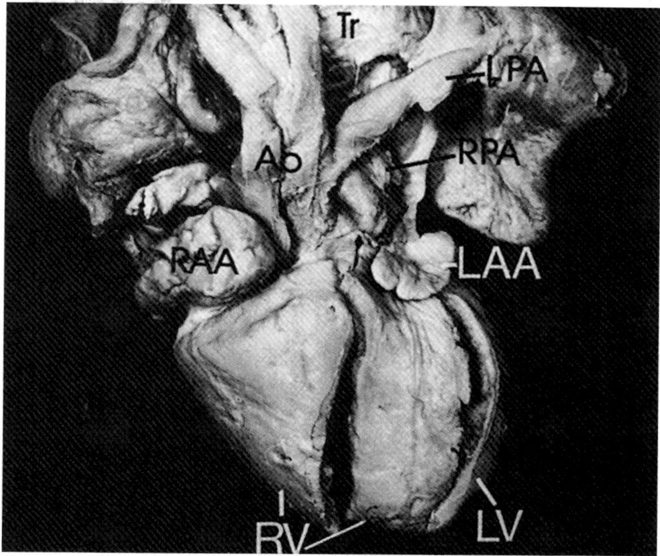

Figure 45-2 Heart specimen from 1-month-old infant viewed from in front. The left pulmonary artery arises from ascending aorta and crosses in front of the dilated right pulmonary artery that arises normally from the pulmonary trunk. This infant had tetralogy of Fallot with absent pulmonary valve. Key: *Ao,* Aorta; *LAA,* left atrial appendage; *LPA,* left pulmonary artery; *LV,* left ventricle; *RAA,* right atrial appendage; *RPA,* right pulmonary artery; *RV,* right ventricle; *Tr,* trachea. (From Calder and colleagues.[C2])

artery.[K11] The RPA origin is rarely stenosed, and the vessel is usually as large as or larger than the normally connected LPA; it is normal in structure, course, and distribution.[G1,K3]

When the RPA arises anomalously from the ascending aorta and no other anomalies are present, pulmonary vascular beds of the two lungs may be similar despite differences in origin of the pulmonary arteries.[C5,H1,M5,P4,R4,R5] Occasionally, pulmonary and tricuspid valves are dilated as a result of right heart failure, and the tricuspid leaflets may be thickened and edges rolled.[G1] Origin of the RPA from the ascending aorta is an isolated lesion in about 20% of cases.[C2,R2] In the remainder, the most common coexisting lesion is patent ductus arteriosus, present in about 50% of cases.[C2,P2]

Other less common associations are with tetralogy of Fallot, ventricular septal defect, aortopulmonary window, coarctation of the aorta, interrupted aortic arch, and atrial septal defect.[C2,C4,C8,F1,G2,K10,M3,M4] Severe contralateral (left) pulmonary vein stenosis may coexist. The vein stenoses are typically tubular, with dilatation of the left pulmonary veins proximal to the stenoses. Also, Sievers and colleagues report coexisting subtotal obstruction of the left pulmonary vein orifices by a membrane that was excised at operation.[S4]

Anomalous Origin of Left Pulmonary Artery

Origin of the LPA from the ascending aorta is rare. It occurs as an isolated lesion in about 40% of cases, usually coexisting with right aortic arch.[C5,H1,K11,R3,S1] In contrast to origin of the RPA from the ascending aorta, the most common associated anomaly is tetralogy of Fallot.[C2,P2] Then, the aortic arch may be left sided.[C2,R3] Tetralogy of Fallot with absent pulmonary valve syndrome is also observed (Fig. 45-2).

Anomalous Origin of Both Pulmonary Arteries

Origin of both RPA and LPA from the ascending aorta has been reported in one patient who had no other cardiac anomaly.[B1] The origin was by way of a short single trunk coming off the posterior aspect of the ascending aorta, with the pulmonary trunk arising normally from the right ventricle and connected only to a patent ductus arteriosus. Repair was attempted unsuccessfully at age 11 days.

CLINICAL FEATURES AND DIAGNOSTIC CRITERIA

When the condition is isolated except for a patent ductus arteriosus, the patient characteristically presents early in infancy with respiratory distress and heart failure.[C5,G1,K4,K6,O1,R1,S7] Frequently the infant is acutely ill. There may be cyanosis from (1) venous admixture in the lungs or (2) reversed shunting through a patent ductus arteriosus or a patent foramen ovale resulting from right heart failure.

There are no typical auscultatory findings, and murmurs may or may not be present.[C7,G1,K4,O1,S7] When present, the murmur is usually systolic and heard along the left sternal border. Rarely, it may be continuous as a result of kinking or stenosis of the artery. The peripheral pulses are jerky or bounding because of rapid runoff from the aorta into the lung and consequent left-to-right shunting. Electrocardiographic findings are not diagnostic and usually indicate biventricular and right atrial enlargement. Cardiomegaly is usually severe on the chest radiograph, with the heart assuming a globular shape.[G1,W2] Pulmonary plethora is usually of similar degree bilaterally.[C5,K3,S7]

When tetralogy of Fallot is present with severe pulmonary stenosis, clinical features are dominated by the tetralogy. The condition may be suspected, however, because the lung supplied by the anomalously arising artery is usually plethoric, whereas the other lung is oligemic.[C2,M4,R3] Since the early 1990s, correct diagnosis and assessment have been adequately made with two-dimensional echocardiography alone, making cardiac catheterization unnecessary[D3,F2,K5,M2,S6] (Fig. 45-3). However, cardiac catheterization and cineangiography

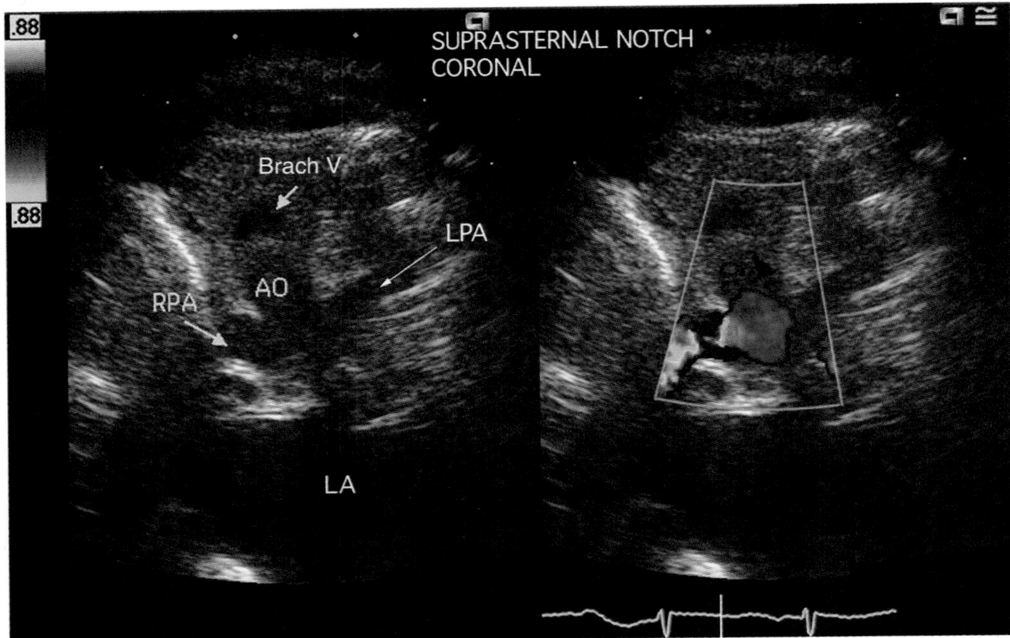

Figure 45-3 Echocardiographic image showing a suprasternal notch coronal view of anomalous origin of right pulmonary artery (RPA) from aorta (AO). Non-color image identifies aorta and both left and right branch pulmonary arteries but does not clearly identify that right branch, but *not* left, arises from aorta. Color image identifies origin of right branch from aorta, with evidence of acceleration of flow into the RPA. Key: *BRACH V,* brachiocephalic vein; *LA,* left atrium; *LPA,* left pulmonary artery.

provide additional information. Pressure in the pulmonary artery arising from the aorta is systemic in almost all cases, because ostial stenosis is rare.[S7] As already noted, pressure in the pulmonary artery that arises normally is usually also elevated to systemic or suprasystemic levels.[B2,S2] Accurate measurement of pulmonary and systemic blood flows is difficult in this situation but not critical, because the infants usually present with clear clinical evidence of increased pulmonary blood flow. Pulmonary vascular resistance in the normally connected lung can be calculated and is a useful guide to operability—and an essential guide in older patients.

Cineangiography is diagnostic, and a right ventriculogram or pulmonary angiogram opacifies only the normally connected pulmonary arteries. Antegrade or retrograde aortography shows the pulmonary artery that arises from the ascending aorta (Fig. 45-4). Cineangiography is also used to define other cardiac anomalies that may be present.[G1,R4]

In neonates and infants in whom catheterization is not critical, computed tomography angiography can confirm morphologic details suspected by echocardiography (Fig. 45-5).

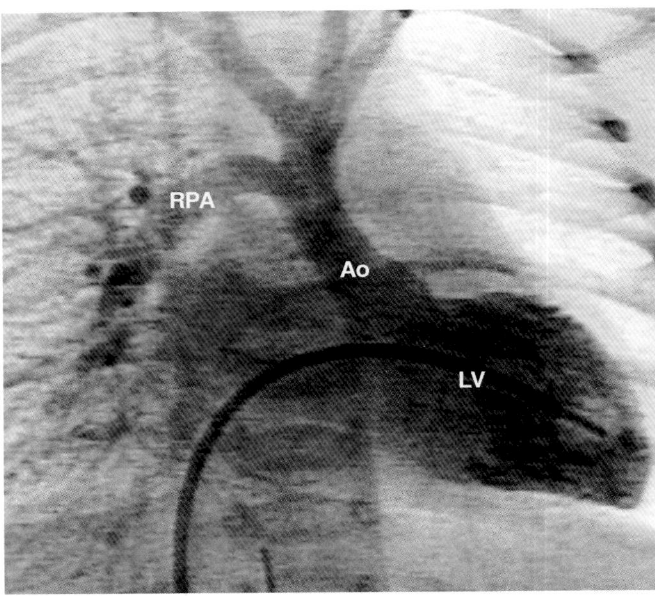

Figure 45-4 Anteroposterior angiographic view of left ventriculogram showing opacification of ascending aorta (AO) and anomalous origin of right pulmonary artery (RPA) from aorta. Key: *LV,* left ventricle.

NATURAL HISTORY

Anomalous origin of a branch pulmonary artery from the ascending aorta is rare, reportedly accounting for 0.12% of all congenital heart defects.[C6] Nearly all cases involve the RPA.[C2,P2] As of 2004, 136 cases of RPA from the aorta had been reported,[P6] and from 2004 to 2010, at least 35 additional cases appeared in the literature.[K2,N2,P1] In 2003, Prifti and colleagues reviewed the reported experience with LPA from the aorta and found 77 cases; however, many of these appear to have had LPA origins from the descending thoracic aorta or from a ductus, with a high association with tetralogy of Fallot, and thus likely represent a different lesion.[P5] It is a lethal condition. About 70% of surgically untreated patients are dead by age 6 months and 80% by age 1 year (Fig. 45-6). Intractable heart failure is the usual mode of death.

Pulmonary hypertension in the anomalous pulmonary artery is uniformly present, and commonly it is also present in the normally connected pulmonary artery. This finding is supported by Pool and colleagues' observation that

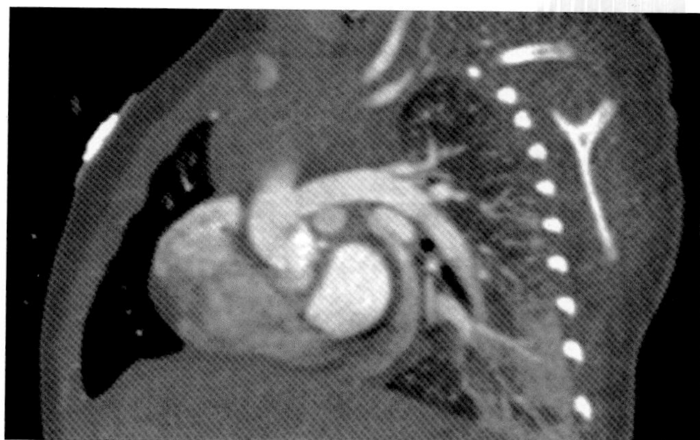

Figure 45-5 Computed tomography (CT) angiographic image performed using electrocardiogram-gated multidetector CT scanner with modulation technique. Sagittal oblique reconstructed image shows left pulmonary artery arising from ascending aorta. (From Diab and colleagues.[D1])

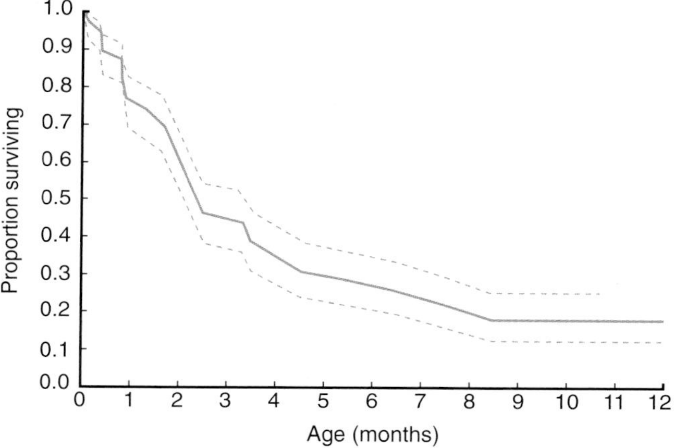

Figure 45-6 Natural history of isolated origin of right pulmonary artery from ascending aorta, with or without patent ductus arteriosus (n = 39). Autopsied nonsurgical cases reported in the literature have been tabulated and analysis made of the proportion alive at any stated age.[B5,C1,D2,F1,G1,K1,K3,K4,K7,K8,K9,M1,O1,P4,R4,S5,S7,T1,T2,V2,V3,W2] Some cases and reports may be missing from this analysis, but the general shape of the relationship is probably correct. Patent ductus arteriosus was present in 26 patients (67%).

pulmonary hypertension develops in 19% of infants born with unilateral absence of a pulmonary artery and no associated malformations, and that ligation of one pulmonary artery within 24 hours of birth in five calves resulted in severe pulmonary hypertension in the opposite lung within 2 months.[P3] Surprisingly, Keane and colleagues report no important obstructive vascular changes in either lung in most patients dying in the first 6 months of life.[K4] This does not mean that pulmonary hypertension was not present, just that pathologic changes were not evident.

Among older patients, pathologic evidence of hypertensive pulmonary vascular disease is usually present, often to a similar extent in the two lungs, sometimes greater in the right and sometimes greater in the left. It is likely that the natural history of isolated origin of the LPA from the ascending aorta is similar, but too few patients have been observed to establish this.

TECHNIQUE OF OPERATION

Preparations for operation, median sternotomy, and cardiopulmonary bypass (CPB) are those normally used (see "Preparation for Cardiopulmonary Bypass" in Section III of Chapter 2), as are the techniques for myocardial management (see "Cold Cardioplegia, Controlled Aortic Root Reperfusion, and [When Needed] Warm Cardioplegic Induction" in Chapter 3). The technique is described for anomalously arising RPA; it is similar when the LPA is affected.

Once the pericardium has been opened, the anomalously originating RPA is visualized coming from either the posterior or right lateral aspect of the ascending aorta (Fig. 45-7, *A*). It passes into the right hemithorax behind the superior vena cava. The aorta is completely dissected from the pulmonary trunk, and the ductus arteriosus is dissected out at this point.

The purse-string sutures and preparation for CPB are made as usual, except that care is taken to place the aortic cannula far enough downstream so that the aorta may be occluded distal to the aortic origin of the RPA (see Fig. 45-7, *A*). A single venous cannula is placed into the right atrium. CPB is established as usual, and as soon as it has begun, a temporary arterial clamp is placed across the RPA.

The ligamentum arteriosum or ductus arteriosum is ligated and specifically divided. Division allows improved mobility of the pulmonary trunk so that the connection to the RPA can be performed with minimal tension. A vent catheter is placed in the left atrium through a purse-string in the right upper pulmonary vein. After the aorta is occluded well distal to the RPA, cold cardioplegia is administered. The clamp is removed from the RPA, which is then thoroughly mobilized beneath the superior vena cava out to the lobar branches.

The pulmonary artery is then disconnected from the ascending aorta (see Fig. 45-7, *A*). The defect left in the ascending aorta is closed by a pericardial patch or other patch material (Fig. 45-7, *B*). In some cases, it may be possible to close the aorta transversely by direct suture. The aorta is rotated anteriorly and leftward. The right side of the pulmonary trunk is pulled out from beneath the aorta (see Fig. 45-7, *B*), and a longitudinal incision is made in it. An anastomosis is made between the end of the well-mobilized RPA and the side of the pulmonary trunk (Fig. 45-7, *C*). A 7-0 polypropylene suture is used, sewing from within the vessels posteriorly and working external to the vessels anteriorly. The completed repair establishes continuity between the RPA and pulmonary trunk, eliminating the shunt (Fig. 45-7, *inset*).

An alternative technique that achieves greater length on the RPA was described by van Son and Hanley[V1] (Fig. 45-8, *A*). After the aorta is occluded, it is incised transversely at the level of RPA origin. The aortic incision is continued posteriorly, leaving a generous cuff of posterior wall around the origin of the RPA. Position of the left coronary artery is noted and its ostium protected from injury. An incision is made in the right lateral wall of the pulmonary trunk so as to create an anteriorly based flap (Fig. 45-8, *B*). An anastomosis of the RPA to the pulmonary trunk is created with the two flaps forming the proximal segment of the RPA (Fig. 45-8, *C*). The ascending aorta is reconstructed by end-to-end anastomosis (Fig. 45-8, *D*).

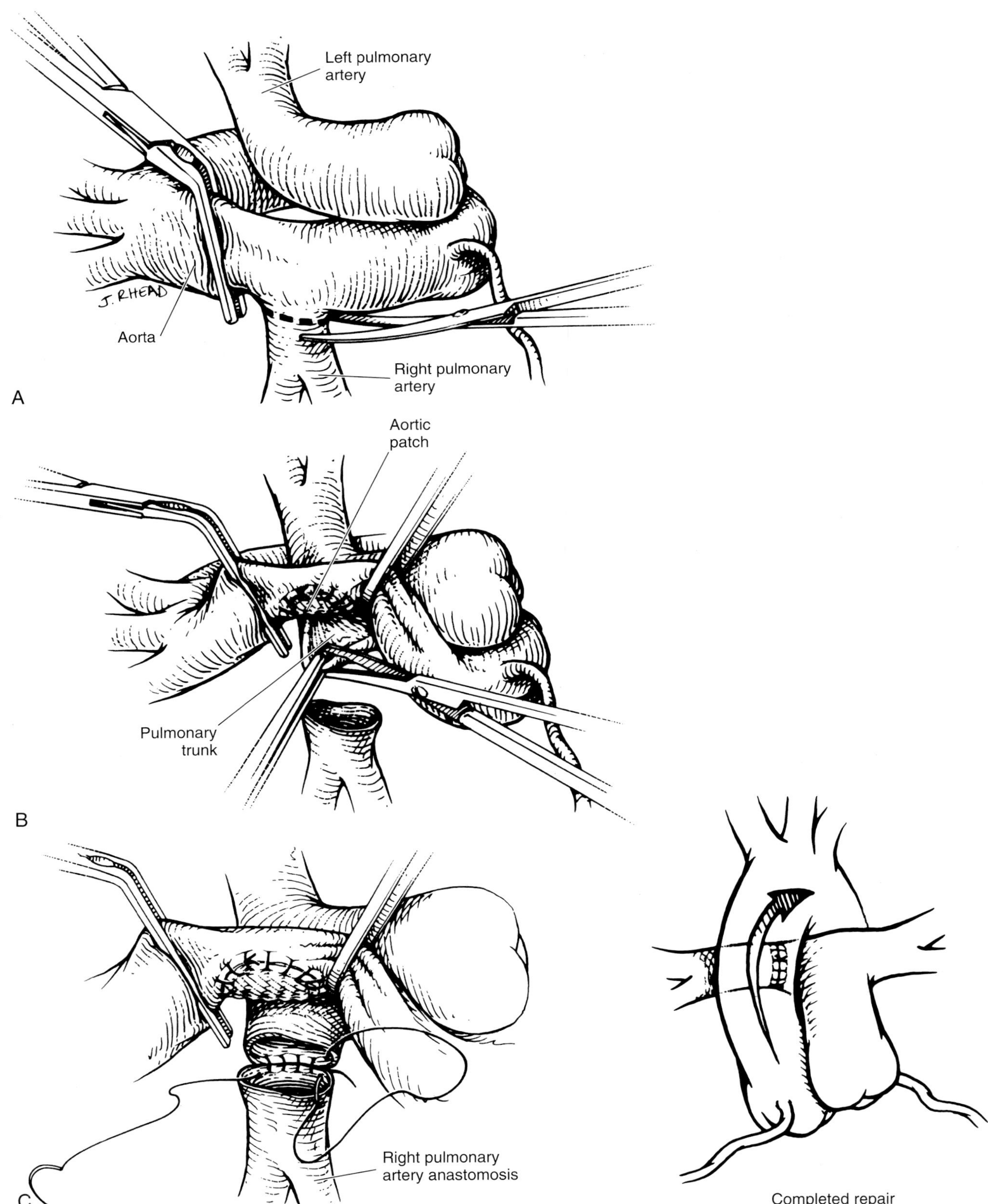

Figure 45-7 Repair of anomalous origin of right pulmonary artery (RPA) from ascending aorta. **A,** Aorta is occluded near origin of brachiocephalic artery above anomalous origin of RPA. This requires cannulating the distal ascending aorta or aortic arch. RPA is removed from aorta *(dashed line)*. **B,** Opening in ascending aorta is repaired by prosthetic patch. Right lateral aspect of pulmonary trunk is mobilized and delivered to the right. An opening is made into the pulmonary trunk. **C,** An end-to-end anastomosis of RPA to pulmonary trunk is constructed using continuous stitches of 6-0 or 7-0 polypropylene or polydioxanone suture. *Inset,* Repair restores normal continuity of pulmonary arteries and eliminates shunting from aorta to RPA.

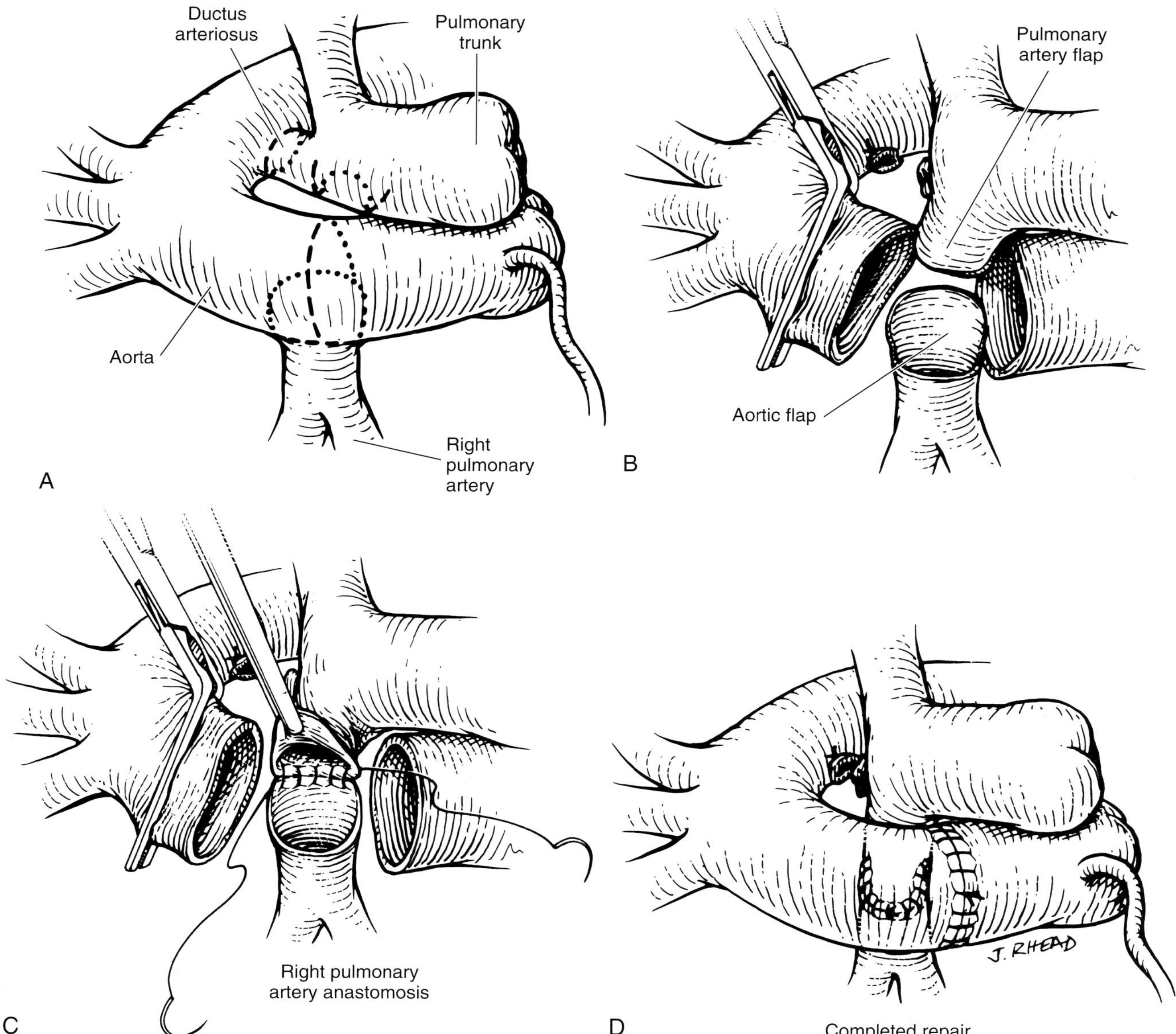

Figure 45-8 Repair of anomalous origin of right pulmonary artery (RPA) from aorta using autogenous flaps of aorta and pulmonary trunk. **A,** Ductus arteriosus is doubly ligated and divided. Aorta is transected at level of anomalous origin of RPA. Dashed line indicates anterior incision of aorta. Posteriorly, as indicated by dotted line, the transection incision separates at midpoint of aorta to encompass origin of RPA, thereby creating a flap of aorta attached to the RPA. Two parallel incisions *(dashed lines)* are made on the pulmonary trunk at proposed site of anastomosis of RPA. Incisions are joined posteriorly *(dotted line)* to create an anteriorly based flap on the pulmonary trunk. **B,** Aortic and pulmonary artery flaps are shown. Sufficient length is created to allow tension-free anastomosis of RPA to pulmonary trunk. **C,** Tissue flaps are anastomosed with continuous stitches of 6-0 polyglyconate suture, creating a proximal extension from pulmonary trunk to RPA. **D,** Aorta is reanastomosed in end-to-end fashion anterior to RPA to complete the repair.

The operation is completed in the usual fashion. It is advisable not only to place left and right atrial pressure catheters but also to insert an additional catheter into the right atrium and advance it across the tricuspid valve for monitoring pulmonary artery pressure during the first 48 or more postoperative hours.

SPECIAL FEATURES OF POSTOPERATIVE CARE

Management usually given to infants after intracardiac surgery is used (see Chapter 5). Pulmonary hypertensive crises can be expected early postoperatively, and the infant is treated accordingly (see "Pulmonary Hypertensive Crises" under Pulmonary Subsystem in Chapter 5).

RESULTS

When origin of the RPA or LPA from the ascending aorta is an isolated condition (apart from patent ductus arteriosus), operation can be a low-risk procedure even in critically ill small infants (Table 45-1).[M2] This has been confirmed in other small individual institutional experiences, each ranging from 1 to 16 cases, with little or no early mortality.[K2,N2,P1,P2,S3] When there are important associated anomalies such as

Table 45-1 Outcome in Six Patients with Anomalous Origin of Right Pulmonary Artery from the Ascending Aorta[a]

Age			Deaths			
			<30 Days			≥30 Days
≤ Days	<	*n*	No.	%	CL(%)	No.
	30	3	0	0		0
30	60	1	0	0		0
60	90	2	0	0		0
90						
TOTAL		6	0	0	0-27	0

[a]These patients were operated on between 1972 and 1995.[M2] Five of six were classified as "simple"; one patient had hypoplastic right pulmonary artery.

tetralogy of Fallot with absence of the pulmonary valve or pulmonary vein stenosis, risk of death increases.

Survivors of repair in infancy, with or without patent ductus arteriosus, have generally done well and have normal pulmonary artery pressure late postoperatively and presumably a normal life expectancy.[B3,K2,K4,P2] Stenosis can occur at the anastomotic site of the RPA.[P7,V4] It can be effectively treated by surgical revision or catheter angioplasty.[K2,N2,T1] Ascending aortic stenosis has been reported at the site of pulmonary artery removal.[K2,N2] Ventilation and perfusion are usually normal in both lungs late postoperatively.[N1]

At least an intermediate-term good result can be obtained in some older patients. Juca and colleagues reported a satisfactory decrease in RPA and LPA pressure in a patient who was 20 years old at operation.[J1,J2] Long and colleagues reported normalization of pulmonary vascular resistance in both lungs in a patient repaired at age 23 years with stenosis of the anomalous pulmonary artery but severe LPA hypertension due to a ductus arteriosus.[L1]

INDICATIONS FOR OPERATION

Diagnosis of origin of RPA or LPA from ascending aorta in infancy is an indication for urgent operation. This is true regardless of pulmonary vascular resistance in the two lungs, because these changes are usually reversible, at least in infants operated on before age 6 to 12 months. In rare cases of presentation beyond infancy, excessive elevation of pulmonary vascular resistance in the normally connected lung is a contraindication to operation.[P2] However, experience is insufficient to state the exact level of pulmonary vascular resistance in the normally connected lung that makes patients inoperable.

If the resistance is normal in the normally connected lung, repair is indicated. The anomalously connected lung will never have infinite resistance, so connecting it to the pulmonary circuit will always lower pulmonary vascular resistance. The difficulty lies in assessing resistance in the anomalously connected lung prior to repair. Pressure and flow to the normally connected lung can be easily measured at catheterization, and thus resistance in that lung can be calculated. Pressure, but not flow, to the anomalously connected lung can be easily measured, thus resistance cannot be calculated. A nuclear medicine lung perfusion scan can be used to estimate the flow ratio to each lung, and when this is combined with other pressure and flow data from catheterization, resistance can be calculated independently in each lung, helping to determine operability.

REFERENCES

A

1. Armer RM, Shumacker HB, Klatte EC. Origin of right pulmonary artery from the aorta: report of a surgically corrected case. Circulation 1961;24:662.

B

1. Beitzke A, Shinebourne EA. Single origin of right and left pulmonary arteries from ascending aorta, with main pulmonary artery from right ventricle. Br Heart J 1980;43:363.
2. Benatar A, Kinsley RH, Milner S, Dansky R, Hummel DA, Levin SE. Surgical correction for one pulmonary artery arising from ascending aorta—report of five cases. Int J Cardiol 1987;16:249.
3. Binet JP, Ribierre M, Dagonnet Y, Le Loch H, Loth P, Planche C, et al. Right pulmonary artery originating from ascending aorta. Reimplantation in an infant of 4 kg. Arch Mal Coeur Vaiss 1975;68:415 (French).
4. Bjork VO, Rudhe U, Zetterqvist P. Aortic origin of the right pulmonary artery and wide patent ductus arteriosus. Scand J Thor Cardiovasc Surg 1970;4:87.
5. Bopp VF. Anormale arterielle Gefassversorgung der rechten Lunge. Zentralbl Allg Pathol 1949;85:155.

C

1. Calazel P, Martinez J. Abnormal origin of 1 of 2 pulmonary arteries from the ascending aorta. Arch Mal Coeur Vaiss 1975;68:397 (French).
2. Calder AL, Brandt PW, Barratt-Boyes BG, Neutze JM. Variants of tetralogy of Fallot with absent pulmonary valve leaflets and origin of one pulmonary artery from the ascending aorta. Am J Cardiol 1980;46:106.
3. Caro C, Lermanda VC, Lyons HA. Aortic origin of right pulmonary artery. Br Heart J 1957;19:345.
4. Carrel T, Pfammatter JP. Interrupted aortic arch, aortopulmonary window and aortic origin of the right pulmonary artery: single stage repair in a neonate. Eur J Cardiothorac Surg 1997;12:668.
5. Caudill DR, Helmsworth JA, Daoud G, Kaplan S. Anomalous origin of left pulmonary artery from ascending aorta. J Thorac Cardiovasc Surg 1969;57:493.
6. Cheng W, Xiao Y, Zhong Q, Wen R. Anomalous origin of left pulmonary artery branch from the aorta with Fallot's tetralogy. Thorac Cardiovasc Surg 2008;56:432-4.
7. Cumming GR, Ferguson CC, Sanchez J. Aortic origin of the right pulmonary artery. Am J Cardiol 1972;30:674.
8. Czarnecki SW, Hopeman AR, Child PL. Tetralogy of Fallot with aortic origin of the left pulmonary artery: radiographic and angiocardiographic considerations. Dis Chest 1964;46:97.

D

1. Diab K, Richardson R, Pophal S, Alboliras E. Left hemitruncus associated with tetralogy of Fallot: fetal diagnosis and postnatal echocardiographic and cardiac computed tomographic confirmation. Pediatr Cardiol 2009;31:534-7.
2. Doering H. Angeborener Defekt der rechten Lungenarterie. Stud Pathol Entwick 1914;2:41.
3. Duncan WJ, Freedom RM, Olley PM, Rowe RD. Two dimensional echocardiographic identification of hemitruncus: anomalous origin of one pulmonary artery from ascending aorta with the other pulmonary artery arising normally from the right ventricle. Am Heart J 1981;102:892.

F

1. Findlay CW, Maier HC. Anomalies of the pulmonary vessels and their surgical significance: with a review of the literature. Surgery 1951;29:604.
2. Fong LV, Anderson RH, Siewers RD, Trento A, Park SC. Anomalous origin of one pulmonary artery from the ascending aorta: a review of echocardiographic, catheter, and morphological features. Br Heart J 1989;62:389.
3. Fraentzel O. Ein fall von abnormer communication der aorta mit der arteria pulmonalis. Virchows Arch [A] 1868;43:420.

G

1. Griffiths SP, Levine OR, Andersen DH. Aortic origin of right pulmonary artery. Circulation 1962;25:73.
2. Gula G, Chew C, Radley-Smith R, Yacoub M. Anomalous origin of the right pulmonary artery from the ascending aorta associated with aortopulmonary window. Thorax 1978;33:265.

H

1. Herbert WH, Rohman M, Farnsworth P, Swamy S. Anomalous origin of the left pulmonary artery from ascending aorta, right aortic arch, and right patent ductus arteriosus. Chest 1973;63:459.

J

1. Juca ER. Origin of right pulmonary artery from ascending aorta (letter). J Thorac Cardiovasc Surg 1984;88:458.
2. Juca ER, Carvalho W Jr, deSousa JR, Araujo JA, Maia F, Karbage JM, et al. Anomalous origin of the right pulmonary artery from the ascending aorta. Arq Bras Cardiol 1979;33:347 (Portuguese).

K

1. Kadoma K, Sugiura S, Saito M, Takao T. Anomalous origin of right pulmonary artery from ascending aorta. Heart 1971;3:786.
2. Kajihara N, Imoto Y, Sakamoto M, Ochiai Y, Kan-o M, Joo K, et al. Surgical results of anomalous origin of the right pulmonary artery from the ascending aorta including reoperation for infrequent complications. Ann Thorac Surg 2008;85:1407-11.
3. Kauffman SL, Yao AC, Webber CB, Lynfield J. Origin of the right pulmonary artery from the aorta: a clinical-pathologic study of two types based on caliber of the pulmonary artery. Am J Cardiol 1967;19:741.
4. Keane JF, Maltz D, Bernhard WF, Corwin RD, Nadas AS. Anomalous origin of one pulmonary artery from the ascending aorta: diagnostic, physiological and surgical considerations. Circulation 1974;50:588.
5. King DH, Huhta JC, Gutgesell HP, Ott DA. Two-dimensional echocardiographic diagnosis of anomalous origin of the right pulmonary artery from the aorta: differentiation from aortopulmonary window. J Am Coll Cardiol 1984;4:351.
6. Kirkpatrick SE, Girod DA, King H. Aortic origin of the right pulmonary artery: surgical repair without a graft. Circulation 1967; 36:777.
7. Kleinschmidt HJ, Lignitz E. Origin of right pulmonary artery from the ascendent aorta. Abnormal pulmonary blood. Zentralbl Allg Pathol 1972;115:547 (German).
8. Kondo M, Sugimoto M, Kano T, Nakata Y, Uesugi M. Origin of the right pulmonary artery from the ascending aorta associated with patent left ductus arteriosus. Kokyu To Junkan 1975;23:637.
9. Kuetel J, Kampmann A, Kyrieleis C. Abnormer ursprung der rechten lungenarterie aus der aszendierenden aorta. Z Kardiol 1972;62:567.
10. Kuers PF, McGoon DC. Tetralogy of Fallot with aortic origin of the right pulmonary artery. J Thorac Cardiovasc Surg 1973;65:327.
11. Kutsche LM, Van Mierop LH. Anomalous origin of a pulmonary artery from the ascending aorta: associated anomalies and pathogenesis. Am J Cardiol 1988;61:850.

L

1. Long MA, Brown SC, de Vries WJ. Anomalous origin of the right pulmonary artery from the ascending aorta: a surgical case study in an adult patient with "irreversible" pulmonary vascular disease. J Card Surg 2009;24:212-5.

M

1. Maier HC. Absence of hypoplasia of a pulmonary artery with anomalous systemic arteries to the lung. J Thorac Surg 1954;28:145.
2. McElhinney DB, Reddy VM, Tworetzky W, Silverman NH, Hanley FL. Early and late results after repair of aortopulmonary septal defect and associated anomalies in infants <6 months of age. Am J Cardiol 1998;81:195.
3. Morgan J, Pitman R, Goodwin JF, Steiner RE, Hollman A. Anomalies of the aorta and pulmonary arteries complicating ventricular septal defect. Br Heart J 1964;24:279.
4. Morgan JR. Left pulmonary artery from ascending aorta in tetralogy of Fallot. Circulation 1972;45:653.
5. Mudd JG, Willman VL, Riberi A. Origin of one pulmonary artery from the aorta. Am Rev Respir Dis 1964;89:255.

N

1. Nashef SA, Jamieson MP, Pollock JC, Houston AB. Aortic origin of right pulmonary artery: successful surgical correction in three consecutive patients. Ann Thorac Surg 1987;44:536.
2. Nathan M, Rimmer D, Piercey G, del Nido PJ, Mayer JE, Bacha EA, et al. Early repair of hemitruncus: excellent early and late outcomes. J Thorac Cardiovasc Surg 2007;133:1329-35.

O

1. Odell JE, Smith JC. Right pulmonary artery arising from ascending aorta. Am J Dis Child 1963;105:87.

P

1. Peng EW, Shanmugam G, Macarthur KJ, Pollock JC. Ascending aortic origin of a branch pulmonary artery–surgical management and long-term outcome. Eur J Cardiothorac Surg 2004;26:762-6.
2. Penkoske PA, Castaneda AR, Fyler DC, Van Praagh R. Origin of pulmonary artery branch from ascending aorta. J Thorac Cardiovasc Surg 1983;85:537.
3. Pool PE, Averill KH, Vogel JH. Effect of ligation of left pulmonary artery at birth on maturation of pulmonary vascular bed. Med Thorac 1962;19:362.
4. Porter DD, Canent RV Jr, Spach MS, Baylin GJ. Origin of the right pulmonary artery from the ascending aorta. Unusual cineangiocardiographic and pathologic findings. Circulation 1963;27:589.
5. Prifti E, Bonacchi M, Murzi B, Crucean A, Bernabei M, Luisi VS, et al. Anomalous origin of the left pulmonary artery from the aorta. Our experience and literature review. Heart Vessels 2003;18: 79-84.
6. Prifti E, Bonacchi M, Murzi B, Crucean A, Leacche M, Bernabei M, et al. Anomalous origin of the right pulmonary artery from the ascending aorta. J Card Surg 2004;19:103-12.
7. Prifti E, Crucean A, Bonacchi M, Bernabei M, Leacche M, Murzi B, et al. Postoperative outcome in patients with anomalous origin of one pulmonary artery branch from the aorta. Eur J Cardiothorac Surg 2003;24:21-7.

R

1. Redo SF, Foster HR Jr, Engle MA, Ehler KH. Anomalous origin of the right pulmonary artery from the ascending aorta. J Thorac Cardiovasc Surg 1965;50:726.
2. Richardson JV, Doty DB, Rossi NP, Ehrenhaft JL. The spectrum of anomalies of aortopulmonary septation. J Thorac Cardiovasc Surg 1979;78:21.
3. Robin E, Silberg B, Ganguley S, Magnisalis K. Aortic origin of the left pulmonary artery. Variant of tetralogy of Fallot. Am J Cardiol 1975;35:324.
4. Rosenberg HS, Hallman GL, Wolfe RR, Latson JR. Origin of the right pulmonary artery from the aorta. Am Heart J 1966;72:106.
5. Rosenburg HS, McNamara DG, Leachman RA, Buzzi RM. The pulmonary vascular structure of children with ventricular septal defect. Arch Pathol 1960;70:141.

S

1. Schillar M, Williams TE Jr, Craenen J, Hosier DM, Sirak HD. Anomalous origin of the left pulmonary artery from the ascending aorta. Vasc Surg 1971;5:126.
2. Semb BK, Björnstad PG. Correction of isolated anomalous origin of the right pulmonary artery from the ascending aorta. Thorac Cardiovasc Surg 1981;29:255.
3. Sibley YD, Roberts KD, Silove ED. Surgical correction of anomalous origin of right pulmonary artery from aorta in a four day old neonate. Br Heart J 1986;56:98.
4. Sievers HH, Lange PE, Radtcke W, Hahne HJ, Heintzen P, Bernhard A. Repair of anomalous origin of the right pulmonary artery from the ascending aorta associated with subtotal left cor triatriatum. Ann Thorac Surg 1985;39:80.
5. Sikl H. Neobvykla malformace arteriosniho trunku: Odstup jedne halvni vetve plicnice z aorty. Cas Lek Cesk 1952;91:1366.
6. Smallhorn JF, Anderson RH, Macartney FJ. Two dimensional echocardiographic assessment of communications between ascending aorta and pulmonary trunk or individual pulmonary arteries. Br Heart J 1982;47:563.

7. Stanton RE, Durnin RE, Fyler DC, Lindesmith GG, Meyer BW. Right pulmonary artery originating from ascending aorta. Am J Dis Child 1968;115:403.

T

1. Tkebuchava T, von Segesser LK, Vogt PR, Bauersfeld U, Jenni R, Kunzli A, et al. Congenital aortopulmonary window: diagnosis, surgical technique and long-term results. Eur J Cardiothorac Surg 1997;11:293.
2. Tobise K, Kobayashi T, Tateda K, Kishi F, Onodera K. Origin of right pulmonary artery from ascending aorta. A case report. Jpn J Intern Med 1973;62:154.

V

1. van Son JA, Hanley FL. Use of autogenous aortic and main pulmonary artery flaps for repair of anomalous origin of the right pulmonary artery from the ascending aorta. J Thorac Cardiovasc Surg 1996;111:675.
2. Vasquez-Perez J, Pereda-Perez RA, Frontera-Izquierdo P. Aortic origin of the right pulmonary artery. Review and report of two cases. Am Esp Pediatr 1976;9:584 (Spanish).
3. Vasquez SF, Trevino CP, Angulo O. Origin of the right pulmonary artery from the aorta and right endocardial fibroelastosis. Report of a case and review of the literature. Arch Dis Cardiol Mex 1966;36:184 (Spanish).
4. Vida VL, Sanders SP, Bottio T, Maschietto N, Rubino M, Milanesi O, et al. Anomalous origin of one pulmonary artery from the ascending aorta. Cardiol Young 2005;15:176-81.

W

1. Wagenvoort CA, Neufeld HN, Birge RF, Caffrey JA, Edwards JE. Origin of right pulmonary artery from ascending aorta. Circulation 1961;23:84.
2. Weintraub RA, Fabian CE, Adams DF. Ectopic origin of one pulmonary artery from ascending aorta. Radiology 1966;86:666.

46 Congenital Anomalies of the Coronary Arteries

INTRODUCTION

Congenital anomalies of the coronary arteries represent a varied group of lesions. Taken together, they are relatively common, seen in 1% to 5% of the population, depending on the method of detection. Many lesions are incidental findings with little or no consequences, but approximately 20% have the potential to cause coronary ischemia and its sequelae.

Box 46-1 presents a useful classification of all congenital coronary artery lesions. Some of these—an anomalous or eccentric location of a coronary artery ostium, multiple ostia, and duplication of coronary arteries—have no physiologic importance but may be important if other cardiac procedures are required. Others lesions such as myocardial bridging, ectasia or aneurysm, and small fistulas may or may not have to be surgically repaired, depending on whether or not they have physiologic consequences.

The most important lesions include large coronary arteriovenous fistula, anomalous connection of a coronary artery to the pulmonary trunk, and anomalous connection of a coronary artery to the wrong aortic sinus. *All* require surgical correction, or occasionally other intervention. This chapter focuses on these three lesions. A discussion of the more minor and incidental lesions outlined in Box 46-1 can be found in the review by Kayalar and colleagues.[K5]

Box 46-1 Classification of Coronary Artery Anomalies

Anomalies of Origin and Course

I. Anomalous location of coronary ostium:
  a. High ostium
  b. Commissural ostium
II. Anomalous origin of coronary artery from opposite sinus with one of four courses:
  a. Interarterial
  b. Transseptal
  c. Retroaortic
  d. Prepulmonic
III. Anomalous origin of coronary artery from pulmonary trunk:
  Type 1: Left coronary artery
  Type 2: Right coronary artery
  Type 3: Circumflex coronary artery
  Type 4: Left and right coronary arteries
IV. Single coronary artery
V. Multiple ostia
VI. Anomalous origin of coronary artery from noncoronary sinus
VII. Duplication of coronary arteries

Anomalies of Intrinsic Coronary Arterial Anatomy

I. Congenital ostial stenoses
II. Coronary artery ectasia or aneurysm
III. Myocardial bridging

Anomalies of Termination

I. Congenital coronary artery fistula
II. Extracardiac termination

Modified from Kayalar and colleagues.[K5]

Section I Coronary Arteriovenous Fistula

DEFINITION

A congenital coronary arteriovenous (AV) fistula is a direct communication between a coronary artery and the lumen of any one of the four cardiac chambers, the coronary sinus or its tributary veins, or the superior vena cava, pulmonary artery, or pulmonary veins close to the heart. Fistulous coronary connections that occur in congenital pulmonary and aortic atresia (see "Right Ventricular Coronary Artery Fistulae" under Morphology in Chapter 40 and "Other Associated Cardiac Anomalies" under Morphology in Chapter 49) are excluded from this chapter.

HISTORICAL NOTE

A congenital coronary AV fistula was first described by Krause in 1865.[K11] The first report in the English literature was that of Trevor in 1912, who described autopsy findings in a case with a fistula from the right coronary artery into the right ventricle. The patient died from associated endocarditis.[T5] Autopsy reports from Blakeway[B9] and from Halpert[H2] followed. The first report of surgical correction was in 1947 by Biorck and Crafoord,[B7] who discovered a fistulous connection to the pulmonary trunk at thoracotomy in a patient presumed to have a patent ductus arteriosus. It was closed with sutures. Probably the first reported case of a fistula that was correctly diagnosed preoperatively was that of Fell and colleagues in 1958,[F2] and the first report of repair using cardiopulmonary bypass (CPB) was that of Swan and colleagues in 1959.[S13] Currarino and colleagues described the use of angiography in diagnosis in 1959.[C15]

MORPHOLOGY

Coronary Artery Site

The right coronary artery or its branches are the site of the fistula in 50% to 55% of cases.[L7,L12] The left coronary artery is involved in about 35%, and both coronary arteries in 5%.[B2] The fistulous artery is almost invariably part of a normally distributed coronary artery with a normal branching pattern. The fistula occurs either in the main vessel that continues beyond the fistula (a side-to-side pattern) or at the termination of the main vessel itself, or at a branch (an end artery).[S5] Rarely, the involved artery is anomalous.[U1] The coronary artery proximal to the fistula is always dilated and elongated and may be serpiginous, and the degree of these changes is roughly proportional to the size of shunt through the fistula. Usually, dilatation is uniform throughout, but it may become aneurysmal anywhere along its course. Rarely, a giant aneurysm occurs involving the whole artery. This is particularly prone to occur in fistulae from the right coronary artery entering either the posterior wall of the left ventricle[L10,O3,W5] or right ventricle[M7] (Fig. 46-1). Although such aneurysms enlarge progressively,[L10] rupture is rare. Should the artery continue beyond the fistula, it reduces abruptly to a diameter smaller than expected. It is probable that in such cases a

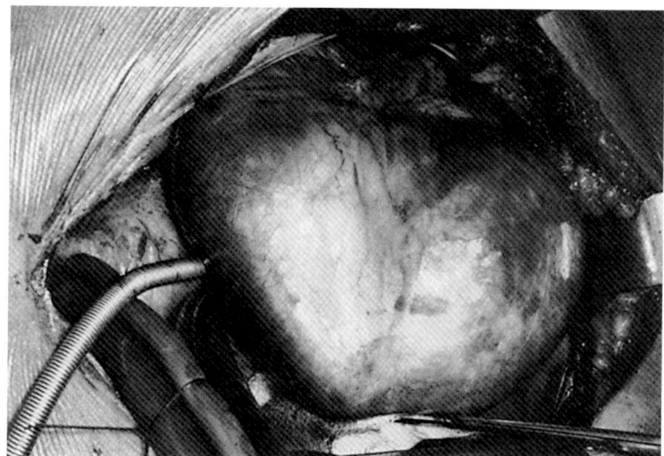

Figure 46-1 Operation on a 43-year-old man with coronary arteriovenous fistula and giant aneurysm of right coronary artery occupying entire surgical field. Fistula was of moderate to large diameter and entered the left ventricle posteriorly, close to interventricular groove and apex.

coronary steal phenomenon occurs.[H9] There is no convincing evidence that these "feeding arteries" are unusually susceptible to developing arteriosclerosis.[J1]

Site of Fistulous Connection

Fistulous connection between the coronary artery and heart may enter any of the four cardiac chambers, the coronary sinus or its tributary veins, or the great arteries or veins adjacent to the heart (pulmonary trunk, proximal pulmonary veins or proximal superior vena cava, or left superior vena cava). There are, however, certain predilections. More than 90% of fistulae open into right heart chambers or their connecting vessels. True AV fistulae to the veins themselves (coronary sinus or its major branches or venae cavae) are uncommon. Thus, about 40% connect to the right ventricle, 25% to right atrium, 15% to 20% to pulmonary artery, 7% to coronary sinus, and only 1% to superior vena cava.[L9,L12]

Fistulae entering the right side of the circulation cause rapid systolic and diastolic runoff from the aorta and a left-to-right shunt. The $\dot{Q}p/\dot{Q}s$ is seldom larger than 1.8 and is often less, and arterial pulse pressure is seldom greatly widened. About 8% of fistulae drain into left heart chambers or their tributaries, usually the left atrium, less often the left ventricle (about 3%), and rarely the proximal pulmonary veins. Left heart fistulae are not, of course, AV fistulae but arterioarterial (arteriocameral,[A3] arteriosystemic) and therefore do not produce a left-to-right shunt. There may be important runoff from the aorta during both systole and diastole when fistulae enter the left atrium, or only during diastole when they enter the left ventricle, because fistulae usually close off during systole, and because there is no pressure gradient. Volume overload on the left ventricle is therefore similar to that produced by aortic regurgitation.

Information on sites of fistulous connections comes in large part from numerous collective reviews of this subject,[H8,L7,L9,L12] and most patients were surgically treated. The right atrium and right ventricle are the most frequent sites of connection for cases requiring surgery. In angiographic series, the most frequent site of connection of small coronary fistulae not requiring surgical therapy was the pulmonary trunk. Fistulae (localized and diffuse) to the left heart are more common in coronary angiographic series than in surgical series.

Size and Multiplicity of Fistulae

In surgically treated cases, the fistulous opening, when single, is seldom larger than 2 to 5 mm (Fig. 46-2) and usually has fibrous margins, although uncommonly it may itself be aneurysmal[U1] as in the first reported case.[B7] Occasionally there may be several openings or a localized angiomatous network of vessels. Among the 58 patients reported from the Texas Heart Institute, multiple fistulae were identified in 16% and an angiomatous lesion in 10%; the fistula was aneurysmal in 19%.[U1] In a number of instances (no doubt many times the number reported in surgical series), the fistula is small and is recognized only because of high-quality cineangiography. As in other sites, most fistulae to the left ventricle are single. In a small group of patients, however, there is a diffuse spongework of tiny connections from a number of, if not most, branches of the left coronary and sometimes also the right coronary artery[A3,C7,R2,S3] (Fig. 46-3). These presumably represent persistence of embryonic trabecular spaces.

Cardiac Chambers

The chamber or vessel into which the fistula connects is variably affected. When the right atrium receives the fistula, it tends to become considerably dilated, whereas the right ventricle and pulmonary trunk show less change (apart from that to be expected from an increase in pulmonary blood flow) until heart failure occurs and they participate in cardiomegaly. Similarly, the left ventricle tends to remain normal in size despite a fistulous connection to it, probably because runoff occurring only in diastole is seldom large and seldom comparable with that occurring in severe aortic regurgitation. Left ventricular hypertrophy may be present. Rarely the left atrium becomes aneurysmally dilated.[F4] The coronary sinus may also become aneurysmal and may rupture; this is the only reported site of preoperative rupture in this condition.[H1] It is possible that runoff through the coronary sinus is limited by the coronary sinus ostium. Arterialization of the coronary sinus occurs, and possibly in relation to this, there is an unusually high prevalence of heart failure in such patients.[O1]

Infective Endocarditis

The fistula is the site of endocarditis in about 5% of cases and is attributed to turbulence.[D2]

Associated Lesions

Most coronary AV fistulae occur as isolated lesions, but there may be coincidental congenital or acquired lesions of almost any type.[B13] In the series reported by Urrutia-S and colleagues, 21 of 58 patients had associated lesions such as atrial septal defect, ventricular septal defect, and acquired valve or coronary disease.[U1]

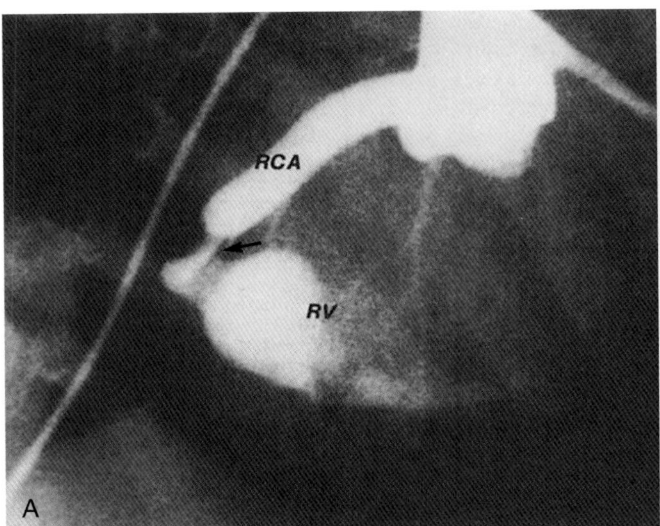

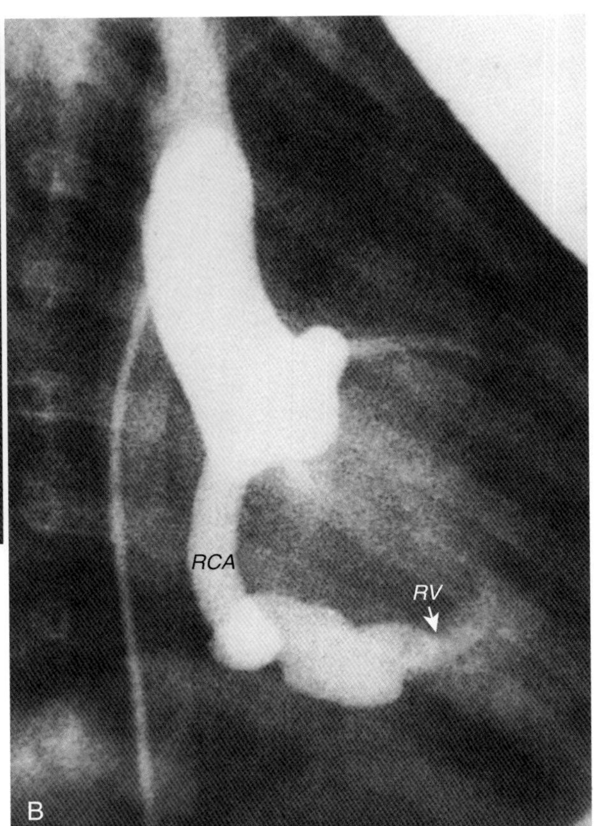

Figure 46-2 Cineangiogram frames in right anterior oblique projection in two patients with coronary arteriovenous fistulae from main right coronary artery (RCA) to right ventricle (RV). **A,** Dilated RCA runs in its usual position in atrioventricular groove, and beyond fistula *(arrow)* it continues around acute margin to divide into posterior descending and inferior left ventricular (posterolateral segment) branches (not seen). **B,** RCA is again shown to be normally positioned and very dilated and tortuous. Fistula *(arrow)* arises from posterior descending branch about halfway along posterior interventricular groove and lies therefore at termination of this vessel.

CLINICAL FEATURES AND DIAGNOSTIC CRITERIA

Age at Presentation

Most patients present late in life, occasionally in childhood, rarely in infancy.

Symptoms

Most patients considered for operation are asymptomatic and present either because of a continuous murmur[O4,R4] or mild cardiomegaly and plethora on chest radiograph. Some 80% of patients under age 20 years are asymptomatic, whereas only 40% of those older are without symptoms.[L9] Patients with small fistulae are being detected because of coronary angiography for other conditions.[G2] They are typically asymptomatic and presumably will continue to be so.

The most common symptoms are *effort dyspnea* and *fatigue* from the left-to-right shunt. Angina is uncommon (about 7%) and myocardial infarction rare (about 3%).[R4] It is postulated that these ischemic symptoms are due to coronary artery steal.

Heart failure occurs in 12% to 15% of patients presenting for operation[D2,L9] but is much more common in older patients, as is angina.[L9] Thus, in the review by Liberthson and colleagues, only 6% of patients under 20 years of age had heart failure, but 19% of those 20 years or older did.[L9] Heart failure can occur in infants with large shunts and in the occasional child with a large right coronary–left ventricular fistula comparable with an aortico–left ventricular tunnel.[D9] The likelihood of older patients having heart failure is not directly related to shunt size; rather, it is presumably related to a long-standing modest left-to-right shunt, as in the case of atrial septal defect. Heart failure is more common in patients with fistulous connection to the coronary sinus (50% vs. 14% in the overall group as reported by Ogden and Stansel).[O1] It may also be more common with onset of atrial fibrillation, which occurs more often when the connection is to the right atrium.[S5]

When infective endocarditis occurs, presentation may be with chills and fever.

Diagnosis

Diagnosis is often strongly suspected from physical signs,[D5] but it may be difficult to distinguish coronary AV fistula from other lesions with rapid aortic runoff and continuous murmurs such as patent ductus arteriosus, ventricular septal defect with aortic regurgitation, ruptured sinus of Valsalva aneurysm, and in infancy, aortico–left ventricular tunnel. In coronary AV fistula, there is usually a continuous murmur that is maximal to the right of the sternum when the fistula enters the right atrium, and usually at the lower left sternal edge when it enters the right ventricle or left ventricle. However, when the pulmonary trunk is involved, the murmur is situated as in a patent ductus arteriosus. When the fistula enters the left ventricle, the murmur is usually only diastolic.

A systolic thrill is occasionally palpable when the fistula lies anteriorly (entry into right atrium or right ventricle). When the shunt and aortic diastolic runoff are large, pulse pressure

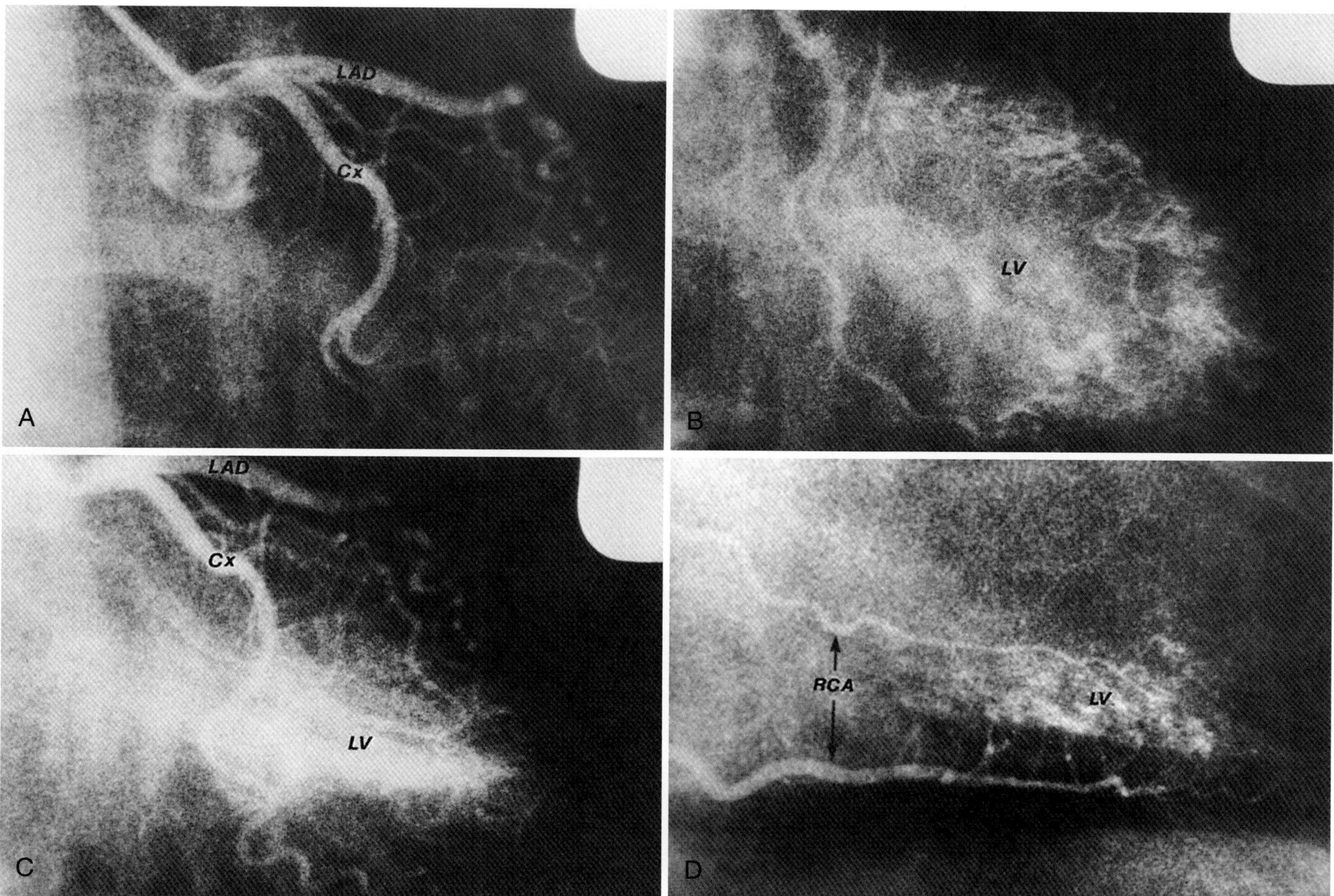

Figure 46-3 Four cineangiogram frames in right anterior oblique projection demonstrating diffuse fistulation from both left and right coronary arteries to cavity of left ventricle (LV). **A** and **B** are diastolic frames (**B** is later in sequence), whereas **C** is a systolic frame that indicates an important shunt to left ventricle; **D** shows similar shunting from branches of right coronary artery (RCA). This 41-year-old woman complained of angina. Key: *Cx,* Circumflex coronary artery; *LAD,* left anterior descending coronary artery.

is wide and the pulse jerky. Rarely, infants with a connection to the left ventricle may present with full-blown signs of severe aortic regurgitation.[D9]

The electrocardiogram (ECG) is entirely normal in about half of surgical patients and shows evidence of right or left ventricular overload in the remainder.[M3] The chest radiograph may also be normal or may show mild cardiomegaly and plethora. Cardiomegaly is more marked when heart failure appears. There may be evidence of right or left atrial enlargement, and occasionally the dilated and tortuous or aneurysmal coronary artery or fistulous site may distort the cardiac silhouette. This is most obvious when a giant aneurysm of the right coronary artery drains to the left ventricle,[L10,O3] although this is rare.

Two-dimensional (2D) echocardiography can detect importantly enlarged coronary arteries and may also confirm specific chamber enlargement.[R10] Thus, diagnosis of a coronary AV fistula can be made by 2D and Doppler echocardiography if the fistula is large enough[A2] (Fig. 46-4). Echocardiography, however, is not definitive.

Cardiac catheterization, aortography, and selective coronary angiography have long been the gold standard for definitive diagnosis and planning of either surgical repair[L7,W2] or coil occlusion by interventional catheterization (Figs. 46-5 and 46-6; also see Figs. 46-2 and 46-3). Left-to-right shunts are calculated, and right heart pressures are measured.

Computed tomography angiography (CTA) can accurately define the morphology of the fistula in both adults and young children[L5,M4]; in cases that will not require hemodynamic measurements to make management decisions, it may be the diagnostic procedure of choice.

NATURAL HISTORY

The natural history of coronary AV fistula is not known precisely, but its general outlines are clear. The fistula, if not present at birth, develops early in life. Likely, small fistulae remain small, and moderate fistulae slowly increase in size, although there may be little change over 10 to 15 years.[J1] Onset of dyspnea, heart failure, and angina can occur in young patients with large fistulae. However, because the shunt is usually only moderate, symptoms often do not appear until later in life consequent to long-standing moderate left ventricular volume overload. Daniel and colleagues found from a review of the literature that if heart failure did not occur early in infancy, it would be virtually unknown until age 20.[D2] The maximum prevalence of heart failure occurs in the fifth and sixth decades.[D2]

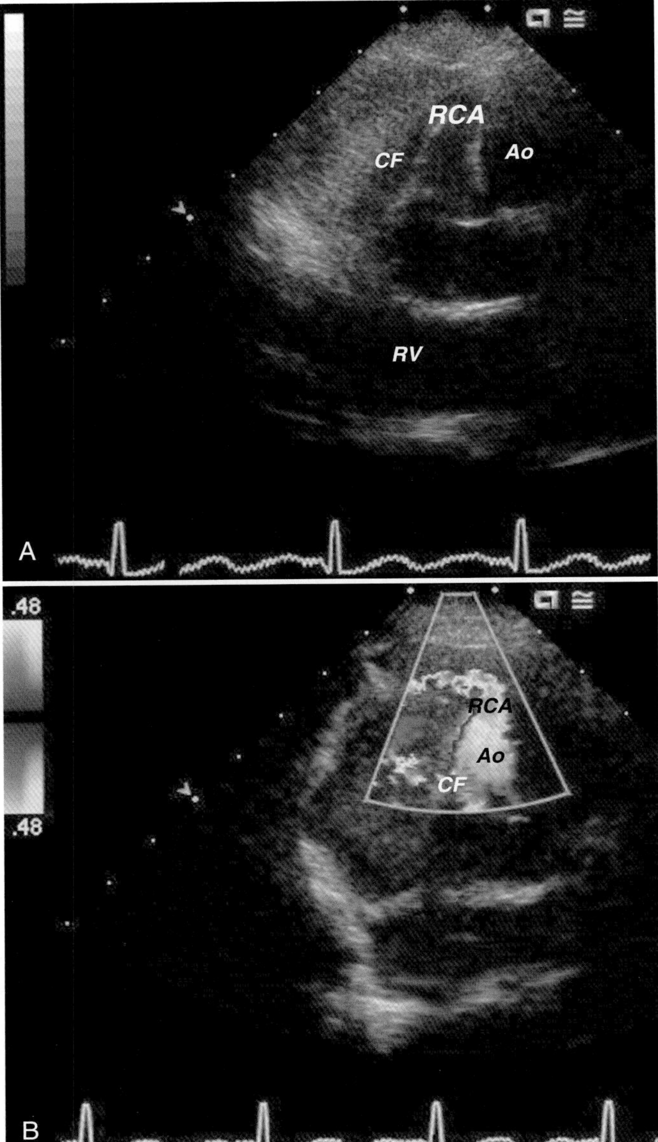

Figure 46-4 Two-dimensional echocardiogram and color-flow Doppler interrogation of coronary artery fistula. **A,** Right coronary artery (RCA) to right ventricular (RV) fistula is demonstrated. Note increased diameter of coronary artery. **B,** Color-flow Doppler signal showing turbulence at fistulous site entering right ventricle. Key: *Ao,* Aorta; *CF,* coronary fistula.

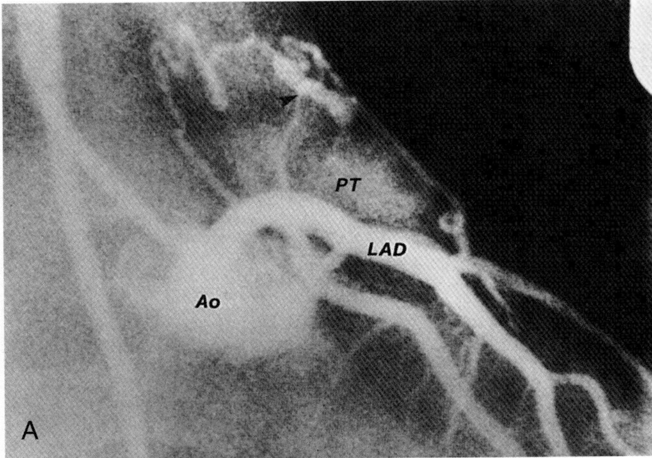

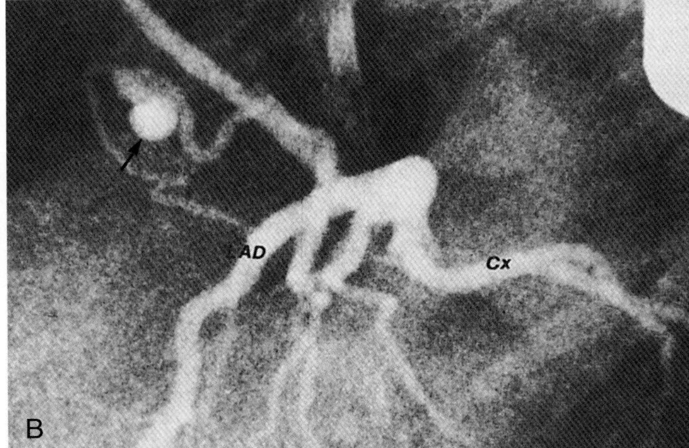

Figure 46-5 Cineangiograms in two patients with small fistulae to pulmonary trunk. **A,** Right anterior oblique projection. Fistula *(arrowhead)* is supplied by small branches from second diagonal and proximal left anterior descending coronary arteries (LAD). Pulmonary trunk (PT) opacifies faintly during part of each cardiac cycle. Operation is not indicated. **B,** Left anterior oblique projection. Fistula *(arrow)* is supplied by two branches from proximal LAD (origin of superior one is overlapped by shadow of cardiac catheter). PT opacified faintly. This lesion was closed at time of atrial septal defect repair. Key: *Ao,* Aorta; *Cx,* circumflex artery.

The other event that may precipitate symptoms and cause premature death is infective endocarditis, which occurs in about 5% of patients and may develop at any age.[D2,S2] Aneurysm formation develops with increasing frequency over time, occurring in 9% of children and 14% to 29% of adults.[S2,S4] Spontaneous rupture is rare,[H1] even though the feeding coronary artery or the fistula itself may become aneurysmal, and as with other aneurysms, there is progressive dilatation of the sac.[L10] Rupture has not been reported in children.[S2] Liberthson and colleagues found that among 173 reported patients with mean age 24 years, fistula-related death occurred in 6%: 1% in those presenting younger than age 20, and 14% in those presenting later (mean age 43 years).[L9] Spontaneous closure of a fistula has been recorded[G5,J1,S2,S9] but is rare.

TECHNIQUE OF OPERATION

Approach in all patients is through a median sternotomy, with preparation made for use of CPB (see "Preparation for Cardiopulmonary Bypass" in Section III of Chapter 2). After opening the pericardium, site of the fistula and location, size, and pathology of the coronary artery leading to it are noted. CPB is indicated:

1. When the artery is dilated and tortuous, to prevent catastrophic hemorrhage during closure of the fistula
2. When the fistula is relatively inaccessible, such as when it is in the left atrioventricular groove or distribution of the circumflex or distal right coronary artery
3. When the fistula is in the course of the coronary artery rather than at its termination, so that the fistula itself can be closed without ligation of the coronary artery
4. When an aneurysm requires excision

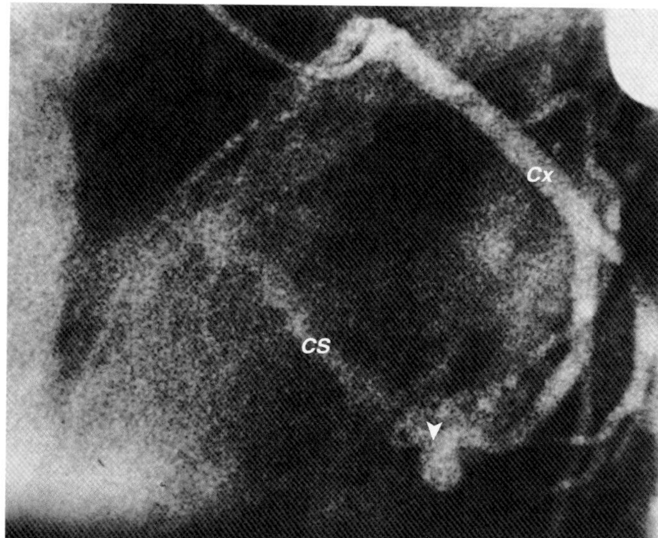

Figure 46-6 Cineangiogram frame in left anterior oblique projection showing a small fistula *(arrowhead)* entering coronary sinus (CS). Feeding left circumflex artery (Cx) is a large vessel that has a small aneurysm at site of fistulous connection. An atrial branch joins with terminal Cx in this area. Shunt is small, and operation is not indicated.

Precise location of the coronary AV fistula is determined and marked with a stitch before establishing CPB, because this is difficult to do later. After establishing CPB, the aorta is clamped. While the fistula is digitally closed, cold cardioplegic solution is administered. When the chamber into which the fistula opens is an atrium or the pulmonary trunk, the chamber is opened and the fistula closed from within with over-and-over sutures supplemented with a pledgeted mattress suture.

Cold cardioplegic solution can be infused both to identify the entry point of the fistula in the opened chamber and to test security of closure. When the fistula enters a ventricle or when the coronary artery is large and continues beyond the fistula, the coronary artery itself is opened and the fistula closed with a running suture, followed by closure of the arteriotomy with 6-0 or 7-0 polypropylene sutures. Use of a running mattress suture beneath the artery through the fistulous site[U1] is not recommended because this may lead to fistula recurrence.

Alternatively, if the fistula enters the right ventricle, right atrium, or pulmonary trunk, once CPB is established, the pulmonary trunk or right atrium, as appropriate, is opened without clamping the aorta. A pressurized blood stream emitted from the fistula makes its identification easy. This technique is especially helpful if the fistula enters the trabeculations of the right atrium or right ventricle. Closure from within the chamber is performed, and elimination of the blood stream confirms efficacy of closure.

When a large aneurysm is present (see Fig. 46-1), it should be excised. If the aneurysm is localized over the fistula site, excision entails trimming away the edges of the dilated vessel and resuturing its walls to create an artery of near-normal size. This is possible because the posterior wall invariably consists of strong tissue. This is necessary only when the artery continues beyond the site of the fistula. When it is an end artery, the aneurysm is completely excised and the vessel remnants oversewn. When the aneurysm involves most of the feeding coronary artery (see Fig. 46-1), there is usually no option but to unroof it completely and close the coronary artery proximal and distal to the sac, the latter closure including the fistula site. In such circumstances, it is always appropriate to consider use of coronary artery bypass grafting (CABG) using either a saphenous vein or internal thoracic artery to the vessel beyond the fistula,[L12] but this may not be possible when the coronary artery is too small.

After completing the repair, if a left-sided chamber has been opened, it is aspirated for air. The remainder of the operation is completed as usual (see "Completing Cardiopulmonary Bypass" in Section III of Chapter 2). Fistulous connection may be safely closed without CPB when it represents the termination of a major coronary artery branch into an easily accessible site and indicators for CPB are absent. In such instances, a suture ligature is placed around the "feeding" coronary artery very close to the fistulous connection. The fistula is then temporarily completely closed (verified by complete ablation of the thrill), and the ECG is monitored for several minutes. If there are no ECG changes, the ligature is tied down and another suture ligature placed for additional security. When the fistula is less clearly localized and consists of multiple vessels, secure closure requires a running suture that encompasses all involved vessels and the underlying wall.

SPECIAL FEATURES OF POSTOPERATIVE CARE

Patients are managed as described in Chapter 5.

RESULTS

Survival

Early (Hospital) Death

Hospital mortality for repair of coronary AV fistula in the *absence* of giant aneurysm formation approaches zero.[B13,H7,L12,U1] A literature review by Liberthson and colleagues indicates a mortality of 4% (CL 2.5%-6.2%) in 173 patients.[L9] Giant aneurysms almost always involve the right coronary artery, necessitating complete aneurysm excision and usually regrafting of the remaining right coronary system; risk of ischemia and arrhythmia increases in this situation. Of 10 reported patients with right coronary artery–left ventricular fistula, 3 (30%; CL 14%-51%) died postoperatively.[D9,L10,M1] Operative complications are rare. Myocardial ischemia, either temporary or with infarction, has been reported in 3% of cases, and fistula recurrence in 4%.[R4] With use of the techniques described here, these complications have become uncommon.

Time-Related Outcomes

Late results of repair are excellent. Edis and colleagues report that essentially all patients in whom the fistula is eradicated remain in New York Heart Association (NYHA) class I.[E1] Lowe and colleagues found no late deaths and no recurrent fistulas among 22 survivors of repair, with a mean follow-up of 10 years.[L12] Although involution of the greatly dilated leading artery can occur when repair is performed in early life,[O4] this is not the case in adults.[J1]

INDICATIONS FOR OPERATION

Some believe that prognosis of a surgically untreated coronary AV fistula is excellent, and operation is indicated only if symptoms are present. However, in view of the probability that at least some of these fistulae will increase in size and therefore eventually produce symptoms and heart failure, the tendency for development of infective endocarditis, the low probability of spontaneous closure, and the safety and efficacy of operation, it is recommended that diagnosis of a coronary AV fistula is an indication for operation unless the shunt is small ($\dot{Q}p/\dot{Q}s < 1.3$).

SPECIAL SITUATIONS AND CONTROVERSIES

Use of various interventional catheter-delivered occluding devices and coils has been reported to treat coronary AV fistulae successfully.[B20,K2,O2,S7] These techniques are increasingly being considered the therapy of choice for appropriately selected patients. In a nationwide survey conducted between 1996 and 2003, 85% of treated patients were managed surgically and 15% with interventional techniques.[S4]

Section II Anomalous Connection of Left Coronary Artery to Pulmonary Trunk

DEFINITION

In anomalous connection of left coronary artery to pulmonary trunk, the whole of the left main coronary artery or only the left anterior descending or circumflex branch connects anomalously to the proximal pulmonary trunk or very rarely to the proximal right pulmonary artery. Branching pattern of the anomalously connecting left coronary artery remains normal. The right coronary artery arises normally from the aorta and has a normal branching pattern. Collaterals from the right coronary artery feed the left coronary artery, in which flow is reversed, so that the left coronary artery drains into the pulmonary artery. Very rarely, both coronary arteries connect to the pulmonary artery by a single trunk.[G3]

HISTORICAL NOTE

In 1886, Brooks in Dublin described, apparently for the first time, anomalous connection of a coronary artery to the pulmonary trunk,[B15] and in 1908, Abbott described anomalous connection of left coronary artery to pulmonary trunk.[A1] Bland, White, and Garland in 1933 described the clinical syndrome associated with the anomaly, based on their experience with a 3-month-old infant who died from it.[B10] The pathophysiology, as suggested by Brooks in his original paper,[B15] is impoverished left ventricular myocardial blood flow—despite good collaterals between right and left coronary arteries—because of retrograde flow from left coronary artery to pulmonary trunk. Edwards supported this hypothesis,[E2] as did Case and colleagues in 1958.[C4] The latter also reported the postmortem observation that radiopaque dye injected into the ascending aorta passed out through the normal right coronary artery and, by collaterals, filled the left coronary artery in retrograde fashion.[C4]

Sabiston and colleagues verified retrograde flow at the first successful operation for the anomaly in 1959 by measuring a striking increase in left coronary artery pressure when its anomalous connection to the pulmonary trunk was occluded.[S1] Actual demonstration of left-to-right shunt into the pulmonary trunk was by Augustasson and colleagues in 1962[A9] and by Rudolph and colleagues in 1963.[R13]

Earliest surgical attempts to ameliorate the condition were indirect. The first attempt was apparently by W.J. Potts, who created an aortopulmonary (AP) fistula to increase saturation in the pulmonary trunk (personal communication, 1955). Kittle and colleagues banded the pulmonary artery,[K9] and Paul and Robbins used pericardial poudrage.[P1] These procedures are obsolete.

Successful ligation of the anomalous left coronary artery connection by Sabiston and colleagues in 1959[S1] was followed by a similar report from Rowe and Young in 1960.[R12] As early as 1953, Mustard reported attempts to anastomose the turned-down left common carotid artery to the anomalous left coronary artery that he detached from the pulmonary trunk together with a button of pulmonary trunk wall.[M14] Apley and colleagues attempted a similar procedure using the left subclavian artery in 1957.[A6] Meyer and colleagues first used this latter procedure successfully to create a two-artery coronary system in 1968,[M6] and others including Pinsky and colleagues reported such a repair.[P2]

In 1966, Cooley and colleagues reported use of coronary artery bypass vein grafting from the aorta to the left main or proximal left anterior descending artery, after closing the left coronary ostium from within the pulmonary trunk.[C14] The next procedure to evolve was translocation of the anomalous coronary artery from pulmonary trunk to ascending aorta. Such a procedure was performed unsuccessfully in 1972 using hypothermic circulatory arrest.[B4] This was first performed successfully for the rare condition of anomalous connection of the right coronary artery to pulmonary trunk (where the artery lies anteriorly and is more readily translocated) by Tingelstad and colleagues in 1971,[T4] and for the left coronary artery by Neches and colleagues in 1974.[N1] The latter also described successful interposition of a free left subclavian artery segment between the left coronary artery and the back of the ascending aorta.

In 1979, use of a tunnel within the pulmonary trunk to connect the ostium of the anomalous coronary artery to the aorta via an AP window was introduced. It was created either of pericardium, as described by Hamilton and colleagues,[H4] or of pulmonary artery wall, as described by Takeuchi and colleagues.[T1] Arciniegas and colleagues modified this concept by placing a free subclavian artery graft inside the pulmonary trunk.[A7] Reconstructive techniques have been devised to permit implanting coronary arteries that are remote from the aorta.[K3,L2,M12,T8] Use of temporary ventricular assistance in infants has been an important adjunct to postoperative management.[C12,D7,V1] The aneurysmal left ventricular wall was excised unsuccessfully in 1960.[B3] This procedure, combined with ligation of the left coronary artery, was subsequently performed successfully by Turina and colleagues in 1973[T7] and Fleming and colleagues in 1975.[F3]

MORPHOGENESIS AND MORPHOLOGY

Morphogenesis

Embryologic information indicates that the proximal coronary arteries grow *from* the peritruncal area *into* the aorta, with formation (normally) of single orifices for both left and right coronary arteries.[B11,B12] Therefore, the phrase "the anomalous artery *arises* from" is inappropriate. For that reason, the former term, *anomalous origin*, has been abandoned in this text for *anomalous connection*.

Morphology

The anomalous left main coronary artery connects most often to the sinus of Valsalva immediately above the left or posterior cusp of the pulmonary trunk and rarely from that above the right cusp.[S12,W1] The left main coronary artery is of variable length, but usually divides into anterior descending and circumflex branches within 5 or 6 mm of its origin. Collateral communications between right and left coronary arteries are always present, but vary in extent and are grossly visible in only a few cases, mainly in adults. Uncommonly, only the circumflex branch connects anomalously to the pulmonary trunk, and rarely only the left anterior descending branch.[E3,R6]

Very rarely, the left main coronary artery or only the circumflex artery connects to the right pulmonary artery near its origin rather than to the pulmonary trunk.[D11,F1,H5,O5] Even more rarely, both the left and right coronary arteries connect to the pulmonary trunk (see "Total Anomalous Connection of Coronary Arteries to Pulmonary Trunk" under Special Situations and Controversies later in this section).

The left ventricle is always hypertrophied and usually greatly dilated, with dilatation often involving primarily the left ventricular apex.[R3] Diffuse left ventricular fibrosis is virtually always present, and patients dying in infancy usually have evidence of recent and old anterolateral myocardial infarction. Fibrosis is most marked in the subendocardial layer. Focal calcification may be present in fibrotic areas. Secondary subendocardial fibroelastosis of variable degree is usually present. However, a considerable amount of left ventricular dysfunction, in infants at least, must be ischemic in origin, in view of the dramatic improvement in left ventricular function that can result from an operation that creates a two-artery coronary system.[B21] Improvement in left ventricular function is not immediate, but occurs over weeks to months. The chronic ischemia accompanying this lesion results in devitalization (or adaptive response) of the myocardium at a cellular and biochemical level. The devitalized myocardium has been termed *hibernating myocardium*[S11] (see "Myocardial Cell Stunning" under Damage from Global Myocardial Ischemia in Chapter 3). The devitalized muscle slowly recovers over the time described once adequate blood flow and oxygen delivery are established.

Several pathologic features may result in mitral valve regurgitation.[W1] There may be extensive fibrosis and sometimes calcification in the papillary muscles, leading to papillary muscle dysfunction. Endocardial fibroelastosis may involve the mitral apparatus, with fusion and shortening of chordae tendineae. Also, papillary muscles may be abnormally positioned, which may lead to mitral regurgitation.[M9,N4] Extensive left ventricular fibrosis can produce left ventricular and mitral anular dilatation and mitral regurgitation.[B22,T2] Reversible left ventricular ischemia must, to some degree, contribute to the mitral valve regurgitation in infants, because in many cases regurgitation has been observed to decrease to an important extent after surgical treatment and creation of a two-artery coronary system.[B21]

CLINICAL FEATURES AND DIAGNOSTIC CRITERIA

Infant Presentation

Symptoms may be recognized within a week or so of birth. When there are no other anomalies, these are seldom severe enough to warrant referral before age 2 months. Presumably, high postnatal pulmonary artery pressure limits runoff into the pulmonary trunk, so there is less coronary steal, and myocardial dysfunction is gradual in onset rather than sudden. Circumoral pallor and blueness are often present. The cardinal symptom is poor feeding. The baby takes the first 2 to 3 ounces well but then stops; there is breathlessness and sweating, and the baby may draw up the knees, arch the back, and uncommonly, cry or scream. The presumed cause is angina. As a result of the feeding problem, weight gain is poor. Few infants with these symptoms improve spontaneously. Usually by age 2 to 3 months, there is overt heart failure with persistent tachypnea and tachycardia. The infant by then is seriously ill and occasionally moribund.

Clinical signs are difficult to distinguish from those of cardiomyopathy or endocardial fibroelastosis. There may be a nonspecific systolic murmur at the base, or a more definite apical pansystolic murmur caused by mitral regurgitation and an apical gallop rhythm. A continuous murmur is not audible in infants. A precordial lift is common in association with marked and frequently gross cardiomegaly. Hepatomegaly also is present, and rales are heard throughout the lungs. The ECG is frequently helpful in diagnosis, because it usually shows anterolateral infarction with Q waves and ST-segment elevation in lateral chest leads[A8] and evidence of left ventricular hypertrophy. However, left ventricular hypertrophy alone may be reflected in the ECG. Myocardial enzymes may be elevated. In addition to cardiomegaly, interstitial pulmonary edema is evident on the chest radiograph.

Echocardiography shows a dilated, poorly contracting left ventricle (with ejection fraction typically <20%) and reveals the functional status and morphology of the mitral valve. In infants otherwise thought to have dilated cardiomyopathy, 2D and pulsed Doppler echocardiography may detect an abnormally large right coronary artery and anomalous connection of the left coronary artery to the pulmonary trunk, with retrograde flow in it[C2,K8] (Fig. 46-7). This technique can also be used to identify an anomalously connecting right coronary artery.[W5]

Although definitive diagnosis is often made by echocardiography, *current practice requires cardiac catheterization and cineangiography.* An aortogram demonstrates the single right coronary artery arising from the aorta, and retrograde filling of the left coronary artery that produces a varying degree of opacification of the pulmonary trunk (Fig. 46-8). A left ventriculogram can be used to assess left ventricular function and degree of mitral regurgitation. It may also demonstrate coronary anatomy, making an aortogram unnecessary. Left ventricular end-diastolic pressure is always elevated but may be lower than anticipated from viewing the typically very poor ejection fraction on echocardiography. Right heart

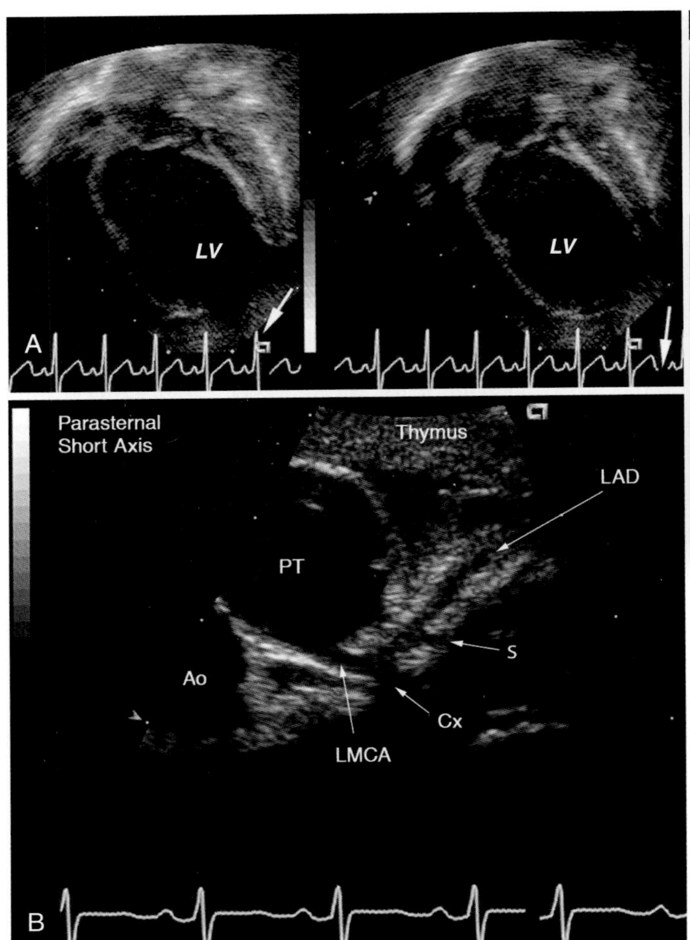

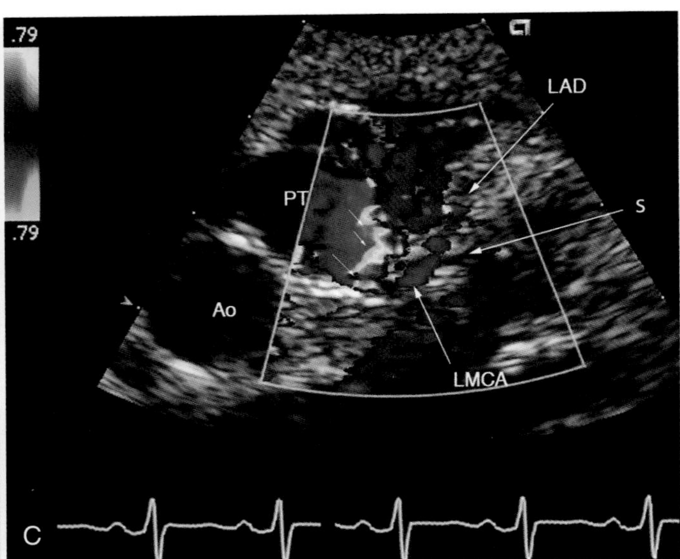

Figure 46-7 Two-dimensional echocardiogram and color-flow Doppler interrogation of anomalous left coronary artery arising from pulmonary trunk. **A,** Apical four-chamber view showing left ventricle (LV) in both diastole and systole. Note markedly dilated LV cavity with severely reduced LV systolic function. **B,** Transthoracic echocardiographic image of anomalous left main coronary artery (LMCA) arising from pulmonary artery. **C,** Color Doppler image of view shown in **B.** Key: *Ao,* Aorta; *Cx,* circumflex coronary artery; *LAD,* left anterior descending coronary artery; *PT,* pulmonary trunk; *S,* septal coronary artery.

catheterization may show an increase in blood oxygen content at pulmonary artery level.

Adult Presentation

Collateral circulation from the right coronary artery is apparently adequate to prevent massive infarction, because few patients presenting later in life report a history of hospitalization in infancy, although there may have been feeding difficulties. When severe symptoms do not occur in infancy, presentation is often delayed to beyond age 20 years.[M10,R8,W4] Some adults remain asymptomatic or complain only of fatigue, dyspnea, or palpitations. About half have effort angina. There usually is a nonspecific systolic murmur, sometimes an apical pansystolic murmur from mitral regurgitation, and occasionally a continuous murmur over the upper left sternal edge due to retrograde flow from the coronary artery into the pulmonary trunk. Occasionally, mitral regurgitation dominates the clinical picture, producing heart failure. In an earlier era, some of these patients were operated on for mitral regurgitation or died without diagnosis of anomalous connection of left coronary artery to pulmonary trunk having been made.[B22,D8,G1,U2]

The resting ECG is virtually always abnormal, with ST-T segment changes or evidence of old anterolateral infarction. Exercise ECG usually shows an abnormal ischemic response, and stress thallium myocardial imaging is usually abnormal.[M10] The chest radiograph may be normal or may show cardiac enlargement. Cineangiography shows more prominent collaterals from the right coronary artery in adults than in infants and usually a near-normal left ventricular ejection fraction, but with anterolateral hypokinesia. Mitral regurgitation occasionally is severe.

Individuals with anomalous left anterior descending or anomalous circumflex coronary artery typically present in adulthood rather than infancy. In the rare case that all coronary arteries arise from the pulmonary artery, death early in life is almost a certainty.[T3]

NATURAL HISTORY

Anomalous connection of the left coronary artery to the pulmonary trunk is rare, occurring in 0.26% of patients with congenital heart disease undergoing cardiac catheterization.[A8] About 65% of infants born with it die during the first year from intractable left ventricular failure[W1] (Fig. 46-9). However, they uncommonly do so in the first 2 months. Explanation for this symptom-free interval is not entirely clear, because extensive left ventricular scarring, particularly of the subendocardium, and evidence of old and recent infarction are usually present by then. It likely results, however, from a combination of initially elevated pulmonary

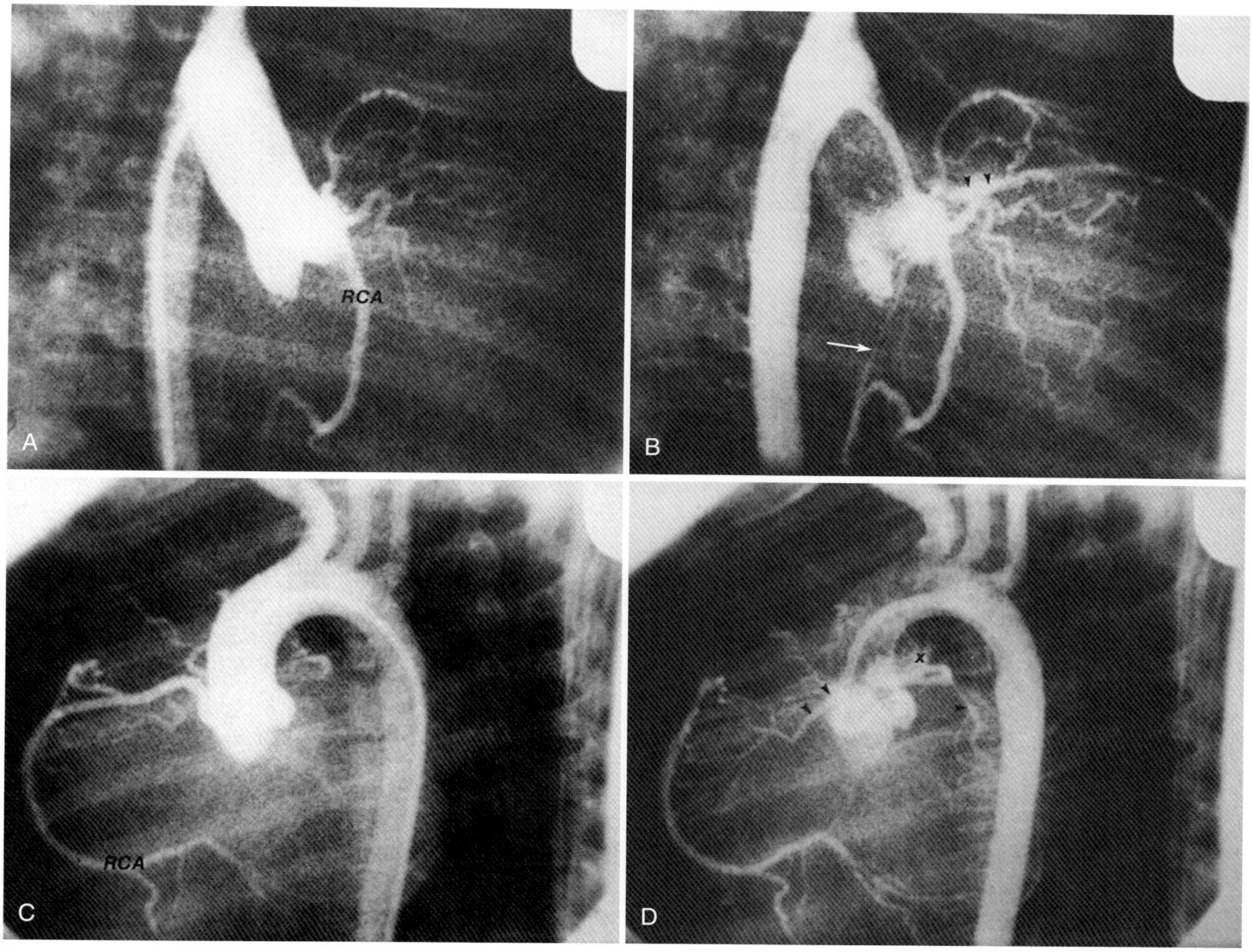

Figure 46-8 Biplane cineangiographic frames in 3-month-old infant with anomalous connection of left coronary artery to pulmonary trunk. **A-B,** In right anterior oblique projection. **C-D,** In left anterior oblique projection. In **A** and **C,** right coronary artery (RCA) fills directly from aorta, and prominent conal branch collaterals are visible. In **B** and **D,** there is delayed retrograde filling of left anterior descending *(double arrowheads)* and circumflex arteries *(single arrow).* Whiff of contrast can be seen in the pulmonary trunk *(x)* in **D.**

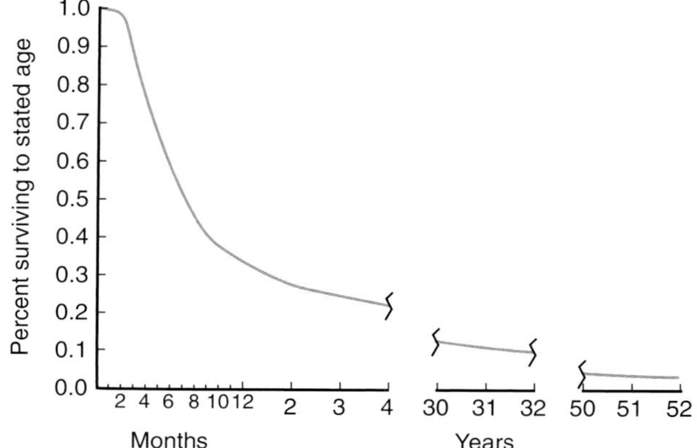

Figure 46-9 Freehand depiction of survival without surgical treatment of patients with anomalous connection of left coronary artery to pulmonary trunk. (Figure is based primarily on collective review of 140 cases by Wesselhoeft and colleagues.[W1])

artery pressure, which limits the runoff, and gradual accumulation of myocyte dysfunction and loss.

If death does not occur during the first year, the hazard lessens considerably and the chronic phase of natural history is reached. Survival to this stage may be related to presence of rich interarterial collaterals, possibly associated with a slightly restrictive opening between left coronary artery and pulmonary trunk. Supporting this is the continuous murmur heard in about 5% of patients. Many such patients are in good health, and a few have normal ECGs.[W1] Survival beyond the first year may also be related to marked right coronary dominance, with this vessel supplying not only the diaphragmatic portion of the left ventricle but also much of the septum and lateral wall.[W1] Patients with this arrangement may occasionally only have papillary muscle ischemia and fibrosis, and mitral regurgitation may dominate the clinical picture.

Most patients who survive infancy continue to be at risk of death from chronic heart failure secondary to ischemic left ventricular cardiomyopathy. Those who survive until the fourth decade are at less risk of death from heart failure (see Fig. 46-9), and those few patients who live to the fifth and sixth decades occasionally die suddenly, as do older patients with long-standing ischemic heart disease (see "Death" under Natural History in Chapter 7). In adult patients, myocardial ischemia and fibrosis are prominent, and occasionally, extensive myocardial calcification develops. However, left ventricular ejection fraction is only moderately depressed or normal in most of these patients.[M10]

TECHNIQUE OF OPERATION

Constructing a Two-Artery Coronary System

Optimally, operation is undertaken with the idea of constructing a two-artery coronary system in all patients. Translocation of the anomalous coronary artery into the aortic root appears to be the most direct and therefore advisable procedure, but it is not always possible. Smith and colleagues found the distance between the midpoint of the empty left aortic sinus and posterior aspect of the anomalously connected coronary artery to vary between 2 and 18 mm.[S12] The longer of these distances probably precludes direct implantation and makes the tunnel (Takeuchi) repair necessary.[T1]

Other methods of creating a two-artery coronary system may be less desirable. In critically ill infants, a case may still be made for use of simple ligation of the anomalously connected coronary artery,[K9] especially if used as a temporary maneuver to resuscitate a patient presenting in cardiac arrest. However, this seems less desirable in an era when mechanical assist devices are available even for the smallest infants. In seriously ill infants, ventricular fibrillation is likely to develop before the heart can be cannulated and CPB commenced. Therefore, vigilance is required to maintain an optimal hemodynamic state during preparations for operation and cannulation for CPB.

Operation is best done with CPB at 18°C to 28°C (see "Preparation for Cardiopulmonary Bypass" in Section III of Chapter 2), although left coronary artery translocation has recently been reported using normothermic CPB and a continuously beating heart.[E4] After sternotomy, the pericardium is opened *without touching the heart,* because even the slightest trauma can induce ventricular fibrillation. Preferably, arterial cannulation of both the aorta and pulmonary trunk is used with a bifurcated system to maximize myocardial perfusion once CPB is started. Single venous cannulation is used. Immediately before commencing CPB, tourniquets are placed around the left and right pulmonary arteries. The tourniquets are tightened as CPB is initiated to prevent perfusion steal into the pulmonary bed from the pulmonary trunk arterial cannula. A left-sided vent is placed through a purse-string in the right upper pulmonary vein.

Myocardial protection during aortic clamping is particularly important for two reasons: the existing compromised state of the myocardium, and the potential for inadequate delivery of cardioplegic solution to the left ventricle. Preferably, cardioplegic solution is delivered simultaneously into the aortic root and pulmonary trunk using a bifurcated cardioplegia delivery system to maximize protection of the left ventricle.

Alternatively, some surgeons use only one arterial cannula (in the aorta) and deliver cardioplegia only into the aortic root. It is critically important to occlude the branch pulmonary arteries at the initiation of CPB and through cardioplegia delivery using this technique.

After completing cardioplegia, the pulmonary trunk cannula and branch pulmonary artery tourniquets are removed. A transverse incision is made in the pulmonary trunk just downstream to the commissure of the pulmonary valve. When the opening of the anomalously connecting left coronary artery is posterior or right-sided, the coronary artery translocation technique is used. When the opening is on the left-sided aspect of the pulmonary trunk, the tunnel operation[T1] should be considered.

Tunnel Operation (Takeuchi Repair)

Taking care to avoid injury to the aortic valve, a button of aortic wall about 5 to 6 mm in diameter is excised at a point at which the left wall of the aorta is in contact with the right side of the pulmonary trunk (Fig. 46-10, *A*). Directly opposite this, a button is excised from the right wall of the pulmonary trunk (Fig. 46-10, *B* [also see *A*]). These openings are sewn together with continuous 7-0 polypropylene to create an aortopulmonary window.

Using a flap of anterior pulmonary trunk wall hinged on the right, the anterior wall of the tunnel is created, completing the tunnel conveying blood from the aortopulmonary window across the back of the pulmonary trunk to the anomalously connecting left coronary artery (Fig. 46-10, *C* [also see *B*]). The large defect in the anterior wall of the pulmonary trunk is reconstructed with a patch of pericardium, pulmonary artery allograft, or polytetrafluoroethylene (PTFE) (Fig. 46-10, *D*). Occasionally, this operation narrows the immediately supravalvar portion of the pulmonary trunk sufficiently to require a transanular patch.

The remainder of the operation is completed in the usual fashion (see "Completing Cardiopulmonary Bypass" in Section III of Chapter 2). Weaning the patient from CPB may require patience, intravenous nitroglycerin, and monitoring left and right atrial pressures.

Left Coronary Artery Translocation

When the left coronary artery connects to the posterior or right-sided aspect of the pulmonary trunk (Fig. 46-11, *A*), the transverse pulmonary trunk incision is continued until the trunk is transected (Fig. 46-11, *B*).[G4,L8,N2,V1] The incision is arranged so that a sizable button of pulmonary artery wall around the coronary ostium is excised (see Fig. 46-11, *B*). The left coronary artery is carefully mobilized for a short distance. An opening is made in the adjacent left posterolateral portion of the aorta (Fig. 46-11, *C*). The button around the coronary ostium is anastomosed to the aorta with 7-0 monofilament absorbable sutures, the pulmonary trunk is reconstructed by end-to-end anastomosis, and the coronary artery explant site is patched (see Fig. 46-11, *C*).

Subclavian–Left Coronary Artery Anastomosis

This procedure may be indicated when the anomalous coronary ostium within the pulmonary trunk is remote from adjacent aorta, making direct coronary translocation impossible and Takeuchi repair difficult. Initial CPB management uses a single aortic cannula, with attention to myocardial perfusion similar to that already described, but because the aortic root is not opened or manipulated, aortic clamping and cardioplegia are not necessary.

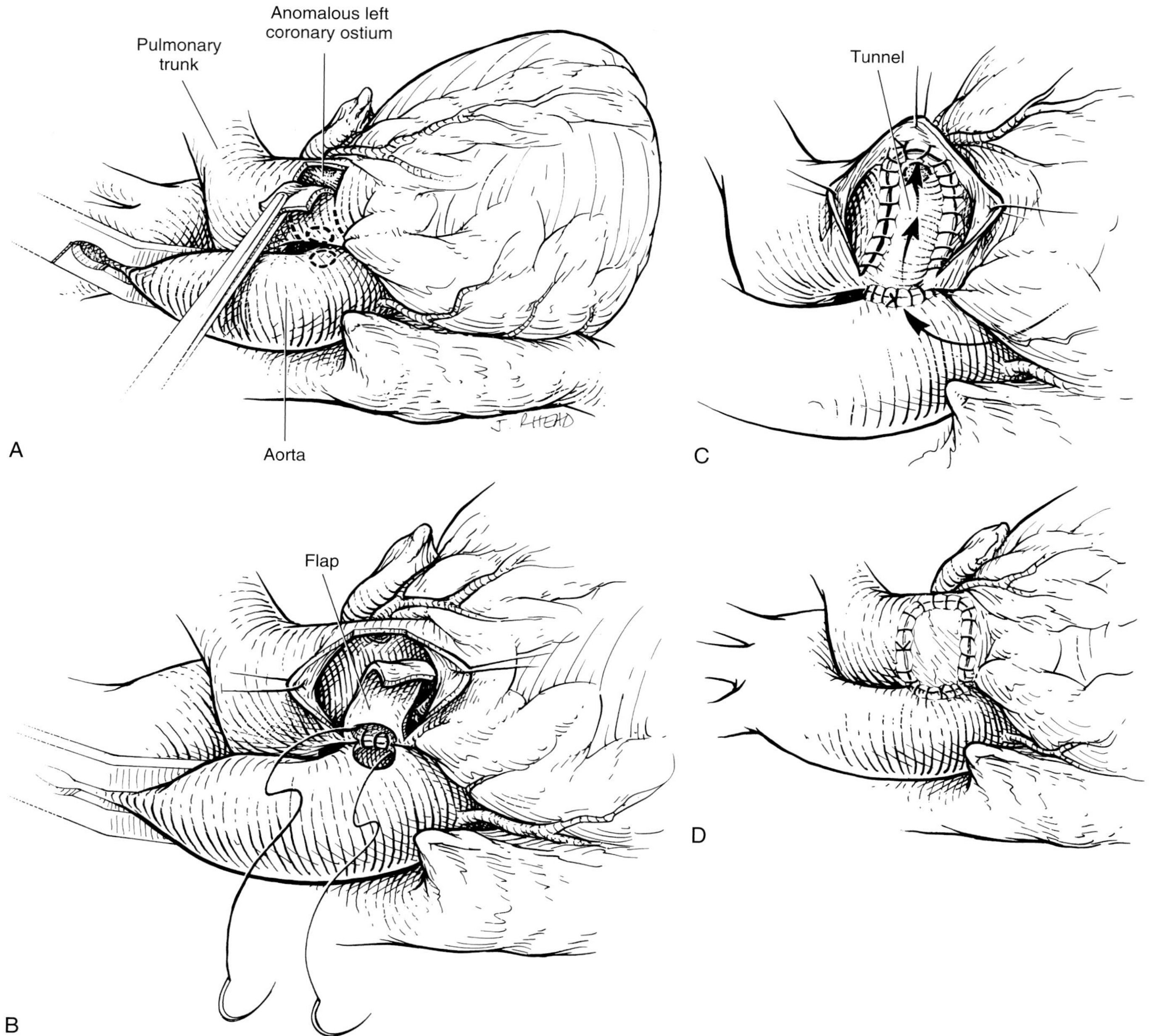

Figure 46-10 Tunnel operation (Takeuchi repair). **A,** After instituting cardiopulmonary bypass using techniques to maximize myocardial preservation, the initially small transverse pulmonary arteriotomy, made to confirm the unfavorable position of the anomalous coronary ostium for direct translocation, is extended to develop an anterior pulmonary arterial wall flap. It is based on the right lateral aspect of the pulmonary trunk. Dotted lines indicate (1) positions of buttons on adjacent aortic and pulmonary arterial wall that are to be removed, and (2) extent of incisions used for anterior pulmonary arterial flap. **B,** Anterior pulmonary arterial wall flap has been fully developed, and aortopulmonary window anastomosis is created using a running 7-0 monofilament absorbable suture. During creation of the aortopulmonary window, care should be taken to avoid direct injury or distortion of the semilunar valve cusps and commissures. **C,** Aortopulmonary window suture line has been completed, and the anterior pulmonary arterial wall flap has been used to create the tunnel connecting aortopulmonary window and remote ostium of anomalous coronary artery. This anastomosis is also performed with a running 7-0 monofilament absorbable suture. Great care should be taken as the suture line approaches the ostium of the coronary artery to avoid distorting the proximal coronary artery. **D,** Remaining defect in the anterior wall of the pulmonary trunk is now reconstructed with an appropriately shaped patch of either glutaraldehyde-treated autologous pericardium, pulmonary artery allograft arterial wall tissue, or polytetrafluoroethylene. A running monofilament nonabsorbable suture is used. Size of patch should be generous to avoid supravalvar pulmonary stenosis.

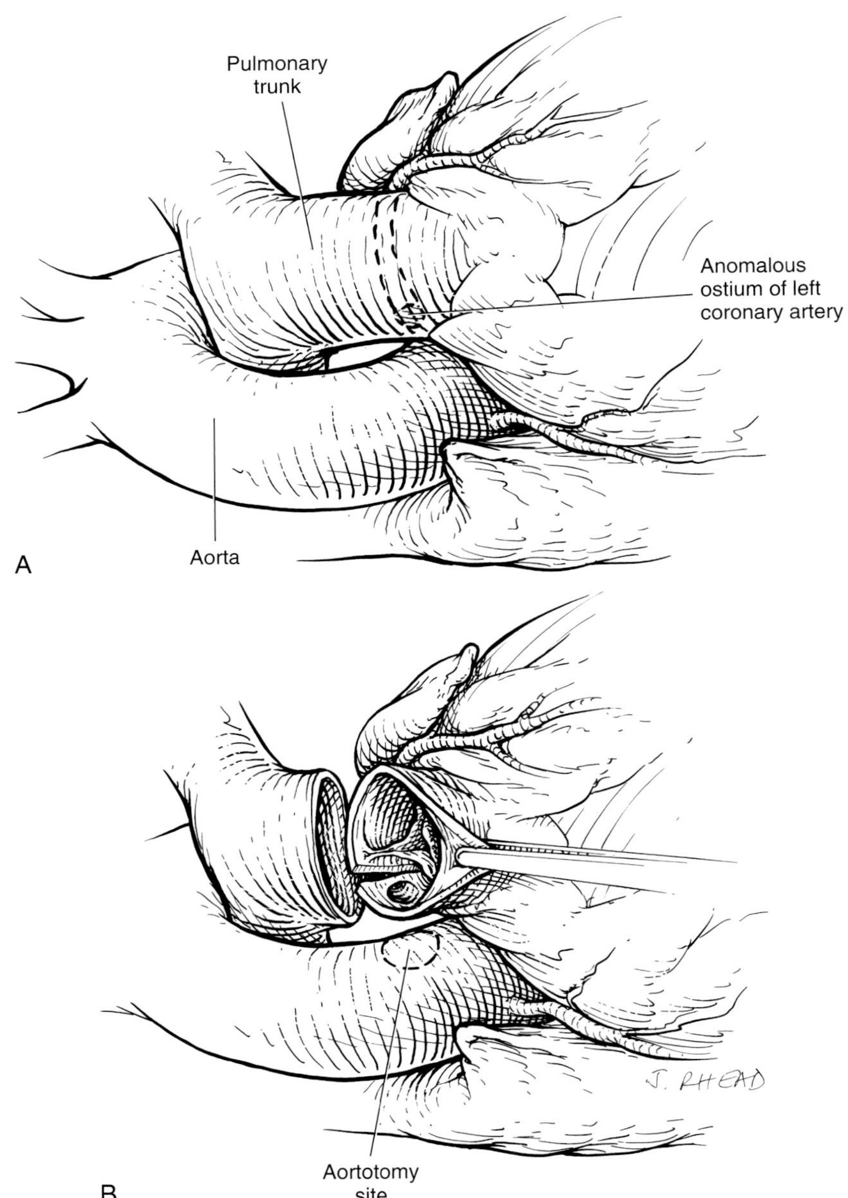

Figure 46-11 Left coronary artery translocation. **A,** Favorable position of anomalous left coronary artery ostium for direct translocation. **B,** Pulmonary trunk has been transected just above sinutubular junction, revealing anomalous coronary origin. Coronary button in the sinus of Valsalva containing the anomalous coronary has been incised. Of note, the button of sinus tissue around the ostium should be made as large as possible without injuring the pulmonary valve. Also shown by dotted line is position of the aortotomy, placed in optimal position for translocating the coronary. Of note, care should be taken in creating the aortotomy not to injure the aortic valve. If there is concern regarding position of the aortotomy in relation to the aortic valve, a separate ascending aortotomy can be performed to determine the aortotomy site relative to the aortic valve cusps.

The left subclavian artery is dissected as far distally as possible and then ligated and divided at this level (Fig. 46-12). It is important that adequate length of left subclavian artery is achieved; otherwise, kinking at the subclavian origin is possible following anastomosis. The connection of the coronary artery to the pulmonary trunk is identified and the coronary mobilized on a generous button of pulmonary sinus tissue. The coronary artery is mobilized appropriately to allow the anastomosis to be performed without tension or kinking. The preferred method of anastomosis is end-to-end connection of subclavian artery to coronary button using a running 7-0 monofilament absorbable suture.

After completing the anastomosis and establishing flow through the reconstructed area, the proximal aspect of the subclavian artery should be examined carefully to ensure that no tension or kinking is present. The coronary explantation site on the pulmonary trunk can be closed primarily or, if preferred, with a small patch of autologous pericardium, pulmonary artery allograft, or PTFE, using a running monofilament nonabsorbable suture. Alternatively, the left coronary

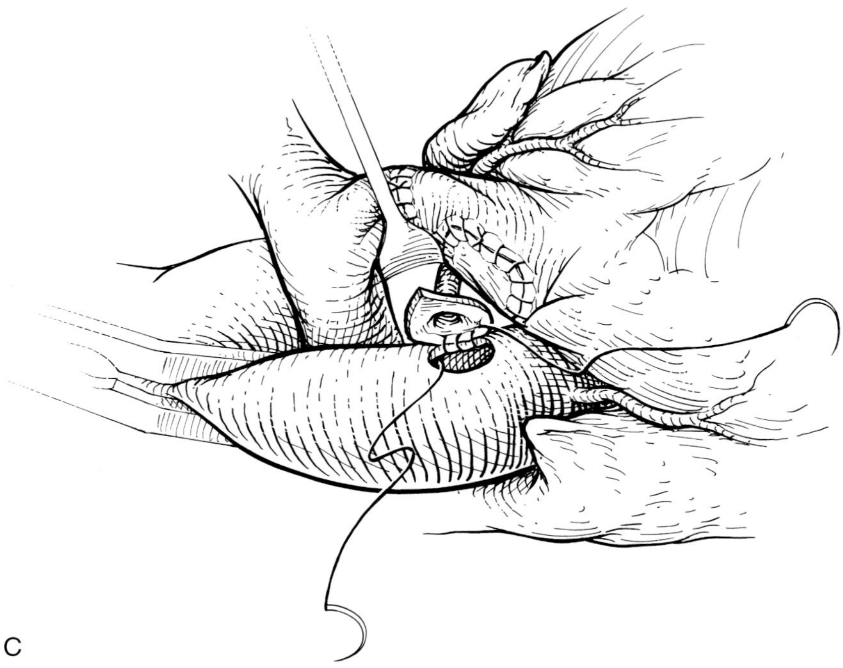

Figure 46-11, cont'd C, The coronary artery is mobilized over an appropriate length so that there is no tension as the artery is brought over to the aortotomy site. A running 7-0 monofilament absorbable suture is used to create the coronary to aortic anastomosis. Also shown is the pulmonary trunk end-to-end reconstruction and reconstruction of the coronary explantation site using a patch of glutaraldehyde-treated autologous pericardium, pulmonary artery allograft, or polytetrafluoroethylene.

artery may be ligated close to the pulmonary trunk and an end-to-side anastomosis used.[K1] The patient's anatomy may not permit this operation to be performed without excessive tension or kinking of the subclavian artery, so the surgeon must always have an alternative procedure in mind.

Other Techniques for Assisting Translocation

A number of techniques have been described to increase the likelihood of translocation of the anomalous coronary into the aorta for coronary arteries remote from the aorta. The coronary artery can be extended by autologous flaps of aorta and pulmonary artery,[K3,M12,T8] or it can be excised with a button of pulmonary artery, mobilized to reach the aorta, and anastomosed within the aortic lumen,[L2] a technique attributed to Yacoub. One such technique is shown in Fig. 46-13.[W6]

Coronary Artery Bypass Grafting

Techniques for CABG are the same as those used for internal thoracic artery grafting in the surgical treatment of arteriosclerotic coronary artery disease (see under Indications for Operation later in this section; see also Technique of Operation in Chapter 7). Even in small patients, the left internal thoracic artery can be used.

Ligation of Left Coronary Artery

This procedure may be carried out in the simplest manner through a limited left anterolateral fourth interspace incision. The pericardium is opened in front of the phrenic nerve after mobilizing the thymus from its upper part. A ligature is tied around the tip of the left atrial appendage to retract it superiorly. The anomalous connection of the left coronary artery is immediately obvious, and is rapidly dissected and ligated close to the pulmonary trunk wall with a single transfixing suture or metal clip. Venous collaterals around the artery may require cautery control. The pericardium is loosely closed and chest closed with or without drainage. The entire procedure can be completed within 30 to 45 minutes.

In the current era, this procedure may be applicable as an interim measure to stabilize critically ill patients before more formal revascularization.[K9] CPB may be used, especially if the anomalous coronary artery connects to the pulmonary trunk posteriorly. Using a single venous cannula, perfusion at 37°C, and no aortic clamping, the pulmonary trunk is opened transversely and the origin of the left coronary artery oversewn with a few simple sutures reinforced with a pledgeted mattress suture. CPB time is approximately 15 minutes.

SPECIAL FEATURES OF POSTOPERATIVE CARE

Care of patients undergoing repair of anomalous connection of left coronary artery to pulmonary trunk is the same as that for other patients undergoing cardiac surgery (see Chapter 5). A left atrial pressure monitoring catheter should be used. In critically ill small infants, low cardiac output can be anticipated during the first few postoperative days, and appropriate measures applied (see "Cardiovascular Subsystem" in Section I of Chapter 5). These measures may include use of temporary left ventricular assistance (see "Temporary Ventricular Assistance" in Section I of Chapter 5).[C12,D7,V1]

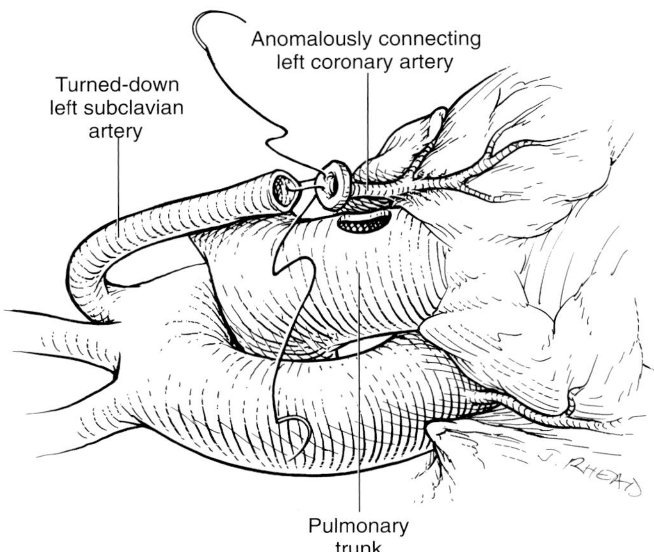

Figure 46-12 Subclavian to left coronary artery anastomosis. This procedure may be indicated when anomalous coronary ostium within the pulmonary trunk is remote from the adjacent aorta, making direct coronary translocation impossible and Takeuchi repair difficult. Approach is through a median sternotomy, using cardiopulmonary bypass (CPB) at normothermic or mildly hypothermic temperatures. CPB involves standard aortic cannulation and a single venous cannula in right atrial appendage. A calcium-supplemented blood prime is used and heart remains beating throughout procedure without utilizing aortic clamping. The left subclavian artery is dissected as far distally as possible and then ligated and divided at this level. It is important that adequate length of left subclavian artery is achieved; otherwise, kinking at the subclavian origin is possible following anastomosis. Connection of the coronary artery is identified and the coronary mobilized on a generous button of pulmonary sinus tissue. The coronary artery is mobilized appropriately to allow the anastomosis to be performed without tension or kinking. The preferred method of anastomosis is end-to-end connection of subclavian artery to coronary button using a running 7-0 monofilament absorbable suture. After completing anastomosis and establishing flow through reconstructed area, careful examination of the proximal aspect of the subclavian artery should be performed to ensure that no tension or kinking is present. Coronary explantation site on pulmonary trunk may be closed primarily or, if preferred, with a small patch of autologous pericardium, pulmonary artery allograft, or polytetrafluoroethylene using a running monofilament nonabsorbable suture.

RESULTS

Survival

Early (Hospital) Death

Early mortality reported for heterogeneous groups of patients is almost valueless because of the powerful effect of risk factors in this setting, the small number of patients in all reported series, and the effect of "patients too sick for operation" on mortality after surgery. These factors also make difficult an appropriate comparison of outcomes after various surgical procedures. There is a suggestion, supported by physiologic arguments, that outcome following simple ligation is not as good as with more formal revascularization (Tables 46-1 and 46-2). Mortality in various subsets from series reported from 1975 to 1980 ranged from 0% to 75%.[A7,A8,B21,C11,D12,L1,M8] Certain trends have emerged over time. Series reported since 1995 emphasize operations that result in a two-artery coronary system and also document excellent survival (mortality 0% to 14%).[A4,B8,C12,I2,L3,R1,S6,T8] Improved postoperative support, including use of temporary ventricular assistance, may play an important role.[C12,D7]

Time-Related Outcomes

Few appropriate studies of long-term survival have been conducted. In one study,[C12] no late deaths were recorded in 21 patients with a mean follow-up of 6.5 years (range 2 months to 18 years) and a total of 145 patient-years of follow-up. Similar midterm results have been reported by others,[I2,L3] supporting the position that most patients survive long term after any of the described procedures.[B21,C11,M10,W4]

Modes of Death

Most hospital deaths result from acute cardiac failure.

Incremental Risk Factors for Premature Death

No formal analysis provides information regarding incremental risk factors for premature death. Presumably, there is an early, rapidly declining hazard phase for death; a low constant phase of hazard follows, conditioned by status of the left ventricular myocardium.

Preoperative status of the left ventricle is also the important risk factor for death during or early after repair, with depressed shortening fraction identified in one analysis of 39 patients.[L3] This status determines functional state of the patient, which is also a powerful risk factor for death.

Important mitral regurgitation is probably also a risk factor[S6] for death early (and perhaps late) after repair, but this is correlated with status of the left ventricle. As with older studies (see Fig. 46-9), more recent reports seem to indicate that deaths are more frequent among infants.[S6]

Functional Status

Functional status is generally good late postoperatively. Of 21 patients assessed by Cochrane and colleagues, 18 were in NYHA class I and 3 in class II at midterm follow-up.[C12] Size of the left ventricle (including cardiothoracic ratio) is nearly always markedly reduced by operation,[B21,L1] and signs of myocardial ischemia are reduced.[D10,M10] Late postoperative functional status in patients operated on in infancy or in adult life appears to depend primarily on status of the left ventricle before operation,[M10] just as it does in arteriosclerotic ischemic heart disease (see "Left Ventricular Function" under Results in Chapter 7). Clearly, however, these patients are not normal. In 11 late survivors, myocardial flow reserve was reduced, and exercise tolerance was lower than normal.[S10]

Left Ventricular Function

Left ventricular function does not change immediately after operation, but it improves strikingly after several months in most surviving patients, as evidenced by reduction in cardiothoracic ratio (Fig. 46-14) and left ventricular end-diastolic and end-systolic volumes, return of left ventricular shape to normal in both diastole and systole, and increase in left

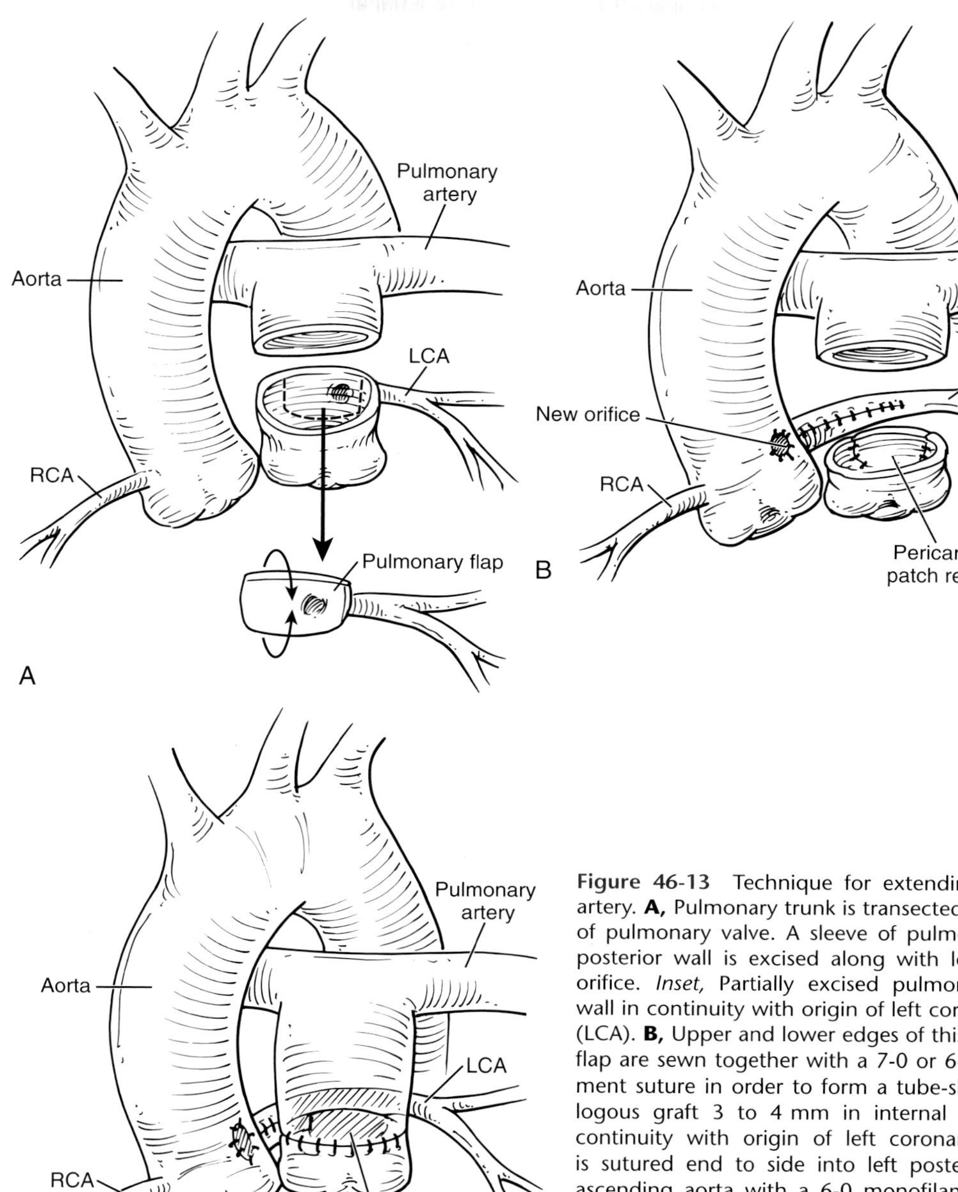

Figure 46-13 Technique for extending coronary artery. **A,** Pulmonary trunk is transected above level of pulmonary valve. A sleeve of pulmonary artery posterior wall is excised along with left coronary orifice. *Inset,* Partially excised pulmonary arterial wall in continuity with origin of left coronary artery (LCA). **B,** Upper and lower edges of this pulmonary flap are sewn together with a 7-0 or 6-0 monofilament suture in order to form a tube-shaped autologous graft 3 to 4 mm in internal diameter in continuity with origin of left coronary. **C,** Graft is sutured end to side into left posterior wall of ascending aorta with a 6-0 monofilament suture. Defect in pulmonary trunk is repaired with a fresh autologous pericardial patch. Key: *RCA,* right coronary artery. (From Wu and colleagues.[W6])

Table 46-1 Age and Hospital Mortality after Operation for Anomalous Connection of Left Coronary Artery to Pulmonary Trunk

Age			Hospital Deaths		
≤ Months	<	*n*	No.	%	CL (%)
3		1	0	0	0-85
3	6	7	2	29	10-55
6	12	4	0	0	0-38
12	24	5	0	0	0-32
24		2	0	0	0-61
TOTAL		19	2	11	4-23

Data from Arciniegas and colleagues.[A7]
Key: *CL,* 70% confidence limits.

Table 46-2 Procedure and Early and Late Mortality after Correction of Anomalous Connection of Left Coronary Artery to Pulmonary Trunk

	Early Mortality				Late Mortality
Procedure	*n*	No.	%	CL (%)	No.
Ligation	10	3	30	14-51	2
Ostial closure	1	0	0	0-86	0
Takeuchi	11	0	0	0-16	0
Ligation/CABG	1	0	0	0-86	—[a]
Thoracotomy	1	1	100	14-100	—
TOTAL	24	4			2

Data from Bunton and colleagues.[B21]
[a]Lost to follow-up evaluation.
Key: *CABG,* Coronary artery bypass grafting (saphenous vein); *CL,* 70% confidence limits.

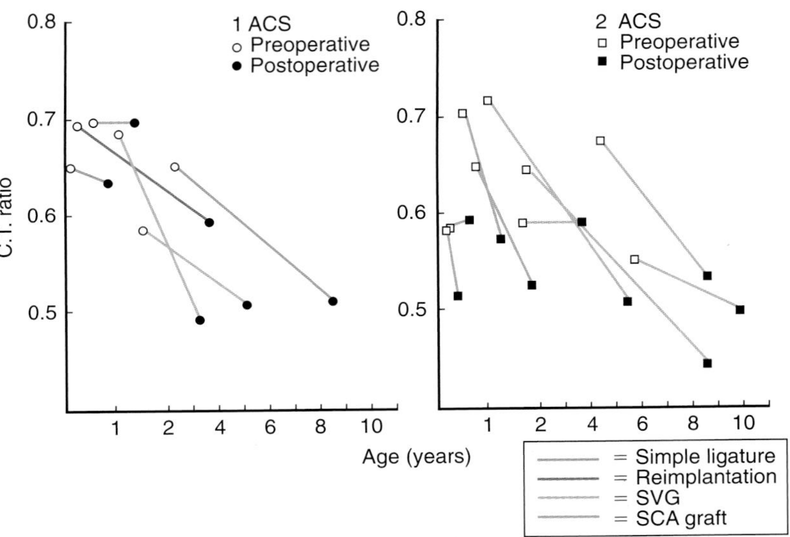

Figure 46-14 Change in cardiothoracic ratio after surgery for anomalous connection of left coronary artery to pulmonary trunk. Along horizontal axis is age in years at time of observation. "1 ACS" *(left graph)* indicates patients with one-artery coronary system postoperatively; "2 ACS" *(right graph)* indicates patients with two-artery coronary system postoperatively. Key: *ACS,* Artery coronary system; *C.T.,* cardiothoracic; *SCA,* subclavian to coronary artery; *SVG,* saphenous vein graft. (From Arciniegas and colleagues.[A7])

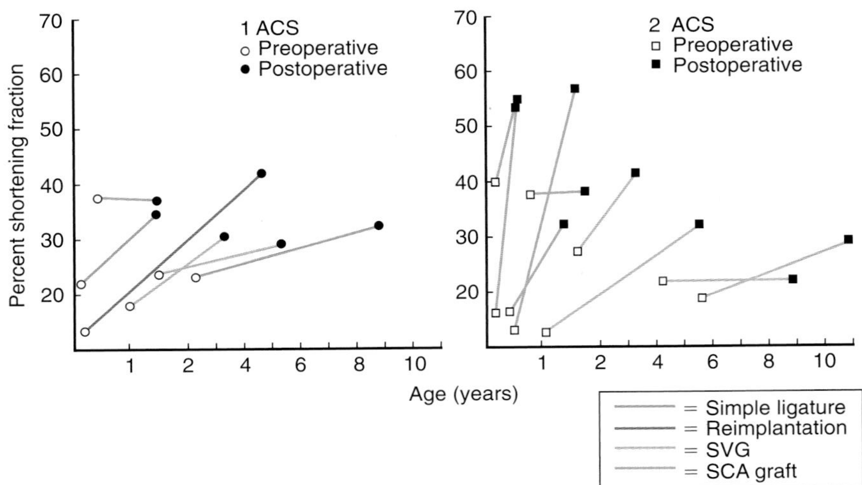

Figure 46-15 Change in left ventricular shortening fraction after surgery for anomalous connection of left coronary artery to pulmonary trunk. Depiction as in Fig. 46-14. Key: *ACS,* Artery coronary system; *SCA,* subclavian to coronary artery; *SVG,* saphenous vein graft. (From Arciniegas and colleagues.[A7])

ventricular ejection fraction and left ventricular shortening during systole[A4,A7,B8,B21,C3,C12,H10,I2,R3,S8] (Fig. 46-15). These findings indicate that in many patients, severe left ventricular dysfunction present preoperatively is due to reversible devitalization of the myocardium, or myocardial *hibernation,* as opposed to myocardial *stunning* (see "Myocardial Cell Stunning" under Damage from Global Myocardial Ischemia in Chapter 3).

Mitral Regurgitation

Mitral regurgitation frequently exists at presentation in patients with anomalous connection of left coronary artery to pulmonary trunk. It is argued by some that the basis for the regurgitation is ischemic and is reversible, and therefore the mitral valve should not be addressed routinely at initial operation for the anomalous coronary artery.[C12] Others routinely perform mitral anuloplasty when regurgitation is severe.[I2] When operation is performed in infancy, even important mitral regurgitation can regress postoperatively, no doubt related to improved left ventricular function.[B21,C12,S8] However, when mitral regurgitation is severe, it may not regress, and reoperation is required for regurgitation a few months to a few years later.[B14,B21,C12,S10] In one study that carefully tracked mitral valve function following surgery, regurgitation did not improve in 38% of cases but remained severe.[S6]

Effect of One-Artery Coronary System

Whether a two-artery coronary system after repair confers a better outcome than a one-artery system remains arguable. Speculatively, a two-artery system would seem to be advantageous, and results of exercise testing in a small number of patients support this view.[M2] Evidently, coronary blood flow is increased either by simple ligation of the anomalous left coronary artery or by creating an aortic origin of left coronary flow. However, coronary perfusion pressure in much of the left ventricle must be greater after the second type of repair, because it is not dependent on collateral flow. As a result, early and long-term results should be better, although magnitude of the difference when all other risk factors are similar remains to be determined.

Conduit Patency after Two-Artery Repair

Conduit patency cannot be assumed because the patient is asymptomatic, as is obvious from the fact that many patients are asymptomatic after a one-artery coronary system repair. The Takeuchi tunnel conduit was found to be obstructed in one of three patients studied late postoperatively by Bunton and colleagues, while four PTFE tubes used in a similar fashion were all patent.[B21] Two of five young patients undergoing left subclavian–left coronary artery anastomosis were found to have occluded conduits 3 to 5 years postoperatively.[K7]

When saphenous vein bypass grafts are used in adults, graft patency may be higher than in arteriosclerotic coronary artery disease. Donaldson and colleagues reported four of five grafts were patent 14 years postoperatively.[D10] When the reports of Moodie and colleagues and Chiariello and colleagues are combined, 11 of 15 grafts were patent.[C11,M10] However, concern remains about the potentially lethal effect of vein graft closure, particularly in view of demonstrated regression of right coronary artery collaterals following successful revascularization.[D10,M10] Anthony and colleagues reported sudden death in a 9-year-old girl 5 months after saphenous vein bypass grafting; at autopsy the graft was occluded and had extensive intimal fibrous hyperplasia.[A5] Similar vein graft obliterative changes were observed by el-Said and colleagues.[E5]

Right Ventricular Outflow Obstruction after Tunnel Repair

Right ventricular outflow obstruction is a risk following Takeuchi tunnel repair,[S6] but use of a generous anterior pulmonary trunk patch apparently reduces risk of serious obstruction.[C12]

INDICATIONS FOR OPERATION

Diagnosis of anomalous connection of left coronary artery to pulmonary trunk in an infant, regardless of clinical status, is an indication for urgent operation. The recommendation that operation be delayed until an older age[D12] is no longer tenable.[K1] Diagnosis is an indication for operation in older patients. Creating a two-artery coronary system may be considered to be indicated in all situations, including critically ill infants,[B1] especially if the option of using left ventricular assistance is available. Proper myocardial management (as described under Technique of Operation in this section) is mandatory.

Translocation of the left coronary artery into the aorta is the optimal operation when anatomy is favorable, with the Takeuchi procedure as the second option in infants. In older patients, internal thoracic artery grafting is a reasonable second alternative when size of the graft permits (see "Internal Thoracic Artery" under Technique of Operation in Chapter 7). Some recommend leaving the mitral valve alone when operation is performed in young patients, even when it is severely regurgitant, because this usually regresses if operation is successful[C12]; however, others routinely perform mitral anuloplasty as part of the initial operation.[I2] In older patients, mitral repair or replacement may be required (see Technique of Operation in Section I of Chapter 11).

SPECIAL SITUATIONS AND CONTROVERSIES

Anomalous Connection of Right Coronary Artery, Circumflex Coronary Artery, or Left Anterior Descending Coronary Artery to Pulmonary Trunk

An anomaly rarer than anomalous connection of left coronary artery to pulmonary trunk is anomalous connection of right coronary artery to pulmonary trunk. As of 2006, 77 cases had been reported.[W3] Undoubtedly, this lesion occurs more frequently and is underdiagnosed because of the relatively benign nature of the lesion compared with anomalous connection of the left coronary artery to pulmonary trunk (Table 46-3). Diagnosis is usually made at autopsy or incidentally in asymptomatic adults. Occasionally the anomaly is associated with symptoms in an older child or adult or with sudden death.[L6] Surgical correction consists of excising the anomalous connection of the right coronary artery to the anterior aspect of the pulmonary trunk, along with a button of pulmonary arterial wall, and translocating it into the anterior aspect of the ascending aorta.[T4]

Anomalous connection of circumflex or left anterior descending coronary artery to pulmonary trunk is also less lethal than anomalous connection of left coronary artery to pulmonary trunk. Both are also rarer than right coronary anomalous connection. Indications for surgery and technique of operation are similar to those for anomalous connection of the right coronary artery.[K4] Operation is indicated at the time of diagnosis for all these variations.

Total Anomalous Connection of Coronary Arteries to Pulmonary Trunk

Rarely, all coronary blood flow originates from the pulmonary trunk, either with a single ostium and trunk from which all branches emerge or from two ostia close together, giving rise to left and right coronary systems.[K6,R5] In less than half the cases reported, this has been an isolated anomaly. In such

Table 46-3 Comparison of Anomalous Right versus Left Coronary Artery Connection to Pulmonary Trunk

	Right Coronary Artery	Left Coronary Artery
Prevalence	0.002%	0.008%
Age at presentation	>2 years	<1 year
Heart failure	No	Yes
Ischemia	No	Yes
Sudden death	Rare	Yes
Physical exam	Murmur	Heart failure, ±systolic murmur
ECG findings	Nonspecific	Ischemia, Q waves in I and aVL >80%
Reimplantation	Yes	Yes

Modified from Williams and colleagues.[W3]
Key: *ECG*, Electrocardiogram.

cases, symptoms appear within a few days of birth, and death follows within 2 weeks.

With the advent of early diagnosis of congenital cardiac anomalies, on rare occasions neonates will appear for surgical consideration with this anomaly. Available pathologic information indicates that either a tunnel (Takeuchi) repair or translocation of the connection to the aortic root is feasible.[H6] Therefore, employing the most protective methods of myocardial management available, urgent operation should be carried out and can surely be successful.

Section III Anomalous Connection of a Main Coronary Artery to Aorta

DEFINITION

This section focuses on a condition in which (1) either the left main coronary artery connects to the aorta in a site other than the left coronary sinus or sinutubular junction (identified by the ridge between the sinus and ascending aorta), or (2) the right coronary artery connects to a site other than the right coronary sinus or sinutubular junction. The anomalously connected artery frequently passes between the aorta and pulmonary trunk *(interarterial course)* before normally distributing to the myocardium, commonly has a proximal course running within the aortic wall *(intramural course),* and occasionally has an ostial stenosis.

All these morphologic variations have been associated with ischemia and clinical events.[K10] Whether the course between the great arteries plays a pathophysiologic role in all clinical events remains controversial. The anomalously connected artery does not always pass between the aorta and pulmonary trunk but may pass in a retroaortic, prepulmonic, or transseptal course.[C10] Rarely the anomalous artery does not arise from the opposite coronary sinus, but rather from the posterior ("noncoronary" sinus). These variations are of concern only when there is ostial stenosis or an intramural course.

HISTORICAL NOTE

Cheitlin and colleagues in 1974 described death from anomalous connection of left main coronary artery to right sinus of Valsalva, with the artery then passing posteriorly between aorta and pulmonary trunk and then behind the trunk before branching into left anterior descending and circumflex arteries.[C9] In 1984, Roberts and colleagues described anomalous connection of right coronary artery to left sinus of Valsalva, with the right coronary artery passing anteriorly between the aorta and pulmonary trunk before passing across the outflow portion of the right ventricle.[R7]

MORPHOLOGY

The morphology of anomalous connection of a main coronary artery to aorta is abnormal in a number of ways beyond connection to the wrong sinus. These abnormalities have important implications with respect to both the likelihood of ischemia-related clinical events and specific surgical management.

Anomalous Connection of Left Main Coronary Artery

Most commonly, two coronary ostia are close together side by side in more or less the center of the right sinus of Valsalva. The ostium of the anomalous left main coronary may be eccentrically placed, however, often high in the right sinus and close to the right-left commissure. Less commonly, there is a single enlarged ostium in the right sinus, giving rise to both the normal right coronary and the anomalous left main coronary arteries. The ostium may have other abnormal characteristics. It may be angulated as it arises from the aorta, its opening may be slitlike, or it may travel in an intramural course, running within the wall of the aorta for up to several centimeters.

The left main coronary artery almost always passes posteriorly in an interarterial course between the aorta and pulmonary trunk, and then behind the pulmonary trunk to branch at the usual site. Much more rarely, the anomalously connecting left main coronary artery passes forward and across the floor of the right ventricle (ventricular septum) to emerge and pass near to its usual point.[I1] Also rarely, it may also pass retroaortically, or anteriorly across the right ventricular free wall. Circulation may be left or right dominant. Finally, anomalous connection of left main coronary artery to non-facing aortic sinus occurs rarely and may be associated with abnormal angulation and slitlike orifice as well.[H3]

Anomalous Connection of Right Coronary Artery

Anomalous connection of right coronary artery to aorta appears to be considerably more common than anomalous aortic origin of left main coronary artery. It may connect to a separate ostium within the left sinus, to a separate ostium just above the commissure between left and right sinuses, or to one just above the sinutubular ridge over the left sinus.[K10] Less commonly, the right coronary artery may connect to a single ostium that also gives origin to the left main coronary artery, and this ostium may lie within the left sinus or over the commissure between left and right sinuses.[K10] The anomalously connecting right coronary artery may have all the other ostial abnormalities described for the anomalously connected left main coronary artery, and always passes forward in an interarterial course between the great arteries. Rarely, one or both coronary ostia may arise from the posterior (the normal noncoronary) sinus.[C5]

CLINICAL FEATURES AND DIAGNOSTIC CRITERIA

Anomalous connection of a coronary artery to the aorta results in no characteristic clinical or ECG features. A meta-analysis using a number of reasonable assumptions suggests that more than 99% are asymptomatic and will remain so (see Natural History).[C8] The true prevalence of this defect is unknown. The most accurate estimate probably comes from a prospective search for the defect in more than 2000 children with normal hearts, in which a prevalence of 0.17% was found, or in other words, about 1 to 2 per 1000 children.[D4] Studies based on cardiac catheterization typically show similar to higher prevalence, probably because of selection bias.[O6,T6]

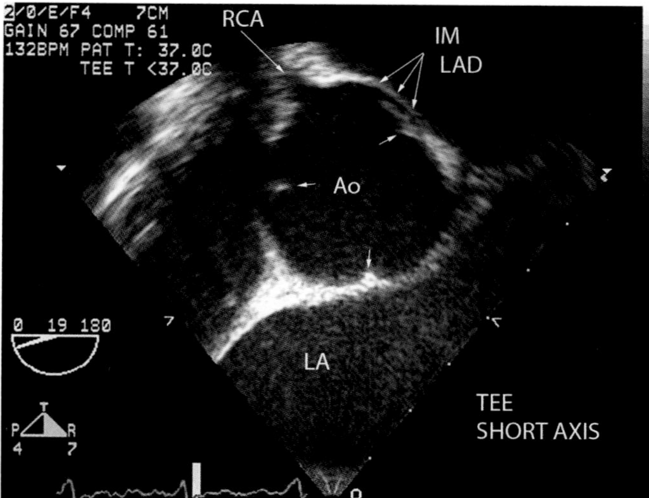

Figure 46-16 Transesophageal echocardiographic (TEE) image of anomalous aortic origin of left main coronary artery from right aortic sinus, with intramural course. Small arrows identify aortic valve commissures. Key: *Ao,* Aorta; *LA,* left atrium; *IM LAD,* intramural left coronary artery; *RCA,* right coronary artery.

Patients who are symptomatic typically present in the second or third decade of life and may complain of angina or syncope, or they may present with sudden death. Rarely, patients present with symptoms as neonates, infants, or in the first decade of life. The anomalous connection is most commonly diagnosed by echocardiography. The ECG may be indicated for other reasons in asymptomatic patients, and the anomalous vessel is identified incidentally. In symptomatic patients, an ECG is typically the initial imaging study.

The purpose of imaging the vessel is to define several clinically relevant morphologic characteristics:

1. Presence of a single ostium or separate ostia
2. Exact position of the ostium within or near the sinus
3. Presence of an intramural course
4. Identification of a slitlike or angulated ostium
5. Identification of an interarterial course, and determination of whether the caliber of the artery is narrowed in this area

Echocardiography can accurately define the ostial position and interarterial course of the vessel. It can also sometimes reveal whether there are one or two ostia and whether there is an intramural course[F5] (Fig. 46-16). However, this modality may have difficulty demonstrating whether there are one or two ostia when these are closely spaced, and whether there is an intramural course when that course is a short segment. Because of these limitations, further imaging is indicated.

Magnetic resonance angiography,[C1,D1] CT,[M5] and angiography at cardiac catheterization all have been used to further characterize the morphology, but available data are insufficient to assess whether these imaging modalities are superior to echocardiography, particularly with respect to defining an intramural course (Fig. 46-17). One study compared the accuracy of catheter-based angiography and CTA in helping determine the origin and proximal course of the anomalous artery. CT was found to be more accurate in revealing the proximal course.[M5] Accurate CT images require gating, so this modality may be of less use in smaller patients because of their faster heart rates.[D6] A search is also made for objective evidence of reversible ischemia. Documentation of compression of the right coronary artery coursing between aorta and pulmonary artery, with the right coronary artery arising from the left main coronary artery, has been demonstrated angiographically in a patient with exertional angina.[L11]

NATURAL HISTORY

The natural history is controversial. A number of cases have been reported in which serious sequelae, including sudden death, have been ascribed to anomalous connection of coronary artery to left sinus of Valsalva (summarized by Berdoff and colleagues[B6] and Mustafa and colleagues[M13]). The relationship between sequelae and anomaly is not conclusive. Asymptomatic patients with the condition were observed by Berdoff and colleagues, with a mean age of 40 to 69 years and with normal segmental wall motion and a left ventricular ejection fraction of 60% to 80%[B6]; no unfavorable events were experienced in a follow-up of 8 to 69 months. Sudden death in neonates may occur in the presence of this defect in rare cases, but causality is difficult to prove.

There are only rare cases of clinical events in individuals once out of the neonatal period, until the second decade is reached. The combined U.S. and Italian registries of sudden deaths in competitive athletes revealed 27 individuals dying with anomalous coronary arteries; all but one death occurred between ages 10 and 32 years. The other individual was 9 years old.[B5] In two thirds of the deaths, there were no previous events and no symptoms. The prevalence of sudden death in competitive athletes is about 1 : 100,000. About 20% of these are due to coronary anomalies; thus, the prevalence of sudden death due to a coronary anomaly is about 2 : 1,000,000 in competitive athletes.

Most clinical events, including sudden death, occur in the second and third decades of life, and more commonly in males. Events are likely to occur during or just after exertion. Sudden death may be the initial event. If an individual lives into the third decade, new onset clinical events are extremely rare.

TECHNIQUE OF OPERATION

Several operations have been developed to relieve ischemia or potential ischemia. The choice of operation depends on the specific morphologic details, emphasizing the importance of accurate preoperative imaging (Fig. 46-18). Translocation of the anomalously connected artery to the correct sinus is indicated in several circumstances. This operation can usually be accomplished and will be effective when there are two reasonably widely spaced ostia, and when there is not an intramural course or angulated or slitlike ostium. The operation effectively removes the vessel from its vulnerable interarterial position. The technique of operation requires standard CPB and cardioplegic arrest. The coronary artery is dissected, mobilized, and translocated using the exact principles outlined for coronary translocation in the arterial switch operation for transposition (see Chapter 52).

Unroofing the proximal coronary artery is indicated when an intramural course is present[M13,N3] (Fig. 46-19). This maneuver may be all that is necessary if the unroofing moves the effective ostium into the appropriate sinus. This

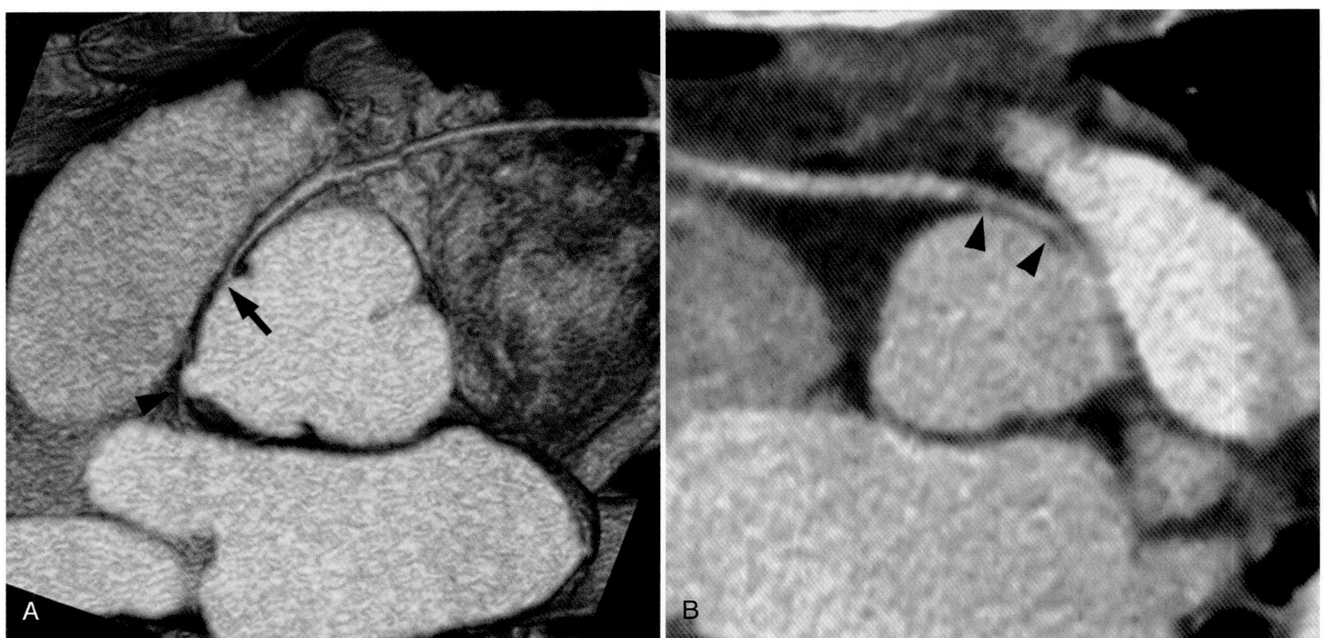

Figure 46-17 Volume-rendered images from cardiac gated computed tomography angiogram (CTA) demonstrating intramural course of right coronary artery. **A,** Image from a 13-year-old boy showing right coronary artery *(arrow)* and left main coronary artery *(arrowhead),* both arising from left coronary sinus at the aortic root. Right coronary artery has an interarterial course. **B,** Short-axis image at aortic root of an 8-year-old boy showing a right coronary artery arising from left coronary sinus. Interarterial portion of right coronary artery is separated from aortic root by a thin wall *(arrowheads),* suggesting an intramural coronary artery. Also, right coronary ostium is small and interarterial segment narrowed.

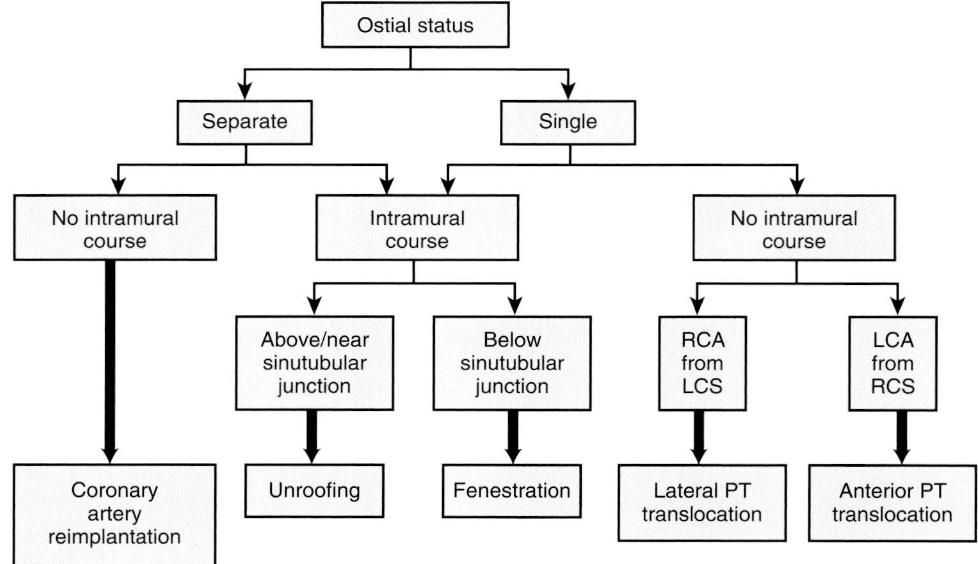

Figure 46-18 Morphology-based surgical management protocol. Key: *LCA,* Left coronary artery; *LCS,* left coronary sinus; *PT,* pulmonary trunk; *RCA,* right coronary artery; *RCS,* right coronary sinus. (From Gulati and colleagues.[G6])

accomplishes two things: It relieves any stenosis in the intramural segment, and it moves the coronary lumen away from the interarterial position. Unroofing can be accomplished whether or not there is a single coronary ostium or separate ostia. Modified unroofing can be performed in some cases to avoid disturbing the commissure of the aortic valve[R11] (Fig. 46-20). In certain cases, both unroofing a short intramural segment and translocation is the appropriate operation. In this case, as in the arterial switch operation, care must be taken to excise the ostium with a button of sinus tissue that fully encompasses the intramural component. Also, in certain cases with an angulated or slitlike ostium but no true intramural element, ostial patching should be performed along with translocation.

When the morphology is that of a single coronary ostium without an intramural element, neither translocation nor

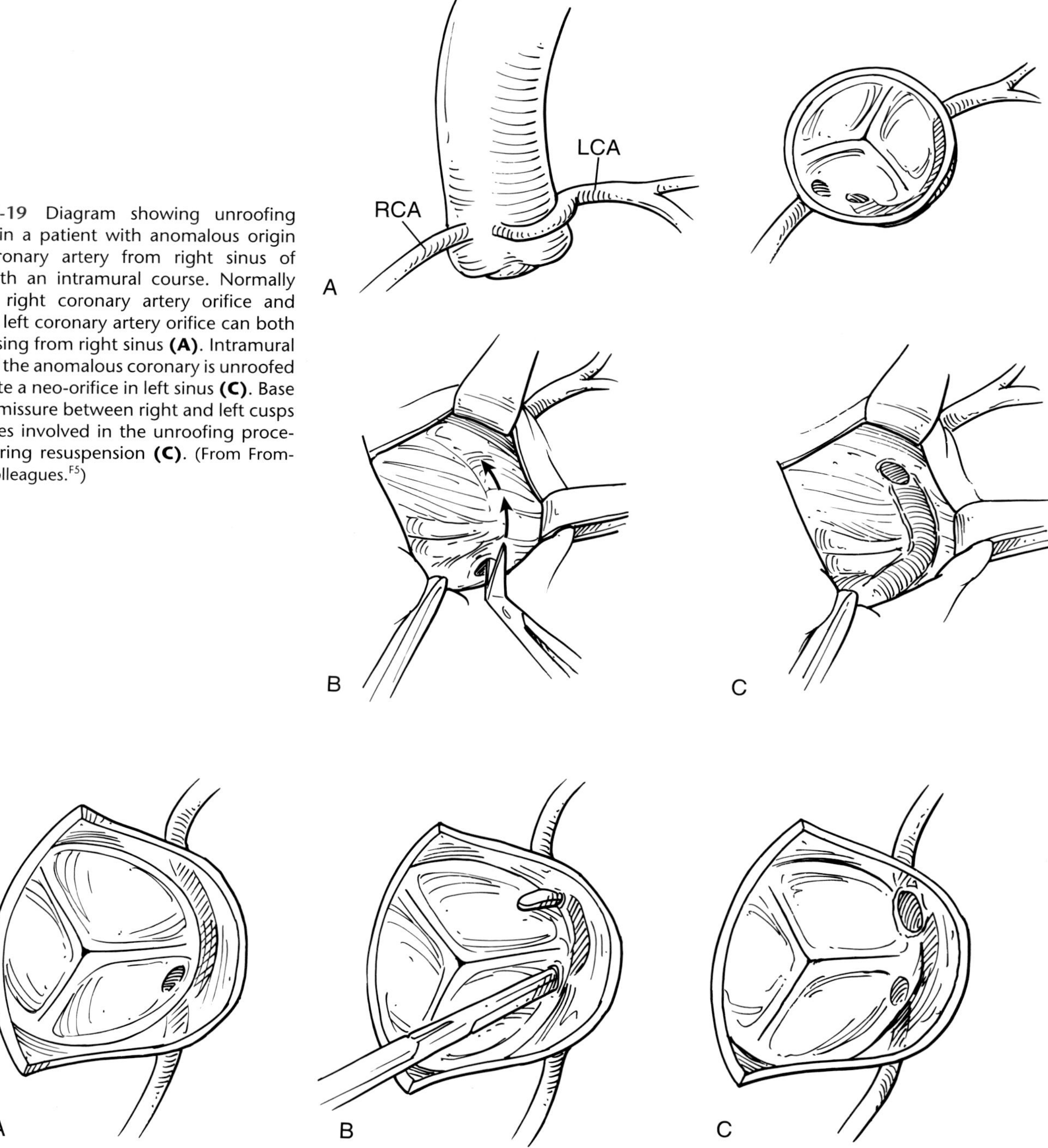

Figure 46-19 Diagram showing unroofing technique in a patient with anomalous origin of left coronary artery from right sinus of Valsalva with an intramural course. Normally positioned right coronary artery orifice and anomalous left coronary artery orifice can both be seen arising from right sinus **(A)**. Intramural segment of the anomalous coronary is unroofed **(B)** to create a neo-orifice in left sinus **(C)**. Base of the commissure between right and left cusps is sometimes involved in the unroofing procedure, requiring resuspension **(C)**. (From Frommelt and colleagues.[F5])

Figure 46-20 Unroofing procedure performed on two of nine patients in whom a neo-ostium was created without taking down the intercoronary commissure. New ostium is created by passing an instrument from native ostium into appropriate sinus. A neo-ostium is created in that sinus at the point at which the artery leaves the aortic wall. (From Romp and colleagues.[R11])

unroofing is possible. The goal of surgery is to eliminate the risk of the interarterial component of the vessel. CABG using the internal thoracic artery or a saphenous vein graft to the anomalously connected artery has been described.[M11] This option, however, is not recommended for several reasons. First, the long-term efficacy of the graft is uncertain in young patients. Second, the graft will be in competition with essentially normal antegrade flow through the anomalously connected artery, raising concern about graft thrombosis or, at the very least, adequacy of the graft when it may be acutely needed during transient compression of the anomalously connected artery. Instead of bypass grafting in this situation, moving the pulmonary trunk away from the aortic root so that the interarterial component of the anomalously connected artery is no longer at risk of compression should be considered.[G6] This can be accomplished in two ways, either translocating the distal pulmonary trunk leftward into the left pulmonary artery (Fig. 46-21), or translocating the right

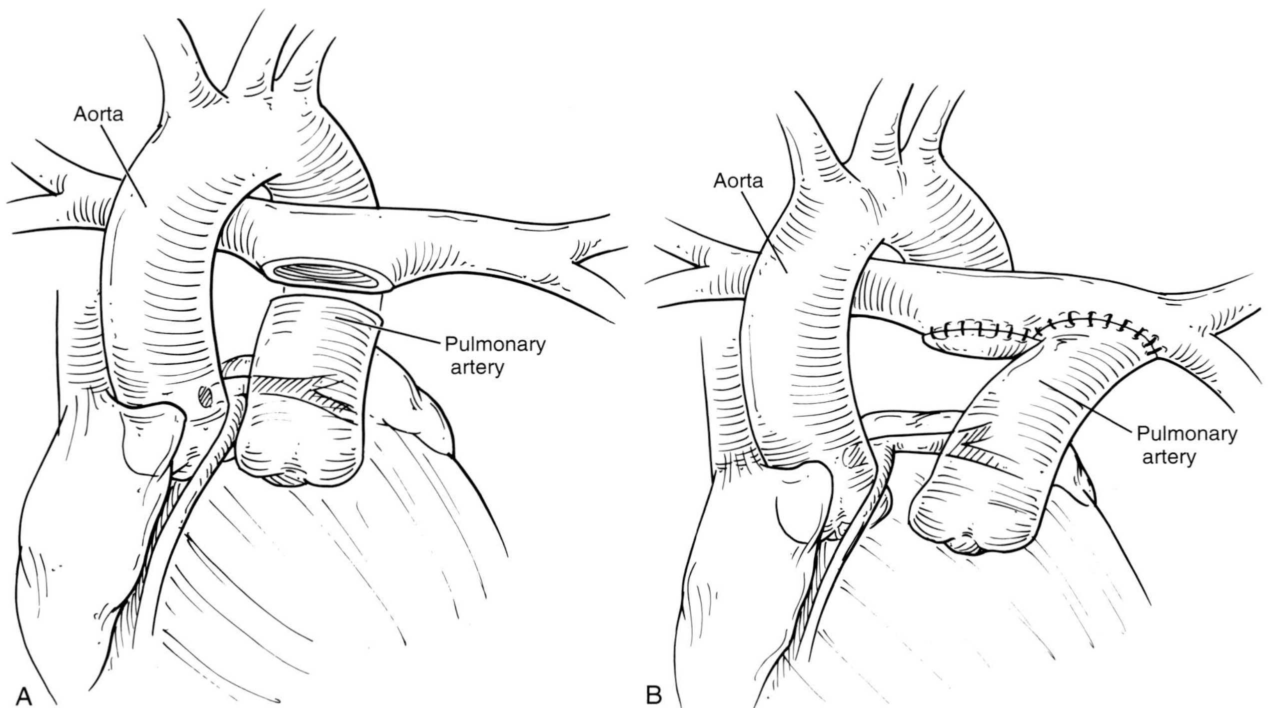

Figure 46-21 Translocation of pulmonary trunk (PT) for single coronary ostium without intramural element. **A,** PT is carefully dissected off its pulmonary bifurcation. Patch augmentation of right pulmonary artery beyond the bifurcation is critical to prevent right pulmonary artery stenosis. Left pulmonary artery is opened toward hilum. PT is translocated toward left hilum and reanastomosed. **B,** Completed translocation of PT toward left hilum to create additional space between it and aorta (Ao). (From Rodefeld and colleagues.[R9])

pulmonary artery branch anterior to the aorta (Fig. 46-22), similar to the Lecompte maneuver in the arterial switch operation for transposition (see Chapter 52).

RESULTS

Early and midterm outcomes are generally excellent regardless of the specific operation, with mortality approaching zero and relief of symptoms in patients who are symptomatic preoperatively.[D3,E6,G6] Romp and colleagues report no mortality and relief of symptoms in nine previously symptomatic patients, all of whom underwent unroofing of an intramural artery.[R11] Of concern, however, despite lack of postoperative symptoms in 24 repaired patients, Brothers and colleagues were able to demonstrate signs of ischemia in almost 40% of patients evaluated with stress echocardiography, exercise stress testing, and stress myocardial perfusion scanning at a mean follow-up of 15 months after surgery.[B18] This same group of investigators also report that exercise capacity and quality of life were normal following surgical repair.[B17]

INDICATIONS FOR OPERATION

Indications for operation remain arguable. Ischemia, whether reversible or not, in the distribution of the anomalously connecting coronary artery is an indication for operation. A syncopal event, angina, or an episode of sudden death with resuscitation is an indication for operation, even if ischemia cannot be demonstrated at evaluation. In fact, ischemia typically is not elicited with stress testing.[B5]

Concerning morphology, such as intramural course, slit-like ostium, or narrowed caliber of the interarterial course, is probably an indication for operation, even in the absence of demonstrable ischemia. Existence of the anomalous connection with an interarterial course, but without symptoms and without other concerning morphologic characteristics, may be an indication for operation in individuals diagnosed in the second and third decades of life but probably not in those diagnosed later. Presence of the anomalous connection without ischemia, symptoms, or concerning morphologic characteristics is probably not an indication for operation in the first decade of life. Effectiveness of operation can be proved by absence postoperatively of any evidence of reversible ischemia.

SPECIAL SITUATIONS AND CONTROVERSIES

Presence of an anomalously connected vessel without other concerning morphologic characteristics in an asymptomatic child under age 10 years is probably not an indication for operation, but it is unclear whether such a patient should undergo operation once the second decade is reached if no clinical events have occurred. A survey of the Congenital Heart Surgeons Society regarding management practices underscores the marked heterogeneity of opinion regarding management of anomalous coronary arteries. There was strong but not unanimous agreement that evidence of ischemia warranted surgery. Less than 80% recommend referral for surgery with symptoms but no objective evidence of ischemia.[B16]

There is no consensus regarding the pathophysiologic importance of the interarterial course, especially when no narrowing of the vessel can be demonstrated in this area during imaging. The concern is that this region of the vessel

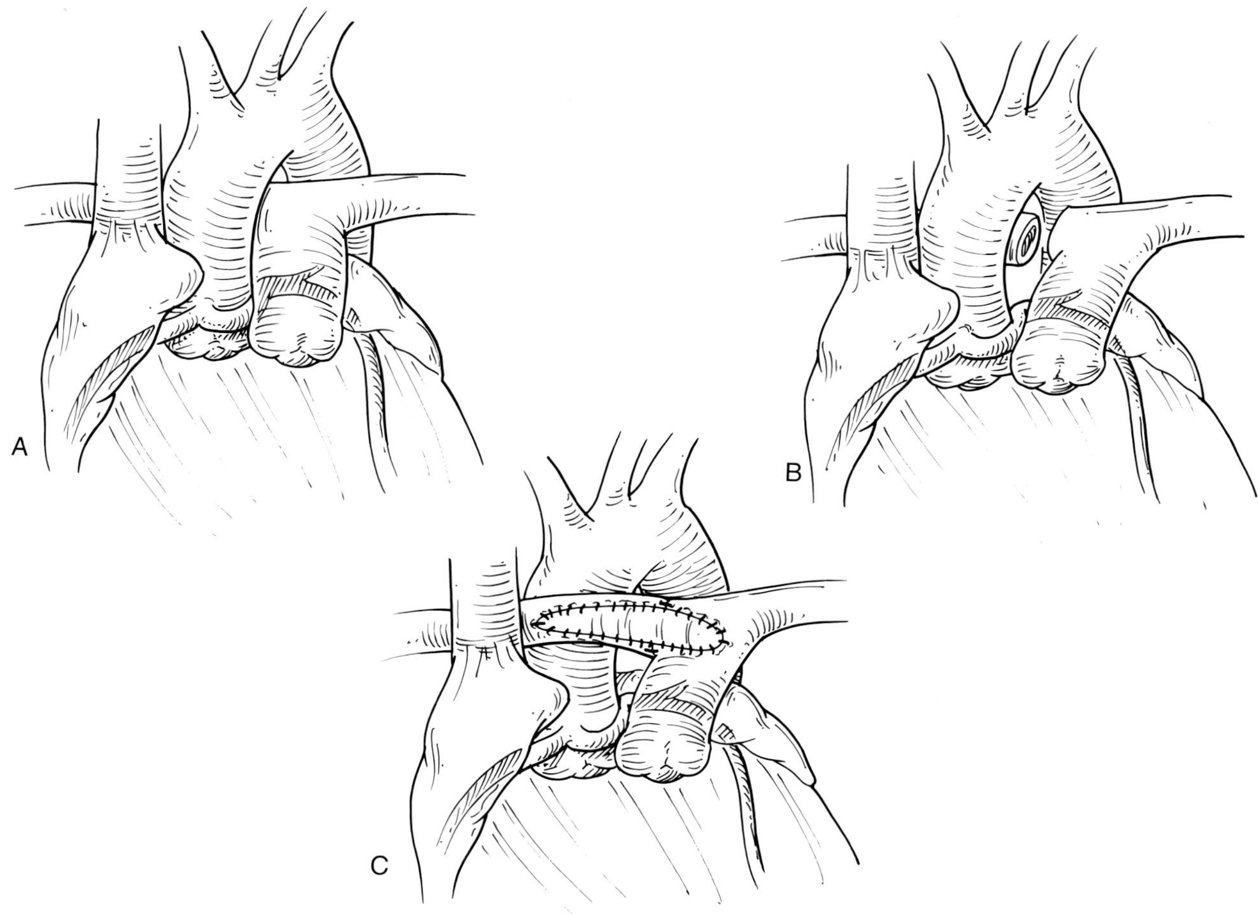

Figure 46-22 Anterior pulmonary artery translocation. **A,** Anomalous left coronary artery from the right coronary sinus (RCS), with single origin and normal proximal course. **B,** Both branch pulmonary arteries are fully mobilized and right pulmonary artery is transected and moved anterior to aorta. **C,** Right pulmonary artery is reattached and a pericardial patch added, as necessary. This moves the pulmonary trunk both anteriorly and leftward, relieving compression on the interarterial portion of anomalous artery. (From Gulati and colleagues.[G6])

is at risk of transient narrowing or stretching during the dynamic conditions of exercise, when the wall tension of both the aorta and pulmonary trunk may increase from pressure and diameter changes. Although not recommended in young patients, use of interventional catheter-based techniques, including coronary artery stenting, has been anecdotally described for various coronary artery anomalies.[L4] These procedures are typically performed in previously undiagnosed adults who present with evolving acute myocardial events at the time of diagnostic, and potentially therapeutic, cardiac catheterization.[A10,C6,C13] CABG is also not recommended in young patients; however, it becomes a more attractive surgical option in older patients, particularly those presenting with symptoms or with associated arteriosclerotic disease. Excellent outcomes can be achieved.[D3] Brothers and colleagues have shown that familial screening in patients with anomalous coronaries yielded positive findings not attributable to chance alone, suggesting a genetic component for this disease.[B16,B19]

REFERENCES

A

1. Abbott ME. Congenital heart disease. In Osler's modern medicine. Vol. IV. Philadelphia, 1927.
2. Agatston AS, Chapman E, Hildner FJ, Samet P. Diagnosis of a right coronary artery-right atrial fistula using two-dimensional and Doppler echocardiography. Am J Cardiol 1984;54:238.
3. Ahmed SS, Haider B, Regan TJ. Silent left coronary artery-cameral fistula: probable cause of myocardial ischemia. Am Heart J 1982; 104:869.
4. Amaral F, Carvalho JS, Granzotti JA, Shinebourne EA. Anomalous origin of the left coronary artery from the pulmonary trunk. Clinical features and midterm results after surgical treatment. Arq Bras Cardiol 1999;72:307.
5. Anthony CL Jr, McAllister HA Jr, Cheitlin MD. Spontaneous graft closure in anomalous origin of the left coronary artery. Chest 1975;68:4.
6. Apley J, Horton RE, Wilson MG. The possible role of surgery in the treatment of anomalous left coronary artery. Thorax 1957;12:23.
7. Arciniegas E, Farooki ZQ, Hakimi M, Green EW. Management of anomalous left coronary artery from the pulmonary artery. Circulation 1980;62:I1.
8. Askenazi J, Nadas AS. Anomalous left coronary artery originating from the pulmonary artery. Report on 15 cases. Circulation 1975;51:976.
9. Augustasson MN, Gasul BM, Lundquist R. Anomalous origin of the left coronary artery from the pulmonary artery (adult type). Pediatrics 1962;29:274.
10. Azzarelli S, Amico F, Giacoppo M, Argentino V, Di Mario C, Fiscella A. Primary coronary angioplasty in a patient with anomalous origin of the right coronary artery from the left sinus of Valsalva. J Cardiovasc Med (Hagerstown) 2007;8: 943-5.

B

1. Backer CL, Stout MJ, Zales VR, Muster AJ, Weigel TJ, Idriss FS, et al. Anomalous origin of the left coronary artery. A twenty-year review of surgical management. J Thorac Cardiovasc Surg 1992; 103:1049.
2. Baim DS, Kline H, Silverman JF. Bilateral coronary artery–pulmonary artery fistulas. Report of five cases and review of the literature. Circulation 1982;65:810.
3. Barratt-Boyes BG. Cardiac surgery in infancy. N Z Med J 1965; 64:17.
4. Barratt-Boyes BG. The technique of intracardiac repair in infancy using deep hypothermia with circulatory arrest and limited cardiopulmonary bypass. In Ionescu MI, Wosler GH, eds. Current techniques in extracorporeal circulation. London: Butterworth, 1976, p. 219.
5. Basso C, Maron BJ, Corrado D, Thiene G. Clinical profile of congenital coronary artery anomalies with origin from the wrong aortic sinus leading to sudden death in young competitive athletes. J Am Coll Cardiol 2000;35:1493-501.
6. Berdoff R, Haimowitz A, Kupersmith J. Anomalous origin of the right coronary artery from the left sinus of Valsalva. Am J Cardiol 1986;58:656.
7. Biorck G, Crafoord C. Arteriovenous aneurysm on the pulmonary artery simulating patent ductus arteriosus botalli. Thorax 1947;2:65.
8. Birk E, Stamler A, Katz J, Berant M, Dagan O, Matitiau A, et al. Anomalous origin of the left coronary artery from the pulmonary artery: diagnosis and postoperative follow up. Isr Med Assoc J 2000;2:111.
9. Blakeway HA. A hitherto undescribed malformation of the heart. J Anat Physiol 1918;52:354.
10. Bland EF, White PD, Garland J. Congenital anomalies of the coronary arteries: report of an unusual case associated with cardiac hypertrophy. Am Heart J 1933;8:787.
11. Bogers AJ, Gittenbergerde Groot AC. The ALCAPA: what's in a name? (letter) J Thorac Cardiovasc Surg 1992;104:527.
12. Bogers AJ, Gittenbergerde Groot AC, Poelmann RE, Peault BM, Huysmans HA. Development of the origin of the coronary arteries, a matter of ingrowth or outgrowth? Anat Embryol 1989;180:437.
13. Bogers AJ, Quaegebeur JM, Huysmans HA. Early and late results of surgical treatment of congenital coronary artery fistula. Thorax 1987;42:369.
14. Bojar RM, Ilbawi MN, DeLeon SY, Riggs TW, Idriss FS. Surgical management of anomalous left coronary artery with mitral insufficiency in infancy: contribution of echocardiography. Pediatr Cardiol 1984;5:35.
15. Brooks SJ. Two cases of an abnormal coronary artery of the heart arising from the pulmonary artery: with some remarks upon the effect of this anomaly in producing cirsoid dilatation of the vessels. J Anat Physiol 1886;20:26.
16. Brothers J, Gaynor JW, Paridon S, Lorber R, Jacobs M. Anomalous aortic origin of a coronary artery with an interarterial course: understanding current management strategies in children and young adults. Pediatr Cardiol 2009;30:911-21.
17. Brothers JA, McBride MG, Marino BS, Tomlinson RS, Seliem MA, Pampaloni MH, et al. Exercise performance and quality of life following surgical repair of anomalous aortic origin of a coronary artery in the pediatric population. J Thorac Cardiovasc Surg 2009; 137:380-4.
18. Brothers JA, McBride MG, Seliem MA, Marino BS, Tomlinson RS, Pampaloni MH, et al. Evaluation of myocardial ischemia after surgical repair of anomalous aortic origin of a coronary artery in a series of pediatric patients. J Am Coll Cardiol 2007;50:2078-82.
19. Brothers JA, Stephens P, Gaynor JW, Lorber R, Vricella LA, Paridon SM. Anomalous aortic origin of a coronary artery with an interarterial course: should family screening be routine? J Am Coll Cardiol 2008;51:2062-4.
20. Brown MA, Balzer D, Lasala J. Multiple coronary artery fistulae treated with a single Amplatzer vascular plug: check the back door when the front is locked. Catheter Cardiovasc Interv 2009; 73:390-4.
21. Bunton R, Jonas RA, Lang P, Rein AJ, Castaneda AR. Anomalous origin of left coronary artery from pulmonary artery. Ligation versus establishment of a two coronary artery system. J Thorac Cardiovasc Surg 1987;93:103.
22. Burchell HB, Brown AL Jr. Anomalous origin of the coronary artery from pulmonary artery masquerading as mitral insufficiency. Am Heart J 1962;63:388.

C

1. Cademartiri F, Runza G, Luccichenti G, Galia M, Mollet NR, Alaimo V, et al. Coronary artery anomalies: incidence, pathophysiology, clinical relevance and role of diagnostic imaging. Radiol Med 2006;111:376-91.
2. Caldwell RL, Hurwitz RA, Girod DA, Weyman AE, Feigenbaum H. Two-dimensional echocardiographic differentiation of anomalous left coronary artery from congestive cardiomyopathy. Am Heart J 1983;106:710.
3. Carvalho JS, Redington AN, Oldershaw PJ, Shinebourne EA, Lincoln CR, Gibson DG. Analysis of left ventricular wall movement before and after reimplantation of anomalous left coronary artery in infancy. Br Heart J 1991;65:218.
4. Case RB, Morrow AG, Stainsby W, Nestor JO. Anomalous origin of the left coronary artery: the physiologic defect and suggested surgical treatment. Circulation 1958;17:1062.
5. Catanzaro JN, Makaryus AN, Catanese C. Sudden cardiac death associated with an extremely rare coronary anomaly of the left and right coronary arteries arising exclusively from the posterior (noncoronary) sinus of Valsalva. Clin Cardiol 2005;28:542-4.
6. Ceyhan C, Tekten T, Onbasili AO. Primary percutaneous coronary intervention of anomalous origin of right coronary artery above the left sinus of Valsalva in a case with acute myocardial infarction. Coronary anomalies and myocardial infarction. Int J Cardiovasc Imaging 2004;20:293-7.
7. Cha SD, Singer E, Maranhao V, Goldberg H. Silent coronary artery–left ventricular fistula: a disorder of the thebesian system? Angiology 1978;29:169.
8. Cheitlin MD. Finding asymptomatic people with a coronary artery arising from the wrong sinus of Valsalva: consequences arising from knowing the anomaly to be familial. J Am Coll Cardiol 2008; 51:2065-7.
9. Cheitlin MD, DeCastro CM, McAlister HA. Sudden death as a complication of anomalous left coronary origin from the anterior sinus of Valsalva. A not-so-minor congenital anomaly. Circulation 1974;50:780.
10. Cheitlin MD, MacGregor J. Congenital anomalies of coronary arteries: role in the pathogenesis of sudden cardiac death. Herz 2009;34:268-79.
11. Chiariello L, Meyer J, Reul GJ Jr, Hallman GL, Cooley DA. Surgical treatment for anomalous origin of left coronary artery from pulmonary artery. Ann Thorac Surg 1975;19:443.
12. Cochrane AD, Coleman DM, Davis AM, Brizard CP, Wolfe R, Karl TR. Excellent long-term functional outcome after an operation for anomalous left coronary artery from the pulmonary artery. J Thorac Cardiovasc Surg 1999;117:332.
13. Conde-Vela C, Sabate M, Quevedo PJ, Hernandez-Antolin R. Primary percutaneous coronary intervention of an anomalous right coronary artery originating from the left sinus of Valsalva. Acute Card Care 2006;8:229-32.
14. Cooley DA, Hallman GL, Bloodwell RD. Definitive surgical treatment of anomalous origin of left coronary artery from pulmonary artery. J Thorac Cardiovasc Surg 1966;52:798.
15. Currarino G, Silverman FN, Landing BH. Abnormal congenital fistulous communications of the coronary arteries. Am J Roentgenol 1959;82:392.

D

1. Danias PG, Stuber M, McConnell MV, Manning WJ. The diagnosis of congenital coronary anomalies with magnetic resonance imaging. Coron Artery Dis 2001;12:621-6.
2. Daniel TM, Graham TP, Sabiston DC Jr. Coronary artery–right ventricular fistula with congestive heart failure: surgical correction in the neonatal period. Surgery 1970;67:985.
3. Davies JE, Burkhart HM, Dearani JA, Suri RM, Phillips SD, Warnes CA, et al. Surgical management of anomalous aortic origin of a coronary artery. Ann Thorac Surg 2009;88:844-8.
4. Davis JA, Cecchin F, Jones TK, Portman MA. Major coronary artery anomalies in a pediatric population: incidence and clinical importance. J Am Coll Cardiol 2001;37:593-7.
5. de Nef JJ, Varghese PJ, Losekoot G. Congenital coronary artery fistula. Analysis of 17 cases. Br Heart J 1971;33:857.
6. Deibler AR, Kuzo RS, Vohringer M, Page EE, Safford RE, Patron JN, et al. Imaging of congenital coronary anomalies with multislice computed tomography. Mayo Clin Proc 2004;79: 1017-23.

7. del Nido PJ, Duncan BW, Mayer JE Jr, Wessel DL, LaPierre RA, Jonas RA. Left ventricular assist device improves survival in children with left ventricular dysfunction after repair of anomalous origin of the left coronary artery from the pulmonary artery. Ann Thorac Surg 1999;67:169.
8. Dietrich W. Ursprung der vorderen Kranzarterie aus der Lungenschlagader mit ungewohnlichen Veranderungen des Herz muskels und der Gefasswande. Virchows Arch [A] 1939;303:436.
9. Dobell AR, Long RW. Right coronary–left ventricular fistula mimicking aortic valve insufficiency in infancy. J Thorac Cardiovasc Surg 1981;82:785.
10. Donaldson RM, Raphael MJ, Yacoub MH, Ross DN. Hemodynamically significant anomalies of the coronary arteries: surgical aspects. Thorac Cardiovasc Surg 1982;30:7.
11. Doty DB, Chandramouli B, Schieken RE, Lauer RM, Ehrenhaft JL. Anomalous origin of the left coronary artery from the right pulmonary artery. J Thorac Cardiovasc Surg 1976;71:787.
12. Driscoll DJ, Nihill MR, Mullins CE, Cooley DA, McNamara DG. Management of symptomatic infants with anomalous origin of the left coronary artery from the pulmonary artery. Am J Cardiol 1981;47:642.

E

1. Edis AJ, Schattenberg TT, Feldt RH, Danielson GK. Congenital coronary artery fistula. Surgical considerations and results of operation. Mayo Clin Proc 1972;47:567.
2. Edwards JE. Functional pathology of congenital cardiac disease. Pediatr Clin North Am 1954;1:13.
3. el Habbal MM, de Leval M, Somerville J. Anomalous origin of the left anterior descending coronary artery from the pulmonary trunk: recognition in life and successful surgical treatment. Br Heart J 1988;60:90.
4. el-Oakley R, al-Saeedi A, al-Faraidi Y, Abou-Zanouna Y, Abdull Hamid J, Jubair K. Reimplantation of anomalous left coronary artery on a beating heart. J Thorac Cardiovasc Surg 1999; 117:395.
5. el-Said GM, Ruzyllo W, Williams RL, Mullins CE, Hallman GL, Cooley DA, et al. Early and late result of saphenous vein graft for anomalous origin of left coronary artery from pulmonary artery. Circulation 1973;48:III2.
6. Erez E, Tam VK, Doublin NA, Stakes J. Anomalous coronary artery with aortic origin and course between the great arteries: improved diagnosis, anatomic findings, and surgical treatment. Ann Thorac Surg 2006;82:973-7.

F

1. Farouk A, Zahka K, Siwik E, Golden A, Karimi M, Uddin M, et al. Anomalous origin of the left coronary artery from the right pulmonary artery. J Card Surg 2009;24:49-54.
2. Fell EH, Weinberg J, Gordon AS, Gasul BM, Johnson FR. Surgery for congenital arteriovenous fistulas. Arch Surg 1958;77:331.
3. Fleming RJ, Marx L, Litwin SB, Gallen WL. Left ventricular aneurysmectomy in a child. Ann Thorac Surg 1975;19:457.
4. Floyd WL, Young WG, Johnsrude IS. Coronary arterial–left atrial fistula. Case with obstruction of the inferior vena cava by a giant left atrium. Am J Cardiol 1970;25:716.
5. Frommelt PC, Frommelt MA, Tweddell JS, Jaquiss RD. Prospective echocardiographic diagnosis and surgical repair of anomalous origin of a coronary artery from the opposite sinus with an interarterial course. J Am Coll Cardiol 2003;42:148-54.

G

1. George JM, Knowlan DM. Anomalous origin of the left coronary artery from the pulmonary artery in an adult. N Engl J Med 1959; 261:993.
2. Goebel N, Gander MP, Steinbrunn W. Small coronary artery fistulae. Ann Radiol 1979;22:277.
3. Goldblatt E, Adams AP, Ross IK, Savage JP, Morris LL. Single-trunk anomalous origin of both coronary arteries from the pulmonary artery. J Thorac Cardiovasc Surg 1984;87:59.
4. Grace RR, Angelini P, Cooley DA. Aortic implantation of anomalous left coronary artery arising from pulmonary artery. Am J Cardiol 1977;39:609.
5. Griffiths SP, Ellis K, Hordof AJ, Martin E, Levine OR, Gersony WM. Spontaneous complete closure of a congenital coronary artery fistula. J Am Coll Cardiol 1983;2:1169.
6. Gulati R, Reddy VM, Culbertson C, Helton G, Suleman S, Reinhartz O, et al. Surgical management of coronary artery arising from the wrong coronary sinus, using standard and novel approaches. J Thorac Cardiovasc Surg 2007;134:1171-8.

H

1. Habermann JH, Howard ML, Johnson ES. Rupture of the coronary sinus with hemopericardium. A rare complication of coronary arteriovenous fistula. Circulation 1963;28:1143.
2. Halpert B. Arteriovenous communication between the right coronary artery and the coronary sinus. Heart 1930;15:129.
3. Hamamichi Y, Okada E, Ichida F. Anomalous origin of the main stem of the left coronary artery from the non-facing sinus of Valsalva associated with sudden death in a young athlete. Cardiol Young 2000;10:147.
4. Hamilton DI, Ghosh PK, Donnelly RJ. An operation for anomalous origin of left coronary artery. Br Heart J 1979;41:121.
5. Hamilton JR, Mulholland HC, O'Kane HO. Origin of the left coronary artery from the right pulmonary artery: a report of successful surgery in a 3-month-old child. Ann Thorac Surg 1986; 41:446.
6. Heifetz SA, Robinowitz M, Mueller KH, Virmani R. Total anomalous origin of the coronary arteries from the pulmonary artery. Pediatr Cardiol 1986;7:11.
7. Holzer R, Johnson R, Ciotti G, Pozzi M, Kitchiner D. Review of an institutional experience of coronary arterial fistulas in childhood set in context of review of the literature. Cardiol Young 2004; 14:380-5.
8. Horiuchi T, Abe T, Tanaka S, Koyamada K. Congenital coronary arteriovenous fistulas. Ann Thorac Surg 1971;11:102.
9. Hudspeth AS, Linder JH. Congenital coronary arteriovenous fistula. Arch Surg 1968;96:832.
10. Hurwitz RA, Caldwell RL, Girod DA, Brown J, King H. Clinical and hemodynamic course of infants and children with anomalous left coronary artery. Am Heart J 1989;118:1176.

I

1. Ishikawa T, Brandt PW. Anomalous origin of the left main coronary artery from the right anterior aortic sinus: angiographic definition of anomalous course. Am J Cardiol 1985;55:770.
2. Isomatsu Y, Imai Y, Shin'oka T, Aoki M, Iwata Y. Surgical intervention for anomalous origin of the left coronary artery from the pulmonary artery: the Tokyo experience. J Thorac Cardiovasc Surg 2001;121:792.

J

1. Jaffe RB, Glancy DL, Epstein SE, Brown BG, Morrow AG. Coronary arterial–right heart fistulae. Long-term observations in seven patients. Circulation 1973;47:133.

K

1. Kakou Guikahue M, Sidi D, Kachaner J, Villain E, Cohen L, Piechaud JF, et al. Anomalous left coronary artery arising from the pulmonary artery in infancy: is early operation better? Br Heart J 1988;60:522.
2. Kassaian SE, Mahmoodian M, Salarifar M, Alidoosti M, Abbasi SH, Rasekh A. Stent-graft exclusion of multiple symptomatic coronary artery fistulae. Tex Heart Inst J 2007;34:199-202.
3. Katsumata T, Westaby S. Anomalous left coronary artery from the pulmonary artery: a simple method for aortic implantation with autogenous arterial tissue. Ann Thorac Surg 1999;68:1090.
4. Kaushal SK, Radhakrisnan S, Dagar KS, Shrivastava S, Iyer KS. Anomalous origin of the left anterior descending coronary artery from the pulmonary artery. J Thorac Cardiovasc Surg 1998;116: 1078.
5. Kayalar N, Burkhart HM, Dearani JA, Cetta F, Schaff HV. Congenital coronary anomalies and surgical treatment. Congenit Heart Dis 2009;4:239-51.
6. Keeton BR, Keenan DJ, Monro JL. Anomalous origin of both coronary arteries from the pulmonary trunk. Br Heart J 1983;49: 397.
7. Kesler KA, Pennington DG, Nouri S, Boegner E, Kanter KR, Harvey L, et al. Left subclavian–left coronary artery anastomosis for anomalous origin of the left coronary artery. (Long-term follow-up.) J Thorac Cardiovasc Surg 1989;98:25.

8. King DH, Danford DA, Huhta JC, Gutgesell HP. Noninvasive detection of anomalous origin of the left main coronary artery from the pulmonary trunk by pulsed Doppler echocardiography. Am J Cardiol 1985;55:608.
9. Kittle CF, Diehl AM, Heilbruun A. Anomalous left coronary artery arising from the pulmonary artery. J Pediatr 1955;47:198.
10. Kragel AH, Roberts WC. Anomalous origin of either the right or left main coronary artery from the aorta with subsequent coursing between aorta and pulmonary trunk: analysis of 32 necropsy cases. Am J Cardiol 1988;62:771.
11. Krause W. Ueber den Ursprung einer accessorischen A. coronaria cordis aus der A. pulmonalis. Z Ratl Med 1865;24:225.

L

1. Laborde F, Marchand M, Leca F, Jarreau MM, Dequirot A, Hazan E. Surgical treatment of anomalous origin of the left coronary artery in infancy and childhood. Early and late results in 20 consecutive cases. J Thorac Cardiovasc Surg 1981;82:423.
2. Laks H, Ardehali A, Grant PW, Allada V. Aortic implantation of anomalous left coronary artery. An improved surgical approach. J Thorac Cardiovasc Surg 1995;109:519.
3. Lambert V, Touchot A, Losay J, Piot JD, Henglein D, Serraf A, et al. Midterm results after surgical repair of the anomalous origin of the coronary artery. Circulation 1996;94:II38.
4. Lawton J, McGrath J, Jones JS, Dehmer GJ. Treatment of coronary artery disease in an anomalous coronary artery by placement of an intracoronary stent. Cathet Cardiovasc Diagn 1997;41:185.
5. Lee CM, Leung TK, Wang HJ, Lee WH, Shen LK, Chen YY. Identification of a coronary-to-bronchial-artery communication with MDCT shows the diagnostic potential of this new technology: case report and review. J Thorac Imaging 2007;22:274-6.
6. Lerberg DB, Ogden JA, Zuberbuhler JR, Bahnson HT. Anomalous origin of the right coronary artery from the pulmonary artery. Ann Thorac Surg 1979;27:87.
7. Levin DC, Fellows KE, Abrams HL. Hemodynamically significant primary anomalies of the coronary arteries. Angiographic aspects. Circulation 1978;58:25.
8. Levitsky S, van der Horst RL, Hastreiter AR, Fisher EA. Anomalous left coronary artery in the infant: recovery of ventricular function following early direct aortic implantation. J Thorac Cardiovasc Surg 1980;79:598.
9. Liberthson RR, Sagar K, Berkoben JP, Weintraub RM, Levine FH. Congenital coronary arteriovenous fistula. Report of 13 patients, review of the literature and delineation of management. Circulation 1979;59:849.
10. Lien CH, Tan NC, Tan L, Seah CS, Tan D. Congenital aneurysm of right coronary artery. Am J Cardiol 1977;39:751.
11. Lopushinsky SR, Mullen JC, Bentley MJ. Anomalous right coronary artery originating from the left main coronary artery. Ann Thorac Surg 2001;71:357.
12. Lowe JE, Oldham HN, Sabiston DC Jr. Surgical management of congenital coronary artery fistulas. Ann Surg 1981;194:373.

M

1. Masuya K, Kusunoki N, Hara S, Funatsu T, Takegoshi N. Congenital right coronary artery fistula communicating with the left ventricle. South Med J 1975;68:1007.
2. McNamara DG, el-Said G. Treatment of anomalous origin of the left coronary artery from the pulmonary artery. Eur J Cardiol 1973;1:497.
3. McNamara JJ, Gross RE. Congenital coronary artery fistula. Surgery 1969;65:59.
4. Meave A, Melendez G, Ochoa JM, Lamothe PA, Calleja R, Alexanderson E. Right coronary artery-to-right ventricle fistula in a pediatric patient evaluated by 64-detector-row computed tomographic coronary angiography. Tex Heart Inst J 2009;36:491-3.
5. Memisoglu E, Hobikoglu G, Tepe MS, Norgaz T, Bilsel T. Congenital coronary anomalies in adults: comparison of anatomic course visualization by catheter angiography and electron beam CT. Catheter Cardiovasc Interv 2005;66:34-42.
6. Meyer BW, Stefanik G, Stiles QR, Lindesmith GG, Jones JC. A method of definitive surgical treatment of anomalous origin of left coronary artery. A case report. J Thorac Cardiovasc Surg 1968;56:104.
7. Meyer MH, Stephenson HE Jr, Keats TE, Martt JM. Coronary artery resection for giant aneurysmal enlargement and arteriovenous fistula. Am Heart J 1967;74:603.
8. Midgley FM, Watson DC Jr, Scott LP 3rd, Kuehl KS, Perry LW, Galioto FM Jr, et al. Repair of anomalous origin of the left coronary artery in the infant and small child. J Am Coll Cardiol 1984;4:1231.
9. Moller JH, Lucas RV Jr, Adams P Jr, Anderson RC, Jorgens J, Edwards JE. Endocardial fibroelastosis: a clinical and anatomic study of 47 patients with emphasis on its relationship to mitral insufficiency. Circulation 1964;30:759.
10. Moodie DS, Fyfe D, Gill CC, Cook SA, Lytle BW, Taylor PC, et al. Anomalous origin of the left coronary artery from the pulmonary artery (Bland-White-Garland syndrome) in adult patients: long-term follow-up after surgery. Am Heart J 1983;106:381.
11. Moodie DS, Gill C, Loop FD, Sheldon WC. Anomalous left main coronary artery originating from the right sinus of Valsalva. Pathophysiology, angiographic definition, and surgical approaches. J Thorac Cardiovasc Surg 1980;80:198.
12. Murthy KS, Krishnanaik S, Mohanty SR, Varghese R, Cherian KM. A new repair for anomalous left coronary artery. Ann Thorac Surg 2001;71:1384.
13. Mustafa I, Gula G, Radley-Smith R, Durrer S, Yacoub M. Anomalous origin of the left coronary artery from the anterior aortic sinus: a potential cause of sudden death. Anatomic characterization and surgical treatment. J Thorac Cardiovasc Surg 1981;82:297.
14. Mustard WT. Anomalies of the coronary arteries. In Pediatric surgery, Vol. 1. Chicago: Year Book, 1953, p. 433.

N

1. Neches WH, Mathews RA, Park SC, Lenox CC, Zuberbuhler JR, Siewers RD, et al. Anomalous origin of the left coronary artery from the pulmonary artery. A new method of surgical repair. Circulation 1974;50:582.
2. Neirotti R, Nijveld A, Ithuralde M, Quaglio M, Seara C, Lubbers L, et al. Anomalous origin of the left coronary artery from the pulmonary artery: repair by aortic reimplantation. Eur J Cardiothorac Surg 1991;5:368.
3. Nelson-Piercy C, Rickards AF, Yacoub MH. Aberrant origin of the right coronary artery as a potential cause of sudden death: successful anatomical correction. Br Heart J 1990;64:208.
4. Noren GR, Raghib G, Moller JH, Amplatz K, Adams P Jr, Edwards JE. Anomalous origin of the left coronary artery from the pulmonary trunk with special reference to the occurrence of mitral insufficiency. Circulation 1964;30:171.

O

1. Ogden JA, Stansel HC Jr. Coronary arterial fistulas terminating in the coronary venous system. J Thorac Cardiovasc Surg 1972;63:172.
2. Ogoh Y, Akagi T, Hashino K, Hayabuchi N, Kato H. Successful embolization of coronary arteriovenous fistula using an interlocking detachable coil. Pediatr Cardiol 1997;18:152.
3. Okuda Y, Tsuneda T, Morishima A, Matsumoto S, Ito Y, Isuzaki M. Right coronary artery to left ventricle fistula. The sixth case in the literature and discussion. Jpn Heart J 1973;14:184.
4. Oldham HN Jr, Ebert PA, Young WG, Sabiston DC Jr. Surgical management of congenital coronary artery fistula. Ann Thorac Surg 1971;12:503.
5. Ott DA, Cooley DA, Pinsky WW, Mullins CE. Anomalous origin of circumflex coronary artery from right pulmonary artery: report of a rare anomaly. J Thorac Cardiovasc Surg 1978;76:190.
6. Ouali S, Neffeti E, Sendid K, Elghoul K, Remedi F, Boughzela E. Congenital anomalous aortic origins of the coronary arteries in adults: a Tunisian coronary arteriography study. Arch Cardiovasc Dis 2009;102:201-8.

P

1. Paul RN, Robbins SG. A surgical treatment prognosed for either endocardial fibroelastosis or anomalous left coronary artery. Pediatrics 1955;47:196.
2. Pinsky WW, Fagan LR, Mudd JF, Willman VL. Subclavian–coronary artery anastomosis in infancy for the Bland-White-Garland syndrome: a three-year and five-year follow-up. J Thorac Cardiovasc Surg 1976;72:15.

R

1. Raanani E, Abramov D, Abramov Y, Birk E, Vidne BA. Individual anatomy demands various techniques in correction of an anomalous origin of the left coronary artery in the pulmonary artery. Thorac Cardiovasc Surg 1995;43:99.
2. Reddy K, Gupta M, Hamby RI. Multiple coronary arteriosystemic fistulas. Am J Cardiol 1974;33:304.
3. Rein AJ, Colan SD, Parness IA, Sanders SP. Regional and global left ventricular function in infants with anomalous origin of the left coronary artery from the pulmonary trunk: preoperative and postoperative assessment. Circulation 1987;75:115.
4. Rittenhouse EA, Doty DB, Ehrenhaft JL. Congenital coronary artery–cardiac chamber fistula. Ann Thorac Surg 1975;20:468.
5. Roberts WC. Anomalous origin of both coronary arteries from the pulmonary artery. Am J Cardiol 1962;10:595.
6. Roberts WC, Robinowitz M. Anomalous origin of the left anterior descending coronary artery from the pulmonary trunk with origin of the right and left circumflex coronary arteries from the aorta. Am J Cardiol 1984;54:1381.
7. Roberts WC, Siegel RJ, Zipes DP. Origin of the right coronary artery from the left sinus of Valsalva and its functional consequences: analysis of 10 necropsy patients. Am J Cardiol 1982;49:863.
8. Roche AH. Anomalous origin of the left coronary artery from the pulmonary artery in the adult. Report of uneventful ligation in two cases. Am J Cardiol 1967;20:561.
9. Rodefeld MD, Culbertson CB, Rosenfeld HM, Hanley FL, Thompson LD. Pulmonary artery translocation: a surgical option for complex anomalous coronary artery anatomy. Ann Thorac Surg 2001;72:2150-2.
10. Rodgers DM, Wolf NM, Barrett MJ, Zuckerman GL, Meister SG. Two-dimensional echocardiographic features of coronary arteriovenous fistula. Am Heart J 1982;104:872.
11. Romp RL, Herlong JR, Landolfo CK, Sanders SP, Miller CE, Ungerleider RM, et al. Outcome of unroofing procedure for repair of anomalous aortic origin of left or right coronary artery. Ann Thorac Surg 2003;76:589-96.
12. Rowe GG, Young WP. Anomalous origin of the coronary arteries with special reference to surgical treatment. J Thorac Cardiovasc Surg 1960;39:777.
13. Rudolph AM, Gootman NL, Kaplan N, Rohman M. Anomalous left coronary artery arising from the pulmonary artery with large left-to-right shunt in infancy. J Pediatr 1963;63:543.

S

1. Sabiston DC, Neill CA Jr, Taussig HB. The direction of blood flow in anomalous left coronary artery arising from the pulmonary artery. Circulation 1960;22:591.
2. Said SA, Lam J, van der Werf T. Solitary coronary artery fistulas: a congenital anomaly in children and adults. A contemporary review. Congenit Heart Dis 2006;1:63-76.
3. Said SA, van der Werf T. Dutch survey of congenital coronary artery fistulas in adults: coronary artery–left ventricular multiple micro-fistulas: multi-center observational survey in the Netherlands. Int J Cardiol 2006;110:33-9.
4. Said SA, van der Werf T. Dutch survey of coronary artery fistulas in adults: congenital solitary fistulas. Int J Cardiol 2006;106:323-32.
5. Sakakibara S, Yokoyama M, Takao A, Nogi M, Gomi H. Coronary arteriovenous fistula. Nine operated cases. Am Heart J 1966;72:307.
6. Schwartz ML, Jonas RA, Colan SD. Anomalous origin of left coronary artery from pulmonary artery: recovery of left ventricular function after dual coronary repair. J Am Coll Cardiol 1997;30:547.
7. Sediq M, Wilkinson JL, Qureshi SA. Successful occlusion of a coronary arteriovenous fistula using an Amplatzer duct occluder. Cardiol Young 2001;11:84.
8. Shrivastava S, Castaneda AR, Moller JH. Anomalous left coronary artery from the pulmonary trunk. Long-term follow-up after ligation. J Thorac Cardiovasc Surg 1978;76:130.
9. Shubrooks SJ Jr, Naggar CZ. Spontaneous near closure of coronary artery fistula. Circulation 1978;57:197.
10. Singh TP, Di Carli MF, Sullivan NM, Leonen MF, Morrow WR. Myocardial flow reserve in long-term survivors of repair of anomalous left coronary artery from pulmonary artery. J Am Coll Cardiol 1998;31:437.
11. Slezak J, Tribulova N, Okruhlicova L, Dhingra R, Bajaj A, Freed D, et al. Hibernating myocardium: pathophysiology, diagnosis, and treatment. Can J Physiol Pharmacol 2009;87:252-65.
12. Smith A, Arnold R, Anderson RH, Wilkinson JL, Qureshi SA, Gerlis LM, et al. Anomalous origin of the left coronary artery from the pulmonary trunk. Anatomic findings in relation to pathophysiology and surgical repair. J Thorac Cardiovasc Surg 1989;98:16.
13. Swan H, Wilson JN, Woodwark G, Blount SG Jr. Surgical obliteration of a coronary artery fistula to right ventricle. AMA Arch Surg 1959;79:820.

T

1. Takeuchi S, Imamura H, Katsumoto J, Hayashi I, Katohgi T, Yozu R, et al. New surgical method for repair of anomalous left coronary artery from the pulmonary artery. J Thorac Cardiovasc Surg 1979;78:7.
2. Talner NS, Halloran KH, Mahdavy M, Gardner TH, Hipona F. Anomalous origin of the left coronary artery from the pulmonary artery: clinical spectrum. Am J Cardiol 1965;15:689.
3. Tavora F, Burke A, Kutys R, Li L, Virmani R. Total anomalous origin of the coronary circulation from the right pulmonary artery. Cardiovasc Pathol 2008;17:246-9.
4. Tingelstad JB, Lower RR, Eldredge WJ. Anomalous origin of the right coronary artery from the main pulmonary artery. Am J Cardiol 1972;30:670.
5. Trevor RS. Aneurysm of the descending branch of the right coronary artery situated in the wall of the right ventricle and opening into the cavity of the ventricle, associated with great dilatation of the right coronary artery and non-valvular infective endocarditis. Proc R Soc Med 1912;5:20.
6. Tuncer C, Batyraliev T, Yilmaz R, Gokce M, Eryonucu B, Koroglu S. Origin and distribution anomalies of the left anterior descending artery in 70,850 adult patients: multicenter data collection. Catheter Cardiovasc Interv 2006;68:574-85.
7. Turina M, Real F, Neier W, Senning A. Left ventricular aneurysmectomy in a 4-month-old infant. J Thorac Cardiovasc Surg 1974;67:915.
8. Turley K, Szarnicki RJ, Flachsbart KD, Richter RC, Popper RW, Tarnoff H. Aortic implantation is possible in all cases of anomalous origin of the left coronary artery from the pulmonary artery. Ann Thorac Surg 1995;60:84.

U

1. Urrutia-S CO, Falaschi G, Ott DA, Cooley DA. Surgical management of 56 patients with congenital coronary artery fistulas. Ann Thorac Surg 1983;35:300.
2. Usman A, Fernandez B, Uricchio JF, Nichols HT. Aberrant origin of left coronary artery combined with mitral regurgitation in an adult. Am J Cardiol 1961;8:130.

V

1. Vouhe PR, Baillot-Vernant F, Trinquet F, Sidi D, de Geeter B, Khoury W, et al. Anomalous left coronary artery from the pulmonary artery in infants. Which operation? When? J Thorac Cardiovasc Surg 1987;97:192.

W

1. Wesselhoeft H, Fawcett JS, Johnson AL. Anomalous origin of the left coronary artery from the pulmonary trunk. Its clinical spectrum, pathology, and pathophysiology, based on a review of 140 cases with seven further cases. Circulation 1968;38:403.
2. Wilde P, Watt I. Congenital coronary artery fistulae: six new cases with a collective review. Clin Radiol 1980;31:301.
3. Williams IA, Gersony WM, Hellenbrand WE. Anomalous right coronary artery arising from the pulmonary artery: a report of 7 cases and a review of the literature. Am Heart J 2006;152:1004.e9-17.
4. Wilson CL, Dlabal PW, McGuire SA. Surgical treatment of anomalous left coronary artery from pulmonary artery: follow-up in teenagers and adults. Am Heart J 1979;98:440.
5. Worsham C, Sanders SP, Burger BM. Origin of the right coronary artery from the pulmonary trunk: diagnosis by two-dimensional echocardiography. Am J Cardiol 1985;55:232.
6. Wu Q, Xu Z. An alternative procedure for correction of anomalous origin of left coronary artery from the pulmonary artery. Ann Thorac Surg 2007;84:2132-3.

47 Congenital Aortic Stenosis

Congenital aortic stenosis is a cardiac anomaly in which narrowing at valvar, subvalvar, supravalvar, or combined (multiple) levels results in a systolic pressure gradient between the inflow portion of the left ventricle (LV) and the aorta beyond the obstruction. A spectrum of defects involves the aortic root, with some overlap of abnormalities. Congenital aortic stenosis in neonates and infants may be part of the constellation of hypoplastic left heart physiology (see "Coarctation as Part of Hypoplastic Left Heart Physiology" under Morphology in Section I of Chapter 48). This association is highly relevant to therapy.

Section I Congenital Valvar Aortic Stenosis

DEFINITION

Congenital valvar aortic stenosis includes defects in which the major malformation involves the aortic valve cusps. An obstruction at valve level is caused by imperfect cusp development with cusp thickening and fusion. Cusp abnormalities can be severe in early life; when they are not, important obstruction may not develop until later in life when calcification occurs.[R10] This chapter discusses congenital valvar aortic stenosis only in the age range from birth to young adult life.

HISTORICAL NOTE

Congenital valvar aortic stenosis has been long recognized by morphologists. Initial efforts to find a surgical solution were made by Carrel and Jeger, who independently attempted experimentally to place conduits between left ventricular apex and aorta.[C3,J3] In 1955, Marquis and Logan reported surgical treatment using dilators introduced through the LV apex, as did Downing in 1956.[D15,M4] Also in 1956, valvotomy was performed by an open technique during inflow stasis with moderate hypothermia induced by surface cooling.[L11,S31,S32] The first report of its treatment by accurate valvotomy during cardiopulmonary bypass (CPB) was by Spencer and colleagues in 1958,[S17] although this had been performed at the Mayo Clinic in 1956 and was reported by Ellis and Kirklin in 1962.[E4,E5]

MORPHOLOGY

Aortic Valve

The prevalences and precise nature of the various types of morphology of severely stenotic aortic valves and coexisting anomalies are incompletely understood for several reasons. First, it is difficult to obtain enough cases to constitute a reasonable sample of the spectrum of severe congenital valvar stenosis in neonates, infants, and children. Second, sources of data range from autopsy studies and surgical studies to echocardiographic and cineangiographic imaging in patients undergoing balloon valvotomy. Third, differing terminology contributes to incompleteness of morphologic data; ideally, not only should the morphologic nature of the cusps be defined, but also that of the sinuses of Valsalva, commissures (upper points of attachment of cusps to the aortic wall), and interleaflet triangles (fibrous or muscular tissue interposed between the sinuses in the subcusp LV outflow tract), as described by Angelini and colleagues for bicuspid valves.[A3]

In patients with stenosis severe enough to require operation in infancy or childhood, the valve is *bicuspid* in about 65% (Table 47-1). The valve usually consists of thickened

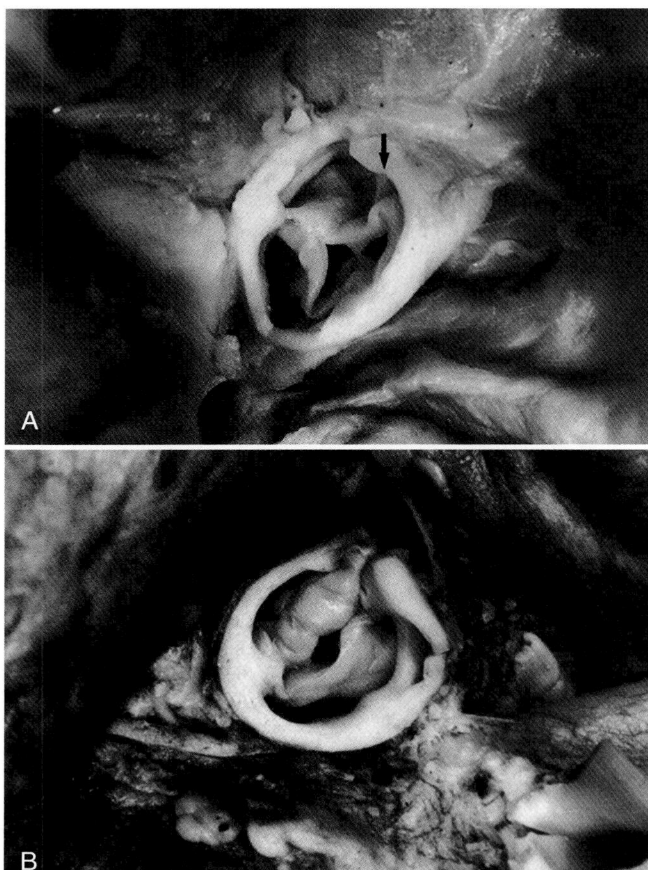

Figure 47-1 Specimens of congenital aortic stenosis with a bicuspid valve. **A,** Bicuspid valve with mild cusp thickening, moderately redundant cusps, and fusion of one commissure. There is a diminutive buttress (commissure) in the anterior cusp *(arrow).* **B,** Bicuspid valve from a neonate with severe aortic stenosis. Cusps are very thickened and obstructive, but there is no commissural fusion or buttress formation.

Table 47-1 Morphology of Congenital Valvar Aortic Stenosis in Surgical Patients Aged 1 Day to 26 Years

Valve	No.	% of 290
Bicuspid	186	64
Tricuspid	89	31
Unicuspid[a]	15	5
TOTAL	290	100

Data from Elkins and colleagues, 1960-1996.[E3]
[a]Frequency may be underestimated because "bicuspid" valve with rudimentary commissures might better be termed *unicuspid.*

right and left cusps in association with anterior and posterior commissures and a slitlike orifice with its long axis in the sagittal plane (Fig. 47-1, *A*). The left cusp is frequently the larger and may contain a transversely placed central thickened ridge, or buttress, representing a rudimentary commissure between normal right and left cusps. Less often, the two cusps are anterior and posterior, and the orifice is then oriented in a coronal plane. There is usually fusion peripherally of one commissure and occasionally of both. However, severe stenosis can occur without fusion, resulting only from thickened cusps and a bicuspid configuration. If free edges of both thickened cusps are taut, they are then equal in length to the diameter of the aortic root and cannot open (Fig. 47-1, *B*).[E1] Most bicuspid valves will show three intercusp triangles on their ventricular side, indicating that three cusps were present in the developing valve.[M1] A bicuspid valve with only two definitive cusps is uncommon and usually is not stenotic early in life, rather presenting later in life with obstruction or regurgitation. A full discussion of the genetics, morphology, natural history, and therapeutic options for adult patients with a congenitally bicuspid aortic valve is found in Chapter 12.

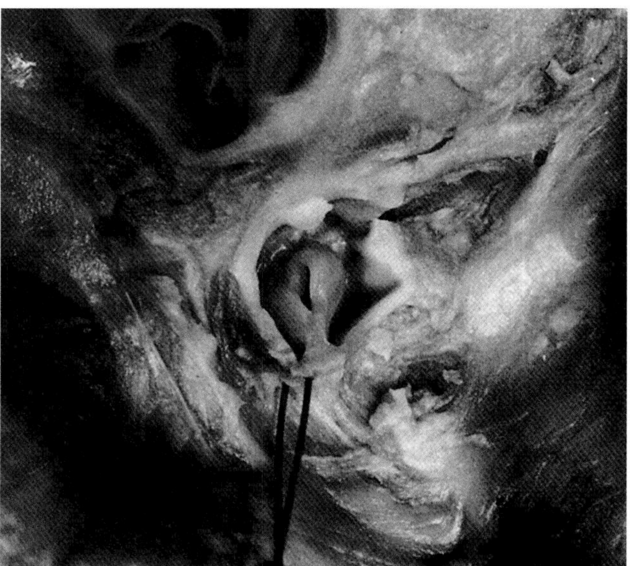

Figure 47-2 Specimen of a unicuspid aortic valve. Single fused commissure is suitable for valvotomy, but cusps cannot be divided elsewhere without producing regurgitation.

In about 30% of patients the valve is ***tricuspid,*** with three thickened cusps of approximately equal size and three recognizable commissures that are fused peripherally to varying degrees, creating a dome with a central stenotic orifice. This type of valve is more favorable for valvotomy because all three commissures can usually be opened.

Less often (5%) the valve may have a ***unicuspid*** configuration with only one commissure (Fig. 47-2). This variety is more common in infants presenting with severe stenosis.[M26] Occasionally, however, the stenosis is not severe, and signs and symptoms develop in later life as the valve thickens and calcifies.[F1] A thickened unicuspid valve is inherently stenotic, whether the commissure is fused or not, unless the cusp is particularly redundant.

The cusps are approximately equal in size in only a small percentage of congenitally bicuspid or stenotic tricuspid valves.[A3] Likewise, the raphae are variable in thickness and length. Number of sinuses may not be the same as number of cusps; most congenitally bicuspid and unicuspid *(unicommissural)* valves have three sinuses and three intercusp triangles.[A3,M1]

Diffuse cusp thickening, most marked at the free cusp edges, contributes importantly to valvar stenosis. Thickening is more extreme in symptomatic neonates and infants, and cusps may be irregular and myxomatous or dysplastic in

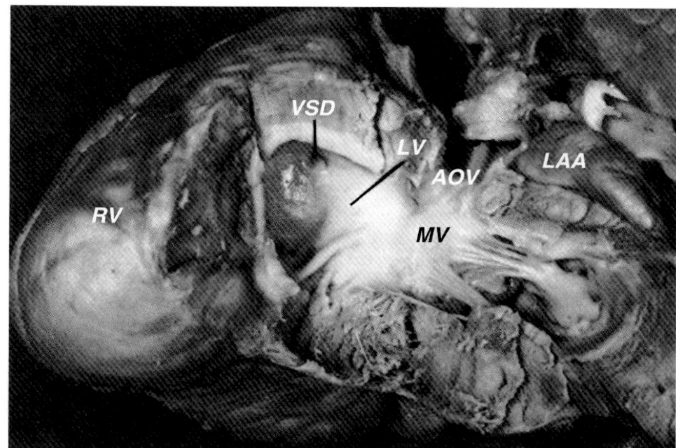

Figure 47-3 Specimen from 10-day-old infant with severe aortic valvar stenosis. Opened left ventricle with thick walls and marked endocardial fibroelastosis is relatively hypoplastic compared with enlarged right ventricle. A small anterior mid-muscular ventricular septal defect is present. Key: *AOV,* Aortic valve; *LAA,* left atrial appendage; *LV,* left ventricle; *MV,* mitral valve; *RV,* right ventricle; *VSD,* ventricular septal defect.

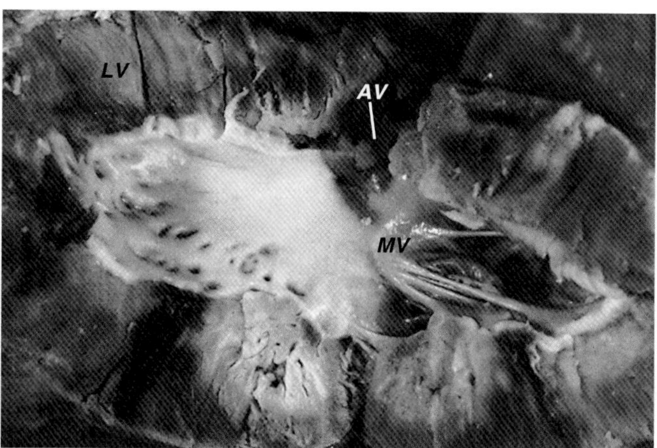

Figure 47-4 Specimen of congenital aortic stenosis from 9-month-old infant. Aortic valve *(AV)* cusps are thickened, nodular, and myxomatous. Opened left ventricle *(LV)* is small and has extreme hypertrophy and moderate endocardial fibroelastosis that also involves the papillary muscles of the mitral valve *(MV)*.

appearance.[C7] In addition, particularly in infants, the aortic "anulus" may be small and stenotic, especially with unicuspid valves,[F12] and frequently in association with other components of hypoplastic left heart physiology such as endocardial fibroelastosis of a hypoplastic left ventricle (Fig. 47-3), coarctation of the aorta, patent ductus arteriosus, and mitral regurgitation or stenosis.[H5,L2]

Left Ventricle

The LV is always concentrically hypertrophied in children with severe aortic stenosis, but in infants hypertrophy may be extreme, with a tiny cavity and extensive fibrosis in the wall (Fig. 47-4). Fibrosis is primarily in the subendocardial region.[C10] Extensive endocardial fibroelastosis may also be present, possibly the result of ischemia of subendocardial layers. In these hearts, the ventricle may be dilated (Fig. 47-5).

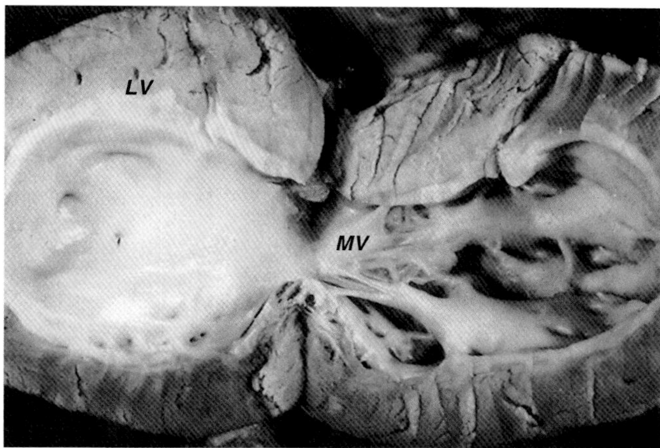

Figure 47-5 Specimen of congenital aortic stenosis from 12-day-old infant. Opened left ventricle *(LV)* is hypertrophied and dilated. Smooth septal surface is due to endocardial fibroelastosis that measures 1.5 mm in thickness. There is associated congenital mitral valve *(MV)* disease, with thickened leaflets and chordae and obliteration of interchordal spaces (see Morphology in Chapter 50).

Coexisting Cardiac Anomalies

Congenital valvar aortic stenosis may be associated with a fibrous subvalvar or supravalvar stenosis, as well as with coarctation of the aorta.[H5]

The various coexisting components of hypoplastic left heart physiology include LV hypoplasia of varying degrees, extreme LV hypertrophy with small cavity size, endocardial fibroelastosis, congenital mitral stenosis or regurgitation, severe coarctation, and subaortic stenosis caused by mitral valve abnormalities (Table 47-2). Patent ductus arteriosus or ventricular septal defect (VSD) as well as pulmonary atresia may also be present.

CLINICAL FEATURES AND DIAGNOSTIC CRITERIA

Symptoms

Neonates and infants with severe valvar aortic stenosis usually present with pallor, perspiration, and inability to feed. Shortness of breath and cyanosis may be present. In children and young adults, even important stenosis may be without symptoms. However, effort dyspnea, effort angina, or effort syncope, singly or in combination, usually indicates a severe lesion.[D16,G10,H13] Dyspnea may be present with moderate stenosis.

Signs

In neonates and infants with severe valvar aortic stenosis, the most striking feature is small pulse volume with pallor, dyspnea, and at times cyanosis. Both the murmur and gradient across the valve may be unimpressive because of a low cardiac output. There also may be a hyperactive right ventricular impulse.

Table 47-2 Coexisting Cardiac Anomalies (Previously or Concurrently Repaired or Left Unrepaired) in Surgical Patients with Congenital Aortic Stenosis[a]

Type of Stenosis	Associated Anomaly	No. of Cases
Valvar (*n* = 78)	Isolated PDA	8
	PDA + ASD	3
	PDA + coarctation	3
	Isolated coarctation	3
	Isolated VSD	1
	PDA + coarctation + VSD	1
	Left SVC	1
TOTAL		20 (26%)
Subvalvar (*n* = 41)	Isolated PDA	2
	PDA + coarctation	1
	Coarctation + congenital mitral stenosis	1
	VSD + important PS	3
	Unroofed coronary sinus syndrome	1
	Left SVC + single coronary orifice	1
	AR (3 mild, 2 important)	5
	VSD	4
TOTAL		18 (44%)
Supravalvar (*n* = 10)	Pulmonary artery stenosis	1
	Left SVC	1
TOTAL		2 (12%)
Combined (*n* = 7)	PDA + coarctation	1
	Congenital mitral stenosis	1
	VSD	1
TOTAL		3 (43%)

[a]Data from 142 patients, UAB experience 1967-1982. Categories are mutually exclusive. Numbers in parentheses are percentages of the *n* of the type.
Key: *AR,* Aortic regurgitation; *ASD,* atrial septal defect; *PDA,* patent ductus arteriosus; *PS,* pulmonary stenosis; *SVC,* superior vena cava; *VSD,* ventricular septal defect.

Clinical signs in children and young adults include an ejection systolic murmur (and thrill) at the base radiating to the carotid vessels, accompanied by a systolic ejection click. An aortic diastolic murmur is uncommon, particularly when compared with patients with discrete subvalvar stenosis. A severe lesion is characterized by palpable pulse of low volume and slow upstroke, single or reversed splitting of second heart sound, apical fourth and sometimes third heart sound, and thrusting LV impulse.

Many investigators have concluded that physical signs are unreliable in assessing severity of valvar stenosis in children.[C16,E6,F13,G10,J8,W1] However, physical signs can be used to differentiate among mild, moderate, and severe lesions in most patients, and severe lesions can always be distinguished from mild ones.[H13]

Electrocardiography

The electrocardiogram (ECG) usually shows severe LV hypertrophy but can be near normal.[H11] Right ventricular hypertrophy on the ECG may be associated with a left-to-right shunt at atrial level through a stretched patent foramen ovale and rarely a reversed shunt at ductus level.[S8]

Chest Radiography

The ascending aorta frequently is prominent in older children but is small in neonates and infants. Increased heart size is seldom seen except in neonates and infants in heart failure, in whom it may be marked. Radiologically demonstrable valvar calcification is rare in patients younger than age 25.

Noninvasive Studies

Two-dimensional echocardiography has become particularly important as a diagnostic tool. In neonates and infants, morphology and severity of narrowing of the valve and size, wall thickness, and contractility of the LV can be assessed.[B14,G9,W6] The congenitally stenotic aortic valve can be continuously reevaluated by Doppler ultrasound measurement of flow velocity across stenotic valves,[H6] which can be used to quantify transvalvar pressure gradient.[S23] Echocardiographic markers are useful for managing fetuses with important aortic stenosis. Serial measurements of fetal cardiac size and function may predict postnatal outcome.[M9]

Estimation of subendocardial oxygen requirements may be helpful in assessing severity of stenosis.[K16,L10]

Cardiac Catheterization and Angiography

A systolic gradient across the aortic valve can be demonstrated at cardiac catheterization, usually through a retrograde aortic approach if possible or otherwise a transseptal approach. Cardiac output can also be measured so that valve area can be calculated. Systolic gradient greater than 75 mmHg or valve area less than 0.5 $cm^2 \cdot m^{-2}$ is indicative of severe stenosis (see "Summary" in text that follows). Measuring gradient and valve area at cardiac catheterization has become less important as echocardiographic measurements have become more accurate. A raised LV end-diastolic pressure indicates LV failure or a fibrotic and noncompliant ventricle.

Angiography demonstrates thickened leaflets that form a dome in systole, with a localized jet of contrast entering the aorta (Fig. 47-6). Although this type of study is not reliable in assessing severity of stenosis, it can assess size of the aortic "anulus" and LV. An aortic root injection allows quantification of aortic regurgitation if present.

Summary

By a combination of clinical and hemodynamic assessments (echocardiography, cardiac catheterization), patients with congenital valvar aortic stenosis can be categorized as having mild, moderate, or severe obstruction.[H13] *Mild* implies that pulse volume and contour are normal, as is the second heart sound. Patients with these findings have an LV-aortic systolic pressure difference less than 40 mmHg at rest, with a mean of 20 mmHg. Patients with *moderate* stenosis have an abnormally small pulse volume on palpation and abnormal contour, and narrow inspiratory splitting of the second heart sound may be present. Such patients generally have systolic gradients less than 75 mmHg, with a mean of 20 to 50 mmHg. Patients with *severe* stenosis have a systolic gradient in excess of 75 mmHg and an abnormal pulse volume and contour, as well as a single second heart sound or reverse splitting. These patients have a mean calculated aortic valve area index of less than 0.5 $cm^2 \cdot m^{-2}$.[H13]

NATURAL HISTORY

Congenital valvar aortic stenosis is three to four times more common in males than in females and occurs in about 5% of Caucasians with congenital heart disease.

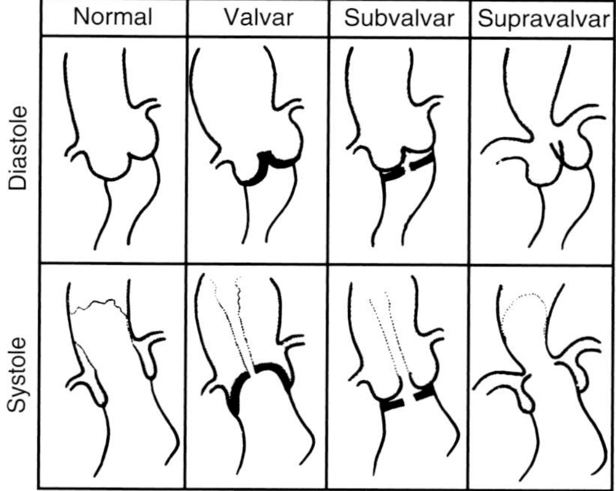

Figure 47-6 Angiographic signs of aortic stenosis. In *valvar stenosis*, there is systolic doming and a jet between thickened cusps. Poststenotic dilatation of aorta is visible. In fibrous *subvalvar stenosis*, a jet may be seen and cusps may not open fully, but doming is absent. The membrane should be visible, and there is often mild aortic regurgitation. In *supravalvar stenosis*, narrowing commencing above aortic cusps is visible. Sinuses of Valsalva are prominent, and coronary arteries are often dilated.

Presentation in Infancy

When neonates and infants present with valvar stenosis, the lesion is typically severe, with rapidly progressive heart failure and death within a few days to a few weeks of birth. Thus, most neonates and young infants come to intervention (currently with percutaneous balloon valvotomy) critically ill and in New York Heart Association (NYHA) class IV or V (Table 47-3). Many have other anomalies associated with the spectrum of the hypoplastic left heart physiology. Ten Harkel and colleagues noted a 5-year survival rate of 73% among patients presenting in infancy.[T2]

Presentation in Childhood

When symptoms are delayed beyond age 1 year, heart failure is rare, and survival without treatment generally is prolonged. Also, associated anomalies are less common. The Second Natural History Study of Congenital Heart Defects includes data on many patients treated for valvar aortic stenosis and followed for 25 years.[K8] Patients were 2 years or older at entry into the study, and 40% managed medically subsequently required surgical management. For patients presenting with LV-aortic pressure gradient greater than 50 mm Hg, 70% required surgical intervention. Almost 40% of patients required a second operation.

Survival is related to (1) sudden death in untreated children and (2) rate of progression of stenosis.

Sudden Death

Occurrence of *sudden death* varies between 1% and 19% of patients.[B19,C2,G10,M4,O2,P2] Of 58 patients younger than 35 years old who died suddenly and were found to have congenital heart disease, three (5%) had aortic valve stenosis.[B3] Analysis of the literature and of a series of 218 patients with congenital valvar stenosis indicates that sudden death directly attributable to aortic stenosis is virtually confined to patients with a severe lesion.[H13] Sudden death in patients with no symptoms and normal physical findings except for the murmur of aortic stenosis has not been documented. Sudden death may occur

Table 47-3 New York Heart Association (NYHA) Functional Class According to Age at First Repair of Congenital Aortic Stenosis[a]

Age at Operation			NYHA Functional Class (mean ± SD)[b]			
≤	Age	<	Valvar (*n* = 78)	Subvalvar (*n* = 41)	Supravalvar (*n* = 16)	Combined (*n* = 7)
Weeks						
		1	4.8 ± 0.45			
1		4	4.1 ± 0.94			
Months						4.0
1		3	4.5 ± 0.71			
3		12	3.0 ± 1.26			
12		48	2.2 ± 0.98	3.2 ± 0.96	1.0	3.0
Years						
4		12	1.7 ± 0.76	1.8 ± 0.94	1.7 ± 0.52	2.0 ± 1.00
12		20	1.7 ± 0.73	1.8 ± 1.19	1.7 ± 0.58	2.5 ± 0.71
20			1.9 ± 0.74	2.8 ± 0.84		

[a]Data from 142 patients, UAB experience 1967-1982.
[b]Patients were categorized into NYHA classes I to V, with class V indicating those undergoing emergency operation because of shock or metabolic acidosis. In the current era, isolated valvar aortic stenosis in newborns and infants is generally treated by percutaneous balloon valvotomy.

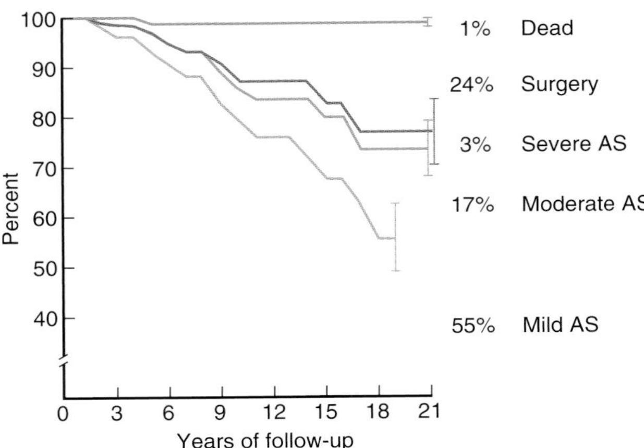

Figure 47-7 Cumulative incidence curves (multiple decrement; see "Competing Risks" in Section IV of Chapter 6) for 153 patients presenting with originally mild congenital valvar aortic stenosis. Vertical bars represent 70% confidence limits. Mean age at presentation was 6.5 years (1 to 25 years) and mean follow-up 8.8 years (1 to 26 years). The one death was caused by infective endocarditis. Patients underwent operation when stenosis was considered severe. Percentages refer to distances between curves. Key: *AS,* Aortic stenosis. (From Hossack and colleagues.[H13])

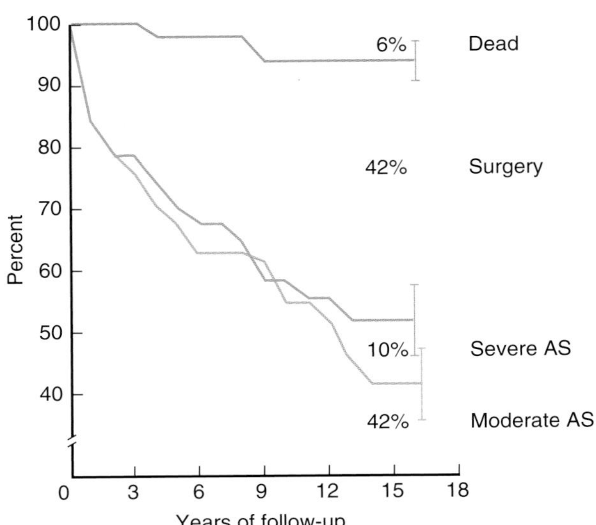

Figure 47-8 Cumulative incidence curves for 54 patients presenting with originally moderate congenital valvar aortic stenosis *(AS).* Vertical bars represent 70% confidence limits. Mean age at presentation was 12 years (1-25 years) and mean follow-up 8.5 years (1-24 years). The two deaths were both sudden, 4 and 9 years after presentation, in association with progression to severe stenosis. Percentages refer to distances between curves. (From Hossack and colleagues.[H13])

in patients with a normal ECG,[H13] but this finding is not incompatible with severe stenosis. Thus, the true prevalence of sudden death in children and adolescents in whom surgery is deferred until the lesion is considered severe on clinical grounds is probably about 1%.

Progression of Stenosis

When congenital aortic valvar deformities are nonobstructive in infancy and childhood, less than 10% progress to mild obstruction within about 10 years. Leech, Mills, and colleagues obtained information on 26 patients aged 1 week to 29 years when first seen, and in whom diagnosis of nonobstructive aortic valve deformity was made based on an isolated aortic ejection sound.[L6] During a 5- to 16-year follow-up, two patients (7%; CL 2%-16%) developed signs of mild stenosis after 7 and 15 years.[M21] As more years pass, an undetermined time-related proportion of patients with deformed (usually congenitally bicuspid) aortic valves develop progressive thickening and calcification and ultimately important stenosis. Vollebergh and Becker suggest that minor inequality of size of tricuspid valves present from birth may lead to formation of senile or degenerative type of aortic valve stenosis presenting in the seventh or eighth decade of life.[V3]

When *mild* stenosis is present at first evaluation in childhood, progression is more rapid. Moderate or severe stenosis develops in about 20% of patients within 10 years and in 45% within about 20 years (Fig. 47-7). Even after this long interval, therefore, 55% of the mild lesions remain mild.

When *moderate* stenosis is present initially, the lesion becomes severe within 10 years in about 60% of patients (Fig. 47-8).

Infective Endocarditis

Spontaneously occurring infective endocarditis appears in less than 1% of patients. The reported incidence is 1.8 to 2.7 episodes per 1000 patient-years.[G7,H13] Infective endocarditis may produce aortic regurgitation and may be a cause of death.

TECHNIQUE OF OPERATION

Percutaneous Balloon Valvotomy

Percutaneous balloon valvotomy is often used for treating congenital valvar aortic stenosis, but a description of this technique is beyond the scope of this text. Its place in treating neonates is discussed under Special Situations and Controversies later in this section.

Valvotomy in Neonates and Critically Ill Infants

Closed techniques and surface cooling for hypothermic circulatory arrest have largely been replaced by aortic valvotomy on CPB using cold cardioplegic myocardial management.

Anesthetic and supportive management must be precise (see Section II of Chapter 4). Drifting downward of body temperature to 32°C to 34°C is probably advantageous. Preparation and median sternotomy are described under "Preparation for Cardiopulmonary Bypass" in Section III of Chapter 2. As the pericardium is being opened, care is taken to touch the heart as seldom as possible because ventricular fibrillation is easily provoked. The purse-string suture is placed for the aortic cannula, the patient heparinized, and the cannula inserted and connected to the arterial tubing. Only then is a purse-string suture placed around the right atrial appendage; if the heart fibrillates, CPB can be established in less than a minute. A single venous cannula is inserted, and CPB is begun with the perfusate at 34°C; the ductus arteriosus is ligated, perfusate taken to 20°C to 28°C, aorta clamped, cold cardioplegia administered, and the perfusate temperature is then taken to 34°C to 36°C. In the presence of aortic regurgitation to a degree that interferes with cardioplegia delivery, cardioplegia can be delivered via small olive tip catheters directly into the coronary ostia, or coronary sinus cardioplegia can be used.

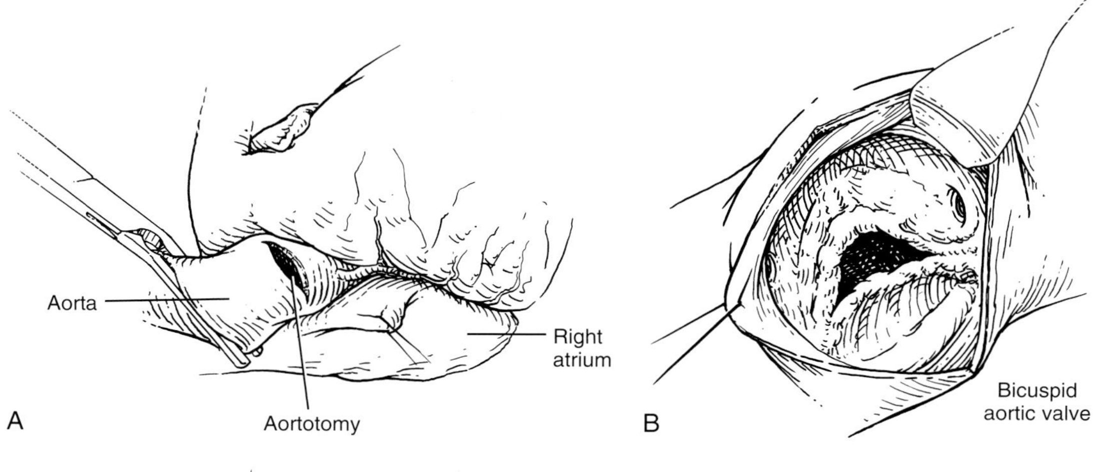

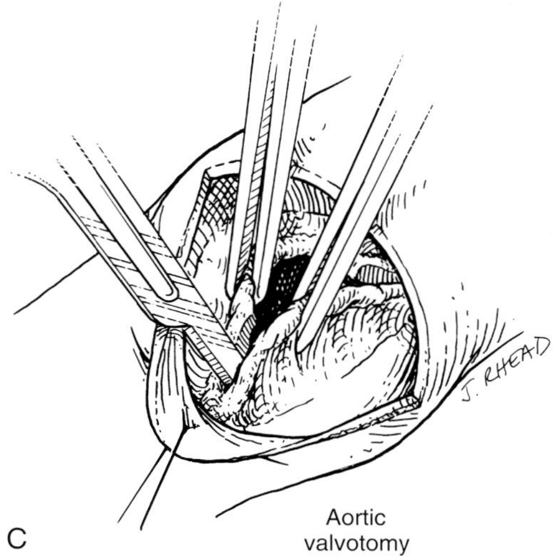

Figure 47-9 Aortic valvotomy. **A,** Operation is performed on cardiopulmonary bypass with aorta occluded. Electromechanical arrest of heart is achieved by infusion of cold cardioplegic solution. A transverse aortotomy is made above sinutubular junction to preserve integrity of aortic root. **B,** Aortic valve is exposed by gentle retraction of aortotomy anteriorly. Valve is inspected to determine optimal location for incision of commissures. Only commissures with adequate cusp attachment to aortic wall are opened; rudimentary commissures (raphe) should not be incised. **C,** Incision of commissure is deepened in stages, and cusps on each side are evaluated for lack of prolapse before further incision; incision is carried no further if prolapse is suspected. Usually, incision may be carried to aortic wall in well-supported commissures.

A transverse aortotomy is made (Fig 47-9, *A*). Two stay sutures are placed on the upstream side of the aortotomy for exposure. The aortic valve is inspected to determine which of the commissures to incise. Only partially formed commissures should be incised; commissurotomy should not be performed where there is only a rudimentary raphe (Fig. 47-9, *B*).

Valvotomy is performed by dividing fused commissures with a knife to within 1 mm of the aortic wall; in neonates the cusps are often gelatinous, but every effort still should be made to identify these commissures. It is important that even tension be placed on the two adjoining cusps so that incision is precise (Fig. 47-9, *C*). Only commissures with adequate cusp/commissural attachment to the aortic wall are opened, because division of rudimentary commissures produces regurgitation. Incisions are deepened in stages, and cusps on each side are evaluated for competence and lack of prolapse before each further incision.[E4] If further incising of the commissure might cause cusp prolapse, the incision is carried no further. Occasionally, myxomatous nodules can be excised from the cusp's free edge, or fibrous thickening can be shaved off the ventricular aspect of one or more cusps. The aortotomy is then closed with a continuous suture. If there is any degree of aortic regurgitation by saline filling of the aortic root, a 6-0 polypropylene suture (Frater stitch) can be placed through the midpoint of each cusp and brought out through the closed aortotomy. The suture is removed when LV contraction begins.

The remainder of the procedure is completed as usual (see "Completing Cardiopulmonary Bypass" in Section III of Chapter 2). A left atrial catheter should be positioned before discontinuing CPB. If the neonate is of suitable size for placing a transesophageal echocardiography (TEE) probe, the repair is evaluated before and after discontinuing CPB. LV and aortic pressures are measured and recorded before closing the chest.

Valvotomy in Older Infants, Children, and Adults

Preparation for operation, the incision, and preparations for CPB are described under "Preparation for Cardiopulmonary Bypass" in Section III of Chapter 2. Using a single venous cannula or caval cannulation, CPB is established at 28°C. A left atrial or LV vent is used. External cardiac cooling may be applied. The aorta is clamped and cold cardioplegic solution infused. The transverse aortotomy is made, and stay sutures applied to edges of the incision for exposure. Commissurotomy is performed as described.

The aortotomy is closed by continuous stitches, and the rest of the operation is completed as usual (see "Completing Cardiopulmonary Bypass" in Section III of Chapter 2).

Cusp Reconstruction

Pericardial cusp extension valvuloplasty procedures (as described by Duran)[D17] to compensate for deficiency of valvar tissue and increase the coaptation surface area have been applied primarily to regurgitant aortic valves (see Chapter 12). More recently, encouraging midterm results with these techniques applied to congenital aortic stenosis support their inclusion as surgical options. *Aortic cusp extension valvuloplasty* may be considered as an adjunctive procedure to primary open valvotomy or in reoperative situations with recurrent aortic stenosis or regurgitation following previous valvotomy. Before proceeding with valve reconstruction, preoperative echocardiographic studies should ascertain the absence of LV subaortic obstruction.

Following a median sternotomy, autologous pericardium is harvested, thoroughly cleaned of all fatty tissue and adhesions, treated with 0.625% glutaraldehyde solution for 3 to 5 minutes, and kept moist with normal saline. CPB, LV venting, and myocardial management are performed as described under "Valvotomy in Older Infants, Children, and Adults."

An oblique aortotomy is made, and the aortic valve evaluated for presence of complete but fused commissures and a raphe in congenitally bicuspid aortic valves. Each cusp is examined for thickness and mobility, free-edge irregularities, and tissue deficiency.

The valve is prepared for cusp extension by first thinning the thickened cusp edges. Fused commissures are incised out to the aortic wall, and subcommissural fusion or scar tissue is released to maximize cusp mobility. Bicuspid valves with a rudimentary raphe are tricupidized by incising through the fused cusp at the raphe all the way to the aortic wall (Fig. 47-10). The pericardial patches are each cut to a length determined by the diameter of the aorta, supplemented with an additional 15% to 20% to account for later pericardial shrinkage. Height of each patch is chosen to extend the line of coaptation of the repaired cusps about 5 mm higher than the highest cusp and to bring the extended cusps into a coaptation point in the center of the valve orifice. The pericardial extensions are sutured to each cusp with continuous 5-0 polypropylene, beginning in the center of the cusp and working toward the commissures. The extensions are attached to the aortic wall, creating neocommissures at the level of the sinutubular junction. Ilbawi and colleagues recommend leaving a little excess pericardial patch at the commissural level, secured with a pledgeted mattress suture through the aortic wall.[P6] With all the patch extensions in place, the newly constructed extensions are trimmed to provide a uniform cusp height and symmetric coaptation surface (see Fig. 47-10). Adequacy of the valve opening is examined, and initial valve competence is assessed by filling the aortic root with saline. Aortotomy closure and discontinuation of CPB are conducted as usual. Evaluation of valve function by TEE is performed before and following discontinuation of CPB. If aortic regurgitation is more than mild or if peak transvalvar gradient by TEE exceeds 30 mmHg,[A2] consideration should be given to reestablishing CPB and revising the valve repair or, if improvement is not feasible, proceeding with valve replacement.

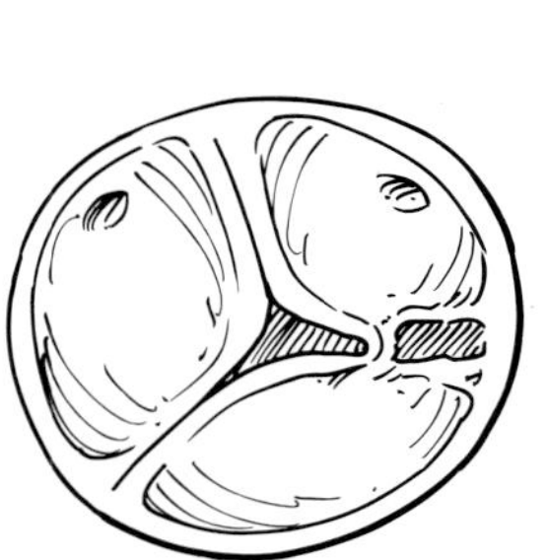

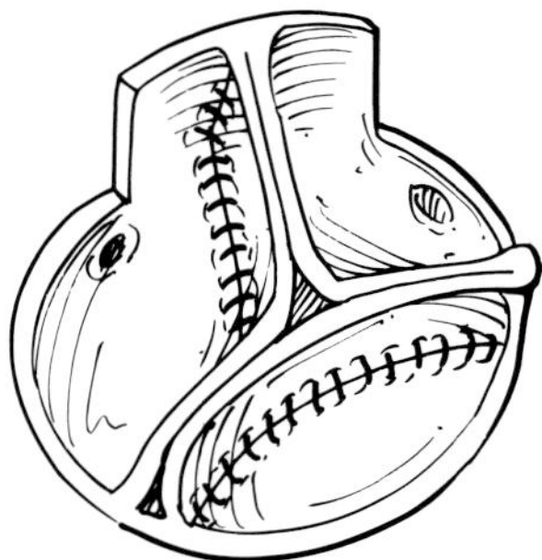

Figure 47-10 Tricuspidization of bicuspid aortic valve. Raphe is split and cusps extended with glutaraldehyde-treated pericardium. (From Pozzi and colleagues.[P7])

Aortic Valve Replacement in Children

When viewed at operation, the congenitally stenotic aortic valve may be too extensively deformed to be opened and remain reasonably competent. However, this situation is rare in primary operations in patients younger than age 10 and uncommon in those younger than 20. It is more common when multiple prior balloon valvotomies have been performed, and particularly when progressive or recurrent stenosis is accompanied by moderate or worse aortic regurgitation.

Aortic valve replacement in older children may be done in a standard fashion using a mechanical prosthesis (see "Isolated Aortic Valve Replacement" under Technique of Operation in Chapter 12). It may also be performed in the standard freehand manner using an aortic valve allograft (see "Allograft Aortic Valve" under Technique of Operation in Chapter 12) or a pulmonary valve autograft (see "Autograft Pulmonary Valve" under Technique of Operation in Chapter 12). Because the aortic root and LV-aortic junction may be quite small in young children who require aortic valve replacement, aortic root enlargement (see "Root-Enlarging Technique" under Technique of Operation in Chapter 12) or replacement (see "Replacement of Aortic Valve and Ascending Aorta, En Bloc" under Technique of Operation in Chapter 12) may be advantageous. An aortic allograft can be used as the replacement device, or a pulmonary autograft may be preferred. The autograft has the advantage of remaining unchanged and uncompromised by host reaction, and it also may grow.

SPECIAL FEATURES OF POSTOPERATIVE CARE

Postoperative care after aortic valvotomy or other procedures discussed in this section are conducted in the manner generally used after intracardiac operations (see Chapter 5).

Whenever valvotomy is performed for congenital valvar aortic stenosis, long-term follow-up is indicated because of possible recurrence of stenosis requiring reoperation.

RESULTS

Early (Hospital) Death

Hospital mortality for surgical treatment of congenital valvar aortic stenosis in heterogeneous groups of patients younger than 20 to 25 years of age is largely an unhelpful value because of the important role of incremental risk factors for death and the selection processes by which treatments (or no treatments) are chosen.

Mortality varies widely among patient subsets, with few or no deaths after valvotomy in children and young adults.[E5,K17,P8] Mortality is higher in neonates, but the potential safety of an open approach in neonates with severe congenital aortic stenosis has been demonstrated.[G6,M19] Still, the current preference in most centers is initial percutaneous balloon valvotomy. Multiple centers have achieved hospital mortalities of 15% or less in neonates.[B1,B28,C15,M20,P3,T8] Again, however, mortality figures in heterogeneous groups of patients, even if all are neonates, are difficult to interpret, as demonstrated by Gaynor and colleagues[G5] and a Congenital Heart Surgeon's Society (CHSS) analysis.[L14] In contrast to many situations in cardiac surgery, nearly all deaths after operation for congenital valvar aortic stenosis occur early postoperatively, most within 48 hours.

Success in salvaging such patients with emergency temporary extracorporeal membrane oxygenator (ECMO) or left ventricular assist device (LVAD) support has not been fully evaluated, but such support is advisable in the face of progressive circulatory failure (see "Treatment of Low Cardiac Output" in Chapter 5).

Hospital mortality after operations for congenital valvar aortic stenosis in patients older than age 1 year approaches zero.

Time-Related Survival

Overall survival up to 40 years is good after the primary operation for congenital valvar aortic stenosis in older infants and children.[D8,T9] In very ill neonates and young infants, however, survival is compromised, primarily by high early risks.[L7]

A CHSS study of 320 neonates with critical aortic stenosis noted 1- and 5-year survival of 72% and 70%, respectively, among those receiving an initial procedure aimed at biventricular repair (Fig. 47-11).

Modes of Death

Almost all early deaths are in acute cardiac failure,[G15] and theoretically most should be preventable by (1) stabilization of critically ill neonates and others (with ECMO or LVAD support if needed) so that operation is not performed in NYHA class V patients as it was in the past,[J2] and (2) proper myocardial management. In neonates and young infants, however, many deaths result from (1) failure to appreciate the importance of coexisting components of the spectrum of the hypoplastic left heart physiology (see "Coarctation as Part of Hypoplastic Left Heart Physiology" under Morphology in Section I of Chapter 48), and (2) nonoptimal selection, in particular of a biventricular pathway rather than a single-ventricle pathway, at least in the present state of knowledge (see Indications for Operation later in this section).[L14]

Deaths occurring late after operation are in various modes, and inferences are made with difficulty. Thus "sudden death" has been reported as the mode of death in 12% of patients included in one long-term follow-up study, but the majority had severe residual or recurrent stenosis or severe aortic regurgitation.[H14] Among neonates for whom staging of repair is necessary for a univentricular pathway, few late deaths now occur between the cavopulmonary shunt stage and completed Fontan.[L14]

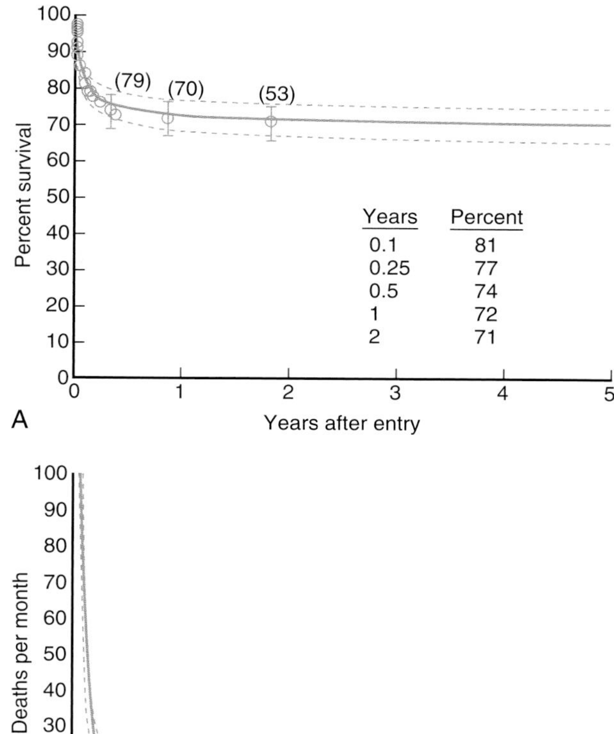

Figure 47-11 Survival of patients with severe left ventricular outflow tract obstruction who had an initial procedure indicating an intended biventricular repair pathway ($n = 116$) after entry into a Congenital Heart Surgeons Society hospital. **A,** Survival. Each circle represents a death positioned according to Kaplan-Meier estimator, vertical bars are 70% confidence limits (CL), and numbers in parentheses are patients remaining at risk. Solid curve enclosed within dashed 70% CLs represents parametric survival estimates. **B,** Hazard function for death (solid line enclosed within 70% CLs). (From Lofland and colleagues.[L14])

Incremental Risk Factors for Premature Death

Coexisting Severe Left-Sided Cardiac Anomalies

Left-sided cardiac defects (components of the spectrum of the hypoplastic left heart physiology, such as small aortic valve diameter, aortic hypoplasia, severe endocardial fibroelastosis, LV hypoplasia, extreme LV hypertrophy with small cavity size, and congenital mitral valve disease[K7]) are associated with high mortality after operation[C17,H5,L14] (Table 47-4). These coexisting major cardiac anomalies, poor preoperative functional class, and young age at admission tend to occur together, and all are risk factors.

The important study by Karl and colleagues from Melbourne, Australia, emphasized the major role of these coexisting important cardiac anomalies in the early postsurgical mortality in neonates.[K3] No deaths (0%; CL 0%-19%) occurred after open valvotomy in neonates with no coexisting anomaly or only a patent ductus, whereas early mortality was 47% (CL 39%-62%) among those with important coexisting cardiac anomalies.

Table 47-4 Incremental Risk Factors for Time-Related Death in Neonates with Critical Aortic Stenosis for Intended Biventricular Repair and for Initial Norwood Procedure

	Risk Factor	Coefficient ± SE[a]	*P*
	Intended Biventricular Repair		
Higher	Grade of endocardial fibroelastosis[b]	0.53 ± 0.23	.02
Lower	Aortic valve diameter *z* score at level of sinuses of Valsalva	0.36 ± 0.109	<.001
Younger	Age at entry[c]	1.49 ± 0.53	.005
	Initial Norwood Procedure		
Smaller	Diameter of ascending aorta[d]	0.95 ± 0.40	.02
	Presence of moderate or severe tricuspid regurgitation	0.86 ± 0.43	.05

Data from Lofland and colleagues.[L14]
[a]Single early hazard phase (see Fig. 47-11, *B*).
[b]Graded subjectively by echocardiographic appearance of left ventricular endocardial brightness and thickness: *0,* None; *1,* involvement of papillary muscles only; *2,* papillary muscle with some endocardial surface involvement; *3,* extensive endocardial surface involvement.
[c]Inverse transformation.
[d]Logarithmic transformation.

Poor Preoperative Functional Class

Advanced symptoms, or NYHA class IV and particularly class V, are associated with a considerably increased risk of death early after operation. Thus, for patients preoperatively in NYHA class I or II (most older infants and children), 15-year survival (all deaths, including those in hospital) after the primary valve operation is about 90%.[A4,B7] In preoperatively very ill neonates and young infants, 10-year survival is about 30%.[P3] However, the risk of death in the constant hazard phase (after about 5 years postoperatively) is no greater in this group than in older patients.

These ideas came from an era when critically ill neonates and young infants were not resuscitated preoperatively by the infusion of prostaglandin E_1 (PGE_1). This risk factor can be neutralized at a cost of only about 5% mortality among neonates by management that includes stabilization on PGE_1 and usually low-dose inotropic support.[J2]

Type of Congenital Valvar Aortic Stenosis

In a few patients, a truly unicuspid or severely dysplastic bicuspid valve may be essentially uncorrectable.[C7] In a few patients, the very small aortic anulus may prevent a satisfactory outcome. Again, these situations usually are found in very sick neonates and young infants. Currently such patients typically are managed by a staged protocol leading to a univentricular repair.[L14]

Young Age

Very young age at operation is associated with a high risk of early death postoperatively.[L7,L14] However, in the past, most patients coming to operation as neonates have been in NYHA functional class IV or V. It is important to recall, however, that with contemporary medical management, survival after operation is possible in critically ill neonates and young infants.[B1,B7,C23,J2,K3,K7,T6]

Table 47-5 Preoperative Functional Class and Functional Class When Last Traced Postoperatively in Patients Undergoing Primary Operation for Congenital Valvar Aortic Stenosis[a]

Follow-up NYHA Class	Preoperative NYHA Class I	II	III	IV	V	Total
I	22	20	5	6	0	53
II	0	2	1	1	0	4
III	0	0	0	0	0	0
IV	0	0	0	0	0	0
Dead	0	2	3	5	10	20
Uncertain	0	1	0	0	0	1
TOTAL	22	25	9	12	10	78

[a]Data from 78 patients, UAB experience 1967-1982.
Key: *NYHA,* New York Heart Association.

Functional Status

Most surviving patients, including those who have had reoperations, are in NYHA class I or II (Table 47-5). Objective evidence of improvement in functional capacity is provided by Whitmer and colleagues, who demonstrated marked regression of exercise-induced ST depression 1 year after operation, as well as an increase in mean total work and peak exercise systolic blood pressure.[W7]

Electrocardiographic Changes

ECG evidence of LV hypertrophy may persist after valvotomy or valve replacement either because of residual stenosis or regurgitation or a progressive secondary cardiomyopathy. Intraoperative damage to the LV or preexisting ischemic myocardial fibrosis exacerbated by delaying operation can contribute to or cause this condition.[E7,M25] Usually, however, LV hypertrophy is reversible.

Left Ventricular Morphology and Function

Preoperative inordinate LV hypertrophy and wall thickness often found in children with congenital valvar aortic stenosis often regresses after successful valvotomy or valve replacement, which reduces LV afterload and increases systolic function.[D11]

Residual or Recurrent Left Ventricular–Aortic Pressure Gradients

Pressure gradient usually is substantially reduced after valvotomy and persists for 5 to 10 years.[J1,L5,M8] Thereafter, the gradient tends to rise steadily, occurring earlier and more frequently when valvotomy was necessary during the neonatal period or in infancy.[K7] In patients with a good initial result, the later rise in gradient is mainly the result of progressive cusp immobility and calcification.[R10] Recurrence and progression of LV-aortic pressure gradient is usually an indication for reintervention with either percutaneous balloon valvotomy or operation.

Following aortic cusp extension procedures with autologous pericardium, long-term durability of repair has been incompletely studied. Alsoufi and colleagues have emphasized the importance of satisfactory relief of aortic stenosis at the time of operation. Among 22 children who underwent this procedure, those with postoperative peak echocardiographic gradients of less than 30 mmHg had stabilization of their peak gradient over the next 2 to 3 years. However, progressive worsening of aortic stenosis was noted in those with early gradients exceeding 30 mmHg (moderate or greater aortic stenosis).

Aortic Regurgitation

Important aortic valve regurgitation is uncommon after valvotomy when the operation has been performed as described (see Technique of Operation earlier in this section). Moderate to severe regurgitation without residual stenosis is present at late follow-up in about 10% of patients, but some regurgitation is combined with moderate or severe residual or recurrent stenosis in an additional 15% to 20%.[H13] Postoperative regurgitation occurs more frequently when valvotomy is radical,[S8] and particularly when an attempt is made to convert a bicuspid into a tricuspid valve.[L5]

Infective Endocarditis

The incidence of endocarditis is not lessened by valvotomy[G7,H13,J7,R6] and may even be somewhat higher than in the natural history.[H13,H14]

Diastolic Heart Failure

Rarely, patients with severe valvar aortic stenosis who undergo surgical or balloon valvotomy as neonates or in infancy develop severe diastolic heart failure years later. Robinson and colleagues at Boston Children's Hospital reported four such patients who presented 14 to 19 years after balloon valvotomy with heart failure and severe diastolic dysfunction.[R11] All had evidence of a confluent layer of LV subendocardial hyperenhancement demonstrated by gadolinium-enhanced magnetic resonance imaging that was documented by histopathology in two patients to be endocardial fibroelastosis (EFE). One patient experienced clinical improvement following aortic valve replacement and extensive EFE resection. Robinson and colleagues hypothesize that EFE may result from early (possibly in utero) and irreversible myocardial damage induced by subendocardial ischemia secondary to persistent pressure overload with decreased ventricular flow, which may gradually progress irrespective of relief of LV outflow obstruction.

Reintervention

As with time-related freedom from death, time-related depictions of freedom from reintervention and aortic valve replacement are of limited value when they are derived from a heterogeneous population.

In general, however, about 85% to 95% of children and young adults (excluding neonates and infants) are free of reintervention (usually valve replacement) for at least 10 years after the initial operation (Figs. 47-12 through 47-14). Then, although constant in the intermediate term, the hazard function (rate of reintervention) begins to rise. By 20 years after initial operation, only 60% of patients will be free of reintervention, and by 40 years only 10% will be free.[D3] The older

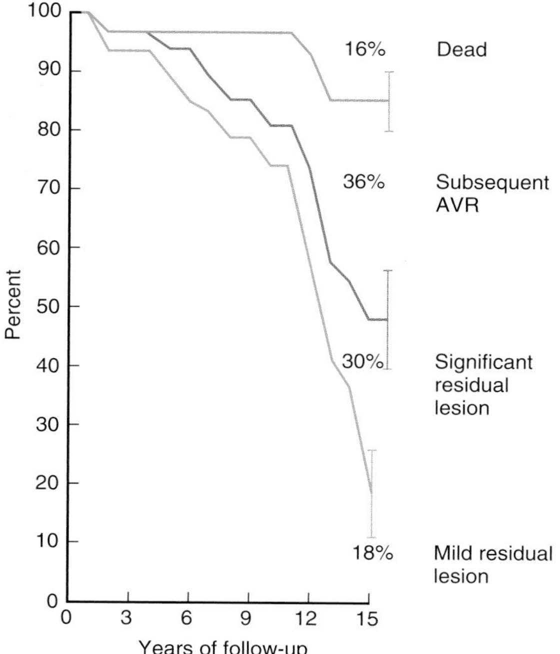

Figure 47-12 Cumulative incidence curves depicting time-related freedom from several unfavorable outcomes in 30 children and young adults (infants excluded) undergoing valvotomy for congenital valvar aortic stenosis. Vertical bars represent 70% confidence limits. Mean follow-up time was 13 years (1-17 years). Percentages refer to distance between curves. Key: *AVR,* Aortic valve replacement. (From Hossackand colleagues.[H13])

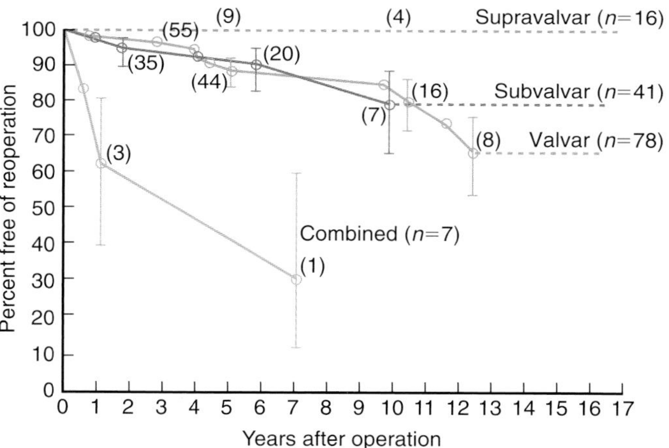

Figure 47-13 Freedom from reoperation on left ventricular or aortic outflow tract after a primary operation for congenital aortic stenosis in 142 patients (UAB experience, 1967-1982).

the patient, the more likely it is that the reintervention will be valve replacement.

Reintervention appears to be required at a shorter interval and in greater prevalence when the initial intervention has been performed in neonatal life or infancy, and is more likely to consist of valvotomy than valve replacement.[B1,B28,G1] Greater frequency of reintervention may be related to generally higher residual gradients in these cases. Reintervention appears to be required more frequently when initial valvotomy has been performed by some method other than an open

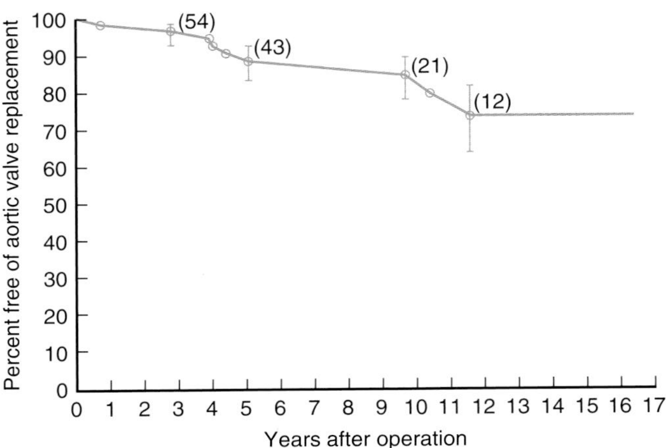

Figure 47-14 Freedom from aortic valve replacement after initial aortic valvotomy in 77 patients with congenital valvar aortic stenosis. Aortic valve replacement may have been after a repeat valvotomy (UAB experience, 1967-1982). Vertical bars represent 70% confidence limits, and numbers in parentheses patients remaining at risk.

operation using CPB.[P3] Reintervention rate increases 15 years after operation from 0.73% per year to 2.3% per year ($P < .0001$).[D8]

Procedures done at reoperation are generally more varied than at initial operation (Table 47-6). A satisfactory repeat valvotomy is sometimes possible, especially when the initial operation has been done in infancy.[K7] At times, an overlooked second level of obstruction is found that requires treatment such as patch graft supravalvar enlargement, a Konno procedure (see Technique of Operation in Section II), or an aortic root replacement (see "Aortic Valve Replacement in Children" under Technique of Operation earlier in this section). These reoperations carry a low risk, but generally carry greater risk than primary operation (see Table 47-6).[S2]

Freedom from further reoperation following aortic valve cusp extension procedures has been variable, with freedom from subsequent aortic valve repair or replacement of 60% to 80% at 5 years and about 50% at 15 years.[D4,P6,P7,Q1] Durability of repair appears greater if a tricuspid valve can be created.[P7]

INDICATIONS FOR OPERATION

Initial Valvotomy

Neonates and Young Infants

In neonates and young infants with severe congenital valvar aortic stenosis, medical treatment is begun on an emergency basis.[K7] When the diagnosis is suspected before transport of a neonate to a cardiac surgical center in the first week or two of life, or as soon as such a patient, usually moribund or in metabolic acidosis, is admitted, prostaglandin E_1 is begun (see Indications for Operation in Chapter 49). This substance usually opens the ductus arteriosus, particularly if the neonate is just a few days old, improves systemic oxygenation, and relieves metabolic acidosis because the right ventricle can support both systemic and pulmonary circulations.[J5,M18] The child's condition should be stable and good before operation is begun.

Before intervention, care must be taken to distinguish the neonates or very young infants with isolated severe congenital valvar aortic stenosis from those whose anomaly is part of the spectrum of hypoplastic left heart physiology. When the anomaly is hypoplastic left heart physiology class III (see Table 48-1 in Chapter 48), the Norwood operation rather than aortic valvotomy is indicated; simple aortic valvotomy is futile.[R8] The criteria for using the more extensive operation are (1) mitral valve area less than 4.75 $cm^2 \cdot m^{-2}$; (2) LV inflow dimension less than 25 mm; (3) small LV, evidenced by a ratio between the apex-to-base dimension of the LV and that of the right ventricle of less than 0.8; or (4) transverse cavitary and aortic "anular" dimension of 6 mm or less.[B28,L3,L9,P3,R8]

In the Congenital Heart Surgeons multi-institutional study of decision making based on 362 neonates, greater intermediate-term survival was obtained by a strategy of an initial Norwood procedure vs. two-ventricle strategy if the arch was small, LV dysfunction was present, or LV outflow tract was small, particularly when less than 4 mm.[H9] Colan and colleagues have also developed and subsequently revalidated a scoring algorithm for decision making in neonates with aortic stenosis and a mitral valve z value of greater than −2.[C17]

In those patients in whom aortic valvotomy alone is indicated, the decision to use percutaneous balloon aortic valvotomy (see Special Situations and Controversies later in this section) or surgical valvotomy remains controversial. Surgical valvotomy may be accomplished by closed transventricular valvotomy,[T6,T7] open surgical valvotomy with CPB, or using hypothermic or normothermic circulatory arrest. The preference is for surgical valvotomy using CPB, as well as more sophisticated methods of myocardial management than have been generally used. However, a large trial may be the only way to determine comparative outcomes in this complex setting.[F8]

Older Infants and Children

Severe congenital valvar aortic stenosis is an indication for operation in older infants and children. Symptoms of angina or syncope always indicate severe stenosis and thus are indications for operation.[D16] Conversely, severe stenosis requiring operation frequently occurs without symptoms, but in such circumstances there will usually be physical signs,[H13] particularly in the pulse and behavior of the second heart sound. Also, the ECG will usually show an LV hypertrophy pattern; an ECG that shows severe hypertrophy (important ST-T depression) is an indication for operation even if the gradient is less than 50 mmHg.

Mild congenital aortic stenosis is not an indication for operation. Because of the natural history, these patients require long-term periodic noninvasive reevaluation and invasive study and operation if indicated.

Older infants and children with moderate stenosis are a controversial group. Many recommend operation,[B7,C18,E5,M29] and others recommend periodic reevaluation of LV-aortic gradient,[C16,E6,F13,W1] subendocardial oxygen requirement,[K16,L10] or valve area. Those against possibly premature operation argue that (1) sudden death is rare in children whose systolic gradient is 50 to 75 mmHg, (2) operation and probable valve replacement will still be necessary, and (3) valve replacement cannot be delayed by early operation. Therefore, operation usually is not recommended in this group, but is advised if stenosis becomes severe on repeated noninvasive follow-up.

Table 47-6 First Reoperation for Congenital Aortic Stenosis, According to Morphologic Category and Procedure at First Operation[a]

Category	Procedure	Prior Procedure	*n*	Hospital Deaths
Valvar	Aortic valvotomy	Aortic valvotomy	2	0
	AVR	Aortic valvotomy	2	0
	AVR + patch ascending aorta	Aortic valvotomy	3	0
	AVR + Konno	Aortic valvotomy	1	0
	AVR + Manougian aortic root enlargement	Aortic valvotomy	2	0
			10	0
Subvalvar	Excision	Excision	1	0
	Excision + myotomy + modified Konno	Excision	1	0
	Myotomy + modified Konno	Excision	1	0
	Excision + patch ascending aorta	Excision	1	0
	AVR + excision + patch ascending aorta	Excision	1	0
	LV-Ao conduit	Excision	1	0
			6	0
Supravalvar	Excision of subvalvar stenosis	Ascending aortic patch	1	0
	Aortic valvotomy + myotomy + ascending aortic patch	Ascending aortic patch	1	0
			2	0
Combined valvar + supravalvar	Excision of subvalvar stenosis	Ascending aortic patch	1	1
	AVR + ascending aortic patch	Valvotomy + ascending aortic patch	1	1
			2	1
Combined valvar + subvalvar	Valvotomy + excision of accessory mitral tissue	Valvotomy	1	0
	AVR + Konno	Valvotomy + excision of subaortic stenosis	1	0
	AVR + excision of fibromuscular stenosis and accessory mitral tissue + Konno	Valvotomy + excision of subaortic stenosis	1	0
			3	0
Combined valvar + subvalvar + supravalvar	Patch ascending aorta + LV-Ao conduit	Excision of subaortic stenosis	1	0

[a]Data from 24 patients undergoing reoperation anywhere after initial operation at UAB, 1967-1982.
Key: *AVR*, Aortic valve replacement; *LV-Ao*, left ventricular to aortic.

Reoperation

When restenosis becomes severe or when symptoms develop with moderate restenosis, reoperation is indicated. Initially, dysplastic valve cusps should not be a contraindication to reoperation, because in a number of patients the cusps have been more normal in appearance at reoperation than in early life.[K7] Although repeat valvotomy or valve replacement is usually required, subvalvar stenosis may have also developed and must not be overlooked. Important subvalvar stenosis is often associated with a small "anulus," as well as some supravalvar narrowing. In this case a Konno operation, aortic root replacement operation, or Ross-Konno operation may be advisable.

SPECIAL SITUATIONS AND CONTROVERSIES

Technique of Operation

Periodic enthusiasm for closed transventricular aortic valvotomy in critically ill neonates and young infants is motivated by high early mortality in this group.[T7] Closed transventricular dilatations have been performed with Hegar dilators and balloon catheters designed for percutaneous use.[B25,T7] Considering the early mortality, need for reintervention, and amount of valvar regurgitation produced, however, no convincing evidence indicates that this method is as good as or superior to the techniques described under Technique of Operation earlier in this section.[P3]

A few groups have preferred to perform valvotomy under inflow stasis at normothermia or mild hypothermia.[C23] Operation under these circumstances is a semiopen one, and forceful stretching or tearing of the valve may result if exposure is not ideal. In children, the method can be used safely, but 7 (26%; CL 17%-37%) of 27 patients followed up to 15 years by Stewart and colleagues had moderate or severe aortic valve regurgitation.[S28] Sink and colleagues reported two (25%; CL 9%-50%) hospital deaths among eight infants, six of whom were neonates.[S14]

Ilbawi and colleagues reported use of extended aortic valvuloplasty in which the commissurotomy incision is extended into the aortic wall around the cusp insertion, mobilizing the valve cusp attachment at the commissures and freeing the aortic insertion of the rudimentary commissure.[I1] They showed reduced aortic valve gradients compared with standard aortic valvotomy at 1.7 years after operation. The method has possible merit, but has not had wide application. Kadri and colleagues, as well as Tolan and colleagues, have described similar operations in which the raphe or fused commissure of the larger cusp of a bicuspid aortic valve is incised, and a triangular piece of pericardium is folded and inserted between the free edges of the incised raphe.[K1,T5] Autologous or bovine pericardium is attached to the free edges of the incised raphe and vertically to the aortic wall.[K1,T5] This procedure produces a tricuspid valve and restores the deficient intercusp triangle, preventing cusp prolapse. Experience with this and other cusp reconstruction procedures (see "Cusp Reconstruction" under Technique of Operation earlier in this section) is limited, so caution should be used in applying these methods until more is known about their efficacy in palliating aortic valve stenosis.

Percutaneous Balloon Aortic Valvotomy in Neonates, Infants, and Children

Percutaneous balloon aortic valvotomy for severe aortic stenosis in neonates was described by Rupprath and Neuhaus in 1985 and Lababidi and Weinhaus in 1986.[L1,R13] A large experience with this technique has accumulated since then, well summarized in the neonatal group by Zeevi and colleagues from Boston Children's Hospital.[Z1] They found no difference when the results were compared with those of surgical valvotomy in a previous era. Similar results have been reported by others.[K4,O1,W10] New technology may improve results still further.[B5,R14]

In the Congenital Heart Surgeons multi-institutional study, 110 neonates for whom the strategy for management was biventricular repair were treated by either surgical (n = 28) or percutaneous balloon (n = 82) aortic valvotomy.[M10] Propensity score adjustment (see "Clinical Studies with Nonrandomly Assigned Treatment" in Section I of Chapter 6) was used to account for procedure selection bias and achieve comparability of patient characteristics. Time-related survival to age 5 years was similar after surgical and percutaneous balloon aortic valvotomy, as was risk of reintervention.

Moore and colleagues studied midterm results of balloon dilatation of congenital aortic stenosis performed at Boston Children's Hospital in 148 children, all more than 1 month old.[M27] Mortality was 0.7% and was successful in 87% of patients, with average peak gradient reduction of 56% ± 20%. At 8 years postoperatively, 95% were alive, but only 50% were free of another intervention (surgical or repeat balloon aortic valvotomy). Aortic valve regurgitation of grade 3 or higher occurred immediately after the procedure in 13% (CL 10%-16%) and was a major factor in determining another intervention.

Gatzoulis and colleagues compared results of balloon aortic valvotomy in 34 children (8 neonates) and surgical valvotomy in 17 children (7 neonates) treated between 1988 and 1993.[G4] Results were equivalent. Two deaths occurred in each group, attributable to small LVs. Peak gradient reduction was equivalent.

Shim and colleagues showed that repeat balloon aortic valvotomy is an effective palliative procedure for children with aortic valve stenosis.[S10] Repeat balloon aortic valvotomy provided immediate gradient reduction comparable with the results reported with initial balloon valvotomy, with no increased risk of developing aortic regurgitation.

Hawkins and colleagues followed 60 patients for 1 to 110 months after balloon aortic valvotomy.[H7] Operation was required in 23 patients (38%), and aortic valve operation was required in 5% to 7% of patients per year after balloon aortic valvotomy. Aortic valve regurgitation was the predominant indication. Aortic valve repair (valvotomy) was possible in 9 of 23 patients requiring operation after balloon aortic valvotomy. Aortic valve replacement was required in the remaining 14 patients.

Sandhu and colleagues showed that balloon aortic valvotomy can be effective in young adults with congenital aortic stenosis.[S1] Of 15 patients aged 16 to 24 years having balloon aortic valvotomy, three required aortic valve replacement for high residual gradient or severe aortic valve regurgitation. Immediate reduction of the pressure gradient by 55% persisted for an average of 1.5 years. Equivalent results were found in 70 children.

Beneficial results of balloon aortic valvotomy in adult patients, especially those with degenerative aortic stenosis, are not long lasting, and restenosis occurs in most patients within 6 months. Wang and colleagues reviewed results of balloon aortic valvotomy in adults, including results from two large registries.[W2] They concluded that long-term survival for adults after balloon aortic valvotomy is similar to the natural history of untreated severe aortic stenosis. Survival for patients having balloon valvotomy alone at 3 years was less than 25%, vs. almost 90% for those having balloon aortic valvotomy followed by aortic valve replacement. Balloon aortic valvotomy is reserved only for those patients who are not candidates for aortic valve replacement because of comorbid illness or advanced age. Balloon aortic valvotomy has not been effective in reducing risk of noncardiac surgery or acting as a bridge to future aortic valve replacement (see Special Situations and Controversies in Chapter 12).

Even with these data, it remains difficult to evaluate balloon aortic valvotomy and determine its effectiveness compared with surgical valvotomy. Immediate, early, and probably midterm results appear to be equivalent to operation in the neonate and child and perhaps in the young adult with congenital aortic stenosis. Long-term results are not currently available. Balloon aortic valvotomy is not effective treatment for adult patients, especially when aortic stenosis is the degenerative type. Application of percutaneous balloon aortic valvotomy seems to be determined by local preference at present.

Section II **Congential Discrete Subvalvar Aortic Stenosis**

DEFINITION

Congenital discrete subvalvar aortic stenosis is an obstruction beneath the aortic valve caused by either a short, localized, fibrous or fibromuscular ridge or a longer diffuse fibrous tunnel. "Diffuse subvalvar aortic stenosis" is a phrase best not used to avoid confusion; it was originally used to distinguish what is now termed *hypertrophic obstructive cardiomyopathy* (HOCM) from congenital aortic stenosis (see Chapter 19).[K13]

Subvalvar aortic stenosis may also be a part of other cardiac anomalies. In these situations, the obstruction may be fibromuscular and indistinguishable from the entity discussed here or may consist of a localized muscular bar or shelf (e.g., in coarctation or aortic arch interruption with VSD) or abnormalities of the mitral valve. In other words, subvalvar aortic stenosis, as well as valvar stenosis, may be part of the spectrum of hypoplastic left heart physiology.

HISTORICAL NOTE

The first description of discrete subvalvar stenosis is attributed to Chevers in 1842.[C8] In 1956, Brock and Fleming from Guys Hospital in London published an early report of diagnosing the condition during life using transventricular puncture to measure LV pressure.[B21] The catheter was then advanced across the aortic valve from below and the level of obstruction demonstrated. Brock reported results of transventricular dilatation in 1959.[B20] Spencer and colleagues published the first substantial report of treatment using CPB in 1960.[S18] The lesion was illustrated clearly in patients operated on at the Mayo Clinic between 1956 and 1960.[E4,E5]

The long fibrous tunnel form of the stenosis was described by Spencer and was later reemphasized by Reis and Morrow and colleagues.[R7] Its effective treatment under difficult circumstances became possible with the introduction of aortoventriculoplasty by Rastan and Koncz, and independently by Konno and colleagues in 1975.[K15,R2,R3] Complete relief of subvalvar stenosis without sacrifice of the aortic valve became possible with the introduction of the modified Konno operation in 1978 (see Technique of Operation later in this section). The aortoseptal approach was introduced by Vouhe and colleagues in 1984.[V5] An alternative form of treatment, LV-aortic conduit, was developed about the same time.[C21,N5]

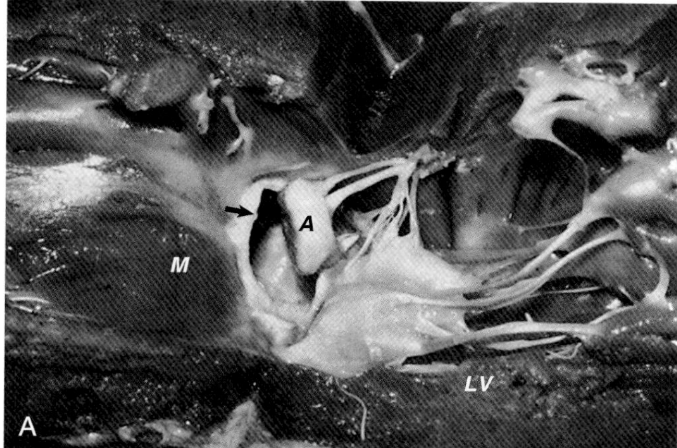

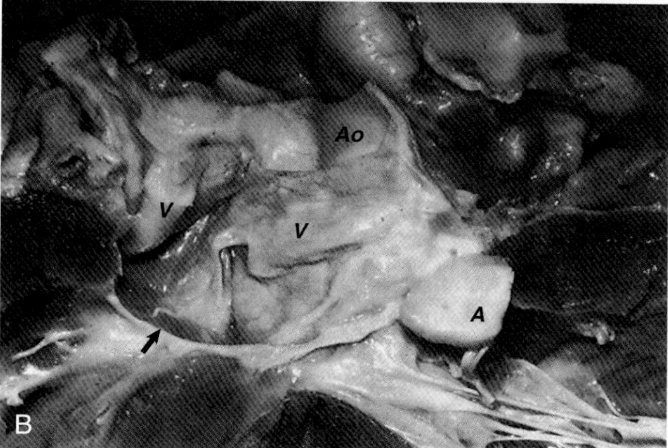

Figure 47-15 Autopsy specimen with medium-level discrete fibrous subvalvar aortic stenosis. **A,** Stenosis viewed intact from below. Note thickness of left ventricular wall *(LV)* and associated muscular hypertrophy *(M)* anteriorly beneath localized fibrous ridge *(arrow)*. **B,** Stenotic zone has been opened into ascending aorta *(Ao)* to show its relationship to aortic valve *(V)*. Accessory mitral leaflet tissue *(A)* contributes to stenosis.

MORPHOLOGY

Left Ventricular Outflow Tract

Localized Subvalvar Aortic Stenosis

The localized form of discrete subvalvar aortic stenosis may be fibrous or fibromuscular. The *fibrous* form involves a spectrum of pathology varying from a discrete short fibrous ridge, a thicker but still discrete fibromuscular shelf, to a long fibrous tunnel. When a fibrous ridge is firmly adherent to a hypertrophied septum anteriorly and to the left, the condition is termed *discrete fibromuscular stenosis*.[K12,N4]

Whether isolated, localized, or only muscular, subvalvar stenosis occurring as an entity separate from HOCM is controversial.

An obstructing localized circumferential fibrous shelf or ridge may be situated at any level between the nadir of the aortic cusps and the free edge of the anterior mitral leaflet, as well as anywhere along the aortic-mitral anulus. An immediately subvalvar fibrous ridge may be adherent to the base of the aortic cusps (only the right or all three[F3]), but more often it is separated from the cusps by several millimeters. Such a high (distal) ridge tends to be narrow, and unless there is severe LV hypertrophy, the remainder of the outflow beneath it remains relatively normal.[K12] A low (proximal) fibrous ridge may be attached almost at the hinge line of the anterior mitral leaflet, but most frequently it occupies an intermediate position well above this and several millimeters below the aortic valve (Fig. 47-15). Usually the ridge is 2 to 3 mm thick and is more prominent anteriorly and laterally than posteriorly on the aortic-mitral anulus. The ridge may be present as a complete fibrous diaphragm, however, and the stenotic orifice may be central and circular or eccentric and slitlike. The aortic-mitral anulus is longer than normal in hearts with discrete subvalvar aortic stenosis, and on average, the diameter of the aortic valve anulus is smaller than normal.[R12] The muscular ventricular septum beneath the right aortic cusp shows a variable degree of hypertrophy and prominence, and in severe cases may contribute importantly to the stenosis.

Tunnel Subvalvar Aortic Stenosis

Much less common, tunnel stenosis presents as a circumferential irregular zone of fibrosis commencing at or close to the LV-aortic junction ("anulus") and extending downward for 10 to 30 mm.[M3,R7,S18] Tunnel stenosis has varying degrees of severity, and its spectrum blends into localized subvalvar aortic stenosis. In its most severe form—the form that requires a special surgical procedure—the stenotic tunnel is long and the diameter of the aortic anulus small, even though aortic valve cusps are normally formed. In patients with less severe disease, the tunnel may be shorter and aortic anulus normal in size; morphology then resembles localized fibromuscular discrete subvalvar aortic stenosis.[K12] These gradations explain the differing prevalences in reported series. Fibrous stenosis is sufficiently long to justify the term *tunnel* in about one fifth of cases of congenital subvalvar aortic stenosis; the full-blown entity with anular hypoplasia is rare.

Aortic Valve

The aortic valve is usually tricuspid and either entirely normal or has some diffuse cusp thickening. Trivial or mild aortic regurgitation is present in about two thirds of patients. The aortic valve, however, may be bicuspid, and congenital commissural fusion may produce varying degrees of valvar stenosis. The valve may have been damaged by endocarditis, a complication of subvalvar stenosis,[M28,M32] which can result in severe regurgitation. Rarely, the subaortic membrane may be infected. Bases of valve cusps are thick when a high-lying fibrous ridge is continuous with them.

Infrequently, supravalvar as well as valvar stenosis coexists with the subvalvar narrowing. This combination is at the mild end of the spectrum of hypoplastic left heart physiology.

Left Ventricle

The LV is usually concentrically hypertrophied. Subendocardial ischemia, and probably fibrosis, occur in subvalvar aortic stenosis as well as in congenital valvar stenosis.[C4] Rarely, there may be excessive hypertrophy of the septum (vs. thickening of the posterior LV wall) and muscle fiber disorientation histologically.[B15,M3] This histology complicates the distinction in a few patients between discrete subvalvar aortic stenosis and HOCM.

Roberts and his group have noted coronary artery luminal narrowing due to structural wall changes of intramural coronary arteries in both humans and dogs with fibrous subvalvar aortic stenosis.[M3,M32] These changes have not been observed in valvar aortic stenosis.

Coexisting Cardiac Anomalies

Discrete subvalvar aortic stenosis occurs as an isolated anomaly in only about half to two thirds of patients coming to operation.[C5,H3,K12] Coexisting anomalies include a VSD that is frequently large,[L4,M2,N4] and the fibromuscular obstruction is then often located immediately below (upstream to) the VSD. When there is aortic arch interruption and patent ductus arteriosus or occasionally coarctation, localized muscular subvalvar stenosis may be associated with a subpulmonary VSD.[F9,V1] Valvar or infundibular pulmonary stenosis[N2] and occasionally tetralogy of Fallot, atrial septal defect, aortopulmonary window, sinus of Valsalva aneurysm, and aneurysm of the membranous ventricular septum may also coexist, occurring more frequently in pediatric surgical patients.

The complex relationship between VSD and discrete subvalvar aortic stenosis is further evidenced by stenosis developing after spontaneous closure or narrowing of the VSD.[C12] Typical discrete subvalvar aortic stenosis may also develop both before and after repair of a complete atrioventricular (AV) septal defect, repair of coarctation, LV-to-aorta internal rerouting in double outlet right ventricle or transposition with VSD, and other forms of congenital cardiac anomalies.[B6,G14,K2,T4]

Other Types of Discrete Subvalvar Aortic Stenosis

Localized subvalvar aortic stenosis may be caused by morphology and mechanisms other than those just described. In an autopsy series that included complex congenital heart disease, Freedom and colleagues found the typical fibrous or fibromuscular variety to be the least common in infancy.[F9] Mitral valve anomalies involving accessory tissue or leaflet malposition (including that found in AV septal defects) may be a cause of obstruction[E2,G12,K19] and may occur in the absence of functional abnormality of the mitral valve or other cardiac anomalies.[M7] Localized muscular obstructions related to abnormal infundibular development or malalignment are frequent and often associated with a VSD and aortic coarctation or interruption.[S13] A developmental complex described by Shone and associates consists of a parachute mitral valve and LV outflow tract obstruction that usually includes localized fibromuscular subaortic stenosis.[S11] Discrete muscular subvalvar aortic stenosis may develop after pulmonary trunk banding for VSD.[F6]

CLINICAL FEATURES AND DIAGNOSTIC CRITERIA

Symptoms

Symptoms of congenital subvalvar aortic stenosis are similar to those of the valvar variety. About 25% of patients requiring operation are asymptomatic despite presence of important obstruction.

Signs

A systolic ejection murmur is heard, but a click is rare. There is an unimpressive aortic diastolic murmur in 65% of patients. It is secondary either to (1) cusp thickening with or without adherence of the fibrous ridge to the cusps or (2) effects of eddy currents produced by the subvalvar stenosis upon aortic valve closure.

When severe stenosis is present, the pulse is slow rising, the second heart sound is single or paradoxically split, a third and occasionally fourth heart sound are audible, and a mid-diastolic murmur may be heard at the apex, usually in association with a fibrotic obstruction that limits anterior mitral leaflet movement.[K12] It is important to recognize, particularly in children, that one or more of these signs may be minimal or absent despite severe obstruction.

Occasionally, aortic regurgitation may be caused by severe congenital cusp deformities or infective endocarditis. When endocarditis occurs on the aortic valve, signs of regurgitation produced by cusp destruction may be less than expected because a tight fibrous stenosis beneath the valve may limit aortic runoff. Moreover, vegetations on the fibrous shelf itself may increase subaortic obstruction.[M32]

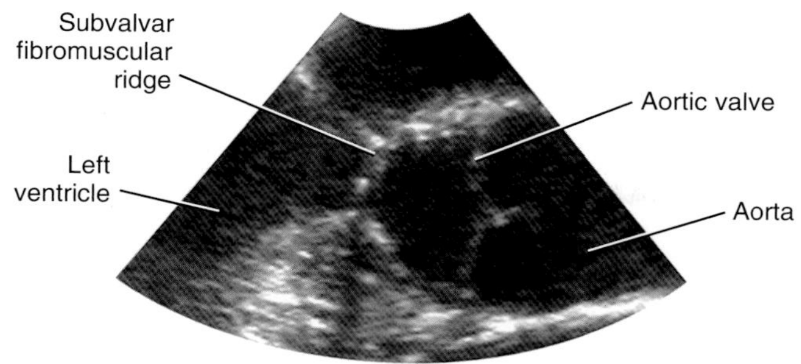

Figure 47-16 Two-dimensional echocardiogram in localized discrete subvalvar aortic stenosis. Fibromuscular ridge is observed narrowing left ventricular outflow tract below aortic valve.

Chest Radiography

The ascending aorta is not usually dilated in the chest radiograph, and valvar calcification is absent. The LV is usually enlarged.

Electrocardiography

The ECG usually shows severe LV hypertrophy.

Echocardiography

Two-dimensional echocardiography can be diagnostic, accurately demonstrating and outlining the obstructing shelf[C12,M3,W5] (Fig. 47-16). The technique is so sensitive that it can demonstrate a subvalvar discrete lesion before a gradient develops. Color flow Doppler imaging sufficiently defines the gradient across the obstruction to allow a definitive decision regarding operation. Siggrusson and colleagues suggested that the angle formed by the septum and aorta (aortoseptal angle) may have prognostic value in patients with discrete subaortic stenosis,[S12] because it is steeper in patients with subaortic stenosis than in normal persons. They suggested this anatomic feature may be causative in development of this condition. M-mode echocardiography is helpful in differentiating this lesion from HOCM.[B15,M3]

Cardiac Catheterization and Cineangiography

Cardiac catheterization shows a systolic pressure gradient below the valve on withdrawal of the catheter across the LV outflow tract. When the fibrous ridge is immediately beneath the valve, the gradient may be apparent at valve level. Postectopic pressure pulse response is normal, and the aortic pulse contour does not show an accessory wave; these features distinguish the lesion from HOCM.

Angiography supports the definitive diagnosis.[H3,K12,M3,N4] The tilted left anterior oblique (LAO) view provides good visualization of the fibrous ridge because it overcomes the foreshortening of the LV outflow tract region present in the conventional LAO projection (Figs. 47-17 through 47-19). Level and thickness of obstruction can be accurately defined in this manner, and additional valvar stenosis and regurgitation also can be evaluated.

Summary

In discrete subvalvar aortic stenosis, features characteristic of HOCM are usually absent. Rarely, however, particularly in severe forms of fibrous subvalvar aortic stenosis,[B15] including the tunnel variety,[M3] there may be abnormal systolic anterior motion (SAM) of the mitral leaflet and an abnormal postectopic response. These signs indicate either a particularly prominent anterior muscular shelf or, in patients who also show an abnormal septal to posterior wall thickness ratio on echocardiography (with disorientation of the muscular pattern of hypertrophy histologically), associated HOCM.

NATURAL HISTORY

Discrete subaortic stenosis is present in 8% to 30% of patients with congenital LV outflow tract obstruction.[B18,K5,K11,M13,N4]

The striking paucity of operations for discrete subvalvar aortic stenosis in the first year of life indicates the difference in life history of patients with congenital subvalvar aortic stenosis compared with patients with valvar stenosis. Typical discrete subvalvar aortic stenosis is rarely a cause of important obstruction in infancy.[F9,H5,N4,S16] Rather, obstruction is often absent in early life and then becomes evident and progressively more severe in childhood or young adulthood.[C11,F10,L8,S7] The subvalvar gradient has first appeared several years after an early study in infancy before VSD and coarctation repair. Also, the lesion appears infrequently after age 30, suggesting that survival beyond this time is rare without surgery or that the lesion gradually takes on the appearance of HOCM.[K16]

Pyle and colleagues provided further support for these concepts in their study of fibrous subaortic stenosis in Newfoundland dogs.[P9] In these animals, subaortic stenosis was never present at birth but was important by 12 weeks of age. Evidence also shows that stenosis might be an inherited trait. A familial occurrence has been reported in humans.[G1,L4,M3] Reports of serial cardiac catheterizations indicate that discrete subvalvar aortic stenosis progresses quite rapidly,[F10,F14,H3,M24,N4] probably more rapidly than valvar stenosis. Such features probably explain why, in published surgical series in which ages of patients are listed, the youngest patients operated on are age 3 to 6 years and surgery is uncommon beyond age 20.[C5,H3,K5,K12,L13,M3,S18]

Aortic regurgitation, often associated with discrete subvalvar aortic stenosis, is progressive and caused by cusp thickening from poststenotic turbulence.[N4] Cusp thickening most likely explains the frequency of endocarditis before and after surgical excision of the membrane.[F5,M28,M32,S30]

TECHNIQUE OF OPERATION

Resection of Localized Subvalvar Aortic Stenosis

Preparation for operation for congenital subvalvar aortic stenosis in children is accomplished as described for valvotomy in Section I. Fig. 47-20 shows anatomic relationships of the subaortic fibromuscular ridge.

A transverse aortotomy is made (Fig. 47-21, *A*). The aortic cusps are retracted and the subvalvar fibrous ridge exposed. Beginning beneath the nadir of the right coronary cusp, a vertical incision is made through the ridge and into the underlying muscle, with depth of incision proportional to estimated septal thickness (Fig. 47-21, *B*). A second incision parallel to the first is made through the ridge below the commissure between right and left aortic valve cusps. Excision of the fibromuscular ridge begins by carrying a vertical incision circumferentially between the parallel incisions

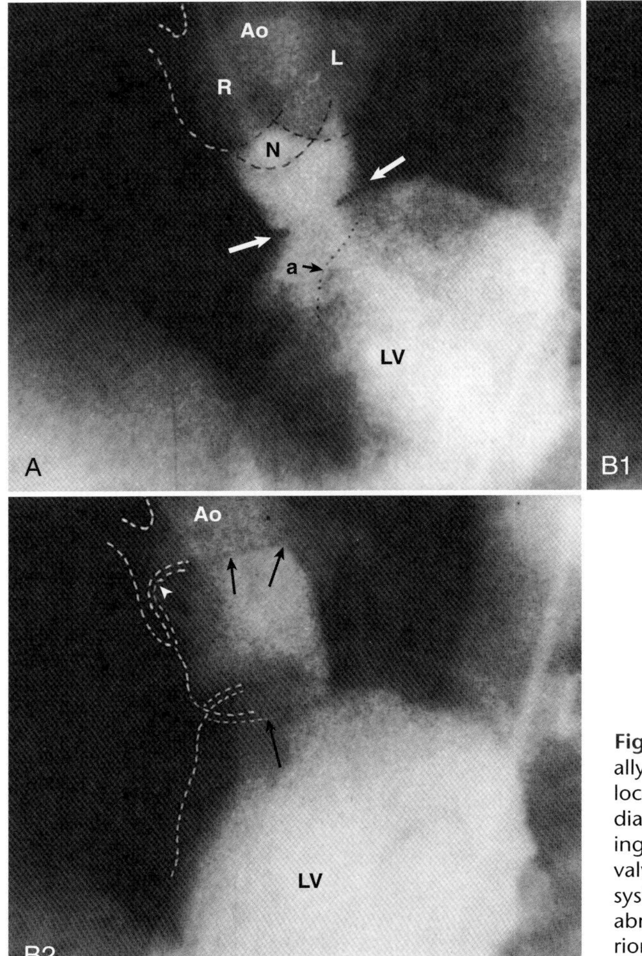

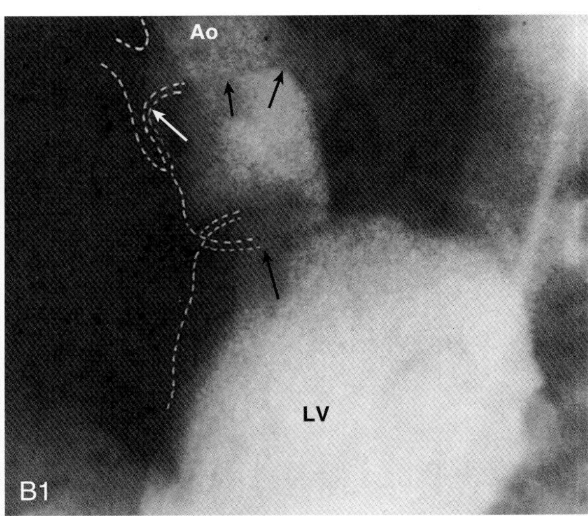

Figure 47-17 Left ventricular cineangiogram in cranially tilted left anterior oblique projection in patient with localized discrete fibrous subvalvar aortic stenosis, in diastole **(A)** and early systole **(B)**. A thin ridge obstructing left ventricular outflow tract about 1 cm below aortic valve is well profiled and indicated by white arrows. In systole, aortic valve is domed *(arrows)*, indicating a valvar abnormality in addition to subaortic ridge. Key: *a,* Anterior mitral leaflet; *Ao,* aorta; *L,* left; *LV,* left ventricle; *N,* noncoronary sinus; *R,* right coronary sinus.

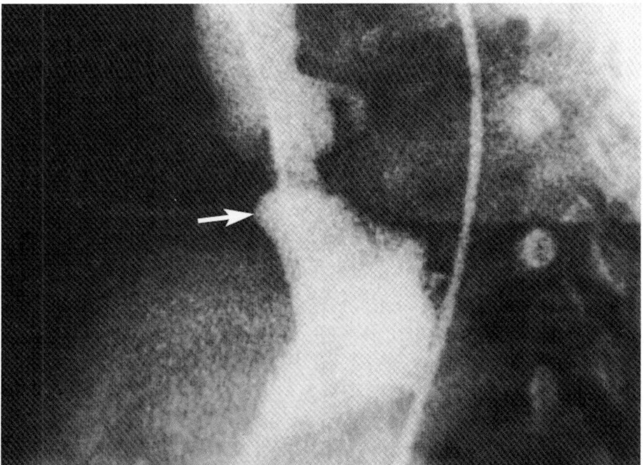

Figure 47-18 Left ventricular cineangiogram in cranially tilted left anterior oblique projection in patient with fibromuscular subvalvar aortic stenosis. Cineangiogram frame in systole shows thick fibromuscular outflow obstruction commencing just beneath aortic valve. Aortic cusps fail to open completely but show no doming. Diverticulum just below obstructing shelf on septal aspect of outflow tract represents a surgically closed ventricular septal defect *(arrow)*.

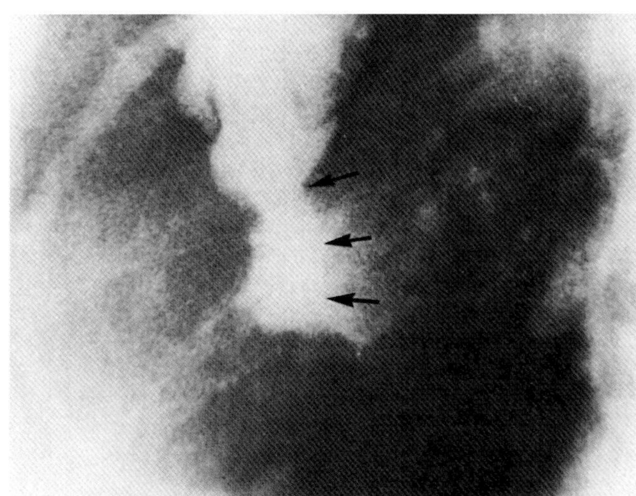

Figure 47-19 Left ventricular cineangiogram in lateral projection in patient with tunnel subvalvar aortic stenosis. Cineangiogram frame in late systole shows outflow tract narrowing 1 cm below aortic ring and extending down into base of left ventricle. Anterior mitral valve leaflet forms posterior margin of stenotic zone *(arrows)* and is prevented from moving back to its normal systolic position. Anterior (septal) margin of outflow tract shows irregular encroachment by obstructing fibromuscular tissue.

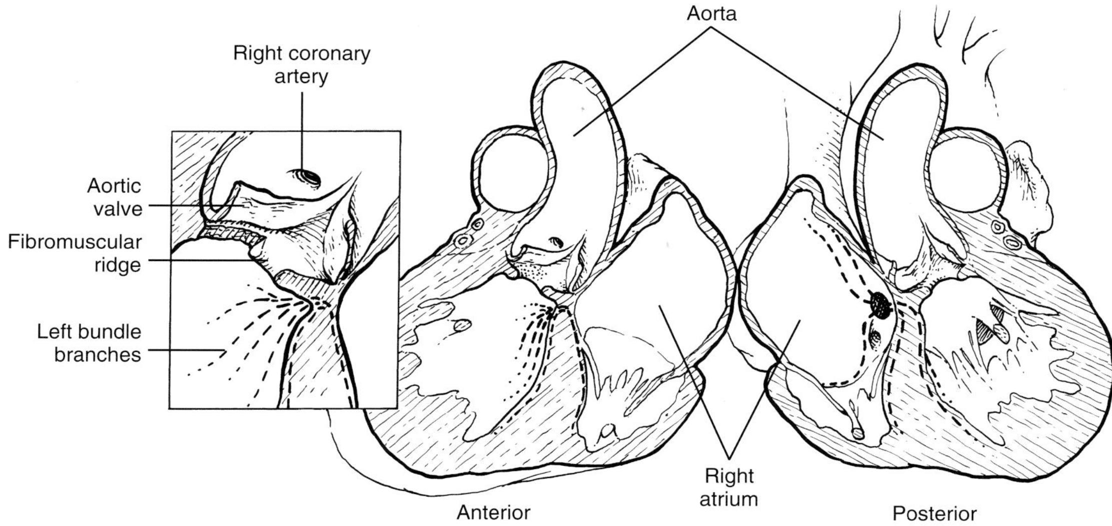

Figure 47-20 Anatomic relations of left ventricular outflow tract in subvalvar aortic stenosis. In this view, heart is bisected; anterior aspect is on left and posterior aspect on right. Inset shows subaortic ridge and left bundle branch of specialized conduction system below the surface of the ventricular septum, with nadir of right coronary cusp marking leftward limit of conduction system. Deep incision of ventricular septum is possible to the left of the midpoint of right coronary cusp.

(Fig. 47-21, *C*), removing fibrous tissue and myocardium deep into the ventricular septum until the mitral apparatus is encountered at the leftward extremity of the LV outflow tract. In this process, care is taken not to penetrate the ventricular septum and produce a VSD. As the dissection is carried down over the anterior mitral leaflet, only the fibrous ridge is removed, shaving it off the leaflet or mitral-aortic anulus with the knife or a Freer septum elevator (Fig. 47-21, *D*). Dissection is carried rightward as far as the mitral leaflet and mitral-aortic anulus extend.

Returning anteriorly, only the fibrous ridge is shaved off the muscular septum to the right of the nadir of the right coronary cusp using a knife or septum elevator (see Fig. 47-21, *D*). The ridge excision is carried rightward over the membranous septum. This technique preserves the integrity of the underlying bundle of His and cores out the entire subvalvar stenosis as a single mass. When the fibromuscular ridge is attached to the undersurface of the belly of one or more of the aortic cusps, it is carefully shaved away from the cusp tissue.

The procedure is not considered complete unless a generous amount of muscle has been removed leftward of the nadir of the right coronary cusp. If only the fibrous component has been enucleated,[G2] a deep trough of muscle is cut from the ventricular septum anteriorly. The trough is centered beneath the commissure between the right and left aortic valve cusps as in the operation for HOCM (see Technique of Operation in Chapter 19). This step is of value even when the fibrous ridge is immediately subvalvar, because the ventricular septum is always hypertrophied.

Yacoub and colleagues propose mobilization of the left and right fibrous trigones along with extensive resection of all components of the subvalvular fibrous ring.[Y1] Their proposition is based on the concept that the aortic and mitral orifices interact, with the fibrous trigones acting as a hinge mechanism for movement of the subaortic curtain and anterior mitral leaflet during the cardiac cycle. The incision to resect the fibrous ring is extended laterally at the location of the left and right fibrous trigones to excise this fibrous tissue in continuity with the obstructing ring. Resection of the left fibrous trigone carries the risk of creating an opening to the outside of the heart or into the anterior mitral leaflet, and injury to the conduction system could occur during resection of the right fibrous trigone. The technique was used in 57 consecutive patients operated on over the course of 25 years without these complications occurring. Pressure gradient over the LV outflow tract after the repair ranged from 0 to 30 mmHg (mean 8 mmHg), and no change in gradient was observed on follow-up assessment.

After determining that the ventricular septum has not been perforated and aortic valve cusps have not been damaged, the aortotomy is closed and the remainder of the procedure accomplished as described under Technique of Operation in Section I for valvotomy.

Ross-Konno Procedure

Aortic valve replacement may be required in some older children or adults when important aortic valve regurgitation coexists with severe subaortic stenosis. Modification of the Ross and Konno procedures is used in these patients (Ross-Konno procedure). CPB is established using either two cannulae for venous uptake (with venae cavae tourniquets) or a single two-stage cannula, with the atrial uptake placed deep in the atrium at the inferior vena cava (see "Preparation for Cardiopulmonary Bypass" in Section III of Chapter 2). Oxygenated blood is returned through a cannula in the ascending aorta. The aorta is occluded and cold cardioplegia administered through a cannula in the coronary sinus (see "Technique of Retrograde Infusion" in Chapter 3), directly into the coronary ostia, or both. The ascending aorta is divided and aortic valve excised. The coronary ostia are mobilized with a rim of sinus aorta, and the noncoronary sinus aorta is removed (see Chapter 12). The pulmonary trunk is removed from the right ventricular (RV) outflow tract in the usual manner for a Ross procedure (see "Autograft Pulmonary

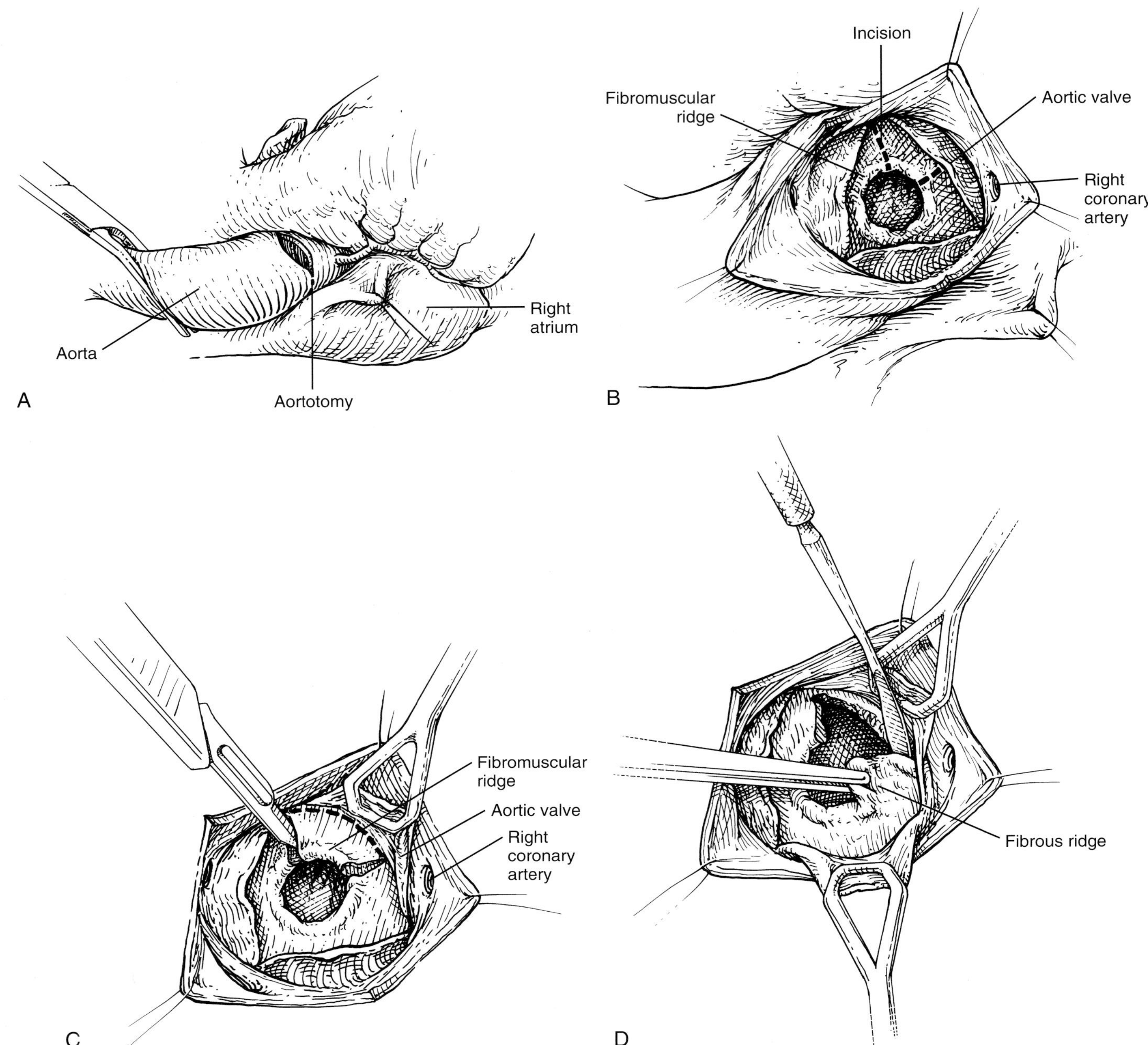

Figure 47-21 Repair of discrete fibromuscular subvalvar aortic stenosis. **A,** Operation is performed on cardiopulmonary bypass with aorta occluded. Cold cardioplegic solution is infused to achieve total electromechanical arrest. A transverse aortotomy is made. **B,** Subaortic ridge is exposed by retracting right coronary cusp. Broken lines indicate proposed incision points. **C,** Scalpel is used to make two incisions through fibromuscular ridge, with one below the commissure between right and left aortic valve cusps and the other parallel to first incision and beneath the nadir of right coronary cusp. Septal myocardium is removed deeply between the two incisions. **D,** Fibrous ridge is dissected from the septum to the right and over anterior leaflet of mitral valve using a Freer septum elevator. Deep incision of ventricular septum carries hazard of heart block. Similarly, deep incision over anterior leaflet of mitral valve risks its perforation.

Valve" under Technique of Operation in Chapter 12). A slightly longer portion of the RV outflow tract below the pulmonary valve may be removed (Fig. 47-22, *A*). A short incision is made through the fibrous tissue of the aortic valve attachment at the nadir of the right coronary sinus into the ventricular septum, as in the Konno procedure (Fig. 47-22, *B*). This incision is not as deep into the septum as in the Konno procedure, however, and should not extend beyond the medial papillary muscle (Lancisi) of the tricuspid valve to avoid injury to the first septal branch of the left anterior descending coronary artery. The fibromuscular subaortic ridge is excised and septal myocardium shaved from the left side to reduce thickness of the hypertrophied ventricular septum in order to widen the LV outflow tract and completely relieve the obstruction (Fig. 47-22, *C*). The pulmonary autograft is then attached to the LV outflow tract (Fig. 47-22, *D*). The lengthened tongue of the attached RV outflow tract is inserted to the depth of the incision in the

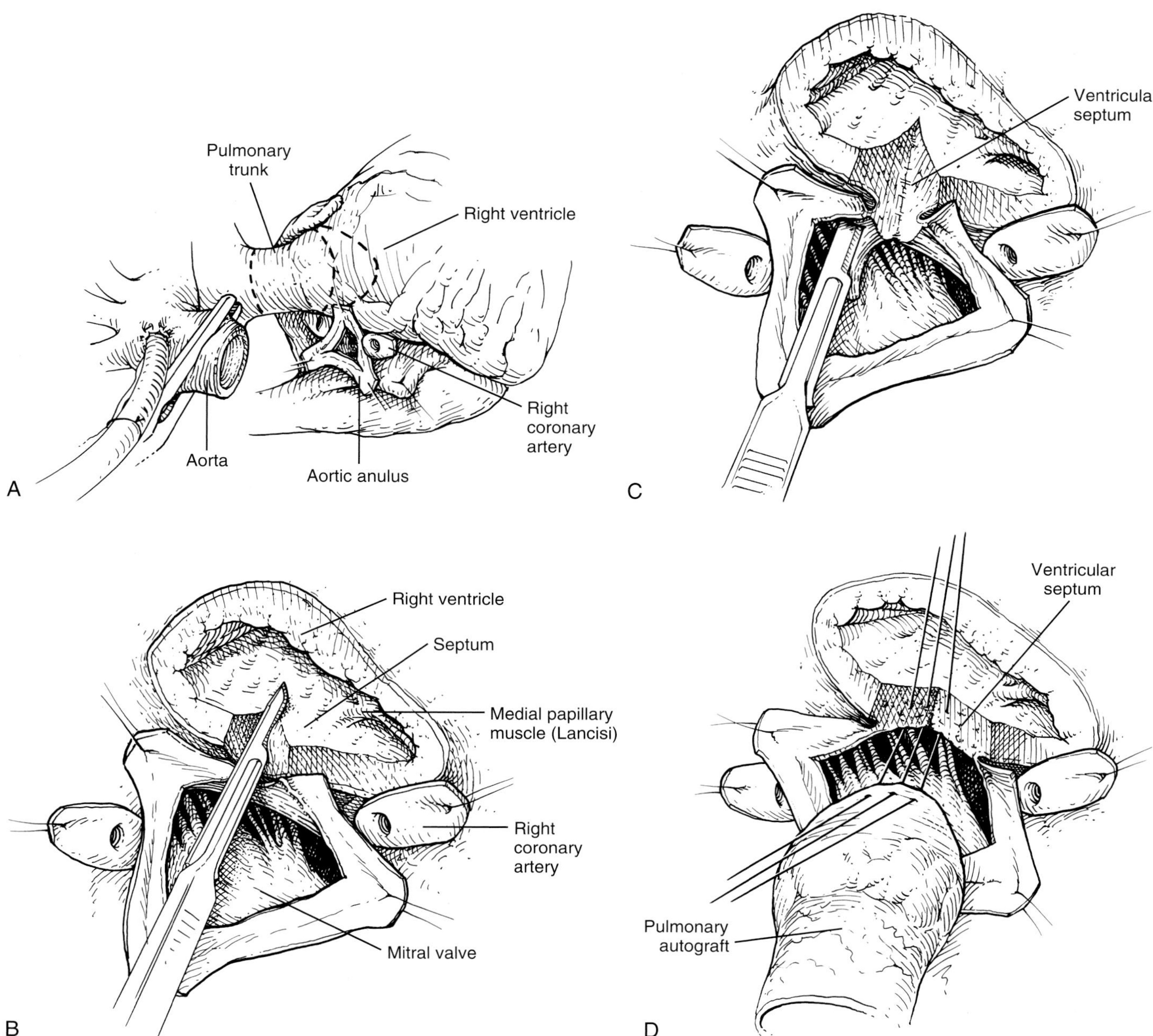

Figure 47-22 Repair of complex subvalvar aortic stenosis requiring aortic valve replacement by pulmonary autograft (Ross-Konno procedure). **A,** Operation is performed on cardiopulmonary bypass with aorta occluded and cold cardioplegia infusion for myocardial management. Aorta is divided and aortic valve excised. Coronary arteries are mobilized with a button of sinus aorta. Rest of sinus aorta is removed. Pulmonary trunk is divided at its bifurcation and removed from right ventricular outflow tract. An extension of the anterior wall of right ventricular outflow tract may be included to fill defect in ventricular septum created by the Konno incision. **B,** An incision is made into ventricular septum (Konno) at the midpoint of right coronary sinus of Valsalva. This incision is not nearly as deep into ventricular septum as in the classic Konno operation, and ordinarily would not pass the depth of the medial papillary muscle (Lancisi) of the tricuspid valve to avoid injury to first septal branch of left anterior descending coronary artery. **C,** Subaortic obstructing ridge is cut away from ventricular septum on left side. Hypertrophied ventricular septum is shaved down on left side to achieve an unobstructed left ventricular outflow tract. **D,** Pulmonary autograft is attached to ventricular septum with interrupted polypropylene stitches. Anterior extension of right ventricular outflow tract may be beneficial when incision of ventricular septum is extensive and deep.

ventricular septum. If no extra length of RV outflow tract has been removed, the pulmonary autograft is simply inserted deeply into the LV outflow tract. The operation is completed as described for the Ross procedure (see "Autograft Pulmonary Valve" under Technique of Operation in Chapter 12).

Repair of Tunnel Stenosis by Aortoventriculoplasty (Konno Operation)

When a tunnel type of subaortic stenosis coexists with hypoplasia and narrowing of the LV-aortic junction, aortoventriculoplasty is a reasonable procedure, using the modification described by Misbach and Ebert and colleagues and others.[K15,M23,R2,R3]

The preliminaries and preparations for CPB are identical to those described earlier for congenital valvar aortic stenosis (see "Preparation for Cardiopulmonary Bypass" in Section III of Chapter 2). CPB is established using two caval cannulae and caval taping, because the RV will be opened. The aorta is occluded, cold cardioplegic solution is infused, and perfusate temperature is stabilized at 20°C to 25°C. Through a small oblique right atriotomy incision, the pump-oxygenator sump sucker is placed across a naturally occurring or surgically created foramen ovale.

Before establishing CPB, position of the right coronary artery must be accurately noted, and a marking stitch placed leftward from this to indicate the RV incision site. A vertical aortotomy is made beginning about 10 mm downstream to the level of the right coronary artery (Fig. 47-23, *A*). The incision is carried well to the left of the right coronary artery and onto the RV over the junction of the contiguous portions of right and left coronary cusps.[D9] The right ventriculotomy may be made first to visualize the pulmonary valve cusps, because these lie near the point of entry of the incision into the RV. After the RV is opened, the scissors are positioned with one blade in the LV through the aortotomy and one in the RV through the ventriculotomy; a scissors cut is made to the left side of the nadir of the right coronary cusp (see Fig. 47-23, *A*). This incision is carried far enough into the two ventricles to gain access below (or upstream to) the tunnel stenosis. The newly created and enlarged anulus is sized, and an appropriately sized mechanical valve prosthesis is chosen. A double-velour collagen or gel-coated polyester graft is fashioned to form an oval-shaped patch. Beginning at the inferior angle of the incision in the ventricular septum, this patch is sewn into place from the RV side out to beyond the aortic anulus and posteriorly through it. A triangular patch of polyester is attached to the primary aortic patch with the anteriorly placed valve stitches (Fig. 47-23, *B*). Horizontal mattress sutures in the anterior aspect of the prosthesis are passed through the patch. The remainder of the polyester patch is sutured into place to enlarge and close the aortotomy (Fig. 47-23, *C*).

The triangular polyester patch is used to close the RV opening (see Fig. 47-23, *C*). The patch must be wide enough to enlarge the RV outflow tract as compensation for projection of the enlarged LV outflow tract into the RV outflow tract. Particular care is taken to anchor the patch at the junction of RV and aorta so that hemostasis is secure in that area.

The left atrial suction device is removed from across the foramen ovale. The foramen is closed, then the right atrium. The remainder of the operation is carried out in the usual manner (see "Completing Cardiopulmonary Bypass" in Section III of Chapter 2).

Aortoventriculoplasty by "Mini" Aortic Root Replacement

Enlarging the subvalvar and valvar area of the LV outflow tract can also be accomplished using biological material, either an ascending aorta valved allograft or a pulmonary artery valved autograft.[C13,C14] The operation is begun in the same manner as the Konno operation, extending the incision into the ventricular septum as far toward the apex as required by the extent of subaortic stenosis; incision into the aorta is kept as short as possible. The aorta is then transected just downstream to the distal extent of the vertical incision, and the coronary ostia with generous buttons of surrounding sinus wall are removed from the aorta. The remnant of aortic root and valve cusps are then excised, leaving a fringe of aortic wall attached to the LV-aortic junction. The V-shaped defect in the ventricular septum is filled in with a polyester patch. This reconstructs and enlarges that portion of the LV outflow tract to which the aortic valved allograft (or pulmonary valved autograft) is attached proximally. The graft is sewn into place, and the coronary buttons are implanted. Finally, the opening in the anterior RV wall is closed with a patch, using a triangular piece of pericardium sutured into the incision and distally onto the anterior aspect of the graft.

The anterior mitral leaflet may be left in place on an aortic valved allograft and used to fill in the ventricular septum. However, this dictates the orientation of the valved cylinder, which may be disadvantageous because the curvature of the aorta is brought anteriorly and to the right. This problem can be overcome by using an aortic allograft with attached anterior mitral leaflet to widen the LV outflow tract posteriorly into the anterior leaflet of the mitral valve, as suggested by Milsom and Doty.[M22] This places the allograft in anatomic position for treating the complex but localized subvalvar aortic stenosis.

Modified Konno Operation

The modified Konno operation, originally described in the first edition of this book, is effective in patients with difficult and complex localized subaortic stenosis or tunnel stenosis when the aortic anulus and valve are normal. This procedure has also been found to be useful in other patients.[C19,D5]

Preparations for operation and establishment of CPB are exactly as described for the Konno operation (see "Repair of Tunnel Stenosis by Aortoventriculoplasty [Konno Operation]" earlier in this section). The aorta is occluded, cold cardioplegic solution infused, and a suction device placed across the foramen ovale (see "Cold Cardioplegia, Controlled Aortic Root Reperfusion, and [When Needed] Warm Cardioplegic Induction" in Chapter 3). Because the Konno operation usually would not be done with a normal-sized anulus and valve, a transverse aortotomy is made just as for the operation for aortic valvotomy (see Section I of this chapter) or resection of discrete subaortic stenosis as described earlier in this section (Fig. 47-24, *A*). When it has been determined that the usual procedures will not enlarge the LV outflow tract sufficiently, the RV is opened through a transverse incision about 2 cm inferior (upstream) to the level of the pulmonary valve cusps. A right-angled clamp is passed

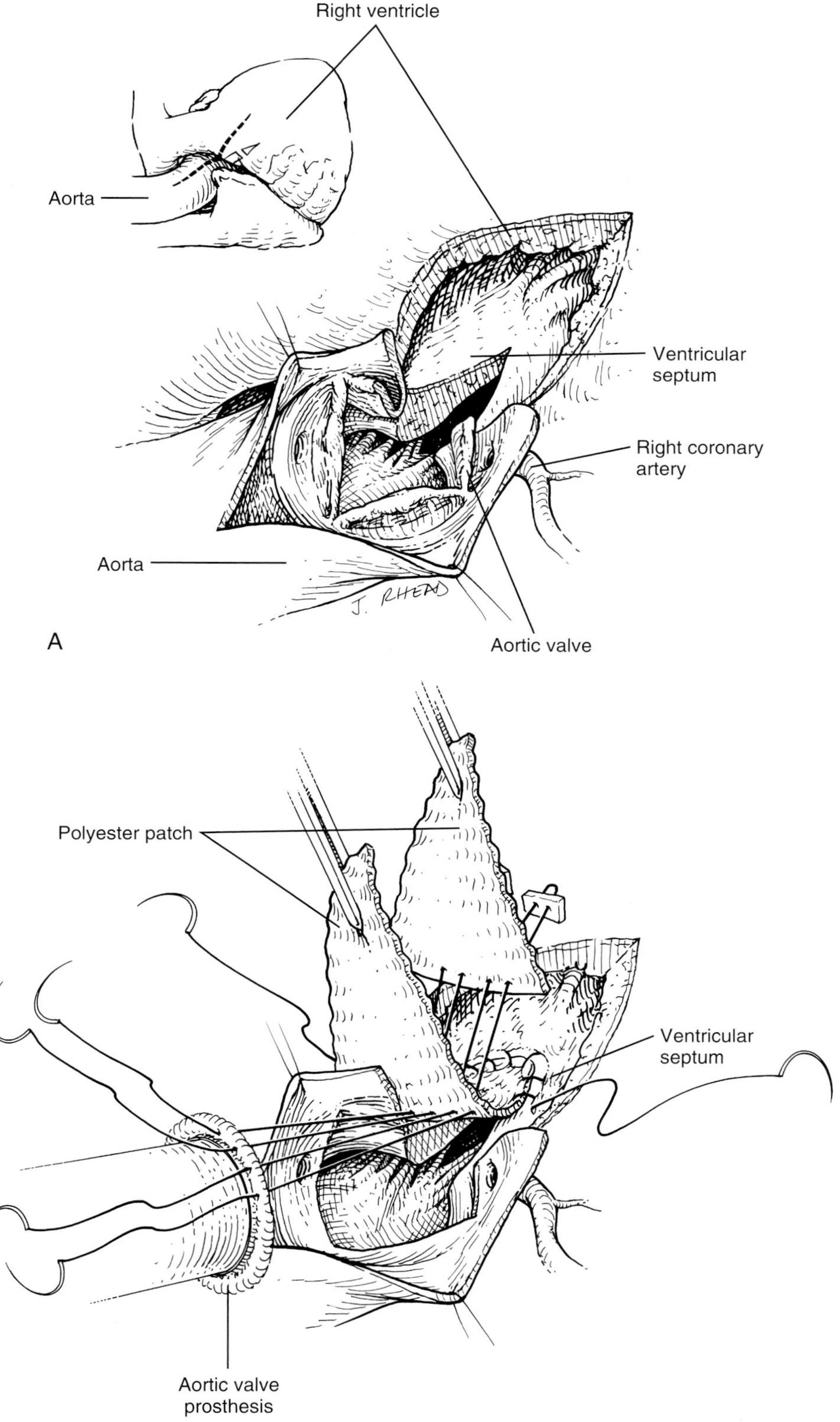

Figure 47-23 Aortoventriculoplasty (Konno operation) and aortic valve replacement. **A,** Vertical aortotomy is directed slightly rightward of the commissure between left and right coronary cusps of aortic valve. As incision is being made, orifice of right coronary artery is visualized, and incision passes clearly leftward of this. Right ventricle (RV) is opened with an oblique incision, pulmonary valve is located, and the two incisions are joined. Before or after excising aortic valve, an incision is made into base of the right coronary cusp just to the left of its nadir. This incision is extended into ventricular septum and toward apex of left ventricle. It is leftward of conduction system. **B,** Patch of collagen-coated polyester is cut into a diamond shape and attached to ventricular septum. A second triangular-shaped patch is fashioned for closing RV outflow tract. This patch and a prosthetic valve are attached to the primary patch at the level of the aortic anulus. A single suture line will suffice for this portion of the reconstruction. Prosthetic valve is attached directly to aortic anulus.

Continued

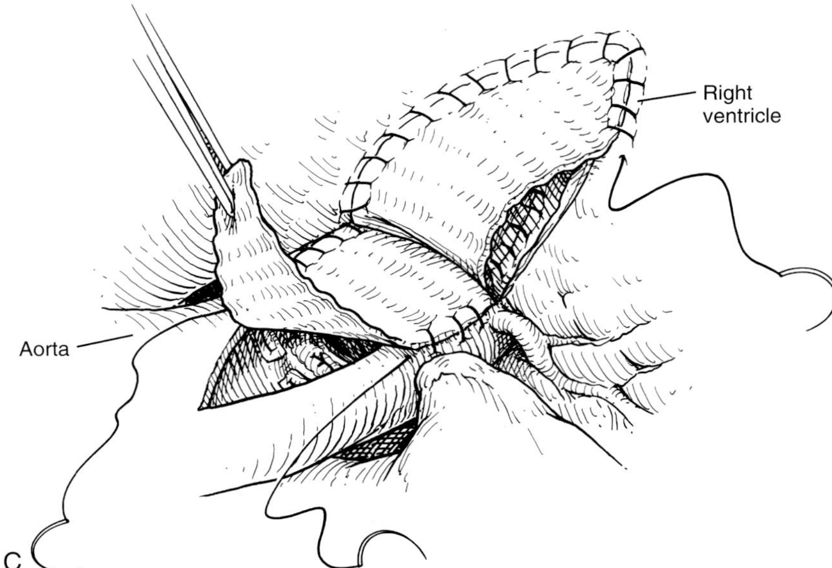

Figure 47-23, cont'd **C,** Primary patch is attached to edges of aortotomy to close aorta. The triangular patch is attached to edges of right ventriculotomy to close RV without obstructing its outflow tract.

from the aortotomy through the aortic valve and into the left side of the LV outflow tract and positioned 1 cm or so upstream to the valve. The tip of the clamp can be palpated through the ventricular septum, and at that point an incision is made in the septum from the RV side (Fig. 47-24, *B*). It is extended inferiorly for about 1 cm, parallel to the LV outflow tract and thus at an angle to the RV outflow tract. The incision through the ventricular septum is now extended superiorly with great care to keep it clearly upstream to the aortic valve (Fig. 47-24, *C*). Hypertrophied myocardium of the ventricular septum is removed to thin it out and relieve obstruction. As described for the Konno operation, an oval patch is trimmed from a double-velour collagen-coated polyester graft. This is sewn into place so as to enlarge the LV outflow tract (Fig. 47-24, *D*). The right ventriculotomy and aortotomy are closed with continuous sutures (Fig. 47-24, *E*).

Valve-Preserving Technique for Enlarging Left Ventricular Outflow Tract and Mitral Anulus

Jonas and colleagues have described an operation for enlarging the LV outflow tract and mitral anulus in patients with tunnel subaortic stenosis, often as a component of Shone syndrome and therefore associated with mitral stenosis and hypoplasia of the mitral anulus.[J4] The aortic valve, if normal, is preserved. The operation consists of an incision from the aorta through the commissure between the left and noncoronary cusps of the aortic valve. The incision is extended into the roof of the left atrium and across the anulus of the mitral valve. The mitral valve is removed and replaced with a mechanical prosthesis. A triangular patch is used to enlarge the mitral anulus and close the left atrium. The aorta is reclosed, preserving the aortic valve. Some regurgitation of the aortic valve may occur, but this is not necessarily negative, because it serves to hasten growth of the aortic anulus.

RESULTS

Early (Hospital) Death

Hospital mortality for repair of *localized* subvalvar aortic stenosis is low but has not quite approached zero. In a combined series of 314 patients compiled from the literature, with operation performed primarily in an earlier era, mortality was 4.8% (CL 3.5%-6.4%).[B7,C5,C9,C18,H3,K5,K12,L13,M13,N4,R7,S18]

Extensive operations, such as aortoventriculoplasty by the Konno or Rastan technique, have a higher mortality.[S3] In older children and young adults, aortoventriculoplasty has been performed with hospital mortalities of 5% to 15%.[B12,D9,M23,R1]

Although experience is limited, results for the Ross-Konno procedure have been good. Reddy and colleagues, Daenen and colleagues, and Brown and colleagues all report mortalities under 10% for series of 11 to 14 patients.[B26,D1,R5] The operation can be successfully accomplished even in neonates.[C1,V2]

Time-Related Survival

About 85% to 95% of heterogeneous groups of children and young adults coming to operation for discrete subvalvar aortic stenosis are alive 15 years later.[A6,B23,M31,N6,S7] Early and late deaths are virtually all related to residual LV outflow tract obstruction or subsequent efforts to relieve it, except for the few patients who die with infective endocarditis.

Incremental Risk Factors for Premature Death

Absence of formal multivariable analysis of a sizable and representative group of patients undergoing appropriate surgical treatment handicaps the effort to identify incremental risk factors in patients with subvalvar aortic stenosis.

However, the *nature of the morphology* is clearly the dominant risk factor. The tunnel form of subvalvar aortic stenosis

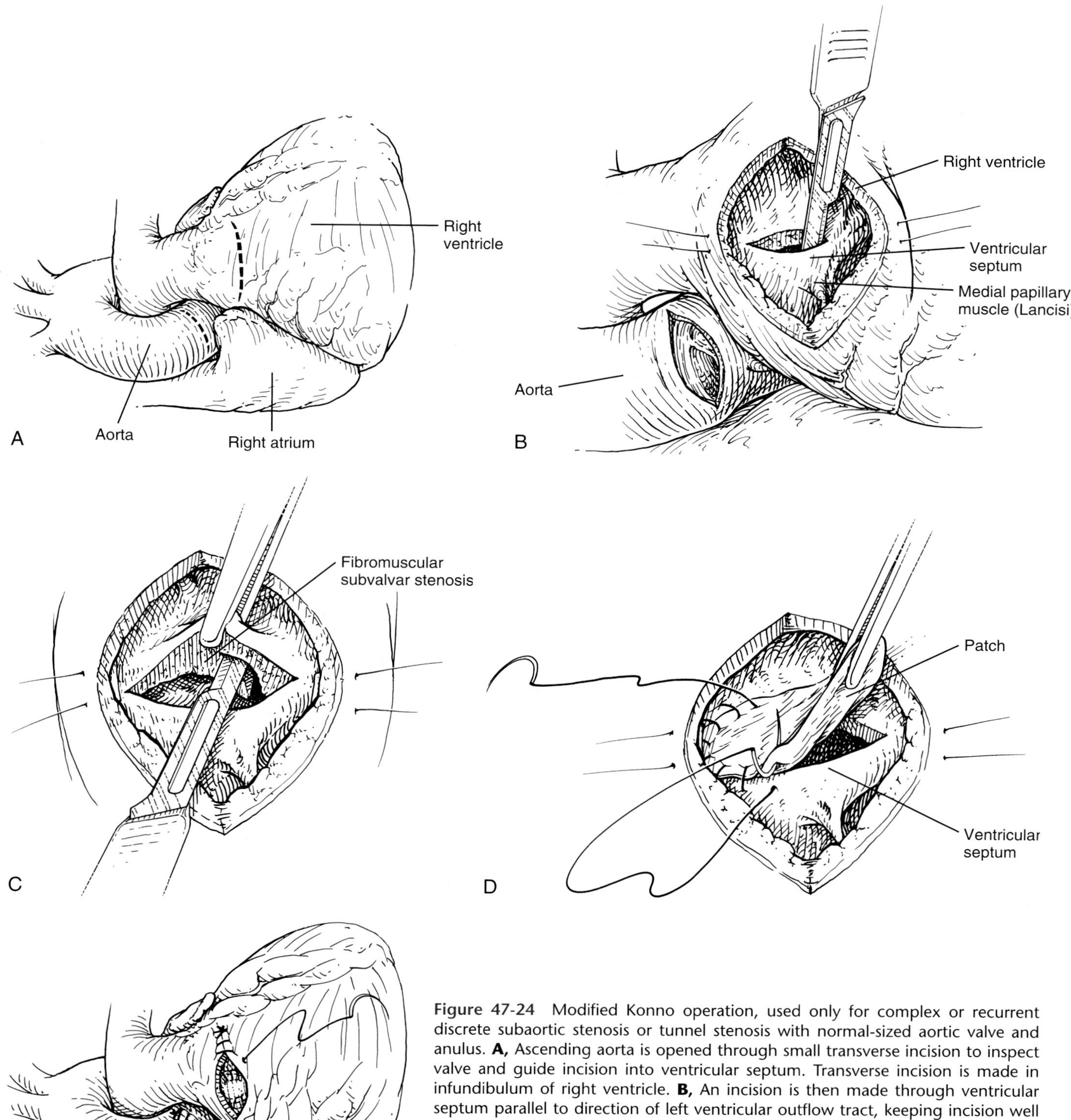

Figure 47-24 Modified Konno operation, used only for complex or recurrent discrete subaortic stenosis or tunnel stenosis with normal-sized aortic valve and anulus. **A,** Ascending aorta is opened through small transverse incision to inspect valve and guide incision into ventricular septum. Transverse incision is made in infundibulum of right ventricle. **B,** An incision is then made through ventricular septum parallel to direction of left ventricular outflow tract, keeping incision well anterior to the level of the muscle of Lancisi (i.e., well to the left) to avoid heart block or central right bundle branch block. Usually a finger or instrument is passed through aortic valve to protect it while making this incision. **C,** Fibromuscular components of subvalvar stenosis are excised as much as possible. Incision in septum is carried to within 1 to 2 mm of aortic valve anulus. **D,** Left ventricular outflow tract is widened by inserting a patch. **E,** Ventriculotomy and aortotomy are closed with continuous sutures.

and small aortic anulus increase the risk of premature death. Increased risk in the early hazard phase after operation is related to more extensive operations required for optimal therapy. Increase in the later hazard phase is related to the tendency of patients with these complex morphologies to have persistent stenosis or develop restenosis that requires complex reoperations.

Morphologic risk factors can be eliminated by using an appropriate but extensive surgical procedure as the initial operation and by making it safe and durable by optimal myocardial management and improved techniques.

Complications

Complications of the resection procedure are rare with current techniques, but include complete heart block, iatrogenic VSD, hemorrhage, and injury to the mitral valve. Reddy and colleagues reported that 1 of 11 patients (9%; CL 1.5%-28%) required a permanent pacemaker after aortoventriculoplasty.[R5]

Functional Status

Functional status of surviving patients is generally good.[B11] Of 38 surviving and traced patients in the UAB experience, 31 (82%; CL 73%-88%) were in NYHA functional class I and six (16%; CL 6%-24%) in NYHA class II. Whitmer and colleagues have shown objective evidence of improved exercise tolerance.[W7]

Hemodynamic Status

Most patients, including those with the less severe forms of tunnel stenosis, have an excellent hemodynamic result late (10 years) postoperatively. The operation usually results in a dramatic immediate gradient reduction, which is sustained or improved over the subsequent 10 years. In a few patients, gradient is mildly increased 5 to 10 years postoperatively compared with measurements in the operating room, but these data are difficult to interpret because of the variability of postrepair operating room measurements.

Sreeram and colleagues suggested that intraoperative echocardiography provides better morphologic information about obstructive lesions of the LV outflow tract and enables immediate assessment of the adequacy of operative repair.[S19] Kuralay and colleagues suggested that use of intraoperative transesophageal echocardiography in adult patients allows optimal resection of the obstruction and reduces complications such as complete heart block and VSD.[K18] Results from simple resection are less good in patients with severe tunnel stenosis.[M31] Wright and colleagues found that in six patients, mean LV-aortic gradient was reduced from 102 to 72 mmHg.[W11] This was a smaller reduction in gradient (30 ± 17 mmHg) than was achieved in patients with discrete subvalvar aortic stenosis (52 ± 40 mmHg) (P for difference $< .05$). The advantages of the Konno or modified Konno procedure in this setting are clear.

Recurrence and Reoperation

Stewart and colleagues found that about half of their patients having operations for localized and diffuse forms of subvalvar aortic stenosis required reoperation, some as long as 17 years after the initial procedure.[S27] The hazard function for reoperation increased at 5 years. Serraf and colleagues analyzed long-term results including risk factors for recurrence and reoperation in 160 patients followed for a median of 13.3 years.[S7] Freedom from reoperation at 15 years was 85%. Recurrence and reoperation were most influenced by coarctation of the aorta and immediate postoperative LV outflow tract gradient.

Brauner and colleagues followed 75 patients an average of 6.7 years after operation for subvalvar aortic stenosis.[B17] They found 18 recurrences in 15 patients (20%). The linearized hazard of recurrence and reoperation was 3.8% per patient-year. When patients had a preoperative LV outflow tract gradient greater than 40 mmHg, risk of reoperation was sevenfold higher, suggesting that early intervention or more extensive operation may prevent recurrence, reoperation, and secondary progressive aortic valve disease. In discussing these findings, Freedom conjectured that the problem of recurrence may be more complex and somehow related to abnormal cellular response in the LV outflow tract.[F7] Recalling earlier work of Ferrans and colleagues in which at least five cell layers are present in resected subvalvar fibrous rings, Freedom called for better understanding of the fundamental mechanisms of mechanical stress and genetic regulation of the endothelial surface of the LV outflow tract in subvalvar aortic stenosis.[F7,F4]

Recurrent discrete subvalvar stenosis is usually indistinguishable morphologically from the primary disease, although its recurrent rather than persistent nature has been documented.[A6] This entity of recurrent discrete subvalvar stenosis is to be clearly distinguished from persistent subvalvar stenosis after an inadequate initial operation, although their effect and treatment are the same.

Aortic Regurgitation

Some investigators have suggested that aortic regurgitation may progress after a satisfactory operation.[C9] Typically, however, aortic regurgitation remains trivial or mild unless endocarditis occurs.[H3,K12] Serraf and colleagues found that relief of subvalvar aortic stenosis improved the degree of aortic regurgitation in 86% of patients (CL 80%-91%) with preoperative aortic regurgitation.[S7]

INDICATIONS FOR OPERATION

Because obstruction from localized congenital subvalvar aortic stenosis tends to progress rather rapidly, and because the propensity for sudden death when it becomes severe is presumably the same as in severe congenital valvar aortic stenosis, operation is advisable whenever the stenosis is moderate (LV-aortic gradient > 50 mmHg) or severe. When the stenosis is severe (gradient > 100 mmHg), operation without delay is indicated. Resection of the subvalvar obstruction is usually the initial procedure of choice.

When the diagnosis has been made but obstruction is mild (LV-aortic gradient less than 50 mmHg), reevaluation with echocardiography is indicated every 6 months because rapid progression can occur. However, some evidence indicates that intervention at an earlier age and at a lower gradient (30 mmHg) may improve late results, depending on the extent of relief of obstruction at the initial operation.[P4,R9]

When discrete subvalvar stenosis is long (tunnel stenosis), and perhaps particularly when it is recurrent, simple resection is usually not effective. In these circumstances, an initial modified Konno operation is indicated.

When there are multiple levels of LV outflow tract obstruction or major associated cardiac anomalies, the general indications previously described pertain, but each patient must be considered with respect to individual morphology and circumstances. The Ross-Konno aortoventriculoplasty is the most generally applicable procedure, because the autograft may grow, and if it does it is the preferred technique in young patients. Either the Konno procedure or the "mini" aortic root replacement may also be used.

SPECIAL SITUATIONS AND CONTROVERSIES

Type of Operation

Simple resection of a discrete subaortic membrane (or shelf) has been recommended by some as equivalent to membrane resection plus transaortic myectomy in terms of likelihood of restenosis.[A5,M15,S26] However, Lupinetti and colleagues and Barkhordarian and colleagues[B2] found that adding septal myectomy to resection of discrete subvalvar aortic stenosis reduced the frequency of reoperation.[L16]

Aortoseptal Approach for Tunnel Stenosis

The modified Konno procedure provides only a limited exposure of the subvalvar area. Vouhe and colleagues have used an "aortoseptal approach" similar to the Konno operation, but without the need to replace the aortic valve.[V4,V5] A longitudinal incision in the aorta is carried obliquely down toward the top of the adjacent portions of right and left aortic cusps. A roughly transverse incision is made in the RV infundibulum, beginning at a point just over this. The aortic and RV incisions come together just over the top of the left anterior fibrous trigone. The aortic "anulus" is now divided through the trigone, going exactly between adjacent extremities of left and right cusps; this can be done without damaging the cusps. This incision is carried well into the ventricular septum, as in the Konno procedure, opening the LV outflow tract widely. After resecting obstructing tissue, the septal incision is closed, the left anterior fibrous trigone reconstructed, and the RV and aortic incisions closed. The authors also describe widening the LV outflow tract with a polyester patch in closing the septal incision, as in the modified Konno procedure. The aortic valve is replaced if it is part of the obstructing process or if it is regurgitant.

Left Ventricular–Aortic Conduit

The LV-aortic conduit (apicoaortic conduit) operation has enjoyed some popularity in the past.[B8,C22] Norwood and colleagues reported a hospital mortality of 22% (CL 8%-45%) with use of this technique in infants.[N6] Complications both early and late postoperatively are common, and 4 (24%; CL 12%-39%) of 17 hospital survivors reported by Brown and colleagues required reoperation, as did 7 (78%; CL 55%-92%) of 9 hospital survivors reported by Di Donato and colleagues.[B24,D10] Currently, few indications exist for the procedure in cases of congenital aortic stenosis. Cooley and colleagues revived interest in apicoaortic conduits with a report of its use in seven patients with complex LV outflow tract obstruction.[C20] They used a transthoracic approach to avoid redo sternotomy and compromise to coronary arteries, the conduction system, and other valves. Two patients died of respiratory insufficiency (29%; CL 10%-55%). The others survived and were improved by operation.

Section III Congenital Supravalvar Aortic Stenosis

DEFINITION

Congenital supravalvar aortic stenosis is an obstruction caused by localized or diffuse narrowing of the aortic lumen commencing immediately above the aortic valve.

HISTORICAL NOTE

The first description of supravalvar aortic stenosis is attributed to Mencarelli in 1930.[M16] It was seldom recognized, however, until Denie and Verheugt emphasized in 1958 that supravalvar stenosis could be differentiated from other varieties of aortic stenosis by retrograde arterial catheterization.[D7] In 1959, Morrow and colleagues pointed out the usefulness of angiography in diagnosis.[M30]

In 1961, Williams, Barratt-Boyes, and Lowe described the association of supravalvar aortic stenosis with unusual "elfin" facies and mental retardation,[W8] a syndrome that was soon confirmed by others.[B9,F2] This constellation of signs and symptoms has since been referred to as *Williams syndrome* or *elfin facies syndrome*. In 1964, Beuren and colleagues reported 10 cases of this syndrome, all associated with multiple peripheral pulmonary artery stenoses.[B10] Watson and Bourassa and Campeau had also noted this association a year earlier.[B16,W3] The similarity between the facies of patients with supravalvar aortic stenosis and severe infantile hypercalcemia was noted in 1963 by Hooft and colleagues and Black and Bonham Carter.[B13,H12] Garcia and colleagues reported the first patient with Williams syndrome and a documented history of infantile hypercalcemia.[G3] The occurrence of a familial form of supravalvar stenosis without elfin facies was reported by Sissman and colleagues in 1959.[S15] Nakanishi and colleagues reported supravalvular aortic stenosis in monozygotic twins without phenotypic features of Williams syndrome.[N1]

Successful operation for supravalvar stenosis using patch graft enlargement of the noncoronary sinus of Valsalva was reported by McGoon and colleagues in 1961,[M14] the first patient being operated on in 1956. Before this publication, successful procedures using a similar technique had been performed.[G13,S24,W8] In 1960, Hara and colleagues successfully performed an excision and end-to-end aortic anastomosis in a patient with supravalvar aortic stenosis,[H2] as did Chard and Cartmill.[C6] Hancock satisfactorily relieved the stenosis by excising the intimal ridge without patch enlargement.[H1] Neither of these procedures is currently recommended.

Most surgeons have placed the patch into the noncoronary sinus of Valsalva,[C24,D2,M14,S24] but in Williams and colleagues' original report, it was placed into the right sinus to relieve any narrowing between the right cusp and aortic wall.[W8] Doty and colleagues recommended using a double-flanged patch that extends into both noncoronary and right sinuses, incising the stenosing ring at points 180 degrees apart. Resecting the remaining stenotic ring above the left coronary sinus may be performed to enhance the repair.[D14,H4] Their report introduced the concept of more anatomic repair of the aortic root and led to a number of modifications of the classic operations for supravalvar aortic stenosis. Subsequent modification of their extended aortoplasty technique[D13] employed incision in the left coronary sinus and repositioning of the commissure between left and right coronary cusps of the aortic valve to achieve a more anatomic repair. Steinberg and colleagues proposed a modification of extended aortoplasty in which an additional separate incision is made across the sinutubular junction into the left coronary sinus of Valsalva to the right of the left coronary ostium.[S25] This incision is closed around an oval-shaped prosthetic patch, and the primary Y-shaped incision is closed with a pantaloon-shaped patch.

Brom introduced an even more symmetric aortoplasty, enlarging all three sinuses of Valsalva by a three-patch technique. The first patient was operated on using this method in 1978, but the technique was not published until 1988.[B22] The aorta is transected distal to the obstruction and incisions made into each of the three sinuses. Pericardial patches are inserted into each of the aortic sinuses to relieve the obstruction while retaining normal geometric relationships of the aortic root.

Myers and Waldhausen and colleagues[M33] described a technique of repair that is symmetric and obviates need for prosthetic patch material. The aorta is divided distal to the obstruction, and incisions are made into each aortic sinus. Distally, three incisions are made in the ascending aorta corresponding to the position of the commissures of the aortic valve. The aorta is mobilized sufficiently to advance the ascending aorta into the incisions in the aortic root.

MORPHOGENESIS AND MORPHOLOGY

Supravalvar Stenosis

Morphogenesis

The vascular pathology of supravalvar aortic stenosis and Williams syndrome results from mutations involving the elastin gene on chromosome 7q11.23.[K10,L12,T1] These mutations include intragenic deletions, translocations, and complete deletion of the elastin gene, suggesting that a quantitative reduction in elastin during vascular development is pathogenically important. Point mutations of the elastin gene (ELN) are especially important in supravalvar aortic stenosis. Stamm and colleagues found Williams syndrome in 61% of patients treated operatively for supravalvar aortic stenosis, and more recently the clinical diagnosis was supported by the chromosome 7q11.23 abnormality.[S20,S21]

Morphology

Stenosis may be localized or diffuse.[P5] Most often the narrowing is *localized* to the supravalvar area of the aorta just above or at the most superior level of the attachments of the valve commissures.[D7,W8] Narrowing of the aorta at this point is usually apparent externally; in association with some dilatation of the sinuses of Valsalva and absence of poststenotic dilatation, this produces an hourglass appearance. In addition, variable intimal thickening in the form of an internal shelf increases the stenosis and may obstruct or even close the ostium of the left main coronary artery (see "Coronary Arteries" later in this section).

Less often, the narrowing is *diffuse*, extending throughout the length of the ascending aorta and even beyond into the arch and into the origins of brachiocephalic arteries.[N3]

Other Aortic Lesions

Supravalvar aortic stenosis should be considered a complex anomaly of the aortic root. Too often the surgeon focuses attention on only the defect at the sinus rim; narrowing and thickening of the sinus rim are fundamental to the morphology, but this defect involves more anomalies. Thickening of the aortic media and intimal hyperplasia reduces aortic circumference at the sinus rim. The morphologic process may not be circumferential but may involve only the sinus rim over one or two sinuses. The sinus of Valsalva beneath the thick and short sinus rim may be abnormal or hypoplastic. Ostia of the coronary arteries may be obstructed not only by the overhanging thick sinus rim, but also by an aortic cusp that becomes bound down or fused to the aorta at the sinus rim.

The aortic valve cusps are reported to be thickened in about 30% of patients with supravalvar aortic stenosis.[D14] True valvar stenosis resulting from leaflet fusion is rare.[R4] The aortic valves are actually involved in every case, because the relationships of the commissures are distorted as they are drawn close together by the shortened and thickened sinus rim. This distortion produces a characteristic buckling of the free edge of the aortic cusp. The free edge of the aortic cusp has normal length in most young patients. It buckles as it accommodates to the shortened space at the sinus rim. The buckled aortic cusps become part of the obstruction within a space too small to accommodate them properly. Thickening of the edges of the aortic cusps, however, is eventually produced by turbulent blood flow from stenosis at the sinus rim. The thickened valve cusps then become an even more important part of the stenosing process.

The aortic anulus may occasionally be hypoplastic.[K9] Subvalvar stenosis of the LV outflow tract may also be part of this total deformity of the aortic root.[D6,K9] McElhinney and colleagues focused attention on the fact that supravalvar aortic stenosis involves not only the supravalvar aorta but the entire aortic root in the 36 patients who were operated on consecutively over 6 years.[M12] Procedures were required on the aortic valve in 39%, which agrees closely with the series reported by Delius and colleagues.[D6] In that series, resection of the subvalvar LV outflow tract was performed in 11 patients, and two patients underwent procedures on the coronary arteries. Four patients had aortic root deformity so severe that the entire root was replaced with a pulmonary autograft (Ross procedure). The authors compared their series to six others and found similar high frequency of associated pathology and LV outflow tract procedures.

Bicuspid aortic valve is common (6 of 15 patients, 40% in the series of Delius and colleagues[D6]).

Coronary Arteries

The aortic valve cusp free edges near the aortic wall may become adherent to the intimal shelf, producing stenosis at the entry into the sinus of Valsalva, thereby obstructing coronary flow. This is more common in the left sinus[D7,P5,R4] but can occur in the right.[W8] When extreme, the proliferative process of the intimal ridge may extend into and narrow or even obstruct the ostium of the left coronary sinus.[M6,T3] Stamm and colleagues found partial adhesion of the leaflets to the stenosing ridge in 54% of patients with supravalvar aortic stenosis.[S22] In 30%, the valve leaflets were thickened and less mobile than normal. The sinuses of Valsalva were enlarged in 75% of cases. Coronary angiography demonstrated evidence of coronary ostial stenosis in 45%. The authors concluded that the entire valvular apparatus is always affected in patients with supravalvar aortic stenosis.

In the absence of obstruction to inflow into the sinus of Valsalva or of ostial stenosis, the coronary arteries are exposed to a high pressure and show dilatation, tortuosity, medial hypertrophy,[N3] and early onset of arteriosclerosis.

Other Cardiac Anomalies

The most common associated anomaly consists of multiple stenoses in the peripheral pulmonary arteries,[B10] which may be severe enough to produce right ventricular hypertension and hypertrophy. Pulmonary valve stenosis occurs infrequently.[B16] Diffuse hypoplasia of the pulmonary trunk may be associated with diffuse hypoplasia of the aorta,[M11,S4,S29] with both arteries showing marked wall thickening and fibromuscular dysplasia histologically in association with disorganization and replacement of the elastic tissue of the media. These patients usually give a familial history, and sudden death in infancy is common.

Less common anomalies include stenosis of the origins of subclavian and carotid and rarely other major systemic arteries, coarctation of the aorta (with or without patent ductus arteriosus), and VSD. Mitral regurgitation occurs rarely, although the mitral valve may be thickened and redundant.[B4] The patient reported by Denie and Verheugt in 1958 had Marfan syndrome,[D7] which has been noted subsequently in about 5% of patients with supravalvar aortic stenosis.[P5]

CLINICAL FEATURES AND DIAGNOSTIC CRITERIA

Symptoms

Symptoms rarely develop in infancy, but appear frequently in childhood, and may appear as late as the second or third decade. They are similar to those of other types of congenital aortic stenosis, although angina may occur more often because of early-onset coronary arteriosclerosis.

Signs

Auscultatory findings are similar to those of congenital valvar aortic stenosis, and the correct diagnosis may not be possible from physical signs. An ejection click is absent, however, and the murmur and thrill tend to be situated higher than in valvar stenosis. An aortic diastolic murmur is uncommon.[L15] Blood pressure may be lower in the left arm than in the right,[C24,K9,W8] resulting from stenosis at the origin of the left subclavian artery or from a jet effect.[F11,G11] Similarly, the left carotid pulse may be diminished.[L15]

A diagnostic clinical feature may be elfin facies (Fig. 47-25), combined with reduced intelligence quotient and failure to thrive.[W8] These retarded children are characteristically small, friendly, and loquacious. Each component of the syndrome varies in severity, however, and the supravalvar stenosis may be mild or occasionally absent in patients with the typical facies.[J6] The disease in this form is always sporadic and the facies identical to severe infantile hypercalcemia. Hypercalcemia has been documented in less than 5% of these infants, although it is more common when the elfin facies is not present.[M5] Less than half of patients with congenital supravalvar aortic stenosis have elfin facies and mental retardation. In the remainder without elfin facies, the disease may be sporadic or familial.

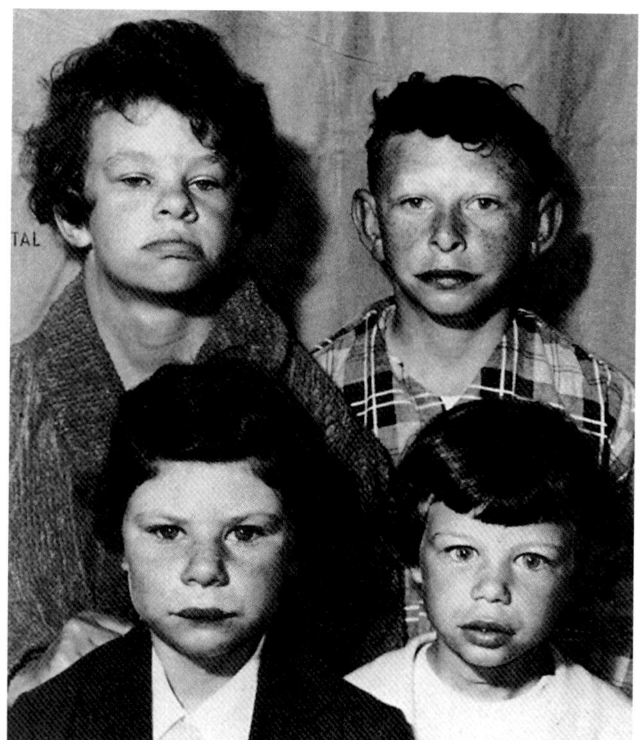

Figure 47-25 Photograph of four children with elfin facies and supravalvar congenital aortic stenosis reported from GLH in 1961. Appearance is characterized by depressed nasal bridge with anteverted nares, thick lips, mandibular recession, short palpebral fissures, and medial eyebrow flare. Dental malocclusion is present. (From Williams and colleagues.[W8])

Echocardiography

Diagnosis and definition of severity can be made with two-dimensional echocardiography and color flow Doppler examination (Fig. 47-26).

Cardiac Catheterization and Angiography

The site of pressure change can be localized on withdrawal of a catheter from LV to aorta. Morphology of the supravalvar stenosis can be outlined on angiography (Fig. 47-26, *C*, and Fig. 47-27), and coexisting anomalies can be identified (Fig. 47-28). For these last reasons, cardiac catheterization and angiocardiography are usually indicated.

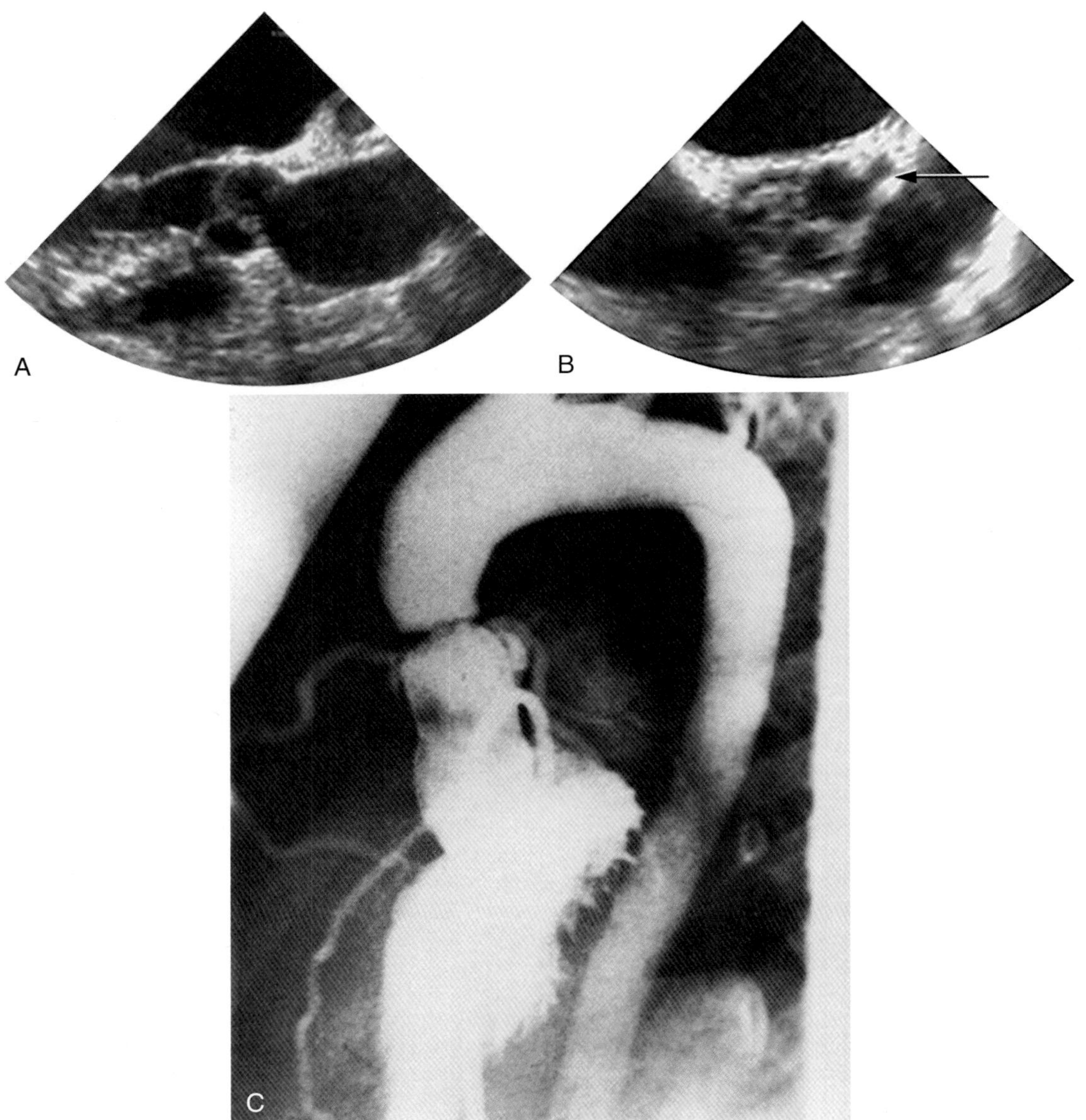

Figure 47-26 Localized supravalvar aortic stenosis. **A,** Two-dimensional echocardiogram demonstrates narrowing of aorta at sinus rim (hourglass deformity). **B,** Free edges of aortic valve are buckled and part of the stenosing process. Left coronary artery appears near stenosed sinus rim *(arrow)*. **C,** Left ventriculogram and aortogram in long-axial position shows stenosis of aorta at sinus rim and close proximity of coronary arteries to the stenosing process.

NATURAL HISTORY

The supravalvar form is the least common type of congenital aortic stenosis. Genders are equally affected.

In infants with elfin facies, mental retardation, and combined congenital supravalvar aortic stenosis and pulmonary stenoses of the diffuse variety, sudden death is common early in life.[S29] Sudden death can occur in all age groups, presumably from severe LV outflow tract obstruction and coronary artery disease.

Progression of supravalvar aortic stenosis may be more rapid and severe than in congenital valvar aortic stenosis.[G8,W9] Because the lesion is uncommon in adults, most untreated patients probably die before reaching adult life.[P1] Death before adult life is particularly likely to occur in those with elfin facies, because they constitute only 11% of adults but 60% of children with the anomaly. Some of the children with elfin facies and the severe form of infantile hypercalcemia die from complications of hypercalcemia. However, a longitudinal study by Hickey and colleagues indicates a more favorable prognosis for children with moderate (mean LV outflow tract systolic gradient 30 mmHg) supravalvar aortic stenosis. Many such children, particularly those with Williams syndrome, show gradual regression of gradient without intervention.[H10]

Kitchiner and colleagues followed 81 patients with supravalvar aortic stenosis from 1 to 29 years (median 8.3 years); 40 patients (49%) had Williams syndrome, 19 (23%) had additional levels of LV outflow tract obstruction, and 47 (58%) had surgical intervention, 20% in the first year after diagnosis.[K14] The data indicated that 88% of the patients would be operated on within 30 years. Predicted survival at 30 years after presentation was 66%.

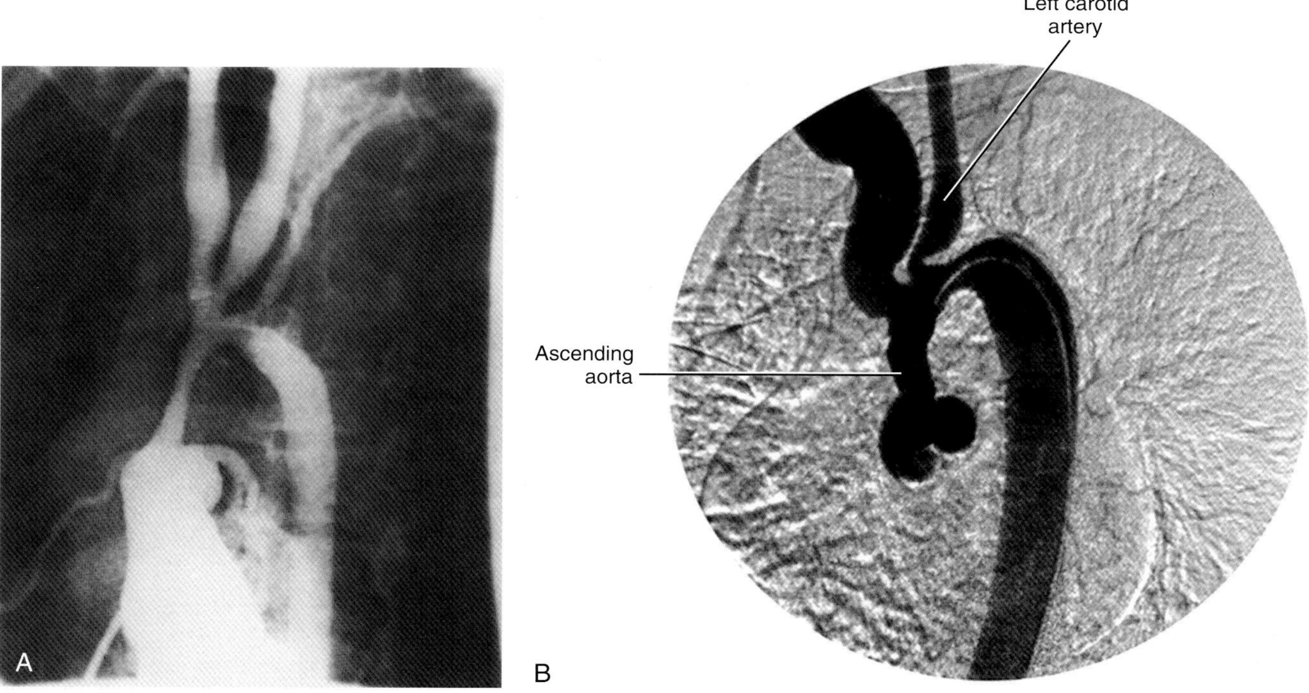

Figure 47-27 Left ventriculogram and aortogram in diffuse supravalvar aortic stenosis. **A,** Ascending aorta becomes diffusely narrow at the level of the aortic valve commissures, just beyond area of right and left coronary arteries. Narrowing extends into transverse arch. **B,** In this patient, diffuse supravalvar stenosis extends through aortic arch. Origin of left carotid artery is stenotic, and left subclavian artery is occluded.

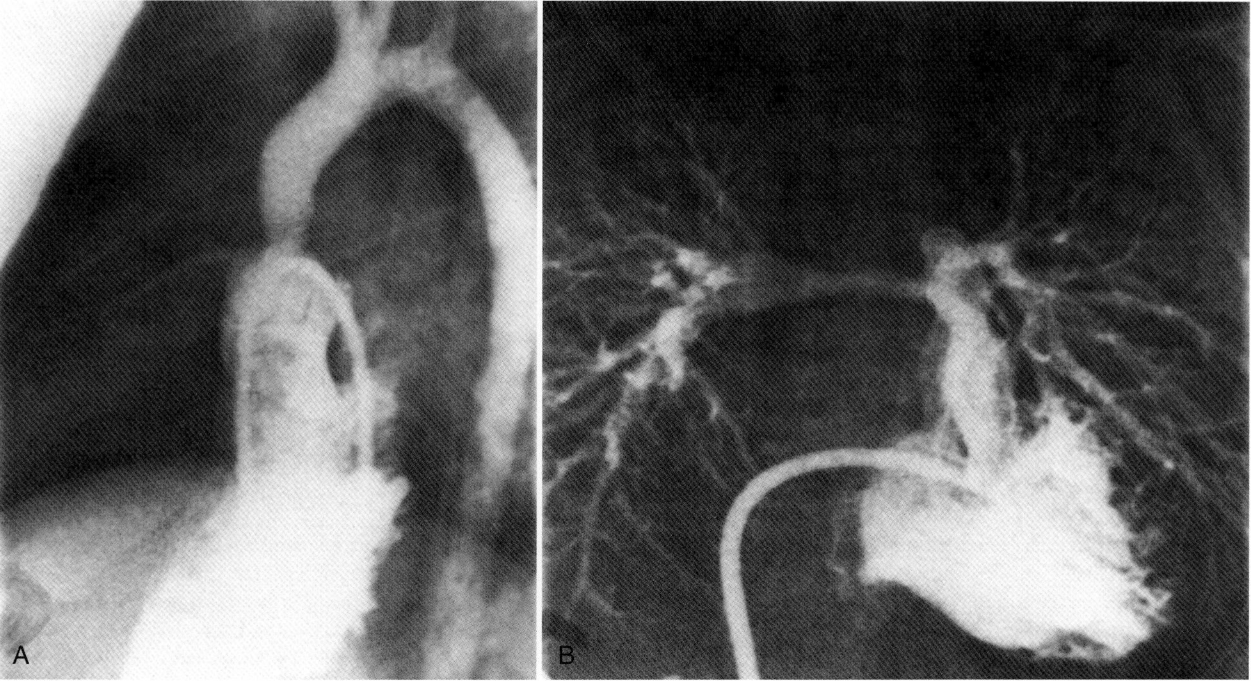

Figure 47-28 Cineangiograms of localized supravalvar aortic stenosis with coexisting diffuse right and left pulmonary artery narrowing. **A,** Left ventriculogram and aortogram in lateral projection in long-axial position. **B,** Right ventriculogram in posteroanterior projection.

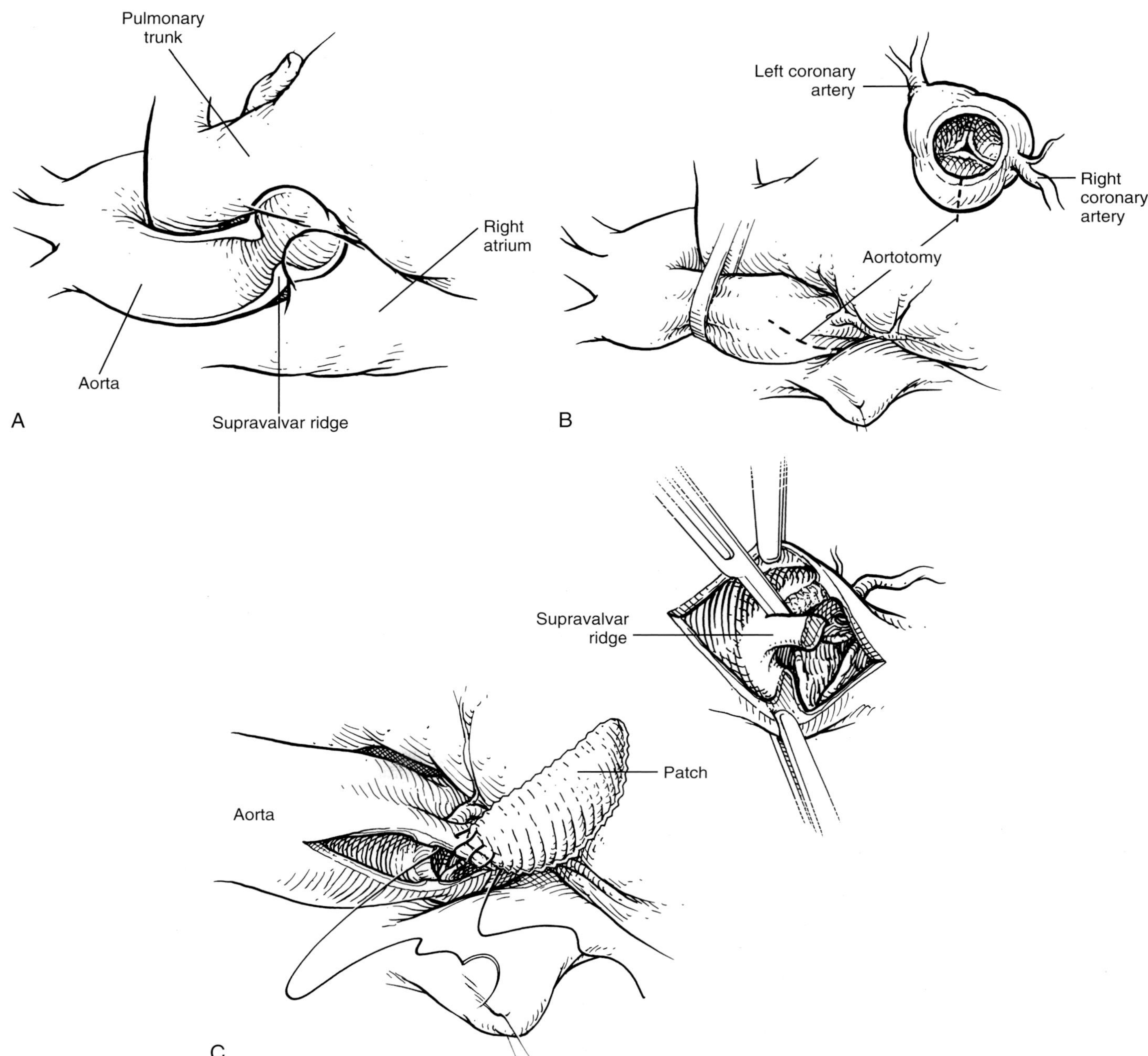

Figure 47-29 Repair of congenital supravalvar aortic stenosis. **A,** External hourglass deformity of aorta is usually less prominent than internal narrowing. **B,** When prominent, as usually occurs, this ridge is excised. **C,** Supravalvar narrowing is eliminated by incorporating an enlarging patch of pericardium (or polyester) into closure of incision.

Interestingly, the peripheral pulmonary stenosis seems to decrease in severity as patients age.[G8,W9]

TECHNIQUE OF OPERATION

Repair of Localized Type

Classic Repair

The external hourglass deformity of the aorta is usually less prominent than the internal narrowing caused by the thick ridge of the sinutubular junction (Fig. 47-29, *A*). The operation is begun exactly as described for the procedure of valvotomy for congenital valvar aortic stenosis in Section I of this chapter. After occluding the aorta and infusing cold cardioplegic solution, the aortotomy is made.

The aorta is opened above the valve and the incision carried into the noncoronary sinus of Valsalva. The aortic valve and subvalvar areas are examined to exclude obstruction at those levels. The intimal shelf is resected (Fig. 47-29, *B*), in part to ensure adequate inflow into the sinuses of Valsalva. A diamond-shaped patch of pericardium or collagen-coated knitted polyester or polytetrafluoroethylene (PTFE) is then incorporated into the incision with a running polypropylene suture (Fig. 47-29, *C*). The patch must be of sufficient size to enlarge the aortic diameter to normal. The remainder of the procedure is completed as usual (see "Completing Cardiopulmonary Bypass" in Section III of Chapter 2).

Pressure is measured in the LV and ascending aorta to determine whether there is any residual gradient across the repair. Intraoperative echocardiography with color flow Doppler examination should be done to assess the degree of turbulence over the repair and determine whether aortic valve regurgitation is present.

Extended Aortoplasty (Doty)

The operation is performed on cardiopulmonary bypass (CPB) using a single two-stage venous uptake cannula, with oxygenated blood returned to a cannula in the ascending aorta (see "Preparation for Cardiopulmonary Bypass" in Section III of Chapter 2). The aorta is occluded and cold cardioplegia infused through a cannula in the coronary sinus (see "Technique of Retrograde Infusion" in Chapter 3). A vent catheter is placed in the right superior pulmonary vein.

An oblique incision is made in the aorta, extending it across the obstructing ridge at the sinutubular junction and into the middle of the noncoronary sinus. The primary incision is also extended to the left to cross the sinutubular junction into the right sinus of Valsalva just anterior to the commissure between the left and right coronary cusps of the aortic valve (Fig. 47-30, *A*). The incisions into the aortic root are nearly directly opposite each other at the sinutubular junction, allowing the aorta to be divided into almost equal portions. The anterior portion of the aortic root that contains the origin of the right coronary artery may move forward (anterior) to widen the space at the sinutubular junction. Buckling of the aortic valve leaflets is relieved as the halves of the aorta are separated anteriorly and posteriorly. The thick ridge of the supravalvar stenosis located above the left coronary sinus is excised (Fig. 47-30, *B*). A crimped tubular polyester graft whose diameter approximates that of the ascending aorta is used for reconstruction. About half of the circumference of the graft is used, and the length should be sufficient to place enough graft into the aortotomy to prevent the anterior portion of the aortic root from being pulled down into the plane of the aorta. A wedge is removed from the graft to accommodate the portion of the aorta containing the right coronary artery. The resulting two limbs of the graft are used to widen both the right and noncoronary sinuses of Valsalva (see Fig. 47-30, *B*) partially closing the aortotomy; the distal end of the graft fills the aortotomy in the ascending aorta.

Entrapment of the left coronary cusp of the aortic valve may be treated not only by resection of the supravalvar thickened rim but also by incision into the left sinus of Valsalva to the left of the left coronary ostium (Fig. 47-30, *C*). This incision mobilizes the commissure between the left and the right coronary cusps and allows the commissure to be moved anteriorly for greater symmetry of the position of the three commissures. The pantaloon-shaped patch is attached to the adventitia of the aorta behind the commissure between the left and right cusps at the anular level. The commissure is attached directly to the patch to achieve equal distance between the three commissures at the sinus rim (see Fig. 47-30, *C*).

Although this operation represents a more symmetric form of repair of supravalvar aortic stenosis than the classic one-patch repair, accurate restoration of the dimensions at the sinutubular junction relative to the aortic anulus is difficult to accomplish.

Three-Patch Repair (Brom)

The operation is performed on CPB using a single two-stage venous uptake cannula and an arterial cannula in the ascending aorta (see "Preparation for Cardiopulmonary Bypass" in Section III of Chapter 2). The aorta is occluded and cold cardioplegia infused (see "Cold Cardioplegia, Controlled Aortic Root Reperfusion, and [When Needed] Warm Cardioplegic Induction" in Chapter 3).

The aorta is divided above the sinutubular junction. Three longitudinal incisions are made through the area of stenosis into the aortic root (Fig. 47-31, *A*). The first is placed in the middle of the noncoronary sinus of Valsalva. The other two are determined by position of the coronary arteries. Incision into the left coronary sinus is usually to the right of the left coronary ostium, and incision into the right sinus is usually to the left of the right coronary ostium. The incisions end about halfway into the sinus aorta, but may go deeper if necessary to achieve good separation of the edges of the aorta at the stenosing ridge. Three triangular patches of autologous pericardium are inserted (Fig. 47-31, *B*). Width of the patch at the sinutubular junction should restore correct dimensions. The diameter at the sinutubular junction should be 10% to 15% less than the diameter at the ventriculoaortic junction ("anulus"). Larger patches achieve a greater diameter but carry the risk of reducing the coaptation area of the aortic valve by lateral displacement of commissural attachments of the valve, possibly resulting in aortic regurgitation. The reconstructed aortic root is anastomosed to the ascending aorta.

Sliding Aortoplasty (Myers-Waldhausen)

The operation is performed on CPB. The aorta is divided above the supravalvar obstruction. Three longitudinal incisions are made through the area of stenosis into the three sinuses of Valsalva as described for the "Three-Patch Repair (Brom)" in the preceding text. Three incisions are made into the ascending aorta distally and correspond exactly to the commissures of the aortic valve (Fig. 47-32, *A*). The ascending aorta is mobilized extensively to allow it to be displaced inferiorly so as to slide the flaps of the ascending aorta into the incisions in the aortic root in a "V-Y" pattern. A continuous stitch of monofilament suture is started at the nadir of each incision in the sinus aorta. The corresponding flap of ascending aorta is attached to the edges of the incision in the sinus aorta by sewing from the nadir to the top of the commissural attachment of the aortic valve (Fig. 47-32, *B*). The diameter of the aortic root at the sinutubular junction will be determined by the diameter of the ascending aorta and should approximate normal dimensions (see "Dimensions of Normal Cardiac and Great Artery Pathways" in Chapter 1). No prosthetic material is employed in this repair.

Repair of Diffuse Type

The operation proceeds as described for the localized type, except that the skin incision is carried about 2 cm more superiorly than usual. The femoral artery is exposed for arterial cannulation. Origins of the brachiocephalic, left common carotid, and left subclavian arteries and the transverse portion

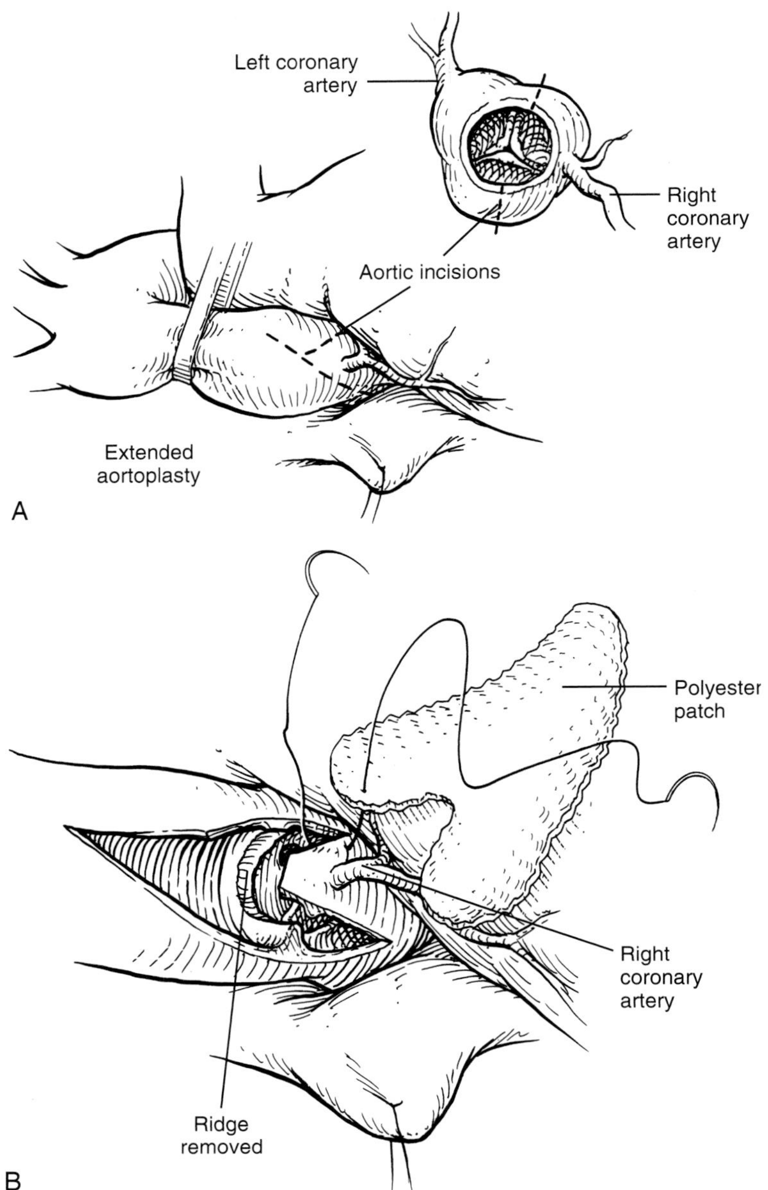

Figure 47-30 Repair of supravalvar aortic stenosis by extended aortoplasty (Doty). **A,** Oblique incision is made in aorta extending across supravalvar ridge into middle of noncoronary sinus of Valsalva. A second incision is made as an inverted "Y" into right sinus, just anterior to commissure between left and right coronary cusps. This divides the stenosing ring at two points almost directly opposite on circumference of ring. **B,** Supravalvar ridge is removed from above left coronary sinus of Valsalva. A patch is fashioned from a tubular polyester graft approximately the diameter of aorta. A wedge is removed to create two limbs on the patch and accommodate position of right coronary ostium (pantaloon patch). Patch is attached to edges of aortotomy in right and noncoronary sinuses of Valsalva and to primary incision in aorta. Sufficient length of graft must be placed into aortotomy to allow portion of aorta containing right coronary ostium to separate anteriorly from primary aortic incision.

of the aortic arch are dissected below and above the left brachiocephalic vein.

CPB is established with arterial inflow to the patient through the femoral artery, and body temperature is taken to 18°C. The operating table is placed with the patient in moderate Trendelenburg position. The aorta is occluded while cold cardioplegia is infused. Aortic reconstruction is done with hypothermic circulatory arrest (see Section IV of Chapter 2).

A longitudinal incision is made in the ascending aorta and carried well down into one or two sinuses of Valsalva, as in repair of the localized form. Any intimal ridge above each sinus of Valsalva is excised as described for the localized type. The incision is carried up the ascending aorta, which is usually thick walled and has a small lumen, and around onto the aortic arch, then if necessary into the upper descending thoracic aorta (Fig. 47-33, *A*). Incisions are made across any stenosis present at the origin of the brachiocephalic and left common carotid arteries, and intimal proliferations dissected away. Thickened interna and media is dissected away from the aortic adventitia by endarterectomy (Fig. 47-33, *B*). A patch of double-velour collagen-coated polyester or PTFE is

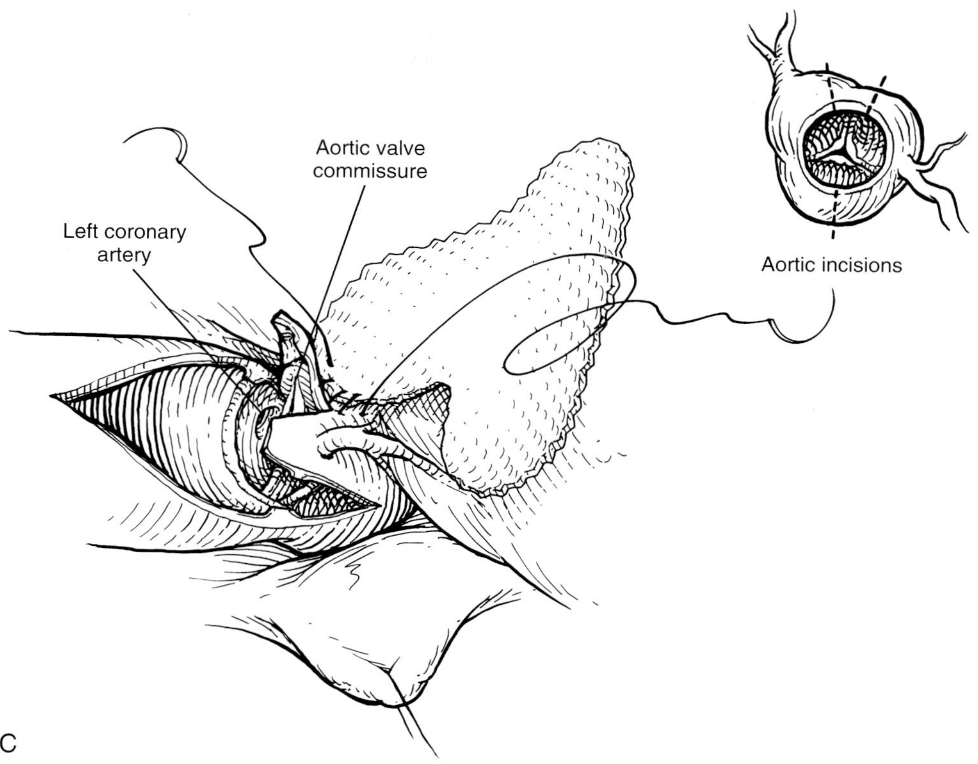

Figure 47-30, cont'd **C,** Greater symmetry of the repair may be accomplished by a third incision into left coronary sinus of Valsalva just posterior to commissure between right and left sinuses. This incision mobilizes the commissure so that it can move anteriorly to achieve better spacing between commissures of aortic valve and to achieve better configuration of left cusp. Pantaloon patch is attached to adventitia of aorta behind commissure at level of "anulus." Commissure is attached directly to inside of patch.

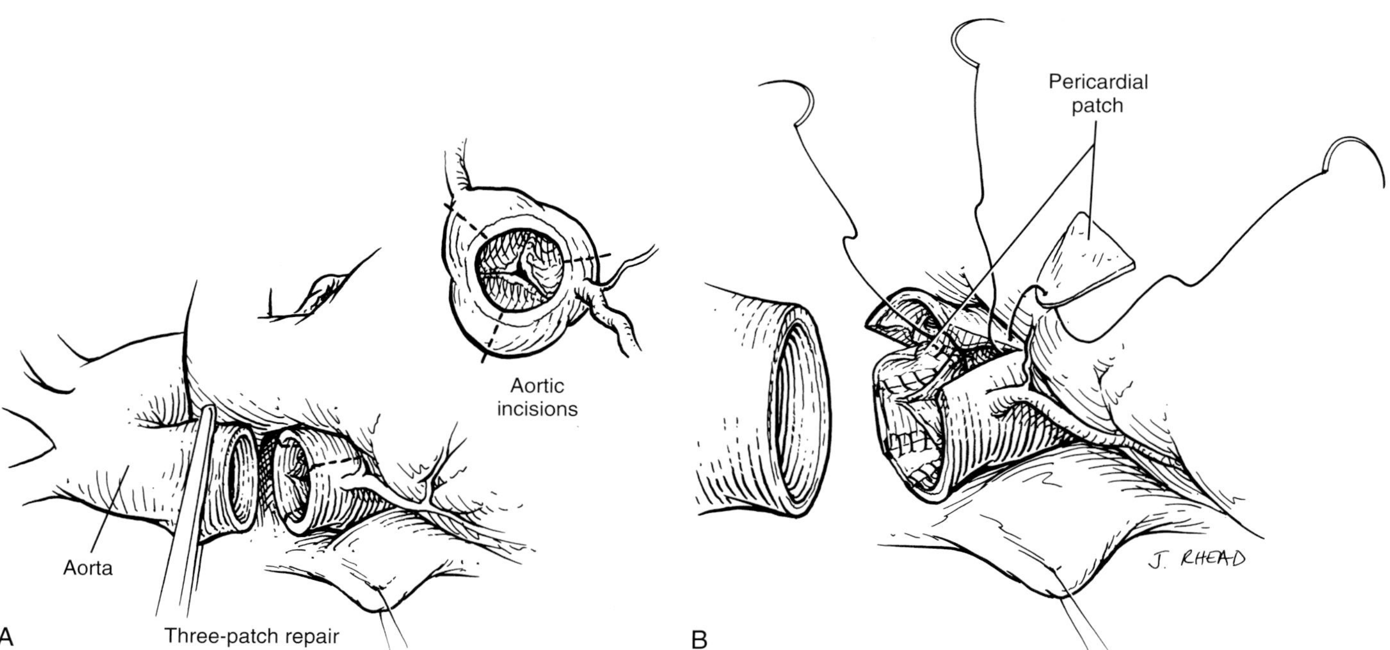

Figure 47-31 Repair of supravalvar aortic stenosis by three-patch technique (Brom). **A,** Aorta is divided above supravalvar stenosing ridge. Three longitudinal incisions are made through the area of stenosis. First is made into middle of noncoronary sinus of Valsalva; second is into left coronary sinus to the right of left coronary ostium; third is into right sinus to the left of right coronary ostium. **B,** Three triangular patches of autologous pericardium are fashioned for insertion to each incision. Width of patches at the top should restore correct dimensions of the sinutubular junction, or 10% to 15% less than the diameter of the ventriculoaortic junction ("anulus"). These patches are attached to aorta by continuous stitches of fine polypropylene suture. Ends of aorta are reanastomosed.

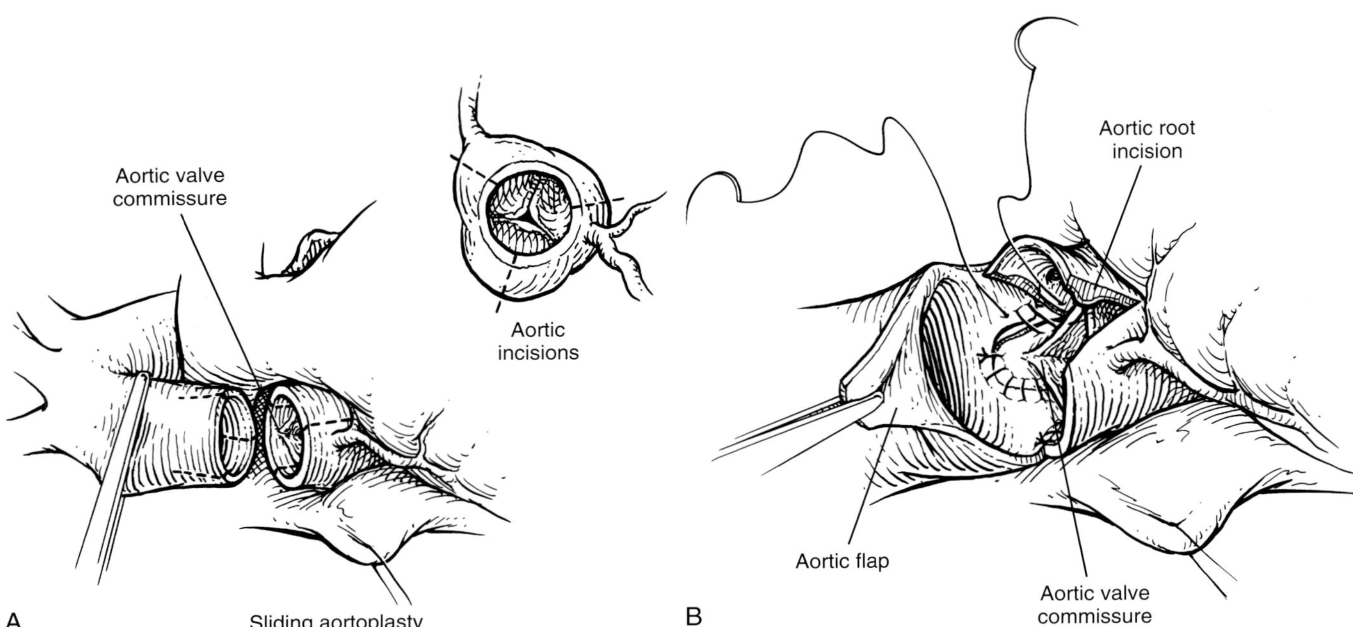

Figure 47-32 Repair of supravalvar aortic stenosis by sliding aortoplasty (Myers-Waldhausen). **A,** Aorta is divided above supravalvar ridge. Three incisions are made in proximal aorta through the stenosing ring into sinuses of Valsalva (see Fig. 47-31). Three incisions are made into distal ascending aorta at points corresponding exactly to position of commissures of aortic valve. Ascending aorta is mobilized to allow it to be displaced inferiorly, sliding the flaps of ascending aorta into the incisions in aortic root in "V-Y" fashion. **B,** Continuous stitch of fine polypropylene suture is started at nadir of each incision in aortic root. Corresponding flap of ascending aorta is attached to edges of incision in aortic sinus by sewing from nadir to top of commissural attachment of aortic valve.

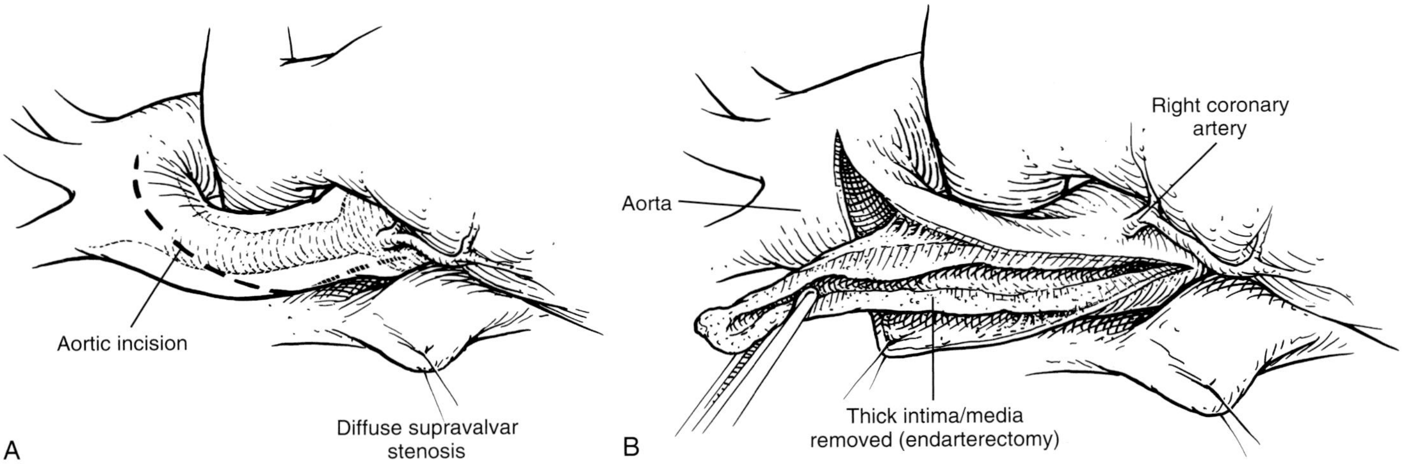

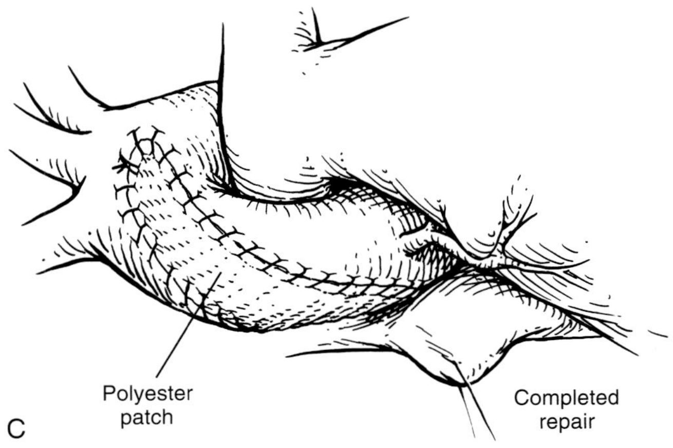

Figure 47-33 Repair of diffuse supravalvar aortic stenosis. **A,** Operation is performed with hypothermic circulatory arrest. Incision is made in ascending aorta extending deep into noncoronary sinus of Valsalva. It is extended distally into aortic arch or even into proximal descending thoracic aorta. **B,** Thickened intima and media is dissected away from aortic adventitia by endarterectomy. **C,** Patch of collagen-coated polyester or polytetrafluoroethylene is used to widen aorta as it is attached to edges of aortotomy.

fashioned to an appropriate size and shape (Fig. 47-33, *C*). In young patients, an allograft of ascending aorta and arch can be used, as in the Norwood operation. Beginning distally, the patch is sutured into place with continuous 4-0 or 5-0 polypropylene. An ear or projection is fashioned into the patch to go across the orifices of the left common carotid and brachiocephalic arteries. Once the arch reconstruction suture lines are into the ascending aorta proximal to origin of the brachiocephalic artery, CPB is reestablished.

A right-angled cannula is inserted through a purse-string suture into the superior vena cava. The vena cava is occluded between the cannula and the right atrium, the cannula is attached to the arterial tubing, and retrograde cerebral perfusion is begun at about 25 mmHg pressure. When air and blood have been flushed out, perfusion through the systemic arterial cannula is reestablished, air is extruded from beneath the patch graft, and the clamp is repositioned on the ascending aorta just proximal to the brachiocephalic artery. Reconstruction of the ascending aorta is continued into the aortic root, attaching the patch to the edges of the aortotomy. Rewarming is accomplished during reconstruction of the ascending aorta and aortic root.

RESULTS

Early (Hospital) Death

Primary repair of isolated *localized* congenital supravalvar aortic stenosis has a low hospital mortality. Early risks are greater in patients with *diffuse* congenital supravalvar aortic stenosis. Sharma and colleagues reported the total experience with operative treatment of supravalvar aortic stenosis at the Texas Heart Institute,[S9] an experience that spanned 29 years and involved 73 patients. Twenty-four patients (32%) had isolated localized supravalvar aortic stenosis and were treated by patch aortoplasty. The results were good, with only one death (4%; CL 0.5%-13%).

Time-Related Survival

Late survival is good. In analyses of 30 to 100 patients, 10-year survival after repair was 88% to 98%, with 20-year survival of 60% to 90%.[B27,H8,S21] Late mortality is more common with complex forms of the anomaly.[S9]

Functional and Hemodynamic Status

Most patients are without symptoms.[M17,S5] Results of treating supravalvar aortic stenosis indicate that pressure gradients from LV to aorta are largely relieved by classic patch aortoplasty for the localized form of the defect.[K9,R4,W4] Keane and colleagues reported that pressure gradients remaining after that operation ranged from 4 to 55 mmHg (mean 27 mmHg).[K9] Good long-term relief of pressure gradients were observed in the Mayo Clinic experience.[R4] Pressure gradient measured intraoperatively after extended patch aortoplasty ranged from 0 to 35 mmHg.[D14] Delius and colleagues reported results in the original cohort of 15 patients followed for 10 to 20 years after extended aortoplasty operation.[D6] The mean immediate postoperative gradient was 20 mmHg (range 0-50 mmHg), and the long-term mean gradient was 32 mmHg (range 6-96 mmHg). A residual gradient is usually caused by overlooked coexisting valvar or subvalvar stenosis.[R4]

Reoperation

Long-term follow-up data on recurrent or residual stenosis requiring reoperation are limited. Of Kitchiner and colleagues' experience with 81 patients followed 1 to 29 years (median 8.3 years), 47 had surgical intervention.[K14] Of those surviving operation, 74% had trivial or mild stenosis at follow-up. Sharma and colleagues reported that 16 of their 73 patients required a second operation during the follow-up period that extended to 22 years.[S9] Brown and colleagues reported that reoperation was required in 14% of 101 patients at a median follow-up of 9.4 years.[B27]

Freedom from reoperation was 69% at 11 years in the study of Delius and colleagues.[D6] Bicuspid aortic valve was a risk factor for reoperation. These data suggest that operations for supravalvar aortic stenosis provide effective long-term relief of the pressure gradient over the sinus rim. The operations are only palliative, however, and many patients will eventually require other operations.

Two studies compare results among the various methods of operative treatment for supravalvar aortic stenosis. Hazekamp and colleagues compared the results of Brom's three-patch technique in 13 patients with 16 patients having other types of repair (14 classic, 1 extended aortoplasty, 1 two-patch repair) for supravalvar aortic stenosis.[H8] No differences in outcome could be demonstrated among the various techniques. All decreased aortic gradient. Mean pressure gradient was less than 10 mmHg in all but four patients, two of whom had the diffuse form of supravalvar aortic stenosis. Two patients required later aortic valve replacement at 2 and 16 years after the initial operation. Stamm and colleagues reviewed 41 years of surgical experience with congenital supravalvar aortic stenosis in 75 patients.[S21] A single patch in the noncoronary sinus was used in 34 patients, an extended aortoplasty to two sinuses of Valsalva in 35 patients, and three-sinus reconstruction in six patients. Multiple-sinus reconstructions (two or three) resulted in superior hemodynamics (lower gradients) and were associated with fewer reoperations ($P = .007$).[S21] The only independent risk factor for reoperation was type of operation ($P < .001$): risk was higher when a single sinus repair was used (approximately 50% by 15 years) compared with two-sinus repair (approximately 15% by 15 years). Similar findings in support of multisinus aortoplasty were reported by Kaushal and colleagues.[K6]

No long-term data are available for the sliding aortoplasty, but the method may retain more of the elastic properties of the aortic root than other repair methods. However, this technique is not suitable for patients with diffuse disease.[S6]

INDICATIONS FOR OPERATION

Operation is advisable in patients with localized or diffuse congenital supravalvar aortic stenosis when peak pressure gradient across the stenosis is 50 mmHg or more. Because of the progressive nature of supravalvar stenosis, operation should be performed without delay at whatever age the criteria for surgery are met.

It can be inferred from the experience reported by Sharma and colleagues that about one third of patients have a simple anomaly that can be treated with a simple operation.[S9] However, nearly half (45% in Sharma and colleagues' experience) have a localized form of supravalvar aortic stenosis plus another obstructive lesion of the LV outflow tract that requires patch aortoplasty plus aortic valvotomy, aortic valve replacement, or subvalvar resection. Therefore, about half of patients with supravalvar aortic stenosis classified as having only localized lesions actually have a complex LV outflow tract anomaly.

Patients with a diffuse form of the defect or with associated cardiac anomalies or infection do less well, with results commensurate with severity and complexity of the defects. Therefore, coexisting diffuse right and left pulmonary arterial stenoses should probably not be approached surgically, because the stenoses usually extend into branches. The possibility of their improvement by percutaneous balloon dilatation[D12] and the tendency for their physiologic effect to decrease as patients age indicate that, in general, their presence should not be a contraindication to surgical relief of supravalvar aortic stenosis.

SPECIAL SITUATIONS AND CONTROVERSIES

Choice of Patch Material

Inserting a patch of prosthetic material or pericardium to enlarge the aortic diameter, combined with resection of the intimal shelf, is a safe and effective procedure.[M14,R4] Theoretically, a false aneurysm may develop at the edge of a polyester onlay patch, similar to when a polyester patch is used in repair of coarctation (see "Late Aneurysm Formation" in Section I of Chapter 48). Polyester graft may also stimulate overgrowth of fibrous tissue (pannus). Pericardium is a more desirable material but might be constrictive, although it does not seem to constrict when applied in the aorta. Tanning with a short exposure to glutaraldehyde may reduce the tendency of pericardium to constrict and makes handling easier during the repair. Glutaraldehyde-fixed bovine pericardium may also have a place in this repair if autologous pericardium is not available. PTFE graft may also be useful.

Al-Halees and colleagues reported using autologous pulmonary artery for the patch in an extended aortoplasty.[A1] The pulmonary trunk above the valve and below the bifurcation was removed and fashioned to provide a pantaloon-shaped patch for reconstructing two aortic sinuses and extending the aorta after resecting the obstructing rim. They suggested that this patch material would grow with the patient.

REFERENCES

A

1. Al-Halees Z, Prabhakar G, Galal O. Reconstruction of supravalvar aortic stenosis with autologous pulmonary artery. Ann Thorac Surg 1998;65:532.
2. Alsoufi B, Karamlou T, Bradley T, Williams WG, Van Arsdell GS, Coles JG, et al. Short and midterm results of aortic valve cusp extension in the treatment of children with congenital aortic valve disease. Ann Thorac Surg 2006;82:1292-300.
3. Angelini A, Ho SY, Anderson RH, Devine WA, Zuberbuhler JR, Becker AE, et al. The morphology of the normal aortic valve as compared with the aortic valve having two leaflets. J Thorac Cardiovasc Surg 1989;98:362.
4. Ankeney JL, Tzeng TS, Liebman J. Surgical therapy for congenital aortic valvular stenosis. J Thorac Cardiovasc Surg 1983;85:41.
5. Ashraf H, Cotroneo J, Dhar N, Gingell R, Roland M, Pieroni D, et al. Long-term results after excision of fixed subaortic stenosis. J Thorac Cardiovasc Surg 1985;90:864.
6. Attie F, Ovseyevitz J, Buendia A, Soto R, Richheimer R, Chavez-Dominguez R, et al. Surgical results in subaortic stenosis. Int J Cardiol 1986;11:329.

B

1. Balaji S, Keeton BR, Sutherland GR, Shore DF, Monro JL. Aortic valvotomy for critical aortic stenosis in neonates and infants aged less than one year. Br Heart J 1989;61:358.
2. Barkhordarian R, Uemura H, Rigby ML, Sethia B, Shore D, Goebells A, et al. A retrospective review in 50 patients with subaortic stenosis and intact ventricular septum: 5-year surgical experience. Interact Cardiovasc Thorac Surg 2007;6:35-8.
3. Basso C, Frescura C, Corrado D, Muriago M, Angelini A, Daliento L, et al. Congenital heart disease and sudden death in the young. Hum Pathol 1995;26:1065.
4. Becker AE, Becker MJ, Edwards JE. Mitral valvular abnormalities associated with supravalvular aortic stenosis. Am J Cardiol 1972; 29:90.
5. Beekman RH, Rocchini AP, Andes A. Balloon valvuloplasty for critical aortic stenosis in the newborn: influence of new catheter technology. J Am Coll Cardiol 1991;17:1172.
6. Ben-Shachar G, Moller JH, Casteneda-Zuniga W, Edwards JE. Signs of membranous subaortic stenosis appearing after correction of persistent common atrioventricular canal. Am J Cardiol 1981; 48:340.
7. Bernhard WF, Keane JF, Fellows KE, Litwin SB, Gross RE. Progress and problems in surgical management of congenital aortic stenosis. J Thorac Cardiovasc Surg 1973;66:404.
8. Bernhard WF, Poirier V, LaFarge CG. Relief of congenital obstruction to left ventricular outflow with a ventricular-aortic prosthesis. J Thorac Cardiovasc Surg 1975;69:223.
9. Beuren AJ, Apitz J, Harmjanz E. Supravalvular aortic stenosis in association with mental retardation and a certain facial appearance. Circulation 1962;26:1235.
10. Beuren AJ, Schulze C, Eberle P, Harmjanz E, Apitz J. The syndrome of supravalvular aortic stenosis, peripheral pulmonary stenosis, mental retardation and similar facial appearance. Am J Cardiol 1964;13:471.
11. Binet JP, Losay J, Demontoux S, Planche C, Langlois J. Subvalvar aortic stenosis. Long-term surgical results. Thorac Cardiovasc Surg 1983;31:96.
12. Bjornstad PB, Rastan H, Keutel J, Beuren AJ, Koncz J. Aortoventriculoplasty for tunnel subaortic stenosis and other obstructions of the left ventricular outflow tract: clinical and hemodynamic results. Circulation 1979;60:59.
13. Black JA, Bonham Carter RE. Association between aortic stenosis and facies of severe infantile hypercalcemia. Lancet 1963;2:745.
14. Blackwood RA, Bloom KR, Williams CM. Aortic stenosis in children: experience with echocardiographic prediction of severity. Circulation 1978;57:263.
15. Bloom KR, Meyer RA, Bove KE, Kaplan S. The association of fixed and dynamic left ventricular outflow obstruction. Am Heart J 1975;89:586.
16. Bourassa MG, Campeau L. Combined supravalvular aortic and pulmonic stenosis. Circulation 1963;28:572.
17. Brauner R, Laks H, Drinkwater DC, Shvarts O, Eghbali K, Galindo A. Benefits of early surgical repair in fixed subaortic stenosis. J Am Coll Cardiol 1997;30:1835.
18. Braunwald E, Goldblatt A, Aygen MM, Rockoff SD, Morrow AG. Congenital aortic stenosis. I. Clinical and hemodynamic findings in 100 patients. Circulation 1963;27:426.
19. Braverman IB, Gibson S. The outlook for children with congenital aortic stenosis. Am Heart J 1957;53:487.
20. Brock R. Aortic subvalvar stenosis with surgical treatment. Guys Hosp Rep 1959;108:144.
21. Brock R, Fleming PR. Aortic subvalvar stenosis. A report of 5 cases diagnosed during life. Guys Hosp Rep 1956;105:391.
22. Brom AG. Obstruction of the left ventricular outflow tract. In: Khonsari S, ed. Cardiac surgery: safeguards and pitfalls in operative technique. Rockville, Md: Aspen, 1988, p. 276.
23. Brown J, Stevens L, Lynch L, Caldwell R, Girod D, Hurwitz R, et al. Surgery for discrete subvalvular aortic stenosis: actuarial survival, hemodynamic results, and acquired aortic regurgitation. Ann Thorac Surg 1985;40:151.
24. Brown JW, Girod DA, Hurwitz RA, Caldwell RL, Rocchini AP, Behrendt DM, et al. Apicoaortic valved conduits for complex left ventricular outflow obstruction: technical considerations and current status. Ann Thorac Surg 1984;38:162.
25. Brown JW, Robison RJ, Waller BF. Transventricular balloon catheter aortic valvotomy in neonates. Ann Thorac Surg 1985; 39:376.

26. Brown JW, Ruzmetov M, Vijay P, Rodefeld MD, Turrentine MW. The Ross-Konno procedure in children: outcomes, autograft and allograft function, and reoperations. Ann Thorac Surg 2006; 82:1301-6.
27. Brown JW, Ruzmetov M, Vijay P, Turrentine MW. Surgical repair of congenital supravalvular aortic stenosis in children. Eur J Cardiothorac Surg 2002;21:50.
28. Burch M, Redington AN, Carvalho JS, Rusconi P, Shinebourne EA, Rigby ML, et al. Open valvotomy for critical aortic stenosis in infancy. Br Heart J 1990;63:37.

C

1. Calhoon JH, Bolton JW. Ross/Konno procedure for critical aortic stenosis in infancy. Ann Thorac Surg 1995;60:S597.
2. Campbell M. The natural history of congenital aortic stenosis. Br Heart J 1968;30:514.
3. Carrel A. On the experimental surgery of the thoracic aorta and the heart. Ann Surg 1910;52:83.
4. Cassels GA, Benjamin JD, Lakier JB. Subendocardial ischemia in patients with discrete subvalvar aortic stenosis. Br Heart J 1978; 40:388.
5. Champsaur G, Trusler GA, Mustard WT. Congenital discrete subvalvular aortic stenosis: surgical experience and long-term follow-up in 20 pediatric patients. Br Heart J 1973;35:443.
6. Chard RB, Cartmill TB, Localized supravalvar aortic stenosis: a new technique for repair. Ann Thorac Surg 1993;55:782.
7. Cheitlin MD, Fenoglio JJ Jr, McAllister HA Jr, Davia JE, DeCastro CM. Congenital aortic stenosis secondary to dysplasia of congenital bicuspid aortic valves without commissural fusion. Am J Cardiol 1978;42:102.
8. Chevers N. Observations on the diseases of the orifice and valves of the aorta. Guys Hosp Rep 1842;387.
9. Chiariello L, Agosti J, Vlad P, Subramanian S. Congenital aortic stenosis: experience with 43 patients. J Thorac Cardiovasc Surg 1976;72:182.
10. Chietlin MD, Robinowitz M, McAllister H, Hoffman JI, Bharati S, Lev M. The distribution of fibrosis in the left ventricle in congenital aortic stenosis and coarctation of the aorta. Circulation 1980;62:823.
11. Choi JY, Sullivan ID. Fixed subaortic stenosis: anatomical spectrum and nature of progression. Br Heart J 1991;65:280.
12. Chung KJ, Fulton DR, Kriedberg MB, Payne DD, Cleveland RJ. Combined discrete subaortic stenosis and ventricular septal defect in infants and children. Am J Cardiol 1984;53:1429.
13. Clarke DR. Extended aortic root replacement for treatment of left ventricular outflow tract obstruction. J Cardiac Surg 1987;2:121.
14. Clarke DR. Extended aortic root replacement with cryopreserved allografts: do they hold up? Ann Thorac Surg 1991;52:669.
15. Cobanoglu A, Dobbs JL. Critical aortic stenosis in the neonate: results of aortic commissurotomy. Eur J Cardiothorac Surg 1996; 10:116.
16. Cohen LS, Friedman WF, Braunwald E. Natural history of mild congenital aortic stenosis elucidated by serial hemodynamic studies. Am J Cardiol 1972;30:1.
17. Colan SD, McElhinney DB, Crawford EC, Keane JF, Lock JE. Validation and re-evaluation of a discriminant model predicting anatomic suitability for biventricular repair in neonates with aortic stenosis. J Am Coll Cardiol 2006;47:1858-65.
18. Cooley DA, Beall AC, Hallman GC, Bucker DL. Obstructive lesions of the left ventricular outflow tract: surgical treatment. Circulation 1965;31:612.
19. Cooley DA, Garrett JR. Septoplasty for left ventricular outflow obstruction without aortic valve replacement: a new technique. Ann Thorac Surg 1986;42:445.
20. Cooley DA, Lopez RM, Absi TS. Apicoaortic conduit for left ventricular outflow tract obstruction: revisited. Ann Thorac Surg 2000;69:1511.
21. Cooley DA, Norman JC, Mullins CE, Grace RR. Left ventricle to abdominal aorta conduit for relief of aortic stenosis. Cardiovasc Dis 1975;2:376.
22. Cooley DA, Norman JC, Reul GJ Jr, Kidd JN, Nihill MR. Surgical treatment of left ventricular outflow tract obstruction with apicoaortic valved conduit. Surgery 1976;80:674.
23. Coran AG, Bernhard WF. The surgical management of valvular aortic stenosis during infancy. J Thorac Cardiovasc Surg 1969; 58:401.
24. Cornell WP, Elkins RC, Criley M, Sabiston DC Jr. Supravalvar aortic stenosis. J Thorac Cardiovasc Surg 1966;51:484.

D

1. Daenen WJ. Repair of complex left ventricular outflow tract obstruction with a pulmonary autograft. J Heart Valve Dis 1995; 4:364.
2. De Bakey ME, Beall AC Jr. Successful surgical correction of supravalvular aortic stenosis. Circulation 1963;27:858.
3. DeBoer DA, Robbins RC, Maron BJ, McIntosh CL, Clark RE. Late results of aortic valvotomy for congenital valvar aortic stenosis. Ann Thorac Surg 1990;50:69.
4. De La Zerda DJ, Cohen O, Fishbein MC, Odim J, Calderon CA, Hekmat D, et al. Aortic valve-sparing repair with autologous pericardial leaflet extension has a greater early re-operation rate in congenital versus acquired valve disease. Eur J Cardiothorac Surg 2007;31:256-60.
5. DeLeon SY, Ilbawi MN, Roberson DA, Arcilla RA, Thilenius OG, Wilson WR, et al. Conal enlargement for diffuse subaortic stenosis. J Thorac Cardiovasc Surg 1991;102:814.
6. Delius RE, Steinberg JB, L'Ecuyer T, Doty DB, Behrendt DM. Long-term follow-up of extended aortoplasty for supravalvular aortic stenosis. J Thorac Cardiovasc Surg 1995;109:155.
7. Denie JJ, Verheugt AP. Supravalvular aortic stenosis. Circulation 1958;18:902.
8. Detter C, Fischlein T, Feldmeier C, Nollert G, Reichart B. Aortic valvotomy for congenital valvular aortic stenosis: a 37-year experience. Ann Thorac Surg 2001;71:1564.
9. De Vivie ER, Hellberg K, Heisig B, Rupprath G, Vogt J, Beuren AJ. Surgical treatment of various types of left ventricular outflow tract stenosis by aortoventriculoplasty: clinical results. Thorac Cardiovasc Surg 1981;29:266.
10. Di Donato RM, Danielson GK, McGoon DC, Driscoll DJ, Julsrud PR, Edwards WD. Left ventricle–aortic conduits in pediatric patients. J Thorac Cardiovasc Surg 1984;88:82.
11. Dorn GW, Donner R, Assey ME, Spann JF Jr, Wiles HB, Carabello BA. Alterations in left ventricular geometry, wall stress, and ejection performance after correction of congenital aortic stenosis. Circulation 1988;78:1358.
12. D'Orsogna L, Sandor GG, Culham JA, Patterson M. Successful balloon angioplasty of peripheral pulmonary stenosis in Williams syndrome. Am Heart J 1987;114:647.
13. Doty DB. Cardiac surgery: operative technique. St Louis: Mosby, 1997, p. 108.
14. Doty DB, Polansky DB, Jenson CB. Supravalvular aortic stenosis: repair by extended aortoplasty. J Thorac Cardiovasc Surg 1977; 74:362.
15. Downing BF. Congenital aortic stenosis: clinical aspects and surgical treatment. Circulation 1956;14:188.
16. Doyle EF, Arumugham P, Lara E, Rutkowski MR, Kiely B. Sudden death in young patients with congenital aortic stenosis. Pediatrics 1974;53:481.
17. Duran CM, Alonso J, Gaite L, Alonso C, Cagigas JC, Marce L, et al. Long-term results of conservative repair of rheumatic aortic valve insufficiency. Eur J Cardiothorac Surg 1988;2:217-23.

E

1. Edwards JE. The congenital bicuspid aortic valve. Circulation 1961;23:485.
2. Edwards JE. Pathology of left ventricular outflow tract obstruction. Circulation 1965;31:586.
3. Elkins RC, Knott-Craig CJ, McCue C, Lane MM. Congenital aortic valve disease: improved survival and quality of life. Ann Surg 1997;225:503.
4. Ellis FH, Ongley PA, Kirklin JW. Results of surgical treatment for congenital aortic stenosis. Circulation 1962;25:29.
5. Ellis FH Jr, Kirklin JW. Congenital valvular aortic stenosis: anatomic findings and surgical techniques. J Thorac Cardiovasc Surg 1962;43:199.
6. El-Said G, Galioto FM Jr, Mullins CE, McNamara DG. Natural hemodynamic history of congenital aortic stenosis in childhood. Am J Cardiol 1972;30:6.
7. Esterly JR, Oppenheimer EH. Some aspects of cardiac pathology in infancy and childhood. Part 4. Myocardial and coronary lesions in cardiac malformations. Pediatrics 1967;39:896.

F

1. Falcone MW, Roberts WC, Morrow AG, Perloff JK. Congenital aortic stenosis resulting from a unicommissural valve. Circulation 1971;44:272.
2. Farrehi C, Dotter CT, Griswold HE. Supravalvular aortic stenosis. Am J Dis Child 1964;108:335.
3. Feigl A, Feigl D, Lucas RV Jr, Edwards JE. Involvement of the aortic valve cusps in discrete subaortic stenosis. Pediatr Cardiol 1984;5:185.
4. Ferrans VJ, Muna WFT, Jones M, Roberts WC. Ultrastructure of the fibrous ring in patients with discrete subaortic stenosis. Lab Invest 1978;39:30.
5. Fontana RS, Edwards JE. Congenital cardiac disease: a review of 357 cases studied pathologically. Philadelphia: WB Saunders, 1962.
6. Freed MD, Rosenthal A, Plauth WH Jr, Nadas AS. Development of subaortic stenosis after pulmonary artery banding. Circulation 1973;47/48:III7.
7. Freedom RM. The long and the short of it: some thoughts about the fixed forms of left ventricular outflow tract obstruction. J Am Coll Cardiol 1997;30:1843.
8. Freedom RM. Neonatal aortic stenosis: the balloon deflated? (Letter.) J Thorac Cardiovasc Surg 1990;100:927.
9. Freedom RM, Dische MR, Rowe RD. Pathologic anatomy of subaortic stenosis and atresia in the first year of life. Ann J Cardiol 1977;39:1035.
10. Freedom RM, Pelech A, Brand A, Vogel M, Olley PM, Smallhorn J, et al. The progressive nature of subaortic stenosis in congenital heart disease. Int J Cardiol 1985;8:137.
11. French JW, Guntheroth WG. An explanation of asymmetric upper extremity blood pressures in supravalvular aortic stenosis: the Coanda effect. Circulation 1970;42:31.
12. Frescura C, Thiene G. Small aortic root in neonates. J Heart Valve Dis 1996;5:II272.
13. Friedman WF, Modlinger J, Morgan JR. Serial hemodynamic observations in asymptomatic children with valvar aortic stenosis. Circulation 1971;43:91.
14. Frommelt MA, Snider AR, Bove EL, Lupinetti FM. Echocardiographic assessment of subvalvar aortic stenosis before and after operation. J Am Coll Cardiol 1992;19:1018.

G

1. Gale AW, Cartmill TB, Bernstein L. Familial subaortic membranous stenosis. Aust NZ J Med 1974;4:576.
2. Gallotti R, Wain WH, Ross DN. Surgical enucleation of discrete subaortic stenosis. Thorac Cardiovasc Surg 1981;29:312.
3. Garcia RE, Friedman WF, Kaback MM, Rowe RD. Idiopathic hypercalcemia and supravalvular aortic stenosis: documentation of a new syndrome. N Engl J Med 1964;271:117.
4. Gatzoulis MA, Rigby ML, Shinebourne EA, Redington AN. Contemporary results of balloon valvuloplasty and surgical valvotomy for congenital aortic stenosis. Arch Dis Child 1995;73:66.
5. Gaynor JW, Bull C, Sullivan ID, Armstrong BE, Deanfield JE, Taylor JF, et al. Late outcome of survivors of intervention for neonatal aortic valve stenosis. Ann Thorac Surg 1995;60:122.
6. Geldein HP, Kleinert S, Weintraub RG, Winkinson JL, Karl TR, Mee RB. Surgical commissurotomy of the aortic valve: outcome of open valvotomy in neonates with critical aortic stenosis. Am Heart J 1996;131:754.
7. Gersony WM, Hayes CJ. Bacterial endocarditis in patients with pulmonary stenosis, aortic stenosis or ventricular septal defect. Circulation 1977;56:I84.
8. Giddins NS, Finley JP, Nanton MA, Roy DL. The natural course of supravalvar aortic stenosis and peripheral pulmonary artery stenosis in Williams's syndrome. Br Heart J 1989;62:315.
9. Glanz S, Hellenbrand WE, Berman MA, Talner NS. Echocardiographic assessment of the severity of aortic stenosis in children and adolescents. Am J Cardiol 1976;38:620.
10. Glew RH, Varghese PJ, Krovetz LJ, Dorst JP, Rowe RD. Sudden death in congenital aortic stenosis: a review of 8 cases with an evaluation of premonitory clinical features. Am Heart J 1969;78:615.
11. Goldstein RE, Epstein SE. Mechanism of elevated innominate artery pressure in supravalvular aortic stenosis. Circulation 1970; 42:23.
12. Gomes AS, Nath PH, Singh A, Lucas RV Jr, Amplatz K, Nicoloff DM, et al. Accessory flaplike tissue causing ventricular outflow obstruction. J Thorac Cardiovasc Surg 1980;80:211.
13. Gordon AS. The surgical management of congenital supravalvular, valvular and subvalvular aortic stenosis using deep hypothermia. J Thorac Cardiovasc Surg 1962;43:141.
14. Gow RM, Freedom RM, Williams WG, Trusler GA, Rowe RD. Coarctation of the aorta or subaortic stenosis with atrioventricular septal defect. Am J Cardiol 1984;53:1421.
15. Gundry SR, Behrendt DM. Prognostic factors in valvotomy for critical aortic stenosis in infancy. J Thorac Cardiovasc Surg 1986;92:747.

H

1. Hancock E. Differentiation of valvular, subvalvular and supravalvular aortic stenosis. Guys Hosp Rep 1961;110:1.
2. Hara M, Dungan T, Lincoln B. Supravalvular aortic stenosis: report of successful excision and aortic reanastomosis. J Thorac Cardiovasc Surg 1962;43:212.
3. Hardesty RL, Griffith BP, Mathews RA, Siewers RD, Neches WH, Park SC, et al. Discrete subvalvular aortic stenosis: an evaluation of operative therapy. J Thorac Cardiovasc Surg 1977;74:352.
4. Harlan JL, Clark EB, Doty DB. Congenital aortic stenosis with hypoplasia of the left sinus of Valsalva: anatomic reconstruction of the aortic root. J Thorac Cardiovasc Surg 1985;89:288.
5. Hastreiter AR, Oshima M, Miller RA, Lev M, Paul MH. Congenital aortic stenosis syndrome in infancy. Circulation 1963;28:1084.
6. Hatle L, Angelsen BA, Tromsdal A. Noninvasive assessment of aortic stenosis by Doppler ultrasound. Br Heart J 1980;43:284.
7. Hawkins JA, Minich LL, Shaddy RE, Tani LY, Orsmond GS, Strutevant JE, et al. Aortic valve repair and replacement after balloon aortic valvuloplasty in children. Ann Thorac Surg 1996; 61:1355.
8. Hazekamp MG, Kappetein AP, Schoof PH, Ottenkamp J, Witsenburg M, Huysmans HA, et al. Brom's three-patch technique for supravalvular aortic stenosis repair. J Thorac Cardiovasc Surg 1999;118:252.
9. Hickey EJ, Caldarone CA, Blackstone EH, Lofland GK, Yeh T, Pizarro C, et al. Critical left ventricular outflow tract obstruction: the disproportionate impact of biventricular repair in borderline cases. J Thorac Cardiovasc Surg 2007;134:1429-37.
10. Hickey EJ, Jung G, Williams WG, Manlhiot C, Van Arsdell GS, Caldarone CA, et al. Congenital supravalvular aortic stenosis: defining surgical and nonsurgical outcomes. Ann Thorac Surg 2008; 86:1919-27.
11. Hohn AR, Van Praagh S, Moore D, Vlad P, Lambert EC. Aortic stenosis. Circulation 1965;32:III4.
12. Hooft C, Vermassen A, Blancquaert A. Observation concerning the evolution of the chronic form of idiopathic hypercalcaemia in children. Helv Paediatr Acta 1963;18:138.
13. Hossack KF, Neutze JM, Lowe JB, Barratt-Boyes BG. Congenital valvar aortic stenosis: natural history and assessment for operation. Br Heart J 1980;43:561.
14. Hsieh KS, Keane JF, Nadas AS, Bernhard WF, Castaneda AR. Long-term follow-up of valvotomy before 1968 for congenital aortic stenosis. Am J Cardiol 1986;58:338.

I

1. Ilbawi MN, DeLeon SY, Wilson WR Jr, Roberson DA, Husayni TS, Quinones JA, et al. Extended aortic valvuloplasty: a new approach for the management of congenital valvar aortic stenosis. Ann Thorac Surg 1991;52:663.

J

1. Jack WD, Kelly DT. Long term follow-up of valvulotomy for congenital aortic stenosis. Am J Cardiol 1976;38:231.
2. Jacobs ML, Blackstone EH, Bailey LL. Intermediate survival in neonates with aortic atresia: a multi-institutional study. The Congenital Heart Surgeons Society. J Thorac Cardiovasc Surg 1998;116:417.
3. Jeger E. Die Chirurgie der Blutgefassen und des Herzens. Berlin: August Hirchwald, 1913.
4. Jonas RA, Keane JF, Lock JE. Aortic valve-preserving procedure for enlargement of the left ventricular outflow tract and mitral anulus. J Thorac Cardiovasc Surg 1998;115:1219.
5. Jonas RA, Lang P, Mayer JE, Castaneda AR. The importance of prostaglandin E_1 in resuscitation of the neonate with critical aortic stenosis. J Thorac Cardiovasc Surg 1985;89:314.

6. Jones KL, Smith DW. The Williams elfin facies syndrome: a new perspective. J Pediatr 1975;86:718.
7. Jones M, Barnhart GR, Morrow AG. Late results after operation for left ventricular outflow tract obstruction. Am J Cardiol 1982; 50:569.
8. Jones RC, Walker WJ, Jahnke EJ, Winn DF. Congenital aortic stenosis: correlation of clinical severity with haemodynamic and surgical findings in 43 cases. Ann Intern Med 1963;58:486.

K

1. Kadri MA, Hovaguimian H, Starr A. Commissurotomy and bileaflet pericardial augmentation–resuspension for bicuspid aortic valve stenosis. Ann Thorac Surg 1997;63:548.
2. Kalfa D, Ghez O, Kreitmann B, Metras D. Secondary subaortic stenosis in heart defects without any initial subaortic obstruction: a multifactorial postoperative event. Eur J Cardiothorac Surg 2007;32:582-7.
3. Karl TR, Sano S, Brawn WJ, Mee RB. Critical aortic stenosis in the first month of life: surgical results in 26 infants. Ann Thorac Surg 1990;50:105.
4. Kasten-Sportes CH, Piechaud JF, Sidi D, Kachaner J. Percutaneous balloon valvuloplasty in neonates with critical aortic stenosis. J Am Coll Cardiol 1989;13:1101.
5. Katz NM, Buckley MJ, Liberthson RR. Discrete membranous subaortic stenosis: report of 31 patients, review of the literature, and delineation of management. Circulation 1977;56:1034.
6. Kaushal S, Backer CL, Patel S, Gossett JG, Mavroudis C. Midterm outcomes in supravalvular aortic stenosis demonstrate the superiority of multisinus aortoplasty. Ann Thorac Surg 2010;89:1371-7.
7. Keane JF, Bernhard WF, Nadas AS. Aortic stenosis in infancy. Circulation 1975;52:1138.
8. Keane JF, Driscoll DJ, Gersony WM, Hayes CJ, Kidd L, O'Fallon WM, et al. Second Natural History Study of Congenital Heart Defects: results of treatment of patients with aortic valvar stenosis. Circulation 1993;87:I16.
9. Keane JF, Fellows KE, La Farge G, Nadas AS, Bernhard WF. The surgical management of discrete and diffuse supravalvar aortic stenosis. Circulation 1976;54:112.
10. Keating MT. Genetic approaches to cardiovascular disease: supravalvular aortic stenosis, Williams syndrome, and long-QT syndrome. Circulation 1995;92:142.
11. Keith JD, Rowe RD, Vlad P. Heart disease in infancy and childhood. 2nd Ed. New York: Macmillan 1967, p. 250.
12. Kelly DT, Wulfsberg E, Rowe RD. Discrete subaortic stenosis. Circulation 1972;46:309.
13. Kirklin JW, Ellis FH Jr. Surgical relief of diffuse subvalvular aortic stenosis. Circulation 1961;24:739.
14. Kitchiner D, Jackson M, Walsh K, Peart I, Arnold R. Prognosis of supravalvar aortic stenosis in 81 patients in Liverpool (1960-1993). Heart 1996;75:396.
15. Konno S, Imai Y, Iida Y, Nakajima M, Tatsuno K. A new method for prosthetic valve replacement in congenital aortic stenosis associated with hypoplasia of the aortic valve ring. J Thorac Cardiovasc Surg 1975;70:909.
16. Krovetz LG, Kurlinski JP. Subendocardial blood flow in children with congenital aortic stenosis. Circulation 1976;54:961.
17. Kugelmeier J, Egloff L, Real F, Rothlin M, Turina M, Senning A. Congenital aortic stenosis: early and late results of aortic valvotomy. Thorac Cardiovasc Surg 1982;30:91.
18. Kuralay E, Ozal E, Bingol H, Cingoz F, Tatar H. Discrete subaortic stenosis: assessing adequacy of myectomy by transesophageal echocardiography. J Card Surg 1999;14:348.
19. Kuribayashi R, Imai T, Yagi Y, Gomi H. Subaortic stenosis caused by an accessory tissue of the mitral valve. J Cardiovasc Surg (Torino) 1979;20:591.

L

1. Lababidi Z, Weinhaus L. Successful balloon valvuloplasty for neonatal critical aortic stenosis. Am Heart J 1986;112:913.
2. Lakier JB, Lewis AB, Heymann MA, Stanger P, Hoffman JI, Rudolph AM. Isolated aortic stenosis in the neonate: natural history and hemodynamic considerations. Circulation 1974;50:801.
3. Latson LA, Cheatham JP, Gutgesell HP. Relation of the echocardiographic estimate of left ventricular size to mortality in infants with severe left ventricular outflow obstruction. Am J Cardiol 1981;48:887.
4. Lauer RM, Du Shane JW, Edwards JE. Obstruction of left ventricular outlet in association with ventricular septal defect. Circulation 1960;22:110.
5. Lawson RM, Bonchek LI, Menashe V, Starr A. Late results of surgery for left ventricular outflow tract obstruction in children. J Thorac Cardiovasc Surg 1976;71:334.
6. Leech G, Mills P, Leatham A. The diagnosis of a non-stenotic bicuspid aortic valve. Br Heart J 1978;40:941.
7. Lees MH, Hauck AJ, Starkey GW, Nadas AS, Gross RE. Congenital aortic stenosis: operative indications and surgical results. Br Heart J 1961;24:31.
8. Leichter DA, Sullivan I, Gersony WM. "Acquired" discrete subvalvular aortic stenosis: natural history and hemodynamics. J Am Coll Cardiol 1989;14:1539.
9. Leung MP, McKay R, Smith A, Anderson RH, Arnold R. Critical aortic stenosis in early infancy: anatomic and echocardiographic substrates of successful open valvotomy. J Thorac Cardiovasc Surg 1991;101:526.
10. Lewis AB, Heymann MA, Stanger P, Hoffman JI, Rudolph AM. Evaluation of subendocardial ischemia in valvar aortic stenosis in children. Circulation 1974;49:978.
11. Lewis FJ, Shumway NE, Niazi SA. Aortic valvulotomy under direct vision during hypothermia. J Thorac Cardiovasc Surg 1956;32:481.
12. Li DY, Toland AE, Boak BB, Atkinson DL, Ensing GJ, Morris CA, et al. Elastin point mutations cause an obstructive vascular disease, supravalvular aortic stenosis. Hum Mol Genet 1997;6:1021.
13. Lillehei CW, Bonnabeau RC Jr, Sellers RD. Subaortic stenosis: diagnostic criteria, surgical approach and late follow-up in 25 patients. J Thorac Cardiovasc Surg 1968;55:94.
14. Lofland GK, McCrindle BW, Williams WG, Blackstone EH, Tchervenkov C, Sittiwangkul R, et al. Critical aortic stenosis in the neonate: a multi-institutional study of management outcomes and risk factors. J Thorac Cardiovasc Surg 2001;121:10.
15. Logan WF, Wyn Jones E, Walker E, Coulshed N, Epstein EJ. Familial supravalvar aortic stenosis. Br Heart J 1965;27:547.
16. Lupinetti FM, Pridjian AK, Callow LB, Crowley DC, Beekman RH, Bove EL. Optimum treatment of discrete subaortic stenosis. Ann Thorac Surg 1992;54:467.

M

1. Maizza AF, Ho SY, Anderson RH. Obstruction of the left ventricular outflow tract: anatomical observations and surgical implications. J Heart Valve Dis 1993;2:66.
2. Manouguian S, Kirckhoff PG, Koncz J, Corovic D, Dahn D. Ventricular septal defect associated with fibrous subvalvar aortic stenosis: diagnostic problems and surgical management. Thoraxchirurgie 1975;23:444.
3. Maron BJ, Redwood DR, Roberts WC, Henry WL, Morrow AG, Epstein SE. Tunnel subaortic stenosis: left ventricular outflow tract obstruction produced by fibromuscular tubular narrowing. Circulation 1976;54:404.
4. Marquis RM, Logan R. Congenital aortic stenosis and its surgical treatment. Br Heart J 1955;17:373.
5. Martin EC, Moseley IF. Supravalvar aortic stenosis. Br Heart J 1973;35:758.
6. Martin MM, Lemmer JH, Shaffer E, Dick M, Bove EL. Obstruction to left coronary artery blood flow secondary to obliteration of the coronary ostium in supravalvular aortic stenosis. Ann Thorac Surg 1988;45:16.
7. Matthewson JW, Riemenschneider TA, McGough EC, Concon VR. Left ventricular outflow tract obstruction produced by redundant mitral valve tissue in a neonate: clinical, angiographic, and operative findings. Circulation 1976;53:198.
8. Mavroudis C, Rees A, Solinger R, Elbl F. The prognostic value of intraoperative pressure gradients with congenital aortic stenosis. Ann Thorac Surg 1984;38:237.
9. McCaffrey FM, Sherman FS. Prenatal diagnosis of severe aortic stenosis. Pediatr Cardiol 1997;18:276.
10. McCrindle BW, Blackstone EH, Williams WG, Sittiwangkul R, Spray TL, Azakie A, et al. Are outcomes of surgical versus transcatheter balloon valvotomy equivalent in neonatal critical aortic stenosis? Circulation 2001;104:I152.
11. McDonald AH, Gerlis LM, Somerville J. Familial arteriopathy with associated pulmonary and systemic arterial stenoses. Br Heart J 1969;31:375.

12. McElhinney DB, Petrossian E, Tworetzky W, Silverman NH, Hanley FL. Issues and outcomes in the management of supravalvar aortic stenosis. Ann Thorac Surg 2000;69:572.
13. McGoon DC, Geha AS, Scofield EL, Du Shane JW. Surgical treatment of congenital aortic stenosis. Dis Chest 1969;55:388.
14. McGoon DC, Mankin HT, Vlad P, Kirklin JW. The surgical treatment of supravalvular aortic stenosis. J Thorac Cardiovasc Surg 1961;41:125.
15. McKay L, Ross DN. Technique for the relief of discrete subaortic stenosis. J Thorac Cardiovasc Surg 1982;84:917.
16. Mencarelli L. Stenosis sopravalvolare aortica and anello. Arch Ital Anat Istol Patol 1930;1:829.
17. Merin G, Copperman IJ, Borman JB. Surgical correction of diffuse supravalvar aortic stenosis involving the branches of the aortic arch. Chest 1976;70:546.
18. Messina L, Turley K, Stanger P, Hoffman JI, Ebert A. Reply to Jonas et al.'s letter to the editor. J Thorac Cardiovasc Surg 1985;89:315.
19. Messina LM, Turley K, Stanger P, Hoffman JI, Ebert PA. Successful aortic valvotomy for severe congenital valvular aortic stenosis in the newborn infant. J Thorac Cardiovasc Surg 1984;88:92.
20. Messmer BJ, Hofstetter R, von Bernuth G. Surgery for critical congenital aortic stenosis during the first three months of life. Eur J Cardiothorac Surg 1991;5:378.
21. Mills P, Leech G, Davies M, Leathan A. The natural history of a non-stenotic bicuspid aortic valve. Br Heart J 1978;40:951.
22. Milsom FP, Doty DB. Aortic valve replacement and mitral valve repair with allograft. J Card Surg 1993;8:350.
23. Misbach GA, Turley K, Ullyot DJ, Ebert PA. Left ventricular outflow enlargement by the Konno procedure. J Thorac Cardiovasc Surg 1982;84:696.
24. Mody MR, Mody GT. Serial hemodynamic observations in congenital valvular and subvalvular aortic stenosis. Am Heart J 1975;89:137.
25. Moller JH, Nakib A, Edwards JE. Infarction of papillary muscles and mitral insufficiency associated with congenital aortic stenosis. Circulation 1966;34:87.
26. Moller JH, Nakib A, Eliot RS, Edwards JE. Symptomatic congenital aortic stenosis in the first year of life. J Pediatr 1966;69:728.
27. Moore P, Egito E, Mowrey H, Perry SB, Lock JE, Keane JF. Midterm results of balloon dilation of congenital aortic stenosis: predictors of success. J Am Coll Cardiol 1996;27:1257.
28. Morrow AG, Fort L 3rd, Roberts WL, Braunwald E. Discrete subaortic stenosis complicated by aortic valvular regurgitation: clinical, hemodynamic and pathologic studies and the results of operative treatment. Circulation 1965;31:163.
29. Morrow AG, Goldblatt A, Braunwald E. Congenital aortic stenosis: surgical treatment and the results of operation. Circulation 1963; 27:450.
30. Morrow AG, Waldhausen JA, Peters RL, Bloodwell RD, Braunwald E. Supravalvular aortic stenosis: clinical, hemodynamic and pathologic observations. Circulation 1959;20:1003.
31. Moses RD, Barnhart GR, Jones M. The late prognosis after localized resection for fixed (discrete and tunnel) left ventricular outflow tract obstruction. J Thorac Cardiovasc Surg 1984;87:410.
32. Muna WF, Ferrans VJ, Pierce JE, Roberts WL. Discrete subaortic stenosis in Newfoundland dogs: association of infective endocarditis. Am J Cardiol 1978;41:746.
33. Myers JL, Waldhausen JA, Cyran SE, Gleason MM, Weber HS, Baylen BG. Results of surgical repair of congenital supravalvular aortic stenosis. J Thorac Cardiovasc Surg 1993;105:281.

N

1. Nakanishi T, Iwasaki Y, Momma K, Imai Y. Supravalvular aortic stenosis, pulmonary artery stenosis, and coronary artery stenosis in twins. Pediatr Cardiol 1996;17:125.
2. Neufeld HN, Ongley PA, Edwards JE. Combined congenital subaortic stenosis and infundibular pulmonary stenosis. Br Heart J 1960;22:686.
3. Neufeld HN, Wagenvoort CA, Ongley PA, Edwards JE. Hypoplasia of ascending aorta: an unusual form of supravalvular aortic stenosis with special reference to localized coronary arterial hypertension. Am J Cardiol 1962;10:746.
4. Newfeld EA, Muster AJ, Paul MH, Idriss FS, Riker WL. Discrete subvalvular aortic stenosis in childhood: study of 51 patients. Am J Cardiol 1976;38:53.
5. Norman JC, Cooley DA, Hallaman GL, Nihill MR. Left ventricular apical–abdominal aortic conduits for left ventricular outflow tract obstructions. Circulation 1977;56:II62.
6. Norwood WI, Lang P, Castaneda AR, Murphy JD. Management of infants with left ventricular outflow obstruction by conduit interposition between the ventricular apex and thoracic aorta. J Thorac Cardiovasc Surg 1983;86:771.

O

1. O'Connor BK, Beekman RH, Rocchini AP, Rosenthal A. Intermediate-term effectiveness of balloon valvuloplasty for congenital aortic stenosis: a prospective follow-up study. Circulation 1991;84:732.
2. Ongley PA, Nadas AS, Paul MY, Rudolph AM, Starkey GW. Aortic stenosis in infants and children. Pediatrics 1958;21:207.

P

1. Pasengrau DG, Kioshos JM, Durnin RE, Kroetz FW. Supravalvular aortic stenosis in adults. Am J Cardiol 1973;31:635.
2. Peckham GB, Keith JD, Evans JR. Congenital aortic stenosis: some observations on the natural history and clinical assessment. Can Med Assoc J 1964;91:639.
3. Pelech AN, Dyck JD, Trusler GA, Williams WG, Olley PM, Rowe RD, et al. Critical aortic stenosis: survival and management. J Thorac Cardiovasc Surg 1987;94:510.
4. Penkoske PA, Collins-Nakai RL, Duncan NF. Subaortic stenosis in childhood: frequency of associated anomalies and surgical options. J Thorac Cardiovasc Surg 1989;98:852.
5. Peterson TA, Todd DB, Edwards JE. Supravalvular aortic stenosis. J Thorac Cardiovasc Surg 1965;50:734.
6. Polimenakos AC, Sathanandam S, Blair C, Elzein C, Roberson D, Ilbawi MN. Selective tricuspidization and aortic cusp extension valvuloplasty: outcome analysis in infants and children. Ann Thorac Surg 2010;90(3)839-46.
7. Pozzi M, Quarti A, Colaneri M, Oggianu A, Baldinelli A, Colonna PL. Valve repair in congenital aortic valve abnormalities. Interact Cardiovasc Thorac Surg 2010;10:587-91.
8. Presbitero P, Somerville J, Revel-Chion R, Ross D. Open aortic valvotomy for congenital aortic stenosis: late results. Br Heart J 1982;47:26.
9. Pyle RL, Patterson DF, Chacko S. Genetics and pathology of discrete subaortic stenosis in the Newfoundland dog. Am Heart J 1976;92:324.

Q

1. Quader MA, Rosenthal GL, Qureshi AM, Mee RB, Mumtaz MA, Joshi R, et al. Aortic valve repair for congenital abnormalities of the aortic valve. Heart Lung Circ 2006;15:248-55.

R

1. Rastan H, Abu-Aishah N, Rastan D, Heisig B, Koncz J, Bjornstad PG, et al. Results of aortoventriculoplasty in 21 consecutive patients with left ventricular outflow tract obstruction. J Thorac Cardiovasc Surg 1978;75:659.
2. Rastan H, Koncz J. Plastische Erweiterung der linken Ausflubahn: Eine neue Operationsmethode. Thoraxchirurgie 1975;23:169.
3. Rastan H, Koncz J. Aortoventriculoplasty: a new technique for the treatment of left ventricular outflow tract obstruction. J Thorac Cardiovasc Surg 1976;71:920.
4. Rastelli GC, McGoon DC, Ongley PA, Mankin HT, Kirklin JW. Surgical treatment of supravalvular aortic stenosis: report of 16 cases and review of literature. J Thorac Cardiovasc Surg 1966;51:873.
5. Reddy VM, Rajasinghe HA, Teitel DF, Haas GS, Hanley FL. Aortoventriculoplasty with the pulmonary autograft: the "Ross-Konno" procedure. J Thorac Cardiovasc Surg 1996;111:158.
6. Reid JM, Coleman EN. The management of congenital aortic stenosis. Thorax 1982;37:902.
7. Reis RL, Peterson LM, Mason DT, Simon AL, Morrow AG. Congenital fixed subvalvar aortic stenosis: an anatomical classification and correlations with operative results. Circulation 1971;43:I11.
8. Rhodes LA, Colan SD, Perry SB, Jonas RA, Sanders SP. Predictors of survival in neonates with critical aortic stenosis. Circulation 1991;84:23.
9. Rizzoli G, Tiso E, Mazzucco A, Daliento L, Rubino M., Tursi V, et al. Discrete subaortic stenosis: operative age and gradient as

predictors of late aortic valve incompetence. J Thorac Cardiovasc Surg 1993;106:95.
10. Roberts WC. The structure of the aortic valve in clinically isolated aortic stenosis: an autopsy study of 162 patients over 15 years of age. Circulation 1970;42:91.
11. Robinson JD, Del Nido PJ, Geggel RL, Perez-Atayde AR, Lock JE, Powell AJ. Left ventricular diastolic heart failure in teenagers who underwent balloon aortic valvuloplasty in early infancy. Am J Cardiol 2010;106:426-9.
12. Rosenquist GC, Clark EB, McAllister HA, Bharati S, Edwards JE. Increased mitral–aortic separation in discrete subaortic stenosis. Circulation 1979;60:70.
13. Rupprath G, Neuhaus KL. Percutaneous balloon valvuloplasty for aortic valve stenosis in infancy. Am J Cardiol 1985;55:1655.
14. Ruzyllo W, Demkow M, Ksiezycka E, Ciszewski M, Szaroszyk W. Stepwise Inoue balloon catheter valvuloplasty for congenital aortic valve stenosis: comparison with standard balloon catheter technique. Pediatr Cardiol 1996;17:15.

S

1. Sandhu SK, Lloyd TR, Crowley DC, Beekman RH. Effectiveness of balloon valvuloplasty in the young adult with congenital aortic stenosis. Catheter Cardiovasc Diagn 1995;36:122.
2. Sandor GG, Olley PM, Trusler GA, Williams WG, Rowe RD, Morch JE. Long-term follow-up of patients after valvotomy for congenital valvular aortic stenosis in children. J Thorac Cardiovasc Surg 1980;80:171.
3. Schaffer MS, Campbell DN, Clarke DR, Wiggins JW Jr, Wolfe RR. Aortoventriculoplasty in children. J Thorac Cardiovasc Surg 1986;92:391.
4. Schmidt RE, Gilbert EF, Amend TC, Chamberlain CR Jr, Lucas RV Jr. Generalized arterial fibromuscular dysplasia and myocardial infarction in familial supravalvular aortic stenosis syndrome. J Pediatr 1969;74:576.
5. Schumacker HB Jr, Mandelbaum I. Surgical considerations in the management of supravalvular aortic stenosis. Circulation 1965;31/32:I36.
6. Scott DJ, Campbell DN, Clarke DR, Goldberg SP, Karlin DR, Mitchell MB. Twenty-year surgical experience with congenital supravalvar aortic stenosis. Ann Thorac Surg 2009;87:1501-8.
7. Serraf A, Zoghby J, Lacour-Gayet F, Houel R, Belli E, Galletti L, et al. Surgical treatment of subaortic stenosis: a seventeen-year experience. J Thorac Cardiovasc Surg 1999;117:669.
8. Shackleton J, Edwards FR, Bickford BJ, Jones RS. Long term follow-up of congenital aortic stenosis after surgery. Br Heart J 1972;34:47.
9. Sharma BK, Fujiwara H, Hallman GL, Ott DA, Reul GJ, Cooley DA. Supravalvar aortic stenosis: a 29-year review of surgical experience. Ann Thorac Surg 1991;51:1031.
10. Shim D, Lloyd TR, Beekman RH. Usefulness of repeat balloon aortic valvuloplasty in children. Am J Cardiol 1997;79:1141.
11. Shone JD, Sellers RD, Anderson RL, Adams P, Lillehei CW, Edwards JE. The developmental complex of parachute mitral valve, supravalvular ring of left atrium, subaortic stenosis and coarctation of aorta. Am J Cardiol 1963;11:714.
12. Sigrusson G, Tacy TA, Vanauker MD, Cape EG. Abnormalities of the left ventricular outflow tract associated with discrete subaortic stenosis in children: an echocardiographic study. J Am Coll Cardiol 1997;30:255.
13. Silverman NH, Gerlis LM, Ho SY, Anderson RH. Fibrous obstruction within the left ventricular outflow tract associated with ventricular septal defect: a pathologic study. J Am Coll Cardiol 1995;25:475.
14. Sink JD, Smallhorn JF, Macartney FJ, Taylor JF, Stark J, de Leval MR. Management of critical aortic stenosis in infancy. J Thorac Cardiovasc Surg 1984;87:82.
15. Sissman NJ, Neill CA, Spencer FC, Taussig HB. Congenital aortic stenosis. Circulation 1959;19:458.
16. Somerville J, Stone S, Ross D. Fate of patients with fixed subaortic stenosis after surgical removal. Br Heart J 1980;43:629.
17. Spencer FC, Neill CA, Bahnson HT. The treatment of congenital aortic stenosis with valvotomy during cardiopulmonary bypass. Surgery 1958;44:109.
18. Spencer FC, Neill CA, Sank L, Bahnson HT. Anatomical variations in 46 patients with congenital aortic stenosis. Am Surg 1960;26:204.
19. Sreeram N, Sutherland GR, Bogers JJ, Stumper O, Hess J, Bos E, et al. Subaortic obstruction: intraoperative echocardiography as an adjunct to operation. Ann Thorac Surg 1990;50:579.
20. Stamm C, Friehs I, Ho SY, Moran AM, Jonas RA, del Nido PJ. Congenital supravalvar aortic stenosis: a simple lesion? Eur J Cardiothorac Surg 2001;19:195.
21. Stamm C, Kreutzer C, Zurakowski D, Nollert G, Friehs, I, Mayer JE, et al. Forty-one years of surgical experience with congenital supravalvular aortic stenosis. J Thorac Cardiovasc Surg 1999; 118:874.
22. Stamm C, Li J, Ho SY, Redington AN, Anderson RH. The aortic root in supravalvular aortic stenosis: the potential surgical relevance of morphologic findings. J Thorac Cardiovasc Surg 1997;114:16.
23. Stamm RB, Martin RP. Quantification of pressure gradients across stenotic valves by Doppler ultrasound. J Am Coll Cardiol 1983;2:707.
24. Starr A, Dotter C, Griswold H. Supravalvular aortic stenosis: diagnosis and treatment. J Thorac Cardiovasc Surg 1961;41:134.
25. Steinberg JB, Delius RE, Behrendt DM. Supravalvular aortic stenosis: a modification of extended aortoplasty. Ann Thorac Surg 1998;65:277.
26. Stellin G, Mazzucco A, Bortolotti U, Tiso E, Daliento L, Maraglino G, et al. Late results after resection of discrete and tunnel subaortic stenosis. Eur J Cardiothorac Surg 1989;3:235.
27. Stewart JR, Merrill WH, Hammon JW Jr, Graham TP Jr, Bender HW Jr. Reappraisal of localized resection for subvalvar aortic stenosis. Ann Thorac Surg 1990;50:197.
28. Stewart JR, Paton BC, Blount SG Jr, Swan H. Congenital aortic stenosis: ten to 22 years after valvulotomy. Arch Surg 1978;113:1248.
29. Strong WB, Perrin E, Liebman J, Silbert DR. Systemic and pulmonary artery dysplasia associated with unexpected death in infancy. J Pediatr 1970;77:233.
30. Sung CS, Price EC, Cooley DA. Discrete subaortic stenosis in adults. Am J Cardiol 1978;42:283.
31. Swan H, Blount SG, Wilkinson RH. Visual repair of congenital aortic stenosis during hypothermia. J Thorac Cardiovasc Surg 1958;35:139.
32. Swan H, Kortz A. Direct vision transaortic approach to the aortic valve during hypothermia: experimental observations and report of a successful clinical case. Ann Surg 1956;144:205.

T

1. Tassabehji M, Metcalfe K, Donnai D, Hurst J, Reardon W, Burch M, et al. Elastin: genomic structure and point mutations in patients with supravalvular aortic stenosis. Hum Mol Genet 1997;6:1029.
2. Ten Harkel AD, Berkhout M, Hop WC, Witsenburg M, Helbing WA. Congenital valvular aortic stenosis: limited progression during childhood. Arch Dis Child 2009;94:531-5.
3. Thistlethwaite PA, Madani MM, Kriett JM, Milhoan K, Jamieson SW. Surgical management of congenital obstruction of the left main coronary artery with supravalvular aortic stenosis. J Thorac Cardiovasc Surg 2000;120:1040.
4. Tokel K, Ozme S, Cil E, Ozkutlu S, Celiker A, Saraclar M, et al. "Acquired" subvalvular aortic stenosis after repair of several congenital cardiac defects. Turk J Pediatr 1996;38:177.
5. Tolan MJ, Daubeney PE, Slavik Z, Keeton BR, Salmon AP, Monro JL. Aortic valve repair of congenital stenosis with bovine pericardium. Ann Thorac Surg 1997;63:465.
6. Trinkle JK, Grover FL, Arom KV. Closed aortic valvotomy in infants: late results. J Thorac Cardiovasc Surg 1978;76:198.
7. Trinkle JK, Norton JB, Richardson JD, Grover FL, Noonan JA. Closed aortic valvotomy and simultaneous correction of associated anomalies in infants. J Thorac Cardiovasc Surg 1975;69:758.
8. Turley K, Bove EL, Iannettoni M, Yeh J, Cotroneo JV, Galdieri RJ. Neonatal aortic stenosis. J Thorac Cardiovasc Surg 1990;99:679.
9. Tveter KJ, Foker JE, Moller JH, Ring WS, Lillehei CW, Varco RL. Long-term evaluation of aortic valvotomy for congenital aortic stenosis. Ann Surg 1987;206:496.

V

1. Van Praagh R, Bernhard WF, Rosenthal A, Parisi LF, Fyler DC. Interrupted aortic arch: surgical treatment. Am J Cardiol 1971;27:200.
2. Van Son JA, Falk V, Mohr FW. Ross-Konno operation with resection of endocardial fibroelastosis for critical aortic stenosis with borderline-sized left ventricle in neonates. Ann Thorac Surg 1997;63:112.

3. Vollebergh FE, Becker AE. Minor congenital variations of cusp size in tricuspid aortic valves: possible link with isolated aortic stenosis. Br Heart J 1977;39:1006.
4. Vouhe PR, Neveux JY. Surgical management of diffuse subaortic stenosis: an integrated approach. Ann Thorac Surg 1991;52:654.
5. Vouhe PR, Poulain H, Bloch G, Loisance DY, Gamain J, Lombaert M, et al. Aortoseptal approach for optimal resection of diffuse subvalvular aortic stenosis. J Thorac Cardiovasc Surg 1984;87:887.

W

1. Wagner HR, Ellison RC, Keane JF, Humphries JO, Nadas AS. Clinical course in aortic stenosis. Circulation 1977;56:I47.
2. Wang A, Harrison JK, Bashore TM. Balloon aortic valvuloplasty. Prog Cardiovasc Dis 1997;40:27.
3. Watson GH. Supravalvular pulmonary and aortic stenosis coexisting. Br Heart J 1963;25:817.
4. Weisz D, Hartmann AF Jr, Weldon CS. Results of surgery for congenital supravalvular aortic stenosis. Am J Cardiol 1976;37:73.
5. Weyman AE, Feigenbaum H, Hurwitz RA, Girod DA, Dillon JC, et al. Cross sectional echocardiography in evaluating patients with discrete subaortic stenosis. Am J Cardiol 1976;37:358.
6. Weyman AE, Fergenbaum H, Hurwitz RA, Girod DA, Dillon JC. Cross-sectional echocardiographic assessment of the severity of aortic stenosis in children. Circulation 1977;55:773.
7. Whitmer JT, James FW, Kaplan S, Schwartz DC, Knight MJ. Exercise testing in children before and after surgical treatment of aortic stenosis. Circulation 1981;63:254.
8. Williams JC, Barratt-Boyes BG, Lowe JB. Supravalvar aortic stenosis. Circulation 1961;24:1311.
9. Wren C, Oslizlok P, Bull C. Natural history of supravalvular aortic stenosis and pulmonary artery stenosis. J Am Coll Cardiol 1990;15:1625.
10. Wren C, Sullivan I, Bull C, Deanfield J. Percutaneous balloon dilatation of aortic valve stenosis in neonates and infants. Br Heart J 1987;58:508.
11. Wright GB, Keane JF, Nadas AS, Bernhard WF, Castaneda AR. Fixed subaortic stenosis in the young: medical and surgical course in 83 patients. Am J Cardiol 1983;52:830.

Y

1. Yacoub M, Onuzo O, Riedel B, Radley-Smith R. Mobilization of the left and right fibrous trigones for relief of severe left ventricular outflow obstruction. J Thorac Cardiovasc Surg 1999;117:126.

Z

1. Zeevi B, Keane JF, Castaneda AR, Perry SB, Lock JE. Neonatal critical valvar aortic stenosis: a comparison of surgical and balloon dilation therapy. Circulation 1989;80:831.

48 Coarctation of the Aorta and Interrupted Aortic Arch

Section I Coarctation of the Aorta

DEFINITION

Coarctation of the aorta is a congenital narrowing of the upper descending thoracic aorta adjacent to the site of attachment of the ductus arteriosus. The aortic lumen may be atretic in the most severe form of this defect, but aortic walls above and below the atresia are in continuity, as distinguished from aortic arch interruption, in which a short distance separates the aortic ends (see Section II). Uncommonly, coarctation occurs more proximally, between the left common carotid and subclavian arteries. Occasional examples of coarctation of the lower thoracic and abdominal aorta are not considered in this chapter.

Coarctation with or without patent ductus arteriosus but without other major associated cardiac anomalies is termed *primary, pure*, or *isolated coarctation*.

HISTORICAL NOTE

Morgagni is credited in 1760 with the first description of an aortic coarctation found at autopsy, and Paris some 30 years later was the first to fully describe its pathologic features.[C12] In 1903, Bonnett suggested dividing the lesion into adult (postductal) and infantile (preductal) types,[B28] a classification that has tended to persist despite its inaccuracy. Regardless of age at presentation, essentially all coarctations are periductal. By 1928, Abbott was able to review 200 autopsy cases in individuals older than 2 years of age.[A1] The natural history of this age group was further elucidated in a collective review of 104 autopsy cases between 1928 and 1946 by Reifenstein, Levine, and Gross.[R14] That coarctation was frequently a cause of death in infancy was not appreciated in these early reports; in the 1950s this aspect was adequately documented.[B6,C19]

Animal experiments designed to develop surgical treatment were published in 1944 by Blalock and Park.[B25] Their procedure involved turndown of the divided left subclavian artery onto the aorta, a technique they recognized would not provide complete relief. Experiments involving excision and end-to-end anastomosis were commenced in 1938 by Gross and Hufnagel.[G13] In their classic article published in 1945, they described the technique of end-to-end anastomosis, including the method of suturing and the design of appropriate clamps.[G13] They also noted that hindquarter paralysis occurring in some of their experimental animals was unlikely to be a problem in humans because of collateral circulation. It seemed to be prevented "by packing the entire back of the animal in ice." They predicted use of aortic allografts when end-to-end anastomosis was not practical.

The first coarctation repair in a patient was performed by Crafoord and Nylin in October 1944.[C24] Gross's first patient was operated on in June 1945.[G11] The procedure was rapidly adopted worldwide. Thus, Clagett in 1948 was able to report the first 21 patients operated on at the Mayo Clinic.[C14] In eight of these, end-to-end anastomosis was not considered wise, and Blalock's left subclavian turndown operation was performed instead. Extending the operation to infants began in 1950 when Burford attempted unsuccessfully to reconstruct an infant aorta using an arterial graft.[C19] A successful end-to-end anastomosis in an infant was reported by Lynxwiler and colleagues in 1951[L21] and by Kirklin and colleagues at the Mayo Clinic in a 10-week-old infant in 1952.[K12] Mustard and colleagues reported a successful result in a 12-day-old infant in 1953.[M37] Repair of coarctation in neonates became more successful after documentation in 1975 to 1977 of the favorable effect of prostaglandin E_1 (PGE_1) in these sick small babies, achieved by maintaining patency of the ductus arteriosus until time of repair.[C1,E6,N4,O2]

Subsequent modifications of surgical technique included use of prosthetic onlay grafts across the coarctation site or of a simple vertical incision and its transverse closure by Vorsschulte in 1957[V17] and subclavian patch aortoplasty by Waldhausen and Nahrwold in 1966.[W2] Use of a prosthetic tube graft as an alternative to the allograft, which was preferred by Gross,[G12] was reported by Morris, Cooley, DeBakey, and Crawford in 1960.[M31]

MORPHOLOGY AND MORPHOGENESIS

Coarctation

Coarctations vary in severity. When stenosis is localized, the lumen must be reduced in cross-sectional area by more than about 50% before there is a hemodynamically important pressure gradient across it, but longer tubular coarctations may be hemodynamically important with lesser narrowing.[G16] Thirty-three percent of autopsy specimens (patients aged 2 years to adulthood) examined prior to the era in which operation was available show moderate luminal narrowing, 42% severe (pinhole) stenosis, and 25% luminal atresia.[G4,R14] Occasionally the adult aorta may be redundant and severely kinked opposite the ligamentum arteriosum, without any pressure gradient; this is called a *pseudocoarctation lesion*.[W10]

The localized morphology of classic coarctation is a shelf, projection, or infolding of the aortic media into the lumen. It is most prominent in that portion of the circumference opposite the ductus arteriosus (the posterior and leftward wall). This inward projection is present also on anterior and posterior walls but absent on the ductal side (inferior or rightward wall). The shelf is usually marked externally by a localized indentation or waisting of the left aortic wall as if a string had been placed around it, pulling the aorta toward the ductus[E3,P9] (Figs. 48-1 and 48-2). External narrowing may be absent in the young infant.[H23] The aorta beyond the narrowing usually shows poststenotic dilatation, and paradoxically the wall beyond the stricture is usually thicker than that just proximal to it where the pressure is higher. The localized shelf or curtain of media and intima lies adjacent to the ductus arteriosus in utero and to the ligamentum arteriosum if the ductus closes. The shelf may be preductal or postductal but is usually periductal.[R26] Hutchins pointed out that the histologic features of this aortic media infolding are identical to those seen at a branch point of the normal aorta.[H27]

In addition to infolding of aortic media, there is usually a localized ridge of intimal hypertrophy *(intimal veil)* that extends the shelf circumferentially and further narrows the lumen.[K10] This, and perhaps other portions of the coarctation area, consists of ductal tissue.[B35,P9] It forms a sling that completely surrounds the periductal aorta,[E7,H23,R27,W8] which may progressively proliferate after birth and cause restenoses after repair of coarctation in neonates and young infants.[B35] It is well documented that use of PGE_1 can result in symptomatic relief of a critical coarctation in some young infants by relaxing the coarctation site without reopening the ductus.[C5,L10]

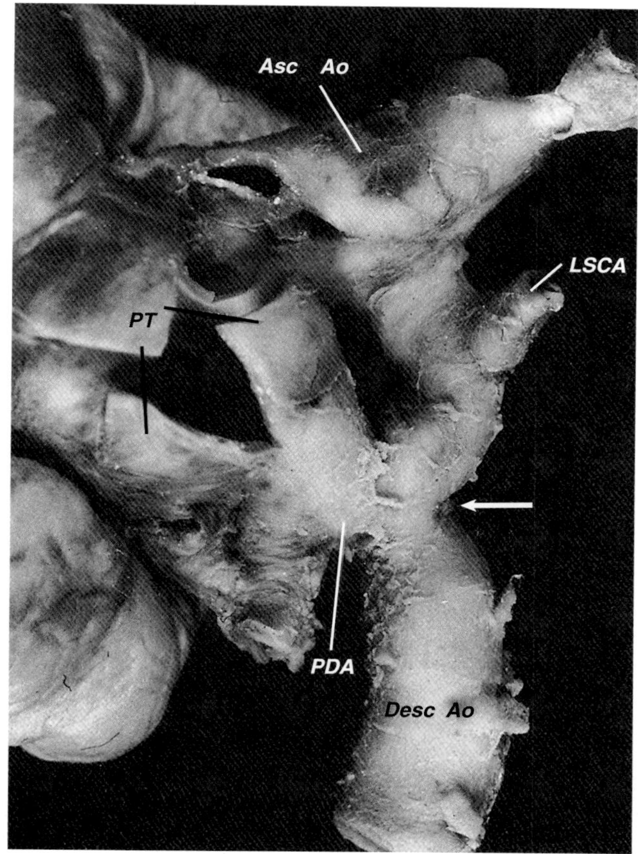

Figure 48-1 Autopsy specimen from 6-week-old girl showing periductal coarctation caused by localized shelf with typical external deformity of aorta at site of narrowing *(arrow)*. Key: *Asc Ao,* Ascending aorta; *Desc Ao,* descending aorta; *LSCA,* left subclavian artery; *PDA,* patent ductus arteriosus; *PT,* pulmonary trunk.

Rodbard has presented experimental and theoretical evidence that lowering of lateral pressure on the aortic wall secondary to the increase in velocity that occurs across a site of narrowing (according to the Bernoulli principle) allows the intimal cells to multiply until probe patency is reached.[R22,R23] Resistance to flow across this stenosis then lowers the velocity so that ingrowth usually stops.

Rudolph and colleagues postulated that prevalence and type of coarctation are related to fetal flow patterns through the ductus and aorta.[R26] These investigators have shown that flow through that portion of the arch between origins of the left common carotid and left subclavian arteries in the normal fetal lamb is approximately half that across the ductus, explaining the normally smaller diameter of the arch compared with the ascending and descending aorta in the normal human newborn.[R26] A localized shelf opposite the ductus may

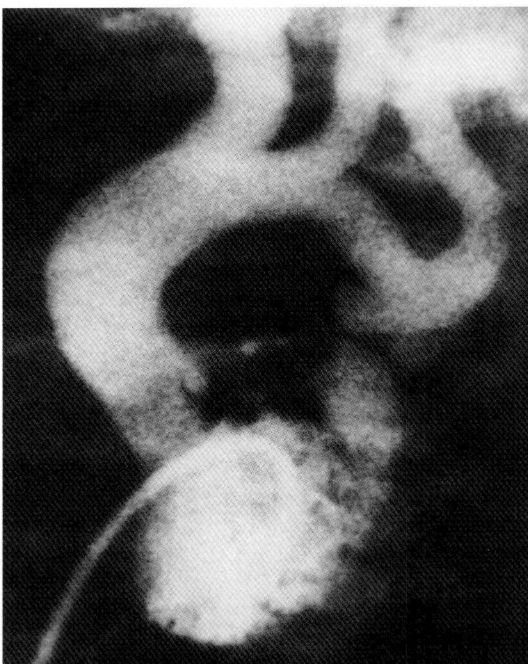

Figure 48-2 Cineangiogram in left anterior oblique view with injection into left ventricle, showing severe coarctation caused by localized shelf opposite an obliterated ductus arteriosus in a 5-day-old neonate. No other cardiovascular anomaly was demonstrated. Note marked angulation of aorta toward mediastinum.

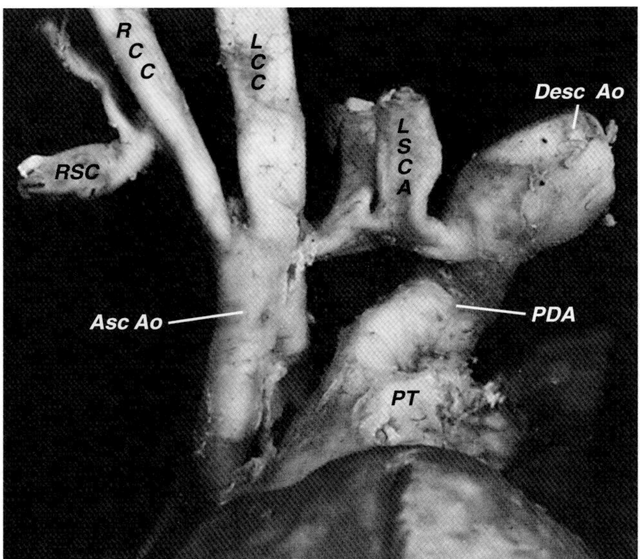

Figure 48-3 Autopsy specimen from 5-day-old neonate with coarctation, demonstrating tubular hypoplasia of aortic arch between left common carotid artery *(LCC)* and patent ductus arteriosus *(PDA)*. Large left vertebral artery arises separately from arch proximal to left subclavian artery *(LSCA)*. This neonate also had perimembranous and muscular ventricular septal defects and mild mitral valve hypoplasia. Key: *Asc Ao,* Ascending aorta; *Desc Ao,* descending aorta; *PT,* pulmonary trunk; *RCC,* right common carotid; *RSC,* right subclavian artery.

result from a reorientation of the angle at which the ductus meets the aorta, which results in abnormal fetal flow patterns in some types of cardiac anomalies. The tendency for a shelf to develop is present when ductal flow is increased more than usual relative to isthmus flow; for example, with a ventricular septal defect (VSD).[H27] However, intrauterine events that account for the relatively frequent association of coarctation with lesions that produce left-to-right shunts postpartum are not fully identified.

Coarctation, as well as isthmus hypoplasia, is more common than usual when ascending aorta flow is diminished during fetal life (and ductal flow is relatively increased) by lesions such as aortic stenosis or atresia (see Chapters 47 and 49), and mitral stenosis or regurgitation (see Chapter 50).[B14,F11,R26,S21,T5,V3] Conversely, prevalence of coarctation is severely reduced and size of the isthmus increased when pulmonary flow and thus right-to-left ductal flow is decreased by lesions such as pulmonary stenosis or atresia, tetralogy of Fallot, and tricuspid atresia.[H27,S21] Coarctation is uncommon when the aortic arch is right sided, presumably because of alteration of ductal and isthmus flow patterns in this situation.[H25,R26]

Distal Aortic Arch Narrowing

Narrowing of the *isthmus*—the segment of aorta between a discrete coarctation and the left subclavian artery—commonly exists with coarctation. Narrowing of the distal aortic arch between the left subclavian and left common carotid arteries also coexists commonly, particularly in neonates and infants (Fig. 48-3). This narrowing appears in some cases to be a transient finding related to prenatal flow pattern (excessive ductal flow extending proximally in the aorta and out the left subclavian artery), which reduces flow in the distal aortic arch between the left subclavian and left common carotid arteries and allows this segment to narrow.[A7,H27,J2] This view leads to the inference that surgical enlargement of the distal arch at the time of coarctation repair is unnecessary because it will, in any event, gradually enlarge after the coarctation is repaired (see under Indications for Operation later in this section). Others believe that the narrowing in this area is a coexisting congenital anomaly and that the narrow area must be widened surgically at the time of coarctation repair. There is evidence that unrepaired arch hypoplasia, at least in some cases, does not grow adequately, requiring repeat surgery.[D4] Whether isolated distal aortic arch narrowing exists as a congenital anomaly in the absence of localized coarctation and results in a pressure gradient is arguable.[A7,D1,R15,S28] It probably does, but uncommonly. In an interesting study comparing 23 patients with coarctation (ranging in age from 1 month to 26 years, median 4.6 years) to normal controls, the proximal arch, distal arch, and isthmus were significantly smaller in the coarctation group; however, the subaortic diameter, aortic root, ascending aorta, and descending aorta were larger.[B13]

Proximal Aortic and Arterial Walls

Although coarctation itself, as well as dimensions of adjacent portions of the aorta, has received considerable attention through the years, only in recent years has evidence emerged to indicate that:

- The wall of the entire aorta proximal to the coarctation is abnormal.

- The abnormalities extend out to all major arteries supplied by the aorta proximal to the coarctation.
- These abnormalities may be primary ones that have developed in utero.[S13]

Coarctation has been documented by fetal echocardiography in utero as early as 21 weeks of gestation,[A7] but it likely exists much earlier. Hypoplasia of the isthmus and, in some patients at least, the distal aortic arch develops during intrauterine development.[A7,M32] It is hypothesized that either the coarctation was present very early in development and the hypoplasia is secondary, or the hypoplasia is related to a primary aortic wall abnormality rather than to the coarctation. Or the hypoplasia and coarctation are a result of altered patterns of blood flow caused by intracardiac abnormalities that lead to decreased flow to the arch and increased flow to the ductus during fetal development.

Degenerative changes occur in the peripheral arterial vasculature proximal to the coarctation, and these changes persist after coarctation repair and can be identified in children. Surrogate markers of arteriosclerosis, such as impaired flow-mediated vasodilatation and increased intima media thickness, were apparent in a study group with a mean age of 12 years.[M26]

Collateral Circulation

Collateral circulation between aorta proximal to the coarctation and that distal to it is one of the striking features of coarctation. When well developed, it is responsible for some of the classic signs of the malformation, such as parascapular pulsations and rib notching. It is usually present to some extent in newborns but increases in size and extensiveness as the patient ages (Fig. 48-4).

Inflow into the collateral circulation is widespread, but is primarily from branches of both subclavian arteries, particularly internal thoracic, vertebral, costocervical, and thyrocervical trunks. *Outflow* from the collateral system is primarily into the upper descending thoracic aorta. The largest *vessels* participating in this outflow are usually the first two pairs of intercostal arteries distal to the coarctation. These are the third and fourth intercostal arteries, and they are greatly enlarged by the large reversed flow (outflow from collateral circulation). This reversed flow into the aorta can be documented by magnetic resonance imaging (MRI)[A19] and has been demonstrated at operation by directional Doppler velocity detector probes.[B7] Flow returns to a normal direction immediately after coarctation repair. Only the intercostals carrying this large *reversed* flow are sufficiently enlarged to

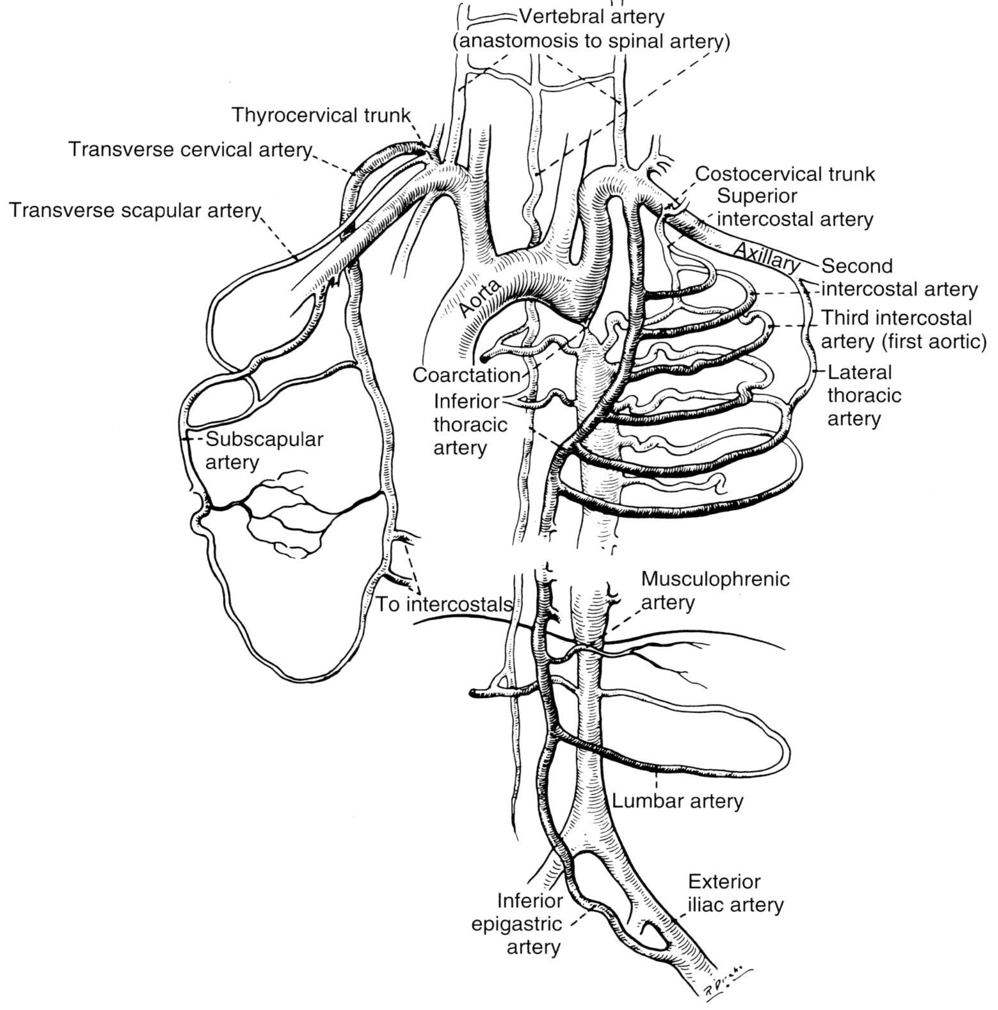

Figure 48-4 Major collateral channels in coarctation of the aorta. (From Edwards and colleagues.[E4])

produce rib notching, which explains lack of notching of the first and second ribs, whose intercostals arise above the coarctation. The lower intercostal arteries provide less outflow from the collateral circulation, as do the inferior epigastric artery and other branches of the abdominal aorta.

Collateral circulation and its clinical manifestations are altered by anatomic variations associated with classic coarctation. Associated stenosis at the origin of the left subclavian artery excludes this artery as an important source of inflow into the collateral circulation; thus, rib notching occurs only on the *right* side. When the right subclavian artery arises as the fourth aortic branch (see Morphology in Section I of Chapter 51) and distal to the coarctation, it does not serve as a source of inflow, and rib notching occurs only on the *left* side.

Aneurysm Formation

Enlarged, tortuous third and fourth intercostal arteries may become aneurysmal,[E4] but this is rare before about age 10 years. Resulting thin-walled *aneurysms* are usually saccular and are most likely to occur at the aortic origin of intercostal arteries. This is a weak point of surgical importance; if an enlarged intercostal artery must be ligated, the ligature should be placed a few millimeters *beyond* its aortic origin.

The aorta itself may become aneurysmal adjacent to the site of maximal narrowing as a result of hemodynamic effects, aortic dissection, or mycotic aneurysm. This is uncommon in young children. Prevalence of aneurysm is about 10% by the end of the second decade of life, 20% by the end of the third decade, and probably even higher in older patients.[S9]

Coronary Arteries

Left ventricular hypertrophy occurring in untreated patients is accompanied by histologic changes in coronary arteries.[V13] In young patients, nonarteriosclerotic lesions are conspicuous in the intimal layer. These consist of degenerative and proliferative changes of the elastic fibers and excess collagenous tissue. The media thickens to about twice normal with a rich elastic fiber network and often hyaline changes. Mean total area of the coronary arteries is increased, so they have greater than normal capacity, presumably in response to increased metabolic requirements of the left ventricle. As a result of prolonged hypertension, arteriosclerotic changes are apt to occur more often and at a younger age. In adolescents and young adults, reduced myocardial perfusion reserve is apparent.[C22]

Atria

In newborn infants it is common for the "valve" of the foramen ovale to be prolapsed, causing left-to-right shunting. This prolapse often resolves after coarctation repair.[J6] A true secundum atrial septal defect (ASD) may also occur with coarctation. Moderate to large ASDs appear to show the same tendency to close when coarctation is present and when it is not.[Y3] In about 10% of patients with ASD, however, intractable heart failure will develop in infancy following coarctation repair, requiring ASD closure. The best predictor of development of heart failure when ASD coexists with coarctation is small mitral valve diameter, not the size of the ASD itself.[S8]

Left Ventricle

Left ventricular hypertrophy without volume increase is present in most patients with coarctation within a few days of birth. This progresses as the patient ages and may be aggravated by associated cardiac anomalies.

The left ventricular outflow tract may be abnormal in patients with arch obstruction, particularly when a VSD coexists.[S23] The left ventricular papillary muscles may be abnormally positioned, typically with a reduced interpapillary distance.[G5]

Aortic Valve

A bicuspid aortic valve is common, although its exact prevalence is uncertain. In two autopsy series, it was 46%[B14] and 27%,[T6] with an additional 6% and 7%, respectively, with congenital valvar stenosis. Tawes and colleagues report that among 250 living children with long-term follow-up, 32 (13%) had clinical evidence of aortic valve disease (mainly stenosis but also regurgitation).[T6] When aortic regurgitation appears in coarctation, it is usually based on a bicuspid aortic valve combined with persistent hypertension. Bicuspid aortic valve is known to be associated with dilatation of the ascending aorta. In one study, presence of coarctation in this setting was not associated with increased magnitude or rate of ascending aortic dilatation.[B12] Another study indicates that patients with coarctation and bicuspid aortic valve have greater aortic root dilatation than those with coarctation and tricuspid aortic valves.[A14] In the presurgical era, aortic dissection was noted to occur in 19% of coarctation patients without bicuspid aortic valve, but in 50% of those with bicuspid aortic valve.[A1,W5]

Intracranial Aneurysm

Coarctation and berry-type intracranial aneurysm coexist in some patients. Some instances of sudden death in untreated as well as treated coarctation are from rupture of the intracranial aneurysm. That coarctation, bicuspid aortic valve, and intracranial aneurysm are associated leads to the inference that coarctation is only one manifestation of a diffuse arteriopathy.[W5]

Coarctation as Part of Hypoplastic Left Heart Physiology

Coarctation (with or without a patent ductus arteriosus, and with or without hypoplasia of the isthmus or distal aortic arch between left common carotid and left subclavian arteries) sometimes coexists with anomalies that also affect left ventricular function and structure directly (see Morphogenesis and Morphology in Chapter 49). This is particularly a problem in symptomatic neonates and infants. These anomalies include:

- Hypoplasia of ascending aorta
- Supravalvar, valvar, subvalvar, and anular aortic stenosis or hypoplasia
- Aortic atresia
- Left ventricular hypoplasia or hypertrophy
- Endocardial fibroelastosis

Table 48-1 Criteria for Hypoplastic Left Heart Class

Class	Criteria
I	Isolated cardiac anomaly[a]
II	Two congenital anomalies affecting left ventricular outflow
III	More than two anomalies, or two with coexisting left ventricular or ascending aortic or aortic arch hypoplasia
IV	Aortic atresia

[a]Anomalies are congenital mitral valve disease, left ventricular hypoplasia (with concordant ventriculoarterial connection), subvalvar or valvar or supravalvar aortic stenosis, ascending aortic or arch hypoplasia, interrupted aortic arch, or coarctation. Hypoplastic left heart *physiology* is said to exist only if the left heart is unable, even with intervention, to independently sustain the systemic circulation (see Chapter 49).

- Mitral stenosis with or without a single papillary muscle (parachute mitral valve)
- Supravalvar mitral ring

When these occur in any of a number of possible combinations, they represent *hypoplastic left heart physiology* (Table 48-1) if the left heart is unable to sustain the systemic circulation (see Chapter 49).

Multiple associated anomalies within the left heart are not unusual even when a functional left heart is present in early infancy. Levine and colleagues[L7] have shown that additional left heart obstructive lesions develop late in more than 20% of patients originally diagnosed in early infancy with isolated coarctation. A predictor of these additional anomalies is mitral valve diameter with a z score less than −1 on the original echocardiogram. A broad spectrum of sizes of important left heart structures can exist without negatively affecting left heart function.[A5,B26,T3]

Coexisting Cardiac Anomalies

When coarctation first presents in older children and young adults (as it did in the early years of cardiac surgery, but uncommonly now), coexisting cardiac anomalies are uncommon. When it presents in neonates, and to some extent in infants, coexisting cardiac anomalies are common (Table 48-2). These associations are explained by the fact that survival beyond infancy is much less likely when coexisting anomalies are present; thus, long-term survivors tend to have simple lesions. Because in the current era most coarctations are diagnosed in neonates or infants, it follows that prevalence of associated anomalies found in neonates with coarctation closely approximates true prevalence.

Patent ductus arteriosus is present in almost 100% of neonates and in most infants with a preductal type of coarctation.[T5] This is considered part of isolated coarctation rather than an additional anomaly. Tubular hypoplasia of the distal aortic arch is also considered to be part of the anomaly of coarctation rather than an associated anomaly. ASD is not considered as an additional anomaly unless large enough to need closure. This excludes the fairly numerous examples of infants presenting with a left-to-right shunt through a stretched patent foramen ovale that may subsequently close. Anomalous right subclavian artery occurs in

Table 48-2 Coexisting Cardiac Anomalies, Exclusive of Obstructive Lesion in the Left Heart–Aorta Complex, in Severely Symptomatic Neonates with Coarctation

Coexisting Cardiac Anomaly	*n*	% of 432
None	171	40
VSD (isolated)	155	36
Single ventricle[a]	32	7
TGA[b]	27	6
AV septal defect[c]	16	4
DORV	9	2
Taussig-Bing heart	12	3
CCTGA	6	1
Truncus arteriosus	1	0.2
Anomalous origin of LCA from PT	1	0.2
TAPVC (with VSD)	1	0.2
PAPVC	1	0.2
SUBTOTAL	432	100
Unknown	3	
TOTAL	435	100

Data from Quaegebeur and colleagues.[Q1]
[a]Univentricular atrioventricular connection (double inlet left ventricle in 12, double inlet right ventricle in one, mitral atresia in 13, tricuspid atresia in 5. common ventricle in 1).
[b]Intact ventricular septum in 3, VSD in 24.
[c]Complete in 14, partial in 2.
Key: *AV,* Atrioventricular; *CCTGA,* congenitally corrected transposition of the great arteries; *DORV,* double outlet right ventricle; *LCA,* left coronary artery; *PAPVC,* partial anomalous pulmonary venous connection; *PT,* pulmonary trunk; *TAPVC,* total anomalous pulmonary venous connection; *TGA,* transposition of the great arteries; *VSD,* ventricular septal defect.

about 1% of cases of coarctation and may be proximal or distal to the coarctation.[D6] This variation does not appear to affect the collateral circulation that develops in any clinically significant way.[D6]

Approximately 82% of individuals born with coarctation have it as an *isolated lesion* (with or without continuing patency of the ductus arteriosus). About 11% have an important coexisting VSD, and approximately 7% have other important coexisting cardiac anomalies. These prevalences are different from those in patients who become symptomatic during neonatal life or infancy and require early intervention (see Table 48-2).

Prevalence of isolated coarctation in patients with an otherwise normal heart appears to be about 40 per 100,000 live births. Persons with pulmonary stenosis or atresia, tetralogy of Fallot, and tricuspid atresia with concordant ventriculoarterial connection have a prevalence of coarctation close to 0 per 100,000. Patients with aortic stenosis and mitral stenosis or regurgitation have a considerably higher prevalence than patients with otherwise normal hearts. Patients with VSD and other lesions such as transposition, double outlet right ventricle, truncus arteriosus, atrioventricular septal defect, and single ventricle who have associated VSD also appear to have a relatively high prevalence of coexisting coarctation. This may relate to altered blood flow patterns within the heart that result in less flow across the aortic isthmus during fetal development.

CLINICAL FEATURES AND DIAGNOSTIC CRITERIA

Mode of presentation and diagnostic criteria depend to a considerable degree on prevalence and severity of coexisting cardiac anomalies, and thus on the patient's age at presentation.

Neonates and Infants

Severe heart failure in a neonate or infant requires that coarctation be considered, especially when a favorable response to medical treatment does not occur promptly.[F15] It may be unsuspected in complex lesions when the baby is in extremis, because even when the ductus is closed, a large left-to-right shunt proximal to the aorta can decrease manifestation of hypertension in the arms. Severe proximal obstructing lesions (aortic or mitral stenosis) can have a similar effect.[F15] Control of heart failure and tachycardia in these situations frequently unmask differential pressures in upper and lower extremities as cardiac output improves.[M6]

Signs and symptoms of coarctation presenting in the neonate are those of heart failure. After a variable period of well-being, tachypnea, feeding problems, and sweating develop. On examination, there is a gallop rhythm and a systolic murmur along the left sternal edge and usually posteriorly over the coarctation site. Femoral pulses are absent or reduced in volume and delayed compared with radial or brachial pulses, although in small, sick infants with tachycardia, pulse delay may be difficult to detect. Blood pressure is higher in the arms than in the legs (by >20 mmHg). Delay in onset of heart failure is probably related, at least in isolated coarctation, to the variable time it takes for the ductus to close. Ductal closure usually commences at the pulmonary end, and generally it is not until the aortic end closes that the periductal aortic shelf produces severe obstruction (see Morphology earlier in this section).[F4,R26,T2] Thus, femoral pulses can be normal at birth but absent at 1 week.[T2]

When the ductus arteriosus remains widely patent and a severe coarctation lies proximal to it (preductal coarctation), there may be a right-to-left shunt into the descending aorta and, classically, cyanosis of the toes and sometimes the left hand while the right hand and lips remain pink (differential cyanosis). Femoral pulses are normal, and there is no ductus murmur. In fact, differential cyanosis is uncommon, either because flow through the coarctation is large or because PO_2 of the pulmonary artery blood is high from an additional intracardiac shunt through a VSD, an interatrial communication, or both. Moreover, despite presence of a severe coarctation proximal to a patent ductus arteriosus, systemic vascular resistance in the lower compartment usually exceeds pulmonary vascular resistance, so the ductal shunt is left to right or bidirectional.[K9]

In infancy, hypertension may be present but is seldom severe, and a collateral circulation is not palpable, although it is usually present angiographically[I1] (Fig. 48-5). Marked cardiomegaly is almost invariable on chest radiograph. The electrocardiogram (ECG) usually shows right ventricular hypertrophy in the first few months of life, even with isolated coarctation.[S28] About two thirds of infants operated on in the first year of life have right ventricular hypertrophy or combined hypertrophy, and fewer than 25% have pure left ventricular hypertrophy.[H7,P7]

Left-to-right shunt through a stretched patent foramen ovale is common in infants with severe coarctation in heart failure. When heart failure disappears, so does the atrial shunt. Congenital aortic stenosis may not be evident clinically (or by catheter withdrawal pressure differential) in infancy, and yet it may be severe enough to require surgical relief at age 2 to 5 years, particularly when it is subvalvar (see Section II in Chapter 47).

Childhood (Age 1 to 14 Years)

Almost all patients who first present at age 1 to 14 years are asymptomatic unless they have important associated anomalies. Tawes and colleagues noted that children with associated anomalies may present in heart failure up to age 3 years,[T5] and Patel and colleagues[P7] noted heart failure in 7 of 65 children (11%) age 1 to 14 years. Subarachnoid hemorrhage from rupture of a berry aneurysm occurs occasionally but is rare in children younger than 7 years,[S20] and spontaneous paresis or paraplegia caused by dilated intercostal arteries compressing the anterior spinal artery or by epidural hemorrhage is even less common.[B34] Hypertension occurs in almost 90% of patients.

The chest radiograph shows cardiomegaly in 33% and rib notching in about 15% (Fig. 48-6), but this feature does not occur before age 3 years.[P7,T5] ECG shows predominantly left ventricular hypertrophy, with right ventricular hypertrophy present only when there is pulmonary hypertension with elevated pulmonary vascular resistance. ECG is normal in about one third of children.

Adolescence (Beyond 14 Years) and Adult Life

Many adolescent and young adult patients remain asymptomatic and are diagnosed at routine examination because femoral pulses are noted to be absent or reduced and delayed in the presence of a cardiac murmur, hypertension, or an abnormal chest radiograph. Hypertension is common and more severe than in younger patients, and heart failure may occur after about age 30 years. Heart failure is preceded by effort dyspnea, cardiomegaly, and important left ventricular hypertrophy on ECG. Headache, nose bleeds, fatigue, and calf claudication occasionally occur. Collaterals are usually palpable or audible posteriorly. Radiographic findings include a "figure-3" sign in the left upper mediastinal shadow (Fig. 48-7) and, almost always, rib notching. (Absence of rib notching in the right chest suggests an anomalous origin of the right subclavian artery and in the left chest a stenosis of the left subclavian artery origin.)

Associated Syndromes

There is an association between *Turner syndrome* and *von Recklinghausen disease* and coarctation.[A6,S42] Rarely, patients with coarctation have *Noonan syndrome* or congenital rubella.[D8]

Special Diagnostic Methods

Two-dimensional echocardiography can visualize coarctation in neonates and small infants (Fig. 48-8) and is usually the definitive study. Associated intracardiac defects can also be defined in detail. Severity of coarctation can often be assessed

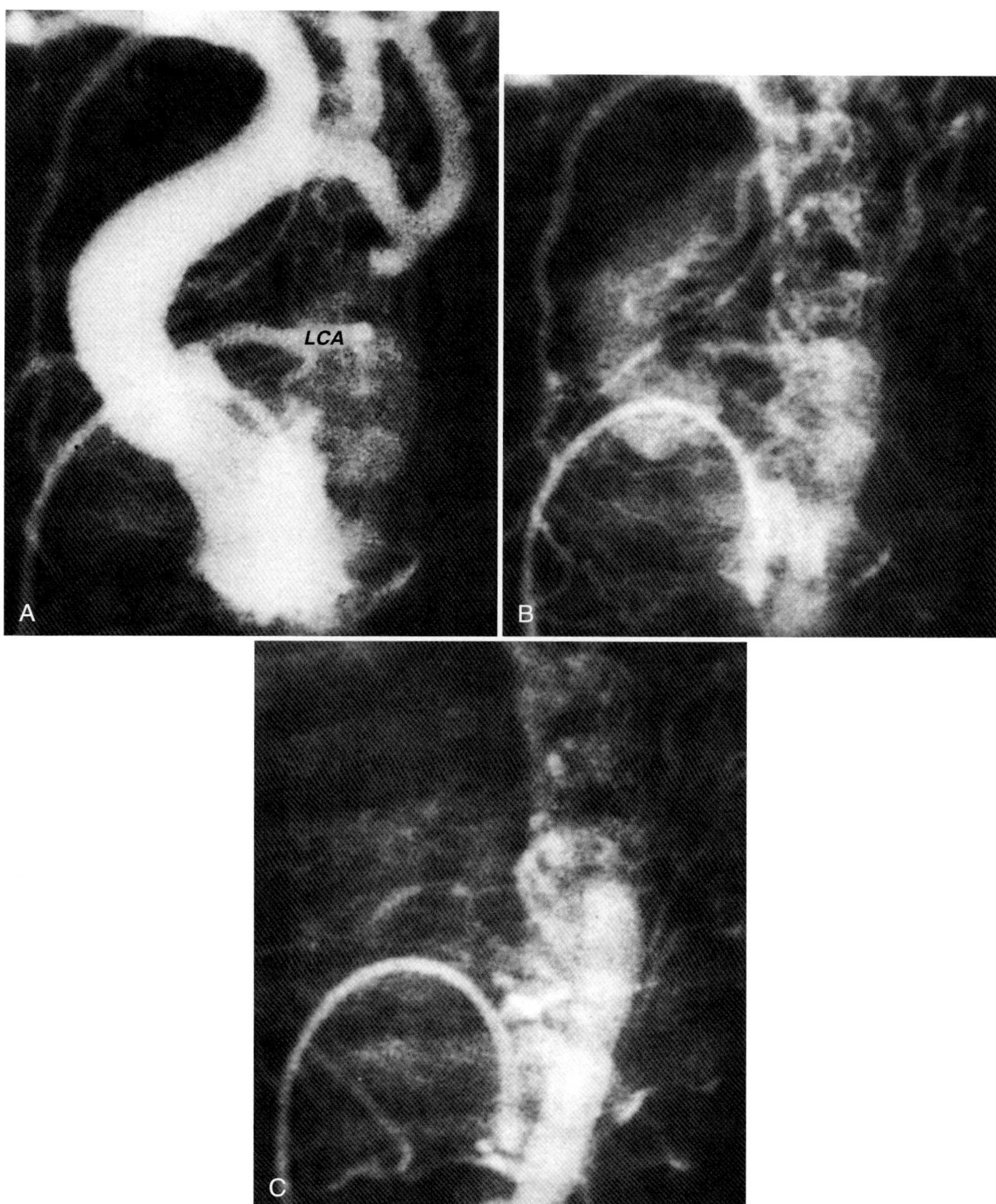

Figure 48-5 Cineangiograms in left anterior oblique view with injection into left ventricle of a severe coarctation 5 mm in length in a 7-week-old infant without other associated anomalies. **A,** Aortic arch and branches are outlined proximal to coarctation, but distal aorta is not opacified. Collateral vessels are visible. **B,** Dense collateral network is visible in this later frame, with contrast in descending aorta below coarctation. **C,** Descending aorta is well outlined, most of its filling coming from collaterals, although a tiny lumen about 5 mm long could be identified connecting the two ends. Key: *LCA,* Left coronary artery.

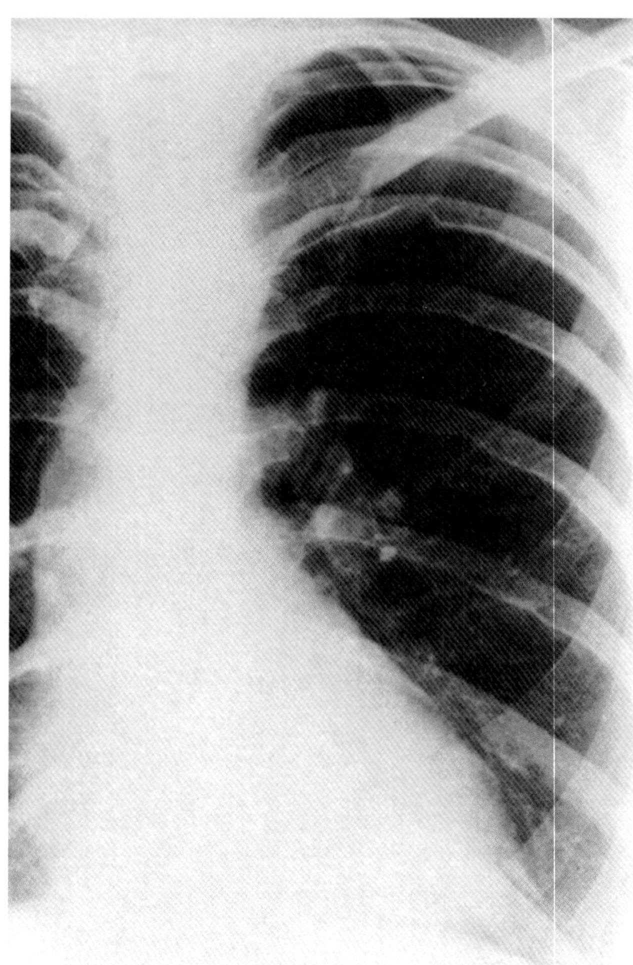

Figure 48-6 Portion of chest radiograph showing severe rib notching in patient with coarctation of the aorta. Note that changes are not present in first two ribs and are typically less severe below the fifth rib.

by characterizing intracardiac and great artery blood flow patterns using color Doppler signaling. Fetal echocardiographic measurements of the *z* value of the aortic isthmus and the isthmus-to-ductus ratio are sensitive indicators of postnatal coarctation.[M15] Outside infancy, echocardiography may still be helpful but is usually not definitive. In moderate or mild coarctation, presence of an open ductus may obscure a coarctation at echocardiographic examination. This is due partly to altered blood flow patterns associated with the patent ductus, but more importantly to the fact that the coarctation itself may evolve as the ductus closes.

MRI and computed tomography (CT) are currently the imaging modalities of choice for coarctation in patients beyond infancy.[B15,C11,G10,R11,R18,S6,S33] Excellent detailed imaging of pertinent vascular structures can be obtained, often exceeding the detail seen with aortography (Fig. 48-9). Three-dimensional rendering can be particularly informative (Fig. 48-10). Post-surgical changes also can be defined in detail (Fig. 48-11). Hemodynamic data can be assessed by MRI and may be particularly useful in older patients with well-developed collaterals, or in patients with restenosis, in whom there may be little or no gradient across the

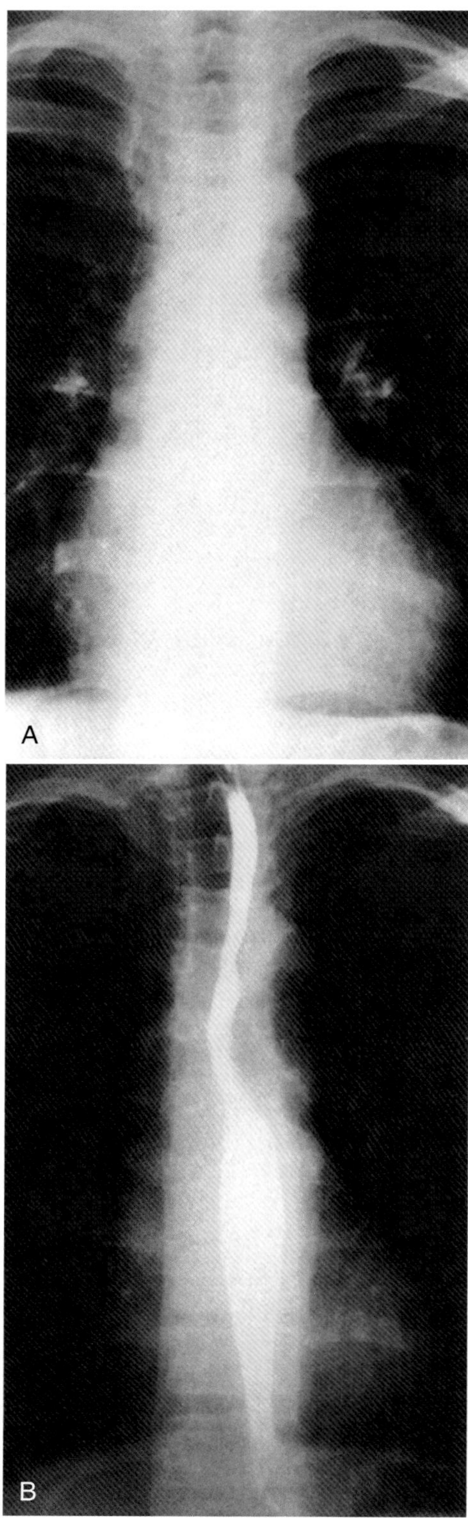

Figure 48-7 Radiographic studies in patient with coarctation, demonstrating classic figure-3 sign present in some patients with coarctation of the aorta. **A,** Chest radiograph. Upper convexity of sign is formed by the aortic isthmus and left subclavian artery, lower convexity by the upper descending aorta at site of poststenotic dilatation. **B,** Barium esophagogram. Note how the two shadows overlap. Isthmus and descending aorta produce upper and lower indentations on leftward margin of barium-filled esophagus.

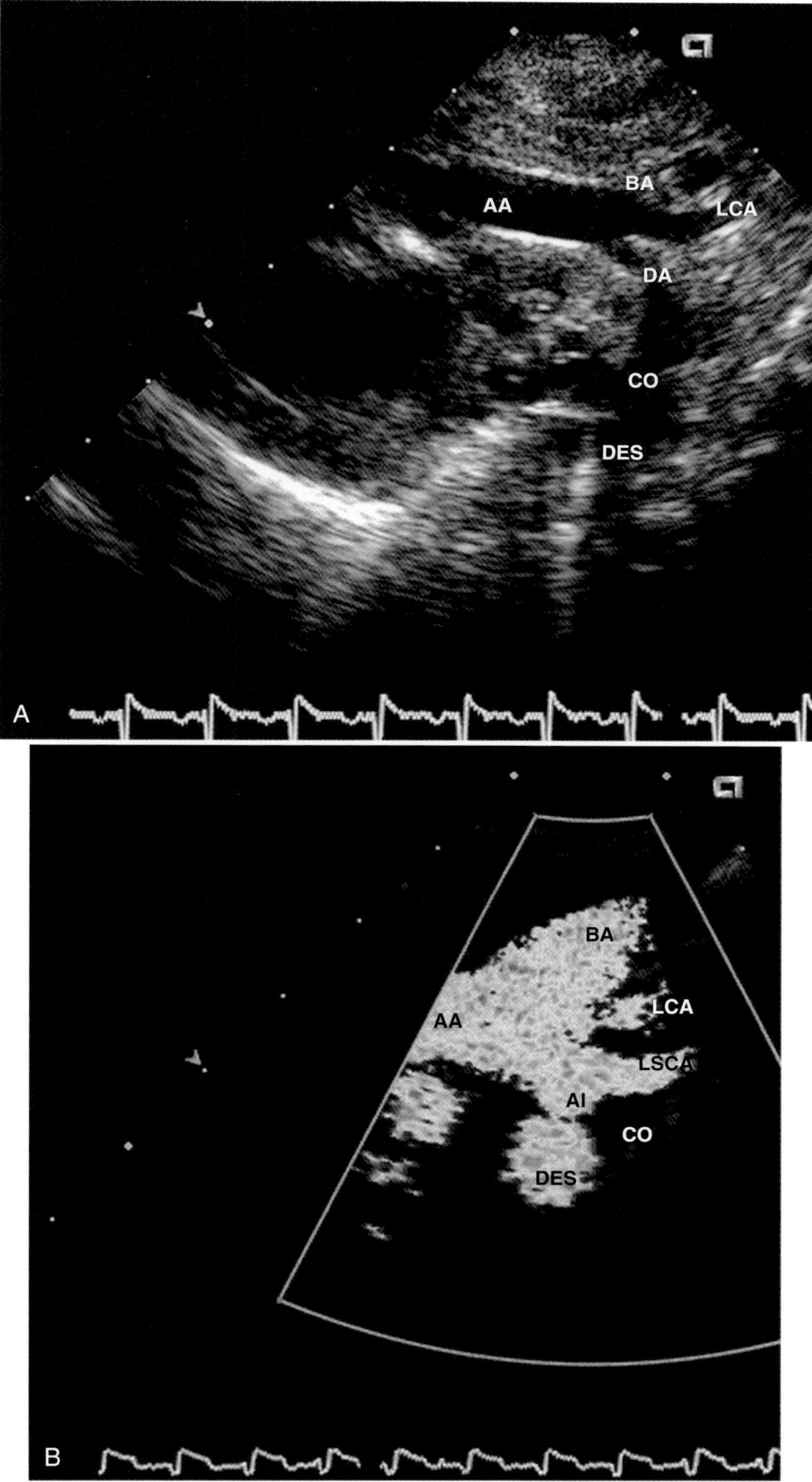

Figure 48-8 Echocardiographic images of neonatal aortic coarctation. **A,** Parasternal view showing small-diameter ascending aorta with origins of brachiocephalic and left carotid arteries, severe hypoplasia of distal aortic arch between left carotid and subclavian arteries, discrete coarctation, and descending aorta. **B,** Color imaging showing discrete narrowing at coarctation site.

Continued

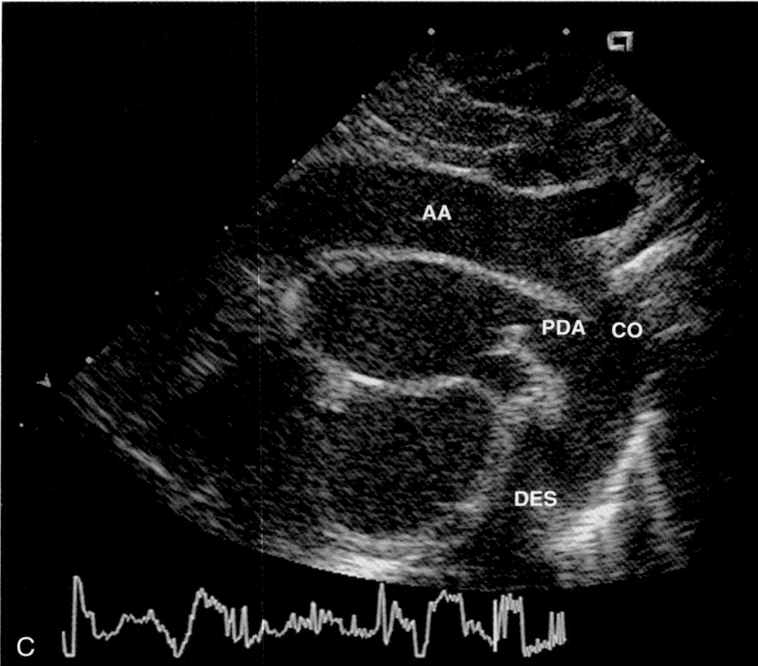

Figure 48-8, cont'd **C,** Image details hypoplasia of distal arch and isthmus, and a large ductus arteriosus entering descending aorta. A discrete coarctation, which was also present in this case, is not seen well in this image. Key: *AA,* Ascending aorta; *AI,* aortic isthmus; *BA,* brachiocephalic artery; *CO,* coarctation; *DA,* distal aortic arch; *DES,* descending aorta; *LCA,* left carotid artery; *LSCA,* left subclavian artery; *PDA,* patent ductus arteriosus.

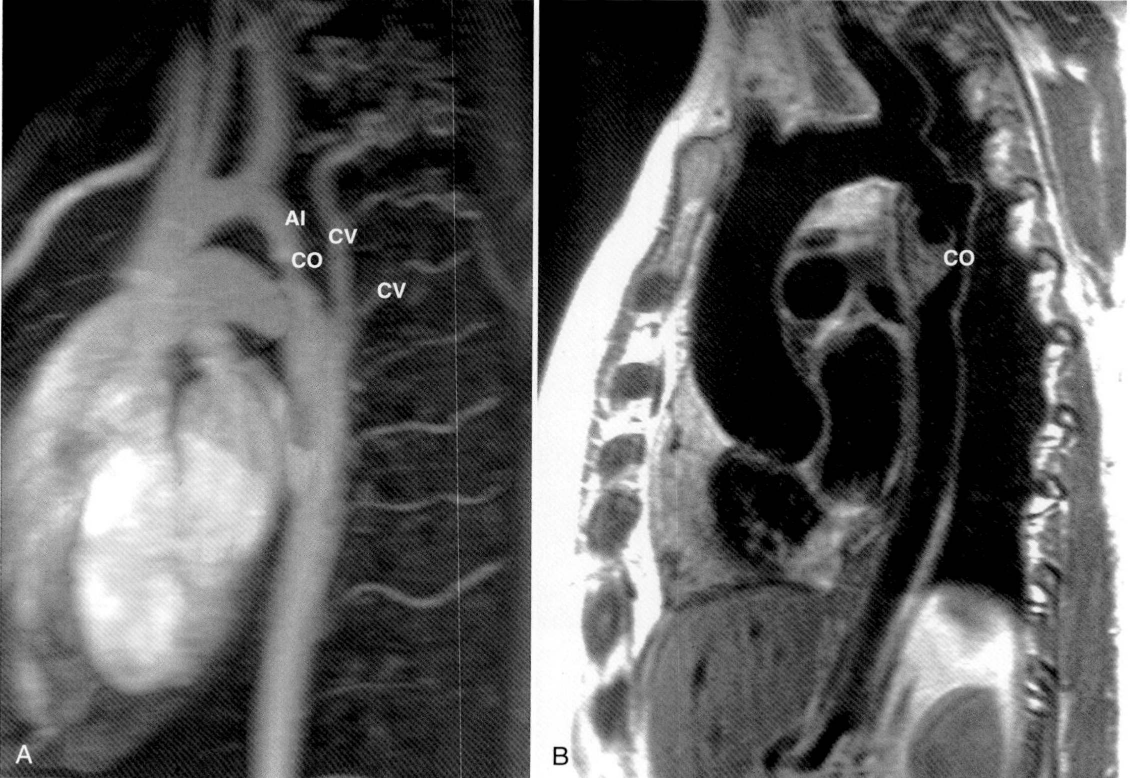

Figure 48-9 Magnetic resonance imaging of coarctation. **A,** Lateral projection (using contrast-enhanced imaging and cardiac gating) of native coarctation in 20-year-old man. Isthmic hypoplasia and collateral vessels are also present. **B,** Lateral projection (using T1-weighted imaging) of recurrent coarctation in 35-year-old woman.

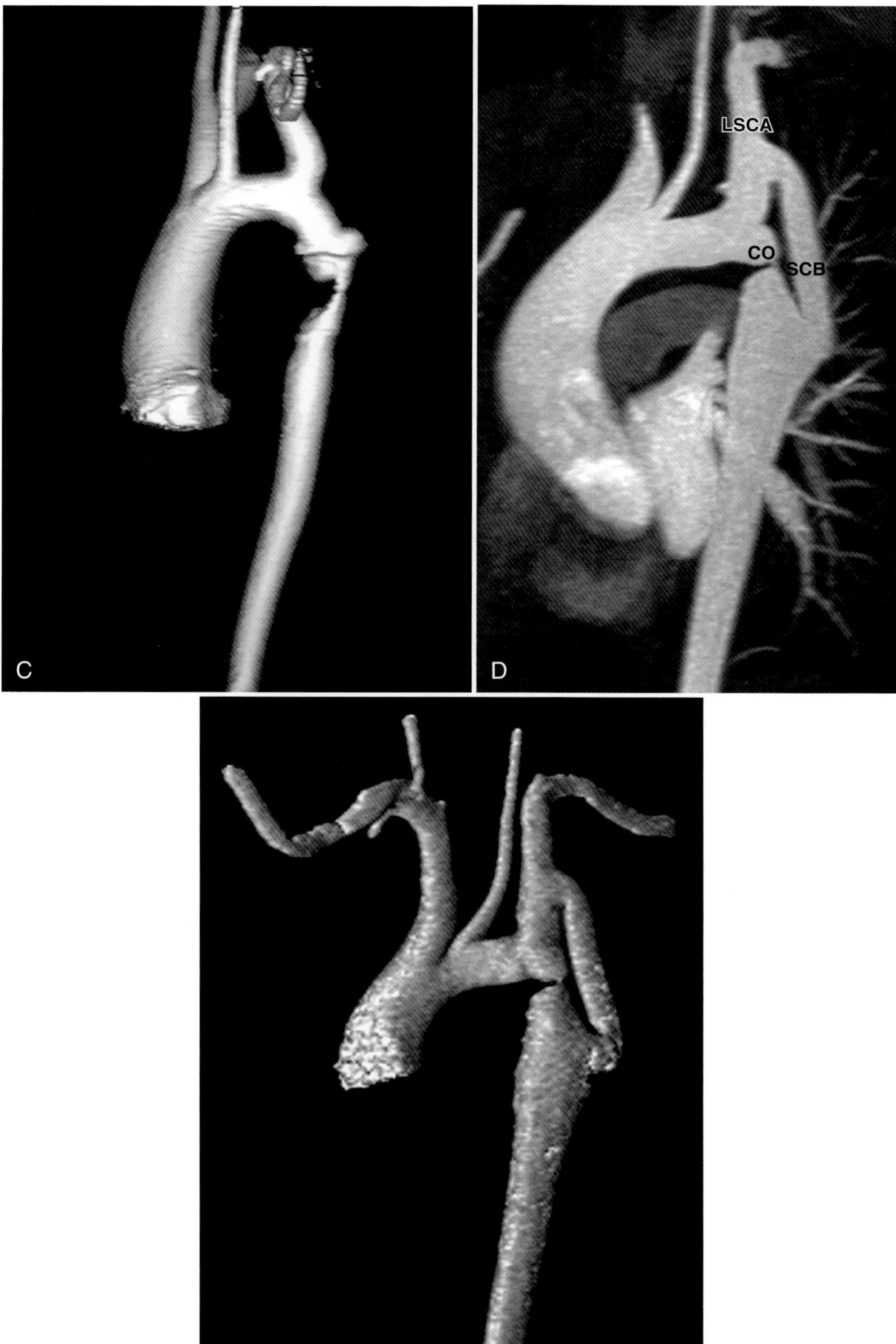

Figure 48-9, cont'd **C,** Three-dimensional rendering of patient shown in **B. D,** Lateral projection (using contrast-enhanced magnetic resonance imaging) of 40-year-old man with recurrent obstruction following childhood creation of left subclavian artery–to–descending aortic synthetic graft bypass of aortic coarctation. **E,** Three-dimensional rendering of recurrent obstruction shown in **D**. Key: *AI,* Aortic isthmus; *CO,* coarctation; *CV,* collateral vessels; *LSCA,* left subclavian artery; *SCB,* subclavian-to-descending aortic bypass.

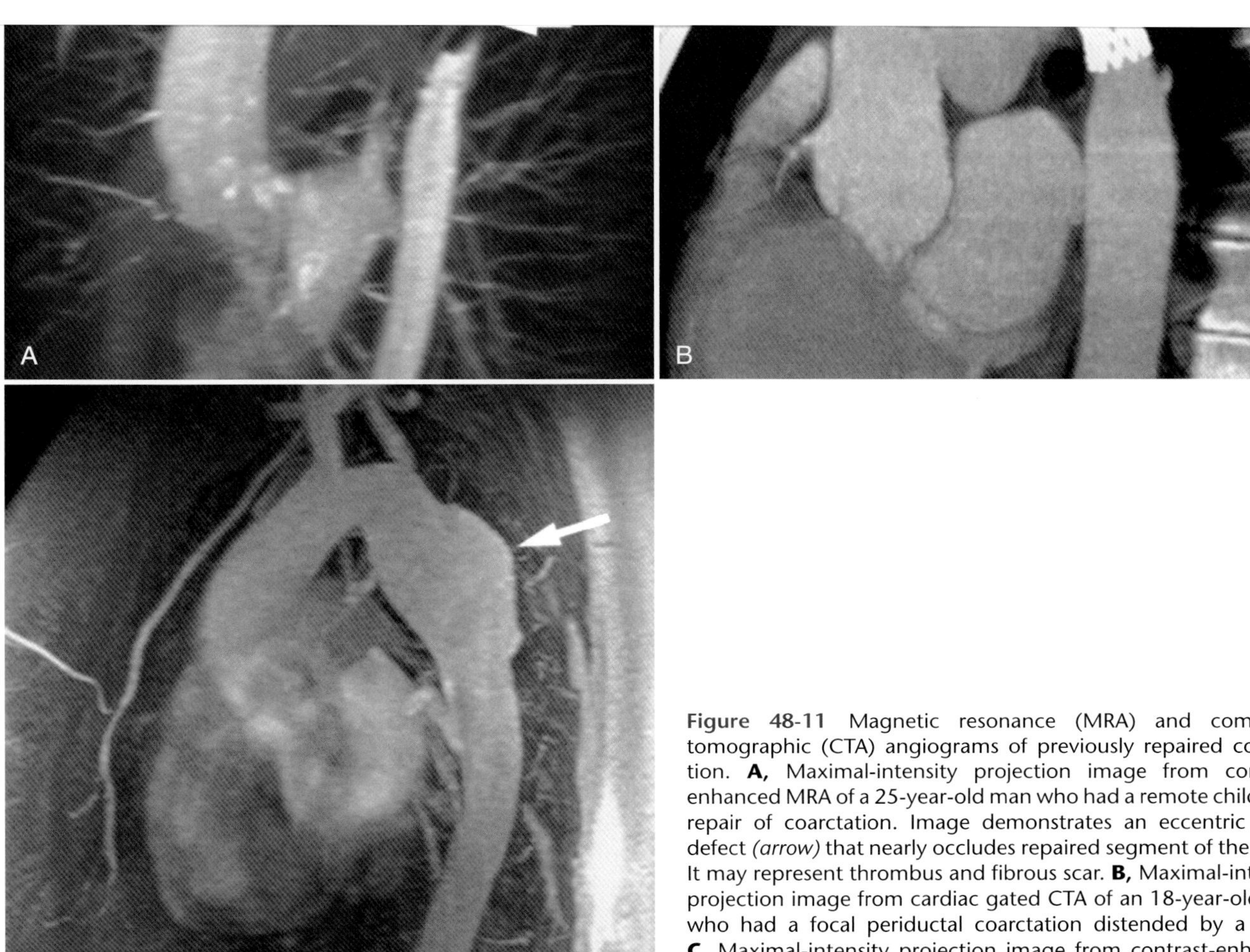

Figure 48-11 Magnetic resonance (MRA) and computed tomographic (CTA) angiograms of previously repaired coarctation. **A,** Maximal-intensity projection image from contrast-enhanced MRA of a 25-year-old man who had a remote childhood repair of coarctation. Image demonstrates an eccentric filling defect *(arrow)* that nearly occludes repaired segment of the aorta. It may represent thrombus and fibrous scar. **B,** Maximal-intensity projection image from cardiac gated CTA of an 18-year-old man who had a focal periductal coarctation distended by a stent. **C,** Maximal-intensity projection image from contrast-enhanced MRA of a 27-year-old woman who developed an aneurysm at site of repaired coarctation.

depressed. Because left ventricular systolic function as reflected in stroke volume and ejection fraction returned to normal after coarctation repair, the mechanism of its preoperative reduction is clearly *afterload mismatch* (see "Increased Ventricular Afterload" in Section I of Chapter 5 and Natural History in Chapter 12) brought about by sudden increase in left ventricular afterload from the rapidly developing coarctation as the ductus closes in the presence of a nonhypertrophied left ventricle. Severe cardiomegaly is present, but it is

Graham and colleagues reported somewhat different findings in the 10% of patients with isolated coarctation presenting with mild or moderate heart failure at 1 to 6 months of age. Left ventricular wall mass was increased in this group (as it is in older children with coarctation[G9]), and left ventricular ejection fraction and stroke volume were only *mildly* decreased. Increased left ventricular thickness had reduced left ventricular afterload (see "Ventricular Afterload" in Section I of Chapter 5); that is, "afterload mismatch" had

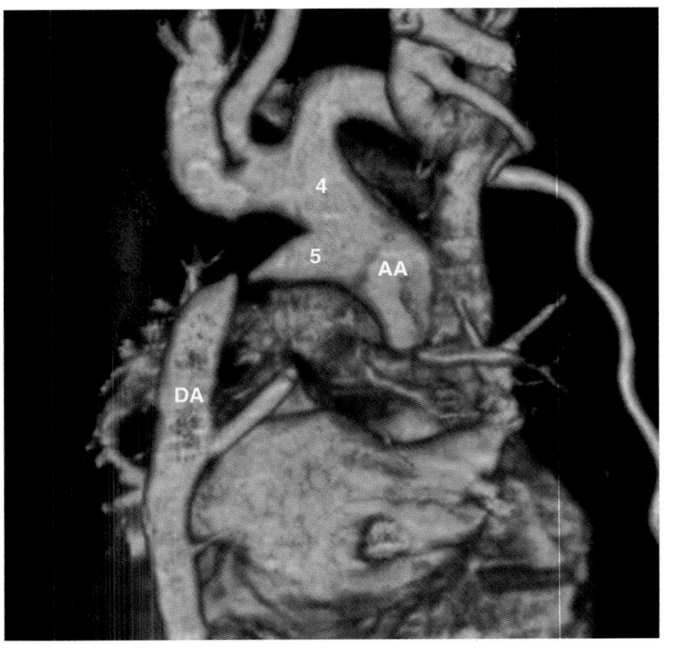

Figure 48-10 Volume-rendered computed tomography angiogram of a 5-year-old girl. Ascending aorta is connected to two proximal aortic arches developed from the fourth branchial arch and the fifth branchial arch. The fifth arch is in continuity with the descending aorta, but with no detectable lumen. Key: *4*, Fourth branchial arch; *5*, fifth branchial arch; *AA*, ascending aorta; *DA*, descending aorta.

coarctation site. Assessment of flow in the collaterals directly, and quantitation of the flow increase in the aorta at the diaphragm compared with the flow in the upper aorta near the coarctation (as a measure of collateral flow), can be more accurate in determining the significance of the coarctation or recoarctation.[A19]

Cardiac catheterization and *aortography*, once the standard for diagnosis in older patients, now play a secondary role and are used mainly when hemodynamic data are important in determining management of the patient. A withdrawal gradient is present at rest across the coarctation, and in borderline cases, measurement of cardiac output and gradient during exercise helps assess severity. Severity of the coarctation can be better assessed on aortography than by catheter withdrawal pressures, mainly because collateral flow may increase the pressure in the aorta distal to the coarctation. Aortography also reveals any hypoplasia of the isthmus or arch, arrangement of the aortic arch branches, degree of collateral circulation, and presence of an aneurysm. Intracardiac hemodynamics can provide important information when

Isolated coarctation is slightly more than twice as common in males as in females, but there is no gender difference in those with important coexisting cardiac anomalies.[S22]

Isolated Coarctation

This category includes patients with or without associated patent ductus arteriosus.

Survival

Coarctation has been surgically correctable since 1944. As a result, information on natural history is difficult to find. Postmortem data from series and case reports published before the era of surgical correction indicate that the median age of death is 31 years, with 76% of deaths attributable to complications of the coarctation.[A1,J5,R14] These reports did not include patients under age 2 years, and therefore neonatal and infant mortality are not accounted for. Among babies born with isolated coarctation, about 10% may be expected to die of acute cardiac failure during the first month of life if untreated. Another 20% may be expected to die later during the first year of life of heart failure or its sequelae. Thus, the true median age of death may be closer to 10 years.

Antemortem series prior to the era of surgical correction indicate that mortality after infancy is about 1.6% per year during the first 2 decades, and then gradually rises to 6.7% per year by the sixth decade.[J5] The most common causes of death, in decreasing order, are heart failure, aortic rupture, infective endocarditis, and intracranial haemorrhage.[J5] The few individuals who survive to age 60 years are usually women, because of their lesser tendency to develop hypertension and arteriosclerosis.[C4]

Heart Failure in Infancy

A number of factors act singly or in combination to produce heart failure in infants with isolated coarctation. *First*, ductal closure, as it progresses from pulmonary to aortic end during the first 7 to 10 days of life, increases the degree of aortic narrowing,[R26,T2] which prior to this event may have been mild and of little functional importance. Consequent development of severe coarctation precipitates left ventricular failure at age 1 to 2 weeks. If the coarctation does not become severe, heart failure does not occur. *Second*, the degree to which collateral circulation is present at birth may also be important. Mathew and colleagues found that all infants with isolated coarctation had collaterals on angiography performed at age 8 days to 15 months, indicating that collaterals developed either during fetal life or, more likely, soon after.[M14] Presumably, collateral development is absent or inadequate as long as the ductus is widely patent and there is pulmonary hypertension.[B6] *Third*, presence of major noncardiac anoma-

about 20% of cases), or rupture of an intracranial aneurysm in about 10%.[A1,R14]

Heart Failure in Childhood and Adult Life

In Reifenstein's series of adolescents and adults, there was only one death from heart failure in a patient younger than 20 years of age; most such deaths occurred in the fourth and fifth decades.[R14] In most instances, there was associated valvar heart disease, usually aortic but occasionally mitral, that combined with hypertension to produce heart failure. Congenitally abnormal aortic valve (bicuspid valves were present in 42% of the hearts[R14]) was the usual cause of stenosis or regurgitation. Heart failure occurs at the extremes of age; about two thirds occurs in infancy. It is uncommon between age 1 and about age 30 and reappears in about two thirds of patients who survive beyond 40 years.[L11]

Infective Endocarditis or Endarteritis

Infective endocarditis or endarteritis causes death at an average age of 29 years and is equally common in the first 5 decades of life. Infection usually occurs on a bicuspid aortic valve and rarely on a mitral valve or in relationship to a VSD. Endarteritis is less common and usually occurs in the poststenotic segment in relationship to the jet lesion on the aortic wall. Mycotic aneurysms can result.

Aortic Rupture

Rupture occurs at an average age of 27 years and is most common in the second and third decades.[A1,R14] It usually involves the ascending aorta and often occurs into the pericardium with tamponade; less often, the aorta immediately beyond the coarctation ruptures at the site of poststenotic dilatation where the wall is dilated and thin. Many of these ruptures are probably true dissecting aneurysms, but pathologic details of the aortic wall are scarce.

Intracranial Lesions

Intracranial lesions caused death at an average age of 28 years in Reifenstein's series and at 30 years in Abbott's series.[A1,R14] Among the 35 patients younger than age 21 years with coarctation and cerebrovascular disease reported in the literature and reviewed by Shearer and colleagues, only three were younger than age 7 years at the time, and in most the incident was fatal.[S20] In the majority of cases, there is a subarachnoid hemorrhage from rupture of a congenital berry aneurysm on the circle of Willis arteries. These lesions are considerably more common in patients with coarctation than in the general population and are more likely to rupture because of associated hypertension.[S20] Other causes of cerebrovascular accidents are arteriosclerosis, particularly in older patients, and emboli, particularly in the presence of infective endocarditis. In the treated series reported by Liberthson and colleagues, a cerebrovascular accident had occurred in only 1 of 91 patients (1.1%; CL 0.1%-3.7%) younger than age 11 years at the time of diagnosis and in 12 of 143 (8%; CL 6%-12%) age 11 to 39 years.[L11] However, in those older than 40 years, 21% (5 of 24; CL 12%-33%) had had a cerebrovascular accident.

presentation so early is uncommon in patients with isolated large VSD (see under Natural History in Section I of Chapter 35). Unless the VSD rapidly diminishes in size, most of these babies die within a few months without surgical treatment. However, in many the VSD rapidly becomes small (see Fig. 35-21 in Chapter 35), and the natural history then becomes essentially that of isolated coarctation.

Coarctation Associated with Other Major Cardiac Anomalies

The combination of coarctation with other major cardiac anomalies nearly always produces severe heart failure during the early weeks of life. Without surgical treatment, from 80% to 100% of such babies die in their first year of life.[F15,L5,S28]

All reported series show a high proportion of associated cardiovascular anomalies in patients with coarctation presenting in infancy[C9,F15,G7,T5] (see Table 48-2). In such infants, isthmus and arch hypoplasia is almost constant as a consequence of disturbed fetal blood flow patterns (see Morphology earlier in this section).[R26] In many of these infants, particularly those with complex and severe intracardiac anomalies, the natural history is primarily that of the associated anomaly. However, associated severe coarctation undoubtedly precipitates early heart failure.

TECHNIQUE OF OPERATION

In general, resection of the coarctation and reconstruction of the aorta should be considered the ideal method of repairing coarctation. For a number of reasons, however, this cannot always be achieved, and alternative methods must be used. The technique of each operation is described in this section.

Preparation, Incision, and Dissection

Neonates and Infants

After anesthetic induction, body temperature is allowed to drift down to a nasopharyngeal temperature of about 35°C. This downward drift is helped by reducing the operating room temperature to about 18°C (65°F) and by using the cooling mode in the heating-cooling pad under the child. Blood pressure in the right arm is monitored by an indwelling radial or brachial artery catheter. Near-infrared spectroscopy can be used to monitor tissue oxygenation both proximal and distal to the coarctation. Substantial changes in tissue oxygen values both above and below the coarctation have been documented with varying technical maneuvers; however, these changes have not yet been correlated with clinical adverse events.[B3,B17]

The patient is positioned in full lateral position, secured with strapping across the hip and onto the operating table, with a sandbag tucked against the front of the chest (Fig. 48-12, *A*). Approach is made through a left posterolateral thoracotomy, with the entry through the fourth intercostal space. For this, the intercostal muscles may be incised in the center of the interspace or entry made via the fifth rib bed, elevating the periosteum from the superior half of this rib and

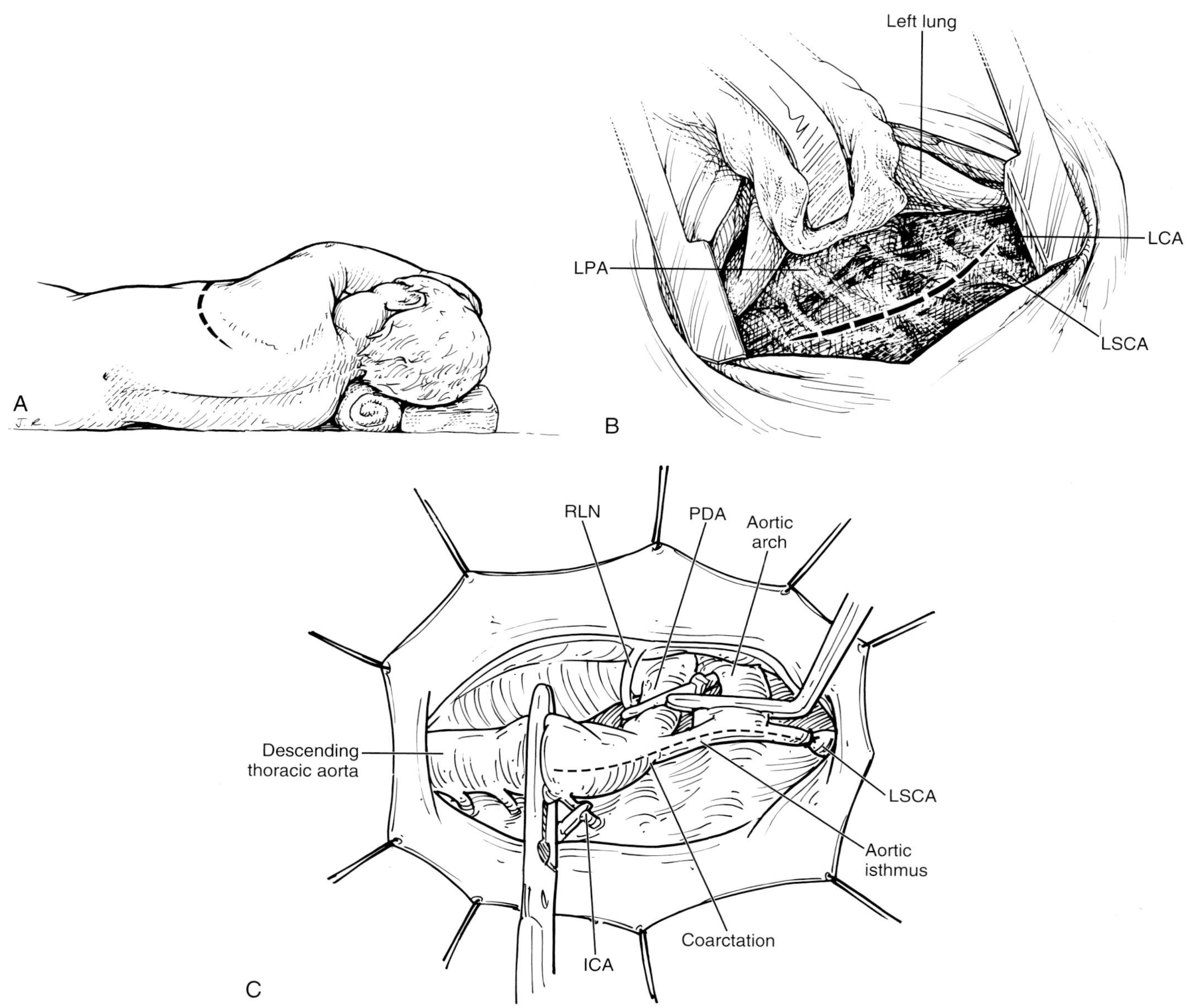

Figure 48-12 Approach, incision, and dissection for coarctation repair. **A,** Patient, often a neonate or infant, is in right lateral decubitus position, and a curving incision is made around the angle of the scapula. In infants, it is usually not necessary to incise the trapezius muscle. **B,** Rib spreader is in place, and lung is retracted anteriorly to expose area of coarctation. Dashed line shows proposed incision in mediastinal pleura. **C,** Mediastinal pleura has been opened and stay sutures placed on the edges for exposures. After dissection is completed (see text), operation proceeds depending on type of repair. For illustration, incision is shown for subclavian flap repair. After left subclavian artery has been ligated just proximal to vertebral artery, a vascular clamp is placed across aortic arch between left common carotid and left subclavian arteries. Distal aortic clamp is placed on descending aorta and may be positioned proximal to the third set of intercostal arteries, or as far distally as just distal to the fourth set of intercostal arteries. A delicate temporary neurovascular clip is placed across ductus arteriosus. Dashed line indicates proposed aortic incision.

Continued

collaterals. In most cases, the trapezius muscle need not be incised. Scoliosis is well documented following left thoracotomy in infants and children[K4]; however, it is not known whether minimizing trauma to chest wall muscles and ribs will reduce this late development.

The rib spreader is inserted and opened in stages to avoid rib fractures (Fig. 48-12, *B*). The lung is retracted anteriorly, and the mediastinal pleura is opened over the aorta downward for several centimeters below the coarctation site and upward to include the distal arch and subclavian artery and, if necessary for arch hypoplasia, all the brachiocephalic arteries. Numerous closely placed stay sutures are placed along each side of the pleural incision, and the ends are gathered into clamps for exposure (Fig. 48-12, *C*). No other retractors are then required. The left superior intercostal vein is ligated and divided.

Keeping dissection in the areolar tissue just superficial to the adventitial aortic coat, the proximal left subclavian artery, the distal transverse arch, and the aortic isthmus are dissected. All dissection is kept close to the aorta, in part because this is the best plane of dissection and in part to minimize the possibility of damage to the thoracic duct. "The Abbott

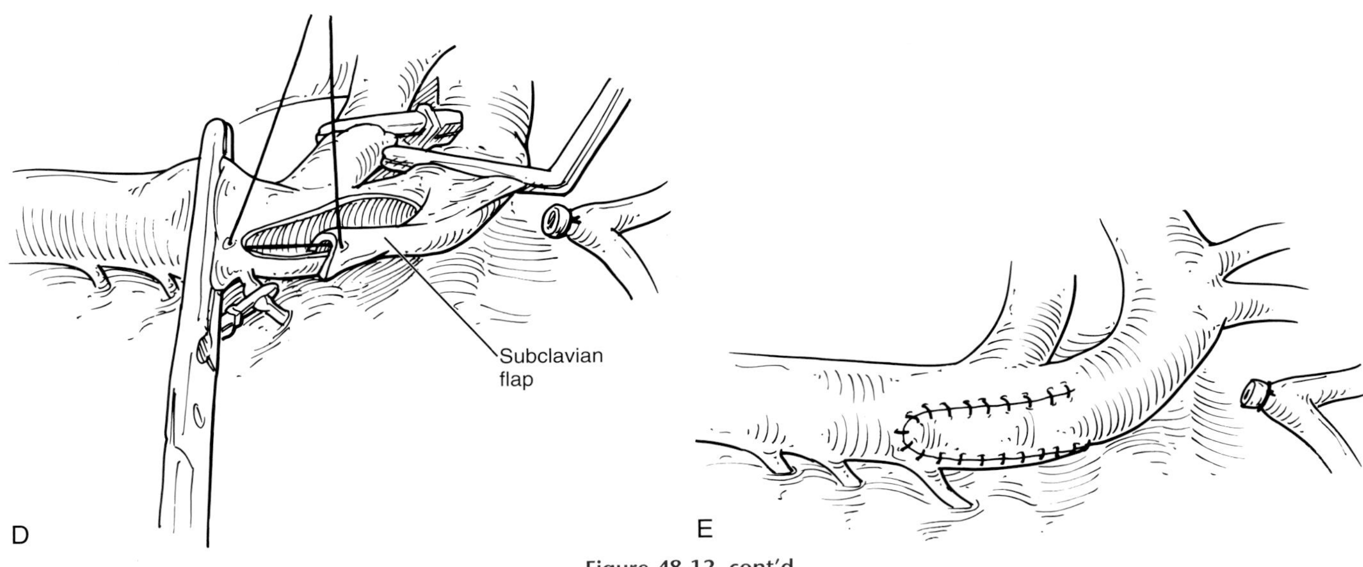

Figure 48-12, cont'd

artery" occasionally arises from the medial aspect of the isthmus and, when present, should be ligated and divided. Next, with great care to avoid damaging the intercostals and bronchial arteries, the aorta beyond the coarctation is dissected. It is occasionally necessary to divide one or more bronchial arteries medially. Finally, the ductus arteriosus or ligamentum arteriosum is dissected. If the nasopharyngeal temperature has not decreased to about 35°C, and especially if the patient is hyperthermic, the left pleural space is lavaged with ice-cold saline for the few minutes required to accomplish the repair (see "Paraplegia after Aortic Clamping" under Special Situations and Controversies in Chapter 24).

Children

The operation is technically more demanding in children than in neonates and infants because collateral circulation is much larger. A long posterolateral thoracotomy incision is made, cutting 1 to 4 cm of the trapezius muscle posteriorly and carrying the incision to the nipple line anteriorly. The pleural space is entered through the top of the bed of the nonresected fifth rib and the rib spreader is opened gradually until a wide exposure is obtained. The mediastinal pleura is opened widely over the upper half of the descending thoracic aorta and subclavian artery. Numerous stay sutures are applied as described for infants (see previous text).

The aortic dissection then proceeds as described for infants; however, it must be done with particular accuracy and precision because of the large intercostal arteries. Even the smallest subadventitial dissection must be scrupulously avoided by keeping dissection in the areolar tissue just superficial to the adventitia. In most cases, after incising the pleura over the aorta and brachiocephalic arteries and dividing the superior intercostal vein, dissection is carried around the aorta just proximal to the coarctation and a tape placed around it. A similarly sharp dissection is made just distal to the coarctation, taking care to avoid damage to a hidden Abbott artery above or an enlarged intercostal artery below. Further dissection is facilitated by gentle traction on the tapes.

The ligamentum arteriosum, the third and sometimes fourth pair of intercostal arteries, Abbott artery if present, and left subclavian and carotid arteries are now completely dissected. The Abbott artery requires ligation and division, as may a bronchial (or esophageal) artery beyond the stricture. All dissection details described for infants are important here as well.

Immediate Post-Repair Management

Following repair by any technique, the distal clamp is removed first. After the proximal clamp has been *slowly* opened, great care is taken to maintain proper ventilation and baseline systemic blood pressure for at least the next 5 minutes as a precaution against sudden development of intractable ventricular fibrillation 3 to 4 minutes after release of the clamp (*de-clamping syndrome*[T5]). It may be necessary for the anesthesiologist to give sodium bicarbonate or an infusion of a pure peripheral vasoconstrictor (or both) just before clamp removal in particularly unstable infants or in those with prolonged clamp times.

After repair, pressures are measured proximal and distal to the repair with fine needles. If there is a systolic gradient of greater than 10 mmHg, clamps are reapplied, sutures removed, and the repair refashioned. In neonates, the residual gradient may reside in the hypoplastic distal aortic arch between left carotid and subclavian arteries. Other causes may be inadequate excision of the intimal flap combined with failure to carry the incision in the aorta far enough distally if the subclavian flap technique is used (see following text), or a poorly formed anastomosis using resection and end-to-end anastomosis.

After the clamps are removed, the heating blanket, warming lamps, a warmed operating room, and warmed and humidified inspired gases are used to warm the infant. Usually the suture line is hemostatic, and the mediastinal pleura can soon be closed over it. A small chest tube is placed through a lateral and inferior stab wound. Incision through the interspace is closed with a few interrupted sutures. Muscles and subcuticular layers are closed with a continuous suture.

The chest tube may be removed in the operating room in neonates and infants after closing the incision. The baby is usually returned to the intensive care unit still intubated.

Resection and Primary Anastomosis

Neonates and Infants

Some form of this operation is currently the preferred technique for young patients. Preparations for operation, incision, and dissection are described previously under "Preparation, Incision, and Dissection." Once the coarctation is resected, there are various options for reconstruction, each of which is described in this section.

When the coarctation is well beyond the origin of the left subclavian artery, the proximal clamp is usually placed across the aorta to include the origin of the left subclavian artery. The distal clamp is placed on the aorta below the third and fourth set of intercostal arteries. The ligamentum arteriosum or ductus arteriousus, which has been tied at its pulmonary end, is transected at its aortic insertion. The aorta is transected proximal to the coarctation at a level that ensures removal of any narrowed portion of the isthmus as well as the coarctation (Fig. 48-13, *A*). Similar transection of the aorta is made beyond the coarctation, where the aortic diameter is usually ample.

The suture line is made with a continuous simple suture of 6-0 or 7-0 absorbable monofilament suture, sewing "from within" for the posterior wall (Fig. 48-13, *B*). After the posterior row of sutures has been placed, the ends of the aorta are approximated by the assistant and the sutures are pulled up snugly. The remainder of the anastomosis is completed by suturing the anterior wall using the other end (Fig. 48-13,

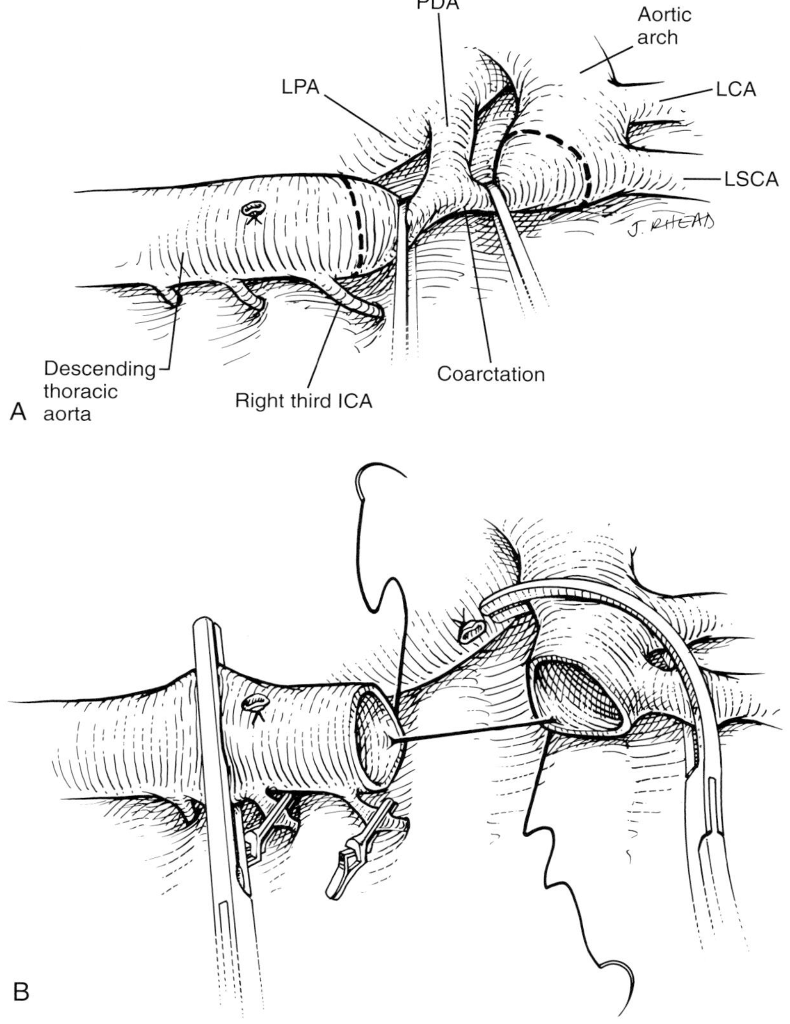

Figure 48-13 Resection and end-to-end anastomosis for repair of coarctation. **A,** With patient in right lateral decubitus position, a curving incision is made around the angle of the scapula, the chest opened, and stay sutures placed on the edges of the mediastinal pleura and held under tension to aid exposure (as shown in Fig. 48-12, but eliminated here for simplicity). After sharply dissecting out the coarctation and contiguous structures, tapes are placed around aorta just above and below coarctation. Traction on tapes elevates aorta anteriorly or posteriorly to provide exposure that facilitates dissection. Dashed lines show levels of aortic transection above and below coarctation site. **B,** Ductus arteriosus (or ligamentum arteriosum) has been ligated and divided, and small bulldog clamps (clips) have been placed on third and fourth pairs of intercostal arteries. Proximal clamp is positioned across aorta and base of subclavian artery to leave ample length for the proximal cuff. Coarctation is excised, getting back to a wide orifice proximally and distally. Running monofilament absorbable suture line is begun at far end of the circumference and progresses along posterior aspect of anastomosis.

Continued

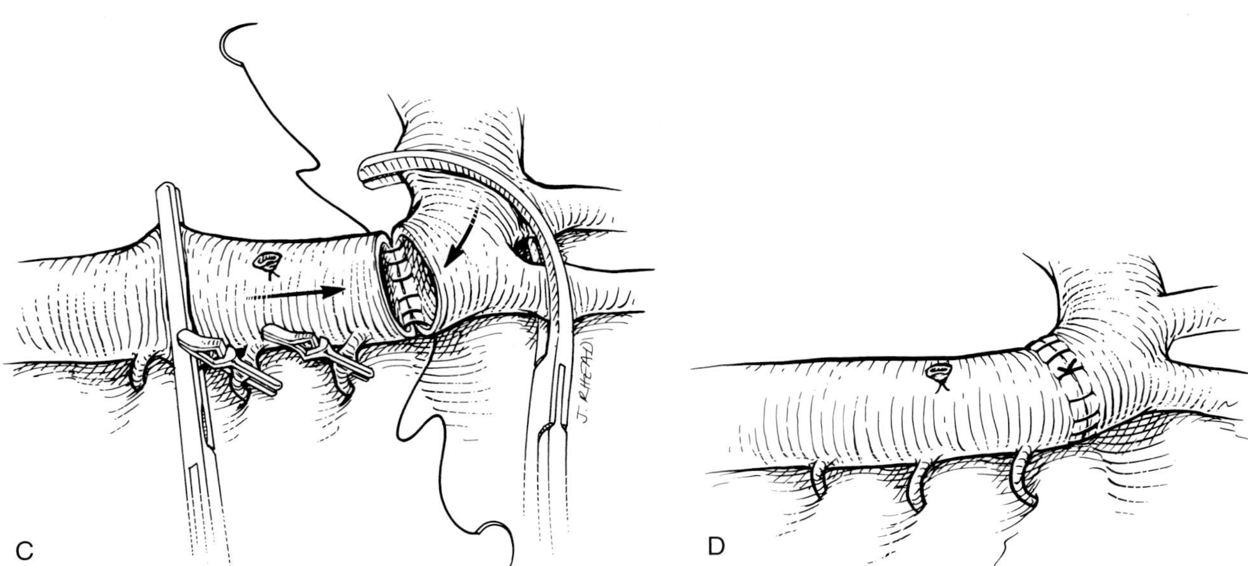

Figure 48-13, cont'd **C,** Aortic ends have been approximated, and posterior circumference suture line is completed. Anterior suture line is begun at far end of the circumference (see text). **D,** Completed anastomosis is shown after removal of clamps. Key: *ICA,* Intercostal artery; *LCA,* left common carotid artery; *LPA,* left pulmonary artery; *LSCA,* left subclavian artery; *PDA,* patent ductus arteriosus.

C). Finally, the clamps are removed as described under "Immediate Post-Repair Management" and the operation completed similarly (Fig. 48-13, *D*).

When the coarctation is near the takeoff of the left subclavian artery, or when the segment between it and the subclavian artery is importantly hypoplastic, proximal transection is begun just beyond the origin of the left subclavian artery.

When the distal portion of the aortic arch between the left common carotid and subclavian arteries is hypoplastic, as it often is in neonates and young infants, the operation may be modified so as to enlarge this area.[A15,L8,R3,V18] In young patients, end-to-end anastomosis is easily accomplished after extended resection, and the distal transverse arch and aorta proximal to the coarctation are widened by the procedure. Alternatively, hypoplasia in the distal arch and even the proximal arch can be managed by placing the curved proximal side-biting clamp to occlude the proximal arch just distal to the brachiocephalic artery origin, occluding both the left carotid and left subclavian arteries, in preparation for performing an end-to-side distal aorta to arch reconstruction (see Fig. 48-14, *A*).[R3] After resecting the discrete coarctation, the isthmus is ligated with a 5-0 polypropylene ligature, and the undersurface of the proximal arch is incised opposite the left carotid artery origin and extended to the point opposite the left subclavian artery origin. The cut end of the descending aorta, trimmed of all ductal tissue, is connected to the incision in the undersurface of the arch with an end-to-side anastomosis using a running suture technique with 6-0 or 7-0 absorbable monofilament suture (Fig. 48-14, *B* and *C*).[R3]

Resection with end-to-end anastomosis can be combined with subclavian flap aortoplasty (see "Subclavian Flap Aortoplasty" in text that follows) if there is concern about the size of the aorta just beyond the subclavian artery.[H26] This problem is better managed by resection with extended end-to-end anastomosis or resection with end-to-side anastomosis, as described earlier; however, the combined operation will be briefly described for completeness. After preparing the subclavian artery and placing clamps as for the standard subclavian flap repair, the coarctation area is excised as described for standard end-to-end anastomosis. The proximal and distal aortic segments are reconstructed with an end-to-end anastomosis, with the exception that the posterior wall and anterior wall continuous suture lines are not tied to each other posterolaterally after their completion. Rather, each suture line is tied to itself posterolaterally, leaving a small posterolateral gap. The subclavian artery is split open longitudinally, and incision is extended into the proximal aortic segment, then carried through the small suture line gap onto the distal aortic segment. The subclavian flap is sewn into position as described previously in the standard subclavian flap method, straddling across the end-to-end anastomosis.

Children and Adults

Operation is carried out in the same steps as in very young patients. However, the vessels are much more friable, intercostal arteries larger and more easily damaged, and the dissection potentially more hazardous. Use of controlled hypotension by the anesthesiologist (see "Coarctation of the Aorta" in Section II of Chapter 4) during dissection is important because it allows dissection to be done more safely and expeditiously. Once the aortic clamps are in place, upper body blood pressure is allowed to increase to moderately hypertensive levels (to promote collateral blood flow, see "Paraplegia after Aortic Clamping" under Special Situations and Controversies in Chapter 24). It is helpful to monitor left ventricular function by transesophageal echocardiography during the aortic clamping. Vasodilatory agents must be withdrawn before the clamps are removed.

Hemorrhage from intercostal arteries or from the Abbott artery can be massive and difficult to control, especially if one of these vessels is damaged early in the dissection before adequate exposure is obtained. Therefore, no effort is made

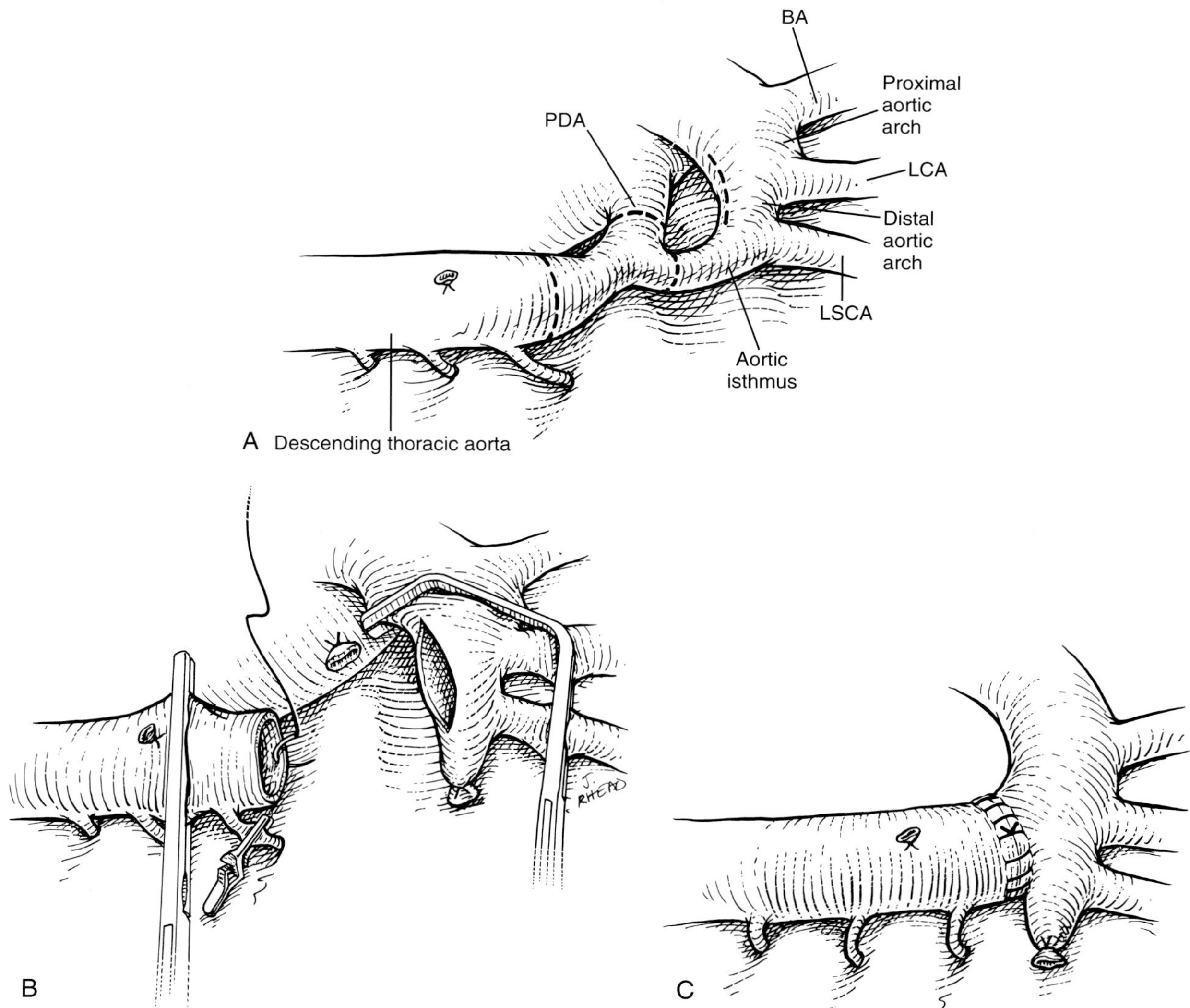

Figure 48-14 Resection and end-to-side aortic anastomosis for aortic coarctation with hypoplasia of isthmus and aortic arch. **A,** Incision and dissection are similar to that described in Fig. 48-12. Dashed lines show transection sites on distal aspect of isthmus, ductus arteriosus, and descending aorta, and incision site on undersurface of proximal aortic arch. **B,** Proximal aortic clamp is placed on aortic arch to include bases of left subclavian and left carotid arteries, with tip of the clamp angled precisely to extend as far proximally as possible without causing obstruction of flow to brachiocephalic artery. Distal aortic clamp is placed between third and fourth sets of intercostal vessels, and the third set of intercostal vessels is controlled with clips. Aortic isthmus is ligated. Ductus arteriosus is ligated at its pulmonary artery end, and coarctation site, including aortic end of ductus, distal aspect of aortic isthmus, and first portion of descending aorta beyond coarctation site, is completely resected along the lines shown in **A**. Incision in undersurface of aortic arch is made such that the length of the incision accommodates entire circumference of the normal aspect of descending aorta. Suture line is begun at far end of the circumference with a running monofilament absorbable suture. **C,** Anastomosis is performed essentially identically as described in the end-to-end anastomosis (see Fig. 48-13), proceeding along the posterior aspect of the circumference and then the anterior aspect. Completed end-to-side distal aorta to arch anastomosis is shown. Key: *BA,* Brachiocephalic artery; *LCA,* left common carotid artery; *LSCA,* left subclavian artery; *PDA,* patent ductus arteriosus.

to dissect these until tapes are around the aorta just above and below the coarctation, left subclavian artery, and in these older patients, aorta distal to the fourth, or if it is large, fifth intercostal artery. With traction on pleural stay sutures in one direction and on aortic tapes in the other, the structures can be liberated gradually by precise sharp dissection. The most inaccessible structures are the right third and fourth intercostal arteries, which must be approached and dissected with particular care. The junction of the enlarged intercostal artery with the aorta is the most fragile and easily damaged point. After dissecting from one side for a time, a sponge can be tucked against the aorta, the tapes swung to the other side, and dissection continued.

It is safer to control the intercostals temporarily with small metal bulldog clamps during resection and anastomosis than it is to ligate and divide them, because delayed hemorrhage can occur from slippage of such a ligature.

Occasionally, because of immobility of the aortic structures in an older patient or because of a long-segment coarctation, end-to-end anastomosis is not possible, and either an interposed polyester tube graft or an augmentation patch is necessary.

Subclavian Flap Aortoplasty

Currently this technique is most frequently used selectively in neonates, when circumstances make resection and reconstruction inappropriate—for example, when it is advantageous to preserve the ductus in the setting of a borderline left ventricle (see Indications for Operation later in this section). PGE_1 infusion is maintained throughout the procedure (see Fig. 48-12, *A* and *B*, which illustrate the exposure). To begin the subclavian flap aortoplasty,[W2] dissection of the subclavian artery is carried distally to expose the branches. It is ligated and divided proximal to all branches, none of which are ligated (Fig. 48-15, *A*). The ductus arteriosus is dissected, and a delicate vascular clamp, such as a temporary neurovascular clip, is placed across the ductus. A delicate vascular clamp is placed across the aortic arch between the left common carotid and left subclavian arteries, and a second clamp is placed well distal to the coarctation but proximal to the intercostal arteries, allowing space above and below the coarctation for the incision, as shown by the dotted line in Fig. 48-15, *A*. Uncommonly, it must be placed beyond the third pair of intercostal arteries (the first set beyond the coarctation), which are then controlled with removable metal clips or vessel loops made from heavy suture material.

The subclavian artery, before its transection, is split open longitudinally along its posterior margin, carrying this incision across the coarctation into the dilated distal aorta for at least 1 cm. Stay sutures are placed on either side at the level of the coarctation. The subclavian artery is transected just proximal to the ligature. Sharp corners at the end of the opened subclavian artery are trimmed; if the subclavian flap is unusually wide, the lateral edge is trimmed so that its width is about 1.5 times the diameter of the aorta. The turned-down subclavian flap may be tacked to the distal opened aorta using a double-ended 6-0 or 7-0 absorbable monofilament suture, which is then carried proximally as a continuous stitch (Fig. 48-15, *B*). Alternatively, the suture line may be started proximally on the medial side and carried just beyond the inferior angle of the aortic incision; another suture line is then started proximally on the lateral side and carried down to the previous one. Absorbable monofilament suture material 6-0 or 7-0 is used.[R9] Angles at either end of the turned-down subclavian flap must lie beyond the level of the coarctation, achieving this when necessary by sliding the flap distally in the process of suturing. In this manner, a proper "cobra head" is achieved. Following completion, the aortic clamps and the neurovascular clamp on the ductus are removed (Fig. 48-15, *C*).

Modifications of the subclavian flap repair have been used successfully.[A8]

Repair of Coarctation Proximal to Left Subclavian Artery

When hypoplasia occurs proximal to the left subclavian artery, the usual methods of repair can be unsatisfactory. When the situation is encountered in infants, a ***reversed subclavian flap aortoplasty*** may be used,[E5,H13,T15] or resection with end-to-side anastomosis as described earlier in this section and shown in Fig. 48-14 can be performed.[R3]

The reverse subclavian flap combined with end-to-end anastomosis is illustrated in Fig. 48-16. After usual exposure and dissection, the left common carotid artery and aortic arch between this and the subclavian artery are completely dissected. Clamps are placed on the left common carotid artery and on the aorta just proximal to this vessel and on the aorta distal to the left subclavian artery. The subclavian artery is ligated and divided distally. The subclavian artery is split down its ***medial side*** and the incision extended proximally onto the arch and the origin of the left common carotid artery (Fig. 48-16, *A*). The subclavian artery is turned down, in reverse to the classic subclavian flap operation, and sewn into place (Fig. 48-16, *B* and *C*). Alternatively, the end-to-side anastomosis of the descending aorta to the arch, as described earlier in this section under "Resection and Primary Anastomosis," can be used.[R3] In addition, when an anomalous right subclavian artery is present, it can be used in the reconstruction to address arch hypoplasia.[H21]

In older patients, ***replacement of the coarcted area*** with an interposed tube graft may be done when the coarctation is severe, but techniques for aneurysms of the distal portion of the transverse aortic arch are necessary (see "Replacement of Aortic Arch" under Technique of Operation in Chapter 26). The simpler palliative placement of a bypassing polyester tube graft between the ascending aorta and lower descending thoracic aorta via a right thoracotomy may be used, but is less satisfactory and should be reserved for particularly complex recurrent arch obstructive problems (see Special Situations and Controversies later in this section for further discussion).[A3,E2]

Repair When Aneurysm Is Present

When an aneurysm is present, either in the intercostal arteries (single or multiple) or aorta (see Morphology earlier in this section), resecting the segment of aorta involved along with the coarctation is required, and continuity is reestablished with an interposed tubular polyester graft. This procedure can be hazardous, particularly in regard to hemostatic control of the large intercostal artery feeding into the aneurysm. Pharmacologically induced hypotension is helpful to dissection. Early placement of the proximal aortic clamp and then ligation and division of the ligamentum arteriosum and placement of a clamp across the coarctation itself allows transection of the aorta proximal to the coarctation. Then gentle forward traction on the clamp across the coarctation allows the distal aorta and posteriorly placed intercostal artery aneurysm to be brought into better view for dissection and management.

Postrepair paraplegia is a greater hazard than usual because of the need to sacrifice intercostal arteries (see "Paraplegia after Aortic Clamping" under Special Situations and Controversies in Chapter 24). Special precautions required for all aneurysm surgery in this area are used (see "Replacement of Descending Thoracic Aorta" under Technique of Operation in Chapter 26).

Repair of Persistent or Recurrent Coarctation

Several options are open to the surgeon. The choice is partly determined by morphologic details of the obstruction and partly by surgeon preference. Resection and primary anastomosis, subclavian flap repair with or without resection, patch aortoplasty, and placing an interposition graft can all be considered. Repeat left thoracotomy is feasible in selected cases with discrete obstruction that does not involve the arch;

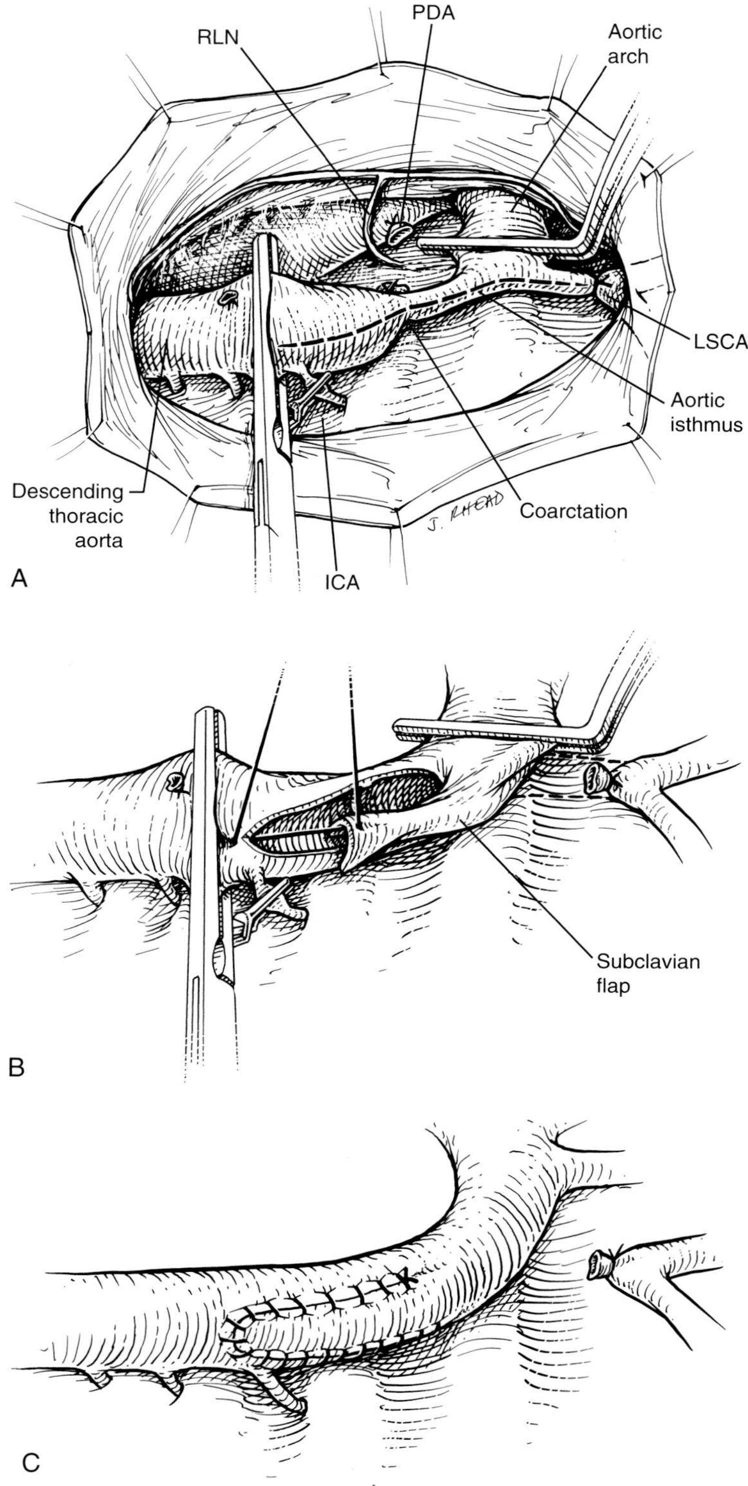

Figure 48-15 Subclavian flap repair for coarctation with preservation of patent ductus arteriosus. Exposure is shown in Fig. 48-12, *A* and *B*. **A,** Mediastinal pleura has been opened and stay sutures placed on the edges for exposure. After dissection is completed (see text) and after left subclavian artery has been ligated just proximal to vertebral artery, a vascular clamp is placed across aortic arch between left common carotid and left subclavian arteries. Distal aortic clamp is placed on descending aorta and may be positioned proximal to the third set of intercostal arteries, or as far distally as just distal to the fourth set of intercostal arteries (see text). A delicate temporary neurovascular clip is placed across the ductus arteriosus. Dashed line indicates proposed aortic incision. **B,** Subclavian artery has been divided distally and turned down for the flap. **C,** Flap sewn into place and aortic clamps and ductal clip removed (see text). Key: *ICA,* Intercostal artery; *LCA,* left common carotid artery; *LPA,* left pulmonary artery; *LSCA,* left subclavian artery; *PDA,* ductus arteriosus; *RLN,* recurrent laryngeal nerve.

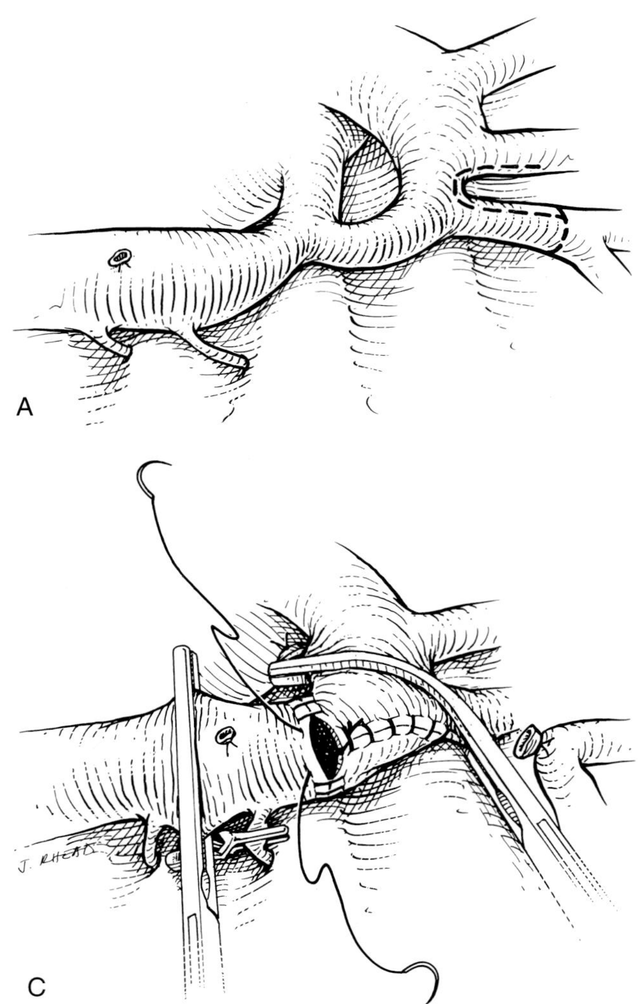

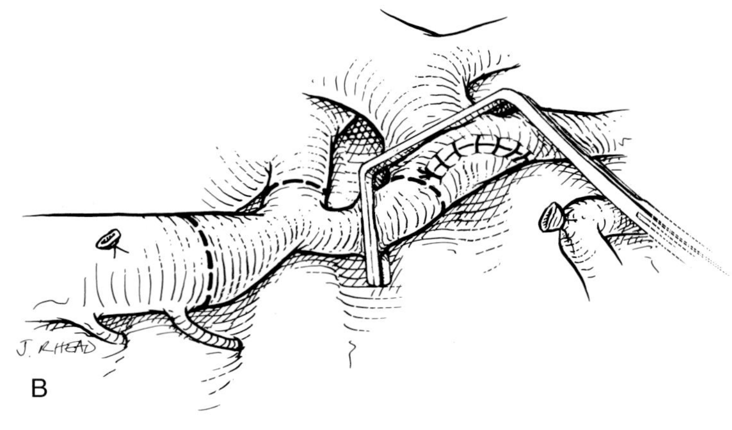

Figure 48-16 End-to-end anastomosis with reverse subclavian flap for aortic coarctation with isthmic and distal arch hypoplasia. **A,** Exposure and dissection is as described in Fig. 48-12, *A* and *B*. Dashed line shows incision along left subclavian and left carotid arteries that is necessary to perform reverse subclavian flap. **B,** A side-biting vascular clamp is placed across the proximal aortic arch to include base of left carotid and left subclavian arteries and also aortic isthmus. Incision shown by dashed line in **A** is performed, and distal subclavian artery is ligated. Using a monofilament absorbable suture, opened subclavian artery is anastomosed to base of left carotid artery to augment distal aortic arch diameter. Dashed lines show points of transection for subsequent end-to-end anastomosis. **C,** Clamp shown in **B** is removed and replaced by arch clamp. Distal aorta is clamped between third and fourth sets of intercostal vessels, and the third set of intercostal vessels is controlled with clips. Ductus arteriosus is ligated and divided, and aortic coarctation resected along dashed lines shown in **B**. End-to-end anastomosis is performed in routine fashion (see Fig. 48-13).

however, most cases require median sternotomy and cardiopulmonary bypass (CPB). Results are excellent.[B29,K1]

In particularly difficult technical situations in older patients, a bypassing polyester tube graft on the left or right side may be all that is possible.[A3,E2] This is most conveniently performed through a right thoracotomy. The end of a properly prepared polyester tube is anastomosed to the side of the intrapericardial portion of the ascending aorta using a side-biting clamp on the aorta. A side-biting clamp is placed on the descending aorta, just above the diaphragm, the tube graft is routed posterior to the right pulmonary hilum, and end-to-side anastomosis is performed. Intermediate-term results are generally good.[S41] Alternative extra-anatomical approaches have been described.[A16,A18,C20,M21,V22]

Repair of Persistent or Recurrent Coarctation with Aneurysm

Aneurysm following coarctation repair is more likely when transverse arch hypoplasia is present.[K19] The aneurysm may be very large and thin walled, with rupture almost a certainty over a 15-year period.[P1,V16] These cases represent a major challenge and must be addressed directly. The option of "indirect management," such as by an extra-anatomical bypass graft, is contraindicated because of the rupture risk. Standardized management techniques have not been established, but they include surgical, interventional, and hybrid techniques.[M8,P1] Optimal outcomes will be achieved with a multidisciplinary team including a cardiac surgeon, interventional cardiologist, and radiologist. The variables that influence treatment strategy include the severity of residual stenosis or hypoplasia, location of the aneurysm relative to the obstruction, suitability of "landing zones" for transcatheter devices, patient age and comorbidity, and likelihood of exclusion of the left subclavian artery or other brachiocephalic artery. Surgical management can vary but typically requires CPB, either via median sternotomy or left thoracotomy, with resection of the aneurysm and obstructive segment and interposition graft insertion. These procedures carry a mortality risk of 14% to 23%, and therefore endovascular management should be considered when anatomic details are favorable.[M8,V16]

Repair from an Anterior Midline Approach

Particularly in neonates and young infants, coarctation of the aorta can be well repaired from an anterior midline approach using CPB. Although use of hypothermic circulatory arrest is advocated by some,[D5,G1,T19,U1,W3] continuous CPB with antegrade cerebral perfusion can be used routinely for this repair[I3,K18,L12,Z1] (Fig. 48-17). The midline approach is particularly useful when concomitant repair of intracardiac defects is contemplated, but it can also be used to advantage when coarctation is accompanied by severe hypoplasia of the proximal transverse arch, or when there is no proximal arch segment because the left carotid and brachiocephalic arteries share a common origin ("bovine" trunk) in association with hypoplasia of the segment between this common brachiocephalic trunk and the left subclavian artery.

Technical and CPB considerations are similar to those involved with repair of interrupted aortic arch (see Section II). The anterior midline approach has also been described for both children and adults with coarctation and other complex arch problems using interposition conduits.[B9,I4]

SPECIAL FEATURES OF POSTOPERATIVE CARE

General

Generally, care of patients after coarctation repair is simple and similar to that accorded any patient after thoracotomy. In neonates and young infants, usual care accorded to small babies who have been critically ill preoperatively is used (see Section IV of Chapter 5).

Managing Systemic Arterial Hypertension

Systemic arterial hypertension is usually present after operation, and its management is controversial. In older patients, mean arterial blood pressure is lowered to about 110 mmHg with nitroprusside for the first 24 hours, and the drug is then rapidly tapered and discontinued (see Appendix 5A in Chapter 5). Thereafter, if systolic blood pressure is greater than 150 mmHg, a β-adrenergic receptor blocking agent or captopril is administered for a few weeks. Care must be taken to avoid a dose that leads to hypotension.

In infants and young children, treatment is given less routinely for postoperative hypertension. Intravenous nitroprusside is the treatment of choice; however, esmolol is also effective.[W9]

Abdominal Pain

Careful interrogation and observation of older patients postoperatively indicate that most have mild abdominal discomfort for a few postoperative days. In 5% to 10% of cases, this is prominent, and abdominal distention with hypoactive bowel sounds may develop.

Treatment consists of bowel decompression via a nasogastric tube and antihypertensive drugs. Antihypertensive therapy is begun and continued until symptoms subside. Intravenous fluids may be required for a day or two. In a study from 1972, Ho and Moss[H22] reported that routine treatment with antihypertensive drugs resulted in fewer (no) instances of laparotomy for abdominal pain than did nontreatment. In current practice, the need for laparotomy for abdominal crisis is rare.

Chylothorax

The nature of chest tube drainage should be observed. Copious serous or milky drainage is probably chyle, a finding in about 5% of patients. The chest tube should be left in place until this stops. If it continues profusely until the sixth or seventh postoperative day, reoperation is indicated.

A chest radiograph is obtained about 7 days after coarctation repair, because chylothorax may develop late and be initially manifested as an unexpected pleural effusion. If present, it should be aspirated. Occasionally, repeated aspirations are required; if the chyle reaccumulates after the third aspiration, reoperation is indicated (see "Chylothorax" under Special Considerations after Cardiac Surgery in Section II of Chapter 5).

RESULTS

Repair of Isolated Coarctation

Survival

Early (Hospital) Death Hospital mortality over the last 20 years has been low (2%-10%) in neonates undergoing operation with or without persisting patency of the ductus arteriosus[T18,Z2] (Table 48-3). In recent years it is not unusual for reports to show early mortality of 0% to 2%.[A8,H2,H26,K8,M23,M24,R3,T13,V10,W13] When repair of coarctation is performed in older infants, children, adolescents, and young adults, early mortality is about 1%.

Time-Related Survival In a heterogeneous group of neonates reported by the Congenital Heart Surgeons Society (CHSS), 12- and 24-month survivals were both 95%.[Q1] In a single-institution study of 191 heterogeneous patients, survival at 2, 5, and 10 years was 92%, 88%, and 88%, respectively. Survival was better at all time points for patients with isolated coarctation[K8] (Fig. 48-18).

Modes of Death When repair is performed in the first few months of life, the few deaths that occur result from continuing heart failure, management errors, or poor preoperative status. Persisting or recurrent hypertension, rupture of intracranial or other aneurysms, acute aortic dissection, acute myocardial infarction, and complications of late-appearing aortic valve disease (related to congenitally bicuspid aortic valve) account for most of these.[B23,M11]

Incremental Risk Factors for Death after Repair There are few well-established risk factors for death except *older age* at operation. Although low birth weight is likely to increase morbidity when repair is performed in the neonatal period,[B2] this has not been extensively evaluated. Coarctation repair has been successfully performed in neonates weighing less than 1 kg.[R12] In one single-institution study, presence of transverse arch hypoplasia was a risk factor for death.[H2]

Hypoplastic left heart class (see Table 48-1) also seems to be related to survival, although most patients with isolated coarctation are in hypoplastic left heart class I (Fig. 48-19; see also Table 48-3). A single-institution study of 55 isolated coarctation repairs with at least one hypoplastic intracardiac left heart structure indicates that outcomes, both early and midterm, are equal to outcomes of patients without associated left heart hypoplasia, and that the hypoplastic intracardiac structures demonstrate somatic growth over time.[W11]

Whether technique of repair is a risk factor for death is arguable.[B20,P11,V4-V6]

Late Postoperative Exercise Capacity

Exercise capacity is lower than normal (80% of predicted) at late follow-up in patients who have had coarctation repair.

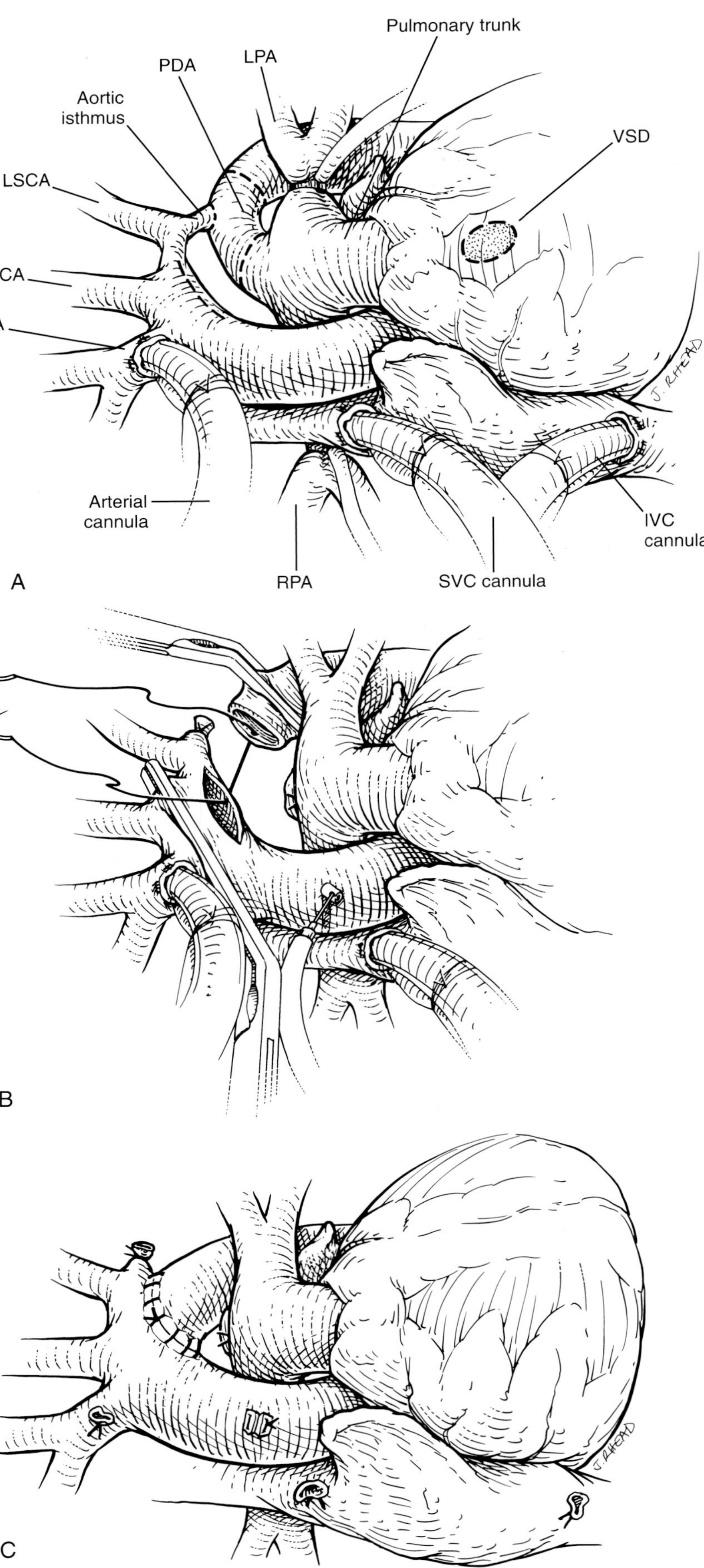

Figure 48-17 Coarctation repair through median sternotomy using cardiopulmonary bypass (CPB). This approach is used when proximal aortic arch obstruction is severe or when an intracardiac procedure (usually a ventricular septal defect) is also repaired. **A,** A standard median sternotomy incision is shown, and great vessels are dissected extensively, similar to that required for neonatal repair of hypoplastic left heart (see Technique of Operation in Chapter 49). After standard preparation for CPB, cannulation is performed with the arterial cannula placed into brachiocephalic artery through a standard purse string, and superior and inferior venae cavae cannulated individually. At institution of CPB, left and right branch pulmonary arteries are temporarily ligated. (See text for details of CPB management.) Dashed lines show incision in proximal aortic arch and transection sites at the distal aspect of hypoplastic aortic isthmus, at the descending aorta, and at the ductus arteriosus. **B,** Cardioplegia needle is placed into mid- ascending aorta, and after clamping the ascending aorta cephalad to the needle, cardioplegic solution is administered (see text for details). After achieving adequate cardiac arrest, the original aortic clamp is moved to base of brachiocephalic and left carotid arteries as shown, allowing continued perfusion into these arteries. The distal aorta is clamped and coarctation site resected along the dashed lines shown in **A**. Aortic isthmus and ductus arteriosus are both ligated, and temporary branch pulmonary artery ligatures are removed. An incision is made in undersurface of proximal aortic arch, and anastomosis is begun at midpoint of posterior aspect of the circumference of descending aorta as shown. A running monofilament absorbable suture is used. **C,** Anastomosis is shown in its completed form, aortic clamps have been removed, and patient is separated from CPB (see Technique of Operation in Section 1 of Chapter 35, and details in text of this chapter for approaches to closure of the ventricular septal defect). Key: *BA,* Brachiocephalic artery; *IVC,* inferior vena cava; *LCA,* left common carotid artery; *LPA,* left pulmonary artery; *LSCA,* left subclavian artery; *PDA,* patent ductus arteriosus; *RPA,* right pulmonary artery; *SVC,* superior vena cava; *VSD,* ventricular septal defect.

Table 48-3 Hospital and Total Deaths after Repair of Isolated Coarctation in Neonates[a]

	Class I[b]						Class II[b]						Class III[b]					
		Hospital Deaths			Total Deaths			Hospital Deaths			Total Deaths			Hospital Deaths			Total Deaths	
Method of Repair	*n*	No.	%	CL (%)	No.	%	*n*	No.	%	CL (%)	No.	%	*n*	No.	%	CL (%)	No.	%
Subclavian flap aortoplasty	27	1	4	0.5-12	2	7												
Resection with end-to-end anastomosis	18	0	0	0-10	1	6	3	1	33	4-76	2	67	1	1	100	15-100	1	100
Resection with end-to-end anastomosis + subclavian aortoplasty	2	0	0	0-61	1	50												
Patch-graft aortoplasty	6	0	0	0-27	0	0	2	1	50	7-93	1	50						
Unknown type of repair	2	0	0	0-61	0	0												
No repair	2	1	50	7-93	1	50												
TOTAL	57	2	4	1-8	5	9	5	2	40	14-71	3	60	1	1	100	15-100	1	100

[a]Data from multiinstitutional study of the Congenital Heart Surgeons Society, 1990 to 1991.
[b]Classes I, II, and III are defined in "Coarctation as Part of Hypoplastic Left Heart Physiology" under Morphology and Morphogenesis and in Table 48-1. One patient in hypoplastic left heart (HLH) III underwent resection and end-to-end anastomosis and died; no patient was in HLH class IV.

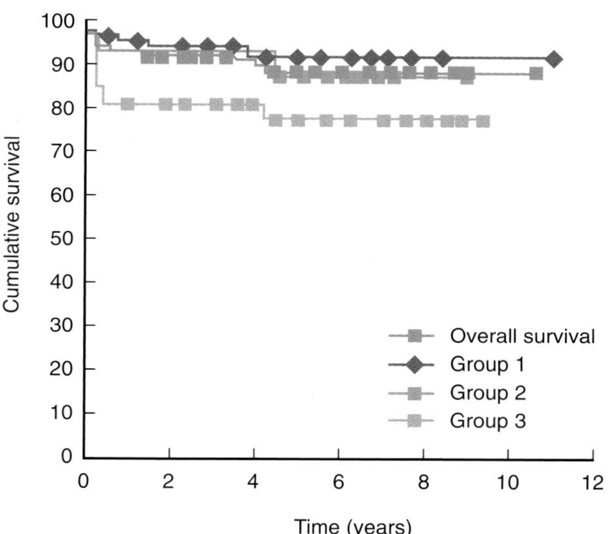

Figure 48-18 Survival of 191 patients undergoing coarctation repair. Group 1 = isolated coarctation. Group 2 = coarctation with ventricular septal defect. Group 3 = coarctation with complex intracardiac anatomy. (From Kaushal and colleagues.[K8])

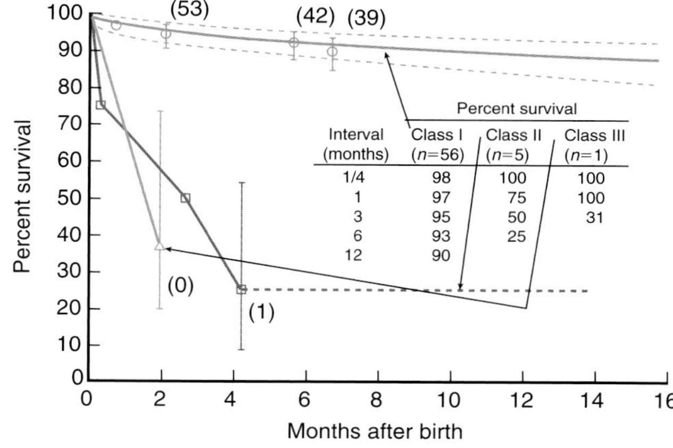

Figure 48-19 Effect of hypoplastic left heart class on survival after repair of otherwise isolated coarctation in 62 neonates. (From multiinstitutional study of the Congenital Heart Surgeons Society, 1990 to 1991.)

This is independent of type or success of repair, age at repair, and presence or absence of upper–lower body blood pressure gradient.[Y2]

Late Postoperative Upper Body Hypertension at Rest and during Exercise

Resting Values About 50% of patients who have undergone coarctation repair have an upper body resting systolic blood pressure higher than the mean value for normal individuals.[F12,H3] The two groups behave differently with exercise as well, with the coarctation group demonstrating exercise-induced hypertension, even in some patients whose blood pressure is normal at rest[H3] (Fig. 48-20). It is important to recall that *systolic hypertension* portends the same prevalence of unfavorable outcome events as diastolic or mean blood pressure hypertension.[L8]

Time course of upper body blood pressure may be generalized as follows. It is often considerably elevated early postoperatively. Thereafter it tends progressively to normalize in most patients such that by 5 years after repair, 80% to 90% of patients have normal upper body systolic and diastolic blood pressures at rest (Fig. 48-21). After 5 years, prevalence of patients with normal blood pressure begins to decline, and by 20 years after operation, only 40% to 50% have normal blood pressure (Fig. 48-22). Prevalence declines still further after that.

The younger the patient is at operation, the longer the period of normotension, or the greater the prevalence of normotension at any given interval after operation (see Figs. 48-21 and 48-22).[N1,S10,S22] However, the differences appear

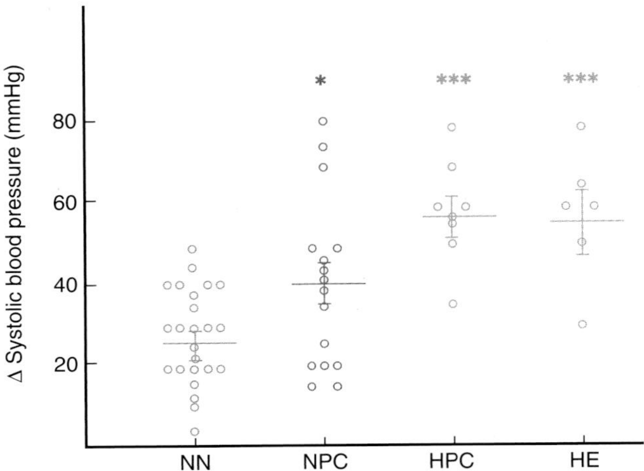

Figure 48-20 Increase (Δ) in upper body systolic blood pressure during standardized exercise testing in patients who have undergone repair of coarctation, and in other patients. (Three asterisks indicate columns that are different from normotensive patients [$P < .01$].) Key: *HE,* Hypertensive patients without coarctation; *HPC,* postcoarctation repair patients with upper body resting hypertension; *NN,* normotensive patients without resting hypertension; *NPC,* postcoarctation repair patients with upper body resting normotension. (From Simsolo and colleagues.[S27])

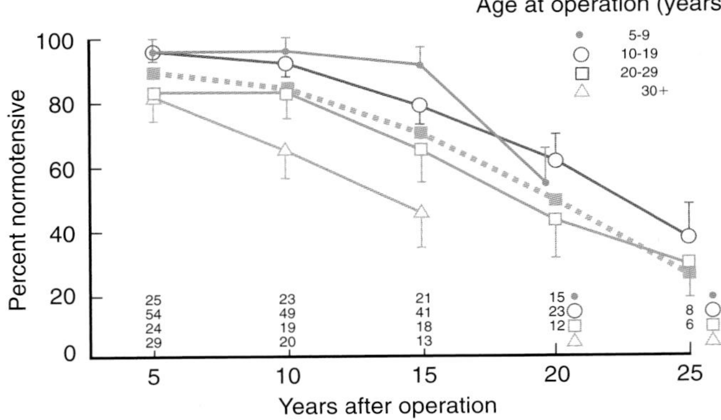

Figure 48-22 Percentage of patients normotensive at various intervals after repair of coarctation, according to age at repair. Dashed line represents all cases combined. Numbers at risk are shown above baseline. (Modified from Clarkson and colleagues.[C15])

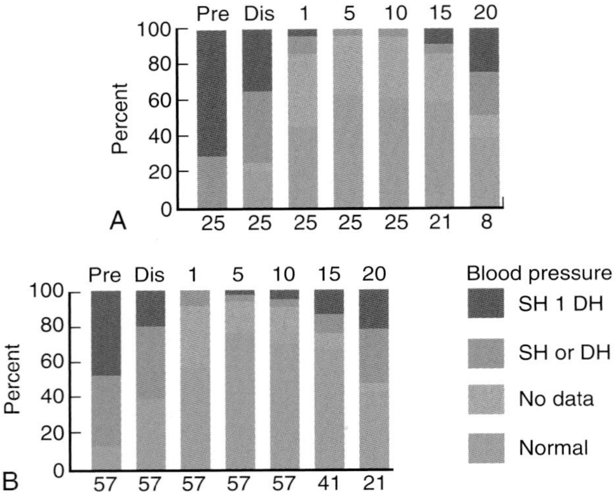

Figure 48-21 Stack plots depicting percent of patients with resting normal blood pressure and with resting hypertension (systolic or diastolic) at various intervals related to age at repair of coarctation. Numbers across top are number of years after repair of coarctation, and numbers beneath bars are number of patients at risk. **A,** Patients 5 to 9 years old at coarctation repair. **B,** Patients 10 to 19 years old at coarctation repair. Key: *DH,* Diastolic hypertension; *Dis,* at discharge from hospital after coarctation repair; *Pre,* preoperatively; *SH,* systolic hypertension. (From Clarkson and colleagues.[C15])

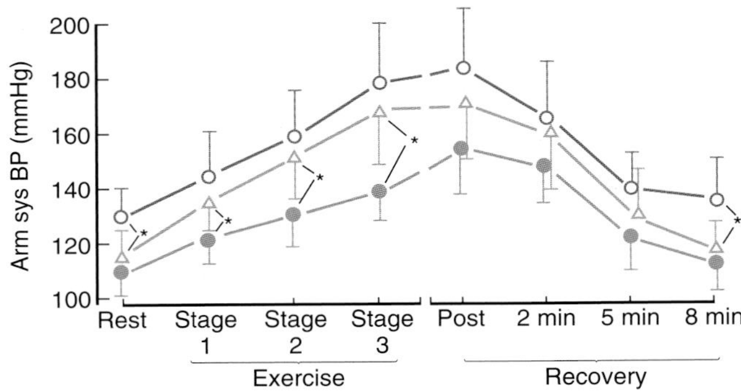

Figure 48-23 Arm systolic blood pressure at rest and during and after exercise in 15 control subjects and 15 patients before and after coarctectomy. Open circles represent preoperative; triangles, postoperative; and closed circles, control subjects. Bars indicate ± 1 SD. * = $P < .01$ postoperative vs. control values. Key: *BP,* Blood pressure; *Post,* post-exercise; *sys,* systolic. (From Pelech and colleagues.[P8])

to be small so long as repair is done before about age 10 years. In patients undergoing coarctation repair as adults (age ≥ 16 years), generally more than half are normotensive; the remainder are on antihypertensive medication, but blood pressure is improved and medication reduced compared with preoperatively.[B22,D11,H15,J3,K23,V15]

Evidence is beginning to emerge that late hypertension is less prevalent in patients who undergo coarctation repair within the first year of life rather than at an older age.[S33] Additionally, method of repair may influence the likelihood of developing hypertension. In two studies evaluating hypertension and compliance of the systemic arterial system a decade or more after coarctation repair, patients undergoing primary resection and end-to-end anastomosis had less hypertension and better vascular compliance than those undergoing subclavian flap aortotplasty.[B10,R21]

Values with Exercise Patients who have undergone coarctation repair experience a considerable increase in upper body blood pressure during exercise, although variability in response is even greater than that at rest (Fig. 48-23; also see Fig. 48-20) and is more variable than that of normal persons, who also experience some increase during exercise (Fig. 48-24; see also Fig. 48-23). The increase with exercise in postcoarctectomy patients with upper body hypertension is similar to that of hypertensive patients without coarctation (see Fig. 48-20). There appears to be an age-related association, with patients operated on after age 1 year having a greater chance of developing exercise-induced hypertension.[S26]

Correlates (Risk Factors) of Upper Body Hypertension Possible basic correlates of an excessive upper body

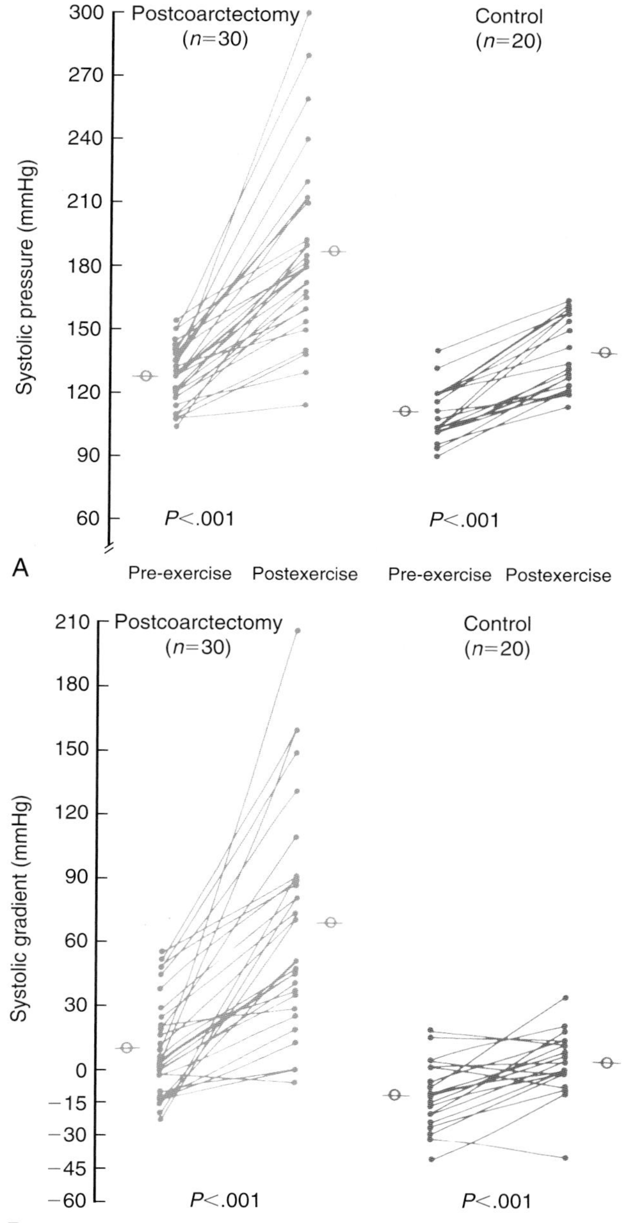

Figure 48-24 Systolic blood pressure before and after exercise in patients after coarctectomy and end-to-end anastomosis and in 20 control subjects. **A,** Arm systolic pressure increased in both groups but more so in coarctectomy patients. **B,** Systolic blood pressure gradient between arm and leg increased, often to high levels, in postcoarctectomy group. Key: θ, Average values. (From Freed and colleagues.[F12])

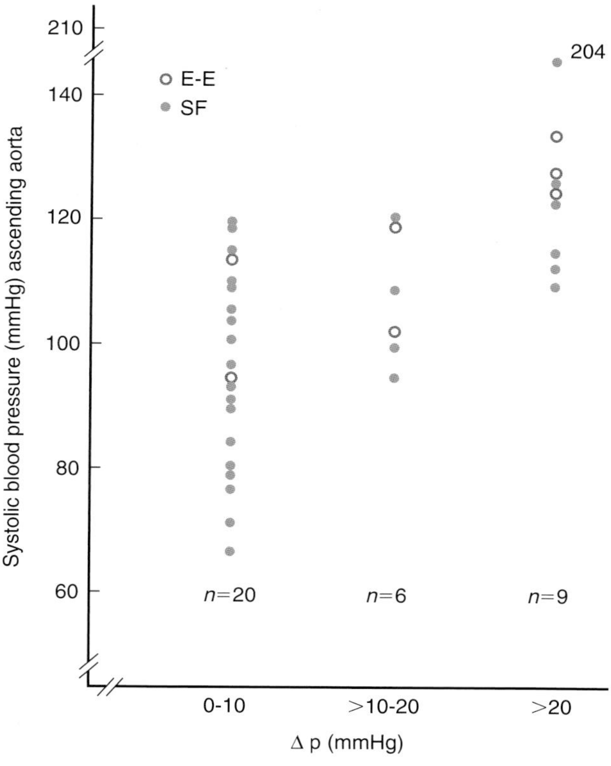

Figure 48-25 Relationship of systolic ascending aortic blood pressure to ascending-to-descending aortic systolic pressure gradient observed at follow-up catheterization 3 months to 9 years after neonatal coarctation surgery. Key: *Δp,* Systolic pressure gradient across repair; *E-E,* end-to-end anastomosis; *SF,* subclavian flap repair. (From Ziemer and colleagues.[Z2])

blood pressure response to rest or exercise in persons who have undergone coarctation repair include:

- Endocrine factors
- Abnormal compliance or reactivity of upper body small blood vessels
- Poorly compliant aorta proximal to coarctation repair
- Morphologically persistent or recurrent coarctation
- Presence of an angulated or "gothic-shaped" arch[O6]

Older age at operation (i.e., >20 years or so) increases prevalence of upper body hypertension after repair of coarctation (described in preceding text), but its effect is probably mediated by one or more basic factors. It is not known whether this prevalence is decreased by operation in very early life.

After repair of coarctation, a positive correlation exists between resting upper body systolic blood pressure (and magnitude of increase with exercise) and the systolic blood pressure gradient between the upper and lower body[M33,Z2] (Fig. 48-25). A positive correlation also exists between resting pulse pressure and development of an upper body–lower body gradient with exercise in repaired coarctation patients who have no resting gradient (Fig. 48-26). There is no such correlation in controls.[M10] This does not identify the cause of the gradient—that is, whether it is true morphologic residual or recurrent coarctation, or whether it is stiffness in the upper body blood vessels. In general, no correlation has been found between width of the anastomosis as determined by aortography and excessive hypertensive tendency.[H11] Thus, it is problematic as to whether a true morphologic narrowing at the surgical site (persistent or recurrent coarctation) can be diagnosed without imaging the operative area to identify or exclude an anatomic narrowing. This is because noncompliance in large-diameter portions of the upper body arterial tree can result not only in hypertension but also in gradients between upper and lower body blood pressure. Urschel and colleagues showed long ago that diversion of

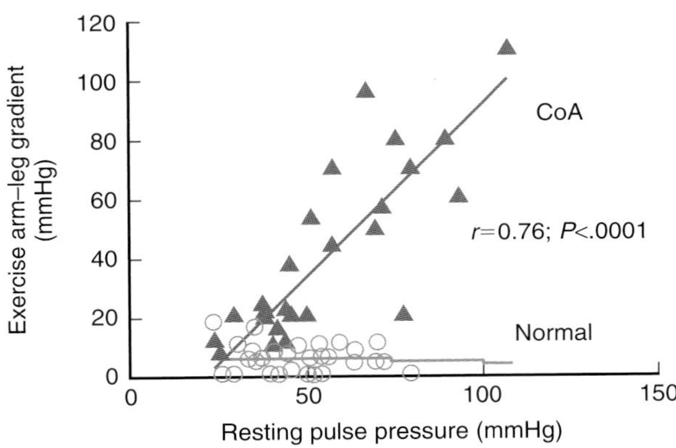

Figure 48-26 Relation between pulse pressure at rest and exercise arm/leg gradient. Coarctation group is represented by triangles, and normal group by circles. (From Markham and colleagues.[M10])

left ventricular output into a rigid tube resulted in increased systolic pressure.[M30,U2]

Poorly compliant upper body aorta and large and small arteries, as discussed earlier in this chapter under Morphology, probably explain these tendencies to hypertension and to developing upper body–lower body systolic pressure gradients during exercise and hypertension of a greater magnitude than in normal individuals.[O5] However, any explanation must account for the fact that upper body hypertension and an exaggerated response to exercise are usually less after coarctation repair. The persisting hypertensive tendency probably explains the persistence of left ventricular hypertrophy in some patients.[P8]

Upper body systolic hypertension appears to be more marked and its exaggeration by exercise greater when a long bypassing tube graft is used for the repair than when end-to-end anastomosis is accomplished.[E2] This may, again, be the effect of a poorly compliant "aortic" segment between the upper and lower body arterial trees.

Studies by Peleck and colleagues, as well as by others, indicate that differences in elaboration of hormones with vasomotor activity or in sensitivity to them do not explain differences in resting and exercise blood pressure in postcoarctectomy patients or between them and normal persons.[P8]

Persisting Upper Body Vascular Abnormalities

Numerous studies in patients many years after coarctation repair have provided convincing evidence for persisting upper body arterial and arteriolar wall abnormalities that produce increased stiffness unrelieved by vasodilating agents.[S4] Whether performing repair in neonates or infants will change this situation is not known. One study suggests that vascular abnormalities are reduced in the postcoarctation arteries, but not in the precoarctation arteries, when repair is performed in infancy, supporting the concept that there is a diffuse developmental defect in the proximal arterial tree.[K22,V19]

Other studies have shown increased reactivity to norepinephrine compared with normal in the blood vessels of the upper body of patients who had received adequate repairs of their coarctation, at least among those with persistent hypertension.[G2]

Persistent or Recurrent Coarctation

Arm/leg gradients commonly develop with exercise in postcoarctation repair patients who have no resting gradient (see Fig. 48-26), but it is uncertain whether this represents a persistent or recurrent coarctation.[M10] The previous discussions make it clear that persistent or recurrent coarctation can be identified with any degree of certainty only by imaging or by examining the repair itself. Reliable information of this type is not widely available.

Many have defined persistent or recurrent coarctation as a postoperative condition characterized by a resting peak pressure gradient exceeding 20 mmHg across the repair area.[B37] Usefulness of this criterion is limited. Freedom from reoperation is not a satisfactory surrogate for known absence of a resting gradient or imaging of the area of repair. It may overestimate or underestimate prevalence of persistent or recurrent coarctation. A ratio of the aortic diameter at the repair site to the aortic diameter at the diaphragm of less than 0.7 has been suggested as a criterion for more than mild aortic narrowing; however, even patients with a higher ratio may exhibit elevated blood pressure and vascular abnormalities.[V23]

It is probable that many early "recoarctations" with luminal narrowings are in fact persistent coarctations.[H14,N1,P5] True recurrent recoarctation probably occurs, although its demonstration by serial aortography has been infrequent. True recoarctation after end-to-end anastomosis has been attributed to lack of growth of the suture line and presence of abnormal mesodermal tissue that proliferates and produces marked intimal and medial hypertrophy.[I1,K11,M35,P4,P5,P10,T20] Remnants of ductal tissue behave in this same way.[B35] Damage to the aorta from the vascular clamps used at repair has also been implicated.[F4] Also, aortic wall mucopolysaccharides in coarctation have an increased chondroitin sulfate fraction, more marked in recoarctation specimens,[B21] a difference that leads to increased wall rigidity (decreased distensibility) that predisposes to or mimics restenosis.[R23]

Technical factors are no doubt responsible for *persistent coarctation*—for example, insufficient resection of a long, narrow segment followed by end-to-end anastomosis, or excessive tension on the suture line due to inadequate mobilization of the aorta above and below the coarctation. Other technical causes include incorrect fashioning of a subclavian flap or polyester onlay patch, failure to resect an obstructing intimal ridge, use of a too-small tube graft in a child, or kinking of such a graft particularly when used as a bypass.

A residual hypoplastic segment of aortic arch, usually between the left subclavian and common carotid arteries (tubular hypoplasia), can possibly contribute to a residual gradient. However, serial aortograms have shown progressive growth of this segment in many cases after coarctectomy, no doubt secondary to restoring normal arch blood flow.[B33,P15] This has been corroborated by Brouwer and colleagues in a well-controlled study; they found that even severely hypoplastic arch segments between the left common carotid and left subclavian arteries substantially increased in size within 6 months of simple repair of coarctation in young infants. Despite the increase, however, *z* values sometimes remain as low as −3, and one early recoarctation has been documented[B36] (Fig. 48-27). To further cloud the picture, in an MRI follow-up evaluation of 65 coarctation repairs, 47% of patients had hypoplasia of the isthmus and arch, and clinical evidence of recoarctation was related to this finding.[J2] Finally, in follow-up of 191 isolated coarctation patients extending to 30 years, recurrent coarctation was noted to

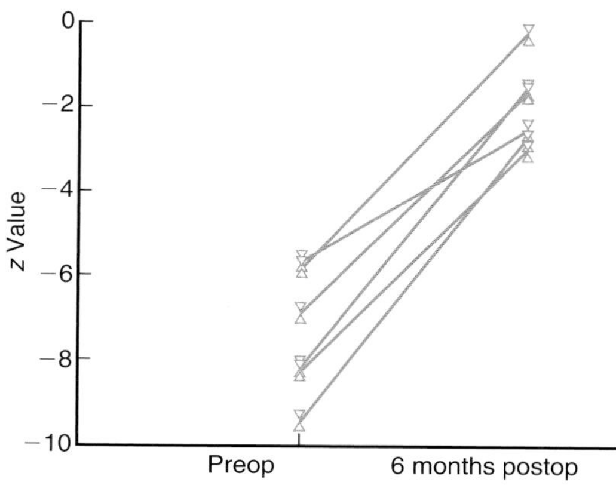

Figure 48-27 The *z* value of diameter of aortic arch between left common carotid and left subclavian arteries in infants younger than age 3 months at time of coarctation repair. Value before operation is shown, as is marked increase, identified by imaging, 6 months after simple end-to-end anastomosis. Key: *Preop,* Preoperatively; *postop,* postoperatively. (From Brouwer and colleagues.[B36])

develop even as late as several decades after repair and was correlated with arch hypoplasia.[S31]

Experimental animal data showing that normal growth of an artery can occur after end-to-end anastomosis[B43,S24] are not necessarily relevant to the situation after coarctectomy if indeed the tissue left behind is abnormal and tends to proliferate and produces excessive scar tissue. Experimental data do not conclusively demonstrate superiority of one suture technique over another for end-to-end anastomosis.[J7]

Recoarctation in children and adults is considerably more common when anatomy of the coarctation is unsuitable for direct end-to-end anastomosis because of a long narrowing or aneurysm formation, necessitating some other type of repair.

Prevalence after End-To-End Anastomosis Prevalence of persisting coarctation or recoarctation after the end-to-end anastomosis technique has been reported as high as about 20% in patients operated on before age 2 years and appears to be related smaller size (weight) at time of repair.[B37,K8] One study indicates that presence of anomalous right subclavian artery is a risk factor for recurrence.[H2] Other studies suggest that prevalence of persistent or recurrent coarctation is much lower, about 2% to 6%, but they have used reoperation-free data as evidence.[C16,H2,K8,T13,W13] Harlan and colleagues interpret their data to indicate a lower prevalence when 7-0 polypropylene rather than silk sutures are used, but they also used reoperation-free data rather than measurement of gradient as their criterion.[H12] Lack of imaging information handicaps drawing appropriate inferences.

More recent studies of infants and neonates in whom more aggressive resection and primary anastomosis techniques were used[B4,R3] indicate a reduction in recurrence, suggesting that eliminating abnormal tissue, rather than suture technique or some other factor, may be the predominant reason for achieving a sustainable unobstructed anastomosis. Prevalence of persistent or recurrent coarctation (a resting postoperative gradient <20 mmHg) of less than 5% has been demonstrated in neonates and infants younger than age 3 months using the technique described by Hanley and colleagues of resection with end-to-side primary anastomosis of the descending aorta to the aortic arch.[R3] Midterm follow-up of 88 patients from this series revealed that at 2 years after operation, 2 of 54 neonatal repairs required reintervention, and none of the non-neonatal repairs did.[O1] End-to-side repair using median sternotomy has also been reported, and outcomes compare favorably with the extended end-to-end technique.[Y6]

Prevalence after Subclavian Flap Aortoplasty The subclavian flap operation may have low prevalence of persistent coarctation in infants.[H8,P13,T11] Hamilton and colleagues reported that of 34 infants younger than age 6 months, none (0%; CL 0%-6%) had residual or recurrent coarctation when followed up to 6 years postoperatively.[H8,H9] The report of Waldhausen and colleagues also indicates zero occurrence (0%; CL 0%-8%) within 6 or more months of operation in 23 infants younger than age 14 months.[W1] Campbell and colleagues reported small gradients (15 and 20 mmHg) in two of four patients studied an average of 42 months after repair in infancy using continuous nonabsorbable suture, and no gradients in seven patients in whom a subclavian flap aortoplasty was made using interrupted or absorbable sutures ($P = .1$).[C2] Penkoske and colleagues at the Toronto Hospital for Sick Children found persisting or recoarctation in 6% (CL 3%-10%) of 81 infants repaired by the subclavian flap, in contrast to 27% using end-to-end anastomosis.[P11] In eight patients studied 4 years after subclavian flap aortoplasty, Fripp and colleagues found a normal arm/leg blood pressure response to exercise.[F16] Growth of the subclavian flap has been demonstrated by Moulton and colleagues.[M34]

The favorable experience reported by Campbell and colleagues included 45 neonates and infants younger than age 8 weeks, as did that of Hamilton and colleagues.[C2,H8] In contrast, Metzdorff and colleagues inferred from their experience that occurrence of persistent or recurrent coarctation is excessive when subclavian flap angioplasty is performed in patients younger than age 8 weeks.[M25] They reported only 75% 2-year freedom from reoperation after subclavian flap aortoplasty in infants younger than age 8 weeks, compared with 100% in older patients.

Finally, Cobanoglu and colleagues reported equally low prevalence of recurrence at 5- and 10-year follow-up using either subclavian flap aortoplasty or resection.[C17] Differences in results in the various series cannot be reconciled, but lack of imaging information probably explains most of them.

Prevalence after End-To-End Anastomosis with Subclavian Flap Aortoplasty Dietl and colleagues reported a lower prevalence of recoarctation in neonates and infants repaired by the combined resection-flap procedure than in those repaired with a subclavian flap or a patchgraft aortoplasty.[D7] This has been confirmed by others using this combined technique.[H26]

Prevalence after Patch Aortoplasty Late results of polyester or polytetrafluoroethylene (PTFE) patch aortoplasty have been variable. Sade and colleagues reported persisting coarctation (mean arm/leg systolic blood pressure difference 33 ± 7.5 mmHg) after end-to-end anastomosis in infants but not after PTFE patch aortoplasty (difference was 5.1 ± 2.3 mmHg).[S2] They also reported growth of both the preoperatively hypoplastic isthmus and the intact posterior aortic wall at the site of repair.[S1] Similar findings were reported by Connor and Baker.[C21] Smith and colleagues found arm/leg pressure gradient during exercise to be only mildly increased over the minimal resting gradient when patch aortoplasty had been used, but it was importantly increased when end-to-end anastomosis was used.[S32] However, Hesslein and colleagues from Houston reported a prevalence of persistent or recoarctation (by the criteria used in this chapter) of 18% with *no* difference for end-to-end anastomosis vs. patch aortoplasty.[H17] Younger patients had a higher prevalence with either operation. Again, the lack of imaging information makes interpretation difficult.

Paraplegia after Repair

A collective review by Brewer and colleagues[B34] identified 51 instances of paraplegia (0.41%; CL 0.35%-0.48%) among 12,532 coarctectomies.

Enough knowledge of the incremental risk factors for paraplegia and their neutralization (see "Paraplegia after Aortic Clamping" under Special Situations and Controversies in Chapter 24) is currently available to make it possible for occurrence of paraplegia after coarctectomy to approach zero. Wherever the collateral circulation typical of coarctation has not developed, risk of paraplegia is increased. This is probably because blood pressure in the distal aorta is lower during aortic clamping when collaterals are poorly developed.[K21]

Situations that may fail to stimulate development of the usual amount of collateral circulation include:

- Coarctation in infants
- Coarctation proximal to the left subclavian artery
- Coarctation with patent ductus arteriosus supplying the descending thoracic aorta
- Coarctation associated with stenosis at the origin of the left subclavian artery
- Coarctation with the right subclavian artery arising as the fourth branch distal to the coarctation
- Something less than severe narrowing at the coarcted area
- Re-repair[B34]

Early Postoperative Hypertension and Abdominal Pain

Nearly all patients, including infants, have some systolic and diastolic hypertension for a variable period after coarctation repair. Many patients, if observed carefully, have mild abdominal discomfort and distention during the first 5 or 6 postoperative days.[H22,R7] In 10% to 20% of cases, this becomes sufficient to produce important discomfort and distention. Then there may be abdominal tenderness, fever, ileus, and leukocytosis. Management should be nonsurgical in virtually all cases (see "Abdominal Pain" under Special Features of Postoperative Care earlier in this section for treatment).

Further discussion of this syndrome is difficult because in the early years of coarctation surgery, many complications that are currently rare were reported as examples of the syndrome. Also, "paradoxical" hypertension is the rule after coarctation repair rather than the hallmark of a special syndrome. However, the syndrome was first described in a single case report by Sealy in 1953.[S11] At laparotomy on the tenth postoperative day, the jejunum and proximal ileum were "edematous and cyanotic but the superior mesenteric arteries and veins were patent." At autopsy, "inflammation of the small arteries and arterioles was confined to the body area below the coarctation," and there were infarcts in liver, spleen, kidney, and intestines. Lober and Lillehei added two cases in 1954,[L14] and Perez-Alvarez and Oudkerk another in 1956.[P12] Ring and Lewis in 1956[R17] considered that the lesion justified the term *syndrome* and that it was due to sudden increase in pulsatile pressures in vessels distal to the coarctation, with acute overdistention of these vessels. In 1957, Sealy and colleagues[S12] linked onset of abdominal pain with presence of paradoxical hypertension, which they described in detail. They noted that following successful coarctectomy, an early systolic hypertension could develop within the first 36 postoperative hours or a more delayed mainly diastolic hypertension could develop after 48 hours that lasted 7 to 14 days. This delayed phase was associated with abdominal pain in 6 of 14 of his patients. This observation was confirmed by many others.[H22,V11] Sealy suggested that the hypertension might be due to an altered baroreceptor response plus an increased excretion of epinephrine or norepinephrine.[G7,S12] Rocchini and colleagues[R20] suggest that the sympathetic nervous system is responsible for the early phase and that the renin-angiotensin system plays a major role in the later phase, although more recent information would indicate that the renin-angiotensin system also plays a role in the early phase.[P3]

Pathologic findings have been described in small arteries and arterioles in vessels below the repaired coarctation[S11] in these patients, and they probably are present to some degree routinely after coarctation repair. They include thrombosis, inflammatory cell infiltration of the entire wall, fragmentation of the internal elastic lamina, and fibroblastic proliferation, as well as marked mesenteric lymphadenitis in the jejunum and proximal ileum.[D10] Rarely there may be infarcts in liver, spleen, and kidneys, and rupture of aneurysms that may have formed on large intraabdominal arteries.[L14]

In a review of the literature up to 1970, Ho and Moss[H22] found the syndrome was reported in 9% (107 of 1193) of patients surviving coarctectomy. It is said to be rare in children younger than age 2 years,[G14,R17,T7,V11] but this is questionable because it is difficult to be sure of its presence or absence in young infants.

Left Arm Function after Subclavian Flap Aortoplasty

Long experience with the Blalock-Taussig shunt showed considerable variability in arm function late after sacrifice of the subclavian artery (see "Interim Events" under Interim Results after Classical Shunting Operations in Section I of Chapter 38). Rarely (<1% of patients) does actual gangrene develop, and preservation of retrograde flow from the vertebral artery may further reduce the prevalence. The affected arm is smaller later in life, but uncommonly is it perceptibly so.[T17] Blood flow to the affected arm is reduced, particularly during stress, but claudication is uncommon.[V7]

Late Aneurysm Formation

A true or false aneurysm may occur late postoperatively. A *true aneurysm* from progressive deterioration of the aortic wall opposite a prosthetic onlay patch has been reported on long follow-up by Knyshov and colleagues,[K14] Vorsschulte,[V17] Bergdahl and colleagues,[B19] Olsson and colleagues,[O3] and Rheuban and colleagues.[R16] Ala-Kulju and colleagues found this to develop in 27% (CL 21%-34%) of 62 patients followed up 2 to 14 years.[A4] Others report a much lower occurrence, 1% to 3% with up to 30 years of follow-up.[V10] One study identifies arch hypoplasia as a risk factor for late aneurysm formation after patch aortoplasty for coarctation.[B5] Another identifies concomitant ridge resection at the time of patch placement.[M16] Presumably, the stiff patch transmits additional tension to the adjacent elastic aortic wall, which thus bears the total burden of the pulse wave and dilates.[B19,O3,S30] This makes the polyester onlay patch technique undesirable in most circumstances. An interposed aortic allograft tube may become aneurysmal, but this is not common on long follow-up.[F9,S9]

A *dissection* may occur occasionally, either in the ascending or descending aorta, proximal or distal to the coarctation repair site. This may lead to late aneurysm formation.

False (suture line) *aneurysms* can be mycotic when they occur early postoperatively,[B19,K13] but they are usually uninfected and have an etiology similar to the false femoral aneurysm that occurs at the distal anastomosis of an aortofemoral prosthetic graft. They may complicate prosthetic tubular grafts as well as prosthetic onlay patches. In the former instance, they are said to be more common at the proximal anastomosis of a bypass tube graft, where the suture line is more oblique in relationship to the transverse forces in the aortic lumen.[O3] They are rare with end-to-end tubular grafts, unless mycotic.

Aneurysms of uncertain type but in the region of the repair have been reported after the subclavian flap repair.[M13] Prevalence of this problem is uncertain.

Valvar Heart Disease

Valvar heart disease may complicate long-term management of patients who have undergone coarctation repair and occasionally prevents a good result.[B18] No doubt a larger number with bicuspid valves will require surgery for calcific aortic stenosis when they reach their fifth and sixth decades of life. Thus, among the 23 patients in Crafoord's original series followed by Bjork and colleagues for more than 26 years, definite aortic valve disease developed in 11 (48%), although operation had not yet been required in four.[B23]

Congenital mitral valve disease has been thought to be infrequent in this setting. Celano and colleagues found coexisting mitral valve anomalies in 12 of 56 (21%) patients with coarctation studied by two-dimensional echocardiography.[C7]

Other Events

Heart failure may occasionally persist postoperatively in older patients who have it preoperatively,[L11] and coronary artery disease with myocardial infarction or angina also occurs but is not common.[M11] *Infective endocarditis* occasionally occurs on the aortic or mitral valve. *Cerebrovascular accidents* are more common in patients with persistent hypertension. Maron and colleagues noted a high prevalence of *conduction defects* in ECGs of their patients.[M11] Bjork and colleagues found *degenerative disease of the hip* joints present in 20% of their 25 patients who had been followed up for 27 to 32 years and who were age 7 to 31 years at coarctectomy.[B23] *Pregnancy* is reasonably well tolerated after coarctation repair, and is even well tolerated in women with unrepaired coarctation. Hypertension, cardiovascular complications, miscarriage, and premature delivery rates are elevated, however.[F1,V20] Late *aortic root and ascending aortic complications including rupture, dissection, aneurysm, and perforation* occur more frequently in patients with repaired coarctation and bicuspid aortic valve than in patients with isolated bicuspid aortic valve or isolated coarctation[C13] (Fig. 48-28).

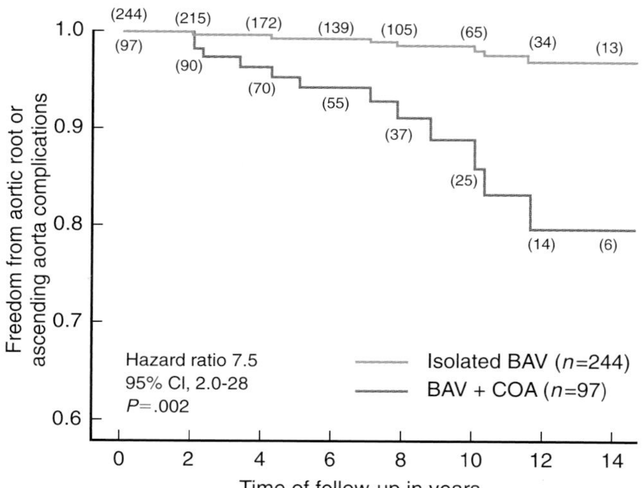

Figure 48-28 Freedom from aortic root or ascending aorta complications for patients with isolated bicuspid aortic valve (244 patients) and patients with associated bicuspid aortic valve and coarctation (97 patients). Numbers in brackets indicate numbers of patients remaining in each period. Key: *BAV,* Bicuspid aortic valve; *COA,* coarctation. (From Ciotti and colleagues.[C13])

Repair of Coarctation and Coexisting Ventricular Septal Defect

Little specific information other than survival is available in this group of patients. The information suggests that similar VSDs have the same tendency to close as when coarctation is not present (see "Spontaneous Closure" under Natural History in Section I of Chapter 35). VSD in patients with coarctation, however, is more likely to be malaligned posteriorly, and malalignment VSDs are less likely to close than those without malalignment. In one study following 23 infants with coarctation and VSDs of various sizes in whom coarctation repair alone was initially performed before 3 months of age, 14 of 23 required subsequent VSD closure, and importantly, size of VSD was not correlated with need for closure.[P2] Other studies indicate that VSD size, as well as other characteristics of the VSD, are important predictors that surgical closure will be required[K5] (see Indications for Surgery for an in-depth discussion of surgical decision making for coarctation with VSD). Among neonates with large VSD undergoing only coarctation repair, by age 12 months 12% of VSDs had become small, and by 24 months 19% had done so in the multiinstitutional study of the CHSS.[Q1] Results of repair of coarctation when VSD coexists, with regard to early, intermediate-term, and late upper body blood pressure, are presumably the same as when the coarctation is isolated, but this has not been confirmed by specific study.

In earlier eras, single-institution studies suggested that early (hospital) mortality tends to be somewhat higher than in patients with isolated coarctation.[B20] More recent single-institution studies, however, suggest that this may no longer be true.[G1,I3] But a difference was found to persist ($P = .01$) in the 1994 multiinstitutional study of the CHSS.[Q1] Also, the hazard function for death may remain higher over time when a VSD is present. Indeed, multiinstitutional data suggest that overall initial risks remain higher in patients with coexisting VSD (Fig. 48-29, *A*). Hazard functions for death in the two groups become similar after about 6 months (Fig. 48-29, *B*).

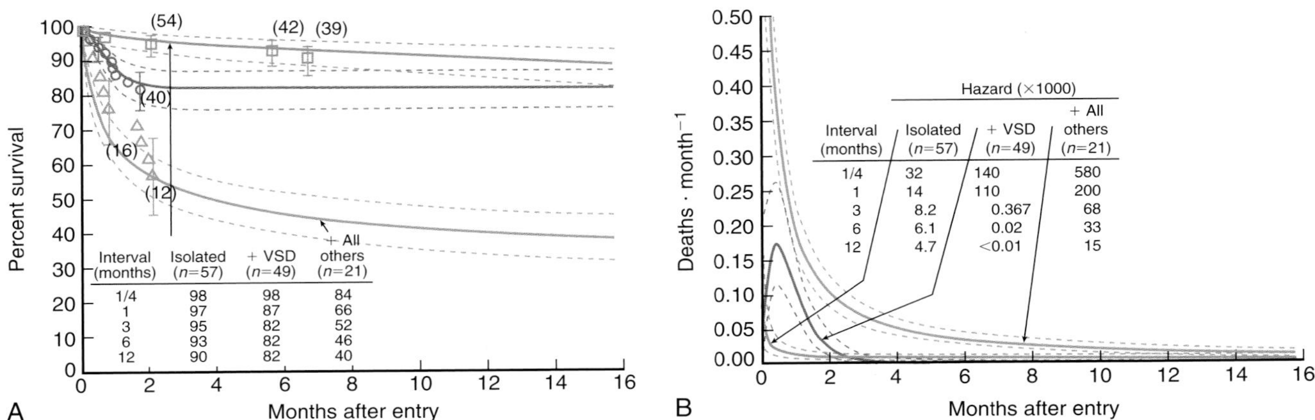

Figure 48-29 Early survival after repair of coarctation of aorta in neonates ($n = 127$) with no other hypoplastic left heart components (hypoplastic left heart class I), according to whether the coarctation is isolated, or with coexisting ventricular septal defect *(VSD)*, or with other important coexisting cardiac anomalies. **A,** Survival. **B,** Hazard function. (From multiinstitutional study of the Congenital Heart Surgeons Society, 1990 to 1991.)

Table 48-4 Hospital and Total Deaths after Repair of Coarctation Coexisting with Ventricular Septal Defect and Presenting in Neonatal Life[a]

	Class I[b]						Class II[b]					
		Hospital Deaths			Total Deaths			Hospital Deaths			Total Deaths	
Method of Repair	*n*	No.	%	CL (%)	No.	%	*n*	No.	%	CL (%)	No.	%
Coarctation alone	25	0	0	0-7	2	8	5	1	20	3-53	1	20
One-stage coarctation + VSD	7	3	43	20-68	3	43	3	1	33	4-76	1	33
Coarctation + PT band with later VSD closure	3	0	0	0-47	0	0	0					
Coarctation + PT band	7	1	14	2-41	1	14	1	0	0	0-85	0	0
Coarctation with later PT band	1	1	100	15-100	1	100	0					
Coarctation with later VSD closure	4	1	25	3-63	1	25	0					
Coarctation + aortic valve commissurotomy	0						1	1	100	15-100	1	100
Coarctation with later VSD closure + aortic valve commissurotomy	0						1	1	100	15-100	1	100
Balloon aortoplasty with later PT band + coarctation resection	1	0	0	0-85	0	0	0					
No repair	1	1	100	15-100	1	100	0					
TOTAL	49	7	14	9-21	9	18	11	4	36	19-56	4	36

[a]Data from multiinstitutional study of the Congenital Heart Surgeons Society, 1990 to 1991.
[b]Classes I, II, and III are defined in Table 48-1. No patient was in class III or IV.
Key: *PT,* Pulmonary trunk; *VSD,* ventricular septal defect.

Again, some single-institution studies indicate that presence of a VSD has no effect on either early or late risk, with excellent early and midterm outcomes reported.[G1,I3,K3,Z2]

A higher proportion of patients with coarctation and VSD may be in hypoplastic left heart class II than is the case in those with isolated coarctation, and survival may be less in those in class II than in class I (Table 48-4).

Current information does not permit comparison of outcomes with different management protocols in a risk-adjusted fashion, although in contrast with interrupted aortic arch and VSD,[J8] the multiinstitutional study of the CHSS found staged repair gave a survival advantage.[Q1] Options include repair of coarctation via thoracotomy with medical management of the VSD, repair of coarctation via thoracotomy with pulmonary trunk banding, and coarctation repair via median sternotomy with VSD closure, using either hypothermic circulatory arrest or continuous perfusion. Excellent results using the midline approach have been reported, employing either continuous perfusion[I3] or hypothermic circulatory arrest.[G1] Although natural history of VSD associated with coarctation is not established, attempts have been made to predict in early infancy the likelihood a VSD associated with coarctation will require surgical closure.[B38] Another approach involves coarctation repair with pulmonary trunk banding using absorbable material (polydioxanone).[B27] Band reabsorption occurred over approximately 6 months in an experience with

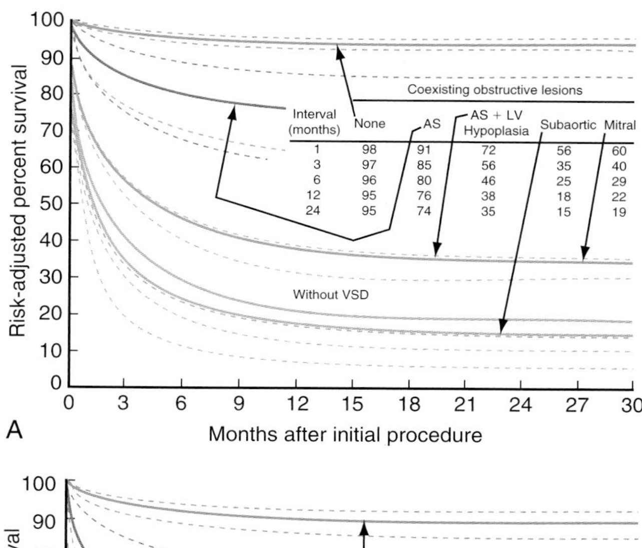

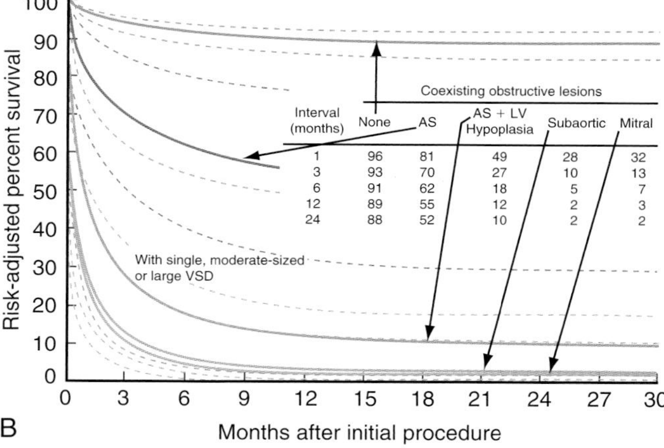

Figure 48-30 Influence of coexisting obstructive lesions of left heart–aorta complex on survival after repair of coarctation of the aorta in neonates. **A,** Isolated coarctation. **B,** Coarctation with single moderate-sized or large ventricular septal defect. Key: *AS,* Aortic stenosis; *LV,* left ventricular; *VSD,* ventricular septal defect. (From Quaegebeur and colleagues.[Q1])

11 selected patients. VSD closure was necessary in only one patient following band reabsorption.

Repair of Coarctation and Other Major Coexisting Intracardiac Anomalies

Early and intermediate-term survival is less good in this group than in others (see Fig. 48-29), particularly when patients are in hypoplastic left heart classes II and III[Q1] (Fig. 48-30). This was a highly heterogeneous group of patients (see Table 48-2), and experience with any one group is small. Individual institutions have recently demonstrated substantially better outcomes in these patient groups, with 5-year survival of more than 70%[S18,T8] for the milder hypoplastic left heart classes and even better outcome for other complex lesions such as *transposition, truncus,* and other *conotruncal* lesions (87% hospital survival and 83% survival at 7 years).[L6,T9]

Difficulties in prospectively (preoperatively) defining a left heart as hypoplastic is discussed in detail in the introductory remarks to Chapter 49 and the footnote to Table 48-1. These difficulties are underscored by the experience of Tani and colleagues,[T4] who performed coarctation repair only in 20 neonates, without mortality, who were designated preoperatively as having a degree of left heart hypoplasia too severe to survive with two-ventricle physiology as judged by a widely used grading system. One confounding factor was that immediate changes in left ventricular cavity size can occur with change in loading conditions after coarctation repair.[K20]

INDICATIONS FOR OPERATION

Isolated Coarctation

Diagnosis of isolated coarctation is an indication for operation, because the probability of survival and a resting upper body normotensive state is greater after repair than in the natural history of the condition.

In the first few months of life, resection with reanastomosis is indicated. Need for enlarging or bypassing a hypoplastic segment of arch between the left common carotid and left subclavian arteries (distal arch) remains arguable, although good results have been reported.[L2,V18] If no arch hypoplasia is present, end-to-end anastomosis is the choice for aortic reconstruction. If distal aortic arch hypoplasia is present, this may be addressed using either a reverse subclavian flap, an extended end-to-end anastomosis, or an end-to-side anastomosis of the descending aorta to the segment of arch between the brachiocephalic and left carotid arteries (proximal arch).[E5,H2,K8,O5,R3]

In critically ill neonates with coarctation, intravenous PGE_1 ($0.1\ mg \cdot kg^{-1} \cdot min^{-1}$) is begun immediately and continued until the situation is remedied at operation.[N4,W1] (For more details about use of PGE_1, see Indications for Operation in Chapter 41.) Response is dramatic in about 80% of infants,[F10] with reappearance of femoral pulses and disappearance of metabolic acidosis from hypoperfusion of the lower body. Operation is then delayed 6 to 12 hours or more until the baby's condition has stabilized in this improved state (for more details, see Indications for Operation in Section II).

Operation (after proper preparation) is indicated when diagnosis is made in neonates and young infants who present in important cardiac failure. If cardiac failure or failure to thrive is not present, urgency of the operation is less; however, surgery should still be considered at the time of presentation, although some prefer to delay it for 3 to 6 months. Argument to proceed at diagnosis is based on recent studies showing a prevalence of persistent or recurrent coarctation that is no different between neonates and older infants. Argument to delay is based on older information showing an apparently higher prevalence of persistent or recurrent coarctation when repair is performed in the first few months of life, and on the absence of any demonstrated lesser probability of long-term survival and a resting upper body normotensive state after repair in neonates than after repair in infants.[V4]

In occasional patients with a mild to moderate degree of left heart hypoplasia in whom it may not be clear that the left heart is adequate to sustain the systemic circulation, the subclavian flap operation can be particularly useful. With this operation, the ductus arteriosus can be preserved, and the PGE_1 can then be weaned slowly to test the adequacy of the left heart once the coarctation is repaired.

In patients presenting beyond early infancy, coarctation resection and aortic reconstruction is also the procedure of choice if there is no proximal hypoplasia.[B36] If important proximal hypoplasia is present, the options available for neonates and young infants are generally not applicable for older patients. The older the patient, the less mobile the aortic tissue becomes, making extensive mobilization of the aorta impossible. If proximal hypoplasia is moderate in severity, patch augmentation of the arch and coarctation site, or graft interposition, are the options of choice. If proximal hypoplasia is severe, graft interposition in indicated.

Coarctation and Coexisting Ventricular Septal Defect

When coarctation coexists with a VSD in a neonate or infant with heart failure, the probability of the VSD closing spontaneously is the major determinant of the treatment protocol. Some have found that if the VSD is larger than small, VSD size is not particularly predictive of spontaneous closure.[P2] Others have found that the likelihood of spontaneous VSD closure is correlated inversely with VSD size.[K5] This same study also suggests that only muscular-type VSDs are likely to close, not perimembranous, outlet, or malalignment types.[K5] Thus, it is reasonable to assume that if the VSD is a large conoventricular one, is large and in the outlet portion of the right ventricle, or is posteriorly malaligned, the probability that it will spontaneously narrow appreciably or close is very small. One-stage repair of the coarctation (by end-to-end anastomosis) and the VSD through a median sternotomy is the procedure of choice for such situations.[T14] There are, however, alternative practices. Coarctation repair alone may be performed,[K5,P2] with later VSD closure if it remains large or the infant has failure to thrive. Also, coarctation repair with concomitant banding of the pulmonary trunk can be performed, with later removal of the band and VSD closure.[K5] Finally, a single-stage repair with two incisions has been described. The arch is repaired using a thoracotomy; the patient is then repositioned, and a median sternotomy is performed for VSD closure using standard CPB techniques.[A13] When the VSD is small or moderate in size, and particularly if it is muscular and occasionally perimembranous, spontaneous reduction in size, and closure, are real possibilities. In this situation the option of coarctation repair alone, with subsequent observation of the VSD and patient, is the preferred treatment protocol.

Whatever the initial procedure, if heart failure persists and the VSD remains large, it is repaired before hospital discharge (see Indications for Operation in Section I of Chapter 35).

Coarctation and Other Major Coexisting Intracardiac Anomalies

When coarctation coexists with other major intracardiac anomalies, the decision to proceed with one-stage repair of both, or to address the coarctation only, is a complex one. This is especially true in cases of single-ventricle physiology in which either a complex cardiac repair or a pulmonary trunk band must accompany coarctation repair. (See Chapter 41 for a more complete discussion of this issue.) With coarctation and truncus arteriosus, both are repaired. With coarctation and transposition, the preferred approach is to repair both, although a staged coarctation repair with subsequent arterial switch can be performed. With coarctation and atrioventricular septal defect, the preferred approach in most cases is to repair the coarctation and defer intracardiac repair for several months.

SPECIAL SITUATIONS AND CONTROVERSIES

Coarctation Proximal to Left Subclavian Artery

Coarctation proximal to the left subclavian artery is rare (≈1% of all cases). Stenosis is localized, and femoral pulses are usually only slightly decreased and systolic pressure gradient across the coarctation mild (<20 mmHg) or moderate. Coarctation is often not detected until young adult life, at which time upper body hypertension is often present. A collateral circulation is generally not well developed.

The natural history of this lesion and its prognosis with antihypertensive medication is not clear, so neither are indications for operation. However, when upper body systolic and diastolic hypertension are severe during moderate exercise, operation is advisable.

A reverse subclavian flap or resection with end-to-side anastomosis is optimal treatment in infants and young children (see Technique of Operation earlier in this section). When a resection and anastomosis is used in older children and adults, either directly or with interposition of a tubular polyester graft, risk of hospital death or a major complication is probably less than 5%.

When an operation is performed in this subset of patients, particular attention must be paid to preventing paraplegia (see "Repair of Coarctation Proximal to Left Subclavian Artery" under Technique of Operation earlier in this section).

Some controversy remains regarding the importance of proximal hypoplasia in the aortic arch in association with coarctation (see Morphology earlier in this section). When it is considered important in association with coarctation, end-to-side reconstruction[R3] or reverse subclavian flap plus coarctation resection and anastomosis are effective solutions.[K4]

Mild and Moderate Coarctation in Classic Position

Uncommonly in infants and older patients, *moderate* coarctation is present in the classic position. Collateral vessels are absent. The natural history of this entity is not clear and thus neither are indications for operation. Degenerative changes are, however, prone to occur in the region of the coarctation, and when calcification is apparent, resection and replacement of this area with a tube graft may be recommended. Surgical techniques are the same as for thoracic aneurysms in this area (see "Replacement of Descending Thoracic Aorta" in Chapter 26).

When coarctation is so *mild* that there is no gradient across the area, in which case the lesion is usually found because of the buckled appearance of the aorta on chest radiography (pseudocoarctation),[N2] operation is advised only when degenerative changes have developed and thus an increased risk of aneurysm formation.

Preventing Paraplegia as a Complication of Repair

Paraplegia does not occur as an operative complication in classic coarctation of the aorta with well-developed collateral circulation. Thus, in preventing paraplegia, great importance attaches to *preoperative* identification of patients with potentially inadequate collateral circulation. In children and adults with periductal coarctation, absence of rib notching on the chest radiograph or of palpable parascapular pulsations suggests that collateral circulation is not well developed. Only mildly diminished femoral pulsations in such patients are often associated with a poorly developed collateral circulation, as are a diminished left radial pulse (usually caused by involvement of the origin of the left subclavian artery in the coarctation) or a diminished right radial pulse (present when the right subclavian artery arises distal to the coarctation). Aortography or CT angiography is indicated under these circumstances, and when adequate collateral arteries are not present, special measures are taken at operation (see "Paraplegia after Aortic Clamping" under Special Situations and Controversies in Chapter 24). If uncertainty remains, pressure can be measured at thoracotomy in the descending aorta with the proximal aortic clamp temporarily in place; if this pressure is less than 50 mmHg, special measures are needed.

Likelihood of paraplegia in very young patients is uncertain, because some collateral circulation is present at birth. However, use of mild hypothermia (35°C nasopharyngeal or tympanic membrane temperature) is a good precaution. This probably allows 30 minutes of safe aortic clamping (see "Subclavian Flap Aortoplasty in Infants" under Technique of Operation earlier in this section). This degree of hypothermia is as protective in older patients as in infants, and a similar technique may be used when the collateral circulation is not well developed. Ice-cold saline lavage may need to be prolonged to about 10 minutes. Instead, a temporary bypass shunt, usually from left subclavian to descending thoracic aorta, or femorofemoral CPB (see "Cardiopulmonary Bypass Established by Peripheral Cannulation" in Section III of Chapter 2) may be used during the period of aortic clamping (see "Paraplegia after Aortic Clamping" under Special Situations and Controversies in Chapter 24). Another alternative is placing a large bypass graft as a permanent method of repair.

Reintervention for Persistent or Recurrent Coarctation

Current indication for reintervention is demonstrating a reduced luminal diameter of greater than 50% at the anastomosis. Under this circumstance, heart failure or upper body hypertension (systolic pressure greater than 140 mmHg in infants and children) is an indication for reintervention.[E9] Currently, percutaneous balloon aortoplasty is generally the treatment of choice (see text that follows), but surgical measures also provide good results.[J1]

Balloon Aortoplasty and Stenting for Coarctation

Percutaneous balloon aortoplasty is controversial as a method of *primary treatment* for aortic coarctation, particularly in small patients. For neonates and young infants, balloon aortoplasty appears to have the same disadvantages as subclavian flap aortoplasty, in that the sling of ductal tissue at the coarctated site is not removed.

Aneurysmal dilatation has developed in some patients treated by balloon angioplasty.[L15] This is not surprising, because the mechanism of gradient relief appears to be tearing of the intima and media.[B33,C3,C6,L17,L18] This process is confirmed in clinical studies by contrast extravasation in 25% of patients at the time of balloon dilatation.[M7] However, some interventional cardiologists[R5] have observed no aneurysms, even when an intimal tear is noted acutely,[S39] whereas others have observed aneurysms in 10% to 20% of patients. An immediate reduction in gradient across the coarctation is usually observed (a decrease from 48 ± 21 to 10 ± 7.3 mmHg was obtained by Rao and colleagues[R5]) and usually persists during the intermediate term.[A10,C23,K2,L1,L16,S37,W12]

The question remains as to whether this result is similar to that obtained by optimal surgical techniques. Several studies directly address this question, although it is acknowledged that there are important difficulties in properly comparing surgical and catheter-based outcomes.[H10] In a recent multicenter study that retrospectively evaluated 80 patients older than age 1 year who were treated either by surgery or transcatheter intervention (balloon angioplasty or stenting), initial relief of the obstruction was similar in the two groups; however, reintervention (32% vs. 0%, $P < .001$) and aneurysm formation (24% vs. 0%, $P < .01$) were both higher after transcatheter therapy.[W4] In a comparison of 57 neonates, retrospective analysis showed that surgery resulted in fewer recurrences and aneurysms, better arch growth, and less need for antihypertensive therapy than did balloon angioplasty.[R24] In a randomized clinical trial of 36 patients between age 3 and 10 years, Shaddy and colleagues showed equal initial outcomes in the surgical and balloon groups, but a significantly greater rate of recurrence and aneurysm formation in the balloon group.[F2]

Arterial occlusion at the site of catheter insertion occurs in some small patients. This is not a trivial complication and can lead to underdevelopment of the ipsilateral leg and claudication, despite good collateral flow.

A detailed multivariable study of risk factors for a poor result from primary balloon dilatation emphasized that age younger than 1 year was particularly associated with a poor result[R6]; recoarctation developed in 71% (CL 45%-90%) of infants. Highest prevalence of recurrence (83%) is found in neonates.[R4] Small size of the aorta between the left subclavian artery and coarctation also was found to predispose patients to a poor result.[P6,Y4]

Recurrent aortic obstruction after surgical treatment is a more favorable situation than primary coarctation for percutaneous balloon angioplasty.[A9,K2] Angioplasty may be most effective for recurrent postsurgical coarctation when it is performed in infancy. Both surgery-free survival and reintervention-free survival after angioplasty for recurrence are higher if the angioplasty occurs beyond infancy[S19] (Fig. 48-31). Excellent initial and intermediate-term results, without aneurysm formation in most patients, appear to be the rule after percutaneous balloon aortoplasty in this setting,[S25,S34] as well as in the setting of recurrent aortic obstruction after repair of interrupted arch and hypoplastic left heart (see "Persistent or Recurrent Aortic Arch Obstruction" under Results in Section II).[S34] Newer data from the Valvuloplasty and Angioplasty of Congenital Anomalies (VACA) Registry, however, indicate that acute suboptimal outcome was present in 25% of recurrent obstruction but only 19% of primary lesions.[M17] On the other hand, arguments have been made that surgical reintervention is preferable to balloon angioplasty for recurrent coarctation, particularly in patients beyond the infancy period and in those with arch hypoplasia.[R13,Z3]

Percutaneous stenting of both native and recurrent coarctation is currently well established, particularly in older

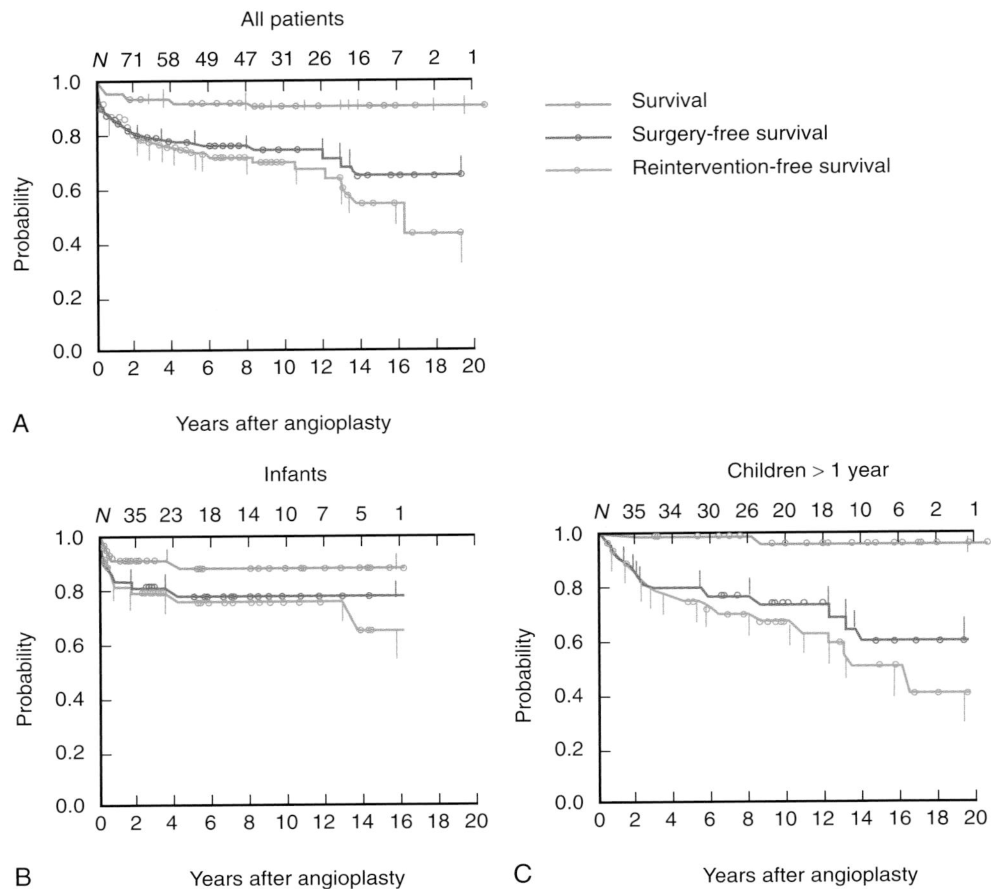

Figure 48-31 Survival and event-free survival in 99 consecutive patients undergoing balloon angioplasty for recurrent coarctation following initial surgical coarctation repair. Outcomes are shown for **(A)** all patients undergoing angioplasty, **(B)** those younger than age 1 year, and **(C)** those older than age 1 year. (From Shaddy and colleagues.[S19])

patients.[B41,B42,E1,M12] Short-term evaluation shows effective relief of obstruction and favorable effects on the myocardium and peripheral vasculature, but longer-term outcome is lacking.[B1,L4,P14,S38] Intimal thickening and luminal reduction were observed in young patients at follow-up, and aneurysm formation was identified in 7%.[M1,S38] In selected adults, complications have generally been lower, and follow-up at 5 years revealed no recurrent obstruction in 46 native and recurrent coarctation patients in one series.[T10] In the 17-institution study of 565 patients (mean age 15 years, all over age 4 years) reported by Forbes and colleagues, 98% had effective relief of obstruction. Acute complications including dissection, intimal tears, aneurysms, cerebrovascular events, and peripheral vascular problems at the insertion site occurred in 14%, and there were two deaths.[F7] A subsequent intermediate-term outcome report on this same multiinstitutional cohort showed that 25% of patients undergoing aortic imaging at a mean follow-up of 19 months had abnormal studies, consisting of dissection, reobstruction, stent fracture, or aneurysm.[F8] Dissection risk may be higher in elderly patients.[F7,V8] Studies examining post-stent hypertension and peripheral vascular abnormalities indicate that similar persistence of these problems occurs as in patients treated surgically.[B11,D3,C10,M38]

Some have taken the position that interventional management is the treatment of choice for native coarctation in older children and adults.[D12] The acute and very early midterm complications noted in the previous paragraph bring into question the validity of this position, because they do not compare favorably with current-era surgical outcomes in similar populations. Furthermore, the truly long-term fate of the aorta after ballooning and stenting is unknown.[M2] Interventional management is not considered the procedure of choice in neonates and infants because of the well-documented extremely high recurrence rate[B39]; however, it may be of benefit as a temporizing maneuver in selected circumstances, such as the presence of profoundly depressed left ventricular function.[B31,L20] Some have recommended temporary stenting in premature infants,[L20,R2,R25] but this is not recommended. Several studies demonstrate that low birth weight is not a risk factor for death or recurrence following surgical repair and that catch-up growth of the arch occurs.[A12,B44,M20]

Finally, the engineering of stents continues to evolve. Covered stents, growth stents, and self-expanding nitinol stents have recently been introduced into clinical practice for coarctation management.[E10,H5,T22]

Coarctation in Adults

Native coarctation diagnosed in adulthood should be treated regardless of age (see Section X in Chapter 29). Excellent results have been achieved with operation in patients older than 50 years (up to 73 years) without mortality and with important improvement of hypertension.[A20,B30,W7] Effective results can be achieved with balloon angioplasty and stenting for uncomplicated native coarctation in adults.[K15] When operation is considered for more complex arch obstructions in adults, extra-anatomical bypass grafting has proved to be a good surgical option.[A18,B39,E2,H16,T12,V22] The procedure can be performed via a median sternotomy[A16,C20] or right thoracotomy.[M21] Other techniques that address the arch directly, using a median sternotomy and CPB, are also effective.[A22] Adults with particular risk of spinal cord injury (i.e., those with either complex anatomy requiring prolonged aortic clamping, or those with mild coarctation [either primary or recurrent] who have poorly developed collaterals) may benefit from partial left heart CPB when a left thoracotomy approach is taken.[F3,H4]

Section II Interrupted Aortic Arch

DEFINITION

Interrupted aortic arch is complete luminal and anatomic discontinuity between two segments of the aortic arch. Those rare specimens that exhibit a fibrous strand connecting two widely separated ends are also included under aortic arch interruption rather than coarctation.

HISTORICAL NOTE

The first description of interrupted aortic arch is attributed to Steidele in 1778.[S36] In this case, the aortic isthmus was absent, so morphology was similar to preductal coarctation. Description of the absence of more proximal portions of the arch occurred later, for the segment between the left subclavian and left common carotid arteries in 1818 by Siedel[S14] and for that between the left common carotid and brachiocephalic arteries by Weisman and Kesten in 1948.[W6] By 1959, Celoria and Patton were able to collect 28 cases that they classified according to the site of obstruction into types A, B, and C (see Morphology and Morphogenesis later in this section).[C8]

The first patient to have successful surgical treatment was a 3-year-old girl operated on by Samson in 1955.[M22] The aortic isthmus was absent between the left subclavian artery and a widely patent ductus arteriosus, but both structures were adjacent, and it was possible to join the divided ductus to the undersurface of the proximal left subclavian artery; the two VSDs were closed 4 years later. Mustard apparently performed a similar successful procedure in a similar patient age 7 months in 1957.[M37] Villalobos and colleagues[V12] and Blake and colleagues[B24] each reported a successful case during the early 1960s, using a prosthetic graft to bridge the gap. Sirak and colleagues[S29] were the first to use the turned-down arch branches successfully (left subclavian or left common carotid artery, or both) for end-to-end anastomosis to the descending aorta (combined with pulmonary trunk banding for the VSD), although this type of operation was attempted as early as 1959.[V2] Sirak's patient was also the first neonate to survive operation, followed by an 18-hour-old boy reported by Norton and colleagues[N5] and an 11-day-old infant operated on in Houston in 1970.[V9] In 1970, a palliative operation consisting of a polyester graft between the pulmonary trunk and descending aorta, combined with pulmonary trunk banding, was used successfully by Litwin and colleagues[L13] in an 11-day-old infant, but this procedure is no longer advocated.

The first simultaneous repair of both interrupted arch and all intracardiac lesions was performed successfully in 1970[B8] in an 8-day-old infant with an interruption distal to the left subclavian artery, a VSD, and total anomalous pulmonary venous connection through a left thoracotomy. The distal end of a 12-mm polyester conduit was anastomosed to the descending aorta; then, through a median sternotomy, the proximal end was anastomosed to the ascending aorta and both intracardiac lesions repaired. The procedure demonstrated that circulatory arrest techniques made an anastomosis to the ascending aorta feasible. In 1973, Murphy and colleagues reported a successful complete repair in a 3-day-old infant of an aortic interruption proximal to the left subclavian artery and a VSD, using circulatory arrest.[M36] They used a segment of the father's basilic vein as the graft between descending and ascending aorta and approached the heart and descending aorta through a median sternotomy with an extension into the third left intercostal space. In 1975, Trusler and Izukawa demonstrated that a median sternotomy alone provided adequate exposure for this procedure in small infants; using circulatory arrest techniques, after excising ductus tissue, they were able to anastomose successfully the descending aorta end to side to the ascending and transverse aortic arch without interposing a graft.[T19] The VSD was also closed. Finally, primary repair via median sternotomy using continuous perfusion cardiopulmonary bypass (CPB) techniques was reported by Asou and colleagues in 1996[A21] and by McElhinney and colleagues in 1997.[M19]

In 1976, the remarkable immediate preoperative improvement produced by the ductus-opening effect of PGE_1 was reported as part of the treatment plan for interrupted aortic arch.[C1,E6,H18,R1]

MORPHOLOGY AND MORPHOGENESIS

Types

The aortic arch may be interrupted at one of three sites (Table 48-5). It may be interrupted just distal to the left subclavian artery (type A of Celoria and Patton[C8]), with blood flowing into the descending aorta from the ductus arteriosus. All forms of interrupted aortic arch display this latter feature, except in rare cases in which the ductus is absent or closes during fetal life. About 40% of cases are type A.[V2] The most common site of interruption (55% of cases) is between the left subclavian and left common carotid arteries (type B). In

Table 48-5 Types of Interrupted Aortic Arch

Type	Definition
A	Interruption located just distal to left subclavian artery
B	Interruption located between left subclavian and left common carotid arteries
C	Interruption located between left common carotid and brachiocephalic artery

only about 5% of cases is the interruption between the left common carotid and brachiocephalic arteries (type C).[V2]

Aortic Arch

Anomalies of the origins of brachiocephalic vessels are frequent in interrupted aortic arch.[R19] Thus, an aberrant right subclavian artery, usually originating as a fourth brachiocephalic branch from the upper descending thoracic aorta, is common in type B but can also occur in type A.[B8] The right subclavian artery may arise high in the neck from the right common carotid artery (cervical origin of right subclavian artery).[K24] A right-sided ductus may persist from the right pulmonary artery and give origin to the right subclavian artery, and the right pulmonary artery may arise from the ascending aorta (see "Anomalous Origin of Right Pulmonary Artery" in Chapter 45). Rarely, interrupted arch occurs with a right aortic arch, and in this instance both the left and right ducts may remain patent and give origin to the subclavian arteries.[R19]

Characteristically, the ascending aorta is about half normal diameter and is straight, dividing into two branches of about equal size (the V sign), and the pulmonary trunk is huge. The descending aorta is a direct continuation of the ductus arteriosus, as in the fetus, and is usually a little larger than the ascending aorta.

In the newborn, there is usually a gap of variable width between the aortic ends, although when the interruption is beyond the left subclavian artery (type A), the gap tends to be wider. Rarely, a fibrous strand connects the two ends. In this situation, the "interruption" should be viewed as a case of severe coarctation and may be distinctly different embryologically. "Interrupted" aortic arch diagnosed beyond infancy as an isolated lesion almost certainly represents coarctation that has progressed to luminal closure.[D2,V21]

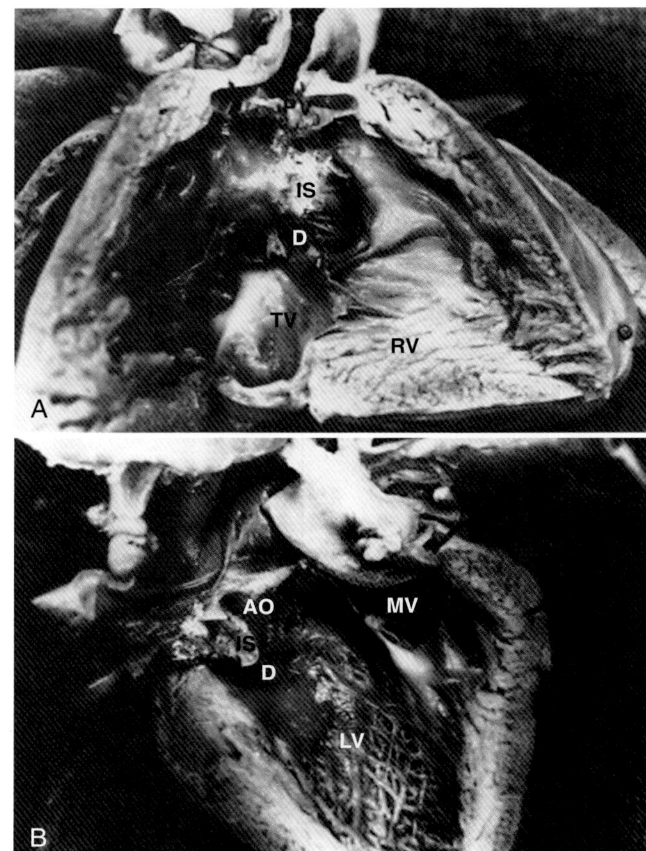

Figure 48-32 Interrupted aortic arch with large conoventricular ventricular septal defect extending toward pulmonary valve and associated with posterior malalignment of infundibular (conal) septum, producing narrowing of left ventricular outflow tract. **A,** Right ventricular view. **B,** Left ventricular view. Key: *AO,* Aortic valve; *D,* ventricular septal defect; *IS,* infundibular septum; *LV,* left ventricle; *MV,* mitral valve, *PV,* pulmonary valve; *RV,* right ventricle; *TV,* tricuspid valve.

Left Ventricular Outflow Anomalies

The aortic valve is bicuspid in 30% to 50% of patients, analogous to coarctation (see Morphology in Section I). Congenital valvar aortic stenosis may be present occasionally, and subaortic stenosis may be present or develop.[F13,I2,V2] Generalized narrowing of the left ventricular outflow tract, conal septal posterior malalignment, the muscle of Moulaert, small aortic anulus, and aortic hypoplasia occur to some degree in most patients with interrupted arch.[A11,B16,B35,H24,S16,V2]

As discussed in Section I for coarctation, interrupted aortic arch may be part of the complex of lesions that constitute hypoplastic left heart physiology.

Coexisting Cardiac Anomalies

A large VSD is present in over 95% of patients, and frequently the infundibular (conal) septum is malaligned and displaced posteriorly and leftward (Figs. 48-32 and 48-33). Most of the VSDs are conoventricular in type, although virtually all types may occur. Some conoventricular defects are also perimembranous, although some may be only juxtatricuspid in position. The malaligned and displaced infundibular septum usually produces subaortic obstruction of variable severity.[F5,F13,H24,S15] This is an important complicating feature. When there are two structurally normal ventricles and inlet valves but no VSD, an aortopulmonary window is typically present. In a multicenter retrospective study of 472 patients with interrupted aortic arch, 4.2% had aortopulmonary window.[A2] Aortopulmonary window may occur with either type A or type B interruption (Fig. 48-34).

Other coexisting lesions are shown in Table 48-6. Pulmonary stenosis rarely if ever occurs as a coexisting lesion. Coexisting lesions occur with equal frequency and with a similar spectrum for interrupted arch types A and B.[G3] Coexisting lesions have been documented with type C as well.[F17]

Morphogenesis and Associated Syndromes

Microdeletion of the q11 segment of chromosome 22 and variable manifestations of velocardiofacial syndrome are common.[L3,L9,L19,M9,M27,R8] Absence of thymic tissue (DiGeorge syndrome) is frequent[C18,F14,V2] and should be sought routinely. Van Mierop and Kutsche found this association only in type B interrupted arch, and they believe this finding has pathogenetic significance.[V1] Up to half of type B cases have DiGeorge syndrome.[G3,L19] However, a population-based regional study indicates that although DiGeorge syndrome is more common in type B interruption, it occurs in type A as

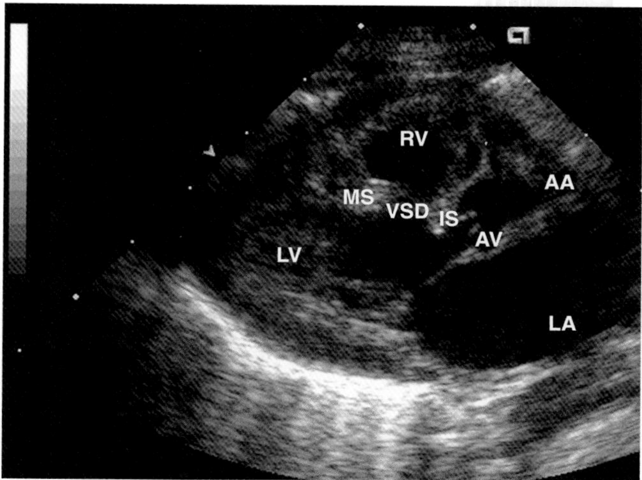

Figure 48-33 Intracardiac image of neonate with interrupted aortic arch and posteriorly malaligned ventricular septal defect. Aortic anulus is mildly hypoplastic, and aortic valve is bicuspid. Infundibular (conal) septum protrudes into left ventricular outflow tract just below aortic valve, narrowing outflow tract substantially. Key: *AA,* Ascending aorta; *AV,* aortic valve; *IS,* infundibular septum; *LA,* left atrium; *LV,* left ventricle; *MS,* muscular septum; *RV,* right ventricle; *VSD,* ventricular septal defect.

Table 48-6 Coexisting Cardiac Anomalies (Exclusive of Other Important Levels of Obstruction in the Left Heart–Aorta Complex) in Interrupted Aortic Arch

Coexisting Cardiac Anomalies	*n*	% of 250
VSD	183	73
Truncus arteriosus	25	10
AP window	10	4
Univentricular AV connection	9[a]	4
TGA with VSD	8	3
DORV	5	2
Taussig-Bing DORV	4	2
Complete AV septal defect	1	0.4
Corrected transposition	1	0.4
None	4	2
TOTAL	250	100

Data from Jonas and colleagues.[J8]
[a]Double inlet left ventricle in three, mitral atresia in four, tricuspid atresia in two.
Key: *AP,* Aortopulmonary; *AV,* atrioventricular; *DORV,* double-outlet right ventricle; *TGA,* transposition of the great arteries; *VSD,* ventricular septal defect.

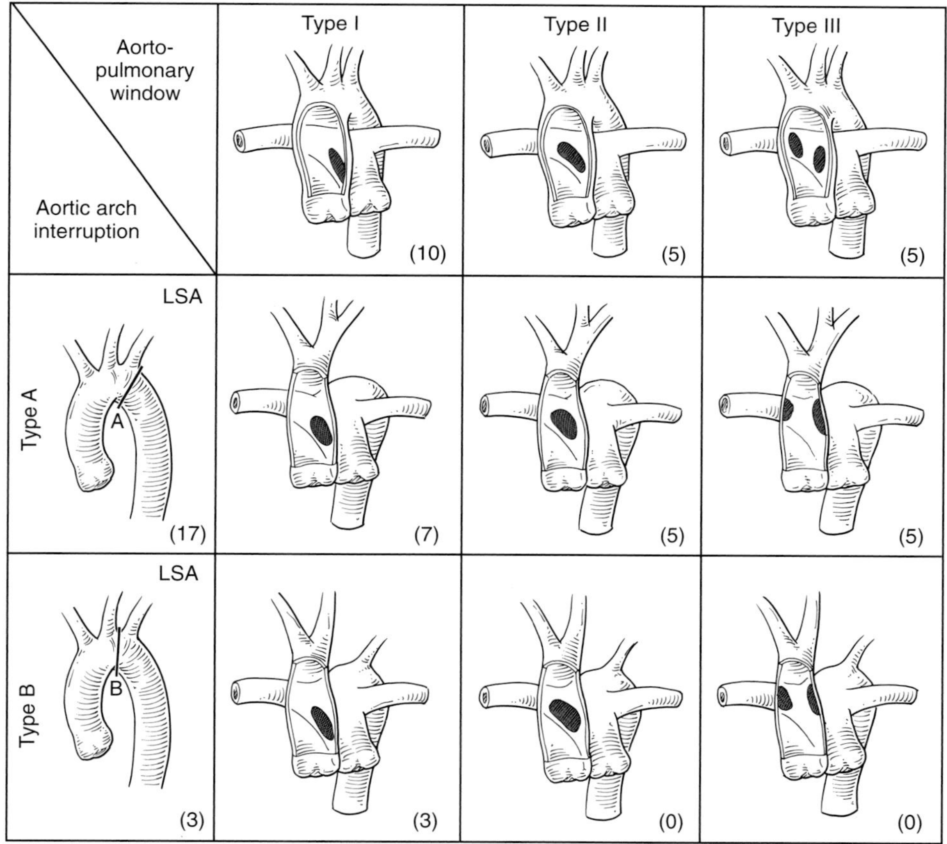

Figure 48-34 Morphologic subtypes of aortopulmonary window and interrupted aortic arch when they occur together. Numbers in parentheses are numbers of patients in each category. (From Akdemir and colleagues.[A2])

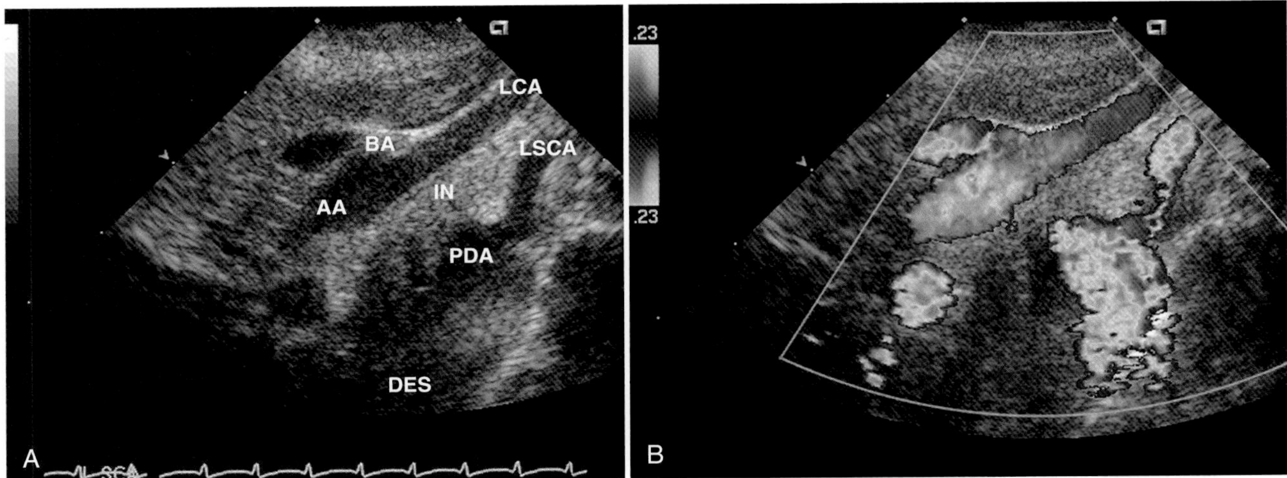

Figure 48-35 Echocardiographic images of neonatal interrupted aortic arch. **A,** Type B interruption. Origin of brachiocephalic artery from ascending aorta is seen, as is origin and entire length of left carotid artery. Interrupted segment is clearly visualized. Ductus arteriosus and descending aorta are also seen, with origin of left subclavian artery arising from descending aorta. **B,** Color-flow imaging of view similar to that seen in **A** helps define length of interrupted segment. Key: *AA,* Ascending aorta; *BA,* brachiocephalic artery; *DES,* descending thoracic aorta; *IN,* interrupted aortic arch; *LCA,* left common carotid artery; *LSCA,* left subclavian artery; *PDA,* patent ductus arteriosus.

well[G6] and has also been reported with type C interruption.[V14] When DiGeorge syndrome is present, hypocalcemia requires treatment,[N5] as do immunologic problems.

CLINICAL FEATURES AND DIAGNOSTIC CRITERIA

Almost all patients with aortic interruption present as critically ill neonates in severe heart failure as a result of the combined effects of volume overload from left-to-right intracardiac shunting and the high afterload imposed by the closing ductus. Metabolic acidosis and anuria develop rapidly.[S15] Femoral pulses become diminished and then impalpable as the ductus closes, and may vary in volume from hour to hour.[H19] When the ductus closes, flow reverses in the vessels distal to the interruption (left subclavian and left common carotid) without recognizable neurologic symptoms developing.[H19] With the ductus still shunting, the expected differential cyanosis between arms and legs is usually not visible, in part because the intracardiac bidirectional shunt minimizes oxygen saturation differences between ascending and descending aorta. Reversed differential cyanosis (blue arms and pink legs) can be obvious, however, when there is associated transposition of the great arteries (see Clinical Features and Diagnostic Criteria in Chapter 52).

Cardiac murmurs are not specific, nor is ECG. The chest radiograph shows gross cardiomegaly and pulmonary plethora. Cardiac catheterization with cineangiography were required for diagnosis in the past.[B8] Currently, enhanced echocardiography usually provides all the necessary diagnostic information relating to both the aortic arch and intracardiac structures[K7,T21] (Fig. 48-35; see also Fig. 48-33). Increasingly, interrupted arch is being diagnosed by fetal echocardiography.[L9] In the unusual case that echocardiography does not provide all the pertinent information, CT angiography provides excellent spatial resolution (Fig. 48-36); thus, cardiac catheterization and contrast studies are unnecessary and disadvantageous.

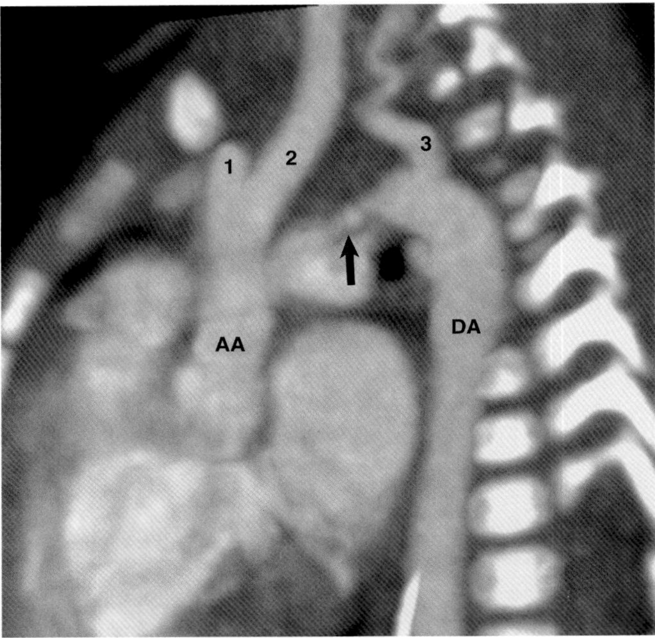

Figure 48-36 Maximal-intensity projection image from a contrast-enhanced computed tomography angiogram of a 2-week-old girl. Ascending aorta *(AA)* supplies brachiocephalic artery *(1)* and left common carotid artery *(2)*. Descending aorta *(DA)* supplies left subclavian artery *(3)*. There is an interruption between left common carotid and left subclavian arteries. Descending aorta is supplied by patent ductus arteriosus *(arrow)* and other collateral arteries.

NATURAL HISTORY

Interrupted aortic arch accounts for 1% to 4% of autopsy cases of congenital heart disease and 1.3% of infants presenting with critical congenital heart disease.[C18,V2] Estimated prevalence is 0.06 per 1000 births.[G3] There is male predominance, and the ratio of type B to type A is 11:4.[G3]

This uncommon anomaly is highly lethal, with median age of death 4 to 10 days; 75% of such babies die within 1 month of birth.[F13,R19,V2] Because the ductus arteriosus is almost always widely patent at birth, collateral circulation does not develop, and death occurs when the ductus closes soon after birth. When the ductus is obliterated in fetal life, collateral circulation is already present at birth[D9] and survival is usual. If the ductus arteriosus stays open, longer survival is possible, but even then, 90% of babies die by age 1 year. In those unusual circumstances in which major associated cardiac anomalies are absent, natural history is similar to that of coarctation without major associated cardiac anomalies.[D9,R10]

TECHNIQUE OF OPERATION

Repair of Interrupted Arch and Ventricular Septal Defect

One-stage repair is considered optimal by some,[H1,H20,R12,S7,S15,T16] and in the multiinstitutional study of the CHSS, one-stage repair gave the best 5-year survival.[J8,M18] Others indicate that little advantage is gained using this technique when compared with staged repair in which the arch is repaired via left thoracotomy, and the VSD is managed by either a concomitant pulmonary trunk band or by subsequent intracardiac closure at a separate operation.[M3] Nevertheless, in institutions experienced with complex neonatal surgery, one-stage repair provides the benefits of immediate normalization of physiology, a single operation, and avoidance of involving the right side of the heart with iatrogenic problems (pulmonary artery stenosis) while achieving good outcomes.

Traditionally, interrupted aortic arch has been repaired using hypothermic circulatory arrest. Recently, CPB techniques have been developed that allow repair to proceed using moderate hypothermia and continuous perfusion.[A21,F6,M19] In a single-institution analysis of 50 patients, mortality using continuous perfusion in 25 patients was 8% (CL 2.8%-18%), and using deep hypothermic circulatory arrest in 25 patients, 32% (CL 21%-44%). By multivariable analysis, however, the difference did not achieve significance.[Y5] Another analysis showed that continuous perfusion, when compared with hypothermic circulatory arrest, was an independent factor *protecting* against death.[M29] In a study of 26 cases focusing on neurodevelopmental outcome at 18 to 24 months following repair, longer hypothermic circulatory arrest time was associated with worse neurodevelopmental outcome.[J9] Both techniques are described in the text that follows.

Repair Using Continuous Perfusion

Operation for a patient with type B interruption and VSD with posteriorly displaced and deficient infundibular septum is described (Fig. 48-37, *A*). Following standard preoperative stabilization and preparation in the operating room, a median sternotomy with slight superior extension is made. The thymus gland is removed except for a small remnant in the neck, and the pericardium is widely opened. The anterior pericardium is removed and fixed in glutaraldehyde. The ascending aorta, pulmonary trunk, ductus arteriosus, all arch vessels, and both venae cavae are dissected. The arch vessels are dissected and mobilized superior to the brachiocephalic vein. A purse-string suture is placed on the brachiocephalic artery midway between its origin and bifurcation; another is placed on the pulmonary trunk. Venous purse strings are placed on the superior and inferior venae cavae. A purse string is place on the right superior pulmonary vein as it merges with the left atrium. After heparin is given, a side-biting clamp is placed on the brachiocephalic artery and a careful arteriotomy is made inside the purse-string suture. A 6F or 8F cannula is then inserted, as allowed by the vessel size, taking care to position the tip of the cannula well within the vessel lumen but not against the back wall of the artery (Fig. 48-37, *B*). A second 8F cannula is placed into the pulmonary trunk. These cannulae are then connected to the bifurcated arterial end of the CPB circuit. Superior and inferior venae cavae are each cannulated with angled metal-tipped 12F venous cannulae connected to the bifurcated venous end of the CPB circuit. CPB is then begun. The branch pulmonary arteries are individually snared. A 10F vent is placed through the right upper pulmonary vein purse string and guided across the mitral valve to decompress the left ventricle. The patient's core temperature is lowered to 25°C over a 15-minute period.

During this time, the distal part of the ductus and the upper descending aorta are dissected. After the target core temperature is reached, perfusion flow rate is reduced to 40 to 50 $mL \cdot kg^{-1} \cdot min^{-1}$, and the arterial cannula in the pulmonary trunk is clamped and removed. A 5-0 polypropylene suture on the ductus arteriosus is tied to occlude the pulmonary artery end of the ductus. A small C clamp is placed on the descending aorta at approximately the second pair of intercostal vessels below the ductus insertion. The left subclavian artery is occluded temporarily with a removable neurovascular clip. The ductus arteriosus is transected near the ligature, and the remaining ductal tissue is removed from the descending aorta, using origins of the intercostal arteries as a landmark indicating normal aortic tissue. The C clamp on the descending aorta prevents backbleeding through the aorta and is also used to manipulate the descending aorta to facilitate its approximation to the ascending aorta at the time of anastomosis.

A small angled clamp is placed obliquely across the arch of the aorta at the base of the brachiocephalic and left carotid arteries, allowing continuous perfusion through the brachiocephalic artery cannula to both of these vessels (Fig. 48-37, *C*). Cardioplegia is introduced in standard fashion through a cannula placed into the midportion of the ascending aorta. Incision is made on the left posterolateral aspect of the distal ascending aorta onto the base of the left carotid artery over a sufficient length to match the circumference of the orifice of the descending aorta. End-to-side anastomosis between descending and ascending aorta is performed using a running suture technique with 7-0 absorbable monofilament suture. Upon completion of the anastomosis, the obliquely placed clamp on the aortic arch and the descending aortic clamp are removed. The ascending aorta is then clamped in standard fashion, allowing perfusion to the entire systemic circulation except the coronary arteries. The perfusion flow rate is increased to 100 $mL \cdot kg^{-1} \cdot min^{-1}$. A repeat dose of cardioplegia is given about this time, and the operation proceeds with VSD closure (see Chapter 35) and, if needed, atrial septal defect (ASD) closure. In the typical case, the VSD is closed via an incision in the pulmonary trunk, and the ASD via right atriotomy. After these defects, the pulmonary trunk incision and atrial incision are closed, and standard maneuvers

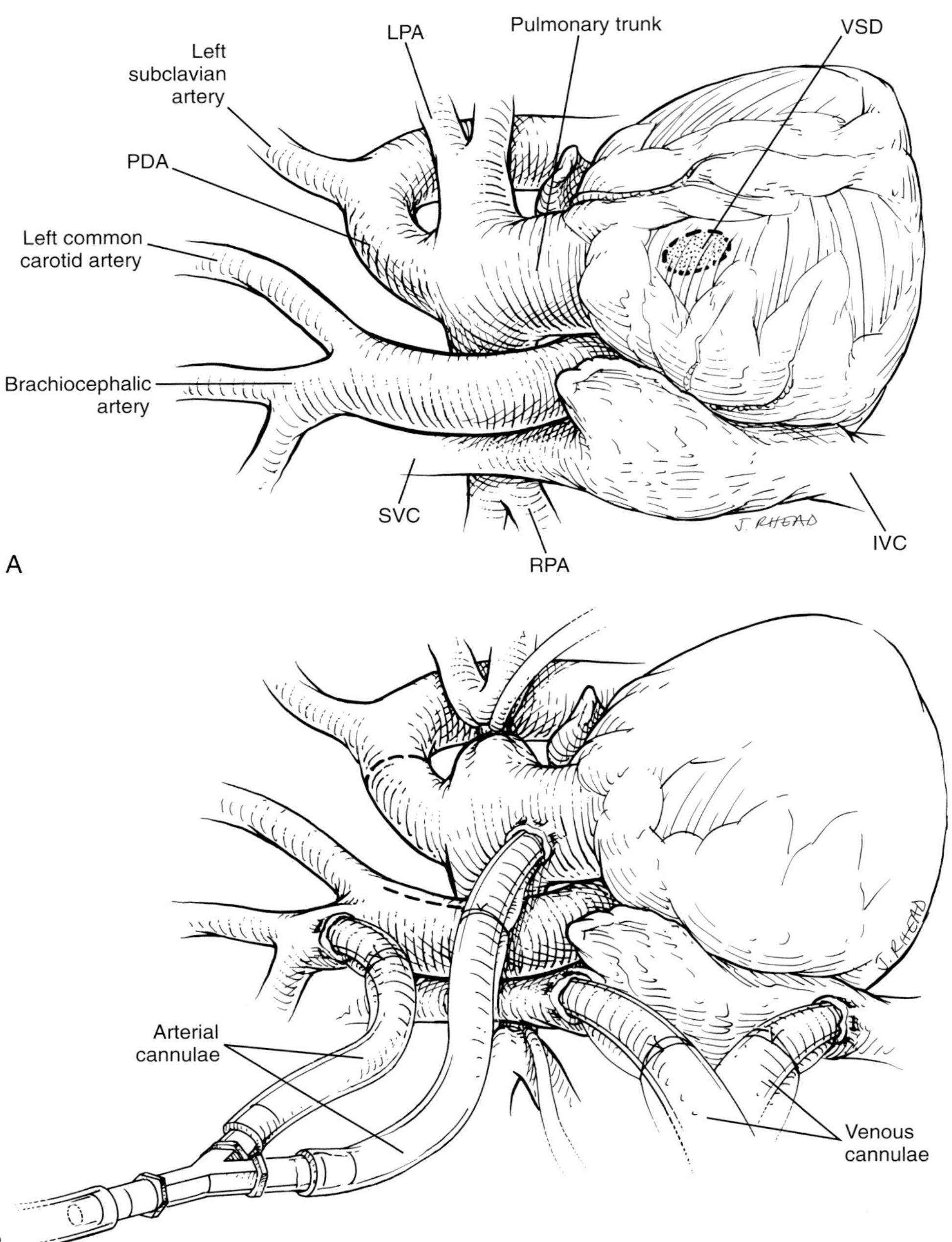

Figure 48-37 Primary repair of interrupted aortic arch using continuous cardiopulmonary bypass (CPB). **A,** Cardiac exposure is through a standard median sternotomy, and preparation and dissection are similar to that used for repair of hypoplastic left heart (see Chapter 49). This figure shows type B aortic arch interruption, with patent ductus arteriosus *(PDA)* and ventricular septal defect *(VSD)*. **B,** Two separate arterial cannulae are used, one introduced into the brachiocephalic artery and the other into the pulmonary trunk. Venous cannulation is performed into superior and inferior venae cavae through standard purse strings. After beginning CPB, branch pulmonary arteries are temporarily occluded (see text for details). Moderate hypothermia and standard cardioplegic myocardial protection are used (see text for details). Dashed lines show points of transection of distal ductus arteriosus and incision in posterolateral aspect of ascending aorta.

for removing the aortic clamp, rewarming, and separation from CPB are implemented (see "Completing Cardiopulmonary Bypass" in Section III of Chapter 2).

Repair Using Circulatory Arrest

After proper stabilization as described under Indications for Operation later in this section, the baby is brought to the operating room, usually with an umbilical artery catheter in place. After usual preliminary steps, primary median sternotomy is made (see Preparation for Cardiopulmonary Bypass in Section III of Chapter 2). Most of the thymus gland, if present, is removed to adequately mobilize branches of the aortic arch. The pericardium is opened widely and stay sutures applied. A portion of the pericardium is prepared in case it is necessary to use it in repairing the ASD. The

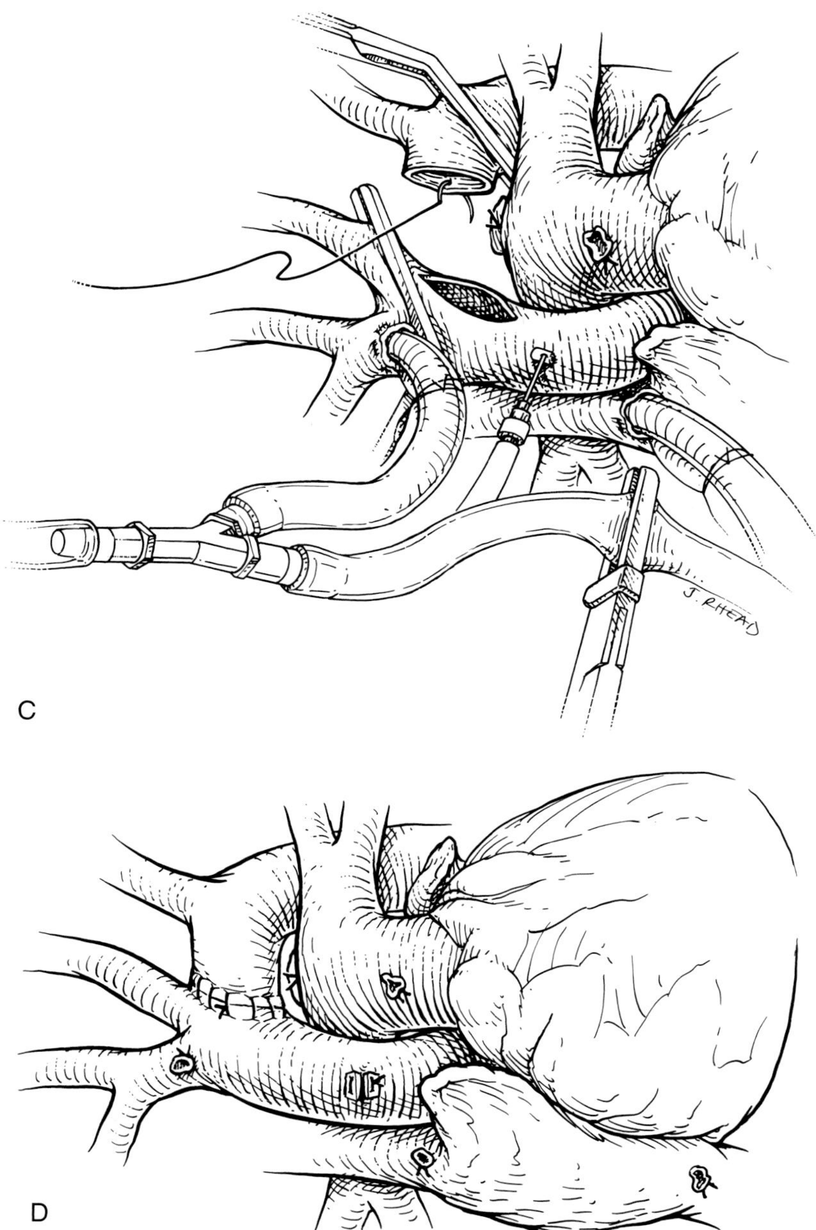

Figure 48-37, cont'd **C,** Cardioplegia has been introduced through a catheter in mid–ascending aorta. Proximal aortic clamp is positioned to allow continued flow through brachiocephalic and left carotid arteries. Arterial cannula in pulmonary trunk has been removed and ductus arteriosus ligated and divided. All ductus tissue has been removed from distal aorta. Incision in posterolateral aspect of ascending aorta has been made. Running suture anastomosis is begun at posterior aspect of circumference of descending aorta. **D,** Completed arch repair. Aortic clamps have been removed and patient separated from CPB (see text for details of methodology for ventricular septal defect closure). Key: *IVC,* Inferior vena cava; *LPA,* left pulmonary artery; *RPA,* right pulmonary artery; *SVC,* superior vena cava.

pulmonary trunk is separated from the ascending aorta, and an elastic snare is placed loosely around the right pulmonary artery. Most of the rest of the dissection is left until CPB is established.

A purse-string suture is placed on the right atrial appendage, somewhat more inferiorly than usual because of the positioning desired for the single right atrial cannula. A purse-string suture is placed on the ascending aorta at a carefully selected place, intended to be just opposite the anastomosis that will be made; this generally means that it is placed slightly more than halfway between the aortic valve and origin of the brachiocephalic artery, toward the right lateral aspect of the ascending aorta. A purse-string suture is placed on the proximal pulmonary trunk at a convenient place.

After heparinizing the patient, a 8F aortic cannula is inserted through the ascending aortic purse string after temporarily placing a side-biting clamp for making the opening. The tip of the cannula must sometimes be shortened if the ascending aorta is diminutive so as to leave only a short segment lying within it. The perfusionist has already arranged the arterial tubing with a Y-connector to accommodate double arterial cannulation. A stopcock is interposed between the aortic cannula and one arm of the arterial tubing, and the arterial tubing is carefully arranged to lie smoothly and as much as possible outside the surgical field. After inserting the aortic cannula, a round-nosed right atrial catheter of appropriate size is introduced through the right atrial appendage and positioned in the orifice of the *superior* vena cava. This allows the cannula and the venous tubing to sweep inferiorly and lie outside the surgical field. CPB is established with the perfusate about 34°C; a second arterial cannula is inserted into the pulmonary trunk through a purse string and is connected to the other arm of the arterial Y; the tip of the cannula remains within the pulmonary trunk. The left pulmonary artery is dissected out promptly and a snare placed and tightened around it, and the snare on the right pulmonary artery is tightened. Cooling of the patient with the perfusate then proceeds. Infusion of PGE_1 is continued during the cooling phase of CPB.

During cooling, the brachiocephalic, right subclavian, right common carotid, left common carotid, and left subclavian arteries are fully mobilized. This step is extremely important to preclude tension on the aortic suture line once it is made. The ductus arteriosus is dissected, and a tie is placed loosely around it. Elastic snares are placed around the right and left common carotid arteries, but not around the subclavian arteries. When the patient's nasopharyngeal (or tympanic membrane) temperature reaches 16° to 18°C, circulatory arrest is established, leaving the venous tubing open until the patient's blood volume has been transferred to the pump-oxygenator. The aorta is clamped just distal to the aortic cannula, and cold cardioplegic solution is infused through the stopcock on the aortic cannula (see Section IV of Chapter 2). All cannulae are then removed from the surgical field, the carotid artery tourniquets tightened, and the aortic clamp removed.

The ductus arteriosus is ligated, taking care to avoid distorting the bifurcation of the pulmonary trunk, and it is transected at its junction with the aorta. As much ductal tissue as possible is removed from the opened aorta, but this cannot be performed in as satisfactory a manner as in discrete coarctation. Particularly in type B interruption, the distal aortic segment is thoroughly mobilized. If the right subclavian artery arises anomalously from the upper descending aorta, it is dissected and divided between ligatures. If the anastomosis cannot be made tension-free in any other manner, the left subclavian artery is also ligated and divided. A small delicate C clamp is placed on the descending aorta so that an assistant can bring it into apposition with the proximal aortic segment without tension. An opening for the anastomosis is made in the left posterolateral aspect of the ascending aorta, as much as possible in its midportion and approximately opposite the arterial cannulation site. An end-to-side anastomosis is made with continuous 7-0 absorbable monofilament suture, beginning along the far side of the inferior angle and sewing so that the stitching in the proximal aorta is from the inside out, because this is the most delicate structure. Five or six of the stitches should be placed before they are carefully pulled up as the aortic segments are brought together; the remainder of the suture line is then completed.

The VSD is repaired. If there is considerable infundibular (conal) septal tissue separating the superior margin of the VSD from the pulmonary valve, the VSD is repaired through the right atrium (see Technique of Operation in Chapter 35). If preliminary echocardiographic studies have shown that the infundibular septum beneath the pulmonary valve is deficient, as is often the case, the VSD is repaired through the pulmonary trunk, which is usually very large in this condition. The foramen ovale, which may have been considerably stretched by a preexisting left-to-right shunt, must be closed. This can be accomplished either primarily or by suturing into place a piece of pericardium using continuous sutures.

Saline is flushed into the left side of the heart before completing closure of the foramen ovale, to emerge through the aortic cannulation site to de-air the left heart. The right atrium is closed. Only the ascending aortic cannula is reinserted, and it is important to have blood gently coming out the cannula as it is inserted into the ascending aorta to prevent air entrapment. After reinserting the right atrial cannula, CPB is begun, the carotid artery tourniquets are released, and rewarming is accomplished. Before removing the aortic cannula, pressure in the ascending aorta can be measured by connecting to a pressure transducer to the stopcock that has previously been placed. It is compared with that recorded from the umbilical artery catheter to assess the status of the aortic anastomosis. The remainder of the procedure is completed in the usual manner (see "Completing Cardiopulmonary Bypass" in Section III of Chapter 2).

Alternative Methods of Arch Repair

Occasionally, other methods of arch repair are indicated when a primary ascending-to-descending aortic anastomosis is not advisable. Methods that preserve growth potential,[H6,M28] such as using the left carotid or subclavian artery, are preferred to interposition grafts. When an anomalous right subclavian artery is present, it can be used for the arch reconstruction.[H21]

Repair of Interrupted Arch and Ventricular Septal Defect and Left Ventricular Outflow Obstruction

Left ventricular outflow tract (LVOT) obstruction occurs to varying degrees with interrupted aortic arch and VSD. The decision to perform a specific procedure to address the LVOT at the initial neonatal operation is a difficult one (see Special Situations and Controversies later in this section). When the LVOT is deemed inadequate, various techniques have been used to address this problem:

- Pulmonary trunk–to-aortic anastomosis (Damus-Kaye-Stansel [DKS] procedure) with arch repair and Rastelli septation (VSD closure and right ventricle–pulmonary trunk conduit)[T1,Y1]
- DKS procedure with arch repair and systemic-to–pulmonary artery shunt, followed by staged Rastelli septation
- Direct muscular or fibromuscular LVOT resection along with arch and VSD repair[S40]
- Norwood operation with Rastelli septation[G15,N3]
- Norwood operation, followed by staged Rastelli septation[E8]
- Ross-Konno operation[R12,S35]

Repair of Interrupted Arch and Other Coexisting Cardiac Anomalies

In general, coexisting cardiac anomalies such as transposition of the great arteries or truncus arteriosus are repaired concomitantly with repair of the interrupted arch, except for those in which a Fontan operation is required.[K6] For these exceptions, the procedures described under Indications for Operation in Chapters 41 and 56 are applicable. Several techniques have been described for one-stage repair of interrupted arch with aortopulmonary window.[K16,K17]

SPECIAL FEATURES OF POSTOPERATIVE CARE

Care is as usual (see Chapter 5). Special attention is paid to the possible occurrence of hypocalcemia if DiGeorge syndrome is present.

Because in this setting appreciable left-to-right shunting is apt to occur through a small residual VSD or ASD (presumably because of some degree of hypoplasia of the left ventricular cavity or outflow obstruction), left-to-right shunting must be carefully sought (see "Risk Factors for Low Cardiac Output" in Section I of Chapter 5). If found in patients whose hemodynamic state is not good, reoperation is indicated.

If extensive atelectasis of the left lung develops, its cause may be left bronchial compression by a directly reconstructed aortic arch. Prevalence of this complication is low when the operation has included wide mobilization as described. However, if this complication occurs, reoperation may be considered if it is believed that the vessels can be further mobilized.

Because the aortic valve is commonly small or bicuspid, and the subvalvar LVOT is small as a result of the posteriorly malaligned infundibular septum, it is common for some degree of LVOT obstruction to be present after repair once the left ventricle ejects a full cardiac output. The degree of obstruction should be assessed immediately after separation from CPB using transesophageal echocardiography. If preoperative assessment and surgical judgment are appropriate, the gradient should be less than 30 mmHg systolic. If the gradient is higher, particularly if there is left ventricular dysfunction or hemodynamic instability, reoperation and alternative reconstruction should be considered (see Special Situations and Controversies later in this section).

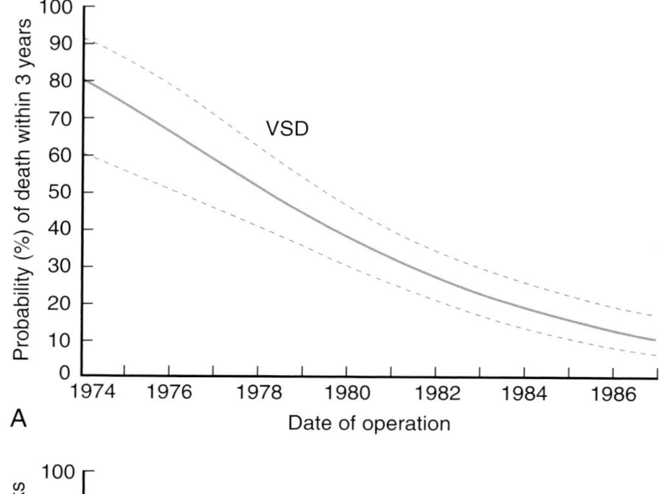

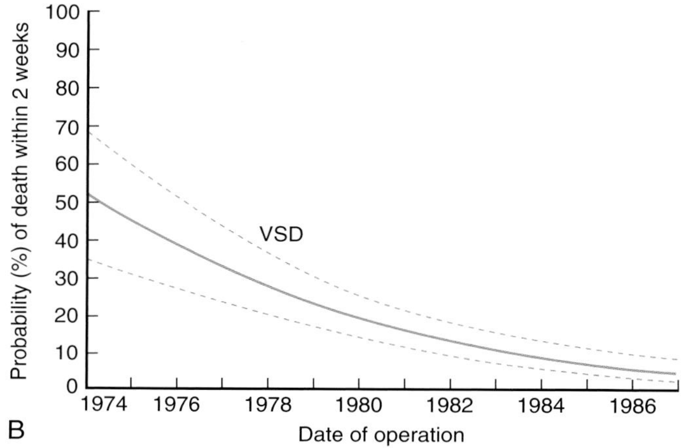

Figure 48-38 Relationship of date of operation to probability of death after repair of interrupted aortic arch with coexisting ventricular septal defect *(VSD)*. Depictions are nomograms of specific solutions of multivariable equations (see original paper for details). **A,** Probability of death within 2 weeks. **B,** Probability of death within 3 years. (From Sell and colleagues.[S15])

RESULTS

Survival

Early (Hospital) Death

Most early reports were based on a small number of patients, and in these mortality ranged from 20% to 80%. However, in patients with interrupted arch and VSD, early mortality in the current era can be 10%[K6,S15] (Fig. 48-38) or less.[F6,H20,M5] In the multiinstitutional study of the CHSS, mortality after optimum repair for type A interruption and VSD was 4% at 30 days; for type B, 11%.[J8]

Time-Related Survival

Realizing that many patients are seriously ill, survival from time of diagnosis (birth), including deaths before operation, is the most realistic evidence of the impact of treatment on the natural history. Overall, 5-year survival after birth can be predicted to be about 45%; rate of dying (hazard function) is rather high immediately after birth but declines rapidly thereafter, reaching a low level by 12 months (Fig. 48-39).

Survival after repair of interrupted aortic arch and VSD in the CHSS multiinstitutional study of a heterogeneous population was 63% at 4 years (Fig. 48-40), and optimal repair in type A interruption with or without coexisting obstructive lesions elsewhere in the left heart was associated with 5-year survival of 93%, and for type B, 83%[J8] (Fig. 48-41). Recent follow-up of this patient cohort indicates that non–risk-adjusted 16-year survival is 59%, and not unexpectedly, it improved the later the date of birth (Fig. 48-42). Single-institution studies from approximately the same era suggest similar 5-year survival of greater than 70%.[F18,L7,M5,S7,S17] Unadjusted survival for interrupted arch with aortopulmonary window (Fig. 48-43) is better than unadjusted survival for interrupted arch with VSD (see Fig. 48-40), and is similar to "optimal repair" survival for interrupted arch with VSD (see Fig. 48-41).[A2]

Modes of Death

Most deaths are with acute or subacute heart failure without or with multiple subsystem failure, although some are related to late reoperations for LVOT obstruction or aortic arch obstruction.

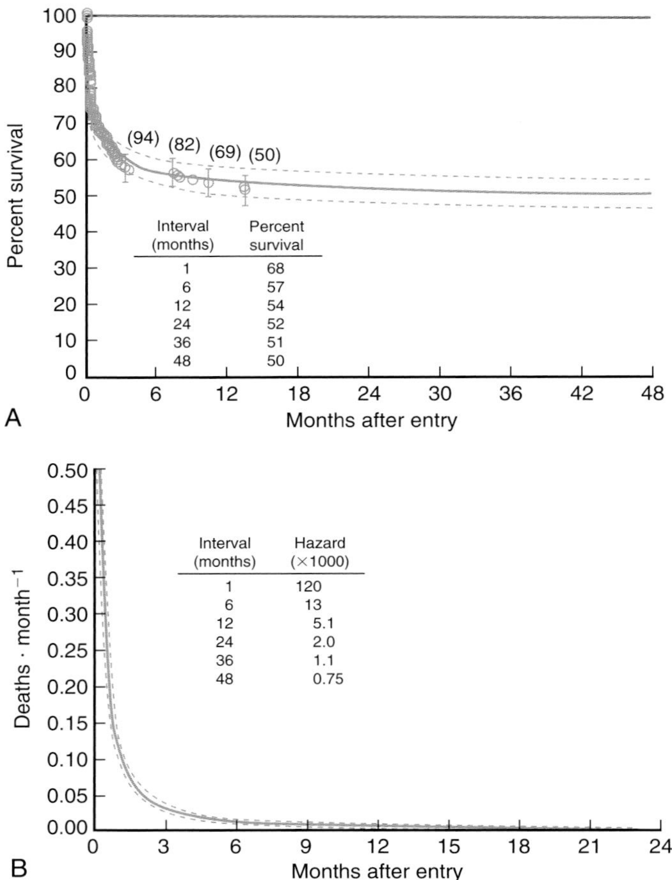

Figure 48-39 Early and intermediate-term survival after entry into treatment institution (essentially at birth) of heterogeneous group of neonates with interrupted arch (n = 168). **A,** Percent survival. **B,** Hazard function for death. (From multiinstitutional study of the Congenital Heart Surgeons Society, 1987 to 1991.)

A — Percent survival; Months after arch repair; (113) (107) (83)

Interval (months)	Percent survival
1	73
6	67
12	65
24	64
36	63
48	63

B — Deaths · month⁻¹; Months after arch repair

Interval (months)	Hazard (×1000)
1	49
6	6.5
12	2.9
24	1.3
36	0.82
48	0.58

Figure 48-40 Early and long-term survival after repair of interrupted aortic arch in heterogeneous group of neonates with interrupted aortic arch and ventricular septal defect. Depiction is as in Fig. 48-39. **A,** Survival. **B,** Hazard function for death. (From Jonas and colleagues.[J8])

Incremental Risk Factors for Premature Death

The 2005 report on the CHSS multiinstitutional study of 472 cases of interrupted aortic arch focuses on risk factors for mortality and reintervention.[M18] A relatively cohesive picture of the risk factors for mortality can be constructed based on this study and a number of other individual institutional studies.

Nature of the *coexisting cardiac anomaly* has been identified as an important risk factor for death, with VSD the most favorable (see Fig. 48-41).[M5] The CHSS study confirms the presence of truncus arteriosus as a risk. Additionally, the CHSS study identifies certain VSD characteristics as risks. Small and moderate VSD and VSDs that are not malaligned are noted to be risks. Several relatively small series showed no association with survival of complexity of coexisting cardiac anomalies.[B40,M4] *Location of the interruption* has its most important effect when it has been between the brachiocephalic and left common carotid artery (type C); this has been a highly lethal but rare lesion.[S15] A smaller difference in survival has been observed between interruptions distal to the left subclavian artery (type A) and those between the left

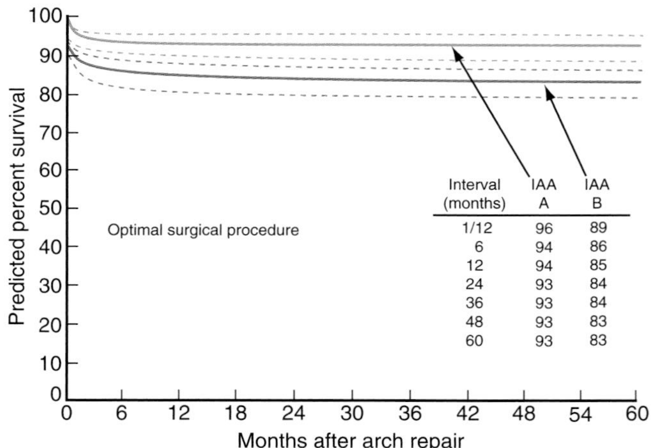

Figure 48-41 Risk-adjusted survival of neonate undergoing single-stage repair at age 7 days of either type A or B interrupted aortic arch *(IAA)* and single large ventricular septal defect. Graph represents nomograms of specific solutions of multivariable equation given in original paper.[J8] Solid lines are point estimates enclosed within 68% confidence limits. (From Jonas and colleagues.[J8])

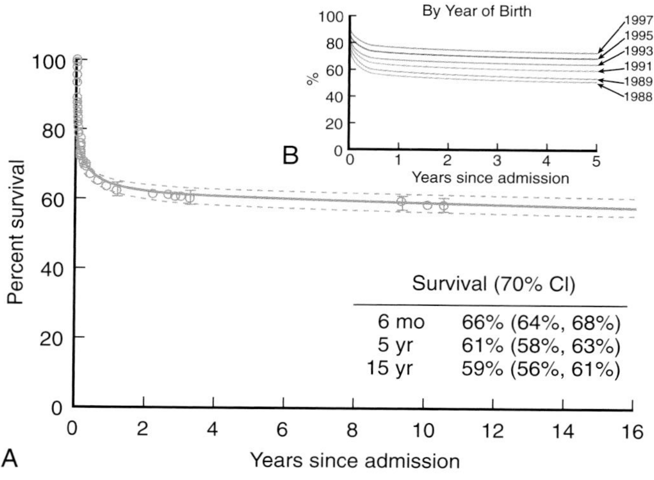

Figure 48-42 Overall time-related survival of 472 neonates with interrupted aortic arch. Time zero is time of initial admission to a Congenital Heart Surgeons Society member institution. Depiction is as in Fig. 48-39. **A,** Overall survival. **B,** Predicted overall survival for first 5 years after admission stratified by year of birth. (From McCrindle and colleagues.[M18])

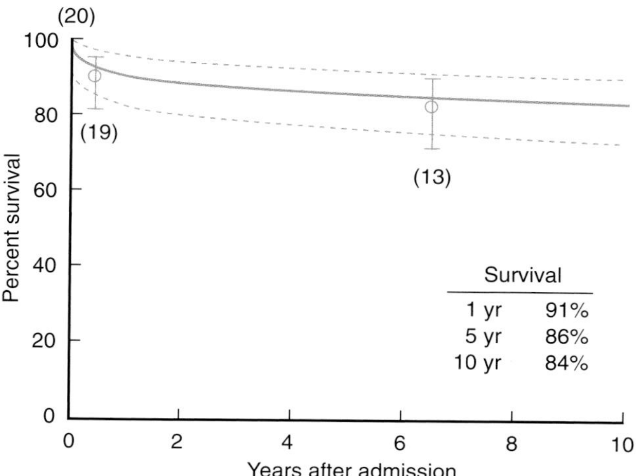

Figure 48-43 Time-related survival of 20 neonates with interrupted aortic arch and aortopulmonary window was characterized by an early hazard phase. Time zero is time of initial admission to a Congenital Heart Surgeons Society member institution. Depiction is as in Fig. 48-39. (From Akdemir and colleagues.[A2])

Table 48-7 Repair of Interrupted Aortic Arch and Ventricular Septal Defect in Neonates, without or with a Concomitant Procedure, and the Non–Risk-Adjusted Total Deaths in Each Group

		Total Deaths				
First Repair	*n*	**No.**	**%**	**CL (%)**		
One-stage repair	116	44	38	33-43	$P(\chi^2) = 0.7$	$P(\chi^2) = 0.5$
Repair IAA + PT band	40	14	35	27-44		
Repair only IAA	17[a]	4	24	12-39		
Transplant	1	0	0	0-85		
Subtotal	174	62	36	32-40		
$P(\chi^2)$			0.6			
No repair of anything	9	9	100	81-100		
TOTAL	183	71	39	35-43		

Data from Jonas and colleagues.[J8]
[a]Seven (zero deaths) had type A interruption, 10 (four deaths) had type B interruption.
Key: *CL,* 70% Confidence limits; *IAA,* interrupted aortic arch; *PT,* pulmonary trunk.

subclavian and left common carotid artery (type B) (see Fig. 48-41). The CHSS study confirms higher risk for types C and B; thus, type A carries the lowest risk.

Type of initial surgical procedure used to address interrupted aortic arch with VSD does not appear to importantly influence outcome, whether the approach is arch repair with VSD closure, arch repair with pulmonary trunk banding, or arch repair alone[M5] (Table 48-7). The CHSS study confirms this as well. As intimated under Technique of Operation earlier in this section, *condition of the patient on entry into the operating room* is important, and a low arterial pH at that time has been a strong risk factor for death (Tables 48-8 and 48-9; Fig. 48-44).

Other levels of LVOT obstruction is a risk factor, and is depicted as decreasing survival as left ventricular aortic junction diameter decreases (see Table 48-8). More complex procedures designed to address this obstruction are identified as carrying greater risk, as is ignoring the obstruction and performing a simple repair of the interruption and VSD closure (see Table 48-9). The CHSS study suggests that a pulmonary trunk to aortic anastomosis (DKS anastomosis) increases risk.

Date of operation has been a powerful risk factor because of great improvements achieved over time (see Fig. 48-38).[M5,Y5] The CHSS study confirms this. Thus, data from earlier eras have little applicability in the current era in institutions prepared for neonatal cardiac surgery.

Low weight at operation is identified as a risk in the CHSS study, as is *lack of augmentation of the arch* at the time of initial arch repair; however, other studies seem to contradict the latter.[M29]

Left Ventricular Outflow Obstruction

Patients with interrupted aortic arch often have at least some degree of hypoplastic left heart physiology as well (see

Table 48-8 Incremental Risk Factors for Time-Related Death at Any Time after Repair of Interrupted Aortic Arch and Ventricular Septal Defect in Neonates

	Incremental Risk Factors for Death (Patient-Specific Variables, Including Institutionally Measured Dimensions)	*P* (Single Hazard Phase)
	Demographic	
Lower	Birth weight	<.0001
Younger	Age at repair	.04
	Morphologic	
	IAA type B	.02
	Outlet or trabecular VSD	.003
Smaller	Size of VSD	.0002
Smaller	Dimension *(z)* of LV-aortic junction	.03

Data from Jonas and colleagues.[J8]
NOTE: For this, the obstructive levels in the left heart–aorta complex were not entered, nor were procedural or institutional variables.
Key: *IAA,* Interrupted aortic arch; *LV,* left ventricular; *VSD,* ventricular septal defect.

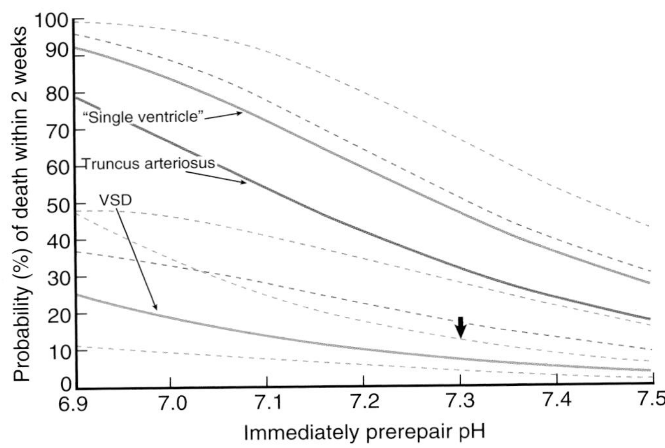

Figure 48-44 Relationship between arterial pH immediately preoperatively and probability of death within 2 weeks of repair of interrupted arch, according to coexisting cardiac anomaly. Depiction is a nomogram of a specific solution of a multivariable equation (see original paper for details). Key: *VSD,* Ventricular septal defect. (From Sell and colleagues.[S15])

Table 48-9 Incremental Risk Factors for Time-Related Death at Any Time after Repair, Entering Patient-Specific, Procedural, and Institutional Variables

	Incremental Risk Factors for Death (Patient-Specific, Procedural, and Institutionally Variables)	*P* (Single Hazard Phase)
	Demographic	
Lower	Birth weight	<.0001
Younger	Age at repair	.0004
	Morphologic	
Higher	Grade of subaortic obstruction (0-5)	.0004
	IAA type B	.04
Smaller	Size of VSD (small, moderate-sized, large)	<.0001
	Procedural	
	PT–Asc Ao anastomosis (DKS anastomosis)	<.0001
	Subaortic myotomy/myectomy and subaortic obstruction (≥grade 2) (interaction term)	.02
	Simple repair and coexisting obstructive lesions elsewhere in the LHA complex (interaction term)	.02
	Institutional	
	Institution B	.006
	Institution H	<.0001

Data from Jonas and colleagues.[J8]
Key: *Asc Ao,* Ascending aorta; *DKS,* Damus-Kay-Stansel; *IAA,* interrupted aortic arch; *LHA,* left heart–aorta; *PT,* pulmonary trunk.

"Coarctation as Part of Hypoplastic Left Heart Physiology" under Morphology in Section I). The specific features all relate to the LVOT, as pointed out several times elsewhere in this section, including:

- Posterior malalignment of infundibular septum
- Hypertrophy of anterolateral muscle bundle of the left ventricle (muscle of Moulaert)
- Bicuspid dysplastic aortic valve
- Narrowness of aortic anulus
- Hypoplasia of ascending aorta and aortic arch; occasionally this is apparent before operation, but more often it becomes evident after repair.

LVOT obstruction has important implications for both short- and long-term prognosis, and for decision making and surgical technique (see Results in following text and Special Situations and Controversies later in this section). In a minority of neonates with interrupted aortic arch and VSD, the LVOT is inadequate, and repair of the arch and VSD alone results in unacceptable obstruction. Although difficult to accomplish, it is best to identify such patients before the initial operation (see Special Situations and Controversies later in this section). In about 40% of patients with a conoventricular VSD, or with a VSD in the outlet portion of the right ventricle, evidence of LVOT obstruction develops at midterm or late follow-up, even when the LVOT was adequate after initial operation[J4,S15] (Fig. 48-45).

Whether the LVOT obstruction *develops* during or sometime after the initial operation, or whether it was *present at birth* and only becomes evident later is uncertain, but both probably occur. Probability that at least the anatomic basis for the obstruction was present at birth is heightened by the shape of the hazard function, which indicates that the rate of recognizing (or developing) LVOT obstruction declines to a constant hazard after about 2 years following initial repair (see Fig. 48-45).

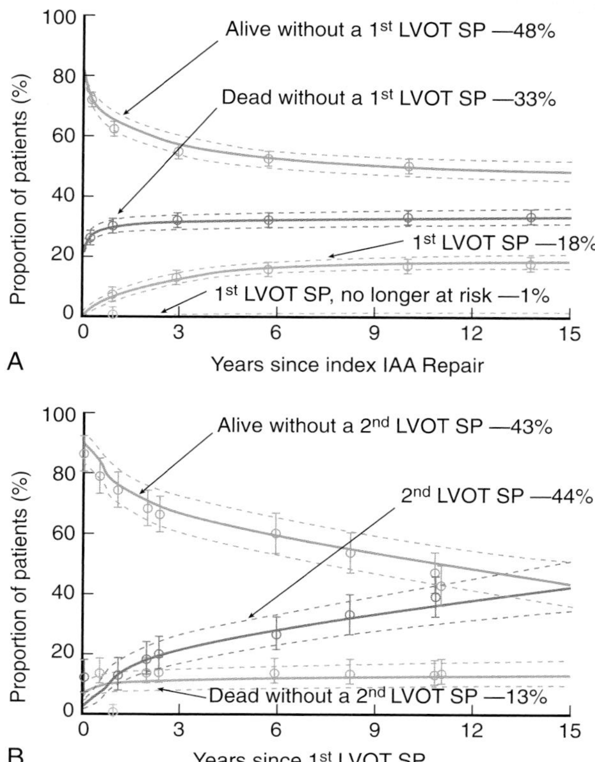

Figure 48-45 Competing risks for first and second subsequent left ventricular outflow tract *(LVOT)* procedures. **A,** All patients began at index interrupted aortic arch *(IAA)* repair (n = 423) and could transition to either subsequent LVOT procedure (still at risk or no longer at risk of additional LVOT procedures) for residual or recurrent obstruction at LVOT or death. **B,** All patients began at time of first subsequent LVOT procedure (n = 67) and could transition to either subsequent LVOT procedure for residual or recurrent obstruction at LVOT or death. Patients considered no longer at risk of LVOT procedures underwent repairs such as the Damus-Kaye-Stansel procedure or heart transplantation and were censored at that point. Solid lines represent parametric point estimates; dashed lines enclose 70% confidence intervals; circles with error bars represent nonparametric estimates. Y-axis represents proportion of patients (expressed as percentage of total) in each category at any given point. Key: *SP,* Subsequent procedure. (From Jegatheeswaran and colleagues.[J4])

Reoperations directed at the most important area of obstruction have been well tolerated, but gradients have not always been eliminated. Intermediate-term survival of patients with this complication has been good, nonetheless,[S15] but long-term survival will probably be adversely affected by presence of this problem.

The CHSS study reveals that 143 of 472 patients (30%) underwent a procedure aimed at addressing either real or perceived LVOT obstruction. The study design was such that it was not possible to identify the decision-making process for performing an LVOT procedure. In 91 of the 143, the procedure was performed at the initial arch repair, and in 52 it was performed later. Risk factors for early LVOT intervention were low birth weight, single ventricle, and type B interruption. Risk factors for late LVOT intervention were single ventricle, anomalous right subclavian artery, and bicuspid aortic valve.

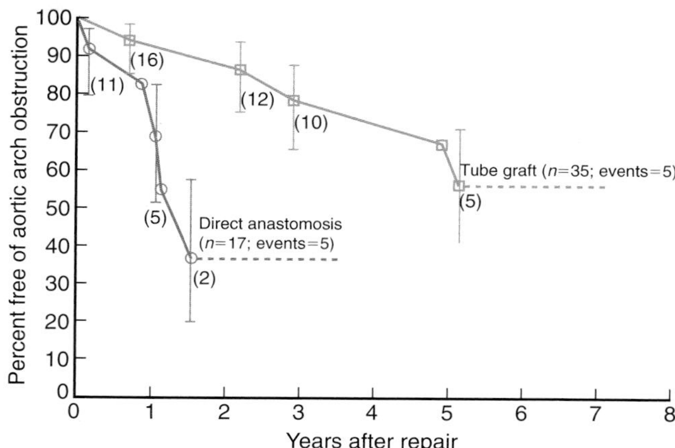

Figure 48-46 Freedom from aortic arch obstruction after repair of interrupted aortic arch, according to whether repair was by direct anastomosis or tube graft reconstruction. Each symbol represents an event, vertical bars are 68% confidence limits, and numbers in parentheses are patients remaining at risk. (From Sell and colleagues.[S15])

Persistent or Recurrent Aortic Arch Obstruction

Persistent or recurrent aortic arch obstruction has in the past been a frequent complication of primary repair with end-to-end anastomosis[M5,O4,S7] (Fig. 48-46), but it usually responds well to percutaneous balloon dilatation.[S5] More recent individual institution studies of routinely advancing the descending aorta to the ascending aorta with direct anastomosis, without use of patch material or brachiocephalic vessel flaps, indicate that recurrent or persistent arch obstruction may be substantially reduced and even eliminated.[M29] This inference is tempered by the fact that follow-up beyond 5 years is not yet available for these more recent series. The CHSS multi-institutional study of 472 patients reported risk factors for arch reintervention.[M18] Overall, by 16 years after entry into the study, 29% of initial repairs required arch reintervention. Early-phase risks include both younger and older age, double outlet right ventricle, and aortopulmonary window. Late-phase risks were truncus arteriosus, use of PTFE in the initial arch repair, and all arch repair techniques other than primary anastomosis with patch augmentation.

Late Reoperation from All Causes

Late reoperation is frequent after neonatal repair of interrupted aortic arch, reflecting the complexity of the underlying lesion. There are multiple reasons for reoperation, including:

- Recurrent arch obstruction
- LVOT obstruction
- Residual VSD
- Bronchial compression
- Diaphragm palsy
- Complete heart block

In a single-institution analysis of 94 patients undergoing initial operation between 1975 and 1999, with follow-up of up to 21 years (mean 6.7 years), reoperation from all causes was 40% at 15 years[S7] (Fig. 48-47). Similar prevalence of

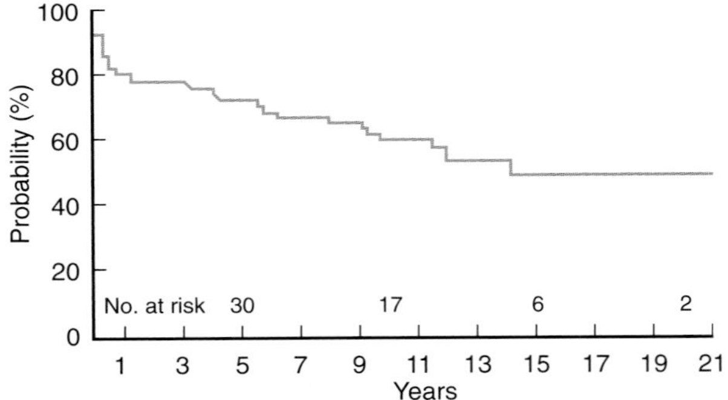

Figure 48-47 Freedom from reoperation from all causes in 94 patients undergoing initial interrupted arch repair between 1975 and 1999. (From Schreiber and colleagues.[S7])

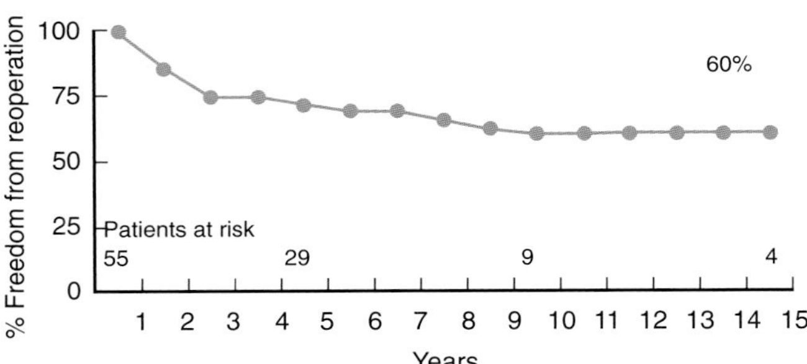

Figure 48-48 Freedom from reoperation from all causes in 65 patients undergoing initial operation for interrupted aortic arch between 1982 and 2005. (From Malhotra and colleagues.[M5])

reintervention was noted in other series from the same period.[O4] Reflecting the general trend that outcomes improve over time, another single-institution analysis of 65 patients undergoing initial operation between 1982 and 2005 showed that reoperation from all causes was 60% at 15 years[M5] (Fig. 48-48).

The cumulative incidence of all types (surgical or catheter-based) reinterventions after repair of interrupted aortic arch exceeds one per patient within about 3 years and approached two per patient by about 25 years (Fig. 48-49). The most common are catheter-based arch procedures (Fig. 48-50).

INDICATIONS FOR OPERATION

Diagnosis of interrupted aortic arch is an indication for operation, no matter what the coexisting cardiac anomaly. Severe chromosomal abnormalities may contraindicate surgical intervention.

Intensive treatment is an essential part of the therapeutic program and begins the moment the diagnosis is suspected, which should be shortly after birth. An infusion of PGE_1 is begun, usually in a dose of 0.05 to 0.1 $\mu g \cdot kg^{-1} \cdot min^{-1}$, and the infant is intubated and appropriately ventilated; high FIO_2 is avoided. If the infant's condition is good in all ways, operation is undertaken at the first convenient time, but not as an emergency. If the infant's condition is not good, then:

- Right-to-left shunting into the descending aorta for augmenting systemic blood flow is encouraged by increasing CO_2 in the inspired gas mixture or mildly hypoventilating the patient so that PaO_2 is about 40 mmHg (to increase pulmonary vascular resistance).
- Cardiac output and renal blood flow are increased by infusing dopamine at 2.5 to 5 $\mu g \cdot kg^{-1} \cdot min^{-1}$.
- Acidosis is corrected by intravenous sodium bicarbonate (see Appendix 5N in Chapter 5).

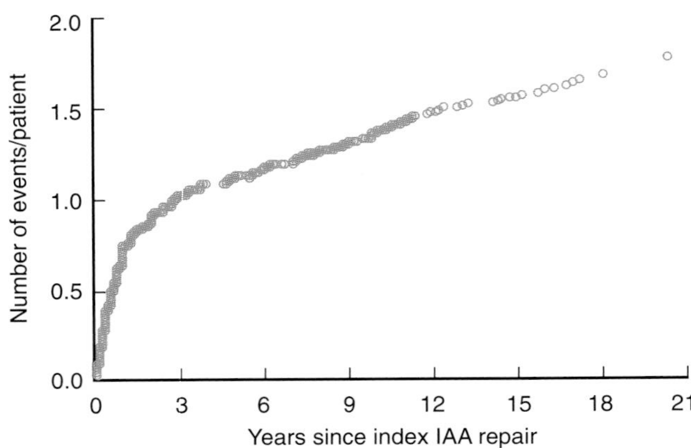

Figure 48-49 Cumulative hazard for subsequent procedures of any type after repair of interrupted aortic arch. Graph demonstrates cumulative number of events per patient at any given point since index procedure. Circles represent any subsequent procedure (n = 436). (From Jegatheeswaran and colleagues.[J4])

Nearly always, the baby can be brought into a good clinical condition by these measures. At that point, operation is performed.

One-stage repair of the interrupted arch and the coexisting anomaly, or repair of the interruption with staged repair of the coexisting anomaly, is carried out, except when some form of single ventricle is the coexisting anomaly. An alternative plan is then necessary (see Section I of Chapter 41).

SPECIAL SITUATIONS AND CONTROVERSIES

Preoperative assessment of adequacy of the LVOT, including the aortic valve and subaortic region, can be challenging in patients with interrupted aortic arch. The aortic valve is frequently bicuspid with some degree of hypoplasia. The subaortic region is often narrowed by a posteriorly malaligned infundibular septum. Preoperative assessment of the LVOT is difficult because preoperative physiologic measurements are unreliable predictors of postoperative physiology. Because flow across the LVOT is typically low preoperatively from the patent ductus with right-to-left shunting, preoperative obstruction is almost never detected, even when the LVOT proves to be inadequate after repair. Therefore, other preoperative measures must be relied on to predict LVOT adequacy after repair. The most difficult assessment is of the subaortic region. Specific criteria for identifying the patient with inadequate LVOT preoperatively have not been widely accepted; currently, individual institutions use various measures to identify these patients. In many cases a subjective intraoperative decision is made by the operating surgeon regarding whether to perform a procedure that addresses the LVOT.[S40] Hanley and colleagues at Stanford (personal communication) have used a simple formula that permits an objectively based

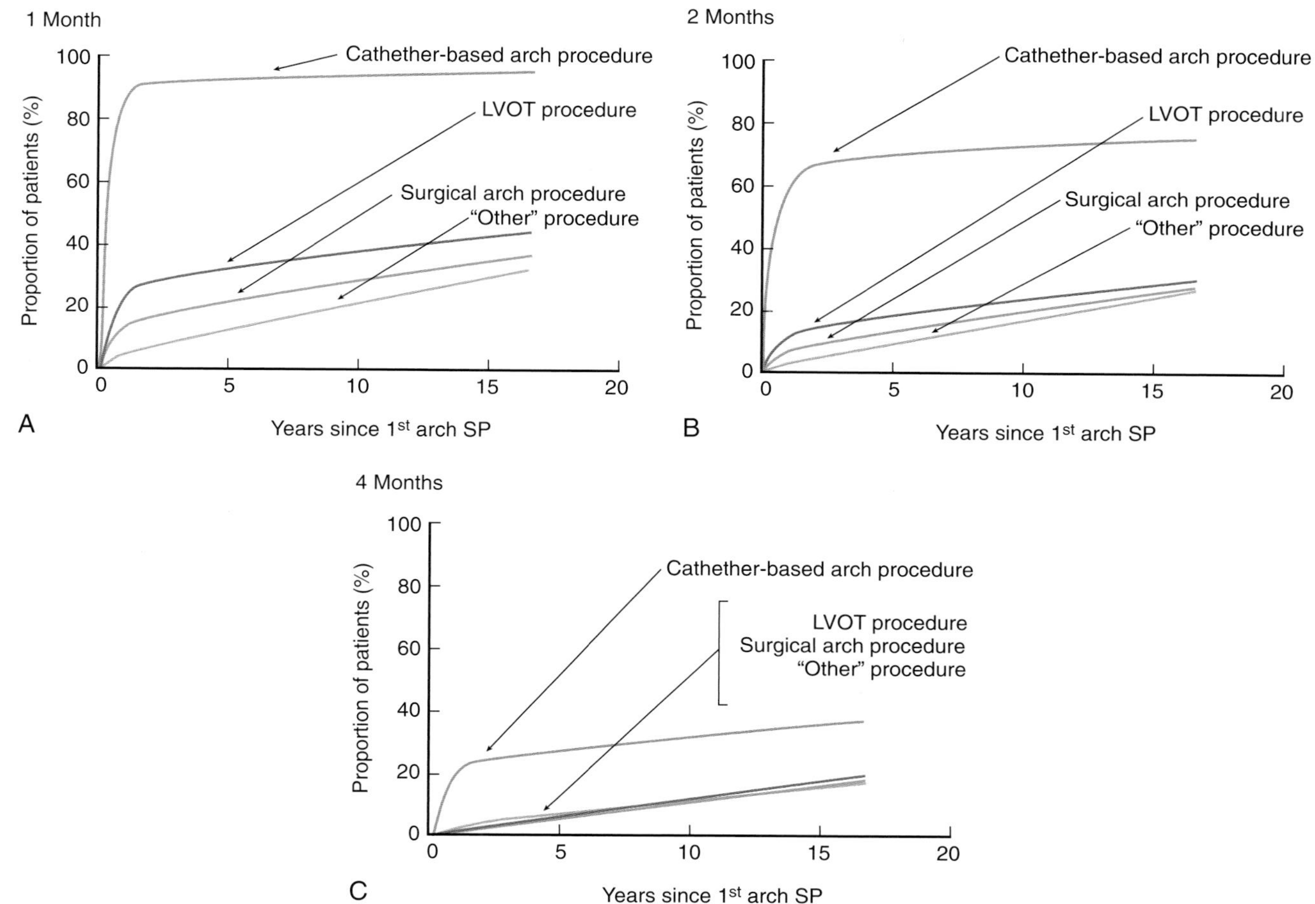

Figure 48-50 Risk of a second subsequent arch procedure stratified by type of most recent procedure (catheter-based arch, "other," surgical arch, left ventricular outflow tract [LVOT] procedure) and interval (1 month **[A]**, 2 months **[B]**, and 4 months **[C]**) from index procedure to most recent arch procedure (in this case the first subsequent arch procedure) for a patient with a particular risk profile. This figure serves to illustrate "risks related to previous procedures" for subsequent arch procedure. A "typical" patient profile was assumed (i.e., one who had interrupted aortic arch without an additional cardiac diagnosis, a birth date near the middle of the study era, an index repair at an average age for patients in the second renewal, an index repair without concomitant LVOT resection, without the use of polytetrafluoroethylene or subclavian artery for arch repair, and without concomitant ventricular septal defect closure and one subsequent arch procedure; see original paper).[J4] These three graphs demonstrate that as interval from index procedure to most recent arch procedure (in this case, first subsequent arch procedure) increases (from 1 to 2 to 4 months), risk of a second subsequent arch procedure decreases, independent of what the most recent procedure had been. Furthermore, risk of a second subsequent arch procedure is generally greatest when most recent procedure was a catheter-based arch procedure, followed by LVOT procedure, surgical arch procedure, and "other" procedure. This finding illustrates the complex, time-dependent interrelationships among subsequent procedures. Key: *Arch,* Aortic arch, *LVOT,* left ventricular outflow tract; *SP,* subsequent procedure. (From Jegatheeswaran and colleagues.[J4])

decision preoperatively. Using echocardiography, if the smallest diameter of the subaortic region (measured in millimeters) is equal to or greater than body weight (measured in kilograms), the LVOT will be adequate, as defined by a postrepair LVOT gradient of less than 20 mmHg. (Others have described different anatomic dimensions used to predict subsequent obstruction.[A17,S3]) Thus, a 4-kg neonate must have a minimum subaortic dimension of at least 4 mm. If this criterion is met, a standard repair involving direct arch reconstruction and VSD closure is performed. If this criterion is not met, an alternative one-stage repair is performed. This involves direct arch reconstruction, DKS procedure, VSD closure allowing the LV to eject to both the aortic and pulmonic valves, and placement of a right ventricle–to–pulmonary trunk valved conduit. Although the 1994 CHSS data indicate that the DKS procedure carries elevated risk,[J8] several single-institution studies suggest that the DKS procedure or similar variants can be performed with low mortality.[E8,G15,N3] Others advocate directly resecting the obstruction in the LVOT at the time of the arch repair and VSD closure[B32,S40]; however, the 1994 CHSS data suggest that attempting to do this is a risk factor for death.[J8]

Finally, the Ross-Konno operation (see Technique of Operation in Section II of Chapter 47) has been applied to this problem.[R12,S35]

REFERENCES

A

1. Abbott ME. Coarctation of the aorta of the adult type. II. A statistical study and historical retrospect of 200 recorded cases with autopsy of stenosis or obliteration of the descending aorta in subjects over the age of two years. Am Heart J 1928;3:574.

2. Akdemir R, Ozhan H, Erbilen E, Yazici M, Gunduz H, Uyan C. Isolated interrupted aortic arch: a case report and review of the literature. Int J Cardiovasc Imaging 2004;20:389-92.
3. Akl BF. Ascending–distal aorta bypass (letter). Ann Thorac Surg 1985;39:196.
4. Ala-Kulju K, Jarvinen A, Maamies T, Mattila S, Merikallio E. Late aneurysms after patch aortoplasty for coarctation of the aorta in adults. Thorac Cardiovasc Surg 1983;31:301.
5. Alboliras ET, Mavroudis C, Pahl E, Gidding SS, Backer CL, Rocchini AP. Left ventricular growth in selected hypoplastic left ventricles: outcome after repair of coarctation of aorta. Ann Thorac Surg 1999;68:549.
6. Albright F, Smith PH, Fraser R. A syndrome characterized by primary ovarian insufficiency and decreased stature. Report of 11 cases with a digression on hormonal control of axillary and pubic hair. Am J Med Sci 1942;204:625.
7. Allan LD, Crawford DC, Tynan M. Evolution of coarctation of the aorta in intrauterine life. Br Heart J 1984;52:471.
8. Allen BS, Halldorsson AO, Barth MJ, Ilbawi MN. Modification of the subclavian patch aortoplasty for repair of aortic coarctation in neonates and infants. Ann Thorac Surg 2000;69:877.
9. Allen HD, Marx GR, Ovitt TW. Balloon angioplasty for coarctation: serial evaluation. J Am Coll Cardiol 1985;5:405.
10. Allen HD, Marx GR, Ovitt TW, Goldberg SJ. Balloon dilatation angioplasty for coarctation of the aorta. Am J Cardiol 1986;57:828.
11. al-Marsafawy HM, Ho SY, Redington AN, Anderson RH. The relationship of the outlet septum to the aortic outflow tract in hearts with interruption of the aortic arch. J Thorac Cardiovasc Surg 1995;109:1225.
12. Almeida de Oliveira S, Lisboa LA, Dallan LA, Abreu FC, Rochitte CE, de Souza JM. Extraanatomic aortic bypass for repair of aortic arch coarctation via sternotomy: midterm clinical and magnetic resonance imaging results. Ann Thorac Surg 2003;76:1962-6.
13. Alsoufi B, Cai S, Coles JG, Williams WG, Van Arsdell GS, Caldarone CA. Outcomes of different surgical strategies in the treatment of neonates with aortic coarctation and associated ventricular septal defects. Ann Thorac Surg 2007;84:1331-7.
14. Aluquin VP, Shutte D, Nihill MR, Lu AY, Chen L, Gelves J, et al. Normal aortic arch growth and comparison with isolated coarctation of the aorta. Am J Cardiol 2003;91:502-5.
15. Amato JJ, Rheinlander HF, Cleveland RJ. A method of enlarging the distal transverse arch in infants with hypoplasia and coarctation of the aorta. Ann Thorac Surg 1977;23:261.
16. Aoyagi S, Fukunaga S, Tayama E, Yoshida T. Extraanatomic aortic bypass for repair of aortic coarctation. J Card Surg 2007; 22:436-9.
17. Apfel HD, Levenbraun J, Quaegebeur JM, Allan LD. Usefulness of preoperative echocardiography in predicting left ventricular outflow obstruction after primary repair of interrupted aortic arch with ventricular septal defect. Am J Cardiol 1998;82:470-3.
18. Arakelyan V, Spiridonov A, Bockeria L. Ascending-to-descending aortic bypass via right thoracotomy for complex (re-) coarctation and hypoplastic aortic arch. Eur J Cardio-thorac Surg 2005;27: 815-20.
19. Araoz PA, Reddy GP, Tarnoff H, Roge CL, Higgins CB. MR findings of collateral circulation are more accurate measures of hemodynamic significance than arm–leg blood pressure gradient after repair of coarctation of the aorta. J Magn Reson Imaging 2003;17:177-83.
20. Aris A, Subirana MT, Ferres P, Torner-Soler M. Repair of aortic coarctation in patients more than 50 years of age. Ann Thorac Surg 1999;67:1376.
21. Asou T, Kado H, Imoto Y, Shiokawa Y, Tominaga R, Kawachi Y, et al. Selective cerebral perfusion technique during aortic arch repair in neonates. Ann Thorac Surg 1996;61:1546.
22. Attenhofer Jost CH, Schaff HV, Connolly HM, Danielson GK, Dearani JA, Puga FJ, et al. Spectrum of reoperations after repair of aortic coarctation: importance of an individualized approach because of coexistent cardiovascular disease. Mayo Clin Proc 2002;77:646-53.

B

1. Babu-Narayan SV, Mohiaddin RH, Cannell TM, Muhll IV, Dimopoulos K, Mullen MJ. Cardiovascular changes after transcatheter endovascular stenting of adult aortic coarctation. Int J Cardiol 2011;149:157-63.
2. Bacha EA, Almodovar M, Wessel DL, Zurakowski D, Mayer JE Jr, Jonas RA, et al. Surgery for coarctation of the aorta in infants weighing less than 2 kg. Ann Thorac Surg 2001;71:1260.
3. Bacha EA, Sawaqed R. Use of the aberrant right subclavian artery in complex aortic arch reconstruction. Ann Thorac Surg 2007; 83:1566-8.
4. Backer CL, Mavroudis C, Zias EA, Amin Z, Weigel TJ. Repair of coarctation with resection and extended end-to-end anastomosis. Ann Thorac Surg 1998;66:1365.
5. Backer CL, Stewart RD, Kelle AM, Mavroudis C. Use of partial cardiopulmonary bypass for coarctation repair through a left thoracotomy in children without collaterals. Ann Thorac Surg 2006;82:964-72.
6. Bahn RC, Edwards JE, DuShane JW. Coarctation of the aorta as a cause of death in early infancy. Pediatrics 1952;8:192.
7. Barnes RW, Rittenhouse EA, Kongtahworn C, Doty DB, Rossi NP, Ehrenhaft JL. Reversed intercostal arterial flow in coarctation of the aorta. Ann Thorac Surg 1975;19:27.
8. Barratt-Boyes BG, Nicholls TT, Brandt PW, Neutze JM. Aortic arch interruption associated with patent ductus arteriosus, ventricular septal defect, and total anomalous pulmonary venous connection. J Thorac Cardiovasc Surg 1972;63:367.
9. Barron DJ, Lamb RK, Ogilvie BC, Monro JL. Technique for extraanatomic bypass in complex aortic coarctation. Ann Thorac Surg 1996;61:241.
10. Bassareo PP, Marras AR, Manai ME, Mercuro G. The influence of different surgical approaches on arterial rigidity in children after aortic coarctation repair. Pediatr Cardiol 2009;30:414-8.
11. Bazan HA. Does stenting of thoracic aortic coarctation induce a late exercise-induced hypertension? Stay tuned. Catheter Cardiovasc Interv 2010;75:262.
12. Beaton AZ, Nguyen T, Lai WW, Chatterjee S, Ramaswamy P, Lytrivi ID, et al. Relation of coarctation of the aorta to the occurrence of ascending aortic dilation in children and young adults with bicuspid aortic valves. Am J Cardiol 2009;103:266-70.
13. Beauchesne LM, Connolly HM, Ammash NM, Warnes CA. Coarctation of the aorta: outcome of pregnancy. J Am Coll Cardiol 2001;38:1728-33.
14. Becker AE, Becker MJ, Edwards JE. Anomalies associated with coarctation of aorta. Particular reference to infancy. Circulation 1970;41:1067.
15. Becker C, Soppa C, Fink U, Haubner M, Muller-Lisse U, Englmeier KH, et al. Spiral CT angiography and 3D reconstruction in patients with aortic coarctation. Eur Radiol 1997;7:1473.
16. Becu LM, Tauxe WN, DuShane JW, Edwards JE. A complex of congenital cardiac anomalies: ventricular septal defects, biventricular origin of the pulmonary trunk, and subaortic stenosis. Am Heart J 1955;50:901.
17. Berens RJ, Stuth EA, Robertson FA, Jaquiss RD, Hoffman GM, Troshynski TJ, et al. Near infrared spectroscopy monitoring during pediatric aortic coarctation repair. Paediatr Anaesth 2006;16:777-81.
18. Bergdahl L, Bjork VO, Jonasson R. Surgical correction of coarctation of the aorta. Influence of age on late results. J Thorac Cardiovasc Surg 1983;85:532.
19. Bergdahl L, Ljungqvist A. Long-term results after repair of coarctation of the aorta by patch grafting. J Thorac Cardiovasc Surg 1980;80:177.
20. Bergdahl LA, Blackstone EH, Kirklin JW, Pacifico AD, Bargeron LM Jr. Determinants of early success in repair of aortic coarctation in infants. J Thorac Cardiovasc Surg 1982;83:736.
21. Berry CL, Tawes RL Jr. Mucopolysaccharides of the aortic wall in coarctation and recoarctation. Cardiovasc Res 1970;4: 224.
22. Bhat MA, Neelakandhan KS, Unnikrishnan M, Rathore RS, Mohan Singh MP, Lone GN. Fate of hypertension after repair of coarctation of the aorta in adults. Br J Surg 2001;88:536.
23. Bjork VO, Bergdahl L, Jonasson R. Coarctation of the aorta. The world's longest follow-up. Adv Cardiol 1978;22:205.
24. Blake HA, Manion WC, Spencer FC. Atresia or absence of the aortic isthmus. J Urol Nephrol 1962;43:607.
25. Blalock A, Park EA. Surgical treatment of experimental coarctation (atresia) of aorta. Ann Surg 1944;119:445.
26. Blaufox AD, Lai WW, Lopez L, Nguyen K, Griepp RB, Parness IA. Survival in neonatal biventricular repair of left-sided cardiac obstructive lesions associated with hypoplastic left ventricle. Am J Cardiol 1998;82:1138.

27. Bonnet D, Patkai J, Tamisier D, Kachaner J, Vouhe P, Sidi D. A new strategy for the surgical treatment of aortic coarctation associated with ventricular septal defect in infants using an absorbable pulmonary artery band. J Am Coll Cardiol 1999;34:866.
28. Bonnett LM. Sur la lesion dite stenose congenitale de laorte dans la region de listhme. Rev Med 1903;23:108.
29. Botta L, Russo V, Oppido G, Rosati M, Massi F, Lovato L, et al. Role of endovascular repair in the management of late pseudo-aneurysms following open surgery for aortic coarctation. Eur J Cardio-thorac Surg 2009;36:670-4.
30. Bouchart F, Dubar A, Tabley A, Litzler PY, Haas-Hubscher C, Redonnet M, et al. Coarctation of the aorta in adults: surgical results and long-term follow-up. Ann Thorac Surg 2000;70:1483.
31. Bouzguenda I, Marini D, Ou P, Boudjemline Y, Bonnet D, Agnoletti G. Percutaneous treatment of neonatal aortic coarctation presenting with severe left ventricular dysfunction as a bridge to surgery. Cardiol Young 2009;19:244-51.
32. Bove EL, Minich LL, Pridjian AK, Lupinetti FM, Snider AR, Dick M 2nd, et al. The management of severe subaortic stenosis, ventricular septal defect and aortic arch obstruction in the neonate. J Thorac Cardiovasc Surg 1993;105:289.
33. Brandt B 3rd, Marvin WJ Jr, Rose EF, Mahoney LT Surgical treatment of coarctation of the aorta after balloon angioplasty. J Thorac Cardiovasc Surg 1987;94:715.
34. Brewer LA 3rd, Fosburg RG, Mulder GA, Verska JJ. Spinal cord complications following surgery for coarctation of the aorta. J Thorac Cardiovasc Surg 1972;64:368.
35. Brom AG. Narrowing of the aortic isthmus and enlargement of the mind. J Thorac Cardiovasc Surg 1965;50:166.
36. Brouwer MH, Cromme-Dijkhuis AH, Ebels T, Eijgelaar A. Growth of the hypoplastic aortic arch after simple coarctation resection and end-to-end anastomosis. J Thorac Cardiovasc Surg 1992;104:426.
37. Brouwer MH, Kuntze CE, Ebels T, Talsma MD, Eijgelaar A. Repair of aortic coarctation in infants. J Thorac Cardiovasc Surg 1991;101:1093.
38. Brouwer RM, Cromme-Dijkhuis AH, Erasmus ME, Contant C, Bogers AJ, Elzenga NJ, et al. Decision making for the surgical management of aortic coarctation associated with ventricular septal defect. J Thorac Cardiovasc Surg 1996;111:168.
39. Brown JW, Ruzmetov M, Hoyer MH, Rodefeld MD, Turrentine MW. Recurrent coarctation: is surgical repair of recurrent coarctation of the aorta safe and effective? Ann Thorac Surg 2009;88:1923-31.
40. Brown JW, Ruzmetov M, Okada Y, Vijay P, Rodefeld MD, Turrentine MW. Outcomes in patients with interrupted aortic arch and associated anomalies: a 20-year experience. Eur J Cardiothorac Surg 2006;29:666-74.
41. Bruckheimer E, Dagan T, Amir G, Birk E. Covered Cheatham-platinum stents for serial dilation of severe native aortic coarctation. Catheter Cardiovasc Interv 2009;74:117-23.
42. Bulbul ZR, Bruckheimer E, Love JC, Fahey JT, Hellenbrand WE. Implantation of balloon-expandable stents for coarctation of the aorta: implantation data and short-term results. Cathet Cardiovasc Diagn 1996;39:36.
43. Bull C, Hoeksema T, Duckworth JA, Mustard WT. An experimental study of the growth of arterial anastomoses. Can J Surg 1963;6:383.
44. Burch PT, Cowley CG, Holubkov R, Null D, Lambert LM, Kouretas PC, et al. Coarctation repair in neonates and young infants: is small size or low weight still a risk factor? J Thorac Cardiovasc Surg 2009;138:547-52.

C

1. Calder AL, Kirker JA, Neutze JM, Starling MB. Pathology of the ductus arteriosus treated with prostaglandins: comparisons with untreated cases. Pediatr Cardiol 1984;5:85.
2. Campbell DB, Waldhausen JA, Pierce WS, Fripp R, Whitman V. Should elective repair of coarctation of the aorta be done in infancy? J Thorac Cardiovasc Surg 1984;88:929.
3. Campbell J, Delorenzi R, Brown J, Girod D, Hurwitz R, Caldwell R, et al. Improved results in newborns undergoing coarctation repair. Ann Thorac Surg 1980;30:273.
4. Campbell M. Natural history of coarctation of the aorta. Br Heart J 1970;32:633.
5. Carroll SJ, Ferris A, Chen J, Liberman L. Efficacy of prostaglandin E1 in relieving obstruction in coarctation of a persistent fifth aortic arch without opening the ductus arteriosus. Pediatr Cardiol 2006;27:766-8.
6. Castaneda-Zuniga WR, Lock JE, Vlodaver Z, Rusnak B, Rysavy JP, Herrera M, et al. Transluminal dilation of coarctation of the abdominal aorta: an experimental study in dogs. Radiology 1982;143:693.
7. Celano V, Pieroni DR, Morera JA, Roland JM, Gingell RL. Two-dimensional echocardiographic examination of mitral valve abnormalities associated with coarctation of the aorta. Circulation 1984;69:924.
8. Celoria GC, Patton RB. Congenital absence of the aortic arch. Am Heart J 1959;58:407.
9. Chang JH, Barrington JD. Coarctation of the aorta in infants and children. J Pediatr Surg 1972;7:127.
10. Chen SS, Donald AE, Storry C, Halcox JP, Bonhoeffer P, Deanfield JE. Impact of aortic stenting on peripheral vascular function and daytime systolic blood pressure in adult coarctation. Heart 2008;94:919-24.
11. Chernoff DM, Derugin N, Rajasinghe HA, Hanley FL, Higgins CB, Gooding CA. Measurement of collateral blood flow in a porcine model of aortic coarctation by velocity-encoded cine MRI. J Magn Reson Imaging 1997;7:557.
12. Christensen NA. Coarctation of the aorta: historical review. Mayo Clin Proc 1948;23:322.
13. Ciotti GR, Vlahos AP, Silverman NH. Morphology and function of the bicuspid aortic valve with and without coarctation of the aorta in the young. Am J Cardiol 2006;98:1096-102.
14. Clagett OT. The surgical treatment of coarctation of the aorta. Mayo Clin Proc 1948;23:359.
15. Clarkson PM, Nicholson MR, Barratt-Boyes BG, Neutze JM, Whitlock RM. Results after repair of coarctation of the aorta beyond infancy: a 10 to 28 year follow-up with particular reference to late systemic hypertension. Am J Cardiol 1983;51:1481.
16. Cobanoglu A, Teply JF, Grunkemeier GL, Sunderland CO, Starr A. Coarctation of the aorta in patients younger than three months. J Thorac Cardiovasc Surg 1985;89:128.
17. Cobanoglu A, Thyagarajan GK, Dobbs JL. Surgery for coarctation of the aorta in infants younger than 3 months: end-to-end repair versus subclavian flap angioplasty: is either operation better? Eur J Cardiothorac Surg 1998;14:19.
18. Collins-Nakai RL, Dick M, Parisi-Buckley L, Fyler DC, Castaneda AR. Interrupted aortic arch in infancy. J Pediatr 1976;88:959.
19. Colodney NM, Carson MJ. Coarctation of the aorta in early infancy. J Pediatr 1950;37:46.
20. Connolly HM, Schaff HV, Izhar U, Dearani JA, Warnes CA, Orszulak TA. Posterior pericardial ascending-to-descending aortic bypass: an alternative surgical approach for complex coarctation of the aorta. Circulation 2001;104:I133-7.
21. Connor TM, Baker WP. A comparison of coarctation resection and patch angioplasty using postexercise blood pressure measurements. Circulation 1981;64:567.
22. Cook SC, Ferketich AK, Raman SV. Myocardial ischemia in asymptomatic adults with repaired aortic coarctation. Int J Cardiol 2009;133:95-101.
23. Cooper RS, Ritter SB, Golinko RJ. Balloon dilatation angioplasty: nonsurgical management of coarctation of the aorta. Circulation 1984;70:903.
24. Crafoord C, Nylin G. Congenital coarctation of the aorta and its surgical treatment. J Thorac Surg 1945;14:347.

D

1. DeBoer A, Grana L, Potts WJ, Lev M. Coarctation of the aorta. Arch Surg 1961;82:801.
2. Decaluwe W, Delhaas T, Gewillig M. Aortic atresia, interrupted aortic arch type C perfused by bilateral arterial duct. Eur Heart J 2005;26:2333.
3. De Caro E, Spadoni I, Crepaz R, Saitta M, Trocchio G, Calevo MG, et al. Stenting of aortic coarctation and exercise-induced hypertension in the young. Catheter Cardiovasc Interv 2010;75:256-61.
4. DeLeon MM, DeLeon SY, Quinones JA, Roughneen PT, Magliato KE, Vitullo DA, et al. Management of arch hypoplasia after successful coarctation repair. Ann Thorac Surg 1997;63:975.
5. DeLeon SY, Idriss FS, Ilbawi MN, Tin N, Berry T. Transmediastinal repair of complex coarctation and interrupted aortic arch. J Thorac Cardiovasc Surg 1981;82:98.

6. DiBardino DJ, Heinle JS, Kung GC, Leonard GT Jr, McKenzie ED, Su JT, et al. Anatomic reconstruction for recurrent aortic obstruction in infants and children. Ann Thorac Surg 2004;78: 926-32.
7. Dietl CA, Torres AR, Favaloro RG, Fessler CL, Grunkemeier GL. Risk of recoarctation in neonates and infants after repair with patch aortoplasty, subclavian flap, and the combined resection–flap procedure. J Thorac Cardiovasc Surg 1992;103:724.
8. Digilio MC, Marino B, Picchio F, Prandstraller D, Toscano A, Giannotti A, et al. Noonan syndrome and aortic coarctation. Am J Med Genet 1998;80:160.
9. Dische MR, Tsai M, Baltaxe HA. Solitary interruption of the arch of the aorta. Am J Cardiol 1975;35:271.
10. Downing DF, Grotzinger PJ, Weller RW. Coarctation of the aorta. The syndrome of necrotizing arteritis of the small intestine following surgical therapy. Am J Dis Child 1958;96:711.
11. Duara R, Theodore S, Sarma PS, Unnikrishnan M, Neelakandhan KS. Correction of coarctation of aorta in adult patients—impact of corrective procedure on long-term recoarctation and systolic hypertension. Thorac Cardiovasc Surg 2008;56:83-6.
12. Duke C, Qureshi SA. Aortic coarctation and recoarctation: to stent or not to stent? J Interv Cardiol 2001;14:283-98.

E

1. Ebeid MR, Prieto LR, Latson LA. Use of balloon-expandable stents for coarctation of the aorta: initial results and intermediate-term follow-up. J Am Coll Cardiol 1997;30:1847.
2. Edie RN, Janani J, Attai LA, Malm JR, Robinson G. Bypass grafts for recurrent or complex coarctations of the aorta. Ann Thorac Surg 1975;20:558.
3. Edwards JE, Christensen NA, Clagett OT, McDonald JR. Pathologic considerations in coarctation of the aorta. Mayo Clin Proc 1948;23:324.
4. Edwards JE, Clagett OT, Drake RL, Christensen NA. The collateral circulation in coarctation of the aorta. Mayo Clin Proc 1948; 23:333.
5. Elgamal MA, McKenzie ED, Fraser CD Jr. Aortic arch advancement: the optimal one-stage approach for surgical management of neonatal coarctation with arch hypoplasia. Ann Thorac Surg 2002;73:1267-73.
6. Elliott RB, Starling MB, Neutze JM. Medical management of the ductus arteriosus. Lancet 1975;1:140.
7. Elzenga NJ, Gittenbergerde Groot AC, Oppenheimer-Dekker A. Coarctation and other obstructive aortic arch anomalies: their relationship to the ductus arteriosus. Int J Cardiol 1986;13:289.
8. Erez E, Tam VK, Kanter KR, Fyfe DA. Successful biventricular repair after initial Norwood operation for interrupted aortic arch with severe left ventricular outflow tract obstruction. Ann Thorac Surg 2001;71:1974-7.
9. Eshaghpour E, Olley PM. Recoarctation of the aorta following coarctectomy in the first year of life: a follow-up study. J Pediatr 1972;80:809.
10. Ewert P, Peters B, Nagdyman N, Miera O, Kuhne T, Berger F. Early and mid-term results with the Growth Stent—a possible concept for transcatheter treatment of aortic coarctation from infancy to adulthood by stent implantation? Catheter Cardiovasc Interv 2008;71:120-6.

F

1. Farouk A, Karimi M, Henderson M, Ostrowsky J, Siwik E, Hennein H. Cerebral regional oxygenation during aortic coarctation repair in pediatric population. Eur J Cardiothorac Surg 2008;34:26-31.
2. Fiore AC, Fischer LK, Schwartz T, Jureidini S, Balfour I, Carpenter D, et al. Comparison of angioplasty and surgery for neonatal aortic coarctation. Ann Thorac Surg 2005;80:1659-65.
3. Fiore AC, Ruzmetov M, Johnson RG, Rodefeld MD, Rieger K, Turrentine MW, et al. Selective use of left heart bypass for aortic coarctation. Ann Thorac Surg 2010;89:851-7.
4. Fishman NH, Bronstein MH, Berman W Jr, Roe BB, Edmunds LH Jr, Robinson SJ, et al. Surgical management of severe aortic coarctation and interrupted aortic arch in neonates. J Thorac Cardiovasc Surg 1976;71:35.
5. Fleming WH, Sarafian LB, Clarke ED, Dooley KJ, Hofshire PJ, Hopeman AR, et al. Critical aortic coarctation: patch aortoplasty in infants less than age 3 months. Am J Cardiol 1979;44:687.
6. Flint JD, Gentles TL, MacCormick J, Spinetto H, Finucane AK. Outcomes using predominantly single-stage approach to interrupted aortic arch and associated defects. Ann Thorac Surg 2010;89:564-9.
7. Forbes TJ, Garekar S, Amin Z, Zahn EM, Nykanen D, Moore P, et al. Procedural results and acute complications in stenting native and recurrent coarctation of the aorta in patients over 4 years of age: a multi-institutional study. Catheter Cardiovasc Interv 2007;70:276-85.
8. Forbes TJ, Moore P, Pedra CA, Zahn EM, Nykanen D, Amin Z, et al. Intermediate follow-up following intravascular stenting for treatment of coarctation of the aorta. Catheter Cardiovasc Interv 2007;70:569-77.
9. Foster JH, Collins HA, Jacobs JK, Scott HW. Long term follow-up of homografts used in the treatment of coarctation of the aorta. J Cardiovasc Surg 1965;19:111.
10. Freed MD, Heymann MA, Lewis AB, Roehl SL, Kensey RC. Prostaglandin E_1 in infants with ductus arteriosus-dependent congenital heart disease. Circulation 1981;64:899.
11. Freed MD, Keane JF, Van Praagh R, Castaneda AR, Bernhard WF, Nadas AS. Coarctation of the aorta with congenital mitral regurgitation. Circulation 1974;49:1175.
12. Freed MD, Rocchini A, Rosenthal A, Nadas AS, Castaneda AR. Exercise-induced hypertension after surgical repair of coarctation of the aorta. Am J Cardiol 1979;43:253.
13. Freedom RM, Bain HH, Esplugas E, Dische R, Rowe RD. Ventricular septal defect in interruption of aortic arch. Am J Cardiol 1977;39:572.
14. Freedom RM, Rosen FS, Nadas AS. Congenital cardiovascular disease and anomalies of the third and fourth pharyngeal pouch. Circulation 1972;46:165.
15. Freundlich E, Engle MA, Goldberg HP. Coarctation of aorta in infancy. Analysis of 10-year experience with medical management. Pediatrics 1961;27:427.
16. Fripp RR, Whitman V, Werner JC, Nicholas GG, Waldhausen JA. Blood pressure response to exercise in children following the subclavian flap procedure for coarctation of the aorta. J Thorac Cardiovasc Surg 1983;85:682.
17. Fujii I, Ueno Y, Kurano R, Goto Y. Interrupted aortic arch type C associated with DiGeorge syndrome in 22q11.2 deletion: first case detected in Japan. Pediatr Int 2005;47:698-700.
18. Fulton JO, Mas C, Brizard CP, Cochrane AD, Karl TR. Does left ventricular outflow tract obstruction influence outcome of interrupted aortic arch repair? Ann Thorac Surg 1999;67:177.

G

1. Gaynor JW, Wernovsky G, Rychik J, Rome JJ, DeCampli WM, Spray TL. Outcome following single-stage repair of coarctation with ventricular septal defect. Eur J Cardiothorac Surg 2000;18:62.
2. Gidding SS, Rocchini AP, Moorehead C, Schork MA, Rosenthal A. Increased forearm vascular reactivity in patients with hypertension after repair of coarctation. Circulation 1985;71:495.
3. Giordano U, Giannico S, Turchetta A, Hammad F, Calzolari F, Calzolari A. The influence of different surgical procedures on hypertension after repair of coarctation. Cardiol Young 2005;15: 477-80.
4. Glancy DL, Roberts WC. Not congenital atresia of the aortic isthmus, but acquired complete occlusion in congenital aortic coarctation. Catheter Cardiovasc Interv 2002;56:103-4; author reply 05.
5. Goldberg SJ, Gerlis LM, Ho SY, Penilla MB. Location to the left papillary muscles in juxtaductal aortic coarctation. Am J Cardiol 1995;75:746.
6. Goldmuntz E. DiGeorge syndrome: new insights. Clin Perinatol 2005;32:963-78.
7. Goodall MC, Sealey WC. Increased sympathetic nerve activity following resection of coarctation of the thoracic aorta. Circulation 1969;39:345.
8. Graham TP Jr, Atwood GF, Boerth RC, Boucek RJ Jr, Smith CW. Right and left heart size and function in infants with symptomatic coarctation. Circulation 1977;56:641.
9. Graham TP Jr, Lewis BW, Jarmakani JM, Canent RV Jr, Capp MP. Left heart volume and mass quantification in children with left ventricular pressure overload. Circulation 1970;41:203.
10. Greenberg SB, Marks LA, Eshaghpour EE. Evaluation of magnetic resonance imaging in coarctation of the aorta: the importance of multiple imaging planes. Pediatr Cardiol 1997;18:345.
11. Gross RE. Surgical correction for coarctation of the aorta. Surgery 1945;18:673.

12. Gross RE. Treatment of certain aortic coarctations by homologous grafts. Ann Surg 1951;134:753.
13. Gross RE, Hufnagel CA. Coarctation of the aorta. Experimental studies regarding its surgical correction. N Engl J Med 1945; 233:287.
14. Groves LK, Effler DB. Problems in the surgical management of coarctation of the aorta. J Thorac Cardiovasc Surg 1960; 39:60.
15. Gruber PJ, Fuller S, Cleaver KM, Abdullah I, Gruber SB, Nicolson SC, et al. Early results of single-stage biventricular repair of severe aortic hypoplasia or atresia with ventricular septal defect and normal left ventricle. J Thorac Cardiovasc Surg 2006;132:260-3.
16. Gupta TC, Wiggens CJ. Basic hemodynamic changes produced by aortic coarctation of different degrees. Circulation 1951;3:17.

H

1. Haas F, Goldberg CS, Ohye RG, Mosca RS, Bove EL. Primary repair of aortic arch obstruction with ventricular septal defect in preterm and low birth weight infants. Eur J Cardiothorac Surg 2000;17:643.
2. Hager A, Kanz S, Kaemmerer H, Hess J. Exercise capacity and exercise hypertension after surgical repair of isolated aortic coarctation. Am J Cardiol 2008;101:1777-80.
3. Hager A, Kanz S, Kaemmerer H, Schreiber C, Hess J. Coarctation Long-term Assessment (COALA): significance of arterial hypertension in a cohort of 404 patients up to 27 years after surgical repair of isolated coarctation of the aorta, even in the absence of restenosis and prosthetic material. J Thorac Cardiovasc Surg 2007;134:738-45.
4. Hager A, Schreiber C, Nutzl S, Hess J. Mortality and restenosis rate of surgical coarctation repair in infancy: a study of 191 patients. Cardiology 2009;112:36-41.
5. Haji-Zeinali AM, Ghazi P, Alidoosti M. Self-expanding nitinol stent implantation for treatment of aortic coarctation. J Endovasc Ther 2009;16:224-32.
6. Hakimi M, Clapp SK, Walters HL 3rd, Lyons JM, Morrow WR. Arch growth after staged repair of interrupted aortic arch using carotid artery interposition. Ann Thorac Surg 1997;64:503.
7. Hallman GL, Yashar JJ, Bloodwell RD, Cooley DA. Surgical correction of coarctation of the aorta in the first year of life. Ann Thorac Surg 1967;4:106.
8. Hamilton DI, Di Eusanio G, Sandrasagra FA, Donnelly RJ. Early and late results of aortoplasty with a left subclavian flap for coarctation of the aorta in infancy. J Thorac Cardiovasc Surg 1978;75:699.
9. Hamilton DI, Medici D, Oyonarte M, Dickinson DF. Aortoplasty with the left subclavian flap in older children. J Thorac Cardiovasc Surg 1981;82:103.
10. Hanley FL. The various therapeutic approaches to aortic coarctation: is it fair to compare? J Am Coll Cardiol 1996;27:471.
11. Hanson E, Eriksson BO, Sorensen SE. Intra-arterial blood pressures at rest and during exercise after surgery for coarctation of the aorta. Eur J Cardiol 1980;11:245.
12. Harlan JL, Doty DB, Brandt B 3rd, Ehrenhaft JL. Coarctation of the aorta in infants. J Thorac Cardiovasc Surg 1984;88:1012.
13. Hart JC, Waldhausen JA. Reversed subclavian flap angioplasty for arch coarctation of the aorta. Ann Thorac Surg 1983;36:715.
14. Hartmann AF Jr, Goldring D, Hernandez A, Behrer MR, Schad N, Ferguson T, et al. Recurrent coarctation of the aorta after successful repair in infancy. Am J Cardiol 1970;25:405.
15. Hashemzadeh K, Hashemzadeh S, Kakaei F. Repair of aortic coarctation in adults: the fate of hypertension. Asian Cardiovasc Thorac Ann 2008;16:11-5.
16. Heinemann MK, Ziemer G, Wahlers T, Kohler A, Borst HG. Extraanatomic thoracic aortic bypass grafts: indications, techniques, and results. Eur J Cardiothorac Surg 1997;11:169.
17. Hesslein PS, McNamara DG, Morriss MJ, Hallman GL, Cooley DA. Comparison of resection versus patch aortoplasty for repair of coarctation in infants and children. Circulation 1981; 64:164.
18. Heymann MA, Berman W Jr, Rudolph AM, Whitman V. Dilation of the ductus arteriosus by prostaglandin E_1 in aortic arch abnormalities. Circulation 1979;59:169.
19. Higgins CB, French JW, Silverman JF, Wexler L. Interruption of the aortic arch: preoperative and postoperative clinical, hemodynamic and angiographic features. Am J Cardiol 1977;39:563.
20. Hirooka K, Fraser CD Jr. One-stage neonatal repair of complex aortic arch obstruction or interruption. Recent experience at Texas Children's Hospital. Tex Heart Inst J 1997;24:317.
21. Hjortdal VE, Khambadkone S, de Leval MR, Tsang VT. Implications of anomalous right subclavian artery in the repair of neonatal aortic coarctation. Ann Thorac Surg 2003;76:572-5.
22. Ho EC, Moss AJ. The syndrome of "mesenteric arteritis" following surgical repair of aortic coarctation. Pediatrics 1972;49:40.
23. Ho SY, Anderson RH. Coarctation, tubular hypoplasia and the ductus arteriosus. Histological study of 35 specimens. Br Heart J 1979;41:268.
24. Ho SY, Wilcox BR, Anderson RH, Lincoln JC. Interrupted aortic arch–anatomical features of surgical significance. Thorac Cardiovasc Surg 1983;31:199.
25. Honey M, Lincoln JC, Osborne MP, de Bono DP. Coarctation of aorta with right aortic arch. Report of surgical correction in 2 cases: one with associated anomalous origin of left circumflex coronary artery from the right pulmonary artery. Br Heart J 1975;37:937.
26. Hovaguimian H, Senthilnathan V, Iguidbashian JP, McIrvin DM, Starr A. Coarctation repair: modification of end-to-end anastomosis with subclavian flap angioplasty. Ann Thorac Surg 1998;65:1751.
27. Hutchins GM. Coarctation of the aorta explained as a branch-point of the ductus arteriosus. Am J Pathol 1971;63:203.

I

1. Ibarra-Perez C, Castaneda AR, Varco RL, Lillehei CW. Recoarctation of the aorta. Nineteen year clinical experience. Am J Cardiol 1969;23:778.
2. Immagoulou A, Anderson RC, Moller JH. Interruption of the aortic arch. Circulation 1962;26:39.
3. Ishino K, Kawada M, Irie H, Kino K, Sano S. Single-stage repair of aortic coarctation with ventricular septal defect using isolated cerebral and myocardial perfusion. Eur J Cardiothorac Surg 2000;17:538.
4. Izhar U, Schaff HV, Mullany CJ, Daly RC, Orszulak TA. Posterior pericardial approach for ascending aorta-to-descending aorta bypass through a median sternotomy. Ann Thorac Surg 2000;70:31.

J

1. Jacob T, Cobanoglu A, Starr A. Late results of ascending aorta-descending aorta bypass grafts for recurrent coarctation of aorta. J Thorac Cardiovasc Surg 1988;95:782.
2. Jahangiri M, Shinebourne EA, Zurakowski D, Rigby ML, Redington AN, Lincoln C. Subclavian flap angioplasty: does the arch look after itself? J Thorac Cardiovasc Surg 2000;120:224.
3. Jaszewski R, Bartczak K. Surgical treatment of aortic coarctation in adults: still open question? Cardiol J 2008;15:491-2.
4. Jegatheeswaran A, McCrindle BW, Blackstone EH, Jacobs ML, Lofland GK, Austin EH 3rd, et al. Persistent risk of subsequent procedures and mortality in patients after interrupted aortic arch repair: a Congenital Heart Surgeons Society study. J Thorac Cardiovasc Surg 2010;140:1059-75.
5. Jenkins NP, Ward C. Coarctation of the aorta: natural history and outcome after surgical treatment. QJM 1999;92:365-71.
6. Jentsch E, Liersch R, Bourgeois M. Prolapsed valve of the foramen ovale in newborns and infants with coarctation of the aorta. Pediatr Cardiol 1988;9:29.
7. Johnson J, Kirby CK. The relationship of the method of suture to the growth of end-to-end arterial anastomosis. Surgery 1950;27:17.
8. Jonas RA, Quaegebeur JM, Kirklin JW, Blackstone EH, Daicoff G. Outcomes in patients with interrupted aortic arch and ventricular septal defect. A multiinstitutional study. Congenital Heart Surgeons Society. J Thorac Cardiovasc Surg 1994;107:1099.
9. Joynt CA, Robertson CM, Cheung PY, Nettel-Aguirre A, Joffe AR, Sauve RS, et al. Two-year neurodevelopmental outcomes of infants undergoing neonatal cardiac surgery for interrupted aortic arch: a descriptive analysis. J Thorac Cardiovasc Surg 2009;138:924-32.

K

1. Kadner A, Dave H, Bettex D, Valsangiacomo-Buechel E, Turina MI, Pretre R. Anatomic reconstruction of recurrent aortic arch obstruction in children. Eur J Cardiothorac Surg 2004;26:60-5.
2. Kan JS, White RI Jr, Mitchell SE, Farmlett EJ, Donahoo JS, Gardner TJ. Treatment of restenosis of coarctation by percutaneous transluminal angioplasty. Circulation 1983;68:1087.

3. Kanter KR, Mahle WT, Kogon BE, Kirshbom PM. What is the optimal management of infants with coarctation and ventricular septal defect? Ann Thorac Surg 2007;84:612-8.
4. Kanter KR, Vincent RN, Fyfe DA. Reverse subclavian flap repair of hypoplastic transverse aorta in infancy. Ann Thorac Surg 2001; 71:1530.
5. Karamlou T, Bernasconi A, Jaeggi E, Alhabshan F, Williams WG, Van Arsdell GS, et al. Factors associated with arch reintervention and growth of the aortic arch after coarctation repair in neonates weighing less than 2.5 kg. J Thorac Cardiovasc Surg 2009; 137:1163-7.
6. Karl TR, Sano S, Brawn W, Mee RB. Repair of hypoplastic or interrupted aortic arch via sternotomy. J Thorac Cardiovasc Surg 1992;104:688.
7. Kaulitz R, Jonas R, van der Velde ME. Echocardiographic assessment of interrupted aortic arch. Cardiol Young 1999;9: 562.
8. Kaushal S, Backer CL, Patel JN, Patel SK, Walker BL, Weigel TJ, et al. Coarctation of the aorta: midterm outcomes of resection with extended end-to-end anastomosis. Ann Thorac Surg 2009; 88:1932-8.
9. Keith JD, Rowe RD, Vlad P. Heart disease in infancy and childhood. New York: Macmillan, 1978, p. 738.
10. Kennedy A, Taylor DG, Durrant TE. Pathology of the intima in coarctation of the aorta: a study using light and scanning electron microscopy. Thorax 1979;34:366.
11. Khoury GH, Hawes CR. Recurrent coarctation of the aorta in infancy and childhood. J Pediatr 1968;72:801.
12. Kirklin JW, Burchell HB, Pugh DG, Burke EC, Mills SD. Surgical treatment of coarctation of the aorta in a ten-week-old infant. Report of a case. Circulation 1952;6:411.
13. Kirsh MM, Perry B, Spooner E. Management of pseudoaneurysm following patch grafting for coarctation of the aorta. J Thorac Cardiovasc Surg 1977;74:636.
14. Knyshov GV, Sitar LL, Glagola MD, Atamanyuk MY. Aortic aneurysms at the site of the repair of coarctation of the aorta: a review of 48 patients. Ann Thorac Surg 1996;61:935.
15. Koerselman J, de Vries H, Jaarsma W, Muyldermans L, Ernst JM, Plokker HW. Balloon angioplasty of coarctation of the aorta: a safe alternative for surgery in adults: immediate and midterm results. Catheter Cardiovasc Interv 2000;50:28.
16. Konstantinov IE, Karamlou T, Williams WG, Quaegebeur JM, del Nido PJ, Spray TL, et al. Surgical management of aortopulmonary window associated with interrupted aortic arch: a Congenital Heart Surgeons Society study. J Thorac Cardiovasc Surg 2006; 131:1136-41 e2.
17. Konstantinov IE, Oka N, d'Udekem Y, Brizard CP. Surgical repair of aortopulmonary window associated with interrupted aortic arch: long-term outcomes. J Thorac Cardiovasc Surg 2010;140:483-4.
18. Kostelka M, Walther T, Geerdts I, Rastan A, Jacobs S, Dahnert I, et al. Primary repair for aortic arch obstruction associated with ventricular septal defect. Ann Thorac Surg 2004;78:1989-93.
19. Kotani Y, Ishino K, Kasahara S, Yoshizumi K, Honjo O, Kawada M, et al. Continuous cerebral and myocardial perfusion during aortic arch repair in neonates and infants. ASAIO J 2006;52: 536-8.
20. Krauser DG, Rutkowski M, Phoon CK. Left ventricular volume after correction of isolated aortic coarctation in neonates. Am J Cardiol 2000;85:904.
21. Krieger KH, Spencer FC. Is paraplegia after repair of coarctation of the aorta due principally to distal hypotension during aortic cross-clamping? Surgery 1985;97:2.
22. Kuhn A, Vogt M. Ascending aortic distensibility is impaired before and after surgical "repair" of coarctation. Ann Thorac Surg 2006;81:2341; author reply 41-2.
23. Kuroczynski W, Hartert M, Pruefer D, Pitzer-Hartert K, Heinemann M, Vahl CF. Surgical treatment of aortic coarctation in adults: beneficial effect on arterial hypertension. Cardiol J 2008;15:537-42.
24. Kutsche LM, Van Mierop LH. Cervical origin of the right subclavian artery in aortic arch interruption: pathogenesis and significance. Am J Cardiol 1984;53:892.

L

1. Lababidi Z, Wu JR. Percutaneous balloon pulmonary valvuloplasty. Am J Cardiol 1983;52:560.
2. Lacour-Gayet F, Bruniaux J, Serraf A, Chambran P, Blaysat G, Losay J, et al. Hypoplastic transverse arch and coarctation in neonates. Surgical reconstruction of the aortic arch. A study of 66 patients. J Thorac Cardiovasc Surg 1990;100:808.
3. Lacour-Gayet F, Serraf A, Galletti L, Bruniaux J, Belli E, Piot D, et al. Biventricular repair of conotruncal anomalies associated with aortic arch obstruction: 103 patients. Circulation 1997;96:II328.
4. Lam YY, Kaya MG, Li W, Mahadevan VS, Khan AA, Henein MY, et al. Effect of endovascular stenting of aortic coarctation on biventricular function in adults. Heart 2007;93:1441-7.
5. Lang HT Jr, Nadas AS. Coarctation of the aorta with congestive heart failure in infancy–medical treatment. Pediatrics 1956;17:45.
6. Lange R, Thielmann M, Schmidt KG, Bauernschmitt R, Jakob H, Hasper B, et al. Spinal cord protection using hypothermic cardiocirculatory arrest in extended repair of recoarctation and persistent hypoplastic aortic arch. Eur J Cardiothorac Surg 1997;11:697.
7. Levine JC, Sanders SP, Colan SD, Jonas RA, Spevak PJ. The risk of having additional obstructive lesions in neonatal coarctation of the aorta. Cardiol Young 2001;11:44.
8. Lew EA. High blood pressure, other risk factors and longevity: the insurance viewpoint. Am J Med 1973;55:281.
9. Lewin MB, Lindsay EA, Jurecic V, Goytia V, Towbin JA, Baldini A. A genetic etiology for interruption of the aortic arch type B. Am J Cardiol 1997;80:493.
10. Liberman L, Gersony WM, Flynn PA, Lamberti JJ, Cooper RS, Stare TJ. Effectiveness of prostaglandin E1 in relieving obstruction in coarctation of the aorta without opening the ductus arteriosus. Pediatr Cardiol 2004;25:49-52.
11. Liberthson RR, Pennington DG, Jacobs MC, Daggett WM. Coarctation of the aorta: review of 234 patients and clarification of management problems. Am J Cardiol 1979;43:835.
12. Lim HG, Kim WH, Jang WS, Lim C, Kwak JG, Lee C, et al. One-stage total repair of aortic arch anomaly using regional perfusion. Eur J Cardiothorac Surg 2007;31:242-8.
13. Litwin SB, Van Praagh R, Bernhard WF. A palliative operation for certain infants with aortic arch interruption. Ann Thorac Surg 1972;14:369.
14. Lobert PH, Lillehei CW. Necrotizing panarteritis following repair of coarctation. Surgery 1954;35:950.
15. Lock JE. Now that we can dilate, should we? Am J Cardiol 1984;54:1360.
16. Lock JE, Bass JL, Amplatz K, Fuhrman BP, Castaneda-Zuniga W. Balloon dilation angioplasty of aortic coarctations in infants and children. Circulation 1983;68:109.
17. Lock JE, Castaneda-Zuniga WR, Bass JL, Foker JE, Amplatz K, Anderson RW. Balloon dilatation of excised aortic coarctations. Radiology 1982;143:689.
18. Lock JE, Niemi T, Burke BA, Einzig S, Castaneda-Zuniga WR. Transcutaneous angioplasty of experimental aortic coarctation. Circulation 1982;66:1280.
19. Loffredo CA, Ferencz C, Wilson PD, Lurie IW. Interrupted aortic arch: an epidemiologic study. Teratology 2000;61:368.
20. Lucas V. Stent treatment of neonatal coarctation: another option for critically ill or extremely small patients with unoperated coarctation or failed surgery. Catheter Cardiovasc Interv 2010;75:562.
21. Lynxwiler CP, Smith S, Babich J. Coarctation of the aorta: report of a case. Arch Pediatr 1951;68:203.

M

1. Magee AG, Brzezinska-Rajszys G, Qureshi SA, Rosenthal E, Zubrzycka M, Ksiazyk J, et al. Stent implantation for aortic coarctation and recoarctation. Heart 1999;82:600.
2. Mahadevan V, Mullen MJ. Endovascular management of aortic coarctation. Int J Cardiol 2004;97(Suppl 1):75-8.
3. Mainwaring RD, Lamberti JJ. Mid-to long-term results of the two-stage approach for type B interrupted aortic arch and ventricular septal defect. Ann Thorac Surg 1997;64:1782.
4. Malec E, Kolcz J, Mroczek T, Zaj c A, Paj k J. Primary reconstruction of interrupted aortic arch—surgical management and results. Scand Cardiovasc J 2000;34:507-10.
5. Malhotra SP, Hanley FL. Routine continuous perfusion for aortic arch reconstruction in the neonate. Semin Thorac Cardiovasc Surg Pediatr Card Surg Annu 2008:57-60.
6. Malm JR, Blumenthal S, Jameson AG, Humphreys GH. Observations on coarctation of the aorta in infants. Arch Surg 1963;86:96.

7. Mann C, Goebel G, Eicken A, Genz T, Sebening W, Kaemmerer H, et al. Balloon dilation for aortic recoarctation: morphology at the site of dilation and long-term efficacy. Cardiol Young 2001;11:30.
8. Marcheix B, Lamarche Y, Perrault P, Cartier R, Bouchard D, Carrier M, et al. Endovascular management of pseudo-aneurysms after previous surgical repair of congenital aortic coarctation. Eur J Cardiothorac Surg 2007;31:1004-7.
9. Marino B, Digilio MC, Persiani M, Di Donato R, Toscano A, Giannotti A, et al. Deletion 22q11 in patients with interrupted aortic arch. Am J Cardiol 1999;84:360.
10. Markham LW, Knecht SK, Daniels SR, Mays WA, Khoury PR, Knilans TK. Development of exercise-induced arm-leg blood pressure gradient and abnormal arterial compliance in patients with repaired coarctation of the aorta. Am J Cardiol 2004;94:1200-2.
11. Maron BJ, Humphries JO, Rowe RD, Mellits ED. Prognosis of surgically corrected coarctation of the aorta: a 20-year postoperative appraisal. Circulation 1973;47:119.
12. Marshall AC, Perry SB, Keane JF, Lock JE. Early results and medium-term follow-up of stent implantation for mild residual or recurrent aortic coarctation. Am Heart J 2000;139:1054.
13. Martin MM, Beekman RH, Rocchini AP, Crowley DC, Rosenthal A. Aortic aneurysms after subclavian angioplasty repair of coarctation of the aorta. Am J Cardiol 1988;61:951.
14. Mathew R, Simon G, Joseph M. Collateral circulation in coarctation of aorta in infancy and childhood. Arch Dis Child 1972;47:950.
15. Matsui H, Mellander M, Roughton M, Jicinska H, Gardiner HM. Morphological and physiological predictors of fetal aortic coarctation. Circulation 2008;118:1793-801.
16. Maxey TS, Serfontein SJ, Reece TB, Rheuban KS, Kron IL. Transverse arch hypoplasia may predispose patients to aneurysm formation after patch repair of aortic coarctation. Ann Thorac Surg 2003;76:1090-3.
17. McCrindle BW, Jones TK, Morrow WR, Hagler DJ, Lloyd TR, Nouri S, et al. Acute results of balloon angioplasty of native coarctation versus recurrent aortic obstruction are equivalent. Valvuloplasty and Angioplasty of Congenital Anomalies (VACA) Registry Investigators. J Am Coll Cardiol 1996;28:1810.
18. McCrindle BW, Tchervenkov CI, Konstantinov IE, Williams WG, Neirotti RA, Jacobs ML, et al. Risk factors associated with mortality and interventions in 472 neonates with interrupted aortic arch: a Congenital Heart Surgeons Society study. J Thorac Cardiovasc Surg 2005;129:343-50.
19. McElhinney DB, Reddy VM, Silverman NH, Hanley FL. Modified Damus-Kaye-Stansel procedure for single ventricle, subaortic stenosis, and arch obstruction in neonates and infants: midterm results and techniques for avoiding circulatory arrest. J Thorac Cardiovasc Surg 1997;114:718.
20. McElhinney DB, Yang SG, Hogarty AN, Rychik J, Gleason MM, Zachary CH, et al. Recurrent arch obstruction after repair of isolated coarctation of the aorta in neonates and young infants: is low weight a risk factor? J Thorac Cardiovasc Surg 2001;122:883-90.
21. McKellar SH, Schaff HV, Dearani JA, Daly RC, Mullany CJ, Orszulak TA, et al. Intermediate-term results of ascending–descending posterior pericardial bypass of complex aortic coarctation. J Thorac Cardiovasc Surg 2007;133:1504-9.
22. Merrill DL, Webster CA, Samson PC. Congenital absence of the aortic isthmus. J Thorac Surg 1957;33:311.
23. Merrill WH, Hoff SJ, Stewart JR, Elkins CC, Graham TP Jr, Bender HW Jr. Operative risk factors and durability of repair of coarctation of the aorta in the neonate. Ann Thorac Surg 1994; 58:399.
24. Messmer BJ, Minale C, Muhler E, von Bernuth G. Surgical correction of coarctation in early infancy: does surgical technique influence the result? Ann Thorac Surg 1991;52:594.
25. Metzdorff MT, Cobanoglu A, Grunkemeier GL, Sunderland CO, Starr A. Influence of age at operation on late results with subclavian flap aortoplasty. J Thorac Cardiovasc Surg 1985;89:235.
26. Meyer AA, Joharchi MS, Kundt G, Schuff-Werner P, Steinhoff G, Kienast W. Predicting the risk of early atherosclerotic disease development in children after repair of aortic coarctation. Eur Heart J 2005;26:617-22.
27. Momma K, Kondo C, Matsuoka R, Takao A. Cardiac anomalies associated with a chromosome 22q11 deletion in patients with conotruncal anomaly face syndrome. Am J Cardiol 1996;78:591.
28. Monro JL, Delany DJ, Ogilvie BC, Salmon AP, Keeton BR. Growth potential in the new aortic arch after non-end-to-end repair of aortic arch interruption in infancy. Ann Thorac Surg 1996; 61:1212.
29. Morales DL, Scully PT, Braud BE, Booth JH, Graves DE, Heinle JS, et al. Interrupted aortic arch repair: aortic arch advancement without a patch minimizes arch reinterventions. Ann Thorac Surg 2006;82:1577-84.
30. Morita S, Kuboyama I, Asou T, Tokunaga K, Nose Y, Nakamura M, et al. The effect of extraanatomic bypass on aortic input impedance studied in open chest dogs: should the vascular prosthesis be compliant to unload the left ventricle? J Thorac Cardiovasc Surg 1991;102:774.
31. Morris GC Jr, Cooley DA, DeBakey ME, Crawford ES. Coarctation of the aorta with particular emphasis upon improved techniques of surgical repair. J Thorac Cardiovasc Surg 1960;40:705.
32. Morrow WR, Huhta JC, Murphy DJ Jr, McNamara DG. Quantitative morphology of the aortic arch in neonatal coarctation. J Am Coll Cardiol 1986;8:616.
33. Moskowitz WB, Schieken RM, Mosteller M, Bossano R. Altered systolic and diastolic function in children after "successful" repair of coarctation of the aorta. Am Heart J 1990;120:103.
34. Moulton AL, Brenner JI, Roberts G, Tavares S, Ali S, Nordenbert A, et al. Subclavian flap repair of coarctation of the aorta in neonates. Realization of growth potential. J Thorac Cardiovasc Surg 1984;87:220.
35. Mulder DG, Linde LM. Recurrent coarctation of the aorta in infancy. Am Surg 1959;25:908.
36. Murphy DA, Lemire GG, Tessler I, Dunn GL. Correction of type B aortic arch interruption with ventricular and atrial septal defects in a three-day-old infant. J Thorac Cardiovasc Surg 1973;65:882.
37. Mustard WT, Rower RD, Keith JD, Sirek A. Coarctation of the aorta with special reference to the first year of life. Ann Surg 1955;141:249.
38. Musto C, Cifarelli A, Pucci E, Paladini S, De Felice F, Fiorilli R, et al. Endovascular treatment of aortic coarctation: long-term effects on hypertension. Int J Cardiol 2008;130:420-5.

N

1. Nanton MA, Olley PM. Residual hypertension after coarctectomy in children. Am J Cardiol 1976;37:769.
2. Nasser WK, Helmen C. Kinking of the aortic arch (pseudocoarctation). Ann Intern Med 1966;64:971.
3. Nathan M, Rimmer D, del Nido PJ, Mayer JE, Bacha EA, Shin A, et al. Aortic atresia or severe left ventricular outflow tract obstruction with ventricular septal defect: results of primary biventricular repair in neonates. Ann Thorac Surg 2006;82:2227-32.
4. Neutze JM, Starling MB, Elliott RB, Barratt-Boyes BG. Palliation of cyanotic congenital heart disease in infancy with E-type prostaglandins. Circulation 1977;55:238.
5. Norton JB Jr, Ullyot DJ, Stewart ET, Rudolph AM, Edmunds LH Jr. Aortic arch atresia with transposition of the great vessels: physiologic considerations and surgical management. Surgery 1970; 67:1011.

O

1. Oliver JM, Alonso-Gonzalez R, Gonzalez AE, Gallego P, Sanchez-Recalde A, Cuesta E, et al. Risk of aortic root or ascending aorta complications in patients with bicuspid aortic valve with and without coarctation of the aorta. Am J Cardiol 2009;104: 1001-6.
2. Olley PM, Coceani F, Bodach E. E-type prostaglandins: a new emergency therapy for certain cyanotic congenital heart malformations. Circulation 1976;53:728.
3. Olsson P, Soderlund S, Dubiel WT, Ovenfors CO. Patch graft or tubular grafts in the repair of coarctation of the aorta. A follow-up study. Scand J Thorac Cardiovasc Surg 1976;10:139.
4. Oosterhof T, Azakie A, Freedom RM, Williams WG, McCrindle BW. Associated factors and trends in outcomes of interrupted aortic arch. Ann Thorac Surg 2004;78:1696-702.
5. O'Rourke MF, Cartmill TB. Influence of aortic coarctation on pulsatile hemodynamics in the proximal aorta. Circulation 1971; 44:281.
6. Ou P, Celermajer DS, Raisky O, Jolivet O, Buyens F, Herment A, et al. Angular (Gothic) aortic arch leads to enhanced systolic wave reflection, central aortic stiffness, and increased left ventricular mass late after aortic coarctation repair: evaluation with magnetic resonance flow mapping. J Thorac Cardiovasc Surg 2008;135:62-8.

P

1. Pacini D, Bergonzini M, Loforte A, Gargiulo G, Pilato E, Di Bartolomeo R. Aneurysms after coarctation repair associated with hypoplastic aortic arch: surgical management through median sternotomy. Ann Thorac Surg 2006;81:758-60.
2. Park JK, Dell RB, Ellis K, Gersony WM. Surgical management of the infant with coarctation of the aorta and ventricular septal defect. J Am Coll Cardiol 1992;20:176.
3. Parker FB Jr, Farrell B, Streeten DH, Blackman MS, Sondheimer HM, Anderson GH Jr. Hypertensive mechanisms in coarctation of the aorta. Further studies of the renin-angiotensin system. J Thorac Cardiovasc Surg 1980;80:568.
4. Parsons CG. Recurrent coarctation of the aorta (editorial). Am Heart J 1967;73:1.
5. Parsons CG, Astley R. Recurrence of aortic coarctation after operation in childhood. Br Med J 1966;5487:573.
6. Patel HT, Madani A, Paris YM, Warner KG, Hijazi ZM. Balloon angioplasty of native coarctation of the aorta in infants and neonates: is it worth the hassle? Pediatr Cardiol 2001;22:53.
7. Patel R, Singh SP, Abrams L, Roberts KD. Coarctation of aorta with special reference to infants. Long-term results of operation in 126 cases. Br Heart J 1977;39:1246.
8. Pelech AN, Kartodihardjo W, Balfe JA, Balfe JW, Olley PM, Leenen FH. Exercise in children before and after coarctectomy: hemodynamic, echocardiographic, and biochemical assessment. Am Heart J 1986;112:1263.
9. Pellegrino A, Deverall PB, Anderson RH, Smith A, Wilkinson JL, Russo P, et al. Aortic coarctation in the first three months of life. An anatomopathological study with respect to treatment. J Thorac Cardiovasc Surg 1985;89:121.
10. Pelletier C, Davignon A, Ethier MF, Stanley P. Coarctation of the aorta in infancy. J Thorac Cardiovasc Surg 1969;57:171.
11. Penkoske PA, Williams WG, Olley PM, LeBlanc J, Trusler GA, Moes CA, et al. Subclavian arterioplasty. Repair of coarctation of the aorta in the first year of life. J Thorac Cardiovasc Surg 1984;87:894.
12. Perez-Alvarez JJ, Oudkerk S. Necrotizing arteritis of the abdominal organs as a postoperative complication following correction of coarctation of the aorta. A case report. Surgery 1955;37:833.
13. Pierce WS, Waldhausen JA, Berman W Jr, Whitman V. Late results of the subclavian flap procedure in infants with coarctation of the thoracic aorta. Circulation 1978;58:1.
14. Pihkala J, Pedra CA, Nykanen D, Benson LN. Implantation of endovascular stents for hypoplasia of the transverse aortic arch. Cardiol Young 2000;10:3.
15. Puchalski MD, Williams RV, Hawkins JA, Minich LL, Tani LY. Follow-up of aortic coarctation repair in neonates. J Am Coll Cardiol 2004;44:188-91.

Q

1. Quaegebeur JM, Jonas RA, Weinberg AD, Blackstone EH, Kirklin JW. Outcomes in seriously ill neonates with coarctation of the aorta. A multiinstitutional study. J Thorac Cardiovasc Surg 1994;108:841.

R

1. Radford DT, Blook KR, Coceani F, Fariello R, Olley PM. Prostaglandin E_1 for interrupted aortic arch in the neonate. Lancet 1976;2:95.
2. Radtke WA, Waller BR, Hebra A, Bradley SM. Palliative stent implantation for aortic coarctation in premature infants weighing <1,500 g. Am J Cardiol 2002;90:1409-12.
3. Rajasinghe HA, Reddy VM, van Son JA, Black MD, McElhinney DB, Brook MM, et al. Coarctation repair using end-to-side anastomosis of descending aorta to proximal aortic arch. Ann Thorac Surg 1996;61:840.
4. Rao PS, Galal O, Smith PA, Wilson AD. Five- to nine-year follow-up results of balloon angioplasty of native aortic coarctation in infants and children. J Am Coll Cardiol 1996;27:462.
5. Rao PS, Najjar HN, Mardini MK, Solymar L, Thapar MK. Balloon angioplasty for coarctation of the aorta: immediate and long-term results. Am Heart J 1988;115:657.
6. Rao PS, Thapar MK, Kutayli F, Carey P. Causes of recoarctation after balloon angioplasty of unoperated aortic coarctation. J Am Coll Cardiol 1989;13:109.
7. Rathi L, Keith JD. Postoperative blood pressures in coarctation of the aorta. Br Heart J 1964;26:671.
8. Ravnan JB, Chen E, Golabi M, Lebo RV. Chromosome 22q11.2 microdeletions in velocardiofacial syndrome patients with widely variable manifestations. Am J Med Genet 1996;66:250.
9. Ray JA, Doddi N, Regula D, Williams JA, Melveger A. Polydioxanone (PDS), a novel monofilament synthetic absorbable suture. Surg Gynecol Obstet 1981;153:497.
10. Reardon MJ, Hallman GL, Cooley DA. Interrupted aortic arch: brief review and summary of an eighteen-year experience. Texas Heart Inst J 1984;11:250.
11. Reddy GP, Higgins CB. Congenital heart disease: measuring physiology with MRI. Semin Roentgenol 1998;33:228.
12. Reddy VM, McElhinney DB, Sagrado T, Parry AJ, Teitel DF, Hanley FL. Results of 102 cases of complete repair of congenital heart defects in patients weighing 700 to 2500 grams. J Thorac Cardiovasc Surg 1999;117:324.
13. Reich O, Tax P, Bartakova H, Tomek V, Gilik J, Lisy J, et al. Long-term (up to 20 years) results of percutaneous balloon angioplasty of recurrent aortic coarctation without use of stents. Eur Heart J 2008;29:2042-8.
14. Reifenstein GH, Levine SA, Gross RE. Coarctation of the aorta. A review of 104 autopsied cases of the "adult type" 2 years of age or older. Am Heart J 1947;33:146.
15. Report of the New England Regional Infant Cardiac Program. Pediatrics 1980;65:375.
16. Rheuban KS, Carpenter MA, Jedeikin R, Dammann JF, Alford BA, Kron IL, et al. Aortic aneurysm after patch angioplasty for coarctation in childhood. J Am Coll Cardiol 1985;55:612.
17. Ring DM, Lewis FJ. Abdominal pain following surgical correction of coarctation of the aorta. A syndrome. J Thorac Surg 1956;31:718.
18. Riquelme C, Laissy JP, Menegazzo D, Debray MP, Cinqualbre A, Langlois J, et al. MR imaging of coarctation of the aorta and its postoperative complications in adults: assessment with spin-echo and cine-MR imaging. Magn Reson Imaging 1999;17:37.
19. Roberts WC, Morrow AG, Braunwald E. Complete interruption of the aortic arch. Circulation 1962;26:39.
20. Rocchini AP, Rosenthal A, Barger AC, Castaneda AR, Nadas AS. Pathogenesis of paradoxical hypertension after coarctation resection. Circulation 1976;54:382.
21. Roclawski M, Sabiniewicz R, Potaz P, Smoczynski A, Pankowski R, Mazurek T, et al. Scoliosis in patients with aortic coarctation and patent ductus arteriosus: does standard posterolateral thoracotomy play a role in the development of the lateral curve of the spine? Pediatr Cardiol 2009;30:941-5.
22. Rodbard S. Vascular modifications induced by flow. Am Heart J 1956; 51:926.
23. Rodbard S. Physical factors in the progression of stenotic vascular lesions. Circulation 1958;17:410.
24. Rodes-Cabau J, Miro J, Dancea A, Ibrahim R, Piette E, Lapierre C, et al. Comparison of surgical and transcatheter treatment for native coarctation of the aorta in patients ≥1 year old. The Quebec Native Coarctation of the Aorta study. Am Heart J 2007;154: 186-92.
25. Rothman A, Galindo A, Evans WN, Collazos JC, Restrepo H. Effectiveness and safety of balloon dilation of native aortic coarctation in premature neonates weighing ≤2,500 grams. Am J Cardiol 2010;105:1176-80.
26. Rudolph AM, Heymann MA, Spitznas U. Hemodynamic considerations in the development of narrowing of the aorta. Am J Cardiol 1972;30:514.
27. Russell GA, Berry PJ, Watterson K, Dhasmana JP, Wisheart JD. Patterns of ductal tissue in coarctation of the aorta in the first three months of life. J Thorac Cardiovasc Surg 1991;102:596.

S

1. Sade RM, Crawford FA, Hohn AR, Riopel DA, Taylor AB. Growth of the aorta after prosthetic patch aortoplasty for coarctation in infants. Ann Thorac Surg 1984;38:21.
2. Sade RM, Taylor AB, Chariker EP. Aortoplasty compared with resection for coarctation of the aorta in young children. Ann Thorac Surg 1979;28:346.
3. Salem MM, Starnes VA, Wells WJ, Acherman RJ, Chang RK, Luciani GB, et al. Predictors of left ventricular outflow obstruction following single-stage repair of interrupted aortic arch and ventricular septal defect. Am J Cardiol 2000;86:1044-7.
4. Samanek M, Goetzova J, Fiserova J, Skovranek J. Differences in muscle blood flow in upper and lower extremities of patients after correction of coarctation of the aorta. Circulation 1976;54:377.

5. Saul JP, Keane JF, Fellows KE, Lock JE. Balloon dilation angioplasty of postoperative aortic obstructions. Am J Cardiol 1987; 59:943.
6. Schaffler GJ, Sorantin E, Groell R, Gamillscheg A, Maier E, Schoellnast H, et al. Helical CT angiography with maximum intensity projection in the assessment of aortic coarctation after surgery. Am J Roentgenol 2000;175:1041.
7. Schreiber C, Eicken A, Vogt M, Gunther T, Wottke M, Thielmann M, et al. Repair of interrupted aortic arch: results after more than 20 years. Ann Thorac Surg 2000;70:1896.
8. Schroeder VA, Pearl JM, Beekman RH, Cripe L, Khoury P, Manning PB, et al. Usefulness of the mitral valve Z score in predicting the need to close moderate- to large-sized atrial septal defects in infants with aortic coarctation. Am J Cardiol 2003;92:480-3.
9. Schuster SR, Gross RE. Surgery for coarctation of the aorta: a review of 500 cases. J Thorac Cardiovasc Surg 1962;43:54.
10. Sciolaro C, Copeland J, Cork R, Barkenbush M, Donnerstein R, Goldberg S. Long-term follow-up comparing subclavian flap angioplasty to resection with modified oblique end-to-end anastomosis. J Thorac Cardiovasc Surg 1991;101:1.
11. Sealy WC. Indications for surgical treatment of coarctation of the aorta. Surg Gynecol Obstet 1953;97:301.
12. Sealy WC, Harris JS, Young WG Jr, Calloway HA Jr. Paradoxical hypertension following resection of coarctation of the aorta. Surgery 1957;42:135.
13. Sehested J, Baandrup U, Mikkelsen E. Different reactivity and structure of the prestenotic and poststenotic aorta in human coarctation. Implications for baroreceptor function. Circulation 1982; 65:1060.
14. Seidel JF. Index Musei Anatomici Kiliensis. Kiel: CF Mohr, 1818, p. 61.
15. Sell JE, Jonas RA, Mayer JE, Blackstone EH, Kirklin JW, Castaneda AR. The results of a surgical program for interrupted aortic arch. J Thorac Cardiovasc Surg 1988;96:864.
16. Sennari E. Morphological study of ventricular septal defect associated with obstruction of aortic arch among Japanese. Jpn Circ J 1985;49:61.
17. Serraf A, Lacour-Gayet F, Robotin M, Bruniaux J, Sousa-Uva M, Roussin R, et al. Repair of interrupted aortic arch: a ten-year experience. J Thorac Cardiovasc Surg 1996;112:1150.
18. Serraf A, Piot JD, Bonnet N, Lacour-Gayet F, Touchot A, Bruniaux J, et al. Biventricular repair approach in ducto-dependent neonates with hypoplastic but morphologically normal left ventricle. J Am Coll Cardiol 1999;33:827.
19. Shaddy RE, Boucek MM, Sturtevant JE, Ruttenberg HD, Jaffe RB, Tani LY, et al. Comparison of angioplasty and surgery for unoperated coarctation of the aorta. Circulation 1993;87:793-9.
20. Shearer WT, Rutman JY, Weinberg WA, Goldring D. Coarctation of the aorta and cerebrovascular accident. A proposal for early corrective surgery. J Pediatr 1970;77:1004.
21. Shinebourne EA, Elseed AM. Relation between fetal flow patterns, coarctation of the aorta and pulmonary blood flow. Br Heart J 1974;36:492.
22. Shinebourne EA, Tam AS, Elseed AM, Paneth M, Lennox SC, Cleland WP, et al. Coarctation of the aorta in infancy and childhood. Br Heart J 1976;38:375.
23. Shiokawa Y, Becker AE. The surgical anatomy of the left ventricular outflow tract in hearts with ventricular septal defect and aortic arch obstruction. Ann Thorac Surg 1998;65:1381.
24. Shumaker HB Jr, Freeman LW, Hutchings IM, Radigan L. Studies in vascular repair: further observations on growth of anastomosis and free vascular transplants in growing animals. Angiology 1951;2:263.
25. Siblini G, Rao PS, Nouri S, Ferdman B, Jureidini SB, Wilson AD. Long-term follow-up results of balloon angioplasty of postoperative aortic recoarctation. Am J Cardiol 1998;81:61.
26. Sigurdardottir LY, Helgason H. Exercise-induced hypertension after corrective surgery for coarctation of the aorta. Pediatr Cardiol 1996;17:301.
27. Simsolo R, Grunfeld B, Gimenez M, Lopez M, Berri G, Becu L, et al. Long-term systemic hypertension in children after successful repair of coarctation of the aorta. Am Heart J 1988;115:1268.
28. Sinha SN, Kardatzke ML, Cole RB, Muster AJ, Wessel HU, Paul MH. Coarctation of the aorta in infancy. Circulation 1969;40:385.
29. Sirak HD, Ressallat M, Hosier DM, DeLorimier AA. A new operation for repairing aortic arch atresia in infancy: report of 3 cases. Circulation 1968;37:II43.
30. Smaill BH, McGiffin DC, Legrice IJ, Young AA, Hunter PJ, Galbraith AJ. The effect of synthetic patch repair of coarctation on regional deformation of the aortic wall. J Thorac Cardiovasc Surg 2000;120:1053.
31. Smith Maia MM, Cortes TM, Parga JR, De Avila LF, Aiello VD, Barbero-Marcial M, et al. Evolutional aspects of children and adolescents with surgically corrected aortic coarctation: clinical, echocardiographic, and magnetic resonance image analysis of 113 patients. J Thorac Cardiovasc Surg 2004;127:712-20.
32. Smith RT Jr, Sade RM, Riopel DA, Taylor AB, Crawford FA Jr, Hohn AR. Stress testing for comparison of synthetic patch aortoplasty with resection and end to end anastomosis for repair of coarctation in childhood. J Am Coll Cardiol 1984;4:765.
33. Soler R, Rodriguez E, Requejo I, Fernandez R, Raposo I. Magnetic resonance imaging of congenital abnormalities of the thoracic aorta. Eur Radiol 1998;8:540.
34. Soulen RL, Kan J, Mitchell S, White RI Jr. Evaluation of balloon angioplasty of coarctation restenosis by magnetic resonance imaging. Am J Cardiol 1987;60:343.
35. Starnes VA, Luciani GB, Wells WJ, Allen RB, Lewis AB. Aortic root replacement with the pulmonary autograft in children with complex left heart obstruction. Ann Thorac Surg 1996;62:442.
36. Steidele RJ. Samml Chir Med Beob, Vol. 2. Vienna: 1778, p. 114.
37. Suarez de Lezo J, Fernandez R, Sancho M, Concha M, Arizon J, Franco M, et al. Percutaneous transluminal angioplasty for aortic isthmic coarctation in infancy. Am J Cardiol 1984;54:1147.
38. Suarez de Lezo J, Pan M, Romero M, Medina A, Segura J, Lafuente M, et al. Immediate and follow-up findings after stent treatment for severe coarctation of aorta. Am J Cardiol 1999; 83:400.
39. Suarez de Lezo J, Pan M, Romero M, Segura J, Pavlovic D, Ojeda S, et al. Percutaneous interventions on severe coarctation of the aorta: a 21-year experience. Pediatr Cardiol 2005;26:176-89.
40. Suzuki T, Ohye RG, Devaney EJ, Ishizaka T, Nathan PN, Goldberg CS, et al. Selective management of the left ventricular outflow tract for repair of interrupted aortic arch with ventricular septal defect: management of left ventricular outflow tract obstruction. J Thorac Cardiovasc Surg 2006;131:779-84.
41. Sweeney MS, Walker WE, Duncan JM, Hallman GL, Livesay JJ, Cooley DA. Reoperation for aortic coarctation: techniques, results, and indications for various approaches. Ann Thorac Surg 1985;40:46.
42. Sybert VP. Cardiovascular malformations and complications in Turner syndrome. Pediatrics 1998;101:E11.

T

1. Takabayashi S, Kado H, Shiokawa Y, Fukae K, Nakano T. Long-term outcome of left ventricular outflow tract after biventricular repair using Damus-Kaye-Stansel anastomosis for interrupted aortic arch and severe aortic stenosis. J Thorac Cardiovasc Surg 2005;130:942-4.
2. Talner NS, Berman MA. Postnatal development of obstruction in coarctation of the aorta: role of the ductus arteriosus. Pediatrics 1975;56:562.
3. Tani LY, Minich LL, Hawkins JA, McGough EC, Pagotto LT, Orsmond GS, et al. Spectrum and influence of hypoplasia of the left heart in neonatal aortic coarctation. Cardiol Young 2000;10:90.
4. Tani LY, Minich LL, Pagotto LT, Shaddy RE, McGough EC, Hawkins JA. Left heart hypoplasia and neonatal aortic arch obstruction: is the Rhodes left ventricular adequacy score applicable? J Thorac Cardiovasc Surg 1999;118:81.
5. Tawes RL Jr, Aberdeen E, Waterston DJ, Carter RE. Coarctation of the aorta in infants and children. A review of 333 operative cases including 179 infants. Circulation 1969;39:I173.
6. Tawes RL Jr, Berry CL, Aberdeen E. Congenital bicuspid aortic valves associated with coarctation of the aorta in children. Br Heart J 1969;31:127.
7. Tawes RL Jr, Bull JC, Roe BB. Hypertension and abdominal pain after resection of aortic coarctation. Ann Surg 1970;171:409.
8. Tchervenkov CI, Tahta SA, Jutras LC, Beland MJ. Biventricular repair in neonates with hypoplastic left heart complex. Ann Thorac Surg 1998;66:1350.
9. Tchervenkov CI, Tahta SA, Jutras L, Beland MJ. Single-stage repair of aortic arch obstruction and associated intracardiac defects with pulmonary homograft patch aortoplasty. J Thorac Cardiovasc Surg 1998;116:897.

10. Thanopoulos BV, Eleftherakis N, Tzanos K, Skoularigis I, Triposkiadis F. Stent implantation for adult aortic coarctation. J Am Coll Cardiol 2008;52:1815-6.
11. Thibault WN, Sperling DR, Gazzaniga AB. Subclavian artery patch angioplasty. Arch Surg 1975;110:1095.
12. Thomka I, Szedo F, Arvay A. Repair of coarctation of the aorta in adults with simultaneous aortic valve replacement and coronary artery bypass grafting. Thorac Cardiovasc Surg 1997;45:93.
13. Thomson JD, Mulpur A, Guerrero R, Nagy Z, Gibbs JL, Watterson KG. Outcome after extended arch repair for aortic coarctation. Heart 2006;92:90-4.
14. Tiraboschi R, Alfieri O, Carpentier A, Parenzan L. One stage correction of coarctation of the aorta associated with intracardiac defects in infancy. J Cardiovasc Surg 1978;19:11.
15. Tiraboschi R, Locatelli G, Bianchi T, Parenzan L. Correction of coarctation of the aorta during the first year of life by means of the subclavian flap technique: 8 cases operated on successfully. Surg Italy 1975;5:244.
16. Tlaskal T, Hucin B, Hruda J, Marek J, Chaloupecky V, Kostelka M, et al. Results of primary and two-stage repair of interrupted aortic arch. Eur J Cardiothorac Surg 1998;14:235.
17. Todd PJ, Dangerfield PH, Hamilton DI, Wilkinson JL. Late effects on the left upper limb of subclavian flap aortoplasty. J Thorac Cardiovasc Surg 1983;85:678.
18. Trinquet F, Vouhe PR, Vernant F, Touati G, Roux PM, Pome G, et al. Coarctation of the aorta in infants: which operation? Ann Thorac Surg 1988;45:186.
19. Trusler GA, Izukawa T. Interrupted aortic arch and ventricular septal defect. Direct repair through a median sternotomy incision in a 13-day-old infant. J Thorac Cardiovasc Surg 1975;69:126.
20. Tucker BL, Stanton RE, Lindesmith GG, Stiles QR, Meyer BW, Jones JC. Recurrent coarctation of the thoracic aorta. Arch Surg 1971;102:556.
21. Tworetzky W, McElhinney DB, Brook MM, Reddy VM, Hanley FL, Silverman NH. Echocardiographic diagnosis alone for the complete repair of major congenital heart defects. J Am Coll Cardiol 1999;33:228.
22. Tzifa A, Ewert P, Brzezinska-Rajszys G, Peters B, Zubrzycka M, Rosenthal E, et al. Covered Cheatham-platinum stents for aortic coarctation: early and intermediate-term results. J Am Coll Cardiol 2006;47:1457-63.

U

1. Ungerleider RM, Ebert PA. Indications and techniques for midline approach to aortic coarctation in infants and children. Ann Thorac Surg 1987;44:517.
2. Urschel CW, Covell JW, Sonnenblick EH, Ross J Jr, Braunwald E. Effects of decreased aortic compliance on performance of the left ventricle. Am J Physiol 1968;214:298.

V

1. Van Mierop LH, Kutsche LM. Interruption of the aortic arch and coarctation of the aorta: pathogenetic relations. Am J Cardiol 1984;54:829.
2. Van Praagh R, Bernhard WF, Rosenthal A, Parisi LF, Fyler DC. Interrupted aortic arch: surgical treatment. Am J Cardiol 1971; 27:200.
3. Van Praagh R, Van Praagh S. The anatomy of common aorticopulmonary trunk (truncus arteriosus communis) and its embryologic implications. Am J Cardiol 1965;16:406.
4. van Son JA, Daniels O, Lacquet LK. Optimal age for repair of aortic coarctation (letter). Ann Thorac Surg 1991;51:344.
5. van Son JA, Daniels O, Vincent JG, van Lier HJ, Lacquet LK. Appraisal of resection and end-to-end anastomosis for repair of coarctation of the aorta in infancy: preference for resection. Ann Thorac Surg 1989;48:496.
6. van Son JA, van Asten WN, van Lier HJ, Daniels O, Skotnicki SH, Lacquet LK. A comparison of coarctation resection and subclavian flap angioplasty using ultrasonographically monitored postocclusive reactive hyperemia. J Thorac Cardiovasc Surg 1990;100:817.
7. van Son JA, van Asten WN, van Lier HJ, Daniels O, Vincent JG, Skotnicki SH, et al. Detrimental sequelae on the hemodynamics of the upper left limb after subclavian flap angioplasty in infancy. Circulation 1990;81:996.
8. Varma C, Benson LN, Butany J, McLaughlin PR. Aortic dissection after stent dilatation for coarctation of the aorta: a case report and literature review. Catheter Cardiovasc Interv 2003;59:528-35.
9. Ventemiglia R, Oglietti J, Wukasch DC, Hallman GL, Cooley DA. Interruption of the aortic arch. J Thorac Cardiovasc Surg 1976;72:235.
10. Venturini A, Papalia U, Chiarotti F, Caretta Q. Primary repair of coarctation of the thoracic aorta by patch graft aortoplasty. A three-decade experience and follow-up in 60 patients. Eur J Cardiothorac Surg 1996;10:890.
11. Verska JJ, De Quattro V, Woolley MM. Coarctation of the aorta. The abdominal pain syndrome and paradoxical hypertension. J Thorac Cardiovasc Surg 1969;58:746.
12. Villalobos MC, Balderrama DP, Lopez JL, Castellanos M. Complete interruption of the aorta. Am J Cardiol 1961;8:664.
13. Vlodaver Z, Neufeld HN. The coronary arteries in coarctation of the aorta. Circulation 1968;37:449.
14. Vogel M, Vernon MM, McElhinney DB, Brown DW, Colan SD, Tworetzky W. Fetal diagnosis of interrupted aortic arch. Am J Cardiol 2010;105:727-34.
15. Vohra HA, Adamson L, Haw MP. Does surgical correction of coarctation of the aorta in adults reduce established hypertension? Interact Cardiovasc Thorac Surg 2009;8:123-7.
16. Vohra HA, Odurny A, Mandal S, Viola N, Kaarne M, Salmon T, et al. Giant aneurysms associated with aortic coarctation: management challenges and options. Pediatr Cardiol 2010;31:521-5.
17. Vorsschulte K. Surgical correction of the aorta by an "isthmus plastic" operation. Thorax 1961;16:338.
18. Vouhe PR, Trinquet F, Lecompte Y, Vernant F, Roux PM, Touati G, et al. Aortic coarctation with hypoplastic aortic arch. Results of extended end-to-end aortic arch anastomosis. J Thorac Cardiovasc Surg 1988;96:557.
19. Vriend JW, de Groot E, de Waal TT, Zijta FM, Kastelein JJ, Mulder BJ. Increased carotid and femoral intima–media thickness in patients after repair of aortic coarctation: influence of early repair. Am Heart J 2006;151:242-7.
20. Vriend JW, Drenthen W, Pieper PG, Roos-Hesselink JW, Zwinderman AH, van Veldhuisen DJ, et al. Outcome of pregnancy in patients after repair of aortic coarctation. Eur Heart J 2005; 26:2173-8.
21. Vriend JW, Lam J, Mulder BJ. Complete aortic arch obstruction: interruption or aortic coarctation? Int J Cardiovasc Imaging 2004;20:393-6.
22. Vriend JW, Mulder BJ, Schoof PH, Hazekamp MG. Median sternotomy for reoperation of the distal aortic arch in postcoarctectomy patients. Ann Thorac Surg 2004;78:e58-60.
23. Vriend JW, Zwinderman AH, de Groot E, Kastelein JJ, Bouma BJ, Mulder BJ. Predictive value of mild, residual descending aortic narrowing for blood pressure and vascular damage in patients after repair of aortic coarctation. Eur Heart J 2005;26:84-90.

W

1. Waldhausen J, Whitman V, Pierce W. Coarctation in infants: management with prostaglandin E_1 and the subclavian flap procedure. Presented at the World Congress of Pediatric Cardiology (abstract). London, 1980.
2. Waldhausen JA, Nahrwold DL. Repair of coarctation of the aorta with a subclavian flap. J Thorac Cardiovasc Surg 1966;51:532.
3. Walhout RJ, Lekkerkerker JC, Oron GH, Hitchcock FJ, Meijboom EJ, Bennink GB. Comparison of polytetrafluoroethylene patch aortoplasty and end-to-end anastomosis for coarctation of the aorta. J Thorac Cardiovasc Surg 2003;126:521-8.
4. Walhout RJ, Suttorp MJ, Mackaij GJ, Ernst JM, Plokker HW. Long-term outcome after balloon angioplasty of coarctation of the aorta in adolescents and adults: is aneurysm formation an issue? Catheter Cardiovasc Interv 2009;73:549-56.
5. Warnes CA. Bicuspid aortic valve and coarctation: two villains part of a diffuse problem. Heart 2003;89:965-6.
6. Weisman D, Kesten HD. Absence of transverse aortic arch with defects of cardiac septums. Report of a case simulating acute abdominal disease in a newborn infant. Am J Dis Child 1948;76:326.
7. Wells WJ, Prendergast TW, Berdjis F, Brandl D, Lange PE, Hetzer R, et al. Repair of coarctation of the aorta in adults: the fate of systolic hypertension. Ann Thorac Surg 1996;61:1168.
8. Wielenga G, Dankmeijer J. Coarctation of the aorta. J Pathol Bacteriol 1968;95:265.
9. Wiest DB, Garner SS, Uber WE, Sade RM. Esmolol for the management of pediatric hypertension after cardiac operations. J Thorac Cardiovasc Surg 1998;115:890.

10. Winer HE, Kronzon I, Glassman E, Cunningham JN Jr, Madayag M. Pseudocoarctation and mid-arch aortic coarctation. Chest 1977;72:519.
11. Wood AE, Javadpour H, Duff D, Oslizlok P, Walsh K. Is extended arch aortoplasty the operation of choice for infant aortic coarctation? Results of 15 years' experience in 181 patients. Ann Thorac Surg 2004;77:1353-8.
12. Wren C, Peart I, Bain H, Hunter S. Balloon dilatation of unoperated aortic coarctation: immediate results and one year follow up. Br Heart J 1987;58:369.
13. Wright GE, Nowak CA, Goldberg CS, Ohye RG, Bove EL, Rocchini AP. Extended resection and end-to-end anastomosis for aortic coarctation in infants: results of a tailored surgical approach. Ann Thorac Surg 2005;80:1453-9.

Y

1. Yamagishi M, Fujiwara K, Yamada Y, Shuntoh K, Kitamura N. A new surgical technique for one-stage repair of interrupted aortic arch with valvular aortic stenosis. J Thorac Cardiovasc Surg 2001;122:392-3.
2. Yamashiro M, Takahashi Y, Ando M, Kikuchi T. End-to-side anastomosis for coarctation of the aorta and type A aortic arch interruption with hypoplastic aortic arch. Jpn J Thorac Cardiovasc Surg 2006;54:273-7.
3. Yeager SB, Keane JF. Fate of moderate and large secundum type atrial septal defect associated with isolated coarctation in infants. Am J Cardiol 1999;84:362-3.
4. Yetman AT, Nykanen D, McCrindle BW, Sunnegardh J, Adatia I, Freedom RM, et al. Balloon angioplasty of recurrent coarctation: a 12-year review. J Am Coll Cardiol 1997;30:811.
5. Yoshida M, Yamaguchi M, Oshima Y, Oka S, Higuma T, Okita Y. Single-stage repair of aortopulmonary window with interrupted aortic arch by transection of the aorta and direct reconstruction. J Thorac Cardiovasc Surg 2009;138:781-3.
6. Younoszai AK, Reddy VM, Hanley FL, Brook MM. Intermediate term follow-up of the end-to-side aortic anastomosis for coarctation of the aorta. Ann Thorac Surg 2002;74:1631-4.

Z

1. Zhang H, Cheng P, Hou J, Li L, Liu H, Liu R, et al. Regional cerebral perfusion for surgical correction of neonatal aortic arch obstruction. Perfusion 2009;24:185-9.
2. Ziemer G, Jonas RA, Perry SB, Freed MD, Castaneda AR. Surgery for coarctation of the aorta in the neonate. Circulation 1986;74:I25.
3. Zoghbi J, Serraf A, Mohammadi S, Belli E, Lacour Gayet F, Aupecle B, et al. Is surgical intervention still indicated in recurrent aortic arch obstruction? J Thorac Cardiovasc Surg 2004;127:203-12.

49 Aortic Atresia and Other Forms of Hypoplastic Left Heart Physiology

DEFINITION

Hypoplastic left heart physiology is defined as inability of the left heart to sustain adequate cardiac output following birth because of underdevelopment of one or more left heart structures despite surgical or medical intervention. Box 49-1 emphasizes four important implications of this definition.

We have chosen to use the term *hypoplastic left heart physiology* rather than the more common and entrenched term *hypoplastic left heart syndrome*, because it more accurately describes the entity. In fact, both terms have important limitations when applied in the clinical setting. In practice, the exact point along the aforementioned continuum where an inadequate left heart is encountered cannot be defined with certainty. This limitation is not intrinsic to the definition of hypoplastic left heart physiology itself, but rather is due to two important factors: (1) tests designed to define morphologic and physiologic characteristics are limited in their ability to accurately predict overall left heart function, and (2) new

Box 49-1 Hypoplastic Left Heart Physiology

1. The term *left heart* refers to the morphologic composite or unit that includes left atrium, mitral valve, left ventricle, aortic valve, and aorta. Each of these plays an important role in determining left heart function.
2. Definition of hypoplastic left heart is physiologic, not morphologic, despite morphologic abnormalities being the underlying cause of left heart inadequacy. A morphologic definition of the hypoplastic left heart is not possible because underdevelopment of a variable number of specific left heart structures, either alone or in various combinations, may be responsible for physiologic inadequacy of the left heart. Some morphologic constellations (e.g., aortic and mitral atresia in combination) essentially always result in hypoplastic left heart physiology, whereas others (e.g., aortic or mitral stenosis) may or may not. Nevertheless, typical morphologic abnormalities that result in hypoplastic left heart physiology can be identified. These include a constellation of atresia or marked hypoplasia of the mitral valve, left ventricle, and aortic valve, in association with hypoplasia of the ascending aorta and aortic arch, aortic coarctation, patent ductus arteriosus, and atrial septal defect. It is important, however, to reemphasize that this constellation does not define hypoplastic left heart physiology; hypoplastic left heart physiology can be present without including all morphologic abnormalities mentioned in this typical example.
3. Hypoplastic left heart physiology is present within a relatively narrow band of the broad continuum of hypoplastic lesions of the left heart. This continuum ranges from isolated simple lesions (e.g., discrete coarctation) at one end of the spectrum to complex multilevel lesions (e.g., combination of aortic atresia, mitral atresia, and absent left ventricle) at the other end. The point along this gradually increasing continuum of left heart abnormalities where hypoplastic left heart physiology is encountered is impossible to pinpoint morphologically. Hypoplastic left heart physiology may be the result of a severe abnormality of a single left heart structure (e.g., mitral atresia) or a combination of several milder abnormalities (e.g., mitral stenosis, left ventricular hypoplasia, and aortic stenosis).
4. Inclusion of the phrase *despite surgical or medical intervention* in its definition is critical to the concept of hypoplastic left heart physiology, because abnormalities such as isolated critical aortic stenosis or isolated severe aortic coarctation may meet the criteria of this physiologic definition before but not after intervention to correct the abnormality. As a result, the lesions cited in the previous sentence are not considered examples of hypoplastic left heart physiology. An important implication of the term *hypoplastic left heart physiology* is that the left heart is incapable of sustaining systemic cardiac output, thereby limiting therapeutic options to (1) reconstructions that use a single (right) ventricular pumping chamber (Norwood procedure, superior cavopulmonary connection, Fontan procedure) or (2) heart transplantation.

developments and reconstructive techniques may allow previously unsalvageable left hearts to function adequately.

The concept of borderline hypoplastic left heart physiology is useful in this context because it emphasizes that it is not possible to define a specific point along the morphologic and physiologic continuum where the left heart becomes unquestionably unsalvageable. *Borderline hypoplastic left heart physiology*, therefore, refers to a zone along this continuum in which it is currently not possible to predict with certainty whether the left heart can be salvaged with surgical reconstructive methods. This concept is of practical importance because it helps characterize the clinical dilemma faced by surgeons who must make a dichotomous decision (reconstructive surgery to salvage the left heart vs. the Norwood procedure or transplantation) in the context of a continuum of morphologic and physiologic left heart compromise. At either pole of this continuum, decision making is straightforward. However, within the zone of borderline hypoplastic left heart physiology, the appropriate management decision requires exquisite attention to many subtle details.

The various malformations that result in hypoplastic left heart physiology together represent a special example of *univentricular atrioventricular connection* (see Chapters 41 and 56). Because of the special clinical and surgical importance of this group of malformations, this subject is discussed separately from other forms of univentricular heart.

HISTORICAL NOTE

The first description of aortic atresia was apparently by Canton in 1850.[C2] Although Abbott had recognized aortic and mitral atresia,[A1] Brockman in 1950 emphasized that in about 50% of cases of mitral atresia, there was coexisting aortic atresia and severe underdevelopment of the left side of the heart.[B15] In 1952, Lev further emphasized the group of congenital heart malformations associated with underdevelopment of the left-sided cardiac chambers and a small ascending aortic arch, articulating for the first time the concept that multiple left-sided structures tended to occur together.[L7] In 1958, Noonan and Nadas brought together the morphologic features of combined aortic and mitral atresia and introduced the phrase "hypoplastic left heart syndrome."[N4] In 1976, Roberts and colleagues further organized the knowledge about this subject by emphasizing that in the presence of a large ventricular septal defect (VSD), aortic atresia can coexist with normal development of the left ventricle and mitral valve.[R7]

The history of attempted reconstructive procedures for hypoplastic left heart physiology dates back to 1970 when Cayler and colleagues described an anastomosis between right pulmonary artery and ascending aorta with placement of bilateral pulmonary artery bands.[C4] Other variations in neonatal reconstructive procedures designed to allow survival without the use of prostaglandins to maintain ductal patency were described by Doty and colleagues in 1977, Norwood and colleagues in 1980, Levitsky and colleagues in 1980, Behrendt and colleagues in 1981, and others.[B11,D6,D7,H3,L3,L6,M11,N6,Y1]

Even though some of these reports noted short-term successes, there is no documentation of long-term survival. In 1983, Norwood and colleagues described for the first time neonatal palliative surgery leading to a subsequent successful Fontan procedure.[N8] Following this report and subsequent reports that systematically documented long-term survival of patients with hypoplastic left heart physiology, it has become widely accepted that many of the technical details of the procedure as described by Norwood are critical to achieving long-term survival. These technical details ensure long-term aortic growth potential, minimize pulmonary valve distortion, address distal arch obstruction, preserve pulmonary artery patency, balance pulmonary and systemic blood flows, and ensure adequate atrial-level mixing. Many of the procedures described before implementation of the Norwood procedure failed to address one or more of these issues critical for long-term survival.

Allograft heart transplantation for hypoplastic left heart physiology dates back to 1985, when Bailey performed the first successful cases as primary therapy in neonates.[B6] Since then, Bailey and colleagues and a limited number of other groups have considered transplantation as one option for treatment, along with reconstructive surgery.

The hybrid procedure for hypoplastic left heart physiology was first developed in 1993 in response to poor outcomes following the Norwood procedure.[G7] The hybrid procedure combines surgical placement of bilateral branch pulmonary artery bands, placement of a stent in the ductus arteriosus, and catheter-based atrial septostomy, avoiding cardiopulmonary bypass (CPB). Initially, it was not widely embraced because of poor interim outcomes; however, more recently it has been used by some programs as an alternative to the Norwood procedure in high-risk patients, and variations of the hybrid procedure have been used as a bridge to transplantation.[C7,D4]

MORPHOGENESIS AND MORPHOLOGY

Morphogenesis

Currently, it is unclear whether the etiology of hypoplastic left heart physiology is similar in all cases. There are genetic factors involved, although these are multiple, complex, and poorly understood at the present time.[G14] Available evidence suggests that a number of primary morphologic etiologies may lead to the end result of hypoplastic left heart physiology. Primary morphologic abnormalities at the aortic valve level, mitral valve level, left ventricular myocardial level, or atrial septal level (intact atrial septum) could all in theory lead ultimately to hypoplasia of the entire left side of the heart as gestation progresses.

Fetal echocardiography has yielded much information regarding progression of hypoplastic left heart physiology. In some cases, critical aortic stenosis with documented forward flow on early fetal echocardiograms progresses to aortic atresia before birth. In such cases, the left ventricle shows evidence of progressive dysfunction and hypoplasia as stenosis proceeds to atresia. Echocardiographic evidence of fetal left ventricular dilated cardiomyopathy progressing to hypoplastic left heart physiology has been reported.[D1,J1] Controversy remains as to whether a closed foramen ovale in utero is a cause or a result of hypoplastic left heart physiology.[S6]

Morphology

In hypoplastic left heart physiology, the heart is enlarged to about twice normal weight for age. Its shape is determined by the large right and small left heart chambers[V1] (Fig. 49-1, *A*). Beyond this, morphologic details vary widely. Four morphologic subtypes of hypoplastic left heart physiology can be defined based on status of the left heart valves:

- Aortic and mitral atresia
- Aortic atresia with mitral stenosis
- Aortic stenosis with mitral atresia
- Aortic and mitral stenosis

Of these, aortic stenosis with mitral atresia is the least common subtype, representing approximately 5% of cases; aortic and mitral atresia is the most common, representing approximately two thirds of cases. Within these subtypes, the status of the atrial septum, size of the left ventricular cavity and muscle mass, ascending aorta and aortic arch, and ductus arteriosus are also important.

Aortic Valve and Ascending Aorta

In aortic atresia, the aortic valve is totally absent. Diminutive aortic sinuses of Valsalva are frequently present, giving origin to relatively normally positioned right and left coronary arteries that have a normal distribution pattern. The ascending aorta is narrow, sometimes as small as 1.5 mm in diameter. The portion of the aorta between the atretic valve and brachiocephalic artery serves only as a conduit for coronary blood flow (Fig. 49-2).

At and beyond the brachiocephalic artery, the aortic arch gradually widens and is joined beyond the origin of the left subclavian artery by a large patent ductus arteriosus. The ductus carries blood from the right ventricle into the descending aorta and retrograde to the brachiocephalic and coronary arteries. A localized aortic coarctation exists in approximately 80% of cases and is usually juxtaductal in location (see Chapter 48).[E1,M10,V5] Prevalence of coarctation is highest in patients with the most severe hypoplasia of the ascending aorta.[A2] In some cases, there may be only mild infolding of the aortic media on the wall opposite the ductal insertion site, or there may be no aortic coarctation whatsoever.

When a patent but hypoplastic aortic valve is present, there may be a variable but still reduced amount of forward flow across the aortic valve (see Chapter 47). The ascending aorta and arch tend to be larger than in aortic atresia, with the diameter of the ascending aorta ranging from 2 to 6 mm. Aortic coarctation is common.

Left Ventricle and Mitral Valve

The left ventricle is severely hypoplastic in 95% of cases of aortic atresia.[S5] In this setting, the ventricular septum is intact.[D8,E2] The mitral valve is either atretic (about one third of patients) or patent but severely hypoplastic (about two thirds of patients)[R7] (see Fig. 49-1, *B* and *C*). When the mitral valve is patent in association with aortic atresia, there may be left ventricular–coronary connections (Fig. 49-3) similar to those present in the right ventricle in cases of pulmonary atresia with intact ventricular septum[B3,O1,S4] (see "Right Ventricle" under Morphology in Chapter 40). It is postulated that these connections serve to decompress the left ventricular chamber. Localized thickening of coronary arteries occurs adjacent to these connections, and there is also a variable degree of endocardial thickening (endocardial fibroelastosis).

Rarely, there is focal calcification and scarring limited to the ventricular subendocardium.[O1] The hypoplastic left ventricle shows myocardial fiber disarray qualitatively similar to that present in hypertrophic obstructive cardiomyopathy (see "Left Ventricle" under Morphology in Section II of Chapter 47), and in the right ventricle in pulmonary atresia with intact ventricular septum[B17] (see "Right Ventricle" under Morphology in Chapter 40).

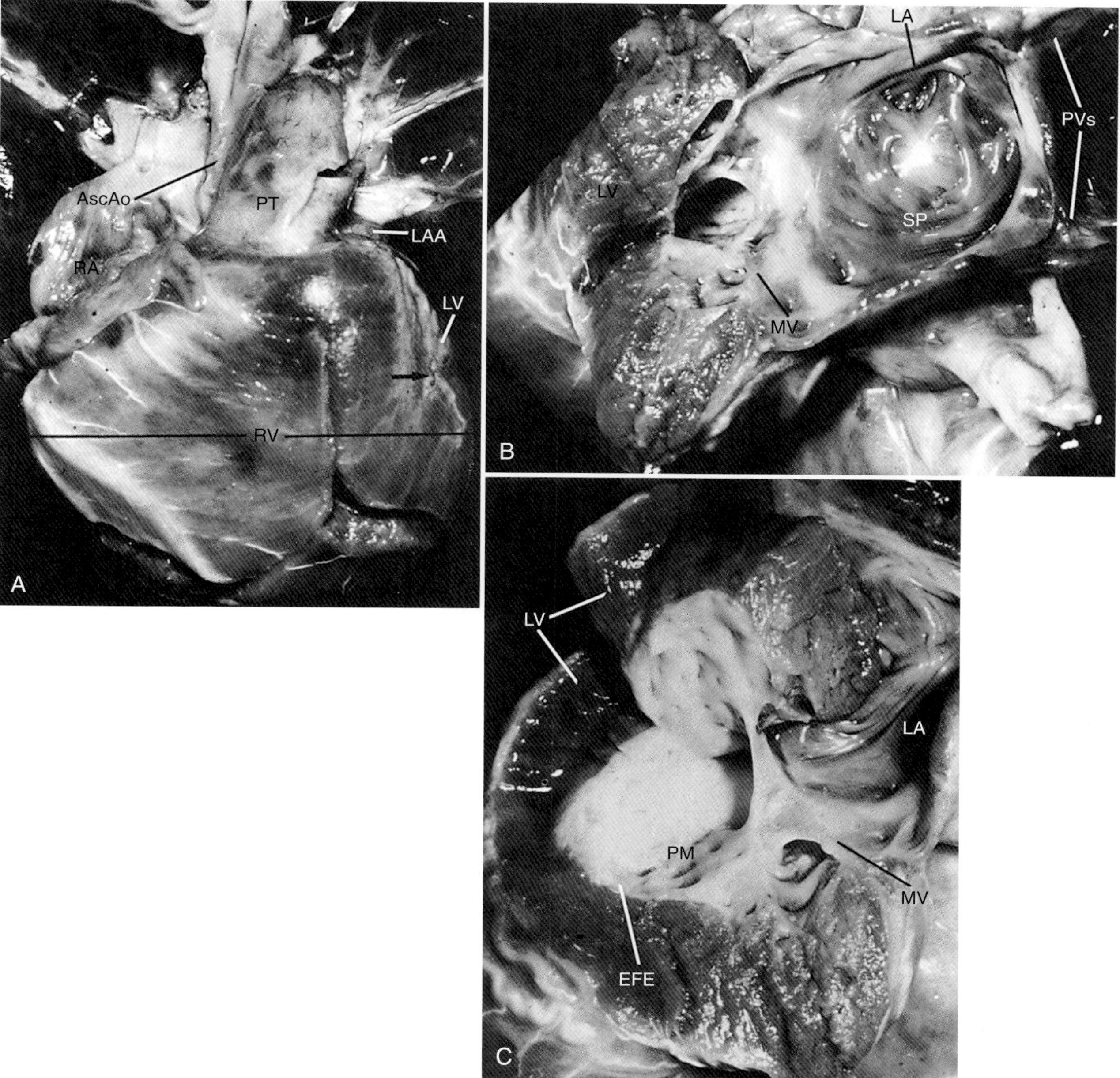

Figure 49-1 Autopsy specimen of aortic atresia and hypoplastic left heart physiology from a 4-day-old neonate. **A,** Globular external shape of heart results from massive right ventricular *(RV)* hypertrophy and enlargement. Pulmonary trunk *(PT)* is large and ascending aorta *(AscAo)* small. Left ventricle *(LV)* is small and displaced posteriorly and does not reach cardiac apex. Arrow points to left anterior descending coronary artery. **B,** Interior of left atrium *(LA)* and partly opened LV. Septum primum (*SP*; fossa ovalis) is thickened and protrudes into right atrium *(RA)*. Mitral valve *(MV)* is hypoplastic and stenotic, and LV wall is grossly thickened. **C,** Interior of fully opened LV. Its cavity is small, and there is marked endocardial fibroelastosis *(EFE)*, which also involves rudimentary papillary muscles *(PM)* of small MV. Key: *LAA,* Left atrial appendage; *PVs,* pulmonary veins.

In approximately 5% of cases of aortic atresia, the left ventricular cavity is near normal size in association with a large VSD. In such cases, there may be mitral valve atresia or a normal mitral valve. In cases of a normal mitral valve, the malformation does not represent hypoplastic left heart physiology, because such patients can undergo two-ventricle repair (see Special Situations and Controversies).

When aortic stenosis rather than atresia is present, the left ventricle tends to be larger than the typically minute, slitlike left ventricle of aortic atresia. Its size may vary widely from extremely hypoplastic with hypertrophic muscle and severe endocardial fibroelastosis to a dilated, thin-walled, poorly functioning chamber. The mitral valve is almost always hypoplastic and may be atretic when severe aortic stenosis is present.

Right Ventricle

The right ventricle is enlarged, with uniform hypertrophy and a marked increase in cavity size (to approximately three times normal).[H2,V1] Both tricuspid and pulmonary valves are larger

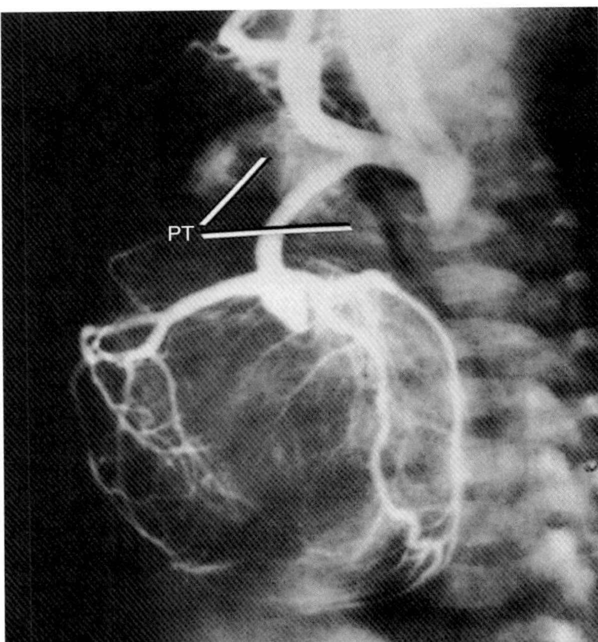

Figure 49-2 Lateral cineangiogram obtained after pressure injection of contrast medium into a brachial artery cannula in a neonate with hypoplastic left heart physiology. (This resulted in marked bradycardia and hypotension and is *not* a recommended technique.) Size of blind ascending aorta, which supplies large coronary arteries, and larger aortic arch and its branches are displayed. Pulmonary trunk *(PT)* is faintly outlined by contrast medium reaching it through the ductus arteriosus.

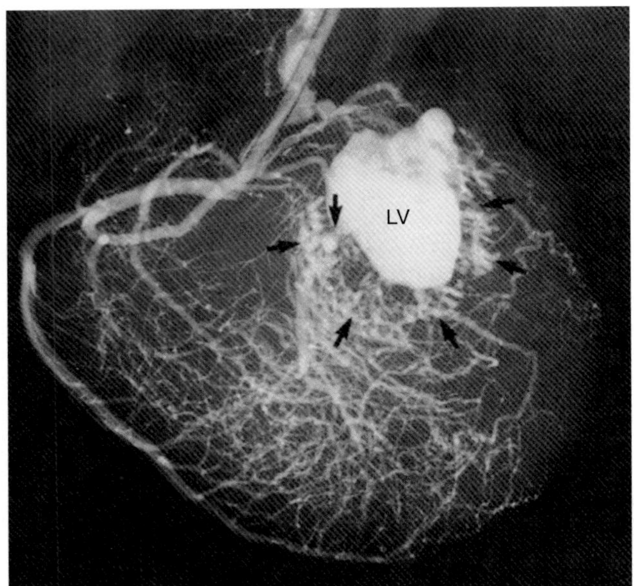

Figure 49-3 Postmortem coronary angiogram obtained by cannulating and injecting contrast medium into a coronary artery ostium in a heart with aortic atresia and hypoplastic left heart physiology. Small left ventricular *(LV)* cavity filled rapidly as contrast medium reached it through numerous coronary-LV connections. These form a prominent network within the thickened LV myocardium *(arrows)*.

than normal, and tricuspid regurgitation of variable degree is common.

Pulmonary Arteries

The pulmonary trunk is large and continues directly into the large patent ductus arteriosus. The right and left branches arise relatively posteriorly and at right angles from the short pulmonary trunk.

Atria and Atrial Septum

The left atrium is relatively small and thick walled, with its long axis directed transversely toward the right atrium. The atrial septum is also thick, making balloon atrial septostomy generally unsatisfactory.[B12,L4] An atrial communication is usually present; in the great majority of cases, this communication is a stretched patent foramen ovale. The septum primum is thickened and stretched so that it herniates into the right atrium and allows left-to-right shunting (see Fig. 49-1, *B*). There may be an aneurysm of the septum primum projecting to the right. The right atrium is larger than normal, with uniform hypertrophy of its walls. When the atrial septum is intact or severely restrictive in association with mitral or aortic atresia or both, there is pulmonary venous hypertension and a variable degree of decompression of pulmonary venous return through connections to the systemic venous system. Pulmonary venous hypertension usually begins in fetal life. This may have important implications for fetal lung development. Dilated pulmonary lymphatic channels form, and these can have an important effect on postnatal lung physiology and surgical outcome.[G9,V4]

Other Associated Cardiac Anomalies

Associated anomalies are uncommon.[F5,M2] Structural abnormalities of the tricuspid and pulmonary valves are rare. Bicuspid pulmonary valve has been described in 4% of specimens; cleft tricuspid valve, tricuspid valve dysplasia, and double orifice tricuspid valve have also been reported.[H3] Other unusual cardiac anomalies include intact atrial septum, total anomalous pulmonary venous connection, levoatrial cardinal vein, coronary sinus atresia, atretic pulmonary veins, complete atrioventricular septal defect, transposition of the great arteries, and interrupted aortic arch.[B2,J3,M6,S7,S15] Coronary artery abnormalities are rare except in patients with aortic atresia and mitral stenosis, in which they occur in approximately 50% of cases.[B3,S4]

Associated Noncardiac Anomalies

Other abnormalities unrelated to the cardiovascular system are found frequently with hypoplastic left heart physiology. Chromosomal abnormalities, genetic defects, and major extracardiac structural malformations, including central nervous system abnormalities, occur in 28% to 40% of patients.[B13,G10,N2]

CLINICAL FEATURES AND DIAGNOSTIC CRITERIA

Presentation is in the newborn period, with mild cyanosis, respiratory distress, and tachycardia. If supportive measures are not undertaken, there can be rapid deterioration, heart failure, and death due to a combination of pulmonary overcirculation and systemic obstruction from ductal closure. Ductal closure is almost inevitable, but its timing varies from

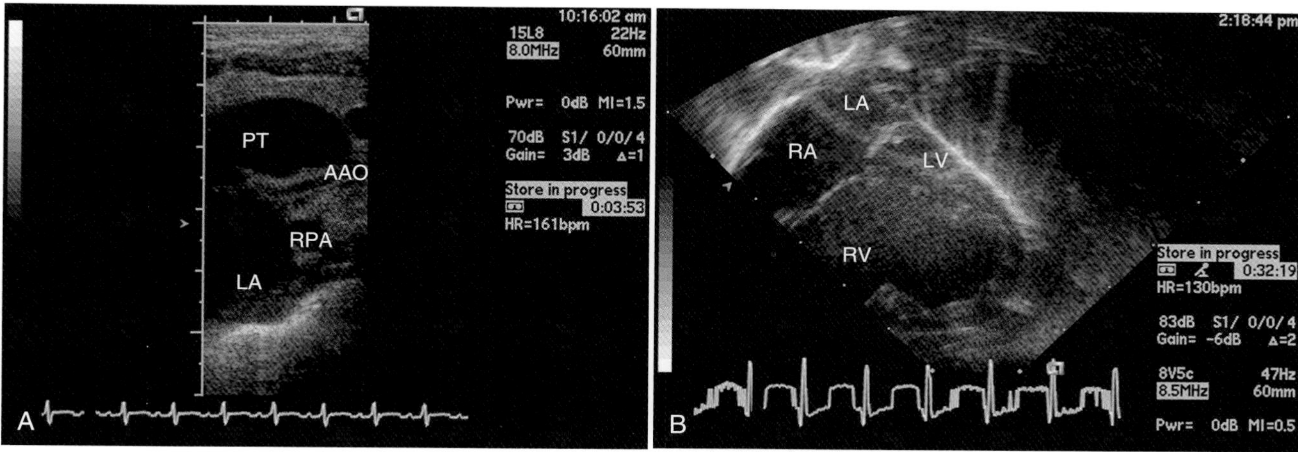

Figure 49-4 Echocardiographic findings in hypoplastic left heart physiology. **A,** Parasternal long-axis view of neonate with aortic atresia, severely hypoplastic ascending aorta *(AAO)*, severely hypoplastic left ventricle, and mitral atresia. In this image, the 1.5-mm-diameter ascending aorta is shown longitudinally. The large pulmonary trunk *(PT)* is also shown. Right pulmonary artery *(RPA)* is visible in cross-section posterior to small ascending aorta. Left atrium *(LA)* is present in this image, but ventricular mass is not shown. **B,** Subcostal image showing four-chamber view of neonate with aortic atresia and mitral atresia, with severely hypoplastic left ventricle *(LV)*. Right atrium *(RA)* and right ventricle *(RV)* are visualized and are markedly enlarged. LA is small, and LV cavity is miniscule. There is no direct communication between LA and hypoplastic LV. Ascending aorta and pulmonary trunk are not visualized in this image.

hours to weeks. This event is followed by rapid circulatory collapse.

On examination, there is a hyperactive right ventricular precordial impulse and a moderate-intensity midsystolic murmur along the left sternal border. The second heart sound is accentuated and single. Heart failure is associated with rales and liver enlargement. In many instances, peripheral pulses and perfusion are poor and blood pressure is low.

The chest radiograph shows moderate cardiomegaly and pulmonary plethora secondary to increased pulmonary blood flow. The electrocardiogram demonstrates right axis deviation and right ventricular hypertrophy and usually no left ventricular forces. However, left ventricular voltages can be present but do not necessarily signify an adequate left ventricular cavity.[F4]

Two-dimensional echocardiography is diagnostic and usually definitive. It demonstrates the large right ventricle, tricuspid valve, and ductus arteriosus and the small or absent left ventricle, aortic and mitral valves, and ascending aorta[M9] (Fig. 49-4). Status of the atrial septum is also easily determined. Doppler color flow signals indicate retrograde flow in the aortic arch and ascending aorta in cases of aortic atresia. Antegrade flow in the ascending aorta in the setting of aortic atresia strongly suggests that left ventricle–to–coronary artery fistulae are present, with left ventricular blood flowing retrograde in the coronary arteries and into the ascending aorta. When the aortic valve is not atretic, forward flow from the left ventricle across the aortic valve is normal. The amount of flow varies widely and may reach as far as the aortic arch. If Doppler color flow indicates substantial forward flow to the level of the arch or bidirectional flow in the patent ductus arteriosus, the patient should be considered to have borderline hypoplastic left heart physiology (see Special Situations and Controversies).

Cardiac catheterization is rarely indicated if it is clear by echocardiographic evaluation that the patient has unequivocal hypoplastic left heart physiology. However, in borderline hypoplastic left heart physiology, cardiac catheterization is often indicated to further characterize the physiology, especially mitral valve gradient and left ventricular end-diastolic pressure. The physiologic information obtained may help determine whether two-ventricle reconstruction is advisable. Catheterization is also indicated when a severely restrictive or intact atrial septum is present, resulting in pulmonary venous hypertension.

Rather than urgently bringing an hours-old infant to surgery under unstable conditions, the atrial septum can be opened by various interventional techniques (e.g., balloon dilatation, blade septostomy, atrial septal puncture with dilatation).

At this writing, computed tomography (CT) and magnetic resonance imaging (MRI) have a limited role in neonates with hypoplastic left heart physiology. CT angiography, however, may play an important role in follow-up, providing precise anatomic detail of aortic arch and pulmonary artery growth and development (Fig. 49-5). MRI can provide quantitative analysis of neoaortic and tricuspid valve regurgitation, and may be helpful in assessing left ventricular size in neonates with borderline left heart physiology in whom two-ventricle reconstruction is being contemplated.[D5]

NATURAL HISTORY

Various morphologic forms of hypoplastic left heart physiology constitute the fourth most common congenital cardiac defect.[F5] About 70% of cases are boys.[N9,R7] Severe heart failure usually develops in the first week of life. Many neonates die within 1 to 2 weeks of birth; only 40% survive the neonatal period, and survival beyond 6 weeks of age is uncommon[B15,F5,L2,R2] (Fig. 49-6). Hypoplastic left heart physiology accounts for 25% of cardiac deaths during the first week of life and 15% of those in the first month of life.[F5,N4]

The ductus arteriosus typically begins to close shortly after birth. In some infants, ductal closure leads to restriction of systemic perfusion, metabolic acidosis, and circulatory

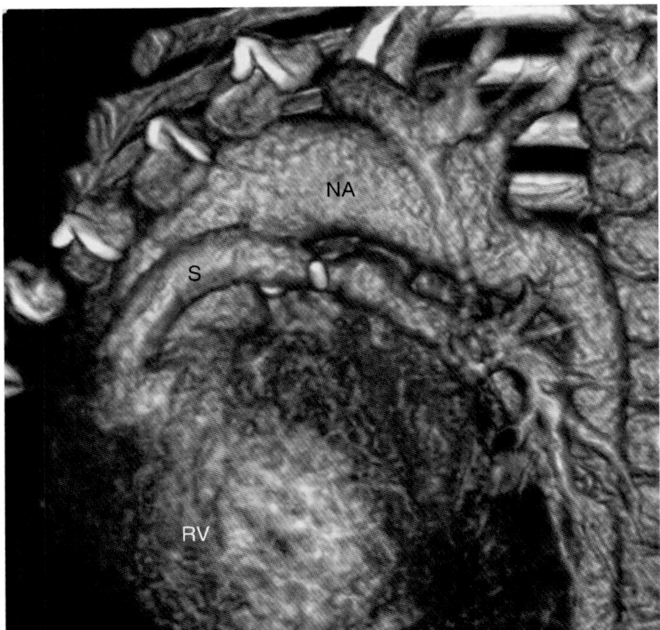

Figure 49-5 Volume-rendered image from a cardiac gated computed tomography angiogram of a 4-month-old boy born with hypoplastic left heart physiology who had undergone a Norwood first-stage repair. A neoaorta *(NA)* is constructed from native pulmonary trunk and connected to descending aorta without obstruction or distortion. Pulmonary circulation is provided through a right ventricular *(RV)*-to–pulmonary trunk small conduit *(S)*. There is mild narrowing in distal conduit as it enters pulmonary trunk.

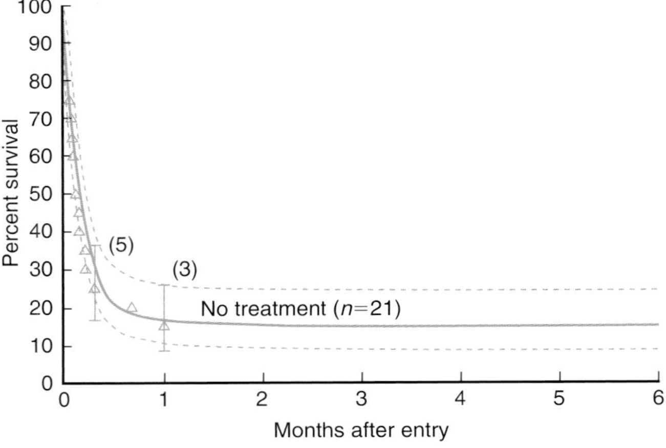

Figure 49-6 Survival of neonates with hypoplastic left heart physiology undergoing no treatment. Each symbol represents a death, positioned at the time of death along the horizontal axis and actuarially along the vertical axis. Vertical bars depict confidence limits equivalent to ±1 standard error. Numbers indicate the number of patients remaining at risk at the time of estimate. Solid lines are parametric estimates of survival, and dashed lines enclose 70% confidence limits. (Modified from Jacobs and colleagues.[J2])

collapse; and death. If the ductus continues to remain patent, a progressive increase in pulmonary circulation and a subsequent decrease in systemic circulation lead to pulmonary edema, coronary hypoperfusion, generalized systemic hypoperfusion, and ultimately death. Rarely, long-term survival will occur if the ductus remains patent and pulmonary vascular resistance (Rp) fails to fall in the perinatal and neonatal period.

TECHNIQUE OF OPERATION

There are two basic surgical options—*reconstruction* and *cardiac transplantation*—for treating hypoplastic left heart physiology. Reconstructive surgery includes the Norwood procedure and its variants, and the hybrid procedure. In a recent survey of practices related to this condition, 86% of 52 institutions recommend as primary treatment the Norwood procedure or one of its variants, and 14% did not make a recommendation, but left the decision solely up to the parents. No institution recommended primary transplantation, the hybrid procedure, or comfort care.[W2]

Reconstructive Surgery

The overall goal of reconstructive surgery is similar to that for any patient with single-ventricle physiology (see Chapter 41)—that is, establishing in the neonatal period an effective mixed circulation in which pulmonary ($\dot{Q}p$) and systemic ($\dot{Q}s$) blood flow are well balanced, followed by one or more operations performed later in infancy or early childhood after Rp has dropped to normal postnatal levels. The purpose of subsequent operations performed outside the neonatal period is to move away from the inefficiency of the completely mixed circulatory state. It should be emphasized that all definitive repairs in hypoplastic left heart physiology are palliative.

The exact form of definitive repair may vary from patient to patient based on the individual's physiologic status. Given the inherently limited reserve of the single right ventricle, it is generally agreed that a completely mixed circulatory state, even one that provides ideal balance between $\dot{Q}p$ and $\dot{Q}s$, is not an acceptable definitive state for hypoplastic left heart physiology. Acceptable definitive repairs include the completed Fontan procedure, the Fontan procedure with fenestration, superior cavopulmonary anastomosis, and superior cavopulmonary anastomosis with additional limited systemic to pulmonary blood flow.

Regardless of the definitive repair, principles of initial surgical management are generally agreed upon. Some variation of the Norwood procedure is considered optimal initial therapy. Its purpose is to provide (1) a completely unobstructed systemic arterial pathway from the right ventricle to all organs, (2) a restrictive connection between the systemic and pulmonary circulations such that $\dot{Q}p$ and $\dot{Q}s$ are adequately balanced, and (3) unobstructed flow of pulmonary venous return across the atrial septum to the right atrium.

Preoperative Management

Perinatal preoperative management is critical to successful outcome. This may include prenatal transport of the mother and fetus to a cardiac center following fetal diagnosis.[C5,J3] Circulatory collapse is usually the result of closure of the ductus arteriosus in the setting of undiagnosed hypoplastic left heart physiology. This may occur when the infant is still in hospital following birth, or after discharge home. If prenatal diagnosis is made and mother and fetus are transferred to an appropriate facility where the infant will undergo surgery, circulatory collapse is all but eliminated.

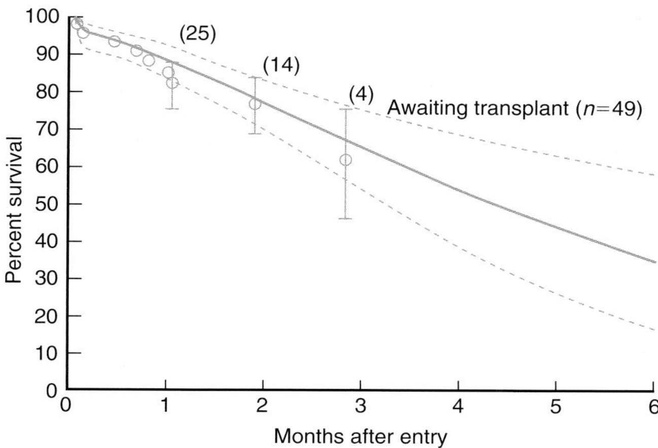

Figure 49-7 Survival of neonates with optimal medical treatment. Format of figure is as in Fig. 49-6. Although estimates represent survival before transplantation, similar survival is achieved with optimal medical treatment prior to reconstruction. (Modified from Jacobs and colleagues.[J2])

After diagnosis, the infant is resuscitated, and prostaglandin E_1 (PGE_1) therapy is initiated.[Y1] Depending on details of the physiologic status of the infant and stability of the infant at initial diagnosis, subsequent preoperative management may vary from essentially no further intervention on the one hand, to maximal intervention on the other. The typical patient, however, shows signs of pulmonary overcirculation, and preoperative management is aimed at reversing or at least controlling this to preserve end-organ and myocardial function.

Supportive therapy in the perinatal and neonatal periods can substantially alter natural history. Judicious use of inotropic support, PGE_1 therapy, nutritional supplementation, and ventilation with 17% or 19% oxygen along with supplemental CO_2 administration may delay the typical physiologic decompensation for a number of weeks[J2] (Fig. 49-7). When indicated, mechanical ventilation can add an extra measure of support. In many cases, the respiratory depression side effect of PGE_1 therapy may warrant mechanical ventilation.

These maneuvers are aimed at achieving a balance of $\dot{Q}p$ and $\dot{Q}s$ and maintaining unobstructed and adequate systemic perfusion. Because flow into the pulmonary circuit is unobstructed, Rp at the microvascular level will determine $\dot{Q}p$. Any maneuver that causes dilatation of the pulmonary microvasculature will result in excessive $\dot{Q}p$. Specifically, avoiding supplemental inspired oxygen is critical to the overall strategy; 21% oxygen or even lower F_{IO_2} helps maintain tone in the pulmonary microvasculature. If this maneuver is not adequate, controlled ventilation through an endotracheal tube achieves moderate elevation of Pa_{CO_2}, causing acidosis, which further constricts pulmonary microvasculature. PGE_1 maintains ductal patency, ensuring unobstructed blood flow to the systemic circulation.

Inotropic agents can be used to enhance cardiac output in the setting of moderate pulmonary overcirculation, but this strategy must be undertaken cautiously because these agents also affect systemic and pulmonary vascular resistances and may unpredictably alter $\dot{Q}p/\dot{Q}s$. Epinephrine and high-dose dopamine, which profoundly increase systemic vascular resistance, should be avoided (see Section IV of Chapter 4). Low- to moderate-dose dopamine and dobutamine should be considered the first-line inotropic agents when supplemental cardiac output is considered necessary.

All these maneuvers are used to create optimal preoperative cardiopulmonary status. Assessing cardiopulmonary status is somewhat indirect. Currently, $\dot{Q}p$ and $\dot{Q}s$ cannot be easily directly measured in the cardiac intensive care unit (ICU). Indirect measures of adequate systemic output include normal peripheral perfusion, adequate urine output, and absence of metabolic acidosis. Evidence of a reasonable balance of $\dot{Q}p$ and $\dot{Q}s$ includes a Pa_{O_2} of about 40 mmHg (Torr) and a systemic diastolic blood pressure greater than 30 mmHg. Even these ideal values do not guarantee that the expected blood flow values in fact do exist. For example, Pa_{O_2} can be influenced by other factors: hemoglobin level, metabolic state, temperature, and presence of sepsis to name a few. Furthermore, the inevitable reduction in Rp that occurs over time commonly thwarts all efforts to maintain systemic output and balanced $\dot{Q}p$ and $\dot{Q}s$. If this occurs, operation should be scheduled immediately.

For the typical neonate diagnosed early after birth and in whom circulatory collapse has not occurred, the ideal time for surgical intervention is about age 2 to 5 days. In this window of time, the infant completes the profound physiologic changes from fetal life to independent life, yet consequences of a continuously increasing $\dot{Q}p$ have not yet taken their toll. If circulatory collapse does occur and end-organ damage results, a longer time before operation is often necessary to allow end-organ recovery.

Although not always advisable, ideally, normal function of renal, hepatic, neurologic, gastrointestinal, and cardiopulmonary systems should be documented following resuscitation prior to proceeding with operation. It is not uncommon for organ systems to recover fairly rapidly but then plateau short of complete recovery. Further delay of operation at that point is usually detrimental.

Although mild obstruction of flow across the atrial septum is typical at the time of Doppler color flow interrogation during diagnostic echocardiography, severe obstruction at the atrial septum may occur, resulting in a clinical presentation similar to that found with obstructive total anomalous pulmonary venous connection (see Chapter 31), with deep cyanosis, pulmonary edema, and eventual hemodynamic instability. This presentation evolves rapidly immediately after birth and must be addressed within hours. Such patients are best managed with percutaneous interventional techniques to create an adequate atrial septal opening, followed by several days of stabilization before proceeding with operation. Management as described earlier continues during transport to the operating room and during surgery until CPB is instituted. The operation can be performed using continuous CPB by way of antegrade cerebral perfusion or using hypothermic circulatory arrest, according to choice of the operating surgeon. Both techniques are described in text that follows.

Neurologic development following operations for hypoplastic left heart physiology is below normal. Although impaired neurologic development is multifactorial, there is little question that circulatory arrest is contributory. Antegrade cerebral perfusion provides the advantage of continuous blood flow and oxygenation to the brain; however, it is possible that this technique also introduces new risks. It is unlikely that techniques of reconstruction that avoid circulatory arrest will result in dramatic changes in short-term survival, because factors related to hypothermia, CPB itself, and myocardial ischemia are not avoided. Long-term benefits related to neurologic development may exist but are yet to be proven.

Norwood Procedure Using Continuous Perfusion

Although several techniques for accomplishing the Norwood procedure using continuous perfusion have been described,[A3,T3] the one presented has been used routinely since 1997 by one of the authors (FLH), with some modifications.[M4,R5]

After median sternotomy, the thymus is subtotally removed and the anterior pericardium opened widely. Aortic arch vessels are dissected well above the brachiocephalic vein. The small aorta is separated from the pulmonary trunk and right pulmonary artery, and the ductus arteriosus, aortic arch, and proximal descending thoracic aorta are dissected.

Marking 7-0 monofilament sutures are placed on adjacent portions of the pulmonary trunk and ascending aorta to indicate the point of eventual pulmonary trunk–to-aorta anastomosis. Positions of these marking sutures are chosen with great care because they will determine the correct orientation of, and incisions in, the aorta and pulmonary trunk necessary to create a functional anastomosis; alignment of this anastomosis is critical for unobstructed coronary blood flow in aortic atresia. The first marking suture is placed in the adventitia of the pulmonary trunk 1 to 2 mm above the sinutubular junction and circumferentially exactly where the small ascending aorta lies against it. The second suture on the aortic adventitia is placed so that its position coincides exactly with the pulmonary trunk suture.

A purse-string suture is placed on the brachiocephalic artery about 5 mm distal to the takeoff of the artery from the arch. It is often necessary to place it above the brachiocephalic vein. Purse-string sutures are placed on the superior and inferior venae cavae. A 5-0 monofilament suture is placed around the pulmonary artery end of the ductus arteriosus.

An 8F (or in patients weighing <3 kg, 6F) arterial cannula is inserted into the brachiocephalic artery, and angled 12F venous cannulae are placed into the venae cavae. Alternatively, a single venous cannula can be used, placed in the right atrial appendage (Fig. 49-8, *A*). Brachiocephalic artery cannulation must be performed accurately; however, experience shows that it can be routinely performed successfully even in patients weighing 3.0 kg or less. Cannulation is best performed by puncturing the artery without using a clamp, and inserting the tip of the cannula to a depth less than the width of the artery, typically 2 to 3 mm.

After venous cannulation and institution of CPB, the ductus arteriosus is immediately ligated (see Fig. 49-8, *A*). Core temperature is reduced to 20°C. During cooling, the pulmonary trunk is transected just above the pulmonary valve in standard fashion (Fig. 49-8, *B*). The distal opening in the pulmonary trunk is then closed directly or patched with an oval piece of pulmonary allograft or other material (see Fig. 49-8, *B*). A clamp is placed across the ascending aorta just proximal to the brachiocephalic artery once the target core temperature has been achieved. Cardioplegia is introduced into the ascending aorta. The ascending aorta is then opened to the level of the transected pulmonary trunk, and the side-to-side anastomosis between proximal pulmonary trunk and ascending aorta is accomplished with interrupted 6-0 or 7-0 monofilament sutures (Fig. 49-8, *C*).

In preparation for arch reconstruction, direct CPB flow is isolated to the brachiocephalic artery only. This is accomplished by clamping the base of the brachiocephalic, left carotid, and left subclavian arteries individually with delicate neurovascular clips, and placing a C-shaped clamp across the descending thoracic aorta approximately 1.5 to 2 cm below the ductal insertion (Fig. 49-8, *D*). Perfusion, now through the distal brachiocephalic artery only, is reduced to 30 to 40 mL · kg^{-1} · min^{-1}, allowing normal brain perfusion.

The original clamp placed across the ascending aorta is removed. The ductus is divided distal to the previously placed suture. The previous incision in the ascending aorta is then continued around the arch, then beyond the ductus, approximately 1.5 cm onto the descending aorta. Ductal tissue is trimmed, and allograft patch reconstruction of the aortic arch, ascending aorta, and pulmonary trunk is performed. The caval cannulae are snared. A right atriotomy is made, and the septum primum is completely removed to create a nonrestrictive interatrial communication. The right atriotomy is closed, and the neurovascular clips on the base of the brachiocephalic artery and the C-clamp on the descending aorta are removed. Total body perfusion is reestablished and increased to normal levels; rewarming is begun.

The last step in the operation is creating a source of pulmonary blood flow. At the choice of the operating surgeon, this can be achieved using either a restrictive systemic arterial–to–pulmonary arterial shunt or a restrictive right ventricular–to–pulmonary arterial conduit. If a shunt is chosen, typically a polytetrafluoroethylene (PTFE) interposition graft is sewn into place from the junction of the brachiocephalic and right subclavian arteries to the proximal portion of the right pulmonary artery (Fig. 49-8, *E*). Both anastomoses are performed using end graft–to–side artery connections with running 7-0 monofilament or PTFE suture. Variation in positioning the PTFE shunt must be considered based on individual patient characteristics to achieve an appropriate balance of $\dot{Q}p$ and $\dot{Q}s$.

In patients weighing less than 3 kg and in those demonstrating very low Rp preoperatively, it may be necessary to perform the systemic connection of the shunt anastomosis at a more distal site on the right subclavian artery. In most cases, a 3.5-mm-diameter PTFE tube graft is used for the shunt procedure; rarely is a larger diameter necessary. Often in patients weighing less than 3 kg, and most frequently in patients weighing less than 2.5 kg, a 3.0-mm-diameter graft should be considered, although risk of shunt thrombosis may increase with a small-diameter shunt. If the right ventricular–to–pulmonary arterial conduit is performed, a PTFE graft of appropriate diameter is chosen. Alternatively, a composite graft consisting of a proximally positioned PTFE tube and a distally positioned small (6- to 7-mm diameter) allograft pulmonary or aortic valve can be used (Fig. 49-8, *F* and *G*).[R5] Regardless of whether a simple conduit or composite conduit is chosen, the diameter of the PTFE tube determines the resistance to flow into the pulmonary arteries. Typically, a 4-mm-diameter graft is used for patients weighing less than 3 kg, a 5-mm-diameter graft for those between 3 and 4 kg, and a 6-mm-diameter graft for those greater than 4 kg.

An incision is made in the infundibular portion of the right ventricle, just below the pulmonary valve. A 5- to 6-mm-diameter circular full-thickness resection of infundibular muscle is then made. It is extremely important that

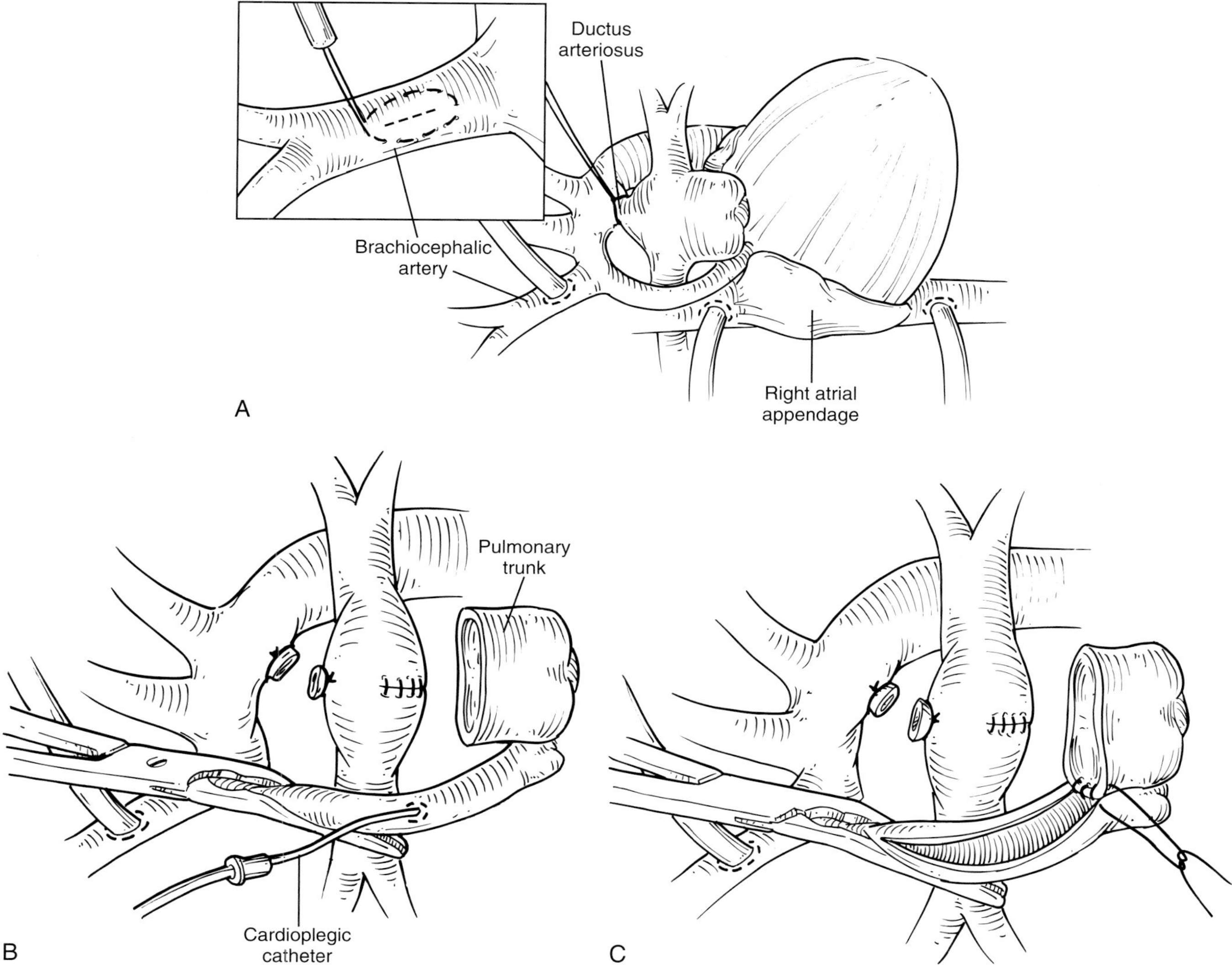

Figure 49-8 Norwood procedure using continuous perfusion. **A,** A 6F or 8F arterial cannula is placed directly into base of brachiocephalic artery for systemic perfusion. Venous cannulation is through the venae cavae. Because of small diameter of the brachiocephalic artery, accuracy is required during this cannulation. Specifically, cannula must not be positioned so deep into the lumen that inflow obstruction occurs because tip of cannula is against back wall of artery. Also, cannula cannot be advanced into proximal or distal artery; such a maneuver increases the chance of unbalanced perfusion. Once perfusion is established, ductus arteriosus is doubly ligated and divided. **B,** During core cooling on cardiopulmonary bypass, pulmonary trunk is transected above sinutubular junction. Distal pulmonary trunk is closed primarily with a running monofilament absorbable 7-0 suture. Once target core temperature is reached, aorta is clamped just proximal to brachiocephalic artery, and cardioplegia is introduced into ascending aorta. **C,** Proximal ascending aorta is then incised down to proximal aorta marking suture, and the side-to-side connection between proximal pulmonary trunk and ascending aorta is accomplished with interrupted 7-0 monofilament suture in standard fashion, paying careful attention to previously placed marking sutures on proximal aorta and proximal pulmonary trunk.

Continued

the caliber of the resulting hole in the infundibulum is maintained transmurally to prevent premature stenosis at this level postoperatively. Using a running 7-0 monofilament suture, the graft is first sewn end to side to the pulmonary trunk, either to the pulmonary artery directly adjacent to the suture line that previously closed the distal pulmonary trunk, or to the center of the patch that was used to close the distal pulmonary trunk. The graft is then positioned to the left of the reconstructed aorta and tailored in length to reach the infundibulotomy. The proximal end of the graft is carefully beveled to the appropriate angle to ensure a smooth course around the large reconstructed aorta. The anastomosis is performed using a running 6-0 monofilament suture.

Once normothermia is achieved, the patient is separated from CPB and decannulated. Management following separation from CPB is described under "Post–Cardiopulmonary Bypass Management" later in this chapter.

Norwood Procedure Using Hypothermic Circulatory Arrest

The heart is exposed by median sternotomy, removal of most of the thymus gland, and opening of the pericardium. If the patient is unstable at this point because of increased $\dot{Q}p$, the right pulmonary artery can be exposed immediately and clamped to reduce overall $\dot{Q}p$ and maintain systemic circulation until CPB is established.

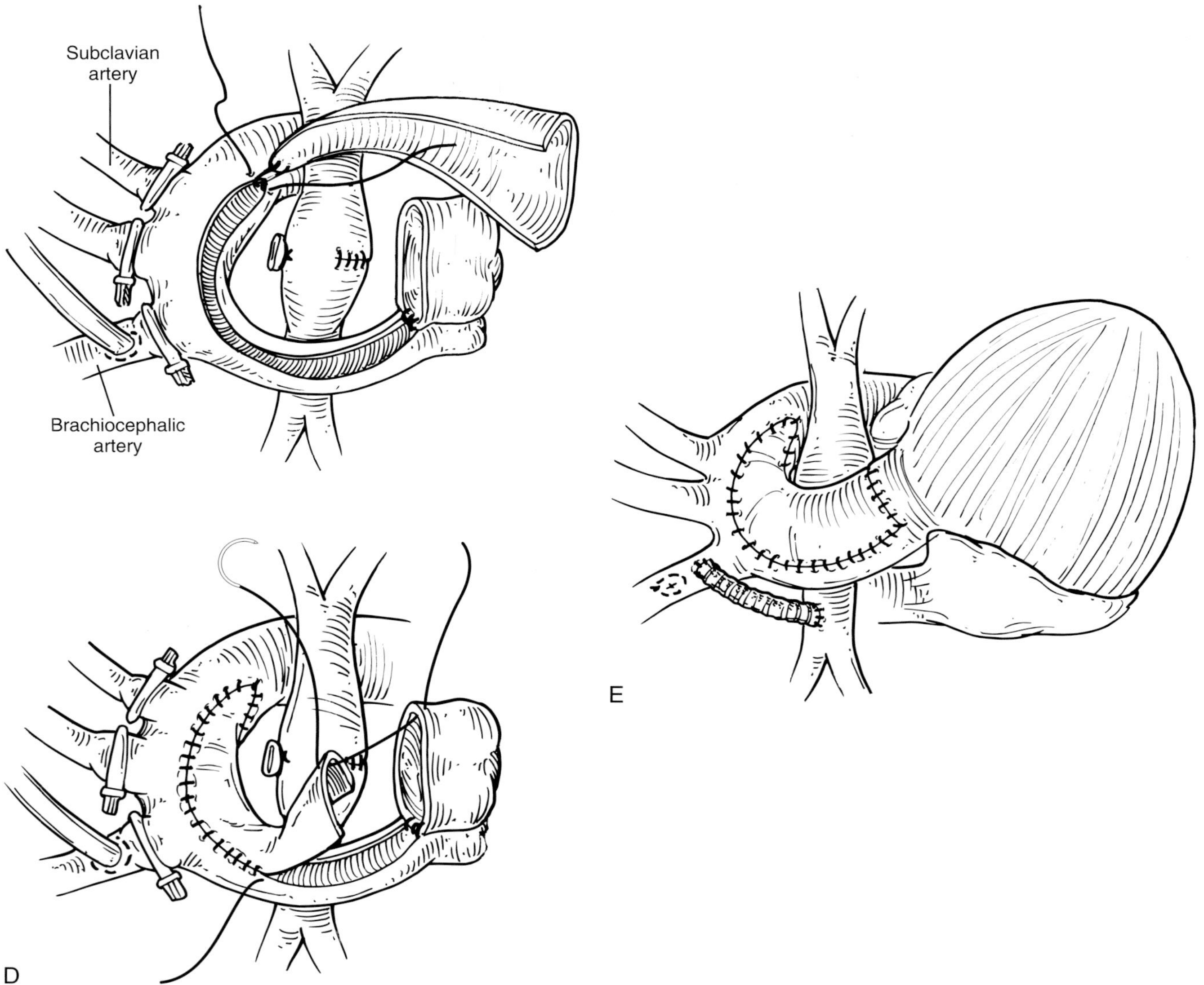

Figure 49-8, cont'd **D,** Small neurovascular clips are placed individually at the bases of brachiocephalic, left carotid, and left subclavian arteries. Additionally, not shown in figure, a clamp is placed on descending aorta beyond ductus arteriosus. Previously created proximal ascending aortic incision is then extended distally around the arch beyond the ductal insertion site, approximately 10 mm onto descending aorta. Aorta is then reconstructed with an allograft patch, beginning distally at end of aortic incision on descending aorta, with posterior suture line followed by anterior suture line, and completing the reconstruction by suturing proximal end of patch around the cut edge of proximal pulmonary trunk. Once aortic reconstruction is completed, vascular clamps are removed, full body perfusion reestablished, and rewarming commenced. **E,** Completed aortic arch reconstruction. To complete the procedure using a systemic-to-pulmonary shunt, an appropriately sized tube of expanded polytetrafluoroethylene (PTFE) is chosen and connected from systemic circulation into pulmonary circulation. Brachiocephalic artery and its branches and right pulmonary artery must be controlled with side-biting vascular clamps.

The patient is prepared for CPB by placing a purse-string suture on the pulmonary trunk just distal to the pulmonary valve. A second purse-string suture is placed around the tip of the right atrial appendage. At that point, if the patient is physiologically stable, the pulmonary trunk is separated from the ascending aorta using either scissors or electrocautery. The ductus arteriosus, aortic arch, and arch vessels are then mobilized using scissors or electrocautery all the way to the first set of intercostal vessels on the descending aorta. Temporary snares are placed around all brachiocephalic arteries.

If the patient becomes physiologically unstable, CPB can be initiated at any time and the great vessel dissection performed with its support. CPB is established using an arterial cannula in the pulmonary trunk and a single venous cannula in the right atrial appendage (Fig. 49-9, *A*). At initiation of CPB, the branch pulmonary arteries are temporarily occluded with clamps or snares to eliminate pulmonary blood flow.

After initiating CPB, while the pulmonary trunk and aorta are still distended with blood, 7-0 monofilament sutures are placed on adjacent portions of the pulmonary trunk and ascending aorta to mark the point of eventual pulmonary trunk–to-aorta anastomosis. Positions of these marking sutures are chosen with great care because they will determine

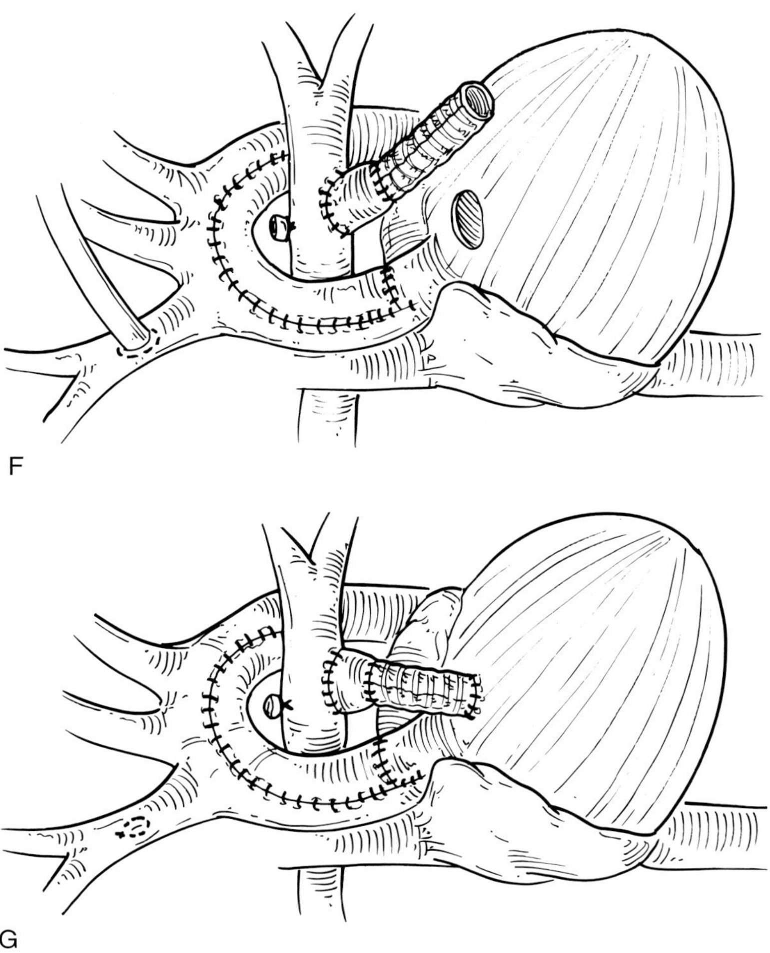

Figure 49-8, cont'd **F,** Completed aortic arch reconstruction. To complete the procedure using a right ventricle to pulmonary artery conduit, an appropriately sized tube of PTFE, or, as shown, composite of PTFE and valved allograft, is used. Prior to placing the conduit, the composite graft is constructed during the initial cooling phase of cardiopulmonary bypass. An aortic or pulmonary allograft valved conduit, either 6- or 7-mm diameter (or a 9- or 10-mm diameter allograft reduced to a bicuspid conduit) is connected end to end to a 3-cm length of PTFE graft. Valved conduit is placed distally within the composite, as shown. A 5- to 6-mm diameter core of infundibular free-wall myocardium is removed from right ventricle just below pulmonary valve. It is critical to remove a uniform full-thickness core of tissue rather than just incise the hypertrophied right ventricle; this prevents stenosis at the inlet to the conduit. Great care should be taken not to injure pulmonary valve or chordae of tricuspid valve (infundibular incision and tissue core removal can, if preferred, be performed before reperfusion of myocardium is initiated; this may provide more controlled conditions). Distal aspect of allograft conduit is connected end to side into transverse pulmonary artery centrally, either near the suture line that closed the distal pulmonary artery stoma created by previous pulmonary trunk transection, or into the patch used to close distal pulmonary artery stoma. This is accomplished with a running suture technique using 7-0 nonabsorbable monofilament suture. Pulmonary arteries are allowed to assume their natural position, and the PTFE proximal portion of the composite is tailored to appropriate length and beveled in preparation for proximal anastomosis of PTFE component to infundibulotomy site. **G,** Proximal anastomosis of conduit to infundibulotomy is performed with a running stitch using 6-0 nonabsorbable monofilament suture.

the correct orientation of, and incisions in, the aorta and pulmonary trunk necessary for creating a functional anastomosis; alignment of this anastomosis is critical for unobstructed coronary blood flow in aortic atresia. The first marking suture is placed in the adventitia of the pulmonary trunk 1 to 2 mm above the sinutubular junction and circumferentially exactly where the small ascending aorta lies against it. The second suture on the aortic adventitia is placed so that its position coincides exactly with the pulmonary trunk suture (see Fig. 49-9, *A*).

When the nasopharyngeal or tympanic membrane temperature reaches 16°C to 18°C after cooling with CPB for an appropriate period (see Section IV of Chapter 2), the snares around the brachiocephalic vessels are tightened and circulatory arrest established. Snares around the left and right pulmonary arteries are removed, and cannulae are removed from the pulmonary trunk and right atrial appendage after draining as much blood volume from the patient into the pump-oxygenator as possible.

Management of myocardial protection is variable. Some experienced centers use no specific cardioplegia and rely on profound hypothermia as the only form of myocardial management. Other experienced institutions use cardioplegia, which can be supplied in several ways. Cannulation of the ascending aorta can be achieved with an appropriately small needle and cardioplegia delivered directly into the aortic

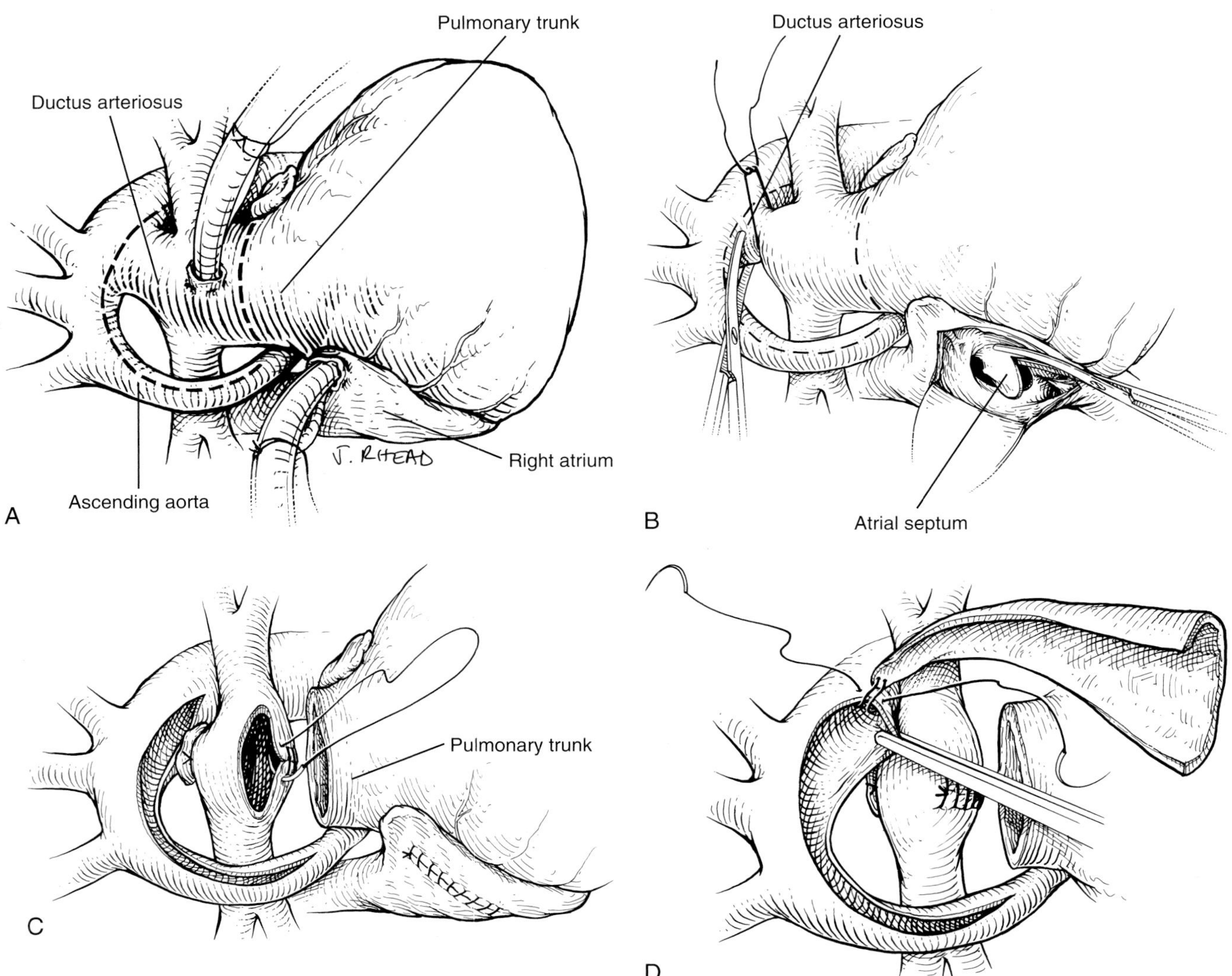

Figure 49-9 Norwood procedure using hypothermic circulatory arrest. **A,** Arterial cannula is placed into pulmonary trunk through a purse-string suture, and the single venous cannula is placed into right atrial appendage. Dashed line on proximal pulmonary trunk shows intended transection site, and dashed line on ascending aorta and aortic arch shows site and extent of intended aortic incision. Marking sutures are placed on pulmonary trunk and ascending aorta precisely where the two dashed lines in this figure converge. After these two marking sutures are placed, aorta and pulmonary trunk should be allowed to assume their natural positions. Under these conditions, examining the two marking sutures with the vessels in their distended state should reveal that these two sutures are touching each other, without even the slightest amount of circumferential or longitudinal offset. As soon as cardiopulmonary bypass (CPB) is instituted, left and right pulmonary arteries must be controlled with either snares or small vascular clamps (not shown in this figure). **B,** After target core temperature is reached, circulatory arrest is instituted and myocardial protection addressed; ductus arteriosus is ligated and transected as shown. It is common practice to temporarily occlude brachiocephalic, left carotid, and left subclavian arteries with snares or small vascular clamps before opening the aorta. Either at this point or following arch reconstruction, atrial septum must be resected. A limited right atriotomy is made and the septum primum identified and resected with scissors. Septum primum should be resected completely, but care taken not to overextend the resection into thickened portion of limbus or conduction area. Right atriotomy is then closed with a running monofilament suture. Dashed lines signify point of pulmonary trunk transection and extent of ascending arch and descending aortic incision. Note that the descending aortic incision extends approximately 5 to 10 mm beyond the ductal insertion site. **C,** Pulmonary trunk has been transected. There is often very little distance between top of pulmonary valve commissures and origin of right pulmonary artery. During pulmonary trunk transection, care should be taken not to injure the commissure of the pulmonary valve or extend incision into orifice of right pulmonary artery. Once transection is completed, the stoma in the distal pulmonary trunk is closed transversely as shown with a running 7-0 absorbable monofilament suture. Incision in aorta is also shown. Proximal extent of this incision is terminated precisely at previously placed marking suture. **D,** Before beginning arch augmentation, allograft patch is tailored to the size of the infant. Patch is roughly triangular in shape; base of triangle will ultimately be sutured to circumference of proximal pulmonary trunk, so width of base should roughly equal circumference of pulmonary trunk. Other two free edges of patch will be anastomosed to posterior and anterior free edges of incised aorta. The edge of the patch that will be sutured to posterior aspect of incised aorta should be shorter than edge that will be sutured to anterior free edge of aorta. If this is not the case, or if entire patch is too long, kinking of reconstruction can result. Also, apical half of the triangularly shaped patch should not be too broad. Patch is sewn into place beginning at most distal aspect of aortic incision, well beyond ductal insertion site. A running 7-0 monofilament nonabsorbable suture is used and posterior suture line is developed first, extending roughly to area opposite brachiocephalic artery origin. Following this, anterior suture line is developed in like fashion.

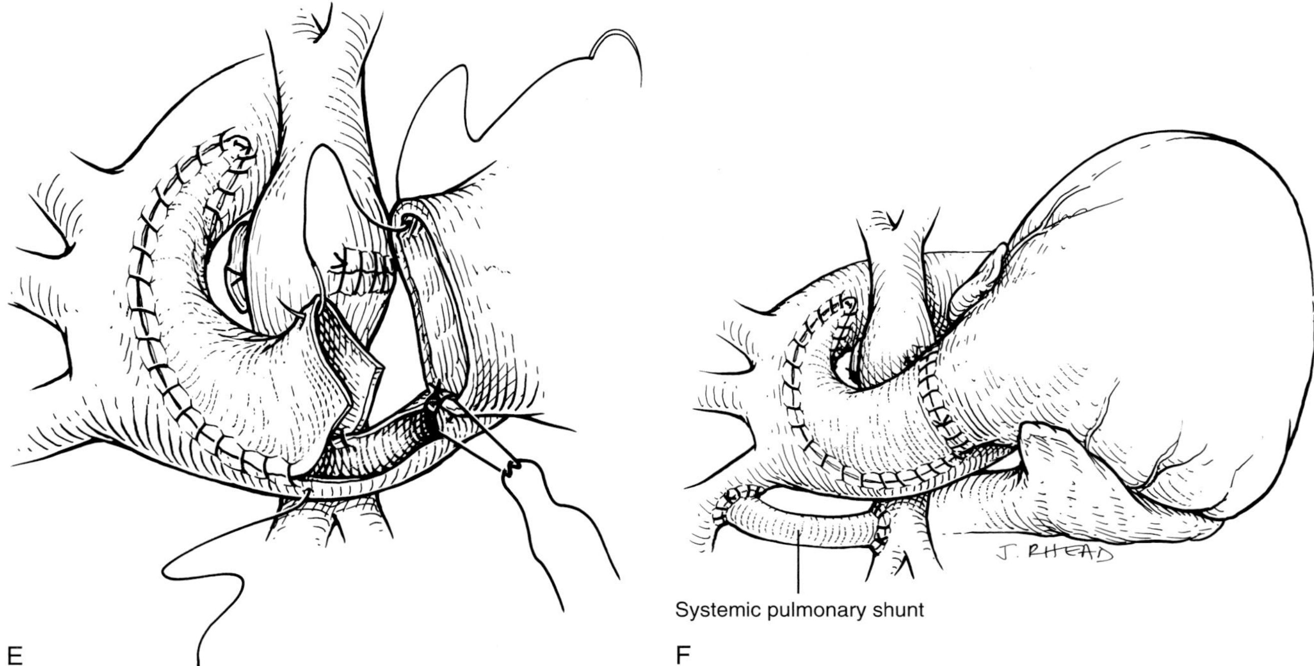

Figure 49-9, cont'd **E,** Distal aspect of patch suture line is completed. Attention is then turned to proximal aspect of aortic incision and to proximal pulmonary trunk. Interrupted 7-0 monofilament nonabsorbable sutures are placed to connect proximal ascending aorta to proximal pulmonary trunk. First suture in this series of five to seven interrupted sutures should be placed precisely at the points of the two previously placed marking sutures. Once this is completed, proximal end of patch is connected to circumference of proximal pulmonary trunk. Prior to final sutures being placed, a probe that can comfortably pass into proximal aorta to the level of coronary arteries is used to confirm patency and appropriate alignment of proximal aorta. **F,** Completed aortic arch reconstruction. To complete procedure using a systemic-to-pulmonary shunt, an appropriately sized tube of expanded polytetrafluoroethylene (PTFE) is chosen and connected from systemic circulation into pulmonary circulation. If shunt is placed during circulatory arrest, vascular clamps generally are not necessary. However, if shunt is placed after reestablishing CPB, brachiocephalic artery and its branches and right pulmonary artery must be controlled with side-biting vascular clamps.
Continued

root. Alternatively, the cardioplegia system can be connected to the arterial cannula in the pulmonary trunk, and cardioplegia delivered into this cannula after circulatory arrest has been established while the brachiocephalic vessel snares and pulmonary artery branch snares are still in place. The only additional maneuver before proceeding with cardioplegia delivery using this method is to clamp the descending aorta distal to the ductal insertion site. The cardioplegic solution is delivered through the arterial cannula into the pulmonary trunk through the ductus and retrograde around the arch to the coronary arteries. All other peripheral runoff through this circuit must be reliably eliminated (see "Methods of Myocardial Management during Cardiac Surgery" in Chapter 3).

After myocardial protection has been addressed and circulatory arrest established, the ductus arteriosus is ligated distal to the origin of the left pulmonary artery. A small atriotomy is made, and through it the entire septum primum is removed to create an unrestrictive intraatrial communication. To avoid conduction problems, care is taken not to extend the resection beyond the septum primum. The atriotomy is closed (Fig. 49-9, *B*).

The pulmonary trunk is divided transversely as proximal as possible without risking damage to the pulmonary valve, leaving the previously placed marking suture proximal to the transection. As the transection is made, particular care is taken to avoid the orifice of the right pulmonary artery. The distal end of the divided pulmonary trunk is then closed with a patch (typically autologous pericardium or pulmonary artery allograft) using continuous 7-0 polypropylene. Alternatively, the distal pulmonary trunk may be closed primarily in transverse fashion (Fig. 49-9, *C*). Direct closure has the advantages of time efficiency and less bulk, and in experienced hands has shown no greater tendency to result in pulmonary trunk stenosis than the patch technique.

The ductus is transected just beyond the previously placed ligature. Redundant ductal tissue is cut away from the distal aorta, leaving a small cuff of ductal tissue at the level of the aortic isthmus. A 5- to 10-mm incision is made from the ductal orifice into the descending aorta to the level of the first set of intercostal vessels (see Fig. 49-9, *C*). A proximal incision is made beginning at the ductal orifice and moving retrograde toward the aortic valve. This incision proceeds along the undersurface of the aortic arch and extends down the hypoplastic ascending aorta to within several millimeters of the atretic or hypoplastic aortic valve, terminating at the same level as the transected pulmonary trunk at the point of the previously placed marking suture (see Fig. 49-9, *C*).

The aorta is then augmented throughout its length from the level of the aortic valve around the arch, to the first set of intercostal vessels, using a patch of pulmonary or aortic allograft tissue (Fig. 49-9, *D*). The patch is tailored to provide adequate but not excessive widening of the aorta. Suturing is begun at the distal end of the incision beyond the isthmus on the upper descending aorta and progresses retrograde until the proximity of the brachiocephalic artery is reached.

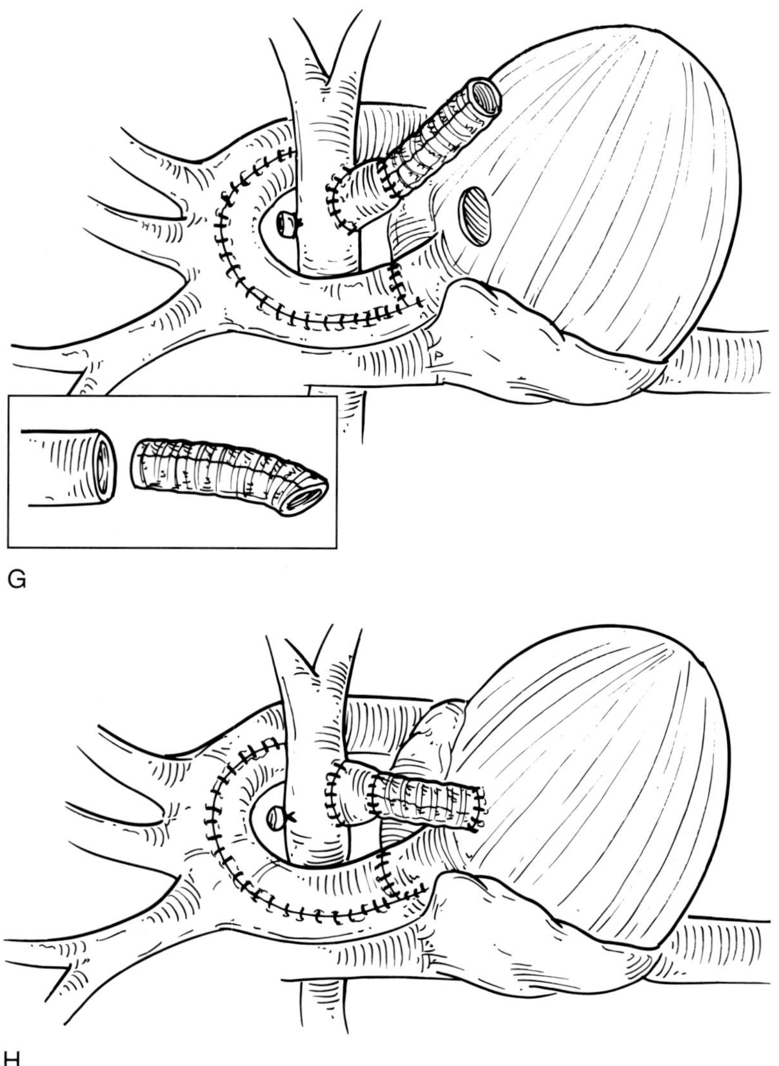

Figure 49-9, cont'd **G,** Completed aortic arch reconstruction. To complete procedure using a right ventricular–to–pulmonary artery conduit, an appropriately sized PTFE tube or, as shown, composite of PTFE and valved allograft is used. Before placing conduit, composite graft is constructed during initial cooling phase of CPB. An aortic or pulmonary allograft valved conduit, either 6- or 7-mm diameter (or a 9- or 10-mm-diameter allograft reduced to a bicuspid conduit) is connected end to end to a 3-cm length of PTFE graft. Valved conduit is placed distally within the composite, as shown. Next part of procedure can be performed either under circulatory arrest or after perfusion has been reestablished. A 5- to 6-mm-diameter core of infundibular free-wall myocardium is removed from right ventricle just below pulmonary valve. To prevent stenosis at the inlet to the conduit, it is critical to actually remove a uniform full-thickness core of tissue rather than just incise the hypertrophied right ventricle. Great care should be taken not to injure pulmonary valve or tricuspid valve chordae. Distal aspect of allograft conduit is connected end to side into transverse pulmonary artery centrally, either near suture line that closed the distal pulmonary artery stoma created by previous pulmonary trunk transaction, or into the patch used to close distal pulmonary artery stoma. This is accomplished with a running suture technique using 7-0 nonabsorbable monofilament suture. Pulmonary arteries are allowed to assume their natural position, and PTFE proximal portion of composite is tailored to appropriate length and beveled in preparation for proximal anastomosis of PTFE component to right ventriculotomy site. **H,** Proximal anastomosis of conduit to infundibulotomy is performed with a running stitch using 6-0 nonabsorbable monofilament suture.

The posterior suture line is developed first, using a running technique and 6-0 or 7-0 nonabsorbable monofilament suture, followed by the anterior suture line.

At this point, the allograft augmentation of the arch is temporarily set aside, and the proximal end of the divided pulmonary trunk is anastomosed side to side to the incised hypoplastic aorta (Fig. 49-9, *E*). This portion of the anastomosis is typically performed with five to seven interrupted 6-0 or 7-0 monofilament nonabsorbable sutures. The first of these connects the end of the aortic incision to the cut edge of the pulmonary trunk exactly where the previously placed marking suture was positioned. On each side of this interrupted suture, two to three other interrupted sutures are placed, attaching first the posterior and then the anterior edge of the longitudinally incised aorta to the circumference of the proximal pulmonary trunk. Care should be taken with small aortas (<3 mm diameter) not to connect them to too broad a segment of pulmonary trunk circumference, because this can stretch the aortic tissue and flatten and obstruct the orifice leading to the coronaries.

Finally, the allograft patch suture line progresses from the level of the brachiocephalic artery down to the aortic-to-pulmonary anastomosis and around the remaining free edge of the proximal pulmonary trunk (Fig. 49-9, *F*). This completes the right ventricular–to–systemic arterial outflow reconstruction.

The last step in the operation is creating a source of pulmonary blood flow. At the choice of the operating surgeon, this can be achieved using either a restrictive systemic arterial–to–pulmonary arterial shunt or a restrictive right ventricle–to–pulmonary arterial conduit. If a shunt is chosen, typically a PTFE interposition graft is sewn into place from the junction of the brachiocephalic and right subclavian arteries on the systemic side to the proximal portion of the right pulmonary artery (see Fig. 49-9, *F*). Both anastomoses are performed using end graft–to–side artery connections with running 7-0 monofilament or PTFE suture. Variation in positioning of the PTFE shunt must be considered, based on individual patient characteristics, to achieve an appropriate balance of $\dot{Q}p$ and $\dot{Q}s$.

In patients weighing less than 3 kg and in those demonstrating very low Rp preoperatively, it may be necessary to perform the systemic pulmonary arterial shunt anastomosis at a more distal site on the right subclavian artery. In most cases, a 3.5-mm-diameter PTFE tube graft is used for the shunt procedure; a larger diameter is rarely necessary. Often in patients weighing less than 3 kg and most frequently in patients weighing less than 2.5 kg, a 3.0-mm-diameter graft should be considered, although risk of shunt thrombosis may increase with a smaller-diameter shunt. If circulatory arrest is prolonged, or by surgeon preference, the shunt may be placed after reestablishing flow on CPB.

If a right ventricular–to–pulmonary arterial conduit is chosen, a PTFE graft of appropriate diameter is selected. Alternatively, a composite graft consisting of a proximally positioned PTFE tube and a distally positioned small (6- to 7-mm diameter) allograft pulmonary or aortic valve can be used[R5] (Fig. 49-9, *G* and *H*). Regardless of whether a simple conduit or composite conduit is chosen, the diameter of the PTFE tube determines the resistance to flow into the pulmonary arteries. Typically, a 4-mm-diameter graft is used for patients weighing less than 3 kg, a 5-mm-diameter graft for those between 3 and 4 kg, and a 6-mm-diameter graft for those greater than 4 kg.

An incision is made in the infundibular portion of the right ventricle, just below the pulmonary valve. A 5- to 6-mm-diameter circular full-thickness resection of infundibular muscle is then made. It is extremely important that the caliber of the resulting hole in the infundibulum is maintained transmurally to prevent premature stenosis at this level postoperatively. Using a running 7-0 monofilament suture, the graft is first sewn end to side to the pulmonary trunk, either to the pulmonary artery directly, adjacent to the suture line that previously closed the distal pulmonary trunk, or to the center of the patch that was used to close the distal pulmonary trunk. The graft is then positioned to the left of the reconstructed aorta and tailored in length to reach the infundibulotomy. The proximal end of the graft is carefully beveled to the appropriate angle to ensure a smooth course around the large reconstructed aorta.

The anastomosis is performed using a running 6-0 monofilament suture. The right atrial and systemic arterial cannulae are reinserted, CPB is reestablished, and rewarming begun. If a systemic-to-pulmonary shunt has been placed, it is occluded with a vascular clamp during the rewarming phase of CPB. When the patient's tympanic membrane or nasopharyngeal temperature reaches 25°C to 30°C, perfusate ionized calcium concentration is measured and calcium chloride added to bring the ionized calcium concentration to a normal level (see Section III of Chapter 2). Separation from CPB is accomplished and decannulation achieved. Details of post-CPB management follow.

Post–Cardiopulmonary Bypass Management

Whether the operation is performed using continuous perfusion or circulatory arrest, post-CPB management is generally the same. Before the patient is separated from CPB, inotropic support is initiated, and particular attention is given to complete reexpansion of both lungs. Endotracheal suctioning by the anesthesiologist is routine. If a systemic-to-pulmonary shunt was used, after complete rewarming has been achieved, approximately 5 minutes before discontinuing CPB, the clamp on the shunt is removed.

Careful attention is given to the mean arterial pressure on CPB at this point; typically a decrease of 10 to 15 mmHg should be expected, indicating adequate runoff into the pulmonary vascular bed. If this decrease is not observed, the cause must be identified. The systemic-to–pulmonary trunk shunt should be immediately assessed for obstruction due to a technical problem. If a right ventricle–to–pulmonary arterial conduit was used, diastolic blood pressure is not affected.

After rewarming has been completed, CPB is discontinued and the aortic and venous cannulae removed. Postoperative care begins immediately (see Special Features of Postoperative Care later in this chapter). Two separate polyvinyl catheters (or a single double-lumen catheter) are placed directly into the right atrial appendage and brought out through the chest wall to continuously monitor atrial pressure and provide reliable access for delivering blood products and pharmacologic support. Atrial and ventricular temporary epicardial pacing wires are placed. Chest drainage tubes are placed appropriately for neonates undergoing CPB (see "Completing Operation" in Section III of Chapter 2).

It may be beneficial to leave the sternum and soft tissue temporarily unapproximated during the early recovery period. This allows for maximal cardiopulmonary function during the first 24 to 48 hours postoperatively and easy accessibility to the mediastinum if aggressive resuscitative measures are necessary. When this "open chest" option is exercised, the skin is sealed with an oval silicone rubber sheet or some other appropriate material. After the patient's cardiopulmonary status has stabilized (48 to 96 hours postoperatively), the sheet is removed under sterile conditions, and the sternum and soft tissues closed in standard fashion. This can be accomplished routinely and effectively in the ICU without returning the patient to the operating room. At some institutions, the "open sternum" option is standard following first-stage reconstruction for hypoplastic left heart physiology.

Technical Modifications of the Norwood Procedure

A number of modifications of the standard ascending aorta and arch reconstruction described in the preceding text have been developed. However, the physiologic principles of providing unobstructed ventricular-to–systemic arterial output and appropriately balanced $\dot{Q}p$ and $\dot{Q}s$ remain the same. Several groups have introduced techniques of reconstructing the ventricular-to–systemic arterial outflow without use of patch material.[B16,F3] Much experience has been obtained, and perioperative outcome and some midterm outcome data are available using these alternative techniques. Theoretical advantages include avoiding foreign patch material and the possibility of a modest reduction in circulatory arrest time. Disadvantages include potential problems with suture line tension, left pulmonary artery and left bronchus compression, and increased resistance to flow to the coronary system.

Currently, there is no clear evidence that these alternative techniques are better or worse than the more standard arch reconstruction technique. Other modifications in the surgical treatment of neonates with hypoplastic left heart physiology have been reported.[G6,T4] The right ventricle–to–pulmonary artery conduit, if used, can be placed to the right side of the reconstructed ascending aorta rather than to the left side as described. This is believed by some to have advantages.[B9]

Hybrid Procedure

Some surgeons prefer the hybrid procedure to the Norwood procedure or one of its variants as a primary procedure in high-risk patients (i.e., those with prematurity, low birth weight, associated genetic or other noncardiac comorbid conditions, extreme shock, or various real or perceived cardiac risk factors, such as severe tricuspid regurgitation, depressed right ventricular function, intact or highly restrictive atrial septum, aortic atresia with mitral stenosis, and very small-diameter ascending aorta). The procedure is ideally performed in a hybrid operating suite, essentially a cardiac catheterization laboratory that also has the dimensions and capability to support major surgery and use of CPB.

Preoperative management is the same as for a patient undergoing a Norwood procedure. The patient is anesthetized, prepped, and draped in the supine position, just as in a formal operating room. CPB support is available. Pulmonary artery branch bands are prepared from segments of PTFE tube grafts. For patients weighing 3 kg or more, 3-mm-diameter grafts are selected. For patients weighing less than 3 kg, 2.5-mm grafts are chosen. The bands are cut to a width of approximately 2 mm.

A median sternotomy incision is made, the pericardium opened, and the branch pulmonary arteries exposed. If the patient is unstable because of pulmonary overcirculation, the right branch pulmonary artery can be temporarily occluded with a delicate neurovascular clip. Care must be taken not to distort the small ascending aorta, particularly if aortic atresia is present. The right and left branch pulmonary arteries are sequentially exposed and banded (Fig. 49-10, *A*). The bands are performed before the ductal stent is placed to prevent migration of the stent during manipulation of the pulmonary artery branches. Position of the bands is confirmed by angiography (Fig. 49-10, *B*). A purse-string suture is placed on the pulmonary trunk immediately proximal to the take-off of the right pulmonary artery, and a 5F or 6F sheath system is inserted through the purse string and advanced over a guidewire through the ductus and into the descending aorta.[P3]

Accurate delineation of the ductal anatomy by angiography is important before deploying the ductal stent. After determining ductal dimensions with angiography, the stent is inserted and deployed (Fig. 49-10, *C*). Another angiogram is performed to assess stent position. If the stent does not cover the entire length of the ductus, ductal narrowing and systemic outflow obstruction may result. If the stent is too long, it could obstruct the origin of the pulmonary arteries or retrograde flow into the proximal arch and ascending aorta, which could be catastrophic in patients with aortic atresia (Fig. 49-10, *D*).

Once position of the stent is confirmed, PGE_1 infusion is discontinued. Based on hemodynamic and echocardiographic data, adequacy of the atrial septal communication is assessed. If deemed restrictive, and depending on the nature of the restriction, a balloon atrial septotomy or deployment of an atrial septal stent is performed. The completed procedure is shown in Fig. 49-10, *E*. Routine echocardiographic assessment is performed on arrival in the ICU and weekly until the patient is discharged. The chest is closed over a single drainage tube. Postoperative care is similar to that after the Norwood procedure.

Alternative techniques have been described for the hybrid procedure. These include a left thoracotomy approach,[B14] different methodology and materials for the pulmonary artery bands,[B14] and use of long-term PGE_1 (avoiding stents) to maintain ductal patency.[S1]

Bidirectional Superior Cavopulmonary Anastomosis (Hemi-Fontan Procedure)

These procedures are performed as a second stage following the Norwood procedure. Bidirectional superior cavopulmonary anastomosis and the hemi-Fontan procedure are described under Technique of Operation in Chapter 41. Because it is generally accepted that there remains substantial risk of mortality in the period between hospital discharge following a successful first-stage reconstruction for hypoplastic left heart physiology and creation of the bidirectional superior cavopulmonary anastomosis,[L8] the second-stage procedure should be performed relatively soon, typically between age 3 and 6 months. Following creation of the bidirectional superior cavopulmonary anastomosis, hemodynamic efficiency is markedly improved and mortality risk substantially reduced.[L8] Data suggest that somatic growth does not occur in patients with first-stage palliation after age 4 months.[G5]

Early construction of the bidirectional superior cavopulmonary shunt has two other advantages:

1. It allows use of a relatively small-diameter systemic-to-pulmonary shunt or right ventricular–to-pulmonary conduit at the time of first-stage reconstruction. This creates an ideal $\dot{Q}p/\dot{Q}s$ ratio during the first months following birth and does not require the initial shunt or conduit to have a life expectancy of more than 6 months. As a result, the initial shunt or conduit does not have to be "oversized" in anticipation of the growing infant requiring increased $\dot{Q}p$ in later infancy. This promotes early hemodynamic stability.
2. It reduces duration of inefficient mixed circulation that is present with a shunt or conduit. This allows maximal preservation of right ventricular function by reducing right ventricular volume work, mortality risk, and chance of distortion of the pulmonary arteries caused by tethering from the PTFE graft.

Comprehensive Second-Stage Procedure Following Hybrid Procedure

This is a complex operation requiring CPB, aortic clamping, and (by preference) either antegrade cerebral perfusion or hypothermic circulatory arrest. Exposure is by median

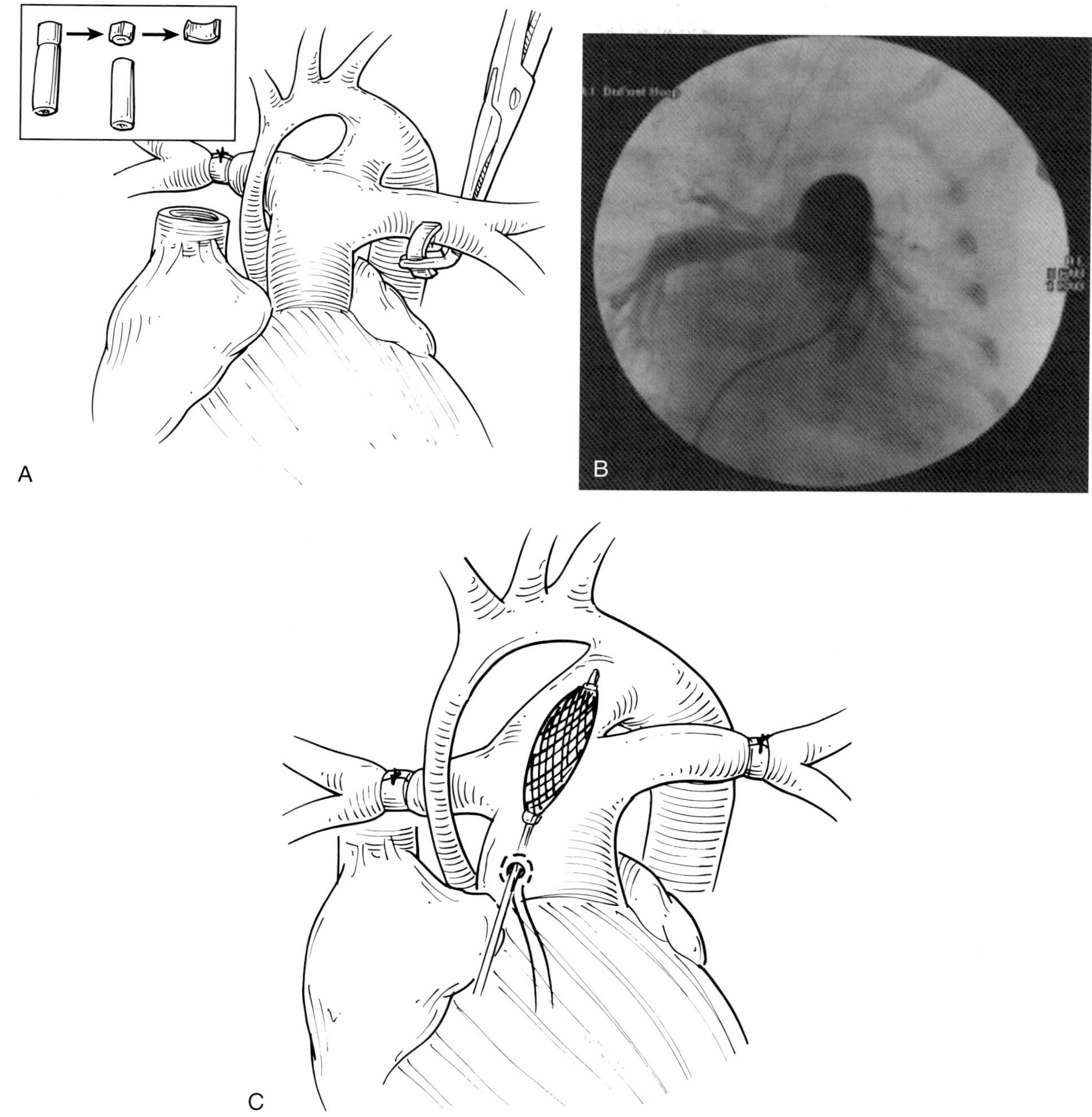

Figure 49-10 Hybrid procedure for first-stage reconstruction. **A,** Inset shows preparation of bands from appropriately sized polytetrafluoroethylene (PTFE) tube grafts. (See text for criteria used to choose correct tube graft diameter). Main figure shows the PTFE band placed on right pulmonary artery. Care must be taken not to place the band too proximal, thereby potentially obstructing the small ascending aorta, and not too distal, thereby potentially distorting upper-lobe branch of right pulmonary artery. Left pulmonary artery band is being positioned, preferably midway between the origin and the lobar arterial branching point. Bands are secured to adventitia of branch pulmonary arteries to avoid migration. **B,** Angiogram confirming positioning of right pulmonary artery band. **C,** Pulmonary artery bands are in place. Purse-string suture of 5-0 polypropylene is placed anteriorly in pulmonary trunk. Using the Seldinger technique, a 5F or 6F sheath system is inserted through purse string and advanced over a guidewire into descending aorta. A hand injection of contrast using a lateral projection is used to demonstrate ductal anatomy. After determining ductal dimensions, a (premounted) Palmaz Genesis stent (Cordis Co., Miami, Fla.) is advanced through the sheath system into position and expanded with the balloon angioplasty catheter.

Continued

sternotomy with dissection of the aortic and pulmonary trunks, aortic arch, brachiocephalic arteries, ductus arteriosus, proximal descending thoracic aorta, and branch pulmonary arteries beyond the band sites. Cannulation technique and CPB management are similar to those used for the Norwood procedure described earlier.

Reconstruction involves removing the ductus arteriosus and stent, Norwood neoaorta and arch reconstruction, removing the pulmonary artery bands with possible branch pulmonary artery reconstruction, atrial septectomy or removal of atrial septal stent, and creating a bidirectional superior cavopulmonary anastomosis. In essence, it embodies most of

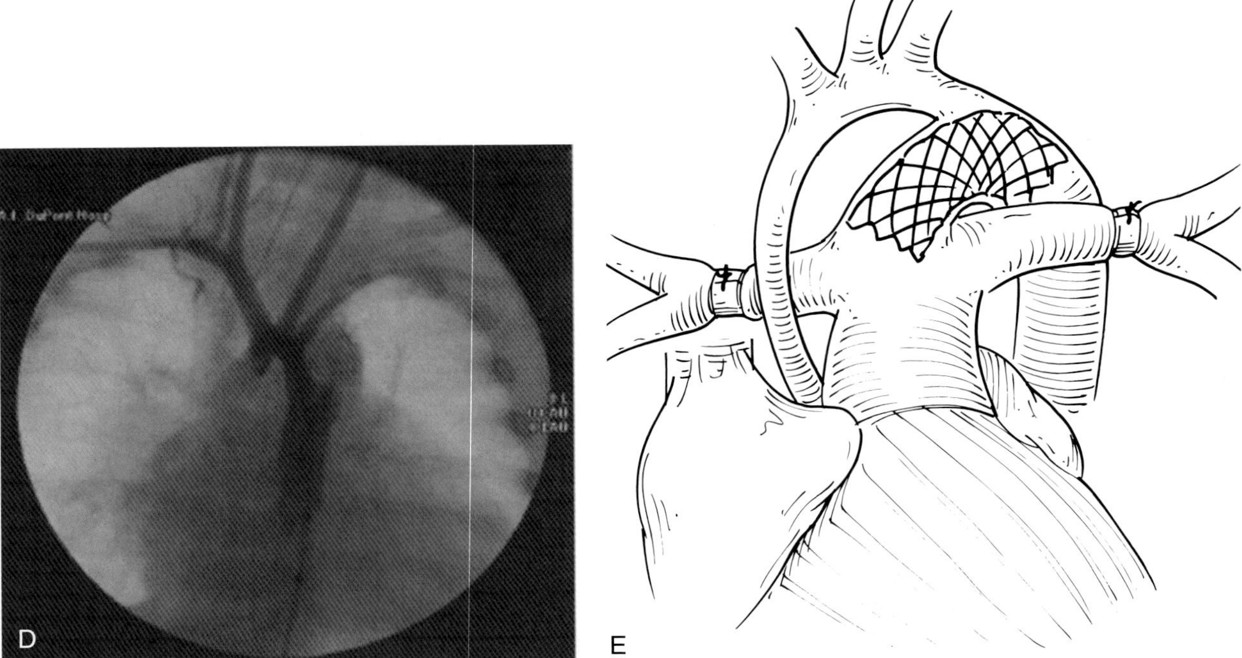

Figure 49-10, cont'd **D,** Angiogram confirming position of ductal stent and patency of arch (in the case of aortic atresia and obligatory retrograde arch flow). **E,** Completed hybrid procedure. (**A** through **D** from Pizarro and colleagues.[P3] **E** from Pizarro and colleagues.[P6])

the technical components of the Norwood operation, with the addition of a reoperative setting. Technical details of the procedure are shown in Fig. 49-11.

Fontan Operation

The Fontan operation is described under Technique of Operation in Chapter 41. Once the bidirectional superior cavopulmonary shunt has been constructed, considerations for completing the Fontan procedure, although somewhat complex, remain no different from those for any other single-ventricle anomaly.

Cardiac Transplantation

Principles of preoperative management are generally similar to those described for reconstructive surgery, but donor hearts are not usually available within the 3- to 5-day period thought to be ideal for performing the Norwood procedure. The waiting period for a donor heart may extend to several weeks or longer. Infants who maintain relatively high Rp can be discharged from the acute care facility, but they must be maintained on a constant infusion of PGE_1 by a portable intravenous pump[J2] (see Fig. 49-7). Infants in whom pulmonary overcirculation with systemic undercirculation develops require constant intensive care with varying degrees of support to maintain cardiopulmonary stability.

General techniques of cardiac transplantation are described under Technique of Operation in Chapter 21. The special methods necessary for patients with forms of hypoplastic left heart physiology have been described as well.[B4,B5,B6] Donor hearts are harvested with the ascending, transverse arch, and upper descending thoracic aorta intact.

After recipients are placed on CPB as described for the Norwood procedure, cooling to 16°C to 18°C is begun. The ductus arteriosus is excised from the aorta as in the Norwood procedure. An aortic incision is made into the descending aorta approximately 1 cm beyond the ductal insertion site and retrograde around the aortic arch to the base of the brachiocephalic artery. Native cardiectomy is performed by transecting the ascending aorta proximal to the brachiocephalic artery and the pulmonary trunk near its bifurcation. The atrial-level incisions are performed in standard fashion.

The donor heart is then implanted. The broadly beveled aorta is anastomosed to the recipient aortic arch beginning at a level opposite the origin of the brachiocephalic artery and extending to the proximal descending aorta beyond the ductal insertion. Donor pulmonary trunk is anastomosed to recipient distal pulmonary trunk. Atrial anastomoses are performed in standard fashion. The transplantation procedure is modified appropriately when the patient has already undergone first-stage reconstruction (Norwood procedure).

SPECIAL FEATURES OF POSTOPERATIVE CARE

Care after first-stage reconstruction is particularly complex and important (see "Management of Hypoplastic Left Heart Physiology" in Section I of Chapter 4 and Section IV of Chapter 5). Many of the same physiologic issues present preoperatively remain. $\dot{Q}p/\dot{Q}s$ must still be balanced; however, an appropriately sized shunt or conduit makes this more manageable postoperatively. Maintaining adequate systemic cardiac output despite well-balanced systemic and pulmonary blood flow distribution is more of a challenge postoperatively because of depressed cardiac function resulting from operation. Aggressive use of inotropic support is usually more warranted postoperatively than preoperatively.

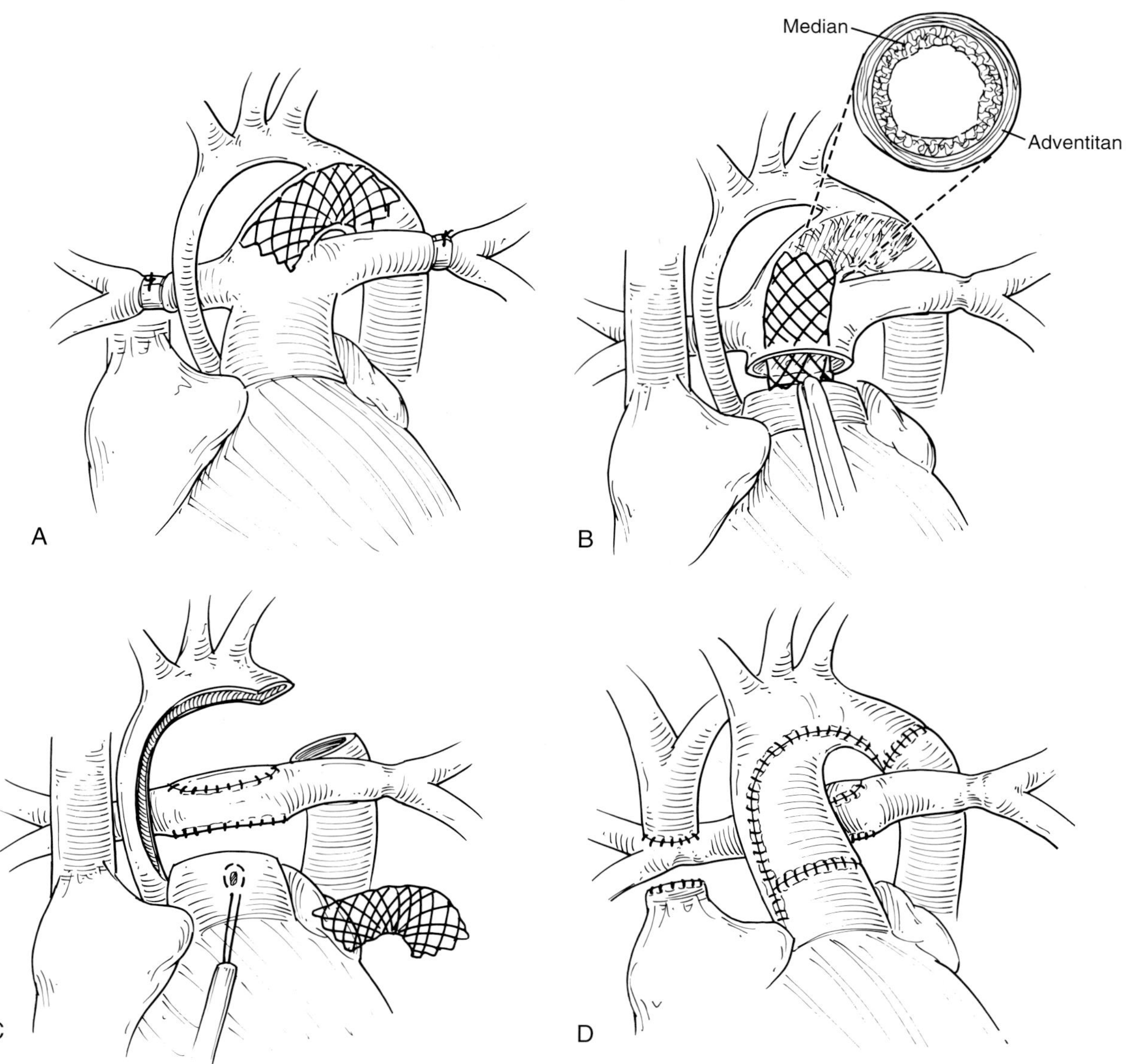

Figure 49-11 Comprehensive second-stage procedure following hybrid reconstruction. **A,** Pre–second-stage illustration showing bilateral pulmonary artery banding and ductal stenting in place. **B,** Excision of ductus and ductal stent en bloc in preparation for aortic arch and neoaortic reconstruction, performed as a standard Norwood arch reconstruction using pulmonary artery allograft patch. Patch closure of distal pulmonary trunk as well as proximal end of ductus is performed using pulmonary artery allograft patch. Pulmonary artery bands have been removed. Note mild distortion at band sites. If stenosis is present at band sites, patch augmentation using pulmonary artery allograft patch is performed (not shown). **C,** Endarterectomy-like removal of ductal stent through transected distal pulmonary trunk. As shown, depending on the time elapsed since initial palliation, partial removal of intima and part of the media is common, without complete disruption of vascular wall, therefore reducing magnitude of reconstruction. **D,** Completed second-stage reconstruction with superior bidirectional cavopulmonary anastomosis. (From Pizarro and colleagues.[P6])

Following transport from the operating room to the cardiac ICU, these infants are managed with aggressive sedation and pharmacologic paralysis for at least 24 hours. Sedation is typically administered using intravenous fentanyl and midazolam, and paralysis is achieved with a continuous infusion of pancuronium. Thus, the infant's metabolic demands are minimized, and complete ventilatory control is possible. Depending on status of $\dot{Q}p/\dot{Q}s$—assessed by clinical evaluation and arterial blood gases—rate of ventilation, tidal volume, and F_{IO_2} can all be manipulated to maximize $\dot{Q}p/\dot{Q}s$ balance. An appropriate combination of tidal volume and ventilatory rate is used to achieve optimal Pa_{CO_2}. If assessment of the infant is that $\dot{Q}p$ is inadequate, either due to a restrictive shunt or conduit or pulmonary hypertension, ventilation is increased to reduce Pa_{CO_2} to approximately 30 to 35 mmHg (Torr). If the assessment is that $\dot{Q}p$ is excessive, ventilation is adjusted to allow Pa_{CO_2} to increase to approximately 45 to 50 mmHg. If $\dot{Q}p$ is assessed to be adequate, Pa_{CO_2} is adjusted to 40 mmHg. Similarly, F_{IO_2} can be adjusted over a range from 17% to 100%, depending on $\dot{Q}p$ and Rp. Higher levels of F_{IO_2} are used when $\dot{Q}p$ is judged to be inadequate, and lower levels if it is judged to be excessive. In a patient whose

$\dot{Q}p$ is considered adequate, FIO_2 is usually reduced to approximately 25% to 30% within several hours after operation.

Some institutions suggest using additional inspired CO_2 both to limit excessive $\dot{Q}p$ and independently improve $\dot{Q}s$. This practice is somewhat controversial.

Use of nitric oxide in the setting of reduced $\dot{Q}p$ should be limited to patients in whom there is clear evidence of an adequately sized shunt or conduit and elevated pulmonary Rp. Use of nitric oxide for a patient with inadequate $\dot{Q}p$ caused by an excessively restrictive shunt or conduit is ineffective and inappropriate. Such a patient should immediately be returned to the operating room for shunt or conduit revision.

A typical level of inotropic support in the early postoperative period includes moderate dopamine (3 to 10 mg · kg^{-1} · min^{-1}, continuous infusion) and milrinone (0.5 mg · kg^{-1} · min^{-1}), with or without addition of low-dose epinephrine (0.03 to 0.05 mg · kg^{-1} · min^{-1}) (see Section IV of Chapter 5). Substantially larger doses of inotropic drugs are as likely to harm as help. Specifically, for the patient who shows evidence of excessive $\dot{Q}p$ and reduced systemic perfusion, increasing inotropic support is likely to exacerbate the physiologic imbalance.

Other maneuvers that maximize oxygen delivery to the systemic tissues include optimizing cardiac output by taking advantage of the Frank-Starling curve (see "Cardiovascular Subsystem" in Section I of Chapter 5). Typically, adjusting atrial filling pressures with volume supplementation to achieve pressures between 6 and 12 mmHg addresses this point. Optimizing oxygen-carrying capacity by adjusting the hematocrit to a minimum of 45% is advised. Despite maximizing cardiac output and balancing $\dot{Q}p$ and $\dot{Q}s$, it is not uncommon for patients to show evidence of marginally inadequate systemic perfusion during the first 24 hours after operation.

Metabolic acidosis with base deficits ranging from 0 to −5 are not uncommon and should be treated aggressively with either intermittent bicarbonate or continuous bicarbonate infusion.

Urine output is also commonly reduced during the first 24 hours (<1 mL · kg^{-1} · h^{-1}), and periods of anuria may occur. If anuria or oliguria persists beyond the first 6 hours postoperatively, serious consideration should be given to placing a peritoneal dialysis catheter (see "Renal Subsystem" in Section I of Chapter 5).

If the infant is returned to the ICU from the operating room with the sternum left open, it should not be closed until hemodynamic status is stabilized. This typically takes 36 to 48 hours. If instability persists, sternal closure can be delayed for as long as 4 to 5 days. If the infant arrives in the ICU from the operating room with the sternal wound completely closed, consideration should be given to opening it in the ICU if hemodynamics are inadequate during the first 24 hours. Substantial cardiac and pulmonary stability can be achieved with this simple maneuver.

After approximately 36 to 48 hours, or after sternal closure, sedation and paralysis can be gradually removed, allowing the patient to take over respiratory function. The weaning process from the ventilator follows the standard principles that apply to all infants following cardiac surgery (see "Pulmonary Subsystem" in Section I of Chapter 5). Prolonged ventilatory support is not unusual following the Norwood procedure and may extend to 5 to 10 days, even in patients who have no definable cardiovascular or pulmonary problem. Under these circumstances, nutrition becomes critical.

Typically, total parenteral nutrition is begun within 48 hours of operation and may be continued or converted to direct enteral feeding using a nasogastric tube. Enteral feeding should be used as soon as cardiovascular stability has been achieved and return of intestinal function is documented.

Some form of antiplatelet therapy is generally recommended to inhibit thrombosis of the shunt or conduit. A typical regimen is to institute aspirin therapy (1 mg · kg^{-1} · d^{-1}) as soon as perioperative hemorrhage is controlled. Care after the bidirectional superior cavopulmonary shunt and Fontan operation is described under Special Features of Postoperative Care in Chapter 41. Postoperative care following transplantation is similar to that for other cardiac transplant patients (see Features of Postoperative Care in Chapter 21).

RESULTS

First-Stage Reconstruction (Norwood Procedure)

Early (Hospital) Death

Early mortality remains variable among institutions.[J2] At institutions with a large experience in neonatal cardiac surgery, mortality following first-stage reconstruction steadily improved in the decades between 1985 and 2005, and then subsequently plateaued, with current hospital mortality of approximately 20%.[G13,K3,M13,N5,R8,T1] In a report from a single institution with a large experience (Mott Children's Hospital, Ann Arbor, Mich.), hospital mortality after first-stage reconstruction was 58% (CL 51%-65%) between 1986 and 1989, and 15% (CL 11%-20%) between 1990 and 1993, reflecting the trend in improved results experienced at most institutions committed to neonatal cardiac surgery.[I1]

Other single-institution studies reporting cases from 2002 to 2005 indicated hospital mortality of 6.2% (2/32; CL 2.2%-14%),[A4] 9.1% (6/66; CL 5.4%-14%),[C11] and 11% (10/88; CL 7.8%-16%).[R5] The Congenital Heart Surgeons Society (CHSS) report of 622 cases performed between 2001 and 2004 indicated early mortality of 17% (CL 16%-19%).[W1] In contrast, at less experienced institutions, hospital mortality still approached 50%. The University Hospital Consortium reported 53% mortality (118/222) among 40 institutions, each performing an average of 7.2 procedures during the 5-year period of the study; however, all cases were performed before 1995.[G16]

Survival following first-stage reconstruction performed in multiple institutions between 1994 and 1997 for patients specifically with aortic atresia is shown in Fig. 49-12.[J2] Survival was about 10% higher at all intervals at the two institutions with the best outcomes in this multicenter study.

Time-Related Survival

Overall, 12-month survival after first-stage reconstruction has been approximately 60%, with nearly all deaths occurring before the second-stage procedure (bidirectional superior cavopulmonary shunt). In one large series, survival was 66% at 1 month, 48% at 12 months, and 44% at 18 months, emphasizing ongoing risk of death even after successful first-stage reconstruction.[M14] In another series, 6 of 41 early survivors (15%) died within 3 to 5 months after operation.[K3] In the recently completed 15-center study conducted by the

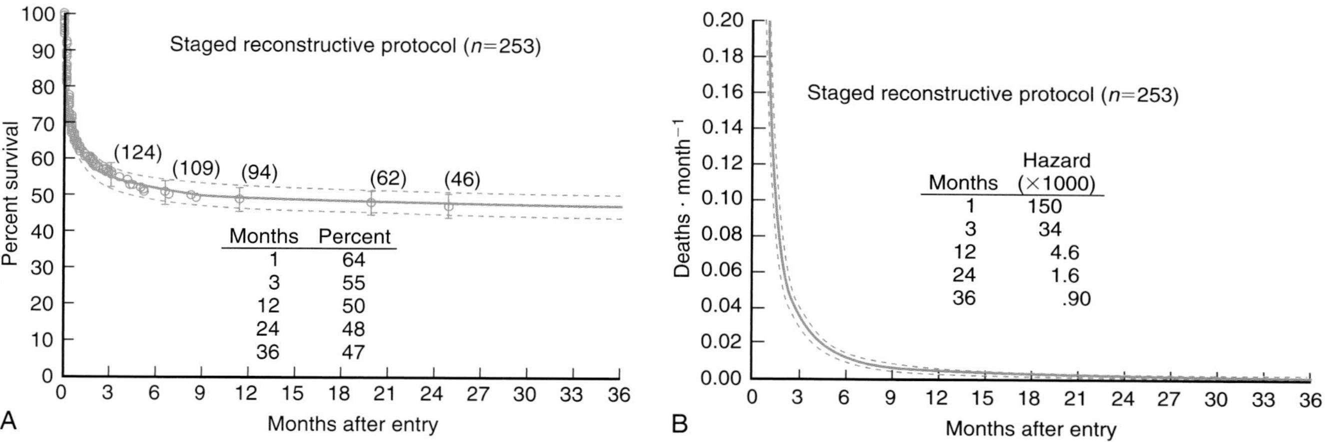

Figure 49-12 Non–risk-adjusted survival and hazard function for 253 patients with hypoplastic left heart physiology initially entered into a protocol of staged reconstructive surgery (Norwood procedure) at multiple institutions. **A,** Survival after entry. **B,** Hazard function for death. Lines, bars, and numbers have representation similar to Fig. 49-6. (From Jacobs and colleagues.[J2])

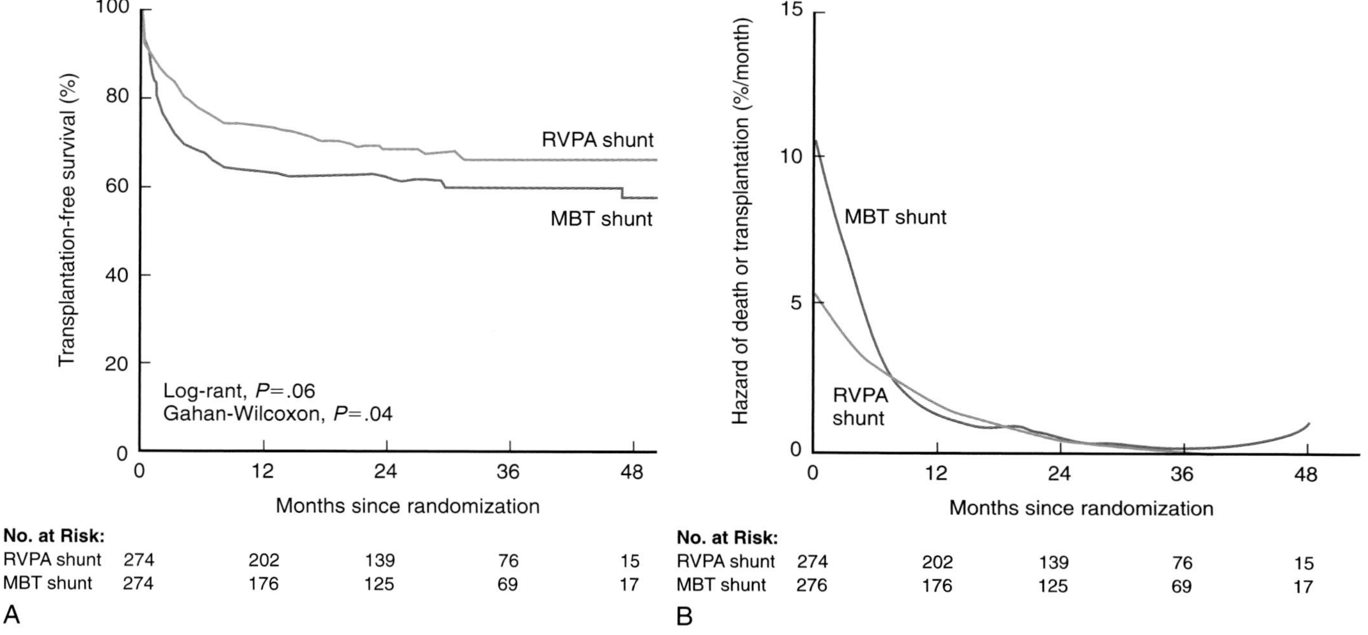

Figure 49-13 Death or transplantation among infants undergoing Norwood procedure, randomized to either modified Blalock-Taussig shunt (MBT shunt) or right ventricle–to–pulmonary artery conduit (RVPA shunt). $P = .02$ for difference in treatment effect for period before and period after 12 months. **A,** Transplantation-free survival. **B,** Hazard function. (From Ohye and colleagues.[O5])

Pediatric Heart Network, 1-year survival was 74% for patients with a right ventricle–to–pulmonary trunk conduit procedure, and 64% for those with a systemic artery–to–pulmonary artery shunt procedure[O5] (Fig. 49-13). Recognition of this pattern of ongoing mortality after hospital discharge has spawned the term *interstage death.* Interstage death of 10%[H4] and 16%[S8] are typical.[G4]

Establishment of home monitoring programs, designed to engage parents and primary cardiologists in recognizing early signs and symptoms of patient destabilization, has substantially decreased mortality between a successful first operation and the anticipated second-stage operation, with some reports showing no interstage deaths.[G4,S11]

Incremental Risk Factors for Death after Operation

Morphologic factors have been associated with risk of death in some series but not in others. In an early study from 1986 by Norwood's group, atrial septal anatomy, preoperative right ventricular hypertrophy, ascending aorta diameter, and coarctation were not correlated with early survival.[H5] Although not supported by the two largest institutional experiences, some institutions suggest that aortic atresia and very small size of the ascending aorta (diameter < 2 mm) may be associated with increased risk for death, both early[M7] and late[J3] after first-stage reconstruction. Intact or highly restrictive atrial septum has been widely associated with increased risk of both early and interstage death.[G9,H4,V4]

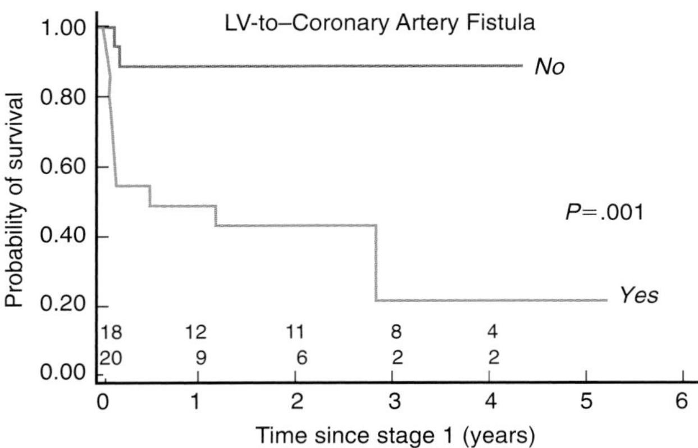

Figure 49-14 Survival after first-stage reconstruction for hypoplastic left heart physiology in anatomic subtype aortic atresia with mitral stenosis. Survival is stratified by presence or absence of echocardiographic or angiographic presence of left ventricle *(LV)*-to–coronary artery fistulae. Risk appears to reside in this subgroup having fistulae because mortality for aortic atresia with mitral stenosis without fistulae is more favorable, similar to other anatomic subtypes. (From Pigula and colleagues.[P2])

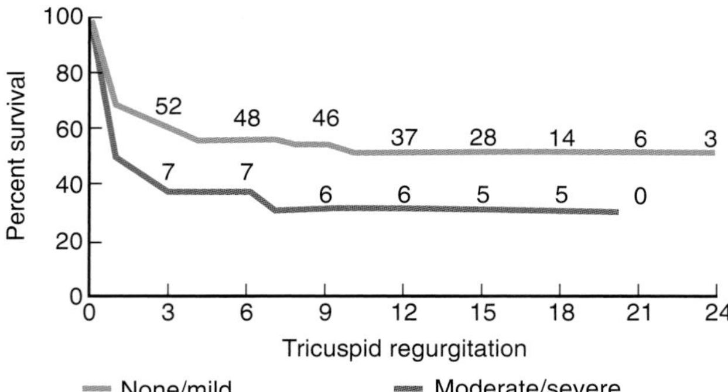

Figure 49-15 Early survival after the first-stage Norwood operation (October 1984–March 1987), according to degree of preoperative tricuspid regurgitation. (From Barber and colleagues.[B8])

The combination of mitral stenosis and aortic atresia has recently been identified as a risk, particularly when left ventricular–to–coronary artery fistulae are present[G8,V3] (Fig. 49-14). In one study, fetal diagnosis has been shown to decrease the risk of death following first-stage reconstruction, suggesting that factors such as prenatal transport and early postnatal stabilization may improve survival.[T6] In another, however, prenatal diagnosis was strongly correlated with superior preoperative clinical status but did not influence surgical outcome.[S9] Moderate or severe tricuspid valve regurgitation preoperatively[B8,S2] (Fig. 49-15) and depressed right ventricular function preoperatively[M7] have correlated with increased risk of death after first-stage reconstruction.

An initially low arterial pH has not correlated with increased risk of deaths in some studies, whereas in others it has.[B7,J3] Small size at operation has been identified as a risk.[M7,S2] Associated noncardiac anomalies (e.g., tracheoesophageal fistula, renal dysplasia, biliary atresia, intracranial abnormalities, pulmonary dysplasia) have been shown to increase risk.[S13] In one large single-institution study, age older than 7 days at time of first-stage reconstruction was a risk factor for interstage death.[H4] In another study, postoperative dysrhythmia and reduced ventricular function were noted to be risks.[S8] A less-than-optimal technical operation has also been identified as a risk factor for death.[K1]

These various studies that identify different risk factors underscore the wide variability among institutions.

Hemodynamic and Morphologic Results

Atrial septectomy performed at first-stage reconstruction usually results in a nonrestrictive opening between the two atria. A gradient in excess of 4 mmHg across the atrial septum develops in about 4% of patients.[C6] About 10% of patients have important (grade 3 or 4) tricuspid valve regurgitation late after first-stage reconstruction.[C6] In interpreting this, the fact that this physiologic variable is a risk factor for death after first-stage operation must be considered.

Systolic pressure gradients are rarely present between right ventricle and reconstructed ascending aorta, indicating that the native pulmonary valve functions well in the setting of systemic outflow. In approximately 10% to 15% of patients, the distal portion of the aortic arch is narrowed such that a systolic pressure gradient greater than 25 mmHg is present. This gradient typically occurs at the distal limit of the allograft patch. It is most likely due to lack of growth potential at this site resulting from a combination of patch material and circumferential ductal tissue in the native aorta.[M1] All patients who have undergone reconstruction for hypoplastic left heart physiology should be evaluated for potential gradients at this site. Aggressive treatment is necessary; often this can be accomplished effectively with percutaneous balloon dilatation.[C6]

Most patients have a $\dot{Q}p/\dot{Q}s$ of 0.8 to 2.0 at the time of cardiac catheterization performed in preparation for the second-stage superior cavopulmonary shunt. Approximately 15% to 20% of patients have elevated Rp greater than 4 Wood units. Pulmonary artery distortion is present in a minority of patients, typically at the central pulmonary trunk site under the aortic arch, or at the shunt or conduit insertion site. Right ventricular end-diastolic pressure is typically somewhat elevated but is greater than 12 mmHg in approximately 10% of patients. A hypoplastic left pulmonary artery has been associated with larger diameter of the reconstructed aorta.[D2]

First-Stage Reconstruction (Hybrid Procedure)

Early (Hospital) Death

Early mortality has been as low as 2.5% (1/40; CL 0.41%-8.2%)[G1] and as high as 29% (6/21; CL 18%-42%),[V2] with other series reporting 5.6% (1/18; CL 0.90%-18%),[S1] 12% (4/33; CL 6.3%-21%),[B14] 18% (2/11; CL 6.3%-38%),[C1] and 20% (2/10; CL 7.0%-41%).[P3]

Time-Related Survival

Time-related survival after the hybrid procedure, which includes interstage survival and survival following comprehensive second-stage surgery, is about 60%. It is influenced by development of obstruction to retrograde flow in the aortic arch caused by the ductal stent in patients with aortic atresia.[S14] Fig. 49-16 shows time-related survival following the hybrid procedure. Other reports confirm a relatively high interstage mortality (21%) and comprehensive second-stage mortality (14%).[P4]

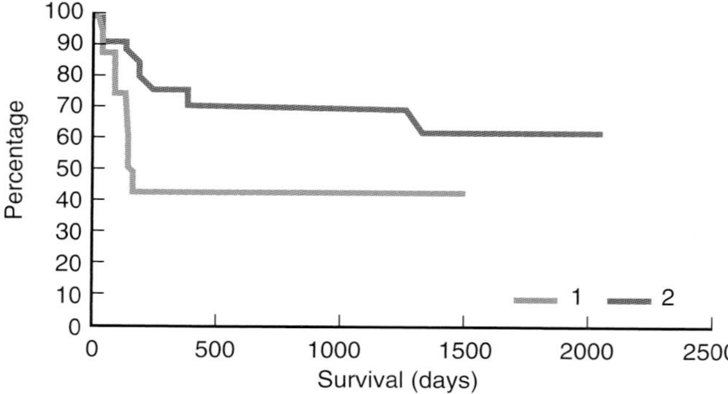

Figure 49-16 Time-related survival in 66 patients after the hybrid procedure for hypoplastic left heart physiology. Group 1 (16 patients) had a predominant prevalence of aortic atresia and obligatory retrograde flow in the aortic arch and developed stent-related obstruction to retrograde flow in the aortic arch. Group 2 (50 patients) had a lesser prevalence of aortic atresia and did not develop stent-related aortic obstruction. (From Stoica and colleagues.[S14])

Incremental Risk Factors for Death after Operation

Aortic atresia with obligatory retrograde flow in the aortic arch appears to be a risk factor for death after the hybrid procedure (see Fig. 49-16).

Hemodynamic and Morphologic Results

About 50% of patients undergoing the hybrid procedure require an interstage catheter-based intervention or surgical intervention before comprehensive second-stage reconstruction.[B10]

Second-Stage Reconstruction (Bidirectional Superior Cavopulmonary Anastomosis)

Outcome following bidirectional superior cavopulmonary anastomosis or hemi-Fontan procedure in hypoplastic left heart physiology is similar to that for patients with other forms of univentricular heart. This naturally follows from the fact that all patients with univentricular heart, including those with hypoplastic left heart physiology, are selected for bidirectional superior cavopulmonary anastomosis based on similar physiologic criteria.

Because a number of institutions with extensive experience with surgery for hypoplastic left heart physiology have reported outcomes, there are ample data on survival following each stage of operation in these patients. These data are supplemented by the more general discussion of outcome following bidirectional superior cavopulmonary anastomosis in all forms of univentricular heart (see Results in Chapter 41).

Although there is probably no difference in survival between hypoplastic left heart physiology patients and other univentricular heart patients *following* bidirectional superior cavopulmonary anastomosis, it is not clear whether hypoplastic left heart physiology patients are as likely as other univentricular heart patients to meet the physiologic criteria necessary to undergo bidirectional superior cavopulmonary anastomosis. Based on a number of factors, including marginal hemodynamics after first-stage reconstruction and ongoing mortality, it is likely that a smaller percentage of these patients will eventually undergo bidirectional superior cavopulmonary anastomosis.

Early (Hospital) Death

Based on results from several institutions with a large experience managing hypoplastic left heart physiology, early mortality following bidirectional superior cavopulmonary anastomosis currently is about 5%[J2,N5] (Fig. 49-17).

Time-Related Survival

Because of the marked improvement in physiologic status following bidirectional superior cavopulmonary anastomosis, mortality following the perioperative period and before the Fontan procedure is generally extremely low[J2] (see Fig. 49-17).

Third-Stage Reconstruction (Fontan Operation)

In theory, there should be no difference in outcome following the Fontan operation for patients with hypoplastic left heart physiology than for patients having other forms of univentricular heart. The logic behind this statement is the same as that given in the previous discussion of outcome following bidirectional superior cavopulmonary anastomosis. This has been confirmed by at least one large single-institution study.[G2] The outcomes discussed here for the Fontan operation in patients with hypoplastic heart physiology should be supplemented by the general discussion of outcomes following the Fontan procedure for all forms of univentricular heart (see Results in Chapter 41).

Early (Hospital) Death

In the early era, mortality after the Fontan operation for hypoplastic left heart physiology was high—8 patients in 50 (16%; CL 11%-23%) reported by Chang and colleagues from Norwood's group.[C6] More recent estimates of hospital mortality in larger patient cohorts from several institutions is about 5%[J2,N5] (see Fig. 49-17).

Time-Related Survival

In the earlier experience of Farrell and colleagues, there was clear evidence of important ongoing mortality following a successful Fontan procedure, with survival of 52% at 4 years.[F1] These patients underwent the Fontan operation in an era before the three-stage protocol (see Chapter 41) was clearly established.

More recent data in the era of the three-stage protocol suggest improved midterm survival for hypoplastic left heart physiology[J2] (see Fig. 49-17). Secure long-term estimates of survival following the Fontan operation for hypoplastic left heart physiology in the era of the three-stage protocol are still lacking. Reasons for improvement in both early and time-related survival following the Fontan procedure are multifactorial and apply not only to hypoplastic left heart physiology but also to all forms of univentricular heart. For a more in-depth discussion of the factors related to Fontan outcome, see Chapter 41. There remain legitimate concerns that the basic morphology of a systemic right ventricle and tricuspid valve will place these patients at increased long-term risk relative to some other morphologic subtypes of single-ventricle physiology.

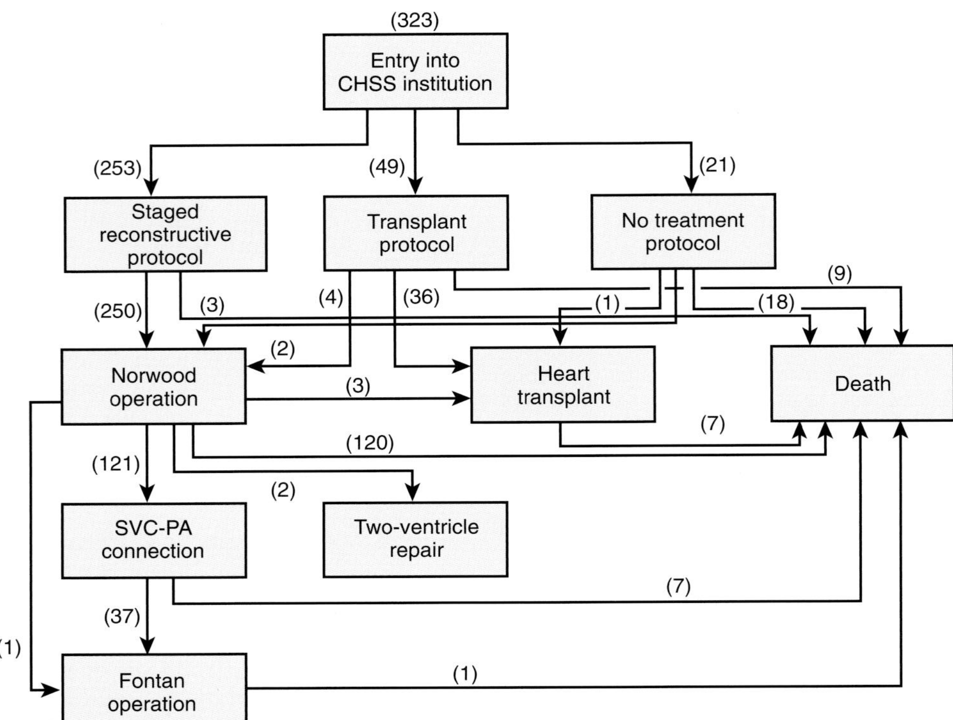

Figure 49-17 Schematic diagram of treatment pathway and fate of 323 patients with hypoplastic left heart physiology after initial assignment to staged reconstructive surgery (Norwood procedure), transplantation, or no treatment. In the staged reconstruction group, death at or after both the superior vena cava–pulmonary artery *(SVC-PA)* connection and the Fontan was approximately 5% or less. Key: *CHSS,* Congenital Heart Surgeons Society. (From Jacobs and colleagues.[J2])

Incremental Risk Factors for Death

Incremental risk factors for death following the Fontan operation are similar in all forms of univentricular heart (see Chapter 41).

Other Commonly Performed Operations

The two most commonly performed additional procedures performed in patients undergoing the standard three-stage protocol are repair of recurrent arch obstruction and tricuspid valve repair for regurgitation. These can be performed either at the time of the second- or third-stage procedure, or separately.

Recurrent arch obstruction can be effectively addressed in most cases with catheter-based balloon dilatation. Typically, recurrent arch obstruction is noted in infancy, and commonly in the first 6 months after the initial Norwood procedure.[C8,S10,T5] It occurs in about 20% of survivors.[C8,T5] Overall risk is low, and gradient relief is excellent. Two single-institution studies revealed no mortality related to the procedure, and gradient relief in all patients, which persisted at midterm follow-up.[C8,T5] One multicenter analysis showed initial success of 89%, with three deaths occurring within 48 hours of the dilatation in patients with poor ventricular function, and freedom from repeat arch intervention of 74% at 18 months.

Tricuspid valve repair can be accomplished with low mortality and midterm (mean 26 months) success (defined as less than moderate residual regurgitation) of 63%.[O3] Patients with poor right ventricular function after valve repair, even if the repair was initially successful, tended to do poorly, with progressive deterioration of the valve over time. Patients with an unsuccessful initial valve repair but preserved ventricular function often benefited from a second valve repair.

Cardiac Transplantation

Experience with cardiac transplantation in neonates with hypoplastic left heart physiology is small relative to the experience with reconstructive surgery and is limited to a few institutions. General information on the results of cardiac transplantation (see Results in Chapter 21) is applicable to this subpopulation. The early concept that neonates receiving cardiac transplants were "privileged hosts" does not appear to have held up. Rejection frequency and severity in neonates appears to be similar to that in the broader cardiac transplantation experience.[B16]

In the Loma Linda experience, 84 neonates have received cardiac transplants, with 13% (CL 7%-23%) early (30-day) mortality and 5-year survival of 82% (CL 71%-88%).[C9] Including patients who died while awaiting transplant, 5-year survival was 61% (CL 52%-70%).[C9]

A recent multicenter study shows similar midterm survival in institutions accomplished with these procedures[J2] (Fig. 49-18). Early in the experience, suppressive immunotherapy included cyclosporine and azathioprine without use of long-term steroid therapy. Steroids and antithymus globulin were used only for early rejection episodes. Currently, suppressive immunotherapy varies somewhat among institutions; however, in general, long-term therapy varies little relative to that given other cardiac transplant recipients (see Chapter 21).

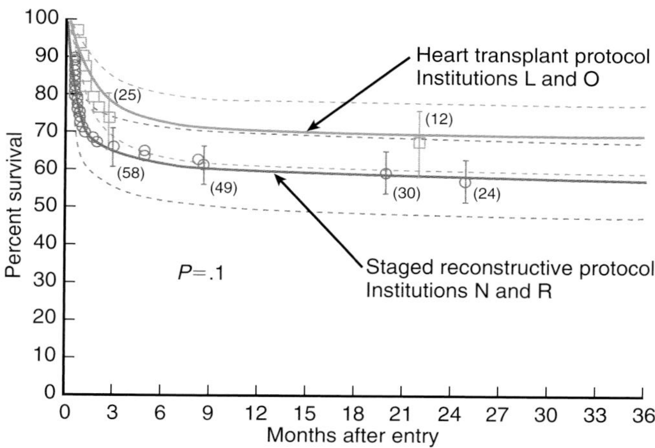

Figure 49-18 Non–risk-adjusted survival of patients with hypoplastic left heart physiology entered into treatment protocols at four experienced institutions, two that followed a staged reconstructive (Norwood procedure) protocol, and two that followed a transplantation protocol. The 70% confidence intervals diverge at a point approximately 1 week after entry and continue to overlap thereafter. The lines, bars, and numbers have representation similar to Fig. 49-6. (From Jacobs and colleagues.[J2])

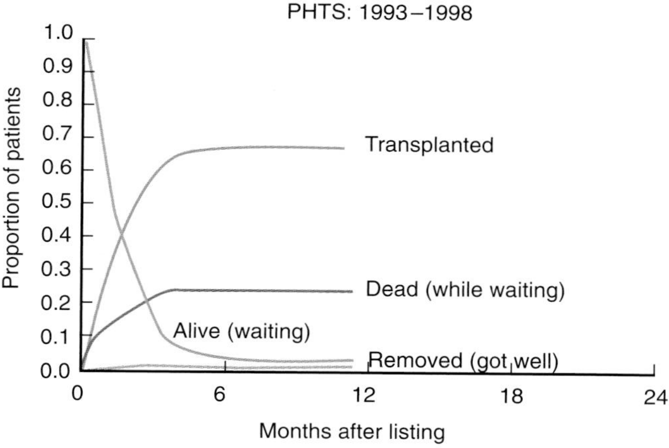

Figure 49-19 Competing outcomes of 262 patients with hypoplastic left heart physiology listed for heart transplantation from 1993 to 1998. Key: *PHTS*, Pediatric Heart Transplant Study Group. (From Chrisant and colleagues.[C10])

High early survival has been the rule following neonatal cardiac transplantation for patients with hypoplastic left heart physiology, based on individual reports of several experienced institutions.[B1,B5,S12] Intermediate-term results have been acceptable and comparable with intermediate-term results for cardiac transplantation in general. On the other hand, surgical mortality (excluding preoperative death) for transplantation was 42% (17/40; CL 34%-52%) among a consortium of institutions infrequently performing this procedure.[G16]

In contrast, the more recent report from the Pediatric Heart Transplant Study Group reports 5-year survival (also excluding preoperative death) of 72%, with most of the deaths occurring in the first 3 months after operation.[C10] When preoperative death is included, survival at 5 years falls to 54%. An important factor that is difficult to quantify is the death rate of neonates born with hypoplastic left heart physiology while awaiting an appropriate donor organ.

Because of limitations of donor heart availability, the typical neonate must wait several weeks to months before receiving a heart. The intrinsic instability of hypoplastic left heart physiology in its natural state can result in mortality during this time. Attempts have been made to quantify recipient mortality while awaiting a donor organ, but reliable information is scarce. In a multicenter study from 1998, 36 of 49 patients (73%) entered into a transplant protocol received a donor heart; the estimate of time-related interim mortality while awaiting transplant is shown in Fig. 49-7.[J2] A more recent multicenter study from the Pediatric Heart Transplant Study group analyzed 262 patients; 25% of listed patients died while awaiting transplantation[C10] (Fig. 49-19). The mean waiting period for those receiving an organ was 1.3 months.

INDICATIONS FOR OPERATION

Hypoplastic left heart physiology is a fatal condition; death usually occurs within 1 month of birth and certainly within 1 year (see Fig. 49-7). Surgical intervention is therefore advisable unless economic conditions or lack of institutional capability deny this possibility, or the patient's legal guardians choose to withhold surgical therapy. Curiously, this latter practice remains relatively widespread, even though current treatment outcomes for hypoplastic left heart physiology are now comparable with outcomes for other cardiac defects for which the option to withhold support is not offered by managing physicians and other healthcare providers.

If intervention is to be accomplished, management should begin as soon as possible, preferably with *prenatal* arrangements for delivery at an institution capable of perinatal resuscitation and subsequent surgical management. Treatment begins at birth or as soon as diagnosis has been made, and consists initially of intensive preoperative therapy. Neonates with hypoplastic left heart physiology usually can be resuscitated and maintained in stable condition with such intervention, and the surgical procedure can be performed as an elective procedure, ideally between 2 and 5 days of life.

Whether staged reconstruction or cardiac transplantation is the treatment of choice remains controversial. Although reconstructive surgery remains the predominant method of managing patients with hypoplastic left heart physiology, there currently are no clear data to recommend reconstruction or transplantation as the procedure of choice. Equivalent outcomes, as judged by early and midterm survival, can be achieved with either treatment.[J2]

SPECIAL SITUATIONS AND CONTROVERSIES

Aortic Atresia with Large Ventricular Septal Defect

Although this lesion includes aortic atresia, it is not representative of hypoplastic left heart physiology. A two-ventricle repair is recommended because such patients commonly have a normal mitral valve and left ventricle. One approach is to perform a typical first-stage reconstruction in the neonatal period, followed by a definitive repair in which the left ventricle is baffled to the pulmonary trunk using a Rastelli-type repair[O4,P1] (see "Rastelli Operation" under Intraventricular Repair in Chapter 52). In this repair, left ventricular outflow is baffled to the pulmonary trunk by an intracardiac patch, a right ventricular to distal pulmonary artery conduit is placed, and takedown of the previously placed systemic–pulmonary trunk shunt is performed.

Alternatively, a one-stage complete repair in the neonate can be accomplished. Anecdotal reports of success with this procedure were reported in the 1980s and 1990s.[A5,F2] In this procedure, the pulmonary trunk and hypoplastic aorta are reconstructed in typical fashion for first-stage reconstruction for hypoplastic left heart physiology. After completing the extracardiac portion of the procedure, the left ventricle is baffled to the pulmonary trunk with a Rastelli-type intracardiac patch. The operation is completed by placing a valved conduit from right ventricle to distal pulmonary arteries. More recently, single-institution series, reporting experience ranging from 11 to 21 cases, indicate that the operation can be performed with very low early and midterm mortality.[G15,M12,N1,O4]

Borderline Hypoplastic Left Heart Physiology

Because of the continuum of morphologic and physiologic compromise among patients with left heart anomalies, clinical decision making can be extremely difficult. Individual patients are positioned along this continuum, yet the surgeon is forced to make a dichotomous management decision. Whether to proceed with a two-ventricle repair or disregard the left-sided structures and perform a single-ventricle repair can be a difficult decision. Although a number of studies have addressed this issue, attempting to quantify the various physiologic and morphologic components of the left heart, the decision remains subjective.[K2,L5,L9,R6]

Pulmonary autograft aortic valve replacement (Ross procedure) in infants and neonates in recent years introduces another factor into this decision-making process (see "Autograft Pulmonary Valve" under Technique of Operation in Chapter 12, and "Repair of Tunnel Stenosis by Aortoventriculoplasty [Konno Operation]" and "Modified Konno Operation" in Section II of Chapter 47). Ability to perform the Ross procedure along with Konno enlargement of the left ventricular outflow tract, in combination with arch reconstruction and resection of left ventricular endocardial fibroelastosis, provides the opportunity to create two-ventricle repairs in patients considered to be poor candidates using older criteria.[R3,R4]

Using aggressive left heart reconstructive techniques, it is possible to physiologically normalize the entire left ventricular outflow tract and improve left ventricular cavity size and diastolic function by resecting the constricting endocardial fibroelastosis. In a small experience of one of the authors (FLH) with such borderline hypoplastic left heart patients, it has been found that the true limiting factor for successful two-ventricle repair is size and function of the mitral valve. Except for the mitral valve, it appears that all morphologic components of the left heart can be adequately addressed surgically using these techniques. Although long-term success has been achieved in a small number of patients, it remains controversial regarding when these aggressive techniques should be applied rather than opting for the single-ventricle approach.

Fetal balloon valvuloplasty provides an additional therapeutic option for patients with a borderline left heart. The sole purpose of the procedure is to convert patients to biventricular physiology who otherwise are destined for single-ventricle physiology. This procedure was first performed in 1989, but only 12 cases were performed between 1989 and 1997. Recently, McElhinney and colleagues reported their experience in 47 cases.[M5] After a learning curve, they currently quote 75% technical success and 10% fetal demise. Thirty percent of those undergoing a technically successful fetal procedure ultimately achieved a two-ventricle circulation. In all of these, additional postnatal, surgical, or interventional procedures were necessary. This experience convincingly demonstrates that fetal balloon valvuloplasty can be technically performed with reasonable safety in the majority of selected patients. However, it is not clear that the procedure plays a causal role in converting patients from a univentricular to a biventricular circulation. The physiologic and morphologic selection criteria for entry into the fetal treatment program were not dissimilar to those of the patients treated by one of the authors, cited earlier, who achieved biventricular repair after a postnatal Ross Konno, arch repair, and endocardial fibroelastosis resection—without fetal intervention.

Use or Avoidance of Circulatory Arrest

When performing the Norwood procedure, the decision to use either hypothermic circulatory arrest or continuous perfusion, most commonly in the form of antegrade cerebral perfusion, is made based on surgeon preference. Surgeon preference is most heavily influenced by personal experience and expert opinion, and less so by objective data.[O2] Hypothermic circulatory arrest techniques have been available for more than 40 years and continue to evolve. Antegrade cerebral perfusion techniques have been available for a little over a decade and are rapidly evolving as well.

Techniques are also now available for reliably performing complex neonatal cardiac surgery, including the Norwood procedure and its variants, without using total body circulatory arrest.[H1,M4,M8,N3,O6] Only limited evidence unequivocally demonstrates that avoiding circulatory arrest is beneficial, but a number of compelling arguments can be made supporting the position that continuous circulation, especially to the brain, should be maintained.

Although numerous maneuvers have been used to minimize unwanted sequelae of controlled cerebral ischemia that attends circulatory arrest, both clinical and animal studies indicate that profound metabolic changes take place within minutes of cessation of blood flow, regardless of temperature of the brain tissue (see Section I of Chapter 2 for details and references). Based on these studies, it is difficult to pinpoint with confidence the threshold for a safe period of circulatory arrest, although several clinical studies have attempted to define that point. The safe period concept is only valid as a tool to be applied prospectively in clinical decision making for individual patients if one assumes that all patients are equally susceptible to cerebral ischemia. There is increasing evidence that this is not the case; it is becoming recognized that genetic polymorphism can influence vulnerability of the brain to ischemic insult from individual to individual.[G3]

Based on data showing that metabolic derangements begin immediately with circulatory arrest, and on carefully conducted animal and clinical studies demonstrating that neurologic sequelae correlate with increasing length of circulatory arrest (see "Safe Duration of Circulatory Arrest" in Section I of Chapter 2), it can be argued that clinical studies failing to show sequelae following circulatory arrest are simply using end-point criteria that are insensitive to subtle cognitive injury that may occur with shorter arrest periods or are underpowered to demonstrate a difference. The strongest justification for using circulatory arrest has been that instrumentation, cannulae, and techniques are not available to allow repair of complex aortic arch problems in neonates using continuous perfusion. This justification, however, no longer exists.[H1,M4,M8,N3,O6] Although it is clear that continuous perfusion can eliminate the metabolic derangements that occur with cessation of cerebral blood flow, potential complications relating to techniques required to maintain ongoing perfusion can also occur, and these must be defined and studied.

Safeguards that are necessary to avoid perfusion-related complications, however, should be no different from those of standard CPB. There are limited data directly comparing continuous perfusion and hypothermic circulatory arrest in patients undergoing the Norwood procedure and its variants. There is a single randomized prospective study comparing it with antegrade cerebral perfusion.[G11] That study did not examine early mortality or morbidity, but focused on neurodevelopmental outcome at midterm follow-up in a single institution; no difference in outcome between the two techniques was demonstrated. This conclusion is of limited value, however, because the methodology used for the antegrade cerebral perfusion group involved periods of hypothermic circulatory arrest, multiple cannulation maneuvers, and baseline perfusion rates (20 mL · kg^{-1} min^{-1}) that many would consider in the low flow range. The critique of this manuscript, which accompanies the publication, emphasizes these limitations and further points out that the compelling theoretical advantages of continuous perfusion must be supplemented by both developing a rigorous physiologic understanding of techniques such as antegrade cerebral perfusion, and standardizing operative techniques that minimize morbidity. The current state-of-the-art of antegrade cerebral perfusion lacks these important components.[N3,S3] Several single-institution studies have established that the Norwood procedure can be performed using continuous perfusion, with early morbidity and mortality comparable with outcomes achieved using hypothermic circulatory arrest.[M4,M8,N3,O6] Some studies indicate an early survival advantage using antegrade cerebral perfusion.[H1]

Comparison of Right Ventricle–to–Pulmonary Trunk Conduit and Systemic-to–Pulmonary Artery Shunt as Source of Pulmonary Blood Flow in First-Stage Reconstruction

For decades, a systemic–pulmonary arterial shunt has been the mainstay for providing regulated $\dot{Q}p$ to the lungs in first-stage reconstruction. The most commonly used procedure for accomplishing this is the modified Blalock-Taussig shunt using a PTFE graft. Its potential disadvantages include excessive volume load, acute thrombosis, and low diastolic blood pressure leading to coronary insufficiency. Although Norwood originally experimented with right ventricle–to–pulmonary artery conduits as the source of pulmonary blood flow in first-stage reconstruction,[N7] this was quickly abandoned.

Over the past decade, the concept of the right ventricle–to–pulmonary trunk conduit as the source of pulmonary blood flow has been reexamined.[I2,K4] These techniques use either a valved or nonvalved conduit between right ventricle and central distal pulmonary trunk. They have several potential advantages, the most important of which is lack of diastolic runoff from the systemic circulation. This provides importantly elevated diastolic blood pressure in the aorta and coronary arteries compared with the systemic-pulmonary shunt, with the potential advantage of promoting more stable cardiac performance by reducing myocardial oxygen supply/demand mismatch that undoubtedly occurs in the standard Norwood operation, in which the single right ventricle has marked pressure and volume load, yet decreased coronary perfusion. Additional potential advantages include (1) improved development of the left pulmonary artery system because the source of pulmonary blood flow enters the pulmonary arteries more centrally, and (2) ability to easily perform second-stage bidirectional superior cavopulmonary anastomosis without need for CPB. The potential disadvantages of this technique are (1) a right ventriculotomy is required to place the conduit, which may lead to ventricular dysfunction and dysrhythmias; (2) damage to the pulmonary valve may occur at the time of the ventriculotomy; (3) excessive thrombosis is theoretically possible because of relative stasis during diastole; and (4) central pulmonary arterial distortion may occur.

One of the authors (FLH) has exclusively used a composite right ventricle–to–pulmonary trunk valved conduit for first-stage reconstruction since January 2002.[R5] With this technique, it is immediately apparent that postoperative diastolic blood pressure is markedly improved (Fig. 49-20) compared with both preoperative diastolic blood pressure and traditional expectations for postoperative diastolic blood pressure using a standard systemic-pulmonary shunt. Early postoperative management is simplified, and hospital mortality as low as 8% can be achieved. Others have also noted these hemodynamic advantages.[I2] Over the past decade, use of the right ventricle–to–pulmonary trunk conduit has increased

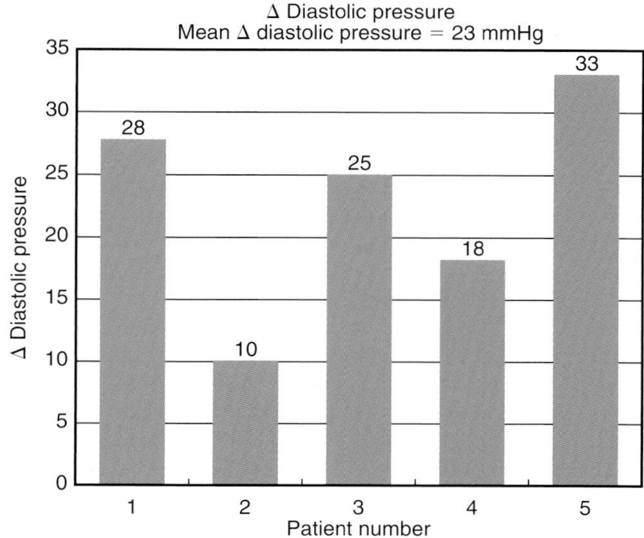

Figure 49-20 Difference in preoperative and early postoperative diastolic blood pressure (Δ diastolic pressure) in five patients undergoing first-stage reconstruction utilizing a valved right ventricle–to–pulmonary artery composite graft. Note marked improvement in diastolic blood pressure in all cases.

steadily, and currently it is chosen about as frequently as the systemic-to-pulmonary artery shunt.

Superiority of one technique over the other has not been unequivocally demonstrated, but a number of studies address this question. Many of these are retrospective single-institution studies and are not randomized; important reports are cited and discussed here. Mair and colleagues retrospectively evaluated 32 patients, 18 with a shunt and 14 with a right ventricle–to–pulmonary artery conduit.[M3] They demonstrated better diastolic blood pressure, lower hospital and interstage mortality, and better ventricular function by catheterization at 3 months in the conduit group. There were no thrombotic events. One concern with this study is that the first 18 patients received shunts, and the last 14 conduits.

In another nonrandomized single-institution study of 66 patients, Cua and colleagues showed no difference in morbidity or mortality in 37 shunt patients and 29 conduit patients.[C11] The conduit group had higher diastolic blood pressure, faster recovery, and shorter hospital stay. Ruffer and colleagues retrospectively analyzed 54 patients, 31 receiving a shunt and 23 a conduit.[R8] Diastolic blood pressure was higher in the conduit group, and mortality was lower (8.7% vs. 19%, P = .12). Hospital length of stay and interstage mortality were similar. Pruetz and colleagues retrospectively report 159 cases, 103 receiving a shunt and 56 a conduit.[P7] Mortality was 42% prior to second-stage surgery in the shunt group, compared with 23% in the conduit group. The left pulmonary artery grew more in the conduit group, but the pulmonary trunk was more likely to be hypoplastic. The conduit group was more likely to need reintervention prior to standard second-stage intervention. Caspi and colleagues showed that the Nakata index for conduit patients was greater (240 ± 18 mm$^2 \cdot$ m^{-2} vs. 190 ± 10 mm$^2 \cdot$ m^{-2}, P = .03), and branch pulmonary arteries were more equal in size than those in shunt patients.[C3]

Graham and colleagues reported similar findings as well as higher diastolic blood pressure and lower right ventricular end-diastolic pressure in conduit patients at catheterization in preparation for second-stage intervention.[G12] Pizzaro and colleagues demonstrated lower operative mortality in the conduit group compared with the shunt group (8% vs. 30%, P = .05) as well as less need for ventilator manipulation, extracorporeal membrane oxygenation, and delayed sternal closure.[P5] Tanoue and colleagues demonstrated that overall ventricular performance was comparable at midterm follow-up in both shunt and conduit groups.[T2] Griselli and colleagues retrospectively evaluated 367 patients and showed lower hospital (15% vs. 31%, $P < .05$) and midterm (22% vs. 41%, $P < .05$) mortality in the conduit group.[G13]

Atallah and colleagues showed lower hospital and 2-year mortality in conduit patients compared with shunt patients, as well as improved psychomotor development; however, shunt patients underwent initial surgery between 1996 and 2002, whereas conduit patients underwent surgery between 2002 and 2005.[A4] In contrast, Tabbutt and colleagues showed similar hospital and midterm survival and hospital length of stay in 149 patients (95 shunts, 54 conduits) but also an increased need for early reintervention in the conduit group.[T1] Lai and colleagues reviewed 80 patients and showed similar early mortality in the conduit and shunt groups, but noted that six of 41 shunt survivors died before second-stage intervention, whereas none of the 29 conduit patients died. Morbidity and mortality associated with second-stage intervention were similar.[L1]

Several studies note the requirement for reintervention for inadequate $\dot{Q}p$ prior to standard second-stage intervention in patients who receive the right ventricle–to–pulmonary trunk conduit.[D3,P7,R5,T1] Whether this is an intrinsic problem with the conduit procedure or part of the learning curve related to a relatively new technique is unclear at this time. When this problem occurs, it can be managed either by surgical or interventional revision of the conduit[D3,P7,T1] or by placing a systemic–to–pulmonary artery shunt, preferably with take-down of the conduit.[H6] The question is whether or not right ventricular function is impaired as a result of the right ventriculotomy or other factors related to the conduit procedure.

Although there are currently no definitive answers, several studies[G12,M3,T2] and the literature review by Raja and colleagues[R1] indicate that there is no evidence that right ventricular function is impaired either early or at midterm follow-up. A single randomized prospective multicenter study comparing the right ventricle–to–pulmonary trunk conduit with the systemic artery–to–pulmonary artery shunt has been performed.[O5] Fifteen institutions enrolled 549 patients. Transplantation-free 1-year survival was higher in the conduit group (74% vs. 64%, P = .01). The hazard function for death is higher for shunt patients from month 1 to month 12 after operation, becomes equal to that for conduit patients from months 13 to 36, then again rises above the hazard for conduit patients from months 36 to 48 (see Fig. 49-13). Unintended reinterventions were higher in the conduit group. Ventricular function was similar in both groups.

To summarize, current evidence suggests that the right ventricle–to–pulmonary trunk conduit is associated with improved early and midterm survival and more favorable early hemodynamics, including diastolic blood pressure and shorter hospital length of stay, and does not negatively affect right ventricular performance at midterm follow-up. Branch pulmonary artery development may be improved. An increased number of unintended procedures have been documented using this technique, but it is likely these will decrease as experience with the technique grows.

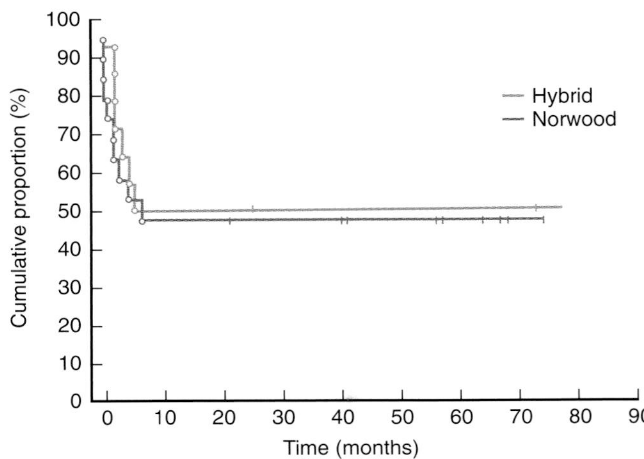

Figure 49-21 Survival according to hybrid and Norwood management strategies in high-risk patients with hypoplastic left heart physiology. (From Pizarro and colleagues.[P4])

Hybrid versus Norwood Procedure

It is difficult to compare these two procedures, mainly because hybrid procedures are usually performed in higher-risk patients. Despite this, a direct comparison of early mortality after neonatal surgery suggests that hybrid outcomes are at least as good as Norwood outcomes. Interstage and second-stage mortality, however, appear to be higher. The only study that examines outcomes following the Norwood procedure and the hybrid procedure in matched high-risk patient cohorts suggests that survival is similar[P4] (Fig. 49-21).

REFERENCES

A

1. Abbott ME. Aortic, mitral, and tricuspid atresia. In Atlas of congenital cardiac disease, New York: American Heart Association, 1936, p. 48.
2. Aiello VD, Ho SY, Anderson RH, Thiene G. Morphologic features of the hypoplastic left heart syndrome—a reappraisal. Pediatr Pathol 1990;10:931.
3. Asou T, Kado H, Imoto Y, Shiokawa Y, Tominaga R, Kawachi Y, et al. Selective cerebral perfusion technique during aortic arch repair in neonates. Ann Thorac Surg 1996;61:1546.
4. Atallah J, Dinu IA, Joffe AR, Robertson CM, Sauve RS, Dyck JD, et al. Two-year survival and mental and psychomotor outcomes after the Norwood procedure: an analysis of the modified Blalock-Taussig shunt and right ventricle-to-pulmonary artery shunt surgical eras. Circulation 2008;118:1410-8.
5. Austin EH, Jonas RA, Mayer JE, Castaneda AR. Aortic atresia with normal left ventricle. Single-stage repair in the neonate. J Thorac Cardiovasc Surg 1989;97:392.

B

1. Backer CL, Idriss FS, Zales VR, Mavroudis C. Cardiac transplantation for hypoplastic left heart syndrome: a modified technique. Ann Thorac Surg 1990;50:894.
2. Backer CL, Zales VR, Harrison HL, Idriss FS, Benson DW Jr, Mavroudis C. Intermediate term results of infant orthotopic cardiac transplantation from two centers. J Thorac Cardiovasc Surg 1991;101:826.
3. Baffa JM, Chen SL, Guttenberg ME, Norwood WI, Weinberg PM. Coronary artery abnormalities and right ventricular histology in hypoplastic left heart syndrome. J Am Coll Cardiol 1992;20:350.
4. Bailey L, Concepcion W, Shattuck H, Huang L. Method of heart transplantation for treatment of hypoplastic left heart syndrome. J Thorac Cardiovasc Surg 1986;92:1.
5. Bailey LL, Assaad AN, Trimm RF, Nehlsen-Cannarella SL, Kanakriyeh MS, Haas GS, et al. Orthotopic transplantation during early infancy as therapy for incurable congenital heart disease. Ann Surg 1988;208:279.
6. Bailey LL, Nehlsen-Cannarella SL, Doroshow RW, Jacobson JG, Martin RD, Allard MW, et al. Cardiac allotransplantation in newborns as therapy for hypoplastic left heart syndrome. N Engl J Med 1986;315:949.
7. Barber G, Chin AJ, Murphy JD, Pigott JD, Norwood WI. Hypoplastic left heart syndrome: lack of correlation between preoperative demographic and laboratory findings and survival following palliative surgery. Pediatr Cardiol 1989;10:129.
8. Barber G, Helton JG, Aglira BA, Chin AJ, Murphy JD, Pigott JD, et al. The significance of tricuspid regurgitation in hypoplastic left-heart syndrome. Am Heart J 1988;116:1563.
9. Barron DJ, Brooks A, Stickley J, Woolley SM, Stumper O, Jones TJ, et al. The Norwood procedure using a right ventricle–pulmonary artery conduit: comparison of the right-sided versus left-sided conduit position. J Thorac Cardiovasc Surg 2009;138:528-37.
10. Barron DJ, Kilby MD, Davies B, Wright JG, Jones TJ, Brawn WJ. Hypoplastic left heart syndrome. Lancet 2009;374:551-64.
11. Behrendt DM, Rocchini A. An operation for the hypoplastic left heart syndrome: preliminary report. Ann Thorac Surg 1981;32:284.
12. Bharati S, Lev M. The surgical anatomy of hypoplasia of aortic tract complex. J Thorac Cardiovasc Surg 1984;88:97.
13. Blake DM, Copel JA, Kleinman CS. Hypoplastic left heart syndrome: prenatal diagnosis, clinical profile, and management. Am J Obstet Gynecol 1991;165:529.
14. Bokeria L, Alekyan B, Berishvili D, et al. A modified hybrid stage I procedure for treatment of hypoplastic left heart syndrome: an original surgical approach. Interact Cardiovasc Thorac Surg 2010;11:142-5.
15. Brockman JL. Congenital mitral atresia. Am Heart 1950;40:301.
16. Bu'Lock FA, Stumper O, Jagtap R, Silove ED, De Giovanni JV, Wright JG, et al. Surgery for infants with a hypoplastic systemic ventricle and severe outflow obstruction: early results with a modified Norwood procedure. Br Heart J 1995;73:456.
17. Bulkley BH, D'Amico B, Taylor AL. Extensive myocardial fiber disarray in aortic and pulmonary atresia. Relevance to hypertrophic cardiomyopathy. Circulation 1983;67:191.

C

1. Caldarone CA, Benson L, Holtby H, Li J, Redington AN, Van Arsdell GS. Initial experience with hybrid palliation for neonates with single-ventricle physiology. Ann Thorac Surg 2007;84:1294-300.
2. Canton M. Congenital obliteration of origin of the aorta. Trans Pathol Soc (Lond) 1850;2:38.
3. Caspi J, Pettitt TW, Mulder T, Stopa A. Development of the pulmonary arteries after the Norwood procedure: comparison between Blalock-Taussig shunt and right ventricular–pulmonary artery conduit. Ann Thorac Surg 2008;86:1299-304.
4. Cayler GG, Smeloff EA, Miller GE Jr. Surgical palliation of hypoplastic left side of the heart. N Engl J Med 1970;282:780.
5. Chang AC, Huhta JC, Yoon GY, Wood DC, Tulzer G, Cohen A, et al. Diagnosis, transport, and outcome in fetuses with left ventricular outflow tract obstruction. J Thorac Cardiovasc Surg 1991;102:841.
6. Chang AC, Farrell PE Jr, Murdison KA, Baffa JM, Barber G, Norwood WI, et al. Hypoplastic left heart syndrome: hemodynamic and angiographic assessment after initial reconstructive surgery and relevance to modified Fontan procedure. J Am Coll Cardiol 1991;17:1143.
7. Chen Q, Parry AJ. The current role of hybrid procedures in the stage 1 palliation of patients with hypoplastic left heart syndrome. Eur J Cardiothorac Surg 2009;36:77-83.
8. Chessa M, Dindar A, Vettukattil JJ, Stumper O, Wright JG, Silove ED, et al. Balloon angioplasty in infants with aortic obstruction after the modified stage I Norwood procedure. Am Heart J 2000;140:227-31.
9. Chiavarelli M, Gundry SR, Razzouk AJ, Bailey LL. Cardiac transplantation for infants with hypoplastic left-heart syndrome. JAMA 1993;270:2944.
10. Chrisant MR, Naftel DC, Drummond-Webb J, Chinnock R, Canter CE, Boucek MM, et al. Fate of infants with hypoplastic left heart syndrome listed for cardiac transplantation: a multicenter study. J Heart Lung Transplant 2005;24:576-82.
11. Cua CL, Thiagarajan RR, Gauvreau K, Lai L, Costello JM, Wessel DL, et al. Early postoperative outcomes in a series of infants with hypoplastic left heart syndrome undergoing stage I palliation operation with either modified Blalock-Taussig shunt or right ventricle to pulmonary artery conduit. Pediatr Crit Care Med 2006;7:238-44.

D

1. Danford DA, Cronican P. Hypoplastic left heart syndrome: progression of left ventricular dilation and dysfunction to left ventricular hypoplasia in utero. Am Heart J 1992;123:1712.
2. Dasi LP, Sundareswaran KS, Sherwin C, de Zelicourt D, Kanter K, Fogel MA, et al. Larger aortic reconstruction corresponds to diminished left pulmonary artery size in patients with single-ventricle physiology. J Thorac Cardiovasc Surg 2010;139:557-61.
3. Desai T, Stumper O, Miller P, Dhillon R, Wright J, Barron D, et al. Acute interventions for stenosed right ventricle–pulmonary artery conduit following the right-sided modification of Norwood-Sano procedure. Congenit Heart Dis 2009;4:433-9.
4. DiBardino DJ, McElhinney DB, Marshall AC, Bacha EA. A review of ductal stenting in hypoplastic left heart syndrome: bridge to transplantation and hybrid stage I palliation. Pediatr Cardiol 2008;29:251-7.

5. Dillman JR, Dorfman AL, Attili AK, Agarwal PP, Bell A, Mueller GC, et al. Cardiovascular magnetic resonance imaging of hypoplastic left heart syndrome in children. Pediatr Radiol 2010; 40:261-74.
6. Doty DB, Knott HW. Hypoplastic left heart syndrome. J Thorac Cardiovasc Surg 1977;74:624.
7. Doty DB, Marvin WJ Jr, Schieken RM, Lauer RM. Hypoplastic left heart syndrome: successful palliation with a new operation. J Thorac Cardiovasc Surg 1980;80:148.
8. Duffy CE, Muster AJ, DeLeon SY, Idriss FS, Ilbawi M, Riggs TW, et al. Successful surgical repair of aortic atresia associated with normal left ventricle. J Am Coll Cardiol 1983;1:1503.

E

1. Elzenga NJ, Gittenbergerde Groot AC. Coarctation and related aortic arch anomalies in hypoplastic left heart syndrome. Int J Cardiol 1985;8:379.
2. Esteban I, Cabrera A. Aortic atresia with normal left ventricle and intact ventricular septum. Chest 1978;73:883.

F

1. Farrell PE Jr, Chang AC, Murdison KA, Baffa JM, Norwood WI, Murphy JD. Outcome and assessment after the modified Fontan procedure for hypoplastic left heart syndrome. Circulation 1992; 85:116.
2. Francois K, Dollery C, Elliott MJ. Aortic atresia with ventricular septal defect and normal left ventricle: one-stage correction in the neonate. Ann Thorac Surg 1994;58:878-80.
3. Fraser CD Jr, Mee RB. Modified Norwood procedure for hypoplastic left heart syndrome. Ann Thorac Surg 1995;60:S546.
4. Freedom RM, Williams WG, Dische MR, Rowe RD. Anatomical variants in aortic atresia—potential candidates for ventriculoaortic reconstitution. Br Heart J 1976;38:821.
5. Fyler DC. Report of the New England Regional Infant Cardiac Program. Pediatrics 1980;65:375.

G

1. Galantowicz M, Cheatham JP, Phillips A, Cua CL, Hoffman TM, Hill SL, et al. Hybrid approach for hypoplastic left heart syndrome: intermediate results after the learning curve. Ann Thorac Surg 2008;85:2063-71.
2. Gaynor JW, Bridges ND, Cohen MI, Mahle WT, Decampli WM, Steven JM, et al. Predictors of outcome after the Fontan operation: is hypoplastic left heart syndrome still a risk factor? J Thorac Cardiovasc Surg 2002;123:237-45.
3. Gaynor JW, Wernovsky G, Jarvik GP, Bernbaum J, Gerdes M, Zackai E, et al. Patient characteristics are important determinants of neurodevelopmental outcome at one year of age after neonatal and infant cardiac surgery. J Thorac Cardiovasc Surg 2007;133: 1344-53.
4. Ghanayem NS, Hoffman GM, Mussatto KA, Cava JR, Frommelt PC, Rudd NA, et al. Home surveillance program prevents interstage mortality after the Norwood procedure. J Thorac Cardiovasc Surg 2003;126:1367-77.
5. Ghanayem NS, Tweddell JS, Hoffman GM, Mussatto K, Jaquiss RD. Optimal timing of the second stage of palliation for hypoplastic left heart syndrome facilitated through home monitoring, and the results of early cavopulmonary anastomosis. Cardiol Young 2006;16 Suppl 1:61-6.
6. Gibbs JL, Wren C, Watterson KG, Hunter S, Hamilton JR. Stenting of the arterial duct combined with banding of the pulmonary arteries and atrial septectomy or septostomy; a new approach to palliation for the hypoplastic left heart syndrome. Br Heart J 1993;69:551.
7. Gibbs JL, Wren C, Watterson KG, Hunter S, Hamilton JR. Stenting of the arterial duct combined with banding of the pulmonary arteries and atrial septectomy or septostomy: a new approach to palliation for the hypoplastic left heart syndrome. Br Heart J 1993;69:551-5.
8. Glatz JA, Fedderly RT, Ghanayem NS, Tweddell JS. Impact of mitral stenosis and aortic atresia on survival in hypoplastic left heart syndrome. Ann Thorac Surg 2008;85:2057-62.
9. Glatz JA, Tabbutt S, Gaynor JW, Rome JJ, Montenegro L, Spray TL, et al. Hypoplastic left heart syndrome with atrial level restriction in the era of prenatal diagnosis. Ann Thorac Surg 2007;84:1633-8.
10. Glauser TA, Rorke LB, Weinberg PM, Clancy RR. Congenital brain anomalies associated with the hypoplastic left heart syndrome. Pediatrics 1990;85:984.
11. Goldberg CS, Bove EL, Devaney EJ, Mollen E, Schwartz E, Tindall S, et al. A randomized clinical trial of regional cerebral perfusion versus deep hypothermic circulatory arrest: outcomes for infants with functional single ventricle. J Thorac Cardiovasc Surg 2007;133:880-7.
12. Graham EM, Atz AM, Bradley SM, Scheurer MA, Bandisode VM, Laudito A, et al. Does a ventriculotomy have deleterious effects following palliation in the Norwood procedure using a shunt placed from the right ventricle to the pulmonary arteries? Cardiol Young 2007;17:145-50.
13. Griselli M, McGuirk SP, Stumper O, Clarke AJ, Miller P, Dhillon R, et al. Influence of surgical strategies on outcome after the Norwood procedure. J Thorac Cardiovasc Surg 2006;131: 418-26.
14. Grossfeld P, Ye M, Harvey R. Hypoplastic left heart syndrome: new genetic insights. J Am Coll Cardiol 2009;53:1072-4.
15. Gruber PJ, Fuller S, Cleaver KM, Abdullah I, Gruber SB, Nicolson SC, et al. Early results of single-stage biventricular repair of severe aortic hypoplasia or atresia with ventricular septal defect and normal left ventricle. J Thorac Cardiovasc Surg 2006;132:260-3.
16. Gutgesell HP, Massaro TA. Management of hypoplastic left heart syndrome in a consortium of university hospitals. Am J Cardiol 1995;76:809.

H

1. Hannan RL, Ybarra MA, Ojito JW, Alonso FA, Rossi AF, Burke RP. Complex neonatal single ventricle palliation using antegrade cerebral perfusion. Ann Thorac Surg 2006;82:1278-85.
2. Hastreiter AR, Van der Horst RL, Dubrow IW, Eckner FO. Quantitative angiographic and morphologic aspects of aortic valve atresia. Am J Cardiol 1983;51:1705.
3. Hawkins JA, Doty DB. Aortic atresia: morphologic characteristics affecting survival and operative palliation. J Thorac Cardiovasc Surg 1984;88:620.
4. Hehir DA, Dominguez TE, Ballweg JA, Ravishankar C, Marino BS, Bird GL, et al. Risk factors for interstage death after stage 1 reconstruction of hypoplastic left heart syndrome and variants. J Thorac Cardiovasc Surg 2008;136:94-9.
5. Helton JG, Aglira BA, Chin AJ, Murphy JD, Pigott JD, Norwood WI. Analysis of potential anatomic or physiologic determinants of outcome of palliative surgery for hypoplastic left heart syndrome. Circulation 1986;74:I70.
6. Hsia TY, Migliavacca F, Pennati G, Balossino R, Dubini G, de Leval MR, et al. Management of a stenotic right ventricle–pulmonary artery shunt early after the Norwood procedure. Ann Thorac Surg 2009;88:830-8.

I

1. Iannettoni MD, Bove EL, Mosca RS, Lupinetti FM, Dorostkar PC, Ludomirsky A, et al. Improving results with first-stage palliation for hypoplastic left heart syndrome. J Thorac Cardiovasc Surg 1994;107:934.
2. Imoto Y, Kado H, Shiokawa Y, Minami K, Yasui H. Experience with the Norwood procedure without circulatory arrest. J Thorac Cardiovasc Surg 2001;122:879.

J

1. Jackson GM, Ludmir J, Castelbaum AJ, Huhta JC, Cohen AW. Intrapartum course of fetuses with isolated hypoplastic left heart syndrome. Am J Obstet Gynecol 1991;165:1068.
2. Jacobs ML, Blackstone EH, Bailey LL. Intermediate survival in neonates with aortic atresia. J Thorac Cardiovasc Surg 1998;116: 417.
3. Jonas RA, Hansen DD, Cook N, Wessel D. Anatomic subtype and survival after reconstructive operation for hypoplastic left heart syndrome. J Thorac Cardiovasc Surg 1994;107:1121.

K

1. Karamichalis JM, Thiagarajan RR, Liu H, Mamic P, Gauvreau K, Bacha EA. Stage I Norwood: optimal technical performance improves outcomes irrespective of preoperative physiologic status or case complexity. J Thorac Cardiovasc Surg 2010;139:962-8.

2. Karl TR, Sano S, Brawn WJ, Mee RB. Critical aortic stenosis in the first month of life: surgical results in 26 infants. Ann Thorac Surg 1990;50:105.
3. Kern JH, Hayes CJ, Michler RE, Gersony WM, Quaegebeur JM. Survival and risk factor analysis for the Norwood procedure for hypoplastic left heart syndrome. Am J Cardiol 1997;80:170.
4. Kishimoto H, Kawahira Y, Kawata H, Miura T, Iwai S, Mori T. The modified Norwood palliation on a beating heart. J Thorac Cardiovasc Surg 1999;118:1130.

L

1. Lai L, Laussen PC, Cua CL, Wessel DL, Costello JM, del Nido PJ, et al. Outcomes after bidirectional Glenn operation: Blalock-Taussig shunt versus right ventricle-to-pulmonary artery conduit. Ann Thorac Surg 2007;83:1768-73.
2. Lambert EC, Canent RV, Hohn AR. Congenital cardiac anomalies in the newborn. A review of conditions causing death or severe distress in the first month of life. Pediatrics 1966;37:343.
3. Lang D, Hofstetter R, Kupferschmid C. Hypoplastic left heart with complete transposition of the great arteries. Br Heart J 1985;53:650.
4. Lang P, Norwood WI. Hemodynamic assessment after palliative surgery for hypoplastic left heart syndrome. Circulation 1983; 68:104.
5. Leung MP, McKay R, Smith A, Anderson RH, Arnold R. Critical aortic stenosis in early infancy. J Thorac Cardiovasc Surg 1991; 101:526.
6. Levitsky S, van der Horst RL, Hasteiter AR, Eckner FA, Bennett EJ. Surgical palliation in aortic atresia. J Thorac Cardiovasc Surg 1980;79:456.
7. Lev M. Pathologic anatomy and interrelationship of hypoplasia of the aortic tract complexes. Lab Invest 1952;1:61.
8. Lofland GK, McCrindle BW, Williams WG, Blackstone EH, Tchervenkov CI, Sittiwangkul R, et al. Critical aortic stenosis in the neonate: a multi-institutional study of management, outcomes, and risk factors. Congenital Heart Surgeons Society. J Thorac Cardiovasc Surg 2001;121:10.
9. Ludman P, Foale R, Alexander N, Nihoyannopoulos P. Cross sectional echocardiographic identification of hypoplastic left heart syndrome and differentiation from other causes of right ventricular overload. Br Heart J 1990;63:355.

M

1. Machii M, Becker AE. Nature of coarctation in hypoplastic left heart syndrome. Ann Thorac Surg 1995;59:1491.
2. Mahowald JM, Lucas RV Jr, Edwards JE. Aortic valvular atresia. Associated cardiovascular anomalies. Pediatr Cardiol 1982;2:99.
3. Mair R, Tulzer G, Sames E, Gitter R, Lechner E, Steiner J, et al. Right ventricular to pulmonary artery conduit instead of modified Blalock-Taussig shunt improves postoperative hemodynamics in newborns after the Norwood operation. J Thorac Cardiovasc Surg 2003;126:1378-84.
4. Malhotra SP, Hanley FL. Routine continuous perfusion for aortic arch reconstruction in the neonate. Semin Thorac Cardiovasc Surg Pediatr Card Surg Annu 2008:57-60.
5. McElhinney DB, Tworetzky W, Lock JE. Current status of fetal cardiac intervention. Circulation 2010;121:1256-63.
6. McGarry KM, Taylor JF, Macartney FJ. Aortic atresia occurring with complete transposition of the great arteries. Br Heart J 1980; 44:711.
7. McGuirk SP, Stickley J, Griselli M, Stumper OF, Laker SJ, Barron DJ, et al. Risk assessment and early outcome following the Norwood procedure for hypoplastic left heart syndrome. Eur J Cardiothorac Surg 2006;29:675-81.
8. McKenzie ED, Andropoulos DB, DiBardino D, Fraser CD, Jr. Congenital heart surgery 2005: the brain: it's the heart of the matter. Am J Surg 2005;190:289-94.
9. Meyer RA, Kaplan S. Echocardiography in the diagnosis of hypoplasia of the left or right ventricles in the neonate. Circulation 1972;46:55.
10. Milo S, Ho SY, Anderson RH. Hypoplastic left heart syndrome: can this malformation be treated surgically? Thorax 1980;35:351.
11. Mohri H, Horiuchi T, Haneda K, Sato S, Kahata O, Ohmi M, et al. Surgical treatment of hypoplastic left heart syndrome. J Thorac Cardiovasc Surg 1979;78:223.
12. Moorthy PS, McGuirk SP, Jones TJ, Brawn WJ, Barron DJ. Damus-Rastelli procedure for biventricular repair of aortic atresia and hypoplasia. Ann Thorac Surg 2007;84:142-6.
13. Mosca RS, Bove EL, Crowley DC, Sandhu SK, Schork MA, Kulik TJ. Hemodynamic characteristics of neonates following first stage palliation for hypoplastic left heart syndrome. Circulation 1995;92:II267.
14. Murdison KA, Baffa JM, Farrell PE Jr, Chang AC, Barber G, Norwood WI, et al. Hypoplastic left heart syndrome. Outcome after initial reconstruction and before modified Fontan procedure. Circulation 1990;82:IV199.

N

1. Nathan M, Rimmer D, del Nido PJ, Mayer JE, Bacha EA, Shin A, et al. Aortic atresia or severe left ventricular outflow tract obstruction with ventricular septal defect: results of primary biventricular repair in neonates. Ann Thorac Surg 2006;82:2227-32.
2. Natowicz M, Chatten J, Clancy R, Conard K, Glauser T, Huff D, et al. Genetic disorders and major extracardiac anomalies associated with hypoplastic left heart syndrome. Pediatrics 1988;82:698.
3. Nelson DP, Andropoulos DB, Fraser CD Jr. Perioperative neuroprotective strategies. Semin Thorac Cardiovasc Surg Pediatr Card Surg Annu 2008:49-56.
4. Noonan JA, Nadas AS. The hypoplastic left heart syndrome: an analysis of 101 cases. Pediatr Clin North Am 1958;5:1029.
5. Norwood WI Jr, Jacobs ML, Murphy JD. Fontan procedure for hypoplastic left heart syndrome. Ann Thorac Surg 1992;54: 1025.
6. Norwood WI, Kirklin JK, Sanders SP. Hypoplastic left heart syndrome. Experience with palliative surgery. Am J Cardiol 1980;45:87.
7. Norwood WI, Lang P, Casteneda AR, Campbell DN. Experience with operations for hypoplastic left heart syndrome. J Thorac Cardiovasc Surg 1981;82:511.
8. Norwood WI, Lang P, Hansen DD. Physiologic repair of aortic atresia–hypoplastic left heart syndrome. N Engl J Med 1983;308:23.
9. Norwood WI, Stellin GJ. Aortic atresia with interrupted aortic arch. J Thorac Cardiovasc Surg 1981;81:239.

O

1. O'Connor WN, Cash JB, Cottrill CM, Johnson GL, Noonan JA. Ventriculocoronary connections in hypoplastic left hearts: an autopsy microscopic study. Circulation 1982;66:1078.
2. Ohye RG, Goldberg CS, Donohue J, Hirsch JC, Gaies M, Jacobs ML, et al. The quest to optimize neurodevelopmental outcomes in neonatal arch reconstruction: the perfusion techniques we use and why we believe in them. J Thorac Cardiovasc Surg 2009; 137:803-6.
3. Ohye RG, Gomez CA, Goldberg CS, Graves HL, Devaney EJ, Bove EL. Repair of the tricuspid valve in hypoplastic left heart syndrome. Cardiol Young 2006;16 Suppl 3:21-6.
4. Ohye RG, Kagisaki K, Lee LA, Mosca RS, Goldberg CS, Bove EL. Biventricular repair for aortic atresia or hypoplasia and ventricular septal defect. J Thorac Cardiovasc Surg 1999;118:648-53.
5. Ohye RG, Sleeper LA, Mahony L, Newburger JW, Pearson GD, Lu M, et al. Comparison of shunt types in the Norwood procedure for single-ventricle lesions. N Engl J Med 2010;362:1980-92.
6. Oppido G, Pace Napoleone C, Turci S, Davies B, Frascaroli G, Martin-Suarez S, et al. Moderately hypothermic cardiopulmonary bypass and low-flow antegrade selective cerebral perfusion for neonatal aortic arch surgery. Ann Thorac Surg 2006;82:2233-9.

P

1. Pearl JM, Cripe LW, Manning PB. Biventricular repair after Norwood palliation. Ann Thorac Surg 2003;75:132-7.
2. Pigula FA, Vida V, Del Nido P, Bacha E. Contemporary results and current strategies in the management of hypoplastic left heart syndrome. Semin Thorac Cardiovasc Surg 2007;19:238-44.
3. Pizarro C, Murdison KA. Off pump palliation for hypoplastic left heart syndrome: surgical approach. Semin Thorac Cardiovasc Surg Pediatr Card Surg Annu 2005:66-71.
4. Pizarro C, Derby CD, Baffa JM, Murdison KA, Radtke WA. Improving the outcome of high-risk neonates with hypoplastic left heart syndrome: hybrid procedure or conventional surgical palliation? Eur J Cardiothorac Surg 2008;33:613-8.
5. Pizarro C, Malec E, Maher KO, Januszewska K, Gidding SS, Murdison KA, et al. Right ventricle to pulmonary artery conduit improves outcome after stage I Norwood for hypoplastic left heart syndrome. Circulation 2003;108:II155-60.

6. Pizarro C, Murdison KA, Derby CD, Radtke W. Stage II reconstruction after hybrid palliation for high-risk patients with a single ventricle. Ann Thorac Surg 2008;85:1382-8.
7. Pruetz JD, Badran S, Dorey F, Starnes VA, Lewis AB. Differential branch pulmonary artery growth after the Norwood procedure with right ventricle–pulmonary artery conduit versus modified Blalock-Taussig shunt in hypoplastic left heart syndrome. J Thorac Cardiovasc Surg 2009;137:1342-8.

R

1. Raja SG, Atamanyuk I, Kostolny M, Tsang V. In hypoplastic left heart patients is Sano shunt compared with modified Blalock-Taussig shunt associated with deleterious effects on ventricular performance? Interact Cardiovasc Thorac Surg 2010;10:620-3.
2. Redo SF, Engle MA, Ehlers KH, Farnsworth PB. Palliative surgery for mitral atresia. Arch Surg 1967;95:717.
3. Reddy VM, Rajasinghe HA, McElhinney DB, van Son JA, Black MD, Silverman NH, et al. Extending the limits of the Ross procedure. Ann Thorac Surg 1995;60:S600.
4. Reddy VM, Rajasinghe HA, Teitel DF, Haas GS, Hanley FL. Aortoventriculoplasty with the pulmonary autograft: the "Ross-Konno" procedure. J Thorac Cardiovasc Surg 1996;111:158.
5. Reinhartz O, Reddy VM, Petrossian E, MacDonald M, Lamberti JJ, Roth SJ, et al. Homograft valved right ventricle to pulmonary artery conduit as a modification of the Norwood procedure. Circulation 2006;114:I594-9.
6. Rhodes LA, Colan SD, Perry SB, Jonas RA, Sanders SP. Predictors of survival in neonates with critical aortic stenosis. Circulation 1991;84:2325.
7. Roberts WC, Perry LW, Chandra RS, Myers GE, Shapiro SR, Scott LP. Aortic valve atresia. A new classification based on necropsy study of 73 cases. Am J Cardiol 1976;37:753.
8. Ruffer A, Danch A, Gottschalk U, Mir T, Lacour-Gayet F, Haun C, et al. The Norwood procedure—does the type of shunt determine outcome? Thorac Cardiovasc Surg 2009;57:270-5.

S

1. Sakurai T, Kado H, Nakano T, Hinokiyama K, Shiose A, Kajimoto M, et al. Early results of bilateral pulmonary artery banding for hypoplastic left heart syndrome. Eur J Cardiothorac Surg 2009;36:973-9.
2. Sano S, Huang SC, Kasahara S, Yoshizumi K, Kotani Y, Ishino K. Risk factors for mortality after the Norwood procedure using right ventricle to pulmonary artery shunt. Ann Thorac Surg 2009;87:178-86.
3. Sasaki T, Tsuda S, Riemer RK, Ramamoorthy C, Reddy VM, Hanley FL. Optimal flow rate for antegrade cerebral perfusion. J Thorac Cardiovasc Surg 2010;139:530-5.
4. Sauer U, Gittenbergerde Groot AC, Geishauser M, Babic R, Buhlmeyer K. Coronary arteries in the hypoplastic left heart syndrome. Circulation 1989;80:I168.
5. Sinha SN, Rusnak SL, Sommers HM, Cole RB, Muster AJ, Paul MH. Hypoplastic left ventricle syndrome. Analysis of thirty autopsy cases in infants with surgical considerations. Am J Cardiol 1968;21:166.
6. Sharland GK, Chita SK, Fagg NL, Anderson RH, Tynan M, Cook AC, et al. Left ventricular dysfunction in the fetus: relation to aortic valve anomalies and endocardial fibroelastosis. Br Heart J 1991;66:419.
7. Shone JD, Edwards JE. Mitral atresia associated with pulmonary venous anomalies. Br Heart J 1964;26:241.
8. Simsic JM, Bradley SM, Stroud MR, Atz AM. Risk factors for interstage death after the Norwood procedure. Pediatr Cardiol 2005;26:400-3.
9. Sivarajan V, Penny DJ, Filan P, Brizard C, Shekerdemian LS. Impact of antenatal diagnosis of hypoplastic left heart syndrome on the clinical presentation and surgical outcomes: the Australian experience. J Paediatr Child Health 2009;45:112-7.
10. Soongswang J, McCrindle BW, Jones TK, Vincent RN, Hsu DT, Kuhn MA, et al. Outcomes of transcatheter balloon angioplasty of obstruction in the neo-aortic arch after the Norwood operation. Cardiol Young 2001;11:54-61.
11. Srinivasan C, Sachdeva R, Morrow WR, Gossett J, Chipman CW, Imamura M, et al. Standardized management improves outcomes after the Norwood procedure. Congenit Heart Dis 2009;4:329-37.
12. Starnes VA, Griffin ML, Pitlick PT, Bernstein D, Baum D, Ivens K, et al. Current approach to hypoplastic left heart syndrome: palliation, transplantation, or both? J Thorac Cardiovasc Surg 1992;104:189.
13. Stasik CN, Gelehrter S, Goldberg CS, Bove EL, Devaney EJ, Ohye RG. Current outcomes and risk factors for the Norwood procedure. J Thorac Cardiovasc Surg 2006;131:412-7.
14. Stoica SC, Philips AB, Egan M, Rodeman R, Chisolm J, Hill S, et al. The retrograde aortic arch in the hybrid approach to hypoplastic left heart syndrome. Ann Thorac Surg 2009;88:1939-47.
15. Suzuki K, Doi S, Oku K, Murakami Y, Mori K, Mimori S, et al. Hypoplastic left heart syndrome with premature closure of foramen ovale: report of an unusual type of totally anomalous pulmonary venous return. Heart Vessels 1990;5:117.

T

1. Tabbutt S, Dominguez TE, Ravishankar C, Marino BS, Gruber PJ, Wernovsky G, et al. Outcomes after the stage I reconstruction comparing the right ventricular to pulmonary artery conduit with the modified Blalock Taussig shunt. Ann Thorac Surg 2005;80:1582-91.
2. Tanoue Y, Kado H, Shiokawa Y, Fusazaki N, Ishikawa S. Midterm ventricular performance after Norwood procedure with right ventricular–pulmonary artery conduit. Ann Thorac Surg 2004;78:1965-71.
3. Tchervenkov CI, Chu VF, Shum-Tim D, Laliberte E, Reyes TU. Norwood operation without circulatory arrest: a new surgical technique. Ann Thorac Surg 2000;70:1730.
4. Tucker WY, McKone RC, Weesner KM, Kon ND. Hypoplastic left heart syndrome: palliation without cardiopulmonary bypass. J Thorac Cardiovasc Surg 1990;99:885.
5. Tworetzky W, McElhinney DB, Burch GH, Teitel DF, Moore P. Balloon arterioplasty of recurrent coarctation after the modified Norwood procedure in infants. Catheter Cardiovasc Interv 2000;50:54-8.
6. Tworetsky W, McElhinney DB, Reddy VM, Brook MM, Hanley FL, Silverman NH. Improved surgical outcome after fetal diagnosis of hypoplastic left heart syndrome. Circulation 2001;103:1269.

V

1. van der Horst RL, Hastreiter AR, DuBrow IW, Eckner FA. Pathologic measurements in aortic atresia. Am Heart J 1983;106:1411.
2. Venugopal PS, Luna KP, Anderson DR, Austin CB, Rosenthal E, Krasemann T, et al. Hybrid procedure as an alternative to surgical palliation of high-risk infants with hypoplastic left heart syndrome and its variants. J Thorac Cardiovasc Surg 2010;139:1211-5.
3. Vida VL, Bacha EA, Larrazabal A, Gauvreau K, Dorfman AL, Marx G, et al. Surgical outcome for patients with the mitral stenosis–aortic atresia variant of hypoplastic left heart syndrome. J Thorac Cardiovasc Surg 2008;135:339-46.
4. Vida VL, Bacha EA, Larrazabal A, Gauvreau K, Thiagaragan R, Fynn-Thompson F, et al. Hypoplastic left heart syndrome with intact or highly restrictive atrial septum: surgical experience from a single center. Ann Thorac Surg 2007;84:581-6.
5. Von Rueden TJ, Knight L, Moller JH, Ewards JE. Coarctation of the aorta associated with aortic valvular atresia. Circulation 1975;52:951.

W

1. Welke KF, Shen I, Ungerleider RM. Current assessment of mortality rates in congenital cardiac surgery. Ann Thorac Surg 2006;82:164-71.
2. Wernovsky G, Ghanayem N, Ohye RG, Bacha EA, Jacobs JP, Gaynor JW, et al. Hypoplastic left heart syndrome: consensus and controversies in 2007. Cardiol Young 2007;17 Suppl 2:75-86.

Y

1. Yabek SM, Mann JS. Prostaglandin E1 infusion in the hypoplastic left heart syndrome. Chest 1979;76:330.

50 Congenital Mitral Valve Disease

DEFINITION

Congenital mitral valve disease is a developmental malformation of one or more of the components of the mitral valve apparatus, including that portion of left atrial wall immediately adjacent to the mitral anulus that produces stenosis or regurgitation or, occasionally, a combined lesion. It often coexists with other cardiac anomalies, particularly those involving the left-sided cardiac chambers and aorta.

Left atrioventricular valve (AV) anomalies associated with AV septal defects (see Chapter 34), aortic atresia and other forms of hypoplastic left heart physiology (see Chapter 49), various forms of AV discordant connection (see Chapter 55), or transposition of the great arteries (see Chapter 52) are special situations discussed in the chapters describing these conditions. Mitral valve anomalies associated with straddling or univentricular AV connections are described in Chapters 35 and 56, respectively. Regurgitation from mitral valve prolapse as part of the syndrome of myxomatous degeneration is described in Chapter 11.

HISTORICAL NOTE

Heterogeneity of congenital mitral valve disease and frequency of its association with other cardiac anomalies make it difficult to trace the historical evolution of knowledge about this entity. However, as early as 1902, Fisher described two cases of congenital disease of the left side of the heart, one of which was a stenotic supravalvar ring.[F1] Parachute mitral valve, another entity in this spectrum, was not described until 1961 and was not fully documented until 1963.[S2,S6]

One of the first reports of surgical treatment of congenital mitral valve disease was that by Starkey in 1959.[S10] In 1962, Creech and colleagues reported repairing congenital mitral regurgitation resulting from a cleft in the posterior leaflet in a 2-year-old girl. Although the child's condition was improved by suturing the cleft, moderate mitral regurgitation persisted.[C10]

MORPHOLOGY

The congenital anomaly may involve any component of the mitral apparatus and may result in stenosis with or without regurgitation or in pure regurgitation. Although only one component may be involved, more often the entire valve is affected.[C2]

Congenital mitral stenosis without or with regurgitation may result from supravalvar, anular, or valvar narrowing and may be accentuated by subvalvar obstruction produced by hypertrophied and misplaced papillary muscles or sheets of fused chordae.[C3] Frequently, stenosis is a result of abnormalities at multiple levels. Although embryologic origins of these complex anomalies are poorly understood, recent studies suggest that abnormal development of a transient left ventricular (LV) structure, a horseshoe-shaped ventricular myocardial ridge, results in various obstructive mitral valve lesions, including parachute mitral valve and formation of asymmetric mitral valves.[O1]

Congenital mitral regurgitation may result from anular dilatation secondary to anterior or posterior leaflet prolapse or to posterior leaflet hypoplasia with chordal shortening. Chordal elongation and valve prolapse may be so severe that chordal rupture can develop even in young children, producing severe regurgitation. Congenital mitral regurgitation may also be produced by clefts, gaps, or perforations in the anterior mitral leaflet, by accessory commissures, or by leaflet hypoplasia at medial or lateral commissures.

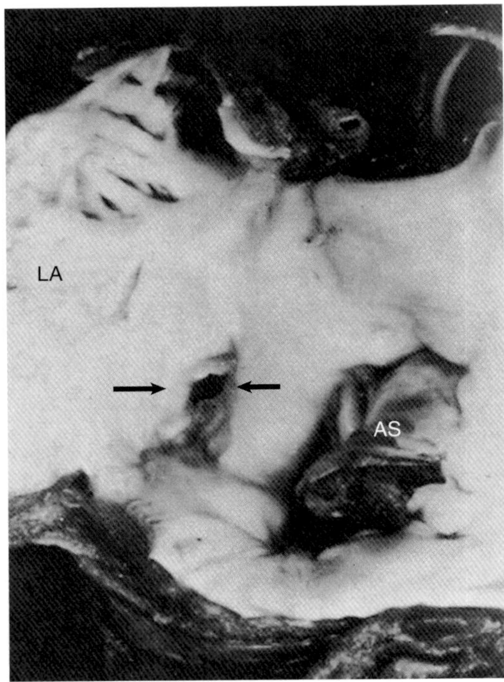

Figure 50-1 Supravalvar ring producing severe obstruction above mitral orifice in an infant dying of heart failure at age 9 months. Arrows indicate small (3 mm) orifice produced by stenosing ring. Key: *AS,* Fossa ovalis atrial septal defect; *LA,* left atrium. (From Davichi and colleagues.[D2])

Supravalvar Ring

A tough fibrous ring may be situated just on the left atrial side of the mitral anulus.[A4] The pulmonary veins and left atrial appendage enter the left atrium above (proximal to) the ring, in contrast to the situation in cor triatriatum (see Chapter 32). The supravalvar ring may be nonobstructive and an incidental finding, or it may protrude into the orifice, producing a variable degree of obstruction.[A4,D2] A ring may also occur on the left atrial aspect of the mitral valve leaflets that, when circumferential, prevents their adequate opening, causing obstruction. This lesion may be particularly difficult to identify echocardiographically.

A supravalvar ring is an isolated lesion in about half the cases in which it contributes importantly to death in the first year of life[D2,S14] (Fig. 50-1). In the other half, it coexists with other cardiac anomalies, particularly with other mitral valve anomalies and with LV outflow tract obstruction.[S6]

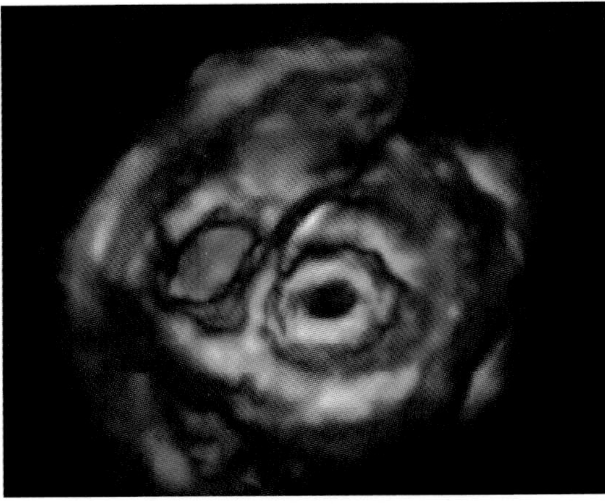

Figure 50-2 Transthoracic real-time three-dimensional echocardiogram: view from left ventricular aspect. Posterior mitral leaflet is immobile and anterior leaflet restricted. Both leaflets are thickened, and well-formed commissures are absent, resulting in a small, circular mitral valve orifice. (From Hamilton-Craig and colleagues.[H2])

Mitral Anulus

The mitral anulus uncommonly is small and obstructive in the absence of severe LV hypoplasia or other valvar abnormalities.[C8] It may be small but not obviously obstructive, particularly in hearts with coarctation of the aorta.[R2] The anulus may be enlarged, usually secondary to mitral regurgitation resulting from some other deformity of the valve. However, the basic valvar anomaly leading to regurgitation may be subtle and difficult to identify. Carpentier and colleagues found essentially isolated anular dilatation in 8 (17%) of 47 cases with congenital mitral valve disease, although some deficiency of commissural tissue is implied by their description.[C3]

Leaflet Anomalies

The orifice through the mitral valve is frequently narrowed by congenital absence of one or both commissures, which are replaced by a continuous sheet of leaflet tissue. Small perforations may be present at what is usually a commissure (Fig. 50-2). The leaflets often then take the form of an inverted

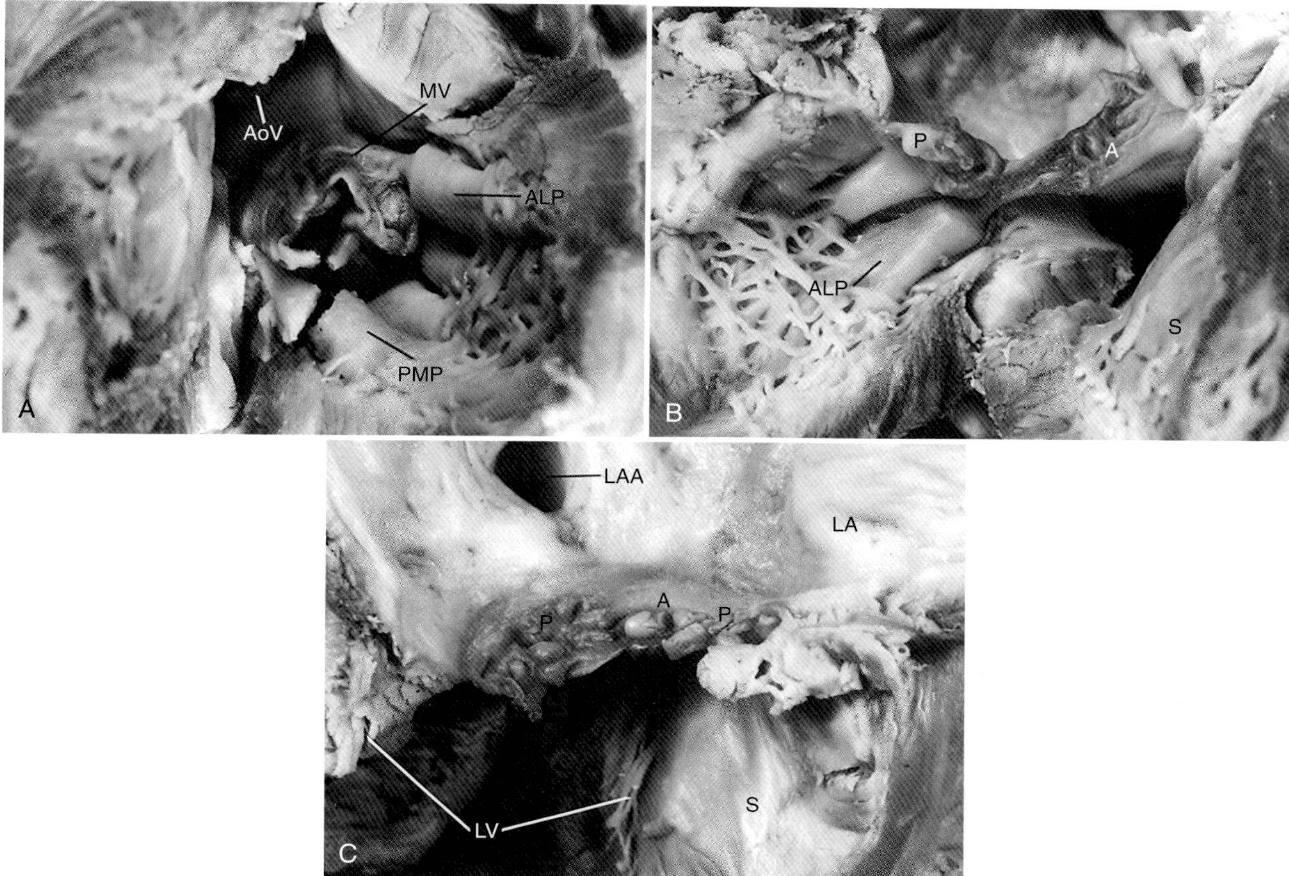

Figure 50-3 Specimen with severe congenital mitral stenosis from an infant dying at age 10 weeks with an associated ventricular septal defect. All components of valve are abnormal and contribute to stenosis. **A,** Viewed from left ventricle (LV) with mitral valve *(MV)* essentially intact. Leaflets are diffusely thickened without commissures, papillary muscles are bulky and almost reach the leaflets, and chordae are thick, fused, and short. **B,** Viewed from LV with mitral anulus divided. **C,** Viewed from left atrium. It is not possible to distinguish anterior from posterior leaflet except by their attachments to anulus. Key: *A,* Anterior mitral leaflet; *ALP,* anterolateral papillary muscle; *AoV,* aortic valve; *LA,* left atrium; *LAA,* left atrial appendage; *LV,* left ventricle; *P,* posterior mitral leaflet; *PMP,* posteromedial papillary muscle; *S,* muscular interventricular septum.

cone; in this circumstance, chordae are usually short and intermixed and the orifice further obstructed by abnormal and hypertrophied papillary muscles beneath it (the so-called hammock valve).[C4] In other cases, there may be congenital leaflet thickening and immobility and consequent orifice narrowing, even though commissures are present (Fig. 50-3).

When congenital mitral regurgitation without important stenosis is the functional lesion, a variety of mitral leaflet anomalies may be responsible. The posterior leaflet may be severely hypoplastic and represented only by tags of fibrous tissue.[C3] In other cases, the anterior leaflet may be long and billowing and the chordae thin, elongated, and occasionally ruptured.[D2,F3] This has been observed as a cause of severe mitral regurgitation in patients as young as age 2 years. It may represent prolapse or myxomatous degeneration of the mitral valve appearing in the very young (see "Mitral Valve Prolapse" under Morphology in Section I of Chapter 11).

Without any stigmata of an AV septal defect, the anterior leaflet or, less commonly, the posterior leaflet may be separated into two leaflets by an accessory commissure or a cleft, with resultant regurgitation through that area.[C10,D4,W1] The abnormality is considered an accessory commissure if there are chordae tendineae associated with it, and a cleft if there are none. Chordae tendineae may pass from the edges of an accessory commissure to ventricular septum or rudimentary papillary muscles (as was the case in two of five cases reported by Carpentier and colleagues[C3]), or the cleft may simply represent leaflet deficiency in that area (Fig. 50-4) without chordal support.[B4,F3] Rarely, there may be a hole in the anterior leaflet.[F3]

Commissural leaflet tissue may be absent at one or the other commissure, resulting in an accessory orifice and mitral regurgitation.[S3]

Chordal Anomalies

Short chordae (often thick and fused) or complete chordal absence bring leaflet tissue down onto the papillary muscles and result in a narrow orifice (Fig. 50-5). Complete absence of chordal development is common in congenital mitral stenosis.[C7] Accessory chordae that attach along the entire free edge of the anterior leaflet rather than leaving its central third free are a cause of restricted leaflet motion and, therefore, stenosis.[R2]

Chordal abnormalities can also result in congenital mitral regurgitation. The most common is chordal elongation,

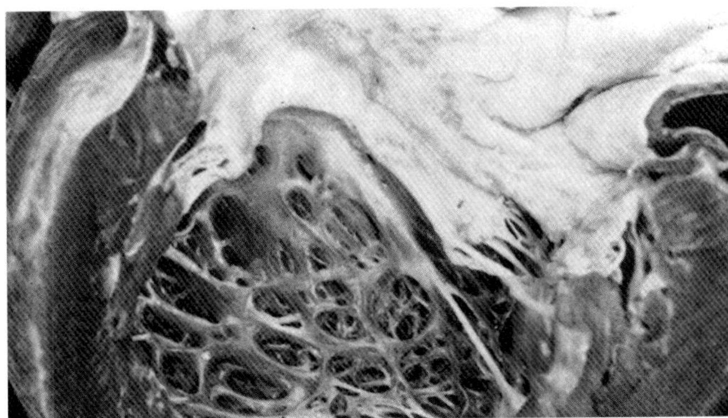

Figure 50-4 Specimen from a 9-year-old boy who died with heart failure from severe mitral regurgitation. There is a large cleft, or gap, without chordae in anterior mitral leaflet. (From Edwards.[E1])

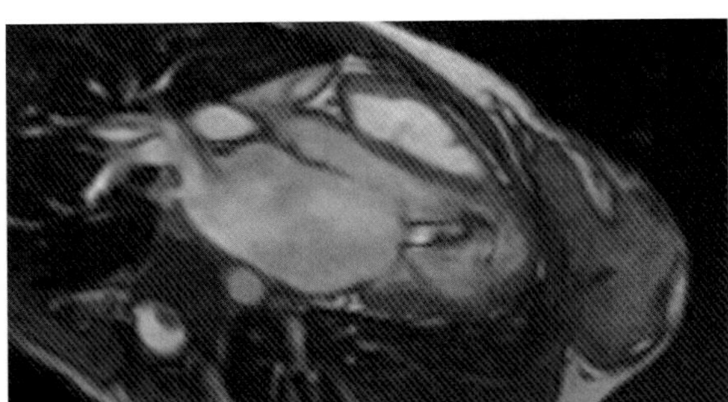

Figure 50-5 Steady-state free precession cardiac magnetic resonance image. Long-axis view demonstrating severe restriction of mitral valve leaflet opening. It confirms insertion of two papillary muscles into the leaflets via abnormally short chordae, along with markedly dilated left atrium. (From Hamilton-Craig and colleagues.[H2])

sometimes with lengthened papillary muscles, the tips of which prolapse along with the leaflet into the left atrium during ventricular systole.[C3]

Papillary Muscle Anomalies

There may be a single large papillary muscle with all chordae attaching to it, the so-called parachute valve described first by Schiebler and colleagues and emphasized by Shone and colleagues[S2,S6] (Figs. 50-6 and 50-7). Usually the chordae are short and thick and limit leaflet movement. This restricts the primary orifice through the opened valve as well as secondary orifices between chordae, resulting in mitral stenosis. In other cases, there is a single large papillary muscle, and near it is a hypoplastic one with only a few chordae attached; the valve orifice is narrowed by the same mechanisms. A parachute valve usually produces only severe stenosis, but it may also produce mitral regurgitation.[G3]

Two hypertrophied and abnormally placed contiguous papillary muscles, usually situated posteriorly, are also a cause of subvalvar obstruction.[C3,C4,D2] Obstruction is often further aggravated by coexistence of short, thick chordae and anomalous thick muscular bands.[R5] In other cases, there are three or more closely placed and hypoplastic or bulky papillary muscles, a situation in which short, thick chordae are often also present and contribute to stenosis. In all these cases, absence of the normal wide interpapillary distance contributes to obstruction in the mitral pathway.

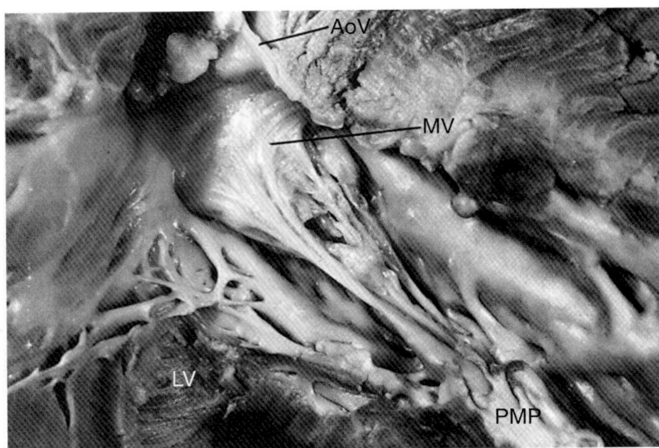

Figure 50-6 Specimen of a heart with congenital mitral stenosis from parachute mitral valve, viewed from left ventricular aspect. Chordae are thickened, and all attach to a single posteromedial papillary muscle. Anterolateral papillary muscle is absent. Key: *AoV,* Aortic valve; *LV,* left ventricle; *MV,* mitral valve; *PMP,* posteromedial papillary muscle.

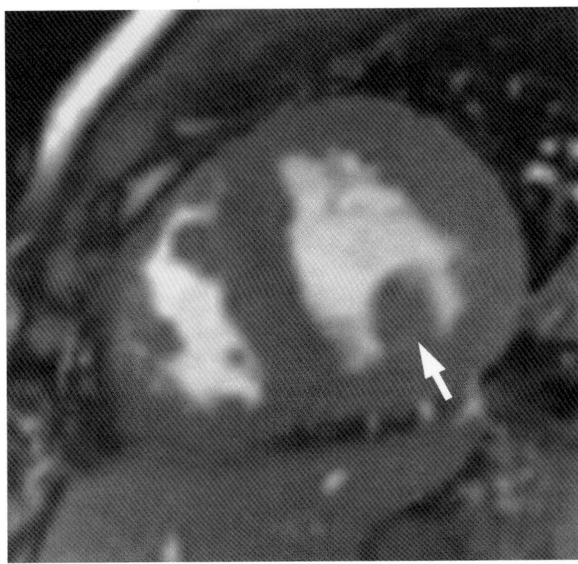

Figure 50-7 Mid-ventricular short-axis view from a magnetic resonance imaging cine sequence of a 4-year-old girl. There is only one papillary muscle, at the posteromedial position, supporting the mitral valve *(arrow)*. Anterolateral papillary muscle is absent.

An anomalous papillary muscle arcade (mitral arcade) formed by a bridge of fibrous tissue running through the free aspect of the anterior mitral leaflet, between the anterolateral and posteromedial papillary muscles, may produce mitral regurgitation[D2,L3] (Fig. 50-8).

Coexisting Cardiac Anomalies

Patients with congenital mitral regurgitation often have coexisting cardiac anomalies, but they tend to be less severe than in congenital mitral stenosis (Table 50-1).

Congenital mitral stenosis is rarely an isolated malformation. In about 30% of cases, it coexists with ventricular septal defect (VSD). In more than 50%, it coexists with one or

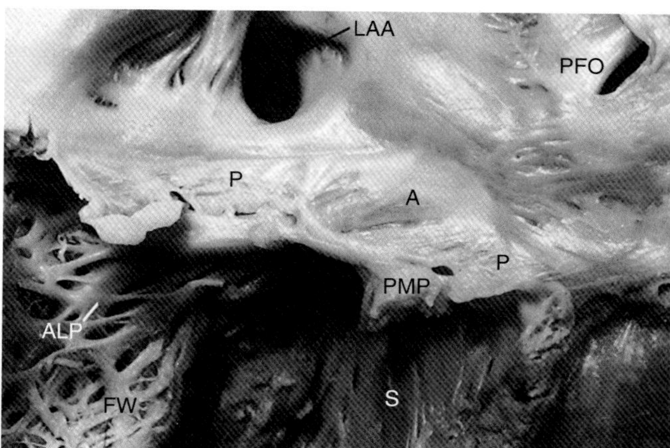

Figure 50-8 Specimen of a heart with mitral arcade producing mitral regurgitation. There is a thick fibrous band stretching between tips of the two papillary muscles along edge of anterior leaflet. Key: *A,* Anterior mitral leaflet; *ALP,* anterolateral papillary muscle; *FW,* left ventricular free wall; *LAA,* left atrial appendage; *P,* posterior mitral leaflet; *PFO,* patent foramen ovale; *PMP,* portion of posteromedial papillary muscle; *S,* muscular septum.

Table 50-1 Coexisting Cardiac Anomalies in Patients Undergoing Operation for Mitral Regurgitation

Anomaly	No.	% of 51
Atrial septal defect	13	25
Ventricular septal defect	12	24
Coarctation of aorta	6	12
Patent ductus	5	10
Constrictive pericarditis	3	6
Subaortic stenosis	3	6
Tricuspid valve regurgitation	3	6
Aortic arch anomaly	1	2
Aortic valve regurgitation	1	2
Aortic valve stenosis	1	2
Coronary artery fistulas	1	2
Pulmonary artery stenosis	1	2
Transposition of the great arteries	1	2

Data from Chauvaud and colleagues.[C6]

Table 50-2 Associated Cardiac Anomalies in Infants with Congenital Mitral Valve Stenosis[a]

Anomaly	No.	% of 85
None	3	4
Subaortic, subvalvar stenosis	47	55
Coarctation	33	39
Ventricular septal defect	28	33
Patent ductus arteriosus	21	25
Atrial septal defect	21	25
DORV	15	18
Small left ventricle	15	18
Tetralogy of Fallot	5	6

Data from Moore and colleagues.[M8]
[a]Age 7.1 ± 6.4 months; weight 5.6 ± 2.3 kg.
Key: *DORV,* Double outlet right ventricle.

another form of LV outflow obstruction, a situation termed *Shone syndrome.*[S6] This may consist only of coarctation or some hypoplasia of the distal aortic arch, with or without patent ductus arteriosus (Table 50-2). LV outflow tract obstruction may be valvar, discrete subvalvar, or combined valvar and subvalvar aortic stenosis, with or without coarctation. Rarely, there is diffuse tunnel subvalvar stenosis, with or without the other forms of LV outflow tract obstruction. The aortic valve may be bicuspid. Frequency of association of LV outflow tract obstruction with congenital mitral valve disease is evidenced by Rosenquist's finding of 31 instances of coexisting important congenital mitral valve anomalies among autopsy specimens from 53 patients whose primary diagnosis in life was coarctation of the aorta.[R2] However, when a large surgical series of coarctation repair is considered that includes adults as well as infants and children, only 2% of patients demonstrate congenital mitral valve disease.[F3] All of this supports considering congenital mitral valve disease as an important component in the entity known as *hypoplastic left heart physiology* (see Chapter 49).

Rare coexistence of a stenosing supravalvar ring with tetralogy of Fallot is noteworthy because, if undetected, it may cause death after tetralogy repair.[B3,C8] Congenital mitral valve disease and subaortic stenosis may rarely coexist with subpulmonary stenosis and intact ventricular septum, subpulmonary stenosis and VSD, or valvar pulmonary stenosis.[B5,G3]

CLINICAL FEATURES AND DIAGNOSTIC CRITERIA

Symptoms and Signs

Isolated Mitral Valve Disease

Symptoms and clinical signs are identical to those of acquired mitral valve disease, the congenital etiology being apparent only when presentation is in infancy or early childhood and there is no rheumatic history (see Clinical Features and Diagnostic Criteria in Section I of Chapter 11). Symptoms of pulmonary venous hypertension include dyspnea, orthopnea or paroxysmal nocturnal dyspnea, and recurrent pulmonary infection.[C8] Pulmonary hypertension is usually present in severe lesions, terminating in heart failure, often with peripheral and central cyanosis.[C8]

Mitral stenosis is associated with a prominent apical mid-diastolic murmur, sometimes with presystolic accentuation, and there may be an opening snap, although the morphologic features commonly resulting in limitation of leaflet movement make this less common than in acquired mitral stenosis.[A4,D1] Mitral regurgitation is evidenced by an apical pansystolic murmur radiating to the axilla, frequently with a third heart sound or a short mid-diastolic murmur and LV overactivity. When there is pulmonary hypertension, the second heart sound is accentuated and there is a right ventricular lift.

Mitral Valve Disease and Left Ventricular Outflow Tract Obstruction

Unless a VSD or patent ductus arteriosus is also present, the mitral signs are usually clinically diagnostic, particularly when the only additional important site of obstruction is a coarctation. When there is severe congenital aortic stenosis, the mitral lesion, unless also severe, may not be clinically obvious, although it worsens the clinical presentation.

Electrocardiography

Electrocardiographic (ECG) evidence of left atrial hypertrophy of greater degree than is usually found in the coexisting cardiac anomaly suggests associated congenital mitral valve disease. Right ventricular hypertrophy is evident on the ECG when there is the usual raised pulmonary vascular resistance and right atrial enlargement, whereas LV hypertrophy is evident on the ECG when there is severe mitral regurgitation or associated LV outflow tract obstruction. Atrial fibrillation is rare.

Chest Radiography

Left atrial enlargement out of proportion to that usually present in any coexisting cardiac anomaly is the most important clue in the chest radiograph of the possible presence of congenital mitral valve disease. There is cardiac enlargement regardless of whether the disease is isolated or complex. Signs of pulmonary venous hypertension and occasionally overt pulmonary edema may be present in severe cases, but pulmonary plethora from a coexisting left-to-right shunt may obscure these signs.

Two-Dimensional Echocardiography

Two-dimensional echocardiography combined with Doppler interrogation can provide a complete analysis of the morphology and function of congenitally abnormal mitral valves[D3,G4,S8,S9,T4,V2] (Fig. 50-9, *A-F*). However, diagnosis by echocardiography of some forms of congenital mitral valve disease, especially supravalvar ring and double orifice mitral valve, requires considerable care and can easily be missed.[S5,S14] Three-dimensional echocardiography can provide important morphologic details that may not be visible with standard imaging (see Fig. 50-2).

Cardiac Catheterization and Cineangiographic Studies

Cardiac catheterization and cineangiographic studies are often performed to evaluate possible associated lesions and define the degree of pulmonary vascular disease.[C2] Morphology of the congenitally abnormal valve can be further evaluated by its cineangiographic appearance.[M1]

Computed Tomography and Magnetic Resonance Imaging

Computed tomography (CT) plays a limited role in evaluating the congenitally abnormal mitral valve, but magnetic resonance imaging (MRI) can provide important morphologic information that may supplement that provided by echocardiography (see Figs. 50-5 and 50-7). In addition, MRI can provide functional information such as quantification of mitral regurgitant fraction and valve area in diastole (Fig. 50-10).

NATURAL HISTORY

Congenital mitral valve disease is a rare congenital cardiac anomaly, occurring in 0.6% of autopsied patients with congenital heart disease and 0.21% to 0.42% of clinical cases of congenital heart disease.[C8]

Natural history is highly variable and depends most importantly on severity of resultant stenosis or regurgitation and on type and severity of coexisting lesions, rather than on the particular morphologic mitral valve lesion itself. For example,

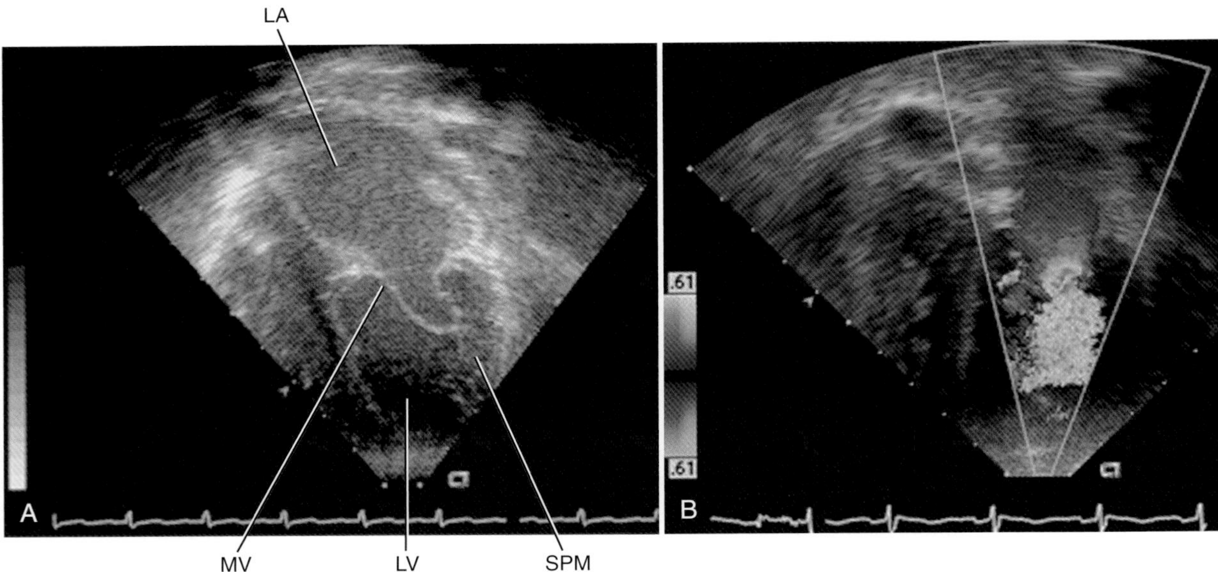

Figure 50-9 Echocardiographic evaluation of congenital mitral valve disease. **A,** Four-chamber view showing mitral stenosis secondary to parachute mitral valve *(MV)*. A single papillary muscle *(SPM)* is present. Note eccentric opening of MV oriented toward SPM. Left atrium *(LA)* is markedly enlarged. **B,** Four-chamber color Doppler view in diastole showing flow disturbance and acceleration at mitral inlet, indicating important mitral stenosis.

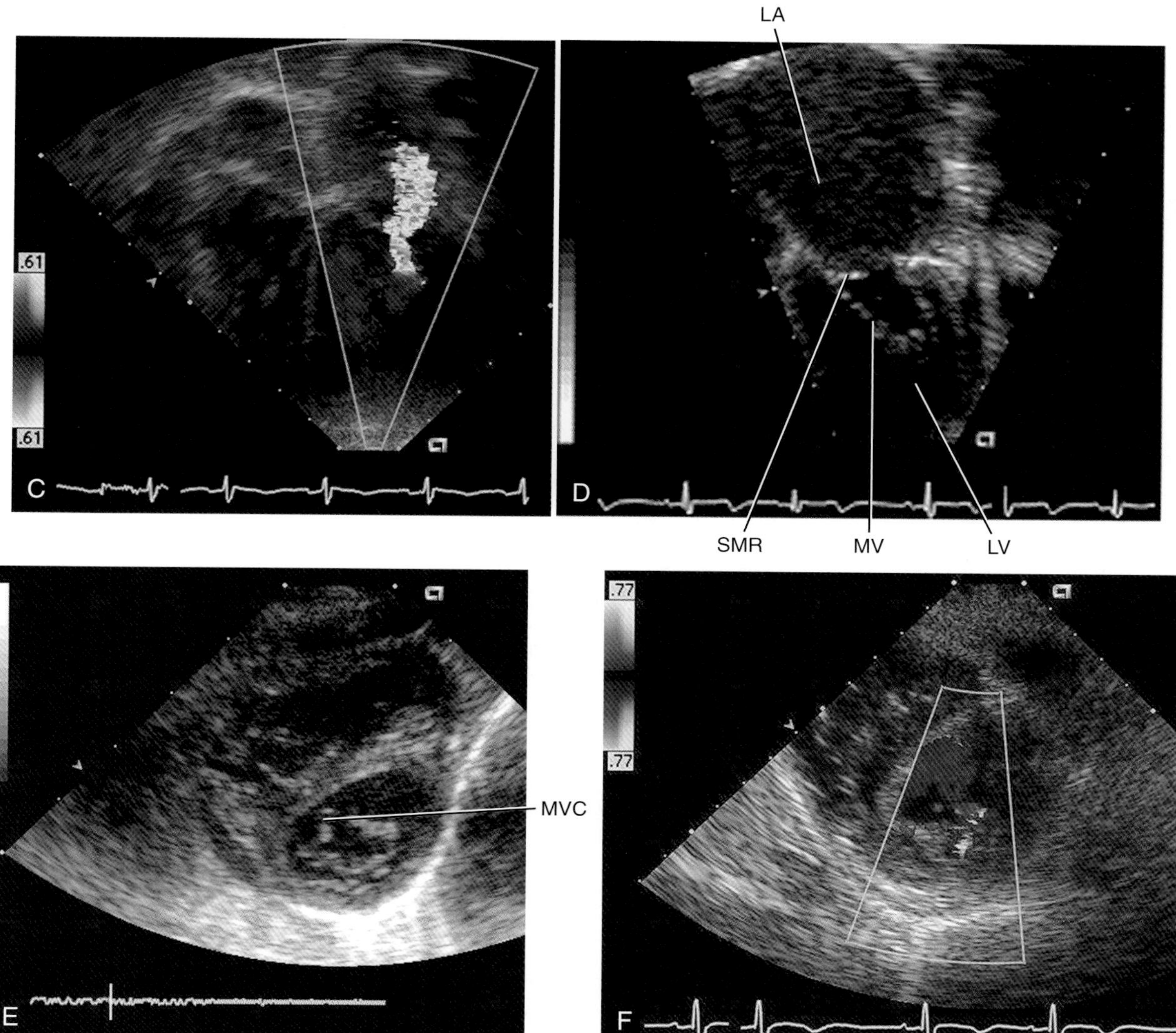

Figure 50-9, cont'd **C,** Four-chamber view with color Doppler in systole, showing mitral regurgitation in setting of congenital mitral stenosis. **D,** Four-chamber echocardiographic image showing supramitral ring *(SMR)* in congenital mitral stenosis. Ring is echo dense and present circumferentially just downstream from MV anulus. Note enlarged LA. **E,** Short-axis view of left ventricle at level of MV orifice, showing cleft in mitral anterior leaflet. **F,** Echocardiographic image with color flow Doppler revealing regurgitant jet through mitral valve cleft *(MVC)*. Key: *LV,* Left ventricle.

in one study, *parachute mitral valve* was associated with 95% freedom from mitral valve surgery at 6 months and 80% freedom at 10 years.[S1] However, associated cardiac defects were present in essentially all cases, particularly LV outflow tract abnormalities, atrial septal defect, VSD, coarctation, and hypoplastic LV; these strongly influence natural history. In another study, only 4% of patients with parachute mitral valve required a procedure on the valve, with intervention dominated by associated cardiac anomalies.[M2] Parachute mitral valve presenting in the adult is rare but does occur and is more likely to be an isolated anomaly than when diagnosed in infants and children. Nine patients have been identified in the literature over the past 50 years; three were asymptomatic without important hemodynamic abnormalities, three presented with stenosis, and three with regurgitation.[H1]

Isolated *congenital mitral stenosis* usually is severe and often produces symptoms and death if untreated during the first 4 to 5 years of life.[C8,V1] When congenital mitral stenosis coexists with other important cardiac anomalies, symptoms occur even earlier. When it is associated with other components of hypoplastic left heart physiology, severe symptoms often develop during the first year of life.

Isolated *congenital mitral regurgitation* is often only moderate in severity in early life, and about half the patients with it do not show development of important symptoms. Symptoms and need for intervention usually come earlier when it coexists with other important cardiac anomalies.

TECHNIQUE OF OPERATION

The overall approach to the neonate, infant, and young child is different from that for older patients. Preservation of the native valve is of paramount importance, even if it means accepting residual valve disease that might otherwise not be considered acceptable in a fully grown patient. The valve must be carefully studied preoperatively and at operation, seeking ways in which it can be repaired rather than replaced. Specific techniques such as rectangular resection, which if unsuccessful will result in obligatory valve replacement as a fallback option, should generally be avoided. Some techniques used for congenital mitral valve disease are the same as those used for older patients with acquired disease, and these are described for both mitral stenosis and regurgitation under Technique of Operation in Section I of Chapter 11. However, many techniques are specific for congenital abnormalities such as supramitral ring (Fig. 50-11), mitral arcade (Fig. 50-12), and single papillary muscle (Fig. 50-13).[C5] In general, repair is possible in 50% to 80% of patients.[C7,S11] Additional comments specific to *congenital* mitral valve disease follow.

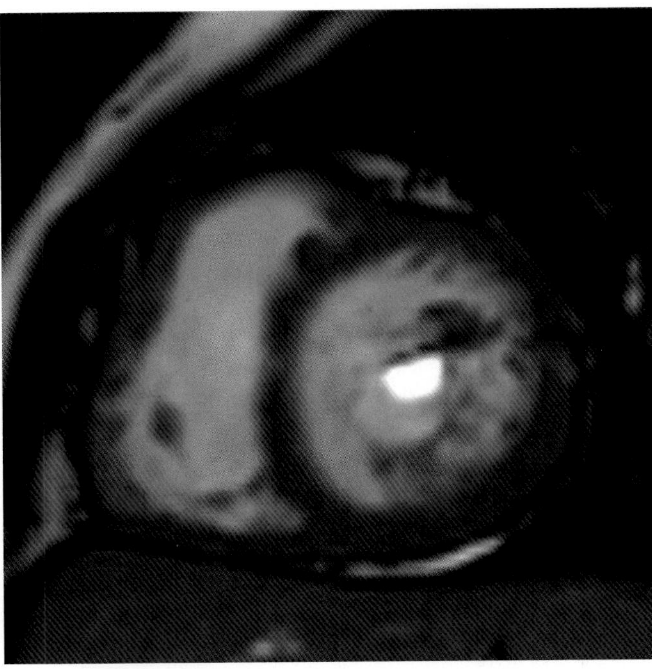

Figure 50-10 Short-axis view at level of mitral valve orifice during diastole: high-velocity mitral inflow is seen as white. During systole, regurgitant jet can be visualized and analyzed, and a regurgitant fraction can be calculated as a percentage of inflow. Mitral orifice area in diastole can be calculated by planimetry and is expressed in square centimeters. Two papillary muscles are demonstrated. (From Hamilton-Craig and colleagues.[H2])

Repair of Congenital Mitral Stenosis

When the valve leaflets are fused into one and are stenotic, leaflet incisions may be made in the areas in which commissures would be expected to have developed. Consideration is given to inserting polyester or polytetrafluoroethylene (PTFE) chordae (see "Repair of Chordae" later in this chapter). At times, fused papillary muscles or chordae may be split or partly excised in an attempt to enlarge the orifice (see Fig. 11-7 in Chapter 11).

Because these maneuvers may result in regurgitation, immediately after discontinuing cardiopulmonary bypass (CPB), a regurgitant mitral jet may first be detected by palpating the posterior left atrial wall and then the superior left atrial wall beneath the aorta. Intraoperative transesophageal echocardiography (TEE) is invaluable at this stage in determining that mitral valve function is sufficiently good to avoid valve replacement. If TEE documents important regurgitation accompanied by high left atrial pressure and a suboptimal hemodynamic state, CPB is reestablished and the valve repaired further or replaced; otherwise, early and late results are unsatisfactory. If hemodynamics are acceptable but regurgitation is moderate to severe, the decision to replace the valve is complex. Importantly, the smaller the patient and mitral anulus, the more likely will be the tendency to

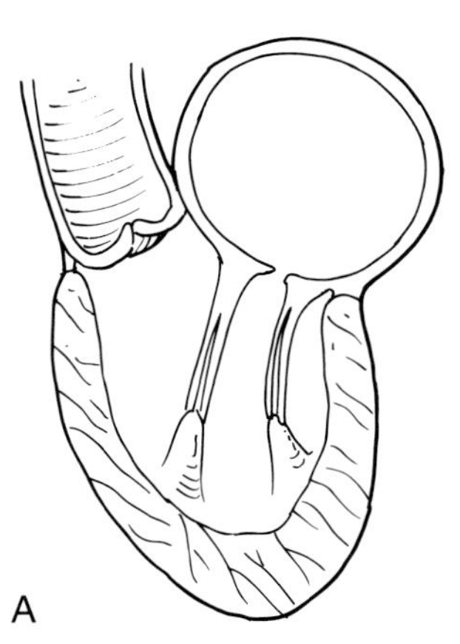

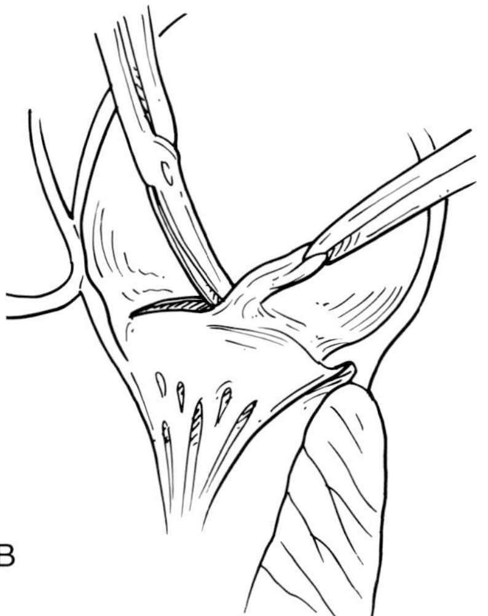

Figure 50-11 Repair of supramitral ring. **A,** Long-axis depiction of left heart showing left atrium, left ventricle, and mitral and aortic valves. A supramitral ring (SMR) is present on mitral valve. **B,** Close-up cutaway view of mitral valve and anulus showing SMR. Ring can be cut away circumferentially using sharp dissection as shown here, but in some cases, it can be peeled away bluntly once the plane between underlying endocardium and ring tissue is established. Ring may be discrete (as shown here) but may also extend to a variable degree onto mitral leaflets, sometimes extending across length of leaflet onto chordal structures, causing thickening, contraction, and immobility. In this case, using both sharp and blunt dissection, as much of the abnormal tissue as possible is removed from leaflet without damaging underlying leaflet tissue. (From Chauvaud.[C5])

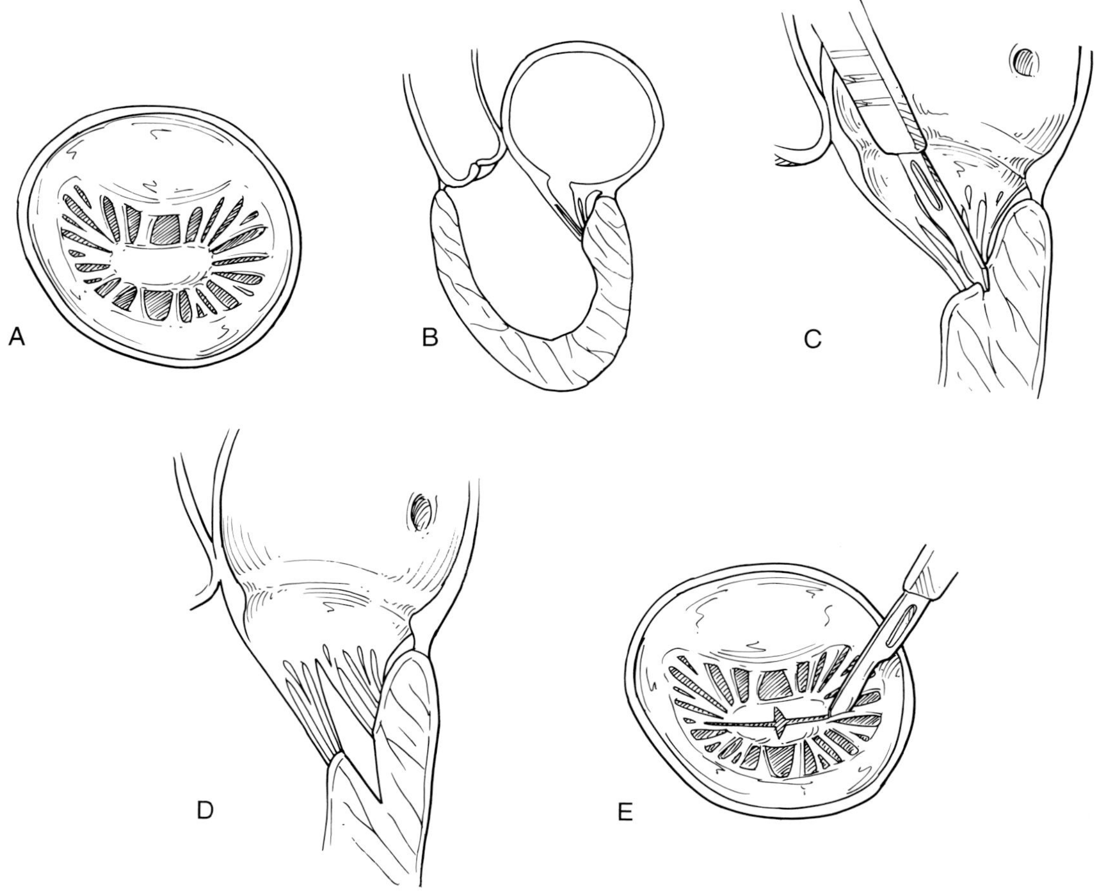

Figure 50-12 Repair of mitral arcade. **A,** En face view of mitral valve with arcade formation of subvalvar mechanism. Note fused, or hammock-like, nature of papillary muscles, and crowded thickened chordal arrangement. **B-E,** Repair involves splitting the lateral attachments between chords, and the papillary muscle between chordal groups. (From Chauvaud.[C5])

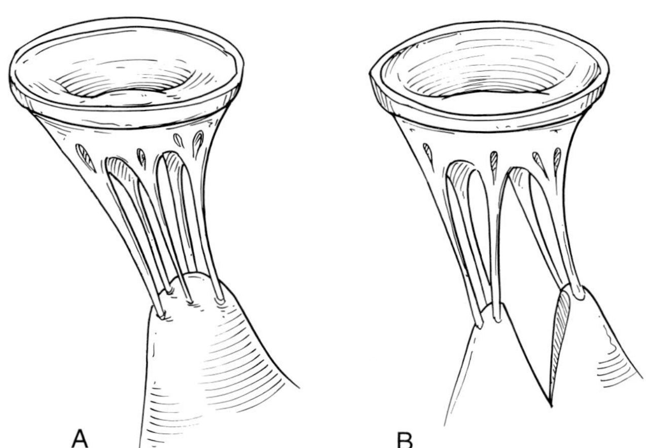

Figure 50-13 Repair of parachute mitral valve. **A,** Note single papillary muscle with all chordal structures attaching to it. **B,** Repair involves splitting the papillary muscle between the two large chordal groups supporting each commissure. Commissural fusion and lateral attachments of chords may also be present, requiring commissurotomy and splitting of lateral chordal attachments. (From Chauvaud.[C5])

accept the result, recognizing that this will be a temporary solution.

Repair of Congenital Mitral Regurgitation

The mitral valve is carefully examined with the possible pathologic bases for congenital mitral regurgitation clearly in mind, because these determine the most appropriate type of operation. Repair based on pathology is performed whenever possible. Specific maneuvers include anuloplasty, repair of cleft leaflet, various forms of chordal repair including shortening, lengthening, and resuspension of ruptured chords, partial leaflet resection, chordal replacement, and partial commissural closure (see Technique of Operation in Section I of Chapter 11).

Anuloplasty

Occasionally, anular dilatation is the dominant pathology even in young children, but it is usually associated with some abnormal thickening and prolapse of a billowing anterior leaflet.[L4] If a reasonable anterior leaflet without ruptured chordae is present, anuloplasty is indicated. Anuloplasty is also appropriate when there is marked hypoplasia or near absence of the posterior leaflet, which probably initially was responsible for the regurgitation and subsequent anular

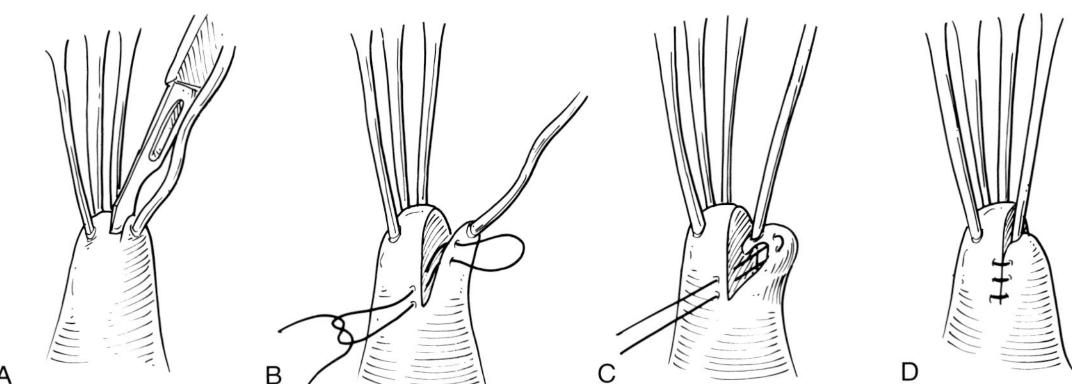

Figure 50-14 Repair of elongated chordae by chordal shortening. **A,** Papillary muscle is split along its length between elongated chord and normal chords. **B-C,** Tip of papillary muscle attached to elongated chord is buried into base of papillary muscle, using a pledgeted suture such that chord is now of proper length. **D,** Papillary muscle is sutured closed. (From Chauvaud.[C5])

dilatation. Following anuloplasty, the mitral valve is essentially converted to a monoleaflet valve.

Although use of an anuloplasty ring is optimal in adults, it is not used in infants and children because it precludes growth of the anulus. Thus, a technique such as the Reed asymmetric measured anuloplasty is chosen (see Fig. 11-15 in Chapter 11).

Repair of Chordae

When regurgitation is caused by ruptured chordae to less than half the posterior leaflet, a rectangular excision and leaflet repair, usually combined with anuloplasty, may be indicated (see Figs. 11-9 and 11-10 in Chapter 11). A result similar to that obtained with rectangular excision can be achieved by simply folding the unsupported component of the leaflet on itself and securing the folds with sutures, rather than excising the leaflet tissue. If the repair attempt is unsuccessful, the folded leaflet tissue can be taken down or unfolded, allowing further valve-sparing reparative maneuvers to be attempted.

A sliding plasty has been used by Carpentier and colleagues to correct congenital elongation of chordae to part of a papillary muscle.[C3] The papillary muscle is incised longitudinally and reconstructed by suturing the halves together asymmetrically, with the part attached to the elongated chordae fixed at a lower level. Elongation of all chordae to a papillary muscle may be treated by chordal shortening[C3] (Fig. 50-14). The extremity of the papillary muscle is incised longitudinally, redundant chordae buried in the trench thus created, and the papillary muscle closed firmly around them by sutures. In these situations, placement of polyester or PTFE chordae can also be useful (see "Repair of Mitral Regurgitation" under Technique of Operation in Section I of Chapter 11).

Chordal repair often involves splitting or separating papillary muscles as well as leaflet commissures. An approach through the LV apex has been described but is not recommended.[B1] Use of artificial chordae for mitral valve reconstruction in children has been described; expanded PTFE sutures are employed in the technique, and early and midterm results have been encouraging.[A1,M4,M9]

Repair of Cleft Mitral Leaflet

When sufficient anterior or posterior mitral leaflet tissue is present on both sides of a cleft leaflet, the cleft is sutured closed with interrupted simple sutures to achieve competence. If there is insufficient leaflet tissue, the cleft closure can be augmented with a patch (Fig. 50-15). A posteromedial (Wooler type) anuloplasty using interrupted simple sutures of monofilament nonabsorbable material, or a Reed anuloplasty, may be helpful.

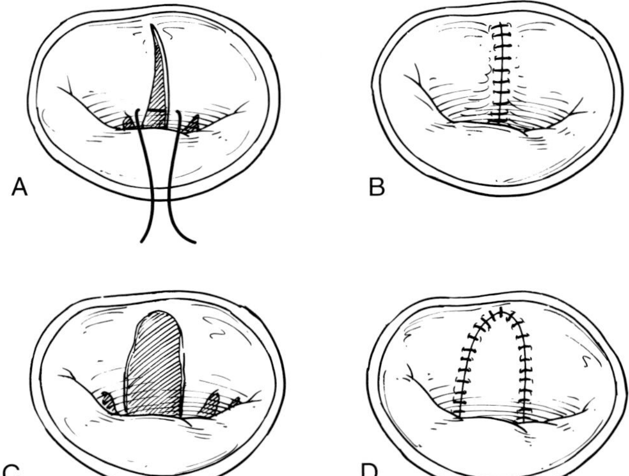

Figure 50-15 Repair of mitral valve cleft. **A,** Cleft is identified over its full extent, with its central limit defined by the first chordal attachments on the leaflet normal edge. A simple suture is placed precisely at this point to appropriately align cleft. **B,** Simple sutures are placed to close remainder of cleft. **C,** If leaflet deficiency is present (as shown here), a patch is used. **D,** Patch has been secured in place using multiple interrupted sutures, again paying close attention to alignment of edges. (From Chauvaud.[C5])

Mitral Valve Replacement

When repair is not possible, mitral valve replacement is performed (see "Mitral Valve Replacement" under Technique of Operation in Section I of Chapter 11). Stent-mounted glutaraldehyde-preserved porcine xenografts are not appropriate in infants and children because of their rapid degeneration and bulk (see "Reoperation," later). The favorable orifice-to-anulus ratio of the St. Jude Medical valve (see "Choice of Device for Valve Replacement" under Indications for Operation, Selection of Technique, and Choice of Device in Section I of Chapter 11) makes it and similar mitral replacement devices the valves of choice in infants and children. A 15-mm-diameter St. Jude Medical valve is available by special order; it can provide a critical advantage in small infants in whom the prosthesis must usually be seated in a supraanular position in the left atrium, immediately downstream from the orifices of the left pulmonary veins.[K2]

SPECIAL FEATURES OF POSTOPERATIVE CARE

The usual practices and protocols are used (see Chapter 5). Patients, even infants, who receive mitral valve replacement with prosthetic valves are maintained on anticoagulation with warfarin using the same general protocols as in adults (see "Special Features of Postoperative Care" in Section I of Chapter 11). Small valves in infants may be prone to dysfunction, either because of thrombosis or leaflet immobility caused by adjacent tissue at or near the small anulus. Placing a left atrial pressure catheter at the time of operation is mandatory, and using intraoperative and postoperative echocardiography to document normal movement of both valve leaflets is important in managing these patients.

RESULTS

Survival

Early (Hospital) Death

In the past, early mortality after operation for mitral valve disease in the pediatric age range was highly variable, ranging between 1% and 50%.[B7,C3,K3,S8,V1] In most reports after 1990, mitral valve surgery in infants and children has a consistently low mortality (0%-10%) for both repair and replacement[A1,B1,C6,H3,H4,M4,M6,O2,S12,S13,U1,Y2] (Table 50-3).

Despite these encouraging reports, the role of patient selection in determining early outcome remains unclear in these complex anomalies. In a series of 31 severely symptomatic patients with mitral stenosis requiring intervention within the first 2 years of life, 18 underwent balloon dilatation and 13 surgical intervention. Early mortality for the surgical patients was 31% (CL 16%-49%).[M8] In a series of seven patients presenting within the first year of life with mitral regurgitation, four required surgical intervention, and three were managed medically. Two of the four surgical patients died in hospital; both required urgent operation. The two survivors underwent elective operation.[G1] Yet, in another study of 17 patients presenting with mitral regurgitation, mitral valve repair was performed in all, and there was no early or late mortality. Mean age was 11 months, with 10 patients younger than age 1 year and 15 in heart failure (3 of whom required preoperative mechanical ventilation).[H4]

Time-Related Survival

In the early surgical era, only about 50% of patients receiving valve repair or replacement for congenital mitral valve disease were alive 10 years later. Many deaths were related to coexisting cardiac anomalies and reoperation. Current results are better.[Z1] In reports after 1990, 5- and 10-year survival appears to be between 80% and 100%[A1,C6,H3,H4,M4,M6,O2,S13,U1,Y2] (Table 50-4). Notably, there has been little or no further improvement in late survival during the last 2 decades.

Table 50-3 Hospital Mortality after Operation for Congenital Mitral Valve Disease

Source	Year	*n*	Hospital Deaths No.	%	CL (%)	Age	Anomaly
Aharon et al.[A1]	1994	79	3	3.8	1.7-7.5	2 m-17 y	5 MS, MR
Chauvaud et al.[C6]	1998	145	7	4.8	3.0-7.4	0.17-12 y; 19 < 2 y	MR
Barbero-Marcial et al.[B1]	1993	12	0	0	0-15	2-74 m	MS
Harada et al.[H3]	1990	28	0	0	0-6.7	4 m-15 y	[a]
Honjo[H4]	2006	17	0	0	0-11	3 m-13 y	MR
Matsumoto et al.[M4]	1999	16	0	0	0-11	5 m-13 y	[b]
McElhinney et al.[M6]	2005	108	7	6.5	4.1-9.9	1 m-18 y	78 MS, 46 MR, 28 PMV, 11 DOMV[c]
Balloon valvuloplasty		64	3	4.7	2.1-9.2		
Surgical valvuloplasty		33	1	3.0	0.5-9.9		
Valve replacement		11	3	27	13-47		
Murakami et al.[M9]	1998	3	0	0	0-47	1.4 y, 4.6 y, 5.1 y	[b]
Oppido et al.[O2]	2008	71	3	4.2	1.9-8.3	3 d-21 y	11 MS, 60 MR
Stellin et al.[S12]	2010	93	7	7.5	4.7-11	5.8 ± 4.9, 13 < 12 m	45 MS, 48 MR
Sugita et al.[S13]	2001	41	0	0	0-4.5	4 < 12 m	MR
Uva et al.[U1]	1995	20	0	0	0-9.2	<1 y	10 MR, 10 MS[d]
Yoshimura et al.[Y2]	1999	56	2	3.6	1.2-8.3	3 m-15 y	Both MS and MR[e]
TOTAL		689	29	4.2	3.4-5.2		

[a]Mitral valve replacement only.
[b]Artificial chordae repair only.
[c]Not mutually exclusive.
[d]Nineteen repairs, 1 replacement.
[e]Thirty-six repairs, 30 replacements.
Key: *DOMV,* Double orifice mitral valve; *m,* months; *MR,* mitral regurgitation; *MS,* mitral stenosis; *PMR,* parachute mitral valve; *y,* years.

Table 50-4 Time-Related Survival after Operation for Congenital Mitral Valve Disease

Source	Year	Operation	*n*	Follow-up Interval	Survival (%) or Mean ± SE
Aharon et al.[A1]	1994	Repair	79	1, 2, 5 y	94, 84, 82
Chauvaud et al.[C6]	1998	Repair	138	10 y	86 ± 8
Chauvaud et al.[C6]	1998	Replacement	7	10 y	51 ± 30
Harada et al.[H3]	1990	Replacement	28	10 y	90
Honjo et al.[H4]	2006	Repair	17	Median 95 m	100
Matsumoto et al.[M4]	1999	Repair	16	26 m	100
McElhinney et al.[M6]	2005	Balloon valvuloplasty Surgical valvuloplasty	33	1, 5, 10 y 1, 5, 10 y	85, 80, 77 95, 85, 85
Oppido et al.[O2]	2008	Repair	71	5 y	94 ± 2.8
Stellin et al.[S12]	2010	Repair	93	5, 10, 20, 30	85, 85, 82, 75
Sugita et al.[S13]	2001	Partial plication	41	Median 15 y	100
Uva et al.[U1]	1995	Artificial chords, 19 repairs, 1 replacement	20	7 y	94 (CL 88-100)
Yoshimura et al.[Y2]	1999	Repair	36	10 y	87 (95% CL 75-99)
Yoshimura et al.[Y2]	1999	Replacement	30	10 y	90 (95% CL 77-100)

Key: *CL*, Confidence limits; *m*, months; *SE*, standard error; *y*, years.

Incremental Risk Factors for Premature Death

Incremental risk factors have been identified in many individual series, but there is little consistency among studies, other than young age, era of surgery, and coexisting cardiac anomalies—all of which appear in multiple analyses. In the analysis of 79 children undergoing mitral valve repair by Aharon and colleagues, no incremental risk factors for early or late death could be identified.[A1] Chauvaud and colleagues in their series of 145 patients undergoing mitral valve repair for regurgitation did not find mitral valve anatomic classification to be an incremental risk factor for early death.[C6] Stellin and colleagues, in a 36-year series of 93 patients undergoing mitral valve repair, identified parachute mitral valve as a risk for early mortality.[S12] Prifti and colleagues identified cardiothoracic ratio > 0.6 and hammock valve morphology as risk factors.[P1]

Caldarone and colleagues, reporting a multicenter study of 139 patients undergoing valve replacement, identified oversized valves relative to patient size as a risk factor, as did Alsoufi and colleagues.[A3,C1] In valve replacement series, supra-anular placement was identified as a risk factor, as was lower body weight and longer CPB time.[K4,S4]

Era

As knowledge about techniques of mitral repair has increased (see "Repair of Mitral Regurgitation" under Technique of Operation in Chapter 11), and as it has been realized that bioprostheses should not be used in young patients, who tolerate mechanical prosthesis and anticoagulation well, results have improved considerably.[A2,B1,C6,C7,H3,M4,M9,U1,Y2]

Coexisting Cardiac Anomalies

Hypoplastic left heart class has a large influence on survival. However, Bolling and colleagues report no deaths (0%; CL 0%-6%) among 30 patients undergoing their first operation for Shone syndrome, although among 17 undergoing a second operation, 4 (24%; CL 12%-39%) died.[B6] Prifti and colleagues report that associated cardiac anomalies are a risk for both reoperation and midterm death after valve repair.[P1] Schaverien and colleagues and Marino and colleagues both report that associated cardiac anomalies are a risk factor for death in patients with parachute mitral valve, even when no surgical procedure on the valve itself is performed.[M2,S1] Caldarone and colleagues, reporting a multicenter study of 139 patients undergoing valve replacement, identified AV septal defect and Shone's complex as risk factors.[C1] Selamet Tierney and colleagues, in a series of valve replacements, identified AV septal defect and, as a surrogate for additional anomalies, additional surgical procedures as risk factors.[S4] Alexiou and colleagues identified AV septal defect as a risk after replacement.[A2]

Preoperative Functional Class

Patients in higher New York Heart Association (NYHA) functional classes are at a considerably greater risk of dying after operation, particularly early postoperatively (Table 50-5). Preoperative cardiothoracic ratio > 0.6 has also been identified as a risk for midterm death after valve repair. This is likely a surrogate for lower functional class.[P1]

Age

A number of studies identify younger age as a risk factor for death after either valve repair or replacement.[S12] Most studies categorize age groups into younger than 2 years or younger than 1 year. Age younger than 2 years was identified as a risk in one study involving predominantly surgical repair and balloon valvotomy.[M6] Age younger than 2 has also been identified as a risk factor following mitral valve replacement.[A3,B2] Prifti and colleagues and Selamet Tierney and colleagues identified age younger than 1 year as a risk for death after repair,[P1,S4] and Alexiou and colleagues identified age younger than 5 years as a risk factor after mechanical valve replacement.[A2]

Mitral Regurgitation versus Stenosis; Repair versus Replacement

Neither of these factors can be definitively related to the probability of death early or late postoperatively.[A1,B1,C7,H3,M4,U1,Y2]

Table 50-5 Hospital Deaths after Operation for Congenital Mitral Valve Disease, According to Preoperative New York Heart Association Functional Class[a]

	UAB				GLH				Total			
		Hospital Deaths				Hospital Deaths				Hospital Deaths		
NYHA Functional Class	*n*	No.	%	CL%	*n*	No.	%	CL%	*n*	No.	%	CL%
I	7	0	0	0-24	0				7	0	0	0-24
II	12	1	8	1-26	1	0	0	0-85	13	1	8	1-24
III	7	1	14	2-41	0				7	1	14	2-41
IV	10	4	40	22-61	8	2	25	9-50	18	6	33	21-48
V[b]	1	1	100	15-100	2	1	50	7-93	3	2	67	24-96
TOTAL	37	7	19	12-28	11	3	27	12-47	48	10	21	15-29
P (logistic)											.01	

[a]Patients are from the surgical experience at GLH and UAB, 1967 to 1984.
[b]NYHA class V indicates emergency operation for shock or metabolic acidosis.
Key: *CL*, 70% confidence limits; *NYHA*, New York Heart Association.

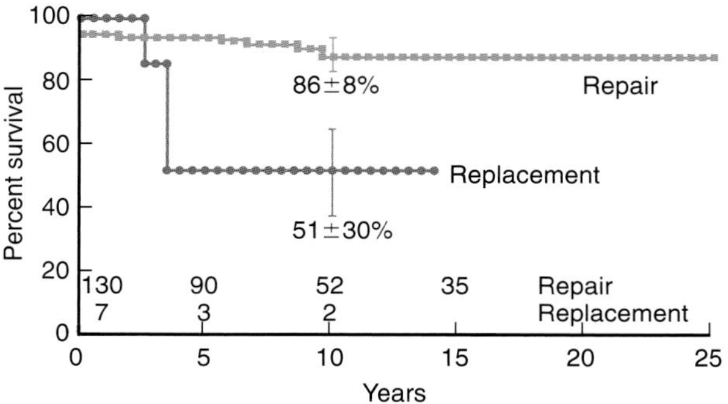

Figure 50-16 Survival after operation for mitral valve regurgitation in children, stratified by type of operation. Patient cohort in replacement group is small. Numbers along horizontal axis are patients at risk. (From Chauvaud and colleagues.[C6])

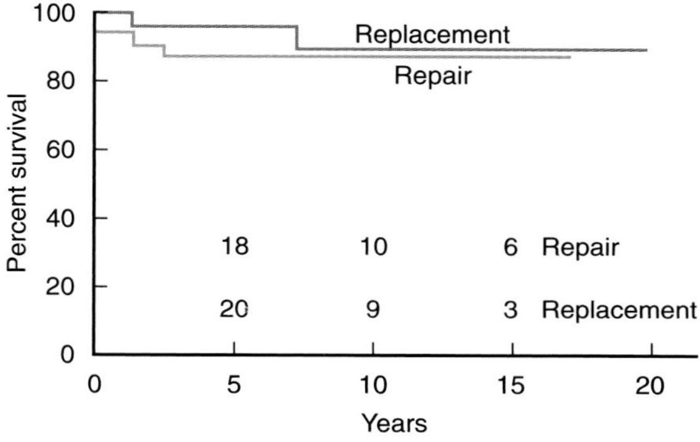

Figure 50-17 Survival after operation for mitral valve disease, stratified by type of operation. Long-term survival is similar in both groups. Numbers along horizontal axis are patients at risk. (From Yoshimura and colleagues.[Y2])

However, outcome is particularly good in patients with mitral stenosis due to a supravalvar ring.[S14]

There is conflicting evidence regarding whether survival is worse after mitral valve replacement than after repair; furthermore, the evidence that can be cited to address this question is indirect. This is understandable for several reasons. First, there are no reports randomizing the two techniques, and second, it is generally acknowledged that repair is preferable to replacement in small patients because of growth reasons, thereby introducing a strong selection bias. One report shows 10-year survival of only 51% (Fig. 50-16) for patients undergoing mitral valve replacement when the primary diagnosis was mitral regurgitation; however, only 7 of the 145 patients underwent initial mitral valve replacement. The study by McElhinney and colleagues was similar, with only 11 of 108 patients undergoing initial valve replacement; replacement carried a higher mortality.[M6] Another report shows that for a primary diagnosis of mitral stenosis, initial mitral valve replacement was an independent predictor of worse survival over time.[M6] However, another study examining patients with primary diagnoses of either stenosis or regurgitation showed no difference between repair and replacement (Fig. 50-17). Other studies with larger numbers of patients undergoing mitral valve replacement have shown that replacement, relative to repair, is not an incremental risk factor for death.[Y2]

There are several large series reporting outcomes exclusively for mitral valve repair or replacement. Repair series tend to show better outcome than replacement series. This is not surprising, for the same reasons stated in the previous paragraph. In one report of 71 repairs, outstanding early and midterm outcome (4.2% early mortality [CL 1.9%-8.3%] and 94% 5-year survival) was demonstrated.[O2] In another report of 94 patients, early mortality was 8.5% (CL 5.5%-13%) and 5-year survival 89%.[P1] Two separate series of mitral repair exclusively for mitral regurgitation showed no early or late mortality.[H4,S13] Both series have fewer associated cardiac anomalies and simpler anomalies than most series with a mixture of stenosis and regurgitation patients.

A number of studies exclusively examine valve replacement. Early mortality ranges from 11% to 36% according to a review by Alsoufi and colleagues, which examined 13 recent institutional series.[A3] Furthermore, from the same review, early mortality is even higher in patients younger than age 2: up to 52%.[A3] In a multicenter study of 139 patients undergoing replacement, 5-year survival was 75% overall, but survival was strongly affected by the ratio of valve size to patient weight, with higher size/weight ratio associated with decreased survival[C1] (Fig. 50-18). In a single-institution study of valve replacement in 25 patients between 1996 and 2006, 5-year survival was 83%.[S4] In 104 valve replacements, Kojori

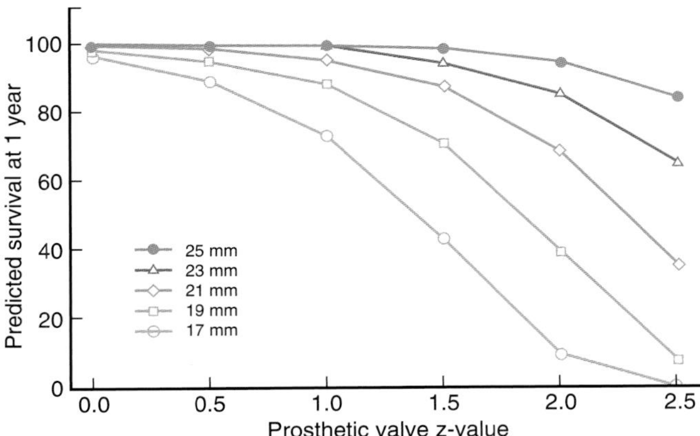

Figure 50-18 Predicted survival at 1 year versus prosthetic valve *z* value after mitral valve replacement, stratified by prosthesis size. Note that as disparity between prosthetic valve size and normal mitral anulus size increases (increasing *z* value), 1-year survival falls precipitously. This effect is greatest at smaller valve sizes. In this analysis, *z* value was based on Rowlatt and colleagues[R4] (formalin fixed; see Chapter 1). (From Caldarone and colleagues.[C1])

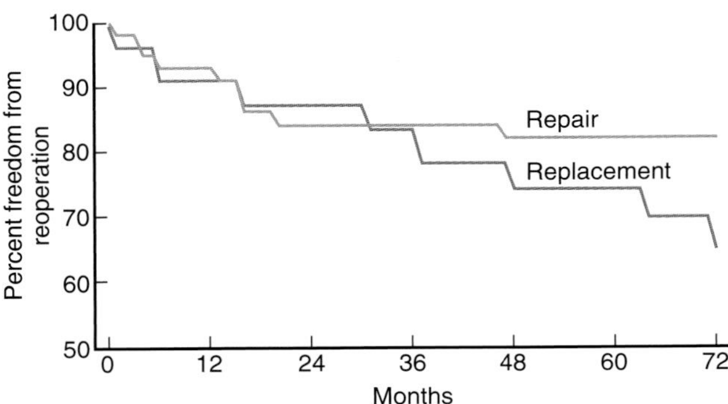

Figure 50-19 Freedom from reoperation after mitral valve repair or replacement. This study included 79 patients, 74 with mitral regurgitation and 5 with mitral stenosis; age ranged from 2 months to 17 years, mean 4.9 years. (From Aharon and colleagues.[A1])

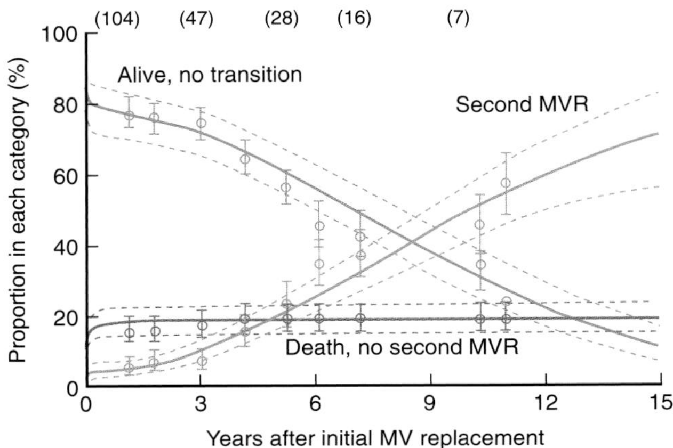

Figure 50-20 Competing-risks analysis for subsequent replacement of the initial replaced mitral valve *(MVR)* or death before subsequent re-replacement. Mechanical valves were used as the initial replacement device in 94 of 104 patients. All patients (mean age, 7.4 years; range, birth to 19 years) began at time of initial MVR (*n* = 104) and could transition to either death or a subsequent replacement. Proportion of patients (expressed as percentage of total) in each of three categories adds to 100% at any given time after initial MVR. Solid lines represent parametric point estimates, dashed lines enclose 70% confidence intervals, and circles with error bars represent nonparametric estimates. Numbers in parentheses represent number of patients at risk. (From Kadoba and colleagues.[K2])

and colleagues showed 6-month, 5-year, and 15-year survival of 83% (CL 79%-86%), 70% (CL 65%-75%), and 62% (CL 56%-68%), respectively.[K4]

Emphasizing the risk of young age on both early and time-related mortality, in another single institution study of 54 patients undergoing replacement, early mortality was 43% (9 of 21; CL 30%-56%) and 10-year survival 33% in patients aged 2 or younger; early mortality was 6.1% (2 of 33; CL 2.1%-14%) and 10-year survival 81% in patients older than age 2.[B2] Masuda and colleagues, however, reported no early mortality (0%; CL 0%-5.0%) and 5 late deaths in 37 patients undergoing valve replacement.[M3] Similarly, for patients undergoing valve replacement after 1990, Alexiou and colleagues reported an early mortality of 3.6% (1 of 28; CL 0.6%-12%) and 10-year survival of 86%.[A2]

Reoperation

In the past, many reoperations were required because of degeneration of bioprostheses. This is part of the incremental risk of young age on bioprosthesis degeneration[S7,T2] (see Fig. 12-42 in Chapter 12). Additionally, small children outgrow both bioprostheses and mechanical prostheses.

Reoperation is much less frequent in the current era—particularly in older children who have little remaining growth potential—first, because mechanical prostheses rather than bioprostheses are used when replacement is necessary; and second, because less-than-perfect repairs are now considered unacceptable.

Reoperation may take one of several forms: repeat repair of a previously repaired valve, replacement of a previously repaired valve, replacement of a previously placed prosthesis, or revision and salvage of a previously placed prosthesis.

Reoperation Following Mitral Valve Repair

Early and midterm freedom from reoperation following mitral valve repair in the current era is high but decreases substantially over time. In one study, freedom from reoperation was 97% at 2 years and 83% at 8 years[A1] (Fig. 50-19). In another, it was 95% (95% CL 90%-98%) at 1 year, 80% (95% CL 71%-87%) at 10 years, and 67% (95% CL 52%-80%) at 15 years.[C6] In still another, it was 76% (CL 70%-82%) after 5 years.[O2]

In a 20-year follow-up study of 56 children, 36 had undergone initial mitral valve repair. Of these, 4 underwent reoperation, with 3 requiring valve replacement for residual mitral regurgitation.[Y2]

Reoperation Following Mitral Valve Replacement

Re-replacement after receipt of an original prosthesis is inversely related to age,[R1] with reoperation inevitable when a prosthetic valve is inserted into the mitral position in a young patient, because the patient outgrows the valve (Fig. 50-20).

Other series examining patients undergoing first valve-replacement surgery at younger than 6 years of age show freedom from re-replacement at 5 years in the range of 70% to 80%, and at 10 years in the range of 25% to 60%.[B2,C1,S4] One reoperation generally suffices because a prosthesis two to three times larger can usually be inserted.[Y2] In older children receiving larger initial valves (≥23 mm), 10- and 15-year freedom from re-replacement is 83% and 83%, respectively.[B2]

Influence of Young Age at Operation

Reoperation was more frequent in a series of 20 patients with mitral valve disease undergoing operation before age 1 year.[U1] Six early reoperations were performed in five patients, with mitral valve replacement in four, a second valve repair in one, and a mechanical prosthesis thrombectomy in one. Late reoperations on the mitral valve were performed five times, with mitral valve repair in two and replacement in three. Overall freedom from reoperation was 58% (CL 47%-69%) at 7 years, and was similar for patients with an original diagnosis of mitral regurgitation and stenosis (Fig. 50-21). As noted under "Reoperation Following Mitral Valve Replacement," in a multicenter study of mechanical prostheses in a cohort of patients younger than age 5, younger age at first valve placement predicted shorter prosthesis longevity.[R1]

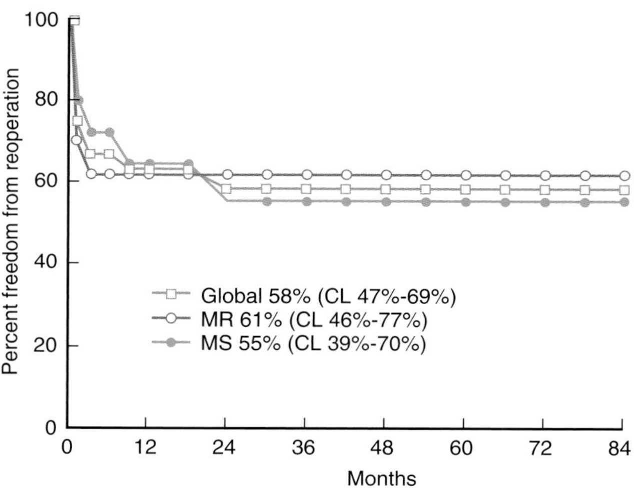

Figure 50-21 Freedom from reoperation among 20 patients (10 with mitral regurgitation and 10 with mitral stenosis) undergoing surgical correction within first year of life. (From Uva and colleagues.[U1])

Reoperation and Use of Artificial Chordae Tendineae

In 16 patients undergoing mitral valve repair using artificial chordae tendineae, no reoperations were required during follow-up of up to 26 months.[M4]

Functional Result

Most patients who have had a reparative operation for congenital mitral stenosis have a lessened diastolic gradient after repair but continue to have a residual gradient up to about 10 mmHg.[C8] An exception is isolated supravalvar ring, in which complete relief of the diastolic gradient may be obtained.[C8,M1,N1]

Most patients with either congenital mitral stenosis or regurgitation have at least some regurgitation after repair. Carpentier and colleagues reported that in 22 of 34 such patients, there was an apical systolic murmur late postoperatively, and only 7 of the 34 showed important decrease in heart size.[C3] Of 12 patients recatheterized, 7 had moderate or severe regurgitation. Flege and colleagues reported a virtually complete repair in only 4 of 13 patients with congenital mitral regurgitation.[F2]

At follow-up to 15 years, 85% to 100% of patients are in NYHA functional class I[A1,B1,C6,H3,U1,Y2] (Table 50-6). Among patients undergoing repair for mitral valve regurgitation, follow-up echocardiography commonly reveals some regurgitation of mild to moderate degree[A1,B1] (see Table 50-6). However, more recent reports suggest improving functional results (see Table 50-6). Among those undergoing mitral valve repair for stenosis, important residual stenosis is uncommon.[B1,U1]

In the series of 33 late-surviving patients following mitral valve repair in whom no reoperation was performed, Yoshimura and colleagues found that eight patients had grade 1+/6+ or 2+/6+ systolic murmurs with echocardiographic findings of trivial or mild mitral regurgitation.[Y2]

The hemodynamic state after *replacement* of a congenitally abnormal mitral valve depends on type and size of the replacement device used (see Table 11-9 in Chapter 11). In general, hemodynamic state and valve function are satisfactory unless a device complication develops. In echocardiographic studies by Uva and colleagues, among patients receiving prosthetic mitral valves, transprosthesis gradient was 6.2 ± 3.7 mmHg.[U1]

Prosthetic valves in children have resulted in no higher incidence of thromboembolism and complications from anticoagulation with warfarin than in adults.[A6,G2] The possible exception to this may be with use of very small mechanical

Table 50-6 Functional and Hemodynamic Status after Operations for Congenital Mitral Valve Disease

Source	*n*	Average Follow-up Time Mean (±SD)	NYHA Class I (%)	Residual or Recurrent Mitral Regurgitation after Repair by Echocardiography
Aharon et al.[A1]	79	4 ± 2.5 y	98	9% moderate, 9% severe
Chauvaud et al.[C6]	145	9 ± 7 y	85	12%
Barbero-Marcial et al.[B1]	12	24 ± 15 m	91	17% moderate MR, 0% MS
Harada et al.[H3]	28	4.2 ± 2.8 y	100	Valve replacement
Uva et al.[U1]	20	68 ± 43 m	95	10% moderate MR
Yoshimura et al.[Y2]	33	92 m	100	6% moderate MR

Key: *m*, Months; *MR*, mitral regurgitation; *MS*, mitral stenosis; *NYHA*, New York Heart Association; *SD*, standard deviation; *y*, years.

prostheses (15- to 17-mm diameter) placed in the supraanular position in infants. Information regarding this observation is, however, anecdotal.

INDICATIONS FOR OPERATION

In view of its natural history, severe symptoms and signs of important pulmonary venous hypertension are an indication for prompt operation in infants with congenital mitral valve disease. A reparative operation is indicated if feasible. These same indications prevail in children and young adults. When symptoms are mild or even moderate, operation is delayed in the hope that when it becomes necessary, and if valve replacement is required, an adult-sized device can be used. Operation is indicated even in the absence of marked symptoms when pulmonary hypertension is severe; in this situation, there may be right-to-left shunting across a patent ductus arteriosus or foramen ovale.

Surgery may be indicated in asymptomatic patients with moderate or worse mitral regurgitation in whom a simple and reliable reparative procedure is anticipated, such as closure of a regurgitant cleft. Delay in repair may lead to progressive damage to the valve, increasing the chance that repair will not be effective.

When repair is performed, long-term follow-up is indicated because of need in some patients for reoperation. When valve replacement is performed in infants, children, and young adults, a bioprosthesis is contraindicated because of its rapid degeneration in these age groups. A mechanical prosthesis is currently the device of choice, with long-term warfarin anticoagulation.

It is important to identify coexisting congenital mitral valve disease in patients being considered for repair of LV outflow tract obstruction, VSD, tetralogy of Fallot, or double outlet right ventricle. When mitral disease is present and is moderate or severe, the mitral disease must also be treated operatively.

SPECIAL SITUATIONS AND CONTROVERSIES

Valved Conduit Bypass of the Mitral Valve

When the mitral anulus is very small, a valved conduit (similar to that used for right ventricular–pulmonary trunk reconstruction) may be placed between the left atrium and LV. Laks and colleagues reported such a procedure (which was unsuccessful) in 1980, and Lansing and colleagues reported a successful case in a 10-year-old girl in 1983.[L1,L2] Others have used this technique with good early results.[C9,M5] Late results are not available.

Pulmonary Autograft Mitral Valve Replacement

Replacing the mitral valve with a pulmonary autograft, sometimes known as the *Ross II operation,* was initially described in 1967.[R3] It is only in the last decade that this procedure has been widely used, primarily in countries with a high prevalence of rheumatic disease, limited financial resources, and poor programs for follow-up anticoagulation monitoring. A 2004 review of worldwide use of the procedure identified 103 cases from 14 reports, with one report accounting for 80 patients.[A5,K1] In that series, 78 of 80 patients had rheumatic disease, and 2 had congenital mitral valve disease; ages of the latter two patients were 4 years (primary mitral stenosis) and 6 years (primary mitral regurgitation). Overall early mortality was 5.0% (4 of 80; CL 2.6%-8.9%), and late mortality 6.25%, but no follow-up specific to the two congenital patients was reported, other than that the 6-year-old developed stenosis of the right ventricle–to–pulmonary artery trunk conduit at 1 year.

Brown and colleagues reported eight patients, four of whom had congenital mitral valve disease[B8]; two of the four had previously placed prosthetic valves that required re-replacement, and two had previously repaired atrioventricular septal defects. Ages of the four ranged from 12 to 22 years at autograft mitral valve replacement. There was no early or late mortality at a mean follow-up of 6.2 months, although one patient required autograft replacement owing to stenosis.

Four other case reports, totaling five patients, describe use of a pulmonary autograft for congenital mitral valve disease in infants ranging from age 2 to 11 months[F4,T1,T3,Y1]; among these, one died (20%; CL 3.2%-53%), one required immediate reoperation, and three survived with no more than short-term follow-up. One other case report describes emergency pulmonary autograft mitral valve replacement in a 36-month-old with a thrombosed mechanical valve originally placed for endocarditis.[M7] Again there was no mid- or long-term follow-up. A pulmonary autograft currently cannot be recommended for congenital mitral valve disease, especially in infants. The experience is limited, and important problems have been demonstrated upon early assessment, with no long-term follow-up available.

Percutaneous Balloon Mitral Valvuloplasty for Congenital Mitral Stenosis

Experience with this technique is small and limited to a few institutions, in contrast to the procedure applied to older patients with rheumatic mitral stenosis. The four reports in the literature total 81 patients, the last one in 2005[G5,K5,L5,M6]; 64 are from one study.[M6] Peak mitral valve gradient was reduced by a median of 33%, but moderate or severe mitral regurgitation was induced in 28% of patients. Procedure-related mortality was 4.7% (3 of 64; CL 2.1%-9.2%) and 5-year survival 74%. One or more reinterventions were needed in 56% of survivors. The procedure is contraindicated when supravalvar mitral stenosis, additional intracardiac anomalies requiring surgery, or important mitral regurgitation are present. Younger age was associated with worse survival and need for more frequent and earlier reintervention.

Because of limited worldwide experience and high prevalence of induced mitral regurgitation, this procedure should be considered unproven and somewhat experimental, especially in young patients.

REFERENCES

A

1. Aharon AS, Laks H, Drinkwater DC, Chugh R, Gates RN, Grant PW, et al. Early and late results of mitral valve repair in children. J Thorac Cardiovasc Surg 1994;107:1262.
2. Alexiou C, Galogavrou M, Chen Q, McDonald A, Salmon AP, Keeton BK, et al. Mitral valve replacement with mechanical prostheses in children: improved operative risk and survival. Eur J Cardiothorac Surg 2001;20:105-13.

3. Alsoufi B, Manlhiot C, McCrindle BW, Al-Halees Z, Sallehuddin A, Al-Oufi S, et al. Results after mitral valve replacement with mechanical prostheses in young children. J Thorac Cardiovasc Surg 2010;139:1189-96.
4. Anabtawi IN, Ellison RG. Congenital stenosing ring of the left atrioventricular canal (supravalvular mitral stenosis). J Thorac Cardiovasc Surg 1965;49:994.
5. Athanasiou T, Cherian A, Ross D. The Ross II procedure: pulmonary autograft in the mitral position. Ann Thorac Surg 2004; 78:1489-95.
6. Attie F, Kuri J, Zononiani C, Renteria V, Buendia A, Ovseyevitz J, et al. Mitral valve replacement in children with rheumatic heart disease. Circulation 1981;64:812.

B

1. Barbero-Marcial M, Riso A, De Albuquerque AT, Atik E, Jatene A. Left ventricular apical approach for the surgical treatment of congenital mitral stenosis. J Thorac Cardiovasc Surg 1993; 106:105.
2. Beierlein W, Becker V, Yates R, Tsang V, Elliott M, de Leval M, et al. Long-term follow-up after mitral valve replacement in childhood: poor event-free survival in the young child. Eur J Cardiothorac Surg 2007;31:860-5.
3. Benrey J, Leachman RD, Cooley DA, Klima T, Lufschanowski R. Supravalvular mitral stenosis associated with tetralogy of Fallot. Am J Cardiol 1976;37:111.
4. Berghuis J, Kirklin JW, Edwards JE, Titus JL. The surgical anatomy of isolated congenital mitral insufficiency. J Thorac Cardiovasc Surg 1964;47:791.
5. Billig DM, Kreidberg MB, Chernoff HL, Khan MA. Mitral stenosis and insufficiency with subaortic and subpulmonic stenosis. J Thorac Cardiovasc Surg 1971;61:121.
6. Bolling SF, Iannettoni MD, Dick M 2nd, Rosenthal A, Bove EL. Shone's anomaly: operative results and late outcome. Ann Thorac Surg 1990;49:887.
7. Borkon AM, Soule L, Reitz BA, Bott VL, Gardner TJ. Five-year follow-up after valve replacement with the St. Jude Medical valve in infants and children. Circulation 1986;74:I110.
8. Brown JW, Ruzmetov M, Rodefeld MD, Turrentine MW. Mitral valve replacement with Ross II technique: initial experience. Ann Thorac Surg 2006;81:502-8.

C

1. Caldarone CA, Raghuveer G, Hills CB, Atkins DL, Burns TL, Behrendt DM, et al. Long-term survival after mitral valve replacement in children aged <5 years: a multi-institutional study. Circulation 2001;104:I143-7.
2. Carney EK, Braunwald E, Rogerts WC, Aygen M, Morrow AG. Congenital mitral regurgitation. Am J Med 1962;33:223.
3. Carpentier A, Branchini B, Cour JC, Asfaou E, Villani M, Deloche A, et al. Congenital malformations of the mitral valve in children. Pathology and surgical treatment. J Thorac Cardiovasc Surg 1976;72:854.
4. Castaneda AR, Anderson RC, Edwards JE. Congenital mitral stenosis resulting from anomalous arcade and obstructing papillary muscles. Report of correction by use of ball valve prosthesis. Am J Cardiol 1969;24:237.
5. Chauvaud S. Surgery of congenital mitral valve disease. J Cardiovasc Surg (Torino) 2004;45:465-76.
6. Chauvaud S, Fuzellier JF, Houel R, Berrebi A, Mihaileanu S, Carpentier A. Reconstructive surgery in congenital mitral valve insufficiency (Carpentier's techniques): long-term results. J Thorac Cardiovasc Surg 1998;115:84.
7. Coles JG, Williams WG, Watanabe T, Duncan KF, Sherret H, Dasmahaptra HK, et al. Surgical experience with reparative techniques in patients with congenital mitral valvular anomalies. Circulation 1987;76:111.
8. Collins-Nakai RL, Rosenthal A, Castaneda AR, Bernhard WF, Nadas AS. Congenital mitral stenosis. A review of 20 years' experience. Circulation 1977;56:1039.
9. Corno A, Giannico S, Leibovich S, Mazzera E, Marcelletti C. The hypoplastic mitral valve. When should a left atrial–left ventricular extracardiac valve conduit be used? J Thorac Cardiovasc Surg 1986;91:848.
10. Creech O, Ledbetter MK, Reemtsma K. Congenital insufficiency with a cleft in the posterior leaflet. Circulation 1962;25:390.

D

1. Daoud G, Kaplan S, Perrin EV, Dorst JP, Edwards FK. Congenital mitral stenosis. Circulation 1963;27:185.
2. Davichi F, Moller JH, Edwards JE. Diseases of the mitral valve in infancy. Circulation 1971;43:565.
3. Di Segni E, Bass JL, Lucas RV Jr, Einzig S. Isolated cleft mitral valve: a variety of congenital mitral regurgitation identified by 2-dimensional echocardiography. Am J Cardiol 1983;51:927.
4. Di Segni E, Edwards JE. Cleft anterior leaflet of the mitral valve with intact septa. A study of twenty cases. Am J Cardiol 1983;51:915.

E

1. Edwards JS. An atlas of congenital anomalies of the heart and great vessels. Springfield, Ill: Charles C Thomas, 1954, p. 41.

F

1. Fisher T. Two cases of congenital disease of the left side of the heart. Br Med J 1902;1:639.
2. Flege JB, Vlad P, Ehrenhaft JL. Congenital mitral incompetence. J Thorac Cardiovasc Surg 1967;53:138.
3. Freed MD, Keane JF, Van Praagh R, Castaneda AR, Bernhard WF, Nadas AS. Coarctation of the aorta with congenital mitral regurgitation. Circulation 1974;49:1175.
4. Frigiola A, Badia T, Pome G, Fesslova V, Russo MG, Iacono C, et al. Pulmonary autograft for mitral valve replacement in infants: the Ross-Kabbani operation. Ann Thorac Surg 2005;79:2150-1.

G

1. Ganeshalingham A, Finucane K, Hornung T. Isolated congenital mitral valve regurgitation presenting in the first year of life. J Paediatr Child Health 2010;46:159-65.
2. Gardner TJ, Roland JM, Neill CA, Donahoo JS. Valve replacement in children. A fifteen-year perspective. J Thorac Cardiovasc Surg 1982;83:178.
3. Glancy DL, Chang MY, Dorney ER, Roberts WC. Parachute mitral valve. Further observations and associated lesions. Am J Cardiol 1971;27:309.
4. Grenadier E, Sahn DJ, Valdes-Cruz LM, Allen HD, Lima CO, Goldbert SJ. Two-dimensional echo Doppler study of congenital disorders of the mitral valve. Am Heart J 1984;107:319.
5. Grifka RG, O'Laughlin MP, Nihill MR, Mullins CE. Double-transseptal, double-balloon valvuloplasty for congenital mitral stenosis. Circulation 1992;85:123-9.

H

1. Hakim FA, Kendall CB, Alharthi M, Mancina JC, Tajik JA, Mookadam F. Parachute mitral valve in adults—a systematic overview. Echocardiography 2010;27:581-6.
2. Hamilton-Craig C, Anscombe R, Platts D, Burstow D, Slaughter R. Congenital mitral stenosis by multimodality cardiac imaging. Echocardiography 2009;26:284-7.
3. Harada Y, Imai Y, Kurosawa H, Ishihara K, Kawada M, Fukuchi S. Ten-year follow-up after valve replacement with the St. Jude Medical prosthesis in children. J Thorac Cardiovasc Surg 1990; 100:175.
4. Honjo O, Ishino K, Kawada M, Akagi T, Sano S. Midterm outcome of mitral valve repair for congenital mitral regurgitation in infants and children. Interact Cardiovasc Thorac Surg 2006;5:589-93.

K

1. Kabbani SS, Jamil H, Hammoud A, Hatab JA, Nabhani F, Hariri R, et al. The mitral pulmonary autograft: assessment at midterm. Ann Thorac Surg 2004;78:60-6.
2. Kadoba K, Jonas RA, Mayer JE, Castaneda AR. Mitral valve replacement in the first year of life. J Thorac Cardiovasc Surg 1990;100:762.
3. Khalil KG, Shapiro I, Kilman JW. Congenital mitral stenosis. J Thorac Cardiovasc Surg 1975;70:40.
4. Kojori F, Chen R, Caldarone CA, Merklinger SL, Azakie A, Williams WG, et al. Outcomes of mitral valve replacement in children: a competing-risks analysis. J Thorac Cardiovasc Surg 2004;128:703-9.

5. Kveselis DA, Rocchini AP, Beekman R, Snider AR, Crowley D, Dick M, et al. Balloon angioplasty for congenital and rheumatic mitral stenosis. Am J Cardiol 1986;57:348-50.

L

1. Laks H, Hellenbrand WE, Kleinman C, Talner NS. Left atrial–left ventricular conduit for relief of congenital mitral stenosis in infancy. J Thorac Cardiovasc Surg 1980;80:782.
2. Lansing AM, Elbl F, Solinger RE, Rees AH. Left atrial–left ventricular bypass for congenital mitral stenosis. Ann Thorac Surg 1983;35:667.
3. Layman TE, Edwards JE. Anomalous mitral arcade. A type of congenital mitral insufficiency. Circulation 1967;35:389.
4. Levy MJ, Varco RL, Lillehei CW, Edwards JE. Mitral insufficiency in infants, children, and adolescents. J Thorac Cardiovasc Surg 1963;45:434.
5. Lo PH, Hung JS, Lau KW, Kim MH, Ku PM, Krayyem M. Inoue-balloon mitral valvuloplasty in double-orifice mitral stenosis. J Invasive Cardiol 2003;15:301-3.

M

1. Macartney FJ, Scott O, Ionescu MI, Deverall PB. Diagnosis and management of parachute mitral valve and supravalvar mitral ring. Br Heart J 1974;36:641.
2. Marino BS, Kruge LE, Cho CJ, Tomlinson RS, Shera D, Weinberg PM, et al. Parachute mitral valve: morphologic descriptors, associated lesions, and outcomes after biventricular repair. J Thorac Cardiovasc Surg 2009;137:385-93.
3. Masuda M, Kado H, Tatewaki H, Shiokawa Y, Yasui H. Late results after mitral valve replacement with bileaflet mechanical prosthesis in children: evaluation of prosthesis-patient mismatch. Ann Thorac Surg 2004;77:913-7.
4. Matsumoto T, Kado H, Masuda M, Shiokawa Y, Fukae K, Morita S, et al. Clinical results of mitral valve repair by reconstructing artificial chordae tendineae in children. J Thorac Cardiovasc Surg 1999;118:94.
5. Mazzera E, Corno A, Di Donato R, Ballerini L, Marino B, Catena G, et al. Surgical bypass of the systemic atrioventricular valve in children by means of a valved conduit. J Thorac Cardiovasc Surg 1988;96:321.
6. McElhinney DB, Sherwood MC, Keane JF, del Nido PJ, Almond CS, Lock JE. Current management of severe congenital mitral stenosis: outcomes of transcatheter and surgical therapy in 108 infants and children. Circulation 2005;112:707-14.
7. Mitchell MB, Maharajh GS, Bielefeld MR, DeGroff CG, Clarke DR. Emergency pulmonary autograft mitral valve replacement in a child. Ann Thorac Surg 2001;72:251-3.
8. Moore P, Adatia I, Spevak PJ, Keane JF, Perry SB, Castaneda AR, et al. Severe congenital mitral stenosis in infants. Circulation 1994;89:2099.
9. Murakami T, Yagihara T, Yamamoto F, Uemura H, Yamashita K, Ishizaka T. Artificial chordae for mitral valve reconstruction in children. Ann Thorac Surg 1998;65:1377.

N

1. Neirotti R, Kreutzer G, Galindez E, Becu L, Ross D. Supravalvular mitral stenosis associated with ventricular septal defect. Am J Dis Child 1977;131:862.

O

1. Oosthoek PW, Wenink AC, Wisse LJ, Gittenbergerde Groot AC. Development of the papillary muscles of the mitral valve: morphogenetic background of parachute-like asymmetric mitral valves and other mitral valve anomalies. J Thorac Cardiovasc Surg 1998;116:36.
2. Oppido G, Davies B, McMullan DM, Cochrane AD, Cheung MM, d'Udekem Y, et al. Surgical treatment of congenital mitral valve disease: midterm results of a repair-oriented policy. J Thorac Cardiovasc Surg 2008;135:1313-21.

P

1. Prifti E, Vanini V, Bonacchi M, Frati G, Bernabei M, Giunti G, et al. Repair of congenital malformations of the mitral valve: early and midterm results. Ann Thorac Surg 2002;73:614-21.

R

1. Raghuveer G, Caldarone CA, Hills CB, Atkins DL, Belmont JM, Moller JH. Predictors of prosthesis survival, growth, and functional status following mechanical mitral valve replacement in children aged <5 years, a multi-institutional study. Circulation 2003;108:II174-9.
2. Rosenquist GC. Congenital mitral valve disease associated with coarctation of the aorta. A spectrum that includes parachute deformity of the mitral valve. Circulation 1974;49:985.
3. Ross DN. Replacement of aortic and mitral valves with a pulmonary autograft. Lancet 1967;2:956-8.
4. Rowlatt UF, Rimoldi IJ, Lev M. The quantitative anatomy of the normal child's heart. Pediatr Clin North Am 1963;10:499-504.
5. Ruckman RN, Van Praagh R. Anatomic types of congenital mitral stenosis: report of 49 autopsy cases with consideration of diagnosis and surgical implications. Am J Cardiol 1978;42:592.

S

1. Schaverien MV, Freedom RM, McCrindle BW. Independent factors associated with outcomes of parachute mitral valve in 84 patients. Circulation 2004;109:2309-13.
2. Schiebler GL, Edwards JE, Burchell HB, DuShane JW, Ongley PA, Wood EH. Congenital corrected transposition of the great vessels. A study of 33 cases. Pediatrics 1961;27:851.
3. Schraft WC, Lisa JR. Duplication of the mitral valve: case report and a review of the literature. Am Heart J 1950;39:136.
4. Selamet Tierney ES, Pigula FA, Berul CI, Lock JE, del Nido PJ, McElhinney DB. Mitral valve replacement in infants and children 5 years of age or younger: evolution in practice and outcome over three decades with a focus on supra-annular prosthesis implantation. J Thorac Cardiovasc Surg 2008;136:954-61.
5. Sethia B, Sullivan ID, Elliott MJ, de Leval M, Stark J. Congenital left ventricular inflow obstruction: is the outcome related to the site of the obstruction? Eur J Cardiothorac Surg 1988;2:312.
6. Shone JD, Sellers RD, Anderson RC, Adams P Jr, Lillehei CW, Edwards JE. The developmental complex of "parachute mitral valve," supravalvular ring of left atrium, subaortic stenosis, and coarctation of aorta. Am J Cardiol 1963;11:714.
7. Silver MM, Pollock J, Silver MD, Williams WG, Trusler GA. Calcification in porcine xenograft valves in children. Am J Cardiol 1980;45:685.
8. Smallhorn J, Tommasini G, Deanfield J, Douglas J, Gibson D, Macartney F. Congenital mitral stenosis. Anatomical and functional assessment by echocardiography. Br Heart J 1981;45:527.
9. Snider AR, Roge CL, Schiller NB, Silverman NH. Congenital left ventricular inflow obstruction evaluated by two-dimensional echocardiography. Circulation 1980;61:848.
10. Starkey GW. Surgical experiences in the treatment of congenital mitral stenosis and mitral insufficiency. J Thorac Surg 1959;38:336.
11. Stellin G, Bortolotti U, Mazzucco A, Faggian G, Guerra F, Daliento L, et al. Repair of congenitally malformed mitral valve in children. J Thorac Cardiovasc Surg 1988;95:480.
12. Stellin G, Padalino MA, Vida VL, Boccuzzo G, Orru E, Biffanti R, et al. Surgical repair of congenital mitral valve malformations in infancy and childhood: a single-center 36-year experience. J Thorac Cardiovasc Surg 2010;140:1238-44.
13. Sugita T, Ueda Y, Matsumoto M, Ogino H, Nishizawa J, Matsuyama K. Early and late results of partial plication annuloplasty for congenital mitral insufficiency. J Thorac Cardiovasc Surg 2001;122:229-33.
14. Sullivan ID, Robinson PJ, de Leval M, Graham TP Jr. Membranous supravalvular mitral stenosis: a treatable form of congenital heart disease. J Am Coll Cardiol 1986;8:159.

T

1. Talwar S, Sinha P, Moulick A, Jonas R. Mitral valve replacement with the pulmonary autograft in children: a word of caution. Pediatr Cardiol 2009;30:831-3.
2. Thandroyen FT, Whitton IN, Pirie D, Rogers MA, Mitha AS. Severe calcification of glutaraldehyde-preserved porcine xenografts in children. Am J Cardiol 1980;45:690.
3. Tireli E, Cetin G, Soyler I, Ozkara A. Mitral valve replacement by a Gore-Tex reinforced pulmonary autograft in a child. J Thorac Cardiovasc Surg 2004;127:1225; author reply -6.
4. Trowitzsch E, Bano-Rodrigo A, Burger BM, Colan SD, Sanders SP. Two-dimensional echocardiographic findings in double orifice mitral valve. J Am Coll Cardiol 1985;6:383.

U

1. Uva MS, Galletti L, Gayet FL, Piot D, Serraf A, Bruniaux J, et al. Surgery for congenital mitral valve disease in the first year of life. J Thorac Cardiovasc Surg 1995;109:164.

V

1. van der Horst RL, Hastreiter AR. Congenital mitral stenosis. Am J Cardiol 1967;20:773.
2. Vitarelli A, Landolina G, Gentile R, Caleffi T, Sciomer S. Echocardiographic assessment of congenital mitral stenosis. Am Heart J 1984;108:523.

W

1. Wenink AC, Gittenbergerde Groot AC, Brom AG. Developmental considerations of mitral valve anomalies. Int J Cardiol 1986; 11:85.

Y

1. Yamagishi M, Shuntoh K, Matsushita T, Fujiwara K, Shinkawa T, Miyazaki T, et al. Mitral valve replacement by a Gore-Tex reinforced pulmonary autograft in a child. J Thorac Cardiovasc Surg 2003;126:1218-9.
2. Yoshimura N, Yamaguchi M, Oshima Y, Oka S, Ootaki Y, Murakami H, et al. Surgery for mitral valve disease in the pediatric age group. J Thorac Cardiovasc Surg 1999;118:99.

Z

1. Zweng TN, Bluett MK, Mosca R, Callow LB, Bove EL. Mitral valve replacement in the first 5 years of life. Ann Thorac Surg 1989;47:720.

51 Vascular Ring and Sling

Section I Vascular Ring

DEFINITION

Vascular ring is a congenital anomaly in which the aortic arch and its branches completely or incompletely encircle and compress the trachea or esophagus or both.

HISTORICAL NOTE

Double aortic arch was apparently first described by Hommel in 1737 (cited by Turner) and a century later by Von Siebold.[T4,V2] Wolman is credited with describing the syndrome of tracheal and esophageal compression produced by a double arch in 1939.[W6] A description of a patient with dysphagia thought to be due to a retroesophageal right subclavian artery was published in 1794 by Bayford, although the vessel was illustrated to pass between the esophagus and trachea rather than in its actual position posterior to the esophagus.[B10,B11]

Modern interest in these anomalies was prompted by the first surgical correction of a double aortic arch by Gross in 1945.[G5] Subsequently, he pioneered surgical treatment of most other forms of vascular ring.[G6,G8,G9] The basis for radiologic diagnosis was initially described by Neuhauser.[N3]

The complex development and regression of the aortic arches during fetal development was elucidated by Congdon in 1922, but until Gross's pioneering surgical work, this information was little used by clinicians.[C6] In 1948, Edwards introduced the hypothetical double aortic arch scheme to conceptualize the numerous anomalies of the arch complex.[E1] This was further elaborated by Kirklin and Clagett in 1950[K3] and by Stewart, Kincaid, and Edwards in 1964.[S6] In 1951, Barry provided a clear anatomic summary and review of Congdon's basic work.[B9] In 1999, Momma and colleagues, followed by McElhinney and colleagues, identified chromosome 22q11 deletions associated with isolated anomalies of laterality or branching of the aortic arch.[M3,M5]

MORPHOLOGY

Variations in arrangement of the ascending, transverse, and descending aorta and its branches are numerous in patients with vascular rings. Several of these may produce compression of the trachea or esophagus, or both, and are of surgical importance. They may be grouped as (1) complete or (2) incomplete vascular rings, including compression by the brachiocephalic artery or left common carotid artery (Box 51-1).[B6] Of 301 patients with vascular ring or sling reported by Backer and Mavroudis, 84% fit into the categories of double aortic arch (30%), right arch with retroesophageal component (27%), and brachiocephalic artery compression syndrome (27%).[B5]

Complete Vascular Ring

Double Aortic Arch

In patients with double aortic arch, the ascending aorta arises normally, but as it leaves the pericardium it divides into two branches, a left and right aortic arch, that join posteriorly to form the descending aorta. The left arch passes anteriorly and to the left of the trachea in the usual position and is joined by the ductus arteriosus (or more often a ligamentum arteriosum), where it becomes the descending aorta. The right aortic arch passes to the right and then posterior to the esophagus to join the left-sided descending aorta, thus completing the vascular ring[E2] (Fig. 51-1). Occasionally the descending aorta is right sided, in which case the left arch (or its remnant) passes behind the esophagus. This was the case in 13 of 19 cases reported by Lincoln and colleagues.[L3] Alternatively, the descending aorta may be essentially a midline structure.

The right arch gives origin to two vessels, the right common carotid and right subclavian arteries, and the left arch gives origin to the left common carotid and left subclavian arteries in that order. The right aortic arch is most often

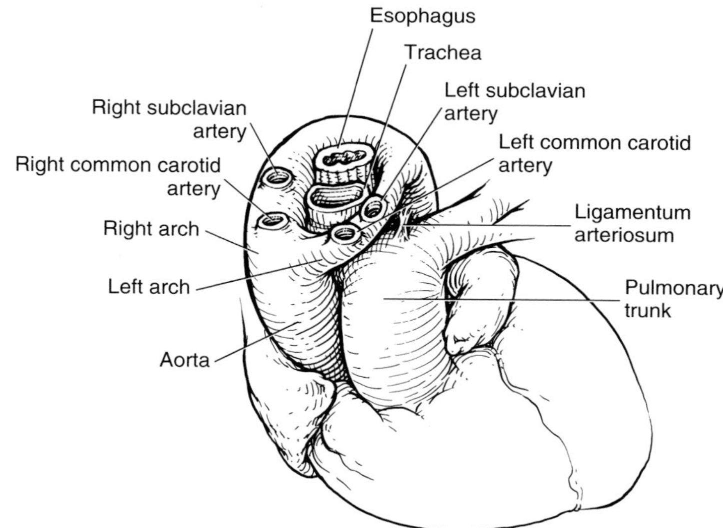

Figure 51-1 Double aortic arch with right dominant arch. Right common carotid and right subclavian arteries arise from right arch. Left common carotid and left subclavian arteries arise from smaller left arch. The two arches join as the descending thoracic aorta, forming a complete vascular ring.

Box 51-1 Classification of Vascular Ring

Complete Vascular Ring
- Double aortic arch
- Right aortic arch with retroesophageal component:
  - Mirror-image branching with retroesophageal ligamentum arteriosum
  - Retroesophageal left subclavian artery with ligamentum arteriosum
  - Retroesophageal left brachiocephalic artery
- Left aortic arch and right descending aorta with right ligamentum arteriosum or patent ductus arteriosus
- Cervical aortic arch complex

Incomplete Vascular Ring
- Left aortic arch and retroesophageal right subclavian artery
- Tracheal compression by brachiocephalic or left common carotid artery
- Ductus arteriosus sling
- Malrotation of heart with patent ductus arteriosus

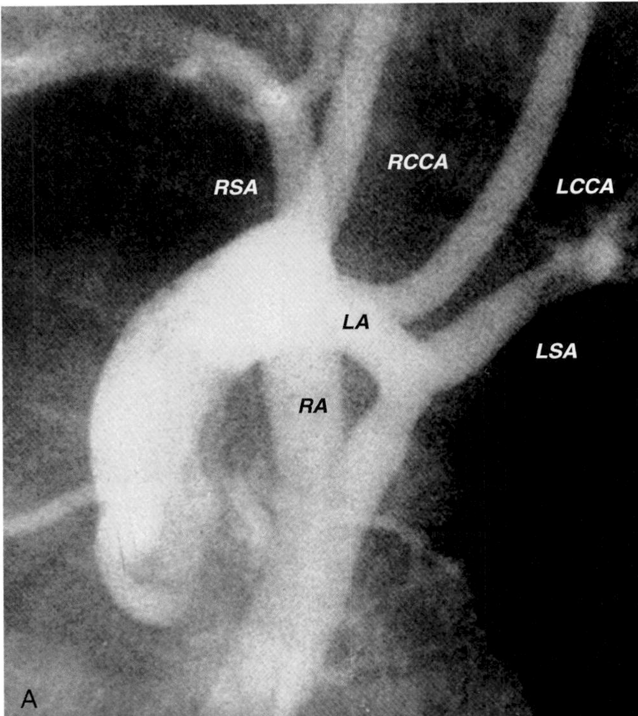

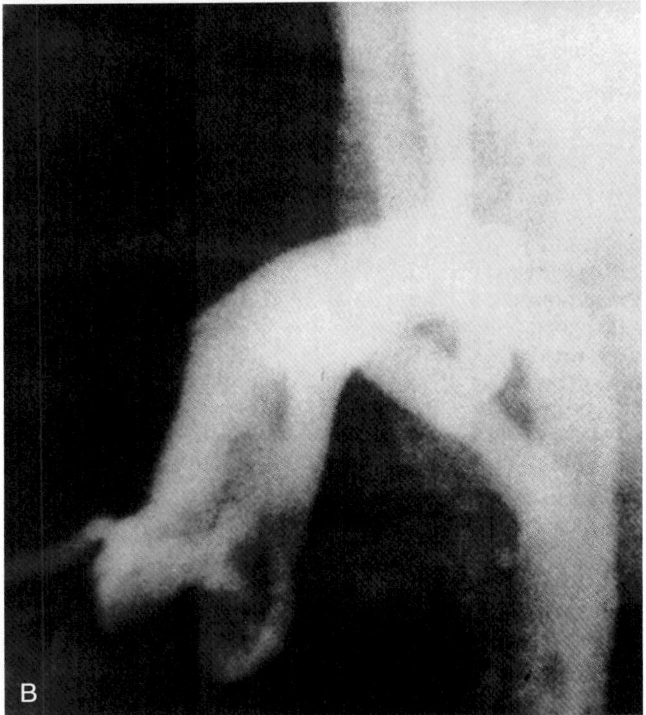

Figure 51-2 Aortogram of right dominant double aortic arch in **(A)** frontal view and **(B)** lateral view with cranial tilt. Left aortic arch is distinctly narrowed beyond origin of left subclavian artery. Key: *LA,* Left arch; *LCCA,* left common carotid artery; *LSA,* left subclavian artery; *RA,* right aortic arch; *RCCA,* right common carotid artery; *RSA,* right subclavian artery.

(75% of cases)[A3] larger (right dominant) than the left, which usually becomes narrow or atretic in its distal part beyond the origin of the left subclavian artery (Fig. 51-2; see also Fig. 51-1). This portion may remain patent or be represented by a fibrous chord that joins the descending aorta,

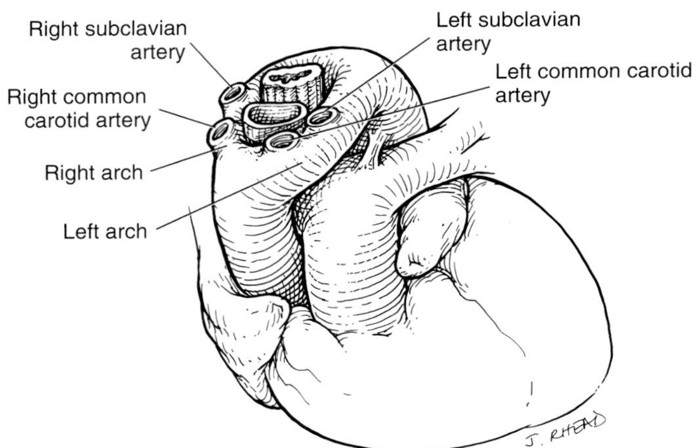

Figure 51-3 Double aortic arch with left dominant arch. Smaller right arch passes posterior to esophagus, forming a complete vascular ring.

often at the site of a diverticulum.[S9] This fibrous chord, at its origin from the base of the left subclavian artery, lies close to the ligamentum arteriosum. The latter structure passes from this point to the adjacent proximal part of the left pulmonary artery (Fig. 51-3; double arch, left dominant). Less commonly (20% of cases) the left aortic arch is larger (left dominant) than the right, which although smaller in its distal part after the origin of the right subclavian artery, is rarely atretic (Fig. 51-4; see also Fig. 51-3). Size of the right and left aortic arches is nearly equal (balanced) in about 5% of cases.[B7]

Associated cardiovascular anomalies are uncommon but include tetralogy of Fallot and transposition of the great arteries.[H7,S6]

Right Aortic Arch with Retroesophageal Component

In the situation of right aortic arch with a retroesophageal vascular or ligamentous component, a vascular ring is usually present, but the anatomic details vary depending on site of regression (interruption) of the embryonic left arch.

In the common situation of right aortic arch without retroesophageal segment, no vascular ring is present. The arch branches arise in mirror image of the normal (Fig. 51-5).[D1] This arrangement is the result of interruption of the embryonic left arch distal to the ductus arteriosus, in which the anterior ligamentum courses from the brachiocephalic artery to the proximal left pulmonary artery (Fig. 51-6, *A*, type 1 right aortic arch). This type is particularly common in tetralogy of Fallot (see Chapter 38) and truncus arteriosus (see Chapter 43).

Mirror-Image Branching and Retroesophageal Ligamentum Arteriosum Interruption of the left arch is proximal (upstream) to the ductus arteriosus (Fig. 51-6, *B*, type 2 right aortic arch). The left-sided ligamentum arteriosum extends from a diverticulum (Kommerell) on the upper descending thoracic aorta, behind the esophagus, forward to the left pulmonary artery. The vascular ring is formed by the ascending portion of the right arch and brachiocephalic artery anteriorly, by the aortic diverticulum posteriorly, and by the ligamentum arteriosum laterally.[K4] In the surgical series reported by Backer and colleagues, this anomaly represented about one third of right arch vascular rings.[B7]

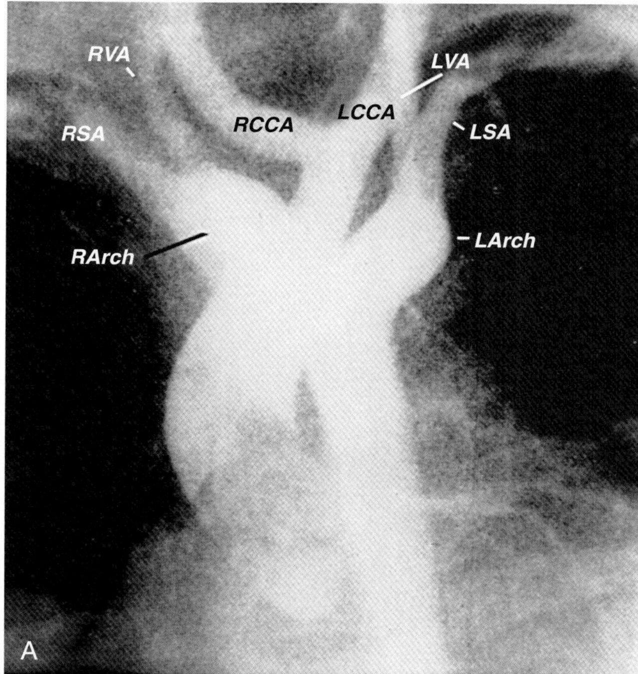

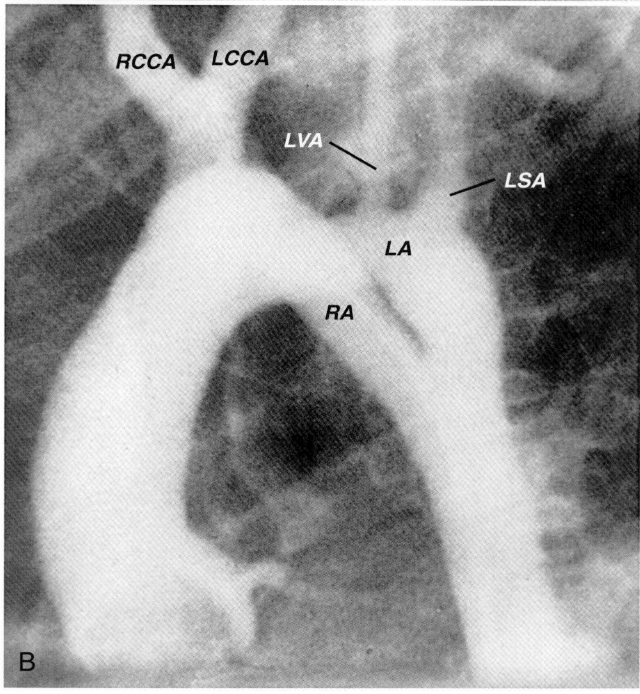

Figure 51-4 Aortogram of balanced double aortic arch in **(A)** frontal and **(B)** lateral views. Right aortic arch is slightly smaller than left (left dominant) where it joins left-sided descending aorta. Right and left common carotid arteries arise from a large common trunk. Key: *LA,* Left arch; *LCCA,* left common carotid artery; *LSA,* left subclavian artery; *LVA,* left vertebral artery; *RA,* right arch; *RCCA,* right common carotid artery; *RSA,* right subclavian artery; *RVA,* right vertebral artery.

Retroesophageal Left Subclavian Artery and Ligamentum (Ductus) Arteriosum Here the interruption of the left arch occurs between the left subclavian and left common carotid arteries (Fig. 51-6, *C*, type 3 right aortic arch). The first branch of the right arch becomes the left common

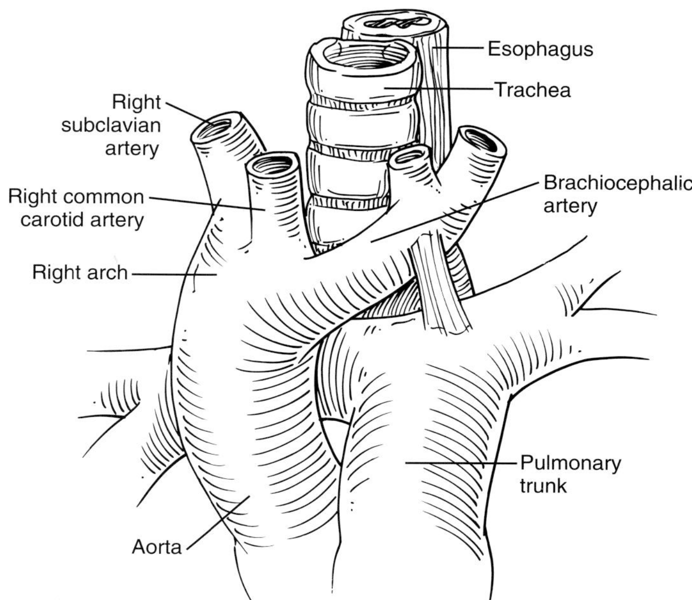

Figure 51-5 Common type of right aortic arch with mirror-image branching. This anomaly is frequently associated with tetralogy of Fallot and truncus arteriosus. Ligamentum arteriosum is anterior, coursing from brachiocephalic artery to pulmonary artery. There is no vascular ring.

carotid artery, and the descending aorta gives origin to the retroesophageal left subclavian artery as the fourth branch. The ductus or ligament arises with the left subclavian artery from an aortic diverticulum or from the left subclavian artery itself near its origin, where the subclavian artery may be narrowed. The descending aorta can be left or right sided.

This is the most common type of vascular ring associated with right arch (see Fig. 51-6, *C*), accounting for about two thirds of right arch vascular rings.[B7] It is usually loose, so compression of either the esophagus or trachea is uncommon. Associated cardiac anomalies are rare.

Retroesophageal Left Brachiocephalic Artery Here interruption occurs between the left common carotid and the right arch (Fig. 51-6, *D*, type 4 right aortic arch). A vascular ring is present, but the anomaly is rare. Bein and colleagues reported a case of long-segment coarctation with this anomaly.[B12]

Left Aortic Arch and Right Descending Aorta

Vascular rings are likely in the uncommon combination of left aortic arch and right descending aorta. The left arch crosses behind the esophagus. In combination with right patent ductus arteriosus or ligamentum arteriosum, a vascular ring is formed.[B14,M8,P1]

Cervical Aortic Arch Complex

Cervical aortic arch is a developmental entity consisting of persistence of the right or left third branchial arch and regression of the fourth branchial arch.[V3] The cervical aortic arch complex consists of a cervical position of the apex of the aortic arch with separate origin of the contralateral carotid artery, a retroesophageal descending aorta coursing contralaterally to the arch, and anomalous origin of the subclavian artery from the descending aorta.[H4] The cervical arch usually

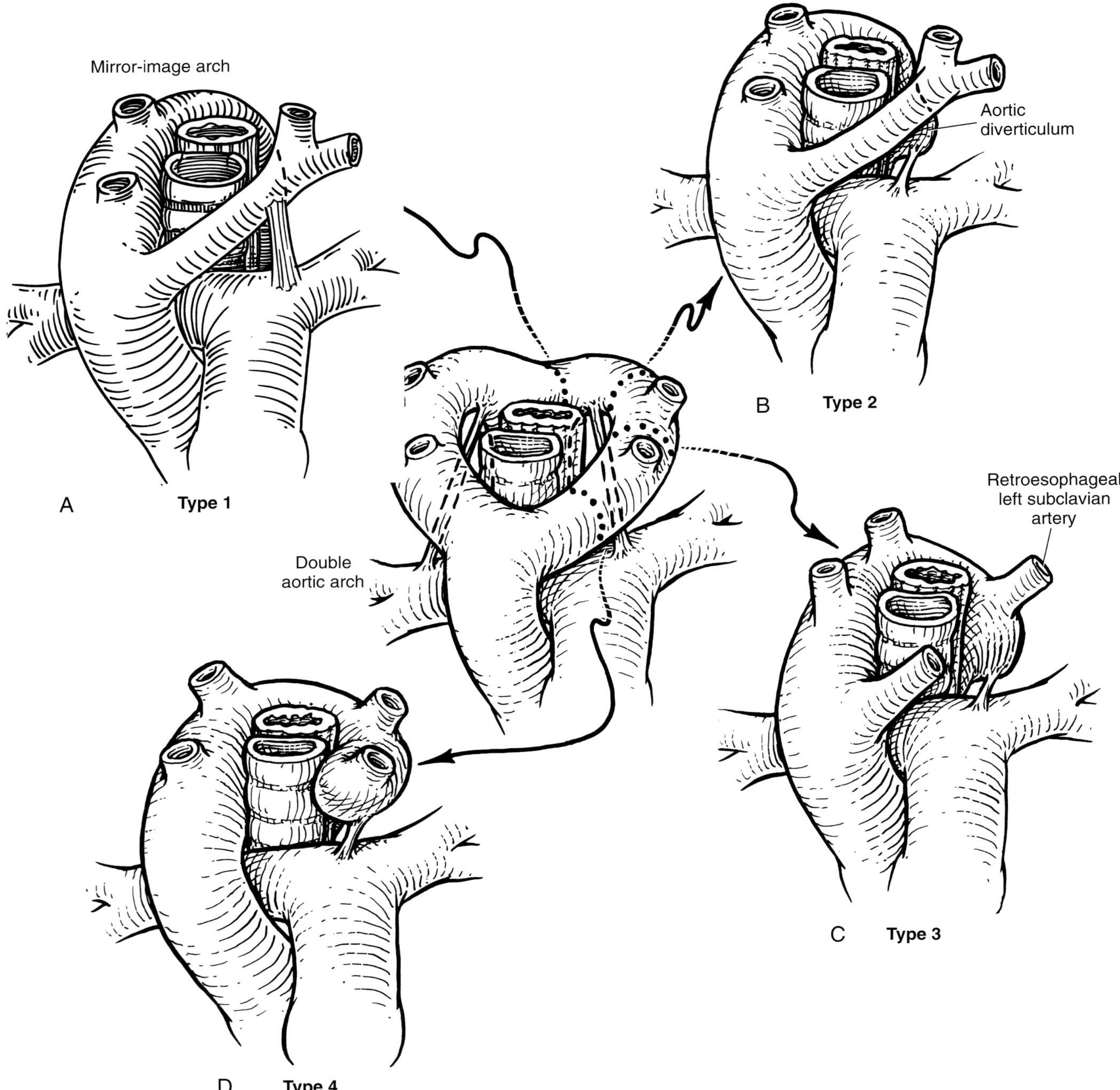

Figure 51-6 Vascular ring associated with right aortic arch. Center drawing depicts a double aortic arch with descending thoracic aorta as a midline or left-sided structure. Ligamentum arteriosum *(dashed line)* is shown originating from junction of right or left arch and descending aorta. Right-sided ligamentum arteriosum to right pulmonary artery usually forms in association with a right-sided descending aorta. Left-sided ligamentum arteriosum is the common configuration connecting midline or left descending thoracic aorta to left pulmonary artery near bifurcation. The four possible sites *(dotted lines)* of regression (interruption) of left arch during fetal development are shown. Various types of right aortic arch are depicted depending on site of interruption. Vascular ring results from a retroesophageal component of left arch giving rise to the ligamentum. **A,** Type 1 right aortic arch. Aortic arch branches arise in mirror image of normal. Anterior ligamentum arteriosum courses from brachiocephalic artery to proximal left pulmonary artery (see Fig. 51-5). There is no vascular ring. **B,** Type 2 right aortic arch. Left arch regresses just distal to left subclavian artery, leaving a retroesophageal aortic diverticulum. Ligamentum (ductus) arteriosum arises posteriorly from descending aorta and courses to left pulmonary artery, completing a vascular ring. **C,** Type 3 right aortic arch. Left arch regresses between left common carotid and left subclavian arteries, leaving a retroesophageal subclavian artery, with ligamentum (ductus) arteriosum forming a complete vascular ring. **D,** Type 4 right aortic arch. Left arch regresses between right arch and left common carotid artery. Complete vascular ring is present in this rare anomaly.

is right sided. The aorta is usually redundant and crosses to the opposite side posterior to the esophagus. The retroesophageal segment of the aorta may be tortuous and severely narrowed.[H4] A vascular ring is formed when there is an aberrant subclavian artery on the side contralateral to the aortic arch and a ligamentum arteriosum. There is considerable variability in anatomic configuration of the aortic arch and its branches.[M7] Abnormalities of brachiocephalic arterial branching and arch laterality are common in patients with cervical aortic arch.[M4] Vascular ring is frequently present, usually formed by the right aortic arch and aberrant left subclavian artery, but occasionally by double aortic arch. Rarely, a left cervical aortic arch, right ligamentum arteriosum, and right descending aorta form the vascular ring (see also discussion under "Left Aortic Arch and Right Descending Aorta").[W3]

Incomplete Vascular Ring

Left Aortic Arch and Retroesophageal Right Subclavian Artery

The relatively common (0.5% of the general population[A1]) retroesophageal right subclavian artery arising as the fourth branch of an otherwise normal aortic arch and passing upward and to the right behind the esophagus was once thought to be a cause of dysphagia (dysphagia lusoria, or "difficulty swallowing due to a trick of nature").[B4,L3,M10] This condition does not form a complete ring and is generally not considered the true cause of vague symptoms related to swallowing. Rarely, a right ligamentum arteriosum passing from the retroesophageal right subclavian artery to the right pulmonary artery forms a vascular ring that is symptomatic.

Tracheal Compression by Brachiocephalic or Left Common Carotid Artery

The brachiocephalic or left common carotid artery may be drawn taut across the anterior wall of the trachea, a potential but uncommon cause of respiratory obstruction.[A2,E3,F1,L3,M9] It is not known why they occasionally compress the trachea. Presumably, the brachiocephalic artery originates more posteriorly from the aortic arch than usual, so it crosses the trachea more posteriorly.[A4]

Ductus Arteriosus Sling

Binet and colleagues described an infant with respiratory obstruction in which an anomalous vessel (presumed to be the ductus arteriosus) originated from the right pulmonary artery, crossed to the left between the esophagus and trachea, and joined the descending aorta adjacent to the origin of a retroesophageal right subclavian artery.[B15]

Severe Malrotation of Heart with Patent Ductus Arteriosus

Compression of the lower trachea can occur with a normal left arch when there is severe malrotation of the heart into the right chest in association with agenesis or hypoplasia of the right lung.[V1,W2] Scherer and Westcott described a patient with dextrocardia and normal lungs in whom the pulmonary trunk lay anterior to the trachea and somewhat to the right. The patent ductus arteriosus connecting with a normally positioned descending aorta pulled the pulmonary trunk backward, compressing the front of the trachea. Compression was relieved by dividing the patent ductus arteriosus.[S3]

CLINICAL FEATURES AND DIAGNOSTIC CRITERIA

Symptoms and Signs

Symptoms of vascular ring relate to the consequences of tracheal and esophageal compression.[A4,M10,W8] Presentation is usually within the first 6 months of life and often within the first month. Inspiratory stridor may be present at birth, often in association with an expiratory wheeze and tachypnea. Stridor may be worse in various positions—for example, when the baby is lying on his or her back rather than side. Often, stridor is relieved by extending the neck. The baby's cry may be hoarse and, in the absence of frank stridor, the breathing noisy. Persistent barking cough is frequently present. There may be episodes of apnea, severe cyanosis, and unconsciousness. When obstruction is severe, subcostal retraction is obvious. Recurrent respiratory infections are common and aggravate the respiratory obstruction; when obstruction is less severe, obstructive symptoms may be apparent only at such times.

The baby often feeds poorly, and there may be obvious difficulty in swallowing liquids, with episodes of choking and increased respiratory obstruction at these times. Dysphagia for solids is common (most severe cases are operated on before the babies are old enough to be offered solid food), with the baby refusing to swallow them or choking and regurgitating.

Dysphagia lusoria is often attributed to retroesophageal origin of the right subclavian artery from the upper descending thoracic aorta.[B4,L3,M10] The artery courses to the right, posterior to the esophagus, producing an indentation of the esophagus that has been blamed for vague symptoms in children, but that is usually not the cause. Should it become ectatic or aneurysmal later in life, difficulty swallowing is more likely.

Symptomatic vascular rings manifesting in adults are rare, and reports often emphasize dysphagia as the predominant symptom. Grathwohl and colleagues[G10] reviewed case reports of 24 adults with vascular rings. Two thirds had symptoms, 63% respiratory. Dysphagia was less prominent, occurring in 33%. Vascular rings occurring in adults may mimic chronic asthma.[H5,P2]

Chest Radiography

Plain chest radiograph in the frontal view is either normal (10%) or shows a right aortic arch (85%).[P5] Anterior tracheal bowing is present on 92% of lateral views, and tracheal narrowing on 77%.

Esophagography

The esophagram is a useful diagnostic measure.[A4,L3] Video esophagography at the time of cineangiography is optimal because it permits a detailed study showing the pulsatile nature of the obstruction and trachea.

With double aortic arch, the esophagram shows left- and right-sided indentations, with that for the right arch usually higher and deeper (Fig. 51-7, *A*). In addition, the retroesophageal component produces a prominent posterior indentation that courses downward and to the left. In contrast, a retroesophageal left subclavian artery arising from the right arch produces a narrower esophageal impression that

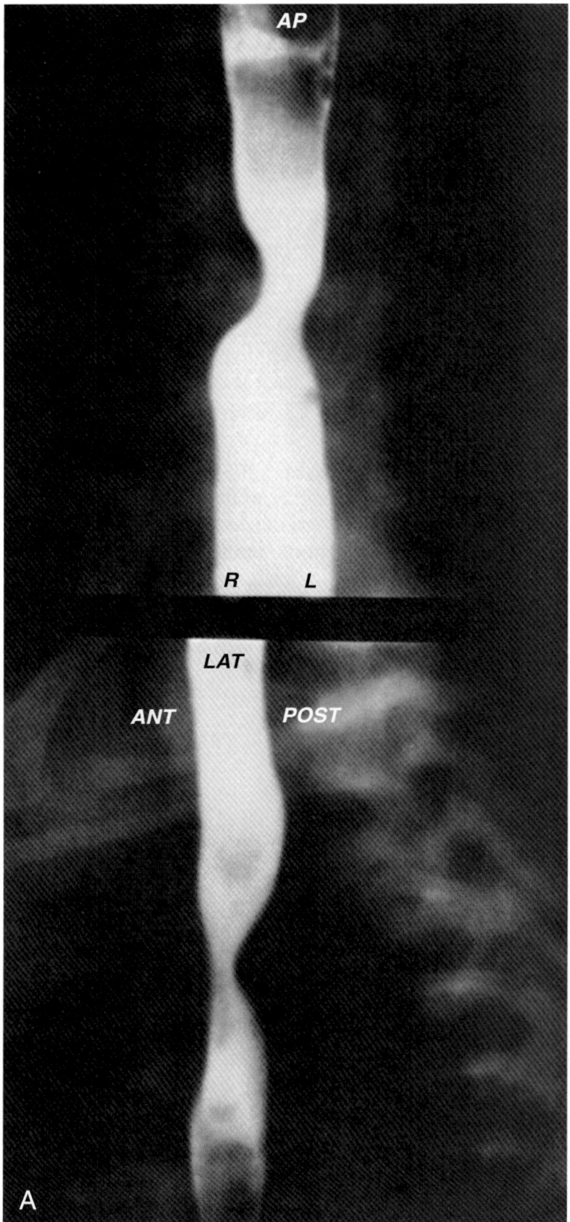

Figure 51-7 Esophagrams in anteroposterior *(AP)* and lateral *(LAT)* projections. **A,** Double aortic arch.

courses upward and rightward. Right arch and left ligamentum arteriosum show more marked right-sided than left-sided indentation (Fig. 51-7, *B*).

Bronchoscopy

Bronchoscopy is rarely done, although it does identify sites of tracheal compression and shows its pulsatile nature.[M10]

Two-Dimensional Echocardiography

Two-dimensional echocardiography is useful in diagnosing vascular ring, at least in neonates and infants, and is critically important for identifying associated cardiac anomalies.[B17] However, it is inferior to computed tomography (CT) in demonstrating details of arch anatomy.

Computed Tomography

CT with contrast usually provides an excellent image of the structures and complements two-dimensional echocardiography. Ultrafast CT with three-dimensional reconstruction provides even greater anatomic detail.[V4] In many institutions, CT has become the standard modality for delineating details of vascular ring anatomy.[B7]

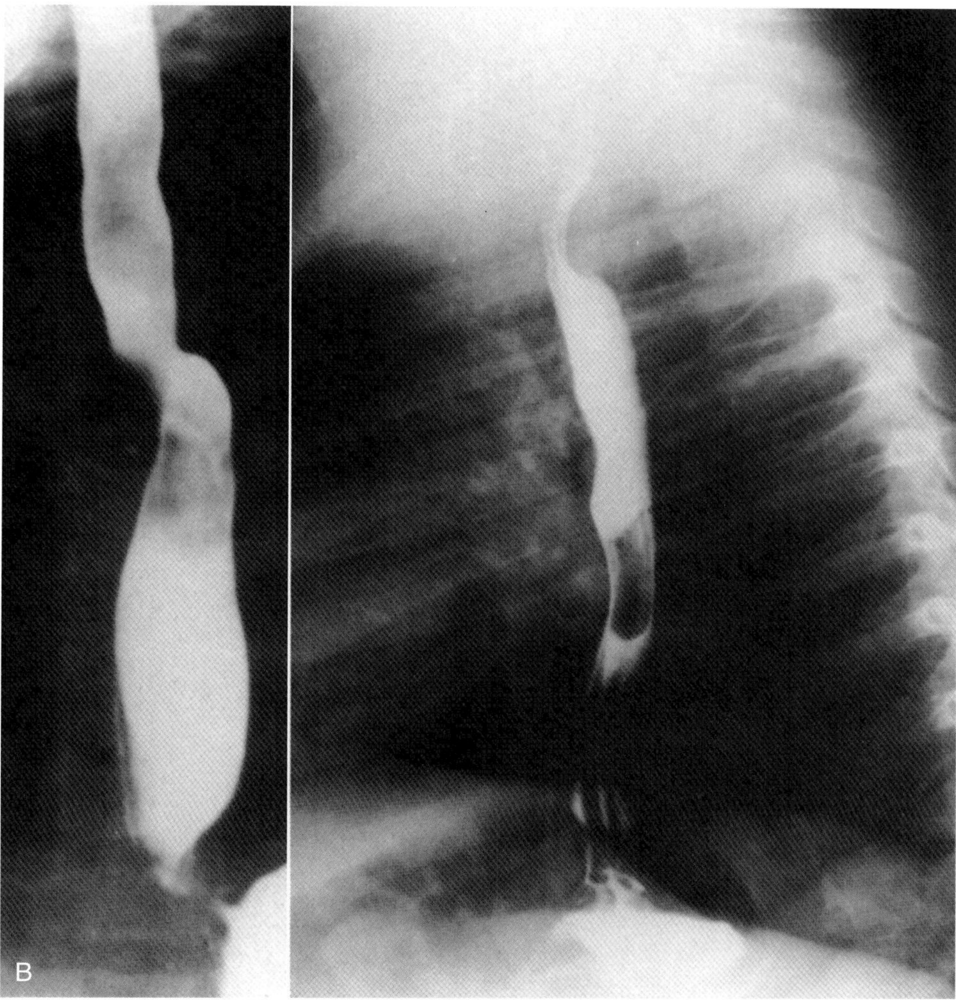

Figure 51-7, cont'd **B,** Right aortic arch with retroesophageal aortic diverticulum giving origin to a retroesophageal left subclavian artery and ligamentum arteriosum. AP views show typical bilateral indentations, lateral views a posterior indentation. Key: *ANT,* Anterior aspect of patient; *L,* left side of patient; *POST,* posterior aspect of patient; *R,* right side of patient.

Magnetic Resonance Imaging

Magnetic resonance imaging (MRI) is diagnostic and delineates severity of tracheal narrowing.[S4]

Aortography

Because of the accuracy of noninvasive imaging, aortography is rarely necessary. Aortography may be performed via a catheter positioned in the ascending aorta and is usually combined with cineangiography to assess associated congenital cardiac anomalies. Using biplane techniques, the first injection depicts both lateral and anteroposterior views, and the second both left and right oblique views. A degree of cranial tilt may separate the arches better in oblique views.[T1] Aortography can establish that the anomaly is a complete double aortic arch and show sites of narrowing in the left or (rarely) right arch (see Figs. 51-2 and 51-4). It cannot distinguish between a double arch with an atretic segment and a right aortic arch with a retroesophageal component. Sharp angulation of one of the brachiocephalic arteries may indicate the site of an atretic segment in a double arch or a constricting ligamentum arteriosum in a right arch with retroesophageal component (Fig. 51-8).

NATURAL HISTORY

Vascular rings of aortic arch origin account for 1% to 2% of cases of congenital heart disease.[N1] Only fragmentary information exists concerning the natural history of these anomalies. Untreated severe respiratory obstruction in the first 6 months of life is presumably fatal before age 1 year, particularly when symptoms are present from birth. Symptoms first appearing after age 6 months are less severe and rarely progressive, except at times of respiratory infection or regurgitation and choking.

When symptoms are of borderline severity, they usually disappear as the child grows. Godtfredsen and colleagues followed 11 patients with symptoms not severe enough to justify surgery.[G3] Of the six who had either double aortic arch or right arch with retroesophageal component, four outgrew their symptoms by age 4 years, and two with persistent symptoms had other anomalies to explain them.

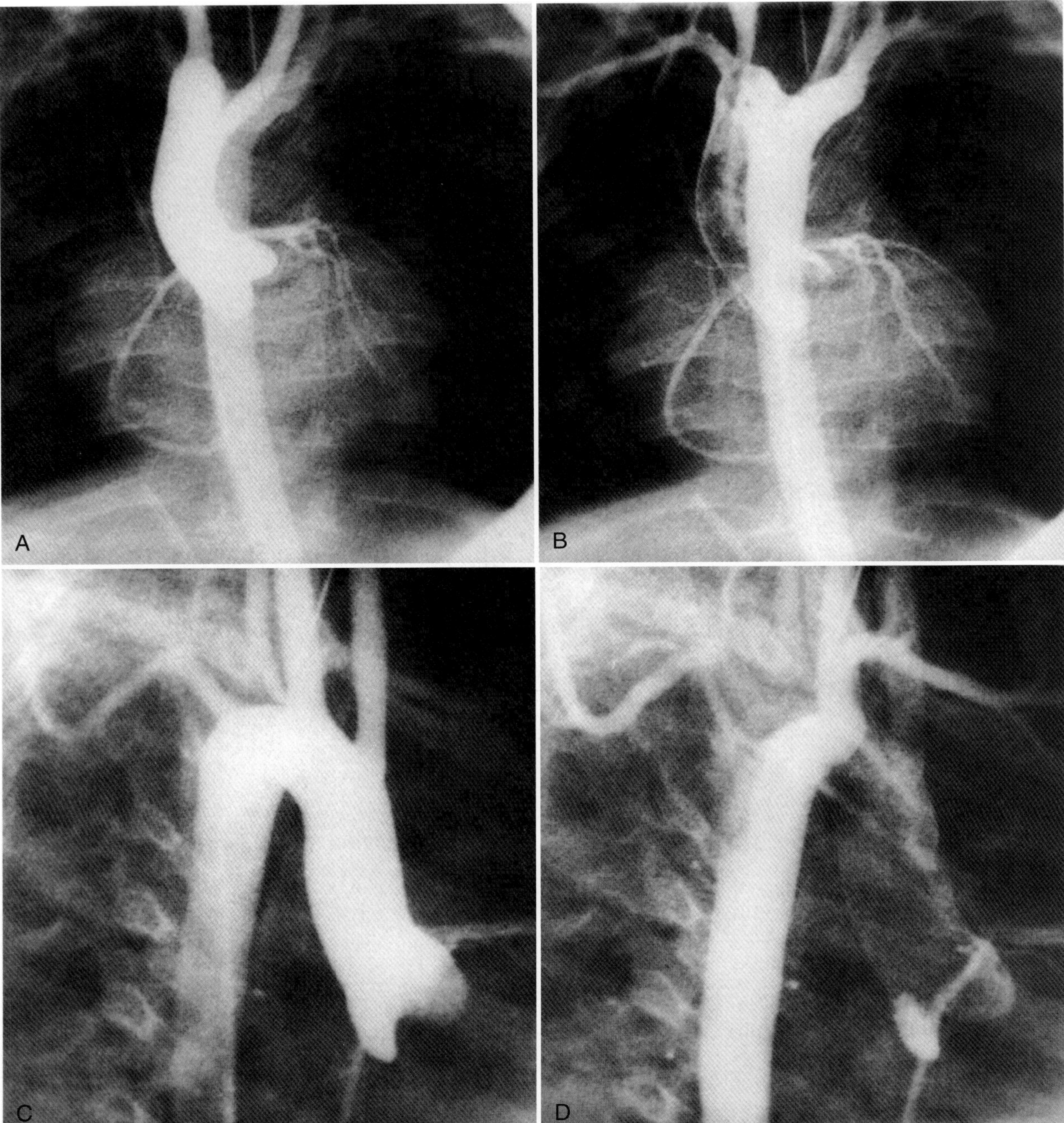

Figure 51-8 Aortogram of right aortic arch with retroesophageal left subclavian artery and ligamentum arteriosum arising from a retroesophageal aortic diverticulum. Frontal views **(A-B)** and right anterior oblique views **(C-D)** are at different phases in cardiac cycle. Angulation at origin of left subclavian artery from diverticulum suggests presence of a ligamentum arteriosum under tension passing forward to left pulmonary artery (as was the case at operation). Angulation is downward in frontal view and anterior in right anterior oblique view. Absence of a similar angulation along course of left common carotid artery suggests that this artery is not connected to the diverticulum by an atretic ligament that forms part of a complete left aortic arch.

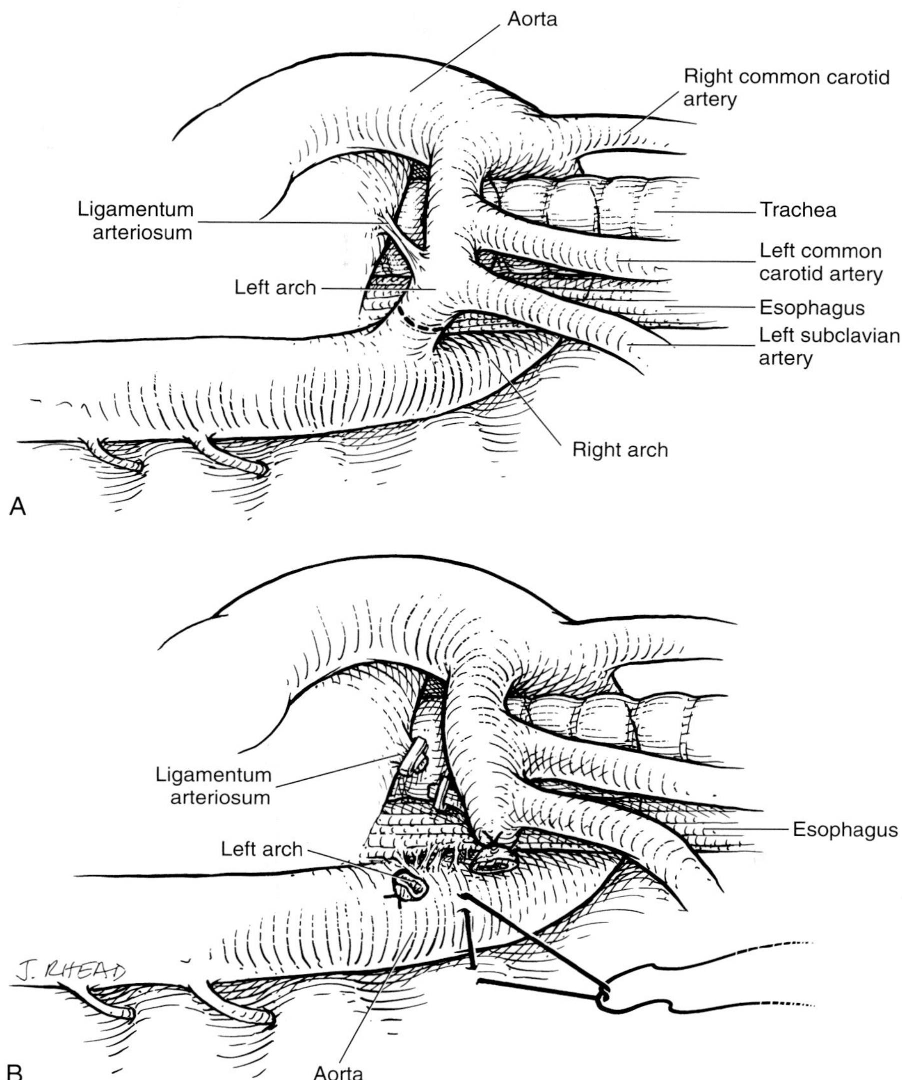

Figure 51-9 Operative repair of vascular ring caused by right dominant double aortic arch. **A,** Surgeon's view of anomaly through left posterolateral thoracotomy. Both arches, their branches, and ligamentum arteriosum are dissected and separated thoroughly from surrounding tissues. Site of division of smaller left arch is shown by dashed line. **B,** Ligamentum arteriosum is divided between surgical clips. Aortic arch is divided and ends ligated or oversewn. Anteromedial surface of aorta is dissected away from esophagus. Adventitia of lateral wall of aorta is sutured to periosteum of an adjacent rib to pull aorta laterally and posteriorly away from esophagus.

Generally, symptoms are milder and of later onset, and dysphagia is less prominent, in patients having right aortic arch with retroesophageal component than in those with double aortic arch.[A4]

TECHNIQUE OF OPERATION

Double Aortic Arch

In all cases of double aortic arch with a left-sided ligamentum, the repair may be approached through a left thoracotomy via the fourth interspace or bed of the nonresected fifth rib, as in the operation for patent ductus arteriosus (see Chapter 37, Fig. 37-3) or coarctation (see Chapter 48, Fig. 48-15). However, a similar approach from the right side may also be used when the left arch is dominant. Median sternotomy may be used when coexisting cardiac anomalies require repair.

When the left arch is dominant, the right arch can be dissected out via a left-sided approach, including the part passing behind the esophagus, and is divided between clamps close to its junction with the descending aorta. Its ends are oversewn with two rows of 4-0 or 5-0 polypropylene sutures. Its mediastinal surface is then dissected further to free it and allow the divided ends to separate. The descending aorta is also mobilized and sometimes sutured to the rib periosteum to keep it away from the esophagus. In this and other operations for relief of vascular rings, "all strands or bands of tissue which form a part of the constricting mechanism" must be dissected away from the trachea or esophagus.[G7] Operation is completed by closing the chest wound in layers after inserting a single intercostal tube for drainage.

More often, the distal left arch is narrowed, and approach is made from the left side. The vascular structures and ligamentum arteriosum are dissected out and separated thoroughly from surrounding structures (Fig. 51-9, *A*). The ligamentum arteriosum is divided, taking care to avoid injury to the recurrent laryngeal nerve. The junction of the left arch with the descending aorta is divided between vascular clamps and the ends oversewn (Fig. 51-9, *B*). The end of the left arch is then further dissected from underlying mediastinal tissues to allow it to retract forward. The medial surface of the descending aorta and distal divided end are also dissected

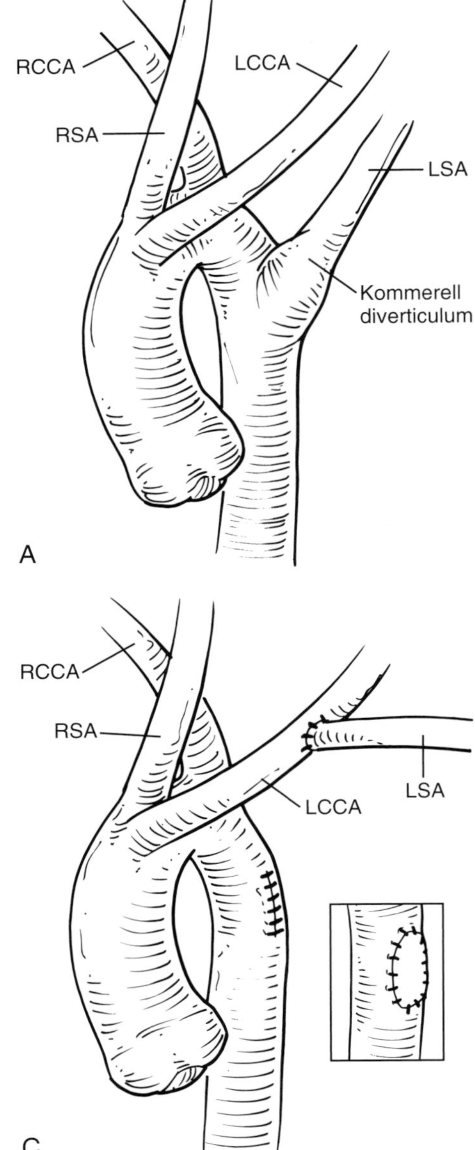

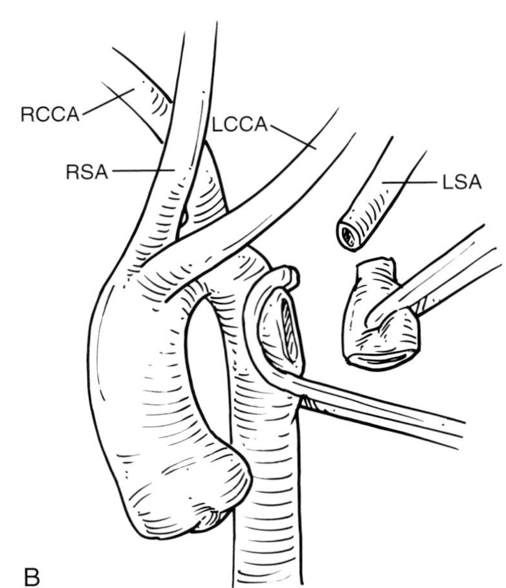

Figure 51-10 Repair of right aortic arch with retroesophageal component. **A,** Anatomy of patient with right aortic arch, retroesophageal left subclavian artery *(LSA)*, and large Kommerell diverticulum (embryologic remnant of left fourth aortic arch). Diameter of Kommerell diverticulum is usually equal to size of descending aorta. Ligamentum arteriosum is not illustrated. **B,** Resection of Kommerell diverticulum through left thoracotomy. Vascular clamp partially occludes descending thoracic aorta at origin of Kommerell diverticulum. Clamp on LSA is not illustrated. Kommerell diverticulum has been completely resected. **C,** Completed repair. Orifice at which Kommerell diverticulum was resected is usually closed primarily or *(inset)* can be patched with polytetrafluoroethylene if necessary. LSA has been implanted into side of left common carotid artery *(LCAA)* with fine running polypropylene sutures. Key: *RCCA,* right common carotid artery; *RSA,* right subclavian artery. (Redrawn from Backer and colleagues.[B7])

away from the esophagus. Adventitia over the lateral wall of the aorta may be sutured to the adjacent rib periosteum to pull it laterally and posteriorly away from the esophagus.

Techniques have been developed to divide vascular rings using video-assisted thoracoscopy.[B18] Compared with standard thoracotomy techniques, it is equally safe (no mortality), and length of stay in the intensive care unit or hospital, duration of intubation, and hospital charges are similar.

Right Aortic Arch with Retroesophageal Component

Right arch with retroesophageal component is generally approached from the left side. After dissection is completed, the ligamentum arteriosum is divided. The aortic diverticulum (Kommerell) is resected when it is large enough to independently compress the esophagus or trachea.[B4] Backer and colleagues recommend routine reimplantation of the left subclavian artery into the left common carotid artery if it arises from the diverticulum (Fig. 51-10). The descending aorta is dissected away from the esophagus and sutured to the periosteum of the rib if necessary to keep it away from the esophagus.

A robotic approach for dividing a left-sided ligamentum has been reported in a type 4 right aortic arch vascular ring.[R2]

Left Aortic Arch

Right-sided thoracotomy is used for left aortic arch and right-sided ligamentum arteriosum[P7,W3] with or without a retroesophageal right subclavian artery (Fig. 51-11). The ligamentum is dissected and divided in the same fashion as for right arch with retroesophageal component.

Tracheal Compression by Brachiocephalic or Left Common Carotid Artery

When the lower trachea is compressed by an anomalous brachiocephalic artery (Fig. 51-12) or a malrotated left aortic

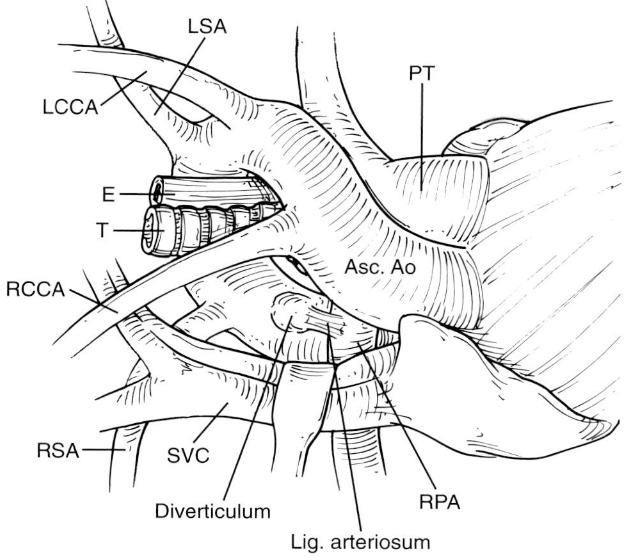

Figure 51-11 Right thoracotomy is necessary to correct the rare case of dominant left arch with right descending aorta and right-sided ligamentum arteriosum passing to right pulmonary artery. Key: *ASC Ao,* Ascending aorta; *LCCA,* left common carotid artery; *Lig.,* ligamentum; *LSA,* left subclavian artery; *PT,* pulmonary trunk; *RCCA,* right common carotid artery; *RPA,* right pulmonary artery; *RSA,* right subclavian artery; *SVC,* superior vena cava. (Redrawn from Jonas.[J1])

arch associated with severe rightward malrotation of the heart, approach may be through a median sternotomy. A short left anterolateral thoracotomy also works well and leaves the sternum intact; the suspending sutures may be passed through the sternum. The anomalous vessel is fully dissected, then suspended from the posterior aspect of the sternum or adjacent ribs with 3-0 or 4-0 polypropylene pledgeted mattress sutures that pick up the adventitia of the vessel.

Hawkins and colleagues have proposed an alternative midline approach in which the brachiocephalic artery is reimplanted more proximally on the ascending aorta and to the right of the trachea.[H2]

SPECIAL FEATURES OF POSTOPERATIVE CARE

Few patients obtain immediate relief of stridor,[L3] but for some the improvement in breathing is prompt and dramatic. Symptoms may worsen in the first postoperative week in some patients. Special respiratory care is therefore required, particularly in small infants. Occasionally, intubation is necessary for several days to allow adequate tracheal aspiration toilet and, if necessary, ventilation. Use of continuous positive airway pressure with the infant breathing spontaneously is often advantageous in this setting.[S7] After extubation, positive pressure is maintained for some days if necessary, using nasal prongs with an appropriate flow of humidified gas. Full humidification and meticulous suctioning techniques are required to keep the airway clear and avoid mucosal damage.

RESULTS

Complete Vascular Ring

In the current era, hospital mortality after repair of vascular ring without major associated lesions should approach zero.[A3,H9,R3,R4] Good functional results are obtained in 90% of surviving patients.[B3] In a 45-year analysis by Backer and colleagues, early mortality was primarily related to major associated cardiac or respiratory anomalies.

Late outcomes after repair of complete vascular ring are generally good, but persistent respiratory symptoms are frequent—54% after repair of double aortic arch in a longitudinal study by Alsenaidi and colleagues,[A3] possibly associated with previous compression-related tracheobronchial damage or maldevelopment. Gastrointestinal symptoms are uncommon.[A3]

Incomplete Vascular Ring

Results are also good in about 90% of patients with incomplete vascular ring.[B3]

Tracheal Compression by Brachiocephalic or Left Common Carotid Artery

Results of arteriopexy for tracheal compression by the brachiocephalic or left common carotid artery were excellent in 93% of a group of 76 patients.[B1] Death occurred in 3 of 79 (3%; CL 1.7%-7.5%) patients.[B4] Similar results have been achieved by the reimplantation technique.[H2]

INDICATIONS FOR OPERATION

Operation is indicated in all patients with important obstructed airway symptoms. Treatment should not be delayed, because hypoxic and apneic spells may occur, as well as further damage to the trachea and bronchi.[B4] Operation is not indicated if symptoms are mild or absent.

SPECIAL SITUATIONS AND CONTROVERSIES

Resection of Kommerell Diverticulum

Most surgeons have routinely left alone a Kommerell diverticulum or performed an aortopexy in the vicinity of the diverticulum by tacking it to the adjacent chest wall. However, Backer and colleagues recommend its routine excision (see Technique of Operation) because of the occasional need to reoperate for symptom recurrence secondary to tracheoesophageal compression by the diverticulum.[B7] Further longitudinal studies are needed to clarify the role of routine diverticular resection.

Section II **Vascular Sling**

DEFINITION

Vascular sling is a congenital anomaly in which the left pulmonary artery (LPA) arises from the right pulmonary artery (RPA) extrapericardially (anomalous LPA), courses to the left

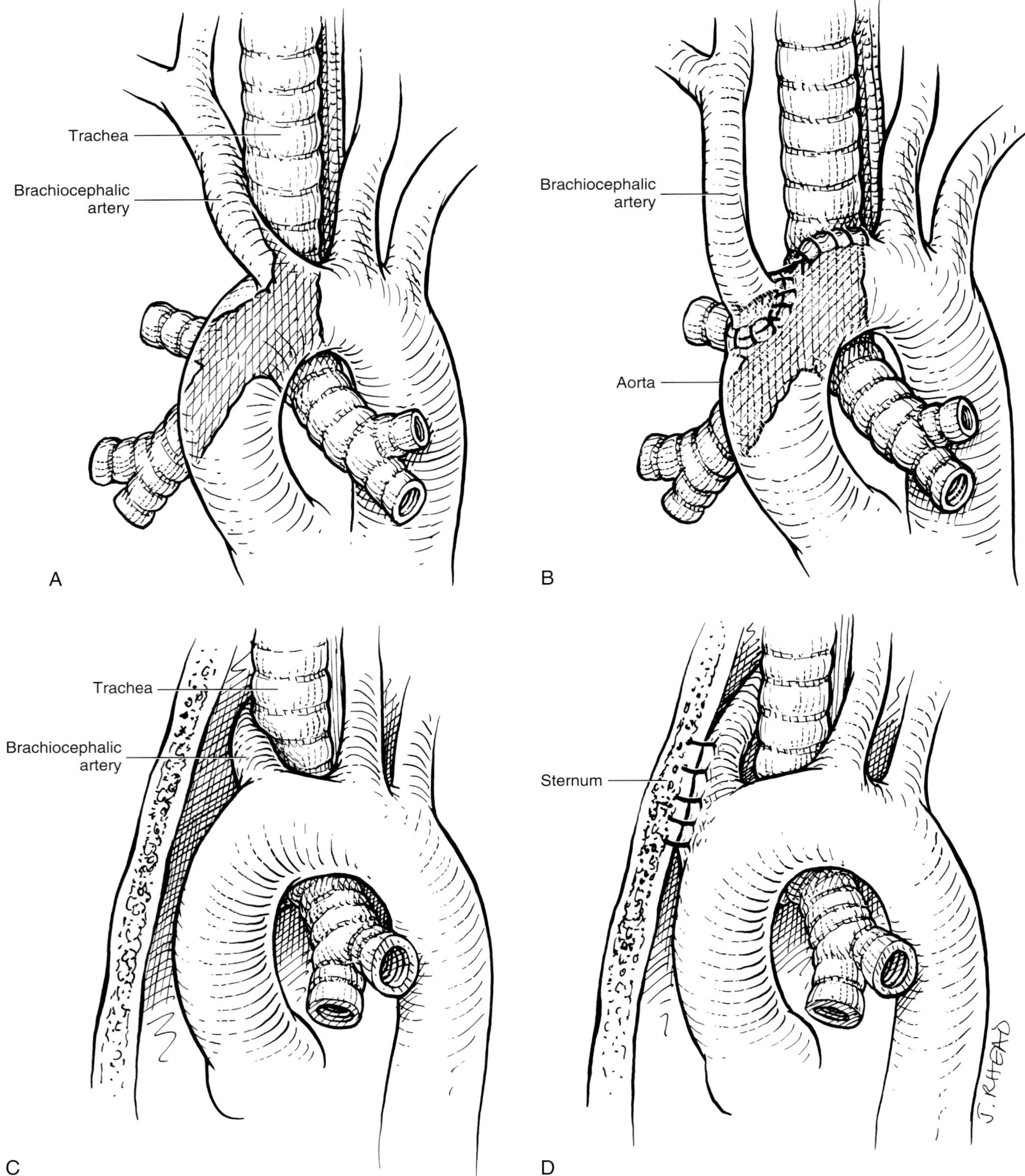

Figure 51-12 Operative repair of tracheal compression by brachiocephalic artery. **A,** Brachiocephalic artery originates from aortic arch more distally than usual, causing compression of trachea. It is shown in midline exposure. **B,** Brachiocephalic artery is disconnected from aorta and its origin closed by suture and reimplanted more proximally on ascending aorta. **C,** Anomaly is approached through a left anterior thoracotomy. Anomalous vessel is completely separated from trachea and attached **(D)** by suture to periosteum of posterior aspect of sternum.

behind the tracheal bifurcation and in front of the esophagus to reach the left lung hilum, and forms a sling around the trachea.

HISTORICAL NOTE

Anomalous LPA was first recognized by Glaevecke and Doehle in 1897 during an autopsy performed on a 7-month-old child who died of asphyxia.[G2] The next report was that of Scheid in 1938, again in the German literature and again from autopsy findings, this time in a 7-month-old child who died of respiratory obstruction.[S2] Description of the anomalous origin and course of the artery is accurate in both reports, but Scheid also described in detail an associated diffuse tracheal stenosis caused by presence of complete cartilaginous rings. This latter condition was again accurately described by Wolman 3 years later.[W7]

Quist-Hanssen from Norway detailed the clinical findings of pulmonary artery sling premortem in 1949, although exact diagnosis was not made until autopsy.[Q1] Welsh and Munro first suggested, based on their autopsy findings, that in this anomaly the barium swallow should show an anterior esophageal indentation; Wittenborg and colleagues soon after accurately defined these features on an esophagram.[W1,W5] In 1980, Stone and colleagues[S8] described diagnosis by CT, and in 1988, Malmgren and colleagues by MRI.[M1]

In 1958, Contro and colleagues coined the term *vascular sling* to distinguish the condition from vascular ring.[C8] Much later, Berdon and colleagues introduced the phrase *ring-sling complex* to emphasize the often coexisting tracheal anomaly.[B13]

In 1954, Potts and colleagues were the first to report successful operation in a patient in whom the anatomy of the malformation was not established before operation. Potts divided the LPA at its origin from the RPA, transferred the vessel in front of the trachea, and reanastomosed it to the proximal stump.[P6] Soon after, Morse and Gladding reported a case diagnosed at right thoracotomy and confirmed at autopsy, in which the anomalous LPA was dissected away (but not divided) from the trachea in an attempt to relieve compression.[M6]

Hiller and Maclean operated successfully on a patient correctly diagnosed by barium swallow and angiography in 1955; after mobilizing and dividing the anomalous LPA, they anastomosed it to the side of the pulmonary trunk (the operation currently practiced). The patient's stridor was relieved completely, and the chest radiograph was normal. However, angiogram 3 weeks later showed LPA occlusion.[H8] In 1962, Mustard and colleagues reported relief of respiratory obstruction following division of the ligamentum arteriosum only.[M10] One year later, Lochard and colleagues reported a case in which the right mainstem bronchus was successfully relocated in front of the anomalous LPA.[L4] Neither of the latter two procedures is practiced currently. An approach through a median sternotomy with cardiopulmonary bypass (CPB) was described by Kirklin in 1986[K2] and subsequently by others.[C7] Single-stage repair of pulmonary artery sling and tracheal stenosis was reported in 1983 by Campbell and colleagues and in 1987 by Hickey and Wood.[H6] Treatment in one stage by excision of tracheal stenosis and simple anterior relocation of the LPA was reported in 1989.[J2]

MORPHOLOGY

Anomalous Left Pulmonary Artery

The anomalous LPA arises extrapericardially from the posterosuperior wall of a normally positioned RPA lying in front of the proximal right main bronchus. The RPA is a direct continuation of the pulmonary trunk, the junction between them marked by attachment of the ligamentum arteriosum (or ductus arteriosus). From its point of origin, the LPA curves upward and backward over the proximal right main bronchus, then to the left behind the lower trachea and its bifurcation at or slightly above the carina[J3] (Fig. 51-13). It courses slightly inferior to lie behind the proximal left mainstem bronchus, then appears immediately superior to it to enter the left lung, and then divides. The left lung hilum is lower than normal in relation to the pulmonary trunk.[C2] The LPA usually indents the posterior wall of the trachea and left main bronchus as it passes behind them and displaces (bows) the distal trachea and carina toward the left. The right main bronchus is bowed anteriorly.[C2] The LPA passes in front of the esophagus, which is usually indented across its entire anterior aspect or, less often, on its leftward anterior surface only.

The anomalous LPA is frequently slightly smaller than normal (see Chapter 1). Rarely, the *right* upper lobe artery comes off the LPA near its origin.[T3] Bamman and colleagues described one case in which the left lung was partly supplied by an LPA in normal position; the anomalous LPA supplied only the left lower lobe and crossed behind the left atrium rather than behind the tracheal bifurcation.[B8]

The ligamentum arteriosum (or ductus arteriosus) follows a normal course from the junction of the pulmonary trunk RPA, passing backward directly superior to the left main bronchus and anomalous LPA (not between them as depicted by Williams and colleagues) to join the descending aorta.[W4] It may participate with the anomalous LPA in forming a vascular ring.

Tracheobronchial and Pulmonary Abnormalities

The trachea near the bifurcation is usually narrowed as a result of posterior compression by the anomalous LPA. This mainly affects the origin of the right main bronchus and trachea just above the carina.[J3] Rarely, the left main bronchus may be narrowed by a similar mechanism.

In about 50% of patients, narrowing of the trachea or proximal main bronchi is secondary to presence of complete ring cartilages (ring-sling complex),[L1,N2] which often are more numerous than normal.[S1,S2] In these areas, the pars membranacea is absent and the lumen is usually severely narrowed. This process may involve the entire length of the trachea or only its proximal or distal portions. The major bronchi may be similarly involved, or their cartilaginous rings may be wide and irregular and the bronchi variable in diameter and length.[C5]

The so-called bronchus suis, consisting of separate high origin from the trachea of the right superior lobar bronchus to the right upper lobe, is more frequent than normal.[A5] It is not itself a cause of obstruction.

When the right main bronchus is selectively narrowed, there is hyperinflation of the right lung (not affecting the right upper lobe when there is a bronchus suis present); when

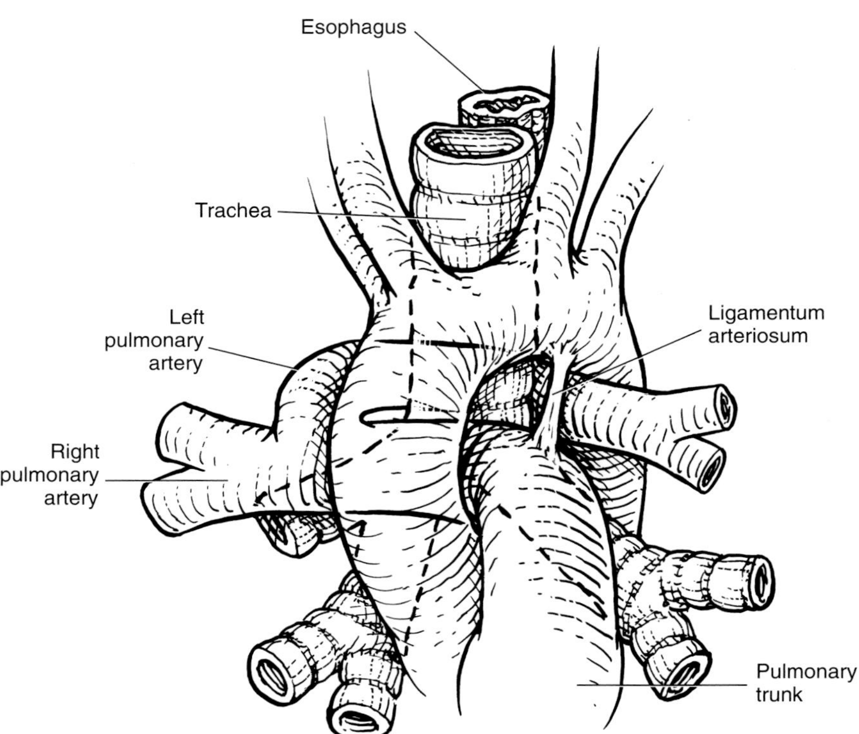

Figure 51-13 Anomalous left pulmonary artery (vascular sling). Left pulmonary artery arises from right pulmonary artery, coursing behind trachea and in front of esophagus to reach hilum of left lung. This produces a sling around trachea just above carina.

the left main bronchus is narrowed, there is hyperinflation of the left lung.[A5] More complete obstruction leads to atelectasis. When obstruction of the right main bronchus is important in utero, there may be retention of fetal fluid in the right lung at birth.

Either the left or right lung may be unilobar.[S1] Rarely, the right lung may be hypoplastic.[H1] The lung hypoplasia may be part of scimitar syndrome.

Other Cardiovascular Anomalies

Other cardiovascular anomalies coexist with half the cases of anomalous LPA.[S1] Most common are left superior vena cava, atrial septal defect, patent ductus arteriosus, and ventricular septal defect. There may also be tetralogy of Fallot, single ventricle, transposition of the great arteries, tricuspid atresia, or aortic arch anomalies.

Noncardiovascular Developmental Anomalies

A variety of noncardiovascular developmental anomalies coexist relatively frequently.[C4]

CLINICAL FEATURES AND DIAGNOSTIC CRITERIA

Symptoms and Signs

Symptoms of vascular sling relate to the consequences of tracheal and esophageal compression.[M10] Up to 90% of patients have important and usually severe symptoms that develop soon after birth.[C4,S1]

The most common presentation is with wheezing and stridor, often with prolongation of the expiratory phase, suggesting asthma, and with a harsh cough and intercostal indrawing. In addition, there may be choking and rapid breathing or apneic spells and associated episodes of cyanosis. Symptoms are episodic, but acute episodes of dyspnea and cyanosis or severe exacerbations of respiratory obstruction are common and may result in unconsciousness, convulsions, or even death. In severe cases, hypercapnia and right lung emphysema requiring mechanical ventilation may be present from birth.[O1]

Symptoms may be precipitated by respiratory infections and are occasionally altered by changes in posture of the infant. They may be made worse by feeding, with or without regurgitation and choking.[Q1,W5] Dysphagia, however, is uncommon.

Chest Radiography

Plain chest radiograph gives important clues to correct diagnosis.[C2] It shows anterior bowing of the right main bronchus and deviation of the lower trachea and carina to the left. In addition, the left lung hilum is lower than normal in relation to position of the pulmonary trunk, and unequal aeration of the lungs frequently is present. Usually the right lung is overinflated, but sometimes the left may be.[A5] When obstruction is more complete, there may be areas of atelectasis. There is mediastinal density between the trachea and esophagus on the lateral view and, in older patients in particular, right-sided mediastinal density opposite the carina in the posteroanterior view.[H8,K1,M2]

In newborns, the initial chest radiograph may show retention of fetal fluid in the right lung, evidenced by a uniform opacity without loss of volume (this is in fact increased) and without an air bronchogram. Once the fetal fluid has been resorbed or suctioned off, the lung will appear hyperinflated.[Z1]

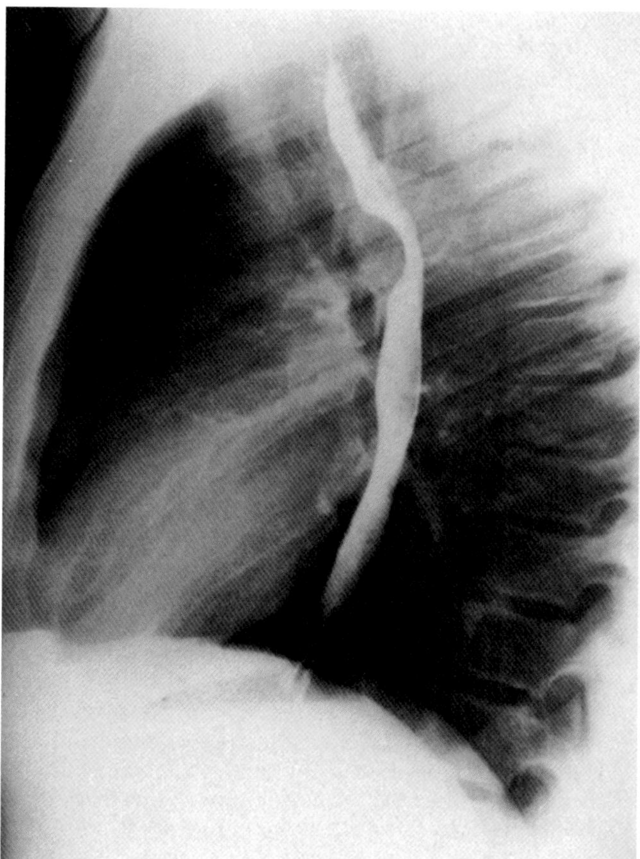

Figure 51-14 Esophagram (lateral) of anomalous left pulmonary artery. Prominent indentation of anterior wall of esophagus is seen immediately above tracheal bifurcation.

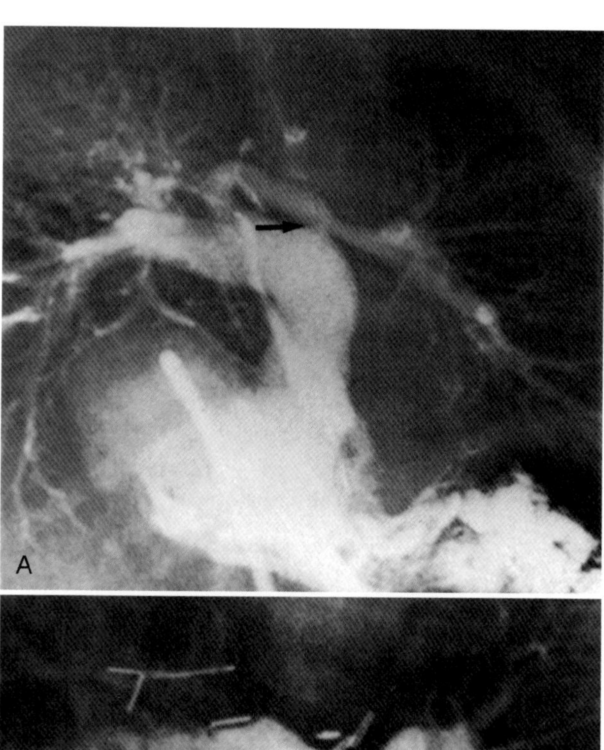

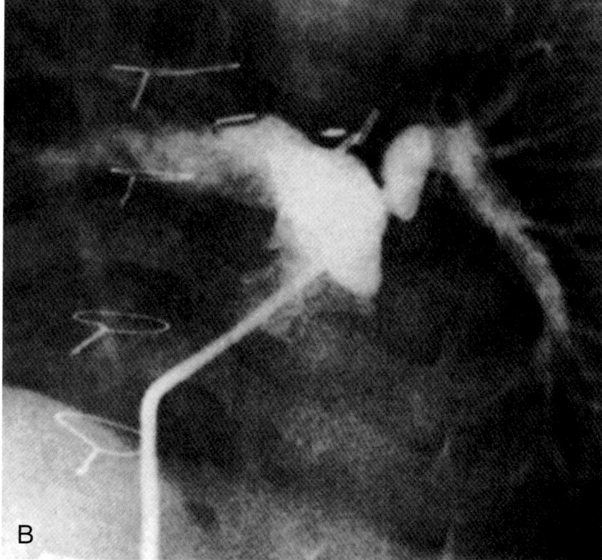

Figure 51-15 Cineangiogram of vascular sling (anomalous left pulmonary artery). **A,** Preoperative study showing left pulmonary artery originating from right pulmonary artery. Small patent ductus arteriosus *(arrow)* is present between distal left pulmonary artery and pulmonary trunk. Concavity apparent in upper surface of left pulmonary artery just lateral to the ductus is impression of descending aorta. **B,** Late postoperative study showing stenosis at anastomosis of left pulmonary artery to pulmonary trunk. This was successfully treated by percutaneous balloon dilatation.

Esophagography

Barium swallow usually shows an anterior indentation of the esophagus in the *lateral* view just above the level of the carina (Fig. 51-14). In the anteroposterior view, there may be no abnormality or a leftward lateral indentation.[G12,S5] The only other conditions known to produce an anterior esophageal indentation at this level are the ductus arteriosus sling (see "Ductus Arteriosus Sling" under Morphology in Section I) and a long, tortuous patent ductus arteriosus.[B15,B16]

In patients with anomalous LPA, these findings are not necessarily present and are variable in their appearance during the esophagram, because they are in part dependent on the phase of the cardiac and respiratory cycles.[B16,D2,W5] High-quality video barium swallow is therefore required. The esophagram can be more difficult to interpret when there is also a retroesophageal subclavian artery passing posterior to the esophagus at a slightly higher level than the LPA.[W5]

Noninvasive Imaging

In most patients, diagnosis can be made by two-dimensional echocardiography, CT with contrast, or MRI.[R1,S8] A tracheogram or a tracheal CT study should be made to evaluate the additional zones of narrowing that are frequently present and influence surgical management.[C2,C3] It is best done in conjunction with video esophageal studies.

Bronchoscopy

Bronchoscopy is required in all patients to evaluate tracheal abnormalities (complete tracheal rings) and identify areas of stenosis that may need surgical repair and affect airway and ventilatory management.

Cardiac Catheterization and Angiography

Cardiac catheterization and angiography display the anomaly well, can confirm diagnosis (Fig. 51-15), and demonstrate associated cardiovascular anomalies. The LPA is visualized best in a cranially tilted frontal view.

NATURAL HISTORY

Vascular sling is a rare condition. The largest series includes 15 patients accumulated over 45 years in a high-volume children's hospital.[B4] Therefore, information about natural history is incomplete.

TECHNIQUE OF OPERATION

Repair is advantageously performed through a median sternotomy using CPB,[K2] although it can be done through a left thoracotomy.[G10,G11]

Reimplantation of Left Pulmonary Artery

With Cardiopulmonary Bypass

After usual preparations and bronchoscopy (if not previously performed) and median sternotomy, the pericardium is opened and retraction sutures applied. The aorta is dissected completely away from both pulmonary arteries. The ligamentum arteriosum, which is often stretched tightly across the carina and is part of the vascular sling, is dissected and divided between ligatures. The decision is then made either to reimplant the LPA or excise a tracheal stenosis (if this exists), move the dissected but undivided LPA anteriorly, and reconstruct the trachea end to end.

When the tracheal rings are normal and no tracheal stenosis or softening is demonstrated, CPB is established using a single venous cannula and a perfusate temperature of about 32°C (see Chapter 2). The left pleural space is opened widely, either then or later. The LPA is identified coming off the RPA. It is dissected out well distally, completely separating it from surrounding structures, including the trachea anteriorly and the esophagus posteriorly. The plane of dissection must be on the adventitia of the LPA to avoid damage to the membranous portion of the trachea (Fig. 51-16, *A*). The LPA is cut away from the RPA, and the defect in the latter is closed with two rows of 5-0 or 6-0 polypropylene sutures. The LPA is then pulled out into the left pleural space. A large window is made in the pericardium behind the phrenic nerve and alongside the pulmonary trunk, and the LPA is brought into the pericardial space through it. An incision is made in the left lateral aspect of the pulmonary trunk. Taking care that the LPA lies nicely without kinking or rotation, its proximal end is anastomosed to the side of the pulmonary trunk with continuous 6-0 or 7-0 polypropylene suture (Fig. 51-16, *B*).

After rewarming the patient, CPB is discontinued and cannulae removed. A polyvinyl pressure-recording catheter may be brought out from the pulmonary trunk via the right ventricle. The remainder of the operation is completed as usual.

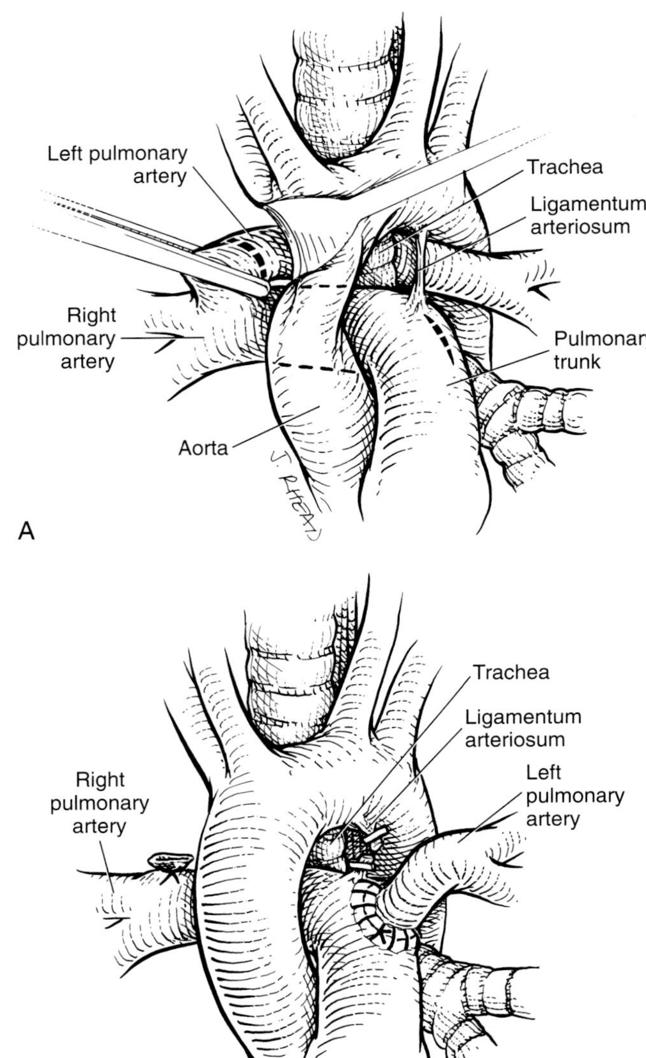

Figure 51-16 Repair of anomalous left pulmonary artery (LPA) using cardiopulmonary bypass. Operation is performed via median sternotomy. **A,** Aorta is mobilized off right pulmonary artery and anomalous origin of LPA, which is extrapericardial, and is retracted toward the left. LPA is divided *(dashed line)*. Arteriotomy is made on left lateral aspect of pulmonary trunk *(dashed line)*. **B,** Proximal end of LPA is ligated or oversewn. Ligamentum arteriosum is divided between clips or ligatures. LPA is completely mobilized from behind trachea out to hilum of left lung, brought through an opening in the pericardial sac, and anastomosed to pulmonary trunk.

Without Cardiopulmonary Bypass

A left posterolateral thoracotomy is made, entering the chest via the fourth interspace or fifth rib bed. Alternatively, some have preferred median sternotomy. The anomalous LPA is identified by dissecting the superior part of the left lung hilum (Fig. 51-17, *A*). The ligamentum arteriosum is divided because this improves exposure and may possibly relieve compression of the left main bronchus.[M10] Dissection of the LPA is continued medially (centrally) and behind the proximal left main bronchus and tracheal bifurcation. The artery is freed completely from the posterior wall of these structures and followed as far as possible into the mediastinum to gain adequate length. Care is taken not to obstruct flow into the RPA by undue tension on the LPA. The patient is given heparin (1.5 mg · kg^{-1}) to obtain systemic anticoagulant effect. The LPA is then divided between vascular clamps, its proximal end on the RPA oversewn with continuous 6-0 or 7-0 polypropylene suture, and the clamp removed (Fig. 51-17, *B*).

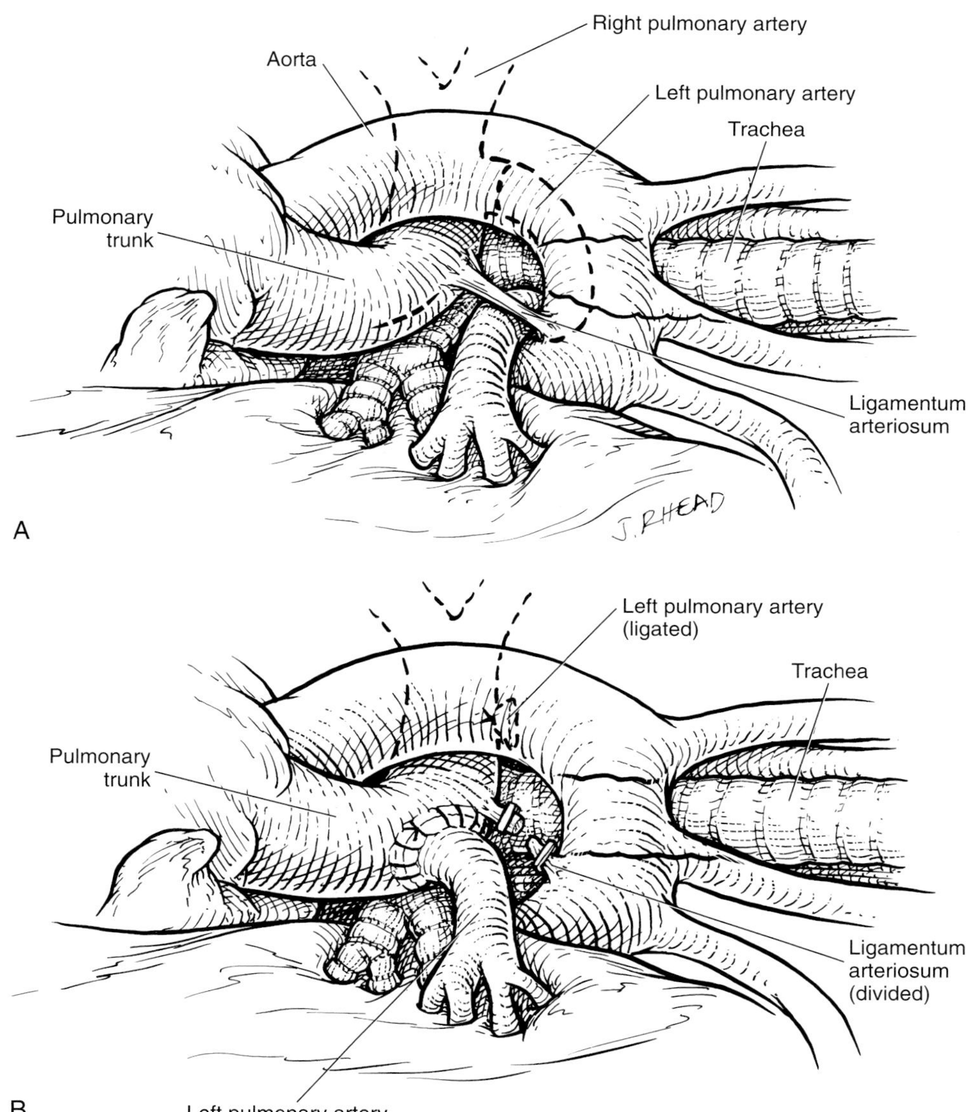

Figure 51-17 Repair of anomalous left pulmonary artery (LPA) without cardiopulmonary bypass. Operation is performed through posterolateral thoracotomy on left side. **A,** Ligamentum arteriosum is mobilized (or divided). Anomalous LPA is dissected from hilum of left lung to its origin from right pulmonary artery, separating it completely from posterior surface of trachea and surrounding tissues. LPA is divided near its origin *(dashed line)* after isolation under a partial occlusion vascular clamp. Arteriotomy *(dashed line)* is made in left lateral aspect of pulmonary trunk, isolated using a partial occlusion vascular clamp (clamp not shown for clarity of illustration). **B,** Proximal end of LPA is ligated or oversewn. Ligamentum arteriosum is ligated and divided. LPA is withdrawn from behind trachea and anastomosed to pulmonary trunk.

The pericardium is opened with a vertical incision anterior to the phrenic nerve to expose the pulmonary trunk, and a second similar incision is made posterior to this structure, through which the distal end of the anomalous LPA is passed. The tip of the left atrial appendage is retracted by a ligature tied to it, and the left wall of the pulmonary trunk is excluded in a curved vascular clamp. The clamp is positioned to allow the LPA to reach the pulmonary trunk without kinking or tension. The excluded portion of the pulmonary trunk is opened and an end-to-side anastomosis performed between it and the LPA (see Fig. 51-17, *B*), refashioning the LPA end obliquely to increase the diameter of the anastomosis. The posterior layer of the anastomosis is performed from within the vessels, using continuous 6-0 or 7-0 polypropylene suture and the anterior layer from outside. Clamps are then removed. Heparin is not reversed.

The pericardium is left open and the chest closed, leaving one intercostal tube for drainage.

Tracheal Resection and Relocation of Left Pulmonary Artery

When there is a localized area of tracheal stenosis, the trachea is minimally mobilized, and the tip of the endotracheal tube is ascertained to lie proximal to the proposed resection. A median sternotomy is performed and CPB established in the manner just described. The anomalous LPA is completely freed from surrounding structures and the stenotic area of

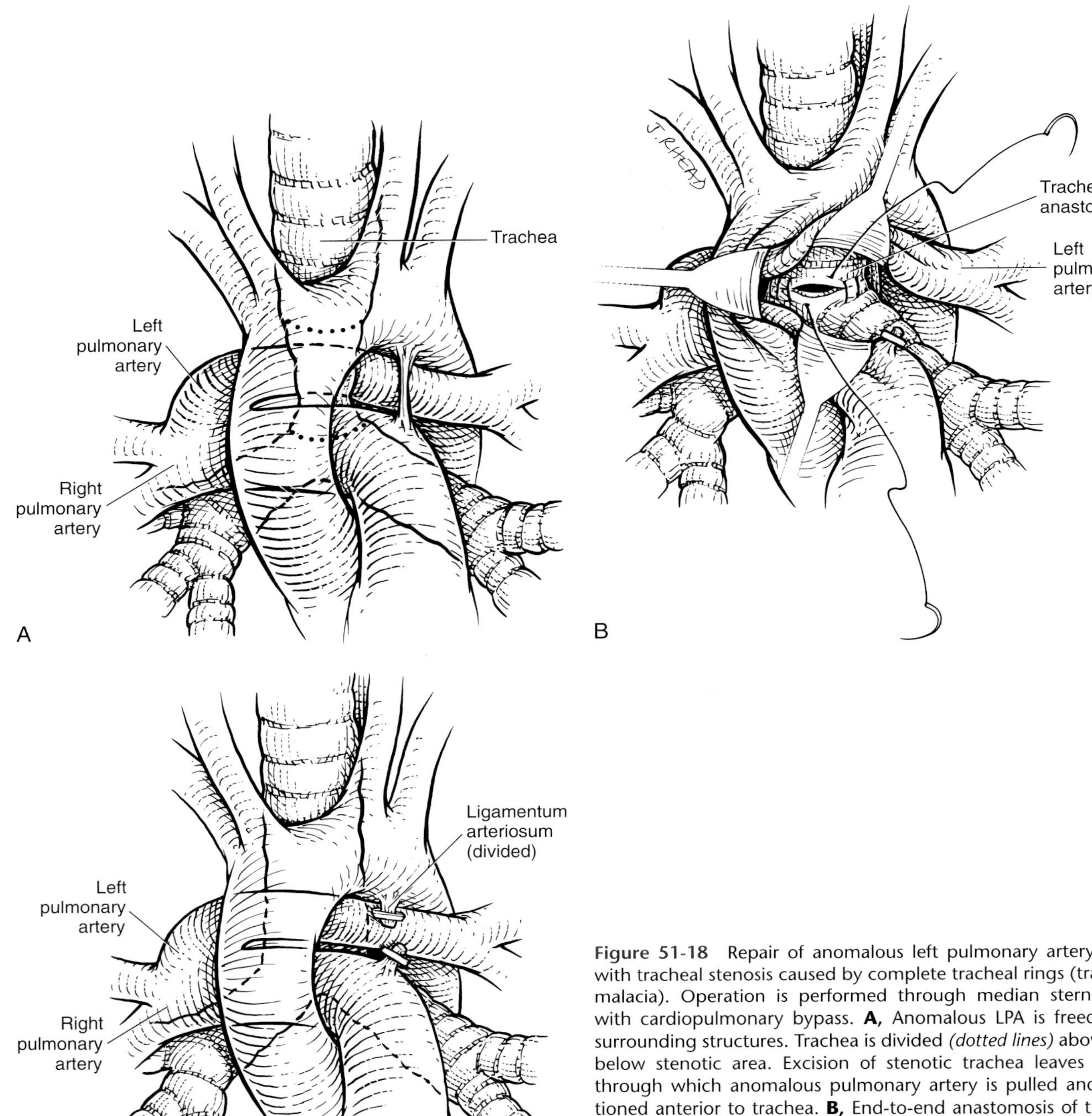

Figure 51-18 Repair of anomalous left pulmonary artery (LPA) with tracheal stenosis caused by complete tracheal rings (tracheomalacia). Operation is performed through median sternotomy with cardiopulmonary bypass. **A,** Anomalous LPA is freed from surrounding structures. Trachea is divided *(dotted lines)* above and below stenotic area. Excision of stenotic trachea leaves a gap through which anomalous pulmonary artery is pulled and positioned anterior to trachea. **B,** End-to-end anastomosis of trachea is constructed using absorbable suture. LPA is shown positioned anterior to trachea. **C,** Completed repair shows LPA still attached anomalously to right pulmonary artery but positioned anterior to trachea to avoid tracheal compression.

trachea excised (Fig. 51-18, *A*). The LPA is brought through the tracheal gap and positioned anterior to the trachea. The patient's neck is flexed if necessary, and an end-to-end tracheal anastomosis is performed (Fig. 51-18, *B* and *C*) using continuous 5-0 or 6-0 polydioxanone suture. CPB is discontinued after the patient has been rewarmed, and the remainder of the operation is completed in the usual manner (see "Completing Cardiopulmonary Bypass" in Section III of Chapter 2). Before muscle relaxants are discontinued in the intensive care unit, the patient is fitted with a back brace to prevent cervical extension.

If tracheal disease is of considerable length and associated with complete tracheal rings, local excision may not be corrective. These longer segments of tracheal stenosis are treated by tracheoplasty.[B4] Using CPB, either a slide tracheoplasty[G4,K5,T2] or a long tracheoplasty with pericardium is performed. For pericardial reconstruction, a vertical anterior incision is made in the trachea through the complete rings under bronchoscopic guidance. A pericardial patch is inserted with polydioxanone suture to widen the trachea. The patch appears to be adequate for enlarging the trachea but does not provide support to it and may collapse during inspiration, partially obstructing the trachea and resulting in noisy respiration for months to a year.[B4] Options that do provide support are a tracheal insert fashioned from costal cartilage[H3] or a prosthesis constructed from prosthetic mesh hardened with cyanoacrylate to which the pericardium is attached with biological glue.

The LPA is transected at its origin, repositioned, and anastomosed to the side of the distal pulmonary trunk to complete the operation.

When major associated cardiac anomalies are present, they can be repaired along with LPA reimplantation on CPB. Tracheal reconstruction, if needed, can be deferred for 2 to 4 days and performed as a separate procedure.

Because of the unavoidable mediastinal contamination from an open trachea, Konstantinov and colleagues recommend placing a pericardial flap between the great vessels and anterior tracheal suture lines.[K5]

SPECIAL FEATURES OF POSTOPERATIVE CARE

Care is as described in Section I. Special attention is required for tracheal care and secretion management if the trachea has been reconstructed.

RESULTS

Survival

Percent survival is not meaningful when derived from the small number of patients known to have been treated surgically. In the series reported by Backer and colleagues, there were no hospital deaths among 12 patients (0%; CL 0%-15%), but two (17%) patients died during the first postoperative year.[B2]

Mode of death is usually respiratory and related to tracheal abnormalities.[S1] When these abnormalities are not present, prognosis is excellent.[B2,D3,G1]

Left Pulmonary Artery Patency

In many groups of patients operated on in an earlier era, usually through a left thoracotomy, the LPA anastomosis frequently was not patent late postoperatively.[C1,P7,S1] With currently used methods, the anastomosis usually remains patent.[B2,D3,L2]

Freedom from Postoperative Respiratory Obstruction

When respiratory obstruction is due only to *compression* of the trachea by an anomalous LPA, relief is virtually always complete after simple reimplantation of the artery. Relief of symptoms has been obtained in a few such patients in whom only the ligamentum arteriosum or a patent ductus arteriosus has been divided.[M10,P3,P4] When *tracheal stenosis* is a component of respiratory obstruction, tracheal resection and relocation of the LPA aided by CPB has provided complete relief of symptoms.[J2] When there is *diffuse anatomic tracheal stenosis associated with complete cartilaginous rings*, relief of respiratory obstruction has been variable, but results after pericardial patch tracheoplasty can be good.[B2]

INDICATIONS FOR OPERATION

When anomalous LPA is present and there are symptoms and radiologic signs of important respiratory obstruction, operation is indicated. When respiratory symptoms are due to tracheal compression without fixed stenosis and without complete tracheal rings, either relocation and reimplantation of the LPA (preferably with CPB) or relocation after tracheal transection and reanastomosis is indicated. When a localized tracheal stenosis is present, resection of the stenosis, relocation of the LPA, and end-to-end anastomosis of the trachea are indicated.

When there is severe diffuse tracheal stenosis with complete cartilaginous rings, the surgical problem is more difficult. Correction of the left pulmonary arterial problem and simultaneous tracheoplasty of some type are indicated, but the outcome has been unpredictable.

REFERENCES

A

1. Abbott ME. Atlas of congenital heart disease. New York: American Heart Association, 1936.
2. Adler SC, Isaacson G, Balsara RK. Innominate artery compression of the trachea: diagnosis and treatment by anterior suspension. A 25-year experience. Ann Otol Rhinol Laryngol 1995;104:924.
3. Alsenaidi K, Gurofsky R, Karamlou T, Williams WG, McCrindle BW. Management and outcomes of double aortic arch in 81 patients. Pediatrics 2006;118:e1336-41.
4. Arciniegas E, Hakimi M, Hertzler JH, Farooki ZQ, Green EW. Surgical management of congenital vascular rings. J Thorac Cardiovasc Surg 1979;77:721.
5. Aytac A, Ozme S, Sarikayalar F, Saylam A. Pulmonary artery sling. Ann Thorac Surg 1976;22:596.

B

1. Backer CL, Holinger LD, Mavroudis C. Innominate artery compression: division and reimplantation vs. suspension (invited letter). J Thorac Cardiovasc Surg 1992;103:817.
2. Backer CL, Idriss FS, Holinger LD, Mavroudis C. Pulmonary artery sling. Results of surgical repair in infancy. J Thorac Cardiovasc Surg 1992;103:683.
3. Backer CL, Ilbawi MN, Idriss FS, DeLeon SY. Vascular anomalies causing tracheoesophageal compression. Review of experience in children. J Thorac Cardiovasc Surg 1989;97:725.
4. Backer CL, Mavroudis C. Vascular rings and pulmonary artery sling. In: Mavroudis C, ed. Pediatric cardiac surgery. St. Louis: Mosby, 1994, p. 645.
5. Backer CL, Mavroudis C. Surgical approach to vascular rings. In: Karp RB, ed. Advances in cardiac surgery, Vol 9. St. Louis: Mosby Year Book, 1997, p. 29.
6. Backer CL, Mavroudis C. Congenital heart surgery nomenclature and database project: vascular rings, tracheal stenosis, pectus excavatum. Ann Thorac Surg 2000;69:S308.
7. Backer CL, Mavroudis C, Rigsby CK, Holinger LD. Trends in vascular ring surgery. J Thorac Cardiovasc Surg 2005;129:1339-47.
8. Bamman JL, Ward BH, Woodrum DE. Aberrant left pulmonary artery. Clinical and embryologic factors. Chest 1977;72:67.
9. Barry A. The aortic derivatives in the human adult. Anat Rec 1951;111:221.
10. Bayford D. An account of a singular case of obstructed deglutition. Mem Med Soc Lond 1794;2:275.
11. Beabout JW, Stewart JR, Kincaid OW. Aberrant right subclavian artery: dispute of commonly accepted concepts. Am J Roentgenol Radium Ther Nucl Med 1964;92:855.

12. Bein S, Saba Z, Patel H, Reinhartz O, Hanley FL. Coarctation of the aorta in the right aortic arch with left aberrant innominate artery. Pediatr Cardiol 2006;27:621-3.
13. Berdon WE, Baker DH, Wung JT, Chrispin A, Kozlowski K, de Silva M, et al. Complete cartilage-ring tracheal stenosis associated with anomalous left pulmonary artery: the ring-sling complex. Radiology 1984;152:57.
14. Berman W Jr, Yabek SM, Dillon T, Neal JF, Akl B, Burstein J. Vascular ring due to left aortic arch and right descending aorta. Circulation 1981;63:458.
15. Binet JP, Conso JF, Losay J, Narcy P, Raynaud EJ, Beaufils F, et al. Ductus arteriosus sling: report of a newly recognized anomaly and its surgical correction. Thorax 1978;33:72.
16. Brandt PW, Clarkson PM, Barratt-Boyes BG, Neutze JM. An unusual esophageal indentation caused by a long tortuous patent ductus arteriosus. Australas Radiol 1973;17:394.
17. Bronshtein M, Lorber A, Berant M, Auslander R, Zimmer EZ. Sonographic diagnosis of fetal vascular rings in early pregnancy. Am J Cardiol 1998;81:101.
18. Burke RP, Rosenfeld HM, Wernovsky G, Jonas RA. Video-assisted thoracoscopic vascular ring division in infants and children. J Am Coll Cardiol 1995;25:943.

C

1. Campbell CD, Wernly JA, Koltip PC, Vitullo D, Replogle RL. Aberrant left pulmonary artery (pulmonary artery sling): successful repair and 24-year follow-up report. Am J Cardiol 1980;45:316.
2. Capitanio MA, Ramos R, Kirkpatrick JA. Pulmonary sling. Roentgen observations. Am J Roentgenol Radium Ther Nucl Med 1971;112:28.
3. Castaneda AR. Pulmonary artery sling (editorial). Ann Thorac Surg 1979;28:210.
4. Clarkson PM, Ritter DG, Rahimtoola SH, Hallermann FJ, McGoon DC. Aberrant left pulmonary artery. Am J Dis Child 1967;113:373.
5. Cohen SR, Landing BH. Tracheostenosis and bronchial abnormalities associated with pulmonary artery sling. Ann Otol Rhinol Laryngol 1976;85:582.
6. Congdon ED. Transformation of the aortic arch system during the development of the human embryo. Carnegie Trust, Washington, DC, Pub No. 277. Contrib Embryol 1922;1:47.
7. Conti VR, Lobe TE. Vascular sling with tracheomalacia: surgical management. Ann Thorac Surg 1989;47:310.
8. Contro S, Miller RA, White H, Potts WJ. Bronchial obstruction due to pulmonary artery anomalies. I. Vascular sling. Circulation 1958;17:418.

D

1. D'Cruz IA, Cantez T, Namin EP, Licata R, Hastreiter AR. Right-sided aorta. Part II. Right aortic arch, right descending aorta and associated anomalies. Br Heart J 1966;28:725.
2. Derrick JR, Stoeckle H. Bronchial obstruction secondary to an aberrant pulmonary artery. AMA J Dis Child 1960;99:830.
3. Dunn JM, Gordon I, Chrispin AR, de Leval MR, Stark J. Early and late results of surgical correction of pulmonary artery sling. Ann Thorac Surg 1979;28:230.

E

1. Edwards JE. Anomalies of the derivatives of the aortic arch system. Med Clin North Am 1948;32:925.
2. Ekstrom G, Sandblom P. Double aortic arch. Acta Chir Scand 1951;102:183.
3. Ericsson NO, Soderlund S. Compression of the trachea by an anomalous innominate artery. J Pediatr Surg 1969;4:424.

F

1. Fineberg C, Stofman HC. Tracheal compression caused by an anomalous innominate artery arising from a brachiocephalic trunk. J Thorac Surg 1959;37:214.

G

1. Gikonyo BM, Jue KL, Edwards JE. Pulmonary vascular sling: report of seven cases and review of the literature. Pediatr Cardiol 1989;10:81.
2. Glaevecke H, Doehle H. Uber eine seltene angeborene Anomalie der Pulmonalarterie. Munch Med Wochenschr 1897;44:950.
3. Godtfredsen J, Wennevold A, Efsen F, Lauridsen P. Natural history of vascular ring with clinical manifestations. A follow-up study of 11 unoperated cases. Scand J Thorac Cardiovasc Surg 1977;11:75.
4. Grillo HC. Slide tracheoplasty for long-segment congenital tracheal stenosis. Ann Thorac Surg 1994;58:613-21.
5. Gross RE. Surgical relief for tracheal obstruction from a vascular ring. N Engl J Med 1945;233:586.
6. Gross RE. Surgical treatment for dysphagia lusoria. Ann Surg 1946;124:532.
7. Gross RE. Arterial malformations which cause compression of the trachea or esophagus. Circulation 1955;11:124.
8. Gross RE, Neuhauser EB. Compression of the trachea or esophagus by vascular anomalies. Surgical therapy in 40 cases. Pediatrics 1951;7:69.
9. Gross RE, Ware PF. The surgical significance of aortic arch anomalies. Surg Gynecol Obstet 1946;83:435.
10. Grothwohl KW, Afifi AY, Dillard TA, Olson JP, Heric BR. Vascular rings of the thoracic aorta in adults. Am Surg 1999;65:1077.
11. Grover FL, Norton JB Jr, Webb GE, Trinkle JK. Pulmonary sling. J Thorac Cardiovasc Surg 1975;69:295.
12. Gumbiner CH, Mullins CE, McNamara DG. Pulmonary artery sling. Am J Cardiol 1980;45:311.

H

1. Han BK, Dunbar JS, Bove K, Rosenkrantz JG. Pulmonary vascular sling with tracheobronchial stenosis and hypoplasia of the right pulmonary artery. Pediatr Radiol 1980;9:113.
2. Hawkins JA, Bailey WW, Clark SM. Innominate artery compression of the trachea: treatment by reimplantation of the innominate artery. J Thorac Cardiovasc Surg 1992;103:678.
3. Hazekamp MG, Koolbergen DR, Kersten J, Peper J, de Mol B, Konig-Jung A. Pediatric tracheal reconstruction with pericardial patch and strips of autologous cartilage. Eur J Cardiothorac Surg 2009;36:344-51.
4. Hellenbrand WE, Kelley MJ, Talner NS, Stansel HC Jr, Berman MA. Cervical aortic arch with retroesophageal aortic obstruction: report of a case with successful surgical intervention. Ann Thorac Surg 1978;26:86.
5. Hickey EJ, Khan A, Anderson D, Lang-Lazdunski L. Complete vascular ring presenting in adulthood: an unusual management dilemma. J Thorac Cardiovasc Surg 2007;134:235-6.
6. Hickey MS, Wood AE. Pulmonary artery sling with tracheal stenosis: one-stage repair. Ann Thorac Surg 1987;44:416.
7. Higashino SM, Ruttenberg HD. Double aortic arch associated with complete transposition of the great vessels. Br Heart J 1968; 30:579.
8. Hiller HG, Maclean AD. Pulmonary artery ring. Acta Radiol (Stockh) 1957;48:434.
9. Humphrey C, Duncan K, Fletcher S. Decade of experience with vascular rings at a single institution. Pediatrics 2006;117:e903-8.

J

1. Jonas RA. Comprehensive surgical management of congenital heart disease. London: Arnold, 2004, p. 500.
2. Jonas RA, Spevak PJ, McGill T, Castaneda AR. Pulmonary artery sling: primary repair by tracheal resection in infancy. J Thorac Cardiovasc Surg 1989;97:548.
3. Jue KL, Raghib G, Amplatz K, Adams P Jr, Edwards JE. Anomalous origin of the left pulmonary artery from the right pulmonary artery. Report of 2 cases and review of the literature. Am J Roentgenol Radium Ther Nucl Med 1965;95:598.

K

1. Kale MK, Rafferty RE, Carton RW. Aberrant left pulmonary artery presenting as a mediastinal mass. Report of a case in an adult. Arch Intern Med 1970;125:121.
2. Kirklin JW, Barratt-Boyes BG. Cardiac surgery. New York: John Wiley & Sons, 1986, p. 1111.
3. Kirklin JW, Clagett OT. Vascular "rings" producing respiratory obstruction in infants. Proc Mayo Clin 1950;25:360.
4. Kommerell B. Verlagerung des osophagus durch eine abnorm verlaufende arteria subclavia dextra (arteria lusoria). Fortschr Geb Rentgenstr 1936;54:59.
5. Konstantinov IE, d'Udekem Y, Saxena P. Interposition pericardial flap after slide tracheoplasty in pulmonary artery sling complex. Ann Thorac Surg 2010;89:289-91.

L

1. Le Bret E, Fauroux B, Sigal-Cinqualbre A, de Labriolle-Vaylet C, Batisse A, Roussin R, et al. Improved lung perfusion with surgical correction of pulmonary artery sling. J Thorac Cardiovasc Surg 2007;133:815-6.
2. Lenox CC, Crisler C, Zuberbuhler JR, Park SC, Neches WH, Mathews RA, et al. Anomalous left pulmonary artery: successful management. J Thorac Cardiovasc Surg 1979;77:748.
3. Lincoln JC, Deverall PB, Stark J, Aberdeen E, Waterston DJ. Vascular anomalies compressing the esophagus and trachea. Thorax 1969;24:295.
4. Lochard J, Vert P, Chalnot P. Trajet aberrant de l'arte're pulmonaire gauche compriment l'origine de la bronche souche droite. Ann Chir Thorac Cardiovasc 1963;17:458.

M

1. Malmgren N, Laurin S, Lundstrom NR. Pulmonary artery sling. Diagnosis by magnetic resonance imaging. Acta Radiol (Stockh) 1988;29:7.
2. Mayer JE Jr, Joyce LD, Reinke D, McGeachie R, Humphrey EW, Varco RL. Aberrant left pulmonary artery presenting as a right paratracheal mass in an adult. J Thorac Cardiovasc Surg 1976;72:571.
3. McElhinney DB, Clark BJ 3rd, Weinberg PM, Kenton ML, McDonald-McGinn D, Driscoll DA, et al. Association of chromosome 22q11 deletion with isolated anomalies of aortic arch laterality and branching. J Am Coll Cardiol 2001;37:2114.
4. McElhinney DB, Thompson LD, Weinberg PM, Jue KL, Hanley FL. Surgical approach to complicated cervical aortic arch: anatomic, developmental, and surgical considerations. Cardiol Young 2000; 10:212.
5. Momma K, Matsuoka R, Takao A. Aortic arch anomalies associated with chromosome 22q11 deletion (CATCH 22). Pediatr Cardiol 1999;20:97.
6. Morse HR, Gladding S. Bronchial obstruction due to misplaced left pulmonary artery. Am J Dis Child 1955;89:351.
7. Mullins CE, Gillette PC, McNamara DG. The complex of cervical aortic arch. Pediatrics 1973;51:210.
8. Murthy K, Mattioli L, Diehl AM, Holder TM. Vascular ring due to left aortic arch, right descending aorta, and right patent ductus arteriosus. J Pediatr Surg 1970;5:550.
9. Mustard WT, Bayliss CE, Fearon B, Pelton D, Trusler GA. Tracheal compression by the innominate artery in children. Ann Thorac Surg 1969;8:312.
10. Mustard WT, Trimble AW, Trusler GA. Mediastinal vascular anomalies causing tracheal and esophageal compression and obstruction in childhood. Can Med Assoc J 1962;87:1301.

N

1. Nadas AS, Fyler DC. Pediatric cardiology. Philadelphia: WB Saunders, 1972, p. 749.
2. Neill CA, Ferencz C, Sabiston DC, Sheldon H. The familial occurrence of hypoplastic right lung with systemic arterial supply and venous drainage "scimitar syndrome." Bull Johns Hopkins Hosp 1960;107:1-21.
3. Neuhauser EB. The roentgen diagnosis of double aortic arch and other anomalies of the great vessels. Am J Roentgenol Radium Ther Nucl Med 1946;56:1.

O

1. Oppido G, Pace Napoleone C, Gargiulo G. Neonatal right lung emphysema due to pulmonary artery sling. Pediatr Cardiol 2008;29:469-70.

P

1. Park SC, Siewers RD, Neches WH, Lenox CC, Zuberbuhler JR. Left aortic arch with right descending aorta and right ligamentum arteriosum. A rare form of vascular ring. J Thorac Cardiovasc Surg 1976;71:779.
2. Parker JM, Cary-Freitas B, Berg BW. Symptomatic vascular rings in adulthood: an uncommon mimic of asthma. J Asthma 2000; 37:275.
3. Phelan PD, Venables AW. Management of pulmonary artery sling (anomalous left pulmonary artery arising from right pulmonary artery): a conservative approach. Thorax 1978;33:67.
4. Philp T, Sumerling MD, Fleming J, Grainger RG. Aberrant left pulmonary artery. Clin Radiol 1972;23:153.
5. Pickhardt PJ, Siegel MJ, Gutierrez FR. Vascular rings in symptomatic children: frequency of chest radiographic findings. Radiology 1997;203:423.
6. Potts WJ, Holinger PH, Rosenblum AH. Anomalous left pulmonary artery causing obstruction to right main bronchus: report of a case. JAMA 1954;155:1409.
7. Price DA, Slaughter RE, Fraser DK. Abnormalities of the aortic arch system compressing the esophagus and trachea. Aust Pediatr J 1982;18:46.

Q

1. Quist-Hanssen S. Mutual compression of the right main bronchus and an abnormal left pulmonary artery as causes of the death of a 7 week old child. Acta Paediatr 1949;37:87.

R

1. Rheuban KS, Ayres N, Still JG, Alford B. Pulmonary artery sling: a new diagnostic tool and clinical review. Pediatrics 1982;69:472.
2. Robinson BL, Nathan M, Brown DW, Baird C, del Nido PJ. Robotic division of an unusual variant of a right aortic arch. Ann Thorac Surg 2007;84:670-3.
3. Roesler M, de Leval M, Chrispin A, Stark J. Surgical management of vascular ring. Ann Surg 1983;197:139.
4. Ruzmetov M, Vijay P, Rodefeld MD, Turrentine MW, Brown JW. Follow-up of surgical correction of aortic arch anomalies causing tracheoesophageal compression: a 38-year single institution experience. J Pediatr Surg 2009;44:1328-32.

S

1. Sade RM, Rosenthal A, Fellows K, Castaneda AR. Pulmonary artery sling. J Thorac Cardiovasc Surg 1975;69:333.
2. Scheid P. Missbildung des Trachealskelettes und der linken Arteria pulmonalis mit Erstickungstod bei 7 Monate Altem Kind. Z Pathol 1938;52:114.
3. Scherer D, Westcott JL. Dextrocardia, left aortic arch and tracheal compression. An unusual type of vascular ring. Radiology 1972;103:383.
4. Soler R, Rodriguez E, Requejo I, Fernandez R, Raposo I. Magnetic resonance imaging of congenital abnormalities of the thoracic aorta. Eur Radiol 1998;8:540.
5. Sprague PL, Kennedy JC. Anomalous left pulmonary artery with an unusual barium swallow. Pediatr Radiol 1976;4:188.
6. Stewart JR, Kincaid OW, Edwards JE. An atlas of vascular rings and related malformations of the aortic arch system. Springfield, Ill.: Charles C. Thomas, 1964.
7. Stewart S 3rd, Edmunds LH Jr, Kirklin JW, Allarde RR. Spontaneous breathing with continuous positive airway pressure after open intracardiac operations in infants. J Thorac Cardiovasc Surg 1973;65:37.
8. Stone DN, Bein ME, Garris JB. Anomalous left pulmonary artery: two new adult cases. Am J Roentgenol 1980;135:1259.
9. Symbas PN, Shuford WH, Edwards FK, Sehdera JS. Vascular ring. J Thorac Cardiovasc Surg 1971;61:149.

T

1. Tonkin IL, Elliott LP, Bargeron LM Jr. Concomitant axial cineangiography and barium esophagography in the evaluation of vascular rings. Radiology 1980;135:69.
2. Tsang V, Murday A, Gillbe C, Goldstraw P. Slide tracheoplasty for congenital funnel-shaped tracheal stenosis. Ann Thorac Surg 1989;48:632-5.
3. Turner AF, Pacuilli JR, Lau FY, Mikity VG, Johnson JL. Partial tracheal obstruction due to anomalous origin of the left pulmonary artery. Calif Med 1971;114:59.
4. Turner W. On irregularities of the pulmonary artery, arch of the aorta and the primary branches of the arch with an attempt to illustrate their mode of origin by reference to development. Br Foreign Med Chir Rev 1962;30:173.

V

1. Van Praagh R, Van Praagh S, Vlad P, Keith JD. Diagnosis of the anatomic types of congenital dextrocardia. Am J Cardiol 1965;15:234.

2. Von Siebold CT. Ringfermiger aorten-bogen bei einem neugeboraen blansuchtigen. Kinde J Geburtsch Faruenzimmer-Kinderkrank 1837;16:294.
3. van Son JA, Bossert T, Mohr FW. Surgical treatment of vascular ring including right cervical aortic arch. J Card Surg 1999;14:98.
4. van Son JA, Starr A. Demonstration of vascular ring anatomy with ultrafast computed tomography. Thorac Cardiovasc Surg 1995;43:120.

W

1. Welsh TM, Munro IB. Congenital stridor caused by an aberrant pulmonary artery. Arch Dis Child 1954;29:101.
2. Wheeler PC, Wolff LJ, Stevens EM. Pseudovascular ring resulting from right lung agenesis, normal aortic arch and patent ductus arteriosus. Am J Roentgenol Radium Ther Nucl Med 1966;98:365.
3. Whitman G, Stephenson LW, Weinberg P. Vascular ring: left cervical aortic arch, right descending aorta, and right ligamentum arteriosum. J Thorac Cardiovasc Surg 1982;83:311.
4. Williams RG, Jaffe RB, Condon VR, Nixon GW. Unusual features of pulmonary sling. Am J Roentgenol 1979;133:1065.
5. Wittenborg MH, Tantiwongse T, Rosenberg BF. Anomalous course of left pulmonary artery with respiratory obstruction. Radiology 1956;67:339.
6. Wolman IJ. Syndrome of constricting double aortic arch in infancy. Report of case. J Pediatr 1939;14:527.
7. Wolman IJ. Congenital stenosis of the trachea. Am J Dis Child 1941;61:1263.
8. Wychulis AR, Kincaid OW, Weidman WH, Danielson GK. Congenital vascular ring: surgical considerations and results of operation. Mayo Clin Proc 1971;46:182.

Z

1. Zumbro GL, Treasure RL, Geiger JP. Respiratory obstruction in the newborn associated with increased volume and opacification of the hemithorax. Ann Thorac Surg 1974;18:622.

52 Complete Transposition of the Great Arteries

DEFINITION

Complete transposition of the great arteries (TGA) is a congenital cardiac anomaly in which the aorta arises entirely or largely from the right ventricle (RV) and in which the pulmonary trunk arises entirely or largely from the left ventricle (LV), known as *ventriculoarterial discordant connection*.[1] Although the phrase *complete transposition of the great arteries* may properly be applied whenever this situation exists, this chapter uses TGA to denote a cardiac anomaly with *atrioventricular concordant connection* as well as ventriculoarterial discordant connection. Thus, the term *TGA* is not applicable to patients with transposed great arteries and tricuspid or mitral atresia or double inlet left or right ventricle (see Chapters 41 and 56) or atrioventricular *discordant* connection (congenitally corrected transposition of the great arteries; see Chapter 55).

[1]The adjectives *left* and *right* used to modify atrium or ventricle always mean *morphologically* left or right. The position of a chamber or valve is referred to as *right-sided* or *left-sided*.

HISTORICAL NOTE

The first morphologic description of TGA is attributed to Baillie in 1797.[B5] The term *transposition of the aorta and pulmonary artery* was coined by Farre when he described the third known case of this anomaly in 1814 using the word *transposition* (*trans*, "across"; *ponere*, "to place"), meaning that the aorta and pulmonary trunk were displaced across the ventricular septum.[F1] In subsequent pathologic descriptions that included attempts to explain its embryologic basis, the word *transposition* was used to describe an anterior position of the aorta relative to the pulmonary trunk, and by the early 1900s, it had become accepted practice to include any abnormal position of the aorta, regardless of its ventricular origin, under this heading.[A1] This broad confusing definition was clarified by Van Praagh and colleagues in 1971, when they strongly advocated return to Farre's original definition of transposition, and introduced the useful term *malposition* to describe those abnormal positions of the aorta in which both great arteries fail to be displaced across the ventricular septum.[V5] This literal meaning of transposition is now accepted by most pathologists and surgeons.

Recognition of TGA during life resulted from observations of Fanconi in 1932 and Taussig in 1938.[T6] Importance of the early appearance of *pulmonary vascular disease*, even when the ventricular septum was intact, was described by Ferguson and colleagues in 1960[F4] and Ferencz in 1966.[F3]

Surgery for TGA commenced in 1950 when Blalock and Hanlon at Johns Hopkins Hospital described a closed method of atrial septectomy[B31] designed to provide mixing of pulmonary and systemic venous return at the atrial level. Edwards, Bargeron, and Lyons modified the Blalock-Hanlon procedure in 1964 by resuturing the septum so as to connect the right pulmonary veins to the right atrium.[E2]

In 1953, Lillehei and Varco described a "partial physiologic correction" (or atrial switch) consisting of anastomosis of right pulmonary veins to right atrium, and inferior vena cava (IVC) to left atrium,[L15] a technique that became known as the "Baffes operation." Baffes incorporated use of an allograft aortic tube to connect the IVC to the left atrium.[B2]

Palliation of TGA was revolutionized when Rashkind and Miller in Philadelphia introduced *balloon atrial septostomy* (BAS) in 1966.[R5,R6] However, in 1971 at Great Ormond Street Hospital in London, Tynan showed that BAS did not allow all babies with TGA to survive until repair.[T18] A modification of this procedure was introduced in 1975 by Park and colleagues with their substitution of a blade rather than a balloon at the end of the catheter.[P6]

Throughout the 1950s there were attempts to correct TGA surgically either at the atrial or the great artery levels. The concept of a physiologic correction at the atrial level by switching the atrial septum so that systemic venous return is directed to the LV and pulmonary venous return to the RV was first proposed by Albert at a meeting of the American College of Surgeons in 1954.[A6] This concept was amplified by Merendino and colleagues in 1957.[M24] The first successful operation of this type was accomplished by Senning in 1959, who refashioned the walls of the right atrium and the atrial septum to accomplish atrial-level transposition of venous return.[S9,S10] Modifications were suggested by many, including Schumaker in 1961[S17] and Bernard and colleagues in 1962.[B21] At the Mayo Clinic the *Senning procedure* was used between 1960 and 1964 with some successes (a few of these patients were still alive and well 30 years later) but with many disappointing results, related in part to the fact that most of the infants and children had a large ventricular septal defect (VSD) and varying degrees of pulmonary vascular disease.[B7,K13]

The *Mustard procedure*, in which the atrial septum is excised and a pericardial baffle used to redirect systemic and pulmonary venous flow, was devised in an attempt to create larger atria than were produced by the Senning procedure[T12] and was successfully introduced at the Toronto Sick Children's Hospital in 1963 and reported in 1964.[M38] (Actually, Wilson and colleagues described essentially the same operation in 1962.[W12]) Mustard's initial results were better than had been achieved with the Senning procedure, at least in part because he had access to a reservoir of young children with TGA and intact ventricular septum who had been palliated by a Blalock-Hanlon operation.

The Mustard technique soon was adopted in almost all cardiac surgical centers. However, a slightly modified Senning repair was reintroduced by Quaegebeur, Rohmer, and Brom in 1977,[Q3] mainly because of persisting problems with baffle obstruction[B19,S25] and arrhythmia[A4,E6,Z1] after the Mustard procedure.

It became conventional to delay this *atrial switch* definitive procedure for 12 to 24 months after BAS. In occasional patients the Mustard procedure was extended to smaller infants by Dillard and colleagues in 1969,[D16] Bonchek and Starr in 1972,[B32] and Subramanian and Wagner in 1975.[S28] The first substantiated proposal that repair was necessary and possible in the first 3 months to avoid considerable pre-repair mortality was by Barratt-Boyes and colleagues.[B8]

TGA with large VSD remained a difficult problem throughout this early era because of high hospital mortality after repair and rapid development of pulmonary vascular disease in many patients. However, enough successes were obtained with the atrial switch procedures to demonstrate the value of continuing to treat patients in this subset surgically. In 1972, Lindesmith and colleagues introduced the use of a *palliative Mustard procedure* in which the VSD was left unclosed for patients with high pulmonary vascular resistance.[L18] The modification in which a large VSD was created in TGA with intact ventricular septum was used by Stark and colleagues in 1976.[S24]

Successes were few in patients with TGA, VSD, and important *left ventricular outflow tract obstruction* (LVOTO) in this early period of intracardiac surgery for TGA. Daicoff and colleagues in 1969 reported a few successful repairs by direct relief of the LVOTO associated with an atrial switch by Mustard's technique.[D2] Later, in 1969, Rastelli and colleagues combined intraventricular tunnel repair (LV to aorta) of the double outlet RV operation (see "Intraventricular Tunnel Repair of Simple Double Outlet Right Ventricle" under Technique of Operation in Chapter 53) with a rerouting valved extracardiac conduit (RV to pulmonary trunk) and closure of the origin of the pulmonary trunk from the LV to produce an anatomic repair of TGA, VSD, and LVOTO.[R7,R8]

Somewhat disappointing results of the atrial switch operation for TGA and large VSD continued to be a stimulus for developing an *arterial switch* operation, particularly because the right (systemic) ventricle sometimes failed late postoperatively in these patients. Much earlier, in 1954, Mustard and colleagues had described unsuccessful attempts to perform an arterial switch operation in seven patients, with transfer of the left coronary ostium to the pulmonary trunk and use of a monkey lung as the oxygenator.[M39] Other reports of unsuccessful operations of this general type were those of Bailey and colleagues in 1954[B3] and Kay and Cross in 1955.[K4] Idriss and colleagues attempted such a procedure in two patients with an intact ventricular septum in 1961 using cardiopulmonary bypass (CPB), transferring the great arteries and a ring of aorta carrying the coronary arteries.[I1] Interest then lagged in many centers, but a few groups persisted with efforts to perfect this approach. Jatene and colleagues in Brazil achieved a major breakthrough in 1975 with the first successful use of an arterial switch procedure *(Jatene procedure)*, applying it in infants with TGA and VSD.[J4,J5] Soon after, Yacoub and colleagues reported successful cases.[Y2] An important technical modification of the original Jatene procedure was the demonstration by Lecompte and colleagues that direct anastomosis of both great arteries without interposition of a tube graft is possible when the pulmonary bifurcation is transferred in front of the distal ascending aortic arch.[L7] Aubert and colleagues successfully used intraarterial baffling and creation of an aortopulmonary tunnel to correct simple TGA by an arterial switch in 1978.[A16]

Yacoub's attempts in London to perform an arterial switch procedure in three infants with TGA and intact ventricular septum were unsuccessful in 1972, but reports by Mauck in 1977 and Abe in 1978 with their colleagues indicated that such a repair was possible in infancy.[A2,M18] However, most infants with TGA and intact ventricular septum did not survive arterial switching. Yacoub approached this problem of the low-pressure LV not being prepared for sustaining systemic pressure by performing pulmonary artery banding as a first stage.[Y3] The matter was resolved when Radley-Smith and Yacoub in London, Quaegebeur in Holland, and Castaneda in Boston with their colleagues demonstrated feasibility and safety of repair of simple TGA in the first few days of life by an arterial switch operation.[C4,Q4,R2]

MORPHOLOGY AND MORPHOGENESIS

Right Ventricle

The RV is normally positioned, hypertrophied, and large in TGA. Its inflow and sinus portions are essentially normal in architecture. In about 90% of cases, there is a subaortic conus, and the aorta is rightward and anterior and ascends parallel to the posterior and leftward pulmonary trunk (Fig. 52-1). Such hearts also have an infundibular septum, which in the absence of a VSD, joins normally with the ventricular septum between the limbs of the trabecula septomarginalis (septal band; TSM). The infundibulum does not deviate to the left as in the normal heart, but projects directly superiorly from the sinus portion of the ventricle (Fig. 52-2).

There is less wedging of the pulmonary trunk between the mitral and tricuspid valves in TGA than of the aorta in normal hearts.[A9] As a result, a larger area of contiguity exists between the mitral and tricuspid valves than normally.[A9] These atrioventricular (AV) valves may be at virtually the same level, and the AV septum and membranous interventricular septum are then smaller than usual or (rarely) absent. The right fibrous trigone of the central fibrous body is abnormally shaped and attenuated.

In about 10% of hearts with TGA and intact ventricular septum,[V5,W9] the subaortic conus in the RV is absent or very hypoplastic. Then the aorta is either directly anterior or anterior and to the left of the pulmonary trunk origin or (rarely) posterior.[V5] In a few cases, however, a posteriorly placed aorta is associated with a subaortic conus.[B49]

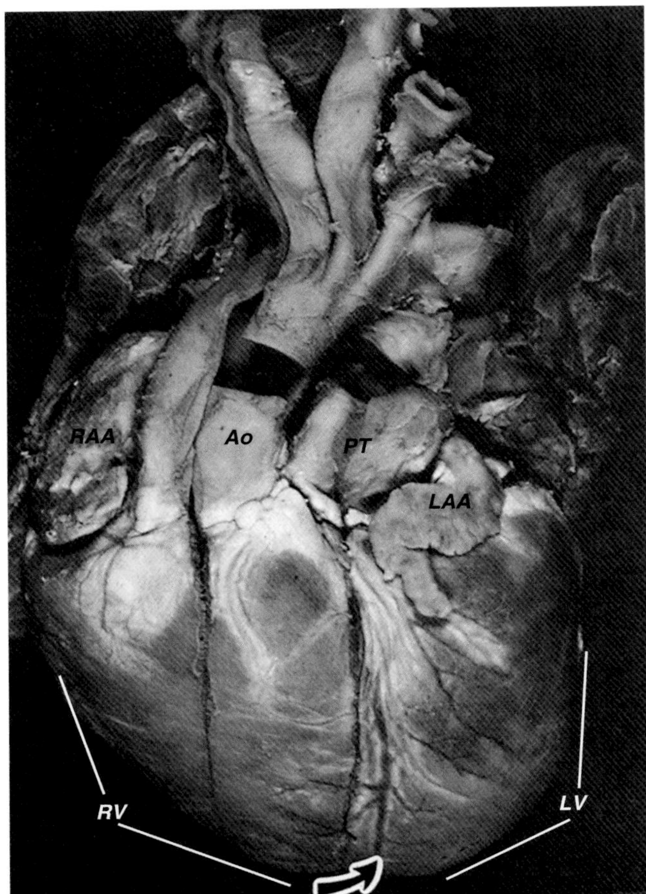

Figure 52-1 Specimen showing external appearance of heart with transposition of great arteries. Infundibulum of morphologically right ventricle extends directly superiorly from sinus portion to give rise to a rightward anterior aorta. Pulmonary trunk lies parallel to aorta in a posterior leftward position and arises from morphologically left ventricle. *Arrow,* Left anterior descending coronary artery. Key: *Ao,* Aorta, *LAA,* left atrial appendage; *LV,* left ventricle; *PT,* pulmonary trunk; *RAA,* right atrial appendage; *RV,* right ventricle.

Left Ventricle

The LV infrequently contains a conus; typically pulmonary-mitral fibrous continuity exists, comparable with aortic-mitral continuity in the normal heart (Fig. 52-3). In about 8% of hearts with TGA, and most often in those with a VSD, a subpulmonary conus is present in the LV.[V2,V5] The subpulmonary conus is frequently stenotic.[G11] In most of these cases, the aorta still lies anteriorly and to the right,[S16] but it may be leftward or posterior.

Ventricular Wall Thickness, Cavity Shape, and Function

In the normal heart, the LV wall is thicker than the RV wall in utero. After birth, LV wall thickness increases progressively, whereas the RV wall becomes relatively thinner.[H18,S20]

In TGA, the RV wall is considerably thicker than normal at birth and increases in thickness with age. When the ventricular septum is intact and no important pulmonary stenosis

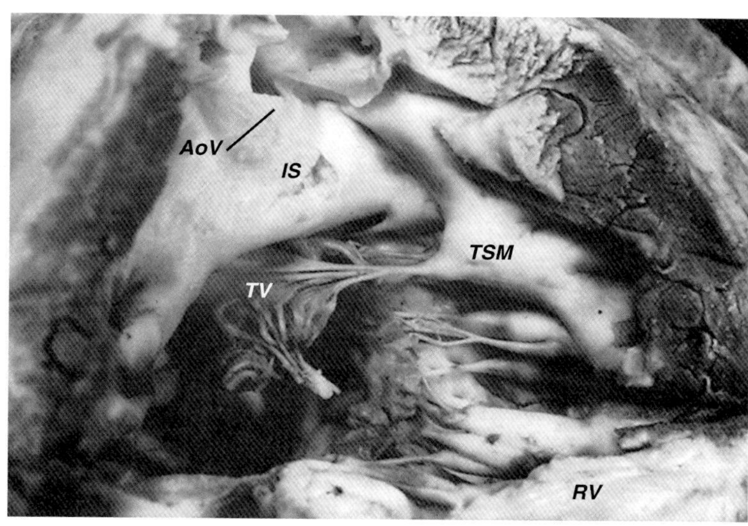

Figure 52-2 Specimen showing interior of right ventricle in heart with transposition of great arteries with an intact ventricular septum. Infundibular (conal) septum inserts in a normal position between the two divisions of trabecula septomarginalis (septal band). These structures and right ventricular free wall are hypertrophied. Infundibulum projects directly superiorly from sinus portion of ventricle rather than superiorly, anteriorly, and leftward as in normal heart, and gives origin to aorta and aortic valve. Key: *AoV,* Aortic valve; *IS,* infundibular septum; *RV,* right ventricle; *TSM,* trabecula septomarginalis; *TV,* tricuspid valve (one chorda has been cut).

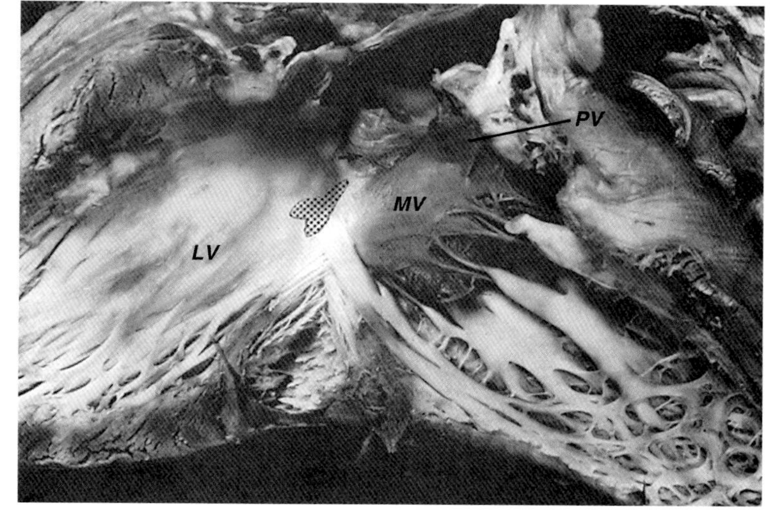

Figure 52-3 Specimen showing interior of left ventricle in heart with simple transposition of great arteries. There is fibrous continuity between mitral and pulmonary valves analogous to aortic-mitral continuity present in normal hearts. Bundle of His penetrates right fibrous trigone *(arrow).* Approximate course of left bundle branch is shown by cross-hatched area. Key: *LV,* Left ventricle; *MV,* mitral valve; *PV,* pulmonary valve.

is present, the LV wall is of normal thickness at birth. Wall thickness remains static, however, leading to less-than-normal thickness within a few weeks of birth and a relatively thin wall by age 2 to 4 months.[B6,C1,D5,M10] When a VSD is present, LV wall thickness increases slightly less than in the normal heart, but remains well within the normal range during the first year of life.[H18,S20] With LVOTO (pulmonary stenosis) the evolution is similar, although when obstruction is severe and the ventricular septum is intact, LV wall thickness eventually exceeds RV wall thickness.[K6] Although not equivalent to LV work potential, LV wall thickness reflects the ventricle's functional capacity.

In infants with TGA, the LV cavity is the usual ellipsoid in shape at birth but soon becomes banana shaped.[B19] Alteration in LV function accompanies this geometric change.

RV function is usually normal in TGA in the perinatal period. Thereafter, when the ventricular septum is intact, RV end-diastolic volume is increased and RV ejection fraction decreased.[G15,J3] Depressed RV ejection fraction is unlikely to be caused by increased afterload or decreased preload and probably results from depressed RV function from relative myocardial hypoxia or the geometry of the chamber.[G15]

LV end-diastolic volume is increased in TGA, and LV ejection fraction is normal. RV/LV end-diastolic volume ratio, normally 1.0, is increased to 1.5 ± 0.33.

Atria

The atria are normally formed in TGA. Right atrial size is usually larger than normal, particularly when the ventricular septum is intact.

Conduction System

The AV node and bundle of His lie in a normal position, although the AV node is abnormally shaped and may be partly engulfed in the right trigone. The left bundle branch originates more distally from the bundle of His than usual and arises as a single cord rather than a sheath. Therefore, damage to the bifurcation of the bundle at VSD closure is

Table 52-1 Position of Great Arteries in Patients with Transposition of the Great Arteries[a]

Position	Number	Percent of 330
Ao anterior 0°	203	62
Ao anterior 30°R	54	16
Ao anterior 60°R	41	12
Ao-PT side-by-side 90°R	24	7
Ao anterior 30°L	6	2
Ao anterior 60°L	2	0.6
Subtotal	330	100
Unknown	183	—
TOTAL	513	

Data from Kirklin and colleagues.[K12]
[a]Data based on 513 neonates with simple transposition of the great arteries (TGA) or TGA with ventricular septal defect undergoing arterial switch operation, 1985 to March 1, 1989, Congenital Heart Surgeons Society multiinstitutional study.
Key: *Ao,* Aorta; *L,* left; *PT,* pulmonary trunk; *R,* right.

Table 52-2 Origin of Coronary Arteries in Hearts with Simple Transposition of the Great Arteries (TGA) and TGA with Ventricular Septal Defect[a]

Origin of Coronary Arteries			
Sinus 1	**Sinus 2**	**No.**	**Percent of 513**
LCx	R[b]	367	72
L	R	1	0.2
LCxR	—	5	1
—	LCxR	36	7
	Single ostium or two very closely placed ostia[c]	26	5
	Two ostia, one far to left and near commissure[d]	10	2
LR	Cx	13	3
LR	LCx	2	0.4
R LCx	—	8	2
L	CxR	75	15
RV LCx	CxR	1	0.2
Malaligned aortic commissures[e]		2	0.4
Unknown		3	1
TOTAL		513	100

Data from Kirklin and colleagues.[K12]
[a]Data based on 513 neonates with simple TGA or TGA with ventricular septal defect undergoing arterial switch operation (see Table 52-1).
[b]Three of the 367 had malaligned pulmonary commissures.
[c]LAD or left main coronary artery passed between aorta and pulmonary artery (intramural) in two (one death) of the 26.
[d]All passed between aorta and pulmonary artery (intramural).
[e]In one, all coronaries arose from a posterior-facing sinus. In one, LCx arose from a posterior-facing sinus, R from a right-sided sinus.
Key: *Cx,* Circumflex artery; *L,* left anterior descending coronary artery; *R,* right coronary artery; *RV,* right ventricle branch.

more likely to produce complete heart block than in the normally structured heart.[B25]

Great Arteries

The aorta is most often directly anterior or slightly to the right (Table 52-1). In the Taussig-Bing heart, great arteries may be side by side, with the aorta to the right (see "Taussig-Bing Heart" under Morphology in Chapter 53). Rarely the aorta is directly posterior.[B49]

Some refer to the aortic sinuses of Valsalva as "left posterior–facing" or "right posterior–facing" sinuses and "nonfacing" sinus. This becomes awkward, however, in the 25% of cases in which positions of the great arteries are different from the usual anteroposterior locations. A more universally applicable scheme is the *Leiden convention*, in which *sinus 1* is on the right of an imagined observer standing in the nonfacing noncoronary aortic sinus of Valsalva looking toward the pulmonary trunk.[G6] Proceeding counterclockwise, the next sinus is *sinus 2.*

In 13% to 30% of patients with TGA, aortic and pulmonary commissures are not precisely aligned because of malalignment of either the aortic or mitral valve.[G6] In one study, commissural malalignment was found in nearly 40% of patients undergoing an arterial switch procedure.[M15] Recognition of commissural malalignment is important in planning the coronary transfer as well as preventing neoaortic valve regurgitation.[K9]

Coronary Arteries

Coronary arteries in TGA usually arise from the aortic sinuses that face the pulmonary trunk, regardless of the interrelationships of the great arteries.[G6] Thus, the noncoronary sinus is usually the anterior one. Most often the *left anterior descending* (LAD) and *circumflex* (Cx) coronary arteries arise as a single trunk (*left main coronary artery* [LCA]) from aortic sinus 1 and distribute in a normal manner, although the Cx system is often small (Table 52-2). The *right coronary artery* (RCA) arises from sinus 2 and follows this artery's usual course.

An almost infinite number of deviations from this usual pattern exist.[K11] Typical patterns are observed when both sinus 1 and sinus 2 give rise to a major coronary artery (Fig. 52-4). Patterns in which the Cx or LCA passes behind the pulmonary trunk deserve special attention by the surgeon (see "Arterial Switch Operation" under Technique of Operation later in this chapter).

All three main coronary arteries may arise from a single sinus (single coronary artery), most frequently, and of utmost concern to the surgeon, from sinus 2. Usually the arteries all arise from a single ostium in the center of the sinus (see Table 52-2). Alternatively, they may arise from a double-barreled ostium consisting of two ostia immediately adjacent to each other and constituting essentially a single ostium. Regardless, often these patients have an infundibular branch arising from sinus 1, making true single RCA uncommon. Coronary artery distribution in this situation has a typical pattern (Fig. 52-5). At times, however (in a pattern not shown in Fig. 52-5), the LCA or LAD passes forward between aorta and pulmonary trunk in an *intramural course* to emerge anteriorly. In this situation, instead of all three main coronary arteries arising from an essentially single, more or less centrally positioned, ostium, the LCA or LAD alone nearly always arises from an entirely separate ostium far to the left of the RCA ostium, adjacent to or just above the valvar commissure between sinus 2 and sinus 1 (Fig. 52-6). An LCA or LAD arising in this

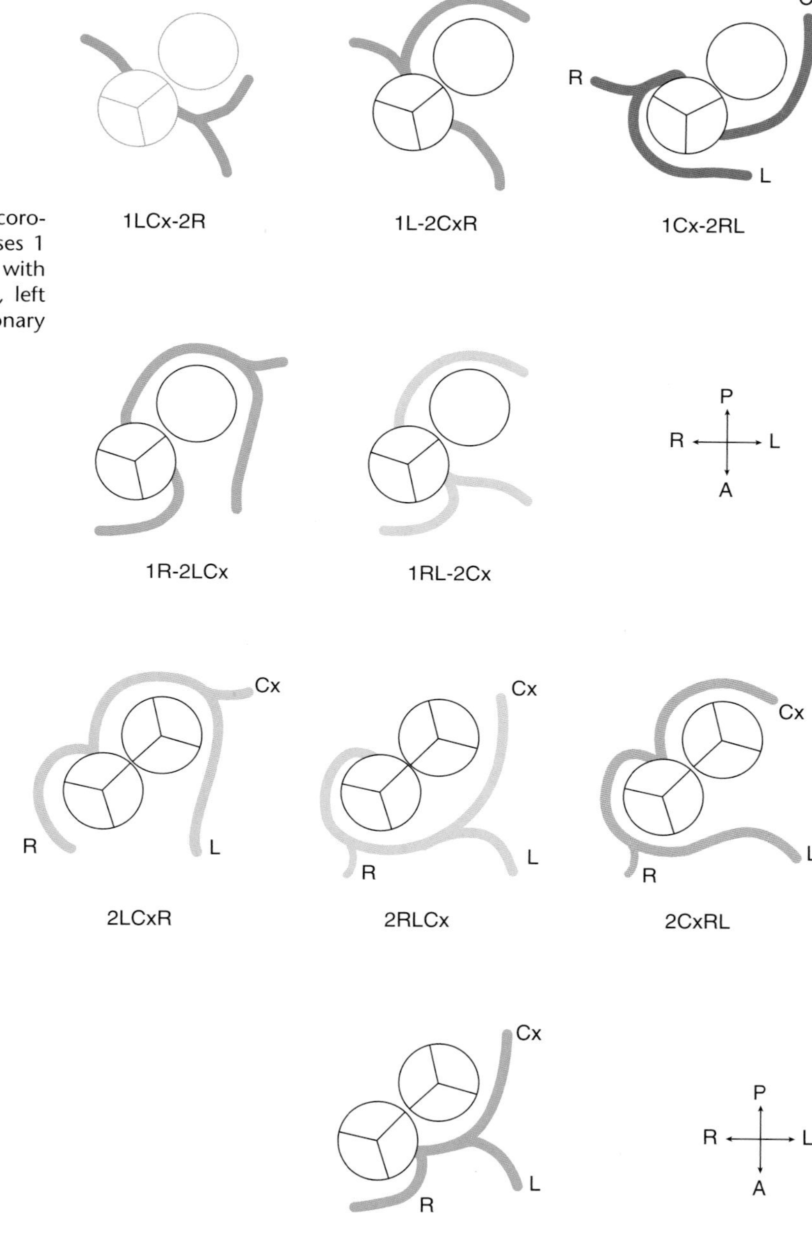

Figure 52-4 Most common patterns of circumflex coronary system when each facing sinus of Valsalva (sinuses 1 and 2) gives origin to a major coronary artery in hearts with transposition of great arteries. Key: *Cx,* Circumflex; *L,* left anterior descending coronary artery; *R,* right coronary artery. (From Quaegebeur.[Q2])

Figure 52-5 Origin of all three major coronary arteries from a single ostium (or a double-barreled ostium) in sinus 2 or sinus 1 in hearts with transposition of great arteries. Key: *Cx,* Circumflex; *L,* left anterior descending coronary artery; *R,* right coronary artery. (From Quaegebeur.[Q2])

location passes forward in an *intramural course* (see Fig. 52-6) and entirely within the aortic wall (Fig. 52-7). It emerges from the aorta anteriorly and has the same appearance externally as when the artery originates from sinus 1.

In patients with situs inversus, the coronary arteries are a mirror image of situs solitus but seem to have a predilection for all coronary arteries to arise from a single sinus.[C12]

Rarely the RCA may be intramural as it passes to the right and forward from its usual origin from sinus 2 in an otherwise typical pattern of "sinus 1: LAD, Cx; sinus 2: RCA" (or 1LCx-2R).

In 88 autopsy specimens, origins of coronary arteries were at or above the level of the sinutubular junction in 20%, paracommissural origin occurred in 3%, and angle of exit from the aortic wall was not orthogonal but tangential in 7%.[L12] Those with high takeoff were all intramural.

A *conus artery* frequently arises separately and from its own ostium in sinus 1. It may supply at least a considerable part of the anterior wall of the infundibulum of the RV.

The course of the *sinus node artery* may be important in the atrial switch (Mustard or Senning) operation. This artery usually arises from the RCA close to its origin and passes superiorly and rightward, usually partly embedded in the most superior portion of the limbus of the atrial septum, where it can be damaged if this portion of the atrial septum is widely excised.[T13] Then the sinus node artery usually passes behind or branches to form an arterial circle around the cavoatrial junction.[A9]

Pulmonary Vascular Disease

Now that repair of simple TGA is usually performed in the first week or two of life, and repair of TGA with VSD is usually performed in the first month or two of life, pulmonary vascular disease has almost disappeared (see Natural History and Results later in this chapter), just as it has in many other types of congenital heart disease. However, it becomes important in many patients with TGA when early surgical treatment is not performed (Table 52-3).[C16,F3,F4,F8,N7,V10]

When pulmonary vascular disease develops in TGA, histologic changes in the pulmonary arteries are comparable with those found in isolated large VSD and can be similarly graded by the Heath-Edwards or Reid criteria (see "Pulmonary Vascular Disease" under Morphology in Section I of Chapter 35). In addition, however, pulmonary microthrombi are present in about 25% of lungs examined at autopsy[N8] or on lung biopsy.[W1] Pulmonary microthrombi produce a variety of intimal lesions, including eccentric cushion lesions and occlusion with recanalization of nonlaminar intimal fibrosis that can result in irregular fibrous septa within vessel lumen. These changes occur with and without laminar and circumferential changes secondary to hypertensive pulmonary vascular disease and are of uncertain etiology and importance. The changes are seldom severe enough to cause an increase in pulmonary vascular resistance (Rp) and occur with equal frequency in TGA with intact ventricular septum, large VSD, and large VSD and LVOTO.[N8] Using lung biopsy specimens, Wagenvoort and colleagues have also described wall thinning and dilatation of pulmonary arteries and, to a lesser extent, pulmonary veins in TGA with intact ventricular septum, particularly when the hematocrit is high.[W1]

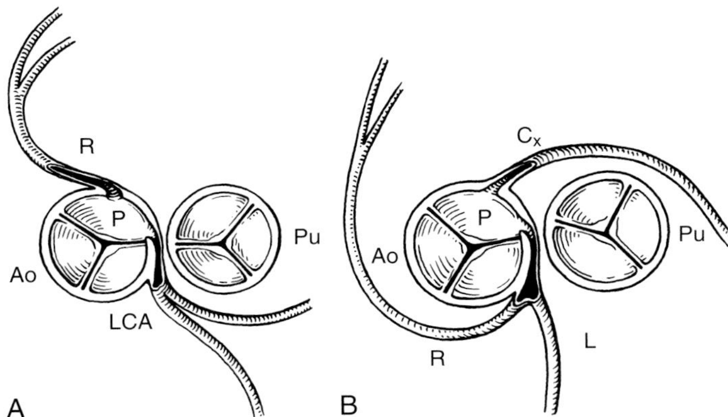

Figure 52-6 Two types of intramural coronary arteries when all major coronary arteries arise from sinus 2 (posterior sinus). **A,** Origin of left coronary artery and right coronary artery from posterior sinus. Aortic and pulmonary orifices have a side-to-side relationship, and there is alignment of interostial commissures. **B,** Origin of coronary arteries from posterior sinus. In this case, left circumflex originates separately, whereas left anterior descending and right coronary arteries initially have a common origin and intramural course. Aortic and pulmonary orifices have a side-to-side relationship. Interostial commissures are not aligned, and sinuses do not completely face one other. Key: *Ao,* Aorta; *Cx,* circumflex; *L,* left anterior descending; *LCA,* left coronary artery; *P,* posterior sinus; *Pu,* pulmonary orifice; *R,* right coronary artery. (From Gittenberger-de Groot and colleagues.[G7])

Coexisting Cardiac Anomalies

About 75% of neonates presenting with TGA have no important coexisting cardiac anomaly other than a patent foramen ovale or an atrial septal defect. About 25% to 40% have a large or small VSD. Only about 5% have associated LVOTO. Some VSDs close spontaneously in the first few weeks or months of life, and some patients without LVOTO during the first few weeks of life develop obstruction later. Also, some with TGA, VSD, and LVOTO are asymptomatic as neonates and present later in life.

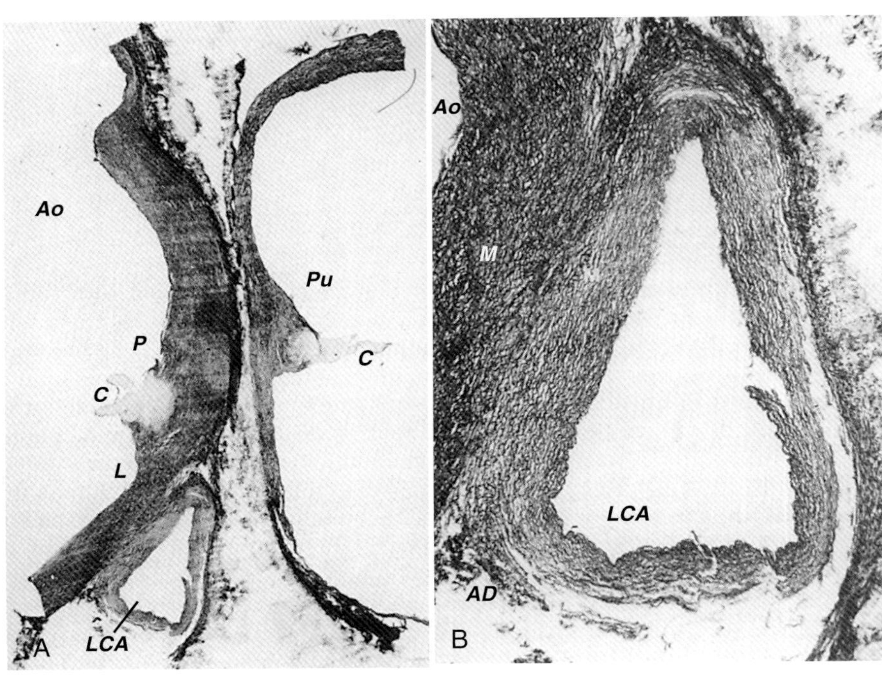

Figure 52-7 Histologic details of an intramural coronary artery. **A,** Cross-section of part of aortic and pulmonary orifices. Left coronary artery, originating from posterior sinus, is at level of left sinus. Interostial commissures of aortic and pulmonary orifices, which lack elastic tissue, are aligned. **B,** Detail of **A.** Media of aorta and coronary artery are continuous, with no intervening loose fibrous tissue of adventitia separating elastic lamellae (van Gieson elastic tissue stain). Key: *AD,* Adventitia; *Ao,* aorta; *C,* commissure; *L,* left sinus; *LCA,* left coronary artery *M,* media of aorta; *P,* posterior sinus; *Pu,* pulmonary orifice. (From Gittenberger-de Groot and colleagues.[G7])

Table 52-3 Prevalence of Important (≥Grade 3 Heath-Edwards) Pulmonary Vascular Disease at Autopsy in Patients with Transposition of the Great Arteries, Age 3 Months and Older

	Intact Ventricular Septum						Large VSD					
		3-12 Months[a]			>12 Months[a]			3-12 Months[a]			>12 Months[a]	
Study	*n*	No.	%	*n*	No.	%	*n*	No.	%	*n*	No.	%
Ferencz[F3]	13[b]	3	23	12	7	58	14	1	7	18	10	56
Vilesetal[V10]	4	1	25	3	2	67	6	3	50	9	9	100
Newfeld et al.[N7]	12	0	0	26	4	15	17	5	29	28	26	93
Clarkson et al.[C16]	6[b]	2	33	9	4	44	7	2	29	5	2	40
TOTAL	35	6	17	50	17	34	44	11	25	60	47	78

[a]Age at death.
[b]Includes patients with small ventricular septal defect.
Key: *VSD,* Ventricular septal defect.

Table 52-4 Types of Ventricular Septal Defect in Hearts with Transposition of the Great Arteries[a]

Type of VSD	No.	% of 81
Conoventricular:	47	58
Without outlet septal malalignment	27	
With outlet septal malalignment:	20	
Displaced to left	10	
Displaced to right	10	
Juxta-aortic	4	5
Juxta-arterial	4	5
Inlet septal (AV canal type)	4[b]	5
Muscular:	22[c]	27
Basal (posterior, inflow)	7	
Midseptal	12	
Apical	1	
Anterior	3	
TOTAL	81	100

[a]Data are based on GLH autopsy study.
[b]These VSDs were also juxtatricuspid.
[c]In 6 of the 22 hearts, VSDs were multiple.
Key: *AV,* Atrioventricular; *VSD,* ventricular septal defect.

Ventricular Septal Defect

The same types of VSD occur with TGA, and with the same definitions, as occur in hearts with a primary VSD, and they occur in about the same proportions (Table 52-4) (see "Location in Septum and Relationship to Conduction System" in Morphology in Section I of Chapter 35). *Conoventricular defects* of the several different varieties are most common and may not necessarily be juxtapulmonary (on LV side) (Fig. 52-8). In some hearts with conoventricular VSDs, the infundibular septum is malaligned and fails to insert within the Y of the TSM. The septum may be displaced leftward, resulting in a variable degree of LVOTO (Figs. 52-9 and 52-10), or rightward, tending to result in RV (subaortic) obstruction (Fig. 52-11).[V5] VSD with malalignment may not be juxtatricuspid, as in tetralogy of Fallot, but the malaligned infundibular septum may be hypoplastic, varying from the usual tetralogy of Fallot (see Morphology in Section I of Chapter 38).

When the infundibular septum is displaced to the right, the pulmonary trunk may be biventricular in origin and over a juxtapulmonary VSD. Hearts with this arrangement are similar to those with double outlet right ventricle and juxtapulmonary VSD[G10,T7,V4] (see "Taussig-Bing Heart" under Morphology in Chapter 53) and may be associated with subaortic stenosis or aortic arch obstruction (arch hypoplasia, coarctation, or interruption).[M31,S6]

Occasionally the VSD is *juxta-aortic* and associated with a malaligned but nondisplaced infundibular septum. The infundibular septum may be absent or almost gone, and the VSD is then *juxta-arterial* (doubly committed) (Fig. 52-12).[H17,L16,V6]

Inlet septal defects that are also juxtatricuspid are slightly more common in hearts with TGA than in those with a concordant ventriculoarterial connection, in which the bundle of His passes from the AV node along the posteroinferior margin of the VSD. The *juxtacrucial type* of inlet septal defect, with its characteristic tricuspid straddling and abnormal AV node position, probably also occurs more often in hearts with TGA than other defects (see "Inlet Septal Ventricular Septal Defect" in Morphology in Section I of Chapter 35).

Most *muscular* VSDs are in the midseptum but may occur in other areas (Fig. 52-13).

Left Ventricular Outflow Tract Obstruction

Development of LVOTO, which produces subpulmonary obstruction, is part of the natural history of many patients with TGA. The obstruction may be dynamic or anatomic. LVOTO occurs in an important way at birth or within a few days in only 0.7% of patients with TGA and intact ventricular septum. Obstruction is present in about 20% of patients born with TGA and VSD. LVOTO may become apparent or develop after birth in other patients, thus reaching an overall prevalence of 30% to 35%.[R8,S1,S14,S16,V3]

Dynamic type of LVOTO, developing in patients with TGA and intact ventricular septum, is the result of leftward bulging of the muscular ventricular septum secondary to higher RV than LV pressure.[N4,S1] Dynamic LVOTO is particularly likely to occur if the aorta lies anterior and more to the left than usual, with increased wedging of the subpulmonary area.[C10] The septum impinges against the anterior mitral leaflet in combination with abnormal systolic anterior leaflet motion (SAM). Thus, the mechanism is similar to that present

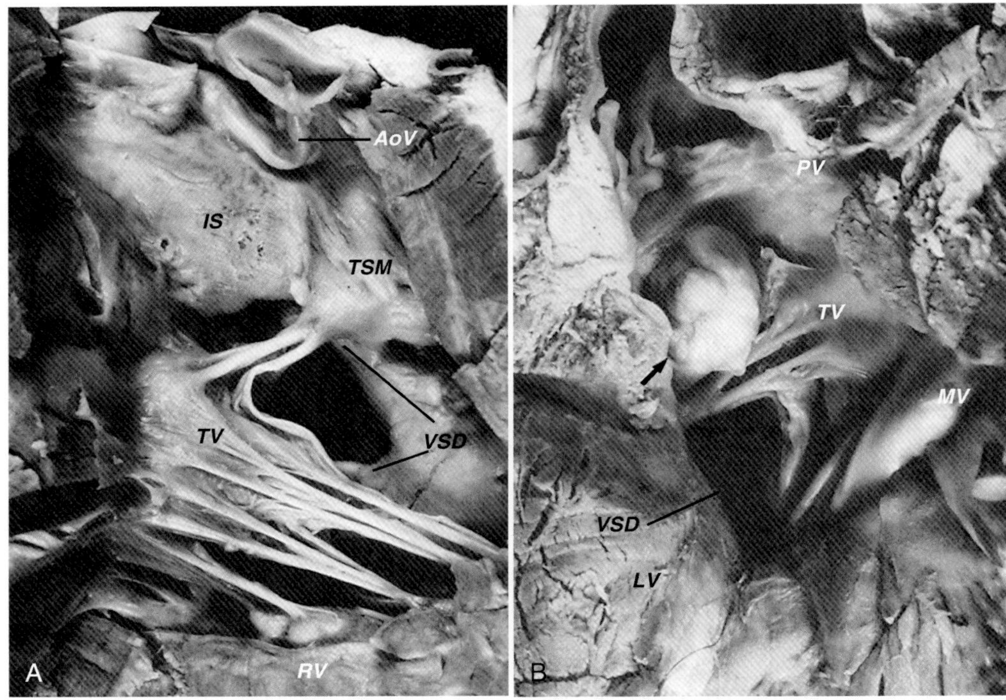

Figure 52-8 Specimen of transposition of great arteries with large conoventricular ventricular septal defect *(VSD)*. **A,** From right ventricular side, VSD is seen to be adjacent to tricuspid valve anulus and extends inferiorly beneath it. Infundibular septum is normally aligned with trabecula septomarginalis. **B,** From left ventricular side, VSD is separated from pulmonary valve in part by an anomalous bulky fibrous pouch *(arrow)* that originates from left side of septal tricuspid leaflet and is a cause of left ventricular outflow tract obstruction. There is mitral-tricuspid continuity across floor of defect. Key: *AoV,* Aortic valve; *IS,* infundibular septum; *LV,* left ventricle; *MV,* mitral valve; *PV,* pulmonary valve; *RV,* right ventricle; *TSM,* trabecula septomarginalis; *TV,* tricuspid valve.

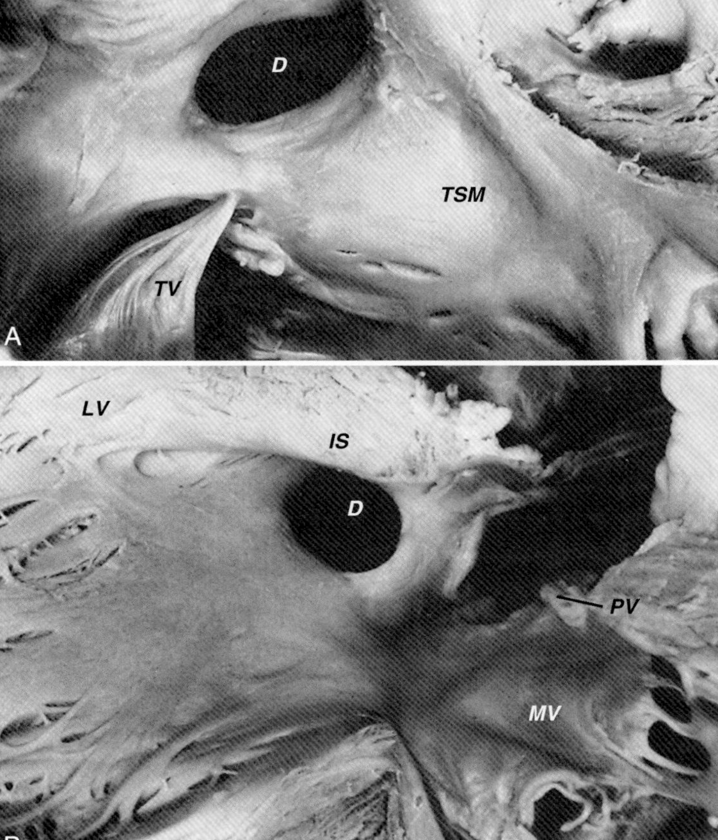

Figure 52-9 Specimen of transposition of great arteries with large conoventricular ventricular septal defect with leftward displacement of infundibular septum. **A,** From right ventricular side. **B,** From left ventricular side, conal septum is fused with left ventricular anterior free wall, with left ventricular outflow tract obstruction only moderate. Key: *Ao,* Aorta; *AoV,* aortic valve; *IS,* infundibular septum; *D,* ventricular septal defect; *LV,* left ventricle; *MV,* mitral valve; *PV,* pulmonary valve; *RV,* right ventricle; *TSM,* trabecula septomarginalis; *TV,* tricuspid valve.

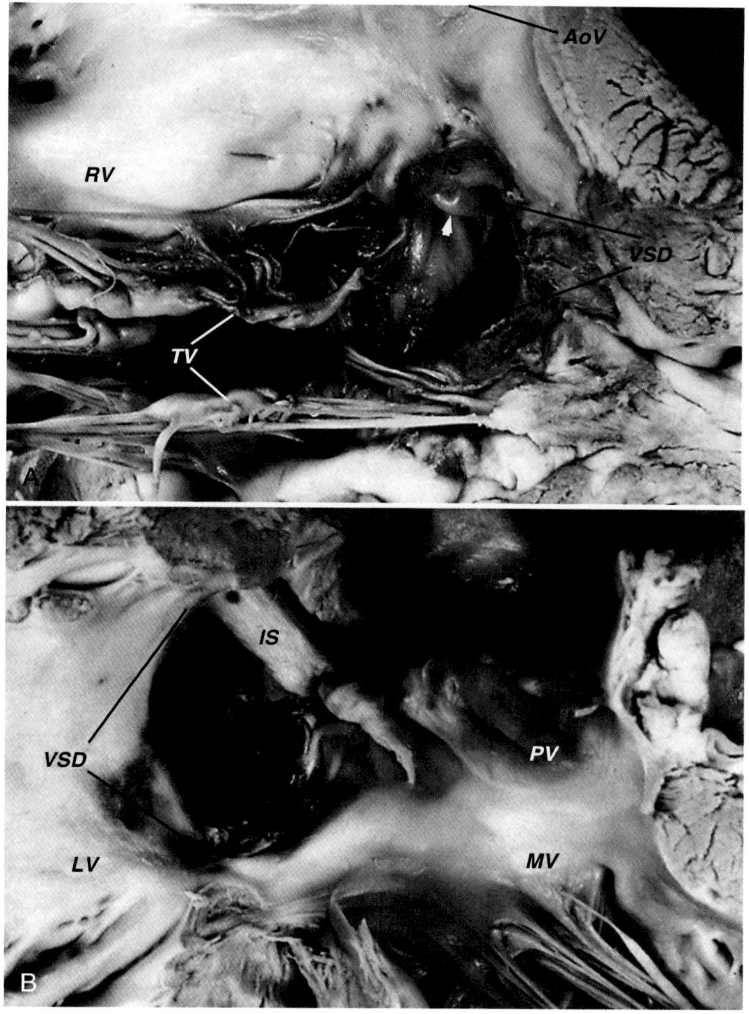

Figure 52-10 Specimen of transposition of great arteries with large conoventricular ventricular septal defect *(VSD)* and leftward displacement of relatively small conal septum. **A,** From right ventricular side, fibrous tag *(arrow),* which also contributes to left ventricular outflow tract obstruction, is seen through VSD. **B,** From left ventricular side. Key: *AoV,* Aortic valve; *IS,* infundibular septum; *LV,* left ventricle; *MV,* mitral valve; *PV,* pulmonary valve; *RV,* right ventricle; *TV,* tricuspid valve; *VSD,* ventricular septal defect.

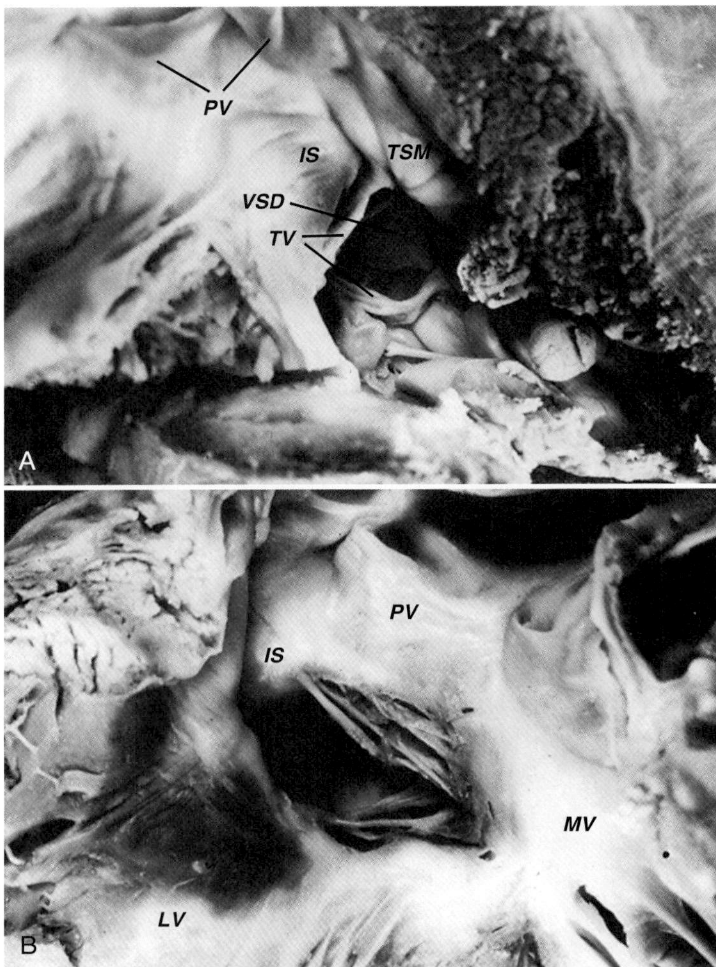

Figure 52-11 Specimen of transposition of great arteries with conoventricular ventricular septal defect *(VSD)* and rightward deviation of infundibular septum that tends to produce subaortic obstruction. **A,** From right ventricular side, VSD is best appreciated by noting deep position of tricuspid valve relative to infundibular septum (compare with Fig. 52-8, *A*). **B,** From left ventricular side, gap between infundibular septum and ventricular septum is obvious. Anomalous tricuspid chordae are attached to edge of VSD. Key: *IS,* Infundibular septum; *LV,* left ventricle; *MV,* mitral valve; *PV,* pulmonary valve; *TSM,* trabecula septomarginalis; *TV,* tricuspid valve.

in hypertrophic obstructive cardiomyopathy (HOCM), but there is no asymmetric septal hypertrophy (see "Dynamic Morphology of Septum and Mitral Valve" under Morphology in Chapter 19). The gradient may be contributed to by the high velocity of blood flow produced by the usually large pulmonary-to-systemic blood flow ratio and the deformation of the LV outflow tract.[A18] When dynamic obstruction is severe, a ridge of endocardial thickening is produced on the septum at its point of contact with the mitral leaflet (Fig. 52-14).[C23] In patients with TGA and intact ventricular septum, rarely a *subvalvar fibrous ridge* may produce LVOTO. The ridge extends onto the anterior mitral leaflet near its hinge. This lesion is analogous to discrete subvalvar aortic stenosis occurring in otherwise normal hearts with ventriculoarterial concordant connection; it is usually localized but may be the tunnel type (see "Tunnel Subvalvar Aortic Stenosis" under Morphology in Section II of Chapter 47). LVOTO in these patients rarely may be caused by *fibrous tags* arising from the mitral apparatus or membranous septum. Valvar stenosis occurs infrequently in this situation, and anular hypoplasia is even less common.[S1,S14]

In patients with TGA and VSD, stenosis is usually subvalvar and valvar. *Subvalvar stenosis* is in the form of a localized fibrous ring, long tunnel-type fibromuscular narrowing, or muscular obstruction related to protrusion of the infundibular septum into the medial or anterior aspect of the LV outflow tract (Figs. 52-15 and 52-16).[V3] An important but fortunately rare form of subvalvar stenosis is attachment of the anterior mitral leaflet to the muscular outflow septum by anomalous fibrous or chordal tissue (Fig. 52-17).[R8,R17,S16] This stenosis can occur in combination with a cleft anterior mitral leaflet with or without overriding or straddling.[M30] Other rare causes of subvalvar pulmonary stenosis are parachute mitral valve,[R8,S16] accessory mitral leaflet tissue, and aneurysm of the membranous ventricular septum. An aneurysm may bulge as a windsock into the LV outflow tract. Its walls are thick, and the VSD is either below the aneurysm or within its sac.[S1,V9] However, most of these "aneurysms" are examples of redundant fibrous tissue prolapsing through the VSD from the tricuspid valve[H17,L5,R13] (see Fig. 52-8) or accessory fibrous tags (see Fig. 52-10) in association with the anterior mitral valve leaflet.

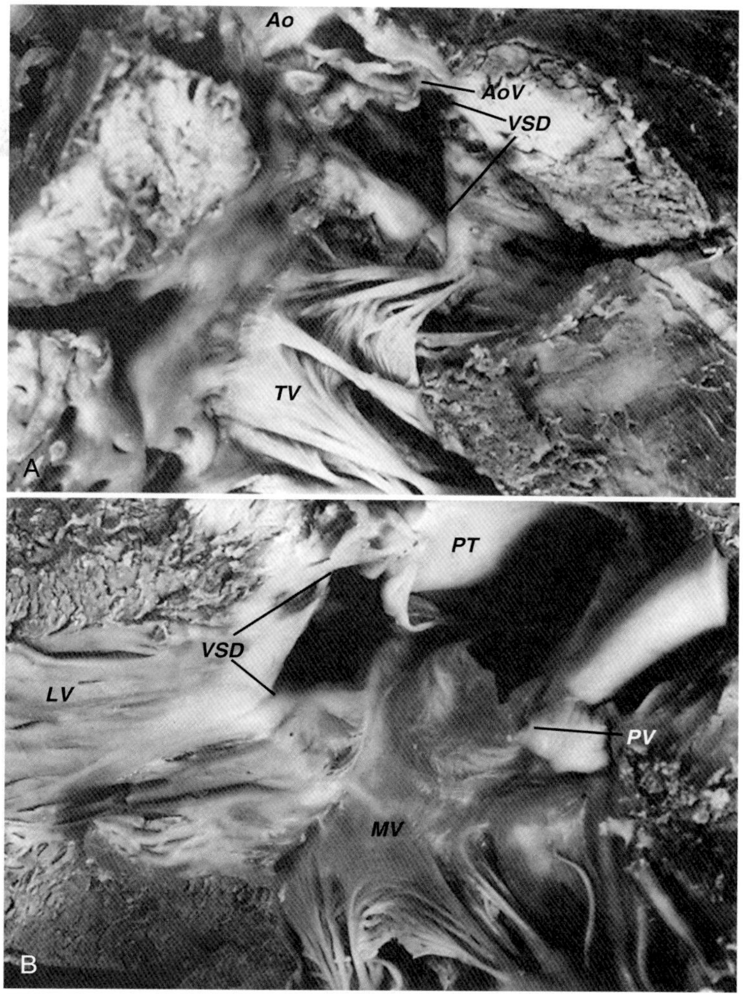

Figure 52-12 Specimen of transposition of great arteries with large juxta-arterial ventricular septal defect (*VSD*). Infundibular septum is absent, and confluent aortic and pulmonary valves form upper margin of VSD. Defect is thus doubly committed. There is mild overriding of pulmonary artery and valve into right ventricle. **A,** From right ventricular side. **B,** From left ventricular side, there is pulmonary-mitral continuity. Key: *Ao,* Aorta; *AoV,* aortic valve; *LV,* left ventricle; *MV,* mitral valve; *PT,* pulmonary trunk; *PV,* pulmonary valve; *TV,* tricuspid valve.

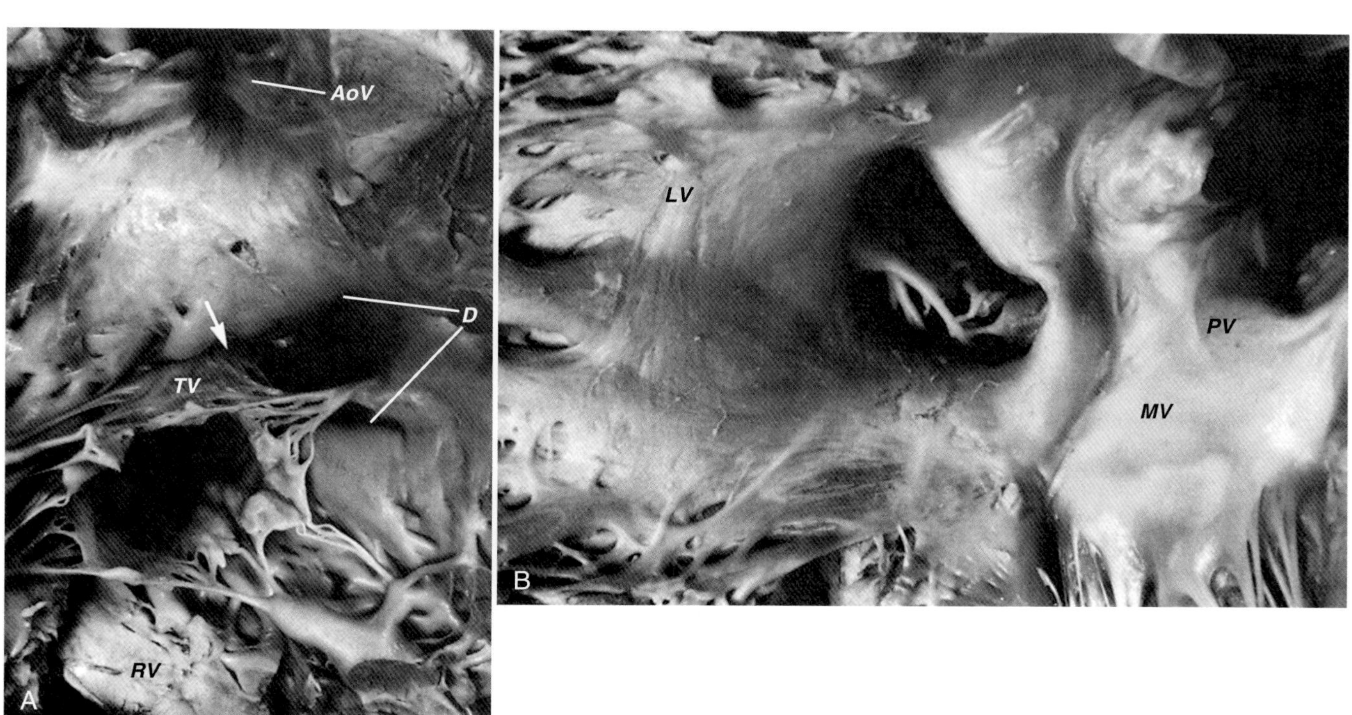

Figure 52-13 Specimen of transposition of great arteries with large inlet muscular ventricular septal defect. This defect could be termed a *conoventricular* ventricular septal defect that is not juxtatricuspid because of a band of muscle separating it from membranous septum and tricuspid ring. **A,** From right ventricular side, muscle band is poorly seen *(arrow)*. **B,** From left ventricular side. Key: *AoV,* Aortic valve; *D,* ventricular septal defect; *LV,* left ventricle; *MV,* mitral valve; *PV,* pulmonary valve; *RV,* right ventricle; *TV,* tricuspid valve.

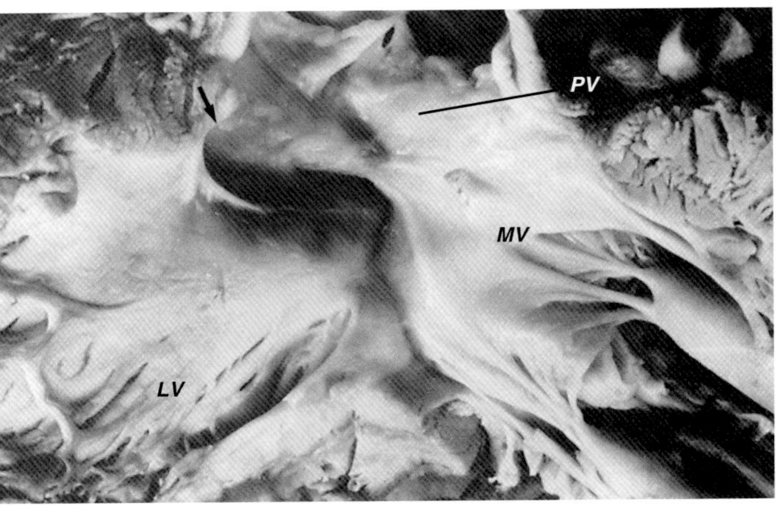

Figure 52-14 Specimen of transposition of great arteries with essentially intact ventricular septum and dynamic muscular form of left ventricular outflow tract obstruction. Arrow points to ridge of endocardial thickening that forms at the point at which mitral leaflet touches septum during diastole. Key: *LV,* Left ventricle; *MV,* mitral valve; *PV,* pulmonary valve.

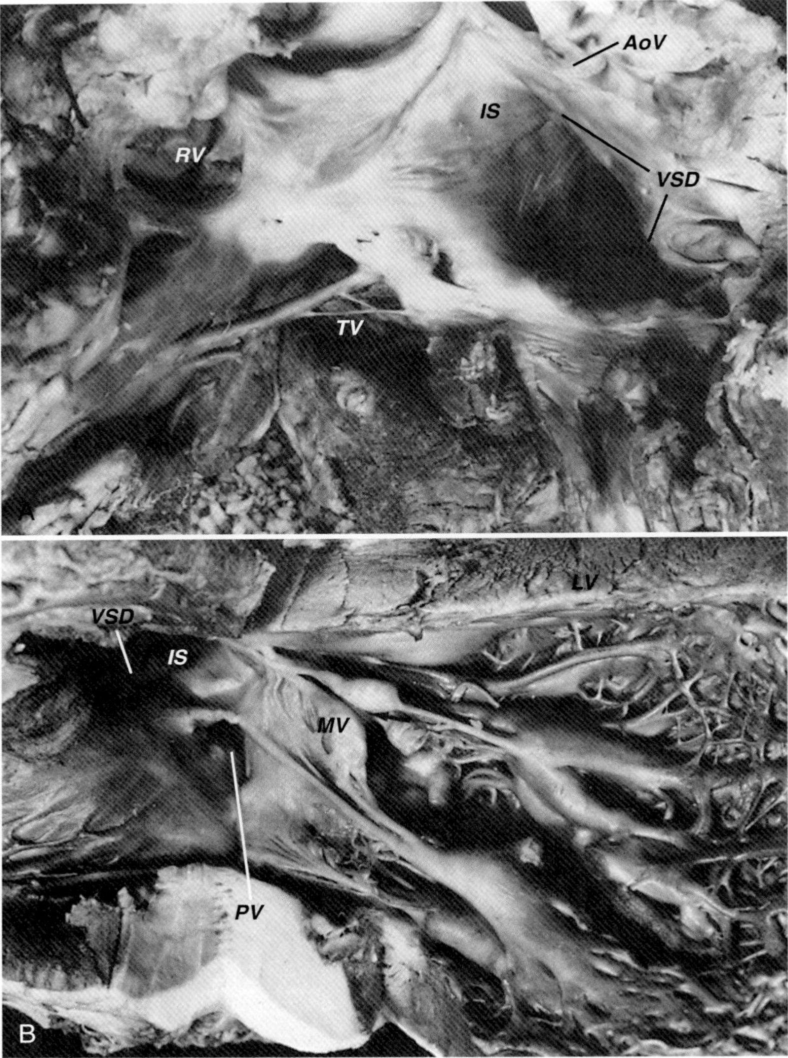

Figure 52-15 Specimen of transposition of great arteries, ventricular septal defect *(VSD),* and left ventricular outflow tract obstruction. VSD is associated with infundibular septal malalignment and leftward displacement into left ventricular outflow tract. **A,** From right ventricular side. **B,** From left ventricular side, infundibular septum has fused with base of anterior mitral valve leaflet, which is cleft *(arrow).* Pulmonary valve ostium is displaced posteriorly and is severely stenotic. Key: *AoV,* Aortic valve; *IS,* infundibular septum; *MV,* mitral valve; *PV,* pulmonary valve ostium; *RV,* right ventricle; *TV,* tricuspid valve.

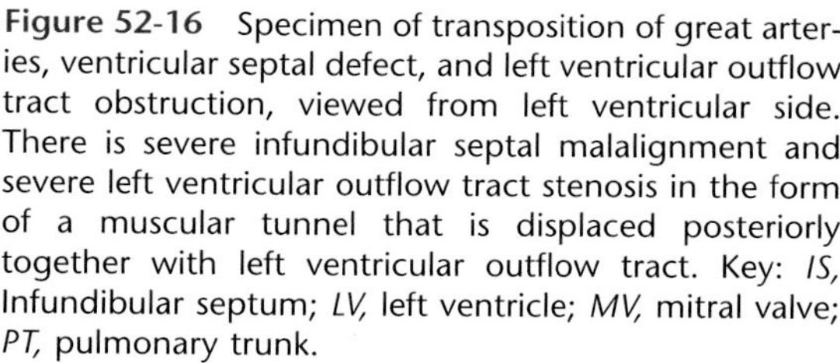

Figure 52-16 Specimen of transposition of great arteries, ventricular septal defect, and left ventricular outflow tract obstruction, viewed from left ventricular side. There is severe infundibular septal malalignment and severe left ventricular outflow tract stenosis in the form of a muscular tunnel that is displaced posteriorly together with left ventricular outflow tract. Key: *IS,* Infundibular septum; *LV,* left ventricle; *MV,* mitral valve; *PT,* pulmonary trunk.

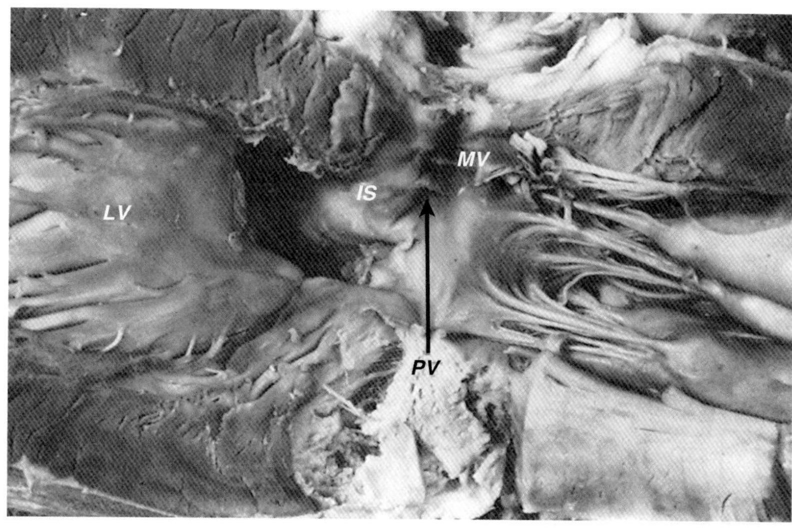

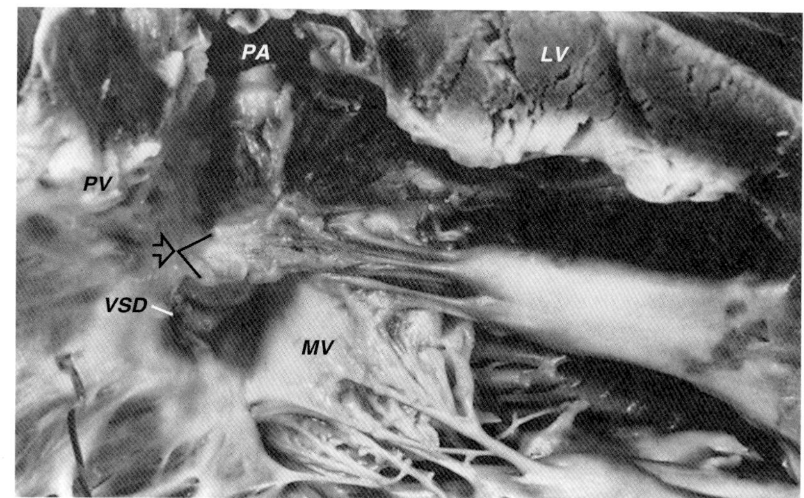

Figure 52-17 Specimen of transposition of great arteries, ventricular septal defect *(VSD),* and left ventricular outflow tract obstruction, viewed from left ventricular side. Left ventricular outflow tract is a stenotic fibrous tunnel formed by bulky fibrous tissue *(arrow)* extending from mitral leaflet to septal surface superior to VSD. Pulmonary valve is in its normal position. Key: *LV,* Left ventricle; *MV,* mitral valve leaflet; *PT,* pulmonary trunk; *PV,* pulmonary valve.

Valvar stenosis is caused by anular hypoplasia and when present is typically associated with subvalvar lesions. The pulmonary valve may be bicuspid. Rarely, there is a stenotic muscular subpulmonary infundibulum.[S1,S16]

Patent Ductus Arteriosus

Patent ductus arteriosus (PDA) is more common in hearts with TGA than in hearts with ventriculoarterial concordant connection. At initial cardiac catheterization at an average age of 2 weeks, Waldman and colleagues found a PDA present in almost half the cases,[W2] but it was functionally (although not necessarily anatomically) closed at 1 month. Persistence of a large PDA for more than a few months is associated with an increased prevalence of pulmonary vascular disease.[N7,W2]

Tricuspid Valve Anomalies

The tricuspid to mitral anulus circumference ratio, normally greater than 1, is less than 1 in 46% of patients (Calder L: personal communication; 1984). This reduced ratio is most marked in hearts with associated coarctation (Fig. 52-18). Functionally important tricuspid valve anomalies are present in only about 4% of surgical patients (Table 52-5). In autopsy studies, however, a considerably higher proportion are found, particularly when there is a VSD.[A8,H17]

Rarely, in hearts with intact ventricular septum, minor tricuspid valve anomalies may lead to severe regurgitation early in life. In hearts with TGA and VSD, anomalous chordal attachments around the edges of conoventricular VSDs are even more common than in isolated VSD. These may complicate transatrial VSD closure and the construction of an intraventricular tunnel in the Rastelli operation.[H17]

The tricuspid leaflets can be redundant and dysplastic in TGA. Accessory tricuspid tissue may prolapse through the VSD and produce LVOTO (see "Left Ventricular Outflow Tract Obstruction" in previous text).

The tricuspid anulus may be dilated, resulting in some regurgitation, or in other cases the valve may be hypoplastic in association with underdevelopment of the RV sinus. Anular overriding or tensor straddling or both can occur, the latter being more common.[A19]

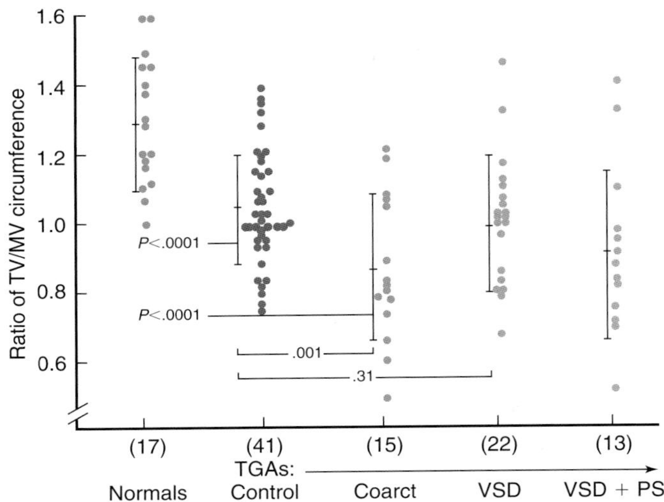

Figure 52-18 Ratio of tricuspid to mitral valve circumference in a series of autopsy hearts with transposition of great arteries *(TGA)* compared with 17 normal hearts. "Control" TGA specimens were those with a completely intact ventricular septum, with or without a small patent ductus arteriosus, atrial septal defect, or patent foramen ovale. Only unoperated specimens and those obtained within 30 days of an intracardiac repair are included. Vertical bars indicate one standard deviation. Individual *P* values are noted. Key: *Coarct,* Coarctation; *PS,* pulmonary stenosis; *TV/MV,* tricuspid to mitral valve; *VSD,* ventricular septal defect. (From Calder L: personal communication; 1984.)

Mitral Valve Anomalies

Important structural anomalies of the mitral valve are present in 20% to 30% of hearts with TGA,[A8,L5,M30,O5,R17] mostly in combination with a VSD, but the majority are not functionally important. There may be slight hypoplasia of the valve ring, often with clockwise rotation (viewed from LV apex). Mitral valve anomalies can be categorized into four groups as those affecting the:

1. Leaflets
2. Commissures
3. Chordae tendineae
4. Papillary muscles

The most important from a surgical standpoint are those of mitral valve overriding or straddling, in which the mitral valve leaflet is frequently also cleft.

Aortic Obstruction

Coexisting aortic obstruction can be discrete (coarctation or less often, interrupted aortic arch) or caused by distal arch hypoplasia. Rarely, it occurs when the ventricular septum is essentially intact, but it occurs in 7% to 10% of patients with TGA and VSD. This coexistence is more frequent when the VSD is juxtapulmonary and the pulmonary trunk is partly over the RV in association with rightward and anterior displacement of the infundibular septum and with some subaortic narrowing.[M27,S6] (Coarctation is also common in the Taussig-Bing type of double outlet right ventricle; see "Taussig-Bing Heart" under Morphology in Chapter 53.) The ductus usually also remains patent to the aorta below the coarctation (preductal coarctation).

Table 52-5 Associated Anomalies in Surgical Series of Patients with Transposition of the Great Arteries[a]

Anomaly	No.	% of 260
No associated anomaly	93	36
Ventricular septal defect:	126	49
Small	31	12
Moderate	30	12
Large	65	25
Multiple	19	7
Patent ductus arteriosus[b]:	37	14
Small[c]	21	8
Moderate	7	3
Large	9	4
Left ventricular outflow tract obstruction[d]:	67	26
Essentially intact ventricular septum	27	10
Ventricular septal defect	40	15
Tricuspid valve anomalies	10	4
Mitral valve anomalies	11	4
Coarctation (or interrupted arch)	11	4
Right ventricular hypoplasia:	8	3
Mild	7	3
Moderate	1	0.4
Large aortopulmonary collateral arteries[e]	1	0.4
Atrial situs inversus	1	0.4
Miscellaneous	4	1.5

[a]Data from series of 260 patients undergoing operation at GLH, 1964-1984. Totals are not cumulative.
[b]Status at time of intracardiac repair.
[c]Excludes 29 patients in whom small patent ductus arteriosus was only possibly present.
[d]Mild in 16, moderate in 20, severe in 31.
[e]Requiring closure.

When there is associated coarctation, underdevelopment of the RV sinus is more common and, as noted earlier, tricuspid-to-mitral anulus circumference is less than in other TGA subsets.

Right Aortic Arch

Right aortic arch occurs in about 5% of patients with TGA.[M4] It is more common when there is an associated VSD than when the ventricular septum is intact and when there is associated leftward juxtaposition of the atrial appendages.[M23]

Leftward Juxtaposition of Atrial Appendages

Leftward juxtaposition of the atrial appendages occurs in about 2.5% of patients with TGA coming to repair.[M23,U2,W16] It is associated with a higher than usual prevalence of important underdevelopment of the RV sinus. Bilateral conus and dextrocardia seem more common in TGA associated with leftward juxtaposition than in TGA generally.

Right Ventricular Hypoplasia

RV hypoplasia was found to some degree in 17% of the autopsy series of TGA reported by Riemenschneider and colleagues.[R14]

Other Anomalies

Rarely, TGA coexists with congenital valvar aortic stenosis,[L5] and very rarely with total anomalous pulmonary venous connection.[S2] TGA can also coexist with complete AV septal defect (see "Complete Atrioventricular Septal Defect" under Morphology in Chapter 34).

CLINICAL FEATURES AND DIAGNOSTIC CRITERIA

When the great arteries are transposed in hearts with AV concordant connection, systemic and pulmonary circulations are in parallel. Unless there is shunting between the two, this defect is incompatible with life for more than a short time. With this arrangement, pulmonary ($\dot{Q}p$) and systemic ($\dot{Q}s$) blood flow can vary independently, and shunting between the two circulations over more than very short periods must be equal in both directions, or eventually all the blood will be in one or the other circulation. Magnitude of bidirectional shunting is highly variable and is referred to as *degree of mixing*.

Symptoms and clinical presentation in patients with TGA depend in large part on degree of mixing between the two parallel circulatory circuits. When there is a high degree of mixing and large $\dot{Q}p$, arterial oxygen saturation (SaO_2) may be near normal, and unless there is pulmonary venous hypertension, symptoms are minimal. When mixing is minimal, SaO_2 is low and symptoms of hypoxia are severe. Adequate mixing can occur only when there are communications of reasonable size at atrial, ventricular, or great artery levels. With adequate-sized communications, mixing tends to be directly related to $\dot{Q}p$. Factors that reduce $\dot{Q}p$, such as LVOTO and increased Rp, reduce mixing and increase cyanosis.

Symptoms and clinical presentation also depend in part on left atrial and pulmonary venous pressure. When $\dot{Q}p$ is even moderately elevated, these pressures tend to become elevated and produce symptoms. Both LV and RV failure usually result.

Clinical features and diagnostic criteria of patients with TGA fall into three groups based on these criteria,[N5] as discussed in the text that follows.

Essentially Intact Ventricular Septum (Poor Mixing)

TGA with essentially intact ventricular septum includes infants without a VSD or with a VSD 3 mm or less in diameter. A patent foramen ovale or naturally occurring atrial septal defect (ASD) is usually present. Cyanosis is apparent in half these infants within the first hour of life and in 90% within the first day[L10] and is rapidly progressive. $\dot{Q}p$ is usually increased to a pulmonary-systemic blood flow ratio ($\dot{Q}p/\dot{Q}s$) of about 2, but because of poor mixing across the small communication, this does not alleviate hypoxia. The baby becomes critically ill with tachypnea and tachycardia and dies from hypoxia and acidosis without appearance of frank heart failure. This rapid downhill course is usually obviated with a naturally occurring ASD of adequate size, because cyanosis is less severe. In surviving infants, appearance of moderate or severe dynamic LVOTO is associated with increasing cyanosis and hypoxic spells even after an adequate atrial septostomy.[A17,T11,Y1]

Clinical signs in most newborns are unimpressive. Generally, patients are of average birth weight and in good general condition, although with severe cyanosis. Clubbing of fingers and toes is absent and generally does not appear unless the infant survives to about age 6 months. There is mild increase in heart and respiratory rates. The heart is not hyperactive, and the liver is barely palpable. A faint mid-systolic ejection-type murmur is present along the midleft sternal edge in less than half these infants. This murmur is more prominent with organic or dynamic LVOTO, first appearing at age 1 or 2 months with the dynamic form and then gradually increasing in intensity. The second heart sound is unremarkable (often apparently single or narrowly split), and the third heart sound and apical mid-diastolic flow murmur are both rare.

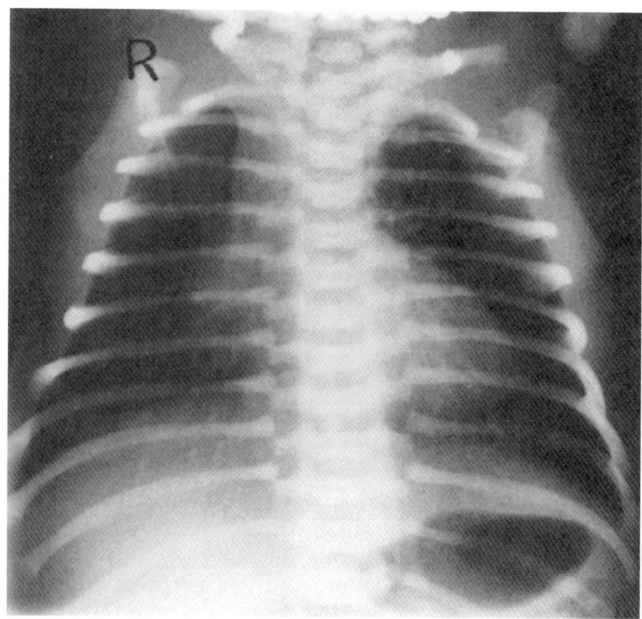

Figure 52-19 Chest radiograph of a 1-day-old neonate with transposition of great arteries and essentially intact ventricular septum, showing typical egg-shaped cardiac silhouette with a narrow superior mediastinum and mild pulmonary plethora.

Chest radiography (Fig. 52-19) has three characteristic features:

1. An oval- or egg-shaped cardiac silhouette with a narrow superior mediastinum
2. Mild cardiac enlargement
3. Moderate pulmonary plethora

In the first week of life, however, the chest radiograph may be normal; occasionally cardiac enlargement may be more marked. The narrow mediastinum is caused in part by the great artery positions and by shrinkage of the thymus, usually associated with stress,[N12] and the plethora is caused by the increase in $\dot{Q}p$. Plethora is less marked when there is important LVOTO.

The *electrocardiogram* (ECG) is often normal at birth, with the usual neonatal RV pattern. By the end of the first week, persistence of an upright T wave in the right precordial leads indicates abnormal RV hypertrophy, and right-axis deviation predominates. The *vectorcardiogram* shows a clockwise horizontal plane loop indicative of a near-normal LV systolic pressure and a dominant RV mass.[M6] When important

LVOTO is present or Rp is elevated, ECG evidence indicates biventricular hypertrophy.

Large Ventricular Septal Defect, Large Patent Ductus Arteriosus, or Both (Good Mixing)

Presentation in this TGA group generally occurs in the latter half of the first month, with mild cyanosis and signs of heart failure resulting from pulmonary venous hypertension and myocardial failure.[C14] Tachycardia, tachypnea, important liver enlargement, and moist lung bases are present. The heart is more active and usually larger than in the poor-mixing group.

A *large VSD* is associated with a moderate-intensity pansystolic murmur along the lower left sternal edge that may not be present initially. There is usually an apical mid-diastolic murmur or gallop rhythm and narrow splitting of the second heart sound with accentuation of the pulmonary component. With a *large PDA,* a continuous murmur, bounding pulses, and an apical mid-diastolic murmur are present in less than half the patients, even when the ventricular septum is intact.[W2] Sudden spontaneous closure of a large PDA when there is no VSD results in an increase in cyanosis (see Natural History later in this chapter).

Chest radiography may show more cardiomegaly, more plethora, and a wider superior mediastinum than in the poor-mixing group. Development of pulmonary vascular disease is associated with reduction in $\dot{Q}p$ and less plethora, particularly in the peripheral lung fields, as well as reduced heart size, but these features generally appear after the neonatal period.

The *ECG* shows biventricular hypertrophy and, when there is a persistent large VSD, a Q wave in V_6. Isolated LV hypertrophy is rare and suggests RV hypoplasia with tricuspid valve overriding.[R14]

When coarctation of the aorta coexists with VSD and PDA, femoral pulses are usually normal because the coarctation is preductal and ductus arteriosus large. Rarely, differential cyanosis can occur, with cyanosis confined to the upper torso. All patients with this combination present early in life in heart failure and respond poorly to decongestive treatment. Isolated LV hypertrophy may be present on ECG because of frequent association of coarctation with RV hypoplasia.[M27]

Large Ventricular Septal Defect and Left Ventricular Outflow Tract Obstruction (Poor Mixing without High Pulmonary Blood Flow)

Large VSD with LVOTO is the least common of the three TGA groups. LVOTO is associated with a decreased $\dot{Q}p$ and poor mixing, but pulmonary venous hypertension and associated symptoms and signs do not develop because of lack of increase in $\dot{Q}p$. Heart failure is therefore not present. Clinical findings are similar to those of tetralogy of Fallot with severe pulmonary stenosis or pulmonary atresia (see Clinical Features and Diagnostic Criteria in Section I of Chapter 38), and cyanosis is severe from birth. The heart is not overactive, and there is a pulmonary ejection murmur and often a single heart sound without an apical gallop or mid-diastolic murmur. Chest radiography shows a near normal–sized heart with normal or ischemic lung fields, and ECG shows biventricular hypertrophy.

Echocardiography

Definitive diagnosis of TGA can be made using two-dimensional (2D) echocardiography.[B28] Two-dimensional echocardiography is also particularly valuable in detecting tricuspid valve abnormalities, including overriding and straddling,[L1] and the varieties of subpulmonary stenosis, including dynamic obstruction.[C9,R15] Echocardiographic features of dynamic LVOTO include leftward deviation of the ventricular septum, abnormal fluttering and premature closure of the pulmonary valve, SAM of the mitral leaflet (about 50% of cases), and prolonged diastolic apposition of the anterior mitral valve leaflet to the septum.[A18,Y1] Echocardiography can also define with reasonable accuracy morphology of the coronary arteries, including number, origin, major branching pattern, and other features such as intramural course (Fig. 52-20).[P11] With two-reader methodology, the sensitivity of echocardiography to detect coronary variants is 86%, with a negative predictive value of 91% (Fig. 52-21).[G16]

Fetal echocardiography may be helpful in identifying abnormalities of the foramen ovale or ductus arteriosus, which is associated with neonatal hypoxia and death, and of the ventricular septum.[M1,T10] Fetal diagnosis may improve perinatal care[K18] and reduce perinatal mortality and postoperative morbidity.[B35]

Cardiac Catheterization

Cardiac catheterization and cineangiography are not performed routinely, particularly in neonates, with major reliance for diagnosis placed on echocardiography.[T19] Nonetheless, knowledge of the information from these studies remains important.

A full study includes calculation of $\dot{Q}p$ and $\dot{Q}s$ and pressures, including those across the LV outflow tract. Because of intracardiac communications in patients with TGA, the Fick method is usually the only practical way of measuring $\dot{Q}p$ and $\dot{Q}s$. Despite complexity of the circulation, standard calculations apply. Meticulous care is required in measuring oxygen consumption using a closed-box technique in infants. Equations are as follows:

$$\dot{Q}p = \frac{\dot{V}O_2}{CpvO_2 - CpaO_2}$$

$$\dot{Q}s = \frac{\dot{V}O_2}{CaO_2 - C\overline{v}O_2}$$

$$\dot{Q}ep = \frac{\dot{V}O_2}{CpvO_2 - C\overline{v}O_2}$$

where

$\dot{Q}p$ = Pulmonary blood flow
$\dot{V}O_2$ = Oxygen consumption, $mL \cdot min^{-1}$
$CpvO_2$ = Pulmonary venous oxygen content, $mL \cdot L^{-1}$
$CpaO_2$ = Pulmonary arterial oxygen content, $mL \cdot L^{-1}$
$\dot{Q}s$ = Systemic blood flow
CaO_2 = Systemic arterial oxygen content, $mL \cdot L^{-1}$
$C\overline{v}O_2$ = Mixed venous oxygen content, $mL \cdot L^{-1}$
$\dot{Q}ep$ = Effective pulmonary blood flow

$\dot{Q}ep$ represents flow of blood from the systemic to the pulmonary circuit at atrial, ventricular, and great arterial levels.

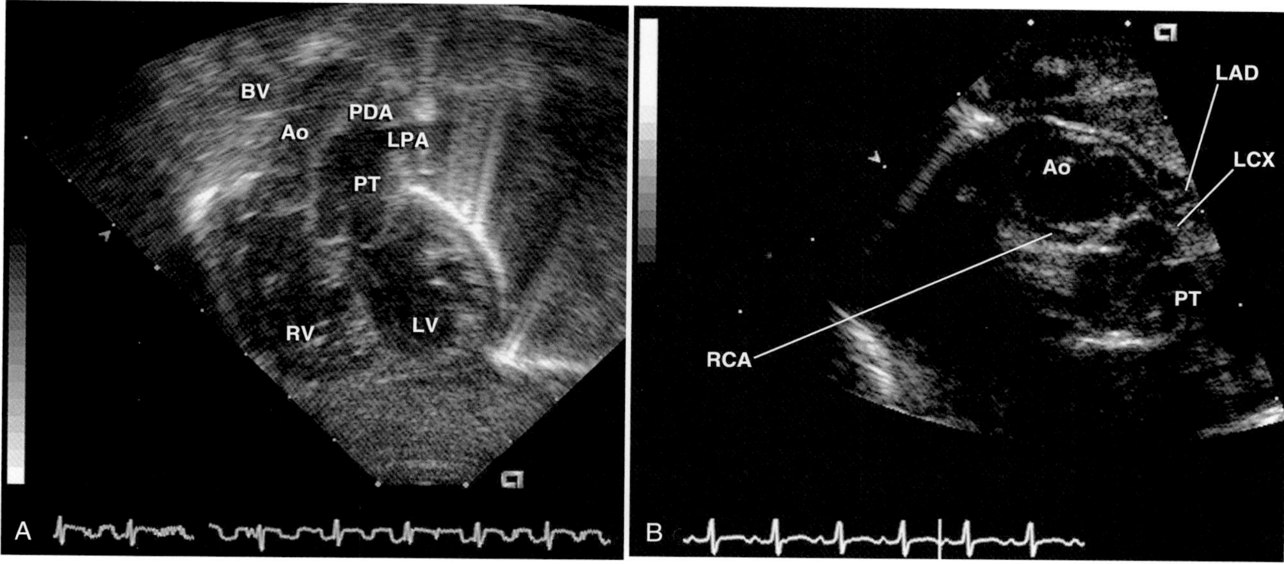

Figure 52-20 Echocardiographic findings in transposition of great arteries. **A,** Subcostal coronal view showing ventricular chambers and great arteries. Pulmonary trunk arises from left ventricle. Left pulmonary artery and ductus arteriosus are also visualized. Aorta arises from right ventricle, and aortic valve is somewhat more superior than pulmonary valve. **B,** Parasternal short-axis view showing two semilunar valves of approximately equal diameter, with aorta anterior and to right. Right coronary artery arises from sinus 1, and left main coronary artery, with its bifurcation into left anterior descending and circumflex arteries, arises from sinus 2. Key: *Ao,* Aorta; *BV,* brachiocephalic vein; *LAD,* left anterior descending coronary artery; *LCX,* left circumflex coronary artery; *LPA,* left pulmonary artery; *LV,* left ventricle; *PDA,* patent ductus arteriosus; *PT,* pulmonary trunk; *RCA,* right coronary artery; *RV,* right ventricle.

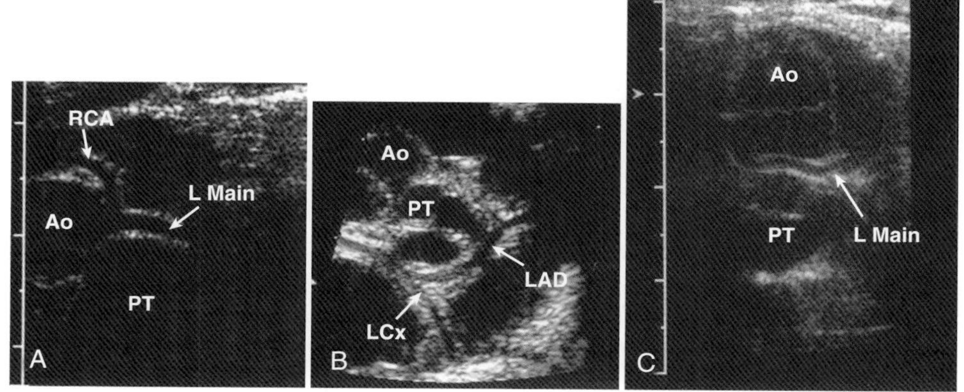

Figure 52-21 Parasternal short-axis echocardiographic views through aortic root showing coronary artery variants. **A,** Single left main coronary artery (LCA): right coronary artery *(RCA)* is first branch that passes anterior to aortic valve and to right, with left main coursing leftward and anterior to pulmonary valve trunk *(PT).* **B,** Single RCA: LCA is seen passing behind pulmonary trunk and bifurcating into left anterior descending artery *(LAD)* and left circumflex artery *(LCx).* **C,** Intramural LCA: there is significant displacement of orifice of LCA arising from right-facing sinus. Proximal LCA runs in wall of aortic root where there is double-border appearance of intramural segment. Key: *Ao,* Aorta; *L Main,* left main coronary artery.

Flow must be equal in the opposite direction (anatomic left-to-right shunt or effective systemic blood flow), or over time one circuit would be deprived of blood.

Inherent errors occur in measuring these flows. When $\dot{Q}p$ is high and therefore pulmonary arterial oxygen saturation ($SpaO_2$) is high, the Fick calculation tends to be inaccurate. This error may be compounded by difficulties in recovering a truly mixed $SpvO_2$. Fortunately, these errors are greatest in patients with a very high $\dot{Q}p$, when concern is minimal about a high Rp. Calculations are more accurate when the $\dot{Q}p$ is low and Rp correspondingly high. Potential for error exists if pulmonary arterial sampling is made proximal to site of entry of sizable systemic (bronchial) collaterals. Truly mixed $SpaO_2$ would then be lower than that measured, and $\dot{Q}p$ correspondingly lower,[L3] but in practice this situation is uncommon.

Thus, with careful technique, Rp in patients with TGA can be calculated with reasonable accuracy. A specific problem arises, however, if hematocrit is particularly high; viscosity of the blood increases sharply when hematocrit is greater than

60%. The effect of viscosity on $\dot{Q}p$ may then become important, and calculated Rp may be higher than that dictated by the pulmonary vascular bed alone.[M4] The only solution to this is to repeat the measurements after lowering the hematocrit by venisection.

$\dot{Q}ep$ is the flow upon which life depends. This flow is relatively fixed, typically only about 1.0 to 1.5 $L \cdot min^{-1} \cdot m^{-2}$. This places a major constraint on oxygen supply to the patient. These relationships become evident in rewriting the Fick equation as follows:

$$\begin{aligned} \dot{V}O_2 &= \dot{Q}ep\,(CpvO_2 - C\bar{v}O_2) \\ &= \dot{Q}ep\,(SpvO_2 - S\bar{v}O_2) \times Hb \times CmaxO_2 \end{aligned}$$

where

$SpvO_2$ = Pulmonary venous oxygen saturation
$S\bar{v}O_2$ = Mixed-venous oxygen saturation
$CmaxO_2$ = Oxygen capacity per gram of Hb
Hb = Hemoglobin concentration, $g \cdot L^{-1}$

On this basis, any reduction in hemoglobin will reduce oxygen uptake, and compensation for it is not possible in patients with TGA.[M9] If stress or exercise increases oxygen requirement, the difference in $CpvO_2$ and $C\bar{v}O_2$ must widen, and because $CpvO_2$ cannot increase, $C\bar{v}O_2$ (and thus tissue PO_2) must fall.

Cineangiography

Using appropriate views, cineangiography demonstrates the cardiac connections and great artery positions (Fig. 52-22), position and number of VSDs (Fig. 52-23), site of any LVOTO (Fig. 52-24), size and function of AV valves, size and function of both ventricles, pattern of the coronary arteries, and presence of other cardiac anomalies.

Computed Tomography and Magnetic Resonance Imaging

Although these newer modalities are more accurate than echocardiography in evaluating anatomy, particularly coronary anatomy, they are not routinely used in the neonate. Cardiac computed tomographic angiography (CTA) and image postprocessing with volume rendering can give an accurate diagnosis of the coronary pattern, even in neonates (Fig. 52-25). These modalities are used more frequently in postoperative patients in whom coronary imaging is indicated.

NATURAL HISTORY

Prevalence

TGA is a common form of congenital heart disease, occurring in 1:2100 to 1:4500 births[G17,L14] and accounting for 7% to 8% of all congenital heart disease. Prevalence might be reduced more than 50% by maternal preconceptional multivitamin use[B39] or may be reduced by avoiding pesticides during the first trimester.[L22] In the Auckland area of New Zealand, prevalence over a 10-year period was 1:2400, whereas in New England (U.S.), it was 1:4000[F12] ($P < .005$). Before the advent of effective treatment, at least 16% of deaths from congenital heart disease during childhood were caused by TGA.[L14]

Male-to-female ratio is 2:1. Male predominance increases to 3.3:1 when the ventricular septum is essentially intact and disappears in complex forms.[L14]

Survival

When patients with all varieties of TGA are considered, 55% survive 1 month, 15% survive 6 months, and only 10% survive 1 year (Fig. 52-26).[A5,K7,K8,L14,M29] Mean life expectancy is 0.65 year, rising to 4 years for those who survive to 12 months and to 6 years for the few who survive for 10 years. Thereafter, life expectancy declines rapidly (see Fig. 52-26).

Survival without treatment is different among subsets. It is particularly poor in untreated patients with *TGA and essentially intact ventricular septum*: 80% at 1 week but only 17% at 2 months and 4% at 1 year.[L14] Survival in this group is better when there is a true ASD (Fig. 52-27).

In patients with *TGA and important VSD*, early survival is higher: 91% at 1 month, 43% at 5 months, and 32% at 1 year.[L14] It is lower when the patient has a very large $\dot{Q}p$ (see Fig. 52-27). The combination of *large VSD and aortic obstruction* (coarctation, interrupted arch) is particularly lethal; all patients die within a few months of birth with severe heart failure. Paradoxically, obstructive pulmonary vascular disease in patients with TGA and VSD improves early survival to 40% at 1 year, but with rapid decline thereafter and none alive by age 5 years.

In patients with *TGA, VSD, and LVOTO*, early survival is still better, reaching 70% at 1 year and 29% at 5 years, because in many patients LVOTO is only moderate initially.

Leibman and colleagues found that PDA increased risk of early death in all subsets of patients.[L14] This is particularly the case when the ductus is large.

Modes of Death

Poor survival in patients with *TGA and essentially intact ventricular septum* is related primarily to hypoxia. Intercurrent pulmonary infections may develop and are particularly lethal because they reduce $\dot{Q}ep$ and lead rapidly to increasing hypoxia, acidemia, and death. Death in this group may also result from cerebrovascular events, usually caused by the polycythemia and increased blood viscosity secondary to severe cyanosis, particularly in association with dehydration. However, hypoxia plus hypochromic microcytic anemia has also been implicated in the etiology of these events.[P16] Nonfatal cerebrovascular events occur in about 6% of patients treated by BAS[P12] and include cerebral abscess.

Patients with *TGA and important VSD* usually die with heart failure. Modes of death described for patients with simple transposition sometimes pertain to this group as well and include frequent intercurrent pulmonary infections.

Hypoxia is the primary cause of morbidity and mortality in patients with *TGA, VSD, and LVOTO.*

Patent Ductus Arteriosus

PDA is present at age 1 week in about half the patients with TGA, but thereafter the prevalence falls rapidly.[P18] When patent, the ductus is small (<3 mm in diameter) in about two

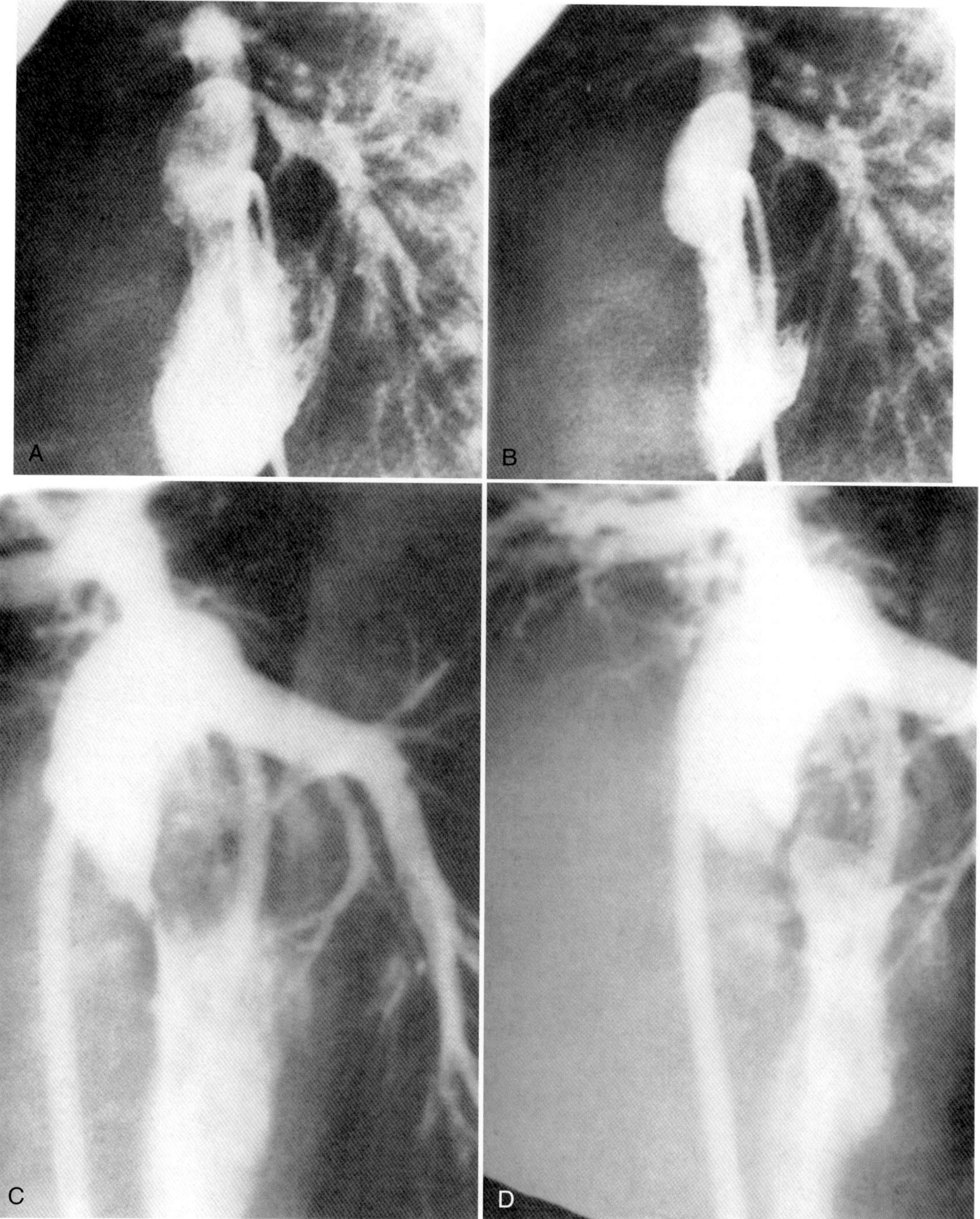

Figure 52-22 Cineangiograms of simple transposition of great arteries. **A-B,** Left ventricular injection, long axial view, in diastole and systole. Left ventricular outflow tract is widely open. Apparent narrowing at origin of left pulmonary artery is frequently seen and, as here, usually disappears during systole. **C-D,** Left ventricular injection, similar views and position, in another infant. Left ventricle gives origin to pulmonary trunk, and there is a long area of subpulmonary left ventricular outflow tract obstruction.

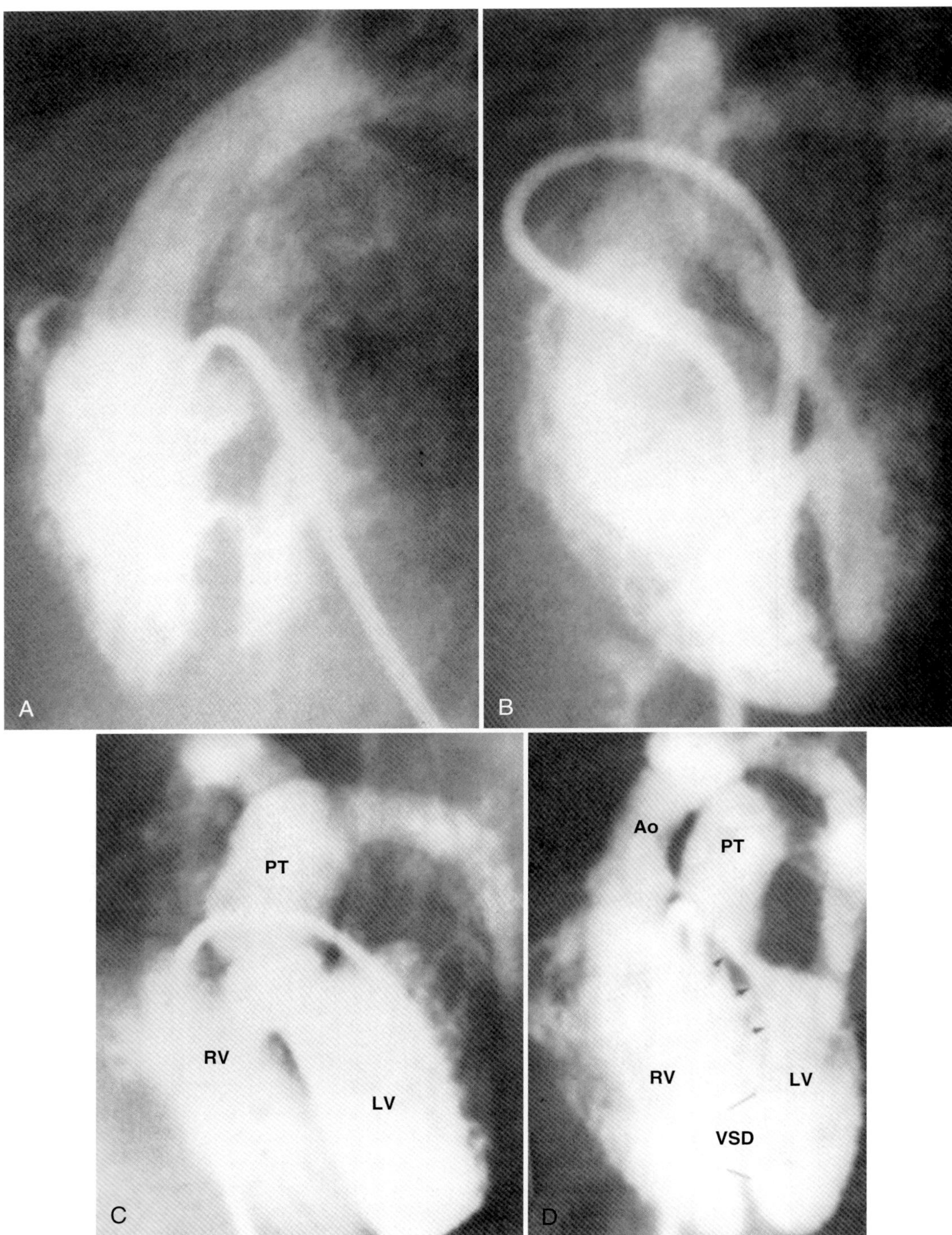

Figure 52-23 Cineangiograms of transposition of great arteries and ventricular septal defect *(VSD).* **A,** Small midmuscular VSD is demonstrated by right ventricular injection in long axial view. **B,** Large VSD in inflow portion of septum is demonstrated by right ventricular injection in four-chamber position. **C,** Large conoventricular VSD is shown with left ventricular ejection in long axial view. **D,** Multiple muscular VSDs are demonstrated with a right ventricular injection in long axial view. Key: *Ao,* Aorta; *LV,* left ventricle; *PT,* pulmonary trunk; *RV,* right ventricle.

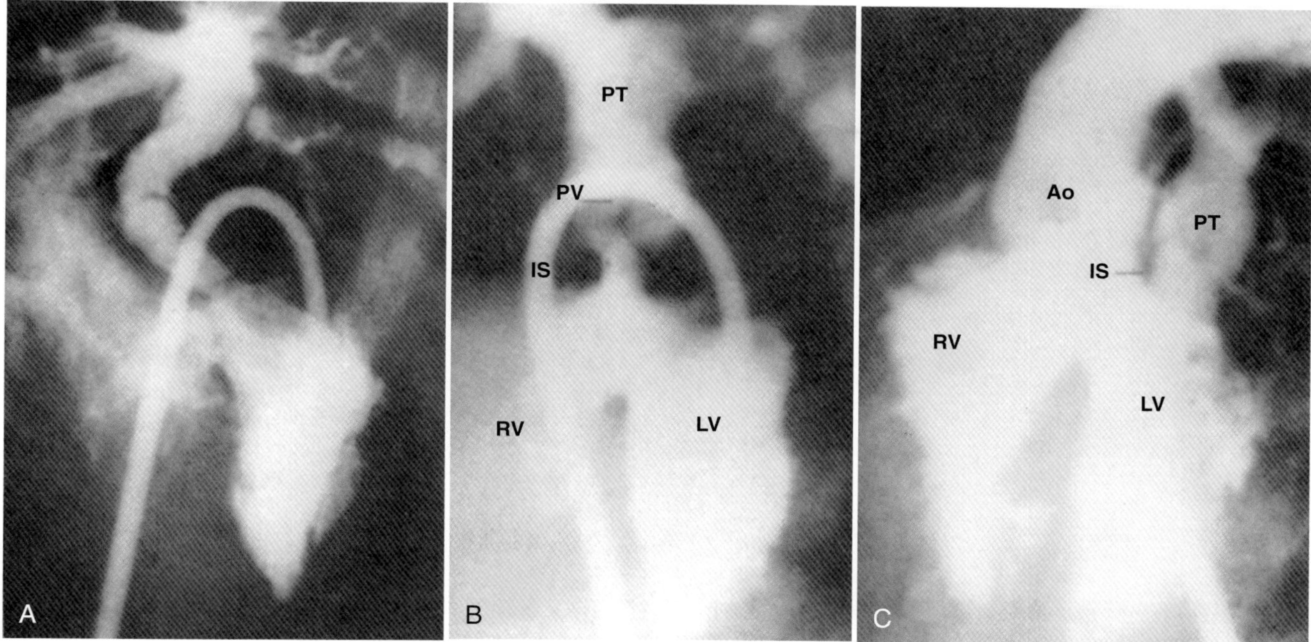

Figure 52-24 Cineangiograms of transposition of great arteries, ventricular septal defect (VSD), and left ventricular outflow tract obstruction (LVOTO). **A,** Subvalvar LVOTO is associated with large conoventricular VSD, as shown by left ventricular injection and four-chamber view. **B,** Long subvalvar LVOTO is associated with large conoventricular VSD, as shown by left ventricular injection and four-chamber view. **C,** Discrete subvalvar LVOTO with large VSD and mild overriding of aorta onto left ventricle, as shown by left ventricular injection and four-chamber view. Key: *Ao,* Aorta; *IS,* infundibular septum; *LV,* left ventricle; *PT,* pulmonary trunk; *PV,* pulmonary valve; *RV,* right ventricle.

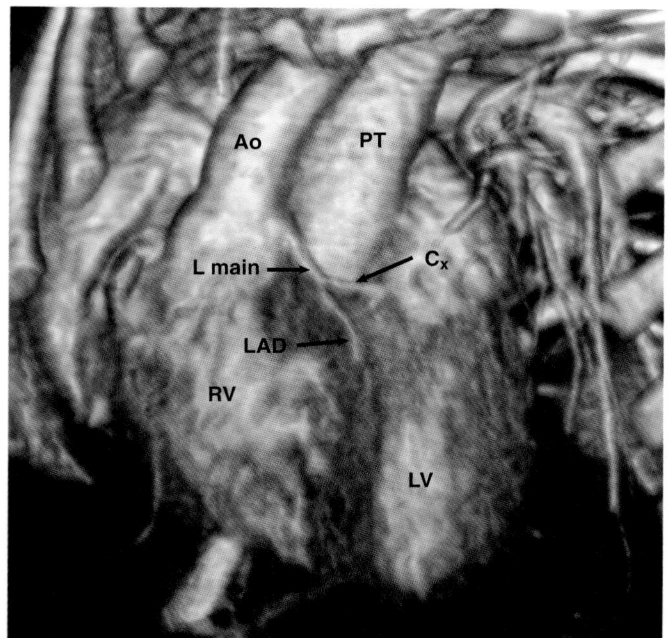

Figure 52-25 Computed tomography volume-rendered image showing left main coronary artery with left anterior descending and circumflex branches arising from left-facing sinus of Valsalva in infant with unrepaired S,D,D transposition of great arteries. Key: *Ao,* Aorta; *Cx,* circumflex coronary artery, *L Main,* left main coronary artery; *LAD,* left anterior descending coronary artery; *LV,* left ventricle *PT,* pulmonary trunk; *RV,* right ventricle.

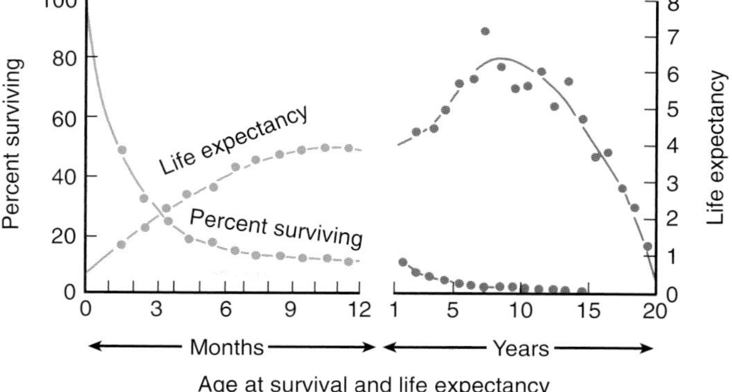

Figure 52-26 Survival and life expectancy of 655 children with transposition of great arteries (TGA) of all types, all of whom died between 1957 and 1964; 73 living children and 14 miscellaneous deaths are excluded. Group is impure in that about 15% of the total had either single ventricle, hypoplasia of left ventricle with mitral stenosis or atresia, or hypoplasia of right ventricle with tricuspid stenosis or atresia. However, trends are representative of patients with TGA. (From Liebman and colleagues.[L14])

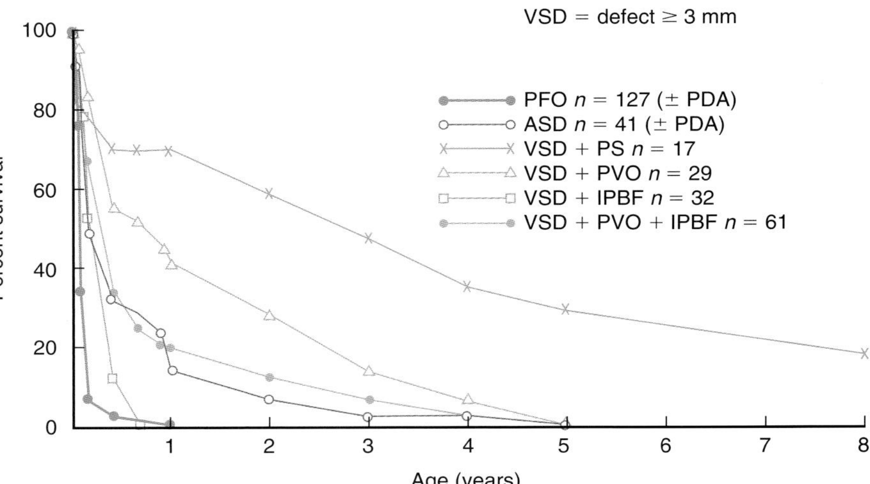

Figure 52-27 Survival of various subsets of patients with transposition of great arteries. Key: *ASD,* Atrial septal defect; *IPBF,* increased pulmonary blood flow; *PFO,* patent foramen ovale; *PS,* pulmonary stenosis; *PVO,* pulmonary vascular obstructive disease; *VSD,* ventricular septal defect. (From Liebman and colleagues.[L14])

thirds of patients and seems to have little influence on natural history.[L14] When it is large, LV output is increased and hypoxia lessens, but heart failure becomes more severe. Under these circumstances, acute and often early closure of the ductus results in sudden increase in hypoxia and clinical deterioration.[P18,W2] This is related not only to decreased mixing at the ductus level but also at the atrial level because of the fall in left atrial pressure that results from decreased pulmonary venous return.[W2]

Atrial Septal Defects

In patients with TGA, the patent foramen ovale tends to close at the usual rate. This is the major cause of the time-related increase in hypoxia and death in patients with TGA and essentially intact ventricular septum without an important PDA. A true ASD, on the other hand, remains unchanged in size and palliates the patient longer.[P18] The same is true for those rare examples of coexisting partial anomalous pulmonary venous connections.

Ventricular Septal Defects

Large VSDs close or narrow in probably a smaller proportion (≈20%) of patients with TGA than in patients with isolated VSD (see "Spontaneous Closure" under Natural History in Section I of Chapter 35). In most cases, however, the closing VSD is initially small and often muscular, and spontaneous closure has been documented to occur as late as the last part of the first decade of life.[P18] This process was rarely documented before the era of BAS, because so few patients survived beyond the first few months of life.[S13]

Left Ventricular Outflow Tract Obstruction

Dynamic LVOTO is not present at birth but can appear within several weeks. It gradually progresses in severity. Awareness of this tendency has increased since the era of BAS, after which LVOTO frequently develops. When dynamic LVOTO becomes important, hypoxia returns and life expectancy is shortened. LVOTO develops infrequently in patients with TGA and important VSD.

Pulmonary Vascular Disease

When TGA occurs as an isolated lesion *(simple TGA)*, pulmonary vascular disease rarely develops in the first few months of life. After about 6 to 24 months, however, its prevalence increases to 10% to 30%.[C16,E3,F1,F4,L3,N8] Its development reduces $\dot{Q}p$ and increases hypoxia.

In patients with TGA and moderate or large VSD, pulmonary vascular disease develops more rapidly than in patients with simple TGA, as it does in those with persistently large PDA. Among those dying at about age 6 months, 25% have developed severe pulmonary vascular disease (≥grade 3), and 50% of infants dying by age 12 months have developed it. These prevalences are much higher than in patients with primary VSD, and mechanisms may include hypoxemia and a prominent bronchopulmonary collateral circulation.[A20,F3,L3,N7,V10,W1]

Increased Blood Flow to Right Lung

At birth in TGA, as in normal patients, slightly more blood flows to the right lung than to the left. In contrast to normal flow, however, flow to the right lung in TGA increases as age increases.[M40,R1,V8] In addition to age, magnitude of the increase is affected by the angle between takeoff of the right pulmonary artery and pulmonary trunk; the wider this angle (and thus the more the pulmonary trunk faces directly into the right pulmonary artery), the greater the blood flow to the right lung. The tendency of infants with intact ventricular septum to develop dynamic LVOTO after the first few months increases the velocity of flow, which increases the momentum effect toward the more directly aligned vessel.

Once right lung flow increases, the right vascular bed grows more and there is a relative increase in Rp and reduced compliance in the left lung, which further reduces left lung flow. It is unlikely that this phenomenon importantly affects the natural history of untreated TGA.

TECHNIQUE OF OPERATION

Currently, the arterial switch operation is advised for most patients with TGA except those with important fixed LVOTO.

An atrial switch operation (Mustard or Senning type) may be appropriate rarely, and in highly selected patients. Patients with poor mixing, typically those with intact ventricular septum and a small ASD, come to the operating room receiving an infusion of prostaglandin E_1 and usually having had BAS.[L4] In current cardiology practice, septostomy is performed through transvenous access using echocardiographic guidance.[J1] These preoperative maneuvers usually result in adequate mixing and a stable patient.

Arterial Switch Operation

Simple Transposition of the Great Arteries with Usual Great Artery and Coronary Patterns

Preparation of the patient for operation, anesthesia, placement of monitoring devices, and details of the median sternotomy and initial dissection are the same as in other operations in neonates and young infants (see "Preparation for Cardiopulmonary Bypass" in Section III of Chapter 2). Positioning of the baby with extension of the neck is particularly important for exposure of the great arteries. Three general types of support systems are in use for arterial switch operation:

1. *Continuous CPB*, usually at 18° to 25°C, with reduced flow rate after reaching the target temperature. In some centers, mild hypothermia or normothermia is used. The IVC and superior venae cavae (SVC) are cannulated directly for venous return.
2. *Near-continuous CPB* at 18° to 20°C and with reduced flow rates (0.5 to 10 $L \cdot min^{-1} \cdot m^{-2}$), but with a single venous cannula inserted through the right atrial appendage (see Sections III and IV in Chapter 2). Hypothermic circulatory arrest is established only for closure of the ASD, which is done through the opening in the tip of the right atrium or a small right atriotomy after removing the venous cannula. After this closure, the venous cannula is reinserted, CPB reinstituted, and full flow restored for rewarming of the patient.
3. Operation primarily is performed during hypothermic circulatory arrest after the patient has been cooled to 18°C by CPB, with rewarming also accomplished by CPB.

Preference for these methods is in the order presented.

Myocardial management is also variable among institutions achieving good results. A prevalent method is infusion into the aortic root through a large-bore needle of a cold, hyperkalemic, sanguineous solution just after clamping the ascending aorta, and no more. Another method is use of the same protocol but with an asanguineous cardioplegic solution.

The aorta and pulmonary trunk must be dissected apart and the ductus arteriosus dissected. The right and left pulmonary arteries are extensively mobilized to their lobar branches and beyond if needed. As much of this as convenient is performed before CPB, but it may be necessary to complete these steps after CPB is established. The aortic purse-string stitch is placed as far downstream as possible to facilitate work on the aortic root and ascending aorta (Fig. 52-28, *A*). When using two venous cannulae, purse-string sutures are placed in the superior and inferior venae cavae as they enter the right atrium. A suture ligature is placed around the aortic end of the ductus (see Fig. 52-28, *A*) Another purse-string stitch is placed in the right superior pulmonary vein as it enters the left atrium (not shown in Fig. 52-28, *A*).

After cannulation is completed, CPB is established and cooling begun. Another suture ligature is placed around the pulmonary end of the ductus and the ductus divided. If the two venae cavae have been directly cannulated, adjustable snares are placed around them and tightened, and a small (13F) angled vent catheter is placed through the purse string in the right superior pulmonary vein, positioning its tip across the mitral valve into the LV. The cardioplegic infusion needle is inserted, the aorta clamped, and infusion given.

The aorta is transected and better exposure is obtained by turning back the proximal segment to facilitate further dissecting apart the great arteries (Fig. 52-28, *B*). The pulmonary trunk is transected just proximal to its bifurcation (Fig. 52-28, *C*). The aortic button around the orifice of the LCA is excised from its sinus, and this is inserted into the left-facing sinus of the neoaorta (originally, pulmonary trunk). The aortic button around the orifice of the right coronary artery is excised and inserted into the right-facing sinus of the neoaorta (Fig. 52-28, *B-D*).

After the Lecompte maneuver (Fig. 52-28, *E*), the neoaorta is constructed by anastomosing the proximal segment of the original pulmonary trunk to the distal aortic segment.

The stretched or torn foramen ovale (or ASD) is closed through an incision in the right atrium, usually with a running stitch. A patch may be used if the ASD is large. The right atrium is closed.

Separate autologous pericardial patches are used to fill in the defects in the proximal neopulmonary trunk. The neopulmonary trunk is then constructed (Fig. 52-28, *F*). All the latter steps involving pulmonary trunk reconstruction may be completed before removing the aortic clamp and beginning reperfusion of the heart, or reperfusion may be started at any point along the way.

A polyvinyl catheter is brought out from the left atrium through the right superior pulmonary vein or left atrial appendage if not already placed, and later, one is brought out from the right atrium. After the neonate has been rewarmed by the perfusate and proper conditions are in place, CPB is discontinued, and the remainder of operation is performed as detailed earlier (see "Completing Cardiopulmonary Bypass" in Section III of Chapter 2). Use of intraoperative echocardiography to assess global and, especially, regional ventricular function is helpful in assessing adequacy of coronary translocation.[S15]

Simple Transposition of the Great Arteries with Origin of Circumflex Coronary Artery from Sinus 2

At times, the Cx coronary artery arises as a branch of the RCA, the ostium of which is in sinus 2 (right-facing sinus). The Cx artery then passes leftward behind the pulmonary trunk and arborizes in the usual fashion (Fig. 52-29, *A*). Less often the LCA arises from sinus 2 (an RCA from sinus 1) and passes leftward behind the pulmonary trunk to bifurcate in the usual manner. In both situations, particular care is required in the transfer of this coronary button from sinus 2.

Operation proceeds in the manner just described until the button of aorta containing the ostium of RCA and Cx has been excised from sinus 2. A trap door opening is made in the right-facing sinus of the proximal neoaorta, cutting this

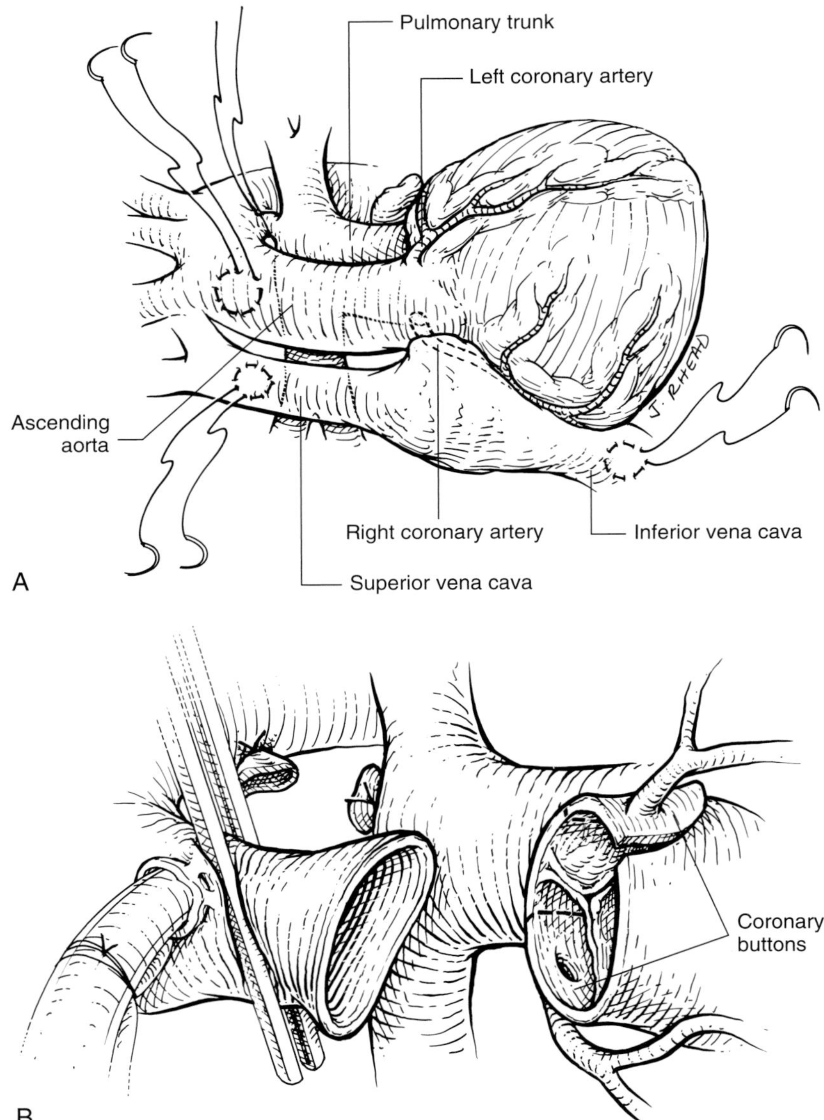

Figure 52-28 Arterial switch operation for transposition of great arteries, with aorta anterior and rightward, and usual coronary artery pattern (1LCx-2R). **A,** Placement of cardiopulmonary bypass (CPB) purse strings is shown in a patient who will undergo operation using continuous bypass and bicaval cannulation. Note that aortic purse string is placed as high on ascending aorta as possible to provide room for great artery manipulation. Venous purse strings are placed directly into superior and inferior venae cavae. A suture ligature has been placed around aortic end of ductus arteriosus. Tissue between great arteries is dissected prior to establishing CPB. A helpful maneuver is to place marking sutures on neoaorta for identifying sites of coronary implantation. Left and right branch pulmonary arteries are mobilized into first-order branching vessels. Cannulation proceeds in standard fashion and ductus arteriosus is immediately ligated. A separate suture ligature is placed on pulmonary artery end of ductus arteriosus and tied, and ductus is transected. A separate purse-string suture is placed in right upper pulmonary vein as it enters left atrium, and a vent catheter is introduced through purse string into left atrium, across mitral valve, and positioned into left ventricle (vent is not shown in this figure). **B,** After target core temperature is achieved, aorta is clamped and cardioplegia introduced into aortic root by one of standard methods. The aorta is transected just above sinutubular junction, and coronary arteries are carefully examined to confirm their positions and to rule out possibility of any unusual variations, such as eccentric coronary ostia or intramural coronary arteries. Using sharp dissection with fine scissors, coronary arteries are removed from their sinuses with at least a 1- to 2-mm cuff of sinus tissue surrounding ostia. Ligated and divided ductus arteriosus is also shown.

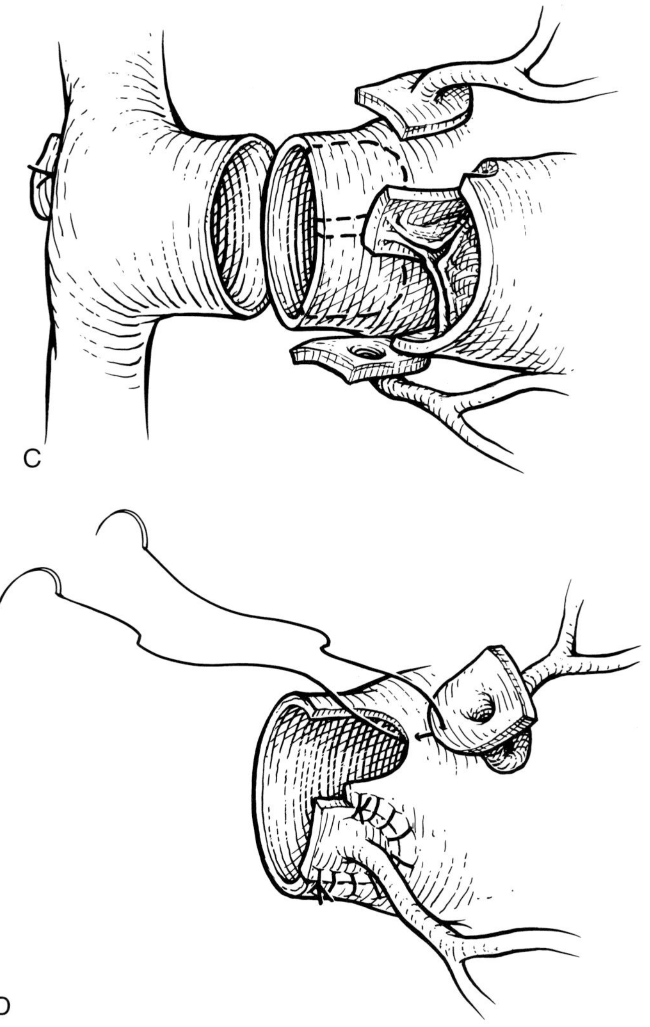

Figure 52-28, cont'd **C,** Coronary buttons have been completely mobilized. Pulmonary trunk is transected at its midportion and sites of coronary implantation (with help of marking sutures, if present) are identified on proximal neoaorta *(dashed lines)*. Various techniques can be used to prepare implantation sites. Most common variation is shown here, in which implantation site is prepared by removing a horseshoe-shaped segment of pulmonary trunk wall. Implantation sites can also be prepared with a simple incision (slit) without resection of any proximal neoaortic tissue. **D,** Coronary implantation is performed sequentially using a running 8-0 or 7-0 monofilament suture. Following implantation, it is important to visualize course of coronary artery and, if any doubt remains as to its patency, a 1- to 1.5-mm probe is passed into its proximal portion to demonstrate patency.

Continued

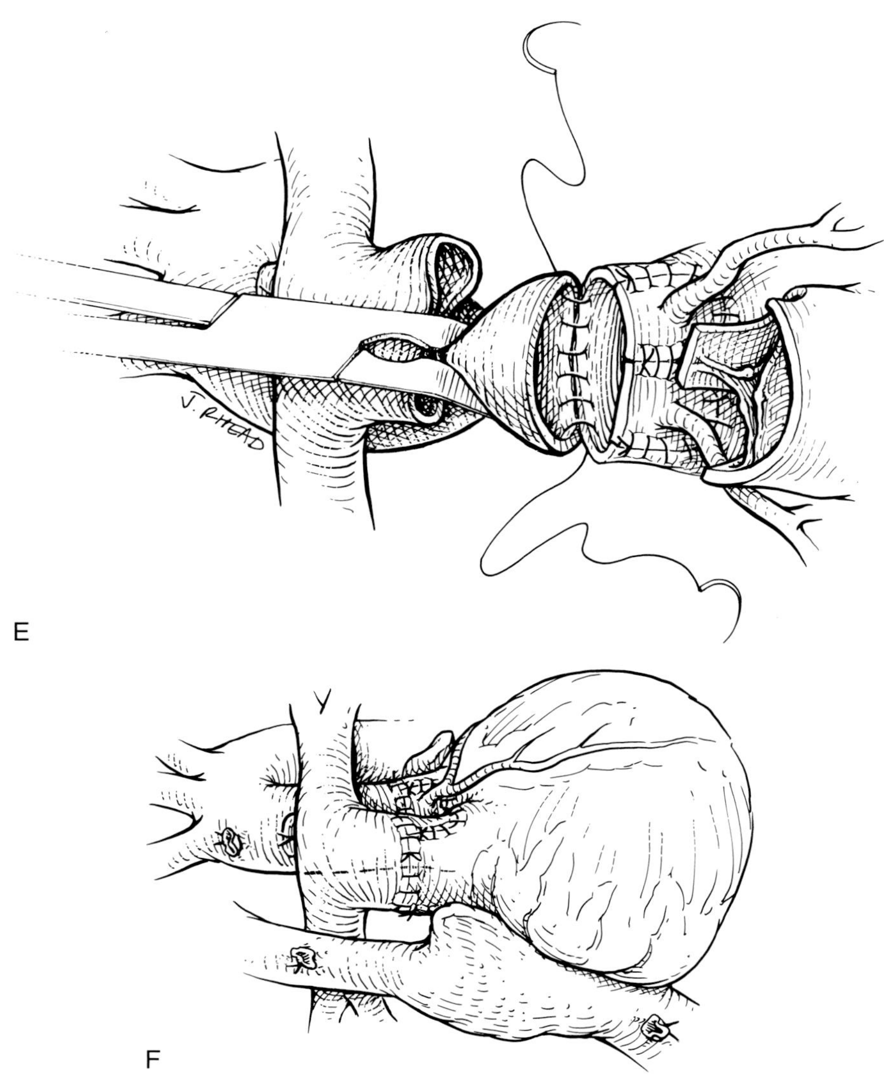

Figure 52-28, cont'd **E,** Coronary arteries are fully implanted. Lecompte maneuver has been performed, as indicated by branch pulmonary arteries now located anterior to aorta. Anastomosis between proximal neoaorta and ascending aorta is performed end to end using a running 7-0 monofilament suture technique. After completing aortic anastomosis, coronary explantation sites on proximal neopulmonary trunk are reconstructed with individual patches of glutaraldehyde-treated autologous pericardium. Individual pericardial patches are tailored to be slightly larger than defects that resulted from coronary explantations. Proximal neopulmonary trunk is then connected to distal pulmonary trunk, end to end, using a running monofilament 7-0 suture technique. **F,** Completed great artery reconstruction is shown, along with closed CPB cannulation sites. Careful examination of proximal coronary arteries and their relation to anteriorly positioned pulmonary trunk and pericardial patches is routinely performed to ensure coronary arteries are not distorted or compressed. (Atrial septal defect [ASD] is closed using standard technique as described in text. ASD can be closed at any point in procedure. The common technique used with continuous CPB is to close ASD after aortic reconstruction is complete, but before embarking on pulmonary trunk reconstruction. In this way, ASD is closed with the aortic clamp still in place, aiding intracardiac visualization. Aortic clamp is then removed prior to performing pulmonary trunk reconstruction, minimizing myocardial ischemia time.)

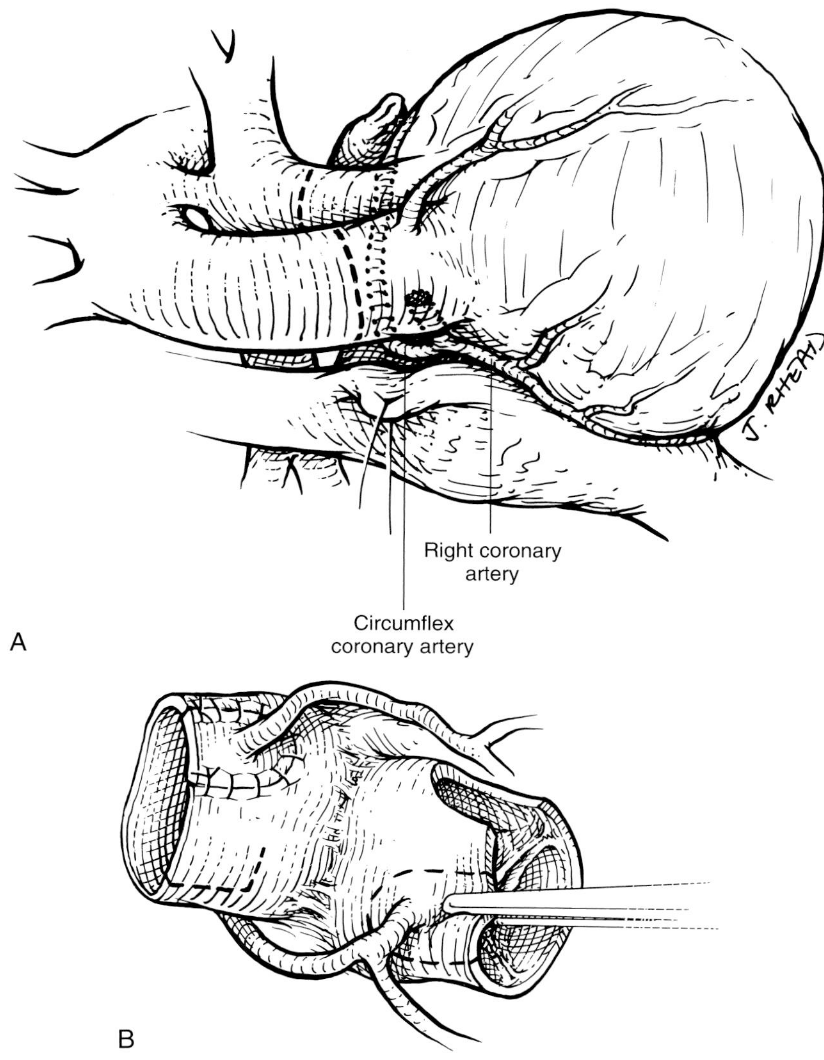

Figure 52-29 Arterial switch operation for transposition of great arteries in patients with second most common coronary artery pattern (1L-2RCx). **A,** Aorta is anterior and slightly to right, as in the usual case. Proposed site of pulmonary trunk transection is as far distal as possible, just before bifurcation, to provide a proper implantation site on proximal neoaorta (native pulmonary trunk) for coronary button from sinus 2. Proposed aortic transection site is slightly more distal than in the case with most common coronary pattern (see Fig. 52-28), to accommodate slightly shorter distal pulmonary trunk segment at time of pulmonary reconstruction. Dashed lines show proposed transected sites of great arteries. Note circumflex coronary artery passing posterior and to left behind great arteries to distribute to its normal myocardial area. **B,** Using standard cardiopulmonary bypass and myocardial protection techniques, operation proceeds in standard fashion until it is necessary to reimplant coronary button from sinus 2. Coronary from sinus 1 has been reimplanted in standard fashion (see Fig. 52-28). Proximal neopulmonary trunk is retracted anteriorly, and tissue between the two great arteries at their bases is fully dissected. Dashed line shows proposed incision to create "trapdoor" flap that serves to orient sinus 2 coronary button after reimplantation such that circumflex artery is neither kinked nor stretched. Because pulmonary trunk was transected as distally as possible, reimplanted coronary also is positioned more cephalad than in usual case. This also minimizes chance of circumflex artery kinking.

Continued

down from the original transection (Fig. 52-29, *B*).[B45] The coronary button from sinus 2 is sutured into place with the same technique as described earlier (Fig. 52-29, *C* and *D*). If a trap door is not used, and the entire ostium containing the RCA and Cx is implanted too far laterally on the circumference of the proximal neoaorta, kinking of the Cx can occur.

Alternatively, a pericardial hood augmentation of the coronary button–to–neoaortic anastomosis can achieve the same result and may be advantageous in situations where the trap door is likely to distort the commissures.[P9]

Simple Transposition of the Great Arteries with Origin of All Coronary Arteries from Sinus 2

When all three major coronary arteries arise from sinus 2, they usually do so from a single ostium (see "Coronary Arteries" under Morphology earlier in this chapter). Operation is performed in the same general manner as described in the preceding text for patients in whom the Cx arises as a branch from the RCA arising from sinus 2.

When all three branches pass to the right and none passes leftward behind the pulmonary trunk, implantation can be into a simple incision in the center of the right-facing sinus.

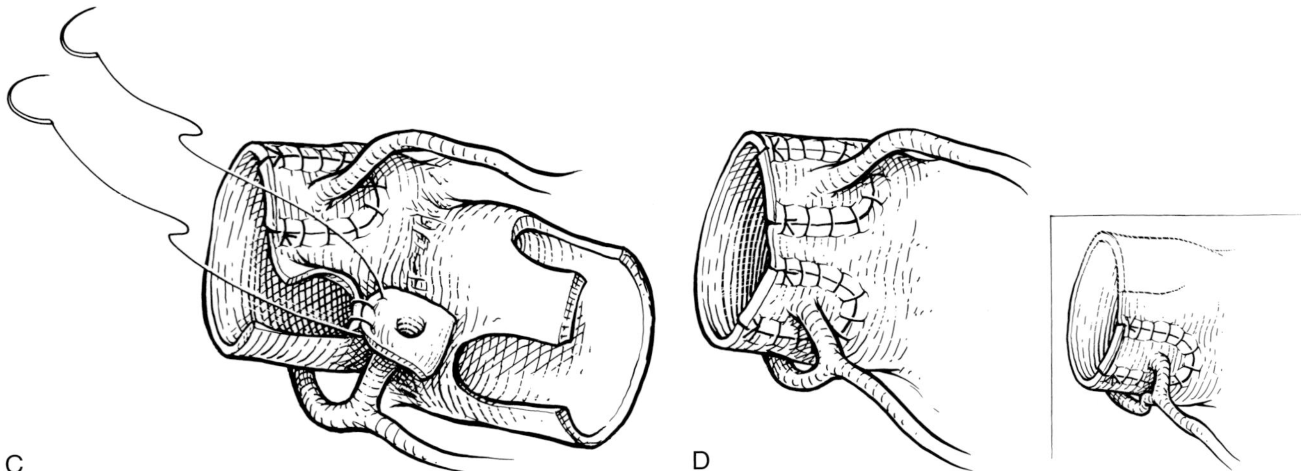

Figure 52-29, cont'd **C,** Coronary button from sinus 2 is sutured into place utilizing "trapdoor" flap. **D,** Trapdoor flap implantation is completed. Note smooth course of circumflex artery passing posterior and to left around great arteries. Inset shows a redundant and kinked circumflex artery that may result from implantation of coronary button too far to right-lateral aspect of circumference of proximal neoaorta. When coronary button is poorly positioned in this manner, in combination with orientation of button that results without using trapdoor flap, circumflex artery is at high risk for obstruction. Other factors that increase likelihood of circumflex artery kinking are placing button too proximally on neoaorta, and inappropriate rotation of coronary button during implantation.

When all three major coronary arteries arise from sinus 2, they may arise infrequently from two ostia, one of which is eccentrically located very near the valve commissure between sinus 2 and sinus 1 (Fig. 52-30, *A*). The LCA or only the LAD typically passes directly forward intramurally within the wall of the aorta. Unless forewarned, the surgeon may not recognize this from external examination after sternotomy, identifying it only after transecting the aorta and examining the interior of the aortic sinuses.

Several techniques have been used successfully to manage this problem.[A15,A16,T2] One involves taking down the adjacent aortic (neopulmonary) valvar commissure (Fig. 52-30, *B*), which is resuspended subsequently on the pericardial patch used for neopulmonary trunk reconstruction. Separate aortic buttons are excised around each orifice, taking pains to include the entire intramural course of the LCA (Fig. 52-30, *B* and *C*). The buttons are inserted into the proximal neoaortic segment in more or less the usual manner. In another technique (Fig. 52-30, *D-F*), both orifices are included in a single aortic button, which is inserted into the proximal neoaortic segment by a special technique that minimizes rotation of the button.

Suzuki provides an excellent summary of different techniques of coronary transfer during the arterial switch operation.[S30]

Transposition of the Great Arteries with More or Less Side-by-Side Great Arteries

The great arteries may be more or less side by side with the aorta to the right, and usually a VSD is present or the cardiac malformation is double outlet right ventricle with juxtapulmonary VSD (Taussig-Bing heart; see "Taussig-Bing Heart" under Morphology in Chapter 53). Prevalence of the various coronary artery patterns is different in this setting, one of the most common being sinus 1LR-2Cx.

Operation is conveniently performed in a somewhat different manner and without the Lecompte maneuver (Fig. 52-31), although some perform the Lecompte maneuver even in this setting. Exact details of configuration and sizes of the great arteries and coronary artery positions may determine advisability of the Lecompte maneuver when more or less side-by-side great arteries are present.

Repair of Coexisting Ventricular Septal Defect

The VSD is repaired with a patch of polyester, polytetrafluoroethylene (PTFE), or autologous pericardium, with due regard for location of the conduction system (see Technique of Operation in Section I of Chapter 35). Approach may be through the right atrium, although for some VSDs access is easier through the proximal aortic (neopulmonary) segment or pulmonary (neoaortic) segment (see "Repair of Taussig-Bing Heart by Arterial Switch Repair" under Technique of Operation in Chapter 53).

Other Techniques

As in most procedures, other techniques are suitable for performing all or parts of the arterial switch operation. In one approach, after transecting the great arteries, the aortic buttons containing the coronary ostia are excised from the proximal aortic segment. Three fine sutures are placed externally on the proximal segment of the neoaorta to mark the site of each valve commissure. The Lecompte maneuver is performed, and the two aortic segments are anastomosed to each other to construct the neoaorta.[B40,P1] The aortic clamp is released momentarily and hemostasis secured. With the clamp open and with due regard for position of commissural marking sutures, sites for implanting the coronary arteries are selected. With aorta again clamped, incisions are made, and the coronary buttons are transferred to the neoaorta. The final steps are closure of the sites from which the coronary buttons were excised and construction of the neopulmonary artery. This method facilitates obtaining hemostasis of the neoaortic anastomosis by examining the suture line after releasing the aortic clamp momentarily and placing any needed additional stitches at that time. Also, the proximal neoaorta is distended, facilitating selection of the site for

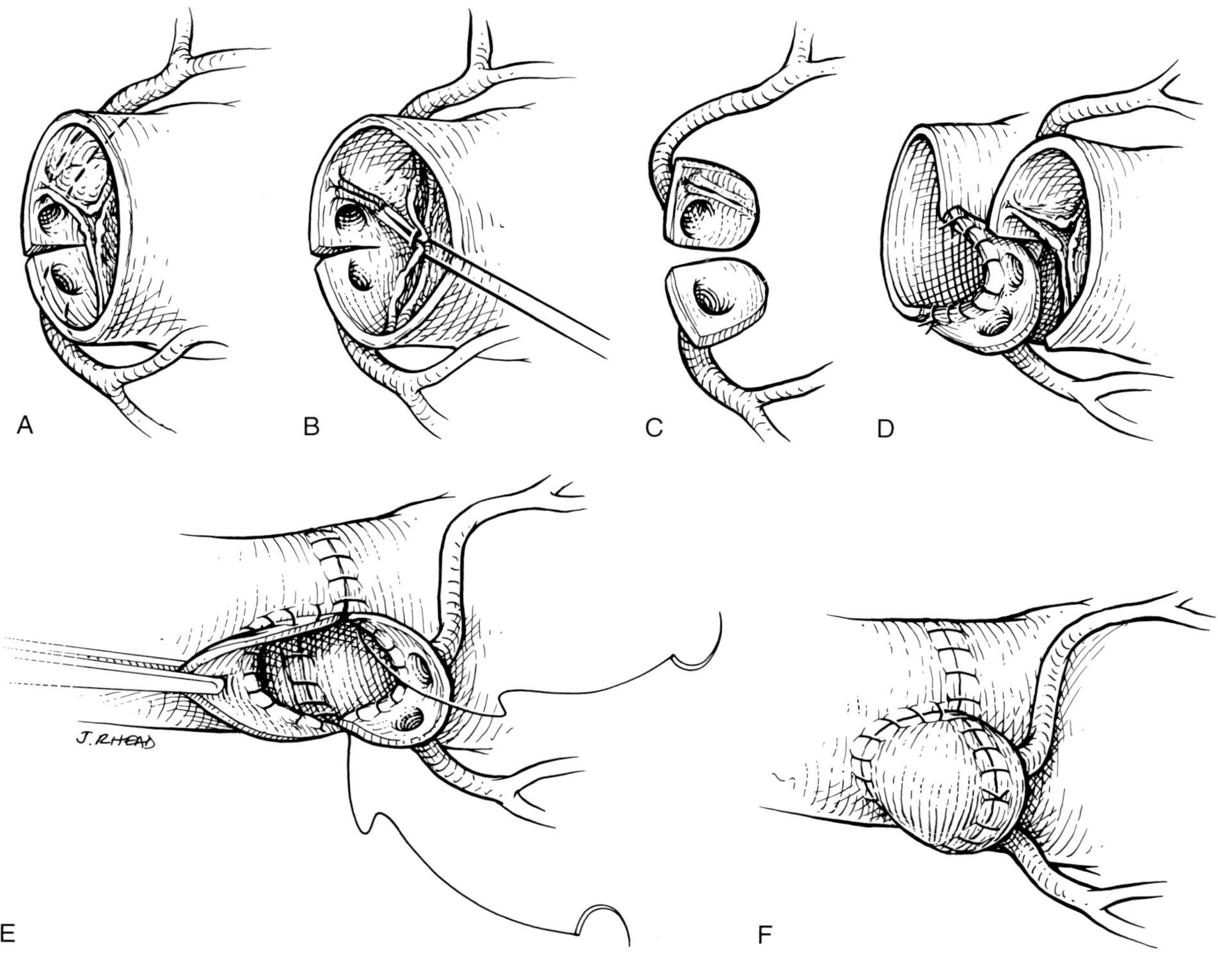

Figure 52-30 Arterial switch operation for transposition of great arteries when all three major coronary arteries arise from sinus 2. In this figure, there are two separate ostia within sinus 2, with an eccentrically placed left main coronary ostium with an intramural left main coronary artery (LCA) course. **A,** Although LCA gives rise to left anterior descending (LAD) and circumflex (Cx) coronary arteries and appears from exterior inspection to be arising from sinus 1, it actually arises from sinus 2 from an eccentrically placed orifice that is distinct from nearby right coronary orifice. LCA orifice is positioned close to commissure between cusps of the two facing sinuses. Proximal aspect of LCA travels circumferentially within wall (intramurally) of neoaorta before emerging from aortic wall to become distinctly separate from it in region of left-facing sinus. Intramural component involves region of commissure between the two cusps of facing sinuses. Several important judgments must be made with this coronary pattern. First, it must be decided whether there is enough tissue separating the two ostia to be able to mobilize coronaries separately. If so, preferred method of management is to mobilize the two coronary buttons separately as shown here. **B,** The second important judgment involves managing intramural component of LCA. Right coronary button is mobilized in standard fashion. If commissure between cusps of two facing sinuses is involved with the intramural component of the LCA, then commissure is stripped away from internal aspect of sinus as shown here, leaving cusps and commissure intact. This then allows for complete mobilization of eccentrically shaped left coronary button. Eccentric shape is necessary for button to contain entire intramural component of LCA. **C,** Two completely mobilized coronary buttons are shown with remnants of commissure present on left coronary button. Each button is then reimplanted in the usual fashion. **D,** If it is determined that the bridge of tissue between the two coronary ostia is either too narrow to allow separating them or is nonexistent (true single ostium), an alternative technique of coronary implantation must be used. Shown here are separate ostia too close together to allow safe mobilization of separate buttons. Also, neither ostia shows an intramural course. In this setting, a single large button encompassing both ostia is mobilized. Proximal neoaorta is prepared for reimplantation by removing an appropriately sized segment of neoaortic wall. Distal aspect of coronary button is then sutured to implantation site. Note that coronary button is rotated minimally. **E,** Proximal neoaorta to ascending aorta anastomosis is performed, completing entire circumference except for that portion that contains coronary button. A small hemisphere-shaped segment of ascending aorta is excised in portion of ascending aorta adjacent to implanted coronary button. A roof of either glutaraldehyde-treated pericardium or pulmonary allograft arterial wall is used to create a convex roof over remaining opening in ascending aorta and remainder of free edge of coronary button. **F,** Completed aortic and coronary reconstruction. Pulmonary trunk reconstruction is performed as usual.

implanting the coronary arteries and creating incisions for receiving them.

In another alternative, the coronary buttons are implanted into incisions made proximal to the transection site. Before creating the neoaortic-aortic anastomosis, incisions into which the coronary buttons will be transferred are made, and the lower halves of the circumference of the buttons are anastomosed into this incision. The upper half is incorporated into the neoaortic-aortic anastomosis, which is made as the next step.[C4] This method puts sites of

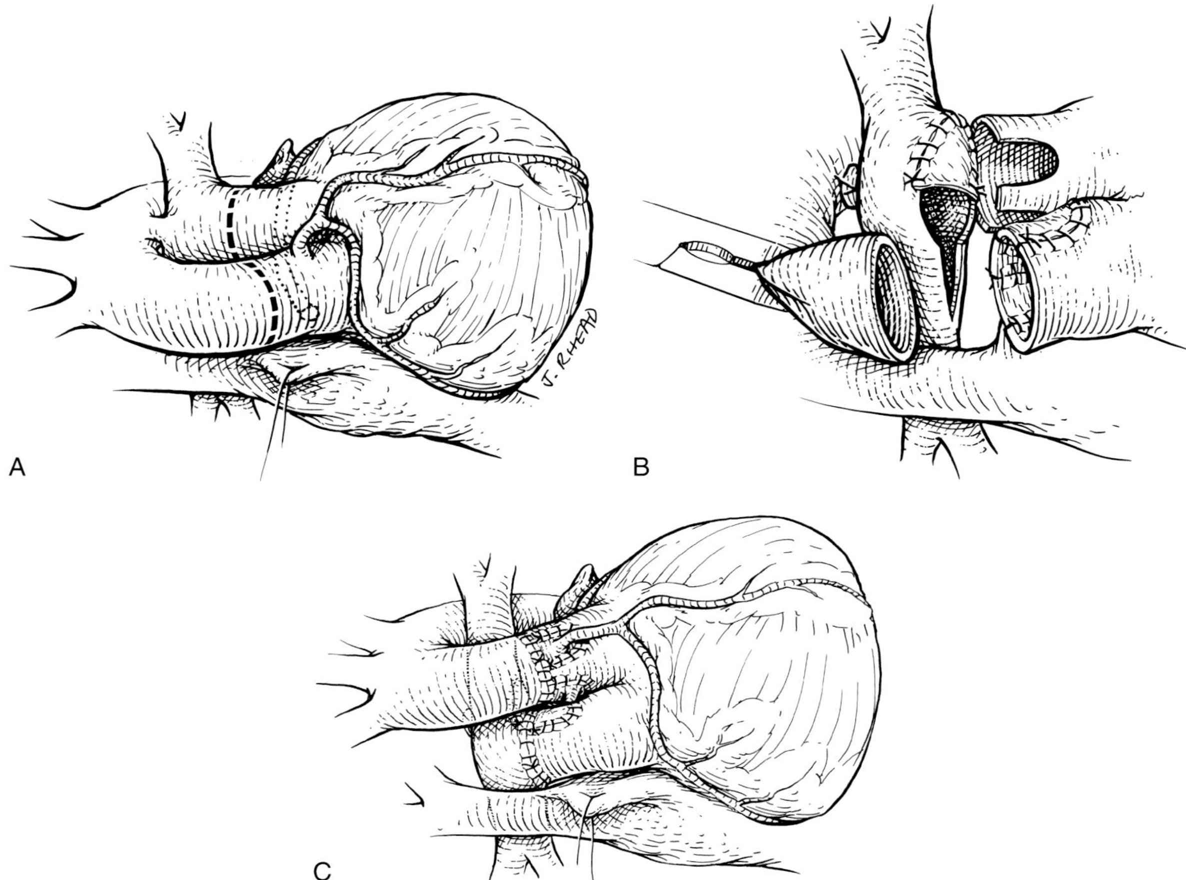

Figure 52-31 Arterial switch operation for transposition of great arteries with side-by-side great arteries and aorta to right, with coronary pattern of 1LR-2Cx. This coronary pattern is common with this great artery orientation. **A,** Dashed lines show proposed transection sites of great arteries. Both arteries are transected high, especially the native aorta, in anticipation of extra length needed for proximal neopulmonary trunk to meet transverse right branch pulmonary artery. **B,** Several important maneuvers required in this variant are shown. Both great arteries have been transected. Lecompte maneuver is not performed. Coronary buttons have been mobilized and coronary implant sites on proximal neoaorta developed. Left-sided aspect of opening in distal pulmonary trunk is partially closed with a semilunar-shaped patch of autologous glutaraldehyde-treated pericardium. Right side of this opening is enlarged into right pulmonary artery as shown. This in effect shifts opening in distal pulmonary trunk to right in preparation for proximal neopulmonary trunk to distal pulmonary trunk reconstruction. This in effect reorients proximal pulmonary trunk to right side away from proximal neoaorta and coronary reimplantation sites. Because proximal neopulmonary trunk is positioned more posterior than usual, access to coronary explantation sites for reconstruction with individual pericardial patches is more difficult. As a result, this part of operation is performed earlier than usual (i.e., before neoaorta reconstruction). Coronary explantation sites can be reconstructed with pericardial patches either before or after coronary reimplantations on proximal neoaorta; however, this component of procedure should be performed before great artery anastomoses are performed. **C,** Completed operation. Coronary artery from sinus 2 is particularly vulnerable. Without Lecompte maneuver, proximal neopulmonary trunk is oriented somewhat posteriorly and can compress posterior reimplanted coronary artery (circumflex artery in this case) over its proximal extent. For this reason, it is critical that proximal neopulmonary trunk be implanted as far right along transverse right pulmonary artery as possible.

coronary implantation somewhat more distally than the other methods. This is a rational approach because the RV infundibulum imposes a more distal position on the original aortic sinuses than is occupied by the original pulmonary sinuses. Use of a trap door rather than a simple incision may be advantageous at times in using this method.[B45] Still other techniques for managing the coronary arteries have been described.[B44,C11,H4,M37,N1,S30,Y4]

As another alternative, defects left in the proximal neopulmonary trunk after excising the coronary ostial buttons may be filled in by a single, somewhat pantaloon-shaped or rectangular pericardial patch, with or without soaking in 0.6% glutaraldehyde for about 7 minutes.[B40,I2] The commissure between sinus 1 and sinus 2 is attached at a proper level to the patch.

Finally, techniques have been described in which neopulmonary artery reconstruction is performed directly without using prosthetic material.[C2]

Arch obstruction in association with transposition can be managed either as a single-stage procedure, combining arch repair with the arterial switch, or in two stages, with arch repair performed via lateral thoracotomy and arterial switch performed via median sternotomy, usually within a week. In recent years, single-stage repair of both lesions has gained favor at many institutions with extensive neonatal experience.[L2,T9]

Atrial Switch Operation

Senning Technique

In the Senning type of atrial switch operation, preparations for operation and median sternotomy incision are performed as usual (see "Preparation for Cardiopulmonary Bypass" in Section III of Chapter 2). Operation may be performed during hypothermic circulatory arrest at about 18°C or, preferably, using CPB and direct caval cannulation. When CPB is used, the patient is cooled to at least 25°C; blood flow is then stabilized at $1.6 \ L \cdot min^{-1} \cdot m^{-2}$ or lower, and if necessary a period of 10 to 15 minutes of low flow or circulatory arrest may be employed. Myocardial management is the same as in the arterial switch operation (see preceding text).

Before CPB is established, specific measurements are made that are critical in subsequent incisions. First, circumferences of the SVC and IVC are determined (by compressing them momentarily with a clamp, measuring length of clamp occupied by compressed cava, and multiplying by 2). Position and superior and inferior extent of proposed left atriotomy are identified at the point of junction of the left atrial–right pulmonary vein wall with the most rightward aspect of the right atrial wall surface. Incision must *not* be extended further superiorly or inferiorly, which would necessitate its being carried leftward and behind the cavae (Fig. 52-32, *A*). The proposed right atriotomy incision is visualized roughly parallel to the left atriotomy incision (see Fig. 52-32, *A*). The superior extent is 3 or 4 mm anterior to the sulcus terminalis, thus anterior to the sinus node, and is anterior to the superior end of the proposed left atriotomy by a distance about two thirds of the SVC circumference. The inferior extent of the proposed right atriotomy is placed anterior to the inferior end of the proposed left atriotomy by a distance equal to two thirds of the IVC circumference. Further right-angled anterior extensions will be needed superiorly and inferiorly so that later a right atrial flap can be created (see Fig. 52-32, *A*).

CPB is established, preferably with direct caval cannulation or with a simple venous cannula for the hypothermic circulatory arrest technique. Initially the interatrial groove on the right side is dissected (see Fig. 52-32, *A*). Care is taken to keep the dissection shallow and not enter the atria.

The left atriotomy is made and pump-oxygenator sump sucker inserted if the patient is on CPB. The right atriotomy and anterior extensions are made (Fig. 52-32, *B*).

The atrial septal flap that will form the anterior wall of the posterior pulmonary venous compartment is fashioned (Fig. 52-32, *B* and *C*). When small, the foramen ovale is closed transversely with a few interrupted sutures, and the flap is created. When the foramen ovale is large, the flap consists solely of superior and posterior aspects of the limbus, but this is quite adequate when the maneuvers described next are used.

After making the septal flap, the coronary sinus is cut down precisely so as to leave anterior and posterior lips (Fig. 52-32, *C* and *D*). If the septal flap is particularly small, the base of the left atrial appendage can be advanced toward the right to meet the anterior superior aspect of the septal flap, and the posterior lip of the cut coronary sinus is used to connect to the anterior inferior aspect of the septal flap. The septal flap is shown being sewn into place without using the posterior coronary sinus lip in Figs. 52-32, *D* and *E*. If not used, the posterior lip may be tacked down (see Fig. 52-32, *E*).

The caval pathway to the mitral valve is formed posteriorly by the repositioned septal flap. The roof of the caval pathway is now completed by suturing the posterior right atrial flap anteriorly to the limbus. Interrupted sutures are used at each end to begin this (Fig. 52-32, *F*), placing these with great care so that the extensions of the cavae will be undistorted. Each suture line is carried toward the midportion of the posterior margin of anterior limbus (see Fig. 52-32, *E*). The sutures are placed along the cut edge of the limbus anteriorly, visualizing and avoiding the position of the AV node (Fig. 52-32, *G*).

The pulmonary venous pathway to the tricuspid valve is now constructed. The anterior extensions of each end of the right atriotomy incision allow the right atrial flap to come to the right and posteriorly with ease (Fig. 52-32, *H*). Suturing is begun superiorly and is completed before beginning the inferior one. This aspect of the reconstruction may be done with 5-0 or 6-0 interrupted or continuous polypropylene sutures. This suture line passes posterior and then superior to the location of the sinus node (Fig. 52-32, *I*). As the superior suture line is developed, the right atrial flap is sutured to the lateral lip of the left atriotomy over the right superior pulmonary vein. A similar suture line is made inferiorly to complete this last step of the operation (Fig. 52-32, *I*).

Alternatively, when a near-linear right atriotomy is made and the anterior right atrial flap does not come easily to the lateral lip of left atrium, the lateral lip of the left atriotomy incision is sutured to the adjacent in situ pericardium. The anterior right atrial flap is then sutured to the pericardium at a convenient distance from the left atrial–pericardial suture line to produce a wide opening between posterior and anterior portions of the pulmonary venous compartment. In essence, the pericardium acts as an augmentation patch for the channel between posterior and anterior portions of the pulmonary venous compartments.

When CPB is used, rewarming is begun about 5 minutes before completing suturing of the right atrial flap. When suturing is completed, and with strong suction on the aortic needle vent, controlled aortic root reperfusion is begun, or the aortic clamp is released. The remainder of the procedure, including de-airing, is completed as usual (see "Completing Cardiopulmonary Bypass" in Section III of Chapter 2).

When hypothermic circulatory arrest is used with a single venous cannula, the cannula is reinserted through the right atrial appendage into the pulmonary venous atrium, CPB is reestablished, and rewarming is begun after removing the aortic clamp (see "Rewarming" in Section IV of Chapter 2). A small puncture may be considered in the most anterior part of the RV just below the aortic valve to allow escape of any entrapped air as the heart begins to contract. When a single venous cannula is used in this manner, pulmonary venous blood is returned to the pump oxygenator, and the circuit is in reality a systemic (right) ventricular bypass only. Thus, it is necessary to massage the heart and inflate the lungs gently to push blood through the lungs until adequate pulmonary (left) ventricular ejection returns. This is required for only a few minutes as a rule. The single venous cannula tip often partially obstructs the caval tunnels beneath the baffle so that caval pressures of 10 to 20 mmHg are usual during rewarming. They usually fall to that in the pulmonary venous atrium after the cannula has been removed. The remainder of the procedure is completed as usual.

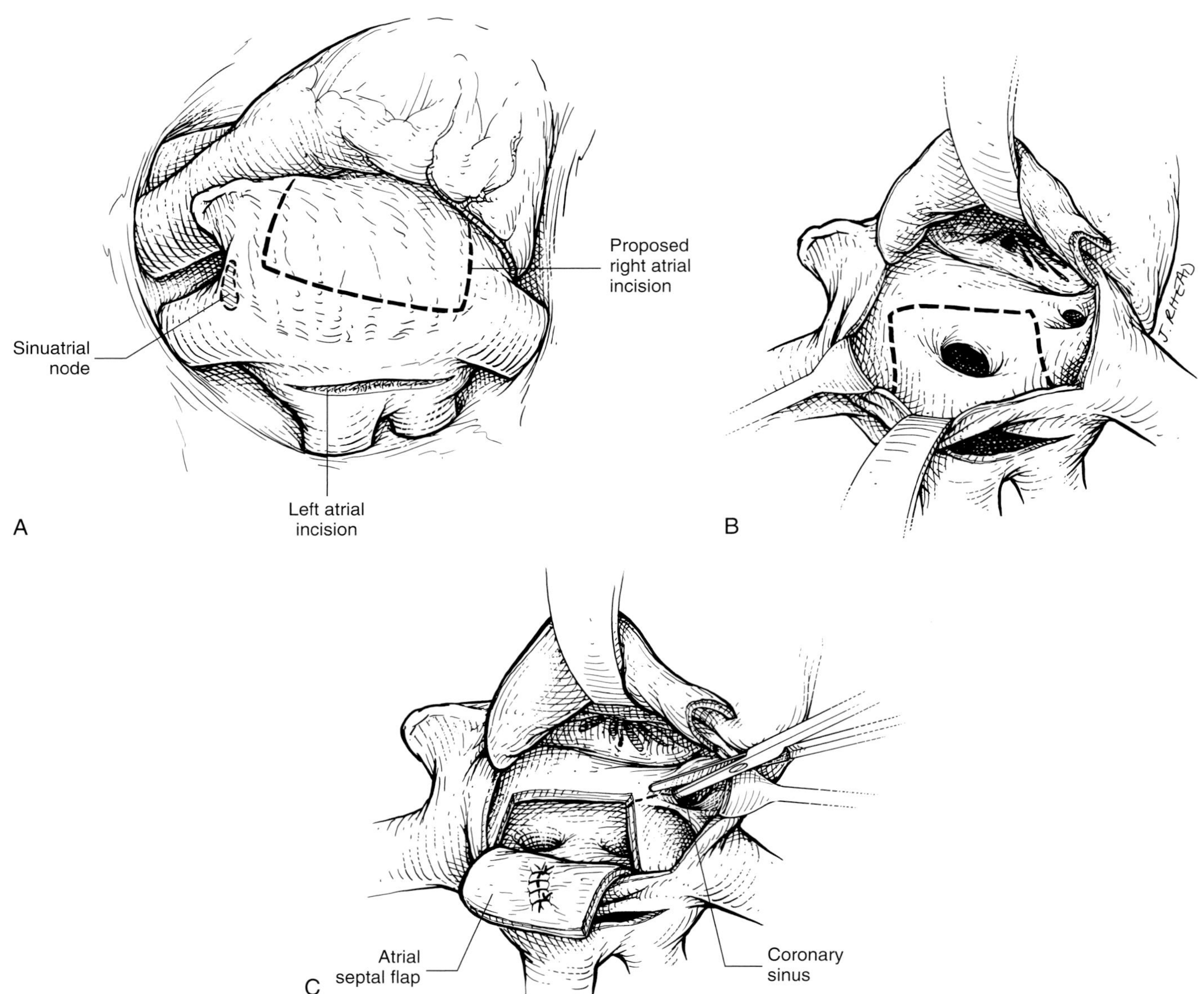

Figure 52-32 Atrial switch operation (Senning technique) for patients with transposition of great arteries. **A,** Dashed line shows approximate position of proposed right atrial incision with two anterior extensions. Also shown is dissection plane in left atrial groove. This shows extent of proposed left atrial incision. Distance between proposed left atrial incision and roughly parallel portion of right atrial incision is carefully measured based on diameters of superior and inferior venae cavae (see text). Note position of sinoatrial node. **B,** After placing patient on cardiopulmonary bypass and providing myocardial protection (see text), left and right atrial incisions are made. Dashed line shows proposed incision in atrial septum. **C,** Atrial septal flap has been developed and patent foramen ovale has been closed primarily within this flap. If there is a true secundum atrial septal defect, it can be closed with a pericardial patch prior to developing septal flap. Coronary sinus is unroofed, with incision shown along dashed line. If atrial septal flap is deficient, posterior lip of incised coronary sinus can be incorporated into subsequent atrial septal flap–left atrial suture line to augment size of pulmonary venous pathway.

With either technique, it is useful to leave a polyvinyl catheter through the right atrial appendage into the pulmonary venous atrium and one through the left atrial appendage into the systemic venous atrium. These catheters, plus an internal jugular catheter and a radial artery catheter placed at the beginning of the operation, allow complete monitoring of the hemodynamic state in the early postoperative period.

Mustard Technique

Preparations for the Mustard type of atrial switch operation and support techniques are the same as when the Senning technique is used.

The most appropriate material, configuration, and size of the atrial baffle to be inserted have been confusing and controversial. *Autologous pericardium* is considered the material of choice because of higher prevalence of baffle complications when polyester is used. If pericardium is not available at a secondary operation, however, allograft or xenograft pericardium, PTFE, or very thin knitted polyester may be used. One concept is to use a relatively small pericardial baffle and sew it snugly in place away from caval orifices in such a manner that as much of the caval pathways as possible is atrial wall rather than baffle. A different concept based on the *Toronto technique*[T13] uses a larger baffle that is sewn into place around

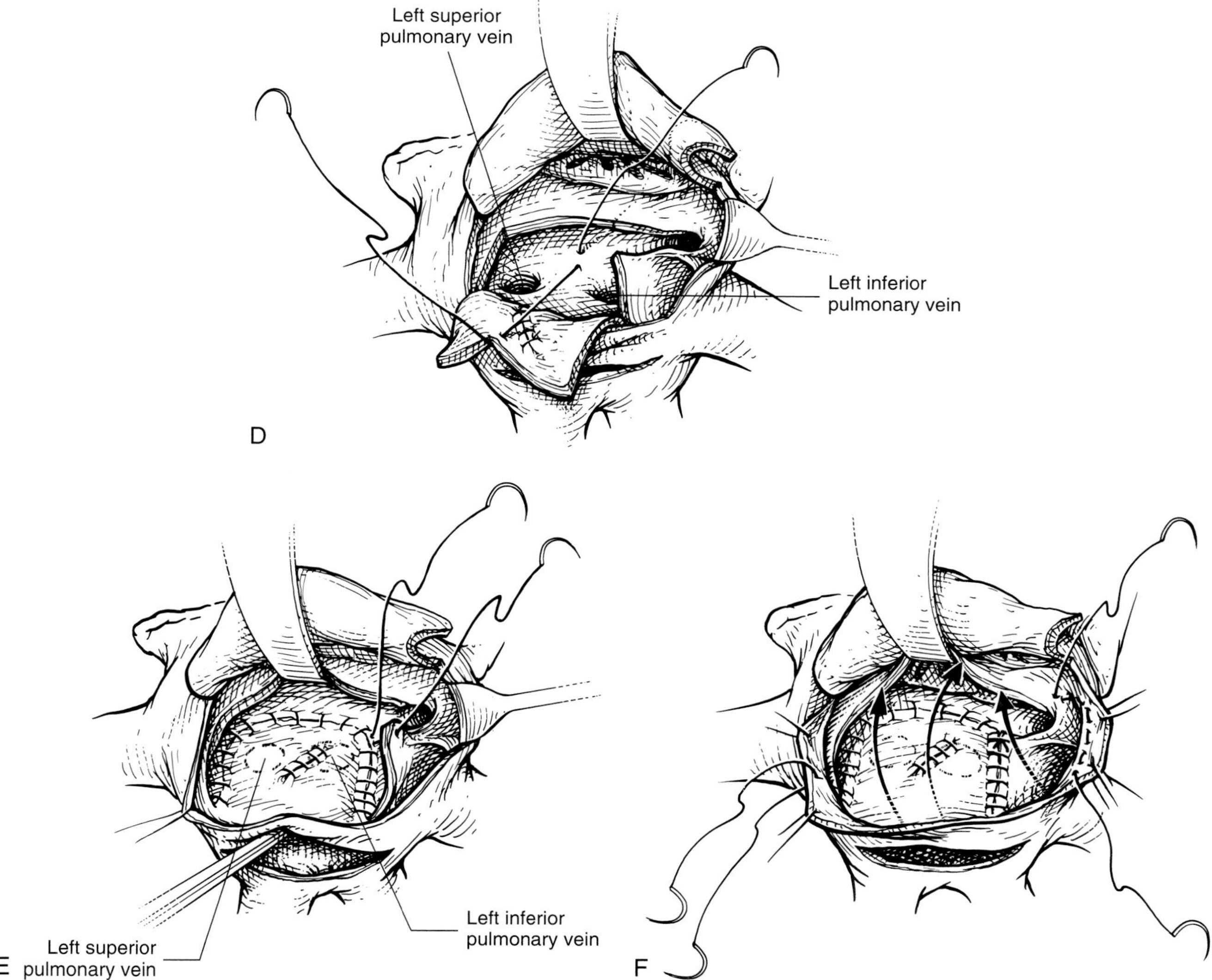

Figure 52-32, cont'd **D,** Atrial septal flap is now repositioned into left atrium and connected to left atrial wall, staying clear of ostia of left pulmonary veins. Suture line is brought anterior and superior to left pulmonary vein and anterior and inferior to left inferior pulmonary vein. **E,** In this illustration, atrial septal flap is well developed and posterior lip of cut coronary sinus is not utilized directly to augment atrial septal flap. After completing atrial septal flap suture line, unused posterior lip of coronary sinus is tacked down to anastomosis. Note position of left superior and left inferior pulmonary veins beneath septal flap *(circular dashed lines).* **F,** Posterior edge of right atrial incision is now approximated to remaining edge of atrial septum. Curved arrows show tissue manipulation required to achieve this. Most critical points in suture line are areas over orifices of superior *(SVC)* and inferior *(IVC)* venae cavae. These two aspects of suture line must be performed with great care to prevent narrowing of cavae at their transition into surgically created tunnel leading to mitral valve. Various techniques can achieve this. As shown at SVC junction, several interrupted sutures can be used to bring the two edges of tissue together over the cava. As shown at region of IVC, a "hemi–purse string" can be used to gather tissue in this area. Alternatively, interrupted simple sutures can also be used at IVC aspect of suture line.

Continued

the caval orifices, with redundancy around the cavae to minimize the chance of narrowing SVC or IVC pathways.

Sternotomy is made, and before the pericardium is opened, it is cleared laterally to within 4 or 5 mm of each phrenic nerve, generally a distance of 5 or 6 cm in a 5-kg infant. Superiorly, the pericardium is cleared nearly to the level of the brachiocephalic vein after reflecting and partially excising the thymus. A longitudinal incision is made in the pericardium a few millimeters anterior to the right phrenic nerve; in a 5-kg infant this incision is about 6.5 cm. Next, a transverse incision is made in the pericardium along the diaphragm, extending to within 4 or 5 mm of the left phrenic nerve, a distance of about 3.5 cm in a 5-kg infant but proportionally longer in a larger patient. Superiorly, a similar but convex incision is made. A left-sided longitudinal incision is made parallel to the left phrenic nerve, but with a mild concavity in its midportion. After the pericardial patch is removed, a similar concavity is made in the midportion of the other long dimension of the rectangle (see Fig. 52-33, *C [inset]*).

After establishing CPB and aortic clamping with cold cardioplegia or establishing hypothermic circulatory arrest, the right atrium is opened through the usual oblique incision (Fig. 52-33, *A*). Atrial stay sutures may be placed for exposure.

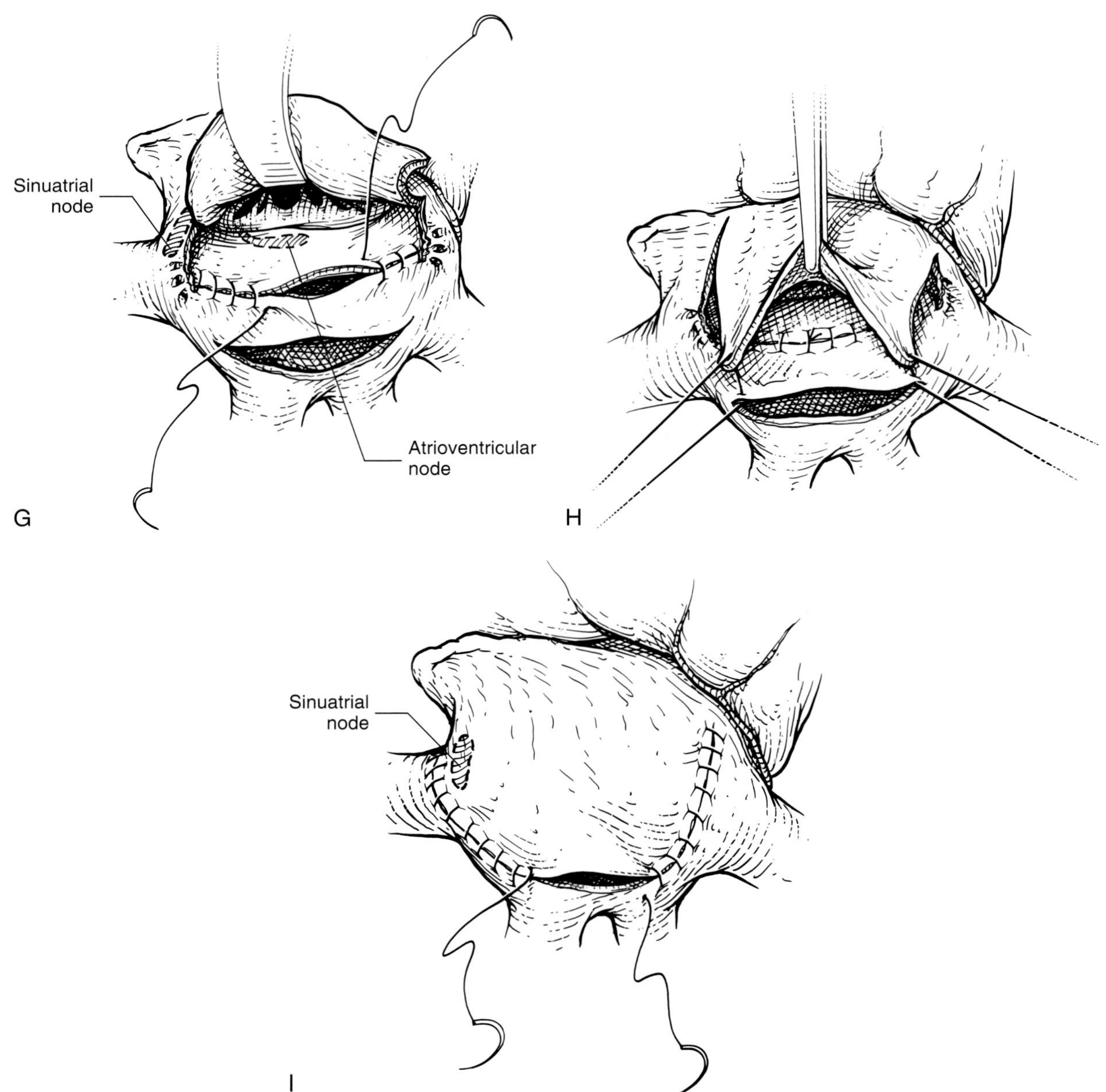

Figure 52-32, cont'd **G,** Remainder of suture line is performed with running monofilament suture to complete systemic venous to mitral valve pathway. Note positions of sinoatrial and atrioventricular nodes. **H,** Anterior edge of right atrial incision is then advanced posteriorly and attached to lateral free edge of left atrial incision. It is critical to utilize the length of anterior cut edge of right atrial incision appropriately such that underlying venae cavae are not constricted. Stay sutures shown here are positioned to allow appropriate length of right atrial flap overlying the two venae cavae. **I,** Suture line has been developed along both its superior and inferior aspects, crossing both cavoatrial junctions, and is completed along lateral edge of left atrial incision. Note that sinoatrial node now lies inside heart within wall of superior limb of systemic venous–to–mitral valve tunnel. Superior limb of the external suture line runs superior to sinoatrial node along superior cavoatrial junction.

The atrial septum is excised, beginning by dividing the limbus superiorly with scissors, centering the cut just to the left of the midpoint of the superior limbus. The incision is carried nearly into the roof of the atrium and then posteriorly beneath the SVC and then inferiorly, removing the thick tissue from behind the SVC and in front of the right pulmonary veins. Occasionally the incision goes outside the atria, and if so, the opening is closed with fine interrupted sutures. Any remnant of the fossa ovalis is completely excised (Fig. 52-33, *B*).

The center of the free wall of the coronary sinus is divided downward with scissors for 7 to 10 mm, exactly as described for the Senning procedure (see Fig. 52-33, *B*). This transfers the coronary sinus opening into the left atrium and widens the area that will be the extension of the IVC toward the mitral valve.

A double-armed 4-0 or 5-0 polypropylene suture is passed through the pericardial baffle, and through the left atrial wall anterior to and between the left superior and inferior pulmonary veins (see Fig. 52-33, *C*). The superior suture line is

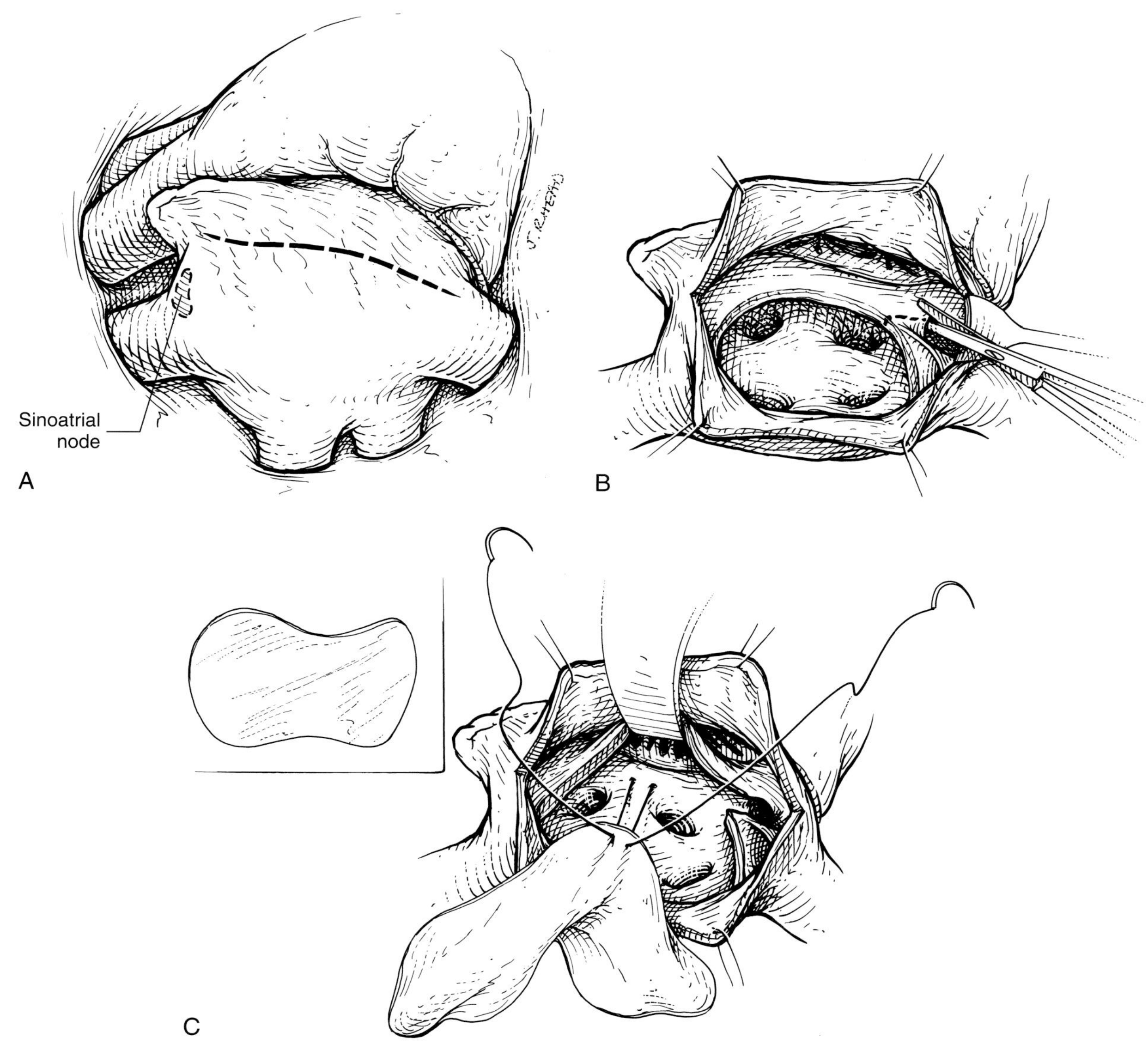

Figure 52-33 Atrial switch operation by Mustard technique (see text). Cardiopulmonary bypass and myocardial protection are similar to those used for Senning technique. **A,** Dashed line indicates proposed atrial incision. **B,** Entire atrial septum is excised as shown, and coronary sinus is cut down similar to Senning procedure *(dashed line)*. **C,** Pericardial patch used to create intraatrial baffle is shown in inset. Shape of this patch is generally that of an oval, with a gradual waist created in its midportion along long axis. Dimensions of patch will vary depending on size of infant. For a newborn infant weighing less than 5 kg, an initial oval patch measuring approximately 7 cm × 3.5 cm will be adequate, and may need to be tailored substantially. Width of patch at waist should be roughly 2.5 cm. Patch is sewn into place, beginning within left atrium, as shown, anterior to left-sided pulmonary veins. *Continued*

made, but as the point just superior to the left superior pulmonary vein is reached, the suture line is carried superiorly to the posterolateral border of the orifice of the SVC and then up around the lateral and anterior margin of the caval orifice (Fig. 52-33, *D*). A larger distance is left between bites on the patch than between those around the caval orifice so as to avoid "purse-stringing" this orifice and to bring a redundant amount of pericardial patch into the area. The inferior suture line is made using the anterior lip of the incised coronary sinus (Fig. 52-33, *D*). The baffle is then sutured to the remnant of atrial septum anteriorly (Fig. 52-33, *E*).

The right atriotomy incision is closed primarily. Alternatively, if there is concern about patency of the pulmonary venous–to–tricuspid valve pathway, the right atrial free wall can be augmented with a patch of pericardium or PTFE.

Repair of Left Ventricular Outflow Tract Obstruction

This discussion refers primarily to the atrial switch operation for TGA with essentially intact ventricular septum, because direct relief of LVOTO is not usually possible in TGA, VSD, and LVOTO.

When obstruction is dynamic and LV systolic pressure is similar to or less than that in the right (systemic) ventricle, nothing is done directly to LVOTO. When LV systolic pressure is considerably higher, surgical relief of LVOTO is

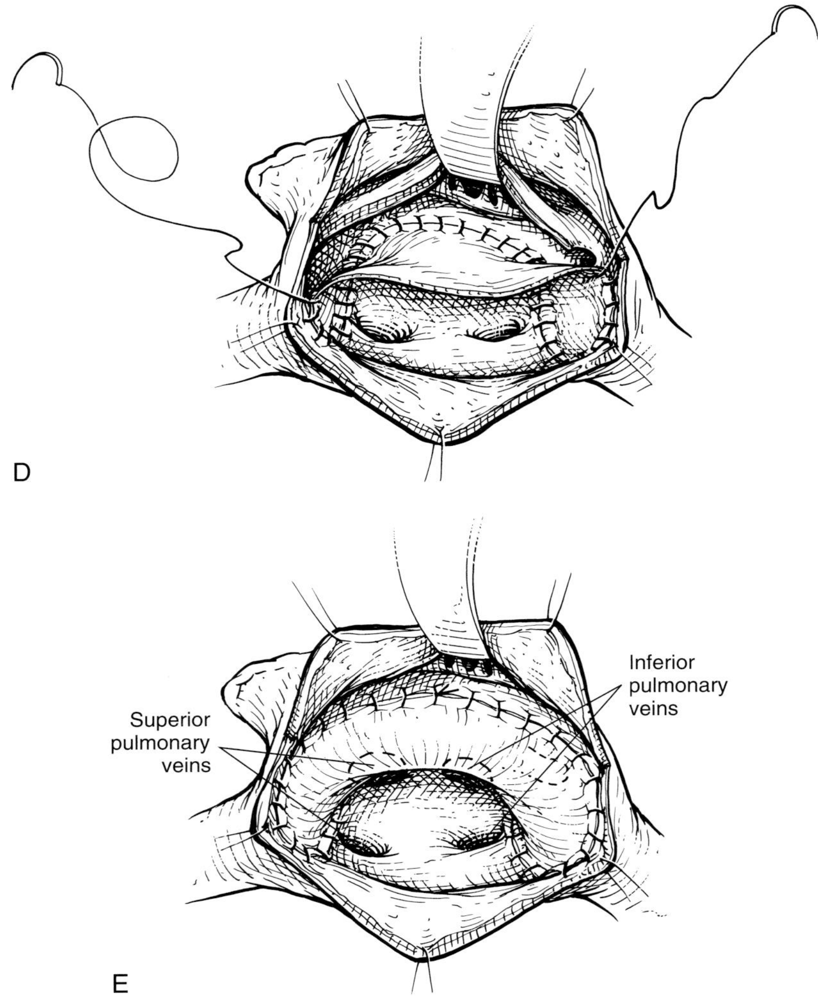

Figure 52-33, cont'd **D,** Suture lines are developed superiorly and inferiorly around orifices of left pulmonary veins and toward superior and inferior caval orifices on their posterior, lateral, and then anterior aspects as shown. Suture line is then transitioned from caval orifices onto cut edge of atrial septum. Eustachian valve (if well developed) and anterior cut lip of coronary sinus can be used to enlarge pathway from inferior vena cava to mitral valve. **E,** Baffle is shown after suture lines are completed. The four pulmonary veins are visible: right-sided pulmonary veins completely, and left-sided ones partially. All pulmonary veins are unobstructed by baffle. Atrial incision, shown here still open, is closed with a running monofilament suture. If pathway from posteriorly positioned pulmonary veins to anteriorly positioned tricuspid valve appears to be narrowed in its midportion as it passes around baffle, right atrial incision can be augmented with pericardial or polytetrafluoroethylene patch.

generally required. This may be in the form of resection of muscle, but in extreme cases a valved extracardiac conduit may be needed (see text that follows).

When the LVOTO is in the form of localized or diffuse fibromuscular obstruction, the obstructive tissue is resected. One approach is through the mitral valve[O2,O3,W8] after creating the septal flap (Senning repair) or excising the atrial septum (Mustard repair). Alternatively, resection is performed through the pulmonary trunk and valve. In the uncommon circumstance of valvar obstruction, valvotomy through the pulmonary trunk is performed.

When LVOTO is severe and cannot be relieved by resection, placing an LV–pulmonary trunk allograft valved conduit is required. (See "Double Outlet Right Ventricle and Pulmonary Stenosis" under Technique of Operation in Section II of Chapter 55 for additional details about placing left ventricular to pulmonary artery conduits.) After the first part of the atrial switch procedure has been completed, a longitudinal incision is made along the left side of the pulmonary trunk; if necessary, the incision is carried onto the left pulmonary artery. The proposed left ventriculotomy, between or beyond the diagonal branches of the LAD and along the anterolateral aspect of the LV near the apex, is marked with 5-0 sutures. The heart is allowed to fall back against the pericardium, and position on the pericardium of the proposed ventriculotomy is noted. Then, with the heart retracted upward and to the right, the proper length of the conduit can be estimated from the curving course between the pulmonary arteriotomy and the designated points on the pericardium. The conduit is trimmed to a proper length. It is cut short (about 5 mm beyond the aortic valve commissures) distally and beveled proximally. The conduit is sewn into position exactly as is done for other ventriculopulmonary trunk conduits (see "Rastelli Operation" later in text). After completing this, the last stages of the atrial switch operation are carried out.

Intraventricular Repair

In hearts with TGA and large VSD, occasionally a completely intraventricular repair can be done by the *intraventricular tunnel technique*.[C21,M21] Its applicability depends on the relationship of the VSD to the great arteries and tricuspid valve. Techniques for doing this are variable and may require enlarging the VSD, but operation is essentially the same as the intraventricular repair that may occasionally be possible in Taussig-Bing heart (see "Intraventricular Tunnel Repair of Taussig-Bing Heart" under Technique of Operation in Chapter 53). In some cases the tunnel may be made superior to the pathway to the pulmonary trunk rather than inferior to it.[M21]

A partially intraventricular repair associated with placing a valved extracardiac conduit between the RV and pulmonary trunk has been described, but in the largest reported series, hospital mortality was high.[P17]

Rastelli Operation

Usual preparations for operation are made when performing the Rastelli operation for TGA, VSD, and LVOTO. A conduit is prepared using an estimate of the largest size of extracardiac conduit that can be comfortably placed within the patient's thorax. A valved conduit is preferred, and options include pulmonary or aortic valved allografts and composite grafts using either woven polyester or PTFE conduits with bioprosthetic valves (see Appendix A in Chapter 12 and Technique of Operation in Section II of Chapter 38).

A median sternotomy incision is made, and if stenoses are present at the pulmonary trunk bifurcation or in proximal portions of right or left pulmonary arteries, a piece of pericardium is removed and set aside. Pericardial stay sutures are placed. The pulmonary trunk in most patients with this anomaly is posterior and to the left of the ascending aorta. Therefore, to avoid conduit compression between the right-sided and anterior ascending aorta and sternum, preparations are made for routing the conduit so that it approaches the pulmonary trunk from the patient's left side. The pulmonary trunk and its bifurcation are dissected completely free of the ascending aorta, and the first portions of left and right pulmonary arteries are also mobilized. Purse-string sutures are placed appropriately (see "Preparation for Cardiopulmonary Bypass" in Section III of Chapter 2). Any previously made systemic–pulmonary arterial anastomotic operations are dissected and closed just after establishing CPB (see "Repair of Tetralogy of Fallot after a Blalock-Taussig or Polytetrafluoroethylene Interposition Shunt" under Technique of Operation in Section I of Chapter 38).

After CPB is established and moderate hypothermia achieved, the aorta is clamped and cold cardioplegia is established (see "Cold Cardioplegia, Controlled Aortic Root Reperfusion, and [When Needed] Warm Cardioplegic Induction" in Chapter 3). The left side of the heart is decompressed using a vent catheter placed through a purse-string suture in the right superior pulmonary vein and positioned across the mitral valve into the left ventricular cavity.

The infundibular free wall of the RV is opened by a moderate-sized vertical ventriculotomy that avoids major coronary artery branches. The incision may have to extend to the midportion of the RV free wall (Fig. 52-34, *A*). Appropriate stay sutures are placed on the ventriculotomy edge (Fig. 52-34, *B*). Origins of the aorta from the RV and pulmonary trunk from the LV are confirmed. It has already been determined by preoperative imaging study that the VSD is a conoventricular perimembranous type in the outflow portion of the ventricular septum, but this is now confirmed visually. The tricuspid valve and its tensor apparatus are usually well away from the pathway between the VSD and aorta, but if not, special measures are required. They may involve detaching tricuspid valve chords, with reattachment onto the intraventricular tunnel material (Hanley FL: personal communication; 2002) or using the conal flap method.[N9] Unless the VSD is clearly large and nonrestrictive, it is enlarged by excising the septum anterior to the defect (see dashed line in Fig. 52-34, *B*). Care is taken that the excision is in the interventricular septum and not the ventricular free wall. Generally this provides considerable enlargement of the VSD, but care should be taken to not injure the septal coronary artery branches.

Intraventricular tunnel repair is now done similarly to that described for simple double outlet right ventricle (see "Intraventricular Tunnel Repair for Simple Double Outlet Right Ventricle" under Technique of Operation in Chapter 53). The LV ejects into the aorta through this tunnel (Fig. 52-34, *C* and *D*).

The pulmonary trunk is divided, and the proximal stump is oversewn at the valve level (see Fig. 52-34, *C*). The distal portion of the trunk and proximal left and right pulmonary arteries are mobilized, allowing the pulmonary trunk to be reoriented for a straightforward end-to-end anastomosis (see Fig. 52-34, *D*). Proximal anastomosis of the conduit to the right ventriculotomy is made (Fig. 52-34, *E* and *F*).

Remainder of the operation includes controlled reperfusion and de-airing procedures (see Chapters 2 and 3). The foramen ovale may be left open; as with tetralogy of Fallot (see Section I of Chapter 38) the right-to-left shunting across it in the early postoperative period augments cardiac output, although at the expense of systemic arterial desaturation. If a true ASD is present, however, it should be closed. Depending on the patient's hemodynamic status, transesophageal echocardiography findings, and surgeon preference, polyvinyl recording catheters may be placed in the right atrium, left atrium, and pulmonary artery for postoperative monitoring.

Lecompte Operation

The alternative method of managing TGA, VSD, and LVOTO, the Lecompte intraventricular repair, is also applicable to other types of ventriculoarterial discordant connections (see "Lecompte Intraventricular Repair" under Technique of Operation in Chapter 53).[R19] Other techniques for reconstructing the RV outflow tract have been described.[D7,M25]

Aortic Root Translocation (Nikaidoh)

For patients with TGA and LVOTO with or without VSD, aortic root translocation has been adopted by some surgeons because of concerns about long-term outcomes of the Rastelli procedure.[N10] In this procedure, the aortic root is detached from the RV along with the coronary arteries and translocated posteriorly after making a septal incision or enlarging the VSD, then patching it, thereby relieving the LVOTO.

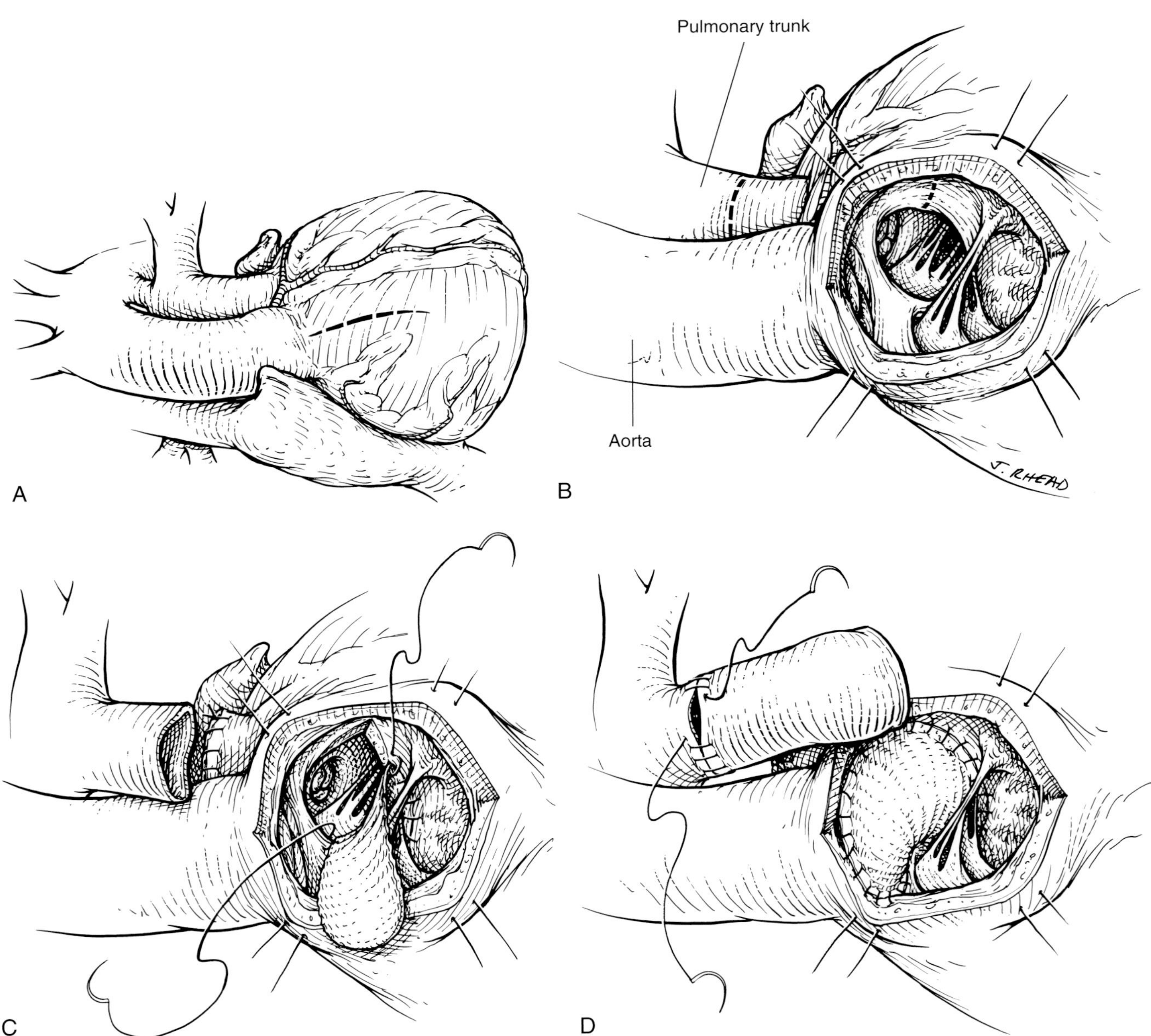

Figure 52-34 Rastelli operation for transposition of great arteries, ventricular septal defect (VSD), and left ventricular outflow tract obstruction. **A,** After standard median sternotomy incision, pulmonary trunk and left and right pulmonary arteries are completely dissected away from aorta and surrounding structures. Dashed line shows site of proposed right ventricular infundibular incision, which is in line with most anterior aspect of aorta. **B,** Standard cardiopulmonary bypass and myocardial protection techniques are used. Right ventricular infundibular incision is made and retraction sutures placed. Through this incision, rightward and anterior ascending aorta can be seen immediately, and leftward and posterior pulmonary valve can be visualized through VSD. Dashed line on rim of VSD shows site of incision on ventricular septum where VSD is enlarged in preparation for left ventricular to aortic baffle. This incision is necessary only when VSD is small (less than 60% aortic diameter). Dashed line on pulmonary trunk indicates proposed site of transection at sinutubular junction. **C,** Pulmonary trunk has been transected and proximal pulmonary trunk oversewn at level of valve. An alternative technique is to close pulmonary valve from within heart, working through infundibular incision and VSD. Using this method, if pulmonary valve anulus is small, it may be closed primarily; otherwise a circular patch is placed around immediately subvalvar tissue. VSD, which has been enlarged by incision, is shown with tunnel from left ventricle to aorta partially constructed. Material for tunnel is fashioned from a tube of polyester with a diameter approximately the size of ascending aorta. After tailoring, this results in a naturally curved baffle that is positioned with convex aspect of baffle facing into right ventricle. Lower aspect of baffle is sewn around rim of VSD, taking standard precautions with respect to inlet valves and conduction system (see “Location in Septum and Relationship to Conduction System” under Morphology in Section I of Chapter 35). Upper aspect of baffle is sewn into place by transitioning suture line away from rim of VSD as patch approaches aortic valve anulus on each side. Baffle is then sewn to immediately subaortic region along lateral aspects, and then finally anterior aspect, of circumference of aorta. A running technique, using nonabsorbable monofilament suture, is used. **D,** Left ventricular to aortic baffle is shown with suture line completed. A valved allograft conduit (or other composite conduit) is used to reconstruct right ventricular outflow tract. Conduit is tailored to appropriate length and is sewn end to end to pulmonary trunk as shown with a running monofilament technique.

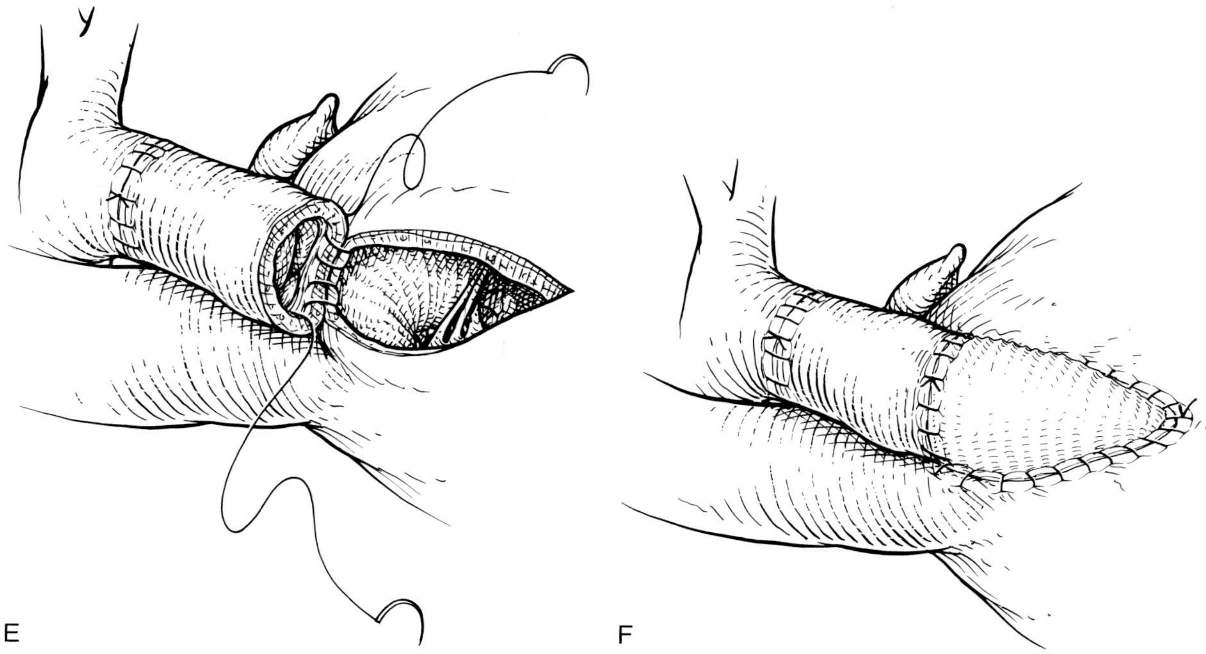

Figure 52-34, cont'd **E,** Proximal end of valved conduit is connected to distal aspect of right ventricular infundibulum incision with a running monofilament suture. This suture line covers approximately 30% of circumference of conduit along its posterior aspect. **F,** A roughly triangular patch of polyester (or allograft arterial wall) is used to close remainder of right ventricular to pulmonary trunk connection. This is sewn into place around lateral and anterior aspects of circumference of proximal edge of conduit, and then around cut edges of infundibular incision. Completed reconstruction is shown.

To avoid kinking or stretching of the coronary arteries, modifications of this procedure with transfer of one or two coronary buttons akin to the arterial switch have been reported (Fig. 52-35).[B9,M33] The pulmonary outflow tract is then reconstructed with an allograft valved conduit or a valveless patch.

Pulmonary Trunk Banding

Pulmonary trunk banding is discussed in detail in Chapter 35 (see "Pulmonary Trunk Banding" under Technique of Operation in Section I), including the Trusler rules for patients with transposition and large VSDs, and in Chapter 41 (see "Pulmonary Trunk Banding" under Technique of Operation in Section II).

Systemic–Pulmonary Arterial Shunting Procedures

Systemic–pulmonary arterial shunting techniques are described in detail in Chapter 38 (see "Technique of Shunting Operations" in Section I), and in Chapter 41 (see "Systemic–Pulmonary Arterial Shunt" under Technique of Operation in Section II). The same guidelines are followed concerning the size and type of shunt as in tetralogy of Fallot and in univentricular hearts.

Repair of Post–Mustard Technique Complications

Caval Obstruction

With caval obstruction after the Mustard procedure, usual preparations for operation through a median sternotomy are made, although others have preferred a right anterolateral thoracotomy.[S32] An oscillating saw is used for the secondary sternotomy, and the usual limited dissection is made (see "Secondary Median Sternotomy" in Section III of Chapter 2) without freeing the front and leftward aspect of the heart.

Tapes are passed around the cavae beyond the caval-atrial junctions, and they are cannulated directly. CPB is commenced and conducted as usual. The aorta is clamped and cold cardioplegic solution infused into the aortic root. The right atrium is opened with a centrally placed transverse or oblique incision.

When obstruction involves only the pathway from the SVC, this portion of the baffle may be enlarged. The baffle is incised vertically at its midpoint with a knife and the incision carried upward to open widely the pathway from the SVC. When this is totally occluded, the SVC–right atrial junction, which is always still patent beneath the baffle, is defined by inserting the tip of a curved forceps through a stab wound in the SVC (avoiding the sinus node area) and cutting down onto the tip of the instrument as it tents the baffle toward the right atrial cavity (pulmonary venous compartment). Alternatively, it may be possible to use the tip of a curved forceps to bluntly dissect the area of obstruction from above downward so that the tip appears below it. The baffle is opened at the point at which it joins the right atrial wall in front of the SVC junction, and fibrous thickening is excised to recontour the baffle and floor of the new tunnel. An elliptical PTFE or polyester patch is now sewn into the baffle incision with continuous 4-0 polypropylene suture to create a new roof to the pathway. An opened, preclotted, knitted or woven double-velour polyester graft of appropriate diameter is used for the patch because it contours toward the pulmonary venous atrium. The patch must not compromise the pulmonary venous channel.

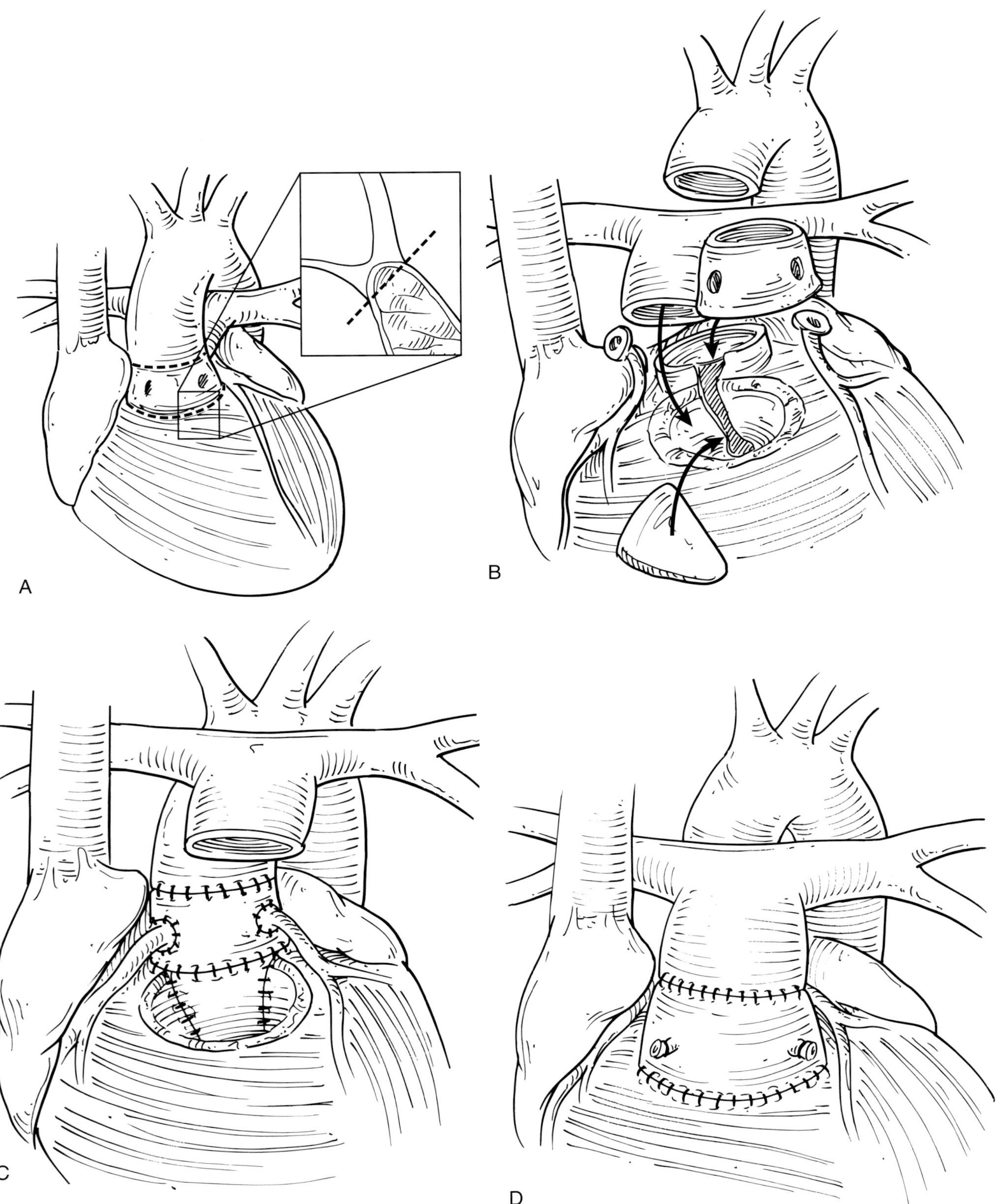

Figure 52-35 Aortic root translocation for transposition of great arteries and left ventricular outflow tract obstruction. **A,** Ventricular and aortic incisions required for aortic autograft excision are shown. Note that infundibular incision is circumferential just below aortic anulus, and as shown in inset depicting cross-section through ventriculoarterial junction, incision is slightly oblique. Coronary ostia are excised as circular buttons from respective sinuses of Valsalva. **B,** Once aortic autograft is excised and coronaries mobilized, pulmonary trunk is transected and an incision is extended across pulmonary valve anulus and septum connecting to ventricular septal defect (VSD), if present. Enlargement of left ventricular outflow tract is then accomplished by inserting a triangular-shaped VSD patch. **C,** Aortic autograft is reinserted into left ventricular outflow tract. It is then rotated 180 degrees so that defects from coronary buttons face anteriorly. Coronaries are then reimplanted. Before reestablishing ascending aortic continuity, branch pulmonary arteries are mobilized and brought anterior to aorta (Lecompte maneuver) in preparation for right ventricular outflow reconstruction. **D,** Right ventricle (RV) to pulmonary trunk continuity is achieved by inserting an interposition allograft connecting RV infundibulum to pulmonary trunk.

Alternatively, the baffle can be removed entirely. When the entire baffle is grossly thickened and distorted, especially if it contains folded polyester and the pathway from the IVC is obstructed, the entire baffle must be excised.[S32] A new baffle is inserted using pericardium, if enough is available, or PTFE or polyester. The remainder of the operation is completed as usual.

As a final alternative for isolated SVC obstruction, a bidirectional superior cavopulmonary anastomosis can be created (see Technique of Operation in Section III of Chapter 41).

Pulmonary Venous Obstruction

With pulmonary venous obstruction after Mustard repair, initial stages of operation and establishing CPB and cold cardioplegia are as described earlier. A transverse incision is made through the right atrial wall and into the anterior pulmonary venous compartment. Incision is carried posteriorly through the waist between anterior and posterior pulmonary venous compartments and directly between the right superior and right inferior pulmonary veins. Excess fibrous tissue surrounding the open stenosis is excised without breaching the baffle. One technique for repair involves closing the transverse atriotomy with continuous 4-0 polypropylene suture to create a vertical atrial suture line in much the same manner as described by Dillard and colleagues as part of the Mustard baffle technique in 1969.[D16] Instead, a V-atrial flap may be created from the lateral right atrial wall anterior to the stenotic site, with the apex of the V advanced posteriorly as a V-Y atrioplasty. Alternatively, a properly sized and shaped preclotted double-velour woven polyester gusset cut from a tube to create a convex contour is sutured into the atriotomy. This approach has the potential disadvantage that the stenosis may recur as the patch thickens,[D15] but this has not yet been reported. The remainder of the operation is completed as usual.

SPECIAL FEATURES OF POSTOPERATIVE CARE

Postoperative care is as usual for patients undergoing all types of intracardiac operations (see Chapter 5), with special considerations after some types of procedures.

When an *arterial switch operation* has been performed, particularly in a neonate, left atrial (or pulmonary artery diastolic) pressure should remain low, less than about 12 mmHg. Because restlessness or agitation increases metabolic demands and cardiac output, neonates and infants are usually kept intubated and sedated for 24 to 48 hours after operation. If cardiac output is less than optimal, particularly when 2D echocardiographic study indicates poor LV function, catecholamine support is used rather than further increasing LV filling pressure.[C22,Q4] Careful study shows that cardiac output falls during the first postoperative day, with lowest values occurring 9 to 12 hours after surgery. This cardiac output profile occurs independently of the perfusion technique used at operation and occurs with and without associated VSD.[W7]

When an *atrial switch operation* has been done, positive end-expiratory pressure (PEEP) is not used because it tends to obstruct the SVC. Infants are nursed in a slightly head-up position. Atrial pressures are kept as low as is compatible with an adequate cardiac output; low-dose (2.5 to 5 mg · kg^{-1} · min^{-1}) dopamine during the early postoperative hours is helpful.

RESULTS

Simple Transposition of the Great Arteries and Transposition of the Great Arteries with Ventricular Septal Defect Using Arterial Switch Operation

Early (Hospital) Death

Currently, in institutions properly prepared for the arterial switch operation in neonates, early (hospital) mortality in both simple TGA and TGA with VSD is about 2% to 7%, a considerable improvement compared with about 15% reported in earlier eras.[B41,B45,B47,C20,D1,K12,L25,Q1,Q4,S4,W6]

Time-Related Survival

Instantaneous risk of death (hazard function) is extremely low by 6 to 12 months after arterial switch repair, and survival declines minimally after that time (Fig. 52-36).[G12,W10] Thus, overall 5-year survival, including hospital mortality, has been 82% among a heterogeneous group of patients operated on in different institutions. In Williams's group, 15-year survival was 81%.[W10] This intermediate-term survival is predicted to

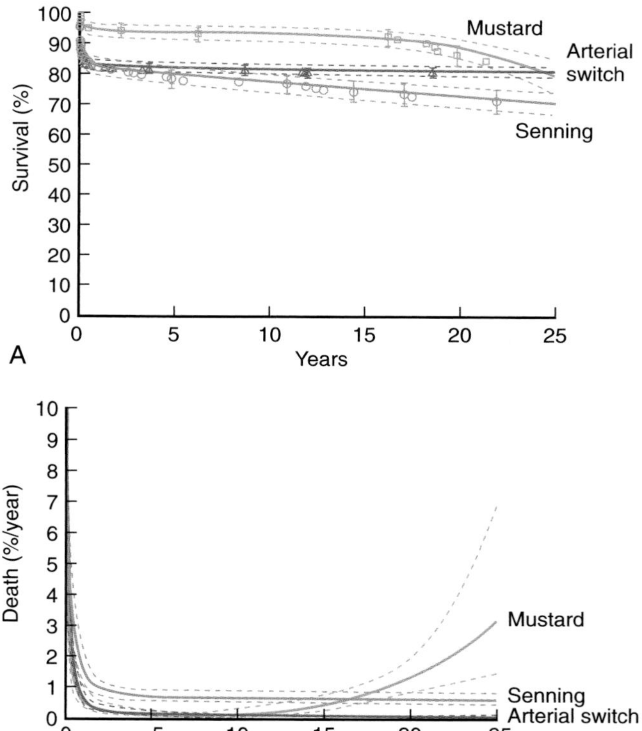

Figure 52-36 Mortality after operation for transposition of great arteries (TGA) in a 24-institution Congenital Heart Surgeons Society study. The 829 neonates were enrolled within the first 2 weeks of life; 516 underwent an arterial switch repair. Experience is stratified by type of repair: arterial switch, Mustard atrial switch, and Senning atrial switch. **A,** Survival. Each symbol represents a death, vertical bars are 68% confidence limits of nonparametric estimates, and solid lines enclosed within 68% confidence bands are parametric estimates. **B,** Instantaneous risk of death (hazard function). Parametric estimates are enclosed within 68% confidence bands. Note: Apparent late increase in risk after the Mustard atrial switch is solely related to general increased risk of death among patients with TGA and ventricular septal defect. (Congenital Heart Surgeons Society data: personal communication, 2011.)

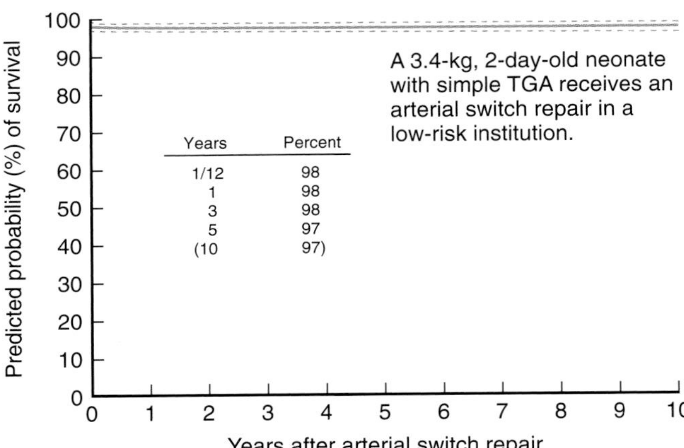

Figure 52-37 Predicted survival after arterial switch repair in neonate with simple transposition of great arteries or transposition of great arteries with ventricular septal defect, operated on in an institution of proven competence ("low risk") in arterial switch repair. Depiction is a specific solution of the multivariable equation described in Appendix 52A, Table 52A-1. Birth weight was entered at 3.4 kg, with usual coronary anatomy (1LCx-2R) and no important coexisting cardiac or noncardiac anomalies. Key: *TGA,* Transposition of great arteries. (From Kirklin and colleagues.[K12])

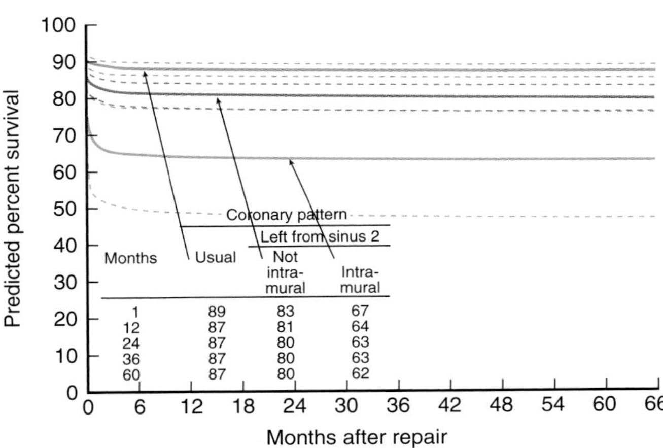

Figure 52-38 Relation between coronary artery pattern and survival after arterial switch operation for simple transposition of great arteries. Depiction is a nomogram of a specific solution of the multivariable equation in Table 52A-3, solved for a neonate weighing 3.4 kg without important coexisting cardiac (including multiple ventricular septal defects) or noncardiac anomalies and without previous pulmonary trunk banding, operated on at 6 days of age. (From Kirklin and colleagues.[K12])

be higher than 95%, however, in uncomplicated cases treated currently in a group of institutions properly prepared for the arterial switch operation (Fig. 52-37). During a comparable era, experiences from single institutions may show outcomes superior to this, with 5-year and even 10-year survival greater than 90% without eliminating high-risk patients.[H1,L24,V11,W6] Long-term (20-year) survival after the arterial switch operation is about 90% in patients operated on in the most experienced institutions.

Modes of Death

Mode of death is usually acute or subacute cardiac failure secondary to ventricular dysfunction resulting from imperfect transfer of coronary arteries to the neoaorta.[L9] This applies to deaths after hospital discharge as well as those during postoperative hospitalization. In the Congenital Heart Surgeons Society's multiinstitutional study, five of six patients dying 6 or more months after the arterial switch operation died with severe ventricular (usually LV) dysfunction.[K12] In one single-institution study, postmortem examination revealed severe proximal coronary artery stenosis caused by fibrocellular intimal thickening in six patients dying after the perioperative period.[T14]

The only other important mode of death occurs with RV dysfunction secondary to severe pulmonary vascular disease, which was not present at operation in a neonate with simple TGA. This mode has occurred in less than 1% of patients.[K12]

Patient-Related Incremental Risk Factors for Death

Coronary Arterial Pattern This has been the most important patient-related risk factor for death, based on multiinstitutional experience during the first decade after introduction of the arterial switch procedure in neonates, with two specific coronary patterns increasing risk. Risk of death is increased when the LCA or either of its branches arises from sinus 2, and risk is further increased when the LCA or LAD passes anteriorly between the two great arteries, a situation typically accompanied by an intramural course of the artery in the aortic wall (see "Coronary Arteries" under Morphology earlier in this chapter) (Fig. 52-38). As is usually the case, these risk factors are particularly strong in situations in which the overall risks are increased. Other unusual coronary patterns, some introduced more recently, have been identified as risk factors for death.[L24,T4,W6]

Coronary arterial pattern is not an immutable risk factor and has been overcome, at least in some institutions, by appropriate techniques of coronary transfer (see "Arterial Switch Operation" under Technique of Operation earlier in this chapter).[Q1] Nevertheless, a recent report of a large single-institution experience cautions that intramural coronary arteries remain associated with increased morbidity and mortality following the neonatal arterial switch operation (Fig. 52-39).[M26]

Multiple Ventricular Septal Defects Multiplicity of VSDs increased the risk of arterial switch repair in the first decade following the procedure's introduction (Fig. 52-40). This risk factor may be neutralized by technical advances,[B46] but this is less certain than in the case of unusual coronary artery patterns. In some studies, presence of a single VSD increases risk of death compared with TGA and intact ventricular septum.[H1]

Older Age at Repair During the initial decade of the neonatal arterial switch experience, the younger the neonate at arterial switch repair, the safer the operation (Fig. 52-41). This age effect was particularly strong in patients with simple TGA and correlated with the magnitude of age-related differences in wall thickness characteristics of the LV of the normal neonatal heart and those of the heart with TGA. This age effect may be neutralized in current practice.[D8,F7]

Arterial switch has been successfully performed beyond the neonatal period—up to age 9 months—in patients with TGA and intact septum, but such patients are more likely to require postoperative mechanical support.[K2]

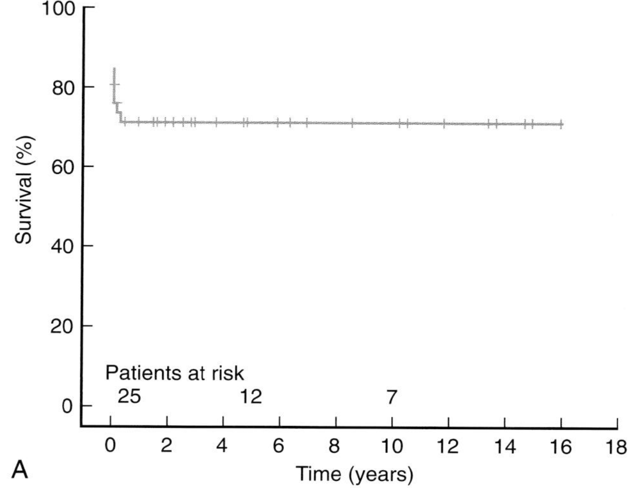

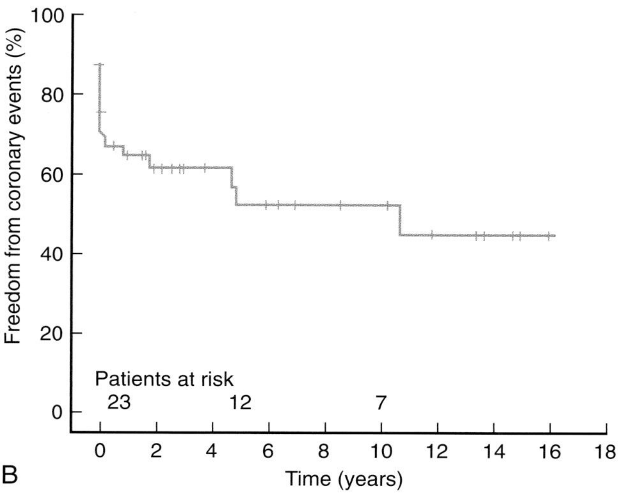

Figure 52-39 Actuarial data in 46 arterial switch patients with an intramural coronary artery, from a single institution. **A,** Survival. All deaths were coronary related. Overall mortality was 28% (13/46), compared with 3.9% for patients without an intramural coronary artery operated on during same period at same institution. **B,** Freedom from coronary events. Overall, 19 of 46 patients (41%) experienced a coronary event. (From Metton and colleagues.[M17])

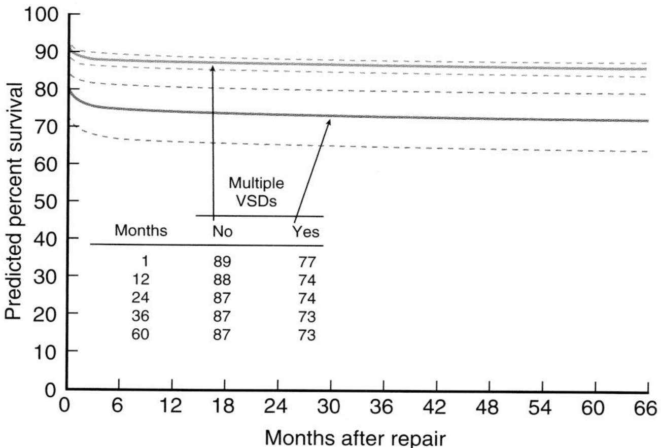

Figure 52-40 Relationship between multiplicity of ventricular septal defects and survival after arterial switch operation. Depiction is a nomogram of a specific solution of the multivariable equation incorporating patient-related risk factors only (see Table 52A-3). Key: *VSD,* Ventricular septal defect. (From Kirklin and colleagues.[K12])

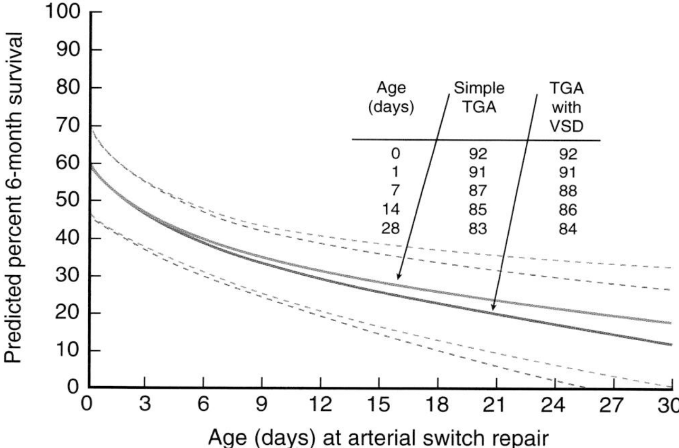

Figure 52-41 Relationship between age at arterial switch operation and probability of survival for at least 6 months postoperatively. Depiction is a nomogram of a specific solution of the multivariable equation incorporating patient-related risk factors only (see Table 52A-3). Key: *TGA,* Transposition of great arteries; *VSD,* ventricular septal defect. (From Kirklin and colleagues.[K12])

Coexisting Cardiac and Noncardiac Congenital Anomalies These anomalies may increase the risk of arterial switch repair, but are fortunately infrequent in patients undergoing repair. The most notable coexisting cardiac anomaly is aortic arch obstruction or interruption.

Operative Support and Procedural Incremental Risk Factors for Death

The support technique (CPB vs. hypothermic circulatory arrest) has not been a risk factor for death[K12] in the experience of some, but duration of circulatory arrest has been found to increase risk by others.[W6] However, longer global myocardial ischemic times have increased probability of death (Fig. 52-42), suggesting that improved methods of myocardial management may improve results of operation. Even in institutions with substantial neonatal experience, CPB time is still a risk factor for early death.[Q1]

Transection of the aorta or the pulmonary trunk at a site different from that described earlier in this chapter under Technique of Operation has been shown to be a risk factor for death (see Table 52A-5, Appendix A). Inferences from various multivariable analyses support the method of management described there (see Table 52A-6).

Growth of Arteries

All currently available information indicates that aortic, pulmonary, and coronary arterial anastomoses grow at a rate comparable with growth of the child.[A14,D6,M14] In one study, the neoaortic root was usually enlarged but with a growth pattern comparable with the normal population. Growth of the neopulmonary anulus was between the fifth and fiftieth percentile of a normal body surface area–matched population.[B42] These relationships reflect the normal disparity between pulmonary and aortic roots (see Chapter 1).

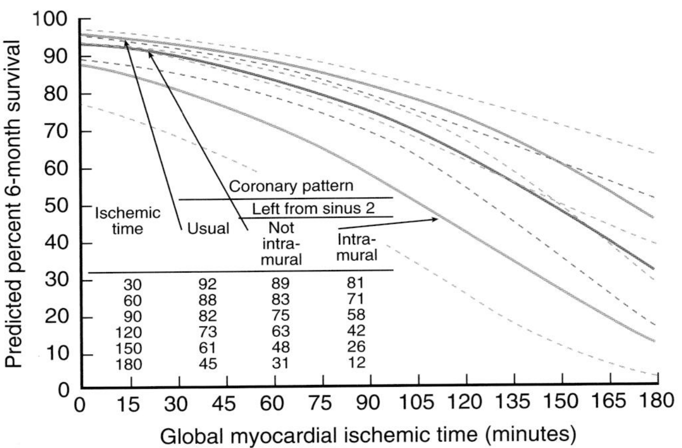

Figure 52-42 Effect of duration of global myocardial ischemia on survival after arterial switch operation for simple transposition of great arteries in 6-day-old patient. Depiction is a nomogram of a specific solution of the multivariable equation incorporating patient-related and support risk factors (see Table 52A-4).

Functional Status

Essentially all surviving patients are fully active and without limitations.[M2,R11] However, decreased exercise capacity has been documented in patients who have undergone an arterial switch procedure as neonates. Residual RV outflow tract obstruction seems to have an effect on exercise capacity. Impaired chronotropic effect also appears to be an important contributor to reduced exercise capacity.[D10,F11,G3,P10]

Ventricular Function

LV function is usually normal after an arterial switch operation. In a study of 12 patients, Borow and colleagues found normal contractility and normal dimensions and wall thickness in 10 of 12 patients studied between 2 and 7 years postoperatively (83%; CL 65%-94%).[B36] However, Hausdorf and colleagues identified 1 patient of 14 studied (7%; CL 1%-22%) late after arterial switch operation in whom LV stiffness was severely increased,[H5] and Okuda and colleagues reported three patients with reduced ejection fractions associated with neoaortic valve regurgitation.[O4] Massin and colleagues found reduced LV function in only 1 of 71 patients at catheterization 1 year after an arterial switch operation, and that patient had had a coronary complication at the time of the arterial switch.[M14] Ventricular function after the arterial switch appears to remain normal at midterm follow-up (mean 3.8 years, maximum 10 years) in a large study,[C19] and with 20-year follow-up, LV dimensions and fractional shortening are within normal limits.[V1]

Interestingly, preoperative dynamic LVOTO, even with a gradient of up to 120 mmHg, disappears after the arterial switch procedure.[W5,Y1]

In a comparative study between the arterial and atrial switch, Backer and colleagues found late postoperatively that systemic ventricular ejection fraction was within the range of normal in 98% of patients with simple TGA undergoing arterial switch repair,[B1] but in 79% of those who underwent an atrial switch repair.

Rhythm Disturbances

Patients with TGA and either intact ventricular septum or VSD treated by the arterial switch operation have been free of supraventricular rhythm disturbances that many patients have after atrial switch procedures. Arensman and colleagues report that this is true whether or not a right ventriculotomy has been made for repair of the VSD.[A13]

Only 3% of patients with simple TGA had arrhythmias after arterial switch repair in one study, compared with 57% after atrial switch repair.[B1,R12] This continues to be the case even in more recent reports of longer-term follow-up.[H7] This casts doubt on the supposition that rhythm disturbances are an inherent part of the malformation of TGA.

Coronary Blood Flow

Positron emission tomography evaluation of coronary blood flow has revealed significantly lower coronary flow reserve in arterial switch patients compared with control subjects,[B16] although these findings are controversial.[Y6] Other studies document exercise-induced perfusion defects and reduced coronary flow reserve at late follow-up[H6]; abnormal autonomic innervation, especially in children undergoing arterial switch at older age[K14]; and small-caliber left coronary systems.[H6,Y7]

Coronary Artery Lesions

Coronary artery obstruction has been documented in a disturbingly high number of asymptomatic TGA patients evaluated prospectively by angiography at 5- to 10-year follow-up. One study showed that 6 of 105 patients (5.7%; 95% CL 1.2%-10.2%) had important coronary lesions.[B33] In patients with perioperative ischemia that subsequently resolved before discharge after arterial switch, coronary obstruction was found in only 1 of 27 patients, whereas in those patients in whom perioperative ischemia persisted, all 10 patients demonstrated coronary obstruction.[B33] In general, coronary patterns involving a major coronary vessel passing behind the pulmonary trunk and operations using unusual techniques of coronary reimplantation demonstrate an increased risk of coronary obstruction.[B33] In other studies, coronary occlusion or stenosis was found in 3.0% to 7.8% of patients at follow-up.[B34,T5]

Coronary artery stenosis continues be higher in complex coronary patterns and in patients with evidence of ischemia.[M26] Also, asymptomatic coronary stenosis remains an ongoing finding with a prevalence similar to earlier reports. Results of both surgical revascularization and percutaneous transluminal angioplasty are acceptable. However, whether or not asymptomatic coronary obstruction with normal ventricular function should be treated remains controversial.[A10,H21,K1,L9,R3] Both CTA and magnetic resonance imaging are useful noninvasive modalities to detect coronary abnormalities and myocardial perfusion defects.[O6,T8] In a recent study using intracoronary ultrasound in 20 patients at 5 to 22 years after arterial switch, Pedra and colleagues found that a disturbingly high proportion of coronary arteries (89%) displayed a variable degree of proximal eccentric intimal proliferation.[P14] All children had coronary artery lesions, with 50% having moderate to severe intimal thickening (>0.3 mm). No risk factors for such abnormalities were encountered, including age, coronary artery pattern, hemodynamics, and follow-up duration. The authors speculate that this suggests early development of arteriosclerosis in reimplanted coronary arteries, which may play a role in the genesis of late coronary events.

Neurodevelopmental Status

At 8-year follow-up in one patient cohort, overall physical and psychosocial health status was similar to that of the general population, according to the Mean Physical Health Summary and the Mean Psychosocial Summary scores; however, increased problems with attention, learning, speech, and developmental delay were reported by parents.[D19] Neurologic testing at age 8 years in this cohort revealed that neurodevelopmental status was below expectation in many respects, including academic achievement, fine motor function, visuospatial skills, working memory, hypothesis generating and testing, sustained attention, and higher-order language skills.[B12] Earlier evaluation in this cohort at age 2.5 years suggested increased problems with expressive language and problem behavior if hypothermic circulatory arrest had been used for the repair.[B11] Others have shown reduced neurologic status in 21% of patients evaluated at age 3.0 to 4.6 years after neonatal arterial switch using circulatory arrest.[H13] In a recent study of 193 late survivors who underwent arterial switch more than 15 years previously, 98% were either attending school or working.[Y5] It is important to realize that the neurodevelopmental alterations in these studies may have as much or more to do with CPB management as they do with the fact that these children had TGA.

Right Ventricular Outflow Tract Obstruction

Right ventricular outflow tract obstruction (RVOTO) was observed as a postoperative complication of arterial switch soon after this technique was introduced.[B27,C4] Whether this is an immutable complication or can be prevented is still not certain.

RVOTO has occurred with sufficient severity to require reintervention in about 10% of patients and in one multi-institutional experience had a peak incidence about 6 months after the arterial switch operation (Fig. 52-43). Others have reported that RVOTO has become evident later after operation.[B43] In one analysis, freedom from reintervention was 94% (95%; CL 64%-99%) at 1 year, and 79% (95%; CL 64%-94%) at 5 years.[N11] Subsequently, others reported much lower need for reintervention, and it is generally believed that this complication occurs less frequently in current practice.[S12] In one large cohort of patients from a single institution, reoperation for RVOTO was 1.5%.[A11] In general it is agreed that adequate mobilization of the branch pulmonary arteries during the Lecompte procedure is necessary to minimize supravalvar pulmonary stenosis. However, there is no consensus on whether a single vs. double patch technique, or use of a certain type of patch material, increases the risk of RVOTO. Smaller neo-PT or complex coronary patterns requiring larger coronary buttons may predispose patients to later RVOTO. Although reintervention for RVOTO shows a declining trend with experience, there still remains a larger number (up to 24%) of patients with mild RVOT gradients who do not necessarily qualify for reintervention, but may have reduced physical performance because of this.[B42]

Usually, obstruction is in the pulmonary trunk. Less frequently, RVOTO is at the bifurcation of the pulmonary trunk, and some have thought that stenosis at this area is the result of the Lecompte maneuver. In a careful analysis of a two-institution experience, however, the Lecompte maneuver could not be identified as a risk factor (Williams WG, Lincoln CL: personal communication; 1992). Occasionally the obstruction is at the RV–pulmonary trunk junction or in the RV infundibulum.

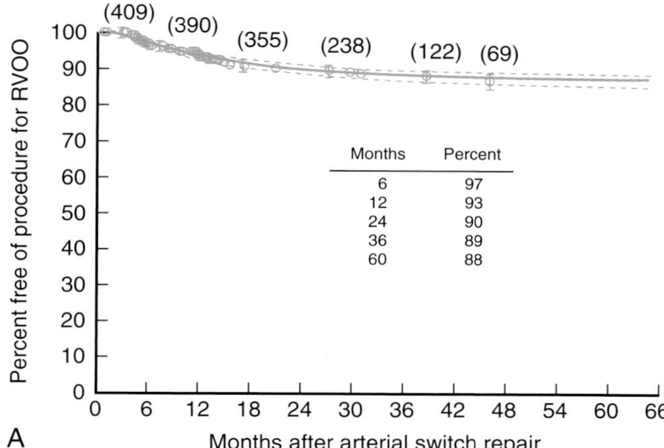

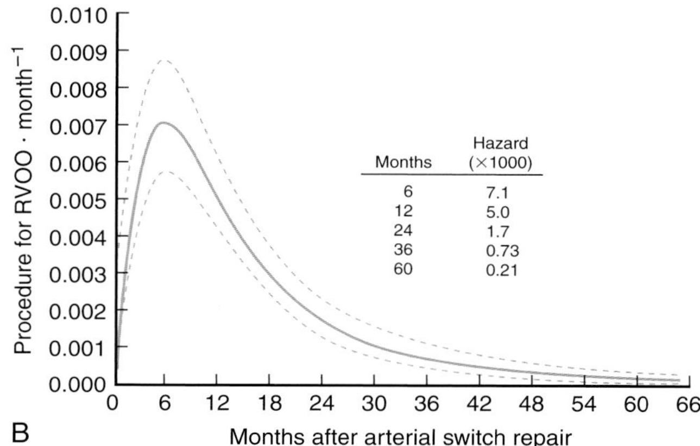

Figure 52-43 Prevalence of reoperation after arterial switch operation for simple transposition of great arteries and transposition of great arteries with ventricular septal defect; right ventricular outflow obstruction. **A,** Time-related freedom from reoperation. Each circle, positioned according to Kaplan-Meier estimator, represents a death; vertical bars represent 70% confidence intervals; numbers in parentheses, patients still at risk; solid line, parametric survival estimate; dashed lines, 70% confidence intervals of parametric estimates. **B,** Hazard function for reoperation. Key: *RVOO,* Right ventricular outflow obstruction. (From Norwood WI, Bove EL, Quaegebeur JM, Blackstone EH, Kirklin JW, Congenital Heart Surgeons Society: personal communication; 1992.)

Neoaortic Valve Regurgitation

The neoaortic valve (pulmonary valve at birth) is competent in about 60% of patients studied several years after the arterial switch operation; mild regurgitation has been found in about 35% of patients and moderate or severe regurgitation in 5% or fewer.[C19,G8,J6,M11] Risk factors for neoaortic regurgitation include older age at time of arterial switch, prior pulmonary trunk banding, presence of VSD, larger discrepancy between neoaortic root and ascending aorta, LVOTO, Taussig-Bing morphology, use of trap door techniques for coronary reimplantation, and implantation of coronary buttons compromising the integrity of the sinutubular junction of the neoaortic root.[C19,F9,H22,J6,L8,L23,M22,S7] Prevalence of neoaortic valve regurgitation in patients at late follow-up is appreciable and progressive over time.[F9,H22,L8,L23,M22,S7] However, need for

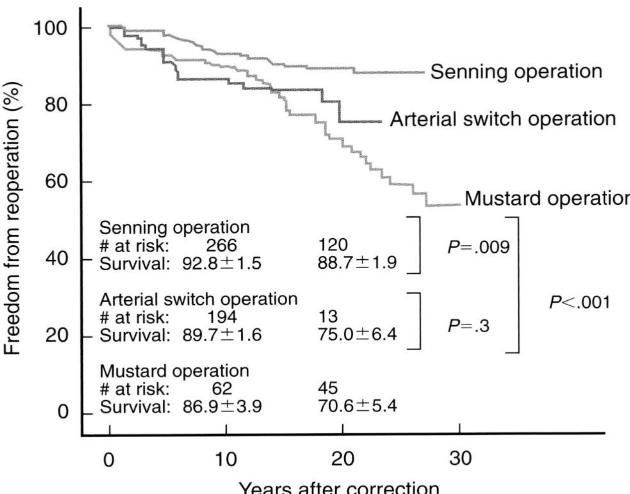

Figure 52-44 Freedom from reoperation among survivors of initial hospitalization after corrective operations for transposition of great arteries, stratified by type of operation.

valve reintervention is less than 2% at current follow-up.[M22] Neoaortic root dilatation and abnormalities in its distensibility have been documented.[M22,M35,S7]

Neopulmonary Valve Regurgitation

Neopulmonary valve regurgitation occurs after an arterial switch operation, but prevalence of important regurgitation has not been well documented. Obstruction at this level is more common, especially in patients with associated aortic coarctation.[H10]

Reoperation

Reinterventions are mainly for RVOTO and LVOTO[H12] after arterial switch. Freedom from reintervention was 75% at 20 years in one large study, with 58% of reoperations involving RVOTO at various levels and 43% involving LVOTO (Fig. 52-44 and Table 52-6). Over a 10-year period, Serraf and colleagues reported that reoperation for supravalvar pulmonary stenosis was necessary in 2.1% of patients, whereas all other indications showed a prevalence of less than 1%.[S12] Some reports document an increase in late reinterventions for coronary artery lesions.[T4,V12] Mortality of reintervention has been low unless reoperation is early following initial operation.

Table 52-6 Reoperations Among 874 Survivors Through Hospitalization after the Mustard, Senning, or Arterial Switch Operation

Procedure	Mustard	Senning	Arterial Switch
All reoperations:			
No. of reoperations	37	38	69
No. of patients	30	33	52
Closure of baffle leak	7 (19%)	11 (29%)	0
Enlargement of systemic venous pathway	24 (65%)	10 (26%)	0
Enlargement of pulmonary venous pathway	18 (49%)	8 (21%)	0
Enlargement of subvalvular pulmonary stenosis	0	0	10 (14%)
Enlargement of valvular pulmonary stenosis	1 (2.7%)	2 (5.3%)	5 (7.2%)
Enlargement of supravalvular pulmonary stenosis	0	0	16 (23%)
Enlargement of pulmonary arterial stenosis	0	0	9 (13%)
Enlargement of left ventricular outflow tract and aortic arch	3 (8.1%)	13 (34%)	19 (28%)
Aortic valve replacement	0	1 (2.6%)	11 (16%)
Banding or debanding of pulmonary artery	2 (5.4%)	7 (18%)	3 (4.3%)
Arterial switch and atrial redirection	0	5 (13%)	0
Tricuspid valve procedure	5 (14%)	4 (10%)	4 (5.8%)
Closure of residual ventricular septal defect	5 (14%)	3 (7.9%)	9 (13%)
Other	2 (5.4%)	2 (5.3%)	5 (7.2%)

Data from Horer and colleagues.[H12]
Percentages refer to percentage of total number of operations in group.

Simple Transposition of the Great Arteries with Atrial Switch Operation

Early (Hospital) Death

Hospital mortality after an atrial switch ranges from 0% to 15%.[A12,C14,E5,L20,M3,M41,T13,U1] Variability in prevalence of risk factors and degree of institutional competence with atrial switch repair are the determining factors.

Atrial switch operations are usually delayed for a few weeks to a few months after birth, in contrast to arterial switch operations, which are usually performed within a few days of birth. Thus, in addition to mortality early after the atrial switch operation, *deaths that occur before operation* must also be considered (Table 52-7). About 10% of uncorrected patients with simple TGA die by age 30 days despite adequate

Table 52-7 Category of Death in Infants with Simple Transposition of the Great Arteries Who Died Before Atrial Switch Repair[a]

Category	No.
NYHA class V on admission and death in continuing hypoxia	4
Cerebral death after late (>12 days old) referral in NYHA class V	6
Associated large PDA and NYHA class IV	3
Intercurrent respiratory infection	1
Escherichia coli sepsis	1
Necrotizing enterocolitis	1
Accident at balloon septostomy	1
TOTAL	17[b]

[a]Data from study of 188 patients with simple transposition of great arteries admitted to GLH, 1970-1984.
[b]Three of the 17 patients died before balloon septostomy.
Key: *NYHA,* New York Heart Association; *PDA,* patent ductus arteriosus.

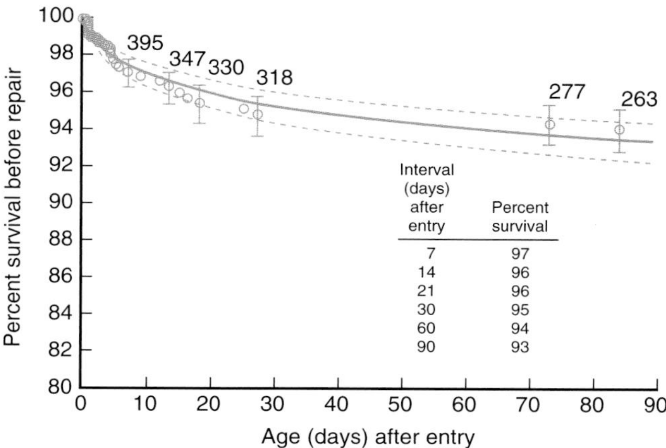

Figure 52-45 Survival before repair of patients with simple transposition of great arteries and transposition of great arteries and ventricular septal defect. Most patients have undergone balloon atrial septostomy. Depiction is as in Fig. 52-43. (From Congenital Heart Surgeons Society experience with 846 patients entered into study during first 2 weeks of life: personal communication; 1992.)

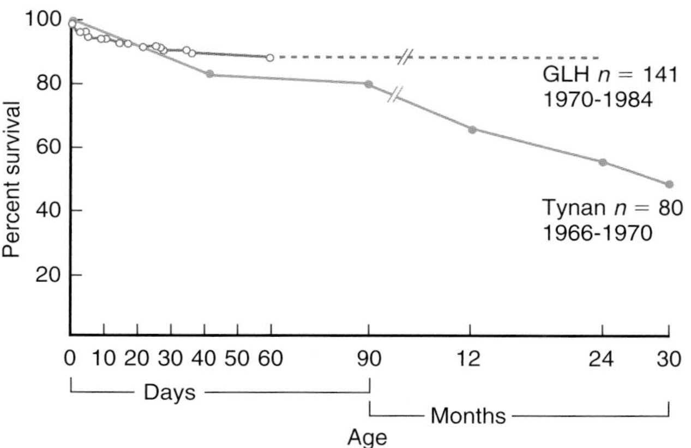

Figure 52-46 Survival to time of atrial baffle repair after initial palliation by balloon atrial septostomy (BAS). Patients were not censored if other palliative procedures were done. Initial palliation in GLH series was BAS (except for five septectomies) and for Tynan's series,[T18] BAS only. GLH series includes only patients with simple transposition of great arteries. Tynan's series also includes those with large ventricular septal defect, but there was no difference in survival before repair between these two subsets.

BAS (Figs. 52-45 and 52-46),[C5] and further deaths occur after 30 days. Death before repair is lower in patients with TGA and VSD. Surgical septectomy may result in better survival until repair[G17,L19,T13,T18] but for many reasons is undesirable. Alternatively, neonatal atrial switch can be performed, and early outcomes can rival outcomes obtained with the arterial switch.[T17]

Time-Related Survival

Survival after the atrial switch operation is strikingly lower in patients with TGA and VSD than in those with simple TGA (Fig. 52-47). This decreased survival is related to higher prevalence of deaths both early after operation and in the months after hospital discharge, as evidenced by hazard functions. Others have documented similar findings, with a 15-year survival after the Mustard procedure of 86% for simple TGA and 64% for complex TGA.[M41]

Time-related survival of patients who have undergone the Mustard operation appears in one multiinstitutional study to be superior to that after the Senning operation, largely attributable to the difference in early mortality (Fig. 52-48). General applicability of this finding is uncertain. Twenty-year follow-up from Senning's group shows a survival of 83%.[T16] In the experience of the Toronto Hospital for Sick Children, however, exclusively using a protocol leading to a Mustard type of atrial switch repair, long-term survival (80% at 20 years) was good. About 10% of patients had symptomatic RV dysfunction,[W11] however, and no late increase in hazard function for death was identified (Fig. 52-49).

Modes of Death

Modes of death after the atrial switch operation are varied (Table 52-8), with low cardiac output being the most common early postoperatively. This mode partly results from the relatively small size of the atria, which makes them perform more as a conduit than a reservoir and results in a lower ventricular filling pressure than normal.[P7]

Forty percent (10 of 25) of late deaths in a 20-year follow-up study were attributable to systemic RV failure.[T16] In the longest follow-up yet available, up to 40 years, from Toronto and Zurich, the most common causes of late death were heart failure and sudden death.[O1] In another long-term study, sudden death occurred with a prevalence of 7% without identifiable risk factors.[W13]

Patient-Related Incremental Risk Factors for Death

Currently, there are few risk factors for death after repair of simple TGA by the atrial switch operation (Table 52-9).

Younger Age at Repair Younger age has often been found in the past to be a risk factor for death after atrial switch repair.[W4] However, some institutions have achieved good results with the Senning atrial switch repair even when performed in the first 2 weeks of life, with hospital mortality in 4 of 26 patients (15%; CL 8%-26%). Several single-institution studies attest to the likelihood that young age can no longer be considered a risk factor for death after atrial switch repair in institutions properly prepared for this type of surgery.[B4,D11,F10]

"Older age" at repair (i.e., >3 years) has been shown to be a risk factor for late death,[G2,W4] as have RV dysfunction and presence of active dysrhythmias.[K10]

Lower Birth Weight As with almost all operations for congenital heart disease, very low birth weight is a risk factor for death after atrial switch repair.

Ventricular Septal Defect or Pulmonary Stenosis

In Senning's long-term follow-up study, late systemic RV failure was three times more common in patients with VSD or pulmonary stenosis compared with patients with simple TGA, and systemic RV failure was found to be the most common cause of late death.[T16]

Electrophysiologic Disturbances

Although much of the information about electrophysiologic disturbances after atrial switch operations comes from patients undergoing the Mustard technique, no evidence indicates that these disturbances are different with the Senning technique.[M12,M13]

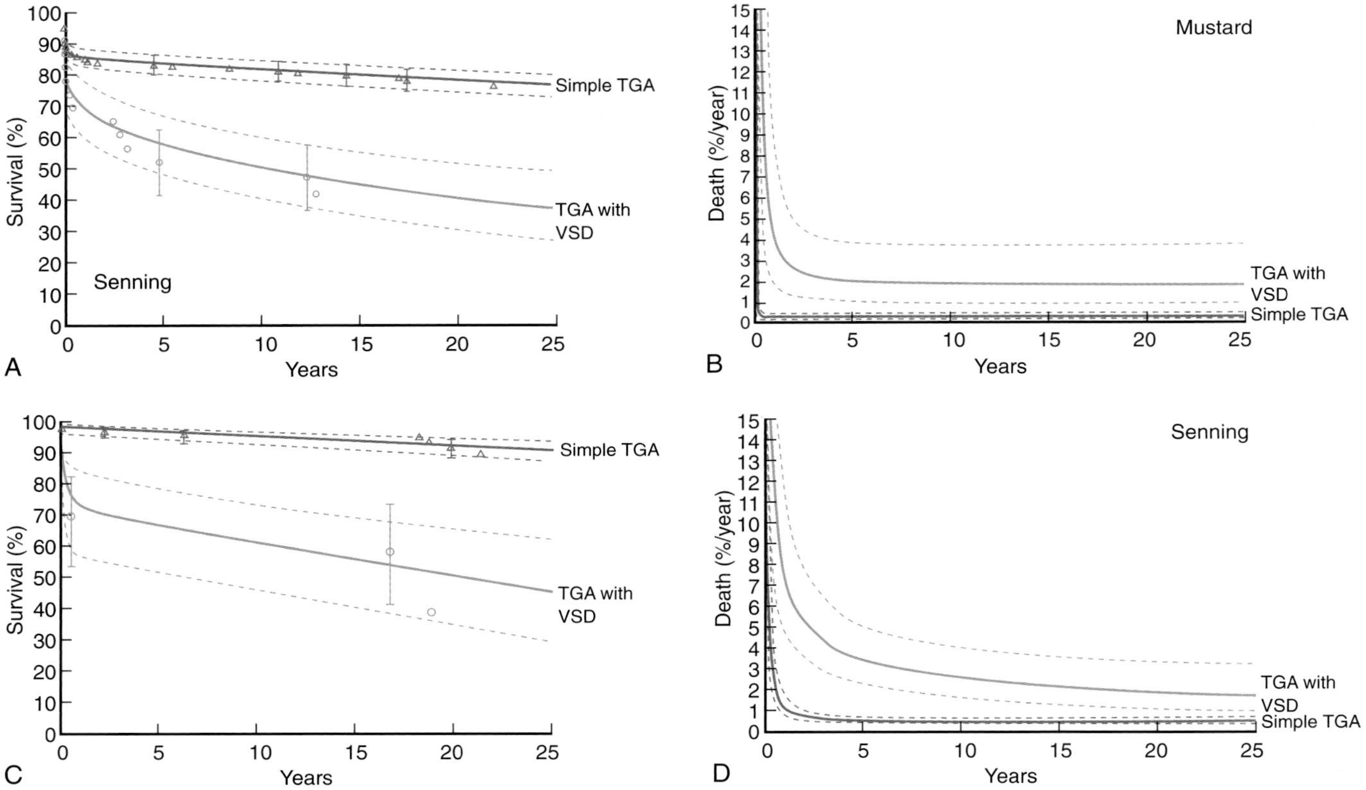

Figure 52-47 Effect of type of transposition of great arteries on mortality after atrial switch operation. Depictions are as in Fig. 52-43. **A,** Survival after Mustard atrial switch. **B,** Instantaneous risk of death (hazard function) after Mustard atrial switch. **C,** Survival after Senning atrial switch. **D,** Instantaneous risk of death (hazard function) after Senning atrial switch. Key: *TGA,* Transposition of great arteries; *VSD,* ventricular septal defect. (Congenital Heart Surgeons Society data: personal communication; 2011.)

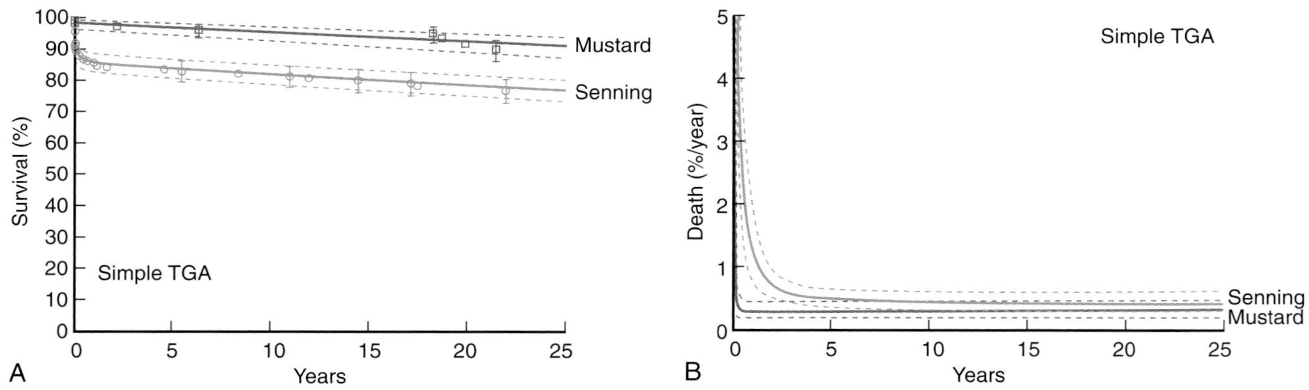

Figure 52-48 Mortality after atrial switch operation for simple transposition of great arteries according to type of operation. Depiction is as in Fig. 52-43. **A,** Survival. **B,** Instantaneous risk of death (hazard function). (Congenital Heart Surgeons Society data: personal communication; 2011.)

The morphologic basis of conduction and rhythm disturbances are understood to some extent. Histologic examination of the sinus node region reveals that the sinus node itself, sinus node artery, and paranodal tissues are frequently abnormal after the Mustard operation.[B26,E4,E6] Acute changes include compression of the sinus node artery by sutures or, less often, intimal thickening or thrombus formation and suture compression, necrosis, or infarction of the sinus node itself with interstitial hemorrhage and edema of nodal tissue and adjacent myocardium. Edwards and Edwards found that in nine patients with sinus node artery compression, the sinus node showed acute infarction in seven.[E4] Chronic changes include marked fibrosis in the node and paranodal tissue, such that in some cases the sinus node can no longer be identified. Surgical maneuvers responsible for this damage include incorrect techniques for SVC cannulation (e.g., too close to the node such that the purse-string suture damages it, use of crushing clamps in this region), damage to the sinus node

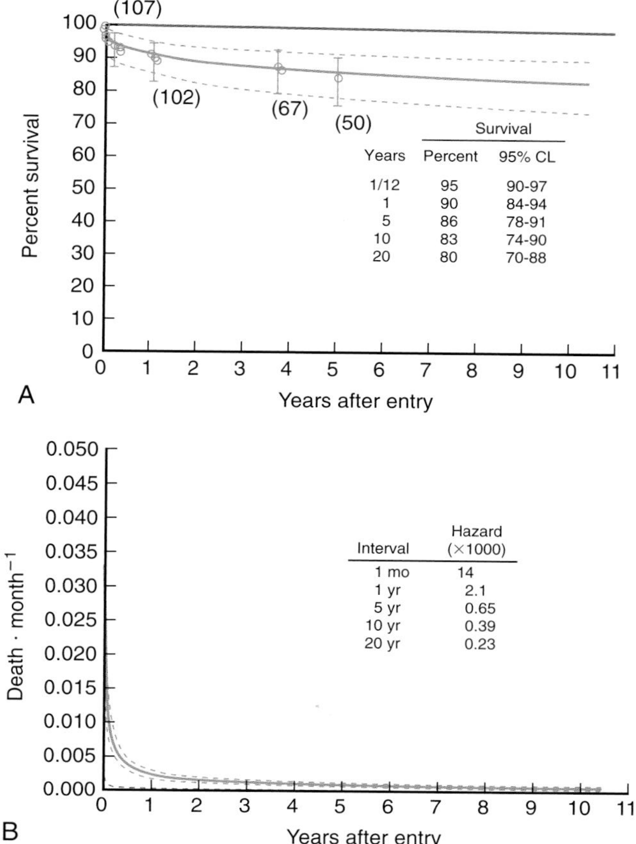

Figure 52-49 Survival and hazard function for death of neonates and infants with simple transposition of great arteries, after entry into hospital and entrance into protocol leading to Mustard-type atrial switch repair. All deaths after entry are included. **A,** Survival (see Fig. 52-43). *Dash-dot-dash line* is survival of age-gender-ethnicity–matched general population. **B,** Hazard function for death. Hazard function for an earlier group of similar patients from same institution and traced for 17 years had no late-rising phase of hazard. Key: *Mo,* Month; *yr,* year. (From Williams WG, Trusler GA, Kirklin JW, Blackstone EH: personal communication; 1986, and Williams and colleagues.[W11])

Table 52-8 Modes of Hospital Death in Patients with Simple Transposition of the Great Arteries[a]

Major Association with Death	Age at Operation	Other Factors
High pulmonary vascular resistance[b]	6, 7, 21 mo	
Low cardiac output	3, 3, 2 mo	NYHA class V in two *Escherichia coli* enteritis in one
Baffle obstruction	19 days	
Respiratory complications	11 days	NYHA class V heart failure, large PDA
Arrhythmia (at 27 days postop)	5 mo[c]	
Chylopericardium (at 26 days postop), tamponade	10 mo[c]	

[a]Data from study of 10 hospital deaths after 141 atrial switch operations for simple transposition of the great arteries at GLH, 1970-1984.
[b]Preoperatively, 8.3, 14, 22 u · m². All showed grade 4 Heath-Edwards changes at autopsy.
[c]Senning repair.
Key: *mo,* Months; *NYHA,* New York Heart Association; *PDA,* patent ductus arteriosus; postop, postoperatively.

Table 52-9 Incremental Risk Factors for Hospital Death after Atrial Switch Operation[a]

Risk Factor	Coefficient ± SD	*P*
Moderate or large VSD	2.2 ± 0.44	<.0001
PDA[b]	0.96 ± 0.49	.05
Age ≤ 30 days	2.3 ± 0.79	.003
Intercept	2.9	

[a]Multivariable logistic analysis is of 38 hospital deaths among 203 patients undergoing atrial switch operation, with or without associated procedures, for all types of transposition of the great arteries at GLH, 1970-1984. Variables entered into analysis are in Appendix 52B.
[b]Small, moderate, or large.
Key: *PDA,* Patent ductus arteriosus; *SD,* standard deviation; *VSD,* ventricular septal defect.

artery by overzealous excision of the limbus and reendothelialization of the bare area so created, and placing suture lines too close to the sinus node.

Although these abnormalities are associated with dysrhythmias and are present in many individuals with late sudden death, it is uncertain whether they explain all late benign arrhythmias after the Mustard and Senning operations. Extensive suture lines within the atria, combined with excision of virtually all the atrial septum, may be related factors.[G5,W15] Although it is no longer believed that atrial conduction occurs through discrete, well-defined internodal tracts[J2] (see "Internodal Pathways" under Conduction System in Chapter 1), preservation of the anterosuperior portion of the limbus may decrease prevalence of dysrhythmia.[C13,T13] In contrast, division of the free wall of the coronary sinus is not detrimental.[C13,T13]

Junctional rhythm becomes progressively more prevalent as the years pass (Fig. 52-50). Usually sinus rhythm is present on standard ECG tracings at hospital discharge after the atrial switch operation for simple TGA.[C13] About 10% of such

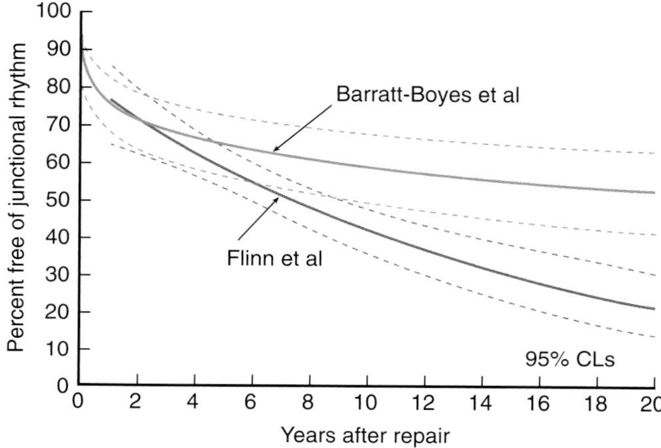

Figure 52-50 Time-related freedom from junctional rhythm after atrial switch operation by Mustard technique. Data from GLH are from same data set as depicted in Table 52-10 and from Flinn and colleagues.[F5] Key: *CL,* Confidence limits. (From Williams and colleagues.[W11])

Table 52-10 Cardiac Rhythm after Mustard Atrial Switch Repair in Patients with Simple Transposition of the Great Arteries[a]

	Prevalence at Hospital Discharge		Rhythm at Last Review					
			Sinus		Junctional[b]		CHB	
Rhythm	**No.**	**%**	**No.**	**%**	**No.**	**%**	**No.**	**%**
Sinus[c]	88	79	59	53	28	25	1	1[d]
Junctional	9[e]	8	2	2	6[f]	5	1	1
Sinus/junctional	12	11	2	2	10	9	0	
Uncertain	3	3	3	3	0		0	
TOTAL	112	100	66	59	44	39	2	2

[a]Data from study of 112 hospital survivors at GLH, 1964-1982; longest follow-up was 17 years.
[b]Among the 28 patients in junctional rhythm, only 4 (19%) later converted to sinus rhythm.
[c]Among the 88 patients in sinus rhythm at discharge, 28 (32%) later converted to junctional rhythm.
[d]Temporary CHB postoperatively.
[e]One known to be present preoperatively.
[f]One with a PR interval of 0.27.
Key: *CHB,* Complete heart block.

patients are in a varying sinus junctional rhythm, and only a few show a pure benign-type junctional rhythm (Table 52-10). Thereafter, there is a gradual decrease in prevalence of sinus rhythm after Mustard-type repair as follow-up continues.[B10,D9,F5] Besides the apparent slight increase in risk of sudden death when a benign junctional rhythm is present, this rhythm appears to have no other importance. In some normal subjects in sinus rhythm, heart rate can fall below 40 beats · min^{-1} during sleep, and rhythm is then usually junctional.[D5,S8,S21]

In patients with *slow junctional rhythm* there is a relatively normal rate response to exercise, often with reversion to sinus rhythm.[H9] Occasionally rapid (accelerated) junctional rhythm can occur. This rhythm, and occasionally supraventricular tachycardias or atrial flutter, can lead to a malignant arrhythmia that reduces cardiac output and requires active measures for control.[E6] Sinus node recovery time after atrial switch operations may be abnormal.[E7,G4,H9] Also, even when in sinus rhythm, maximal exercise heart rate response and postexercise recovery rate may be abnormal.[H9]

Twenty-four-hour *Holter monitoring* after both the Mustard and Senning procedures may reveal dysrhythmias that are infrequent enough to be overlooked on standard ECGs, even when these are repeated on many occasions.[M12] This technique allows frequency of rhythm disturbances to be assessed, as well as their categorization as a normal or probably abnormal variant. Holter studies that fail to make this latter differentiation overstate dysrhythmia prevalence.[B10] Before a postoperative dysrhythmia can be categorized as resulting from the surgical procedure, it is necessary to know that the abnormal rhythm was not present on a preoperative Holter monitor recording.[S22] Using these criteria, dysrhythmias do not occur often before atrial switch procedures. Thus, 24 patients with TGA aged 1 to 10 months had preoperative monitoring; using the criteria in Table 52-11, only one was abnormal (frequent atrial premature beats), although five patients showed abnormalities within the normal range.[S22]

Postoperative Holter monitoring reveals additional dysrhythmias (Table 52-12), particularly when the patient is in junctional rhythm. If standard ECG always shows sinus rhythm, however, in about two thirds of patients the Holter study is normal. Rarely is an important abnormality in rhythm disclosed for the first time on Holter monitoring. Dysrhythmias that predispose to sudden death in this context are as yet unknown.

Table 52-11 Criteria of Normality and Abnormality of Arrhythmias Observed on 24-Hour Ambulatory Electrocardiographic Monitoring in Normal Infants and Children

Arrhythmia	Normal Criteria	Abnormal Criteria
Junctional (nodal)	Rare, unsustained	Frequent, sustained
Accelerated junctional (>100 · min^{-1})	Unsustained (<6 beats)	Prolonged, repetitive
Tachycardias/ bradycardias	Occasional	Frequent episodes
Sinus pauses	50%-99% duration[a]	50%-99% duration[a] when ≥10 · h^{-1}
	Infrequent (<10 · h^{-1})	≥100% duration, total pause ≥ 1800 ms
Premature beats	Infrequent (<10 · h^{-1})	≥10 · h^{-1}
Atrial bi/trigeminy	Infrequent (<3 episodes)	Repetitive
	Unsustained	Sustained
Supraventricular tachycardia[b]	Unsustained (<6 beats)	Sustained, chaotic, repetitive

[a]PP (or RR) interval length of sinus pause beat compared with preceding normal beat.
[b]Some are caused by atrial flutter.

Rhythm monitoring during maximal exercise testing may provide additional information, although at present its prognostic implications are also unknown. Mathews and colleagues noted that of 15 patients in sinus rhythm at rest who underwent exercise testing a mean of 9 years after Mustard repair, nine developed either premature atrial or ventricular contractions or junctional rhythm during exercise.[M16] This finding contrasted with a control group, none of whom developed a dysrhythmia.[M16]

Sudden death may well be related to some of these dysrhythmias. This complication was emphasized during early

Table 52-12 Arrhythmias on 24-Hour Ambulatory Electrocardiographic Monitoring of Patients after Mustard Atrial Switch Procedure[a]

	Persistent SR			Persistent JR		
		Abnormal		Normal	Abnormal	
Rhythm on Holter Monitor	**Normal**	**No.**	**% of 19**		**No.**	**% of 17**
SR	16	0	0	3	0	0
JR	0	3	16	1	14	82
Accelerated JR	1	0	0	1	2	12
Tachy/bradycardias	0	0	0	1	1	6
Sinus pauses[b]:						
50%-99%	5	6	32	4	6	35
≥100%	0	3	16	0	2	12
≥1800 ms	0	0	0	0	2	12
APBs	9	2	11	2	7	41
VPBs	3	1	5	0	3	18
Bi/trigeminy	0	0	0	2	2	12
SVT	0	1	5	2	2	12
Total Arrhythmias[c]	18	13		16	27	
Total Patients	11	8	42 CL 29%-57%	0	17	100 CL 89%-100%

[a]Data from a study at GLH, 1970-1984. Criteria are given in Table 52-11.
[b]See Table 52-11.
[c]Excluding junctional rhythm.
Key: *APBs,* Atrial premature beats; *CL,* 70% confidence limits; *JR,* junctional rhythm; *SR,* sinus rhythm; *SVT,* supraventricular tachycardia; *VPBs,* ventricular premature beats.

development of the atrial switch operation by Aberdeen.[A3] Sudden death occurs in about 5% of hospital survivors over 10 to 20 years. Sudden death is rare in patients who remain in sinus rhythm postoperatively and when pacemaker recovery times are normal.[E7,G4,H9] Risk of sudden death in patients in junctional rhythm is 7%. No other risk factors for sudden death could be identified in a collaborative study of 372 patients.[F5] In a prospective 8-year study of 100 Senning and Mustard patients, progressive loss of a stable sinus rhythm was noted in more than 60% of patients at a mean follow-up of 7 years. However, rhythm disturbance identified by ECG or Holter monitoring did not identify patients at risk for sudden death.[D9]

Changes in P-wave amplitude and contour are virtually constant after Mustard repair.[C13,E6] Postoperatively, the P wave is greatly diminished in amplitude and is frequently bifid in shape. The mean frontal plane P-wave axis, however, is unchanged.

At late follow-up (23 years post-Mustard procedure), prevalence of atrial fibrillation or flutter is approximately 20% and seems to be a marker of reduced RV function.[G1,L13,P19] Episodes of supraventricular tachycardia occur in 3% to 5% of hospital survivors of the Mustard-type atrial switch procedure. In a 27-year follow-up of survivors of Senning procedures, 78% were in sinus rhythm, and freedom from pacemaker implantation for hospital survivors was 81 ± 5.9% at 25 years.[H11] In the 20-institution study of the Congenital Heart Surgeons Society, 94% and 91% of patients were free of pacemaker insertion 5 and 9 years after atrial switch repair, with risk factors being TGA and VSD vs. simple TGA and Senning versus Mustard type of repair.[W4]

Growth and Functional Status

Most patients appear to be asymptomatic after an atrial switch procedure, although at 9 to 12 years of follow-up in a large multiinstitutional study, only 60% were in New York Heart Association (NYHA) class I, and most of the rest in class II.[H16,T11,W4] However, graded exercise testing has shown that up to 80% have reduced exercise capacity associated with lower maximal oxygen consumption values compared with normal.[P13,R10] Normal hemodynamic state is present in only one third of patients who claim to be asymptomatic and functionally normal.[B29] These abnormalities are more prominent in patients operated on at an older age[D17,M16] and are often accompanied by abnormal cardiac rhythms (see preceding text).

Patients found to have normal or near-normal exercise capacity tend to have a normal response of RV systolic function to exercise.[M36] Functional capacity may be better in patients receiving the Senning rather than the Mustard type of atrial switch procedure; Bjornstad and colleagues found atrial function to be superior with the Senning operation.[B30,D17,M16] Abnormal lung function has been implicated in reduced exercise capacity.[H14]

Height and weight increase considerably after an atrial switch repair, particularly in those with importantly decreased height and weight preoperatively.[L11] Return to normal height and weight may be achieved within 2 years of operation.

Coronary Arteries

Abnormalities in the caliber of proximal coronary arteries have been noted in patients after the atrial switch procedure. Diameter of the RCA is larger and that of LCA smaller in symptomatic patients compared with either asymptomatic or non-TGA patients.[A7]

Venous Pathway Obstruction

The complex problem of obstructed venous pathway is discussed in detail under Special Situations and Controversies later in this chapter.

Right Ventricular Function

Ventricular function after atrial switch repair of transposition is often discussed by analogy with function of the ventricles in congenitally corrected TGA. Contrary to traditional beliefs, right (systemic) ventricular function is demonstrably abnormal only during stress, and then only mildly (see "Ventricular Function" under Natural History in Chapter 55). This finding suggests that more severe abnormalities in ventricular function found after an atrial switch repair are related primarily to abnormalities in ventricular filling patterns and other post–atrial switch effects.[P15]

RV systolic function, usually studied by measuring ejection fraction at rest or during exercise or another form of stress, is usually reduced after atrial switch repair in patients with simple TGA.[B14,B15,D13,G14,H3,M36] However, at least some patients have reduced ejection fraction preoperatively, and it is uncertain whether further reduction postoperatively is common.[G14] When RV systolic function decreases after an atrial switch procedure, it is usually associated with increased RV end-diastolic volume.[H3]

During exercise, RV ejection fraction may increase, remain unchanged, or decrease; patient age at operation, time of study, and the postoperative interval are not predictive of the change.[B17,M36,P8,R4] In a group of patients averaging 10 years of follow-up after an atrial switch operation, cardiac output response to submaximal exercise was abnormally reduced compared with non-TGA subjects.[P2] Other reports support this finding.[M17] Limitation in cardiac output may have complex etiologies. Dobutamine-induced increases in systemic RV contractility may not be attended by increased stroke volume, possibly because of limited ventricular filling caused by rigid atrial baffles or decreased RV compliance caused by hypertrophy.[P2,T15] More recent studies examining this stroke volume effect suggest that, in fact, atrial transport is responsible.[D14]

Further evidence about a possible decrease in RV function after atrial switch repair was obtained by Borow and colleagues.[B37] The systemic RVs in patients in whom the procedure was performed during the first year of life responded to afterload stress (methoxamine infusion) with a smaller increase in minute work index than did ventricles in normal patients or patients after repair of isolated VSD or tetralogy of Fallot. Parrish and colleagues found a similar impairment of systemic RV response in patients with congenitally corrected transposition.[P8] The reasons for this finding are not entirely evident. Myocardial fiber arrangement in the RV may differ from that in the LV, which may render it less able to function systemically.[S27] Possibly the RV cannot benefit from the septal component of ejection because of bellowslike action of the ventricular free wall.[B17] Benson and colleagues suggest that a mismatch may exist between RV coronary blood supply and demand.[B17] In a study of 22 patients at a mean of 15 years post–atrial switch, all showed evidence of either fixed or reversible perfusion defects in the RV.[M28]

In any event, progressive deterioration of RV function is uncommon after the atrial switch procedure in patients with simple TGA, although serial evaluations of RV function suggest worsening of function over time.[H19] Thus, obvious RV failure with marked hypokinesis and increased end-diastolic volume and signs and symptoms of heart failure[B14] is rare.[C15,P4] Frank RV dysfunction is more common in patients with associated large VSD that also requires repair.[G14,P8] In a 27-year single-institution follow-up of 314 survivors of the Senning operation (82 with VSD), freedom from reoperation for systemic RV failure at 25 years was 96% ± 1.2%.[H11]

Left Ventricular Function

LV function at rest is often normal late after atrial switch operations.[H3] In some patients, however, LV ejection fraction fails to increase with exercise.[M36]

Tricuspid Valve Regurgitation

Important (moderate or severe) tricuspid regurgitation occurs infrequently after the atrial switch procedure for simple TGA. Exceptional patient groups with a prevalence of up to 15% have been reported,[H2] but reasons for this variability are not evident. Trivial and mild regurgitation occasionally occur.[C15,G9,M3,M34]

Left Ventricular Outflow Tract Obstruction

When an atrial switch procedure is performed for patients with simple TGA and dynamic LVOTO (see Morphology earlier in this chapter), obstruction rarely progresses thereafter.[P4] In fact, LVOTO usually regresses to some degree, whether or not a myotomy or myectomy is performed (Fig. 52-51).

Results of direct relief of the other types of LVOTO are also reasonably good (Fig. 52-52). When direct relief has not been possible, bypassing the obstruction with an LV–pulmonary trunk valved conduit provides good relief.[C23]

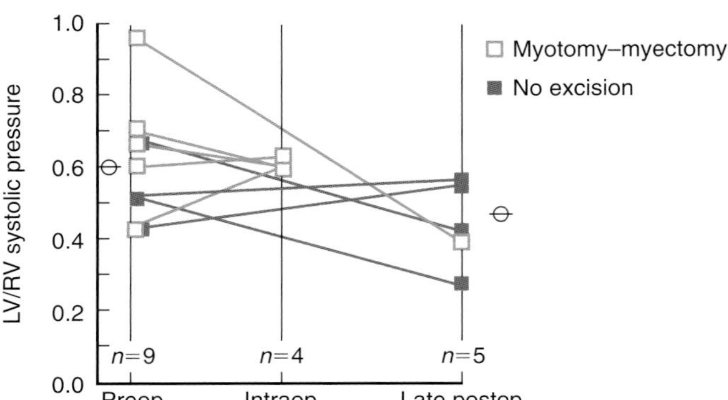

Figure 52-51 Preoperative, intraoperative, and late postoperative (mean 35 months) pressure measurements in patients with simple transposition of great arteries and dynamic type of left ventricular outflow obstruction undergoing an atrial switch procedure (GLH, 1964-1984). Follow-up time is 23 to 134 months (mean 56 months). When myotomy or myectomy was performed, approach was through pulmonary trunk. Key: *Intraop,* Intraoperative; *LV/RV,* left ventricular/right ventricular; *Postop,* postoperative; *Preop,* preoperative.

Residual Atrial Shunting

Trivial leaking at the baffle suture line occurs in about a fourth of patients (26%; CL 24%-29% in 390 collected cases).[A12,G9,G13,H2,M3,M34,P4,S29,T1,T13]

Severe leaks requiring reoperation are uncommon, occurring in 12 (3%; CL 2%-4%) of the 390 collected cases. Leaks are most common in the trabeculated upper portion of the atrium.

Pulmonary Vascular Disease

When an atrial switch operation is performed in the first 3 months for patients with TGA and essentially intact ventricular septum, new and progressive pulmonary vascular disease is uncommon; Mahoney and colleagues found no instances (0%; CL 0%-7%) in 28 patients undergoing operation during the first 100 days of life.[M3] However, when repair is done after age 3 months, some patients (5%-10%) with normal Rp preoperatively develop pulmonary vascular disease postoperatively (Table 52-13).[N8,R16] The disease often progresses and causes death.[B20] More recent studies confirm that pulmonary hypertension can develop and progress in patients documented as having normal pulmonary artery pressure postoperatively.[E1]

Infants with simple TGA with evidence of elevated Rp preoperatively to levels less than about 12 U · m² may experience a satisfactory fall in resistance late postoperatively.[C16] Some of this fall is related to reduction in hematocrit that occurs postoperatively.[C16,D12,H5] In some patients, however, preexisting pulmonary vascular disease may progress postoperatively and be a cause of late mortality (Table 52-14).[M5] The occasional neonate with TGA who manifests evidence of pulmonary vascular disease may have antenatal constriction of the ductus arteriosus.[K17]

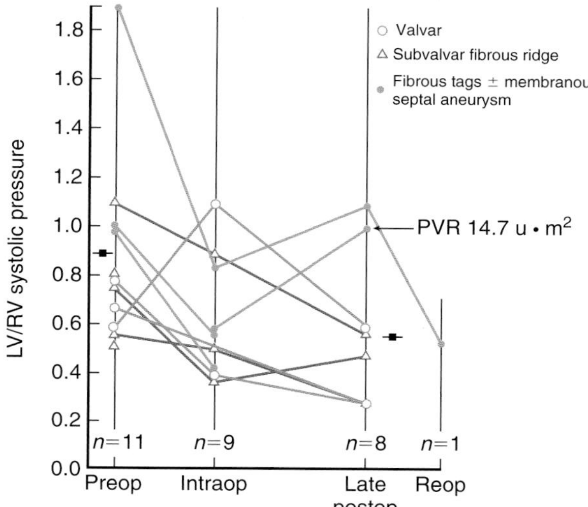

Figure 52-52 Depiction is as in Fig. 52-51, except left ventricular outflow obstruction was morphologic rather than dynamic (GLH, 1964-1984). Obstruction was relieved through a pulmonary trunk approach. Follow-up time is 16 to 55 months (mean 35 months). Key: *Intraop,* Intraoperative; *LV/RV,* left ventricular/right ventricular; *Postop,* postoperative; *Preop,* preoperative; *PVR,* pulmonary vascular resistance; *Reop,* reoperative.

Transposition of the Great Arteries, Ventricular Septal Defect, and Left Ventricular Outflow Tract Obstruction

Early (Hospital) Death

In the early years of their use, early mortality after both the Rastelli and Lecompte operations (see "Lecompte Intraventricular Repair" under Technique of Operation in Chapter 53) was high: 20% to 30%.[B38,L6] In more recent times, however, mortality after both types of repairs has been reduced to less than 5%.[K15,V13] Contemporary early mortality after Rastelli, Lecompte, or Nikaidoh operations are comparable.[H15]

Time-Related Survival

Including early in-hospital mortality, 10-year predicted survival of patients undergoing surgery during the 1980 to 1991

Table 52-13 Pulmonary Vascular Resistance after Atrial Switch Operation[a]

Preoperative Study		Operation	Postoperative Study		
Age (months)	Rp (u · m²)	Age (months)	Age (months)	Rp (u · m²)	Comments
3	2.0	4	57	35	
		3[b]	21	15	
		5	45	9.2	
		35	103	8.9	(Late death): small PDA; grade 4 PVD
		24	44	8.1	
		43	102	7.7	Large PDA
4	1.6	4	49	6.7	Large baffle leak (reoperation)
		45	98	7.2	
		38	47	6.2	
		26	45	4.2	
		46[c]	78	4.0	

[a]Data are from patients with simple transposition of great arteries operated on at age 3 or more months; GLH, 1964-1984. Patients for whom no data are available preoperatively are presumed to have then had normal resistance.
[b]Mild fibrous left ventricular outflow tract obstruction.
[c]Mild dynamic left ventricular outflow tract obstruction.
Key: *PDA,* Patent ductus arteriosus; *PVD,* pulmonary vascular disease; *Rp,* pulmonary vascular resistance.

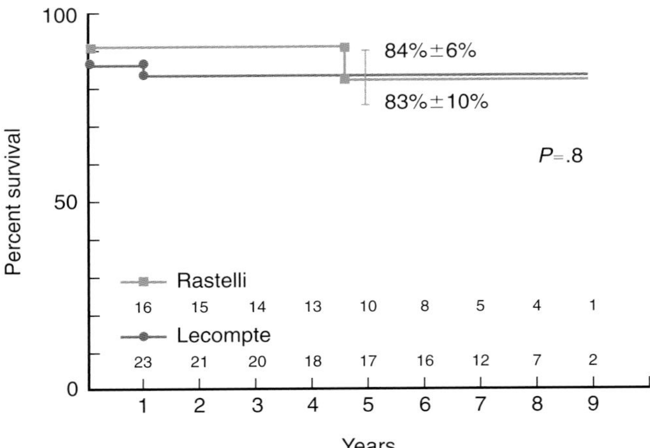

Figure 52-53 Survival (Kaplan-Meier method), including hospital deaths, after Rastelli and Lecompte operations for transposition of great arteries, ventricular septal defect, and left ventricular outflow tract obstruction. Numbers indicate traced patients at each time interval. (From Vouhe and colleagues.[V13])

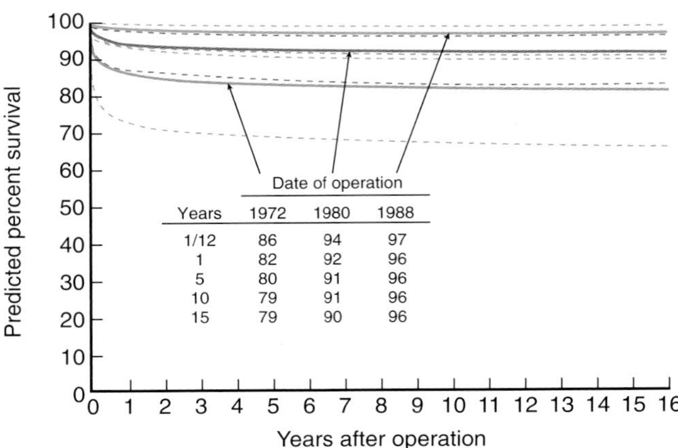

Figure 52-54 Improvement across time of early and late survival of reasonably good-risk patients after Rastelli operation for transposition of great arteries, ventricular septal defect, and left ventricular outflow tract obstruction. Depiction is a nomogram of a specific solution of the multivariable equation in Table 52-15. New York Heart Association class was entered as grade II.

Table 52-14 Pulmonary Vascular Resistance in Patients with Preoperatively Moderate or Severe Pulmonary Vascular Disease[a]

Preoperative Study		Operation	Postoperative Study (or Autopsy)	
Age (months)	Rp (u · m²)	Age (mo)		Rp (u · m²)
5[b]	22	5	(HD)	Gr4 PVD
6[c]	14	7	(HD)	Gr4 PVD
10	11	12		3.6
57	10	58		4.2
19	8.3	20	(HD)	Gr4 PVD
		20	(HD)	Gr4 PVD
		40	(HD)	Gr4 PVD
		37	(HD)	Gr4 PVD
30	7.8	32		3.1
		32	(HD)	Gr2 PVD

[a]Data from patients with simple transposition of great arteries who were aged 3 months or older at time of an atrial switch operation at GLH, 1964-1984.
[b]Small patent ductus arteriosus.
[c]Moderate patent ductus arteriosus.
Key: *Gr,* Grade; *HD,* hospital death; *PVD,* pulmonary vascular disease; *Rp,* pulmonary vascular resistance.

Table 52-15 Incremental Risk Factors for Premature Death after Rastelli Operation for Transposition of the Great Arteries, Ventricular Septal Defect, and Left Ventricular Outflow Tract Obstruction[a]

	Single Hazard Phase	
Risk Factor	**Coefficient ± SD**	***P***
Earlier date of operation (months since 1/1/67)	−0.14 ± 0.085	.10
NYHA functional class	0.6 ± 0.42	.14
Intercept	0.112	

[a]Analysis is of 57 patients (22 deaths, including hospital and later deaths) operated on at UAB, 1967-1984. See Appendix 52C for variables entered into analyses.
Key: *NYHA,* New York Heart Association; *SD,* standard deviation.

period was 80% to 85%, with no difference attributed to whether the Rastelli or Lecompte operation was done[V13] (Fig. 52-53). Predicted 10-year survival for patients operated on in the latter part of that period was even higher—about 95% (Fig. 52-54). Recently, 15- and 20-year follow-ups have been reported after the Rastelli operation.[K15] In this experience, 10-year follow-up was comparable with that just described, but 15- and 20-year survival dropped to 68% and 52%, respectively. Based on very small numbers, late survival appears to be similar for the Nikaidoh operation.[H15]

Incremental Risk Factors for Death

Few if any patient-related risk factors for death have been identified for TGA, VSD, and LVOTO repair, but advanced disability has been (Table 52-15), probably in part because it is usually associated with severe cyanosis, polycythemia, advanced ventricular hypertrophy, and heart failure. Young age at operation has not been found to be a risk factor with the Lecompte operation; Vouhe and colleagues reported no deaths (0%; CL 0%-21%) among infants undergoing this operation,[V13] although the youngest patient was 4 months old. Straddling tricuspid valve has been identified as a risk factor for early death in at least one series.[K15]

Earlier date of operation has been a risk factor for death after repair, but results have been better in recent years (see Table 52-15).

Procedural risk factors for premature death have not yet been identified. Survival is similar after the Rastelli and Lecompte procedures.[V13] Reports on the Nikaidoh procedure or modifications thereof have yielded comparable early results, although numbers are small.[B9,B24,M33,N10]

Functional Status

Functional status of most patients undergoing repair of TGA, VSD, and LVOTO by either the Rastelli or Lecompte method is good. Vouhe and colleagues report that 98% of patients undergoing these operations were in NYHA class I or II.[V13]

Complete Heart Block

Complete heart block may occur with slightly greater frequency than after repair of simple primary VSD. Vouhe and colleagues report one such patient (2%; CL 2%-5%) among 62.[V13]

Reoperation

Reoperation is in general ultimately inevitable when an extracardiac conduit is used. When the Rastelli operation is properly performed, however, placing the conduit to the left of the ascending aorta rather than to the right as originally described by Rastelli,[R8] reoperation occurs with the same prevalence as when it is used in other operations (see "Reoperation and Other Reinterventions for Right Ventricular Outflow Problems" in Section I of Chapter 38).

Patients have not been entirely free of reoperation for RVOTO after the Lecompte operation for TGA, VSD, and LVOTO; 7% (CL 2%-15%) of 30 surviving patients had reoperation over a 5-year period.[V13] However, the proportion of patients having either reoperation for this problem, or the problem itself but as yet without reoperation, was lower in those undergoing the Lecompte operation (26%) than in those undergoing the Rastelli operation (67%; $P = .005$).[V13]

Reoperation for obstruction in the subaortic region within the surgically created tunnel between the LV and aorta may occur in as many as 35% to 40% of patients undergoing the Rastelli operation or one of its variants.[R10] Risk factors are not clearly defined but may include small VSD size and early age at operation. Other factors such as surgical technique and ventricular geometric changes may also be important. At medium term, the need for intervention for LVOTO may be higher after the Rastelli operation compared with the Lecompte and Nikaidoh operations; however, again the numbers are very small.[L8] Resection of the infundibular septum and adequate enlargement of the VSD may be the reason for this. Nevertheless, mortality with reintervention is currently far better than previously reported. Although the Nikaidoh operation has theoretical advantages, concern about developing translocated aortic valve regurgitation is very high.

INDICATIONS FOR OPERATION

Simple Transposition of the Great Arteries in Neonates

Presence of the malformation is an indication for operation. If cyanosis and symptoms are severe, BAS is performed as soon as possible. A less attractive alternative is immediate arterial switch.

When indicated, an arterial switch operation should be performed within the first week of life, and at least within the first 30 days of life. Increased Rp at this stage is not a contraindication to repair.[C7] LVOTO, which is typically dynamic in this setting, is also not a contraindication regardless of its imaged appearance.[W5] Risk of operation is probably lowest when it is performed in the first week of life (see Fig. 52-41), and there is the additional advantage of minimizing exposure time of the brain to the hypoxia of uncorrected TGA.[N6]

Excellence of results to date favors the arterial switch over the atrial switch operation (see Fig. 52-37).

Simple Transposition of the Great Arteries Presenting after Age 30 Days

Primary arterial switch operation may carry a higher risk for infants with simple TGA who are beyond age 1 month, because by then the LV has usually become morphologically adapted to supporting the low-pressure pulmonary circulation. Davis and colleagues have taken exception to this and, based on their favorable experience, recommend a *primary* arterial switch operation unless the infant is older than age 8 weeks.[D8] Arterial switch has been successfully performed beyond the neonatal period and up to 9 months of age in patients with intact septum, but such patients are more likely to require postoperative mechanical support.[K2] Based on these experiences and similar observations by others, there is a willingness in most cases to perform primary arterial switch in infants younger than 8 weeks of age, and in some cases even in older infants with persisting large PDA, as long as mechanical assistance can be provided (see "Temporary Ventricular Assistance" in Section I of Chapter 5). If mechanical assistance is not available, or if primary arterial switch is not undertaken for some other reason, the options are:

- Pulmonary trunk banding with concomitant systemic–pulmonary artery shunting, followed within 1 or 2 weeks by arterial switch operation[B22,J7,Y3]
- Atrial switch operation

Because the first approach appears to carry only slightly more risk than a primary atrial switch operation in a neonate in institutions properly prepared for this surgery, it is the more desirable of the two procedures.[J7]

When arterial switch operation is delayed for a month or more after banding, risk of postoperative death may be considerably increased,[K12] although others have shown no increased risk in waiting up to 4 months after banding.[N3] In institutions not well prepared for this type of surgery, an atrial switch operation may be more appropriate.

Transposition of the Great Arteries with Ventricular Septal Defect

TGA with VSD is an indication for arterial switch operation and repair of the VSD. It is indicated at the time the patient is first seen, with the procedure performed within the first few weeks of life.

Transposition of the Great Arteries with Ventricular Septal Defect and Left Ventricular Outflow Tract Obstruction

Diagnosis of TGA with VSD and LVOTO is an indication for operation, but type and timing of the definitive procedure remain controversial.

Many babies born with TGA, VSD, and LVOTO are not sufficiently cyanotic in early life to require urgent surgical intervention. Although the youngest age at which the Lecompte operation can be performed is not certain, it can be performed in infants older than age 6 months with a reasonably low mortality. The Lecompte procedure is probably the indicated operation in patients with this anomaly who appear for surgical repair between age 6 months and 4 to 5 years. When cyanosis and symptoms are important before age 6 months, either a systemic–pulmonary artery shunt, followed by a Lecompte operation within 6 to 18 months, or a primary

Lecompte operation, is indicated. The choice is best made in individual institutions according to their capabilities and experience.

In children age 3 to 5 years, either the Lecompte or Rastelli operation provides good results. In special situations, the Nikaidoh[B24,N10] procedure may be considered as an alternative to the Rastelli or Lecompte operation.

SPECIAL SITUATIONS AND CONTROVERSIES

Arterial Switch Repair

Transposition of the Great Arteries with Posterior Aorta

The unusual posterior aorta variant of TGA, described in 1971 by Van Praagh and colleagues,[V5] had been considered a contraindication to the arterial switch operation until a successful case was reported by Tam, Murphy, and Norwood.[T3] They repaired the conoventricular VSD through the aorta after transecting the great arteries, and transplanted the coronary ostia just as in the routine approach. Switch of the great arteries was accomplished without the Lecompte maneuver. Benatar and colleagues had previously reported treating a patient with this morphology by an arterial switch repair, but the patient died on the fifth postoperative day.[B13]

Straddling Atrioventricular Valves

Serraf and colleagues have shown that straddling AV valves, either tricuspid or mitral, do not represent a contraindication to two-ventricle repair in TGA.[S11] When appropriate, the arterial switch operation can be combined with AV valve repair in most patients, with good outcome.

Other Techniques

Current surgical techniques for the arterial switch operation (see Technique of Operation earlier in this chapter) have evolved from original descriptions of Jatene and of Yacoub, in which a synthetic tube was used to aid in reconstruction of the neopulmonary artery. This approach is now rarely necessary.

The Damus-Kaye-Stansel type of arterial switch procedure has also been used in patients with TGA and large VSD.[D3,D4,D6,K5,S23] The pulmonary trunk is transected near its bifurcation and the proximal end anastomosed end-to-side to the ascending aorta. A valved extracardiac conduit is placed between the RV and distal pulmonary trunk and the VSD closed. RV (pulmonary) systolic pressure falls to about 30 mmHg, and aortic pressure, which is above 100 mmHg, keeps the aortic valve closed. Some have recommended suturing the aortic valve closed. Mortality in this relatively simple and theoretically attractive operation has been considerable; Ceithaml and colleagues from the Mayo Clinic report 10 deaths (53%; CL 38%-66%) among 19 patients.[C6] However, if patients younger than 1 year of age or those with severe pulmonary vascular disease or LV systolic pressure less than two-thirds systemic are excluded, hospital mortality was 1 in 7 patients (14%; CL 2%-41%). Patients have been clinically well after repair. Over time, an increasing prevalence of regurgitation of the original aortic valve has been observed.[J6] The Damus-Kaye-Stansel repair is now rarely used for patients with TGA and VSD.

Atrial Switch Complications

Superior Vena Caval Obstruction

SVC pathway obstruction appears late postoperatively in 5% to 10% of survivors of the Mustard type of atrial switch procedure[C15] (Table 52-16). Prevalence appears to be unrelated to age at repair, although Cobanoglu and colleagues reported that freedom from reoperation was 59% in patients younger than 7 months of age at operation, compared with 95% in those older than 1 year.[C17] A Congenital Heart Surgeons Society multiinstitutional study found that the highest hazard for reintervention (operative or percutaneous intervention) for pathway obstruction was in the first 6 months after repair, followed by a constant low risk of 0.018% per year thereafter. At 1 and 9 years, freedom from such reinterventions was 97% and 95%, respectively.[W4]

SVC obstruction is maximal at the site of excision of the superior remnant (limbus) of the atrial septum beneath the

Table 52-16 Incidence of Superior Vena Caval (Upper Systemic Venous Compartment) Obstruction after Mustard Operation[a]

Age at Operation			SVCO (Moderate/Severe)[b]			
≤ Months	<	Hospital Survivors	No.	%	Reoperation No.	Late Death No.
	1	3	—	0		
1	3	26	3[c]	12	3	1
3	6	57	4	7	2	3[d]
6	12	48	3	6	2	0
12	24	14	0			
24		18	2	11	2	0
TOTAL		166	12	7	9	4 (2%)
$P(\chi)^2$					.8	

[a]Data from analysis based on 166 hospital survivors of Mustard operation for transposition of great arteries of all types at GLH, 1964 to July 1981.
[b]Pressure gradients ranged between 9 and 22 mmHg.
[c]One patient had associated significant lower venous compartment obstruction.
[d]Two of these three deaths occurred without reoperation (one from associated severe pulmonary venous compartment obstruction, the other from noncardiac causes).
Key: *SVCO,* Superior vena caval obstruction.

upper baffle compartment, and thus lies within the right atrium rather than at the SVC–right atrial junction. This location was first described by Mazzei and Mulder in 1971.[M20] The venous pathway may be totally occluded for over 1 cm or more in this area, or there may be only a localized zone of narrowing. Baffle shape, size, and composition are each important in its production, as is the position of suture lines within the atrium. Because it has proven impossible to eliminate this problem after the Mustard procedure, despite intense study, the exact mechanism is not understood.

Prevalence of late SVC obstruction after a Senning operation is probably lower than after a Mustard operation,[B14,F2,P3,W18] although some have found no difference.[B14,F2,H8,P3,W18] Geometry of the pathway is, on average, better with the Senning-type repair, and the entire compartment is composed of viable atrial wall. Chin and colleagues, however, found SVC obstruction present in 2 of 28 (7%; CL 2.4%-16%) recatheterized patients after Senning repair.[C8]

Clinical Features The patient may be asymptomatic. Venables and colleagues found that although symptoms could be present with an SVC mean pressure as low as 10 mmHg, they were not constant until it rose above 16 mmHg.[V7]

The least conspicuous clinical feature, but one that suggests diagnosis, is *ruddiness* of the cheeks. Puffiness of the eyelids, face, and neck can mask fixed distention of the jugular veins. Tortuous subcutaneous venous collaterals can occur[P4] but are uncommon. A bilateral or right-sided pleural effusion may be present, sometimes chylous. On chest radiograph, there may be bilateral cervical and axillary lymphadenopathy and paramediastinal densities caused by tortuous collaterals.[M20]

Less common features are increasing head circumference and hydrocephalus associated with widening of the cranial sutures in children younger than age 18 months (the upper age limit for normal closure of the cranial sutures), which is a response to increased intracranial venous pressure.[M3,R18,S19,S31,V7] Children older than age 3 may develop pseudotumor cerebri.[R18] There may also be protein-losing enteropathy,[K16,M32] presumably caused by interference with the normal return of intestinal lymph to the venous system secondary to a high venous pressure (this is more common with IVC obstruction).[M32]

Time of Onset SVC obstruction is usually apparent within 12 months of operation, although asymptomatic patients may not be discovered until they are investigated later. The appearance between 12 and 18 months after operation of a new stenosis has not been convincingly documented, although slow progression of a mild to severe stenosis has been. Prevalence is 9% at 4 years, with no further events up to 17 years postoperatively (Fig. 52-55).

Diagnosis Diagnosis can be made noninvasively using 2D echocardiography,[C8,S19] Doppler ultrasound,[W17] pulse Doppler echocardiography,[S26] or radionuclide angiography.[H20] However, cardiac catheterization and cineangiography are advisable before reoperation. In severe cases, these modalities demonstrate a striking difference in waveform between SVC and systemic venous atrium, similar to a situation that may be present at the end of operation,[P7] and a high mean pressure in the SVC (Fig. 52-56). Large amplitudes of phasic pressure in the systemic venous atrium due to its small volume, which can cause a rapid rise in pressure as the chamber fills, are followed by a rapid fall when it empties into a more compliant LV.[P7,V7] These abnormal waveforms are not necessarily present

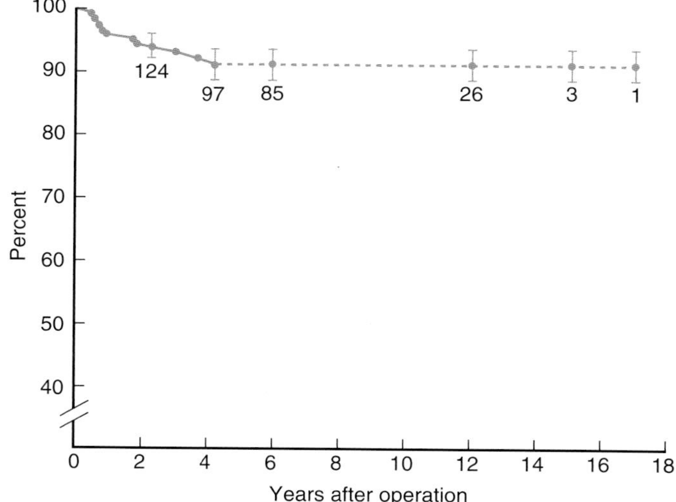

Figure 52-55 Freedom from superior vena caval obstruction in hospital survivors of Mustard-type atrial switch operation (GLH, 1964-1981). Time of appearance of obstruction is taken as time of postoperative cardiac catheterization (n = 10) or recognition of an increase in head circumference (>2 SD of expected mean for age) at 6 and 9 months postoperatively. Obstructions documented as appearing after 1 year postoperatively were either without symptoms at an earlier stage or, in one patient, had serial cardiac catheterization showing progression of a mild stenosis. Of 166 patients, 94 had late postoperative cardiac catheterization. Each closed circle up to 4 years is an event, vertical bars represent 68% confidence limits, and numbers are traced patients.

late postoperatively (Fig. 52-57), nor is there necessarily a gradient,[C15] but they are common.[S18,V7] When SVC obstruction is mild, the striking feature is the damped waveform in the SVC tracing.

Obstruction severe enough to become apparent clinically is associated with an SVC mean pressure above about 15 mmHg and an SVC–systemic venous atrium gradient of at least 10 mmHg.[M3,P4,V7] In 19 patients with severe obstruction, Silove and Taylor recorded a mean gradient of 17 ± 9.0.[S18] SVC pressure tends to be higher when there is also IVC obstruction.[V7] Occasionally the SVC tracing may show tall *a* waves caused by contraction of the right atrial appendage (when it lies above the site of stenosis); in this situation the blood refluxes up the SVC (see Fig. 52-56).[S18]

Angiography shows either complete obstruction or severe stenosis.

Treatment When symptoms are present, reoperation is indicated (see Technique of Operation earlier in this chapter). Reoperation is also indicated in any child who shows progressive increase in head size beyond the normal range. Balloon expandable stents delivered using interventional cardiologic techniques have been successful in relieving some obstructions.[B50,W3] Alternatively, if Rp is acceptably low, a bidirectional superior cavopulmonary anastomosis can be performed.

Inferior Vena Caval Obstruction

Although an important occurrence of IVC pathway obstruction was reported in the early series of Stark and associates[S25] and Venables and colleagues[V7] using polyester baffles, current prevalence is low (1%-2%).[A12,C6,G13,M3,P4,T13] This complication

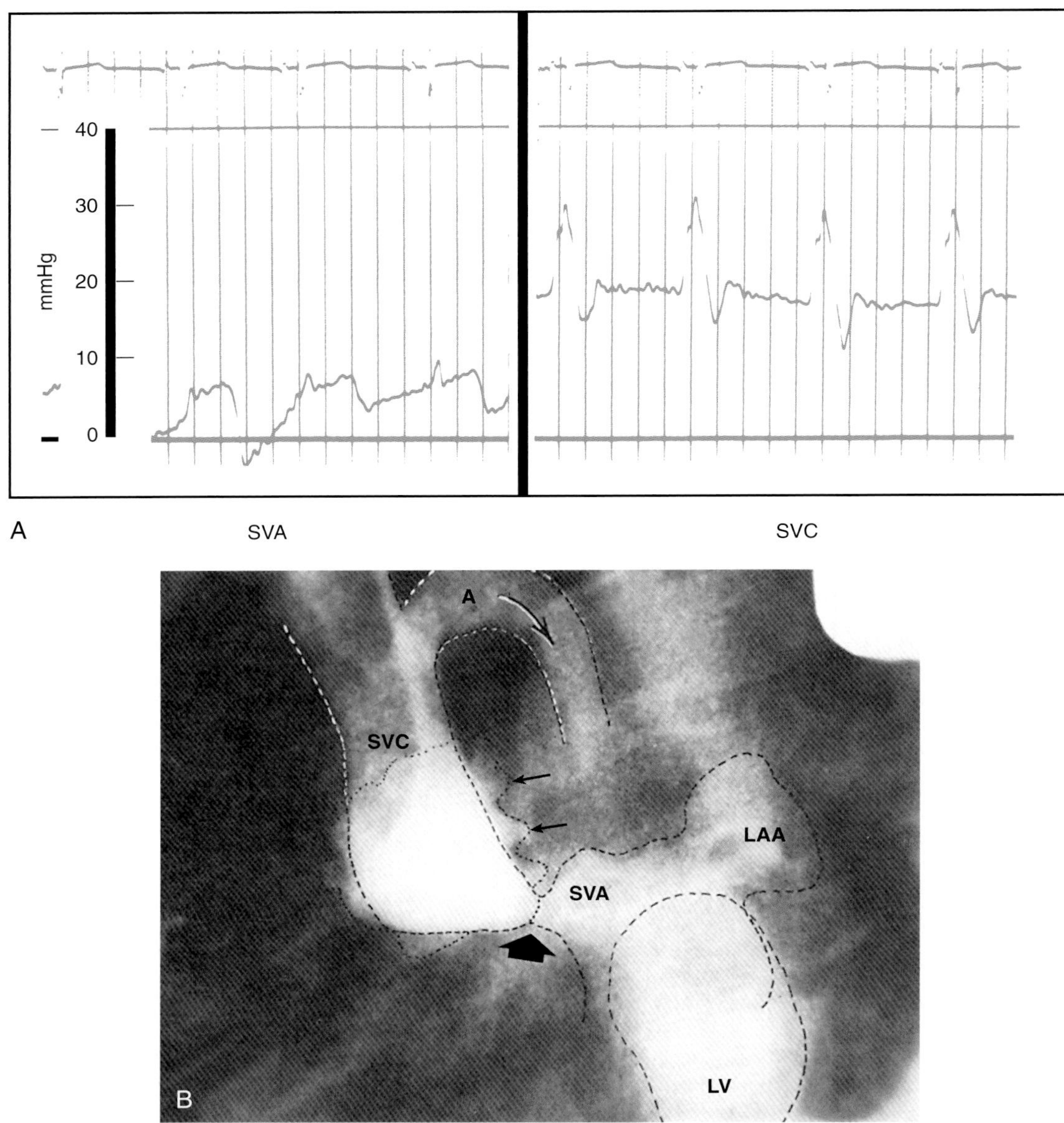

Figure 52-56 Data from postoperative cardiac catheterization in patient who had undergone Mustard repair and developed severe obstruction to superior vena caval *(SVC)* flow into systemic venous atrium *(SVA)*. **A,** Phasic withdrawal pressures from SVA to SVC. Mean pressures were 5 and 20 mmHg, respectively. Note dominant *a* wave in SVC tracing, caused by contraction of portion of right atrial appendage that lies above site of obstruction. **B,** Cineangiogram after injection into SVC, in 20-degree left anterior oblique projection. Heavy arrow marks site of obstruction. Fine dotted lines *(small arrows)* outline that portion of original right atrial appendage that lies in upper venous compartment beneath baffle and above site of obstruction. There is retrograde flow into azygos vein. Key: *A,* Azygos vein; *LAA,* left atrial appendage; *LV,* left ventricle. (From Clarkson and colleagues.[C15])

can be minimized when at the atrial switch procedure, the coronary sinus is opened down into the left atrium (see Technique of Operation earlier in this chapter).

Postoperative IVC obstruction, as with SVC obstruction, occurs within the heart at about the midpoint of the lower portion of the systemic venous compartment adjacent to the coronary sinus ostium. Patients with important IVC obstruction usually are symptomatic, with liver enlargement, ascites, and leg edema. A protein-losing enteropathy may occur more frequently than with SVC obstruction,[M32] and particularly when combined with some degree of SVC obstruction, there may be low cardiac output and premature late death.

Diagnostic techniques used in obstructed IVC are similar to those for SVC obstruction. Pressure gradients are also similar, averaging 18 ± 8.8 mmHg in the series reported by Silove and Taylor.[S18]

Reoperation with insertion of a new baffle is always indicated for IVC obstruction (see Technique of Operation earlier in this chapter). Balloon expandable stents have been used for IVC as for SVC obstruction.[B48,B50]

Pulmonary Venous Obstruction

Pulmonary venous obstruction is a less common but more lethal type of venous pathway obstruction. It is more common

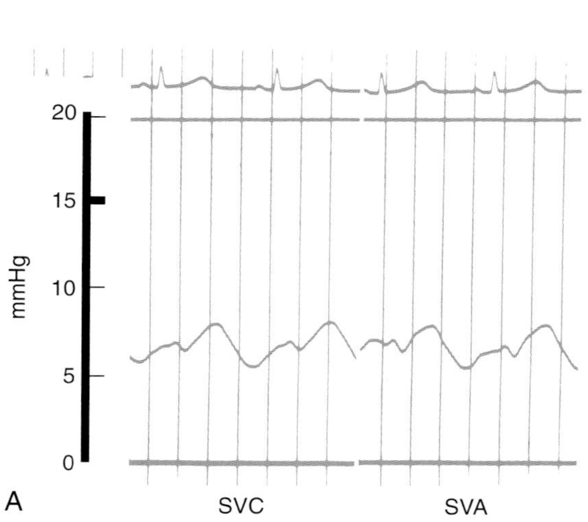

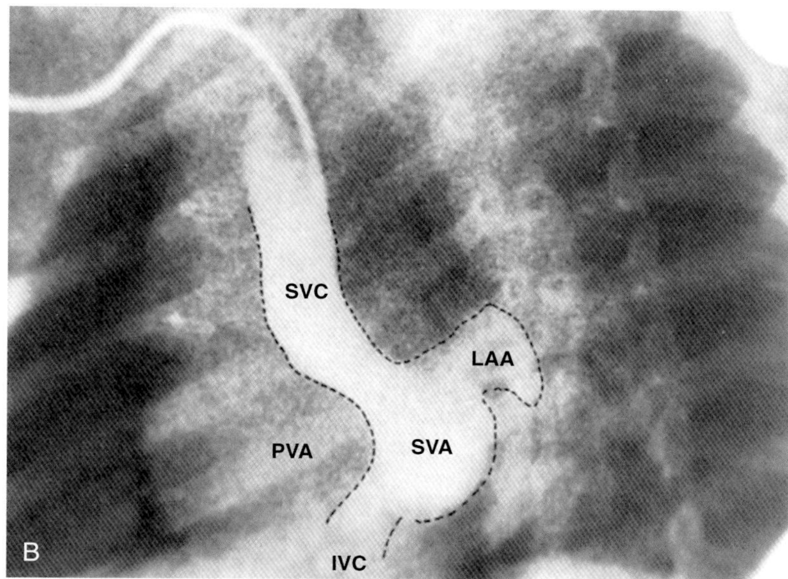

Figure 52-57 Data from postoperative cardiac catheterization in patient who had undergone Mustard-type atrial switch operation and who has unrestricted systemic venous drainage. **A,** Phasic withdrawal pressures. **B,** Cineangiogram (see Fig. 52-56). Key: *IVC,* Inferior vena cava; *LAA,* left atrial appendage; *PVA,* pulmonary venous atrium; *SVA,* systemic venous atrium; *SVC,* superior vena cava. (From Clarkson and colleagues.[C15])

when a polyester baffle is used in a Mustard repair.[D18,R9] It has been reported after Senning repair as well.[C8,S5]

Pulmonary venous obstruction usually occurs at the waist of the pulmonary venous atrium, which lies just anterior to entry of the right pulmonary veins between the crista terminalis on the lateral right atrial wall and the center of the baffle in the Mustard operation. In severe stenosis, there is a circular fibrotic ostium at this point, which is less than 10 mm in diameter, that divides the pulmonary venous atrium into two almost equal compartments of adequate size. The right pulmonary vein ostia are usually not stenotic. Rare examples of isolated left pulmonary vein stenosis or occlusion have been reported, presumably secondary to placing the baffle suture line too close to these ostia,[L21,T13] although rarely, congenital pulmonary vein stenosis coexists with TGA.

Symptoms Pulmonary venous obstruction produces pulmonary venous hypertension and symptoms of progressive dyspnea with cough, fatigue, and at times cyanosis. Pulmonary venous congestion is visible on plain chest radiography and may progress to interstitial pulmonary edema. These signs are unilateral when only the left pulmonary veins are stenotic. A continuous murmur with diastolic accentuation may be heard along the lower left sternal edge.[B18,D18,P5]

Time of Onset Time of onset is similar to that of caval obstruction and is usually within 6 to 12 months of operation, but occasional cases of late onset up to 10 years postoperatively have been documented by serial cardiac catheterizations.[B18,D18] However, mild early obstruction does not necessarily progress.

Diagnosis Diagnosis is confirmed by cardiac catheterization, when ideally the catheter is passed retrogradely across the stenosis to the posterior pulmonary venous compartment to obtain a withdrawal gradient. If this is impossible, a comparison is made between pulmonary artery wedge pressure and RV diastolic pressure. Gradient greater than 10 mmHg is important, although it is frequently higher.[D18] Pulmonary hypertension and usually an elevation of the calculated Rp are present. Normal pulmonary artery and LV systolic pressures argue against important stenosis. On cineangiography, narrowing of the pulmonary venous atrium waist can be seen best in lateral projection.[C15] Diagnosis is also possible using 2D echocardiography.[C8,S5]

Treatment Urgent reoperation is indicated.

Palliative Operations for Patients with Severe Pulmonary Vascular Disease

Palliative operations may be indicated when Rp is elevated beyond about 10 U · m^2.[M8] However, more recent experience suggests that full repair can be achieved with good long-term outcome, including regression of pulmonary hypertension, even when initial Rp calculations show levels of 10 to 20 U · m^2.[N2] Thus, in the current era, with general improvements in preoperative and postoperative care and the availability of pulmonary vasoactive agents such as nitrous oxide, palliative procedures are rarely indicated. Palliation consists of an atrial (or preferably an arterial) switch procedure without closing an existing VSD or creating a VSD when one is not present.

Technique of Operation

When the ventricular septum is essentially intact, a large VSD is created in the apex of the ventricular septum through a limited apical left ventriculotomy. After the ventriculotomy is made, a finger is inserted through the tricuspid valve through the previously made right atriotomy to tent the ventricular septum toward the left, and a limited opening is made with a knife onto the finger. The opening is then progressively enlarged (up to 20 mm) using the knife, avoiding damage to the inferior papillary muscle. (Hegar dilators are used to measure the size of the created defect.) The ventriculotomy is closed, and the switch procedure completed.

Special Features of Postoperative Care

SaO_2 in TGA depends on the relative proportions of systemic venous and pulmonary venous blood reaching the aorta, and on SvO_2.[M7] After palliative switch repair, the effective systemic flow is greatly increased, with the ratio usually changing from 1:3 to approximately 2:1. Decrease in the proportion of systemic venous blood entering the aorta is also influenced by the rise in systemic arteriolar resistance that follows the rise in SaO_2, because the increase in systemic vascular resistance decreases the right-to-left shunting of systemic venous blood through the open VSD. Finally, doubling of effective systemic flow results in an important increase in SvO_2 despite concomitant reduction in hemoglobin concentration. As a result of these complex interactions, there is an absolute increase in SaO_2 of approximately 20% in most patients after a palliative switch operation[M7]; the increase ranged from 6% to 48% (mean = 24%) in the report by Byrne and colleagues.[B51] The only preoperative variable that correlates with postoperative SaO_2 is pulmonary arteriovenous oxygen difference: A higher arteriovenous oxygen difference is associated with a higher postoperative SaO_2.[B51]

Results

Hospital mortality after a palliative switch operation has been surprisingly low. Lindesmith and colleagues report no deaths in 10 patients with VSD,[L17] Byrne and colleagues report no deaths in 23 patients (20 with VSD, 3 with created VSD[B51]), and Bernhard and colleagues report one death in 8 patients.[B23]

Staged Conversion of Atrial Switch to Arterial Switch for Systemic Right Ventricular Failure

Late failure of the systemic RV occurs in up to 10% of patients after the atrial switch procedure. Because ample evidence suggests lesser degrees of RV dysfunction in a much greater percentage of patients with the atrial switch procedure,[H19,K3] it seems likely that late RV failure will become an increasingly common problem as longer follow-up is obtained.

When the systemic RV fails, treatment options include lesion-specific surgical intervention (e.g., tricuspid valve repair or replacement), medical management, transplantation, and conversion from atrial to arterial switch.[C3] Escalation of medical management may be effective in the short term, but this form of therapy should be seen as limited in a young individual with progressive systemic RV failure. Nevertheless, this form of therapy, followed by cardiac transplantation when end-stage ventricular failure develops, represents an effective therapeutic plan. Tricuspid valve repair is difficult when the valve is in the systemic position and is generally not indicated. Valve replacement is indicated in highly selected patients who have good systemic RV function. An alternative plan is to intervene earlier in the course of systemic RV failure by performing a staged conversion to the arterial switch. Indications for embarking on the staged conversion are not clearly defined; however, it is generally accepted that the process should begin well before end-stage heart failure is present. Relative indications include worsening functional status, progressive loss of RV function, and progressive tricuspid valve regurgitation. Besides end-stage heart failure, biventricular dysfunction and severe rhythm disturbances are contraindications.

There are two general controversies related to this topic. First, the choice of management between (1) medical management followed by transplantation and (2) staged conversion; and second, if staged conversion is considered, the timing of the intervention in the gradual course of progressive RV dysfunction. The conversion process carries substantial risk. Initiation of the process too late in the course of progressive failure results in unacceptable outcome, whereas initiation of the process at the first signs of RV dysfunction or tricuspid regurgitation, although effective in minimizing the risk of the conversion process, may be premature. Adding to the uncertainty, only limited experience and data are available to define the ideal interval between pulmonary trunk banding and the arterial switch, or the preferred methodology for determining when the LV is adequately prepared. The subject of LV training and conversion to arterial switch in atrial switch patients with failing RV is discussed in more detail under "Transposition of the Great Arteries" in Chapter 29. Pulmonary trunk banding alone as a treatment for isolated progressive tricuspid valve regurgitation has resulted in a decrease in regurgitation in some cases, but the evidence is only anecdotal. In one study, banding did not improve the severity of regurgitation at follow-up, but did improve symptoms in a cohort of patients.[W14]

Occasionally, LV-to–pulmonary trunk obstruction is already present. If LV peak pressure is greater than 75% of systemic pressure, it is possible to proceed with conversion immediately. It should be emphasized that the biomechanics of the unconditioned LV are poorly appreciated.[F6]

Technical details of the staged conversion have been described and outcomes reviewed.[C18] Operative mortality was 12.5% (CL 4%-27%) and 1-year survival 80% (CL 62%-92%) in one series.[C18] In that series, age younger than 16 years was thought to increase the chance of successful conversion. In another study, early mortality was 33% (2 of 6 patients).[M19] In the experience of one of the authors (FLH), of 31 patients entering a banding protocol, 52% met criteria to proceed to conversion. Survival after conversion was 75% at mean follow-up of 5 years. Age at banding did not influence outcome. The experience of Winlaw and colleagues was similar.[W14] Nine of 20 banded patients (45%) underwent conversion, with 6 successful midterm outcomes (67%).[W14] Another study suggests that conversion may be more appropriate for Mustard than for Senning patients; however, most studies show no difference based on the type of former atrial procedure.[S3] Important differences in outcome among these studies is not surprising, considering the small number of patients, lack of consensus regarding patient selection, and lack of a universal protocol for LV training.

52A Multivariable Risk Factor Equations for Death after Arterial Switch Operation for Simple Transposition of the Great Arteries and Transposition of the Great Arteries with Ventricular Septal Defect

Table 52A-1 Congenital Heart Surgeons Society Equation for Death after Arterial Switch Repair Incorporating Patient-Related Risk Factors and "High-Risk" vs. "Low-Risk" Institutions and Institutional Experience (in Years)[a]

	Incremental Risk Factors	Single Hazard Phase *P*
	Patient	
(Lower)	Birth weight[b]	.05
	LCA, LAD, or Cx arising from sinus 2[c]	.007
	Intramural course of LCA or LAD[d]	.07
	Coexisting cardiac anomalies (including multiple VSDs)	.07
	Coexisting noncardiac anomalies	.07
	PT banding > 1 month previously[e]	.009
	Institutional	
(Lesser)	Interval since first switch operation[f]:	
	In "low-risk" institutions	<.0001
	In "high-risk" institutions	.0004

Data from Kirklin and colleagues.[K12]
[a]Only patient and institutional ("high-risk" vs. "low-risk" and experience) potential risk factors were analyzed; $n = 513$ patients with simple TGA or TGA with VSD.
[b]Active only in simple TGA in "low-risk" institutions.
[c]Applies to arteries without or with an intramural course.
[d]Active only in "high-risk" institutions; added an increment of risk to "origin from sinus 2."
[e]Active only in "low-risk" institutions.
[f]In this equation, "interval since the first arterial switch repair" was specific for each patient.
Key: *Cx,* Circumflex artery; *LAD,* left anterior descending coronary artery; *LCA,* left coronary artery; *PT,* pulmonary trunk; *VSD(s),* ventricular septal defect(s).

Table 52A-2 Congenital Heart Surgeons Society Equation for Death after Arterial Switch Repair Incorporating Patient-Related Risk Factors and "High-Risk" and "Low-Risk" Institutions and Institutional Experience (in Number of Cases)[a]

	Incremental Risk Factors	Single Hazard Phase *P*
	Patient	
(Older)	Age at operation[b]	.06
	LCA, LAD, or Cx arising from sinus 2:	
	In "low-risk" institutions	.09
	In "high-risk" institutions	.0007
	Intramural course of LCA or LAD[c]	.002
	Coexisting cardiac or noncardiac anomalies	.06
	PT banding > 1 month previously[d]	.002
	Institutional	
	Number of cases since first switch operation[e]:	
	In "low-risk" institutions	.001
	In "high-risk" institutions	<.0001

Data from Kirklin and colleagues.[K12]
[a]Only patient and institutional ("high-risk" vs. "low-risk" and experience) potential risk factors were entered into analysis for this parsimoniously derived equation; $n = 513$ patients with simple TGA or TGA with VSD. The experience was in terms of number of arterial switch operations performed on CHSS patients.
[b]Applies only to patients with simple TGA who have not undergone pulmonary trunk banding >1 month previously.
[c]Active only in "high-risk" institutions.
[d]Active only in "low-risk" institutions.
[e]In this equation, "number of cases since the first arterial switch repair" was specific for each patient.
Key: *Cx,* Circumflex artery; *LAD,* left anterior descending coronary artery; *LCA,* left coronary artery; *PT,* pulmonary trunk; *TGA,* transposition of great arteries; *VSD,* ventricular septal defect.

Table 52A-3 Congenital Heart Surgeons Society Equation for Death after Arterial Switch Repair, Incorporating Only Patient-Related Risk Factors[a]

	Incremental Risk Factors for Death[b]	Single Hazard Phase *P*
(Older)	Age at repair[c]:	.08
	In simple TGA[d]	.07
	LCA, LAD, or Cx arising from sinus 2[e]:	.05
	Without an intramural course of LCA or LAD[f]	.02
	With an intramural course of LCA or LAD[f]	.02
	Coexisting noncardiac anomalies	.02
	PT banding > 1 month previously	.097

Data from Kirklin and colleagues.[K12]
[a]Only patient potential risk factors were entered into the parsimonious analysis ($n = 513$ patients with simple TGA or TGA with VSD).
[b]The ratio between size of the pulmonary trunk and that of the ascending aorta was not entered into the analysis because the value was available in only 140 patients, but univariable ratios of <1.2 and >2.3 were associated with lower survival ($P = .09$).
[c]This variable was active only in patients without pulmonary trunk banding >1 month previously.
[d]An increment in risk was added when the patient had simple TGA (an interaction term) rather than TGA with VSD.
[e]Among the 12 patients classified as having an "intramural course," in 1 the artery to the left system arose from the midportion of sinus 2 and juxtaposed to the right coronary artery. The left artery coursed anteriorly between aorta and pulmonary trunk but could possibly not have had an intramural course.
[f]These are mutually exclusive variables.
Key: *Cx,* Circumflex artery; *LAD,* left anterior descending artery; *LCA,* left coronary artery; *PT,* pulmonary trunk; *TGA,* transposition of great arteries; *VSD,* ventricular septal defect.

Table 52A-4 Congenital Heart Surgeons Society Equation for Death after Arterial Switch Repair, Incorporating Patient-Related and Support Technique Risk Factors[a]

	Incremental Risk Factors for Death	Single Hazard Phase *P*
	Patient	
(Older)	Age at repair[b]:	.31
(Older)	In simple TGA[c]	.02
	LCA, LAD, or Cx arising from sinus 2:	
	Without an intramural course of LCA or LAD	.10
	With an intramural course of LCA or LAD	.06
	Multiple VSDs	.02
	Coexisting noncardiac anomalies	.01
	PT banding >1 month previously	.23
	Support	
(Longer)	Myocardial ischemic time	.001

Data from Kirklin and colleagues.[K12]
[a]Patient-specific and support risk factors were entered into the nonparsimonious analysis of 513 patients as described for Appendix Tables 52A-1, 52A-2, and 52A-3. Risk factors identified in the previous analyses in this sequential series were forced to remain in the equation, even though the *P* value was >.1.
[b]This variable was active only in patients without PT banding >1 month previously.
[c]An increment in risk was added when the patient had simple TGA (an interaction term) rather than TGA and VSD.
Key: *CA,* Coronary artery; *Cx,* circumflex artery; *LCA,* left coronary artery; *PT,* pulmonary trunk; *TGA,* transposition of great arteries; *VSD,* ventricular septal defect.

Table 52A-5 Congenital Heart Surgeons Society Equation for Death after Arterial Switch Repair, Incorporating Patient-Related and Procedural Risk Factors[a]

	Incremental Risk Factors	Single Hazard Phase *P*
	Patient	
	LCA, LAD, or Cx arising from sinus 2:	
	Without intramural course of LCA or LAD	.099
	With intramural course of LCA or LAD	.02
	Multiple VSDs	.01
	Coexisting noncardiac anomalies	.09
	PT banding >1 month previously	.7
(Older)	Age at repair[b]:	.11
	In simple TGA[c]	.21
	Procedure	
	Aorta transected distally	.002
	PT transected proximally or at midportion	.06
	No Lecompte maneuver	.0003
	Coronary implantation not at transection site	.05

Data from Kirklin and colleagues.[K12]
[a]Patient-related and procedural risk factors were entered into nonparsimonious analysis as in Table 52A-4. Risk factors identified in the previous analyses in this sequential series were forced to remain in the equation, even though $P > .1$.
[b]Active only in patients without PT banding >1 month previously.
[c]Increment in risk was added when the patient had simple TGA (an interaction term) rather than TGA and VSD.
Key: *Cx,* Circumflex artery; *LAD,* left anterior descending coronary artery; *LCA,* left coronary artery; *PT,* pulmonary trunk; *TGA,* transposition of great arteries; *VSD(s),* ventricular septal defect(s).

Table 52A-6 Congenital Heart Surgeons Society Equation for Death after Arterial Switch Repair, Incorporating Patient-Related, Support, and Procedural Risk Factors[a]

	Incremental Risk Factors	Single Hazard Phase *P*
	Patient	
	LCA, LAD, or Cx arising from sinus 2:	
	Without intramural course of LCA or LAD	.15
	With intramural course of LCA or LAD	.03
	Multiple VSDs	.01
	Coexisting noncardiac anomalies	.03
	PT banding >1 month previously	.9
(Older)	Age at repair[b]:	.5
	In simple TGA[c]	.07
	Support	
(Longer)	Myocardial ischemic time	.0005
	Procedural	
	Aorta transected distally	.0006
	PT not transected proximally or at midportion	.09
	No Lecompte maneuver	.001
	Coronary implantation not at transection site	.08

Data from Kirklin and colleagues.[K12]
[a]Patient-related, support, and procedural risk factors were entered into the nonparsimonious analysis as in Table 52A-4. Risk factors identified in the previous analyses in this sequential series were forced to remain in the equation, even though $P > .1$.
[b]Active only in patients without PT banding >1 month previously.
[c]Increment in risk was added when the patient had simple TGA (an interaction term) rather than TGA with VSD.
Key: *Cx,* Circumflex artery; *LAD,* left anterior descending coronary artery; *LCA,* left coronary artery; *PT,* pulmonary trunk; *TGA,* transposition of great arteries; *VSD(s),* ventricular septal defect(s).

52B Multivariable Analysis of Risk Factors for Death after Atrial Switch Operation

Variables entered into the multivariable logistic regression analysis of hospital deaths in patients with TGA at Green Lane Hospital between 1970 and 1984 after atrial switch repair were as follows:

- Age at operation
- Date of operation
- Atrial septal defect creation (none, septostomy, repeat septostomy, septectomy)
- Other palliation (Blalock-Taussig, Waterston, banding, ductus ligation, coarctation repair)
- Atrial septal defect size at repair (none, small, moderate, large)
- Ventricular septal defect size (small, moderate, large)
- Additional ventricular septal defects (yes/no)
- Left ventricular outflow tract obstruction (yes/no) and type (valvar, fibrous, muscular)
- Coarctation (yes/no)
- Right ventricular size (moderate or severe hypoplasia: yes/no)
- Urgency of operation (elective, New York Heart Association class IV, semi-urgent, urgent)
- Type of operation (standard Mustard, V-Y Mustard, Senning)
- Technique of cardiopulmonary bypass (standard/profound hypothermia; circulatory arrest)
- Preoperative pulmonary vascular resistance (or lung histology) in patients aged 3 months or older

- Early reoperation (for bleeding, baffle obstruction, baffle leak, infection)
- Discharge electrocardiogram (sinus, junctional, complete heart block)
- Patent ductus arteriosus (absent/small, moderate, large in various combinations)
- Operation (baffle repair) at age 30 days or younger (yes/no)
- Early operation (repair or palliation) at age 30 days or younger (yes/no)
- Preoperative growth patterns (normal, third percentile, well below third percentile, always below third percentile but steady, always below third percentile but declining, and various combinations)

Additional variables considered in Cox's proportional hazard model for late mortality in the same data set are as follows:

- Upper systemic venous compartment obstruction (none/mild, moderate, severe)
- Lower systemic venous compartment obstruction (same criteria)
- Pulmonary venous compartment obstruction (same criteria)
- Baffle leak (same criteria)
- Residual left ventricular outflow tract obstruction
- Residual ventricular septal defect (yes/no)

52C Multivariable Analysis of Risk Factors for Death after Rastelli Operation

Risk factors entered into the multivariable analysis of death, in the hazard function domain, after Rastelli operation (UAB experience) are as follows:

- Demographic: gender, age at operation, body surface area
- Clinical: New York Heart Association functional class, hematocrit
- Morphology: juxtaposition of atrial appendages
- Surgical: cardioplegia; aortic clamp time in cardioplegic group; type of valved conduit; enlargement of ventricular septal defect

REFERENCES

A

1. Abbott ME. Congenital cardiac diseases. In: Osler W, McCrae T, eds. Modern medicine. Vol. 4. 3rd Ed. Philadelphia: Lea & Febiger, 1927.
2. Abe T, Kuribayashi R, Sato M, Nieda S, Takahashi M, Okubo T. Successful Jatene operation for transposition of the great arteries with intact ventricular septum. A case report. J Thorac Cardiovasc Surg 1978;75:64.
3. Aberdeen E. Correction of uncomplicated cases of transposition of the great arteries. Br Heart J 1971;33:66.
4. Aberdeen E, Waterston DJ, Carr I, Graham G, Bonham-Carter RE, Subramanian S. Successful "correction" of transposed great arteries by Mustard's operation. Lancet 1965;192:1233.
5. Abrams HL, Kaplan HS, Purdy A. Diagnosis of complete transposition of the great vessels. Radiology 1951;57:500.
6. Albert HM. Surgical correction of transposition of the great vessels. Surg Forum 1954;5:74.
7. Amin Z, McElhinney DB, Moore P, Reddy VM, Hanley FL. Coronary arterial size late after the atrial inversion procedure for transposition of the great arteries: implications for the arterial switch operation. J Thorac Cardiovasc Surg 2000;120:1047.
8. Ammirati A, Arteaga M, Garcia-Pelaez I, Maitre MJ, Marcelletti C, Bosman C, et al. Congenital mitral valve anomalies in transposition of the great arteries. Jpn Heart J 1989;30:187.
9. Anderson RH, Becker AE, Lucchese FE, Meier MA, Rigby ML, Soto B. Morphology of congenital heart disease. Baltimore: University Park Press, 1983.
10. Angeli E, Formigari R, Pace Napoleone C, Oppido G, Ragni L, Picchio FM, et al. Long-term coronary artery outcome after arterial switch operation for transposition of the great arteries. Eur J Cardiothorac Surg 2010;38:714-20.
11. Angeli E, Raisky O, Bonnet D, Sidi D, Vouhe PR. Late reoperations after neonatal arterial switch operation for transposition of the great arteries. Eur J Cardiothorac Surg 2008;34:32-6.
12. Arciniegas E, Farooki ZQ, Hakimi M, Perry BL, Green EW. Results of the Mustard operation for dextro-transposition of the great arteries. J Thorac Cardiovasc Surg 1981;81:580.
13. Arensman FW, Bostock J, Radley-Smith R, Yacoub MH. Cardiac rhythm and conduction before and after anatomic correction of transposition of the great arteries. Am J Cardiol 1983;52:836.
14. Arensman FW, Sievers HH, Lange P, Radley-Smith R, Bernhard A, Heintzen P, et al. Assessment of coronary and aortic anastomoses after anatomic correction of transposition of the great arteries. J Thorac Cardiovasc Surg 1985;90:597.
15. Asou T, Karl TR, Pawade A, Mee RB. Arterial switch: translocation of the intramural coronary artery. Ann Thorac Surg 1994;57:461-5.
16. Aubert J, Pannetier A, Couvelly JP, Unal D, Rouault F, Delarue A. Transposition of the great arteries. New technique for anatomical correction. Br Heart J 1978;40:204.
17. Aziz KU, Paul MH, Idriss FS, Wilson AD, Muster AJ. Clinical manifestations of dynamic left ventricular outflow tract stenosis in infants with d-transposition of the great arteries with intact ventricular septum. Am J Cardiol 1979;44:290.
18. Aziz KU, Paul MH, Muster AJ. Echocardiographic assessment of left ventricular outflow tract in d-transposition of the great arteries. Am J Cardiol 1978;41:543.

12. DeLeon VH, Hougen TJ, Norwood WI, Lang P, Marx GR, Castaneda A. Results of the Senning operation for transposition of the great arteries with intact ventricular septum in neonates. Circulation 1984;70:I21.
13. Derrick GP, Josen M, Vogel M, Henein MY, Shinebourne EA, Redington AN. Abnormalities of right ventricular long axis function after atrial repair of transposition of the great arteries. Heart 2001;86:203.
14. Derrick GP, Narang I, White PA, Kelleher A, Bush A, Penny DJ, et al. Failure of stroke volume augmentation during exercise and dobutamine stress is unrelated to load-independent indexes of right ventricular performance after the Mustard operation. Circulation 2000;102:III154.
15. Dickinson DF, Scott O. Ambulatory electrocardiographic monitoring in 100 healthy teenage boys. Br Heart J 1984;51:179.
16. Dillard DH, Mohri H, Merendino KA, Morgan BC, Baum D, Crawford EW. Total surgical correction of transposition of the great arteries in children less than six months of age. Surg Gynecol Obstet 1969;129:1258.
17. Douard H, Labbe L, Barat JL, Broustet JP, Baudet E, Choussat A. Cardiorespiratory response to exercise after venous switch operation for transposition of the great arteries. Chest 1997;111:23.
18. Driscoll DJ, Nihill MR, Vargo TA, Mullins CE, McNamara DG. Late development of pulmonary venous obstruction following Mustard's operation using a Dacron baffle. Circulation 1977;55:484.
19. Dunbar-Masterson C, Wypij D, Bellinger DC, Rappaport LA, Baker AL, Jonas RA, et al. General health status of children with D-transposition of the great arteries after the arterial switch operation. Circulation 2001;104:I138.

E

1. Ebenroth ES, Hurwitz RA, Cordes TM. Late onset of pulmonary hypertension after successful Mustard surgery for d-transposition of the great arteries. Am J Cardiol 2000;85:127.
2. Edwards WS, Bargeron LM, Lyons C. Reposition of right pulmonary vein in transposition of the great vessels. JAMA 1964;188:522.
3. Edwards WD, Edwards JE. Hypertensive pulmonary vascular disease in alpha-transposition of the great arteries. Am J Cardiol 1978;41:921.
4. Edwards WD, Edwards JE. Pathology of the sinus node in d-transposition following the Mustard operation. J Thorac Cardiovasc Surg 1978;75:213.
5. Egloff LP, Freed MD, Dick M, Norwood WI, Castaneda AR. Early and late results with the Mustard operation in infancy. Ann Thorac Surg 1978;26:474.
6. El-Said G, Rosenberg HS, Mullins CE, Hallman GL, Cooley DA, McNamara DG. Dysrhythmias after Mustard's operation for transposition of the great arteries. Am J Cardiol 1972;30:526.
7. El-Said GM, Gillette PC, Mullins CE, Nihill MR, McNamara DG. Significance of pacemaker recovery time after the Mustard operation for transposition of the great arteries. Am J Cardiol 1976;38:448.

F

1. Farre JR. Pathological researches. Essay 1: On malformation of the human heart. London: Longman, Hurst, Rees, Orme, Brown, 1814, p. 28.
2. Feder E, Meisner H, Buhlmeyer K, Struck E, Sebening F. Operative treatment of TGA: comparison of Senning's and Mustard's operation in patients under 2 years of age. Thorac Cardiovasc Surg 1980;28:7.
3. Ferencz C. Transposition of the great vessels. Pathophysiologic considerations based upon a study of the lungs. Circulation 1966;33:232.
4. Ferguson DJ, Adams P, Watson D. Pulmonary arteriosclerosis in transposition of the great vessels. Am J Dis Child 1960;99:653.
5. Flinn CJ, Wolff GS, Dick M 2nd, Campbell RM, Borkat G, Casta A, et al. Cardiac rhythm after the Mustard operation for complete transposition of the great arteries. N Engl J Med 1984;310:1635.
6. Fogel MA, Gupta K, Baxter BC, Weinberg PM, Haselgrove J, Hoffman EA. Biomechanics of the deconditioned left ventricle. Am J Physiol 1996;271:1193.
7. Foran JP, Sullivan ID, Elliott MJ, de Leval MR. Primary arterial switch operation for transposition of the great arteries with intact ventricular septum in infants older than 21 days. J Am Coll Cardiol 1998;31:883.
8. Forenz C, Greco JM, Libi-Sylora M. Variability of pulmonary vascular disease in certain malformations of the heart. In: Kidd BS, Keith JD, eds. The natural history and progressive treatment of congenital heart defects. Springfield: Charles C. Thomas, 1971, p. 300.
9. Formigari R, Toscano A, Giardini A, Gargiulo G, Di Donato R, Picchio FM, et al. Prevalence and predictors of neoaortic regurgitation after arterial switch operation for transposition of the great arteries. J Thorac Cardiovasc Surg 2003;126:1753-9.
10. Fortune RL, Paquet M, Collins-Nakai RL, Duncan NF. Intracardiac repair of dextro-transposition of the great arteries in the newborn period. J Thorac Cardiovasc Surg 1983;85:371.
11. Fredriksen PM, Pettersen E, Thaulow E. Declining aerobic capacity of patients with arterial and atrial switch procedures. Pediatr Cardiol 2009;30:166-71.
12. Fyler DC. Report of the New England regional infant cardiac program. Pediatrics 1980;65:375.

G

1. Gatzoulis MA, Walters J, McLaughlin PR, Merchant N, Webb GD, Liu P. Late arrhythmia in adults with the mustard procedure for transposition of great arteries: a surrogate marker for right ventricular dysfunction? Heart 2000;84:409.
2. Genoni M, Vogt P, von Segesser L, Seifert B, Arbenz U, Jenni R, et al. Extended follow-up after atrial repair for transposition of the great arteries: a younger age at surgery improves late survival. J Card Surg 1999;14:246.
3. Giardini A, Khambadkone S, Rizzo N, Riley G, Pace Napoleone C, Muthialu N, et al. Determinants of exercise capacity after arterial switch operation for transposition of the great arteries. Am J Cardiol 2009;104:1007-12.
4. Gillette PC, El-Said GM, Sivarajan N, Mullins CE, Williams RL, McNamara DG. Electrophysiological abnormalities after Mustard's operation for transposition of the great arteries. Br Heart J 1974;36:186.
5. Gillette PC, Kugler JD, Garson A Jr, Gutgesell HP, Duff DF, McNamara DG. Mechanisms of cardiac arrhythmias after the Mustard operation for transposition of the great arteries. Am J Cardiol 1980;45:1225.
6. Gittenberger-de Groot AC, Sauer U, Oppenheimer-Dekker A, Quaegebeur J. Coronary arterial anatomy in transposition of the great arteries: a morphologic study. Pediatr Cardiol 1983;4:15.
7. Gittenberger-de Groot AC, Sauer U, Quaegebeur J. Aortic intramural coronary artery in three hearts with transposition of the great arteries. J Thorac Cardiovasc Surg 1986;91:566.
8. Gleason MM, Chin AJ, Andrews BA, Barber G, Helton JG, Murphy JD, et al. Two-dimensional and Doppler echocardiographic assessment of neonatal arterial repair for transposition of the great arteries. J Am Coll Cardiol 1989;13:1320.
9. Godman MJ, Friedli B, Pasternac A, Kidd BS, Trusler GA, Mustard WT. Hemodynamic studies in children four to ten years after the Mustard operation for transposition of the great arteries. Circulation 1976;53:532.
10. Goor DA, Lillehei CW. In: Congenital malformations of the heart. Orlando, Fla: Grune & Stratton, 1975, p. 210.
11. Goor DA, Lillehei CW. In: Congenital malformations of the heart. Orlando, Fla: Grune & Stratton, 1975, p. 215.
12. Gorler H, Ono M, Thies A, Lunkewitz E, Westhoff-Bleck M, Haverich A, et al. Long-term morbidity and quality of life after surgical repair of transposition of the great arteries: atrial versus arterial switch operation. Interact CardioVasc Thorac Surg 2011; 12:569-74.
13. Graham TP Jr. Hemodynamic residua and sequelae following intraatrial repair of transposition of the great arteries. A review. Pediatr Cardiol 1982;2:203.
14. Graham TP Jr, Atwood GF, Boucek RJ Jr, Boerth RC, Bender HW Jr. Abnormalities of right ventricular function following Mustard's operation for transposition of the great arteries. Circulation 1975;52:678.
15. Graham TP Jr, Atwood GF, Boucek RJ Jr, Boerth RC, Nelson JH. Right heart volume characteristics in transposition of the great arteries. Circulation 1975;51:881.
16. Gremmels DB, Tacy TA, Brook MM, Silverman NH. Accuracy of coronary artery anatomy using two-dimensional echocardiography in d-transposition of great arteries using a two-reviewer method. J Am Soc Echocardiogr 2004;17:454-60.

17. Gutgesell HP, Garson A, McNamara DG. Prognosis for the newborn with transposition of the great arteries. Am J Cardiol 1979;44:96.

H

1. Haas F, Wottke M, Poppert H, Meisner H. Long-term survival and functional follow-up in patients after the arterial switch operation. Ann Thorac Surg 1999;68:1692.
2. Hagler DJ, Ritter DG, Mair DD, Davis GD, McGoon DC. Clinical, angiographic, and hemodynamic assessment of late results after Mustard operation. Circulation 1978;57:1214.
3. Hagler DJ, Ritter DG, Mair DD, Tajik AJ, Seward JB, Fulton RE, et al. Right and left ventricular function after the Mustard procedure in transposition of the great arteries. Am J Cardiol 1979;44:276.
4. Han JJ, Lee YT, Park YK, Hong SN, Kim SH. Left subclavian artery bypass graft in complicated arterial switch operation. Ann Thorac Surg 1996;61:1523.
5. Hausdorf G, Gravinghoff L, Sieg K, Keck EW, Radley-Smith R, Yacoub MH. Left ventricular performance after anatomic correction of D-transposition of the great arteries. J Am Coll Cardiol 1985;5:479.
6. Hauser M, Bengel FM, Kuhn A, Sauer U, Zylla S, Braun SL, et al. Myocardial blood flow and flow reserve after coronary reimplantation in patients after arterial switch and Ross operation. Circulation 2001;103:1875.
7. Hayashi G, Kurosaki K, Echigo S, Kado H, Fukushima N, Yokota M, et al. Prevalence of arrhythmias and their risk factors mid- and long-term after the arterial switch operation. Pediatr Cardiol 2006;27:689-94.
8. Helbing WA, Hansen B, Ottenkamp J, Rohmer J, Chin JG, Brom AG, et al. Long-term results of atrial correction for transposition of the great arteries: comparison of Mustard and Senning operations. J Thorac Cardiovasc Surg 1994;108:363.
9. Hesslein PS, Gutgesell HP, Gillette PC, McNamara DG. Exercise assessment of sinoatrial node function following the Mustard operation. Am Heart J 1982;103:351.
10. Hirata Y, Chen JM, Quaegebeur JM, Mosca RS. Should we address the neopulmonic valve? Significance of right-sided obstruction after surgery for transposition of the great arteries and coarctation. Ann Thorac Surg 2008;86:1293-8.
11. Horer J, Karl E, Theodoratou G, Schreiber C, Cleuziou J, Prodan Z, et al. Incidence and results of reoperations following the Senning operation: 27 years of follow-up in 314 patients at a single center. Eur J Cardiothorac Surg 2008;33:1061-8.
12. Horer J, Schreiber C, Cleuziou J, Vogt M, Prodan Z, Busch R, et al. Improvement in long-term survival after hospital discharge but not in freedom from reoperation after the change from atrial to arterial switch for transposition of the great arteries. J Thorac Cardiovasc Surg 2009;137:347-54.
13. Hovels-Gurich HH, Seghaye MC, Sigler M, Kotlarek F, Bartl A, Neuser J, et al. Neurodevelopmental outcome related to cerebral risk factors in children after neonatal arterial switch operation. Ann Thorac Surg 2001;71:881.
14. Hruda J, Sulc J, Radvansky J, Hucin B, Samanek M. Good exercise tolerance and impaired lung function after atrial repair of transposition. Eur J Cardiothorac Surg 1997;12:184.
15. Hu SS, Liu ZG, Li SJ, Shen XD, Wang X, Liu JP, et al. Strategy for biventricular outflow tract reconstruction: Rastelli, REV, or Nikaidoh procedure? J Thorac Cardiovasc Surg 2008;135:331-8.
16. Hucin B, Voriskova M, Hruda J, Marek J, Janousek J, Reich O, et al. Late complications and quality of life after atrial correction of transposition of the great arteries in 12 to 18 year follow-up. J Cardiovasc Surg 2000;41:233.
17. Huhta JC, Edwards WD, Danielson GK, Feldt RH. Abnormalities of the tricuspid valve in complete transposition of the great arteries with ventricular septal defect. J Thorac Cardiovasc Surg 1982; 83:569.
18. Huhta JC, Edwards WD, Feldt RH, Puga FJ. Left ventricular wall thickness in complete transposition of the great arteries. J Thorac Cardiovasc Surg 1982;84:97.
19. Hurwitz RA, Caldwell RL, Girod DA, Brown J. Right ventricular systolic function in adolescents and young adults after Mustard operation for transposition of the great arteries. Am J Cardiol 1996;77:294.
20. Hurwitz RA, Papanicolaou N, Treves S, Keane JF, Castaneda A. Radionuclide angiocardiography in evaluation of patients after repair of transposition of the great arteries. Am J Cardiol 1982; 49:761.
21. Hutter PA, Kreb DL, Mantel SF, Hitchcock JF, Meijboom EJ, Bennink GB. Twenty-five years' experience with the arterial switch operation. J Thorac Cardiovasc Surg 2002;124:790-7.
22. Hwang HY, Kim WH, Kwak JG, Lee JR, Kim YJ, Rho JR, et al. Mid-term follow-up of neoaortic regurgitation after the arterial switch operation for transposition of the great arteries. Eur J Cardiothorac Surg 2006;29:162-7.

I

1. Idriss FS, Goldstein IR, Grana L, French D, Potts WJ. A new technic for complete correction of transposition of the great vessels: an experimental study with a preliminary clinical report. Circulation 1961;24:5.
2. Idriss FS, Ilbawi MN, DeLeon SY, Duffy CE, Muster AJ, Berry TE, et al. Arterial switch in simple and complex transposition of the great arteries. J Thorac Cardiovasc Surg 1988;95:29.

J

1. Jamjureeruk V, Sangtawesin C, Layangool T. Balloon atrial septostomy under two-dimensional echocardiographic control: a new outlook. Pediatr Cardiol 1997;18:197.
2. Janse MJ, Anderson RH. Specialized internodal atrial pathway: fact or fiction. Am J Cardiol 1974;2:117.
3. Jarmakani JM, Canent RV Jr. Preoperative and postoperative right ventricular function in children with transposition of the great vessels. Circulation 1974;50:II39.
4. Jatene AD, Fontes VF, Paulista PP, de Souza LC, Neger F, Galantier M, et al. Successful anatomic correction of transposition of the great vessels. A preliminary report. Arq Bras Cardiol 1975; 28:461.
5. Jatene AD, Fontes VF, Paulista PP, Souza LC, Neger F, Galantier M, et al. Anatomic correction of transposition of the great vessels. J Thorac Cardiovasc Surg 1976;72:364.
6. Jenkins KJ, Hanley FL, Colan SD, Mayer JE Jr, Castaneda AR, Wernovsky G. Function of the anatomic pulmonary valve in the systemic circulation. Circulation 1991;84:III173.
7. Jonas RA, Giglia TM, Sanders SP, Wernovsky G, Nadal-Ginard B, Mayer JE Jr, et al. Rapid, two-stage arterial switch for transposition of the great arteries and intact ventricular septum beyond the neonatal period. Circulation 1989;80:I203.

K

1. Kampmann C, Kuroczynski W, Trubel H, Knuf M, Schneider M, Heinemann MK. Late results after PTCA for coronary stenosis after the arterial switch procedure for transposition of the great arteries. Ann Thorac Surg 2005;80:1641-6.
2. Kang N, de Leval MR, Elliott M, Tsang V, Kocyildirim E, Sehic I, et al. Extending the boundaries of the primary arterial switch operation in patients with transposition of the great arteries and intact ventricular septum. Circulation 2004;110:II123-7.
3. Kato H, Nakano S, Matsuda H, Hirose H, Shimazaki Y, Kawashima Y. Right ventricular myocardial function after atrial switch operation for transposition of the great arteries. Am J Cardiol 1989; 63:226.
4. Kay EB, Cross FS. Surgical treatment of transposition of the great vessels. Surgery 1955;38:712.
5. Kaye MP. Anatomic correction of transposition of great arteries. Mayo Clin Proc 1975;50:638.
6. Keane JF, Ellison RC, Rudd M, Nadas AS. Pulmonary blood flow and left ventricular volumes in transposition of the great arteries and intact ventricular septum. Br Heart J 1973;35:521.
7. Keith JD, Neill CA, Vlad P, Rowe RD, Chute AL. Transposition of the great vessels. Circulation 1953;7:830.
8. Kidd BS. The fate of children with transposition of the great arteries following balloon atrial septostomy. In: Kidd BS, Rowe RD, eds. The child with congenital heart disease after surgery. Mount Kisco, N.Y.: Futura, 1976, p. 153.
9. Kim SJ, Kim WH, Lim C, Oh SS, Kim YM. Commissural malalignment of aortic-pulmonary sinus in complete transposition of great arteries. Ann Thorac Surg 2003;76:1906-10.
10. Kirjavainen M, Happonen JM, Louhimo I. Late results of Senning operation. J Thorac Cardiovasc Surg 1999;117:488.
11. Kirklin JW, Barratt-Boyes BG. Cardiac surgery. 1st Ed. New York: John Wiley & Sons, 1985, p. 1136.

12. Kirklin JW, Blackstone EH, Tchervenkov CI, Castaneda AR, and The Congenital Heart Surgeons Society. Clinical outcomes after the arterial switch operation for transposition. Patient, support, procedural, and institutional risk factors. Circulation 1992;86:1501.
13. Kirklin JW, Devloo RA, Weidman WH. Open intra-cardiac repair for transposition of the great vessels: 11 cases. Surgery 1961;50:58.
14. Kondo C, Nakazawa M, Momma K, Kusakabe K. Sympathetic denervation and reinnervation after arterial switch operation for complete transposition. Circulation 1998;97:2414.
15. Kreutzer C, De Vive J, Oppido G, Kreutzer J, Gauvreau K, Freed M, et al. Twenty-five-year experience with Rastelli repair for transposition of the great arteries. J Thorac Cardiovasc Surg 2000;120:211.
16. Krueger SK, Burney DW, Ferlic RM. Protein-losing enteropathy complicating the Mustard procedure. Surgery 1977;81:305.
17. Kumar A, Taylor GP, Sandor GG, Patterson MW. Pulmonary vascular disease in neonates with transposition of the great arteries and intact ventricular septum. Br Heart J 1993;69:442.
18. Kumar RK, Newburger JW, Gauvreau K, Kamenir SA, Hornberger LK. Comparison of outcome when hypoplastic left heart syndrome and transposition of the great arteries are diagnosed prenatally versus when diagnosis of these two conditions is made only postnatally. Am J Cardiol 1999;83:1649.

L

1. La Corte MA, Fellows KE, Williams RG. Over-riding tricuspid valve: echocardiographic and angiographic features. Am J Cardiol 1976; 37:911.
2. Lacour-Gayet F, Serraf A, Galletti L, Bruniaux J, Belli E, Piot D, et al. Biventricular repair of conotruncal anomalies associated with aortic arch obstruction: 103 patients. Circulation 1997;96:II328.
3. Lakier JB, Stanger P, Heymann MA, Hoffman JI, Rudolph AM. Early onset of pulmonary vascular obstruction in patients with aortopulmonary transposition and intact ventricular septum. Circulation 1975;51:875.
4. Lang P, Freed MD, Bierman FZ, Norwood WI Jr, Nadas AS. Use of prostaglandin E_1 in infants with d-transposition of the great arteries and intact ventricular septum. Am J Cardiol 1979;44:76.
5. Layman TE, Edwards JE. Anomalies of the cardiac valves associated with complete transposition of the great vessels. Am J Cardiol 1967;19:247.
6. Lecompte Y, Neveux JY, Leca F, Zannini L, Tu TV, Duboys Y, et al. Reconstruction of the pulmonary outflow tract without prosthetic conduit. J Thorac Cardiovasc Surg 1982;84:727.
7. Lecompte Y, Zannini L, Hazan E, Jarreau MM, Bex JP, Tu TV, et al. Anatomic correction of transposition of the great arteries. J Thorac Cardiovasc Surg 1981;82:629.
8. Lee JR, Lim HG, Kim YJ, Rho JR, Bae EJ, Noh CI, et al. Repair of transposition of the great arteries, ventricular septal defect and left ventricular outflow tract obstruction. Eur J Cardiothorac Surg 2004;25:735-41.
9. Legendre A, Losay J, Touchot-Kone A, Serraf A, Belli E, Piot JD, et al. Coronary events after arterial switch operation for transposition of the great arteries. Circulation 2003;108:II186-90.
10. Levin DL, Paul MH, Muster AJ, Newfeld EA, Waldman JD. The clinical diagnosis of D transposition of the great vessels in the neonate. Arch Intern Med 1977;137:1421.
11. Levy RJ, Rosenthal A, Castaneda AR, Nadas AS. Growth after surgical repair of simple D-transposition of the great arteries. Ann Thorac Surg 1978;25:225.
12. Li J, Tulloh RM, Cook A, Schneider M, Ho SY, Anderson RH. Coronary arterial origins in transposition of the great arteries: factors that affect outcome. A morphological and clinical study. Heart 2000;83:320.
13. Li W, Somerville J. Atrial flutter in grown-up congenital heart (GUCH) patients. Clinical characteristics of affected population. Int J Cardiol 2000;75:129.
14. Liebman J, Cullum L, Belloc NB. Natural history of transposition of the great arteries. Anatomy and birth and death characteristics. Circulation 1969;40:237.
15. Lillehei CW, Varco RL. Certain physiologic, pathologic and surgical features of complete transposition of the great vessels. Surgery 1953;34:376.
16. Lincoln C, Hasse J, Anderson RH, Shinebourne E. Surgical correction in complete levotransposition of the great arteries with an unusual subaortic ventricular septal defect. Am J Cardiol 1976;38:344.
17. Lindesmith GG, Stanton RE, Lurie PR, Takahashi M, Tucker BL, Stiles QR, et al. An assessment of Mustard's operation as a palliative procedure for transposition of the great vessels. Ann Thorac Surg 1975;19:514.
18. Lindesmith GG, Stiles QR, Tucker BL, Gallaher ME, Stanton RE, Meyer BW. The Mustard operation as a palliative procedure. J Thorac Cardiovasc Surg 1972;63:75.
19. Litwin SB, Plauth WH Jr, Jones JE, Bernhard WF. Appraisal of surgical atrial septectomy for transposition of the great arteries. Circulation 1971;43:I7.
20. Locatelli G, Benedetto GD, Villani M, Vanini V, Bianchi T, Parenzan L. Transposition of the great arteries. Successful Senning's operation in 35 consecutive patients. J Thorac Cardiovasc Surg 1979;27:120.
21. Lock JE, Lucas RV Jr, Amplatz K, Bessinger FB Jr. Silent unilateral pulmonary venous obstruction. Occurrence after surgical correction of transposition of the great arteries. Chest 1978;73:224.
22. Loffredo CA, Silbergeld EK, Ferencz C, Zhang J. Association of transposition of the great arteries in infants with maternal exposures to herbicides and rodenticides. Am J Epidemiol 2001;153:529.
23. Losay J, Touchot A, Capderou A, Piot JD, Belli E, Planche C, et al. Aortic valve regurgitation after arterial switch operation for transposition of the great arteries: incidence, risk factors, and outcome. J Am Coll Cardiol 2006;47:2057-62.
24. Losay J, Touchot A, Serraf A, Litvinova A, Lambert V, Piot JD, et al. Late outcome after arterial switch operation for transposition of the great arteries. Circulation 2001;104:I121.
25. Lupinetti FM, Bove EL, Minich LL, Snider AR, Callow LB, Meliones JN, et al. Intermediate-term survival and functional results after arterial repair for transposition of the great arteries. J Thorac Cardiovasc Surg 1992;103:421.

M

1. Maeno YV, Kamenir SA, Sinclair B, van der Velde ME, Smallhorn JF, Hornberger LK. Prenatal features of ductus arteriosus constriction and restrictive foramen ovale in d-transposition of the great arteries. Circulation 1999;99:1209.
2. Mahle WT, McBride MG, Paridon SM. Exercise performance after the arterial switch operation for D-transposition of the great arteries. Am J Cardiol 2001;87:753.
3. Mahony L, Turley K, Ebert P, Heymann MA. Long-term results after atrial repair of transposition of the great arteries in early infancy. Circulation 1982;66:253.
4. Mair DD. Effect of markedly elevated hematocrit level on blood viscosity and assessment of pulmonary vascular resistance. J Thorac Cardiovasc Surg 1979;77:682.
5. Mair DD, Danielson GK, Wallace RB, McGoon DC. Long-term follow-up of Mustard operation survivors. Circulation 1974;50:II46.
6. Mair DD, Macartney FJ, Weidman WH, Ritter DG, Ongley PA, Smith RE. The vectorcardiogram in complete transposition of the great arteries: correlation with anatomic and hemodynamic findings and calculated left ventricular mass. J Electrocardiol 1970;3:217.
7. Mair DD, Ritter DG. Factors influencing intercirculatory mixing in patients with complete transposition of the great arteries. Am J Cardiol 1972;30:653.
8. Mair DD, Ritter DG, Danielson GK, Wallace RB, McGoon DC. The palliative Mustard operation: rationale and results. Am J Cardiol 1976;37:762.
9. Mair DD, Ritter DG, Ongley PA, Helmholz HF Jr. Hemodynamics and evaluation for surgery of patients with complete transposition of the great arteries and ventricular septal defect. Am J Cardiol 1971;28:632.
10. Maroto E, Fouron JC, Douste-Blazy MY, Carceller AM, van Doesburg N, Kratz C, et al. Influence of age on wall thickness, cavity dimensions and myocardial contractility of the left ventricle in simple transposition of the great arteries. Circulation 1983; 67:1311.
11. Martin RP, Ettedgui JA, Qureshi SA, Gibbs JL, Baker EJ, Radley-Smith R, et al. A quantitative evaluation of aortic regurgitation after anatomic correction of transposition of the great arteries. J Am Coll Cardiol 1988;12:1281.
12. Martin TC, Smith L, Hernandez A, Weldon CS. Dysrhythmias following the Senning operation for dextro-transposition of the great arteries. J Thorac Cardiovasc Surg 1983;85:928.
13. Marx GR, Hougen TJ, Norwood WI, Fyler DC, Castaneda AR, Nadas AS. Transposition of the great arteries with intact ventricular

septum: results of Mustard and Senning operations in 123 consecutive patients. J Am Coll Cardiol 1983;1:476.
14. Massin MM, Nitsch GB, Dabritz S, Messmer BJ, von Bernuth G. Angiographic study of aorta, coronary arteries, and left ventricular performance after neonatal arterial switch operation for simple transposition of the great arteries. Am Heart J 1997;134:298.
15. Massoudy P, Baltalarli A, de Leval MR, Cook A, Neudorf U, Derrick G, et al. Anatomic variability in coronary arterial distribution with regard to the arterial switch procedure. Circulation 2002;106:1980-4.
16. Mathews RA, Fricker FJ, Beerman LB, Stephenson RJ, Fischer DR, Neches WH, et al. Exercise studies after the Mustard operation in transposition of the great arteries. Am J Cardiol 1983;51:1526.
17. Matthys D, De Wolf D, Verhaaren H. Lack of increase in stroke volume during exercise in asymptomatic adolescents in sinus rhythm after intraatrial repair for simple transposition of the great arteries. Am J Cardiol 1996;78:595.
18. Mauck HP Jr, Robertson LW, Parr EL, Lower RR. Anatomic correction of transposition of the great arteries without significant ventricular septal defect or patent ductus arteriosus. J Thorac Cardiovasc Surg 1977;74:631.
19. Mavroudis C, Backer CL. Arterial switch after failed atrial baffle procedures for transposition of the great arteries. Ann Thorac Surg 2000;69:851.
20. Mazzei EA, Mulder DG. Superior vena cava syndrome following complete correction (Mustard repair) of transposition of the great vessels. Ann Thorac Surg 1971;11:243.
21. McGoon DC. Intraventricular repair of transposition of the great arteries. J Thorac Cardiovasc Surg 1972;64:430.
22. McMahon CJ, Ravekes WJ, Smith EO, Denfield SW, Pignatelli RH, Altman CA, et al. Risk factors for neo-aortic root enlargement and aortic regurgitation following arterial switch operation. Pediatr Cardiol 2004;25:329-35.
23. Melhuish BP, Van Praagh R. Juxtaposition of the atrial appendages. A sign of severe cyanotic congenital heart disease. Br Heart J 1968;30:269.
24. Merendino KA, Jesseph JE, Herron PW, Thomas GI, Vetto RR. Interatrial venous transposition. A one-stage intracardiac operation for the conversion of complete transposition of the aorta and pulmonary artery to corrected transposition. Surgery 1957; 42:898.
25. Metras D, Kreitmann B, Riberi A, Yao JG, el-Khoury E, Wernert F, et al. Extending the concept of the autograft for complete repair of transposition of the great arteries with ventricular septal defect and left ventricular outflow tract obstruction: a report of ten cases of a modified procedure. J Thorac Cardiovasc Surg 1997;114:746.
26. Metton O, Calvaruso D, Gaudin R, Mussa S, Raisky O, Bonnet D, et al. Intramural coronary arteries and outcome of neonatal arterial switch operation. Eur J Cardiothorac Surg 2010;37:1246-53.
27. Milanesi O, Thiene G, Bini RM, Pellegrino PA. Complete transposition of great arteries with coarctation of aorta. Br Heart J 1982;48:566.
28. Millane T, Bernard EJ, Jaeggi E, Howman-Giles RB, Uren RF, Cartmill TB, et al. Role of ischemia and infarction in late right ventricular dysfunction after atrial repair of transposition of the great arteries. J Am Coll Cardiol 2000;35:1661.
29. Miller RA. Complete transposition of the great arteries. In: Morse DP, ed. Congenital heart disease, pathogenetic factors, natural history, diagnosis, and surgical treatment. Philadelphia: FA Davis, 1962, p. 74.
30. Moene RJ, Oppenheimer-Dekker A. Congenital mitral valve anomalies in transposition of the great arteries. Am J Cardiol 1982;49:1972.
31. Moene RJ, Oppenheimer-Dekker A, Bartelings MM. Anatomic obstruction of the right ventricular outflow tract in transposition of the great arteries. Am J Cardiol 1983;51:1701.
32. Moodie DS, Feldt RH, Wallace RB. Transient protein-losing enteropathy secondary to elevated caval pressures and caval obstruction after the Mustard procedure. J Thorac Cardiovasc Surg 1976;72:379.
33. Morell VO, Jacobs JP, Quintessenza JA. Aortic translocation in the management of transposition of the great arteries with ventricular septal defect and pulmonary stenosis: results and follow-up. Ann Thorac Surg 2005;79:2089-93.
34. Morgan JR, Miller BL, Daicoff GR, Andrews EJ. Hemodynamic and angiocardiographic evaluation after Mustard procedure for transposition of the great arteries. J Thorac Cardiovasc Surg 1972;64:878.
35. Murakami T, Nakazawa M, Momma K, Imai Y. Impaired distensibility of neoaorta after arterial switch procedure. Ann Thorac Surg 2000;70:1907.
36. Murphy JH, Barlai-Kovach MM, Mathews RA, Beerman LB, Park SC, Neches WH, et al. Rest and exercise right and left ventricular function late after the Mustard operation: assessment by radionuclide ventriculography. Am J Cardiol 1983;51:1520.
37. Murthy KS, Cherian KM. A new technique of arterial switch operation with in situ coronary reallocation for transposition of great arteries. J Thorac Cardiovasc Surg 1996;112:27.
38. Mustard WT. Successful two-stage correction of transposition of the great vessels. Surgery 1964;55:469.
39. Mustard WT, Chute AL, Keith JD, Sivek A, Rowe RD, Vlad P. A surgical approach to transposition of the great vessels with extracorporeal circuit. Surgery 1954;36:39.
40. Muster AJ, Paul MH, Van Grondelle A, Conway JJ. Asymmetric distribution of the pulmonary blood flow between the right and left lungs in d-transposition of the great arteries. Am J Cardiol 1976;38:352.
41. Myridakis DJ, Ehlers KH, Engle MA. Late follow-up after venous switch operation (Mustard procedure) for simple and complex transposition of the great arteries. Am J Cardiol 1994;74:1030.

N

1. Nair KK, Chan KC, Hickey MS. Arterial switch operation: successful bilateral internal thoracic artery grafting. Ann Thorac Surg 2000;69:949.
2. Nakajima Y, Momma K, Seguchi M, Nakazawa M, Imai Y. Pulmonary hypertension in patients with complete transposition of the great arteries: midterm results after surgery. Pediatr Cardiol 1996; 17:104.
3. Nakazawa M, Oyama K, Imai Y, Nojima K, Aotsuka H, Satomi G, et al. Criteria for two-staged arterial switch operation for simple transposition of the great arteries. Circulation 1988;78:124.
4. Nanda NC, Gramiak R, Manning JA, Lipchik EO. Echocardiographic features of subpulmonic obstruction in dextro-position of the great vessels. Circulation 1975;51:515.
5. Neutze JM. Transposition of the great vessels in infancy. N Z Med J 1965;64:13.
6. Newburger JW, Silbert AR, Buckley LP, Fyler DC. Cognitive function and age at repair of transposition of the great arteries in children. N Engl J Med 1984;310:1495.
7. Newfeld EA, Paul MM, Muster AJ, Idriss FS. Pulmonary vascular disease in complete transposition of the great arteries: a study of 200 patients. Am J Cardiol 1974;34:75.
8. Newfeld EA, Paul MH, Muster AJ, Idriss FS. Pulmonary vascular disease in transposition of the great vessels and intact ventricular septum. Circulation 1979;59:525.
9. Niinami H, Imai Y, Sawatari K, Hoshino S, Ishihara K, Aoki M. Surgical management of tricuspid malinsertion in the Rastelli operation: conal flap method. Ann Thorac Surg 1995;59:1476.
10. Nikaidoh H. Aortic translocation and biventricular outflow tract reconstruction. A new surgical repair for transposition of the great arteries associated with ventricular septal defect and pulmonary stenosis. J Thorac Cardiovasc Surg 1984;88:365.
11. Nogi S, McCrindle BW, Boutin C, Williams WG, Freedom RM, Benson LN. Fate of the neopulmonary valve after the arterial switch operation in neonates. J Thorac Cardiovasc Surg 1998;115:557.
12. Nogrady MB, Dunbar JS. Complete transposition of the great vessels: re-evaluation of the so-called "typical configuration" on plain films of the chest. J Can Assoc Radiol 1969;20:124.

O

1. Oechslin E, Jenni R. 40 years after the first atrial switch procedure in patients with transposition of the great arteries: long-term results in Toronto and Zurich. Thorac Cardiovasc Surg 2000;48:233.
2. Oelert H, Borst HG. Transmitral resection of subpulmonary stenosis in transposition of the great arteries. Thorac Cardiovasc Surg 1979;27:58.
3. Oelert H, Stegmann T, Leitz KH, Luhmer I, Reichelt W, Borst HG. Transposition of the great arteries, ventricular septal defect, and left ventricular outflow obstruction: results of conservative correction. Thorac Cardiovasc Surg 1979;27:219.
4. Okuda H, Nakazawa M, Imai Y, Kurosawa H, Takanashi Y, Hoshino S, et al. Comparison of ventricular function after Senning

and Jatene procedures for complete transposition of the great arteries. Am J Cardiol 1985;55:530.
5. Otero-Coto E, Quero Jimenez M, Deverall PB, Bain H. Anomalous mitral "cleft" with abnormal ventriculo-arterial connection: anatomical findings and surgical implications. Pediatr Cardiol 1984;5:1.
6. Ou P, Mousseaux E, Azarine A, Dupont P, Agnoletti G, Vouhe P, et al. Detection of coronary complications after the arterial switch operation for transposition of the great arteries: first experience with multislice computed tomography in children. J Thorac Cardiovasc Surg 2006;131:639-43.

P

1. Pacifico AD, Stewart RW, Bargeron LM Jr. Repair of transposition of the great arteries with ventricular septal defect by an arterial switch operation. Circulation 1983;68:II49.
2. Page E, Perrault H, Flore P, Rossignol AM, Pironneau S, Rocca C, et al. Cardiac output response to dynamic exercise after atrial switch repair for transposition of the great arteries. Am J Cardiol 1996;77:892.
3. Parenzan L, Locatelli G, Alfieri O, Villani M, Invernizzi G. The Senning operation for transposition of the great arteries. J Thorac Cardiovasc Surg 1978;76:305.
4. Park SC, Neches WH, Mathews RA, Fricker FJ, Beerman LB, Fischer DR, et al. Hemodynamic function after the Mustard operation for transposition of the great arteries. Am J Cardiol 1983; 51:1514.
5. Park SC, Weiss FH, Siewers RD, Neches WH, Zuberbuhler JR, Lenox CC. Continuous murmur following Mustard operation for transposition of the great arteries. A sign of pulmonary venous obstruction. Circulation 1976;54:684.
6. Park SC, Zuberbuhler JR, Neches WH, Lenox CC, Zoltun RA. A new atrial septostomy technique. Cathet Cardiovasc Diagn 1975;1:195.
7. Parr GV, Blackstone EH, Kirklin JW, Pacifico AD, Lauridsen P. Cardiac performance early after interatrial transposition of venous return in infants and small children. Circulation 1974;50:II2.
8. Parrish MD, Graham TP Jr, Bender HW, Jones JP, Patton J, Partain CL. Radionuclide angiographic evaluation of right and left ventricular function during exercise after repair of transposition of the great arteries. Comparison with normal subjects and patients with congenitally corrected transposition. Circulation 1983; 67:178.
9. Parry AJ, Thurm M, Hanley FL. The use of "pericardial hoods" for maintaining exact coronary artery geometry in the arterial switch operation with complex coronary anatomy. Eur J Cardiothorac Surg 1999;15:159-65.
10. Pasquali SK, Marino BS, McBride MG, Wernovsky G, Paridon SM. Coronary artery pattern and age impact exercise performance late after the arterial switch operation. J Thorac Cardiovasc Surg 2007;134:1207-12.
11. Pasquini L, Parness IA, Colan SD, Wernovsky G, Mayer JE, Sanders SP. Diagnosis of intramural coronary artery in transposition of the great arteries using two-dimensional echocardiography. Circulation 1993;88:1136.
12. Paul MH. Transposition of the great arteries. In: Adams FH, Emmanouilides GC, eds. Heart disease in infants, children and adolescents. 3rd Ed. Baltimore: Williams & Wilkins, 1983, p. 296.
13. Paul MH, Wessel HU. Exercise studies in patients with transposition of the great arteries after atrial repair operations (Mustard/Senning): a review. Pediatr Cardiol 1999;20:49.
14. Pedra SR, Pedra CA, Abizaid AA, Braga SL, Staico R, Arrieta R, et al. Intracoronary ultrasound assessment late after the arterial switch operation for transposition of the great arteries. J Am Coll Cardiol 2005;45:2061-8.
15. Peterson RJ, Franch RH, Fajman WA, Jones RH. Comparison of cardiac function in surgically corrected and congenitally corrected transposition of the great arteries. J Thorac Cardiovasc Surg 1988; 96:227.
16. Phornphutkul C, Rosenthal A, Nadas AS, Berenberg W. Cerebrovascular accidents in infants and children with cyanotic congenital heart disease. Am J Cardiol 1973;32:329.
17. Pitlick P, French J, Guthaner D, Shumway N, Baum D. Results of intraventricular baffle procedure for ventricular septal defect and double outlet right ventricle or d-transposition of the great arteries. Am J Cardiol 1981;47:307.
18. Plauth WH Jr, Nadas AS, Bernhard WF, Fyler DC. Changing hemodynamics in patients with transposition of the great arteries. Circulation 1970;42:131.
19. Puley G, Siu S, Connelly M, Harrison D, Webb G, Williams WG, et al. Arrhythmia and survival in patients >18 years of age after the Mustard procedure for complete transposition of the great arteries. Am J Cardiol 1999;83:1080.

Q

1. Qamar ZA, Goldberg CS, Devaney EJ, Bove EL, Ohye RG. Current risk factors and outcomes for the arterial switch operation. Ann Thorac Surg 2007;84:871-9.
2. Quaegebeur JM. The arterial switch operation. Rationale, results, and perspectives. Thesis; Leiden University, The Netherlands; 1986.
3. Quaegebeur JM, Rohmer J, Brom AG. Revival of the Senning operation in the treatment of transposition of the great arteries. Preliminary report on recent experience. Thorax 1977;32:517.
4. Quaegebeur JM, Rohmer J, Ottenkamp J, Buis T, Kirklin JW, Blackstone EH, et al. The arterial switch operation. An eight-year experience. J Thorac Cardiovasc Surg 1986;92:361.

R

1. Rabinovitch M, Rosenthal A, Sade RM, Castaneda AR, Treves S, Nadas AS. Regional lung function studies and radionuclide angiography in D-transposition of the great arteries. Pediatr Res 1977;11:1117.
2. Radley-Smith R, Yacoub MH. One stage anatomic correction of simple complete transposition of the great arteries in neonates. Br Heart J 1984;51:685.
3. Raisky O, Bergoend E, Agnoletti G, Ou P, Bonnet D, Sidi D, et al. Late coronary artery lesions after neonatal arterial switch operation: results of surgical coronary revascularization. Eur J Cardiothorac Surg 2007;31:894-8.
4. Ramsay JM, Venables AW, Kelly MJ, Kalff V. Right and left ventricular function at rest and with exercise after the Mustard operation for transposition of the great arteries. Br Heart J 1984;51:364.
5. Rashkind WJ, Miller WW. Creation of an atrial septal defect without thoracotomy: a palliative approach to complete transposition of the great arteries. JAMA 1966;196:991.
6. Rashkind WJ, Miller WW. Transposition of the great arteries. Results of palliation by balloon atrioseptostomy in thirty-one infants. Circulation 1968;38:453.
7. Rastelli GC. A new approach to "anatomic" repair of transposition of the great arteries. Mayo Clin Proc 1969;44:1.
8. Rastelli GC, Wallace RB, Ongley PA. Complete repair of transposition of the great arteries with pulmonary stenosis. A review and report of a case corrected by using a new surgical technique. Circulation 1969;39:83.
9. Reul GJ Jr, Cooley DA, Sandiford FM, Hallman GL. Complications following the contoured Dacron baffle in correction of transposition of the great arteries. Surgery 1974;76:946.
10. Reybrouck T, Dumoulin M, Van der Hauwaert LG. Cardiorespiratory exercise testing after venous switch operation in children with complete transposition of the great arteries. Am J Cardiol 1988;61:861.
11. Reybrouck T, Eyskens B, Mertens L, Defoor J, Daenen W, Gewillig M. Cardiorespiratory exercise function after the arterial switch operation for transposition of the great arteries. Eur Heart J 2001;22:1052.
12. Rhodes LA, Wernovsky G, Keane JF, Mayer JE Jr, Shuren A, Dindy C, et al. Arrhythmias and intracardiac conduction after the arterial switch operation. J Thorac Cardiovasc Surg 1995;109:303.
13. Riemenschneider TA, Goldberg SJ, Ruttenberg HD, Gyepes MT. Subpulmonic obstruction in complete (D) transposition produced by redundant tricuspid tissue. Circulation 1969;39:603.
14. Riemenschneider TA, Vincent WR, Ruttenberg HD, Desilets DT. Transposition of the great vessels with hypoplasia of the right ventricle. Circulation 1968;38:386.
15. Riggs TW, Muster AJ, Aziz KU, Paul MH, Ilbawi M, Idriss FS. Two-dimensional echocardiographic and angiocardiographic diagnosis of subpulmonary stenosis due to tricuspid valve pouch in complete transposition of the great arteries. J Am Coll Cardiol 1983;1:484.
16. Rosengart R, Fisbein M, Emmanouilides GC. Progressive pulmonary vascular disease after surgical correction (Mustard procedure)

of transposition of the great arteries with intact ventricular septum. Am J Cardiol 1975;35:107.
17. Rosenquist GC, Stark J, Taylor JF. Congenital mitral valve disease in transposition of the great arteries. Circulation 1975;51:731.
18. Rosman NP, Shands KN. Hydrocephalus caused by increased intracranial venous pressure: a clinicopathological study. Ann Neurol 1978;3:445.
19. Rubay J, Lecompte Y, Batisse A, Durandy Y, Dibie A, Lemoine G, et al. Anatomic repair of anomalies of ventriculo-arterial connection (REV). Results of a new technique in cases associated with pulmonary outflow tract obstruction. Eur J Cardiothorac Surg 1988;2:305.

S

1. Sansa M, Tonkin IL, Bargeron LM Jr, Elliott LP. Left ventricular outflow tract obstruction in transposition of the great arteries: an angiographic study of 74 cases. Am J Cardiol 1979;44:88.
2. Sapsford RN, Aberdeen E, Watson DA, Crew AD. Transposed great arteries combined with totally anomalous pulmonary veins. A report of a successful correction. J Thorac Cardiovasc Surg 1972; 63:360.
3. Sarkar D, Bull C, Yates R, Wright D, Cullen S, Gewillig M, et al. Comparison of long-term outcomes of atrial repair of simple transposition with implications for a late arterial switch strategy. Circulation 1999;100:II176.
4. Sarris GE, Chatzis AC, Giannopoulos NM, Kirvassilis G, Berggren H, Hazekamp M, et al. The arterial switch operation in Europe for transposition of the great arteries: a multi-institutional study from the European Congenital Heart Surgeons Association. J Thorac Cardiovasc Surg 2006;132:633-9.
5. Satomi G, Nakamura K, Takao A, Imai Y. Two-dimensional echocardiographic detection of pulmonary venous channel stenosis after Senning's operation. Circulation 1983;68:545.
6. Schneeweiss A, Motro M, Shem-Tov A, Neufeld HN. Subaortic stenosis: an unrecognized problem in transposition of the great arteries. Am J Cardiol 1981;48:336.
7. Schwartz ML, Gauvreau K, del Nido P, Mayer JE, Colan SD. Long-term predictors of aortic root dilation and aortic regurgitation after arterial switch operation. Circulation 2004;110:II128-32.
8. Scott O, Williams GJ, Fiddler GI. Results of 24-hour ambulatory monitoring of electrocardiogram in 131 healthy boys aged 10 to 13 years. Br Heart J 1980;44:304.
9. Senning A. Surgical correction of transposition of the great vessels. Surgery 1959;45:966.
10. Senning A. Surgical correction of transposition of the great vessels. Surgery 1966;59:334.
11. Serraf A, Nakamura T, Lacour-Gayet F, Piot D, Bruniaux J, Touchot A, et al. Surgical approaches for double-outlet right ventricle or transposition of the great arteries associated with straddling atrioventricular valves. J Thorac Cardiovasc Surg 1996;111:527.
12. Serraf A, Roux D, Lacour-Gayet F, Touchot A, Bruniaux J, Sousa-Uva M, et al. Reoperation after the arterial switch operation for transposition of the great arteries. J Thorac Cardiovasc Surg 1995;110:892.
13. Shaher RM, Fowler RS, Kidd BS, Moes CA, Keith JD. Spontaneous closure of a ventricular septal defect in a case of complete transposition of the great vessels. Can Med Assoc J 1965;93:1037.
14. Shaher RM, Puddu GC, Khoury G, Moes CA, Mustard WT. Complete transposition of the great vessels with anatomic obstruction of the outflow tract of the left ventricle. Surgical implications of anatomic findings. Am J Cardiol 1967;19:658.
15. Shankar S, Sreeram N, Brawn WJ, Sethia B. Intraoperative ultrasonographic troubleshooting after the arterial switch operation. Ann Thorac Surg 1997;63:445.
16. Shrivastava S, Tadavarthy SM, Fukuda T, Edwards JE. Anatomic causes of pulmonary stenosis in complete transposition. Circulation 1976;54:154.
17. Shumacker HB Jr. A new operation for transposition of the great vessels. Surgery 1961;50:773.
18. Silove ED, Taylor JF. Haemodynamics after Mustard's operation for transposition of the great arteries. Br Heart J 1976;38:1037.
19. Silverman NH, Snider AR, Colo J, Ebert PA, Turley K. Superior vena caval obstruction after Mustard's operation: detection by two-dimensional contrast echocardiography. Circulation 1981;64:392.
20. Smith A, Wilkinson JL, Arnold R, Dickinson DF, Anderson RH. Growth and development of ventricular walls in complete transposition of the great arteries with intact septum (simple transposition). Am J Cardiol 1982;49:362.
21. Southall DP, Johnston F, Shinebourne EA, Johnston PG. 24-hour electrocardiographic study of heart rate and rhythm patterns in population of healthy children. Br Heart J 1981;45:281.
22. Southall DP, Keeton BR, Leanage R, Lam L, Joseph MC, Anderson RH, et al. Cardiac rhythm and conduction before and after Mustard's operation for complete transposition of the great arteries. Br Heart J 1980;43:21.
23. Stansel HC Jr. A new operation for d-loop transposition of the great vessels. Ann Thorac Surg 1975;19:565.
24. Stark J, de Leval MR, Taylor JF. Mustard operation and creation of ventricular septal defect in two patients with transposition of the great arteries, intact ventricular septum and pulmonary vascular disease. Am J Cardiol 1976;38:524.
25. Stark J, Silove ED, Taylor JF, Graham GR. Obstruction to systemic venous return following the Mustard operation for transposition of the great arteries. J Thorac Cardiovasc Surg 1974;68:742.
26. Stevenson JG, Kawabori I, Guntheroth WG, Dooley TK, Dillard D. Pulsed Doppler echocardiographic detection of obstruction of systemic venous return after repair of transposition of the great arteries. Circulation 1979;60:1091.
27. Streeter DD Jr, Spotnitz HM, Patel DP, Ross J Jr, Sonnenblick EH. Fiber orientation in the canine left ventricle during diastole and systole. Circ Res 1969;24:339.
28. Subramanian S, Wagner H. Correction of transposition of the great arteries in infants under surface-induced deep hypothermia. Ann Thorac Surg 1973;16:391.
29. Sunderland CO, Henken DP, Nichols GM, Dhindsa DS, Bonchek LI, Menashe VD, et al. Postoperative hemodynamic and electrophysiologic evaluation of the interatrial baffle procedure. Am J Cardiol 1975;35:660.
30. Suzuki T. Modification of the arterial switch operation for transposition of the great arteries with complex coronary artery patterns. Gen Thorac Cardiovasc Surg 2009;57:281-92.
31. Sweeney MF, Bell WE, Doty DB, Schieken RM. Communicating hydrocephalus secondary to venous complications following intra-atrial baffle operation (Mustard procedure) for d-transposition of the great arteries. Pediatr Cardiol 1982;3:237.
32. Szarnicki RJ, Stark J, de Leval M. Reoperation for complications after inflow correction of transposition of the great arteries: technical considerations. Ann Thorac Surg 1978;25:150.

T

1. Takahashi M, Lindesmith GG, Lewis AB, Stiles QR, Stanton RE, Meyer BW, et al. Long-term results of the Mustard procedure. Circulation 1977;56:II85.
2. Takeuchi S, Katogi T. New technique for the arterial switch operation in difficult situations. Ann Thorac Surg 1990;50:1000-1.
3. Tam S, Murphy JD, Norwood WI. Transposition of the great arteries with posterior aorta. Anatomic repair. J Thorac Cardiovasc Surg 1990;100:441.
4. Tamisier D, Ouaknine R, Pouard P, Mauriat P, Lefebvre D, Sidi D, et al. Neonatal arterial switch operation: coronary artery patterns and coronary events. Eur J Cardiothorac Surg 1997;11:810.
5. Tanel RE, Wernovsky G, Landzberg MJ, Perry SB, Burke RP. Coronary artery abnormalities detected at cardiac catheterization following the arterial switch operation for transposition of the great arteries. Am J Cardiol 1995;76:153.
6. Taussig HB. Complete transposition of the great vessels; clinical and pathologic features. Am Heart J 1938;16:728.
7. Taussig HB, Bing RJ. Complete transposition of aorta and levoposition of pulmonary artery. Am Heart J 1949;37:551.
8. Taylor AM, Dymarkowski S, Hamaekers P, Razavi R, Gewillig M, Mertens L, et al. MR coronary angiography and late-enhancement myocardial MR in children who underwent arterial switch surgery for transposition of great arteries. Radiology 2005;234:542-7.
9. Tchervenkov CI, Tahta SA, Cecere R, Beland MJ. Single-stage arterial switch with aortic arch enlargement for transposition complexes with aortic arch obstruction. Ann Thorac Surg 1997; 64:1776.
10. Tometzki AJ, Suda K, Kohl T, Kovalchin JP, Silverman NH. Accuracy of prenatal echocardiographic diagnosis and prognosis of fetuses with conotruncal anomalies. J Am Coll Cardiol 1999; 33:1696.
11. Tonkin IL, Sansa M, Elliott LP, Bargeron LM Jr. Recognition of developing left ventricular outflow tract obstruction in complete transposition of the great arteries. Radiology 1980;134:53.

12. Trusler GA, Bull RC, Hoeksema T, Mustard WT. The effect on cardiac output of a reduction in atrial volume. J Thorac Cardiovasc Surg 1963;46:109.
13. Trusler GA, Williams WG, Izukawa T, Olley PM. Current results with the Mustard operation in isolated transposition of the great arteries. J Thorac Cardiovasc Surg 1980;80:381.
14. Tsuda E, Imakita M, Yagihara T, Ono Y, Echigo S, Takahashi O, et al. Late death after arterial switch operation for transposition of the great arteries. Am Heart J 1992;124:1551.
15. Tulevski II, Lee PL, Groenink M, van der Wall EE, Stoker J, Pieper PG, et al. Dobutamine-induced increase of right ventricular contractility without increased stroke volume in adolescent patients with transposition of the great arteries: evaluation with magnetic resonance imaging. Int J Card Imaging 2000;16:471.
16. Turina MI, Siebenmann R, von Segesser L, Schonbeck M, Senning A. Late functional deterioration after atrial correction for transposition of the great arteries. Circulation 1989;80:I162.
17. Turley K, Verrier ED. Intermediate results from the period of the Congenital Heart Surgeons Transposition Study: 1985 to 1989. Congenital Heart Surgeons Society Database. Ann Thorac Surg 1995;60:505.
18. Tynan M. Survival of infants with transposition of great arteries after balloon atrial septostomy. Lancet 1971;1:621.
19. Tworetzky W, McElhinney DB, Brook MM, Reddy VM, Hanley FL, Silverman NH. Echocardiographic diagnosis alone for the complete repair of major congenital heart defects. J Am Coll Cardiol 1999;33:228.

U

1. Ullal RR, Anderson RH, Lincoln C. Mustard's operation modified to avoid dysrhythmias and pulmonary and systemic venous obstruction. J Thorac Cardiovasc Surg 1979;78:431.
2. Urban AE, Stark J, Waterston DJ. Mustard's operation for transposition of the great arteries complicated by juxtaposition of the atrial appendages. Ann Thorac Surg 1976;21:304.

V

1. Vandekerckhove KD, Blom NA, Lalezari S, Koolbergen DR, Rijlaarsdam ME, Hazekamp MG. Long-term follow-up of arterial switch operation with an emphasis on function and dimensions of left ventricle and aorta. Eur J Cardiothorac Surg 2009;35:582-8.
2. Van Doesburg NH, Bierman FZ, Williams RG. Left ventricular geometry in infants with d-transposition of the great arteries and intact interventricular septum. Circulation 1983;68:733.
3. Van Gils FA, Moulaert AJ, Oppenheimer-Dekker A, Wenink CG. Transposition of the great arteries with ventricular septal defect and pulmonary stenosis. Br Heart J 1978;40:494.
4. Van Praagh R. What is the Taussig-Bing malformation? Circulation 1968;38:445.
5. Van Praagh R, Perez-Trevino C, Lopez-Cuellar M, Baker FW, Zuberbuhler JR, Quero M, et al. Transposition of the great arteries with posterior aorta, anterior pulmonary artery, subpulmonary conus and fibrous continuity between aortic and atrioventricular valves. Am J Cardiol 1971;28:621.
6. Van Praagh R, Weinberg PM, Calder L, Buckley LF, Van Praagh S. The transposition complexes: How many are there? In: Davila JC, ed. Second Henry Ford Hospital International Symposium on Cardiac Surgery. E. Norwalk, Conn: Appleton & Lange, 1977, p. 207.
7. Venables AW, Edis B, Clarke CP. Vena caval obstruction complicating the Mustard operation for complete transposition of the great arteries. Eur J Cardiol 1974;1:401.
8. Vidne BA, Duszynski D, Subramanian S. Pulmonary blood flow distribution in transposition of the great arteries. Am J Cardiol 1976;38:62.
9. Vidne BA, Subramanian S, Wagner HR. Aneurysm of the membranous ventricular septum in transposition of the great arteries. Circulation 1976;53:157.
10. Viles PH, Ongley PA, Titus JL. The spectrum of pulmonary vascular disease in transposition of the great arteries. Circulation 1969;40:31.
11. von Bernuth G. 25 years after the first arterial switch procedure: mid-term results. Thorac Cardiovasc Surg 2000;48:228.
12. Vouhe PR, Haydar A, Ouaknine R, Albanese SB, Mauriat P, Pouard P, et al. Arterial switch operation: a new technique of coronary transfer. Eur J Cardiothorac Surg 1994;8:74-8.
13. Vouhe PR, Tamisier D, Leca F, Ouaknine R, Vernant F, Neveux JY. Transposition of the great arteries, ventricular septal defect and pulmonary outflow tract obstruction: Rastelli or Lecompte procedure? J Thorac Cardiovasc Surg 1992;103:428.

W

1. Wagenvoort CA, Nauta J, van der Schaar PJ, Weeda HW, Wagenvoort N. The pulmonary vasculature in complete transposition of the great vessels, judged from lung biopsies. Circulation 1968;38:746.
2. Waldman JD, Paul MH, Newfeld EA, Muster AJ, Idriss FS. Transposition of the great arteries with intact ventricular septum and patent ductus arteriosus. Am J Cardiol 1977;39:232.
3. Ward CJ, Mullins CE, Nihill MR, Grifka RG, Vick GW 3rd. Use of intravascular stents in systemic venous and systemic venous baffle obstructions. Short-term follow-up results. Circulation 1995;91:2948.
4. Wells WJ, Blackstone E. Intermediate outcome after Mustard and Senning procedures: a study by the Congenital Heart Surgeons Society. Semin Thorac Cardiovasc Surg Pediatr Card Surg Annu 2000;3:186.
5. Wernovsky G, Jonas RA, Colan SD, Sanders SP, Wessel DL, Castaneda AR, et al. Results of the arterial switch operation in patients with transposition of the great arteries and abnormalities of the mitral valve or left ventricular outflow tract. J Am Coll Cardiol 1990;16:1446.
6. Wernovsky G, Mayer JE Jr, Jonas RA, Hanley FL, Blackstone EH, Kirklin JW, et al. Factors influencing early and late outcome of the arterial switch operation for transposition of the great arteries. J Thorac Cardiovasc Surg 1995;109:289.
7. Wernovsky G, Wypij D, Jonas RA, Mayer JE Jr, Hanley FL, Hickey PR, et al. Postoperative course and hemodynamic profile after the arterial switch operation in neonates and infants. Circulation 1995;92:2226.
8. Wilcox BR, Henry GW, Anderson RH. The transmitral approach to left ventricular outflow tract obstruction. Ann Thorac Surg 1983;35:288.
9. Wilkinson JL, Arnold R, Anderson RH, Acerete F. "Posterior" transposition reconsidered. Br Heart J 1975;37:757.
10. Williams WG, McCrindle BW, Ashburn DA, Jonas RA, Mavroudis C, Blackstone EH. Outcomes of 829 neonates with complete transposition of the great arteries 12-17 years after repair. Eur J Cardiothorac Surg 2003;24:1-10.
11. Williams WG, Trusler GA, Kirklin JW, Blackstone EH, Coles JG, Izukawa T, et al. Early and late results of a protocol for simple transposition leading to an atrial switch (Mustard) repair. J Thorac Cardiovasc Surg 1988;95:717.
12. Wilson HE, Nafrawi AG, Cardozo RH, Aguillon A. Rational approach to surgery for complete transposition of the great vessels: analysis of the basic hemodynamics and critical appraisal of previously proposed corrective procedures with a suggested approach based on laboratory and clinical studies. Ann Surg 1962;155:258.
13. Wilson NJ, Clarkson PM, Barratt-Boyes BG, Calder AL, Whitlock RM, Easthope RN, et al. Long-term outcome after the Mustard repair for simple transposition of the great arteries. 28-year follow-up. J Am Coll Cardiol 1998;32:758.
14. Winlaw DS, McGuirk SP, Balmer C, Langley SM, Griselli M, Stumper O, et al. Intention-to-treat analysis of pulmonary artery banding in conditions with a morphological right ventricle in the systemic circulation with a view to anatomic biventricular repair. Circulation 2005;111:405-11.
15. Wittig JH, Stark J. Intraoperative mapping of atrial activation before, during and after the Mustard operation. J Thorac Cardiovasc Surg 1977;73:1.
16. Wood AE, Freedom RM, Williams WG, Trusler GA. The Mustard procedure in transposition of the great arteries associated with juxtaposition of the atrial appendages with and without dextrocardia. J Thorac Cardiovasc Surg 1983;85:451.
17. Wyse RK, Haworth SG, Taylor JF, Macartney FJ. Obstruction of superior vena caval pathway after Mustard's repair. Reliable diagnosis by transcutaneous Doppler ultrasound. Br Heart J 1979; 42:162.
18. Wyse RK, Macartney FJ, Rohmer J, Ottenkamp J, Brom AG. Differential atrial filling after Mustard and Senning repairs. Detection by transcutaneous Doppler ultrasound. Br Heart J 1980; 44:692.

Y

1. Yacoub MH, Arensman FW, Keck E, Radley-Smith R. Fate of dynamic left ventricular outflow tract obstruction after anatomic correction of transposition of the great arteries. Circulation 1983;68:II56.
2. Yacoub MH, Radley-Smith R, Hilton CJ. Anatomical correction of complete transposition of the great arteries and ventricular septal defect in infancy. Br Med J 1976;1:1112.
3. Yacoub MH, Radley-Smith R, Maclaurin R. Two-stage operation for anatomical correction of transposition of the great arteries with intact ventricular septum. Lancet 1977;1:1275.
4. Yaku H, Nunn GR, Sholler GF. Internal mammary artery grafting in a neonate for coronary hypoperfusion after arterial switch. Ann Thorac Surg 1997;64:543.
5. Yamazaki A, Yamamoto N, Sakamoto T, Ishihara K, Iwata Y, Matsumura G, et al. Long-term outcomes and social independence level after arterial switch operation. Eur J Cardiothorac Surg 2008;33:239-43.
6. Yates RW, Marsden PK, Badawi RD, Cronin BF, Anderson DR, Tynan MJ, et al. Evaluation of myocardial perfusion using positron emission tomography in infants following a neonatal arterial switch operation. Pediatr Cardiol 2000;21:111.
7. Yatsunami K, Nakazawa M, Kondo C, Teshima H, Momma K, Takanashi Y, et al. Small left coronary arteries after arterial switch operation for complete transposition. Ann Thorac Surg 1997;64:746.

Z

1. Zuberbuhler JR, Bauersfeld SR. Unusual arrhythmias after corrective surgery for transposition of the great vessels. Am Heart J 1967;73:752.

53 Double Outlet Right Ventricle

DEFINITION

Double outlet right ventricle (DORV) is a congenital cardiac anomaly in which both great arteries arise wholly or in large part from the right ventricle.[1] It is a type of ventriculoarterial connection (see "Cardiac Connections" under Terminology and Classification of Heart Disease in Chapter 1).

In this chapter, DORV with *atrioventricular (AV) concordant connection* is discussed in detail. DORV also occurs in other settings (Fig. 53-1), but when the AV connection is discordant, that becomes the surgically more important feature, and patients with this combination (commonly called *congenitally corrected transposition of the great arteries*) are better considered along with others with AV discordant connection (see Chapter 55). DORV may also occur in patients with univentricular AV connections (see "Ventriculoarterial Connections" under Morphology in Chapter 56). It is a frequent occurrence in patients with atrial isomerism (see "Ventriculoarterial Connections" under Morphology in Chapter 58).

One or both great arteries may directly overlie the ventricular septal defect (VSD) and thus arise biventricularly.[U1] For purposes of categorization, the great artery so arising is assigned to the ventricle it overlies by more than 50% on morphologic examination. Thus, when one great artery arises wholly or nearly so from the right ventricle (RV) and the other more than 50% from it, the condition is termed *DORV*. Uncommonly, both great arteries arise biventricularly in association with a doubly committed juxta-arterial VSD (see Chapter 35, Figs. 35-8 and 35-9). One option is to arbitrarily assign each great artery to the ventricle above from which more than 50% arises and categorize the anomaly accordingly; the alternative is to term the malformation *double outlet both ventricles*.

Tetralogy of Fallot is an entity characterized by a variable amount of dextroposition of the aorta. When the aorta arises more than 50% from the RV, the anomaly may be categorized as *tetralogy of Fallot with DORV* or as *DORV with pulmonary stenosis*. Edwards uses still different criteria for distinguishing between these two conditions.[E1] Taussig-Bing heart (see description under Morphology later in this chapter) is an entity with variability in the origin of the *pulmonary artery*. This diagnosis may be made when the pulmonary artery arises wholly or nearly so from the RV (in which case, it is a type of DORV), equally from right and left ventricles, or more than 50% but not entirely from the left ventricle (LV; in which case, it is not a type of DORV). When it arises entirely or essentially so from the LV, the assignment is to *transposition of the great arteries with VSD*.

Because of this differing terminology, surgical reports must clearly describe the entities under discussion.

[1]The adjectives *left* and *right* used to modify atrium or ventricle mean *morphologically* left and right, respectively. Position of the chamber is referred to as *right-sided* or *left-sided*.

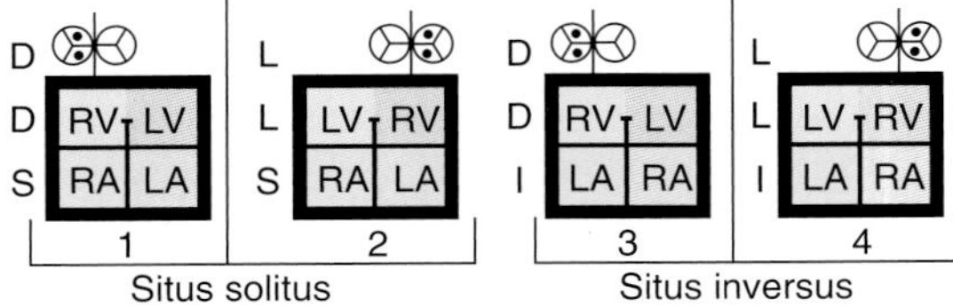

Figure 53-1 Model of the four basic hearts as they occur in double outlet right ventricle, with usual great artery positions (aorta lateral to pulmonary trunk). Models 2 and 3 show atrioventricular discordant connection. The Van Praagh symbolic convention is used (see "Symbolic Convention of Van Praagh" under Terminology and Classification of Heart Disease in Chapter 1). Key: *LA*, Left atrium; *LV*, left ventricle; *RA*, right atrium; *RV*, right ventricle.

HISTORICAL NOTE

When Kirklin performed the first repair of DORV (which was of the simple type with a subaortic VSD) in May 1957 at the Mayo Clinic, the anomaly was virtually unknown, and the preoperative diagnosis was large VSD with high pulmonary blood flow.[K7] Diagnosis was correctly made at operation, the term *double outlet right ventricle* or *origin of both great vessels from the right ventricle* coined in the operating room, position of the His bundle deduced, and intraventricular tunnel repair performed in much the same manner as is done today.[K7] An identical sequence occurred at GLH in September 1958.[B3] Earlier, in 1952, Braun and colleagues reported what was clearly a case of DORV with pulmonary stenosis and used the phrase *double outlet ventricle*, but the title of their paper was confusing, and it escaped notice.[B13] About the time of the first repair, the first morphologic paper with the title "Double Outlet Right Ventricle" was published by Witham[W3]; subsequently, other early descriptions of the morphology appeared.[C2,E4,E5,N1] In 1963, Redo and colleagues also reported repair of this entity.[R1]

Taussig-Bing heart was described in 1949, but its place in the spectrum of DORV was not recognized until later.[H3,N2,T1,V1] Many early papers understandably referred to it under the heading *Transposition*.[A9,B5,C4] Lev and colleagues recognized it as a form of DORV with subpulmonary VSD.[L4] They and earlier workers did not clearly state, however, that Taussig-Bing heart is different from the heart with classic DORV with subaortic VSD, not only with respect to relationships of the VSD but also with respect to position and interrelations of great arteries and infundibular (outlet) septum.[A4,A7,W2] Early reports of successful surgical treatment were published in 1967 and 1969.[D1,H2] Other early reports were by Patrick and McGoon in 1968 and by Kawashima and colleagues in 1971.[K3,P3]

The other types of DORV with AV concordant connection began to be clarified in the classic paper by Lev and colleagues in 1972.[L4] Successful correction of unusual forms was reported in the 1970s and early 1980s.[K6,P6,S13]

MORPHOLOGY AND MORPHOGENESIS

Although controversies developed concerning categorization of hearts with DORV and their basic morphologic features, these are now straightforward because of numerous detailed morphologic and clinical studies. The basic categorization of Lev and colleagues forms the basis of most surgical thought about this anomaly, but the terms they used, such as "subaortic" and "subpulmonary," are relational ones.[L4] Confusion arises when their terms are used as morphologic ones for actual location of the VSD (see "Location in Septum and Relationship to Conduction System" under Morphology in Section I of Chapter 35).

Actual categorization of DORV and related conditions (specifically, Taussig-Bing heart, transposition of the great arteries with VSD, and double outlet left ventricle) is less important than a generalized surgical plan for their management.[S1] Even so, development of a valid body of knowledge concerning surgical methods and outcomes requires accurate categorization of morphologic details and other patient characteristics. Even with the goal of accurate morphologic categorization and description, problems remain. Although a *conus* (or *infundibulum*) is easy to define as the presence of muscle between a semilunar and AV valve, the muscle strip may vary from a few millimeters to a few centimeters wide. An aorta that is to the right and side by side with the pulmonary trunk may seem essentially normal in position to one observer or in D-malposition to another. These matters complicate categorization accuracy and precision.

Morphogenesis

Complex categorization points to a unifying hypothesis of morphogenesis put forth in a series of papers by the Van Praaghs, summarized recently by Richard Van Praagh.[V2] He hypothesizes that "the distal or subsemilunar part of the infundibulum or conus arteriosus performs an arterial switch during cardiogenesis," with the development stage similar to the Taussig-Bing heart. The developmental steps that avoid double outlet right ventricle relate to asymmetric conal free wall enlargement. Van Praagh proposes that failure of this morphologic step leads to such entities as double outlet right and left ventricle, various transposition entities, and isolated atrial and ventricular discordant connections.

Ventricular Septal Defect

The VSD is usually large, but in about 10% of cases it is smaller than the aortic root and flow restrictive.[D1,L1,M2,M4,S4] It may be multiple; rarely, it is absent.[A2,M7,S11]

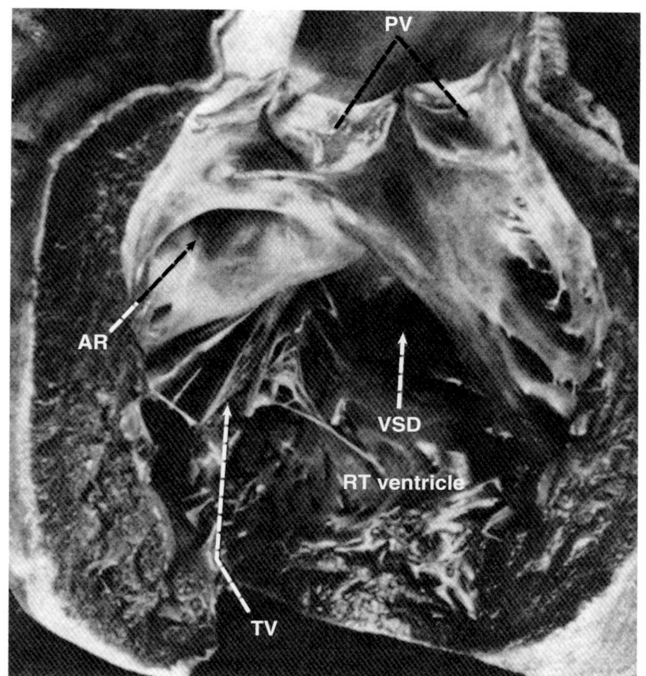

Figure 53-2 Autopsy specimen of simple double outlet right ventricle with subaortic ventricular septal defect *(VSD)*. There is a prominent subaortic conus and a well-developed infundibular septum separating pulmonary valve *(PV)* from aorta, tricuspid valve *(TV)*, and VSD. Key: *AR,* Aortic root (conus); *RT,* right. (From Kirklin and colleagues.[K7])

In most DORV hearts, the VSD is conoventricular, lying between the limbs of the trabecula septomarginalis (TSM; septal band).[C1,T1] However, such defects vary in their relationships with the great arteries. Therefore, the VSD is discussed in *relational categories.*[A5,L4]

Subaortic Ventricular Septal Defect

The subaortic VSD and TSM lie more posteriorly in the ventricular septum than subpulmonary and doubly committed VSDs, and are tucked beneath the infundibular (conal) septum (Fig. 53-2). Distance between the VSD and aortic valve varies, depending on presence and length of the subaortic conus (infundibulum); this determines whether the aorta overrides the VSD and hence whether the VSD is juxtaaortic.

When there is aortic-mitral fibrous continuity, absence of a subaortic conus, and a typical juxtaaortic VSD, the posterosuperior margin of the VSD is formed by the left aortic cusp or base of the anterior mitral leaflet, depending on degree of overriding. The ventriculoinfundibular fold and rightward posterior division of the TSM may form the posterior margin of the VSD. Alternatively, the VSD may reach the tricuspid anulus (opposite the anteroseptal leaflet commissure), resulting in mitral-tricuspid continuity, and the VSD is perimembranous[H4,W2] (see "Perimembranous Ventricular Septal Defect" under Morphology in Section I of Chapter 35). In this event, the rightward posterior division of the trabecula septomarginalis is deficient, and the bundle of His lies along the posteroinferior border of the VSD and is at risk during surgical repair[A4,A5] (Fig. 53-3). Occasionally

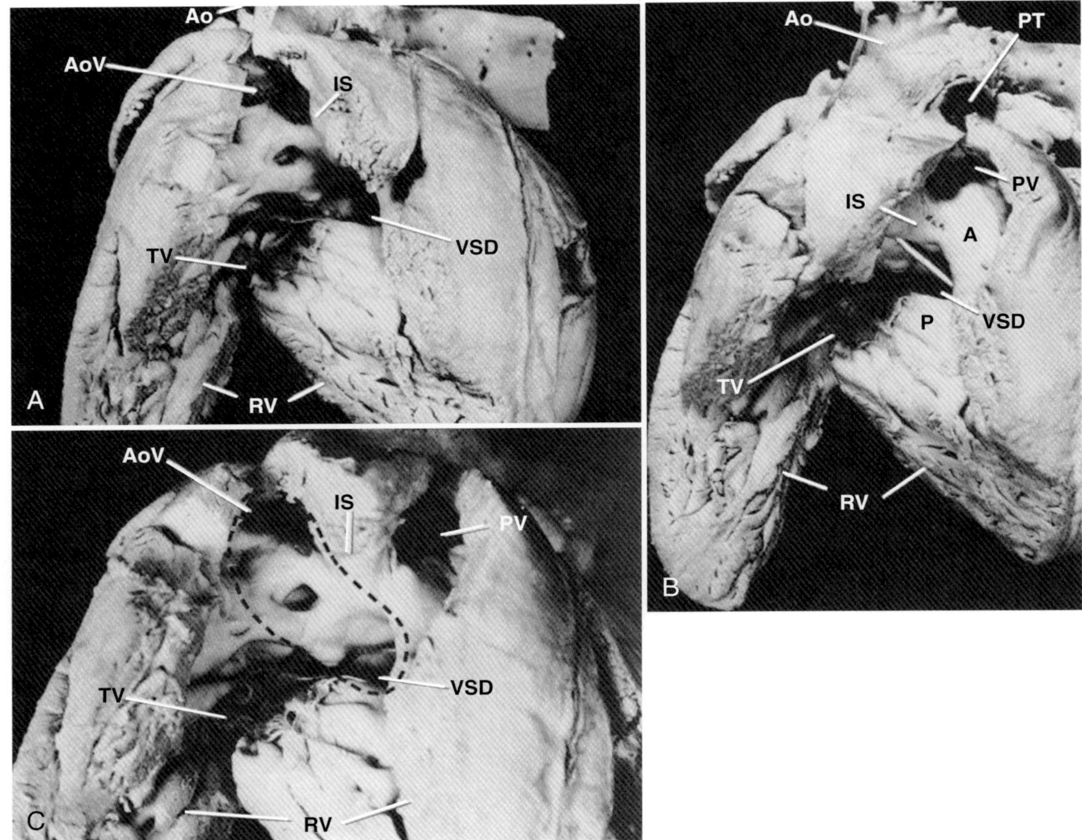

Figure 53-3 Three specimens of double outlet right ventricle with subaortic ventricular septal defect *(VSD)*. Right ventricle *(RV)* has been opened. **A,** Infundibular (conal) septum has been displaced to left to reveal aortic valve *(AoV)* and aorta *(Ao)*. A broad band of subaortic conal muscle separates aortic from tricuspid valve *(TV)*. **B,** Infundibular septum and adjacent portion of anterior wall to which it attaches have been swung to the right to reveal the pulmonary outflow, valve *(PV)*, and trunk *(PT)*. VSD lies between the two limbs of the trabecula septomarginalis (TSM) and reaches the tricuspid anulus inferiorly (probe through VSD passes out the aorta). The infundibular septum inserts behind left anterior division of TSM, and its leftward end contributes to the interventricular septum in front of the VSD. **C,** Close-up view of right ventricular outflow to both great arteries. Posterior and leftward insertions of infundibular (conal) septum are clearly seen. Dashed line shows position of suture line for patch used in an intraventricular tunnel repair. Key: *A,* Left anterior division of septal band; *IS,* infundibular (conal) septum; *P,* right posterior division of trabecula septomarginalis. (From Barratt-Boyes and Calder.[B2])

the VSD may extend farther inferiorly beneath the septal leaflet of the tricuspid valve.[S13] Inferiorly, the VSD is bordered by the trabecula septomarginalis and anteriorly by the infundibular septum.

Chordal attachments of anterior and septal tricuspid leaflets are variable; they may be anomalously attached around the edge of the VSD and seriously interfere with placing of the tunnel patch[B2,S5] (Fig. 53-4).

When DORV is associated with L-malposition of the aorta, the VSD is usually juxtaaortic and thus also subaortic. VSD and TSM, within whose limbs the VSD is cradled, lie more anteriorly and superiorly than when the aorta is to the right.[V3] The TSM and its limbs form inferior and posterior margins of the defect, as does the aortic valve superiorly. The VSD occasionally extends to the tricuspid anulus and is perimembranous.

Subpulmonary Ventricular Septal Defect

Taussig-Bing heart is the typical example of DORV and subpulmonary VSD.[H3,L5,S12,T1,V1] It may be considered a form of DORV in which the VSD is subpulmonary and associated with malalignment of the infundibular septum.

The VSD and TSM lie more superiorly and anteriorly in the ventricular septum, directly beneath the pulmonary conus or valve, than they do in subaortic VSD with right-sided aorta, but in a position similar to that of subaortic VSD with aortic L-malposition. If there is a subpulmonary conus, infundibular (conal) muscle forms the superior margin of the defect. If there is no subpulmonary conus, there is pulmonary-mitral and occasionally pulmonary-tricuspid continuity, and the VSD is juxtapulmonary with the pulmonary valve overriding it (Fig. 53-5). The posterosuperior margin of the VSD is formed by the zone of fibrous continuity or by the pulmonary cusps, depending on degree of pulmonary valve overriding, or by the subpulmonary conus if present. As with subaortic VSD, the defect may extend to the tricuspid anulus posteroinferiorly and be perimembranous (see Fig. 53-5), but often it does not. The infundibular septum is usually sagittally oriented and is then not a part of the interventricular septum.[H2,Y1]

Doubly Committed Ventricular Septal Defect

In doubly committed VSD, an uncommon variant, the VSD and TSM lie more superiorly in the septum than subaortic or

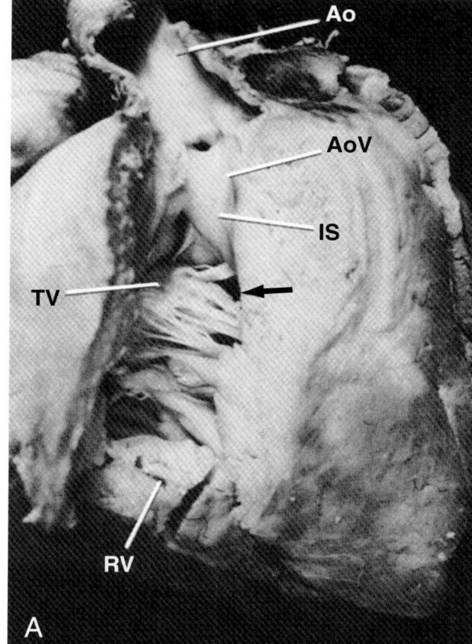

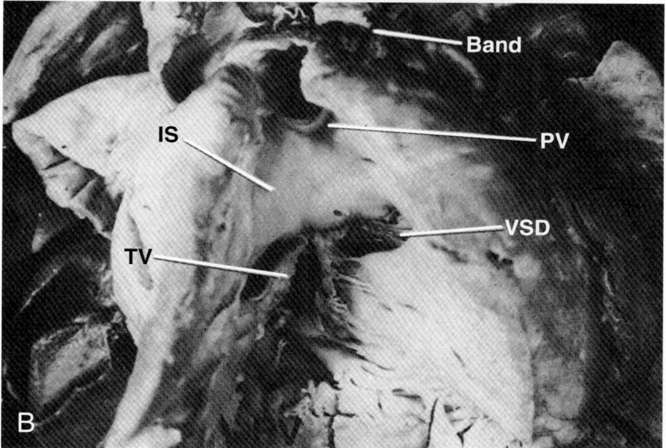

Figure 53-4 Specimen of double outlet right ventricle *(RV)* with bilateral conus and subaortic ventricular septal defect *(VSD)* in a patient with a pulmonary trunk band. **A,** Right ventricular outflow tract has been opened as has aortic valve *(AoV)* and aorta *(Ao)*. VSD *(arrow)* is only just visible, because it is partly overlaid by anomalously attached chordae from the tricuspid valve *(TV)*, which may interfere with placing an intraventricular tunnel patch. **B,** Infundibular (conal) septum *(CS)* displaced to right to reveal pulmonary valve *(PV)* and extensive subpulmonary conus. Infundibular septum inserts posteriorly and is unrelated to interventricular septum. In some respects, this VSD is intermediate between a subaortic and a subpulmonary defect and illustrates the difficulties of accurate and precise categorization. (From Barratt-Boyes and Calder.[B2])

subpulmonary VSDs. This, plus absence (or severe hypoplasia) of the infundibular septum and consequent confluence of the aortic and pulmonary valves, place the defect in a juxtaarterial position.[A4,B2] The semilunar valves are related to posterior and superior boundaries of the defect. Anterior and inferior boundaries are formed by the TSM and its left anterior division; posteroinferior boundaries are formed by the posterior division. This muscle band usually separates the VSD from the tricuspid valve anulus. There is usually no conus, but if present it is very narrow, and there may be aortic-tricuspid and pulmonary-mitral continuity (Fig. 53-6).

The VSD and its relationships resemble those of isolated juxtaarterial VSD (see Chapter 35), tetralogy of Fallot with juxtaarterial VSD (see Chapter 38), and some types of double outlet left ventricle (see Chapter 54). Both semilunar valves usually lie over the RV, but it can be difficult to decide whether this is the case or whether they lie mostly over the LV. At times, they may arise equally over both ventricles, a condition that can be called *double outlet both ventricles*.[B11]

Noncommitted or Remote Ventricular Septal Defect

Trabecular VSDs are not related to the TSM and its divisions, as are VSDs of most hearts with DORV, and they are clearly away from the semilunar valves.[L4] However, an inlet septal VSD (see Morphology in Section I of Chapter 35) may be sufficiently remote from the great arteries as to be considered noncommitted[L11] (Fig. 53-7).

Infundibulum

In general, hearts with DORV may have bilateral conuses, one beneath the aortic valve and one beneath the pulmonary valve, or a single conus beneath either semilunar valve, or no conus. About three fourths of hearts with subaortic VSD have bilateral conuses, and about one fourth have only a subpulmonary conus (Table 53-1). An operative experience, however, may reflect a nonrepresentative prevalence of morphologic features. For example, in 350 patients operated on at Madras Medical Mission, the distribution of conal morphology was weighted far more toward absent conus (86%); prevalence of subaortic VSD was 57% (KM Cherian; personal communication, 2000) (Table 53-2). Hearts with subpulmonary VSD (Taussig-Bing hearts) have either bilateral conus or a single conus beneath the aortic valve, in about equal proportions. Hearts with doubly committed VSDs may have a single common conus beneath the two semilunar valves ("doubly committed"), or there may be fibrous continuity between one of the semilunar valves and one of the AV valves, associated with absence of a conus.

There is a pattern of relations between conus and position of the great arteries[V2] (Table 53-3). As a general rule, presence of conus beneath a semilunar valve tends to result in an anterior position of the valve and great artery. Absence of conus links semilunar valve and artery to the mitral valve with fibrous continuity, resulting in a posterior position of valve and artery. As a result, degree of conal development beneath the aortic and pulmonary valves fairly well predicts position and relationship of the great arteries. This can be inferred from the Madras experience (see Table 53-2), in which there is a high prevalence of normally related great arteries and subaortic or absent conus. Anterior position (D-malposition) of the aorta is uncommon (26%) when there are bilateral conuses, but common (67%) when there is only a subaortic conus. An anterior position has not been observed to occur with only subpulmonary conus or with no conus. An aorta side by side with or posterior to the pulmonary trunk occurs in all conal patterns.

Great Arteries

Both great arteries may lie over the RV in their entirety in the rare instances of DORV with intact ventricular septum and noncommitted VSD. This is often the situation as well when the VSD is subaortic. When the VSD is doubly

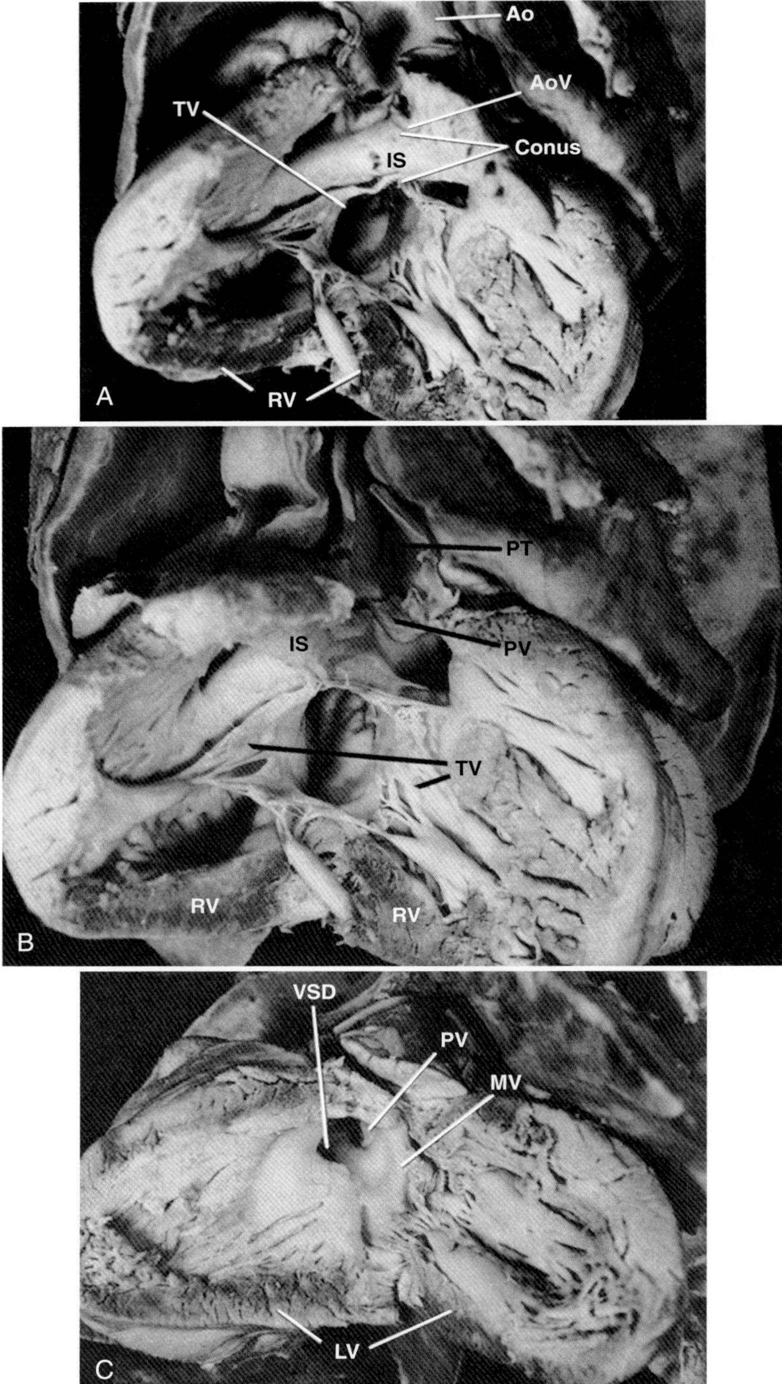

Figure 53-5 Specimen of double outlet right ventricle *(RV)* with subpulmonary ventricular septal defect *(VSD)* (Taussig-Bing heart). **A,** Right ventricular outflow tract, aortic valve *(AoV)*, and aorta *(Ao)* have been opened. The subaortic conus separates aortic from tricuspid valve *(TV)*. Rightward aspect of infundibular (conal) septum is visible. **B,** Infundibular septum and adjacent portion of free wall are displaced toward aorta to reveal opened RV outflow tract, pulmonary valve *(PV)*, and pulmonary trunk *(PT)*. Infundibular septum lies in a sagittal plane and has no attachment to the ventricular septum; moreover, it separates VSD from aortic valve. VSD lies directly above trabecula septomarginalis (TSM), but because the rightward posterior division of the TSM is deficient, it reaches the tricuspid anulus and is perimembranous. PV overrides VSD onto left ventricle *(LV)*. There is no subpulmonary conus. Aorta is to the right and slightly anterior to pulmonary trunk. **C,** View from opened LV. Overriding PV is in direct fibrous continuity with anterior leaflet of mitral valve (MV). (From Barratt-Boyes and Calder.[B2])

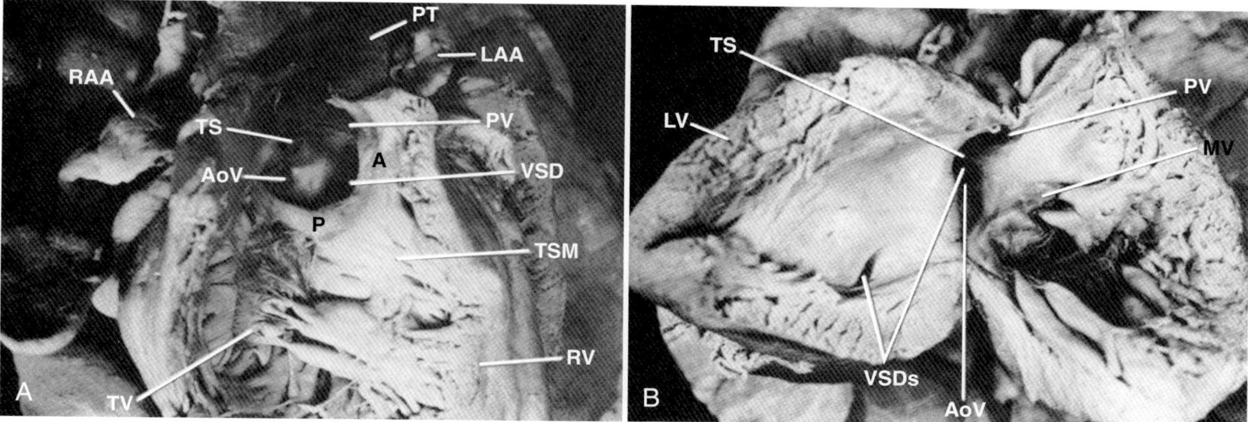

Figure 53-6 Specimen of double outlet right ventricle *(RV)* with doubly committed ventricular septal defect *(VSD)*. **A,** Right ventricular outflow tract. Both great arteries override ventricular septum. Aortic *(AoV)* and pulmonary valves *(PV)* are in fibrous continuity because there is no infundibular (conal) septum. Aortic valve lies rightward and posterior to pulmonary valve, making a tunnel repair possible. VSD lies between the two divisions of the trabecula septomarginalis *(TSM)*. Persistence of the right posterior division of the septal band prevents aortic–tricuspid valve *(TV)* continuity. **B,** View from opened left ventricle *(LV)*. Pulmonary and aortic valves are in tenuous fibrous continuity with the mitral valve *(MV)* because there is no conus. There is an additional slitlike VSD in the sinus septum. Key: *A,* Left anterior division of trabecula septomarginalis; *LAA,* left atrial appendage; *P,* right posterior division of septal band; *PT,* pulmonary trunk; *RAA,* right atrial appendage. (From Brandt and colleagues.[B11])

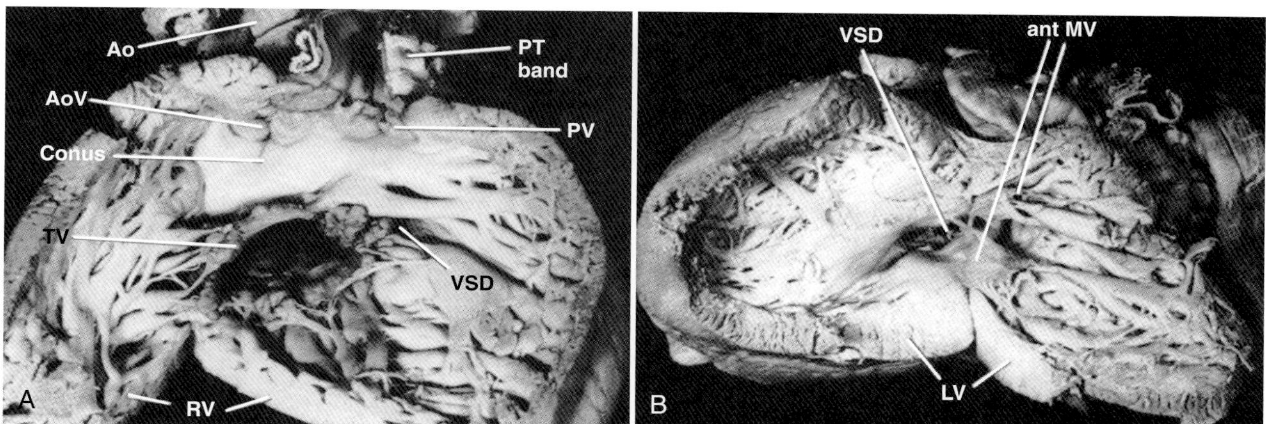

Figure 53-7 Specimen of double outlet right ventricle *(RV)* with noncommitted ventricular septal defect *(VSD)*. **A,** Right ventricular outflow tract, opened through pulmonary valve *(PV)* and banded pulmonary trunk *(PT)* and aortic valve *(AoV)*. A well-developed subsemilunar conus separates aortic and pulmonary valves from tricuspid valve *(TV)* and VSD, which is partly obscured by tricuspid valve. Aortic and pulmonary valves are joined (i.e., infundibular [conal] septum is absent). Aorta *(Ao)* and pulmonary trunk *(PT)* lie side by side, with their valves at the same level. **B,** View from opened left ventricle *(LV)*. The only exit is via the VSD (which is of inlet septal type) through which tricuspid valve tissue can be seen. Anterior mitral valve leaflet is cleft. Key: *ant MV,* Anterior mitral leaflet. (From Barratt-Boyes and Calder.[B2])

committed or subpulmonary, there is usually a variable degree of overriding of one or both great arteries over the VSD.

Positional interrelationships of the great arteries are variable in hearts with DORV. Interrelationships are normal or near-normal in most patients with DORV, with the aorta located rightward and posterior relative to the pulmonary trunk[A4,H4,P6] (Table 53-4). Less often, the great arteries are side by side, with the aorta to the right. D-malposition may be present in hearts with DORV, with the aorta anterior and to the right of the pulmonary trunk or at times directly anterior. Rarely, it is anterior and to the left. Occasionally there is L-malposition, with aorta to the left but side by side with the pulmonary trunk.

Although in 77% of hearts with subaortic VSD the aorta is to the right and either side by side or posterior to the pulmonary trunk (more or less normally related), it is anterior (D-malposition) in 23% of cases (see Table 53-4). Furthermore, more or less normally related great arteries are not unique to hearts with subaortic VSD; those with subpulmonary VSD have normally related great arteries in similar frequency (P for difference = .8).

Only in hearts with noncommitted VSD is the frequency of more or less normally related great arteries less (33%) (P for difference = .06; see Table 53-4). Although *D-malposition of the aorta* may be considered characteristic of ordinary transposition (see "Great Arteries" under Morphology in Chapter 52) and by implication Taussig-Bing heart, hearts with DORV and subpulmonary VSD are associated with typical D-malposition in a minority of cases (see Table 53-4).

Table 53-1 Relationship of Ventricular Septal Defect and Conus Pattern in Double Outlet Right Ventricle[a]

		Type of Conus											
		Bilateral			Subpulmonary Only			Subaortic Only			Absent		
Relationship of VSD	*n*	No.	% of *n*	CL (%)	No.	% of *n*	CL (%)	No.	% of *n*	CL (%)	No.	% of *n*	CL (%)
Subaortic	22	17	77	64-87	5	23	13-36	0	0	0-8	0	0	0-8
			(63	51-74)		(100	68-100)		(0	0-19)		(0	0-85)
Subpulmonary	11	5	45	27-65	0	0	0-16	6	55	35-73	0	0	0-16
			(19	11-29)		(0	0-32)		(67	44-85)		(0	0-85)
Doubly committed	3	2	67	24-96	0	0	0-47	0	0	0-47	1	33	4-76
			(7	2-17)		(0	0-32)		(0	0-19)		(100	15-100)
Noncommitted	6	3	50	24-76	0	0	0-27	3	50	24-76	0	0	0-27
			(11	5-21)		(0	0-32)		(33	15-56)		(0	15-100)
TOTAL	42	27	64	55-73	5	12	7-19	9	21	15-30	1	2	0.3-8
$P(\chi^2)$[b]			.3			.16			.0007				

Note: In parentheses are percentages and confidence limits of various VSD locations within each type of conus.
[a]Data based on study at GLH of 42 autopsy specimens. Specimens with atrial isomerism or L-malposition of the aorta are excluded.
[b]*P* values along bottom of table refer to difference in prevalence of type of conus within the various relationships of the VSD.
Key: *CL,* 70% confidence limits; *VSD,* ventricular septal defect.

Table 53-2 Cardiac Morphology of 350 Patients with Double Outlet Right Ventricle[a]

VSD Position	No.	%	Conus	No.	%	Position of Aorta in Relation to Pulmonary Trunk	No.	%
Subaortic	199	57	Subaortic	32	9.1	Normal	232	66
Subpulmonary	37	11	Subpulmonary	6	1.7	D-Malposed	51	15
Doubly committed	21	6	Bilateral	10	2.9	L-Malposed	29	8.3
Noncommitted	93	27	Noconus	302	87	Anteroposterior	38	11

[a]Data from study of 350 patients with double outlet right ventricle operated on at the Institute for Cardiovascular Disease, Madras Medical Mission, 1989-2000. (Cherian KM; personal communication, 2000.)
Key: *VSD,* Ventricular septal defect.

Table 53-3 Type of Conus and Position of Great Arteries in Double Outlet Right Ventricle[a]

		Aortic Position Relative to Pulmonary Trunk						
		Side by Side or Posterior[b]			Anterior[c]			
Type of Conus	*n*	No.	% of *n*	CL	No.	% of *n*	CL	*P*[d]
Bilateral	27	20	74	63-83	7	26	17-37	
			(69	58-79)		(54	36-71)	.3
Subpulmonary only	5	5	100	68-100	0	0	0-32	
			(17	10-28)		(0	0-14)	.14
Subaortic only	9	3	33	15-56	6	67	44-85	
			(10	5-20)		(46	29-64)	.009
Absent	1	1	100	15-85	0	0	0-85)	
			(3	0.4-11)		(0	0-14)	.7
TOTAL	42	29	69	60-77	13	31	23-40	
$P(\chi^2)$			.04			.4		

[a]Data and presentation are as described for Table 53-1.
[b]*Side by side* or *posterior* refers to aorta being to the right and beside or slightly posterior to pulmonary trunk, with the great arteries more or less normally interrelated.
[c]*Anterior* refers to D-malposition, with aorta anterior and more or less to the right.
[d]*P-value column* refers to difference in occurrence of the given VSD position in the two great artery positions.
Key: *CL,* 70% confidence limits.

Table 53-4 Relationship of Ventricular Septal Defect and Position of Great Arteries in Double Outlet Right Ventricle[a]

		Aortic Position Relative to Pulmonary Trunk						
		Side by Side or Posterior[b]			Anterior[c]			
Relationship of VSD	***n***	**No.**	**% of *n***	**CL (%)**	**No.**	**% of *n***	**CL (%)**	***P***
Subaortic	22	17	77	64-87	5	23	13-36	$P = .8^d$
			(59	47-69)		(38	23-57)	.2
Subpulmonary	11	8	73	53-88	3	27	12-47	
			(28	18-39)		(23	10-41)	.8
Doubly committed	3	2	67	24-96	1	33	4-76	
			(7	2-16)		(8	1-24)	.7
Noncommitted	6	2	33	12-62	4	67	38-88	
			(7	2-16)		(31	16-49)	.06
TOTAL	42	29	69	60-77	13	31	23-40	

[a]Data and presentation are as described for Table 53-1.
[b]*Side by side* or *posterior* refers to aorta being to the right and beside or slightly posterior to pulmonary trunk, with the great arteries more or less normally interrelated.
[c]*Anterior* refers to D-malposition, with aorta anterior and more or less to the right.
[d]Refers to difference in occurrence of subaortic and subpulmonic VSDs in DORV with anteriorly placed aorta.
Key: *CL,* 70% confidence limits; *VSD,* ventricular septal defect percent of 42.

Hearts with doubly committed VSD tend to have more or less normally related great arteries. Observing great artery position at cineangiography or operation does not permit a reasonably accurate inference as to the position and category of the VSD (see Table 53-4). There is no greater certainty that the VSD is subaortic when the great arteries are more or less normally interrelated than when in D-malposition ($P = .2$). When the aorta is in D-malposition, there is no greater certainty that the VSD will be subpulmonary than subaortic ($P = .8$).

Pulmonary Stenosis

Pulmonary stenosis is common in hearts with a subaortic VSD. It is most often infundibular (Fig. 53-8), but it may be valvar, with or without a small pulmonary valve ring. Thus, all types of pulmonary stenosis observed in hearts with tetralogy of Fallot may be seen in DORV. Rarely, infundibular stenosis may be of the isolated low-lying variety, producing a two-chambered RV.[J2,M4]

Pulmonary stenosis is also common in hearts with doubly committed VSD (five of five in the GLH experience). It is uncommon in association with Taussig-Bing heart and in hearts with a noncommitted VSD.[L4,L9]

Conduction System

The AV node is in its normal position in the AV septum, and the bundle of His penetrates the right fibrous trigone in the usual way. Thus, the course of the bundle of His relative to the VSD is the same as in primary VSD and in tetralogy of Fallot (see Chapters 35 and 38). The bundle is at risk of damage during repair when the defect reaches the tricuspid anulus (and becomes perimembranous). This is true whether the defect is subaortic or subpulmonary and whether the ascending aorta is right or left sided.[A5,B8,L8] However, as in other conditions with clockwise rotation and dextroposition of the aorta, the bundle is more on the LV side of the septum than usual.[B8] Furthermore, the trigone is often attenuated in DORV when there is a subaortic conus, which removes the aortic anulus from the central fibrous skeleton of the heart.

When a complete AV septal defect coexists, the node and bundle course are altered accordingly (see "Conduction System" under Morphology in Chapter 34).

Coronary Arteries

Coronary artery pattern depends on position of the great arteries. In most varieties of DORV, it is similar to normal except that the aortic sinuses are rotated in a clockwise direction (viewed from below), such that the right coronary arises anteriorly and the left coronary posteriorly.[E3] When the aorta is anterior and rightward, the pattern is usually similar to that in transposition of the great arteries (see "Coronary Arteries" under Morphology in Chapter 52), with the right coronary artery arising from sinus 2 (right posterior facing sinus).[L3,U2] In 15% of cases, a single coronary ostium may arise either anteriorly or posteriorly that supplies left and right sides of the heart.[G2,W2] The branching pattern is also usually normal, except for occasional origin of the left anterior descending from the right coronary artery, with this vessel crossing the RV outflow from right to left as in tetralogy of Fallot (see Chapter 38). This anomaly was found in 25% of the DORV hearts reported in the early Mayo Clinic series, but it was not encountered in 42 GLH autopsy cases.[G2]

When the aorta is to the left in L-malposition, the right coronary artery passes to the right from the anterior sinus of the leftward anterior aorta to reach the AV groove in front of the pulmonary trunk. Its position prohibits extensive anterior patching across the pulmonary "anulus."

Associated Anomalies

Major associated cardiac anomalies, in addition to pulmonary stenosis of the tetralogy of Fallot type, may coexist. Coarctation of the aorta may be present, particularly in Taussig-Bing

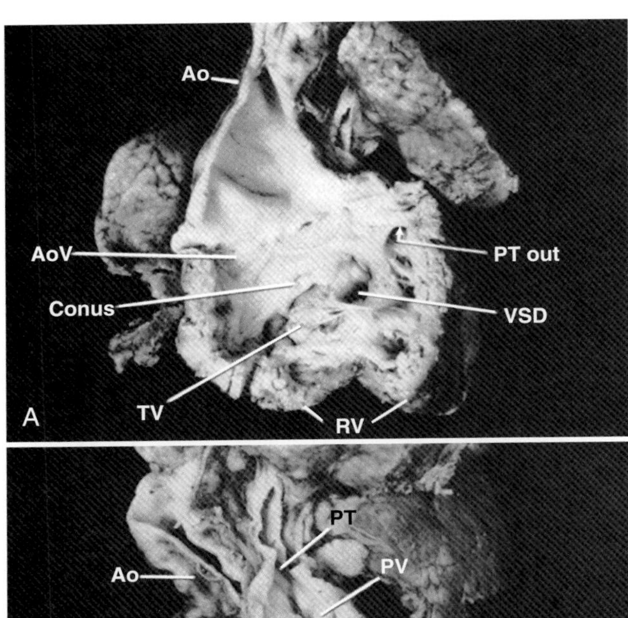

Figure 53-8 Specimen of double outlet right ventricle *(RV)* with subaortic ventricular septal defect *(VSD)* and infundibular pulmonary stenosis. **A,** Right ventricular outflow tract is opened to aortic valve *(AoV)* and aorta *(Ao)*. A subaortic conus separates aortic and tricuspid valves *(TV)*. Poorly expanded subpulmonary conus narrows outflow tract. **B,** Infundibular (conal) septum is displaced to reveal opened pulmonary outflow tract. Pulmonary valve *(PV)* is bicuspid, and it and the pulmonary trunk *(PT)* are smaller than normal. Aorta is slightly anterior to pulmonary trunk. A probe passes through VSD and into aorta. Key: *PT out,* Pulmonary outflow. (From Barratt-Boyes and Calder.[B2])

variant, and may require repair in the neonatal period; rarely, discrete subvalvar aortic stenosis may coexist.[G1,S9] Various other cardiac anomalies coexist in about 30% of patients coming to intracardiac repair of DORV with a subaortic or doubly committed VSD[P6] (Tables 53-5 and 53-6).

Table 53-5 Associated Cardiac Anomalies (Exclusive of Pulmonary Stenosis and Atrioventricular Septal Defect) in Patients Undergoing Surgical Correction of Double Outlet Right Ventricle with Subaortic or Doubly Committed Ventricular Septal Defect[a]

Associated Cardiac Anomalies	No.	Percentage of Total ($n = 70$)
Multiple VSDs	9	13
Patent ductus arteriosus	8	11
Pulmonary artery distribution deficiencies or post-shunt stenoses	9	13
Pulmonary atresia	2	3
LV hypoplasia + MV hypoplasia or regurgitation	2	3
Congenital mitral stenosis	1	1.4
Subaortic stenosis	2	3
Tricuspid regurgitation (severe)	2	3
Unroofed coronary sinus syndrome	3	4
Azygos continuation of IVC	1	1.4
Right aortic arch	1	1.4
Aberrant right subclavian artery	1	1.4
Origin of right coronary from left coronary artery	1	1.4
Juxtaposed atrial appendages	1	1.4
Situs inversus totalis (Van Praagh S,L,L)	2	3
No associated anomalies	41	59

[a]Data combine the experience at UAB (1967-1982; $n = 42$) and GLH (1958-1984; $n = 28$). Because some patients had multiple anomalies, total is not cumulative, nor is list mutually exclusive.
Key: *IVC,* Inferior vena cava; *LV,* left ventricular; *MV,* mitral valve; *VSD,* ventricular septal defect.

Morphologic Syndromes of Double Outlet Right Ventricle

Simple Double Outlet Right Ventricle

The phrase *simple DORV* connotes the commonly occurring and easily repaired type of DORV in which the VSD is subaortic and the aorta is to the right, usually by the side of the pulmonary trunk or slightly posterior to it, or which in about 20% of cases is somewhat anterior to the pulmonary trunk (see Table 53-4). The aorta may spiral around the pulmonary trunk as it leaves the heart, or the great arteries may course parallel to each other.[A4] Usually there is a conus (infundibulum) beneath both the aorta and pulmonary valve, but in some cases there may be no subaortic conus (see Table 53-1). Coronary arterial anatomy is normal.

In borderline cases, this type of DORV merges with the type in which a perimembranous VSD demonstrates inlet extension and appears to be noncommitted and, on the other hand, the type in which the VSD demonstrates outlet extension and appears to be doubly committed.

Taussig-Bing Heart

In the most representative cases, the Taussig-Bing heart is similar from heart to heart. The VSD is anterior and superior and subpulmonary. The left main coronary artery is anterior to the pulmonary trunk. The pulmonary trunk arises biventricularly over the VSD, and the aorta is to the right and slightly anterior to or alongside it (see Table 53-4). The first portions of aorta and pulmonary trunk are parallel rather than tending to spiral as do normally positioned great arteries.[A4,A7,D4] The infundibular septum is in the sagittal plane and is not part of the interventricular septum. Lev and colleagues were able to use specific morphologic features within the RV as the hallmark of Taussig-Bing heart, but this is rarely possible clinically or surgically.[L5]

Subaortic stenosis, from narrowing of the subaortic infundibulum, may develop in Taussig-Bing heart.[Y1] Pulmonary stenosis is uncommon.[L9] The mitral valve may straddle across the subpulmonary VSD, and in such cases the LV may be hypoplastic.[K9,M10] Associated coarctation of the aorta is

Table 53-6 Associated Cardiac Anomalies in Patients with Varieties of Double Outlet Right Ventricle Other Than Those with Subaortic or Doubly Committed Ventricular Septal Defects[a]

Associated Cardiac Anomalies	*n*	Percentage of Total (*n* = 15)	Hospital Deaths
Hypoplasia of LV and MV	1	7	1
Congenital mitral stenosis	1	7	1
Two-storied heart	2	13	1
Dextrocardia	2	13	0
Juxtaposed atrial appendages	3	20	1
LSVC to CS	3	20	1
Coarctation of aorta	1	7	0
MV override or straddling	1	7	1
TV override or straddling	1	7	0
Hypoplastic RV and TV	1	7	0
AV discordant connection (Van Praagh S,L,L)	3	20	0
Multiple VSDs	2	13	2
ASD (moderate or large)	6	40	2
No associated anomalies (apart from PS or small ASD)	5	33	1

[a]Data from experience with surgical correction at GLH (1964-1984; *n* = 15). Because most patients had multiple anomalies, total is not cumulative, nor is list mutually exclusive.
Key: *ASD*, Atrial septal defect; *AV*, atrioventricular; *CS*, coronary sinus; *LSVC*, left superior vena cava; *LV*, left ventricle; *MV*, mitral valve; *PS*, pulmonary stenosis; *RV*, right ventricle; *TV*, tricuspid valve; *VSD*, ventricular septal defect.

common (about 50% of cases).[N2,P2,S9,Y1] This contrasts with the 6% prevalence in transposition with VSD.[P2]

In borderline cases, this type of DORV merges with transposition of the great arteries and large VSD and, on the other hand, may merge with DORV and noncommitted VSD of the trabecular type.

Double Outlet Right Ventricle with Doubly Committed Ventricular Septal Defect
In DORV with doubly committed VSD, an uncommon syndrome, the VSD is immediately beneath both aorta and pulmonary trunk and is juxta-arterial.

Double Outlet Right Ventricle with Noncommitted Ventricular Septal Defect
When the VSD is in the trabecular septum and clearly far removed from the great arteries, the anomaly is easily categorized into this subset. When the VSD is in the inlet septum and up against the tricuspid valve, categorization as DORV with noncommitted VSD can be questioned, but at least the defect is further removed from the aorta than in most hearts with DORV and subaortic VSD.

Double Outlet Right Ventricle with L-Malposition
DORV with L-malposition usually has a subaortic VSD (rarely extending back to the tricuspid anulus) and pulmonary stenosis and presents a rare but distinctive clinical and surgical syndrome.[D2,L7,L8,P4,V3] Rarely the VSD may be perimembranous and extend up toward the pulmonary valve, or it may be truly subpulmonary.[S6,W1,Y2] The VSD may, contrariwise, extend into the inlet septum and be noncommitted.[A6] Mehrizi has reported DORV with L-malposition and doubly committed VSD.[M8]

Double Outlet Right Ventricle with Complete Atrioventricular Septal Defect
In cases of DORV with complete AV septal defect, the interventricular communication is large and usually extends deeply beneath a bridging left superior leaflet (see "Atrioventricular Valves" under Morphology in Chapter 34) to be subaortic in position.[S10] Occasionally, however, the interventricular communication does not extend in this manner and is noncommitted.[B7]

Double Outlet Right Ventricle with Superior-Inferior Ventricles
In most hearts with this ventricular position, there is a ventricular L-loop, atrial situs solitus, and AV discordant connection (see Chapter 55). Uncommonly, in DORV with atrial situs solitus, AV concordant connection, and D-ventricular loop, there is a positional anomaly termed *superior-inferior ventricles* *(over-and-under ventricles, upstairs-downstairs ventricles)* (see "Cardiac and Arterial Positions" under Terminology and Classification of Heart Disease in Chapter 1). The RV is superior (and sometimes a little posterior) and the LV inferior. There may be D- or L-malposition of the aorta. The VSD is usually perimembranous and in the inlet portion of the septum. The right AV valve is usually more superiorly placed than usual relative to the left AV valve, and either AV valve may straddle the VSD (see "Ventricular Septal Defect with Straddling or Overriding Tricuspid Valve" under Morphology in Chapter 35). Severe LV hypoplasia may be present, and pulmonary stenosis is common.

CLINICAL FEATURES AND DIAGNOSTIC CRITERIA

Pathophysiology

Clinical features of patients with this morphologically highly variable anomaly are necessarily also highly variable. In general, patients with a large VSD and no pulmonary stenosis or severe pulmonary vascular disease are not clinically cyanotic. This is because pulmonary blood flow ($\dot{Q}p$) is high and the resultant mixture of blood in the RV has a high enough oxygen saturation to prevent clinically evident cyanosis; however, there is some arterial desaturation.

Streaming of Blood Flow
SaO_2 is also affected by streaming of blood within the RV, which is determined by the relationship of the semilunar valves to the VSD and the position and presence of the infundibular septum.[N2,S11] Thus, in simple DORV, flow of highly oxygen-saturated LV blood through the VSD is directed preferentially beneath the infundibular septum into the adjacent aorta (particularly when the subaortic conus is short or absent), whereas systemic venous blood passes largely out of the pulmonary trunk. As a result, patients with this arrangement present in infancy with high $\dot{Q}p$ in heart failure without cyanosis and cannot be clinically distinguished from infants with a large VSD (see Clinical Features and Diagnostic Criteria in Section I of Chapter 35).

When the VSD is subpulmonary, as in Taussig-Bing heart, flow through it of highly saturated LV blood is directed into the adjacent pulmonary trunk by the vertically positioned infundibular septum. $SpaO_2$ is then higher than SaO_2, with systemic venous blood from the RV tending to flow more into the aorta.[W1] This situation is aggravated when there is overriding of the pulmonary trunk onto the LV. Thus, these infants present in a fashion similar to patients with transposition of the great arteries with large VSD in heart failure with mild cyanosis (see "Large Ventricular Septal Defect, Large Patent Ductus Arteriosus, or Both [Good Mixing]" under Morphology in Chapter 52).

Pulmonary Vascular Disease

Pulmonary vascular disease may be more rapid in onset in patients with DORV without pulmonary stenosis than in patients with simple large VSD, particularly in Taussig-Bing heart (see "Pulmonary Vascular Disease" under Natural History in Section I of Chapter 35).[S13] The resultant reduction in $\dot{Q}p$ has a more marked influence on SaO_2 than in simple VSD, because it reduces the amount of highly saturated blood in a common mixing chamber.

Pulmonary Stenosis

When important pulmonary stenosis is present, cyanosis becomes severe, and the clinical features and presentation are similar to those of patients with tetralogy of Fallot (see Chapter 38).

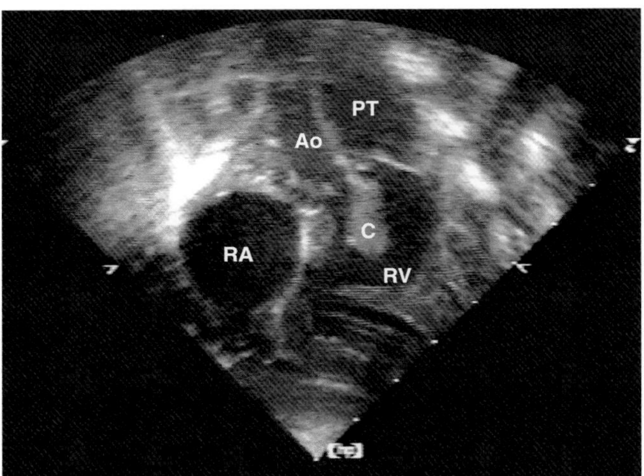

Figure 53-9 Echocardiogram (subxiphoid view) in double outlet right ventricle *(RV)* of the Taussig-Bing type. There is side-by-side relation of the great arteries such that the vessel closest to the left ventricle is the pulmonary trunk *(PT)*. The VSD is subpulmonary. There is a prominent subarterial conus *(C)*. The aorta *(Ao)* is smaller than the pulmonary trunk, suggesting an aortic arch abnormality. Key: *RA,* Right atrium.

Examination

On physical examination, no clinical signs distinguish patients with DORV with and without pulmonary stenosis from the conditions that they mimic. The electrocardiogram (ECG) is not diagnostic, nor is the chest radiograph. However, in those uncommon instances in which there is L-malposition of the aorta, the aorta may be evident on the posteroanterior chest radiograph as it ascends vertically from the cardiac silhouette in the left upper mediastinum[L8,V3]; this finding is not specific, however (see Clinical Features and Diagnostic Criteria in Chapter 57).

Echocardiography

Two-dimensional echocardiography provides a considerable amount of information regarding size of the VSD, relationship of the VSD to the semilunar valves, presence of subvalvar conus, and AV valve abnormalities.[H1,S2,S11] Position of the great arteries and conus are usually apparent[M1] (Fig. 53-9). The coronary arterial anatomy can also generally be defined accurately in neonates and infants by echocardiography alone.

Cardiac Catheterization and Cineangiography

Because echocardiographic assessment of morphology is reliable, cardiac catheterization before surgical intervention is not routinely required in neonates and young infants. In older infants and children, it may be needed to assess hemodynamics such as pulmonary vascular resistance and ventricular end-diastolic pressure, and to define extracardiac morphology such as the peripheral pulmonary vasculature and presence of aortopulmonary collateral vessels. Cineangiography can be used when necessary to define intracardiac morphology (Fig. 53-10). The whole of the ventricular septum must be profiled so that its upper part can be projected cranially. In this way, great vessel positions can be assessed relative to the two ventricles, and location of the VSDs determined.[B1,B2] VSD size can be judged (Fig. 53-11) and subsets such as Taussig-Bing heart identified (Fig. 53-12). Cineangiography is of particular value in assessing the complex interrelationships present in DORV with superior-inferior ventricles and criss-cross hearts.[B12]

NATURAL HISTORY

The natural history of patients with DORV and AV concordant connection is highly variable, but some general trends can be identified.

The natural history of simple DORV is similar to that of simple large VSD (see Natural History in Section I of Chapter 35); this is probably also true for patients with DORV whose VSD is doubly committed or noncommitted. The exception is that spontaneous VSD closure, which is fatal rather than curative, is rare in DORV.[M3]

When the VSD is subpulmonary, as in Taussig-Bing heart, the natural history is similar to that for transposition and large VSD, but it is even more unfavorable (see "Ventricular Septal Defects" under Natural History in Chapter 52). This is in part because severe pulmonary vascular disease occurs early in life. Poor prognosis for these patients may also be related to frequent occurrence of left-sided cardiac and extracardiac malformations such as coarctation of the aorta and LV and mitral valve hypoplasia (see "Coarctation as Part of Hypoplastic Left Heart Physiology" under Morphology in Section I of Chapter 48).

When pulmonary stenosis or atresia is present in DORV with subaortic VSD, and probably in those with doubly committed or noncommitted VSD as well, the natural history is indistinguishable from that of patients with tetralogy of Fallot and pulmonary stenosis or atresia (see Chapter 38).

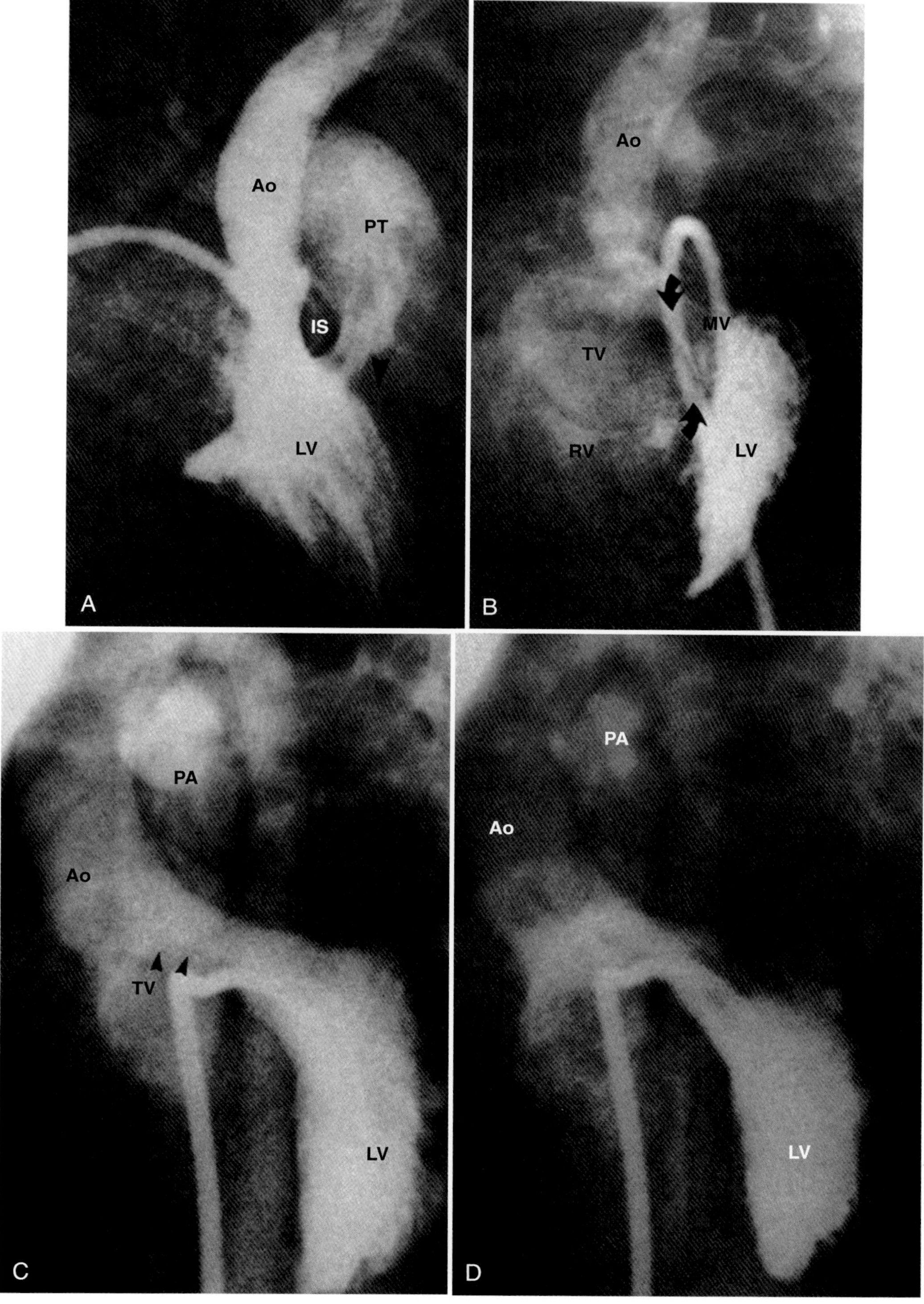

Figure 53-10 Cineangiograms of simple double outlet right ventricle (DORV) with conoventricular ventricular septal defect (VSD). **A,** Left ventriculogram in elongated right anterior oblique view. Infundibular septum is well shown. **B,** Four-chambered view. VSD is also perimembranous and abuts tricuspid valve *(TV)*. **C,** Left ventriculogram in four-chamber view of another patient in whom VSD is separated from the tricuspid valve *(arrowheads)* by a bar of muscle. **D,** This is from the same cineangiogram a few frames later.

Continued

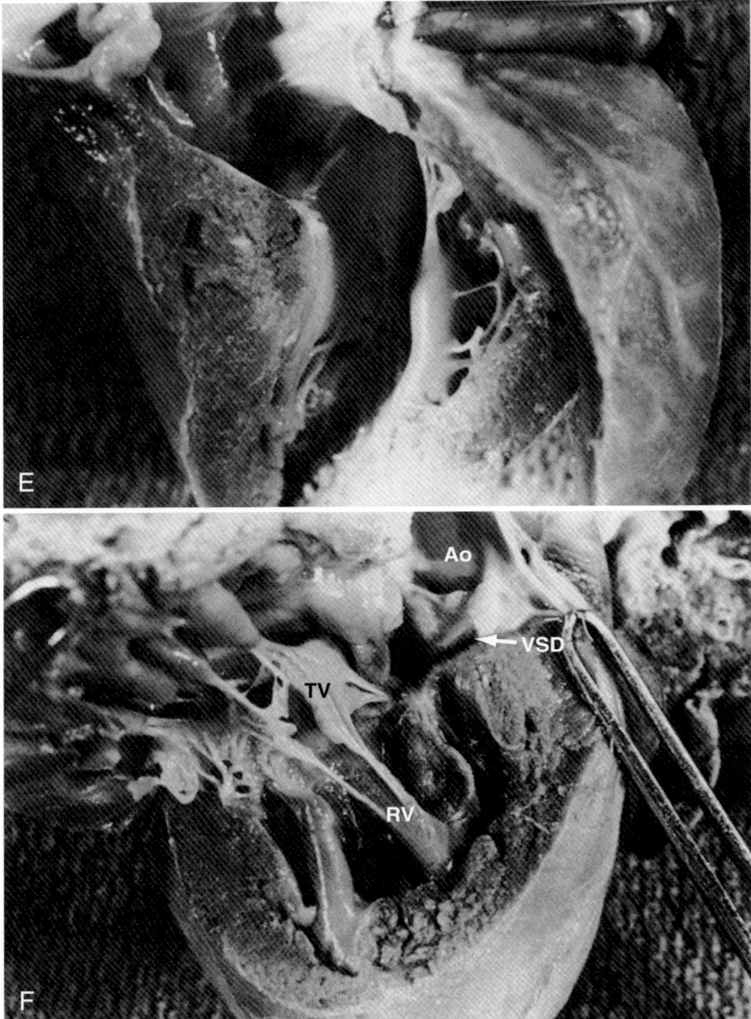

Figure 53-10, cont'd **E,** Specimen illustrating DORV of a type similar to that shown in **C** and **D**, viewed from left ventricular aspect. **F,** Same specimen viewed from right ventricular aspect. Note rim of muscle between VSD and tricuspid valve, such that the VSD is conoventricular but not perimembranous. Key: *Ao,* Aorta; *IS,* infundibular (conal) septum; *LV,* left ventricular; *MV,* mitral valve; *PT,* pulmonary trunk; *RV,* right ventricle.

The natural history in some patients is dominated by an associated cardiac anomaly, such as a complete AV septal defect (see Natural History in Chapter 34).

TECHNIQUE OF OPERATION

The type of operation selected depends in part on position of the VSD, relationship of the great arteries, size of the patient, and adequacy of the resulting ventricles and their respective outflows after closing or baffling the VSD. In general:

- Subaortic VSD with an adequate tricuspid to pulmonary valve distance is treated by simple intraventricular baffling that directs LV blood through the VSD to the aorta (intraventricular tunnel repair).
- Subpulmonary VSD, as in Taussig-Bing heart, without pulmonary stenosis is treated with an arterial switch procedure with simple VSD closure that directs blood from the LV to the neoaortic valve.
- Blood flow in doubly committed VSDs is usually baffled using a more complex patch from LV to aorta.
- Noncommitted VSD may be treated by baffling of blood through the VSD to the aorta, accompanied by myocardial flap reinsertion of the straddling tricuspid valve or by a Fontan type of procedure.

Various surgical procedures are described, but description does not imply recommendations. Indications are described later in this chapter under Indications for Operation. Only the general methods are described here, and each patient may be sufficiently unique to require an individual approach.

Intraventricular Tunnel Repair of Simple Double Outlet Right Ventricle

Preparation for operation, draping, arrangement for cardiopulmonary bypass (CPB), median sternotomy, and placing stay sutures and sutures for cannulation are as usual (see Section III in Chapter 2). The pericardium is cleared in case

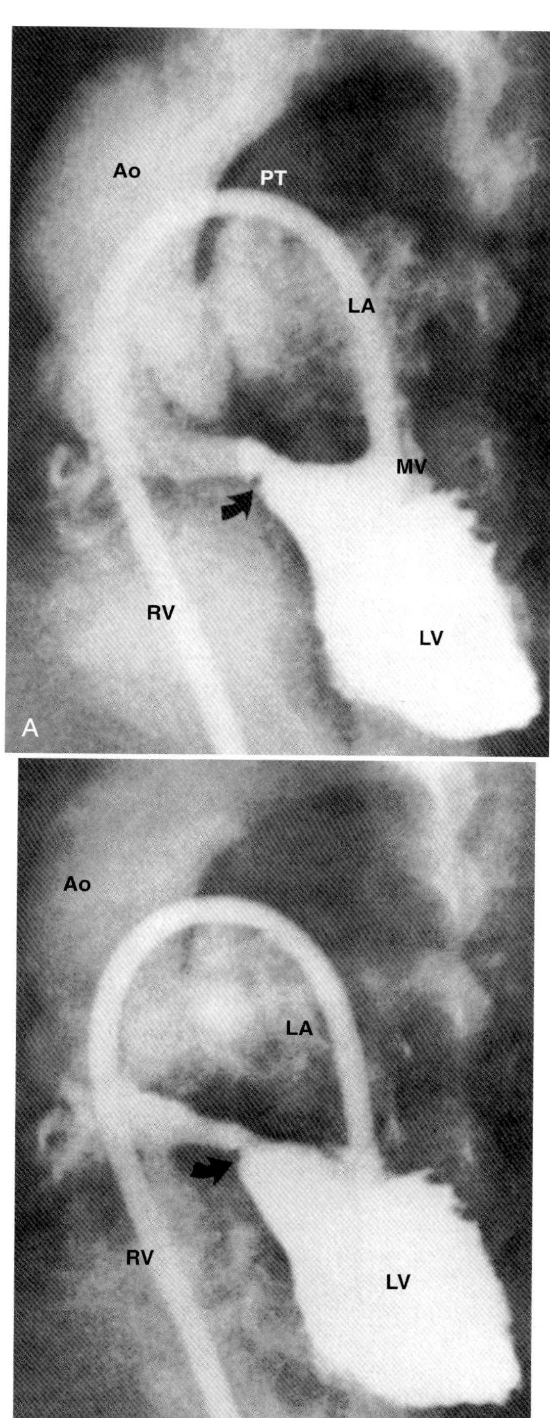

Figure 53-11 Cineangiogram of simple double outlet right ventricle with restrictive subaortic ventricular septal defect (VSD). Early phase **(A)** and late phase **(B)** of cineangiogram made in long axial projection after injection of contrast into left ventricle. Key: *Ao,* Aorta; *LA,* left atrium; *LV,* left ventricle; *MV,* mitral valve; *PT,* pulmonary trunk; *RV,* right ventricle.

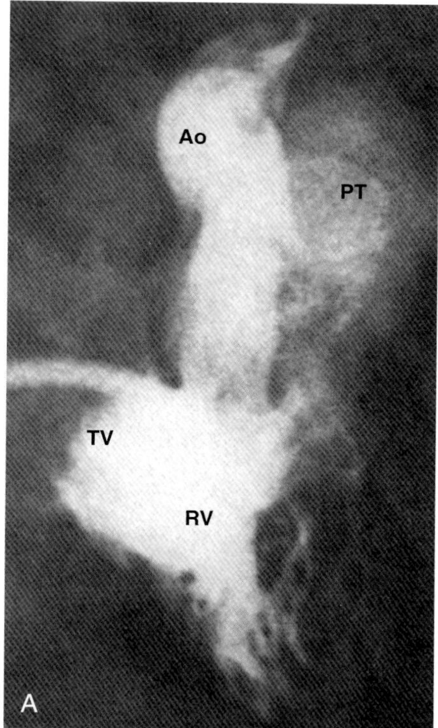

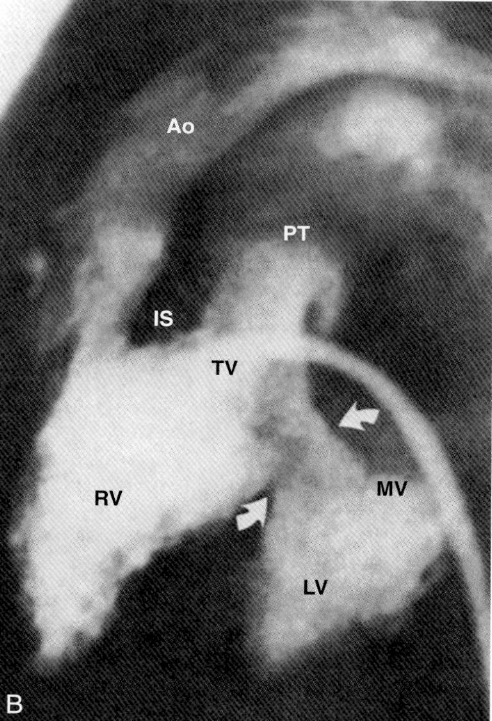

Figure 53-12 Cineangiogram made in an elongated right anterior oblique view **(A)** and in a long axial view **(B)** of a Taussig-Bing heart. The prominent infundibular septum is seen between aorta *(Ao)* and pulmonary trunk *(PT),* but it is clearly **(B)** not interventricular in position. The ventricular septal defect is between the arrows, and the pulmonary trunk somewhat overrides it. Key: *IS,* Infundibular (conal) septum; *LV,* left ventricle; *MV,* mitral valve; *RV,* right ventricle; *TV,* tricuspid valve.

it is needed, and a double velour woven polyester tube (see "Decision and Technique for Transanular Patching" under Technique of Operation in Section I of Chapter 38) whose diameter is about 20% larger than that of the aorta is preclotted, or a collagen-impregnated polyester tube is selected (see "Grafts for Use in Aortic Surgery" in Chapter 24). The intrapericardial anatomy is carefully evaluated.

Support technique and myocardial management are chosen from the usually available alternatives (see "Cold Cardioplegia, Controlled Aortic Root Reperfusion, and [When Needed] Warm Cardioplegic Induction" in Chapter 3). If two venous cannulae are used, after placing the aortic clamp, the right atrium is opened through a small incision, and a pump-oxygenator sump sucker is placed across the natural or surgically created foramen ovale. A single venous cannula can be used if the operation is to be performed through the RV. Operation is performed at 25°C with continuous CPB at a flow of $1.6\ L \cdot min^{-1} \cdot m^{-2}$, or at 18°C to 20°C with low CPB flow rate and circulatory arrest when needed for improved exposure. If the desire is to perform the operation entirely during hypothermic circulatory arrest, that technique may be chosen (see Section IV of Chapter 2).

A thorough examination of the intraventricular anatomy can usually be made through the tricuspid valve, and based on this examination, the repair is planned. Repair of simple DORV can be accomplished through the right atrium, although the most superior part of the repair must sometimes be made through a radial incision along the base of the tricuspid anterior and septal leaflets[C3,G3,I1] (see Fig. 35-26 in Chapter 35). Through the atrial approach, it is more difficult to be certain that the geometry of the intraventricular tunnel is exactly correct; lacking firm evidence for increased safety of the atrial approach to repair of isolated VSD (see Chapter 35) or tetralogy of Fallot (see Chapter 38), the RV approach may be equally satisfactory.

An intraventricular tunnel is created within the RV that conducts LV blood through the VSD to the aorta. For the transatrial approach, the right atrium is opened in a cephalad-caudad direction near the AV groove. Stay sutures are placed as for the approach for closure of an isolated VSD or as for transatrial repair of tetralogy of Fallot (see Technique of Operation in Section I of Chapters 35 and 38). The anterior tricuspid valve leaflet is elevated by fine stay sutures. For the RV approach, a transverse ventriculotomy is made low in the RV outflow tract, unless the distance between the left anterior descending coronary artery (LAD) on the left and the right coronary artery (RCA) on the right is inadequate, in which case a vertical infundibular incision is used. Special care is required if there is an anomalous origin of the LAD from the RCA. For exposure, stay sutures are placed on the ventriculotomy. The anatomy is carefully assessed, verifying anatomic details of the diagnosis. Location and size of the VSD are noted, and particularly whether it abuts the tricuspid valve or has a rim of muscle along its posterior border (Fig. 53-13). This latter determines the relationship of the bundle of His to the posterior margin of the VSD.

Small size of the VSD does not alone negate the possibility of an adequate intraventricular tunnel between LV and aorta. The possibility of enlarging it and creating a tunnel of adequate size and configuration depends primarily on the distance between the tricuspid and pulmonary valves.[S1] Sakata, Lecompte, and colleagues estimate that when this distance is less than the diameter of the aorta, a tunnel placed posterior to the pulmonary trunk will be stenotic; they recommend that in such a case, the tunnel be placed anterior to the orifice of the pulmonary trunk.[S1] However, in simple DORV, this distance is usually long (see Figs. 53-2 and 53-4), making this malformation suited for intraventricular tunnel repair, with the tunnel posterior to the orifice of the pulmonary trunk.

As a first step, the VSD is enlarged anteriorly if it is clearly restrictive to flow into a tunnel from the LV. Before this is done, the area of the proposed enlargement is carefully examined to be certain that it is interventricular septum and not hypertrophied and trabeculated anterior ventricular wall. Cutting into the latter imposes the risks of damaging the LAD and developing an LV false aneurysm.[E2] Generally, a simple incision into the interventricular septum from the VSD gapes open widely and suffices, but occasionally some muscle must be excised. In doing this, the mitral valve must be kept out of harm's way.

The VSD patch is then cut from a polyester tube (see Fig. 53-13). Geometry of the patch is crucial in preventing subaortic stenosis after the repair. The patch will form the anterior half of the tunnel connecting the VSD to the aortic orifice; the posterior half of the tunnel will be heart tissue, and experience indicates that this provides adequately for growth of the tunnel. Thus, initial trimming is made to retain about half to two thirds of the circumference of the tube graft that was selected, so as to have a diameter about 20% greater than that of the ascending aorta. The patch is then trimmed so that its *length* is the distance from the anterior angle of the VSD to the anterior edge of the subaortic conus or, if this is hypoplastic, LV-aortic junction (aortic valve "anulus").

The technique for inserting the patch is analogous to that for inserting the patch in isolated VSD (see Fig. 35-24 in Chapter 35) or tetralogy of Fallot (see Chapter 38). Because correct orientation of the patch is essential to creating a geometrically correct tunnel, a marking stitch is placed at the most anterior part of the repair, and another is placed through the patch at a corresponding point. A similar marking stitch is placed over the midportion of the aorta anteriorly and in the patch. The first pledgeted mattress stitch is passed from the atrial to ventricular side through the base of the tricuspid commissural tissue between the anterior and septal leaflets (see Fig. 53-13). If the approach is through the right atrium and tricuspid valve, the suture is usually begun anteriorly at the most caudal aspect of the VSD. (If a bar of muscle separates the VSD from the tricuspid anulus, the sutures may be placed just on the right side of the edge of this muscle, as in a similar anatomic situation in tetralogy of Fallot; see Chapter 38.) Suturing is carried leftward for a short distance between the patch and tricuspid leaflet tissue and after a few stitches between the patch and ventriculoinfundibular fold and up along the right side of subaortic infundibulum. When the marking stitch is reached, the suture is held. With the other arm of the suture, the patch is sewn to the RV side of the septum, 5 to 7 mm back from the edge of the VSD, proceeding rightward, anteriorly, and then superiorly (see Fig. 53-13). When the repair is completed, the contoured polyester patch forms the anterior portion of an unobstructed intraventricular tunnel between the VSD and aorta.

Rewarming the patient by the perfusate is commenced, and the interatrial communication is closed with a few sutures, but not tied until there is effective ventricular contraction (to

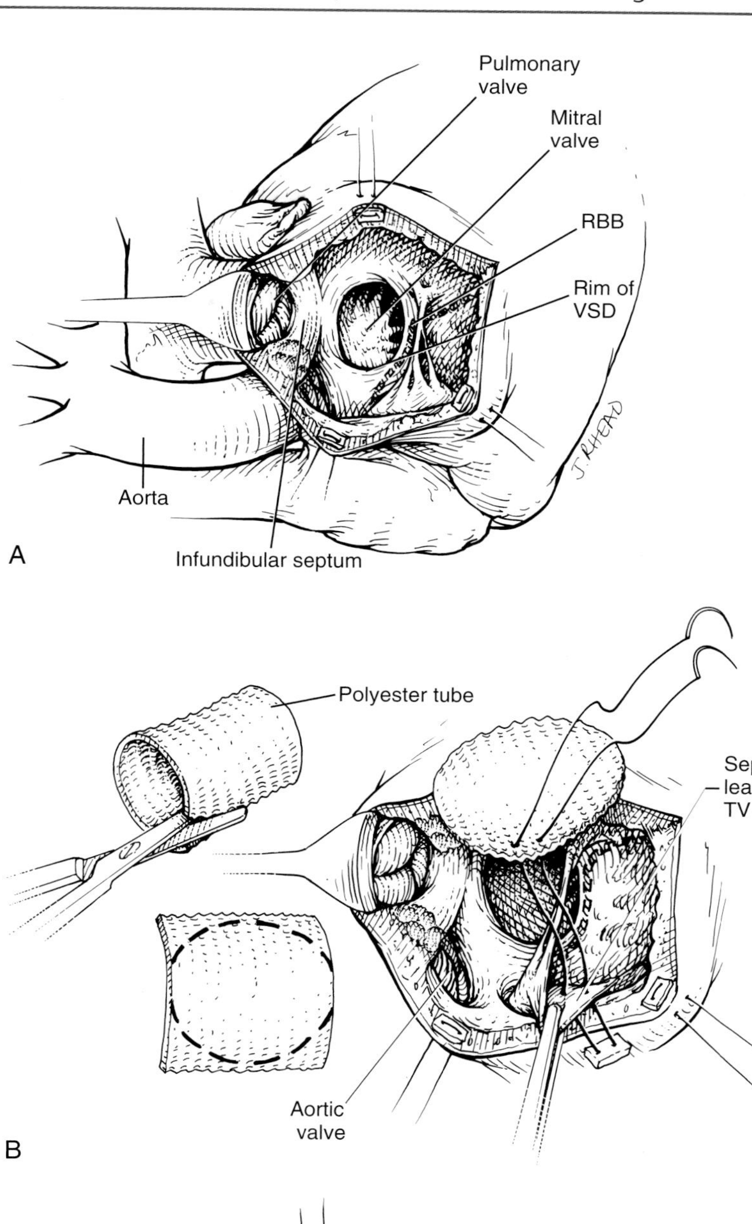

Figure 53-13 Intraventricular tunnel repair for simple double outlet right ventricle with subaortic ventricular septal defect *(VSD)*. **A,** Pulmonary and aortic valves are at nearly the same level. The perimembranous VSD has been exposed through a right ventriculotomy. There is moderate hypertrophy of the parietal band, which is mobilized and partially resected. **B,** A polyester tube of diameter about 20% larger than that of the aortic root has been cut to a length that is the same as the distance from the anterior border of the VSD to the aortic valve. About three-fifths circumference of the tube is used and is contoured as shown. Corrugations in the polyester patch assist the surgeon in maintaining proper orientation of the patch as it is being sewn in place. A pledgeted mattress suture is placed through the base of the commissure between septal and anterior tricuspid leaflets to begin the tunnel repair. **C,** Suturing has been carried to the left along the ventriculoinfundibular fold and up over the subaortic conus. With the other arm of the suture, inferior and superior portions of the repair are completed. The contoured tunnel offers no obstruction to flow from left ventricle to aorta. Key: *RBB,* Right bundle branch; *TV,* tricuspid valve.

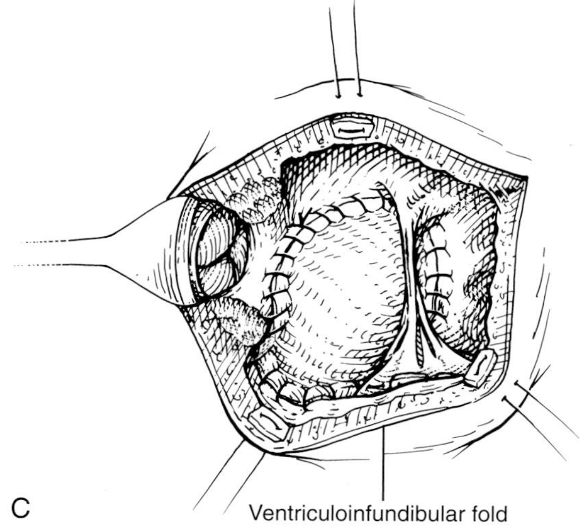

avoid LV distension). The left atrium is filled with saline via a blunt needle and the aortic clamp removed with strong suction on the aortic needle vent.

If an RV approach is used, it is closed either primarily or with a small patch; a patch is used when there is infundibular pulmonic stenosis (as for tetralogy of Fallot) or if the intraventricular tunnel bulges anteriorly, potentially obstructing RV outflow. The remainder of the operation is carried out as usual (see Section III in Chapter 2). The repair is evaluated by transesophageal echocardiography just before and after discontinuing CPB. In addition to the usual measurements, LV and aortic pressures are measured to exclude any gradient across the baffle; when the repair is done as described, no gradient is present.

Repair of Double Outlet Right Ventricle with Subaortic Ventricular Septal Defect and Pulmonary Stenosis

Repair is essentially that for tetralogy of Fallot, as described in "Technique of Operation" in Section I of Chapter 38. The only difference is the intraventricular tunnel repair, as just described, rather than simple VSD closure.

Repair of Taussig-Bing Heart by Arterial Switch Repair

The usual Taussig-Bing type of DORV with subpulmonary VSD is best treated by closure of the VSD in such a manner that the LV ejects into the neoaorta, and by an arterial switch (see "Arterial Switch Operation" under Technique of Operation in Chapter 52).

Approach to repair of the VSD is varied, and the decision is best made before operation, based on the following considerations (Quaegebeur JM; personal communication, 1991):

- When the VSD is perimembranous or juxta-tricuspid, and particularly when it extends toward the inlet septum, repair is probably most effectively accomplished from the right atrium.
- When the VSD extends toward the RV outlet and the pulmonary trunk does not override the VSD, repair is most easily accomplished through the proximal aortic (neopulmonary) segment after removing the aortic buttons containing coronary ostia. The landmarks and techniques are identical to those used when a VSD is repaired through a right ventriculotomy.
- When the pulmonary trunk is large and overrides the VSD, as is usually the case, an approach to the VSD through the proximal pulmonary (neoaortic) segment is convenient.[O1] However, the posteroinferior portion of the insertion of the patch to close the VSD (performed so that the LV ejects into the pulmonary trunk [neoaorta]) is approached from the RV aspect as a protection against damaging the conducting tissue.

The arterial switch is then performed (see "Arterial Switch Operation" under Technique of Operation in Chapter 52). Because the great arteries are often side by side, suitable adjustments are made in the operation (see Chapter 52, Fig. 52-28). If arch hypoplasia is present, it is addressed surgically with one of several possible approaches. Either a standard interrupted arch repair technique is used (see Technique of Operation in Section II of Chapter 48) or the relatively hypoplastic ascending aorta can be reoriented from its vertical position to a horizontal position and anastomosed end to end to the descending aorta, followed by anastomosis of the proximal pulmonary trunk (neoaorta) to the transversely positioned ascending aorta.[L6] When arch hypoplasia is present, there is a high likelihood of hypoplasia of the RV outflow tract, and clinically important postoperative infundibular obstruction is common. Therefore, the RV outflow tract should be addressed surgically when arch obstruction is present. In this setting, the VSD is best repaired through a vertical infundibular incision, with infundibular resection and patching.

Intraventricular Tunnel Repair of Taussig-Bing Heart

Although the place of the intraventricular tunnel repair of Taussig-Bing heart is not securely established, small series of successful operations have been reported.[A1,K3,M6,P1,P3,S14,Y1]

Initial stages of operation are the same as in other operations for Taussig-Bing heart. After CPB and cold cardioplegia have been established and the right atrium opened, morphology within the RV is studied through the tricuspid valve. Distance from tricuspid to pulmonary valves is estimated; if this distance is too short, the LV-to–pulmonary trunk tunnel will probably need to pass anterior to the pulmonary valve (see "Intraventricular Tunnel Repair of Simple Double Outlet Right Ventricle" earlier in this chapter); alternatively, an arterial switch operation is used.[L2,R3] Any attachment of tricuspid chordae to septal edges of the malaligned infundibular septum is noted because special measures are needed for these. Straddling or overriding of the mitral valve is of considerable importance because this may make the planned operation impossible. Usually, after completing the examination from the right atrium, a transverse right ventriculotomy is made for the repair, although sometimes repair may be accomplished from the right atrial approach.

Ideally, the surgically created intraventricular tunnel is fashioned to lie posterior to the pulmonary trunk (Kawashima method), but this depends on availability of space between the tricuspid and pulmonary valves, as noted earlier[K3] (Fig. 53-14). Adequate space is more likely to be available when the great arteries are side by side rather than in an anteroposterior position. Generally the VSD is enlarged anteriorly, and at least a portion of infundibular septum is excised. It may be helpful to open the pulmonary trunk and pass a Hegar dilator through the pulmonary valve to expose the infundibular septum and protect the mitral apparatus (see "Lecompte Intraventricular Repair" in text that follows). As this is being done, care is taken to avoid damaging the aortic valve cusps and chordae from the tricuspid valve. If these chordae attach alongside an area that requires enlargement, that portion is not excised but instead is turned up as a flap. After creation of the intraventricular tunnel, the flap of infundibular septum is sutured in place over the tunnel.[B9] The polyester patch is trimmed to an appropriate size and configuration (see Fig. 53-13) and sewn into place with the usual care to avoid damaging the conduction system (see Fig. 53-14).

When the aorta is directly anterior, there is usually insufficient space between the tricuspid and pulmonary valves for a posterior position of the intraventricular tunnel. If an intraventricular tunnel repair is performed, the VSD is enlarged appropriately and the tunnel created *anterior* to the

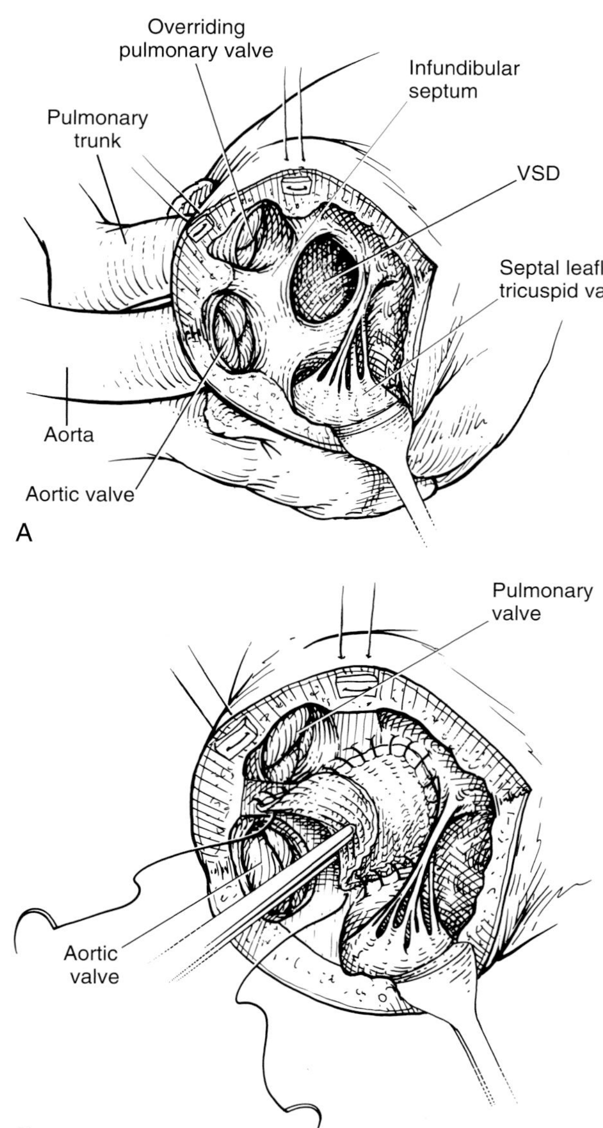

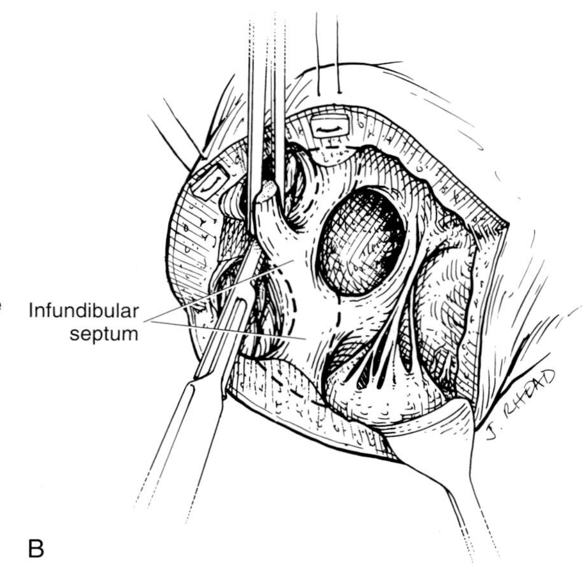

Figure 53-14 Intraventricular tunnel repair of Taussig-Bing heart (Kawashima method). In the illustration, great arteries are side by side, with aorta to the right of the pulmonary trunk and with an adequate distance between tricuspid and pulmonary valves. **A,** Right ventricle is opened through a vertical or transverse incision. The tricuspid valve apparatus is away from the infundibular septum and ventricular septal defect *(VSD)*, which facilitates intraventricular repair. **B,** VSD is enlarged by excising ventricular septum anteriorly, and the infundibular septum is partially cut away to provide better access of intraventricular tunnel to aortic orifice *(dashed lines)*. Often, only an incision is required. **C,** The intraventricular tunnel repair is performed using an appropriately sized and shaped patch made from a polyester tube (see Fig. 53-12) and placed with continuous suture, sometimes supplemented with interrupted stitches. Tunnel conducts blood from left ventricle to aorta.

pulmonary orifice (Patrick-McGoon method)[M9,P1,P3] (Fig. 53-15). In some cases, if this technique is used, a prosthetic tube (rather than a patch) is needed for part of the pathway, and part of the tube is incorporated into the closure of the right ventriculotomy.[D7]

Lecompte Intraventricular Repair

Although the role of this operation, which Lecompte calls *REV* (réparation à l'étage ventriculaire), is not yet certain, its concepts and results mandate consideration. In this operation, the LV is connected to the aorta and the RV to the pulmonary trunk by a technique that does not require an extracardiac conduit.[B9,L2,R3,S1,V4] It is designed for patients in whom a simple intraventricular tunnel repair is not possible, nor is an arterial switch operation combined with repair of the VSD in such a manner that the LV is connected to the proximal pulmonary trunk (neoaortic) segment. The reason for the latter is usually coexisting important pulmonary (LV outflow) stenosis. The diagnosis may be some form of DORV or transposition with VSD and LV outflow obstruction. The Lecompte operation has also been demonstrated to be applicable to double outlet LV in infancy, thus avoiding need for a valved extracardiac conduit (Bailey LL; personal communication, 1991).

Initial stages of operation are the same as for intraventricular repair. After CPB and cold cardioplegia have been established, and after the preliminary examination from the right atrium is accomplished, a vertical right ventriculotomy is made and extended as far cephalad as possible. After thorough assessment of intraventricular anatomy and great arteries, the aorta and pulmonary trunk are transected (Fig. 53-16, *A*). All interventricular and infundibular septal tissue between the VSD and great arteries is resected. A Hegar dilator introduced through the pulmonary trunk helps with exposure during resection (Fig. 53-16, *B*). Cusps of the aortic valve

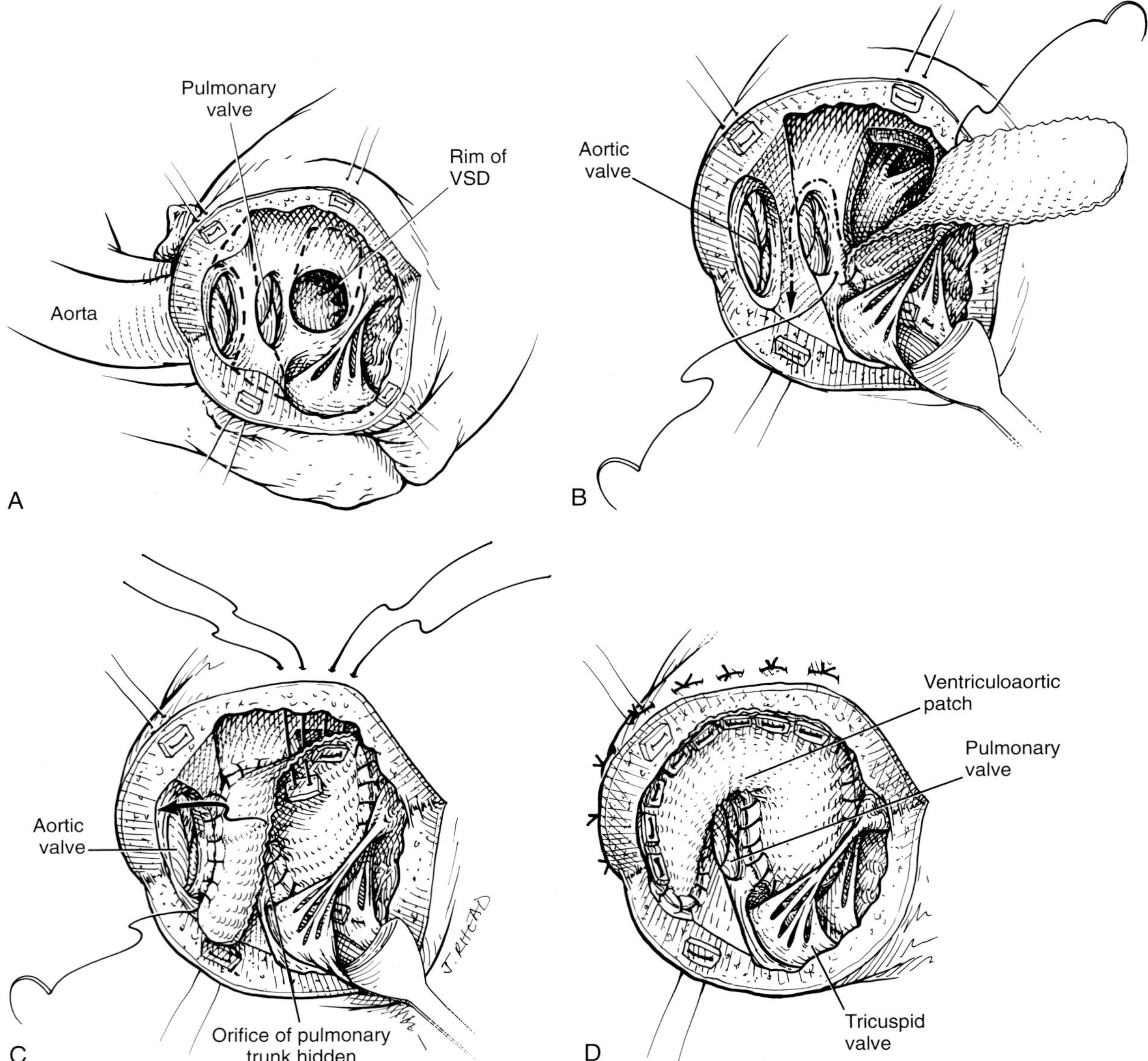

Figure 53-15 Repair of double outlet right ventricle with subpulmonary ventricular septal defect *(VSD)* (Taussig-Bing heart) when there is only a short distance between tricuspid and pulmonary valves (Patrick-McGoon method[M9,P1,P3]). Aorta is usually anterior to pulmonary trunk. **A,** Through a transverse right ventriculotomy, the VSD is enlarged and much of the inlet septum excised *(dashed line).* **B,** A contoured polyester (or polytetrafluoroethylene) patch is cut from a tube graft whose diameter is about 20% larger than that of the aorta. Initial suturing is performed in the usual manner, preventing damage to the bundle of His. A continuous suture is used, often supplemented by interrupted stitches. **C,** With the leftward arm of the continuous suture, suture line is continued leftward along the posterior and then leftward margin of the ventriculopulmonary trunk junction, and finally along the anterior margin of this junction *(dashed line).* With the other arm of the suture, the patch is sutured inferior to the VSD, to the right side of the septum, and then anterior to the defect. **D,** Insertion of spiraled patch has been completed. Left ventricular blood now passes beneath the patch to the aorta, while right ventricular blood passes to the pulmonary trunk behind the tunnel.

must be visualized to protect them from damage in the course of resection. The excision is kept away from regions occupied by the bundle of His and its primary branches. When tricuspid chordae are attached to a portion of the infundibular or ventricular septum, this portion is raised as a flap with chordae attached.[B9] After completing the intraventricular repair, the flap is sutured to the roof of the tunnel, more or less in its original position.

The intraventricular tunnel repair is performed by suturing a polyester or polytetrafluoroethylene (PTFE) patch into place to form the roof of the LV-aortic pathway (Fig. 53-16, *C*).

The proximal segment of the pulmonary trunk is closed (for details, see "Bidirectional Superior Cavopulmonary Shunt" under Technique of Operation in Chapter 41). Because this repair is generally performed in patients in whom the aorta is anterior to the pulmonary trunk, the pulmonary trunk and its bifurcation are usually translocated anterior to the aorta. For this, the aortic clamp is repositioned, and the distal aortic segment is brought behind the bifurcation of the

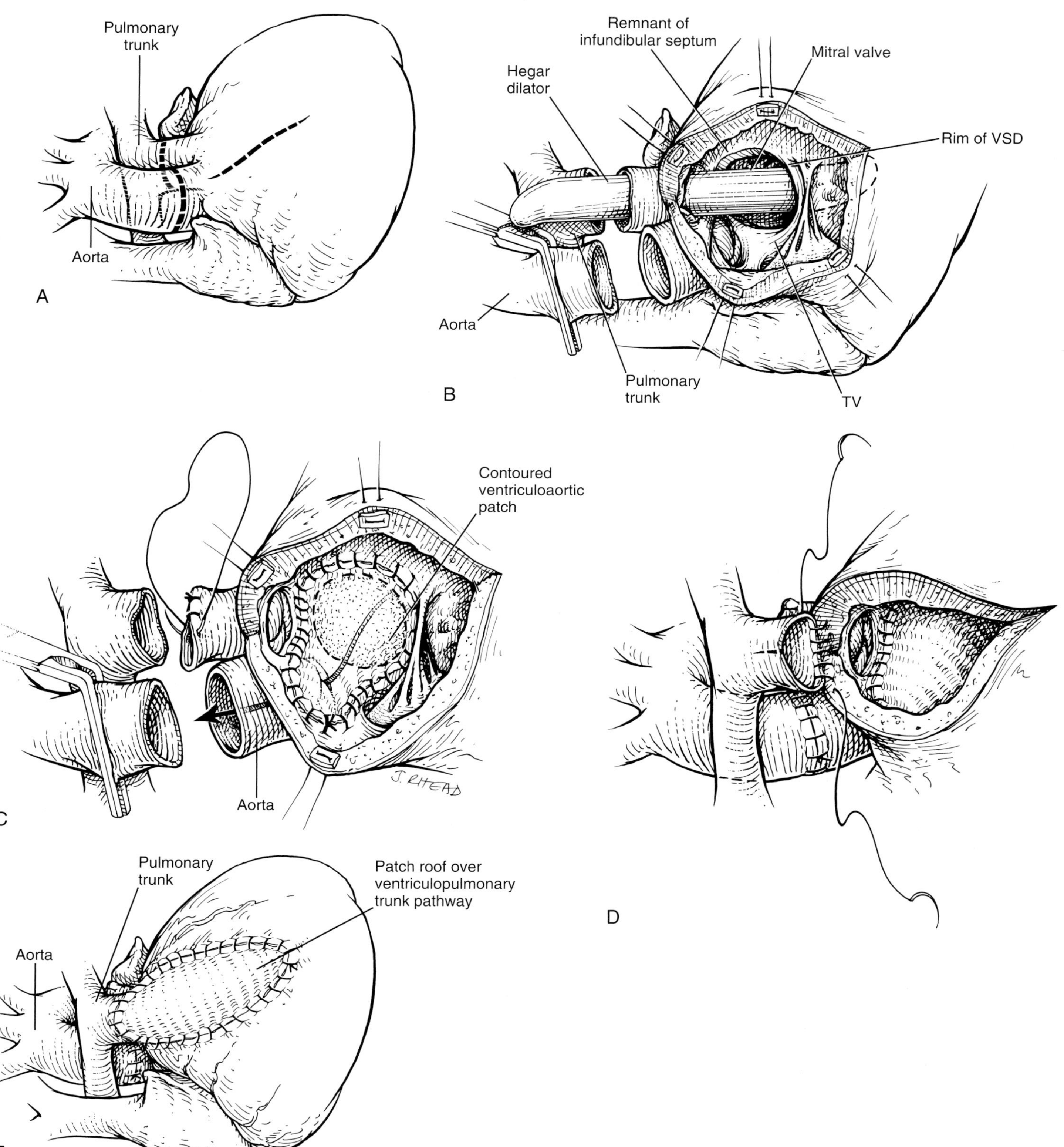

Figure 53-16 Lecompte operation for double outlet right ventricle with pulmonary stenosis and for other abnormalities of ventriculoarterial connection and ventricular septal defect *(VSD)*, including transposition of the great arteries with VSD and left ventricular outflow tract obstruction. **A,** Dashed lines indicate sites for transecting aorta and pulmonary trunk and for the right ventriculotomy. **B,** Right ventriculotomy has been made, great arteries have been transected, a Hegar dilator has been passed down through the proximal segment of the pulmonary trunk and into the left ventricle to improve exposure (and protect the mitral valve), VSD has been enlarged, and infundibular (conal) septum has been resected. **C,** Polyester patch has been sewn into place to form anterior portion of newly created left ventriculoaortic pathway, using the same general technique shown in Fig. 53-13. Proximal pulmonary trunk stump is oversewn. **D,** Aorta has been repositioned behind pulmonary trunk bifurcation and reconstructed. Pulmonary trunk has been enlarged by an incision anteriorly and its posterior wall anastomosed to the right ventriculotomy. **E,** Repair is completed with a polyester (or polytetrafluoroethylene or pericardial) patch placed as a roof over the right ventriculopulmonary trunk pathway, using the same principles as in placing a transanular patch in repair of tetralogy of Fallot (see Fig. 38-29 in Chapter 38).

pulmonary trunk (Fig. 53-16, *D*), as in the Lecompte maneuver for the arterial switch operation (see "Arterial Switch Operation" under Technique of Operation in Chapter 52). The aorta is reconstructed behind and to the right of the distal pulmonary trunk segment.

The posterior lip of the distal segment of the pulmonary trunk is anastomosed to the cephalad margin of the right ventriculotomy. The right ventricular–pulmonary trunk pathway is completed by suturing a roof of pericardium, polyester, or PTFE into place (Fig. 53-16, *E*). Lecompte incorporates a monocusp valve beneath the patch.

Nikaidoh Aortic Translocation and Right Ventricular Outflow Reconstruction

The first step in this procedure is to core out the intact aortic root from the RV, including aortic valve and coronary arteries, as described earlier by Bex and colleagues[B6,N3] (Fig. 53-17). The pulmonary trunk is transected, and an incision in the interventricular septum between the VSD and lumen of the proximal stump of the pulmonary trunk opens this area widely. This allows the VSD (and through it the LV) to be joined to the aorta by a roofing patch, which is similar to that

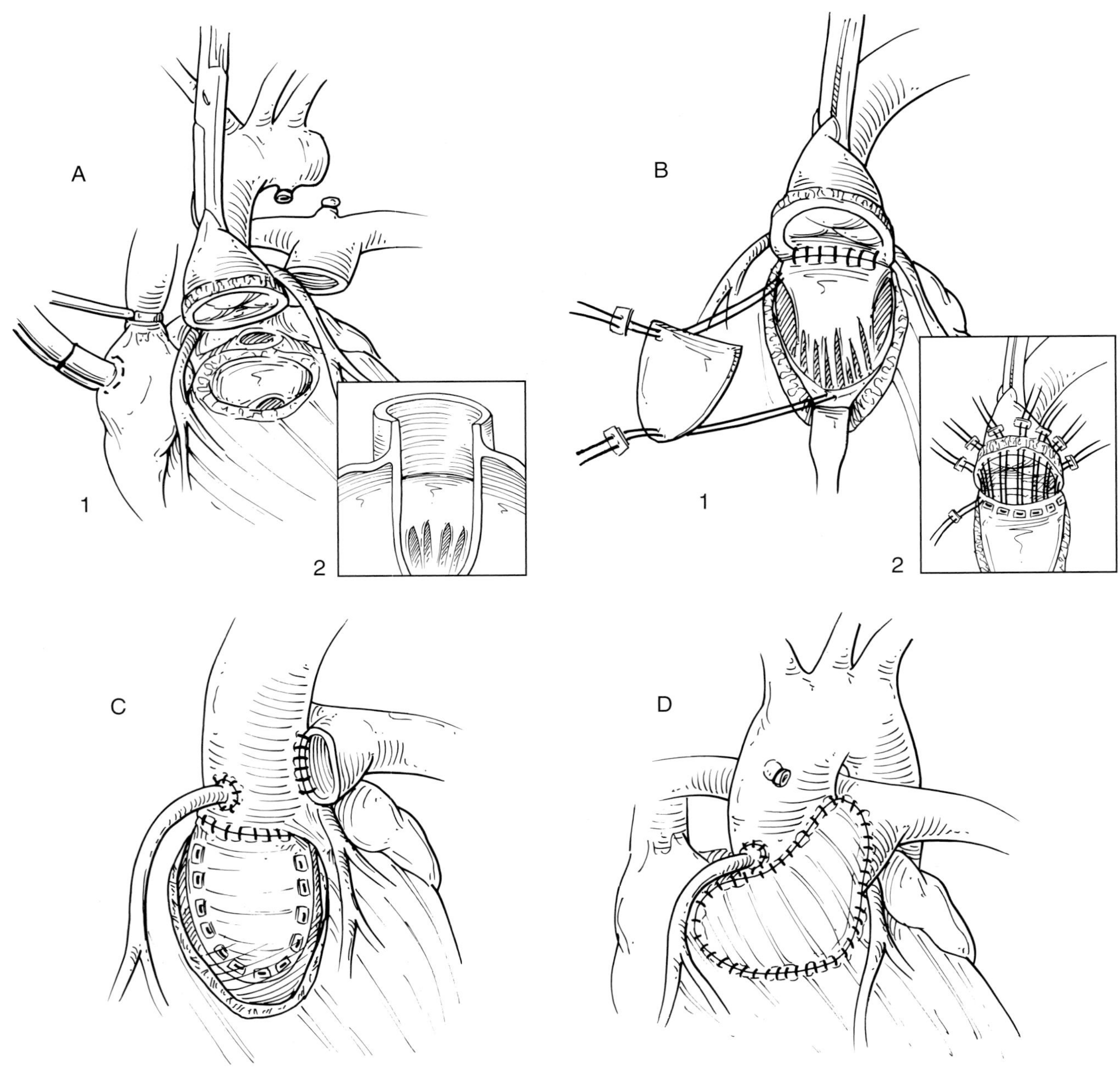

Figure 53-17 Nikaidoh aortic translocation and right ventricular outflow tract reconstruction. **A1,** Anteriorly located aortic root is fully mobilized beneath the valve and both coronaries skeletonized. **A2,** Division of pulmonary trunk and infundibular (conal) septum (when present). Pulmonary-mitral continuity is demonstrated. **B1,** Anastomosis of aorta to open pulmonary "anulus" after posterior translocation. Ventricular septal defect (VSD) patch will be anastomosed to apical rim of VSD. **B2,** Anastomosis of superior portion of VSD patch to anterior rim of mobilized aortic root. **C,** Right ventricular outflow tract (RVOT) is reconstructed by anchoring right lateral wall of pulmonary trunk to aortic root and overlaying a patch of pericardium to cover aortic root, right ventriculotomy, and pulmonary trunk. **D,** Large pericardial patch is used to reconstruct RVOT. Care must be taken to avoid RVOT obstruction. A flat patch is required to curve longitudinally (along axis of aorta) and from anterior to posterior (to reach distal pulmonary trunk). (From Yeh 2006.[Y3])

placed in the other intraventricular tunnel repairs. The pulmonary trunk is then joined to the RV outflow tract as described for the Lecompte intraventricular repair.

Repair of Taussig-Bing Heart by Atrial Switch Procedure

Operation is begun through the atrial incision mandated by the venous switch procedure to be used (see "Atrial Switch Operation" under Technique of Operation in Chapter 52). Working through the tricuspid valve, the VSD is repaired so that the LV ejects into the pulmonary trunk.[H2] An atrial switch procedure is done. When important LV outflow obstruction is present, an allograft valved extracardiac conduit is also placed between the LV and pulmonary trunk.

Intraventricular Tunnel Repair of Double Outlet Right Ventricle with Doubly Committed Ventricular Septal Defect

After CPB and cold cardioplegia are established, a transverse right ventriculotomy is made. A slightly modified tunnel repair is done, very much as described under "Intraventricular Tunnel Repair of Simple Double Outlet Right Ventricle" earlier in this chapter. However, when the two semilunar valves lie side by side and the pulmonary "anulus" is the larger, contouring the patch to achieve this may be difficult without obstructing flow into the pulmonary trunk. This problem can be minimized by enlarging the VSD anteriorly as much as possible before placing the patch.

Intraventricular Tunnel Repair of Double Outlet Right Ventricle with Noncommitted Ventricular Septal Defect

When the noncommitted VSD is of the inlet septal type (see Morphology in Section I of Chapter 35), it extends beneath the tricuspid septal leaflet rather than anteriorly or superiorly. It may be possible to enlarge this defect anteriorly and superiorly so that a tunnel repair can be performed that connects the LV to the aorta (Fig. 53-18). The precautions used against damaging the conduction system are those used for repair of inlet septal VSD (see Fig. 34-20 in Chapter 34). If the tunnel obstructs access to the pulmonary valve, an allograft (or other biological) valved conduit is placed from the RV to the pulmonary trunk.

Other Operations for Double Outlet Right Ventricle with Noncommitted Ventricular Septal Defect

In some patients with an inlet septal type of noncommitted VSD, tricuspid valve chordae may overhang the defect; in these cases, its enlargement as described is not possible, and a tunnel repair cannot be carried out. The same situation may exist when there is a large single or multiple muscular VSDs in the trabecular septum.

When pulmonary stenosis coexists, a Fontan operation is performed. The technique of total cavopulmonary connection (see discussion under Technique of Operation in Chapter 41) is particularly suited to this situation because nothing has to be done to the AV valves or within the ventricle except to enlarge the VSD if it is restrictive.

When the tunnel repair cannot be made and *pulmonary stenosis is not present*, the situation should be identified very early in life, and a pulmonary trunk band should be placed (see "Pulmonary Trunk Banding" under Technique of Operation in Chapter 35). Subsequently a Fontan operation should be performed.

Repair of Double Outlet Right Ventricle with Complete Atrioventricular Septal Defect

Technique of repair is similar to that for repair of complete AV septal defect and tetralogy of Fallot as described under Technique of Operation in Chapter 34. However, the situation becomes considerably more complex in the setting of heterotaxy syndromes, in which anomalous pulmonary venous connection is common and the VSD of the AV septal defect may be remote from the aortic valve in the presence of a muscular subaortic infundibulum (conus) (see Chapter 58).

Repair of Double Outlet Right Ventricle with L-Malposition of the Aorta

In nearly all surgical patients in this subset, the VSD is subaortic and pulmonary stenosis coexists. The heart is opened by a vertical incision in the RV. Usually, the VSD is easily visualized anterosuperiorly in the ventricular septum and well away from the tricuspid anulus. An intraventricular tunnel repair with a contoured patch may not be necessary, and a simple polyester or PTFE patch may be used to close the VSD in such a way that the LV ejects into the aorta. Stitches may be placed along the edge of the VSD posteriorly unless the defect abuts the tricuspid valve. An allograft valved extracardiac conduit is usually placed between the RV and pulmonary trunk, because of associated severe valvar and subvalvar pulmonary stenosis (see Figs. 38-68 and 38-70 in Chapter 38).

Repair of Double Outlet Right Ventricle with Discordant Atrioventricular Connections

A complete discussion of discordant AV connections is found in Chapter 55. In DORV with discordant AV connections, three major options are available:

- Traditional or physiologic repair in which the morphologic RV is retained as the systemic ventricle
- Anatomically corrective operations that leave the morphologic LV as the systemic ventricle
- Single-ventricle strategies ending in the Fontan operation

Traditional repairs that use the RV as the systemic ventricle include VSD closure and the Rastelli procedure, or VSD closure with baffling of LV to pulmonary trunk, with or without relief of LV outflow tract obstruction to the pulmonary trunk. *Anatomic repairs* include the "double switch" procedure (atrial switch procedure and arterial switch combined with VSD closure to direct blood from LV to neoaortic valve) and atrial switch procedure with rerouting of blood from LV through VSD to aortic valve, with or without a Rastelli procedure.

Palliative Operations

Shunting operations are described in Chapter 38 (see "Technique of Shunting Operations" under Technique of Operation in Section I) and pulmonary trunk banding in Chapter 35 (see "Pulmonary Trunk Banding" under Technique of Operation in Section I).

SPECIAL FEATURES OF POSTOPERATIVE CARE

Care after corrective or palliative operations for DORV is described in Chapter 5.

RESULTS

Survival

Early (Hospital) Death

Even intraventricular tunnel repair of *simple DORV* in heterogeneous patient populations has had a hospital mortality through the years of about 20%.[K8] This figure is not relevant, however, to the current era (see "Incremental Risk Factors for Premature Death" later in this chapter), a fact verified by multivariable and univariable analyses[K8] in widely separated institutions (Fig. 53-19) and more recent data reported by Kleinert and colleagues,[K10] all indicating a current hospital mortality of less than 2%. In 148 patients having biventricular repair, overall mortality was 8.1% (CL 5.8%-11%). Belli and colleagues reported similar results in 154 patients in the present era (9.8%; CL 7.2%-13%).[B4] Brown and colleagues reported results of various repairs for DORV in 124 patients operated on between 1980 and 2000.[B14] Depending on complexity of the anatomy and location of the VSD, four types of repair were used: intraventricular baffle ($n = 53$), baffle plus conduit ($n = 20$), arterial switch ($n = 16$), and Fontan procedures ($n = 33$). Hospital mortality was 4.8% (CL 2.9%-7.7%).

Overall hospital mortality following the various types of repair of *Taussig-Bing heart* has been even higher in the past, about 50%.[K8] This again is not relevant to the current era, in which the arterial switch procedure is used for most of these patients (see Fig. 52-37 in Chapter 52). For example, employing the arterial switch operation for DORV with subpulmonary VSD, Masuda and colleagues reported one death in 27 patients (3.7%; CL 0.5%-12%) ranging in age from 10 days to 5 years (median 0.4 years).[M5]

Given the frequency of coexisting coarctation and the possible application of preliminary pulmonary trunk banding for Taussig-Bing hearts, controversy exists regarding the advisability of initial repair of coarctation only vs. one-stage correction using the arterial switch operation. In the current era, low mortality (<5%) has been reported both with initial repair of coarctation through a left thoracotomy followed by subsequent arterial switch[G4,R2] and with single-stage repair via sternotomy.[A3]

Kawashima and colleagues used an interventricular rerouting repair with extensive resection of the infundibular septum in 10 of 41 patients with Taussig-Bing heart (average age 2 years), with no deaths (0%; CL 0%-17%).[K4]

Estimating overall early mortality after repair of *DORV with doubly committed VSD* is difficult because of the small number of reported cases, but in general it has been about the same as after repair of simple DORV.[K8] The same difficulty is true of *DORV with noncommitted VSD*, exacerbated by the variety of operations used and the uncertainty of categorization of many patients in this group. Early mortality has probably been about 50%. The Fontan operation should be expected to yield the same mortality as in patients with univentricular AV connection, which is less than 5% in appropriately selected patients (see Chapter 41).

Time-Related Survival

Long-term survival after repair of simple DORV exceeds 95% at 15 years (see Fig. 53-19).

Incremental Risk Factors for Premature Death

An analysis based on the UAB experience between 1967 and July 1984 probably still serves reasonably well for simple DORV and DORV with doubly committed VSD, but not for varieties of DORV in which the arterial switch operation is now performed.[K8]

Age at Repair

Currently, and in contrast to an era before about 1980, *young age* at operation is not a risk factor for death early or late after repair of simple DORV and probably of DORV with doubly committed VSD.[L10] In fact, *older age* at operation is now the risk factor, and it is a particularly strong risk factor in the constant hazard phase (see Fig. 53-19). These relationships, and indeed survival in general, are similar to those obtained after repair of primary isolated VSD, and they probably are explained largely by absence or presence and severity of pulmonary vascular disease. Currently, patients undergoing repair of simple DORV during the first 6 months of life have about a 99% chance of 1-month survival and a 95% chance of long-term survival and surgical cure.

Among patients with Taussig-Bing heart, age greater than about 6 months is a risk factor for mortality, likely related to pulmonary vascular disease. However, Feng and colleagues found similar survival among a small group of patients with transposition and VSD and those with Taussig-Bing heart who underwent an arterial switch operation and VSD closure before or after age 6 months.[F1]

Type of Double Outlet Right Ventricle

Simple DORV and *DORV with doubly committed VSD* and no pulmonary stenosis are particularly favorable types of DORV with regard to survival after repair and are not risk factors for death.

In the past, *DORV with subpulmonary VSD* was a strong risk factor for death early or late after repair, largely related to combining repair of the VSD with an atrial switch procedure.[K8] Early and long-term survival after repair of the VSD combined with an arterial switch procedure are similar to those after the arterial switch repair of transposition of the great arteries and VSD[K1,M5,Q1,Q2] (see Chapter 52, Fig. 52-37).

In the past, survival after repair of *DORV with noncommitted VSD* has been less than that of any other group, but assignment of patients to this group is almost by exclusion. This makes it the least homogeneous group morphologically; also, a number of different kinds of repairs are used. The anatomic subset is sufficiently uncommon, the categorization of patients into it sufficiently arguable, and operations for

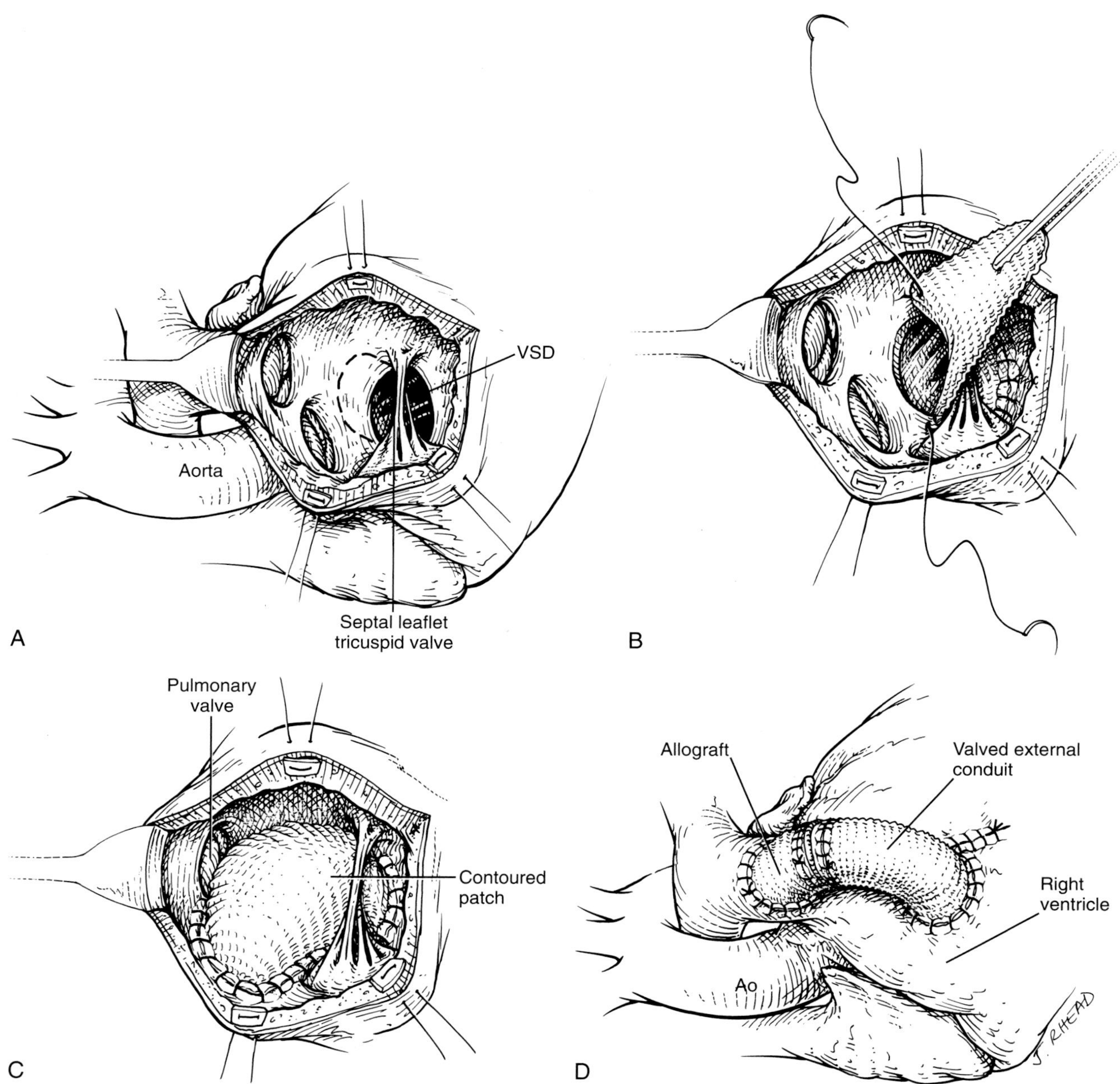

Figure 53-18 Repair of double outlet right ventricle with noncommitted inlet septal ventricular septal defect *(VSD)*. **A,** VSD is noncommitted, but typically is not far from being either subaortic or subpulmonary. It is enlarged anteriorly *(dashed line)* after visualizing the mitral apparatus, being certain not to damage the anterior free wall or anterior descending coronary artery with the enlargement. **B,** An intraventricular tunnel repair is made. In the case illustration, the pulmonary trunk is left on the right ventricular side, but the tunnel partially obstructs approach to it. In some patients, an appropriate tunnel cannot be made except by leaving the pulmonary trunk on the left ventricular side of the tunnel; entry into the pulmonary trunk is closed off before making the tunnel repair, or the pulmonary trunk is divided when the conduit is placed. Right ventriculopulmonary artery continuity is established with a xenograft **(C)** or allograft valved extracardiac conduit **(D)**.

correcting it sufficiently variable that some time may elapse before early and intermediate-term survival are known with a reasonable degree of certainty. When known, it may indicate more frequent use of the Fontan group of operations in this subset of patients.

Major Associated Cardiac Anomalies

Pulmonary stenosis coexists with DORV in many patients, and its presence often requires creating a nonvalved or valved connection to the pulmonary trunk. Related to this, the presence of pulmonary stenosis is probably an incremental risk factor for death, because both procedures increase mortality.[S13]

Complete AV septal defects, straddling AV valves, hypoplasia of a ventricular chamber, mitral valve abnormalities, and other coexisting anomalies increase risk.[B4] This has usually been related to persisting in an attempt to perform an optimal operation rather than accepting the need for a more appropriate and often simpler procedure such as the Fontan group of operations.

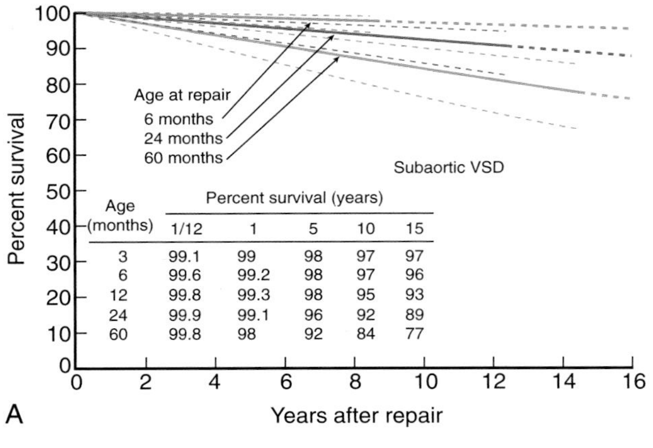

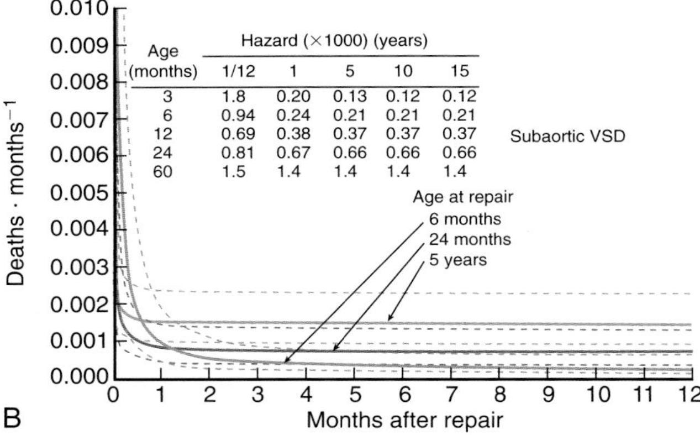

Figure 53-19 Relationship between age at operation and early and long-term survival after repair of simple double outlet right ventricle. Depiction is a nomogram of a specific solution of a multivariable risk factor equation.[K4] Solid lines represent continuous point estimates, and dashed lines enclose 70% confidence intervals. **A,** Percent survival. **B,** Hazard function for death. Key: *VSD,* Ventricular septal defect. (From Kirklin and colleagues.[K8])

Surgical Era

Earlier date of operation has been clearly identified as a risk factor for death by several studies.[K8] This indicates that outcomes after repair of all types of DORV are currently better than at any time in the past, and this difference is quantifiable.

Type of Operation

Atrial Switch Operation Use of an atrial switch operation in conjunction with an intraventricular tunnel repair has given poor results in general, including hospital mortalities of 30% to 40%. In this setting, the atrial switch repair is at least as strong a risk factor as it is in transposition of the great arteries and VSD (see Chapter 52). For this reason, it is no longer used.

Complex Intraventricular Tunnel Repair A simple intraventricular tunnel repair, such as that performed for DORV with subaortic VSD, has no more demonstrable risk than repair of a large primary isolated VSD with a patch (see Chapter 35). This is the reason for excellent outcome after repair of simple DORV in early life.

A somewhat more complex intraventricular tunnel repair, such as that used to redirect LV outflow in the Rastelli operation (see "Rastelli Operation" under Technique of Operation in Chapter 52) but with minimal excision of septal tissue and a resultant straight and relatively short pathway leading to the aorta, has little demonstrable incremental risk. This is supported by the current low early mortality after the Rastelli operation and by the low prevalence of complications from the tunnel itself late postoperatively. When used under proper circumstances for Taussig-Bing malformation, early and intermediate-term survival has been good and comparable to that obtained with the arterial switch repair.[S3]

More complex intraventricular tunnel repairs appear to be incremental risk factors, although this idea has not been properly tested by analysis. Hospital mortality has been 10% to 15% after such procedures but may currently be less than 5%.[K4,P1,V4] However, late morality may be affected by baffle obstruction and patch dehiscence with complex tunnels.[P1]

Transanular Patches and Extracardiac Conduits Use of transanular patches and extracardiac conduits has increased the risk of operations for DORV, but at times their use is inescapable.[K8,S13] As in other situations, controversy exists as to whether absence of a valve in the RV–pulmonary trunk connection adds to risk. Whether the risk of these procedures is any different from that imposed by the type of RV–pulmonary artery connection used in the Lecompte operation (REV) remains to be determined.

Operations for Double Outlet Right Ventricle with Atrioventricular Discordant Connections A variety of operations have been successfully applied to this subset of DORV. No single strategy has proved superior in terms of long-term survival and freedom from reoperation. Shin'oka and colleagues found no significant difference in late survival 15 to 20 years after operation according to procedure performed,[S7] whether traditional repair, anatomic repair, or Fontan procedure was employed.

Complications of Intraventricular Tunnel Repair

Need for reoperation for complications of the tunnel repair (leakage or obstruction primarily) is directly related to complexity of the tunnel. Thus, in simple intraventricular tunnel repair for DORV and subaortic VSD, only 1% of patients have had catheterization evidence of tunnel leakage or obstruction, or reoperation for it.[K8] By contrast, 18% or more of patients with complex intraventricular tunnel repairs have required reoperation for important obstruction or leakage, or have had evidence of these problems ($P = .005$).[I2,K8] An analysis by Fujii and colleagues indicated that length of the intraventricular tunnel is predictive of mortality. Among patients in whom the length between the top of the interventricular septum and aortic valve was less than 80% of normal LV end-diameter, event-free survival at 7 years was 89%, vs. 26% when it was greater than 80%.[F3] Late tunnel obstruction of complex intraventricular tunnel repairs may be more likely to develop when performed in young infants.[P1]

The likelihood of reoperation for LV outflow tract (LVOT) obstruction also relates to presence of potentially obstructing infundibular muscle in the new LVOT under the patch. Dearani and colleagues have emphasized the importance of VSD enlargement and infundibular septal resection when performing the Rastelli operation.[D3] Similarly, Rubay and colleagues emphasized the importance of conal resection in the REV procedure.[R3,Y3] Yeh and colleagues have reported the advantages of the Nikaidoh procedure in preventing late LVOT obstruction. In the setting of Taussig-Bing heart with valvar or subvalvar pulmonary stenosis of sufficient severity to preclude the arterial switch operation, identification of the optimal procedure to maximize early and late survival and minimize occurrence of LVOT obstruction awaits further long-term studies.

Complications after Taussig-Bing Repair

Complications of complex intraventricular tunnel repair have been detailed in the preceding discussion. Reoperations following the arterial switch operation have also been common, most notably RV outflow tract (RVOT) obstruction, both supravalvar—likely related to insufficient mobilization of the pulmonary arteries in preparation for the Lecompte maneuver, pericardial patch shrinkage, or inadequate patch size (see Chapter 52)—and subvalvar. Alsoufi and colleagues reported a 10-year freedom from RVOT obstruction of 55%.[A3] They indicate that alterations in constructing the patch for pulmonary trunk reconstruction have reduced supravalvar obstruction. More complete resection of the subaortic RV outlet has reduced occurrence of RVOT obstruction requiring reoperation.[A3,S8] Further studies are needed to clarify the importance of these problems with current techniques.

INDICATIONS FOR OPERATION

Much of the previous information on outcomes after surgical repair of DORV is not applicable to patient care decisions in the current era, except that it permits developing equations that take into account the change in outcomes related to more recent dates of operation. Greater safety of intracardiac operations done early in life and good results of the arterial switch operation are two important factors in the improvement of current results. Improvements in myocardial management, support techniques, and intensive care unit management of neonates and infants undoubtedly play a role as well.

Recommendations for specific operations can only be general, and some cases may require special consideration. Representative strategies based on location of the VSD are presented in Table 53-7.

Simple Double Outlet Right Ventricle with Subaortic Ventricular Septal Defect

Simple DORV can be diagnosed very early in life, often by echocardiography alone. Repair should be electively planned by age 3 to 6 months, or sooner if signs of heart failure or failure to thrive persist. The operation should be intraventricular tunnel repair performed via a right atrial or, more frequently, RV approach.

When important pulmonary stenosis coexists, indications for operation and the operation are the same as for tetralogy of Fallot (see Indications for Operation in Section I of Chapter 38). Essentially, repair is advisable whenever important symptoms develop or electively, according to the same principles that apply to tetralogy of Fallot.

Double Outlet Right Ventricle with Subpulmonary Ventricular Septal Defect (Taussig-Bing Heart)

Taussig-Bing heart should be repaired by closure of the VSD so that the LV ejects into the pulmonary trunk (neoaorta), combined with an arterial switch repair. Operation should be performed during the first month of life or as soon as possible thereafter. Some surgeons continue to prefer the Kawashima procedure when the great arteries are side by side,[K2,K4] but many currently apply the arterial switch operation irrespective of great artery position.[A3,R2]

There is possibly no longer an indication for one of the intraventricular repairs for this anomaly unless there is coexisting subpulmonary obstruction of such a type and severity as to contraindicate arterial switch repair. Under these circumstances, an intraventricular tunnel repair (Kawashima) is indicated, supplemented by RV–pulmonary trunk valved conduit or a reconstruction of the type described under "Lecompte Intraventricular Repair." Nikaidoh aortic translocation and RV outflow reconstruction can also be considered in this setting. The atrial switch type of operation no longer has a place in managing this group of patients.

Operations other than those including the arterial switch repair but including an extracardiac conduit should ideally be deferred until about 3 to 6 years of age. However, if more than a single systemic-pulmonary shunt appears to be necessary in the interim, it is preferable to proceed prematurely with complete repair (see Indications for Operation in Section II of Chapter 38).

Double Outlet Right Ventricle with Doubly Committed Ventricular Septal Defect

Generally this malformation is uncomplicated by coexisting cardiac anomalies, and the rationale and timing of repair are the same as for simple DORV.

Double Outlet Right Ventricle with Noncommitted Ventricular Septal Defect

Placing a patient in the subset of DORV with noncommitted VSD is often controversial, complicating the discussion of indications. When the malformation truly seems to be of this type, repair should consist of appropriately enlarging the VSD if possible so that an intraventricular tunnel can be created to direct LV blood to the aorta. When the pulmonary trunk is obstructed by the tunnel, a RV–pulmonary trunk valved extracardiac conduit or the Lecompte procedure is added. Hu and colleagues have reported using the translocation technique for this anomaly, with a double root translocation procedure.[H5] When the anatomy dictates that the tunnel be directed to the pulmonary trunk, and if pulmonary stenosis

Table 53-7 Type of Operation for Double Outlet Right Ventricle by Ventricular Septal Defect Relation

Relationship of VSD	IVR	ASW	Senning	Fontan
Subaortic	80	0	0	4
Subpulmonary	2	27	10[a]	6
Noncommitted	14	4	0	11
AV septal defect	6	0	0	10
Doubly committed	5	0	0	0
TOTAL	107	35	6	31

From Kleinert and colleagues.[K10]
[a]Four of these patients later converted to arterial switch.
Key: *ASW,* Arterial switch operation; *AV,* atrioventricular; *IVR,* intraventricular tunnel repair; *VSD,* ventricular septal defect.

is not present, the tunnel is made and an arterial switch operation added. Alternatively, pulmonary trunk banding early in life and a subsequent Fontan operation may be considered.

SPECIAL SITUATIONS AND CONTROVERSIES

Single-Ventricle Strategy versus Biventricular Repair for Complex Double Outlet Right Ventricle

There is controversy regarding the optimal treatment strategy for certain forms of complex DORV related to the most reliable approach to achieve long-term survival, maintain good functional outcome, and minimize reoperation. Evidence-based recommendations are confounded by the large variety of anatomic variants within specific morphologic subsets (and potential importance of such variants for the conduct of and outcome after specific operations), the small number of specific operations for these anatomic variants at any given institution, the duration of follow-up needed to fully evaluate newer surgical procedures, and "philosophical" differences among institutions regarding single versus biventricular approaches. The controversial aspects relate primarily to two areas: hypoplasia of mitral valve or LV[B10,P7] and nonsubaortic VSDs that are not reparable with the arterial switch operation and simple baffling of the LV to the neoaortic valve. Bradley and colleagues have drawn attention to this controversy with an elegant analysis of nearly 400 patients[B10] in which they conclude that extending biventricular repair in "borderline anatomic candidates" may be of questionable long-term benefit compared with the Fontan pathway. Similar observations have been made by others.[D5]

In favor of the Fontan approach is its current low operative risk, low risk of reoperation, and excellent functional outcomes in most patients.[K5] This may be especially relevant given the improved results with the Fontan approach in the presence of two functioning ventricles.[J1,P5] The major limitations of the Fontan operation relate to the increasing hazard of ventricular dysfunction and heart failure after 15 to 18 years.[F2] Whether this risk will be decreased or neutralized by more current energy-efficient methods of Fontan constructions remains to be determined.[J1] It is also important to consider the reality that certain components of these "borderline anatomic variants" (e.g., modest elevation of pulmonary vascular resistance, ventricular hypertrophy, AV valve regurgitation) may represent risk factors for the Fontan operation.

The increasing late risk for reoperation and mortality after Rastelli-type operations for DORV have been well documented.[B10,K11] Late morbidity and mortality relate not only to RVOT and extracardiac conduit obstruction but also to progressive LVOT obstruction in the setting of complex intraventricular baffles (see preceding text under Results). However, encouraging early and midterm results are emerging from newer procedures such as the REV procedure,[L2] Nikaidoh procedure,[N3] and single and double root translocation operations (see also previous discussions under Technique of Operation and Results), as well as modifications of baffling techniques,[D6] that provide some optimism for improved late survival and freedom from reoperation.[A8] For example, Devaney and colleagues[D6] reported biventricular repairs in 12 patients with AV septal defect with an interventricular communication remote from the aortic valve in the presence of a muscular subaortic infundibulum. There were 11 early and 10 late survivors. Infundibular resection and a complex extended intraventricular baffle contributed to absence of late LV outflow obstruction.

Until appropriate short- and longer-term outcome analyses are available, coupled with experiential insights, selection of one- or two-ventricle strategies for many of these complex variants will remain a function of institutional bias and surgeon preference.

REFERENCES

A

1. Agarwala B, Doyle EF, Danilowicz D, Spencer FC, Mills NM. Double outlet right ventricle with pulmonic stenosis and anteriorly positioned aorta (Taussig-Bing variant). Am J Cardiol 1973;32:850.
2. Ainger LE. Double outlet right ventricle, intact ventricular septum, mitral stenosis and blind left ventricle. Am Heart J 1965;70:521.
3. Alsoufi B, Cai S, Williams WG, Coles JG, Caldarone CA, Redington AM, et al. Improved results with single-stage total correction of Taussig-Bing anomaly. Eur J Cardiothorac Surg 2008;33:244-50.
4. Anderson RH, Becker AE, Wilcox BR, Macartney FJ, Wilkinson JL. Surgical anatomy of double-outlet right ventricle—a reappraisal. Am J Cardiol 1983;52:555.
5. Anderson RH, Ho SY, Wilcox BR. The surgical anatomy of ventricular septal defect part IV: double outlet ventricle. J Card Surg 1996;11:2.
6. Anderson RH, Pickering D, Brown R. Double outlet right ventricle with L-malposition and uncommitted ventricular septal defect. Eur J Cardiol 1975;3/2:133.
7. Angelini P, Leachman RD. Spectrum of double outlet right ventricle: an embryologic interpretation. Card Dis Bull Texas Heart Inst 1976;3:127.
8. Artrip JH, Sauer H, Campbell DN, Mitchell MB, Haun C, Almodovar MC, et al. Biventricular repair in double outlet right ventricle: surgical results based on the STS-EACTS International Nomenclature classification. Eur J Cardio-thorac Surg 2006;29: 545-50.
9. Azevedo de AC, Toledo AN, deCarvalho AA, Rowbach R. Transposition of the aorta and levoposition of the pulmonary artery (Taussig-Bing syndrome). Am Heart J 1956;52:249-56.

B

1. Baron MG. Radiologic notes in cardiology: angiographic differentiation between tetralogy of Fallot and double outlet right ventricle. Circulation 1971;43:451.
2. Barratt-Boyes BG, Calder AL. Double outlet ventricle: classification and surgical management. In: Davila JC, ed. Second Henry Ford Hospital International Symposium on Cardiac Surgery. East Norwalk, Conn: Appleton & Lange, 1977, p. 49.
3. Barratt-Boyes BG, Lowe JB, Watt WJ, Cole DS, Williams JC. Initial experiences with extracorporeal circulation in intracardiac surgery. BMJ 1960;2:1826.
4. Belli E, Serraf A, Lacour-Gayet F, Prodan S, Piot D, Losay J, et al. Biventricular repair for double outlet right ventricle: results and long-term follow-up. Circulation 1998;98:II360.
5. Beuren A. Differential diagnosis of the Taussig-Bing heart from complete transposition of the great vessels with a posterior overriding pulmonary artery. Circulation 1960;21:1071.
6. Bex JP, Lecompte Y, Baillot F, Hazan E. Anatomical correction of transposition of the great arteries. Ann Thorac Surg 1980;29:86.
7. Bharati S, Kirklin JW, McAllister HA Jr, Lev M. The surgical anatomy of common atrioventricular orifice associated with tetralogy of Fallot, double outlet right ventricle and complete regular transposition. Circulation 1980;61:1142.
8. Bharati S, Lev M. The conduction system in double outlet right ventricle with subpulmonic ventricular septal defect and related hearts (the Taussig-Bing group). Circulation 1976;54:459.
9. Borromee L, Lecompte Y, Batisse A, Lemoine G, Vouhe P, Sakata R, et al. Anatomic repair of anomalies of ventriculoarterial connection associated with ventricular septal defect. II. Clinical results in 50 patients with pulmonary outflow tract obstruction. J Thorac Cardiovasc Surg 1988;95:96.

10. Bradley TJ, Karamlou T, Kulik A, Mitrovic B, Vigneswaran T, Jaffer S, et al. Determinants of repair type, reintervention, and mortality in 393 children with double-outlet right ventricle. J Thorac Cardiovasc Surg 2007;134:967-73.
11. Brandt PS, Calder AL, Barratt-Boyes BG, Neutze JM. Double outlet left ventricle: morphology, cineangiography, diagnosis, and surgical treatment. Am J Cardiol 1976;38:897.
12. Brandt PW. Cineangiography of atrioventricular and ventriculo-arterial connections. In: Pediatric cardiology. Vol. 4. London: Churchill Livingstone, 1981, p. 191.
13. Braun K, De Vries A, Feingold DS, Ehrenfeld NE, Feldman J, Schorr S. Complete dextroposition of the aorta, pulmonary stenosis, interventricular septal defect, and patent foramen ovale. Am Heart J 1952;43:773.
14. Brown JW, Ruzmetov M, Okada Y, Vijay P, Turrentine MW. Surgical results in patients with double outlet right ventricle: a 20-year experience. Ann Thorac Surg 2001;72:1630.

C

1. Capuani A, Uemura H, Ho SY, Anderson RH. Anatomic spectrum of abnormal ventriculoarterial connections: surgical implications. Ann Thorac Surg 1995;59:352.
2. Cheng TO. Double outlet right ventricle: diagnosis during life. Am J Med 1962;32:637.
3. Cherian KM, John TA, Abraham KA. Transatrial correction of origin of both great vessels from right ventricle with pulmonary hypertension. J Thorac Cardiovasc Surg 1982;84:783.
4. Chiechi MA. Incomplete transposition of the great vessels with biventricular origin of the pulmonary artery (Taussig-Bing complex): report of 4 cases and review of the literature. Am J Med 1957; 22:234.

D

1. Daicoff GR, Kirklin JW. Surgical correction of Taussig-Bing malformation. Report of three cases (abstract). Am J Cardiol 1967;19:125.
2. Danielson GK, Ritter DG, Coleman HN III, DuShane JW. Successful repair of double-outlet right ventricle with transposition of the great arteries (aorta anterior and to the left), pulmonary stenosis, and subaortic ventricular septal defect. J Thorac Cardiovasc Surg 1972;63:741.
3. Dearani JA, Danielson GK, Puga FJ, Mair DD, Schleck CD. Late results of the Rastelli operation for transposition of the great arteries. Semin Thorac Cardiovasc Surg Pediatr Card Surg Annu 2001;4:3-15.
4. de la Cruz MV, Berrazueta JR, Artega M, Attie F, Soni J. Rules for diagnosis of atrioventricular discordance and spatial identification of ventricles. Br Heart J 1976;38:341.
5. Delius RE, Rademecker MA, de Leval MR, Elliott MJ, Stark J. Is a high-risk biventricular repair always preferable to conversion to a single ventricle repair? J Thorac Cardiovasc Surg 1996;112: 1561-9.
6. Devaney EJ, Lee T, Gelehrter S, Hirsch JC, Ohye RG, Anderson RH, et al. Biventricular repair of atrioventricular septal defect with common atrioventricular valve and double-outlet right ventricle. Ann Thorac Surg 2010;89:537-43.
7. Doty DB. Correction of Taussig-Bing malformation by intraventricular conduit. J Thorac Cardiovasc Surg 1986;91:133.

E

1. Edwards WD. Double-outlet right ventricle and tetralogy of Fallot. Two distinct but not mutually exclusive entities (editorial). J Thorac Cardiovasc Surg 1981;82:418.
2. Edwards WD, Wilcox WD, Danielson GK, Feldt RH. Postoperative false aneurysm of left ventricle and obstruction of left circumflex coronary artery complicating enlargement of restrictive ventricular septal defect in double-outlet right ventricle. J Thorac Cardiovasc Surg 1980;80:141.
3. Elliott LP, Amplatz K, Edwards JE. Coronary arterial patterns in transposition complexes: anatomic and angiocardiographic studies. Am J Cardiol 1966;17:362.
4. Engle MA, Holswade GR, Campbell WG, Goldberg HP. Ventricular septal defect with transposition of aorta masquerading as acyanotic ventricular septal defect (abstract). Circulation 1960;22:745.
5. Engle MA, Steinberg I. Angiocardiography in diagnosis of transposition of aorta with subaortic ventricular septal defect (origin of both great vessels from right ventricle) (abstract). Circulation 1961;24:927.

F

1. Feng B, Liu Y, Hu S, Shen X, Wang X, Wang H, et al. Arterial switch for transposition of the great vessels and Taussig-Bing anomaly after six months of age. Ann Thorac Surg 2009;88: 1948-51.
2. Fontan F, Kirklin JW, Fernandez G, Costa F, Naftel DC, Tritto F, et al. Outcome after a "perfect" Fontan operation. Circulation 1990;81:1520-36.
3. Fujii Y, Kotani Y, Takagaki M, Arai S, Kasahara S, Otsuki S, et al. The impact of the length between the top of the interventricular septum and the aortic valve on the indications for a biventricular repair in patients with a transposition of the great arteries or a double outlet right ventricle. Interact Cardiovasc Thorac Surg 2010;10:900-5.

G

1. Golan M, Hegesh J, Massini C, Goor DA. Double-outlet right ventricle associated with discrete subaortic stenosis. Pediatr Cardiol 1984;5:157.
2. Gomes MM, Weidman WH, McGoon DC, Danielson GK. Double-outlet right ventricle without pulmonic stenosis: surgical considerations and results of operation. Circulation 1971;43:I31.
3. Goor DA, Massini C, Shem-Tov A, Neufeld HN. Transatrial repair of double-outlet right ventricle in infants. Thorax 1982;37:371.
4. Griselli M, McGuirk SP, Ko CS, Clarke AJ, Barron DJ, Brawn WJ. Arterial switch operation in patients with Taussig-Bing anomaly—influence of staged repair and coronary anatomy on outcome. Eur J Cardiothorac Surg 2007;31:229-35.

H

1. Hagler DJ, Tajik AJ, Seward JB, Mair DD, Ritter DQ. Double outlet right ventricle. Wide angle two-dimensional echocardiographic observations. Circulation 1983;63:419.
2. Hightower BM, Barcia A, Bargeron LM, Kirklin JW. Double-outlet right ventricle with transposed great arteries and subpulmonary ventricular septal defect: the Taussig-Bing malformation. Circulation 1969;49/50:I207.
3. Hinkes P, Rosenquist GC, White RI Jr. Roentgenographic reexamination of the internal anatomy of the Taussig-Bing heart. Am Heart J 1971;81:335.
4. Howell CE, Ho SY, Anderson RH, Elliott MJ. Fibrous skeleton and ventricular outflow tracts in double-outlet right ventricle. Ann Thorac Surg 1991;51:394.
5. Hu S, Xie Y, Li S, Wang X, Yan F, Li Y, et al. Double-root translocation for double-outlet right ventricle with noncommitted ventricular septal defect or double-outlet right ventricle with subpulmonary ventricular septal defect associated with pulmonary stenosis: an optimized solution. Ann Thorac Surg 2010;89:1360-5.

I

1. Ionescu MI, Scott O, Wooler GH. Surgical treatment of acyanotic double-outlet right ventricle. Thorax 1976;22:336.
2. Iwai S, Ichikawa H, Fukushima N, Sawa Y. Left ventricular outflow tract after Kawashima intraventricular rerouting. Asian Cardiovasc Thorac Ann 2007;15:367-70.

J

1. Jacobs ML, Norwood WI Jr. Fontan operation: influence of modifications on morbidity and mortality. Ann Thorac Surg 1994;58: 945-52.
2. Judson JP, Danielson GK, Ritter DG, Hagler DJ. Successful repair of coexisting double-outlet right ventricle and two-chambered right ventricle. J Thorac Cardiovasc Surg 1982;84:113.

K

1. Kanter K, Anderson R, Lincoln C, Firmin R, Rigby M. Anatomic correction of double-outlet right ventricle with subpulmonary ventricular septal defect (the "Taussig-Bing" anomaly). Ann Thorac Surg 1986;41:287.
2. Kawahira Y, Yagihara T, Uemura H, Ishizaka T, Yoshikawa Y, Yoshizumi K, et al. Ventricular outflow tracts after Kawashima intraventricular rerouting for double outlet right ventricle with

subpulmonary ventricular septal defect. Eur J Cardiothorac Surg 1999;16:26-31.

3. Kawashima Y, Fujita T, Miyamoto T, Manabe H. Intraventricular rerouting of blood for the correction of Taussig-Bing malformation. J Thorac Cardiovasc Surg 1971;62:825.
4. Kawashima Y, Matsuda H, Yagihara T, Shimazaki Y, Yamamoto F, Nishigaki K, et al. Intraventricular repair for Taussig-Bing anomaly. J Thorac Cardiovasc Surg 1993;105:591-7.
5. Kirklin JK, Brown RN, Bryant AS, Naftel DC, Colvin EV, Pearce FB, et al. Is the "perfect Fontan" operation routinely achievable in the modern era? Cardiol Young 2008;18:328-36.
6. Kirklin JK, Castaneda AR. Surgical correction of double-outlet right ventricle with noncommitted ventricular septal defect. J Thorac Cardiovasc Surg 1977;73:399.
7. Kirklin JW, Harp RA, McGoon DC. Surgical treatment of origin of both vessels from right ventricle, including cases of pulmonary stenosis. J Thorac Cardiovasc Surg 1964;48:1026.
8. Kirklin JW, Pacifico AD, Blackstone EH, Kirklin JK, Bargeron LM Jr. Current risks and protocols for operations for double-outlet right ventricle. J Thorac Cardiovasc Surg 1986;92:913.
9. Kitamura N, Takao A, Ando M, Imai Y, Konno S. Taussig-Bing heart with mitral valve straddling. Circulation 1974;49:761.
10. Kleinert S, Sano T, Weintraub RG, Mee RB, Karl TR, Wilkinson JL. Anatomic features and surgical strategies in double outlet right ventricle. Circulation 1997;96:1233.
11. Kreutzer C, De Vive J, Oppido G, Kreutzer J, Gauvreau K, Freed M, et al. Twenty-five-year experience with rastelli repair for transposition of the great arteries. J Thorac Cardiovasc Surg 2000; 120:211-23.

L

1. Lavoie R, Sestier F, Gilbert G, Chameides L, Van Praagh R, Grondin P. Double outlet right ventricle with left ventricular outflow tract obstruction due to small ventricular septal defect. Am Heart J 1971;82:290.
2. Lecompte Y, Neveux JY, Leca F, Zannini L, Tu TV, Duboys Y, et al. Reconstruction of the pulmonary outflow tract without prosthetic conduit. J Thorac Cardiovasc Surg 1982;84:727.
3. Lev M, Bharati S. Transposition of the arterial trunks in levocardia. In: Sommers SC, ed. Cardiovascular pathology decennial 1966-1975. East Norwalk, Conn: Appleton & Lange, 1975, p. 30.
4. Lev M, Bharati S, Meng CCL, Liberthson RR, Paul MH, Idriss F. A concept of double-outlet right ventricle. J Thorac Cardiovasc Surg 1972;64:271.
5. Lev M, Rimoldi HJ, Eckner FA, Melhuish BP, Meng L, Paul MH. The Taussig-Bing heart: qualitative and quantitative anatomy. Arch Pathol 1966;81:24.
6. Liddicoat JR, Reddy VM, Hanley FL. New approach to great-vessel reconstruction in transposition complexes with interrupted aortic arch. Ann Thorac Surg 1994;58:1146.
7. Lincoln C. Total correction of D-loop double-outlet right ventricle with bilateral conus, L-transposition, and pulmonic stenosis. J Thorac Cardiovasc Surg 1972;64:435.
8. Lincoln C, Anderson RH, Shinebourne EA, English TA, Wilkinson JL. Double outlet right ventricle with L-malposition of the aorta. Br Heart J 1975;37:453.
9. Lopez FN, Dobben GG, Rabinowitz M, Ferguson LA, Reisler H, Cassels DE, et al. Taussig-Bing complex with pulmonary stenosis. Dis Chest 1966;50:1.
10. Luber JM, Castaneda AR, Lang P, Norwood WI. Repair of double-outlet right ventricle: early and late results. Circulation 1983;68:II144.
11. Luisi VS, Pasque A, Verunelli F, Eufrate S. Double outlet right ventricle, non-committed ventricular septal defect and pulmonic stenosis. Anatomical and surgical considerations. Thorac Cardiovasc Surg 1980;28:368.

M

1. Macartney FJ, Rigby ML, Anderson RH, Stark J, Silverman NH. Double outlet right ventricle. Cross sectional echocardiographic findings, their anatomical explanation, and surgical relevance. Br Heart J 1984;52:164.
2. Marin-Garcia J, Neches WH, Park SC, Lenox CC, Zuberbuhler JR, Bahnson HT. Double-outlet right ventricle with restrictive ventricular septal defect. J Thorac Cardiovasc Surg 1978;76:853.
3. Marino B, Loperfido F, Sardi CS. Spontaneous closure of ventricular septal defect in a case of double outlet right ventricle. Br Heart J 1983;49:608.
4. Mason DT, Morrow AG, Elkins RC, Friedman WF. Origin of both great vessels from the right ventricle associated with severe obstruction to left ventricular outflow. Am J Cardiol 1969;24: 118.
5. Masuda M, Kado H, Shiokawa Y, Fukae K, Kanegae Y, Kawachi Y, et al. Clinical results of arterial switch operation for double-outlet right ventricle with subpulmonary stenosis. Eur J Cardiothorac Surg 1999;15:283.
6. Mavroudis C, Backer CL, Munster AJ, Rocchini AP, Rees AH, Gevitz M. Taussig-Bing anomaly: arterial switch versus Kawashima intraventricular repair. Ann Thorac Surg 1996;61:1330.
7. McMahon JE, Lips M. Double outlet right ventricle with intact ventricular septum. Circulation 1964;30:745.
8. Mehrizi A. The origin of both great vessels from the right ventricle. I. With pulmonic stenosis. Clinico-pathological correlation in 18 autopsied cases; 11 without pulmonic stenosis. Clinico-pathological correlation in 13 autopsied cases. Bull Johns Hopkins Hosp 1965;117:75.
9. Metras D, Coulibaly AO, Ouattara K. Successful intraventricular repair of Taussig-Bing anomaly in infancy. Report of a case. J Thorac Cardiovasc Surg 1984;88:311.
10. Muster AJ, Bharati S, Aziz KU, Idriss FS, Paul MH, Lev M, et al. Taussig-Bing anomaly with straddling mitral valve. J Thorac Cardiovasc Surg 1979;77:832.

N

1. Neufeld HN, DuShane JW, Wood EH, Kirklin JW, Edwards JE. Origin of both great vessels from the right ventricle. I. Without pulmonary stenosis. Circulation 1961;23:399.
2. Neufeld HN, Lucas RV, Lester RG, Adams P, Anderson RC, Edwards JE. Origin of both great vessels from the right ventricle without pulmonary stenosis. Br Heart J 1962;24:393.
3. Nikaidoh H. Aortic translocation and biventricular outflow tract reconstruction. A new surgical repair for transposition of the great arteries associated with ventricular septal defect and pulmonary stenosis. J Thorac Cardiovasc Surg 1984;88:365.

O

1. Ottino G, Kugler JD, McNamara DG, Hallman GL. Taussig-Bing anomaly: total repair with closure of ventricular septal defect through the pulmonary artery. Ann Thorac Surg 1980;29:170.

P

1. Pacifico AD, Kirklin JK, Colvin EV, Bargeron LM Jr. Intraventricular tunnel repair for Taussig-Bing heart and related cardiac anomalies. Circulation 1986;74:153.
2. Parr GV, Bharati S, Lev M, Waldhausen JA. Fetal coarctation in complete transposition of the great arteries with ventricular septal defect vs. Taussig-Bing group of hearts. Surgical significance (abstract). Circulation 1982;66:II195.
3. Patrick DL, McGoon DC. Operation for double-outlet right ventricle with transposition of the great arteries. J Cardiovasc Surg 1968;9:537.
4. Paul MH, Van Praagh S, Van Praagh R. Transposition of the great arteries. In: Watson H, ed. Paediatric cardiology. London: Lloyd-Luke, 1968, p. 576.
5. Pearl JM, Laks H, Drinkwater DC, Capouya ER, George BL, Williams RG. Modified Fontan procedure in patients less than 4 years of age. Circulation 1992;86:II100-5.
6. Piccoli G, Pacifico AD, Kirklin JW, Blackstone EH, Kirklin JK, Bargeron LM Jr. Changing results and concepts in the surgical treatment of double-outlet right ventricle: analysis of 137 operations in 126 patients. Am J Cardiol 1983;52:549.
7. Pitkanen OM, Hornberger LK, Miner SE, Mondal T, Smallhorn JF, Jaeggi E, et al. Borderline left ventricles in prenatally diagnosed atrioventricular septal defect or double outlet right ventricle: echocardiographic predictors of biventricular repair. Am Heart J 2006;152:163.

Q

1. Quaegebeur JM. The optimal repair for the Taussig-Bing heart (editorial). J Thorac Cardiovasc Surg 1983;85:276.

2. Quaegebeur JM, Bartelings M, Gittenberger-DeGroot AC. Double outlet right ventricle with subpulmonary ventricular septal defect: an anatomical basis for surgical repair. Pediatr Cardiol 1984;5:234.

R

1. Redo SF, Engle MA, Holswade GR, Goldbert HP. Operative correction of ventricular septal defect with origin of both great vessels from the right ventricle. J Thorac Cardiovasc Surg 1963;45:526.
2. Rodefeld MD, Ruzmetov M, Vijay P, Fiore AC, Turrentine MW, Brown JW. Surgical results of arterial switch operation for Taussig-Bing anomaly: is position of the great arteries a risk factor? Ann Thorac Surg 2007;83:1451-7.
3. Rubay J, Lecompte Y, Batisse A, Durandy Y, Dibie A, Lemoine G, et al. Anatomic repair of anomalies of ventriculo-arterial connection (REV). Eur J Cardiothorac Surg 1988;2:305.

S

1. Sakata R, Lecompte Y, Batisse A, Borromee L, Durandy Y. Anatomic repair of anomalies of ventriculoarterial connection associated with ventricular septal defect. I. Criteria of surgical decision. J Thorac Cardiovasc Surg 1988;95:90.
2. Sanders SP, Bierman FZ, Williams RG. Conotruncal malformations: diagnosis in infancy using subxiphoid two-dimensional echocardiography. Am J Cardiol 1982;50:1361.
3. Serraf A, Lacour-Gayet F, Bruniaux J, Losay J, Petit J, Touchot-Kone A, et al. Anatomic repair of Taussig-Bing hearts. Circulation 1991;84:III200.
4. Serraf A, Lacour-Gayet F, Houyel L, Bruniaux J, Sousa-Uva MS, Roux D, et al. Subaortic obstruction in double-outlet right ventricles. Surgical considerations for anatomic repair. Circulation 1993;88:II177.
5. Serraf A, Nakamura T, Lacour-Gayet F, Piot D, Bruniaux J, Touchot A, et al. Surgical approaches for double-outlet right ventricle or transposition of the great arteries associated with straddling atrioventricular valves. J Thorac Cardiovasc Surg 1996;111:527.
6. Shafer AB, Lopez JF, Kline IK, Lev M. Truncal inversion with biventricular pulmonary trunk and aorta from right ventricle (variant of Taussig-Bing complex). Circulation 1967;36:783.
7. Shin'oka T, Kurosawa H, Imai Y, Aoki M, Ishiyama M, Sakamoto T, et al. Outcomes of definitive surgical repair for congenitally corrected transposition of the great arteries or double outlet right ventricle with discordant atrioventricular connections: risk analyses in 189 patients. J Thorac Cardiovasc Surg 2007;133:1318-28.
8. Sinzobahamvya N, Blaschczok HC, Asfour B, Arenz C, Jussli MJ, Schindler E, et al. Right ventricular outflow tract obstruction after arterial switch operation for the Taussig-Bing heart. Eur J Cardiothorac Surg 2007;31:873-8.
9. Sondheimer HM, Freedom RM, Olley PM. Double outlet right ventricle: clinical spectrum and prognosis. Am J Cardiol 1977; 39:709.
10. Sridaromont S, Feldt RH, Ritter DG, Davis GD, McGoon DC, Edwards JE. Double-outlet right ventricle associated with persistent common atrioventricular canal. Circulation 1975;52:933.
11. Sridaromont S, Ritter DG, Feldt RH, Davis GD, Edwards JE. Double-outlet right ventricle. Anatomic and angiocardiographic correlations. Mayo Clin Proc 1978;53:555.
12. Stellin G, Zuberbuhler JR, Anderson RH, Siewers RD. The surgical anatomy of the Taussig-Bing malformation. J Thorac Cardiovasc Surg 1987;93:560.
13. Stewart RW, Kirklin JW, Pacifico AD, Blackstone EH, Bargeron LM Jr. Repair of double outlet right ventricle. An analysis of 62 cases. J Thorac Cardiovasc Surg 1979;78:502.
14. Stewart S. Double-outlet right ventricle (S,D,D), VSD related to pulmonary artery, and pulmonic stenosis absent. Correction with an intraventricular conduit in infancy. J Thorac Cardiovasc Surg 1977;74:70.

T

1. Taussig HB, Bing RJ. Complete transposition of the aorta and a levoposition of the pulmonary artery. Am Heart J 1949;37:551.

U

1. Ueda M, Becker AE. Classification of hearts with overriding aortic and pulmonary valves. Int J Cardiol 1985;9:357.
2. Uemura H, Yagihara T, Kawashima Y, Nishigaki K, Kamiya T, Ho SY, et al. Coronary arterial anatomy in double-outlet right ventricle with subpulmonary VSD. Ann Thorac Surg 1995;59:591.

V

1. Van Praagh R. What is the Taussig-Bing malformation? (editorial). Circulation 1968;38:445.
2. Van Praagh R. Normally and abnormally related great arteries: what have we learned? World J Pediatr Congenital Heart Surg 2010;1:364-85.
3. Van Praagh R, Perez-Trevino C, Reynolds JL, Moes CA, Keith JD, Roy DL, et al. Double outlet right ventricle (S,D,L) with subaortic ventricular septal defect and pulmonary stenosis. Pediatr Cardiol 1975;35:42.
4. Vouhe PR, Tamisier D, Leca F, Ouaknine R, Vernant F, Neveux JY. Transposition of the great arteries, ventricular septal defect and pulmonary outflow tract obstruction: Rastelli or Lecompte procedure? J Thorac Cardiovasc Surg 1992;103:428.

W

1. Wedemeyer AL, Lucas RV Jr, Castaneda AR. Taussig-Bing malformation, coarctation of the aorta, and reversed patent ductus arteriosus. Circulation 1970;42:1021.
2. Wilcox BR, Ho SY, Macartney FJ, Becker AE, Gelis LM, Anderson RH. Surgical anatomy of double-outlet right ventricle with situs solitus and atrioventricular concordance. J Thorac Cardiovasc Surg 1981;82:405.
3. Witham AC. Double outlet right ventricle: a partial transposition complex. Am Heart J 1957;53:928.

Y

1. Yacoub MH, Radley-Smith R. Anatomic correction of the Taussig-Bing anomaly. J Thorac Cardiovasc Surg 1984;88:380.
2. Yamaguchi M, Horikoshi K, Toriyama A, Kimura K, Mito H, Tei G, et al. Successful repair of double-outlet right ventricle with bilateral conus, L-transposition of great arteries (S,D,L), and subpulmonary ventricular septal defect. J Thorac Cardiovasc Surg 1976;71:366.
3. Yeh T Jr, Ramaciotti C, Leonard SR, Roy L, Nikaidoh H. The aortic translocation (Nikaidoh) procedure: midterm results superior to the Rastelli procedure. J Thorac Cardiovasc Surg 2007;133: 461-9.

54 Double Outlet Left Ventricle

DEFINITION

Double outlet left ventricle (DOLV) is a cardiac anomaly in which both great arteries arise from the left ventricle (LV).[1] The great arteries are assigned to one or the other ventricle by the rules described under Definition in Chapter 53.

DOLV may occur with atrioventricular (AV) concordant or discordant connection, as does double outlet right ventricle (DORV; see Chapter 53). DOLV with AV discordant connection is discussed in Chapter 55. DOLV, like DORV, may also occur in patients with univentricular AV connections (see Chapter 56) and in those with atrial isomerism (see Chapter 58).

HISTORICAL NOTE

Marechal is credited with describing the first case of DOLV in 1819, but this was in a heart with double inlet LV with an infundibular outlet chamber.[M1] The first reported case in a heart with two ventricles and without pulmonary stenosis was that of Sakakibara and colleagues in 1967, for which they performed a successful intraventricular repair.[S1] DOLV is therefore another congenital cardiac anomaly that remained, for all practical purposes, undescribed until the advent of intracardiac surgery. It is also of interest that the first case reported by Potts and colleagues as tetralogy of Fallot and receiving a side-to-side aortopulmonary artery anastomosis[P3] underwent subsequent repair for well-documented DOLV with pulmonary stenosis (John Kirklin: personal communication; 1983). A unique case of DOLV with an intact ventricular septum was reported by Paul and colleagues in 1970, establishing with certainty the existence of the entity.[P2] Subsequent reports expanded the surgical possibilities by reporting reconstruction of the pulmonary pathway in cases in which a completely intraventricular repair was not possible, usually by a valved extracardiac conduit from the right ventricle to pulmonary trunk.[K1,P1] Anderson and colleagues reported the sixth case of DOLV in 1974.[A1] Sharratt and colleagues in 1976 reported use of a Fontan-type procedure in hearts with DOLV and severe right ventricular hypoplasia.[S2]

Five cases were added to the literature in 1976.[B3] Additional cases have been reported by Urban and colleagues and Stegmann and colleagues.[S4,U1]

MORPHOLOGY AND MORPHOGENESIS

As with DORV, there is great variability among hearts with DOLV and AV concordant connection. Because of its rarity, generalizations are even more difficult than for DORV.

[1]The adjectives *left* and *right* used to modify atrium or ventricle mean *morphologically* left and *morphologically* right. *Position* of the chamber is referred to as *right-sided* or *left-sided*.

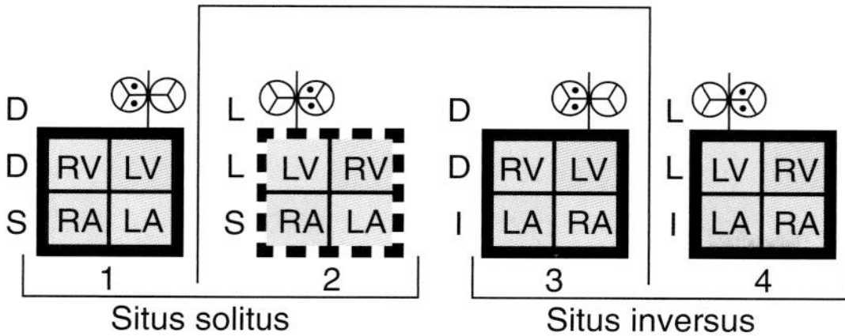

Figure 54-1 Models of the four basic hearts as they occur in double outlet left ventricle, depicting usual positions of great arteries (aorta medial to pulmonary trunk). Models 2 and 3 depict atrioventricular discordant connection. In the Van Praagh convention, first letter (S or I) refers to atrial position (solitus or inversus), second letter (D or L) to ventricular loop (right or left), and third letter to position of origin of aorta relative to origin of pulmonary trunk (see Appendix 1H in Chapter 1). Key: *LA,* Left atrium; *LV,* left ventricle; *RA,* right atrium; *RV,* right ventricle.

Diagnosis can be ambiguus, because some override of one of the great arteries is commonly present. Defining a DOLV based on 50% or more of great arterial override may result in a substantially higher number of cases being reported. Many patients with complete transposition of the great arteries with subaortic ventricular septal defect (VSD), pulmonary stenosis, and a variable degree of aortic override have been misclassified as having DOLV. An exclusive or near-exclusive origin of both great arteries from the left ventricle (<20% override) will identify the classic form of DOLV and prevent misdiagnosis.[M4] Although it was initially thought bilateral absent conus was a prerequisite for the diagnosis of DOLV, all possible conal configurations have been described: subpulmonic, subaortic, bilaterally present, and bilaterally absent. When present, the length of conus under either great artery is typically relatively short and is an important factor in causing the great artery to embryologically align with the left ventricle.[V1]

A segmental approach is necessary for complete understanding of this malformation (see "Terminology and Classification of Heart Disease" in Chapter 1).[B3,V2] DOLV occurs in each of the four basic hearts (Fig. 54-1) but is most common in hearts with atrial situs solitus and ventricular right-handedness or D-loop (S,D,D).[B2,M4] Morphologic characteristics of the VSD and its relationship to the great arteries at the level of the semilunar valves are similar to those in DORV and described by terms defined in "Ventricular Septal Defect" under Morphology in Chapter 53. Subaortic VSD is the most common, followed by subpulmonic, and then by doubly committed. VSD remote from the great arteries is rare[M4] (Table 54-1). Absence of a VSD (intact ventricular septum) is also rare but has been described.[B1]

Atrial Situs Solitus and Ventricular Right-Handedness (D-Loop) (Atrioventricular Concordant Connection)

In this subset, the aorta is usually in D-malposition (S,D,D), but examples occur with it in L-malposition (S,D,L) (see "Symbolic Convention of Van Praagh" in Chapter 1). In the former, the great arteries may appear in relatively normal position (aorta to the right and somewhat posterior to pulmonary trunk), side to side, or with aorta somewhat anterior to the pulmonary trunk.[B2]

Table 54-1 Double Outlet Left Ventricle with Situs Solitus and Atrioventricular Concordance in 71 Patients

Type	Frequency (%)
Subaortic VSD:	73
Right anterior aorta with pulmonary stenosis	49
Left anterior aorta with pulmonary stenosis	24
Subpulmonary VSD with right anterior aorta	15
Doubly committed VSD with right anterior aorta	10
Remote VSD with left anterior aorta	1

Data from Menon and Hagler.[M4]
Key: *VSD,* Ventricular septal defect.

Ventricular Septal Defect

The ventricular septum is rarely intact.[P2] Usually, a large VSD is present and lies between the limbs of the trabecula septomarginalis (septal band).

Most commonly, the VSD is *subaortic* in position (Fig. 54-2; see Table 54-1). It may extend back to the tricuspid anulus, or it may be separated from the anulus by a muscular bridge.[B2] When the aorta overrides the VSD and arises in part from the right ventricle, the VSD is *juxtaaortic,* and this entity begins to merge with transposition of the great arteries.

When the VSD is subpulmonary, it is usually more anterior and well separated from the tricuspid valve by a rather wide band of muscle. In some cases, the pulmonary trunk origin overrides the VSD and lies in part over the right ventricle. Malalignment of conal septum may be present and can cause aortic outflow obstruction and be associated with aortic arch hypoplasia.[M4]

Occasionally the VSD is juxtaarterial and lies immediately below both great arteries (*doubly committed;* see Chapter 53, Fig. 53-6). The VSD is typically very large, and there is absence or near absence of conus bilaterally, resulting in aortic-mitral and pulmonary-mitral fibrous continuity and side-by-side great arteries. It is frequently difficult to decide whether DOLV or DORV is present, in which case the term *double outlet both ventricles* is appropriate.[B3]

Conal Pattern

Most often there is absence of a subaortic conus and presence of aortic-mitral fibrous continuity and a subpulmonary conus displaced into the LV (Fig. 54-3). Rarely, bilaterally absent conus permits aortic-mitral-tricuspid and pulmonary-tricuspid fibrous continuity (see Fig. 54-2). In this event, both semilunar valves arise at the same level. Very rarely, only a subaortic conus is present. There may be a conus bilaterally.

Pulmonary Stenosis

Pulmonary stenosis is present in most cases and is either valvar (sometimes with anular stenosis) or subvalvar when it is due to a restrictive subpulmonary conus with secondary fibrosis of the ostium. When the VSD is subaortic and there is infundibular pulmonary stenosis, the great arteries are usually relatively normally interrelated.[B2]

Right Ventricular and Tricuspid Valve Hypoplasia

There is a tendency for the right ventricular sinus and tricuspid valve to be at least somewhat hypoplastic.[B2] The

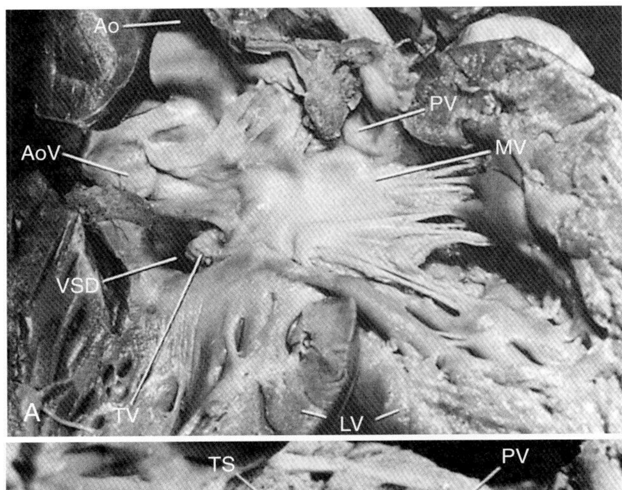

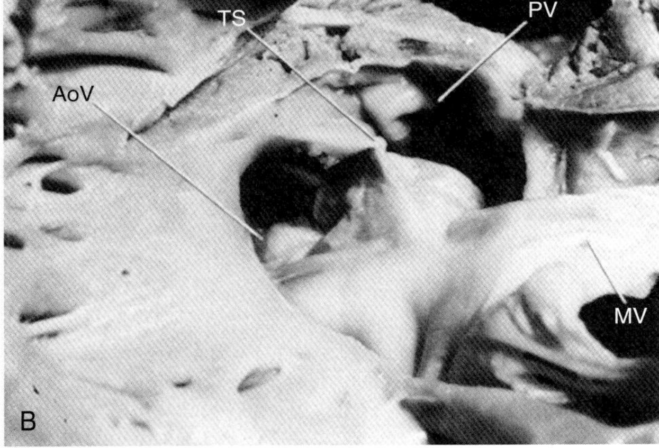

Figure 54-2 Specimen of double outlet left ventricle and atrioventricular concordant connection. **A,** Viewed from opened left ventricle *(LV)* and aorta *(Ao)*. Aortic valve *(AoV)* is bicuspid but otherwise normal. Ventricular septal defect *(VSD)* is subaortic, with its upper margin separated from AoV by 4 mm. Tricuspid valve *(TV)* is visible through VSD (Ebstein anomaly of tricuspid valve is present). **B,** Close-up of LV outflow tract before aorta was opened. Pulmonary valve *(PV)* is not stenotic, and AoV and PV are in continuity, separated only by a thin fibrous ridge called the *truncal septum (TS)*. There is both PV and aortic–mitral valve *(MV)* fibrous continuity (i.e., conus is absent bilaterally). (From Brandt and colleagues.[B3])

extreme example is coexistence of tricuspid atresia, with the two reported cases having ventricular right-handedness (S,D,D).[V2,V3] Rarely, the tricuspid valve may show an Ebstein anomaly.[B3]

Left Ventricle

The LV is usually well formed. One case of mitral atresia with large LV and infundibular outlet chamber (S,D,D segmental arrangement) has been reported.[V2]

Conduction System

Position of AV node and bundle of His is normal. Thus, the bundle penetrates from a normally positioned posterior AV node through the right trigone in the region of the commissure between tricuspid septal and anterior leaflets and at the base of the noncoronary aortic cusp, and its two branches distribute in normal fashion. Whether it is at risk during repair depends on the relationship of the lower VSD margin to the tricuspid anulus (see "Location in Septum and Relationship to Conduction System" under Morphology in Section 1 of Chapter 35).

Atrial Situs Inversus and Ventricular Left-Handedness (L-Loop) (Atrioventricular Concordant Connection)

Both I,L,L and I,L,D arrangements have been reported (i.e., aorta to the left or right), although both are rare. Usually the VSD is subaortic, and pulmonary stenosis coexists.

CLINICAL FEATURES AND DIAGNOSTIC CRITERIA

Pathophysiology

In hearts with DOLV and AV concordant connection, the LV is a common mixing chamber, receiving pulmonary venous blood through the mitral valve and caval blood through the right ventricle and VSD. Clinical presentation, however, is dominated by varying degrees of cyanosis due to a combination of the frequent occurrence of pulmonary stenosis and streaming caused by the variable malposition of the great arteries and their relationship to the VSD. Thus, streaming of desaturated right ventricular blood into the aorta may occur when the VSD is subaortic, leading to unexpectedly severe cyanosis. In the absence of pulmonary stenosis, heart failure often develops early in life because of large pulmonary blood flow.

In hearts with DOLV and AV discordant connection, the LV receives caval blood through the mitral valve, and pulmonary venous blood through the right ventricle and VSD. The tendency to develop severe cyanosis is more likely than in AV concordant connection.

Examination

Physical findings, chest radiograph, and electrocardiogram are not diagnostic, but reflect cardiopulmonary physiology in each case.

Echocardiography

Echocardiography with color flow imaging may be diagnostic, and associated morphologic lesions are readily detected.[M2,M5] The main challenge is to distinguish DOLV from other, more common conotruncal anomalies such as transposition of the great arteries and DORV (Fig. 54-4). The focus is on defining the VSD and the relationship of the VSD to the two great arteries, presence or absence of conus under each great artery, presence or absence of pulmonary stenosis, and positioning of the two great arteries in relation to each other. Coronary artery pattern is also important because some surgical repair techniques used for DOLV require specific knowledge of coronary artery course. Other imaging studies are not usually performed unless clinical presentation indicates that specific and quantitative knowledge of physiology of the pulmonary vasculature is important in formulating the management plan. Even with increased recognition of DOLV by echocardiography, diagnosis may be elusive. In a recent experience with six patients with both echocardiography and cardiac catheterization available, diagnosis was made preoperatively in four patients and intraoperatively in two.[M3]

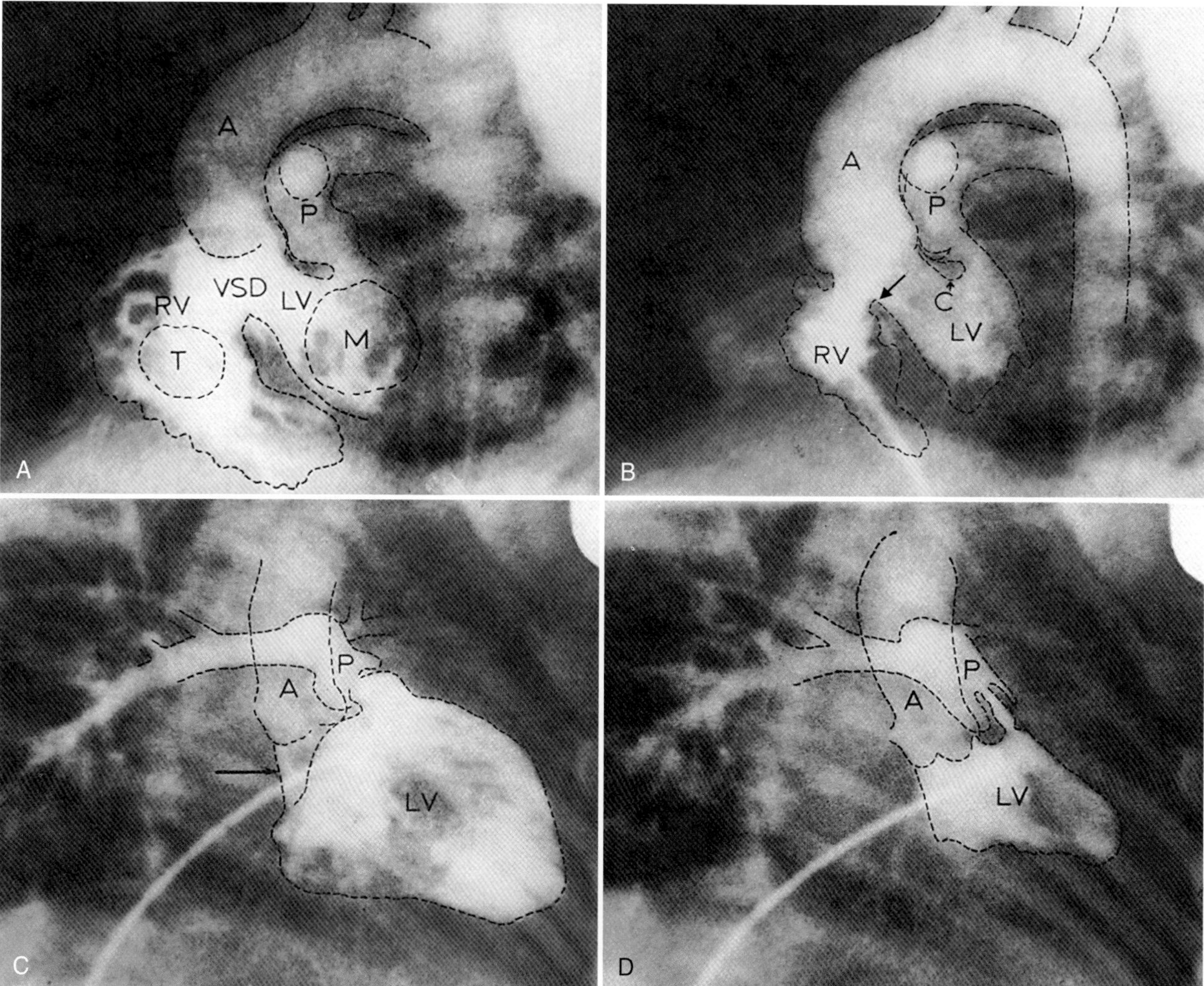

Figure 54-3 Cineangiograms of normally positioned heart and atrioventricular concordant connection, double outlet left ventricle (DOLV), subaortic ventricular septal defect *(VSD)*, and pulmonary stenosis. **A,** Diastolic frame in left anterior oblique (LAO) projection. Non-opaque flow outlines tricuspid *(T)* and mitral *(M)* valves opening into their respective ventricles. Tricuspid anulus is smaller than mitral anulus, but right ventricle *(RV)* is not hypoplastic compared with left ventricle *(LV)*. Distance between aortic and mitral valves in this view is within normal range and consistent with aortic-mitral fibrous continuity. **B,** Systolic LAO frame confirms subaortic position of VSD. Position of upper margin of basal septum (i.e., lower margin of VSD; *large arrow*) indicates that aorta *(A)* arises from LV, except for rightward anterior sinus, which arises from RV free wall. Conal septum *(C)* is entirely within LV. **C,** Diastolic frame in right anterior oblique (RAO) projection with LV injection of contrast. Low position of aortic root showing a normal relationship to intact atrioventricular septum *(arrow)* suggests a normal deficiency of subaortic conus. Overlap of aorta *(A)* indicates (by correlating with LAO views) that it is to the right and slightly anterior to pulmonary *(P)* trunk. **D,** Systolic RAO frame shows severe narrowing of subpulmonary conus, indicating its muscular nature. (From Brandt and colleagues.[B3])

Cardiac Catheterization and Cineangiography

Biplane cineangiography, selecting injection sites and projections suited to the individual problem, is diagnostic but provides little additional morphologic information beyond that obtained by echocardiography.[B3] Because DOLV is rare, cineangiography was once performed to support a diagnosis made by echocardiography, but this role has now been overtaken by magnetic resonance imaging (MRI). Cardiac catheterization, however, remains the only way to obtain specific hemodynamic and oxymetric data if it is necessary to define the physiology of the pulmonary vasculature.

When catheterization is performed, both left and right ventricular injections are desirable.[B3,K1] With appropriate projections, angiography can confirm the diagnosis of DOLV and rule out other conotruncal anomalies, but it is rarely necessary in current practice. Angiography can also define the position and number of VSDs, presence and site of pulmonary and aortic stenosis, and size of the right ventricle and tricuspid valve relative to the LV and mitral valve (see Fig. 54-3).

Magnetic Resonance and Computed Tomography Imaging

Computed tomography provides no specific advantages over MRI in diagnosing DOLV and thus is not routinely used. MRI may be used to supplement the intracardiac

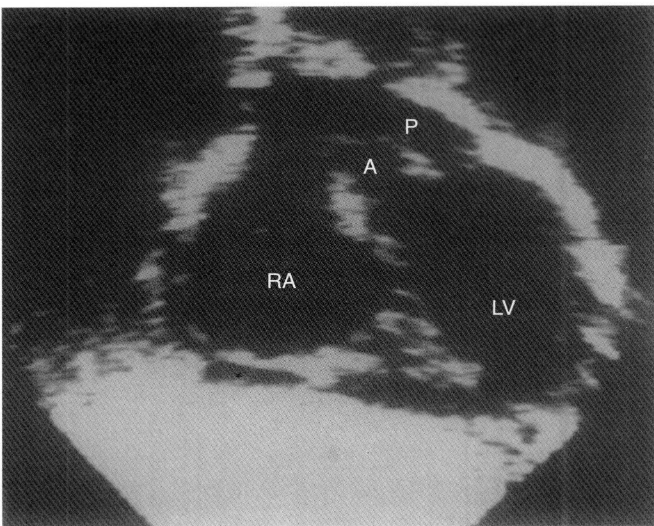

Figure 54-4 Two-dimensional echocardiographic image of double outlet left ventricle. Subcostal right oblique view showing anterior and leftward position of pulmonary trunk *(P)* and aorta *(A)* arising from left ventricle *(LV)*. Key: *RA*, Right atrium. (From Marino and Bevilacqua.[M2])

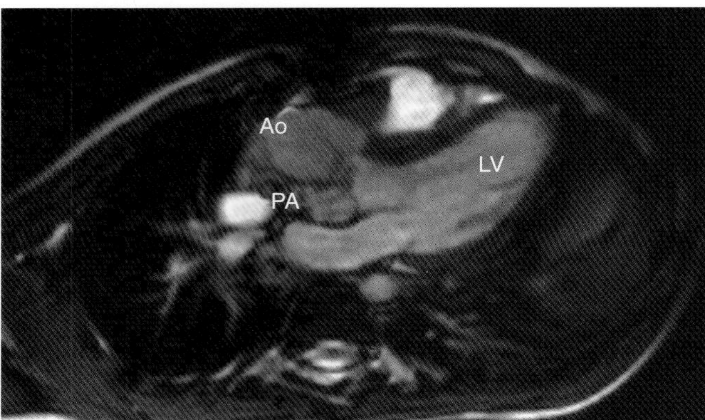

Figure 54-5 Magnetic resonance imaging, axial scan, in double outlet left ventricle. Intracardiac anatomy of left ventricle *(LV)* and aortic *(Ao)* and pulmonary trunk *(PT)* outflow tracts are visualized in detail. There is mild subaortic stenosis. Pulmonary trunk is posterior to aorta and is hypoplastic. (From Lilje and colleagues.[L1])

morphologic information obtained by echocardiography (Fig. 54-5).

NATURAL HISTORY

Natural history of patients with DOLV without pulmonary stenosis appears to be similar to that of patients with isolated large VSD (see Natural History in Section 1 of Chapter 35), except that progressive VSD narrowing and closure has not been documented in DOLV. Cyanosis may be present because of the common mixing chamber beneath the great arteries, but considerable streaming of flow is often present and accounts for significant variability in arterial oxygen levels.

Natural history of patients with DOLV and pulmonary stenosis is similar to that of patients with tetralogy of Fallot (see Natural History in Section 1 of Chapter 38), and in both entities the degree of hypoxia and clinical course are directly related to severity of pulmonary stenosis.

TECHNIQUE OF OPERATION

Identification of Morphology

There are no clues to the specific diagnosis of DOLV from external examination of the heart when it is exposed at operation. Generally, only AV connection—concordant or discordant—can be confirmed by external observation. For this reason, detailed and complete preoperative imaging must be performed to identify all aspects of the anomaly. Even when this has been done, relation of the great arteries to VSD, and VSD to AV valves, may be different from that anticipated from preoperative imaging. Thus, when the heart is opened, accurate evaluation must be made of all aspects of morphology.

When the AV connection is *concordant*, finding a large VSD located far downstream (distally) and anterosuperiorly in the ventricular septum mandates thorough consideration of all diagnostic possibilities associated with a VSD in this position, including not only DOLV but also ordinary subpulmonary VSD with ventriculoarterial concordant connection, tetralogy of Fallot with subpulmonary VSD (if pulmonary stenosis coexists), anterosuperior VSD with complete transposition of the great arteries, DORV with doubly committed VSD, and Taussig-Bing–type DORV (which has its VSD in this same position, but an aorta far removed from the VSD and clearly originating from the right ventricle alone).

When the AV connection is *discordant*, the same detailed observations must be made. These generally reveal findings similar to those of congenitally corrected transposition of the great arteries (see Chapter 55), but in DOLV, the aorta as well as the pulmonary trunk arise entirely or in large part from the right-sided (in atrial situs solitus) LV.

Repair of Double Outlet Left Ventricle and Atrioventricular Concordant Connection

Preparations for operation, sternotomy, and placement of purse-string sutures are those generally used (see "Preparation for Cardiopulmonary Bypass" in Section 3 of Chapter 2). Cardiopulmonary bypass (CPB) is established, perfusate temperature lowered to 25°C, the aorta clamped, and usual techniques of myocardial management instituted (see "Cold Cardioplegia, Controlled Aortic Root Reperfusion, and [When Needed] Warm Cardioplegic Induction" in Chapter 3). The usual oblique right atriotomy is made (see Chapter 30, Fig. 30-14, *A*), and the interior of the right ventricle is inspected through the tricuspid valve. It can usually be confirmed from the right atrium that neither great artery arises wholly or in large part from the right ventricle, and that the VSD is in the outlet portion of the ventricular septum.

Usually, repair is made through a vertical incision in the distal portion of the right ventricle. After placing stay sutures, position of VSD, origin of aorta and pulmonary trunk from LV and their relationships to the VSD, and the nature of any pulmonary stenosis are verified.

With Pulmonary Stenosis

When pulmonary stenosis is present in a DOLV, it is usually not possible to relieve it directly and do a completely intraventricular repair, as is described for patients with no coexisting pulmonary stenosis. However, if examination of the pulmonary valve through a vertical anterior incision in the pulmonary trunk or through the ventricle shows it to be widely patent and the subvalvar fibromuscular obstructing ring localized, the ring may be excised satisfactorily, permitting a completely intraventricular repair.

Usually the pulmonary anulus is small and the subvalvar stenosis too long and narrow for a simple intraventricular repair to be effective. It is not possible to place a transanular patch, because the left anterior descending coronary artery is immediately in front of the pulmonary anulus, and a valved extracardiac conduit or a variant of the Lecompte operation (réparation à l'étage ventriculaire [REV]) is necessary. In the former, the pulmonary trunk is transected at the sinutubular junction, and the proximal pulmonary trunk stump is oversewn by placing two rows of continuous polypropylene sutures at the level of the valve. Then the VSD is closed by suturing into place a patch, taking the usual precautions to avoid damaging the bundle of His (Fig. 54-6, *A*). An

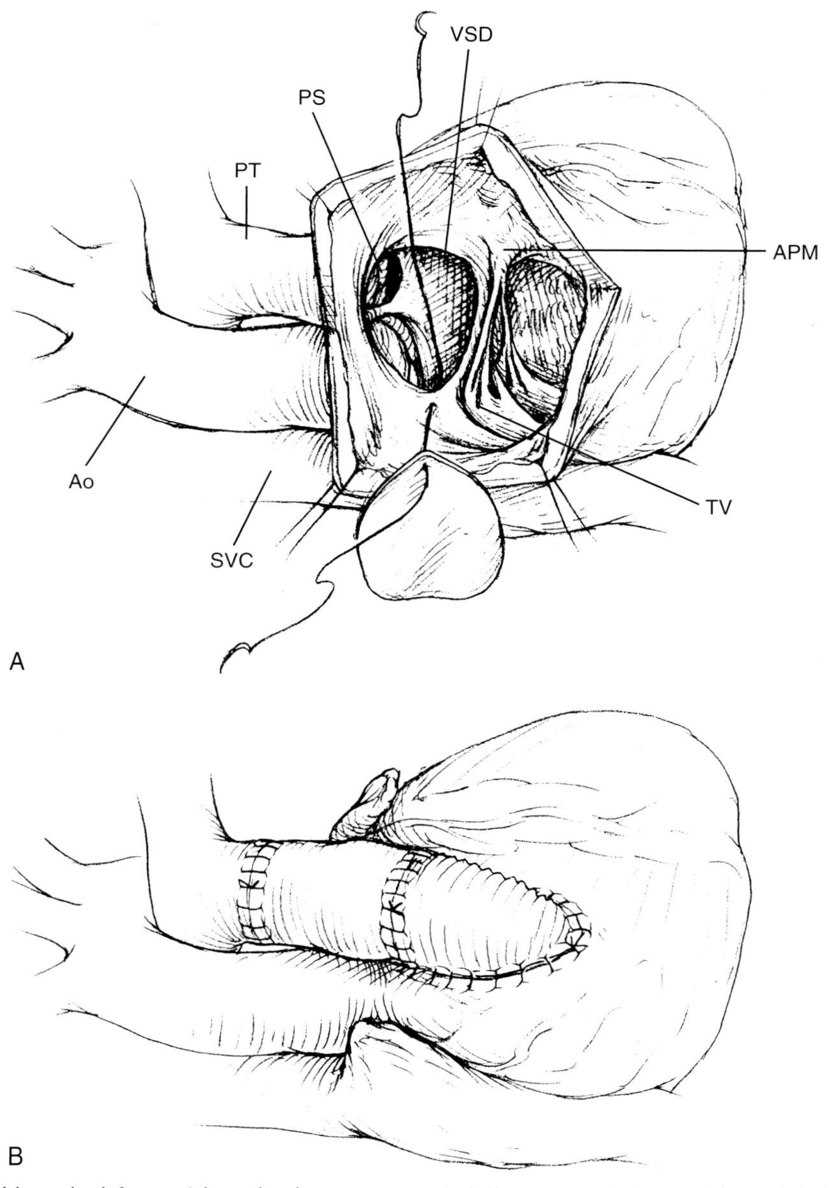

Figure 54-6 Repair of double outlet left ventricle and pulmonary stenosis *(PS)*. **A,** Aorta *(Ao)* is to right and slightly posterior to pulmonary trunk *(PT)*. Right ventricle (RV) has been opened by a vertical incision. Ventricular septal defect *(VSD)* is closed with a patch. In this example, a band of muscle lies between VSD and tricuspid valve *(TV)*, so bundle of His is away from posterior border of VSD, and sutures for patch closure can be placed in muscular border of defect. **B,** Repair is completed by placing an allograft-valved conduit between RV and PT. Distal anastomosis is performed end to end between conduit and distal portion of transected PT. Pulmonary artery is transected at sinutubular junction (not shown), and proximal PT stump is oversewn with a two-layer running polypropylene suture at level of pulmonary valve. (It is important to avoid a blind pouch of proximal PT, as this may serve as a nidus for thrombus.) This suture line should be constructed with particular caution; it is at systemic pressure and relatively inaccessible following conduit placement. Proximal conduit to RV anastomosis is then performed in a fashion similar to that for tetralogy with pulmonary atresia (see Technique of Operation in Section II of Chapter 38). Key: *APM,* Anterior papillary muscle; *SVC,* superior vena cava.

allograft-valved extracardiac conduit is prepared (see Figs. 38-77 and 38-78 in Chapter 38) and sutured distally to the pulmonary trunk and proximally to the right ventriculotomy (Fig. 54-6, *B*). Returning to the right atrium, the foramen ovale is closed, and the remainder of the operation is completed in the usual manner.

Alternatively, a Lecompte operation (REV) can be performed (see "Lecompte Intraventricular Repair" under Technique of Operation in Chapter 53). This has the great advantage of not requiring an extracardiac conduit. Transfer of the pulmonary trunk to the right ventricle can be accomplished without the need to transect and reconstruct the aorta.[C1,D1]

Patch augmentation of the right ventricular outflow tract may be possible in selected cases of DOLV with pulmonary stenosis. For this to be possible, the pulmonary trunk must be either anterior or side by side relative to the aorta, and the coronary arteries must course behind the pulmonary root[S3] (Fig. 54-7).

Without Pulmonary Stenosis

When pulmonary stenosis is not present, the morphologic arrangements may allow intraventricular tunnel repair. A contoured patch is placed into the VSD so that the right ventricle ejects into the pulmonary trunk while the LV continues to eject into the aorta. The VSD may have to be enlarged anteriorly and superiorly before this is done. When an intraventricular tunnel repair is not possible, the pulmonary orifice is closed off from within the ventricle or from within the pulmonary trunk, or the pulmonary trunk is divided; the VSD is closed, leaving the aorta coming off the LV; and an allograft-valved extracardiac conduit is placed between the right ventricle and pulmonary trunk. Alternatively, the pulmonary trunk can be connected to the right ventricle by the Lecompte operation (REV). If the pulmonary valve is relatively normal in size (with or without subpulmonic stenosis), the pulmonary root, including the valve, can be translocated to the right ventricle in the same fashion. This has been described in patients with DOLV who have a subpulmonic conus.[C1,D1] Additionally, the intact pulmonary valve and root can be translocated to the right ventricle even when a subpulmonary conus is absent, as described by Hanley and colleagues[M3] (Fig. 54-8). Pulmonary root translocation in the presence of severe pulmonary stenosis, using a monocusp valve and patch augmentation of the small pulmonary anulus, has also been described.[O1]

Rarely, in the absence of pulmonary stenosis, are these types of repair not possible. It may then be possible to close the VSD with a contoured patch so the right ventricle ejects into the aorta and the LV into the pulmonary trunk, and to

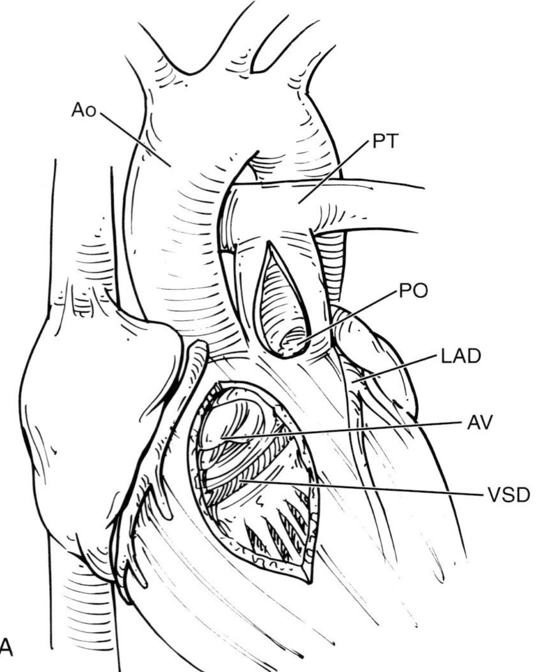

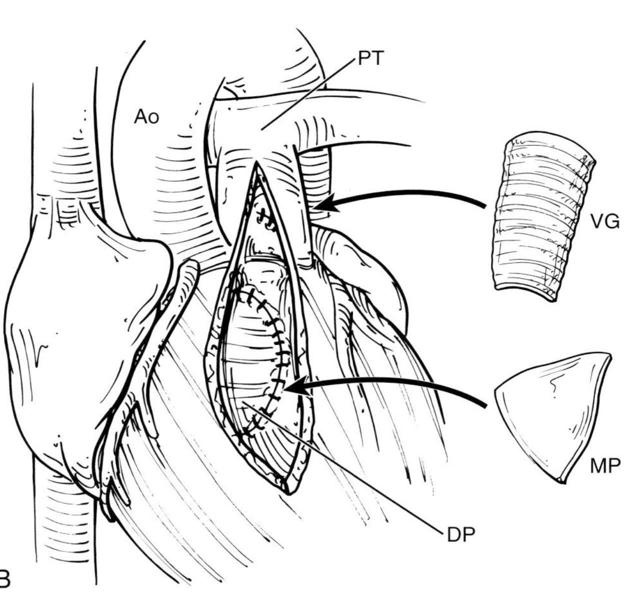

Figure 54-7 Patch augmentation of right ventricular (RV) outflow tract in double outlet left ventricle with pulmonary stenosis. **A,** Great arteries are side by side, with aorta *(Ao)* to right of pulmonary trunk *(PT)*. Right coronary artery arises anteriorly from aorta, and left anterior descending coronary artery *(LAD)* is shown, with left main coronary artery arising posteriorly and passing behind PT. Right ventriculotomy is performed overlying subaortic ventricular septal defect *(VSD)*. Pulmonary arteriotomy is also performed to expose stenotic pulmonary valve orifice *(PO)*. **B,** Bridge of muscle between right ventriculotomy and pulmonary arteriotomy has been incised to create continuity between these two openings. VSD has been closed with a Dacron patch *(DP)*. Various options for RV outflow reconstruction can be used, but stenotic native pulmonary valve opening is always closed from within pulmonary artery. In this illustration, a monocusp valve is used. Triangular-shaped patch is sutured to edges of ventriculotomy, serving as a monocusp valve. Woven Dacron vascular graft patch *(VG)* is placed to construct a roof for RV outflow tract. Alternatively (not shown), vascular graft roof can be used without monocusp prosthesis, or a full prosthetic valve can be positioned within RV outflow tract underneath the roof. Key: *AV,* aortic valve; *MP,* monocusp patch. (Redrawn from Sohn and colleagues.[S3])

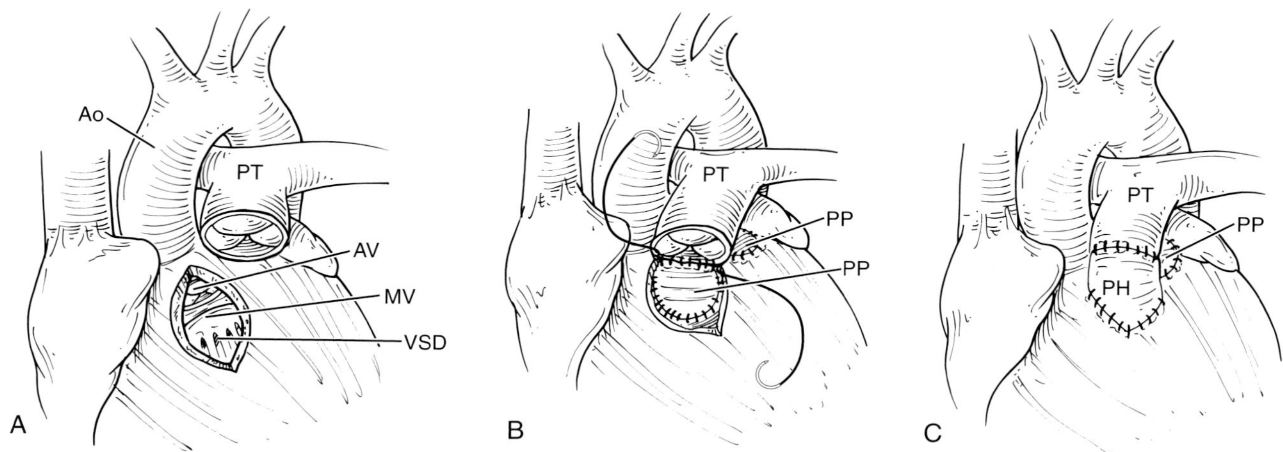

Figure 54-8 Repair of double outlet left ventricle (DOLV) without pulmonary stenosis: pulmonary root translocation. **A,** Pulmonary root (including intact pulmonary valve) *(PT)*, positioned to left and slightly posterior to aorta *(Ao)*, being excised. Care is taken to separate pulmonary valve from any attachments to central fibrous body or mitral valve anulus. Through a right ventriculotomy and ventricular septal defect *(VSD)*, aortic *(AV)* and mitral *(MV)* valves can be visualized in LV. **B,** Two separate polytetrafluoroethylene patches *(PP)* have been used to close VSD and defect in LV created from excision of pulmonary root. If pulmonary-mitral fibrous continuity is present, patch on LV will be partially sewn to anterior mitral leaflet hinge point. Posterior rim of mobilized pulmonary root *(PT)* is sutured to superior aspect of right ventriculotomy. **C,** Procedure is completed by creating a hood *(PH)* across anterior aspect of anastomosis. (Redrawn from Menon and Hagler.[M4])

complete the operation by performing an arterial switch procedure (see "Arterial Switch Operation" under Technique of Operation in Chapter 52).

Double Outlet Left Ventricle with Atrioventricular Concordant Connection and Important Hypoplasia of Right Ventricle and Tricuspid Valve

An important degree of hypoplasia of the right ventricle and tricuspid valve (see later text on Indications for Operation) makes the types of repair described in the preceding text inadvisable. A Fontan operation may be performed (see Technique of Operation and Indications for Operation in Chapter 41), or one combining an intracardiac septation with a bidirectional cavopulmonary anastomosis ("one-and-a-half" ventricle repair; see Chapter 40).

SPECIAL FEATURES OF POSTOPERATIVE CARE

Postoperative care follows the usual protocols (see Chapter 5).

RESULTS

Survival

Early (Hospital) Death

In the current era, hospital mortality is expected to be about 5%, based on recent reports of patients doing well after surgical correction.[C1,D1,M3] Total number of surgically managed cases reported, however, is only several dozen. The experience of McElhinney and colleagues has been updated to include six patients undergoing intracardiac repair, with no early or midterm deaths (FL Hanley: personal communication; 2002).[M3]

Time-Related Survival

The number of cases is so small, and variability of the anomaly and repairs so great, little useful information is available about time-related survival and risk factors for death. However, these are probably similar to those for DORV (see Fig. 53-19 in Chapter 53) and transposition, VSD, and LV outflow obstruction (see Figs. 52-53 and Figs. 52-54 in Chapter 52).

Other Outcome Events

The small number of patients and variability in the morphology and surgical procedures mitigate against obtaining sufficient information in this area to draw reasonable inferences.

When an allograft-valved extracardiac conduit is used, reoperation will probably be necessary at some time (see "Reoperation" under Results in Section II of Chapter 38).

INDICATIONS FOR OPERATION

Diagnosis of DOLV is an indication for operation. When pulmonary stenosis coexists, Lecompte intraventricular repair (REV; see Chapter 53) may be considered optimal, and in this case, young age is not a contraindication. Conduit repair may be performed in infancy, accepting the need for early reoperation and conduit replacement. Classic shunting operations (see Chapter 38) remain an alternative. Arguments for and against this approach are similar to those outlined for tetralogy of Fallot (see Chapter 38).

In the absence of pulmonary stenosis, corrective operation should usually be performed in the first 6 months of life if preoperative imaging studies support the likely success of a completely intraventricular repair. Alternatively, but less desirably, pulmonary trunk banding may be performed if the patient has heart failure or if pulmonary vascular resistance is rising, and repair delayed until later in life. Ideal timing of the subsequent repair may be influenced by morphology. If preoperative imaging studies suggest that a completely intraventricular repair will be straightforward, repair can be pursued at age 1 to 2 years. If morphology is more challenging for a completely intraventricular repair, some believe it may be of benefit to delay repair beyond age 2 years to maximize the likelihood of success. The logic underlying this approach is not proven, but the argument is that a complex intracardiac baffle is more likely to remain unobstructed over time if operation is performed in a more fully grown patient.

When there is right ventricular and tricuspid valvar hypoplasia, with z value for diameter of the tricuspid valve less than −2, a Fontan operation (see Chapter 41) or, alternatively, the "one-and-a-half" ventricle repair (see Chapter 40) should be considered. Usual indications, timing, and techniques of the Fontan operation are used (see Chapter 41).

REFERENCES

A

1. Anderson R, Galbraith R, Gibson R, Miller G. Double outlet left ventricle. Br Heart J 1974;36:554.

B

1. Beitzke A, Suppan C. Double outlet left ventricle with intact ventricular septum. Int J Cardiol 1984;5:175-183.
2. Bharati S, Lev M, Stewart R, McAllister HA Jr, Kirklin JW. The morphologic spectrum of double outlet left ventricle and its surgical significance. Circulation 1978;58:558.
3. Brandt PW, Calder AL, Barratt-Boyes BG, Neutze JM. Double outlet left ventricle. Morphology, cineangiocardiographic diagnosis and surgical treatment. Am J Cardiol 1976;38:897.

C

1. Chiavelli M, Boucek MM, Bailey LL. Arterial connection of double-outlet left ventricle by pulmonary artery translocation. Ann Thorac Surg 1992;53:1098.

D

1. DeLeon SY, Ow EP, Chiemmongkoltip P, Vitullo DA, Quinones JA, Fisher EA, et al. Alternatives in biventricular repair of double-outlet left ventricle. Ann Thorac Surg 1995;60:213.

K

1. Kerr AR, Barcia A, Bargeron LM Jr, Kirklin JW. Double-outlet left ventricle with ventricular septal defect and pulmonary stenosis: report of surgical repair. Am Heart J 1971;81:688.

L

1. Lilje C, Weiss F, Lacour-Gayet F, Razek V, Ntalakoura K, Weil J, et al. Images in cardiovascular medicine. Double-outlet left ventricle. Circulation 2007;115:e36-7.

M

1. Marechal. Confirmation vicieuse du coeur d'un infant affecte de la maladie bleue. J Gen Med 1819;69:354.
2. Marino B, Bevilacqua M. Double-outlet left ventricle: two-dimensional echocardiographic diagnosis. Am Heart J 1992;123:1075-1077.
3. McElhinney DB, Reddy VM, Hanley FL. Pulmonary root translocation for biventricular repair of double-outlet left ventricle with absent subpulmonic conus. J Thorac Cardiovasc Surg 1997;114:501.
4. Menon SC, Hagler DJ. Double-outlet left ventricle: diagnosis and management. Curr Treat Options Cardiovasc Med 2008;10:448-452.
5. Mohan JC, Agarwala R, Arora R. Double outlet left ventricle with intact ventricular septum: a cross-sectional and Doppler echocardiographic diagnosis. Int J Cardiol 1991;33:447.

O

1. Ootaki Y, Yamaguchi M, Oshima Y, Yoshimura N, Oka S. Pulmonary root translocation for biventricular repair of double-outlet left ventricle. Ann Thorac Surg 2001;71:1347-1349.

P

1. Pacifico AD, Kirklin JW, Bargeron LM Jr, Soto B. Surgical treatment of double-outlet left ventricle. Report of four cases. Circulation 1973;47/48:III19.
2. Paul MH, Muster AJ, Sinha SN, Cole RB, Van Praagh R. Double-outlet left ventricle with an intact ventricular septum: clinical and autopsy diagnosis and developmental implications. Circulation 1970;41:129.
3. Potts WJ, Smith S, Gibson S. Anastomosis of the aorta to a pulmonary artery. JAMA 1946;132:627.

S

1. Sakakibara S, Takao A, Arai T, Hashimoto A, Nogi M. Both great vessels arising from the left ventricle. Bull Heart Inst Jpn 1967:66.
2. Sharratt GP, Sbokos CG, Johnson AM, Anderson RH, Monro JL. Surgical "correction" of solitus-concordant, double-outlet left ventricle with L-malposition and tricuspid stenosis with hypoplastic right ventricle. J Thorac Cardiovasc Surg 1976;71:853.
3. Sohn S, Kim HS, Han JJ. Right ventricular outflow patch reconstruction for repair of double-outlet left ventricle. Pediatr Cardiol 2008;29:452-454.
4. Stegmann T, Oster H, Bissenden J, Kallfelz HC, Oelert H. Surgical treatment of double-outlet left ventricle in 2 patients with D-position and L-position of the aorta. Ann Thorac Surg 1979;27:121.

U

1. Urban AE, Anderson RH, Stark J. Double outlet left ventricle associated with situs inversus and atrioventricular concordance. Am Heart J 1977;94:91.

V

1. Van Praagh R. Normally and abnormally related great arteries: what have we learned? World J Pediatr Congen Heart Surg 2010;1:2010.
2. Van Praagh R, Weinberg PM. Double outlet left ventricle. In Adams FH, Emmanouilides GC, eds. Heart disease in infants, children, and adolescents. 3rd Ed. Baltimore: Williams & Wilkins, 1983, p. 370.
3. Vaseenon I, Diehl AM, Mattioli L. Tricuspid atresia with double outlet left ventricle and bilateral conus. Chest 1978;74:676.

55 Congenitally Corrected Transposition of the Great Arteries and Other Forms of Atrioventricular Discordant Connection

Section I Congenitally Corrected Transposition of the Great Arteries

DEFINITION

Congenitally corrected transposition of the great arteries is a congenital cardiac anomaly with ventriculoarterial discordant connection (transposition of the great arteries) and atrioventricular (AV) discordant connection, the right atrium connecting to left ventricle and left atrium connecting to right ventricle.[1] Circulatory pathways are therefore in series. The condition occurs in atrial situs solitus and atrial situs inversus. Ventricles may lie in any position.

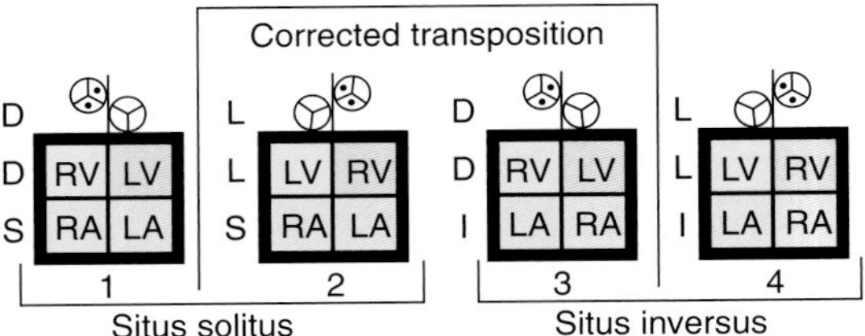

Figure 55-1 Diagrammatic models of the four basic hearts (see Appendix 1H in Chapter 1) as they occur in transposition of the great arteries (ventriculoarterial discordant connection), with most common great arterial positions indicated. Degree of elevation of great arteries above their respective ventricles corresponds to usual type of conal development. Models 1 and 4 are complete transposition of the great arteries, and models 2 and 3 are congenitally corrected transposition of the great arteries. Key: *LA,* Left atrium; *LV,* left ventricle; *RA,* right atrium; *RV,* right ventricle.

HISTORICAL NOTE

Rokitansky probably was first to describe a case of congenitally corrected transposition of the great arteries (CCTGA) in 1875.[R6] After that, pathologists recognized the condition easily but considered it rare.[L7] With advent of cardiac surgery, interest and knowledge expanded rapidly, and papers by Anderson and colleagues[A8] from the University of Minnesota in 1957 and by Schiebler and colleagues[S4] from the Mayo Clinic in 1961 established the clinical syndromes associated with it.

Monckenberg (1913)[M14] and later Uher (1936)[U1] described the anterior position of the AV node, its usual location in CCTGA. In 1931, Walmsley[W1] recognized fundamental differences in cardiac structure in such hearts, including a different coronary arterial pattern and altered morphology in the central fibrous body and conduction system. In 1963, Lev and colleagues[L2] again described the anomalous position of the AV node and His bundle. Clinicians, however, remained unaware of these observations until Anderson and colleagues confirmed the unusual position of the AV node and extended knowledge of the pathway of the bundle of His.[A12,A13]

First repairs of a cardiac malformation associated with CCTGA were reported in 1957 by Anderson, Lillehei, and Lester from the University of Minnesota.[A8] This repair and others reported from the Mayo Clinic[B14,M3] resulted in the morphologic right ventricle serving the systemic circulation. In 1990, Ilbawi and colleagues introduced the *double switch concept* in which the morphologic left ventricle serves the systemic circulation.[I1]

MORPHOLOGY

In atrial situs solitus, the most common arrangement of CCTGA is ventricular L-loop and L-malposition of the aorta (S,L,L; see "Symbolic Convention of Van Praagh" under Terminology and Classification of Heart Disease in Chapter 1) (Fig. 55-1). The left ventricle (LV) usually lies to the right side and right ventricle (RV) to the left side. The mitral valve then lies to the right side and tricuspid valve to the left side. The LV is usually slightly posterior and inferior to the RV. Mirror-image relationships pertain when there is atrial situs inversus (I,D,D). In rare cases, unusual twisting of the heart

[1]The adjectives *left* and *right* used to modify atrium or ventricle always mean *morphologically* right or left. Position of the chamber is referred to as *right-sided* or *left-sided*.

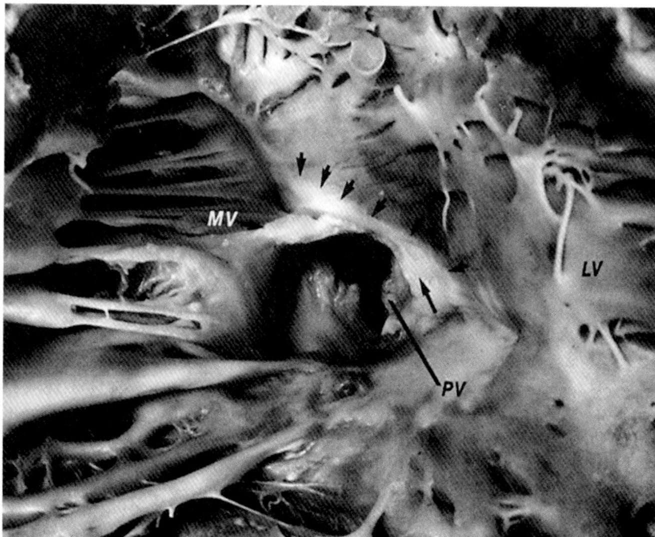

Figure 55-2 Specimen of a heart with congenitally corrected transposition of the great arteries and atrial situs solitus viewed from below, showing outflow tract of right-sided left ventricle (LV). Septal leaflet of right-sided mitral valve (MV) has been swung to the right. A fibrous subvalvar membrane is visible *(large arrows)* and is continuous with anterior part of ventriculopulmonary junction ("anulus"). Part of the membrane was removed at operation, and fused, thickened pulmonary valve (PV) cusps were divided. Bundle of His is visible as a raised pale ridge crossing anterior wall of outflow tract just beneath valve anulus *(small arrows)*. This heart had a large inlet septal ventricular septal defect (not shown).

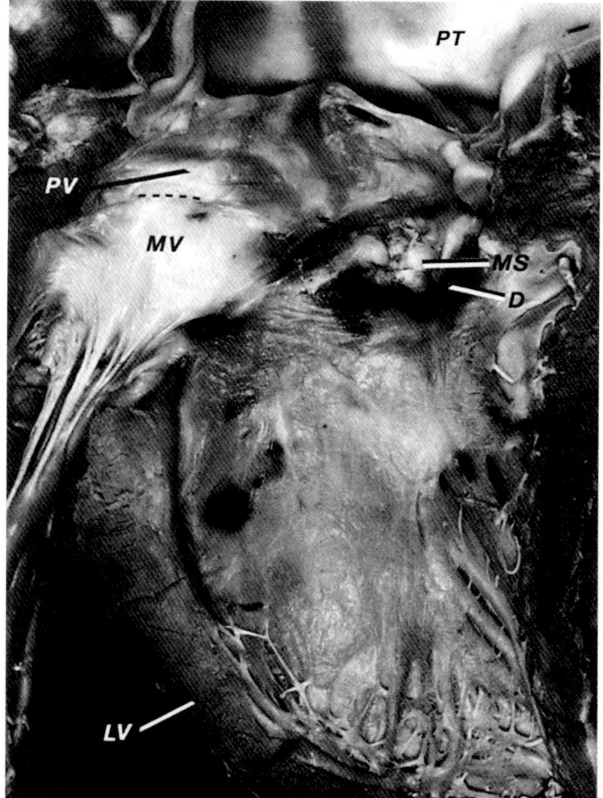

Figure 55-3 Specimen of a heart with congenitally corrected transposition of the great arteries with opened right-sided left ventricle (LV) and pulmonary trunk (PT). Exposed ventricular septal surface is smooth and has fine apical trabeculations. There is a moderate-sized aneurysm of the membranous ventricular septum (MS) bulging into left ventricular outflow tract, associated with an infundibular ventricular septal defect (D). There is pulmonary (PV)–mitral valve (MV) fibrous continuity, the pulmonary cusp reaching to dashed line.

along its long axis occurs, resulting in atypical topology *(criss-cross heart)*. For example, in atrial situs solitus, there may be a discordant AV connection, but the ventricles are D-loop; similarly, discordant AV connection in atrial situs inversus will have L-loop ventricles.[D12]

Ventricles

Usually there is fibrous continuity in the right-sided LV between the right-sided mitral and pulmonary valves and a well-developed left-sided RV infundibulum separating left-sided tricuspid and aortic valves. However, rare cases have been described with bilateral conus or bilaterally deficient conus.[V3]

The LV outflow tract beneath the pulmonary valve lies between the septal (pulmonary) leaflet of the mitral valve on the right and muscular ventricular septum on the left (Fig. 55-2). In its anterior part, there is often a prominent recess.[A13] Ventricular outflow tracts do not cross, and ascending aorta and pulmonary trunk are parallel.

In atrial situs solitus, the apex of the heart is usually to the left and is formed by the RV. Dextrocardia exists in about 25% of cases, and occasionally mesocardia.[C2] In atrial situs inversus, there is nearly always dextrocardia.

Other bizarre rotational anomalies occasionally occur in this and other hearts with AV discordant connections (see Morphology in Section II later in this chapter).

Pulmonary Outflow Tract

The pulmonary valve lies in a transverse plane and arises from the right-sided LV in a wedged position between the mitral and tricuspid valves. Wedging of the pulmonary valve is said to be more marked in corrected than in complete transposition (see Morphology in Chapter 52) and more marked than that of the aorta in the normal heart[L7] (see Chapter 1). The pulmonary valve lies to the right and posterior to the aortic valve. Axis of the AV valves is partway between transverse and sagittal planes as in the normal heart.

The long axis of pulmonary outflow from the right-sided LV is obliquely oriented[A14] and potentially restrictive, particularly when there is LV hypertrophy. Obstruction is organic in about half the hearts,[A6,A14] and in at least 25% it is hemodynamically important.[L7]

Pulmonary valve cusps may be thickened and fused or occasionally bicuspid or unicuspid. When valve stenosis is present, the pulmonary trunk may be narrowed by valve tethering, as in tetralogy of Fallot (see "Pulmonary Valve" under Morphology in Section I of Chapter 38). There may be pulmonary atresia with or without confluence between right and left pulmonary arteries. There may be subvalvar narrowing due either to a membrane that is adherent on its right (laterally) with the right-sided anterior mitral leaflet (see Fig. 55-2) or to an aneurysmal bulging of the membranous septum into the posterior part of the outflow tract with or without a ventricular septal defect (VSD)[A6,K12] (Fig. 55-3). Less severe obstruction is usually due to fibrous tags (valvar excrescences) attached to the LV–pulmonary trunk junction, membranous septum, or right-sided mitral valve or due to valvar excrescences projecting through a VSD from the left-sided tricuspid valve leaflet.[L4,W6] In about 1% of cases, pulmonary atresia is associated with arborization abnormalities of the branch pulmonary arteries and presence of major aortopulmonary collateral arteries.

Atrial Septum

Atrial and ventricular septa are malaligned except where pulmonary, mitral, and tricuspid valves lie in close proximity and are joined by the right fibrous trigone. Elsewhere, atrial septal attachment to the fibrous skeleton of the heart is moved to the right of ventricular septal attachment.[A13,B5] These alignment differences are usually severe enough in hearts with atrial situs solitus to prevent the normally positioned (regular) AV node (known as *posterior, inferior,* or *lateral node*) from reaching the underlying ventricular septum.

Mitral Valve

The right-sided mitral valve lies at the entrance to the right-sided LV. Because of the wedged position of the pulmonary valve, the mitral anulus extends anterior to the pulmonary anulus so that the pulmonary valve is tucked beneath (to the left of) the septal mitral valve leaflet (see Fig. 55-2). The mitral valve is rotated so that its usual septal leaflet, which is in fibrous continuity with the pulmonary valve and can therefore be called the *pulmonary leaflet,* is posterior and its mural leaflet anterior (see Fig. 55-3). The smaller papillary muscle arises from the anterolateral free wall of the ventricle, where it can be damaged by left ventriculotomy. Its position is frequently marked by direct coronary artery branches crossing the front of the LV from the anterior descending coronary artery.[A6] The larger papillary muscle arises from the posterolateral LV free wall. Mitral valve abnormalities are common, having been found in 55% of an autopsy series[G2] (Fig. 55-4).

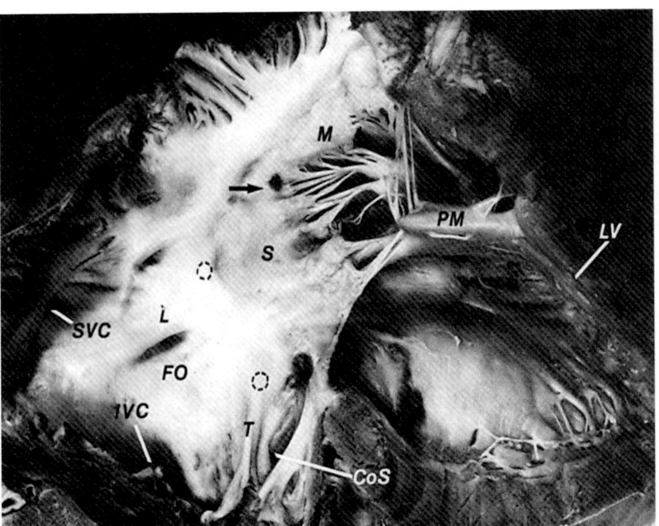

Figure 55-4 Specimen with congenitally corrected transposition of the great arteries in which right atrium and right-sided left ventricle have been opened, the incision passing across the inferior mitral valve commissure. Arrow marks superior commissure between septal (right-sided) mitral leaflet and mural leaflet. Likely positions of the two atrioventricular nodes are shown by dotted lines. Large posterolateral papillary muscle is well seen. Key: *CoS,* coronary sinus; *FO,* fossa ovalis; *IVC,* inferior vena cava; *L,* limbus; *LV,* left ventricle; *M,* mural leaflet; *PM,* papillary muscle; *S,* septal mitral leaflet; *SVC,* superior vena cava; *T,* tendon of Todaro.

Aortic Valve

The aortic valve, usually normal, is over the RV infundibulum, and it and the aorta are usually in a leftward and anterior position (S,L,L). Occasionally the aorta lies to the right and anterior to the pulmonary artery (S,L,D), associated with infundibular rotation in this direction.[A6] In atrial situs inversus, the aorta is virtually always to the right (I,D,D).

Subaortic obstruction rarely occurs in the left-sided RV outflow tract.

Tricuspid Valve

The left-sided tricuspid valve lies at the entrance to the left-sided RV, which has usual coarse trabeculations, a trabecula septomarginalis (septal band), and an infundibular septum. The valve is positioned almost in a sagittal plane and has the usual three leaflets but with the septal leaflet more medial and anterior than normal. According to some, it is nearly always structurally abnormal (90% of cases according to Allwork et al.[A6]). Others report fewer structural abnormalities, ranging from 23% to 43%.[A1,H8] In most instances, there is leaflet dysplasia with abnormal thickened chordal attachments of the septal and posterior leaflets,[B7,B18] and in a minority there is a true Ebstein anomaly with downward displacement of origins of septal and posterior leaflets. Ebstein anomaly often differs from that in a heart with normal connections in three respects[A7]:

- The anterior leaflet is normal in size rather than large and sail-like.
- The anulus is not dilated.
- The RV sinus is not enlarged.

In about 30% of hearts, morphologic changes make the tricuspid valve regurgitant or, rarely, stenotic. There may be a thinned, dilated atrialized portion of the RV[A7,L7] with a variable degree of hypoplasia.[E3]

Atrioventricular Node and Bundle of His

The AV node and bundle of His in CCTGA (and in most, if not all, hearts with atrial situs solitus and AV discordant connection) differ from normal.[B10] Although a regular (posterior) AV node is present in front of the coronary sinus ostium in the apex of the triangle of Koch, the penetrating bundle of His usually does not extend from it because of septal malalignment. In exceptions in which the regular (posterior) AV node gives rise to the penetrating bundle, septal malalignment is mild. Degree of septal malalignment is influenced by size of the pulmonary trunk. Thus, presence of either pulmonary atresia or severe pulmonary stenosis results in less septal malalignment and an increased chance that the posterior AV node will align with the penetrating bundle.[A10,H9]

In contrast, in atrial situs inversus, the penetrating bundle of His most commonly extends from the regular (posterior) node.[D5,M3,T5,W5] The bundle of His arising from the regular AV node then lies adjacent to the posteroinferior margin of the VSD.[D5] An anterior AV node is generally also present but without a connection to a bundle of His. It has been suggested that in those cases of situs inversus in which pulmonary atresia or severe pulmonary stenosis has been present and the conduction system studied, there was only a minor degree of septal malalignment; therefore, this biased case selection may be the reason the penetrating bundle is said to "always" arise from the regular AV node in atrial situs inversus.[A10] Indeed, there are many exceptions to the rule that the AV node and penetrating bundle are abnormal in situs solitus CCTGA and normal in situs inversus CCTGA.[S8]

In situs solitus, the second anterior (superior) node is located adjacent to the right AV orifice beneath the ostium of the right atrial appendage at its junction with the anterior atrial wall where the anterior horn of the limbus of the atrial septum joins the AV anulus (see Fig. 55-4). It is from this node that the penetrating bundle of His most commonly arises. Immediately beneath the node is the right fibrous trigone through which the penetrating bundle passes to lie immediately inferior (caudad) to the pulmonary anulus in the anterior LV free wall (see Fig. 55-2). It then passes over the anulus and descends away from it onto the anterior part of the infundibular septum.[A12,A13] The bundle descends for some distance before branching, lying between membranous and muscular portions of the septum. It is subendocardial in position and frequently visible as a pale ridge of tissue (see Fig. 55-2). A cordlike right branch penetrates across the crest of the muscular septum to reach the left-sided RV septal surface near the origin of the papillary muscle of the conus and passes downward on the surface of the septal band to reach the moderator band. The sheetlike left bundle branch continues downward on the LV septal surface from the branching bundle. Occasionally, penetrating bundles pass from both regular and anterior AV nodes to form a sling of conducting tissue surrounding the pulmonary valve orifice.[A13,B9,S14]

The encircling portion of the AV bundle is prone to fibrosis in older people,[A13] a feature that may explain spontaneous occurrence of complete heart block. Occasionally, when there is congenital complete heart block, anatomic discontinuity has been demonstrated between the node and either the bundle of His[B11,L2] or a sling of conduction tissue in the ventricular septum.[B12,W3] In cases with Wolff-Parkinson-White syndrome, accessory pathways are present (see Section III in Chapter 16).[B12,S14]

Ventricular Septum

In the absence of positional anomalies, most of the muscular sinus septum lies in a sagittal plane and is therefore profiled in the anteroposterior view (rather than left anterior oblique) on cineangiography.[L7] However, the left-sided RV cavity is circular in cross-section, and the lower-pressure LV wraps around it.

Septal malalignment and separation result in enlargement of the membranous septum and filling of the gap between atrial, ventricular, and infundibular septa. The degree of septal malalignment is thought to be influenced by size of the pulmonary trunk.[A10,H9] The AV part of the membranous septum lies between left atrium and LV (rather than right atrium and LV as in the normal heart), and its interventricular portion lies beneath the posterior part of the pulmonary anulus. An aneurysm of this portion of the septum is common with or without a VSD (see Fig. 55-3) and can be a cause of LV outflow tract obstruction.[A6,A7,K12] When a VSD is present, the aneurysm lies along its superior margin.

Ventricular Septal Defect

VSD is the most common coexisting anomaly and is present in about 80% of hearts.[A6] Usually it is large, subpulmonary, and associated with virtual absence of the membranous septum (infundibulum). The pulmonary valve commonly overrides the VSD to arise in part from the left-sided RV. As viewed from the right (LV) side (Fig. 55-5), the VSD is bounded superiorly by the pulmonary anulus or pulmonary valve itself, depending on degree of overriding. There may be membranous septal remnants along this margin (see Fig. 55-3). Posteriorly, it is bounded by that part of the right-sided mitral anulus from which the septal leaflet arises, and anteriorly and inferiorly by infundibular and muscular interventricular septa, respectively. Its posteroinferior margin may extend to the mitral anulus with a zone of mitral-pulmonary-tricuspid fibrous continuity. It is frequently narrowed or nearly closed by an aneurysm of the membranous septum (see Fig. 55-3) or valvar excrescences from the left-sided tricuspid valve (see Section IV in Chapter 38).[A6]

Viewed from the RV (left) side, this perimembranous VSD lies, as usual, within the Y of the trabecula septomarginalis and beneath the infundibular septum; the VSD, in other words, is infundibular in type and is often accompanied by some malalignment of the infundibular septum that

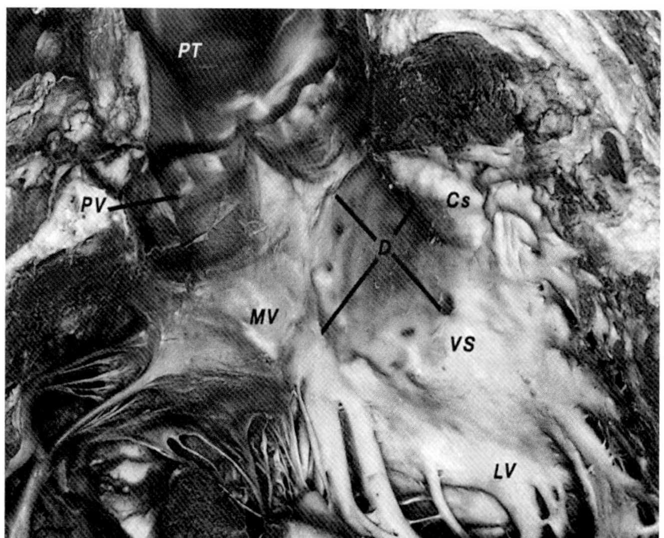

Figure 55-5 Specimen of a heart with congenitally corrected transposition of the great arteries in which a large conoventricular ventricular septal defect had been closed with a polyester patch 4 years before death. Right-sided left ventricle and pulmonary trunk have been opened. Limits of patch are easily discerned. Defect is bounded superiorly by the pulmonary anulus, posteriorly by the mitral ring, anteriorly by the infundibular (conal) septum, and inferiorly by the muscular ventricular septum. Key: *Cs,* Infundibular (conal) septum; *D,* ventricular septal defect closed by a patch; *LV,* left ventricle; *MV,* septal mitral valve leaflet; *PT,* pulmonary trunk; *PV,* normal pulmonary valve; *VS,* ventricular septum.

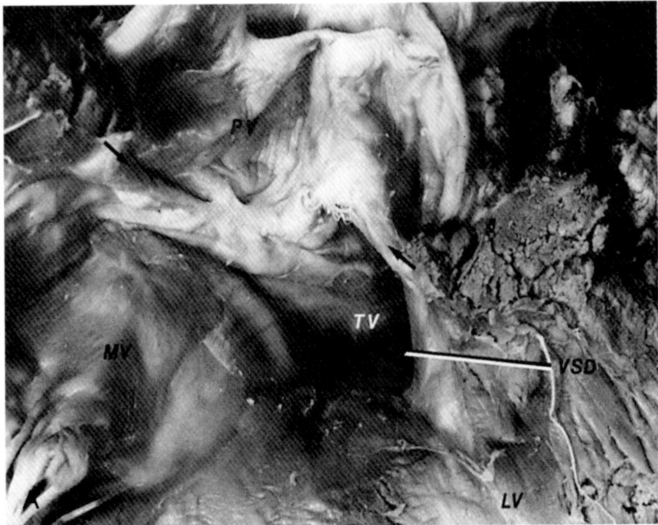

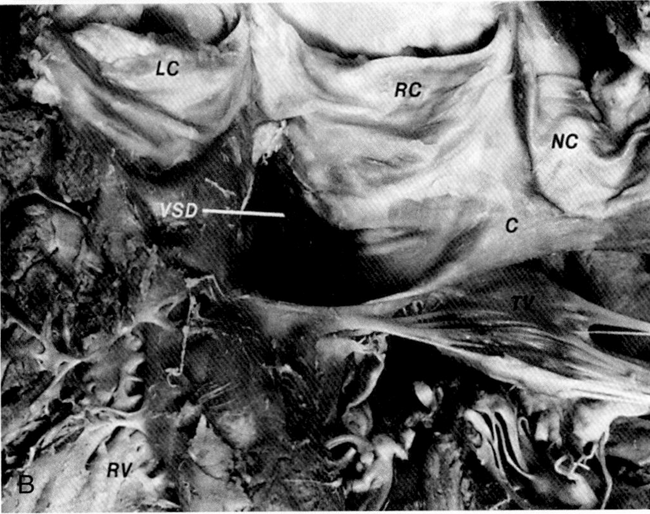

Figure 55-6 Specimen of a heart with congenitally corrected transposition of the great arteries and doubly committed subarterial ventricular septal defect (VSD). **A,** Viewed from right-sided left ventricle (LV). There is a partially obstructing subpulmonary fibrous membrane present *(arrows)*. **B,** Viewed from left-sided right ventricle (RV). Infundibular septum is absent, but there is a relatively short subaortic conus and tricuspid-mitral-pulmonary fibrous continuity through VSD. Key: *C,* Subaortic conus; *LC,* left coronary (right-sided) aortic cusp; *MV,* mitral valve; *NC,* non-coronary (anterior) aortic cusp; *PV,* pulmonary valve; *RC,* right coronary (left-sided) aortic cusp; *TV,* tricuspid valve.

contributes to subpulmonary stenosis. The bundle of His courses along its anterior margin on the LV (right) side in a subendocardial position and bifurcates at its anteroinferior angle with the right bundle branch crossing this angle of the defect to reach the RV.

In about 10% of cases (more often in Japanese patients),[O2] the VSD lies within the infundibular septum; when it completely replaces it, it is immediately below both great arteries (doubly committed, juxta-arterial) (Fig. 55-6). Uncommonly, it is muscular, lying in the sinus (trabecular) septum. A large, typical inlet septal VSD may uncommonly occur. Also, there may be multiple VSDs.

Coronary Arteries

Coronary arteries demonstrate anatomy appropriate to their ventricles. Thus, the right-sided left coronary artery (coronary artery to right-sided LV) with its left anterior descending and circumflex branches supplies the LV, and the right coronary artery and its conal and posterior descending branches supplies the RV. Aortic origins are, however, peculiar to the malformation. The anterior sinus is the noncoronary one; the right-sided left coronary artery arises from the right posterior sinus and passes directly in front of the pulmonary valve to divide into left anterior descending and circumflex branches, the latter passing in front of the right atrial appendage in the AV groove; the left-sided right coronary artery arises from the left posterior sinus and runs in the AV groove and in front of the left atrial appendage, terminating posteriorly as the posterior descending artery. Lev and Rowlatt used the terms "right sided" and "left sided" to describe these vessels.[L3] The most common major variation from this arrangement is for a single coronary artery to arise from the right sinus and divide into right and left main branches; this occurs in less than 10% of cases. Other minor variations occur.[D1,M7]

Other Associated Anomalies

Only 1% to 2% of hearts with CCTGA have no coexisting anomalies.[A6,A16,L7] Coexisting anomalies other than those described in the preceding text include a supravalvar left atrial ring, which may be a cause of left-sided (tricuspid) valve stenosis,[A6] and coarctation of the aorta in association with a VSD.[C8,M4] Coarctation may be particularly common when severe forms of Ebstein anomaly are present.[C4] A patent ductus arteriosus is sometimes present, as is a true atrial septal defect in about 20% of cases.

Overriding or straddling of AV valves is more common when there are positional anomalies, as is hypoplasia of one or other ventricle.[E3] The left-sided tricuspid valve may override or straddle a VSD,[L5] which is at times associated with hypoplasia of the left-sided RV and at times with superior-inferior ventricles (see "Positional Anomalies" under Ventricular Position and Rotation in Section II of this chapter and "Cardiac and Arterial Positions" under Terminology and Classification of Heart Disease in Chapter 1). The left-sided tricuspid valve straddles the posterior part of the ventricular septum, which is then prevented from reaching the crux, and the conduction tissue passes anterior to the pulmonary anulus.[M11] More rarely, the right-sided mitral valve may behave similarly (as it does at times in AV discordant connection with double outlet right ventricle [see Section II]); invariably this is associated with LV hypoplasia and superior-inferior ventricles.[B6,S9] The mitral valve straddles the anterior part of the septum so that it does not extend to the crux, and a regular posterior node only may be present, with the bundle passing posterior to the pulmonary anulus.[B6]

CLINICAL FEATURES AND DIAGNOSTIC CRITERIA

Clinical features depend solely on the presence and combination of associated cardiovascular lesions. The rare patient with no associated lesions will be asymptomatic for years or decades and may present with left-sided RV failure after several decades or more. More commonly, clinical features are dominated by a large VSD associated with some restriction of

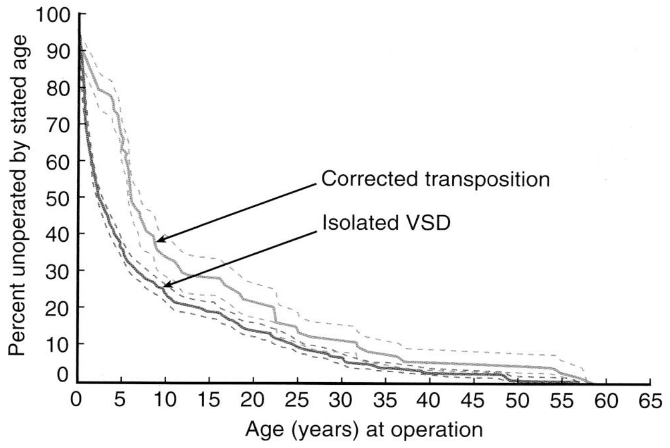

Figure 55-7 Cumulative distribution of age at operation of patients with congenitally corrected transposition of the great arteries (CCTGA) and ventricular septal defect (VSD) with or without pulmonary stenosis, compared with patients with concordant atrioventricular (AV) connection having isolated VSD repair. Dashed lines enclose 70% confidence limits. Note that only 67% of those with isolated VSD are without operation by age 1 year, whereas 88% of those with CCTGA remain without operation by that age. (Data regarding patients with VSD and CCTGA are from the UAB experience, 1967-1983; depiction of patients with "isolated VSD" [i.e., VSD in hearts with concordant AV connection] is from Rizzoli and colleagues.[R4])

pulmonary blood flow attributable to morphology of the subpulmonary LV outflow tract. Therefore, symptoms from sequelae of large pulmonary blood flow occur in only about 30% of cases[F5] (Fig. 55-7), in contrast to an isolated large VSD (see "Clinical Features and Diagnostic Criteria" in Section I of Chapter 35).

It is uncommon for pulmonary stenosis to be severe enough to require a shunting procedure in the first year of life. Friedberg and Nadas found only 30% of their patients presented in the first year of life with cyanosis, although cyanosis was present at some time during the course of the disease in two thirds of patients.[F5]

Most often, presentation is in childhood or in the second decade because of growth failure and exercise intolerance from a left-to-right shunt or, if there is important pulmonary stenosis, mild or moderate cyanosis or effort intolerance. Left-sided tricuspid valve regurgitation may complicate the other anomalies present or occur as an isolated finding. Regurgitation seems to worsen with time, and therefore patients with it occasionally present first in the third, fourth, or fifth decade of life; however, occasionally a neonate or infant will present in heart failure with severe left-sided tricuspid valve regurgitation.

The clinical feature bringing some patients to medical attention is bradycardia from congenitally complete heart block (present from birth or soon after), which occurs in 10% to 30% of cases.[C1,F5,L2] Complete heart block at times is episodic and induced temporarily by cardiac catheterization, anesthesia, exercise, or sternotomy.[S4] First- or second-degree heart block is found in an additional 20% to 30% of patients,[B14,S4] many of whom earlier had normal AV conduction,[F5] and this degree of heart block may be a prelude to developing complete heart block (see Natural History later in this section). Wolff-Parkinson-White syndrome, either type A or B, coexists occasionally (see Section III in Chapter 16).[B11,G7,S4,S13]

Physical findings are generally not diagnostic,[F5] but finding a loud second heart sound at the second left intercostal space is suggestive because it may represent closure of the leftward and anterior aortic valve.[H4,S4]

Although chest radiography may suggest that a congenital cardiac malformation has AV discordant connection by an ascending aortic shadow appearing along the left upper cardiac silhouette, this is not diagnostic because there are many other anomalies with the aorta in L-malposition (see Clinical Features and Diagnostic Criteria in Chapter 57). Electrocardiography (ECG) may suggest a correct diagnosis when there is reversal of precordial Q-wave pattern with deep Q waves in leads V_2 and aVR, and QS complexes in leads V_3 and aVF in right precordial leads. Congenital or developing complete heart block is also suggestive of CCTGA.[L7]

Echocardiography provides accurate diagnosis of CCTGA.[A19,H1,S13] When spatial orientation of the ventricular septum is abnormal, the left-sided AV valve inserts more toward the apex than the right-sided one and has direct chordal attachments to the inlet septum. There is also continuity between the right-sided AV valve and the posterior (pulmonary) semilunar valve.[L7] Additional findings of transposed great arteries with aorta anterior and to the left, and a left-sided ventricle containing a coarsely trabeculated endocardial surface and moderator band, help confirm the diagnosis (Fig. 55-8). Presence of VSDs, valve function, and venous connections can all be defined.

Computed tomography (CT) and magnetic resonance imaging (MRI) provide excellent delineation of the morphology of CCTGA[C5,K1] (Fig. 55-9), but in neonates and infants, these imaging modalities add little to echocardiography with respect to making the diagnosis and identifying associated cardiac anomalies. These additional studies can be extremely helpful, however, in providing additional information that may be important in complex management decisions that eventually must be made for many of these patients. MRI can be particularly helpful in quantitating ventricular volumes and valve regurgitant fraction (Fig. 55-10). It can also be helpful in quantitating LV mass and determining the ventricular septal position in cases being evaluated for a double switch procedure (Fig. 55-11). Volume-rendered CT imaging is capable of showing excellent spatial resolution of the coronary arteries and is particularly helpful in demonstrating the interrelationships between the coronary arteries and adjacent structures (Fig. 55-12).

Cardiac catheterization and biplane cineangiography provide confirmatory diagnostic data (Fig. 55-13). Pressure and flows are measured to quantify severity of pulmonary stenosis and any intracardiac shunt. Angiographic views must profile the ventricular septum and establish morphology of various chambers and sites of systemic and pulmonary venous connection and, thus, cardiac connections present. They can define location and number of VSDs, nature of the pulmonary stenosis and of tricuspid valve function, and other associated anomalies.[B16,L7,S10] Catheterization is rarely used in modern practice to define morphology, because echocardiography, CT, and MRI adequately provide these details in essentially all cases. Catheterization is indispensable if pulmonary vascular resistance, shunt fractions, or ventricular end-diastolic pressure is required for decision making.

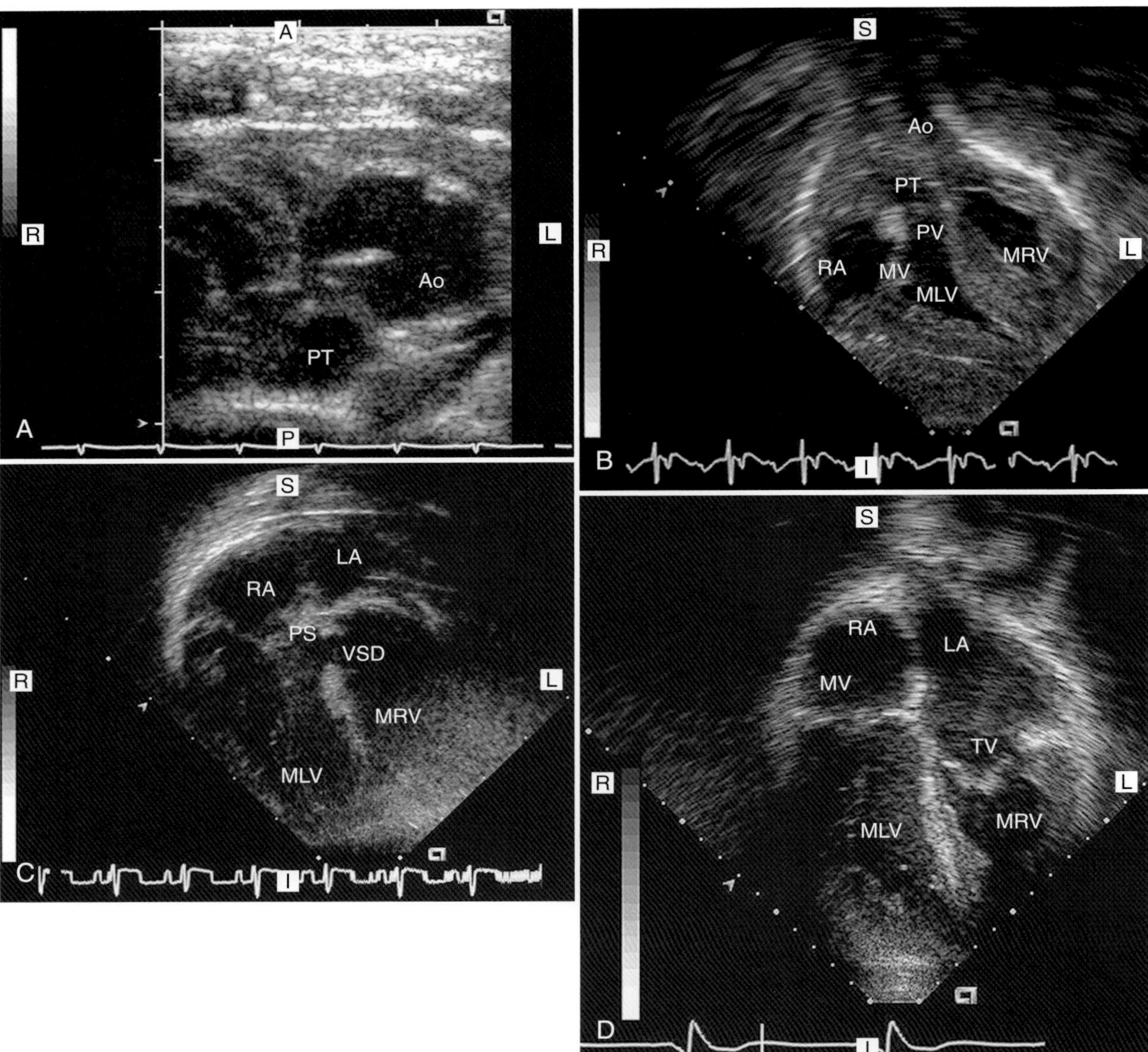

Figure 55-8 Echocardiographic findings in congenitally corrected transposition of the great arteries (CCTGA). **A,** Position of the great arteries. Aorta (Ao) is positioned anterior and to the left, with pulmonary trunk (PT) posterior and to the right. The typical size discrepancy commonly found in CCTGA is demonstrated in this case, with the pulmonary valve and pulmonary trunk approximately 50% the diameter of the aortic root. **B,** Subcostal coronal image. Note bowing of ventricular septum from the left-sided morphologic right ventricle (MRV) into right-sided morphologic left ventricle (MLV). MRV is identified by typical course trabeculations noted here at the apical portion of the chamber. Clearly seen is right atrium (RA) connecting through mitral valve (MV) to MLV, and the ventricular outflow through pulmonary valve (PV) to PT. Note fibrous continuity between somewhat thickened PV and MV. There is no important subpulmonic stenosis. Aorta is seen arising from left-sided MRV. **C,** Apical four-chamber view of CCTGA with ventricular septal defect (VSD) and subpulmonic stenosis. VSD is of moderate size, and there is important fibromuscular obstruction in the right-sided MLV outflow tract just below PV. **D,** Apical four-chamber view of patient with CCTGA and Ebstein anomaly of tricuspid valve (TV). Note septal attachments and displacement of left-sided TV into left-sided MRV chamber. This is contrasted to the normally positioned right-sided mitral valve (MV) between right atrium and right-sided MLV. Key: *A,* Anterior; *I,* inferior; *L,* left; *LA,* left atrium; *P,* posterior; *PS,* subpulmonic and subpulmonic stenosis; *R,* right; *RA,* right atrium; *S,* superior.

NATURAL HISTORY

Heart Block

About 5% to 10% of infants with CCTGA or other types of AV discordant connection (see Section II) have complete heart block at birth.[C1,F5,L2] This proportion slowly increases at about 2% per year to reach a prevalence of about 10% to 15% by adolescence and 30% by adulthood.[H13] Block may be in the AV node or in single or multiple sites more distally. In some infants born with complete heart block, bundle of His potentials are not recordable,[G4] and morphologic evidence of a connection between an AV node and more distal parts of the His bundle cannot be found.

At least 40% to 50% of patients with AV discordant connection are born with first- or second-degree AV block.[B14] As time passes, prolongation of the PR interval often develops, even in those with originally normal intervals.[F5] Thus, Gillette and colleagues[G4] found normal AV conduction at age 6 to 7 years in only 38% (CL 29%-47%) of 40 patients with CCTGA. Progressive prolonging of the PR interval may eventuate in

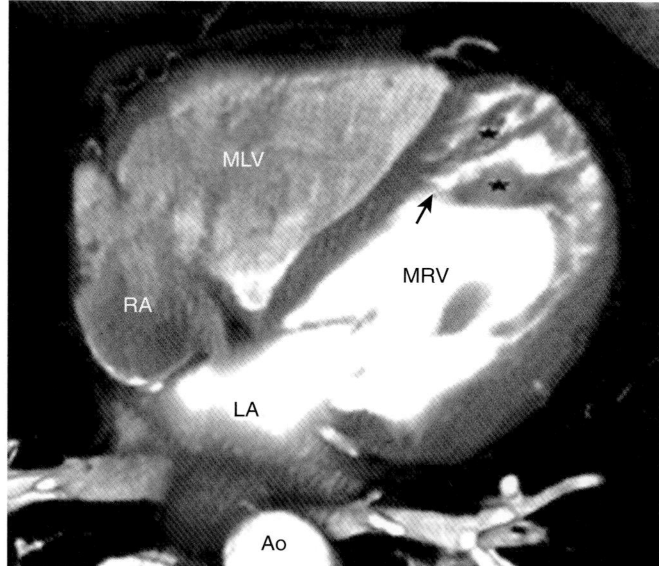

Figure 55-9 Computed tomography (CT) image of corrected transposition of the great arteries. Axial maximum intensity projection CT image shows the right atrium (RA) connects to the morphologic left ventricle (MLV), and the left-sided ventricle shows prominent trabeculation *(stars)* with a thickened moderator band *(arrow)*, which are characteristic of a morphologic right ventricle (MRV). Key: *Ao,* Aorta; *LA,* left atrium. (From Kantarci and colleagues [Fig. 1].[K1])

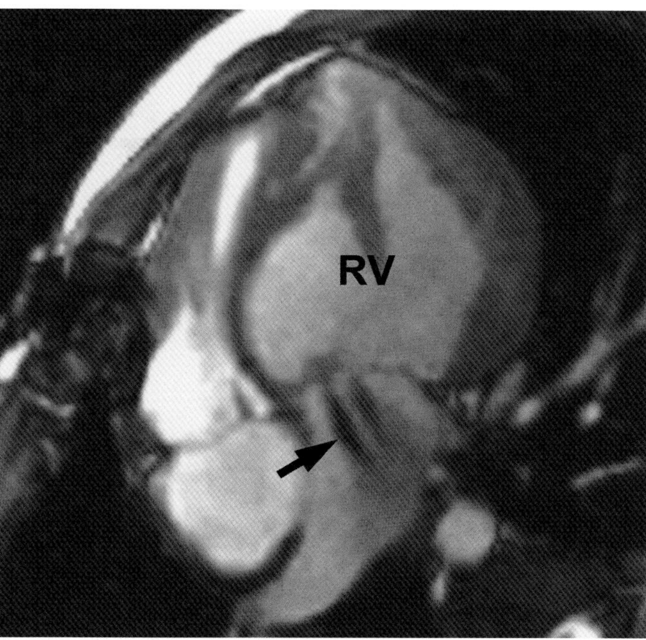

Figure 55-10 Four-chamber view from magnetic resonance imaging (MRI) cine sequence of a 33-year-old man with congenitally corrected transposition of the great arteries. The patient has symptoms of heart failure. The right ventricle (RV) is enlarged, with reduced ejection fraction. Tricuspid anulus enlargement caused multiple tricuspid regurgitant jets *(arrow)*, which worsen the volume loading of the right ventricle.

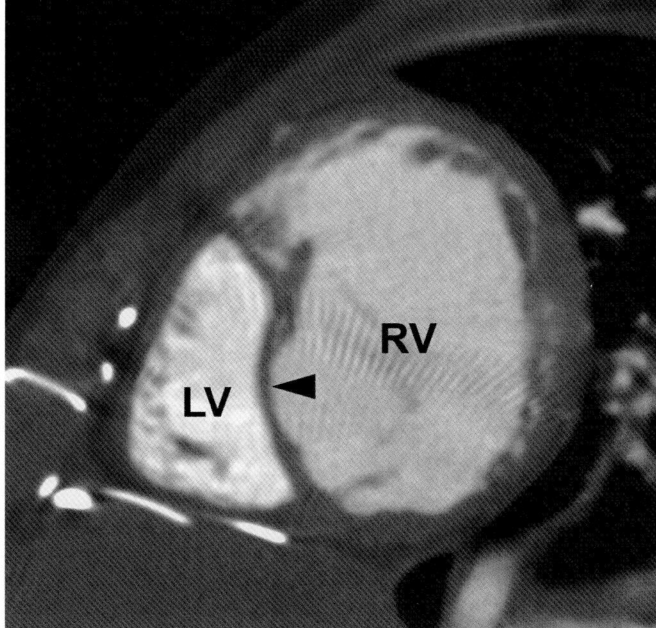

Figure 55-11 Mid–short-axis view from a cardiac gated computed tomography angiogram (CTA) of a 4-year-old girl with congenitally corrected transposition of the great arteries without ventricular septal defect or pulmonary stenosis. Note the thin left ventricular (LV) wall and bulging of the septum *(arrowhead)* from right ventricle (RV) to the LV because the RV is pumping at systemic pressure. RV is hypertrophied and dilated. LV wall and septum are thin. Patient underwent this study as a baseline evaluation in preparation for placing a pulmonary artery band for LV retraining in anticipation of performing a double switch procedure.

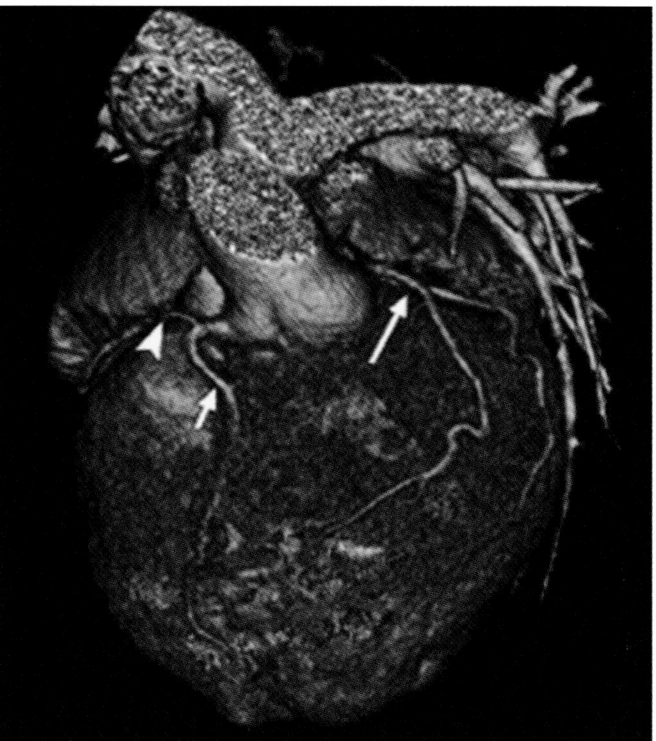

Figure 55-12 Three-dimensional volume-rendered computed tomography image shows spatial relationship of great arteries, with ascending aorta anterior and to left of pulmonary trunk. Anterior descending artery *(short arrow)* and circumflex artery *(arrowhead)* arise from common left anterior descending coronary artery off anterior aortic sinus. Right coronary artery *(long arrow)* arises from posterior aortic sinus. (From Chang and colleagues [Fig. 1F].[C5])

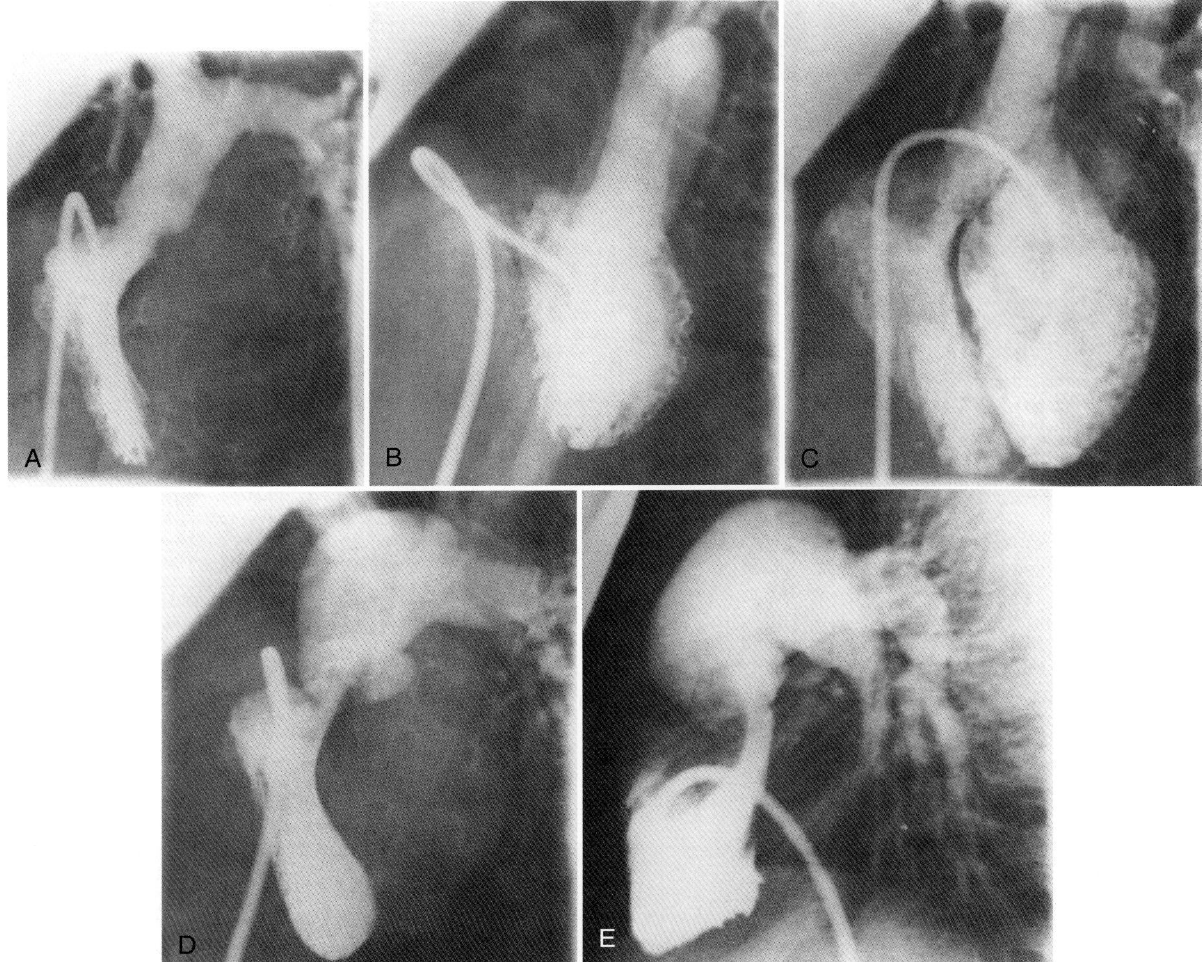

Figure 55-13 Cineangiograms in congenitally corrected transposition of the great arteries. **A,** Left ventricular injection in four-chamber position, anteroposterior (AP) projection. Pulmonary trunk arises from right-sided left ventricle (RV). Note concavity into low-pressure left ventricle (LV) produced by the nonopacified high-pressure left-sided RV. **B,** RV injection in four-chamber position, AP projection. Aorta arises from left-sided RV. **C,** In another patient, RV injection in four-chamber position, AP projection. In this patient, in contrast to the first one, a ventricular septal defect allows dye to pass into right-sided LV and out pulmonary trunk. Pulmonary trunk and ascending aorta are superimposed. **D,** In a patient with coexisting subvalvar pulmonary stenosis, LV injection in four-chamber position, AP projection. Severe subvalvar narrowing is evident as well as poststenotic dilatation of the pulmonary trunk. **E,** LV injection, lateral projection. The long severe subvalvar narrowing is evident.

episodic or permanent complete heart block.[S4] However, about 40% of patients with AV discordant connection retain normal PR intervals and QRS durations throughout their lives.

Ventricular Function

General outlines of the truth about systemic (morphologic right) and pulmonary (morphologic left) ventricular function are gradually becoming apparent, although many of the details are missing (see Special Situations and Controversies later in this section). Ventricular function is not normal but is sufficiently good that a large proportion of patients maintain essentially normal functional status well into adult life.[D7,K5] In 12 adults with CCTGA, many with associated anomalies, followed longitudinally for 10 years, ventricular ejection fraction did not change.[D7] However, systemic ventricular function (function of the RV) tends to gradually deteriorate during and after the second decade of life[G6]; isolated reports of survival into the seventh, eighth, and ninth decades do exist.[M13,R5,S2]

In the unusual circumstance of CCTGA without other cardiac anomalies, an adequate cardiac index is usually sustained during exercise,[P3] but increase in heart rate accounts for this, and stroke volume is not increased. Response of the systemic (right) ventricular ejection fraction to exercise is variable, the ejection fraction increasing in some patients[B8] but not in others.[P1,P3] Systemic (right) ventricular end-systolic and end-diastolic volumes also behave variably during exercise, but on the average do not change, whereas in normal individuals, systemic (left) ventricular end-systolic volume decreases with exercise.[P3]

Pulmonary (left) ventricular ejection fraction usually increases with exercise in patients with CCTGA without other cardiac anomalies.[P3] Other indices do not change systematically with exercise, as is also the case in normal individuals.

Etiology of ventricular dysfunction is poorly understood. Myocardial perfusion plays a role. Perfusion defects at rest are common in the morphologic RV in CCTGA, and their extent correlates inversely with ejection fraction.[E4,H6,H7]

Women of childbearing age seem to tolerate pregnancy and delivery moderately well, with some increased risk of maternal complications and fetal loss.[C7,T4]

Effect of Coexisting Cardiac Anomalies

Because of the high prevalence of coexisting cardiac anomalies, survival free from cardiac intervention is less than 30% at 36 months after birth.[W2] Even without coexisting anomalies, the likelihood of developing heart block and reduced systemic (right) ventricular function probably adversely affects natural history; coexisting cardiac anomalies further affect it. A multicenter study involving 182 patients confirms these points: By age 45 years, 25% of patients without coexisting anomalies developed heart failure, and 67% of those with associated anomalies did.[G5] Other studies link heart failure in this setting to increased risk of death.[P4]

The natural history of CCTGA patients whose only coexisting lesion is a large VSD tends to be slightly better than that of patients with isolated large VSDs (see Fig. 55-7); this may be because their VSDs are smaller than in patients presenting with isolated VSDs. (This difference was not apparent in the report of Friedberg and Nadas,[F5] possibly related to their inclusion of patients with univentricular AV connection [single ventricle] in their study.) Chronic symptoms of effort intolerance and growth failure are common in patients with CCTGA in the first 2 decades of life, but death is infrequent. Although estimates of survival are unavailable, presumably death from chronic heart failure occurs with increasing frequency during the third, fourth, and fifth decades of life.

When important pulmonary stenosis coexists with VSD, cyanosis appears in early life, and the natural history may be similar to that of tetralogy of Fallot (see Natural History under Section I of Chapter 38). However, compared with tetralogy of Fallot, lack of a subpulmonic infundibulum in CCTGA may substantially alter the likelihood of a dynamic muscular component of pulmonary obstruction.

The natural history of the left AV valve in patients with CCTGA and other types of AV discordant connection is unclear. Occasionally the valve may be importantly regurgitant from early in life, but more commonly there is little or no regurgitation initially, and then its prevalence and magnitude increase progressively during the second through fifth decades. The exception is Ebstein anomaly of the left-sided tricuspid valve, when regurgitation is commonly present from birth.

In atrial situs inversus, VSD and pulmonary stenosis are more likely to be present than in atrial situs solitus. However, there is less likelihood of developing spontaneous complete heart block, because of the considerably higher prevalence of the penetrating bundle connecting to a normally positioned AV node.[A18]

TECHNIQUE OF OPERATION

Repair of Coexisting Ventricular Septal Defect

Preparations for operation, median sternotomy, and placing pericardial stay sutures are as usual (see "Preparation for Cardiopulmonary Bypass" in Section III of Chapter 2). Placing purse-string sutures for aortic cannulation and cannulation itself are more difficult than usual because of aortic L-malposition. These procedures are facilitated by grasping aortic adventitia with one or two small curved hemostats and retracting them inferiorly and rightward. Usual purse-string sutures are placed for aortic cannulation and the cardioplegic catheter; caval tapes and purse-string sutures are also placed. In atrial situs solitus and dextrocardia, right atrium and venae cavae are hidden behind the ventricle, making cannulation difficult, although difficulty of direct caval cannulation is not increased.

Through Right-Sided Mitral Valve

Cardiopulmonary bypass (CPB) is established in the usual manner, as are cardioplegia and controlled reperfusion (see "Cold Cardioplegia, Controlled Aortic Root Reperfusion, and [When Needed] Warm Cardioplegic Induction" in Chapter 3). The right atrium is opened through an oblique incision (Fig. 55-14). A pump-oxygenator sump sucker is introduced through the right superior pulmonary vein across the left-sided AV valve into the left-sided ventricular chamber.

The VSD is examined through the right-sided mitral valve (Fig. 55-15, *A*). Although it does not permit quite as free access to the interior of the ventricle as the normal right-sided tricuspid valve, in most cases the VSD can be repaired through the intact mitral valve. When exposure is suboptimal, an incision is made in the base of the mitral valve septal leaflet near the superior commissure and through the base of the

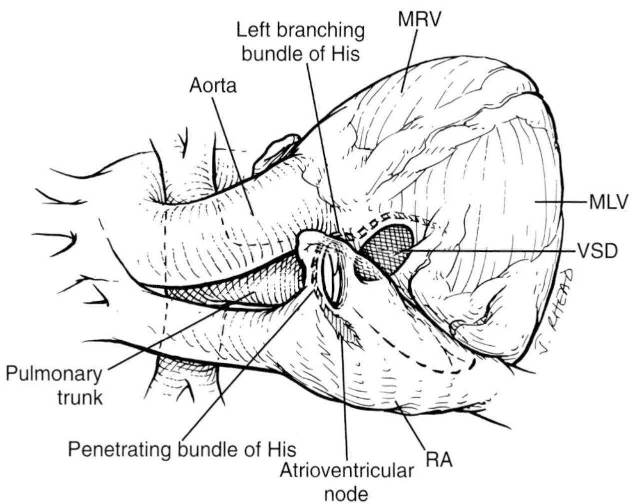

Figure 55-14 Morphologic characteristics and conduction system in situs solitus congenitally corrected transposition of the great arteries and ventricular septal defect (VSD). Dashed line on free wall of right atrium (RA) shows site of incision used for VSD closure. Note superior placement of atrioventricular (AV) node, in contrast to the normal heart in which the AV node is located more inferiorly within the triangle of Koch in proximity to coronary sinus. Penetrating bundle of His passes anterior to pulmonary valve anulus, and branching bundles are in proximity to superior and anterior edges of VSD when viewed through the right-sided mitral valve. Left branching bundle of His is shown here on left ventricular side of septum. The mitral valve that guards the opening between right atrium and morphologic left ventricle (MLV) is not shown in this figure so that relationships among conduction system, pulmonary valve anulus, and VSD can be illustrated more clearly. Key: *MRV*, morphologic right ventricle.

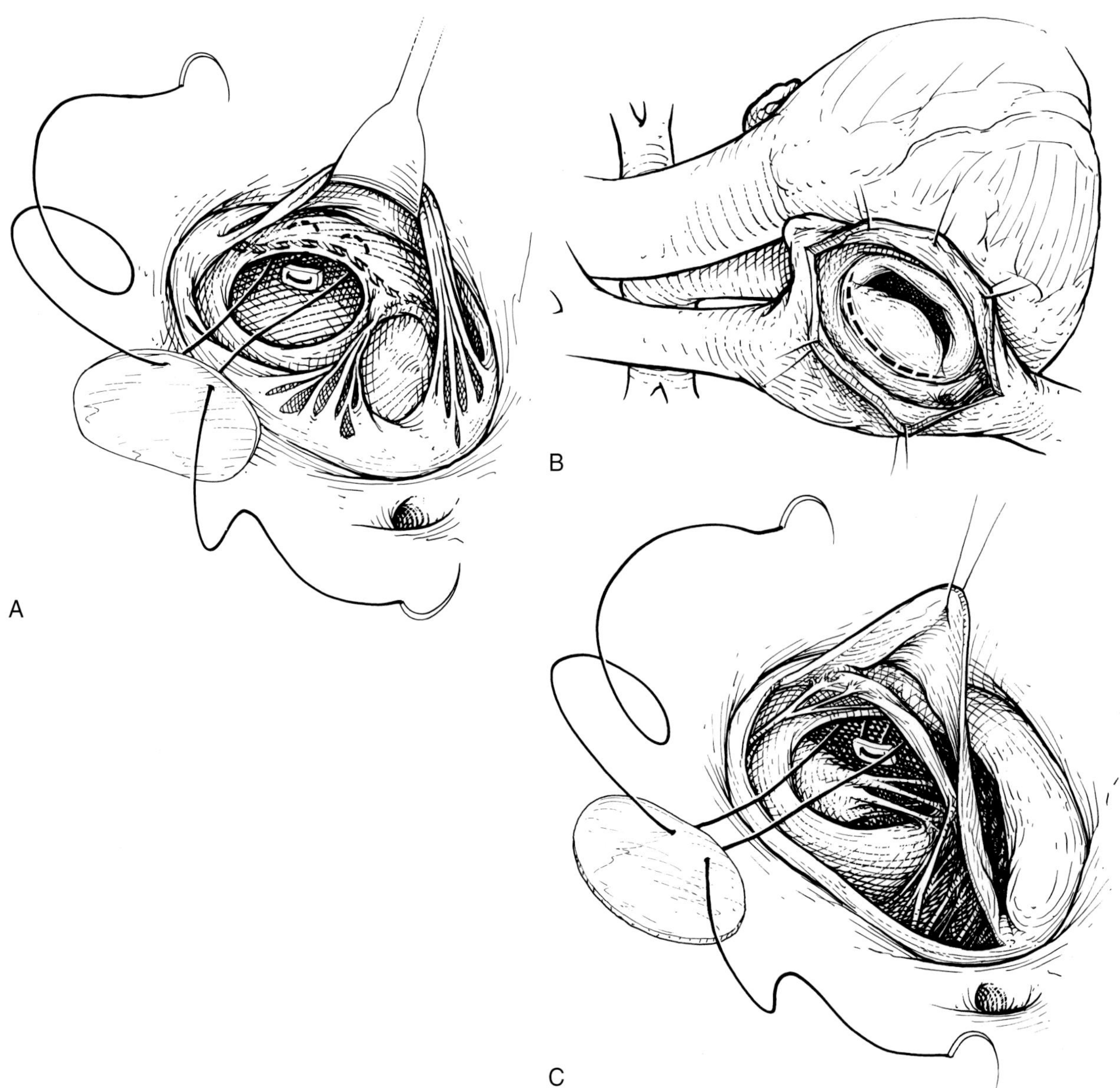

Figure 55-15 Repair of ventricular septal defect (VSD) in patient with situs solitus, congenitally corrected transposition of the great arteries, and VSD. **A,** Close-up view of VSD through intact mitral valve. Intracardiac exposure is gained through a right atrial incision as shown in Fig. 55-14. Exposure of a typical conoventricular VSD is more difficult working through the mitral valve orifice compared with a similar defect in a patient with atrioventricular concordant connection working through tricuspid valve. However, VSD can be exposed and closed in most circumstances without incising the posterior leaflet. The retractor is used to move aside anterior aspect of mitral valve anulus and anterior valve leaflet. In this case, the VSD patch is sewn into place with a running monofilament nonabsorbable suture, beginning at the most anterior aspect of the rim of the VSD. To avoid injury to the conduction system, sutures must be placed on morphologic right ventricular side of VSD rim along its anterior and superior aspects. Here, a single felt pledget is positioned on morphologic right ventricular side of septum to initiate the suture line. Two dashed lines to left and right of pledget represent partial thickness suture placement on morphologic right ventricular side of defect along its anterior aspect. Branching bundle of His is shown coursing along anterior aspect of VSD. **B,** If VSD cannot be adequately exposed through the mitral valve orifice, it may be beneficial to incise the posterior mitral valve leaflet 1 to 2 mm from its anular attachment as shown by dashed lines. **C,** Incised posterior leaflet of mitral valve has been retracted anteriorly, allowing direct exposure of conoventricular VSD. VSD patch is then sewn into place exactly as described in **A.**

commissural tissue into the mural leaflet (Fig. 55-15, *B-C*). The technique is similar to that used occasionally for inlet septal VSD. Working through the aperture created, VSD repair can be accomplished nicely (Fig. 55-15, *D-E*). However, the alternative of repairing the VSD through the aorta should be considered when approach through the right atrium is not optimal (see text that follows).

Margins of the VSD are studied (see Fig. 55-15, *A* and *C*). Location of the anterior AV node and bundle of His arching over the subpulmonary outflow tract and passing anterior to the VSD are conceptualized (in fact, the bundle often can be seen as a thin, pale line as shown in Fig. 55-14). Electrophysiologic mapping is unnecessary. The left-sided tricuspid valve can usually be seen through the

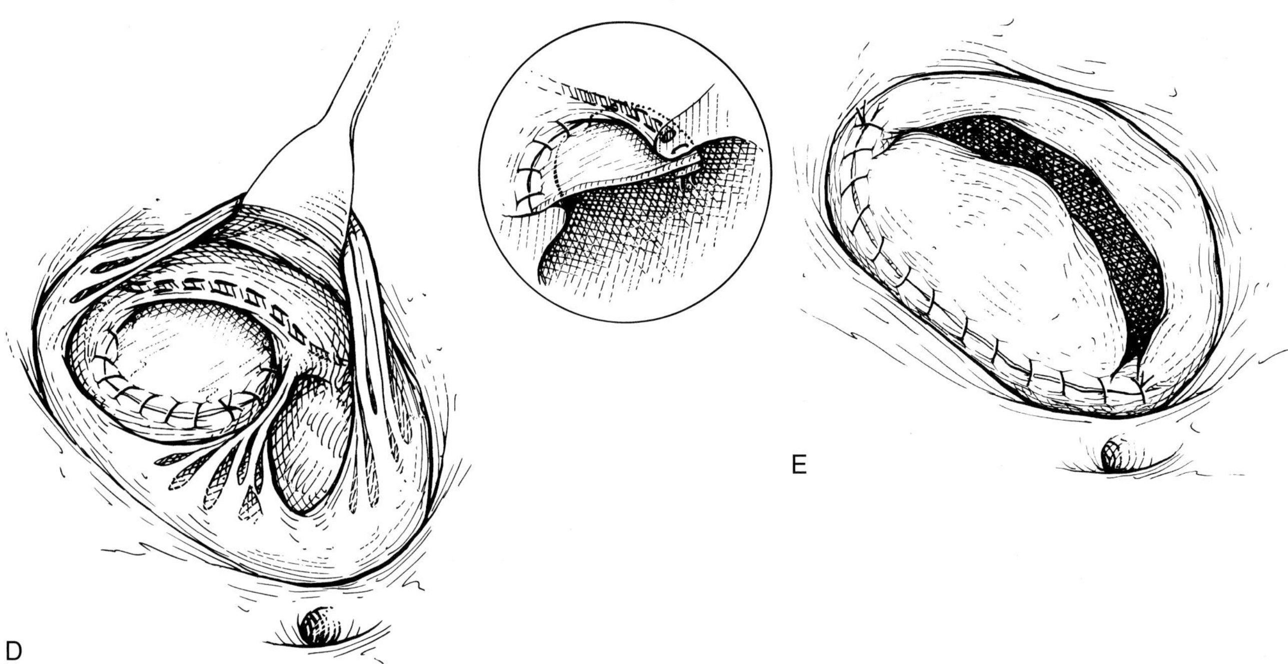

Figure 55-15, cont'd **D,** Completed VSD patch closure is shown in a case with the mitral valve posterior leaflet left intact. Note that patch is placed on morphologic right ventricular aspect of VSD rim along the anterior and superior components, and then on the edge, or if convenient, the left ventricular aspect of rim along the posterior and inferior aspects where conduction tissue is not of concern. The inset shows section through a plane perpendicular to ventricular septum, illustrating transition of VSD patch from right to left side in relation to the branching bundle of His. **E,** If incision of posterior leaflet of mitral valve is necessary, repair of the leaflet is performed using a fine running monofilament suture, attaching leaflet to anulus.

VSD, and some of its chordae often attach to the inferior VSD border.

VSD repair is made by sewing into place a properly sized patch of either glutaraldehyde-treated autologous pericardium or double-velour knitted polyester, keeping sutures on the left (RV) side of the defect anterosuperiorly, anteriorly, and as much as possible inferiorly (see Fig. 55-15, *A* and *D*). Chordae from the left-sided tricuspid valve, often attached to the inferior edge of the VSD, limit this possibility inferiorly. Continuous polypropylene suture, ranging from 6-0 to 4-0 depending on the size of the patient, is used, or interrupted pledgeted mattress sutures when exposure is difficult because of overlying chordal structures. After VSD repair is complete, if a circumferential incision has been made in the mitral leaflets, this incision is closed with continuous polypropylene suture using previously placed fine stay sutures to keep the closure properly oriented so valve distortion is avoided (Fig. 55-15, *E*). If a patent foramen ovale or atrial septal defect is present, it is closed.

The subpulmonary (LV outflow) tract is examined. Unless the pulmonary valve itself is stenotic or valvar excrescences obstruct the subvalvar area, little can be done to improve the variable degree of narrowing usually present (see Results). Only placing an LV–pulmonary trunk valved extracardiac conduit provides good relief. However, if pulmonary blood flow has been large (>2.0 preoperatively), even a 50-mmHg gradient does not necessarily indicate need for a conduit. With elimination of left-to-right shunt by closing the large VSD, right-sided LV pressure usually decreases appreciably.

The usual de-airing procedures are accomplished (see "De-airing the Heart" in Section III of Chapter 2). The aortic clamp is removed, and the right atrial incision is closed with a continuous polypropylene suture. The remainder of the procedure, including placing temporary atrial and ventricular pacing wires, is carried out in the usual manner (see "Placing Epicardial Pacemaker Leads" later in this section and "Completing Cardiopulmonary Bypass" in Section III of Chapter 2).

Through Aorta

An attractive alternative approach is closing the VSD through the aorta, which allows the patch to be sutured into place from the RV (left-sided) aspect of the septum.[M5] Experience of Russo and colleagues suggests this may reduce the prevalence of perioperative complete heart block.[R7] This approach is more attractive than that through the pulmonary trunk, which some advocate.[O3]

Through Left-Sided Tricuspid Valve

When isolated dextrocardia complicates CCTGA and VSD, the VSD can be repaired through a left-sided incision in the usually large left-sided left atrium. Exposure through the left-sided tricuspid valve usually allows good exposure, and surgically induced heart block should be avoidable because suturing is all on the RV (left) side of the septum.[F3]

Repair of Coexisting Ventricular Septal Defect and Pulmonary Stenosis

The main decision-making challenge is determining whether satisfactory repair can be accomplished without a valved extracardiac conduit. When the pulmonary valve is stenotic, it is approached through a pulmonary arteriotomy during moderately hypothermic CPB and cold cardioplegia, and valvotomy is performed as for isolated pulmonary valve stenosis (see Fig. 39-10 in Chapter 39). The pulmonary arteriotomy is best closed with a patch and continuous suture. Obstructing fibrous subvalvar tags are excised, bearing in mind the His bundle position (see Fig. 55-14). A subvalvar fibrous membrane can be excised with utmost care if it is at the anteroinferior angle. Aneurysm of the membranous ventricular septum is excised and the deficiency closed as part of VSD repair. If other excrescences are present, they are first examined to ensure they are not functioning parts of the AV valves or subvalvar mechanisms; then they are sharply resected.

Muscle must never be removed from the rightward (medial) aspect of the right-sided LV outflow tract or from the anterior part adjacent to the pulmonary anulus, because the His bundle lies there. Then Hegar dilators are used to measure the resulting orifice and the z value estimated (see "General Plan and Details of Repair Common to All Approaches" under Technique of Operation in Section I of Chapter 38). Valvotomy may be inadequate because of a bicuspid valve, supravalvar pulmonary trunk narrowing (tethering) at the level of commissural attachment, or (most commonly) a narrow subpulmonary LV outflow tract. However, if the z value is greater than -1, the pulmonary trunk is repaired, usual de-airing and other procedures carried out, and CPB discontinued.

Pressures are measured before removing the cannulae. Relationship between the postvalvotomy left-to-right ventricular pressure ($P_{LV/RV}$) in the operating room and that the next morning and late postoperatively is not known. However, it has seemed reasonable not to revert to CPB and place a valved extracardiac conduit if $P_{LV/RV}$ in the operating room is less than about 0.85, considering that the right-sided ventricle and valve are a morphologic LV and mitral valve. On the other hand, pulmonary stenosis usually represents a fixed resistance, and the LV-to–pulmonary trunk gradient will increase with exercise.

A polyvinyl catheter is placed in the right-sided LV and, if possible, threaded into the pulmonary trunk. LV pressure is remeasured the next morning in the intensive care unit with this catheter, and if calculated $P_{LV/RV}$ is less than about 0.7, the patient is not returned to the operating room for placing a valved extracardiac conduit.

Placing Valved Extracardiac Conduit

When pulmonary stenosis is so severe that the patient is cyanotic preoperatively, or when simple procedures to relieve the stenosis are unsatisfactory (see earlier) or postrepair $P_{LV/RV}$ is too high, a valved extracardiac conduit is used.[E1] After VSD repair, working through the right atrium, a site is chosen for attaching the conduit to the right-sided LV by examining the LV interior through the mitral valve. A site is chosen on the anterior wall, but rather inferior and away from any papillary muscles and major coronary artery branches. Left ventriculotomy is then made. If there is reasonable flow across the native LV–pulmonary trunk outflow tract, it can be left intact, creating an end-to-side anastomosis of conduit to pulmonary trunk. This results in LV ejection via two routes: native tract and conduit. More commonly when a conduit is required, obstruction is severe; therefore the pulmonary trunk is transected at the valve level, the proximal stump oversewn, and the conduit connected end to end to the distal pulmonary trunk (Fig. 55-16).

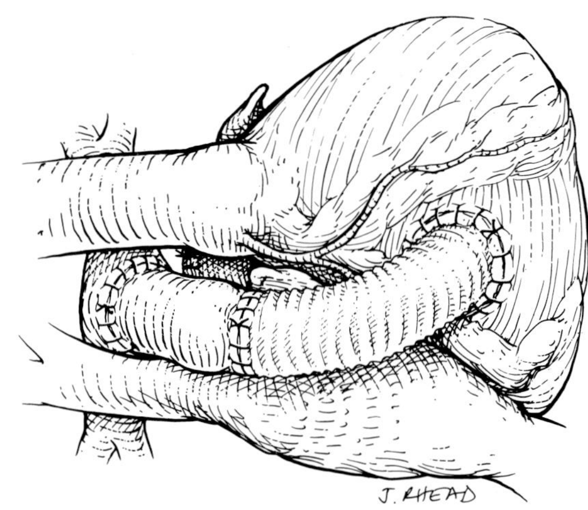

Figure 55-16 Standard repair of situs solitus congenitally corrected transposition of the great arteries, ventricular septal defect (VSD), and pulmonary stenosis. Repair of VSD proceeds as shown in Fig. 55-15. Placing valved conduit from morphologic left ventricle to pulmonary trunk is shown. Pulmonary trunk, lying to the right of and posterior to the aorta, has been transected and the proximal stump of the stenotic pulmonary valve oversewn at valve level with a two-layer running monofilament suture. Morphologic left ventriculotomy site is chosen before right atrium is closed following VSD repair in order to visualize internal papillary muscle structure prior to ventriculotomy. Typically the ventricle is incised and a limited excision of free wall is performed. Exact site of left ventriculotomy is chosen based on several considerations. Primarily, papillary muscle position and major epicardial coronary artery branches are judiciously avoided. The secondary consideration is to create the ventriculotomy at a site that keeps the proximal conduit away from the sternum as much as possible. Typically the conduit is positioned to right side of the midline and ascending aorta, as illustrated. Conduit is usually much longer than that required in tetralogy of Fallot with pulmonary atresia (see Section II of Chapter 38). A composite conduit is usually constructed using a distal valved allograft and a proximal polytetrafluoroethylene or polyester tube. Distal position of valved conduit component within the composite allows the valve to be positioned more posteriorly in mediastinum, thereby avoiding compression and distortion of valve with sternal closure.

Reconstruction can be accomplished in a number of ways. An allograft-valved conduit has previously been prepared by extending it proximally with a woven polyester tube (see Fig. 55-16). Alternatively, proximal extension may be with an aortic allograft, or the allograft aortic valve and ascending aorta may be left long distally, and proximal anastomosis augmented with a pericardial hood (see "Placement of Valved Conduit" in Section II of Chapter 38). These extensions are particularly necessary in this situation because the conduit must be of sufficient length to prevent kinking, and the valve must lie away from the LV so that it is not distorted. Estimating length and lie of the conduit is important to avoid its compression by the sternum.

The conduit is trimmed to size, cutting the distal end square but leaving more of the ascending aorta beyond the aortic valve than in the case of tetralogy, because this facilitates a smooth conduit contour and limits length of the polyester extension. The proximal polyester end of the conduit is trimmed to make a cobra head, the distal allograft end anastomosed end to end to the distal pulmonary trunk, and the proximal polyester end anastomosed to the ventriculotomy. The conduit most commonly is placed to the right around the right atrium and atrial appendage (see Fig. 55-16), although extreme deviations in cardiac position may influence conduit position, occasionally making a left-sided placement appropriate. Aeba and colleagues describe placing the conduit from the apex of the LV to the pulmonary trunk to avoid the well-known problem of sternal compression.[A2]

Transanular Patch

Doty and colleagues[D10] proposed using a posteriorly placed transanular patch across the pulmonary valve anulus in this situation. However, average gradient across the repair was 40 mmHg.

Correction for Regurgitant Left-Sided Tricuspid Valve

When important left-sided tricuspid valve regurgitation coexists, repair and anuloplasty are only occasionally successful but should be attempted if it seems feasible.[W6] If replacement is required, the same considerations apply to the replacement device as in ordinary left-sided mitral valve replacement (see "Choice of Device for Valve Replacement" in Section I of Chapter 11). Valve replacement is the same as for a left-sided mitral valve, including choice of venous cannulae and approach through the right side of the left atrium (see "Mitral Valve Replacement" in Section I of Chapter 11 and Fig. 11-19). The replacement device is either sewn in with interrupted pledgeted mattress sutures or simple interrupted sutures. A continuous suture technique is not desirable when there is absence of a well-defined anulus in some areas, as may occur when there is downward displacement into the ventricle of some of the left-sided tricuspid valve leaflets, as in Ebstein anomaly.

Double Switch Procedures

Because of concern over long-term fate of the morphologic RV and tricuspid valve in the systemic circulation, some suggest placing the morphologic LV and mitral valve into the systemic circulation. This requires switching both venous return and arterial outflow (double switch) by one of several procedures, all of which are technically substantially more complex than those already described. The double switch concept was originally suggested by Ilbawi and colleagues for patients with CCTGA, VSD, and pulmonary stenosis.[I1] In this setting, the morphologic LV is connected to the aorta by creating an intraventricular baffle (which also closes the VSD); an extracardiac conduit is placed from morphologic RV to pulmonary trunk, and a Mustard or Senning intraatrial transposition of venous return is performed. The concept was subsequently applied to CCTGA without pulmonary stenosis, with or without VSD. In this setting, an arterial switch is performed to correct the ventriculoarterial discordant connection. (All of these reconstructive procedures used in combination in the double switch procedures are individually described in detail in Chapter 52.) Aortic translocation has also been used for selected cases of CCTGA with VSD and pulmonary stenosis.[D2,H10,K14]

If these procedures are being considered for patients without VSD in whom the morphologic LV is working at low pressure, the same considerations must be addressed as in simple transposition of the great arteries (TGA) with unprepared LV (see "Simple Transposition of the Great Arteries Presenting after Age 30 Days" under Indications for Operation in Chapter 52).

Both major double switch procedures are performed using a standard median sternotomy incision, CPB with moderate hypothermia using bicaval venous cannulation through purse-string sutures placed directly on the venae cavae, aortic cannulation at the base of the brachiocephalic artery, and venting of the systemic ventricle by way of a cannula introduced through the right upper pulmonary vein. Multiple doses of cold cardioplegic solution are used for these extensive procedures (see "Methods of Myocardial Management" under Neonates and Infants in Chapter 3). Individual components of the two major double switch procedures are as follows:

1. The *atrial baffle procedure*, which is performed exactly as for simple TGA (see "Mustard Technique" and "Senning Technique" under Technique of Operation in Chapter 52). It is not uncommon in CCTGA of both the S,L,L and the I,D,D types for cardiac positioning abnormalities such as mesocardia or apicocaval juxtaposition to be present. In these cases, the free wall of the systemic venous atrium is likely to be deficient, making the Mustard technique preferable to the Senning. Atrial baffle placement may be more difficult than in simple TGA, because the left-sided tricuspid valve is positioned much more posteriorly across the atrial septum in relation to the vena cavae.
2. For patients with VSD and pulmonary stenosis, the *morphologic LV–to-aortic intracardiac baffle procedure*, which is accomplished through a subaortic incision in the infundibulum of the morphologic RV as described under "Intraventricular Repair" in Chapter 52, for S,D,D transposition with VSD and pulmonary stenosis or atresia. The morphologic RV-to–pulmonary trunk conduit is placed as described under "Rastelli Operation" in Chapter 52. This procedure is shown in Fig. 55-17, *A* to *E*.
3. For patients without pulmonary stenosis, the *arterial switch procedure* is performed using the same techniques described under "Arterial Switch Operation" in Chapter 52 for simple TGA. If a VSD is present, it is closed as described earlier under "Repair of Coexisting Ventricular Septal Defect." This procedure is shown in Fig. 55-18, *A* to *D*.

Double Switch Procedures Combined with Bidirectional Superior Cavopulmonary Anastomosis

Bidirectional superior cavopulmonary anastomosis may provide substantial advantages in the setting of both double switch procedures. It reduces complexity of the intraatrial procedure, because only the inferior vena cava is baffled to the tricuspid valve. This reduces myocardial ischemia time because (1) the cavopulmonary anastomosis can be performed during rewarming after the aortic clamp is removed and myocardial reperfusion is established, and (2) the simplified inferior vena cava baffling can be accomplished much more quickly than a full Mustard or Senning procedure. An additional advantage is that recognized complications of the full Mustard or Senning procedure (e.g., superior caval obstruction, pulmonary venous obstruction, sinus node dysfunction) are eliminated.

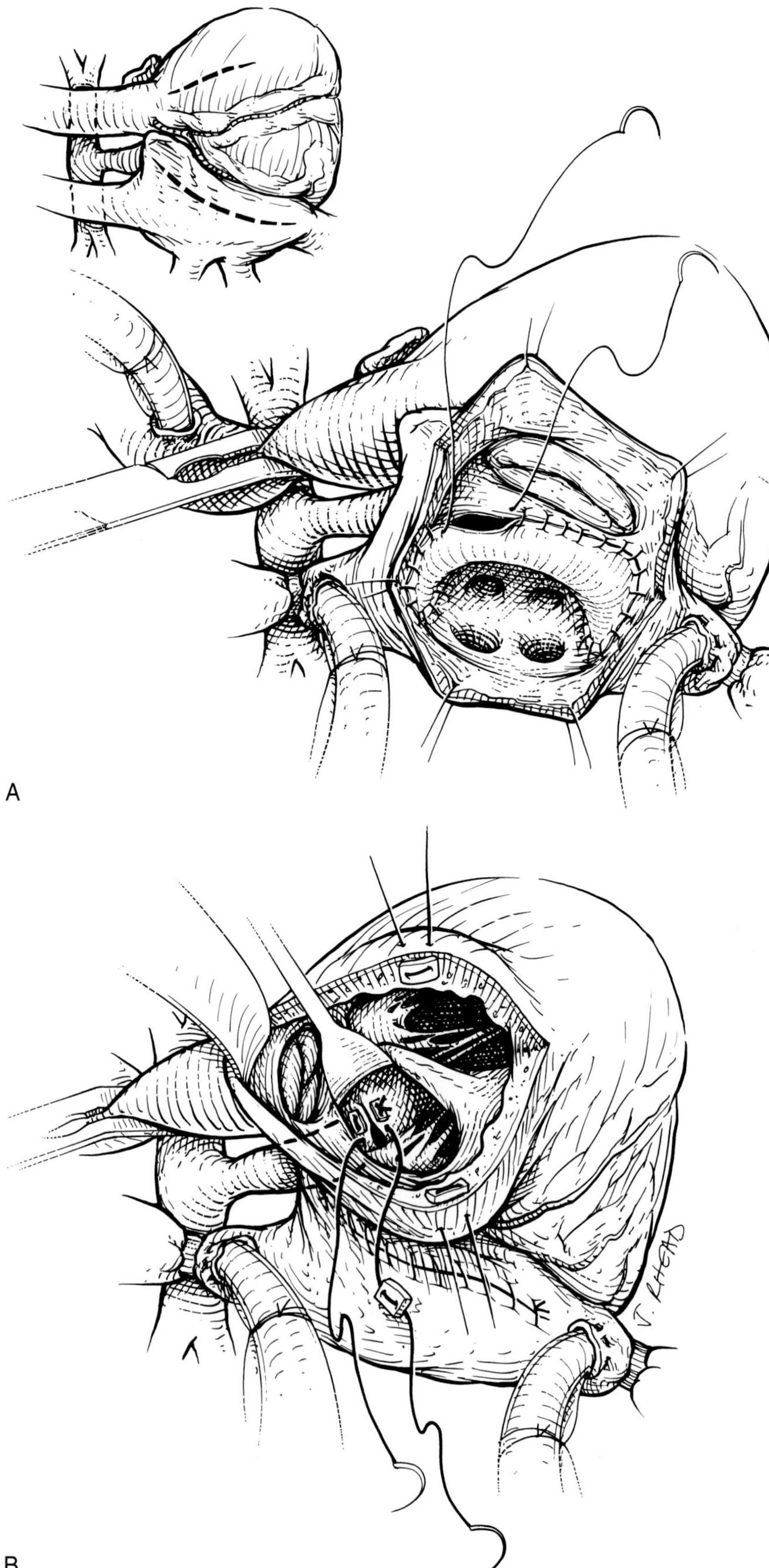

Figure 55-17 Double switch concept using a Rastelli morphologic left ventricle–aortic intraventricular tunnel and an intraatrial Mustard baffle. **A,** Dashed lines on inset show the two incisions used for this procedure; one is along right atrial free wall, the other along subaortic infundibulum of left-sided morphologic right ventricle (MRV). Routine cardiopulmonary bypass techniques and myocardial protection are used. After cardiac arrest, right atrium is opened and Mustard intraatrial baffle constructed. As illustrated, baffle suture line is almost completed. Details of Mustard procedure are provided in Chapter 52. The only important difference when the Mustard procedure is performed in congenially corrected transposition is that the surgeon must be aware of superior displacement of the atrioventricular node. **B,** After completing Mustard intraatrial baffle, the right atriotomy is closed with a running monofilament suture. The left-sided MRV infundibular incision is made, and exposure to intraventricular morphology is aided by a combination of stay sutures and retractors. In this case, the stenotic pulmonary valve and subpulmonic morphologic left ventricular (MLV) outflow tract are identified and closed internally with doubly pledgeted interrupted mattress sutures. Pulmonary anulus and subpulmonic region are exposed by gently retracting superior anterior aspect of rim of the ventricular septal defect (VSD) with a vein retractor, as illustrated.

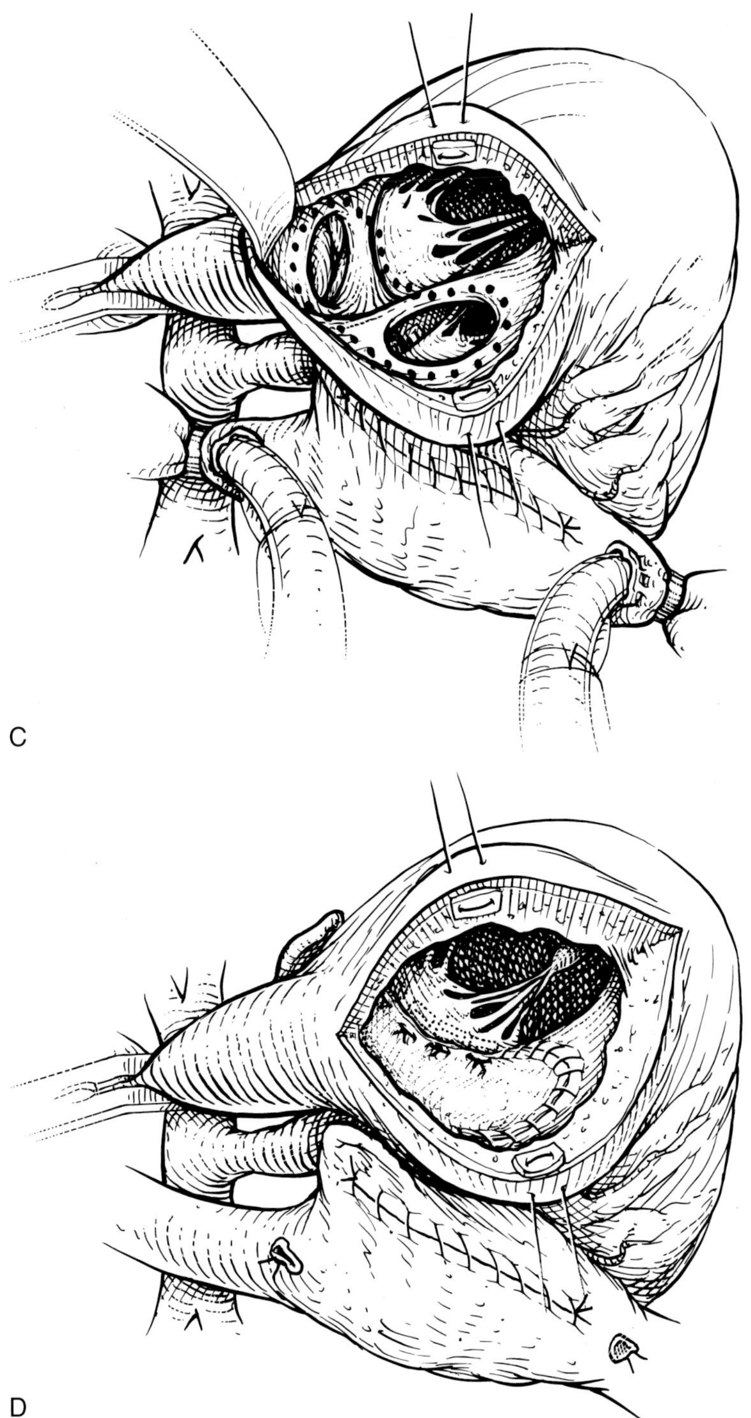

Figure 55-17, cont'd **C,** Vein retractor on rim of VSD has been removed. Dotted line shows suture line used to create intraventricular baffle that will establish a pathway from the right-sided posterior MLV through VSD to left-sided anterior aorta. Note that exposure through this incision in MRV allows the surgeon to directly view MRV aspect of the ventricular septum, making it easy to place all sutures on right ventricular aspect of the rim of VSD, thereby avoiding direct injury to conduction system. It is important to realize that from this perspective on the MRV side, the vulnerable area for conduction injury is now at posterior and inferior aspect of VSD. **D,** A polyester tube graft of diameter approximately equal to that of the aorta is used to create MLV-to-aortic baffle. Natural curvature of resulting baffle patch is placed such that it is seen as convex when viewed through infundibular incision in MRV. Typically a running monofilament suture technique is used to place baffle. Routine care must be taken with respect to the conduction system along posterior inferior rim of VSD (see Chapter 35). Aortic end of baffle is sewn into place along the immediate subaortic musculature (see text for further details). As can be seen from **C,** there is potential for an hourglass deformity in the pathway from MLV to aorta at its midportion as the baffle passes the tricuspid valve anulus. Obstruction at this level can be avoided by attending to several factors. The baffle itself should be made particularly wide at its midportion. Additionally, the suture line should be placed into anulus of tricuspid valve at this level in order to maximize width of the pathway. Finally, judicious resection of muscle along floor of pathway in subpulmonic region at the upper rim of VSD may be helpful. It is critical to perform this resection with absolute knowledge of the position of conduction system. *Continued*

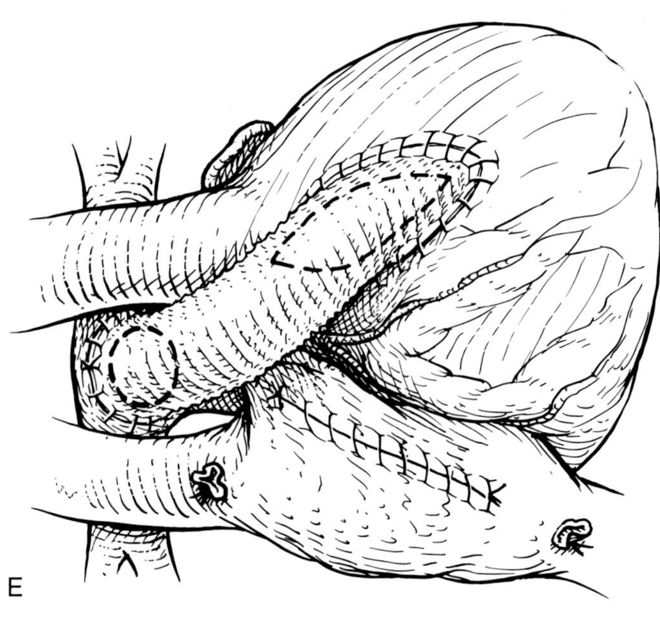

Figure 55-17, cont'd **E,** Procedure is completed by placing an external valved conduit from left-sided anterior MRV to pulmonary trunk. In this instance, the subpulmonic area was closed previously during the intracardiac portion of the operation **(B)**. Conduit is placed from infundibular incision in the MRV, coursing either to left or right side of aortic valve and ascending aorta. Positioning of conduit in this operation is somewhat more problematic than placing conduit from right-sided MLV to pulmonary trunk, as described in the "standard repair" in Fig. 55-16. Ventricular incision in MRV is more anterior and much more likely to be immediately substernal, increasing risk of compression. Whether to place the conduit to left or right of aortic valve and ascending aorta is an individual decision based on particular details of cardiac position within chest cavity. The principle is to place conduit in such a way that minimizes sternal compression. In this case, a composite graft of polyester and a bioprosthetic valve is used. Again, length of conduit is typically much longer than in cases of tetralogy of Fallot with pulmonary atresia. Similar to the situation described in Fig. 55-16, the valve is placed distally within the conduit, close to conduit to pulmonary trunk anastomosis.

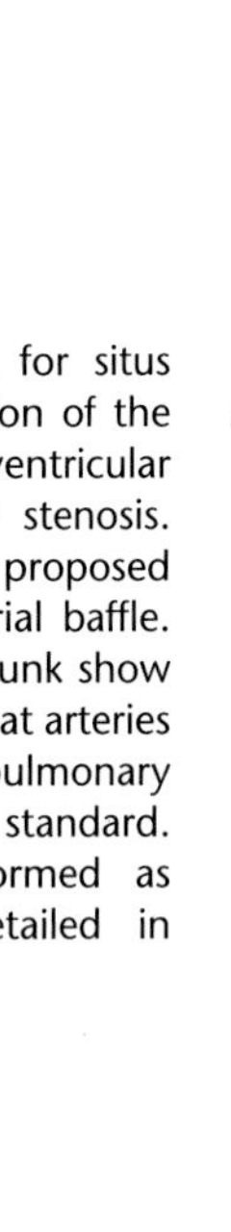

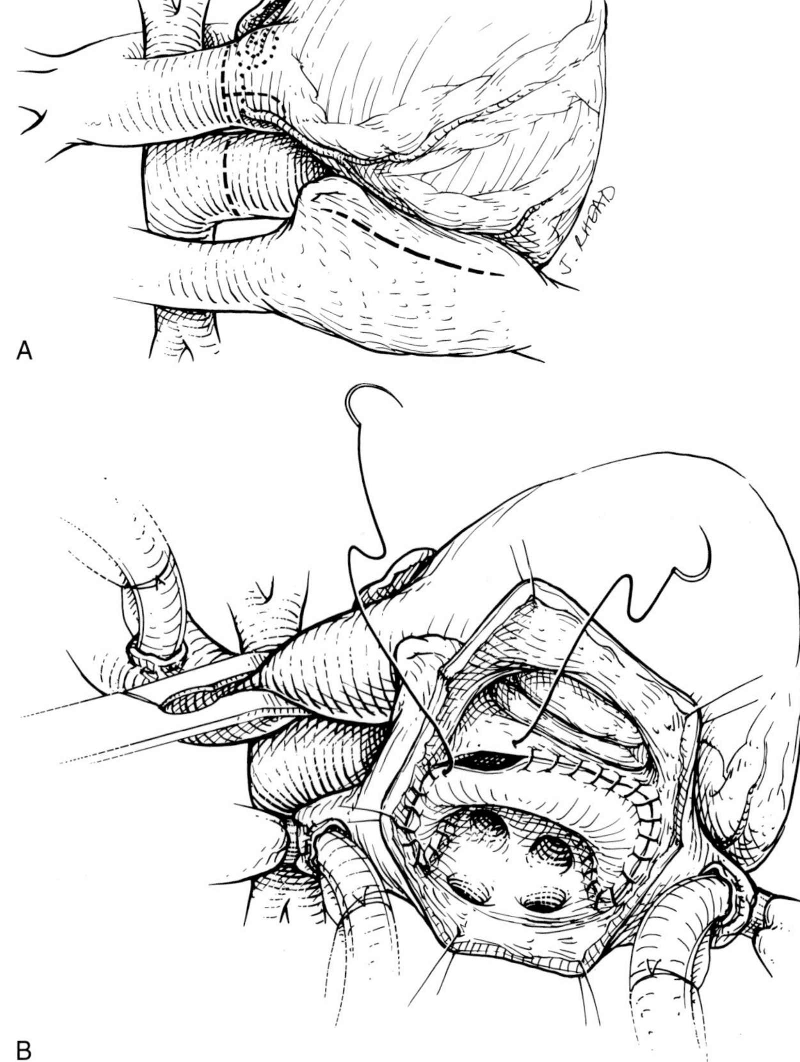

Figure 55-18 Double switch concept for situs solitus congenitally corrected transposition of the great arteries (CCTGA), with or without ventricular septal defect, and without pulmonary stenosis. **A,** Dashed line on right atrium shows proposed incision for performing Mustard intraatrial baffle. Dashed lines on aorta and pulmonary trunk show proposed incisions for transecting the great arteries and mobilizing coronary arteries. Cardiopulmonary bypass and myocardial protection are standard. **B,** Mustard intraatrial baffle is performed as described in Fig. 55-17 and as detailed in Chapter 52.

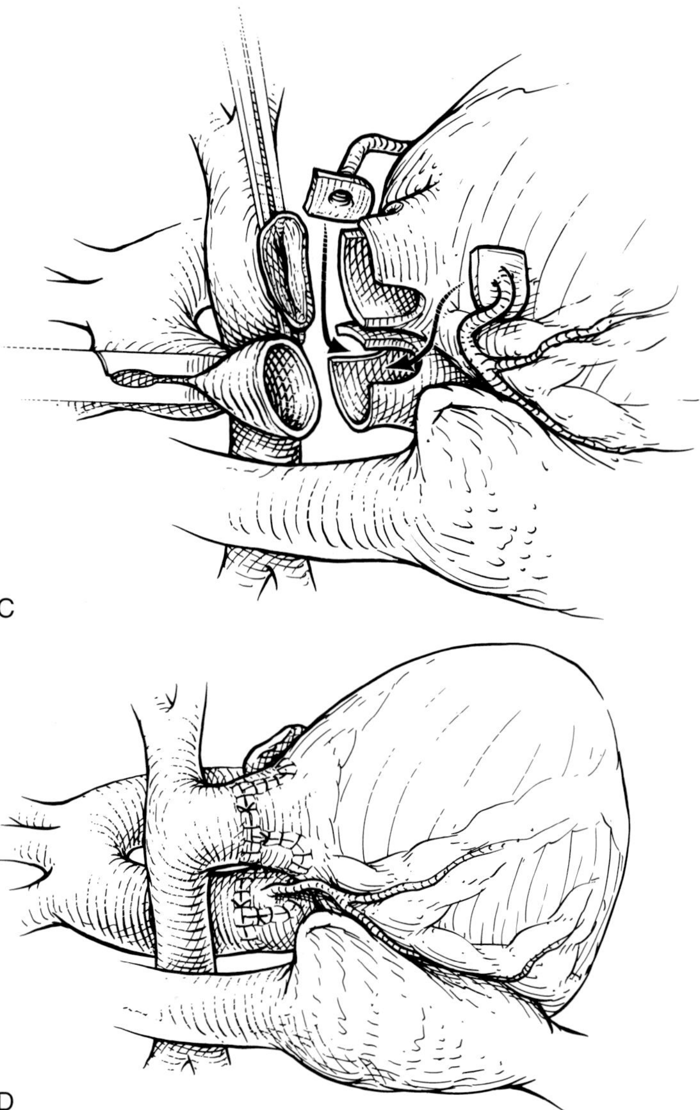

Figure 55-18, cont'd **C,** Arterial switch component of procedure proceeds essentially exactly as described in detail in Chapter 52 for simple transposition of the great arteries (TGA). Although the great arteries in CCTGA are typically L-transposed, as compared with D-transposed in simple TGA, in principle there are no differences between the two situations. In CCTGA, the Lecompte maneuver is usually performed because the native pulmonary trunk is positioned posterior to the aorta. **D,** Completed arterial switch component.

Other advantages exist specifically in CCTGA with VSD and pulmonary stenosis. If an extracardiac conduit is necessary owing to severe pulmonary stenosis, its longevity will be extended because of reduced volume of flow it carries. This may be particularly pertinent in a small growing child. Additionally, if the morphologic RV size is reduced, either because of intrinsic reasons or as a result of a large morphologic LV–aortic baffle occupying part of its cavity, the bidirectional superior cavopulmonary anastomosis may provide superior hemodynamics. Finally, in patients with positional abnormalities such as situs solitus with mesocardia or dextrocardia, or with situs inversus, simplicity of the "hemi-Mustard" procedure makes it preferable to the full Mustard or Senning procedure.

For these reasons, bidirectional superior cavopulmonary anastomosis with hemi-Mustard procedure has become the preferred technique for performing the atrial component of the operation in both forms of the double switch for at least one of the authors.[M1] The procedure is performed as described in Chapter 41 under "Bidirectional Superior Cavopulmonary Shunt." The double switch procedure, inferior vena cava–to–tricuspid valve atrial baffle (hemi-Mustard), and bidirectional superior cavopulmonary anastomosis are shown in Fig. 55-19.

Placing Epicardial Pacemaker Leads

When complete heart block has been present intermittently or permanently preoperatively, or when it has developed intraoperatively, permanent epicardial atrial and ventricular pacemaking leads are placed, and a permanent pacemaker pulse generator is placed subcutaneously (see "Technique of Intervention" in Section I of Chapter 16).

SPECIAL FEATURES OF POSTOPERATIVE CARE

Patients are managed with protocols generally used after cardiac surgery (see Chapter 5). In patients with AV discordant connection such as these, particular attention is paid to the cardiac rhythm. When complete heart block is present, AV sequential pacing augments cardiac output and is therefore used routinely.

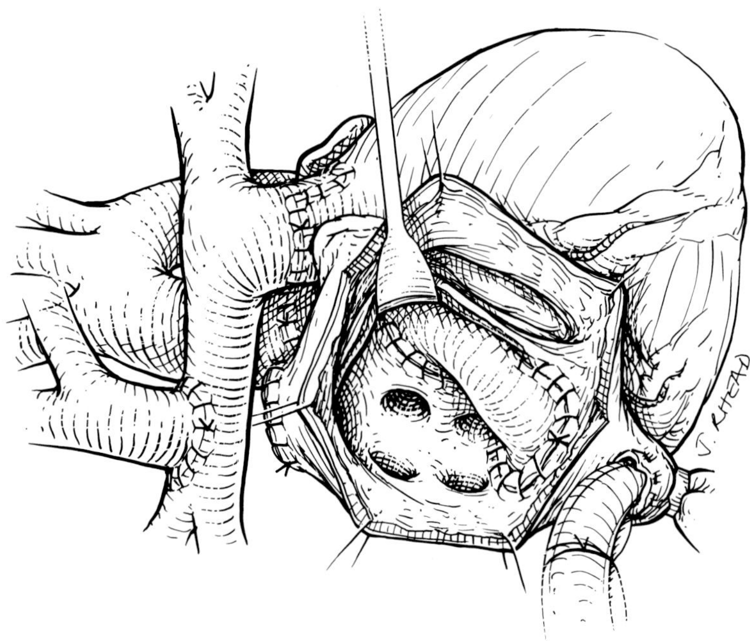

Figure 55-19 Bidirectional superior cavopulmonary anastomosis and "hemi-Mustard" modification for double switch procedure for congenitally corrected transposition of the great arteries. As in all double switch variations, atrial and arterial components can be performed in any order desired. In certain circumstances (see text), modifying the atrial component by performing a hemi-Mustard connection of the inferior vena cava to the tricuspid valve in combination with a bidirectional superior cavopulmonary anastomosis, rather than the full Mustard procedure, is beneficial. When this procedure is elected, the simplified intraatrial baffle can be performed either before or after the great artery component, whether that be a formal arterial switch or a Rastelli morphologic left ventricle–aortic intraventricular baffle. It is advantageous, however, to perform the bidirectional superior cavopulmonary anastomosis as the last component of the operation after removing the aortic clamp and establishing myocardial reperfusion. The intraatrial component of this procedure proceeds by performing a formal atrial septectomy (see "Mustard Technique" under Technique of Operation in Chapter 52). It may be advantageous in some cases to further enlarge the intraatrial opening by incising superiorly into the limbus of the atrial septum. The intraatrial baffle is much simplified, in essence constructing only inferior vena caval limb of Mustard baffle. Shape of baffle patch used is circular. Diameter of patch is equal to the straight-line distance measured from most superior limit of tricuspid valve anulus to orifice of inferior vena cava. Suture line follows exact details of the standard Mustard patch around inferior vena cava orifice. Superior aspect of baffle is sewn around tricuspid valve orifice. Bidirectional superior cavopulmonary anastomosis is performed exactly as described in Chapter 41.

RESULTS

Survival

Morphologic Right Ventricle Supporting Systemic Circulation

Early (Hospital) Death When operation is performed for CCTGA and VSD, hospital mortality has been 5% to 10%. When performed for CCTGA with coexisting VSD and important pulmonary stenosis, it has been 10% to 20%. When performed for coexisting left-sided tricuspid valvar regurgitation requiring valve replacement, it has been 15% to 25%.[A1,B13,D3,L8,M8,S1,T3,W4,W6,Y4] Reducing hospital mortality is surely possible and has been documented in studies showing a reduction from 21% (17/82; CL 16%-26%) for operations performed prior to 1987 to 3.4% (1/29; CL 0.6%-11%) for those performed between 1987 and 1996.[B13]

Time-Related Survival The 1-month and 1-, 5-, 10-, and 20-year survivals after repair of important coexisting cardiac anomalies in heterogeneous groups of patients with CCTGA repaired over the past 35 years have been about 88%, 80%, 76%, and 46%, respectively, including hospital deaths.[H12,Y4] In more recent experience, close to 90% 10-year survival has been demonstrated in a risk-unadjusted population of patients undergoing surgery for CCTGA.[S8,V8] When a late-rising phase of hazard will become evident in patients operated on in the current era is not yet known.

Hraska and colleagues suggest that time-related survival is best when a Fontan procedure is performed (100% at 5 years), with lower survival in septated patients undergoing VSD closure (75% at 5 years) and even lower survival in septated patients undergoing tricuspid valve surgery (55% at 5 years).[H11] It should be emphasized that their patients underwent surgery between 1963 and 1996. Hörer and colleagues found similar long-term outcomes in patients undergoing septation and those undergoing a Fontan procedure.[H5]

Morphologic Left Ventricle Supporting Systemic Circulation

Early (Hospital) Death Early outcomes appear to be as good or better with more complicated double switch procedures ("anatomic repair") that assign the morphologic LV to the systemic circulation than with the "physiologic" procedures just described. Jahangiri and colleagues reported no mortality in the anatomic repair group (0 of 19 patients; 0%; CL 0%-10%), and 7% mortality in the physiologic repair group (5 of 70 patients; CL 4%-12%), $P = .3$.[J1] Yeh and colleagues reported equivalent outcomes.[Y4]

In a group of patients with structurally abnormal tricuspid valves, mortality was 11% (1 of 9 patients; CL 1%-33%) following anatomic repair and 33% (5 of 15 patients; CL 19%-50%) following physiologic repair (P for difference = .2).[A1]

Table 55-1 Causes of Early and Late Death in 151 Patients

	Physiologic Repair (n = 67)			Anatomic Repair (n = 84)			Fontan (n = 38)		
Cause	No.	%	CL (%)	No.	%	CL (%)	No.	%	CL (%)
Low-output syndrome	4	6.0	3.1-11	3	3.6	1.6-7.0	4	11	5.4-18
Heart failure	8	12	7.8-17	3	3.6	1.6-7.0	0	0	0-4.9
Pulmonary hypertension	0	0	0-2.8	1	1.2	0.2-4.0	0	0	0-4.9
Infection	2	3.0	1.0-6.9	3	3.6	1.6-7.0	1	2.6	0.4-8.6
Arrhythmia/sudden death	1	1.5	0.2-5.0	5	6.0	3.3-10	1	2.6	0.4-8.6
Noncardiac	1	1.5	0.2-5.0	1	1.2	0.2-4.0	0	0	0-4.9
Gastrointestinal bleeding	0	0	0-2.8	1	1.2	0.2-4.0	0	0	0-4.9
Cerebral damage	1	1.5	0.2-5.0	1	1.2	0.2-4.0	0	0	0-4.9
Unknown	1	1.5	0.2-5.0	1	1.2	0.2-4.0	1	2.6	0.4-8.6

Adapted from Shin'oka and colleagues (Table E1).[S8]

Results reported from 10 single institutional experiences between 1993 and 2002 reveal that early mortality for procedures placing the morphologic LV in the systemic circulation compares favorably with that of simpler, more classic repairs. In these 10 studies, early mortality ranged from 0% to 14%. Each experience was small, with a combined total of 150 patients with 11 early deaths (7.3%; CL 5.1%-10%).[I2,I3,I5,K2,M9,R2,S5,S11,Y1,Y2]

Reports between 2002 and 2010 have larger numbers of patients and confirm that early mortality can be low. In three recent large single-institution studies, early mortality was 0% (46 patients; CL 0%-4.0%),[D11] 2.1% (1 of 48 patients; CL 0.3%-6.8%),[M1] and 6.8% (3 of 44 patients; CL 3.0%-13%).[B15] These studies included both the arterial switch type and the Rastelli type of double switch. In another study focusing on 20 patients with the arterial switch type of double switch only, there was no early mortality.[L9] Other large series report early mortality of about 15%.[S7] Most studies show similar early mortality of the two major double switch operations, but Gaies et al. found a difference, with 94% early survival (33 of 35 patients; CL 87%-98%) in the arterial switch type and 77% survival (23 of 30 patients; CL 66%-85%) in the Rastelli type.[G1]

Time-Related Survival Recent data suggest midterm survival is excellent. Two studies with follow-up extending to 15 years (mean 5 years) show no intermediate mortality.[L9,M1] Another shows 15-year survival of 75% in patients with the arterial switch type of double switch and 80% in patients with the Rastelli type.[S8] Still another study of 45 patients (38 underwent the Rastelli type and 7 the arterial switch type) showed survival of 84% at 5 years and 78% at 10 years.[K6] As with early mortality, most studies show similar time-related survival of the two major double switch operations, but the Gaies group reported a substantial difference, with 10-year survival of 91% in the arterial switch type and 55% in the Rastelli type.[G1]

Modes of Death

Some patients die suddenly.[M8,W6] This has even been noted when operation places the morphologic LV as the systemic ventricle[M13]; however, one large study suggests that it is more common following anatomic repair than physiologic repair.[S8] Whether this is due to sudden appearance of complete heart block with ventricular asystole or fibrillation or to pacemaker failure or change in conductance of leads is unknown. Well-documented progression of morphologic RV dysfunction and tricuspid valve regurgitation when these structures are in the systemic circulation no doubt play a role, particularly in those dying from low-output state and heart failure.[S1] Table 55-1 shows cause of death in one series of 151 patients.[S8]

Incremental Risk Factors for Death

Systemic tricuspid valve regurgitation is a risk factor for death.[H12,R8,S8] Studies identifying Ebstein anomaly and tricuspid valve replacement as risk factors are probably identifying the same underlying problem of systemic tricuspid valve regurgitation.[H11] Risk factors for death following anatomic repair have been identified and include left ventricular training using a pulmonary artery band and severe preoperative RV failure.[Q2,S8] Inclusion of a bidirectional cavopulmonary anastomosis as part of the repair has a survival benefit.[S8]

Reasons for lower survival in patients with CCTGA than that observed after repair of VSD, AV septal defect, tetralogy of Fallot, or transposition with AV concordant connection are not evident, even after risk adjustment. Speculatively, the major reasons may be abnormalities of the conduction system, imperfection of methods used to prevent and manage heart block, and abnormalities of systemic (right) ventricular function. It follows that patients receiving anatomic repair, although subject to the same conduction risks, would not have the additional risk of the systemic RV. In an analysis of 40 patients with a mean follow-up of 20 years, important regurgitation of the systemic tricuspid valve was found to be the major risk factor for death.[P6] In another study,[A1] presence of an abnormal systemic tricuspid valve resulted in early mortality of 33% (5 of 15 patients; CL 19%-50%) when the morphologic RV was assigned to the systemic circulation. Another study examining both anatomic and physiologic repair identified tricuspid regurgitation as a risk factor for physiologic but not anatomic repair patients.[S8] Subsequent studies show both early and late survival after anatomic repair to be similar to survival following repair of the other index lesions mentioned.[B15,D11,L9,M1] This improvement is probably due to multiple factors including presence of a systemic LV,

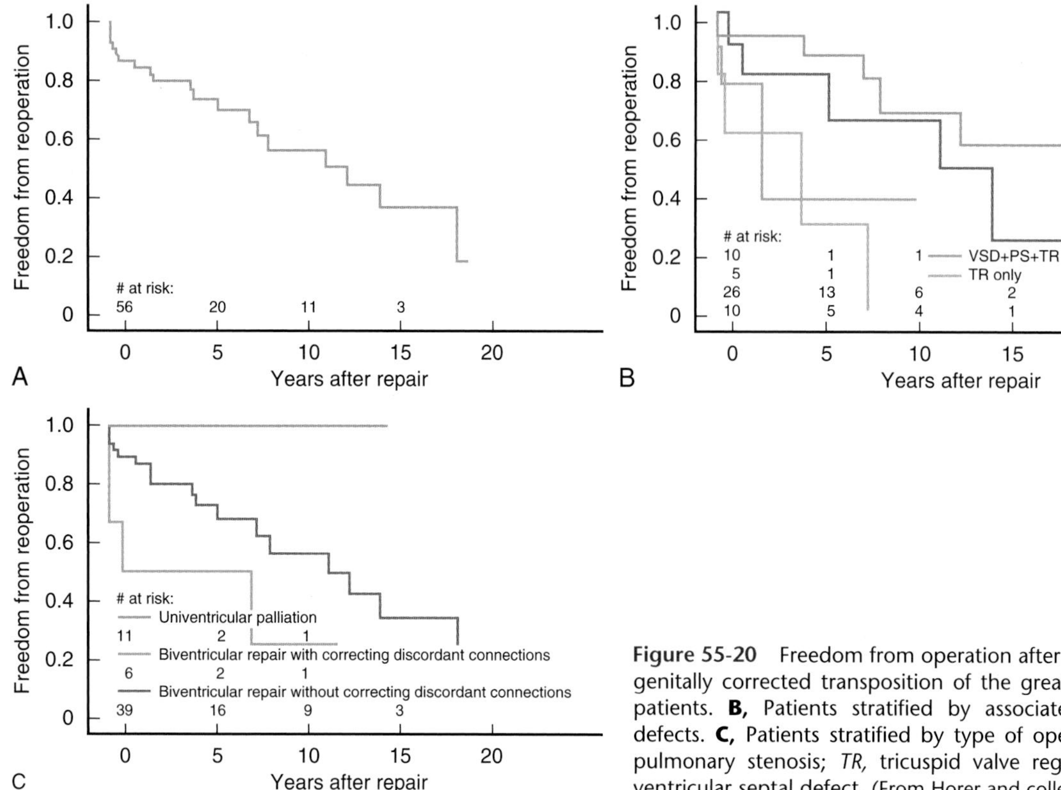

Figure 55-20 Freedom from operation after surgery for congenitally corrected transposition of the great arteries. **A,** All patients. **B,** Patients stratified by associated morphologic defects. **C,** Patients stratified by type of operation. Key: *PS,* pulmonary stenosis; *TR,* tricuspid valve regurgitation; *VSD,* ventricular septal defect. (From Horer and colleagues [Fig. 4].[H5])

increased experience with the complex procedures involved in anatomic repair, and improved management of conduction problems. In the meta-analysis performed by Alghamdi and colleagues, anatomic repair—in particular anatomic repair of the Rastelli type—had a beneficial effect on early survival compared with physiologic repair.[A5]

Reoperation

Reoperation is common after all types of surgery for CCTGA except for the Fontan operation. The morphology of associated cardiac defects and the type of operation both influence the prevalence of reoperation (Fig. 55-20). Common causes for reoperation are those to be expected: heart block, ventricular-to–pulmonary trunk conduit obstruction or regurgitation, and systemic tricuspid valve regurgitation.

Postrepair Complete Heart Block

It was anticipated that a repair (see Technique of Operation earlier) based on secure knowledge of location of the cardiac conduction system would eliminate complete heart block as a complication of VSD repair in patients with CCTGA.[D3] Such has not been the case. In all reported series, prevalence has been 15% to 30%[H14] (Table 55-2). This is very different from the near-zero prevalence after repair of VSD in hearts with AV concordant connection. Patients with atrial situs inversus have a lower prevalence of postoperative complete heart block, but it also does not approach zero.[D6]

PR interval is generally not lengthened by repair in patients in whom heart block does not develop perioperatively.[C3] However, delayed intraventricular conduction, particularly to the left-sided RV, develops in about half of patients.

Multivariable analysis indicates that chordal straddling or insertion on the septal crest (usually from the left-sided tricuspid valve) increases the probability of producing complete heart block at the time of VSD repair (Table 55-3). This arrangement may prevent surgeons from placing sutures precisely where they prefer them. Presumably, placing the LV in the systemic circulation should have little effect on these rhythm complications. Malhotra and colleagues noted that 21% of patients developed complete heart block following surgery in a series of 48 double switches.[M1]

In patients with complete heart block and systemic RV failure, improved ventricular function has been demonstrated in selected individuals by upgrading the pacing system to a biventricular system to achieve cardiac resynchronization.[K8,K11]

Development of Tricuspid Valve Regurgitation

Immediately after simple classic repair of CCTGA with VSD, left-sided tricuspid valve regurgitation sometimes appears. Fox and colleagues[F2] reported this to have occurred immediately after repair in 6 of 14 patients (43%; CL 27%-60%) in whom it was not present before operation. Westerman and colleagues[W4] observed the same phenomenon. Its mechanism is not completely understood, but as best as can be determined, regurgitation does not result from direct damage to valvar tissue or chordae. Rather, its mechanism when the tricuspid valve is abnormal is primarily related to decreased morphologic LV pressure after VSD closure, resulting in shifting of the ventricular septum toward the morphologic LV side.[A1,J1] It seems likely a similar mechanism is involved when the tricuspid valve is normal.

Operations assigning the morphologic LV to the systemic circulation result in improved tricuspid valve function,

Table 55-2 Heart Block after Operation in Patients with Congenitally Corrected Transposition of the Great Arteries[a]

Operation	*n*	Preoperative Complete Heart Block	Postoperative Permanent Complete Heart Block		
			No.	% of (*n* – Preoperative Block)	CL (%)
Repair VSD	16	2	2	14	5-31
Repair VSD + PS	15	1	3	21	10-38
Repair VSD + valved extracardiac conduit to PT	26	3[b]	6	26	16-39
Tricuspid valve repair	1	0		0	0-85
Tricuspid valve replacement				21	15-28
Isolated	5	1		0	0-38
With VSD repair	8	2		17	2-46
With VSD + PS repair	1	1			
With VSD repair + CABG	1	0		0	0-85
Repair ASD	1	0		0	0-85
Fontan-type operation	1	0		0	0-85
TOTAL	75	10 13 (CL 9–9)	12	18	13-25

Data from McGrath and colleagues.[M6]
[a]Heart block developed in 0 (0%; CL 0%-24%) of 7 patients whose repair did not include closure of a VSD and in 12 (21%; CL 15%-28%) of 58 who had a VSD closed as part of the procedure (*P*(Fisher) = .22).
[b]In one, complete heart block preoperatively was episodic and was permanent after repair.
Key: *ASD,* Atrial septal defect; *CABG,* coronary artery bypass grafting; *CL,* 70% confidence limits; *PS,* pulmonary stenosis; *PT,* pulmonary trunk; *VSD,* ventricular septal defect.

Table 55-3 Incremental Risk Factors for Development of Complete Heart Block in Patients with Atrioventricular Discordant Connection Undergoing Closure of a Ventricular Septal Defect[a]

	Incremental Risk Factors	Logistic Coefficient ± SD	*P*
(Older)	Age at repair	1.0 ± 0.38	.009
	Morphology other than CCTGA	1.0 ± 0.62	.10
	Chordae straddling or attaching to edge of VSD	1.6 ± 0.66	.01

Data from McGrath and colleagues.[M6]
[a]Patients with complete heart block before repair were excluded. Excluded also were patients (*n* = 9) in whom repair did not include either closure of the VSD or an intraventricular tunnel repair, because developed heart block was limited to these two groups.
Key: *CCTGA,* Congenitally corrected transposition of the great arteries; *VSD,* ventricular septal defect.

probably for two reasons: the pressure in the morphologic RV is markedly reduced, and the ventricular septum is shifted toward the morphologic RV.[A1,J1,J2,M1] This hypothesis is further supported by the work of Kollars and colleagues, who showed not only that systemic tricuspid valve regurgitation improved by increasing LV pressure with pulmonary artery banding but also that tricuspid regurgitation became worse in patients in whom LV pressure was reduced to less than half of systemic levels with an LV-to–pulmonary trunk conduit.[K10] It also may be associated with development of complete heart block.[W4]

Tricuspid regurgitation may be sufficiently severe to require later valve replacement. Attempts at valve repair when the valve is in the systemic circulation are usually futile.[A1,S3] In one series of 52 patients with up to 10 years of follow-up, tricuspid valve regurgitation was severe enough to require reoperation in 12 (24%).[T3] When the RV is placed in the pulmonary circulation, tricuspid valve function typically improves, often without specifically surgically addressing the valve.[I3,I5,J2,M1]

Functional Status

In the study by Malhotra and colleagues in which all patients underwent anatomic repair, 91% were in New York Heart Association (NYHA) class I postoperatively.[M1] Similar functional outcome has been reported by others following anatomic repair.[D11] In the multicenter study of Graham and colleagues of patients with physiologic or no repair, 60% of those with associated defects were in NYHA class I, and 70% of patients without associated defects were in NYHA class I.[G5] Despite these functional class findings, the same study showed that by age 45 years, clinical heart failure was present in 67% of those with associated lesions and 25% of those without associated lesions; moderate or severe systemic RV dysfunction was present in 56% and 32%, respectively.[G5] Hraska and colleagues showed that only 40% of physiologically repaired patients were free of RV failure at 15 years.[H11]

Ventricular Function

The preponderance of evidence suggests that the systemic RV functions abnormally in unoperated patients at rest, even if they are asymptomatic.[G5] If some form of physiologic repair has been performed, these preoperative abnormalities are more severe. Ischemia appears to play an underlying role in deterioration in most cases, along with other hemodynamic stresses such as volume overload from tricuspid regurgitation. Systemic RVs commonly show evidence of deterioration over time. Giardini and colleagues studied 34 patients at a mean age of 25 years with either CCTGA not undergoing anatomic repair or simple TGA following atrial baffle surgery.[G3] The groups were similar. Abnormal myocardial fibrosis, determined by late gadolinium enhancement at MRI, was found in 41%. These findings were associated with RV dysfunction, poor exercise tolerance, arrhythmias, and progressive clinical deterioration. However, normal systemic RV systolic function late postoperatively has been found in some patients.[H14] The rule is that after physiologic repair, even asymptomatic adult patients demonstrate abnormalities of the systemic RV, including reduced resting and stress ejection fraction, large ventricular volumes, and regional wall motion abnormalities.[D8,G5,T7] Asymptomatic patients also demonstrate a neurohormonal profile typical of heart failure.[K9] Additionally, systemic RV coronary flow reserve is reduced, even in unoperated patients and those with isolated CCTGA, with both ischemic and persistent perfusion defects.[H2]

When surgery involves placing the morphologic LV in the systemic circulation, early and midterm follow-up studies demonstrate both well-maintained LV and RV function.[I2,M1,M9,R2] However, late systemic LV dysfunction has been observed, mostly in association with prior LV training and in patients with complete heart block requiring pacemakers.[B3,Q2]

INDICATIONS FOR OPERATION

CCTGA per se is not a definitive indication for a reparative operation. On the other hand, the natural history of the morphologic RV in the systemic circulation presents enough concern that the question of performing a double switch procedure should be left open. When VSD coexists, indications for operation are those for repair of VSD in otherwise normal hearts (see Indications for Operation in Section I of Chapter 35).

When VSD and important pulmonary stenosis coexist, repair may require an allograft-valved extracardiac conduit; surgical indications and staging are therefore the same as described for tetralogy of Fallot with pulmonary atresia (see Indications for Operation in Section II of Chapter 38). When important left-sided tricuspid regurgitation coexists, indications for operation are the same as those described for acquired mitral regurgitation (see Indications for Operation in Section I of Chapter 11). When complete heart block develops, indications and techniques for pacemaker intervention are those described in Technique of Intervention in Section I of Chapter 16.

Certain morphologic characteristics may increase difficulty of the various septation procedures described in this chapter: (1) presence of straddling tricuspid chordae—increasing complexity of the surgery and risk of postoperative complete heart block, (2) AV septal defect, and (3) non-committed VSD with pulmonary stenosis. These, among others, may be considered by some to be indications for a Fontan rather than a biventricular repair. Whatever the initial interventions, patients may ultimately develop a situation in which only cardiac transplantation can be effective.

SPECIAL SITUATIONS AND CONTROVERSIES

Anatomic versus Physiologic Repair

Definitive data are unavailable to determine whether long-term outcome is better in CCTGA with the morphologic RV or LV in the systemic circulation. A multicenter retrospective study of 167 patients undergoing repair did, however, show that long-term systemic AV valve function and systemic ventricular function were better in patients undergoing a double switch type operation compared with those undergoing physiologic repair (Fig. 55-21).[L6] Surgical procedures are simpler technically when the morphologic RV is assigned to the systemic circulation, in theory reducing both short- and long-term complications related to reconstruction. However, available data from the same study[L6] indicate that surgically induced arrhythmias and reoperation are not higher in the more complex anatomic repair group (Fig. 55-22). Operative, midterm, and late mortalities following procedures placing the LV in the systemic circulation have been well documented over the past decade and are excellent.[L6,M1]

Even prior to 1998, superiority of the anatomic repair was evident. The meta-analysis of 11 different studies (in which all dates of operation were 1998 or earlier) performed by Alghamdi and colleagues showed that anatomic repair of the Rastelli type had superior outcomes to physiologic repair.[A5]

In a limited study of nine patients who underwent a procedure assigning the morphologic LV to the systemic circulation and six who underwent a procedure assigning the morphologic RV to the systemic circulation, exercise capacity was equivalent,[O1] but this does not mean exercise capacity was normal. Other studies testing patients after both anatomic and physiologic repair reveal that oxygen uptake, exercise duration, heart rate responses, and other variables measured are subnormal.[T2,Y3]

Left Ventricular Training

An important variable that must be considered when assessing long-term outcome following the double switch is whether it is necessary to train the morphologic LV with a pulmonary artery band. This situation arises only when the double switch is being considered in patients in whom the LV myocardial mass has involuted because it has been functioning at low pressure—that is, when CCTGA is present without VSD or pulmonary stenosis.

Although definitive evidence is lacking that trained LVs are functionally different from normal, there is concern and some suggestion that when placed in the systemic circulation, involuted LVs trained with a band may not perform as well as those that never involuted. Comparing trained LVs and those not requiring training, Quinn and colleagues showed that the early outcome after the double switch was similar for mortality and LV function, but there was increased risk of LV deterioration and death or transplantation over time in the trained LV group.[Q2] Lim and colleagues[L6] suggest that LV training is a risk factor for death after anatomic repair. However, Bautista-Hernandez and colleagues showed that after anatomic repair, there was no reduction in LV function and no deaths at midterm follow-up in the cohort of patients who had received LV training with a band.[B3]

An important factor that limits drawing definitive conclusions about the adequacy of the trained LV is that there are currently no standardized criteria for defining when an LV is trained. Thus, any reduction in function of trained LVs following anatomic repair may represent an intrinsic limitation of the trained LV itself, or the fact that an adequate training protocol was not in place. It is clear that some LVs do not respond to training, and these patients never become candidates for a double switch procedure.[Q2] (See Chapter 52 for more in-depth discussion of LV training.)

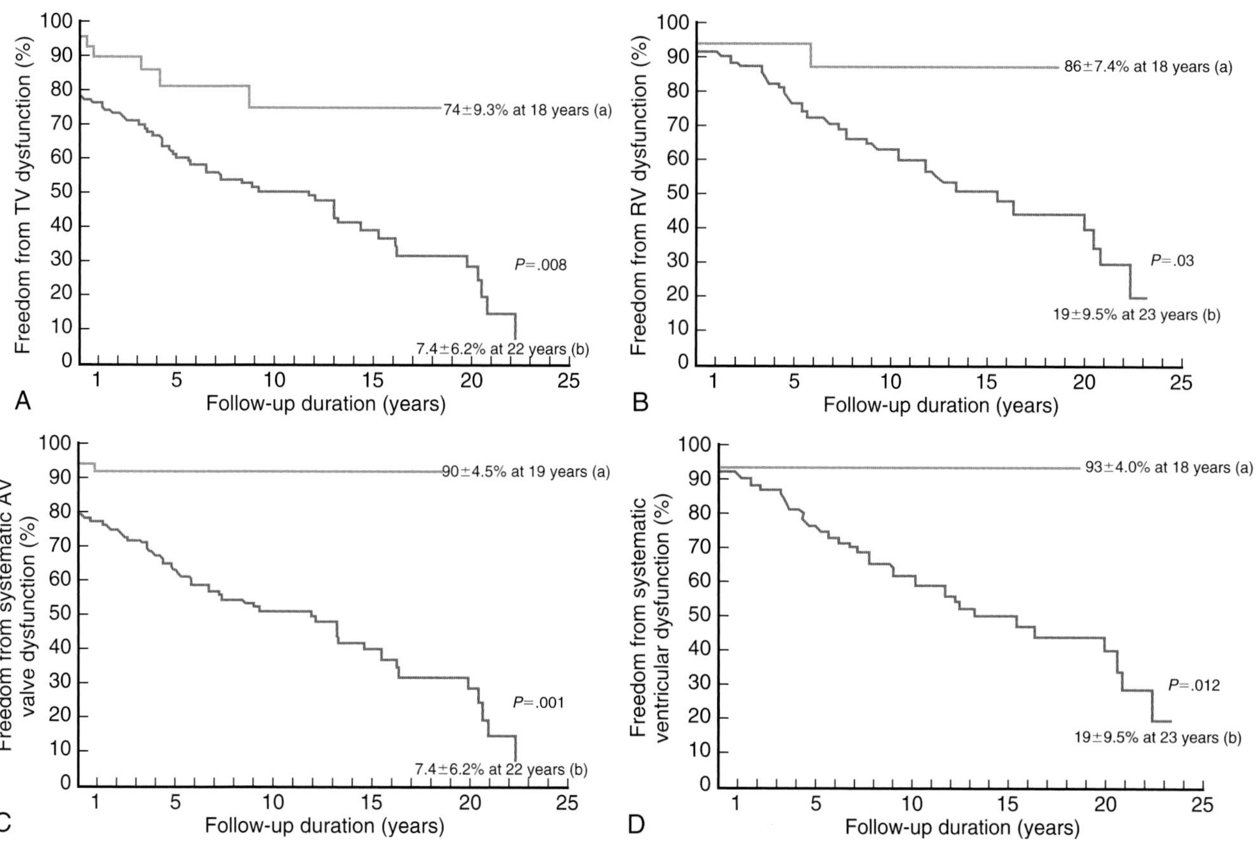

Figure 55-21 Freedom from atrioventricular (AV) valve and ventricular dysfunction in 167 patients undergoing either physiologic or anatomic repair for congenitally corrected transposition. **A,** Freedom from tricuspid valve (TV) dysfunction. **B,** Freedom from right ventricular (RV) dysfunction. **C,** Freedom from systemic AV valve dysfunction. **D,** Freedom from systemic ventricular dysfunction. AV dysfunction was defined as regurgitation of grade 2 and more; ventricular dysfunction was defined as mild to moderate dysfunction and worse. Solid lines: anatomic repair. Broken lines: physiologic repair. (From Lim and colleagues [Fig. 2].[L6])

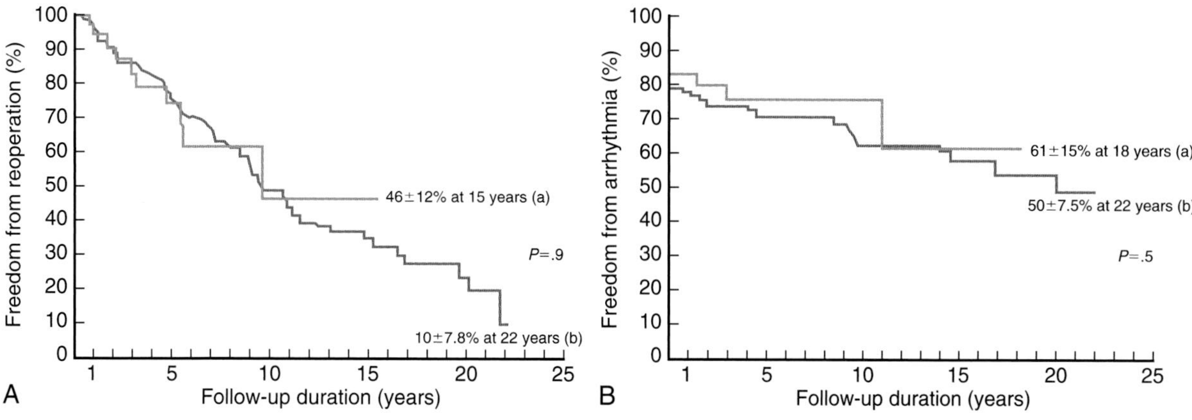

Figure 55-22 Reoperation and arrhythmia in 167 patients after undergoing repair for congenitally corrected transposition. **A,** Freedom from reoperation. **B,** Freedom from arrhythmia. Solid lines: Anatomic repair. Broken lines: Physiologic repair. (Modified from Lim and colleagues [Fig. 1].[L6])

Use of Bidirectional Superior Cavopulmonary Anastomosis

Use of the bidirectional superior cavopulmonary anastomosis with hemi-Mustard atrial baffle, either selectively or exclusively, as part of operations for CCTGA when the morphologic LV is placed in the systemic circulation has a number of specific advantages[L6,M1]:

- It may benefit the small or poorly functioning RV.
- It importantly reduces complexity of the atrial baffle procedure.
- It eliminates complications related to the superior limb of the atrial baffle.
- It reduces flow across an RV–pulmonary trunk conduit.
- It likely increases conduit longevity.

The study by Malhotra and colleagues documents that RV–pulmonary artery conduits have increased longevity when a bidirectional superior cavopulmonary anastomosis is used.[M1] Lim and colleagues have demonstrated improved survival when it is used.[L6] In some cases with VSD and moderate pulmonary stenosis, a bidirectional superior cavopulmonary anastomosis may allow use of the small native pulmonary valve as an adequate structure for RV outflow, avoiding a prosthetic conduit. In this operation, the native pulmonary valve and anulus, in continuity with the pulmonary trunk, are removed from the LV outflow tract intact and transposed onto the RV infundibulum. The resulting opening in the LV outflow tract is closed with a patch, and the LV is baffled to the aorta with an intraventricular tunnel.[M1] The bidirectional cavopulmonary anastomosis and hemi-Mustard can also be helpful when constructing a full atrial baffle is difficult, such as in patients with juxtaposition of the ventricular apex and inferior vena cava, as found in mesocardia or dextrocardia with situs solitus. The bidirectional superior cavopulmonary anastomosis can also be used in specific cases when physiologic repair is performed.[B1,L6]

Fontan versus Intracardiac Repair

After weighing the benefits and risks of performing the complex procedures described in this chapter versus those of a Fontan operation, one study concludes that the Fontan operation is advisable.[D4] Many surgeons disagree, and recent outcomes after any of the various procedures that use the double switch concept or physiologic repair concept support their position.[L6,M1] Reoperation is almost certainly higher after operations (both anatomic and physiologic) that septate the heart in CCTGA than for the Fontan, at least up to midterm follow-up (see Fig. 55-20).

Neonatal Congenitally Corrected Transposition of the Great Arteries without Associated Cardiac Anomalies

The era of anatomic repair presents an interesting possibility for patients with CCTGA without associated lesions. Compared with normal control subjects, these patients are considered to have a reasonable prognosis without intervention, but a number of studies document that abnormal systemic RV function and even RV failure with systemic AV valve regurgitation are much more likely to occur over time, usually over decades. The question arises whether anatomic repair would benefit them. Although there is no evidence available to answer this question, it has been posed by many in the field.

If it is hypothesized that anatomic repair is beneficial, it can be argued that the neonatal period would be the optimal time for surgery to take advantage of the prepared LV. Allowing the LV to involute, followed by retraining with a pulmonary artery band, before anatomic repair is much less attractive because of concerns about the function of a retrained LV. To date, there are no reports of elective neonatal anatomic repair in asymptomatic patients with this anatomic profile. Bautista-Hernandez and colleagues report successful neonatal anatomic repair in two patients with Ebstein-like changes of the systemic AV valve and severe regurgitation with severe heart failure.[B4]

An alternative to neonatal anatomic repair in asymptomatic patients without associated cardiac anomalies is neonatal placement of a band, thereby preventing LV involution. Metton and colleagues have placed bands in 11 asymptomatic neonates and infants with isolated CCTGA.[M10] Some degree of systemic AV valve regurgitation was present preoperatively in eight patients and depressed systemic RV function in two. The band procedure was performed without mortality, but five patients required inotropic support. There was one late death. In the remainder, there was no progression of systemic AV valve regurgitation in seven and improvement in three. Only one patient has undergone anatomic repair, successfully. The others are candidates, having preserved LV mass and function.

Section II Other Forms of Atrioventricular Discordant Connection

DEFINITION

Atrioventricular discordant connection is a congenital cardiac anomaly in which the right atrium connects to the LV and the left atrium connects to the RV (see "Cardiac Chambers and Major Vessels" in Chapter 1).[2] When AV discordant connection occurs in atrial situs solitus, there is ventricular L-loop (left handedness of the ventricular internal architecture)[A9,V1,V6]; when it occurs in atrial situs inversus, there is ventricular D-loop (right handedness).

Conditions with AV discordant connection (other than CCTGA, covered earlier) are discussed together in this section. Were accumulated experience large enough, each of the other subsets would deserve separate chapters, just as in the setting of AV concordant connection.

HISTORICAL NOTE

History of development of knowledge and surgical treatment of CCTGA is discussed in Section I. The time of first recognition of AV discordant connection associated with double outlet right ventricle (DORV) is not clear, but as late as 1960 the entity was not distinguished from DORV with concordant AV connection. Ruttenberg and colleagues described DORV coexisting with AV discordant connection in 1964.[R9] In 1965, this type of DORV (with VSD and pulmonary stenosis) was recognized and repaired using an extracardiac conduit for rerouting pulmonary blood flow, perhaps for the first time.[K4] Double outlet left ventricle (DOLV) associated with AV discordant connection is rare; the first surgical case was reported in 1976 by Brandt and colleagues.[B17]

Isolated ventricular inversion was named by Van Praagh in 1966 when he described one such case,[V4] but a similar malformation had been reported by Ratner, Abbott, and Beattle in 1921[R1] and by Lev and Rowlatt in 1961.[L3] In 1975, Quero-Jimenez and colleagues reviewed six reported cases,

[2]As noted in Section 1 of this chapter, the adjectives *left* and *right* used to modify atrium or ventricle always mean *morphologically* right or left. Position of the chamber is referred to as *right-sided* or *left-sided*.

including two of their own.[Q1] *Isolated atrial inversion* was named when the first such case was reported in 1972.[C6]

MORPHOLOGY

Among hearts with AV discordant connection, there is great variability in ventriculoarterial connections and in many other morphologic details.[A4]

Ventricular Architecture

The ventricles are said to be inverted, but because many ventricular positional anomalies occur, the term *ventricular inversion* is not very useful; it is necessary to describe the internal architecture of each ventricle more specifically. A convenient way of doing this is with Van Praagh's terms *ventricular D-loop* and *ventricular L-loop*, defined in Chapter 1 (see "Situs of the Ventricles" under Terminology and Classification of Heart Disease in Chapter 1), or *right handedness* and *left handedness*,[A9,V1,V6] also defined in Chapter 1.

Ventricular Position and Rotation

In patients with atrial situs solitus, the RV is generally left sided and the LV lies side by side and to the right of it. The entire length of the ventricular septum is usually visualized in profile in an anteroposterior view during diagnostic imaging. However, there are variations in anterosuperior orientation of the ventricles and variations in their rotation (see "Cardiac and Arterial Positions" under Terminology and Classification of Heart Disease in Chapter 1).

Positional Anomalies

An extreme variation of anterosuperior position occurs in so-called superior-inferior ventricles ("over-and-under" or "upstairs-downstairs" ventricles). The septum is not vertically oriented, as is usual in AV discordant connection, but horizontal, and the LV lies inferiorly and RV superiorly. This may have been described first by Kinsley and colleagues.[K3] When ventricles are positioned in this manner, there is usually AV discordant connection, an inlet VSD, and DORV.[H3,O4] One chamber may be hypoplastic, and there may be AV valve straddling. Rarely, superior-inferior ventricle position is associated with AV concordant connection and DORV (see "Double Outlet Right Ventricle with Superior-Inferior Ventricles" under Morphology in Chapter 53).

Rotational Anomalies

When rotational anomalies are present, even more bizarre situations occur. Although the LV inlet portion generally remains on the right side in patients with atrial situs solitus, trabecular and outlet portions may be left sided and present a confusing picture.[S9] Generally, however, the ventricular septum is in the coronal plane, the LV is posterior, and the RV anterior. In the domain of these extreme rotational anomalies, criss-cross pathways occur in which inflow pathways of the ventricles appear to cross rather than being parallel.[A15,F3,F4,S14,T6] Then the question arises as to whether an AV discordant connection necessarily implies ventricular L-loop (or left handedness) in atrial situs solitus, and D-loop or (right handedness) in atrial situs inversus. In this text, the assumption is made that it does, although this may not always be the case.[D12]

Ventricular Size

Varying degrees of hypoplasia of the left-sided RV may be present.[E3] When the ventricles are in a superior-inferior position, the LV may be hypoplastic. Ventricular hypoplasia is frequently associated with straddling and overriding of the AV valve of the hypoplastic ventricle.

Cardiac Position

Dextrocardia occurs in about 25% of cases with atrial situs solitus, and rarely levocardia exists when the atrial situs is inverted.[C2]

Ventriculoarterial Connection

Discordant Connection

The morphology of congenitally corrected transposition of the great arteries (AV discordant connection and ventriculoarterial discordant connection) is described in Section I.

Double Outlet Right Ventricle

Double outlet left-sided RV may coexist with situs solitus and AV discordant connection (L-loop), and in nearly all cases VSD and pulmonary stenosis coexist. Because the left-sided RV is the systemic ventricle, cyanosis is not a necessary result of the ventriculoarterial connection, but of associated pulmonary stenosis. The apex of the heart may point to the right (dextrocardia with atrial situs solitus and ventricular L-loop).[K4] The aorta is usually in L-malposition but may be in any position. The VSD is usually very distal in the septum and beneath the adjacent great arteries (usually pulmonary) but can be anywhere.

The pulmonary trunk is not in a wedged position. Probably related to this, location of the conduction system tends to be different from that in corrected transposition (see "Atrioventricular Node and Bundle of His" later).[L7]

This entity is closely related to corrected transposition with VSD in which the pulmonary trunk partially overrides the VSD and partly arises over the left-sided RV. Corrected transposition is the appropriate diagnosis when there is fibrous continuity between the pulmonary and mitral valves. When there is lack of continuity between these valves, there is subpulmonic conus muscle, and the case is assigned the diagnosis of *AV discordant connection with DORV*. In most cases of DORV and AV discordant connection, the pulmonary trunk is nearly completely over the left-sided RV.

Double Outlet Left Ventricle

DOLV may coexist with AV discordant connection.[B17,S12,V5] Because the right-sided LV is the pulmonary ventricle, cyanosis is the necessary result. The VSD is in a position similar to that in DORV with AV discordant connection, but the aorta overrides the VSD to such an extent that it emerges wholly or in large part from the right-sided LV. This may occur in patients with atrial situs inversus.[A3]

Concordant Connection

Ventriculoarterial concordant connection is unusual in AV discordant connection and is of two types: isolated ventricular inversion[Q1,V3] and isolated atrial inversion.[C6] The systemic and pulmonary circulations are parallel, and the physiology is that of ordinary transposition of the great arteries (see "Essentially

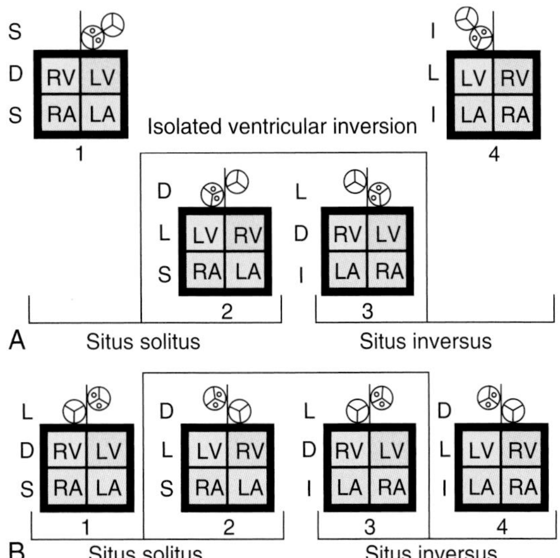

Figure 55-23 Models illustrating isolated ventricular inversion and anatomically corrected malposition of the great arteries.[V2] **A,** Models of isolated ventricular inversion (2, 3) (models 1 and 4 are the normal heart, with origin of the pulmonary trunk indicated by spiraled vertical extension of partition line). Similarities between models 2 and 3 here and in **B** are apparent. Isolated ventricular inversion is a cyanotic condition because of atrioventricular discordant connection. **B,** Models of anatomically corrected malposition of the great arteries. In this text, it is considered that only models 1 and 4 represent anatomically corrected malposition of the great arteries. Key: *LA,* Left atrium; *LV,* left ventricle; *RA,* right atrium; *RV,* right ventricle.

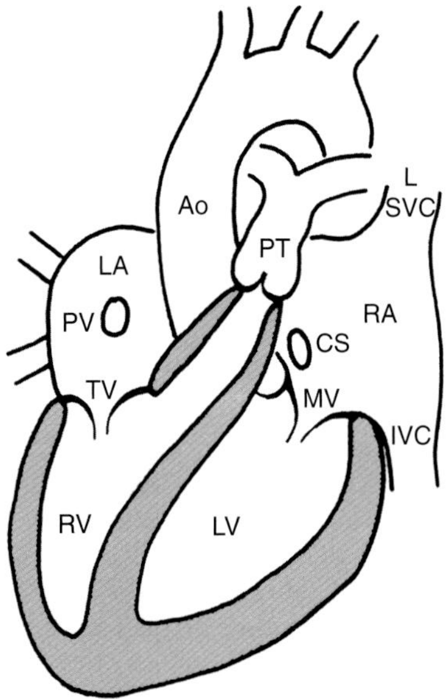

Figure 55-24 Line drawing of exact relationships of cardiac chambers and great arteries in isolated atrial inversion. Right superior vena cava and left pulmonary veins are not shown. Key: *Ao,* Aorta; *CS,* coronary sinus; *IVC,* inferior vena cava; *LA,* left atrium; *LSVC,* left superior vena cava; *LV,* left ventricle; *MV,* mitral valve; *PT,* pulmonary trunk; *PV,* pulmonary valve; *RA,* right atrium; *RV,* right ventricle; *TV,* tricuspid valve. (From Clarkson and colleagues.[C6])

Intact Ventricular Septum [Poor Mixing]" under Clinical Features and Diagnostic Criteria in Chapter 52), and cyanosis results.

In isolated ventricular inversion with atrial situs solitus, as originally defined,[V3] the aortic origin lies to the right and posterior to the pulmonary trunk origin, and there is aortic-mitral fibrous continuity and a muscular subpulmonary infundibulum (conus), as in the normal heart. However, there is AV discordant connection, and the aorta arises from a right-sided LV; for this reason, both great arteries are parallel. Other variations exist and are due to positioning of the great arteries and presence or absence of a subaortic and subpulmonic conus.[K7] A VSD may be present; pulmonary stenosis is generally absent.[Q1] When there is situs inversus, a mirror-image pattern occurs.[A11,L1]

As in CCTGA, the inverted ventricles in patients with isolated atrial or ventricular inversion usually lie side by side with the ventricular septum in a sagittal plane and have a coronary artery distribution pattern similar to that in CCTGA (see Morphology in Section I). It is important surgically to note that in isolated ventricular inversion, the right-sided left coronary artery does *not* cross in front of the pulmonary outflow, so its enlargement anteriorly is feasible. Although Losekoot and colleagues have suggested that the conduction tissue will be as for CCTGA,[L7] position of cardiac conduction tissue in this condition is at present uncertain.

In isolated atrial inversion, there is atrial situs inversus with ventricular D-loop and dextrocardia with fibrous aortic-mitral continuity and a subpulmonary conus (Fig. 55-23, *A*, model 3). However, in a case reported by Clarkson[C6] (Fig. 55-24), the great arteries crossed in a virtually normal fashion, with the morphologic RV lying to the right and posterior to the morphologic LV. The unusual feature of this heart was visceroatrial discordance, with abdominal organs in situs solitus position and the atria (and their venous connections) inverted. This rare additional feature did not alter the circulatory pathways from those present in isolated ventricular inversion.

In addition to the heart just described, there are others with identical connections but conal development that is the reverse of that described in isolated ventricular inversion (see Fig. 55-23, *B*, models 2 and 3). That is, the aorta arises from the morphological LV and lies, in a situs solitus heart, to the right of the pulmonary trunk, but it is separated from the mitral valve by a muscular subaortic conus. Under these circumstances, there is usually pulmonary-tricuspid fibrous continuity, but a subpulmonary conus may also (rarely) be present. These hearts can be considered to have anatomically corrected malposition of the great arteries,[V2] or contrariwise (as in this text) a variant within the general category of AV discordant connection and ventriculoarterial concordant connection.

Atrioventricular Node and Bundle of His

The AV conduction tissue is abnormal in most patients with AV discordant connection and typically so in the subset of CCTGA with atrial situs solitus, where an anterior AV node gives rise to the bundle of His (see "Atrioventricular Node and Bundle of His" under Morphology in Section I).

When DORV coexists and left-sided RV wedging of the pulmonary trunk is not present, both anterior and posterior AV nodes usually persist, connected by a sling of conduction tissue around the VSD, which continues on as the branching bundle.[L7] However, only the anterior AV node or the regular posterior one gives rise to the penetrating bundle.[L7] This variability may predispose patients to surgically induced complete heart block.

When there is DOLV, the AV node connecting to the penetrating bundle is usually the anterior one. Duplicated, or twin, AV nodes may exist, especially in the presence of malaligned AV septal defect. Reciprocating tachycardia may then be present.[E2] Position of conduction tissue is uncertain in patients with isolated ventricular or atrial inversion.

Accessory Conduction Pathways

Kent bundles may occur, particularly in those with CCTGA, and may give rise to preexcitation and the Wolff-Parkinson-White syndrome (see "Wolff-Parkinson-White Syndrome" in Section III of Chapter 16).[B12,S14] Kent bundles may be in the posterior wall of the left-sided RV or posterolateral wall of the right-sided LV. It is presumed by Bharati and colleagues that the relative frequency of these findings is associated with the high prevalence of Ebstein anomaly of the left-sided tricuspid valve in these cases.[B12]

Coronary Arteries

Coronary arteries are abnormal, but appropriate terminology for describing them is controversial. The simple terms *right-sided* and *left-sided* seem best.[L3] The right-sided coronary artery, arising from the right posterior coronary sinus and analogous to the normal left coronary artery, gives rise to the anterior descending coronary artery, coursing from right to left, and circumflex artery. The left-sided coronary artery arises from the left posterior aortic sinus and passes around the left-sided tricuspid orifice, usually to become the posterior descending artery on the back of the heart.[L7]

Atrioventricular Valves

The right-sided mitral valve typically has two leaflets and usually is in fibrous continuity with the pulmonary valve. As in the normal heart, it has no septal attachments but rather has typically paired papillary muscles.

The left-sided tricuspid valve consists of three leaflets. The septal leaflet, and often the posterior (inferior) leaflet, is displaced more than normally into the ventricle, but the deformity is not typically an Ebstein malformation (see "Tricuspid Valve" under Morphology in Section I).

The AV valves may, uncommonly, straddle and override the ventricular septum. When overriding is greater than 50%, by convention the diagnosis is *univentricular AV connection with straddling and overriding AV valve* (see Morphology in Chapter 56). When overriding is less than this, the diagnosis is *AV discordant connection with straddling AV valve.* A left-sided tricuspid valve may override and straddle a VSD[L5] and is at times associated with hypoplasia of the left-sided RV and at times with a superior-inferior position of the ventricles. More rarely, the right-sided mitral valve straddles and overrides a VSD[B6,S9]; this is invariably associated with hypoplasia of the LV and superior-inferior position of the ventricles.[B6] When an AV valve straddles, the ventriculoarterial connection may be discordant, in which case the AV node is still anterior but is even farther anteriorly along the superior aspect of the right-sided mitral valve.[B6] The penetrating bundle descends directly onto the ventricular septum without passing anterior to the pulmonary outflow tract. The ventriculoarterial connection may also be DORV.

CLINICAL FEATURES AND DIAGNOSTIC CRITERIA

The clinical features of patients with AV discordant connection vary widely, depending on ventriculoarterial connection and associated cardiac anomalies, most commonly VSD or pulmonary stenosis. Thus, there is no typical clinical picture.[A19]

Congenitally Corrected Transposition of the Great Arteries

In this condition, pulmonary and systemic circulations are in series. Most commonly, both VSD and pulmonary and subpulmonary stenosis are present, so it is not uncommon for the presentation to be during the first year of life from sequelae of a large $\dot{Q}p$. The clinical features and diagnostic criteria of this subset are fully discussed in Section I.

Double Outlet Right Ventricle and Double Outlet Left Ventricle

There is no characteristic presentation of either DORV or DOLV coexisting with AV discordant connection. However, because with DORV there is usually coexisting pulmonary stenosis, cyanosis is usually evident; and because in this setting with DOLV the aorta arises from the ventricle receiving systemic venous blood (see Morphology earlier in this section), cyanosis is evident. Diagnosis is made by the same methods as described for CCTGA (see Section I). Echocardiography can usually define the morphology definitively, even in very complex cases.[O4]

Isolated Ventricular or Atrial Inversion

Patients present similarly to those with complete transposition of the great arteries (see Clinical Features and Diagnostic Criteria in Chapter 41). When the ventricular septum is intact, there is severe cyanosis in infancy[C2]; when there is a large VSD, moderate cyanosis is accompanied by heart failure and cardiomegaly.[Q1] Pulmonary stenosis adds to degree of cyanosis. Diagnosis is made by the same methods as described for corrected transposition (see Section I). Cineangiography has been important in the past for definitive diagnosis (Fig. 55-25), but now two-dimensional echocardiography is extremely reliable, even in this complex setting.[P2]

NATURAL HISTORY

Most of the information concerning natural history drawn from patients with CCTGA is discussed in Section I. Other morphologic findings may affect natural history. For example, patients with situs inversus are more likely to have DORV and tetralogy of Fallot physiology, but less likely to have systemic AV valve regurgitation and heart block than patients with situs solitus.[M12]

TECHNIQUE OF OPERATION

Except for CCTGA, most malformations associated with AV discordant connection require complex and often unique operations, and only their general nature can be described.

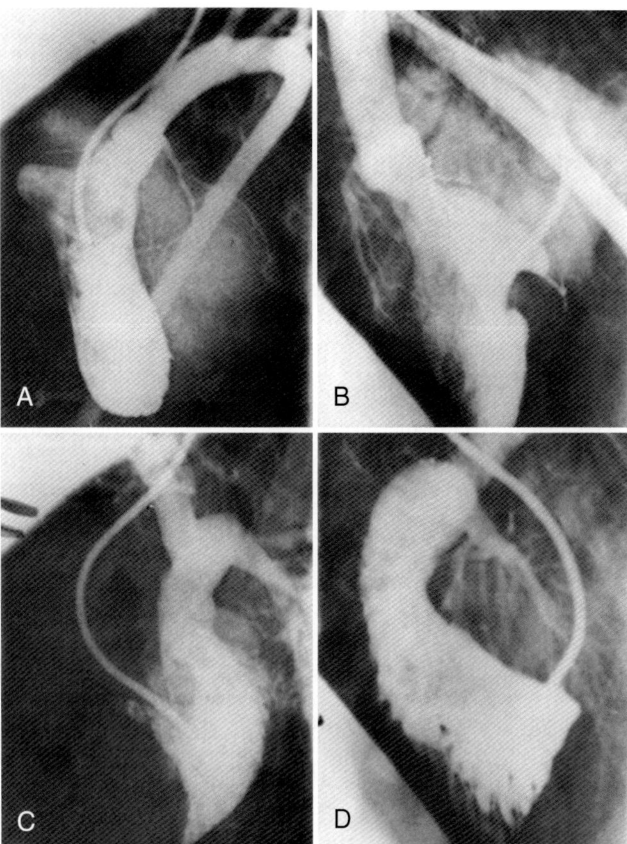

Figure 55-25 Cineangiogram in isolated ventricular inversion (atrioventricular discordant connection and ventriculoarterial concordant connection). **A,** Left ventricular injection, four-chamber position, anteroposterior projection. Aorta arises from right-sided left ventricle. **B,** Lateral projection. **C,** Right ventricular injection, four-chamber position, anteroposterior projection. Pulmonary trunk arises from left-sided right ventricle. **D,** Lateral projection.

When approaching such an operation, the surgeon must preoperatively obtain the best three-dimensional concept of the morphology, including probable location of the conduction system, and carefully plan the procedure using many of the principles described under Technique of Operation in Chapters 52, 53, and 54 and in Section I of this chapter. When single ventricle physiology coexists, techniques and principles described in Chapter 41 apply.

Congenitally Corrected Transposition of the Great Arteries

See Section I of this chapter.

Double Outlet Right Ventricle and Pulmonary Stenosis

Because the RV receives pulmonary venous blood (see Morphology earlier in this chapter), origin of the aorta from it is physiologically appropriate. The pulmonary trunk must be repositioned so as to receive blood from the LV if simple repair is chosen.

The proper approach to repair is less certain than it is in CCTGA because information about the conduction system is less complete. Further, there is controversy as to whether a completely intraventricular repair is adequate or whether a valved extracardiac conduit between LV and the pulmonary trunk is usually necessary.[K4,V7] In part because of the data presented by Tabry and colleagues[T1,T5] and in part because important subpulmonary stenosis is usually present, use of a valved extracardiac conduit has been preferred. However, the concepts underlying the Lecompte, or REV *(réparation à l'étage ventriculaire),* operation (see "Lecompte Intraventricular Repair" under Technique of Operation in Chapter 53) may well be applicable in this and other subsets of AV discordant connection and would avoid use of an extracardiac conduit. Also, various double switch operations may be applicable (see Technique of Operation in Section I).

Double Outlet Left Ventricle

The preferred surgical option consists of leaving the aorta with the right-sided LV, connecting pulmonary trunk to RV with a conduit, and performing an atrial switch operation[S12] utilizing the double switch concept described under Technique of Operation in Section I.

The alternative physiologic repair, an intraventricular tunnel repair, may be used (see "Intraventricular Tunnel Repair of Simple Double Outlet Right Ventricle" in Chapter 53) and constructed so as to conduct blood from the left-sided RV (in atrial situs solitus) through the VSD and then to the aorta. Sutures between the polyester patch for the tunnel and the ventricular septum are placed with due regard for location of the conducting tissue (see "Double Outlet Right Ventricle and Pulmonary Stenosis" earlier in this section). On occasion, it may be possible to do this repair without obstructing LV access to the pulmonary trunk. However, if access is compromised or if pulmonary stenosis is present, an allograft-valved extracardiac conduit is placed between the LV and the pulmonary trunk (see Technique of Operation in Section I) or a Lecompte procedure (REV) performed (see "Lecompte Intraventricular Repair" under Technique of Operation in Chapter 53).

Isolated Ventricular or Atrial Inversion

When the ventricular septum is intact, balloon septotomy is required in infancy, followed by an atrial switch operation (see Technique of Operation in Chapter 52). This returns the circulation functionally and anatomically to normal, because the LV is the systemic ventricle.[C6]

When there is a large VSD, it is closed through the left-sided RV in a fashion similar to that for primary VSD (presuming the bundle lies on the LV side) or from the right atrium.[B2] An atrial switch operation is then performed.[A17]

Placing Epicardial Pacemaker Leads

When complete heart block is present preoperatively or develops intraoperatively, and when in sinus rhythm the PR interval is long, permanent epicardial atrial and ventricular pacemaking leads are placed and connected to a permanent pacemaker pulse generator placed subcutaneously (see Technique of Intervention in Section I of Chapter 16 for the details of the technique).

SPECIAL FEATURES OF POSTOPERATIVE CARE

Patients are managed with protocols generally used after cardiac surgery (see Chapter 5). Particular attention is paid to cardiac rhythm. When complete heart block is present, AV sequential pacing is advantageous to cardiac output and therefore is used routinely.

RESULTS

Survival

Early (Hospital) Death

Hospital mortality after intracardiac repair of coexisting cardiac anomalies in patients with CCTGA was discussed in detail in Section I. In series reported prior to 1985, mortality was generally higher in patients with AV discordant connection and other types of ventriculoarterial connections such as DORV, DOLV, and isolated ventricular inversion.[A3,T1] This is probably related to complexity of the operations required for these conditions, often involving intraventricular rerouting and extracardiac conduits. However, increased knowledge about congenital heart disease, improved surgical techniques, and improved techniques for cardiopulmonary bypass and myocardial management currently allow lower mortalities.[H3,I4,M9,S6,S15,Y2,Y4] This has been verified by recent studies indicating that when either classical repair techniques or the double switch concept are used, outcomes are comparable whether the associated morphology is transposition (CCTGA) or one of the other ventriculoarterial connections.[B13,S8]

Time-Related Survival

Among all patients with AV discordant connection undergoing intraventricular repair prior to 1985, long-term survival has been compromised by a slowly rising late phase of hazard.[M6] The long-term outcome concerns are supported by data from Yeh and colleagues, who show survival of 48% at 20 years.[Y4] It is not yet certain that deaths occurring late postoperatively can be prevented as effectively as those occurring early after operation, nor has it yet been demonstrated that the double switch concept benefits long-term outcome.

Modes of Death

In the past, most patients dying after early operation had acute or subacute cardiac failure.[M6] Although abnormal ventricular architecture probably contributed to this, current methods, including improved methods of myocardial management, should considerably reduce the prevalence of this mode of death.

Some deaths late postoperatively have been sudden.[M6,M8,W6] Whether this is due to sudden appearance of unidentified complete heart block with ventricular asystole, ventricular fibrillation related to myocardial dysfunction, or pacemaker failure is unknown.

Incremental Risk Factors for Death

Probably AV discordant connection itself is a risk factor for death after intracardiac repair (see "Incremental Risk Factors of Death" in Section I). This is the result of abnormal ventricular architecture (see "Ventricular Function" under Natural History in Section I), abnormalities in the conduction system, problems associated with the tricuspid valve being a part of the systemic circulation, and relative unfamiliarity of even experienced congenital heart surgeons with approach and exposure to the surgical procedures required for this type of congenital heart disease.

Although early-era experience suggested that ventriculoarterial connections other than discordant ones (CCTGA) were risk factors for premature death,[M6] more recent experience does not support the position that ventriculoarterial connections other than discordant ones are risk factors.[H3,I4,M9,Y2]

Postrepair Complete Heart Block

It is disappointing that reasonably secure knowledge of the location of the bundle of His has not allowed complete heart block to disappear as a postoperative complication of repairing a VSD or constructing an intraventricular tunnel. There is about a 20% risk of developing complete heart block after repair of a VSD (Table 55-4; see also "Postrepair Complete Heart Block" under Results in Section I).

Table 55-4 Development of Postoperative Complete Heart Block after Intracardiac Repair in Patients with Discordant Atrioventricular Connection

Ventriculoarterial Connection	n	Preoperative Complete Heart Block			n	Developed Postoperative Complete Heart Block		
		No.	%	CL (%)		No.	%	CL (%)
Discordant[a]	75	10	13	9-19	65	15	23	17-30
DORV	14	0	0	0-13	13[c]	5	38	23-57
DOLV	4	1	25	3-63	3	2	67	24-96
Concordant[b]	2	0	0	0-61	2	1	50	7-93
SORV	4	0	0	0-38	4	0	0	0-38
TOTAL	99	11	11	8-15	87	23	26	21-32
$P(\chi^2)$			45				.21	

Data from McGrath and colleagues.[M6]
[a]Congenitally corrected transposition of the great arteries.
[b]Isolated ventricular inversion.
[c]Heart transplant patient not considered at risk.
Key: *CL*, 70% confidence limits; *DOLV*, double outlet left ventricle; *DORV*, double outlet right ventricle; *SORV*, single outlet right ventricle.

Abandoning ECG monitoring of each stitch[F2] in favor of a repair[D9] based on knowledge of morphology during cold cardioplegic cardiac arrest has not increased the risk of heart block.[M6] Prevalence of surgically induced heart block was not demonstrated to have been reduced by electrophysiologic mapping at surgery.[F2,M3]

Risk factors for developing complete heart block are discussed in Section I of this chapter.

Other Outcome Events

The discussions of developing left-sided tricuspid valve regurgitation, functional status, and ventricular function after repair of CCTGA (see Results in Section I) apply to all subsets of patients with AV discordant connection undergoing repair. When indications for cardiac transplantation are present, the procedure should be carried out.[D9,R3]

Outcome of valved extracardiac conduits frequently used in repairs for this group of anomalies appears to be the same as for their use in general (see "Reoperations" under Results in Section II of Chapter 38).

INDICATIONS FOR OPERATION

The diagnoses of DORV, DOLV, and isolated ventricular or atrial inversion in patients with AV discordant connection are indications for operation, but each has special considerations.

Isolated ventricular and atrial inversion have unrepaired pathophysiology and prognosis similar to that of patients with complete transposition of the great arteries (see "Essentially Intact Ventricular Septum [Poor Mixing]" in Chapter 52). Therefore, repair is indicated, and it should be performed as early in life as possible.

DORV and DOLV in the setting of AV discordant connection usually require a valved extracardiac conduit (or the Lecompte operation [REV]) for repair. Thus, there are advantages to deferring repair until age 3 to 4 years when an adult-sized conduit can be inserted, even though a palliative shunt or pulmonary trunk banding may be required in the interim. Alternatively, primary repair may be done in early life, accepting the likelihood of early conduit replacement. Knowledge of the concepts and techniques of Lecompte and others (see "Lecompte Intraventricular Repair" under Technique of Operation in Chapter 53) may, in some cases, allow repair without an extracardiac conduit, and this permits repair earlier in life.

When one ventricle is importantly hypoplastic, a Fontan operation can provide the same result as in other single-ventricle patients (see Chapter 41).[P5]

When myocardial function has deteriorated severely, cardiac transplantation can provide the same result as in patients with AV concordant connection. Abnormal positions of the great arteries are not contraindications.

SPECIAL SITUATIONS AND CONTROVERSIES

Many of the controversies surrounding management of CCTGA apply to all subsets of AV discordant connection (see Special Situations and Controversies in Section I).

Intraoperative Electrophysiologic Mapping

The bundle of His can often be identified during cardiac operations by electrophysiologic mapping techniques[F1,K13,M2] that usually (but not always) allow localization of the bundle and, by implication, locus of the AV node. However, the procedure is cumbersome surgically because the heart must be open but perfused and beating during mapping, which means the patient must be on CPB at a normal or near-normal temperature with the aorta not clamped for more than a few minutes (unless controlled aortic root perfusion is used during mapping). Risk of air embolization exists, and the CPB time is prolonged by 5 to 20 minutes. In the Mayo Clinic[M3] and UAB experiences,[F2] mapping did not reduce prevalence of complete heart block during VSD repair in patients with CCTGA, so intraoperative mapping is not routinely used at present.

Routine Placement of Permanent Epicardial Pacemaker Leads

A selective approach to placing permanent epicardial pacemaking leads is followed, but some prefer to routinely place such leads. Should heart block develop, the transvenous route of placement (usually through the subclavian vein[H3]) is simple. Difficulty with stability of the intraventricular endocardial pacemaker lead has not been encountered, despite the relatively smooth interior of the right-sided morphologic LV.[E2] Placing prophylactic epicardial myocardial leads at operation without connecting them to a pacemaker pulse generator would seem irrational, so unless a clear indication of need exists, this appears to be unwise. One important indication for placing prophylactic epicardial leads is if the cardiac repair involves use of a bidirectional cavopulmonary anastomosis, because transvenous access is not possible.

REFERENCES

A

1. Acar P, Sidi D, Bonnet D, Aggoun Y, Bonhoeffer P, Kachaner J. Maintaining tricuspid valve competence in double discordance: a challenge for the paediatric cardiologist. Heart 1998;80:479.
2. Aeba R, Katogi T, Koizumi K, Iino Y, Mori M, Yozu R. Apico-pulmonary artery conduit repair of congenitally corrected transposition of the great arteries with ventricular septal defect and pulmonary outflow tract obstruction: a 10-year follow-up. Ann Thorac Surg 2003;76:1383-7; discussion 87-8.
3. Akagawa H, Yoshioka F, Isomura T, Ohishi K, Hirata K, Kato H, et al. Surgical treatment of double-outlet left ventricle in situs inversus [I,D,D]. Ann Thorac Surg 1984;37:337.
4. Albuquerque de AT, Rigby ML, Anderson RH, Lincoln C, Shinebourne EA. The spectrum of atrioventricular discordance. A clinical study. Br Heart J 1984;51:498.
5. Alghamdi AA, McCrindle BW, Van Arsdell GS. Physiologic versus anatomic repair of congenitally corrected transposition of the great arteries: meta-analysis of individual patient data. Ann Thorac Surg 2006;81:1529-35.
6. Allwork SP, Bentall HH, Becker AE, Cameron H, Gerlis LM, Wilkinson JL, et al. Congenitally corrected transposition of the great arteries: morphologic study of 32 cases. Am J Cardiol 1976; 38:910.
7. Anderson KR, Danielson GK, McGoon DC, Lie JT. Ebstein's anomaly of the left-sided tricuspid valve. Pathological anatomy of the valvular malformations. Circulation 1978;58:I87.
8. Anderson RC, Lillehei CW, Lester RG. Corrected transposition of the great vessels of the heart. Pediatrics 1957;20:626.
9. Anderson RH. Criss-cross hearts revisited: a question of definition. Pediatr Cardiol 1982;3:305.

10. Anderson RH. The conduction tissues in congenitally corrected transposition. Ann Thorac Surg 2004;77:1881-2.
11. Anderson RH, Arnold R, Jones RS. D-bulboventricular loop with L-transposition in situs inversus. Circulation 1972;46:173.
12. Anderson RH, Arnold R, Wilkinson JL. The conducting system in congenitally corrected transposition. Lancet 1973;1:1286.
13. Anderson RH, Becker AE, Arnold R, Wilkinson JL. The conducting tissues in congenitally corrected transposition. Circulation 1974;50:911.
14. Anderson RH, Becker AE, Gerlis LM. The pulmonary outflow tract in classically corrected transposition. J Thorac Cardiovasc Surg 1975;69:747.
15. Anderson RH, Shinebourne EA, Gerlis LM. Criss-cross atrioventricular relationships producing paradoxical atrioventricular concordance or discordance. Their significance to nomenclature of congenital heart disease. Circulation 1974;50:176.
16. Anselmi G, Munoz S, Machado I, Blanco P, Espino-Vela J. Complex cardiovascular malformations associated with the corrected type of transposition of the great vessels. Am Heart J 1963; 66:614.
17. Arciprete P, Macartney FJ, de Leval M, Stark J. Mustard's operation for patients with ventriculoarterial concordance. Report of two cases and a cautionary tale. Br Heart J 1985;53:443.
18. Attie F, Cerda J, Richheimer R, Chavez-Dominguez R, Buendia A, Ovseyevitz J, et al. Congenitally corrected transposition with mirror-image atrial arrangement. Int J Cardiol 1987;14:169.
19. Attie F, Ovseyevitz J, Llamas G, Buendia A, Vargas J, Munoz L. The clinical features and diagnosis of a discordant atrioventricular connexion. Int J Cardiol 1985;8:395.

B

1. Backer CL, Stewart RD, Mavroudis C. The classical and the one-and-a-half ventricular options for surgical repair in patients with discordant atrioventricular connections. Cardiol Young 2006; 16(Suppl 3):91-6.
2. Baudet EM, Hafez A, Choussat A, Roques X. Isolated ventricular inversion with situs solitus: successful surgical repair. Ann Thorac Surg 1986;41:91.
3. Bautista-Hernandez V, Marx GR, Gauvreau K, Mayer JE Jr, Cecchin F, del Nido PJ. Determinants of left ventricular dysfunction after anatomic repair of congenitally corrected transposition of the great arteries. Ann Thorac Surg 2006;82:2059-66.
4. Bautista-Hernandez V, Serrano F, Palacios JM, Caffarena JM. Successful neonatal double switch in symptomatic patients with congenitally corrected transposition of the great arteries. Ann Thorac Surg 2008;85:e1-2.
5. Becker AE, Anderson RH. Conditions with discordant atrioventricular connexions—anatomy and conductive tissues. In Anderson RH, Shinebourne EA, eds. Pediatric cardiology, 1977. London: Churchill Livingstone, 1978, p. 184.
6. Becker AE, Ho SY, Caruso G, Milo S, Anderson RH. Straddling right atrioventricular valves in atrioventricular discordance. Circulation 1980;61:1133.
7. Becu LM, Swan HF, Du Shane JW, Edwards JE. Ebstein malformation of the left atrioventricular valve in corrected transposition of the great vessels with ventricular septal defect. Mayo Clin Proc 1955;30:483.
8. Benson LN, Burns R, Schwaiger M, Schelbert HR, Lewis AB, Freedom RM, et al. Radionuclide angiographic evaluation of ventricular function in isolated congenitally corrected transposition of the great arteries. Am J Cardiol 1986;58:319.
9. Bharati S, Lev M. The course of the conduction system in dextrocardia. Circulation 1978;57:163.
10. Bharati S, Lev M, Kirklin JW. Cardiac surgery and the conduction system, 2nd Ed. Mount Kisco, N.Y.: Futura, 1992.
11. Bharati S, McCue C, Tingelstad JB, Mantakas M, Shiel F, Lev M. Lack of connection between the atria and the peripheral conduction system in a case of corrected transposition with congenital atrioventricular block. Am J Cardiol 1978;42:147.
12. Bharati S, Rosen K, Steinfield L, Miller RA, Lev M. The anatomic substrate for preexcitation in corrected transposition. Circulation 1980;62:831.
13. Biliciler-Denktas G, Feldt RH, Connolly HM, Weaver AL, Puga FJ, Danielson GK. Early and late results of operations for defects associated with corrected transposition and other anomalies with atrioventricular discordance in a pediatric population. J Thorac Cardiovasc Surg 2001;122:234.
14. Bonfils-Roberts EA, Guller B, McGoon DC, Danielson GK. Corrected transposition—surgical treatment of associated anomalies. Ann Thorac Surg 1974;17:200.
15. Bove EL, Ohye RG, Devaney EJ, Kurosawa H, Shin'oka T, Ikeda A, et al. Anatomic correction of congenitally corrected transposition and its close cousins. Cardiol Young 2006;16(Suppl 3):85-90.
16. Brandt PW. Cineangiography of atrioventricular and ventriculoarterial connections. In Godman MJ, ed. Pediatric cardiology, Vol. 4. London: Churchill Livingstone, 1981, p. 191.
17. Brandt PW, Calder AL, Barratt-Boyes BG, Neutze JM. Double outlet left ventricle. Morphology, cineangiocardiographic diagnosis and surgical treatment. Am J Cardiol 1976;38:897.
18. Brenner JI, Bharati S, Winn WC Jr, Lev M. Absent tricuspid valve with aortic atresia in mixed levocardia (atria situs solitus. L-loop). A hitherto undescribed entity. Circulation 1978;57:836.

C

1. Cardell BS. Corrected transposition of the great vessels. Br Heart J 1956;18:186.
2. Carey LS, Ruttenberg HD. Roentgenographic features of congenital corrected transposition of the great vessels. AJR Am J Roentgenol 1964;92:623.
3. Castagna RC, Bastos P, de Leval M, Stark J, Taylor JF, Anderson RH, et al. Changes in ventricular depolarization in patients in sinus rhythm following closure of ventricular septal defect associated with atrioventricular discordance. Thorac Cardiovasc Surg 1981;29:148.
4. Celermajer DS, Cullen S, Deanfield JE, Sullivan ID. Congenitally corrected transposition and Ebstein's anomaly of the systemic atrioventricular valve: association with aortic arch obstruction. J Am Coll Cardiol 1991;18:1056.
5. Chang DS, Barack BM, Lee MH, Lee HY. Congenitally corrected transposition of the great arteries: imaging with 16-MDCT. AJR Am J Roentgenol 2007;188:W428-30.
6. Clarkson PM, Brandt PW, Barratt-Boyes BG, Neutze JM. Isolated atrial inversion. Visceral situs solitus, visceroatrial discordance, discordant ventricular D loop without transposition, dextrocardia: diagnosis and surgical correction. Am J Cardiol 1972;29:877.
7. Connolly HM, Grogan M, Warnes CA. Pregnancy among women with congenitally corrected transposition of great arteries. J Am Coll Cardiol 1999;33:1692.
8. Craig BG, Smallhorn JF, Rowe RD, Williams WG, Trusler GA, Freedom RM. Severe obstruction to systemic blood flow in congenitally corrected transposition (discordant atrioventricular and ventricu-loarterial connexions): an analysis of 14 patients. Int J Cardiol 1986;11:209.

D

1. Dabizzi RP, Barletta GA, Caprioli G, Baldrighi G, Baldrighi V. Coronary artery anatomy in corrected transposition of the great arteries. J Am Coll Cardiol 1988;12:486.
2. Davies B, Oppido G, Wilkinson JL, Brizard CP. Aortic translocation, Senning procedure and right ventricular outflow tract augmentation for congenitally corrected transposition, ventricular septal defect and pulmonary stenosis. Eur J Cardiothorac Surg 2008;33:934-6.
3. de Leval MR, Bastos P, Stark J, Taylor JF, Macartney FJ, Anderson RH. Surgical technique to reduce the risks of heart block following closure of ventricular septal defect in atrioventricular discordance. J Thorac Cardiovasc Surg 1979;78:515.
4. Delius RE, Rademecker MA, de Leval MR, Elliott MJ, Stark J. Is a high-risk biventricular repair always preferable to conversion to a single ventricle repair? J Thorac Cardiovasc Surg 1996; 112:1561.
5. Dick M, Van Praagh R, Rudd M, Folkerth T, Castaneda AR. Electrophysiologic delineation of the specialized atrioventricular conduction system in two patients with corrected transposition of the great arteries with situs inversus (I,D,D). Circulation 1977;55:896.
6. Di Donato RM, Wernovsky G, Jonas RA, Mayer JE Jr, Keane JF, Castaneda AR. Corrected transposition in situs inversus. Biventricular repair of associated cardiac anomalies. Circulation 1991; 84:III193.
7. Dimas AP, Moodie DS, Sterba R, Gill CC. Long-term function of the morphologic right ventricle in adult patients with corrected transposition of the great arteries. Am Heart J 1989;118:526.
8. Dodge-Khatami A, Tulevski II, Bennink GB, Hitchcock JF, de Mol BA, van der Wall EE, et al. Comparable systemic ventricular function in healthy adults and patients with unoperated congenitally

corrected transposition using MRI dobutamine stress testing. Ann Thorac Surg 2002;73:1759-64.
9. Doty DB, Renlund DG, Caputo GR, Burton NA, Jones KW. Cardiac transplantation in situs inversus. J Thorac Cardiovasc Surg 1990;99:493.
10. Doty DB, Truesdell SC, Marvin WJ Jr. Techniques to avoid injury of the conduction tissue during the surgical treatment of corrected transposition. Circulation 1983;68:II63.
11. Duncan BW, Mee RB, Mesia CI, Qureshi A, Rosenthal GL, Seshadri SG, et al. Results of the double switch operation for congenitally corrected transposition of the great arteries. Eur J Cardiothorac Surg 2003;24:11-20.
12. Duncan WJ, Wong KK, Freedom RM. A criss-cross heart with twisted atrioventricular connections, "perfect streaming," and double discordance. Pediatr Cardiol 2006;27:604-7.

E

1. Egloff L, Rothlin M, Schneider J, Arbenz U, Schonbeck M, Senning A, et al. Congenitally corrected transposition of the great arteries: a clinical and surgical study. Thorac Cardiovasc Surg 1980;28:228.
2. Epstein MR, Saul JP, Weindling SN, Triedman JK, Walsh EP. Atrioventricular reciprocating tachycardia involving twin atrioventricular nodes in patients with complex congenital heart disease. J Cardiovasc Electrophysiol 2001;12:671.
3. Erath HG Jr, Graham TP Jr, Hammon JW Jr, Smith CW. Hypoplasia of the systemic ventricle in congenitally corrected transposition of the great arteries. Preoperative documentation and possible implications of operation. J Thorac Cardiovasc Surg 1980;79:770.
4. Espinola-Zavaleta N, Alexanderson E, Attie F, Castellanos LM, Duenas R, Rosas M, et al. Right ventricular function and ventricular perfusion defects in adults with congenitally corrected transposition: correlation of echocardiography and nuclear medicine. Cardiol Young 2004;14:174-81.

F

1. Fiddler GI, Maloney JD, Danielson GK, McGoon DC, Ritter DG. Intraoperative identification of the conduction system in dextrocardia with complex congenital heart disease. Am J Cardiol 1977; 39:301.
2. Fox LS, Kirklin JW, Pacifico AD, Waldo AL, Bargeron LM Jr. Intracardiac repair of cardiac malformations with atrioventricular discordance. Circulation 1976;54:123.
3. Franco-Vazquez JS, Perez-Trevino C, Gaxiola A. Corrected transposition of the great arteries with extreme counter-clockwise torsion of the heart. Acta Cardiol 1973;28:636.
4. Freedom RM, Culham G, Rowe RD. The criss-cross and superoinferior ventricular heart: an angiocardiographic study. Am J Cardiol 1978;42:620.
5. Friedberg DZ, Nadas AS. Clinical profile of patients with congenital corrected transposition of the great arteries. A study of 60 cases. N Engl J Med 1970;282:1053.

G

1. Gaies MG, Goldberg CS, Ohye RG, Devaney EJ, Hirsch JC, Bove EL. Early and intermediate outcome after anatomic repair of congenitally corrected transposition of the great arteries. Ann Thorac Surg 2009;88:1952-60.
2. Gerlis LM, Wilson N, Dickinson DF. Abnormalities of the mitral valve in congenitally corrected transposition (discordant atrioventricular and ventriculoarterial connections). Br Heart J 1986;55:475.
3. Giardini A, Lovato L, Donti A, Formigari R, Oppido G, Gargiulo G, et al. Relation between right ventricular structural alterations and markers of adverse clinical outcome in adults with systemic right ventricle and either congenital complete (after Senning operation) or congenitally corrected transposition of the great arteries. Am J Cardiol 2006;98:1277-82.
4. Gillette PC, Busch U, Mullins CE, McNamara DG. Electrophysiologic studies in patients with ventricular inversion and "corrected transposition." Circulation 1979;60:939.
5. Graham TP Jr, Bernard YD, Mellen BG, Celermajer D, Baumgartner H, Cetta F, et al. Long-term outcome in congenitally corrected transposition of the great arteries: a multi-institutional study. J Am Coll Cardiol 2000;36:255.
6. Graham TP Jr, Parrish MD, Boucek RJ Jr, Boerth RC, Breitweser JA, Thompson S, et al. Assessment of ventricular size and function in congenitally corrected transposition of the great arteries. Am J Cardiol 1983;51:244.
7. Grolleau R, Baissus C, Puech P. Corrected transposition of the great vessels and preexcitation syndrome (apropos of 2 cases). Arch Mal Coeur Vaiss 1977;70:69.

H

1. Hagler DJ, Tajik AJ, Seward JB, Edwards WD, Mair DD, Ritter DG. Atrioventricular and ventriculoarterial discordance (corrected transposition of the great arteries). Mayo Clin Proc 1981;56:591.
2. Hauser M, Bengel FM, Hager A, Kuehn A, Nekolla SG, Kaemmerer H, et al. Impaired myocardial blood flow and coronary flow reserve of the anatomical right systemic ventricle in patients with congenitally corrected transposition of the great arteries. Heart 2003;89:1231-5.
3. Hibino N, Imai Y, Aoki M, Shin'oka T, Hiramatsu T. Double switch operation for superior-inferior ventricles. Ann Thorac Surg 2001;72:2119.
4. Honey M. The diagnosis of corrected transposition of the great vessels. Br Heart J 1963;25:313.
5. Horer J, Schreiber C, Krane S, Prodan Z, Cleuziou J, Vogt M, et al. Outcome after surgical repair/palliation of congenitally corrected transposition of the great arteries. Thorac Cardiovasc Surg 2008;56:391-7.
6. Hornung TS, Bernard EJ, Celermajer DS, Jaeggi E, Howman-Giles RB, Chard RB, et al. Right ventricular dysfunction in congenitally corrected transposition of the great arteries. Am J Cardiol 1999; 84:1116.
7. Hornung TS, Bernard EJ, Jaeggi ET, Howman-Giles RB, Celermajer DS, Hawker RE. Myocardial perfusion defects and associated systemic ventricular dysfunction in congenitally corrected transposition of the great arteries. Heart 1998;80:322.
8. Horvath P, Szufladowicz M, de Leval MR, Elliott MJ, Stark J. Tricuspid valve abnormalities in patients with atrioventricular discordance: surgical implications. Ann Thorac Surg 1994;57:941.
9. Hosseinpour AR, McCarthy KP, Griselli M, Sethia B, Ho SY. Congenitally corrected transposition: size of the pulmonary trunk and septal malalignment. Ann Thorac Surg 2004;77:2163-6.
10. Hraska V. Anatomic correction of corrected transposition {I,D,D} using an atrial switch and aortic translocation. Ann Thorac Surg 2008;85:352-3.
11. Hraska V, Duncan BW, Mayer JE Jr, Freed M, del Nido PJ, Jonas RA. Long-term outcome of surgically treated patients with corrected transposition of the great arteries. J Thorac Cardiovasc Surg 2005;129:182-91.
12. Huhta JC, Danielson GK, Ritter DG, Ilstrup DM. Survival in atrioventricular discordance. Pediatr Cardiol 1985;6:57.
13. Huhta JC, Maloney JD, Ritter DG, Ilstrup DM, Feldt RH. Complete atrioventricular block in patients with atrioventricular discordance. Circulation 1983;67:1374.
14. Hwang B, Bowman F, Malm J, Krongrad E. Surgical repair of congenitally corrected transposition of the great arteries: results and follow-up. Am J Cardiol 1982;50:781.

I

1. Ilbawi MN, DeLeon SY, Backer CL, Duffy CE, Muster AJ, Zales VR, et al. An alternative approach to the surgical management of physiologically corrected transposition with ventricular septal defect and pulmonary stenosis or atresia. J Thorac Cardiovasc Surg 1990; 100:410.
2. Ilbawi MN, Ocampo CB, Allen BS, Barth MJ, Roberson DA, Chiemmongkoltip P, et al. Intermediate results of the anatomic repair for congenitally corrected transposition. Ann Thorac Surg 2002;73:594.
3. Imai Y. Double-switch operation for congenitally corrected transposition. Adv Card Surg 1997;9:65.
4. Imai Y, Sawatari K, Hoshino S, Ishihara K, Nakazawa M, Momma K. Ventricular function after anatomic repair in patients with atrioventricular discordance. J Thorac Cardiovasc Surg 1994;107:1272.
5. Imamura M, Drummond-Webb JJ, Murphy DJ Jr, Prieto LR, Latson LA, Flamm SD, et al. Results of the double switch operation in the current era. Ann Thorac Surg 2000;70:100.

J

1. Jahangiri M, Redington AN, Elliott MJ, Stark J, Tsang VT, de Leval MR. A case for anatomic correction in atrioventricular

discordance? Effects of surgery on tricuspid valve function. J Thorac Cardiovasc Surg 2001;121:1040.

2. Jahangiri M, Redington AN, Elliott MJ, Stark J, Tsang VT, de Leval MR. A case for anatomic correction in atrioventricular discordance? Effects of surgery on tricuspid valve function. J Thorac Cardiovasc Surg 2001;121:1040-5.

K

1. Kantarci M, Koplay M, Bayraktutan U, Gundogdu F, Ceviz N. Congenitally corrected transposition of the great arteries: MDCT angiography findings and interpretation of complex coronary anatomy. Int J Cardiovasc Imaging 2007;23:405-10.
2. Karl TR, Weintraub RG, Brizard CP, Cochrane AD, Mee RB. Senning plus arterial switch operation for discordant (congenitally corrected) transposition. Ann Thorac Surg 1997;64:495.
3. Kinsley RH, McGoon DC, Danielson GK. Corrected transposition of the great arteries: associated ventricular rotation. Circulation 1974;49:574.
4. Kiser JC, Ongley PA, Kirklin JW, Clarkson PM, McGoon DC. Surgical treatment of dextrocardia with inversion of ventricles and double-outlet right ventricle. J Thorac Cardiovasc Surg 1968;55:6.
5. Kishon Y, Shem-Tov AA, Schneeweiss A, Neufeld HN. Corrected transposition of the great arteries without associated defects—study of 10 patients. Int J Cardiol 1983;3:112.
6. Koh M, Yagihara T, Uemura H, Kagisaki K, Hagino I, Ishizaka T, et al. Intermediate results of the double-switch operations for atrioventricular discordance. Ann Thorac Surg 2006;81:671-7.
7. Konstantinov IE, Lai L, Colan SD, Williams WG, Li J, Jonas RA, et al. Atrioventricular discordance with ventriculoarterial concordance: a remaining indication for the atrial switch operation. J Thorac Cardiovasc Surg 2004;128:944-5.
8. Kordybach M, Kowalski M, Hoffman P. Heart failure in a patient with corrected transposition of the great arteries. When is biventricular pacing indicated? Acta Cardiol 2009;64:673-6.
9. Kozelj M, Prokselj K, Berden P, Jan M, Osredkar J, Bunc M, et al. The syndrome of cardiac failure in adults with congenitally corrected transposition. Cardiol Young 2008;18:599-607.
10. Kral Kollars CA, Gelehrter S, Bove EL, Ensing G. Effects of morphologic left ventricular pressure on right ventricular geometry and tricuspid valve regurgitation in patients with congenitally corrected transposition of the great arteries. Am J Cardiol 2010;105:735-9.
11. Krishnan K, Avramovitch NA, Kim MH, Trohman RG. Cardiac resynchronization therapy: a potential option for congenitally corrected transposition of the great vessels. J Heart Lung Transplant 2005;24:2293-6.
12. Krongrad E, Ellis K, Steeg CN, Bowman FO Jr, Malm JR, Gersony WM. Subpulmonary obstruction in congenitally corrected transposition of the great arteries due to ventricular membranous septal aneurysms. Circulation 1976;54:679.
13. Kupersmith J, Krongrad E, Gersony WM, Bowman FO Jr. Electrophysiologic identification of the specialized conduction system in corrected transposition of the great arteries. Circulation 1974;50:795.
14. Kwak JG, Lee CH, Lee C, Park CS. Aortic root translocation with atrial switch: another surgical option for congenitally corrected transposition of the great arteries with isolated pulmonary stenosis. J Thorac Cardiovasc Surg 2010;139:1652-3.

L

1. Leijala MA, Lincoln CR, Shinebourne EA, Nellen M. A rare congenital cardiac malformation with situs inversus and discordant atrioventricular and concordant ventriculoarterial connections: diagnosis and surgical treatment. Am Heart J 1981;101:355.
2. Lev M, Fielding RT, Zaeske D. Mixed levocardia with ventricular inversion (corrected transposition) with complete A-V block. Am J Cardiol 1963;12:875.
3. Lev M, Rowlatt UF. The pathologic anatomy of mixed levocardia. A review of thirteen cases of atrial or ventricular inversion with or without corrected transposition. Am J Cardiol 1961;8:216.
4. Levy MJ, Lillehei CW, Elliott LP, Carey LS, Adams P Jr, Edwards JE. Accessory valvular tissue causing subpulmonary stenosis in corrected transposition of great vessels. Circulation 1963;27:494.
5. Liberthson RR, Paul MH, Muster AJ, Arcilla RA, Eckner FA, Lev M. Straddling and displaced atrioventricular orifices and valves with primitive ventricles. Circulation 1971;43:213.
6. Lim HG, Lee JR, Kim YJ, Park YH, Jun TG, Kim WH, et al. Outcomes of biventricular repair for congenitally corrected transposition of the great arteries. Ann Thorac Surg 2010;89:159-67.
7. Losekoot TG, Anderson RH, Becker AE, Danielson GK, Soto B. Congenitally corrected transposition. New York: Churchill Livingstone, 1983.
8. Lundstrom U, Bull C, Wyse RK, Somerville J. The natural and "unnatural" history of congenitally corrected transposition. Am J Cardiol 1990;65:1222.
9. Ly M, Belli E, Leobon B, Kortas C, Grollmuss OE, Piot D, et al. Results of the double switch operation for congenitally corrected transposition of the great arteries. Eur J Cardiothorac Surg 2009; 35:879-84.

M

1. Malhotra SP, Reddy VM, Qiu M, Pirolli TJ, Barboza L, Reinhartz O, Hanley FL. The hemi-Mustard/bidirectional Glenn atrial switch procedure in the double-switch operation for congenitally corrected transposition of the great arteries: rationale and midterm results. J Thorac Cardiovasc Surg 2011;141:162.
2. Maloney JD, Ritter DG, McGoon DC, Danielson GK. Identification of the conduction system in corrected transposition and common ventricle at operation. Mayo Clin Proc 1975;50:387.
3. Marcelletti C, Maloney JD, Ritter DG, Danielson GK, McGoon DC, Wallace RB. Corrected transposition and ventricular septal defect: surgical experience. Ann Surg 1980;191:751.
4. Marino B, Sanders SP, Parness IA, Colan SD. Obstruction of right ventricular inflow and outflow in corrected transposition of the great arteries {S,L,L}: two-dimensional echocardiographic diagnosis. J Am Coll Cardiol 1986;8:407.
5. Matsuda H, Kawashima Y, Hirose H, Nakano S, Shirakura R, Shimazaki Y, et al. Transaortic closure of ventricular septal defect in atrioventricular discordance with pulmonary stenosis or atresia. Results in five patients. J Thorac Cardiovasc Surg 1984;88:776.
6. McGrath LB, Kirklin JW, Blackstone EH, Pacifico AD, Kirklin JK, Bargeron LM Jr. Death and other events after cardiac repair in discordant atrioventricular connection. J Thorac Cardiovasc Surg 1985;90:711.
7. McKay R, Anderson RH, Smith A. The coronary arteries in hearts with discordant atrioventricular connections. J Thorac Cardiovasc Surg 1996;111:988.
8. Metcalfe J, Somerville J. Surgical repair of lesions associated with corrected transposition. Br Heart J 1983;50:476.
9. Metras D, Kreitmann B, Fraisse A, Riberi A, Wernert F, Nassi C, et al. Anatomic repair of corrected transposition or atrioventricular discordance: report of 8 cases. Eur J Cardiothorac Surg 1998;13: 117.
10. Metton O, Gaudin R, Ou P, Gerelli S, Mussa S, Sidi D, et al. Early prophylactic pulmonary artery banding in isolated congenitally corrected transposition of the great arteries. Eur J Cardiothorac Surg 2010;38:728.
11. Milo S, Ho SY, Macartney FJ, Wilkinson JL, Becker AE, Wenink AC, et al. Straddling and overriding atrioventricular valves—morphology and classification. Am J Cardiol 1979;44:1122.
12. Mishra S, Kothari SS, Saxena A, Juneja R, Rajani M. Atrioventricular discordance in situs inversus. Indian Heart J 1999;51:422.
13. Misumi I, Kimura Y, Hokamura Y, Yamabe H, Ueno K. Congenitally corrected transposition of the great arteries with a patent foramen ovale in an 81-year-old man—a case report. Angiology 1999;50:75.
14. Monckeberg JG. Zur Entwicklungsgeschichte des Atrioventrijularystems. Verh Dtsch Pathol [In Centralblatt Allg Pathol Anat 24.] 1913;16:228.

O

1. Ohuchi H, Hiraumi Y, Tasato H, Kuwahara A, Chado H, Toyohara K, et al. Comparison of the right and left ventricle as a systemic ventricle during exercise in patients with congenital heart disease. Am Heart J 1999;137:1185.
2. Okamura K, Konno S. Two types of ventricular septal defect in corrected transposition of the great arteries: reference to surgical approaches. Am Heart J 1973;85:483.
3. Olinger GN, Maloney JV Jr. Trans-pulmonary artery repair of ventricular septal defect associated with congenitally corrected transposition of the great arteries. J Thorac Cardiovasc Surg 1977;73:353.

4. Ozkutlu S, Elshershari H, Akcoren Z, Ondergolu LS, Tekinalp G. Visceroatrial situs solitus with atrioventricular alignment discordance double outlet right ventricle and superoinferior ventricles: fetal and neonatal echocardiographic findings. J Am Soc Echocardiogr 2002;15:749.

P

1. Parrish MD, Graham TP Jr, Bender HW, Jones JP, Patton J, Partain CL. Radionuclide angiographic evaluation of right and left ventricular function during exercise after repair of transposition of the great arteries: comparison with normal subjects and patients with congenitally corrected transposition. Circulation 1983;67:178.
2. Pasquini L, Sanders SP, Parness I, Colan S, Keane JF, Mayer JE Jr, et al. Echocardiographic and anatomic findings in atrioventricular discordance with ventriculoarterial concordance. Am J Cardiol 1988;62:1256.
3. Peterson RJ, Franch RH, Fajman WA, Jones RH. Comparison of cardiac function in surgically corrected and congenitally corrected transposition of the great arteries. J Thorac Cardiovasc Surg 1988;96:227.
4. Piran S, Veldtman G, Siu S, Webb GD, Liu PP. Heart failure and ventricular dysfunction in patients with single or systemic right ventricles. Circulation 2002;105:1189.
5. Prasad K, Balram A, Iyer KS, Murthy KS, Shrivastava S, Rajani M, et al. Surgical treatment of major intracardiac lesions associated with discordant atrioventricular connexion. Int J Cardiol 1990;26:191.
6. Prieto LR, Hordof AJ, Secic M, Rosenbaum MS, Gersony WM. Progressive tricuspid valve disease in patients with congenitally corrected transposition of the great arteries. Circulation 1998; 98:997.

Q

1. Quero-Jimenez M, Raposo-Sonnenfeld I. Isolated ventricular inversion with situs solitus. Br Heart J 1975;37:293.
2. Quinn DW, McGuirk SP, Metha C, Nightingale P, de Giovanni JV, Dhillon R, et al. The morphologic left ventricle that requires training by means of pulmonary artery banding before the double-switch procedure for congenitally corrected transposition of the great arteries is at risk of late dysfunction. J Thorac Cardiovasc Surg 2008;135:1137-44.

R

1. Ratner B, Abbott ME, Beattie WW. Rare cardiac anomaly. Cor triloculare biventriculare in mirror-picture dextrocardia with persistent omphalomesenteric bay, right aortic arch and pulmonary artery forming descending aorta. Am J Dis Child 1921;22:508.
2. Reddy VM, McElhinney DB, Silverman NH, Hanley FL. The double switch procedure for anatomical repair of congenitally corrected transposition of the great arteries in infants and children. Eur Heart J 1997;18:1470.
3. Reitz BA, Jamieson SW, Gaudiani VA, Oyer PE, Stinson EB. Method for cardiac transplantation in corrected transposition of the great arteries. J Cardiovasc Surg (Torino) 1982;23:293.
4. Rizzoli G, Blackstone EH, Kirklin JW, Pacifico AD, Bargeron LM Jr. Incremental risk factors in hospital mortality rate after repair of ventricular septal defect. J Thorac Cardiovasc Surg 1980;80:494.
5. Roffi M, de Marchi SF, Seiler C. Congenitally corrected transposition of the great arteries in an 80 year old woman. Heart 1998; 79:622.
6. Rokitansky CF von. Die Defecte der Scheidewande des Herzens. Vienna: Wilhelm Braumuller, 1875.
7. Russo P, Danielson GK, Driscoll DJ. Transaortic closure of ventricular septal defect in patients with corrected transposition with pulmonary stenosis or atresia. Circulation 1987;76:III88.
8. Rutledge JM, Nihill MR, Fraser CD, Smith OE, McMahon CJ, Bezold LI. Outcome of 121 patients with congenitally corrected transposition of the great arteries. Pediatr Cardiol 2002;23:137.
9. Ruttenberg HD, Anderson RC, Elliott LP, Edwards JE. Origin of both great vessels from the arterial ventricle: a complex with ventricular inversion. Br Heart J 1964;26:631.

S

1. Sano T, Riesenfeld T, Karl TR, Wilkinson JL. Intermediate-term outcome after intracardiac repair of associated cardiac defects in patients with atrioventricular and ventriculoarterial discordance. Circulation 1995;92:II272.
2. Sasaki O, Hamada M, Hiasa G, Ogimoto A, Ohtsuka T, Suzuki M, et al. Congenitally corrected transposition of the great arteries in a 65-year-old woman. Jpn Heart J 2001;42:645.
3. Scherptong RW, Vliegen HW, Winter MM, Holman ER, Mulder BJ, van der Wall EE, et al. Tricuspid valve surgery in adults with a dysfunctional systemic right ventricle: repair or replace? Circulation 2009;119:1467-72.
4. Schiebler GL, Edwards JE, Burchell HB, Dushane JW, Ongley PA, Wood EH. Congenital corrected transposition of the great vessels: a study of 33 cases. Pediatrics 1961;27:II849.
5. Sharma R, Bhan A, Juneja R, Kothari SS, Saxena A, Venugopal P. Double switch for congenitally corrected transposition of the great arteries. Eur J Cardiothorac Surg 1999;15:276.
6. Sharma R, Marwah A, Shah S, Maheshwari S. Isolated atrioventricular discordance: surgical experience. Ann Thorac Surg 2008; 85:1403-6.
7. Sharma R, Talwar S, Marwah A, Shah S, Maheshwari S, Suresh P, et al. Anatomic repair for congenitally corrected transposition of the great arteries. J Thorac Cardiovasc Surg 2009; 137:404-12.
8. Shin'oka T, Kurosawa H, Imai Y, Aoki M, Ishiyama M, Sakamoto T, et al. Outcomes of definitive surgical repair for congenitally corrected transposition of the great arteries or double outlet right ventricle with discordant atrioventricular connections: risk analyses in 189 patients. J Thorac Cardiovasc Surg 2007;133: 1318-28.
9. Sieg K, Hagler DJ, Ritter DG, McGoon DC, Maloney JD, Seward JB, et al. Straddling right atrioventricular valve in criss-cross atrioventricular relationship. Mayo Clin Proc 1977;52:561.
10. Soto B, Bargeron LM Jr, Bream PR, Elliott LP. Conditions with atrioventricular discordance—angiographic study. In Anderson RH, Shinebourne EA, eds. Pediatric cardiology; 1977. London: Churchill Livingstone, 1978, p. 207.
11. Stumper O, Wright JG, De Giovanni JV, Silove ED, Sethia B, Brawn WJ. Combined atrial and arterial switch procedure for congenital corrected transposition with ventricular septal defect. Br Heart J 1995;73:479.
12. Subirana MT, de Leval M, Somerville J. Double-outlet left ventricle with atrioventricular discordance. Am J Cardiol 1984; 54:1385.
13. Sutherland GR, Smallhorn JF, Anderson RH, Rigby ML, Hunter S. Atrioventricular discordance. Cross-sectional echocardiographic-morphological correlative study. Br Heart J 1983;50:8.
14. Symons JC, Shinebourne EA, Joseph MC, Lincoln C, Ho Y, Anderson RH. Criss-cross heart with congenitally corrected transposition: report of a case with D-transposed aorta and ventricular preexcitation. Eur J Cardiol 1977;5:493.
15. Szufladowicz M, Horvath P, de Leval M, Elliott M, Wyse R, Stark J. Intracardiac repair of lesions associated with atrioventricular discordance. Eur J Cardiothorac Surg 1996;10:443.

T

1. Tabry IF, McGoon DC, Danielson GK, Wallace RB, Davis Z, Maloney JD. Surgical management of double-outlet right ventricle associated with atrioventricular discordance. J Thorac Cardiovasc Surg 1978;76:336.
2. Tay EL, Frogoudaki A, Inuzuka R, Giannakoulas G, Prapa M, Li W, et al. Exercise intolerance in patients with congenitally corrected transposition of the great arteries relates to right ventricular filling pressures. Int J Cardiol 2011;147:219.
3. Termignon JL, Leca F, Vouhe PR, Vernant F, Bical OM, Lecompte Y, et al. "Classic" repair of congenitally corrected transposition and ventricular septal defect. Ann Thorac Surg 1996;62:199.
4. Therrien J, Barnes I, Somerville J. Outcome of pregnancy in patients with congenitally corrected transposition of the great arteries. Am J Cardiol 1999;84:820.
5. Thiene G, Nava A, Rossi L. The conduction system in corrected transposition with situs inversus. Eur J Cardiol 1977;6:57.
6. Todd DB, Anderson RC, Edwards JE. Inverted malformations in corrected transposition of the great vessels. Circulation 1985;32:298.
7. Tulevski II, Zijta FM, Smeijers AS, Dodge-Khatami A, van der Wall EE, Mulder BJ. Regional and global right ventricular dysfunction in asymptomatic or minimally symptomatic patients with congenitally corrected transposition. Cardiol Young 2004;14: 168-73.

U

1. Uher V. Zur Pathologie des Reizleitungsstems bei kongenitalen Herza-nomalien. Frankfurter Z Pathol 1936;49:347.

V

1. Van Praagh R, David I, Gordon D, Wright GB, Van Praagh S. Ventricular diagnosis and designation. In Godman MJ, ed. Pediatric cardiology, Vol. 4. London: Churchill Livingstone, 1981, p.153.
2. Van Praagh R, Durnin RE, Jockin H, Wagner HR, Korns M, Garabedian H. Anatomically corrected malposition of the great arteries (S,D,L). Circulation 1975;51:20.
3. Van Praagh R, Layton WM, Van Praagh S. The morphogenesis of normal and abnormal relationships between the great arteries and the ventricles: pathologic and experimental data. In Van Praagh R, Takao A, eds. Etiology and morphogenesis of congenital heart disease. Mount Kisco, N.Y.: Futura, 1980, p. 282.
4. Van Praagh R, Van Praagh S. Isolated ventricular inversion. Am J Cardiol 1966;17:395.
5. Van Praagh R, Weinberg PM. Double outlet left ventricle. In Moss AJ, Adams FH, Emmanoulides GC, eds. Heart disease in infants, children and adolescents, 2nd Ed. Baltimore: Williams & Wilkins, 1977, p. 367.
6. Van Praagh S, La Corte M, Fellows KE, Bossina K, Busch JH, Beck EW, et al. Superior-inferior ventricles: anatomic and angiocardiographic findings in 10 postmortem cases. In Van Praagh R, ed. Etiology and morphology of congenital heart disease, Mount Kisco, N.Y.: Futura, 1980, p. 317.
7. Villani M, Ross DN. Successful surgical repair of solitus, dextrocardia, atrioventricular discordance, and double outlet right ventricle with L-malposition of the aorta. Eur J Cardiol 1978;3:105.
8. Voskuil M, Hazekamp MG, Kroft LJ, Lubbers WJ, Ottenkamp J, van der Wall EE, et al. Postsurgical course of patients with congenitally corrected transposition of the great arteries. Am J Cardiol 1999;83:558.

W

1. Walmsley T. Transposition of the ventricles and the arterial stems. J Anat 1931;65:528.
2. Wan AW, Jevremovic A, Selamet Tierney ES, McCrindle BW, Dunn E, Manlhiot C, et al. Comparison of impact of prenatal versus postnatal diagnosis of congenitally corrected transposition of the great arteries. Am J Cardiol 2009;104:1276-9.
3. Wenink AC. Congenitally complete heart block with an interrupted Monckeberg sling. Eur J Cardiol 1979;9:89.
4. Westerman GR, Lang P, Castaneda AR, Norwood WI. Corrected transposition and repair of associated intracardiac defects. Circulation 1982;66:I197.
5. Wilkinson JL, Smith A, Lincoln C, Anderson RH. Conducting tissues in congenitally corrected transposition with situs inversus. Br Heart J 1978;40:41.
6. Williams WG, Suri R, Shindo G, Freedom RM, Morch JE, Trusler GA. Repair of major intracardiac anomalies associated with atrioventricular discordance. Ann Thorac Surg 1981;31:527.

Y

1. Yagihara T, Kishimoto H, Isobe F, Yamamoto F, Nishigaki K, Matsuki O, et al. Double switch operation in cardiac anomalies with atrioventricular and ventriculoarterial discordance. J Thorac Cardiovasc Surg 1994;107:351.
2. Yamagishi M, Imai Y, Hoshino S, Ishihara K, Koh Y, Nagatsu M, et al. Anatomic correction of atrioventricular discordance. J Thorac Cardiovasc Surg 1993;105:1067.
3. Yasuda K, Ohuchi H, Ono Y, Yagihara T, Echigo S. Cardiorespiratory responses to exercise after anatomic repair of atrioventricular discordance with abnormal ventriculoarterial connection. Pediatr Cardiol 2007;28:14-20.
4. Yeh T Jr, Connelly MS, Coles JG, Webb GD, McLaughlin PR, Freedom RM, et al. Atrioventricular discordance: results of repair in 127 patients. J Thorac Cardiovasc Surg 1999;117:1190.

56 Double Inlet Ventricle and Atretic Atrioventricular Valve

DEFINITION

Double inlet ventricle is a congenital cardiac malformation in which both atria connect to only one ventricular chamber by either two separate atrioventricular (AV) valves or a common AV valve. Closely related to double inlet ventricle are cardiac malformations in which both atria connect to only one ventricular chamber because of atresia of one AV valve that is imperforate or absent. As a group, double inlet ventricles and those with an atretic AV valve are appropriately considered as having a *single ventricle* or *univentricular AV connection,* although these phrases are not appropriate for describing morphology of an individual heart.[A4]

The ventricular mass in these settings rarely consists only of a solitary ventricle. When, as is usual, there are two ventricles, one is usually incomplete (rudimentary) and hypoplastic. Often the incomplete ventricle is connected to an atrium by overriding of an AV valve. Such arrangements are termed *double inlet ventricle* only if more than 50% of the overriding valve lies over the main (dominant) ventricle.

Classic tricuspid atresia (univentricular AV connection with atrial situs solitus, ventricular D-loop, single inlet left ventricular main chamber, right-sided AV valve [tricuspid] atresia, and ventriculoarterial [VA] concordant or discordant connection)[A7,E4] is separately discussed in Chapter 41.[1] Most

[1]The adjectives *left* and *right* used to modify atrium or ventricle mean *morphologically* left or right. *Position* of a chamber or valve is referred to as *right sided* or *left sided.*

morphologic variants of left-sided AV valve (mitral) atresia with patent aortic outlet are included in this chapter. Mitral atresia in association with either aortic atresia or aortic stenosis, intact ventricular septum, and concordant AV and VA connections represent two of the four classic morphologic forms of hypoplastic left heart physiology and are discussed in Chapter 49.

HISTORICAL NOTE

One of the earliest descriptions of a variety of this congenital anomaly was by Holmes, who in 1824 noted that it was intermediate between a normal heart and one with a solitary ventricular chamber.[H1] It is believed that Peacock described a heart with "both auricles opening into the left ventricle" in 1854. Rokitansky described and illustrated a case of double inlet left ventricle in 1875, as did Mann in 1907, describing the heart as *cor triloculare biatriatum*.[M3,R6] Taussig described "single ventricle with a diminutive outlet chamber" in 1939.[T1] Lev and colleagues have listed a number of other descriptions of "single (primitive) ventricle" that were published more than 100 years ago.[L4]

An important contribution by Van Praagh and colleagues in 1964 at the Mayo Clinic was clear definition of the entity as one in which both AV valves empty into the same ventricle.[V2] About the same time, Elliott and colleagues expressed the view, now accepted, that hearts with atresia of one AV valve (and thus a single AV valve) have much in common with hearts with double inlet ventricle.[E4] Anderson and colleagues introduced the phrase *univentricular AV connection* to collate this group of malformations.[A2,A3,A4,A7,S10,W5]

Lev clearly established as a different entity hearts with a huge ventricular septal defect (VSD) or common ventricle, in which one side of the common chamber was morphologically right ventricle and the other left ventricle; he thereby excluded them from the single-ventricle category.[L4]

Surgical palliation of double inlet ventricle without pulmonary stenosis began with the original description of pulmonary trunk banding by Muller and Damman in 1952.[M10] Palliation of double inlet ventricle with pulmonary stenosis has as its basis the original Blalock-Taussig shunt; its application to patients with double inlet ventricle and pulmonary stenosis was only a matter of time.[B6] Redo and colleagues may have been the first to show the favorable effect of a Blalock-Hanlon atrial septectomy in patients with left-sided (mitral) valve atresia.[R4]

Septating the main chamber to establish two circulations in series emerged from the Mayo Clinic experience of unexpectedly encountering a patient with double inlet ventricle in 1956.[M5] Preoperative diagnosis was corrected transposition with VSD, but correct diagnosis was made after opening the ventricle. Septation was accomplished, but the patient died about 6 months after operation, probably during a Stokes-Adams episode. This concept lay dormant for some years, but in 1972 it was further developed by Sakakibara and colleagues and in 1973 by Edie, Malm, and colleagues, who reported four successful septation repairs.[E3,S2] Three long-term survivors of septation were reported in 1973 by Arai, Sakakibara, and colleagues, and one was reported by Ionescu and colleagues.[A10,I2] McGoon, Danielson, and colleagues began to report successful results from the Mayo Clinic about this same time.[M5] The right atrial approach to septation was suggested and applied by Doty and colleagues in 1979.[D2]

A different surgical concept—using the main (dominant) ventricular chamber for generating systemic blood flow and allowing the vis a tergo of the systemic venous system to generate pulmonary blood flow—was stimulated by the work of Fontan and Baudet (published in 1971 and known as the *Fontan operation*) and by the work of Kreutzer and colleagues.[F2,K6,K7] Application of this concept to surgical treatment of double inlet ventricle was reported by Yacoub and Radley-Smith in 1976.[Y1]

Subaortic stenosis became apparent as a major problem when experience with the Fontan operation increased during the early 1970s.[N3,R1] In 1973, Neches and colleagues applied the concept of placing the main chamber in direct communication with the aorta by performing an anastomosis of pulmonary trunk to aorta.[N3,P2] Others have accomplished this by an anastomosis of the proximal segment of the divided pulmonary trunk to the side of the ascending aorta, a part of a Damus-Kaye-Stansel (DKS) operation.[J1,N3,Y1] This concept has been revitalized more recently by extensive augmentation of the usually hypoplastic aortic arch in conjunction with the DKS operation in the Norwood I operation and by using the arterial switch operation for this purpose, first by Freedom, Williams, Trusler, and colleagues in 1980 and in neonates by Karl and colleagues in 1991.[F5,J1,K1,R8] Penkoske and colleagues approached the problem directly by enlarging the VSD in 1984.[P4]

Application of cardiac transplantation to this group of patients was a natural evolution in managing patients with univentricular AV connections and myocardial failure.

MORPHOLOGY

Generalizations

Ventricular Mass

The main (dominant) chamber making up the ventricular mass in double inlet ventricle with two ventricles may have a left ventricular internal architecture, a right ventricular internal architecture, or an indeterminate architecture. Main chamber volume is largest when there is no pulmonary stenosis but considerably smaller when pulmonary stenosis is present.[K4] This is related to the fact that main chamber volume is positively correlated with pulmonary-to-systemic flow ratio ($\dot{Q}p/\dot{Q}s$).[S7] The nondominant, incomplete (rudimentary) hypoplastic chamber, when present, is always opposite architecture to the dominant chamber. Ventricular topology in double inlet ventricles may be either right-handed (D-loop), left-handed (L-loop), or indeterminate (Tables 56-1 and 56-2). (See "Symbolic Convention of Van Praagh" under Terminology and Classification of Heart Disease in Chapter 1.)[V1]

The nondominant chamber is called *incomplete* (or *rudimentary*) because it lacks one or more of its component parts, usually the inlet portion but occasionally also the outlet, leaving only the apical trabeculated part. The incomplete chamber is always smaller than the dominant chamber and is connected to the dominant chamber by a VSD. The VSD is sometimes called a *bulboventricular foramen,* but this term applies only when the incomplete chamber is of right ventricular morphology. Rarely, such as when there is double inlet to one chamber and double outlet from the other, both chambers are incomplete. The ventricular septum is malaligned

Table 56-1 Ventricular Architectural Pattern and Atrial Situs in Double Inlet Ventricles[a]

Atrial Situs	n	Solitary Ventricle	Two Ventricles		
		Indeterminate	Right-Handed (D-Loop)	Left-Handed (L-Loop)	Undetermined Loop
Solitus	101 (87) + <u>89</u>	15	32 + <u>89</u>	50	4
Inversus	2 (2)	0	2	0	0
Ambiguus:	12 (10)	7	5	0	0
Bilateral right-sidedness	8 (7)	5	3		
Bilateral left-sidedness	4 (3)	2	2		
Unknown	1 (1)	1	0	0	0
TOTAL	116 + <u>89</u> = 205	23 (20)	39 (34) + <u>89</u>	50 (43)	4

Data from Stefanelli and colleagues.[S14]
[a]Cases of classic tricuspid atresia (n = 89) are included and underlined.
Key: ( ), Percentage of 116.

Table 56-2 Morphologic Findings in 189 Patients with Double Inlet or Common Inlet Ventricle

	DIRV (n = 31)	DILV (n = 45)	CIRV (n = 93)	CILV (n = 20)
Atrial Arrangement				
Usual	19 (61%)	40 (89%)	—	2 (10%)
Mirror image	1 (3%)	1 (2%)	—	—
Right isomerism	8 (26%)	4 (9%)	89 (96%)	16 (80%)
Left isomerism	3 (10%)	—	4 (4%)	2 (10%)
Ventricular Loop				
D-loop	21 (68%)	18 (40%)		
L-loop	10 (32%)	27 (60%)		
Ventriculoarterial Connections				
SORV	18 (58%)	5 (11%)	42 (45%)	7 (35%)
DORV	12 (39%)	1 (2%)	39 (42%)	6 (30%)
DOLV	—	2 (4%)	—	2 (10%)
Discordant	1 (3%)	30 (67%)	8 (9%)	4 (20%)
Concordant	—	7 (16%)	4 (4%)	1 (5%)
Pulmonary Pathway				
Pulmonary atresia with nonconfluent PA	5 (16%)	—	3 (3%)	1 (5%)
Pulmonary atresia with confluent PA	13 (42%)	5 (11%)	39 (42%)	6 (30%)
Pulmonary stenosis	6 (19%)	16 (36%)	43 (46%)	9 (45%)
No obstruction	7 (23%)	24 (53%)	8 (9%)	4 (20%)
Aortic Pathway				
Coarctation/interruption	2 (6%)	4 (9%)	1 (1%)	1 (5%)
No obstruction	29 (94%)	41 (91%)	92 (99%)	19 (95%)

Modified from Kitamura and colleagues.[K4]
Key: *CILV,* Common inlet left ventricle; *CIRV,* common inlet right ventricle; *DILV,* double inlet left ventricle; *DIRV,* double inlet right ventricle; *DOLV,* double outlet left ventricle; *DORV,* double outlet right ventricle; *PA,* pulmonary arteries; *SORV,* aorta arising from right ventricle with pulmonary atresia.

and incomplete in nearly all hearts with double inlet ventricle, or is completely absent.

Some consider a solitary ventricle with double inlet to be an indeterminate ventricle, and some consider it to be a right ventricle.[V3,W4]

Atria

Any type of atrial situs can be present. However, with double inlet left ventricle, there is usually atrial situs solitus, and with double inlet right and indeterminate ventricles, about half have situs solitus and half have a heterotaxy pattern, right atrial isomerism predominating (see Chapter 58).[A8] Situs inversus (mirror image) is unusual (see Tables 56-1 and 56-2).

Atrioventricular Connection

There are usually two perforate AV valves positioned entirely in the dominant ventricle. Their morphologic characteristics are frequently indeterminate, neither tricuspid nor mitral, and it is therefore best to call them *left-sided* (draining the

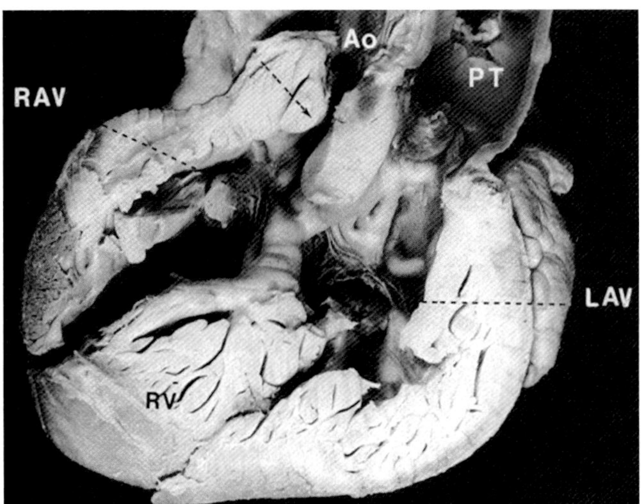

Figure 56-1 Interior view of a specimen of double inlet right ventricle with anterior portion removed. There are separate right-sided and left-sided atrioventricular valves entering a thick-walled large ventricular chamber with right ventricular morphology. Ventriculoarterial connection is double outlet with aorta rightward and anterior above a prominent conus that is producing subaortic obstruction *(arrow)*. Key: *Ao,* Aorta; *LAV,* left-sided atrioventricular valve; *PT,* pulmonary trunk; *RAV,* right-sided atrioventricular valve; *RV,* right ventricle.

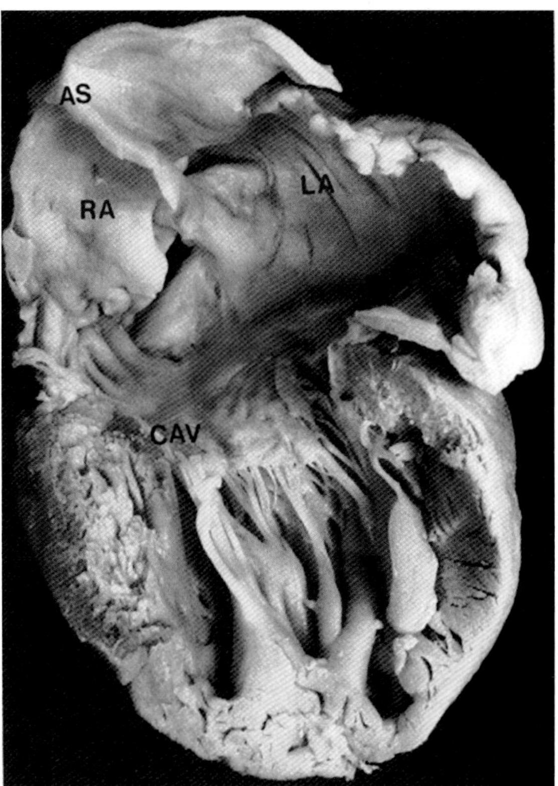

Figure 56-2 Interior view of specimen of double inlet right ventricle, opened to expose structures as they would appear in a four-chamber imaged view. There is a common atrioventricular valve (CAV) entering the large right ventricular chamber and a large ostium primum atrial septal defect (complete atrioventricular septal defect). Key: *AS,* Atrial septum; *LA,* left atrium; *RA,* right atrium.

left-sided atrium) and *right-sided* (draining the right-sided atrium)[R5] (Fig. 56-1). Alternatively, there may be a common AV valve (Fig. 56-2), although this is rare in double inlet left ventricle.[A5] When the AV valve is a common one, valvar abnormalities are common, including important regurgitation.[S11]

In about 20% of cases, one of the perforate valves or the common valve overrides the remnant of ventricular septum, or the tension apparatus of one or both valves straddles the septum.[A5] Rarely, a common patent AV valve overrides or straddles the septum.[H2]

Atresia of an AV valve usually involves total absence of the AV connection, but occasionally there is an imperforate membrane with a miniature tension apparatus beneath it.[A9,R2,T4] Typically (as in classic tricuspid atresia; see Morphology in Chapter 41) the small, incomplete ventricular chamber is on the same side as the atretic valve, but it may be on the opposite side.

Ventriculoarterial Connections

VA connections can be of any type, except in the case of a solitary ventricle, where there can only be a single or double outlet. In double inlet left ventricle, the most frequent connection is discordant, with aorta and subaortic incomplete right ventricle (outlet chamber) to the left, but sometimes to the right, of the pulmonary trunk; concordant, double outlet, and single outlet connections occur (Table 56-3).

Conduction Tissue

Morphology of the AV node and conduction system is abnormal. Position of the AV node is determined primarily by whether the ventricular septal remnant reaches the crux (see "Atrioventricular Node" under Conduction System in Chapter 1). From the surgeon's standpoint, it is important to know that the AV node can be anywhere around the perimeter of the right-sided AV valve.

Coronary Arteries

Terminology of the coronary artery branches is arguable. Left and right coronary arteries usually arise from the two aortic sinuses facing the pulmonary trunk. There are usually prominent descending branches (encircling coronary arteries) that indicate points of attachment of septum to free ventricular wall, and therefore the boundaries of the incomplete ventricle.[L4,R7]

Types

Double Inlet Left Ventricle

In double inlet left ventricle, the most common double inlet connection, the dominant ventricle is of left ventricular morphology.[L3,V1,V3] Apical trabeculations beyond insertions of the papillary muscles display a delicate criss-cross pattern. The septal surface is typically smooth in its superior half, and the crescentic margin bounding the VSD is smooth (Fig. 56-3). VSD morphology, however, can be variable. Of 46 patients with double inlet left ventricle carefully evaluated by Bevilacqua and colleagues, 24 had VSDs separated from the semilunar valves and completely surrounded by muscle (muscular defects), 19 had VSDs adjacent to the anterior semilunar valve (subaortic defect) in association with malalignment or

Table 56-3 Summary of Morphologic Features of the Ventriculoarterial Connections in 97 Specimens of Double Inlet Left Ventricle

Feature	Right Ventricle Leftward	Right Ventricle Rightward
Ventriculoarterial Connection[a]		
Concordant	2	13
Discordant	51	16
Double outlet RV	1	3
Aorta from RV/pulmonary atresia	6	1
Double outlet LV	2	1
Aorta from LV/pulmonary atresia	—	1
Infundibular Morphology		
Subpulmonary	2	13
Subaortic	58	17
Subpulmonary and subaortic	1	3
Markedly attenuated	1	2
Aortic Valve in Relation to Pulmonary Valve		
Right posterior	2	14
Right anterior	2	17
Right side-by-side	2	3
Left anterior	54	—
Left side-by-side	2	1
Arterial Trunks		
Spiraling	2	14
Parallel	60	21

Modified from Uemura and colleagues.[U1]
[a]For overriding of the aortic or pulmonary valve, the so-called 50% rule was applied.
Key: *LV,* Left ventricle; *RV,* right ventricle.

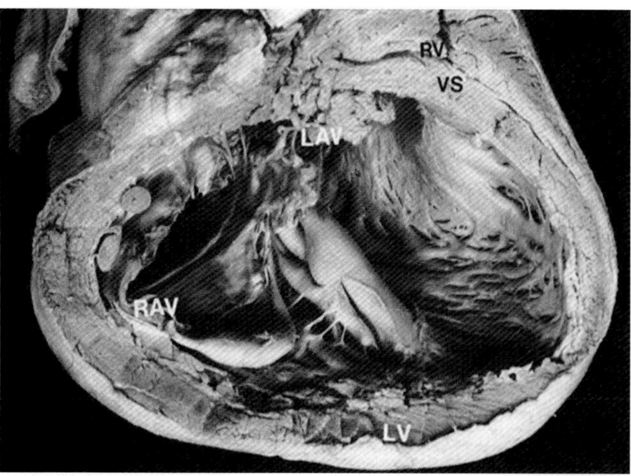

Figure 56-3 Interior view of specimen of double inlet left ventricle. Right-sided atrioventricular valve (RAV) is larger than the left-sided one (not completely visualized). The large ventricle has left ventricular morphology, with fine trabeculations near the apex and a smooth surface to the superior half of the ventricular septum (VS). There is a smooth crescentic lower margin bounding the ventricular septal defect. The incomplete right ventricle (RV) lies superiorly and leftward (L-loop). Key: *LAV,* Left-sided atrioventricular valve; *LV,* left ventricle.

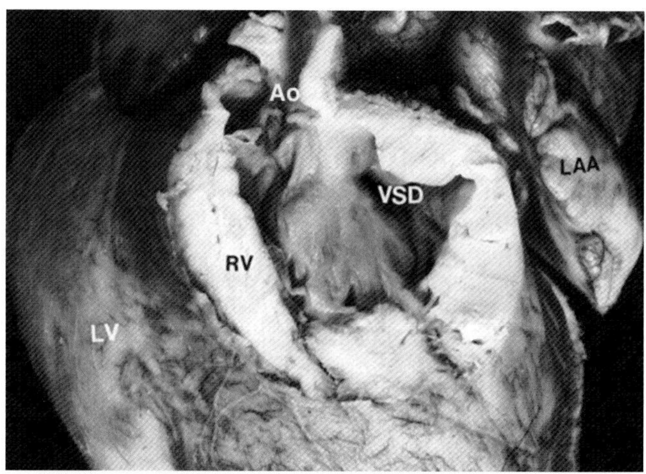

Figure 56-4 Specimen of double inlet left ventricle with L-loop. Incomplete right ventricle (RV) has been opened, showing coarse trabeculae present in its inferior part and a restrictive ventricular septal defect (VSD). The aorta (Ao) arises from this chamber. Key: *LAA,* Left atrial appendage; *LV,* left ventricle.

hypoplasia of the infundibular septum, and 3 had multiple muscular defects.[B3]

The small incomplete (rudimentary) ventricle is of right ventricular morphology, with coarse apical trabeculations and frequently a recognizable trabecula septomarginalis (septal band) bounding the VSD anteriorly. A smooth-walled infundibulum is present when one or both great arteries arise from this chamber (Fig. 56-4). Otherwise, and rarely, the chamber exists as a blind pouch. It is always positioned on the anterosuperior shoulder of the dominant left ventricle (Fig. 56-5), usually to the left but sometimes to the right. The septum thus lies obliquely and never extends to the crux.

The typical morphology of double inlet left ventricle, with ventricular L-looping, left-sided incomplete right ventricle, and VA discordant connections, occurs in about half of all cases, with a wide variety of VA connections in the remainder[U1] (see Table 56-3). The relatively uniform internal cardiac architecture of the AV valves and myocardium in typical double inlet left ventricle may be more variable when double outlet right ventricle occurs with it.[S3] Atrial situs is usually solitus, occasionally ambiguus, but rarely situs inversus.

Two variants of double inlet left ventricle warrant further description: (1) double inlet left ventricle with ventricular L-loop, left-sided incomplete right ventricle, and VA discordant connection and (2) double inlet left ventricle with ventricular D-loop, right-sided incomplete right ventricle, and VA concordant connection.

With Ventricular L-Loop, Left-Sided Incomplete Right Ventricle, and Ventriculoarterial Discordant Connection This is the largest subset of hearts with double inlet ventricle, comprising half the cases (see Figs. 56-3 through 56-5). The large left ventricular main chamber lies to the right and receives left-sided and right-sided AV valves, which usually are of tricuspid and mitral morphology, respectively, although both may be bicuspid. There may be some straddling and overriding (but <50%) of the AV valves. The majority of AV valves function normally, but the most common abnormality is stenosis of the left-sided "tricuspid" valve.[B3] A heavy trabecula often separates insertion of the papillary muscles into the diaphragmatic free wall of the left

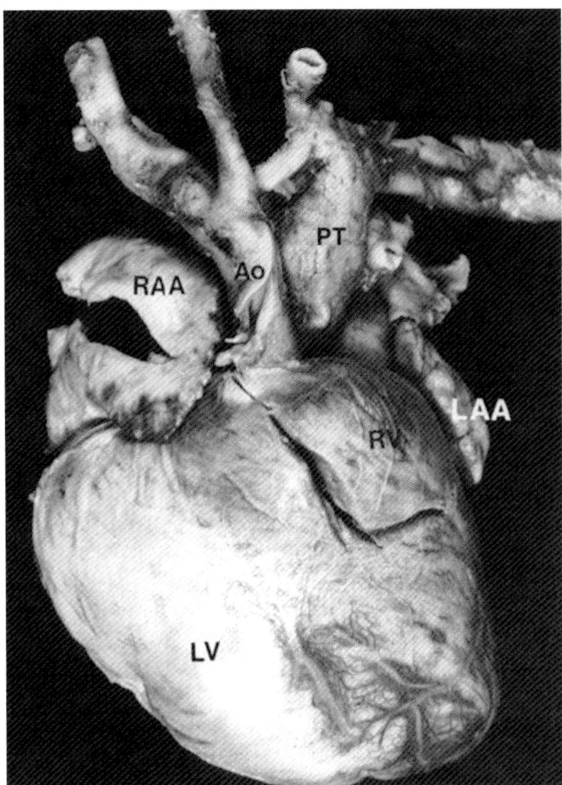

Figure 56-5 Frontal view of heart with double inlet left ventricle and L-loop. Specimen is the same as in Fig. 56-4. Incomplete right ventricle (RV) lies superiorly and to the left (on the shoulder) of the dominant left ventricle (LV). There is severe coarctation with hypoplasia of the transverse arch. Key: *Ao,* Aorta; *LAA,* left atrial appendage; *PT,* pulmonary trunk; *RAA,* right atrial appendage.

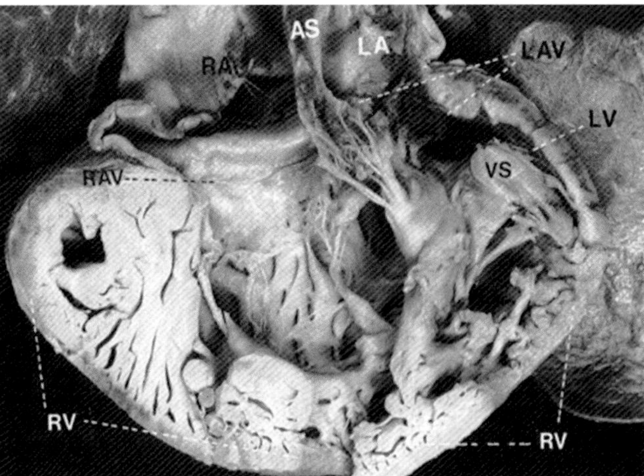

Figure 56-6 Interior view of specimen with double inlet right ventricle and ventricular D-loop. There are two atrioventricular valves. The larger chamber has typical right ventricular morphology, and the diminutive incomplete left ventricle (LV) lies posteriorly and to the left (in the hip pocket). The ventricular septum (VS) is small. Key: *AS,* Atrial septum; *LA,* left atrium; *LAV,* left-sided atrioventricular valve; *RA,* right atrium; *RAV,* right-sided atrioventricular valve; *RV,* right ventricle.

ventricle. The left-sided tricuspid valve commonly has attachments of the subvalvar tension apparatus to the ventricular septum.[D1]

The aorta arises above the short infundibulum of the incomplete left-sided right ventricle (see Fig. 56-4). The pulmonary trunk arises from the base of the left ventricle, anterior and superior to the right-sided AV ("mitral") valve, usually with pulmonary-mitral fibrous continuity. Subvalvar and valvar pulmonary stenoses occur but are not common, and pulmonary atresia occurs only occasionally.

The VSD is usually large and lies beneath the infundibular septum, but it may be restrictive, producing subaortic stenosis (see "Subaortic Stenosis" later under Natural History). As noted, the VSD may be in an atypical position within the apical septal trabeculations, and occasionally it is multiple. Muscular defects are more likely than subarterial defects to be restrictive.[B5]

The AV node is anterior and away from the atrial septum, lying in the right atrial wall adjacent to the superior commissural tissue between anterior and posterior leaflets of the right-sided AV valve.[A3,B4,E5] This arrangement also pertains to ventricular D-loop when the left ventricle is the main chamber, because again there is no ventricular septum extending to the crux. The bundle of His passes anterior to the pulmonary valve to reach the ventricular septum (see later Figs. 56-19 and 56-21).[A3,B2,B4]

Configuration of coronary arteries is similar to that in congenitally corrected transposition of the great arteries (see "Atrioventricular Node and Bundle of His" and "Coronary Arteries" under Morphology in Section I of Chapter 55).

With Ventricular D-Loop, Right-Sided Incomplete Right Ventricle, and Ventriculoarterial Concordant Connection This occurs in about 10% of cases and most resembles the normal heart. The large left ventricle lies to the left and posteriorly, and the small right ventricle lies to the right, anteriorly and superiorly. It was first described by Holmes and is often called the *Holmes heart.*[A6,H1]

There are usually two AV valves (often with the right-sided one straddling but with less than 50% override) or a common valve. The incomplete right ventricle is similar to that present in classic tricuspid atresia, with an extensive infundibulum leading to a pulmonary valve that is normally related to the aortic valve. Pulmonary stenosis is common, and the VSD may be restrictive.

The AV node is again anterior at about the 11-o'clock position relative to the right AV valve, as seen by the surgeon from the right atrium. The bundle of His descends from the anteriorly positioned AV node directly onto the ventricular septum without coming into relation with the ventricular outflow tract.[E6,W3] Rarely the AV node and bundle encircles the anterior aspect of the right AV orifice.[A6]

Double Inlet Right Ventricle

In double inlet right ventricle, both atria connect to a morphologically right ventricle. Apical trabeculations are coarse, and the trabecula septomarginalis is recognizable on the septal surface, with the VSD contained between its anterior and posterior limbs. The incomplete left ventricle is always positioned posteriorly and inferiorly ("in the hip pocket") in relation to the main chamber and usually lies to the left (D-loop; Fig. 56-6) or rarely to the right (L-loop). More often than not, it is very small and slitlike, communicating with the main chamber by a tiny VSD, with no connection to a great artery.[K3,S11] In other cases, the left ventricle is of reasonable size and the obliquely placed septum is well

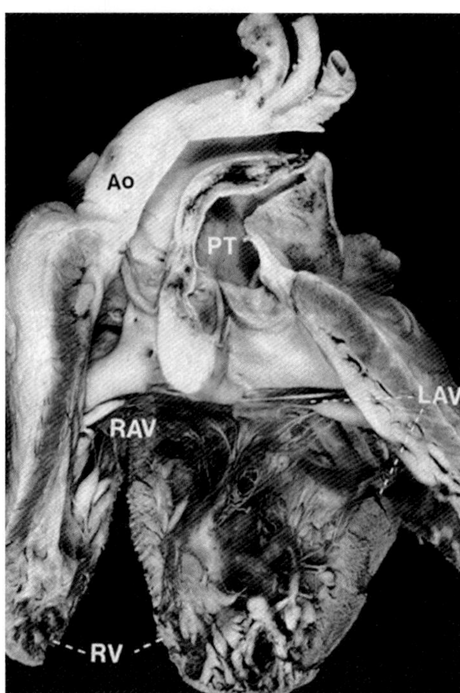

Figure 56-7 Specimen of double inlet right ventricle and double outlet right ventricle. Arguably, the main chamber can be considered of indeterminate type rather than right ventricular. Key: *Ao*, Aorta; *LAV*, left-sided atrioventricular valve; *PT*, pulmonary trunk; *RAV*, right-sided atrioventricular valve; *RV*, right ventricle.

formed; in contrast to that in double inlet left ventricle, it extends superiorly to the crux. In these cases, fine apical trabeculations are recognizable, and the superior septal surface beneath the VSD is smooth.

The VA connection is usually double outlet or single outlet (pulmonary atresia) from the right ventricle (Fig. 56-7; see also Fig. 56-1). A concordant connection sometimes occurs, with the aorta arising from the incomplete left ventricle. Pulmonary stenosis can be present.[S9]

Two AV valves may enter the large right ventricle, with the left one straddling, or frequently a common AV valve. Atrial situs inversus, and particularly right atrial isomerism, is more common in double inlet right ventricle than in double inlet left ventricle. Double inlet right ventricle associated with right atrial isomerism seems to be particularly prevalent in the Chinese.[W1]

In the presence of a D-loop and a ventricular septum reaching the crux, the AV node has its usual posterior position in the atrial septum with its normal relation to the ostium of the coronary sinus.[W6] The perforating bundle of His passes through the AV anulus and on to ventricular myocardium, either on the ventricular septum or on a trabecula on the posterior ventricular wall. In rare L-loop, the conduction system is variable, but a conventionally located AV node may be present, as well as a more rudimentary node located more anteriorly and superiorly along the right-sided AV anulus.[E5] The nonbranching bundle then descends onto a free-running trabecula in the main chamber.

Double Inlet Indeterminate Ventricle

Double inlet indeterminate ventricle includes hearts in which both atria connect to a solitary ventricle.[W4] Prevalence of this subset depends on the care with which a search is made for the possibility that the malformation is actually double inlet right ventricle, because a tiny isolated accessory ventricular chamber may be missed by cardiac imaging and may be found only on careful autopsy examination. Even when the ventricle is truly solitary, it may represent a morphologically right ventricle without a rudimentary left ventricle, because apical trabeculations are always coarse, and there may be a free-standing column posteriorly reminiscent of the trabecula septomarginalis (see Fig. 56-7).[V3]

There is a higher prevalence of heterotaxy in double inlet indeterminate ventricle than in the other types of double inlet ventricle. With it, as well as with atrial situs solitus and inversus, two perforate AV valves are usually present. The only VA connection possible is double or single (pulmonary atresia) outlet ventricle. Pulmonary stenosis is common. The great arteries are often more or less normally related.

The AV node is usually posterior when there is a rudimentary ridge in the ventricle and distinct papillary muscles to both AV valves. In this case, the AV node passes down a free-running trabecula.[W4] When a ridge is absent, the AV node is usually situated laterally (away from the atrial septum) and anteriorly, and the nonbranching bundle descends into the right parietal wall of the indeterminate ventricle.[W4]

Common Ventricle

Rarely an apparently common (solitary) ventricle has no ventricular septum or a diminutive apical ridge, but importantly, one side of the ventricular mass is morphologically right ventricle and the other morphologically left. Lev and colleagues consider this to be a heart with a huge VSD rather than double inlet common ventricle.[L4]

Left Atrioventricular (Mitral) Valve Atresia and Patent Aortic Outlet

Left-sided AV (mitral) valve atresia with patent aortic outlet has a widely varying morphology.[R5,T4] All variants are discussed here, with one exception: mitral atresia with patent aortic outlet (aortic stenosis) with intact ventricular septum, atrial situs solitus, levocardia, single inlet right ventricle with D-loop, and hypoplasia of all left cardiac segments, together with VA concordant connection. This variant is considered one of the four classic morphologic variants of hypoplastic left heart physiology, along with mitral atresia–aortic atresia, mitral stenosis–aortic atresia, and mitral stenosis–aortic stenosis (see "Left Ventricle and Mitral Valve" under Morphogenesis and Morphology in Chapter 49).

The atretic valve may be imperforate, in which case there is a hypoplastic membrane, sometimes with a miniature chordal apparatus beneath it; or the AV connection may be absent, with the floor of the atrium being separated from the ventricle by fibrofatty tissue.[A9,T4] In a study of 23 patients with patent aortic outlet and atresia of the left AV valve, 15 had absence of the left AV connection, 5 had an imperforate left AV valve, and 3 had atrial isomerism. Those with imperforate left AV valve demonstrated concordant AV connections.[A11]

The patent right-sided AV valve may occasionally override the remnant of ventricular septum,[K5] but with more than 50% of the anulus committed to the larger right ventricular chamber. The tension apparatus may straddle the septum, which reaches the crux.[H2]

In this most common arrangement ("mitral" atresia), there is atrial situs solitus, ventricular D-loop, and a dominant right ventricle connected to the right atrium by a patent right-sided (usually tricuspid) AV valve and a small and incomplete left ventricle lying posteriorly and to the left (Figs. 56-8 and 56-9).[G2] The left ventricle may be a blind chamber connecting to the right ventricle by a small VSD (in which case the VA connection is either double or single outlet right ventricle), but more commonly it functions as an outlet chamber giving origin to the aorta (concordant VA connection) and rarely to the pulmonary artery.[T4] The left ventricle is often smaller than suggested by the position of the left anterior descending coronary artery (see Fig. 56-9). Characteristically, when the aorta arises from the small left ventricle, the VSD is restrictive and the aorta small in association with coarctation or aortic arch hypoplasia.[T4] Interatrial obstruction is also common.

Alternatively, and less commonly, the arrangement is atrial situs solitus and ventricular L-loop with single inlet and more or less right-sided left ventricle, in which case the right atrium

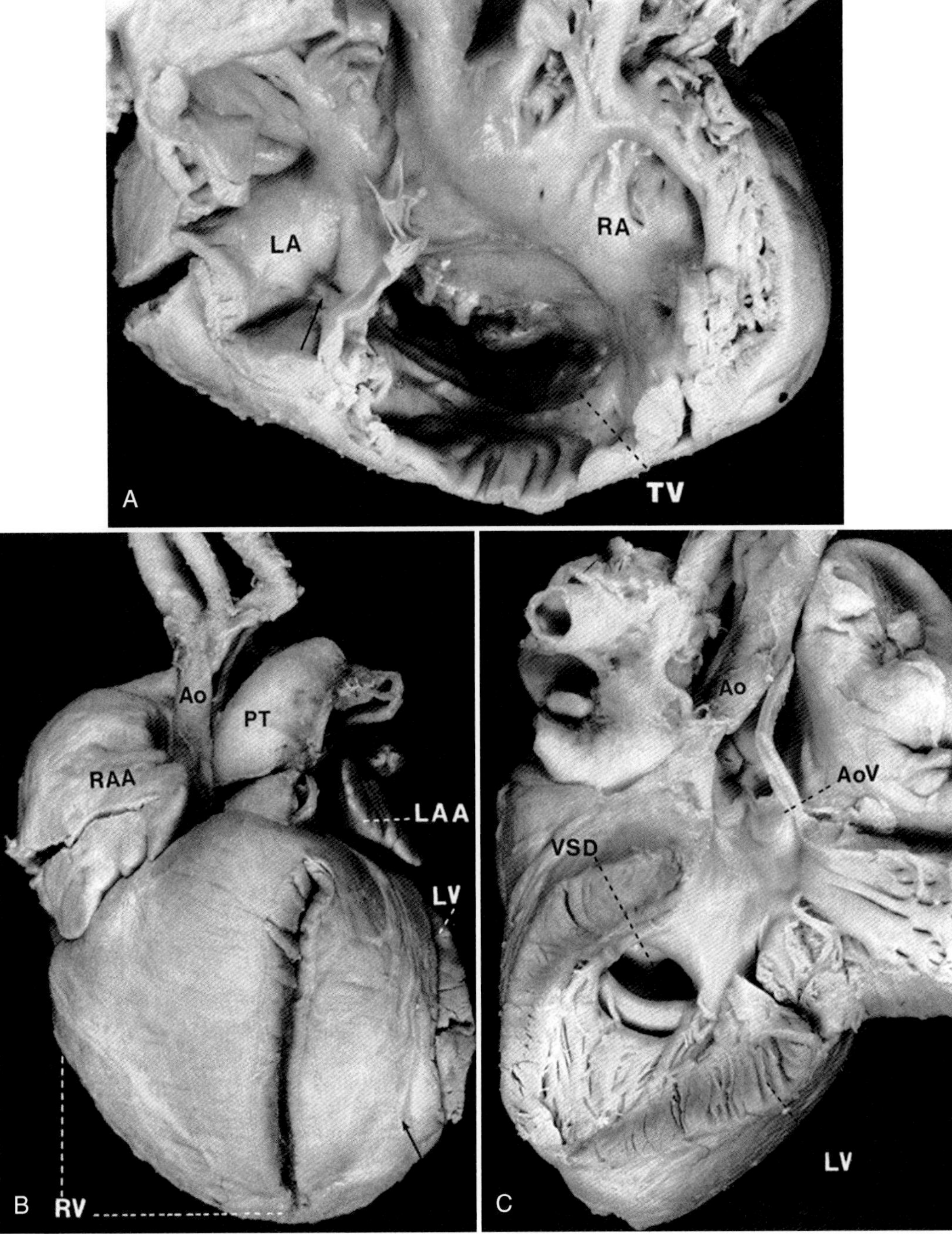

Figure 56-8 Specimens of hearts with left-sided mitral atresia but no aortic atresia in hearts with ventricular D-loop. **A,** Posterior view of the atria, with atrial walls and septum displaced anteriorly and superiorly, except for septum primum. Arrow indicates site of atretic mitral valve. **B,** External frontal view of another heart. Enlarged right ventricle (RV) is demarcated by anterior descending coronary artery *(arrow)*, although large branches extend over RV. Left ventricle (LV) is underdeveloped. **C,** View of opened LV in same specimen as in **B.** Midmuscular ventricular septal defects (VSD) and normally connected aorta (Ao) are seen.

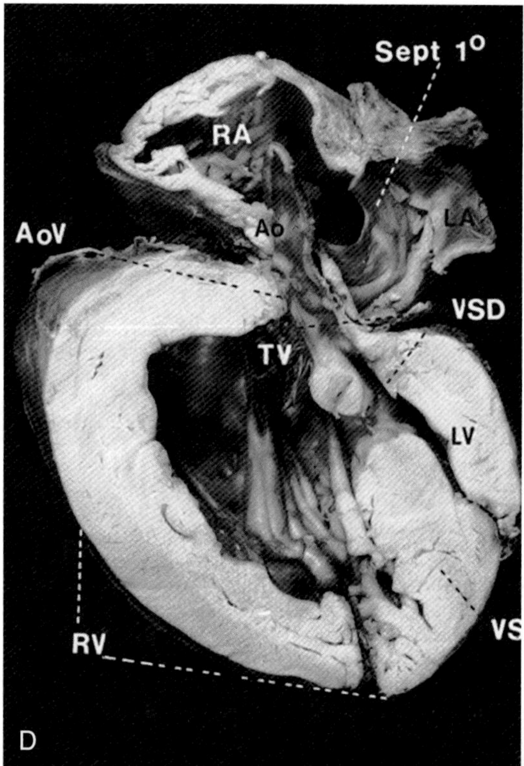

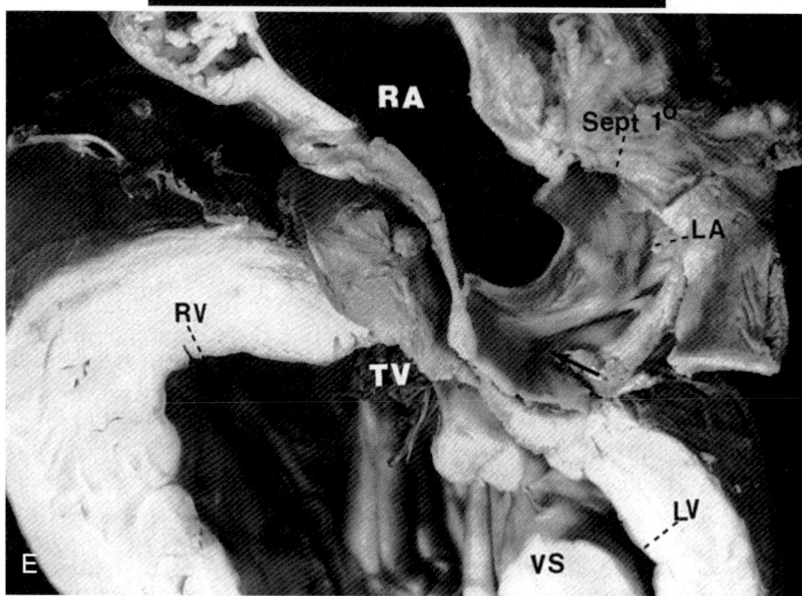

Figure 56-8, cont'd **D,** Heart specimen opened to expose structures as they would be seen in a four-chamber view. Conoventricular and midmuscular VSDs are present. Ascending aorta and aortic valve (AoV) are normally connected to hypoplastic LV cavity. RV is enlarged and hypertrophied. **E,** Close-up view of same specimen as in **D.** Dimple at site of atretic mitral valve is indicated by arrow. Thickened septum primum is evident. Key: *LA,* Left atrium; *LAA,* left atrial appendage; *PT,* pulmonary trunk; *RA,* right atrium; *RAA,* right atrial appendage; *Sept 1°,* septum primum; *TV,* right-sided tricuspid valve; *VS,* ventricular septum.

is connected to the dominant left ventricle by a patent AV valve with either mitral or indeterminate morphology. There is an incomplete left-sided right ventricle situated anteriorly and to the left, above which is the atretic left-sided AV valve, and the VSD may be restrictive. The septum does not reach the crux. The usual VA connection is discordant with the right ventricle giving origin to the aorta, but double outlet left ventricle also occurs.

Right Atrioventricular (Tricuspid) Valve Atresia

Excluding cases of classic right-sided (tricuspid) valve atresia (see Chapter 41), right-sided AV valve atresia can occur with single inlet and more or less left-sided right ventricle (ventricular L-loop). Right AV valve atresia has also been reported in association with an indeterminate solitary ventricle.[A9] The patent left-sided AV valve may occasionally override the septum and may have multiple leaflets.[K5]

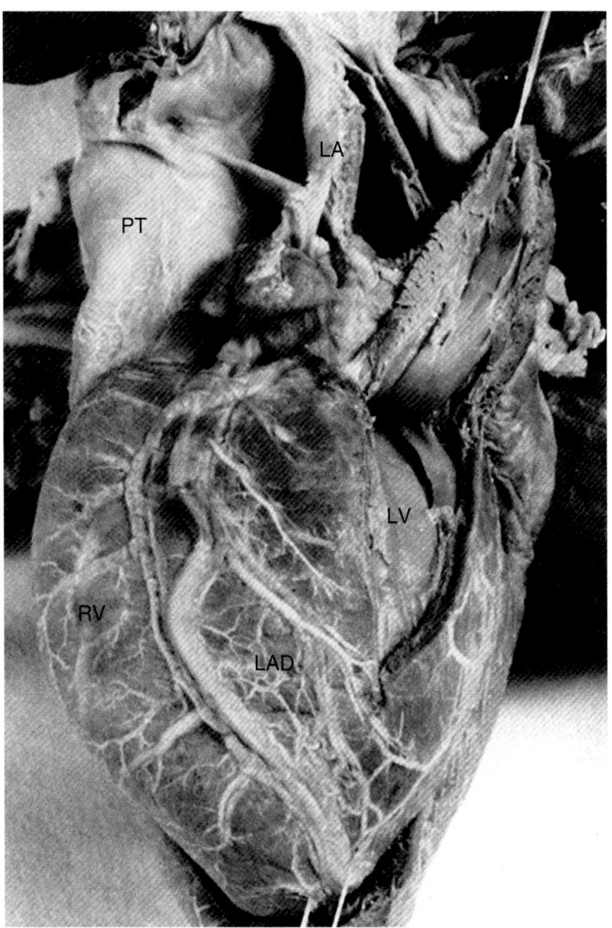

Figure 56-9 Relation of left anterior descending coronary artery (LAD) to ventricular septum in hearts with mitral atresia and patent aortic root. Note that in this heart, the clearly visible artery is the LAD, which does not closely relate to the left ventricular (LV) cavity. Key: *LA,* Left atrial cavity; *PT,* pulmonary trunk; *RV,* right ventricle. (From Gittenberger-de Groot and colleagues.[G2])

Associated Cardiac Anomalies

Associated cardiac anomalies occur in at least one third of patients with double inlet ventricle. AV valve malformations are common and include leaflet dysplasia, leaflet cleft and tags, and anular hypoplasia, in addition to straddling.[Q1,Q2] These can produce either valvar regurgitation or stenosis. The pulmonary valve may be stenotic from anular hypoplasia and leaflet thickening, or it may be atretic. Subvalvar pulmonary stenosis is common and results from either infundibular narrowing (muscle hypertrophy, hypoplasia, or occasionally a deviated septum) (see Fig. 56-1) or, more commonly, a restrictive VSD leading to an outflow chamber from which the pulmonary trunk arises (see Fig. 56-4). Aortic arch anomalies (coarctation, aortic arch interruption, or arch hypoplasia) also sometimes coexist with single ventricle (see Table 56-2). Multiple VSDs are not rare.

Subaortic stenosis is one of the most important coexisting cardiac anomalies. Because of the variable time of its appearance, it is discussed later under Natural History.

CLINICAL FEATURES AND DIAGNOSTIC CRITERIA

Clinical manifestations vary with morphology. Patients without pulmonary stenosis or atresia, about one third of the total, present in a manner similar to those with tricuspid atresia and normally related great vessels without pulmonary stenosis or atresia (see Clinical Features and Diagnostic Criteria in Chapter 41).

When mild or moderate pulmonary stenosis coexists, early years of life may be without important symptoms. A $\dot{Q}p/\dot{Q}s$ of approximately 2 or less results in only moderate cardiomegaly and mild pulmonary overcirculation on the chest radiograph and good functional status, albeit with mild cyanosis. Presentation in early or middle childhood rather than in infancy is common and is usually precipitated by cyanosis, a cardiac murmur, or typical findings on a chest radiograph. Clinical presentation is similar to that of tricuspid atresia and normally related great arteries with mild to moderate pulmonary stenosis (see Chapter 41).

When pulmonary stenosis is severe or pulmonary atresia is present, important cyanosis usually results in presentation in the early days or weeks of life, similar to that of tricuspid atresia and normally related great vessels with severe pulmonary stenosis or pulmonary atresia.

Atresia of the left-sided AV valve, when combined with a restrictive foramen ovale, results in severe pulmonary venous hypertension with its typical chest radiographic appearance and severe respiratory distress in early life. The presentation can mimic that of classic hypoplastic left heart physiology with restrictive or intact atrial septum (see Chapter 49). This situation may be masked initially by pulmonary stenosis and small pulmonary blood flow, only to become apparent after a systemic–pulmonary artery shunt is created. Severe AV valve regurgitation results in elevated atrial pressure and early appearance of heart failure.

Double inlet single left ventricle with AV and VA discordant connections, restrictive VSD (bulboventricular foramen), and aortic arch hypoplasia typically mimics hypoplastic left heart physiology in its presentation (see Chapter 49).

The electrocardiogram and chest radiograph may raise suspicion of the presence of double inlet ventricle, but echocardiography usually is the first definitive diagnostic procedure. Absence of the posterior (inlet) septum between the AV valves, one of the hallmarks of double inlet ventricle, can usually be diagnosed from the echocardiogram, particularly when associated with apposition of the unsupported septal leaflets of the two AV valves.[B1,C1,F1] Echocardiography with Doppler color flow imaging can provide all the necessary diagnostic information (Figs. 56-10 and 56-11).[H4,L2]

Cineangiography may be performed (Figs. 56-12 and 56-13) but currently is not necessary for planning therapy in the neonate or infant, and may be disadvantageous to the condition of the patient. It should be recalled that the Holmes heart is easily misdiagnosed as tetralogy of Fallot.[S1] Cardiac catheterization and cineangiography can provide important information about the patient presenting in older infancy or later, or about the patient who has previously undergone surgery, primarily by defining pulmonary vascular resistance and morphology of the branch pulmonary arteries.

Magnetic resonance imaging and computed tomography have little diagnostic role in the neonate.

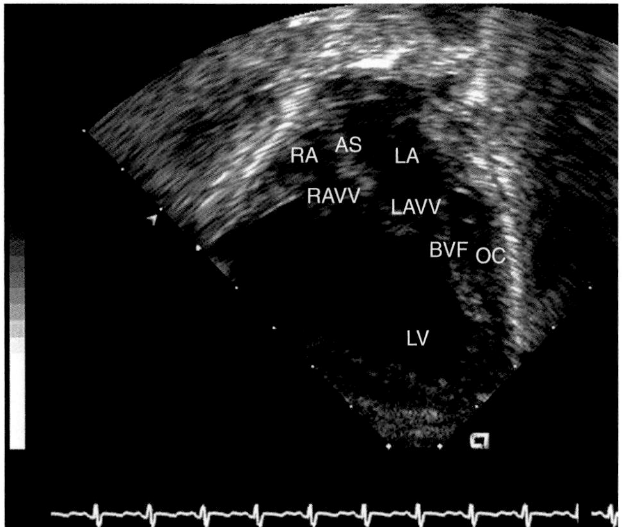

Figure 56-10 Four-chamber echocardiographic view demonstrating S,L,L double inlet left ventricle (see "Symbolic Convention of Van Praagh" in Chapter 1). Atrial septum is intact, and right-sided atrioventricular valve (RAVV) is smaller than left-sided one (LAVV). The dominant ventricle shows features of a morphologic left ventricle and is positioned to right side and posteriorly. The small outlet ventricular chamber is positioned to the left side and anteriorly. This image views the posterior aspect of the heart, so the great arteries, which are L-transposed with the aorta arising from the incomplete ventricle, are not seen. There is a communication between main and incomplete ventricular chambers (ventricular septal defect, or bulboventricular foramen). Key: *AS,* Atrial septum; *BVF,* bulboventricular foramen or ventricular septal defect; *LA,* left atrium; *LV,* left ventricle; *OC,* outlet ventricular chamber, or incomplete right ventricle; *RA,* right atrium.

NATURAL HISTORY

Double Inlet Ventricle

Estimated overall survival without treatment is about 57% at 1 year and 45% at 5 years[F3,G1,M1,M9] (Fig. 56-14). The monumental study by Franklin and colleagues documented the relatively favorable prognosis of certain subsets. Specifically, patients with atrial situs solitus and double inlet left ventricle, ventricular L-loop, discordant VA connection without systemic outflow obstruction, $\dot{Q}p/\dot{Q}s$ of about 1 to 2 (due to mild to moderate pulmonary stenosis), and presentation between 14 and 60 days of age have about a 90% chance of surviving for at least 10 years without intervention (Fig. 56-15). Estimated survival without intervention of other commonly encountered subsets is illustrated in Figs. 56-15 and 56-16. Although the natural history impact of differing AV connections has not been clearly defined, evidence exists that differences in left ventricular function are present depending on whether the inlet connection has two patent valves or one (Fig. 56-17).[R3]

Presentation with severe acidosis and low cardiac output has been a particularly severe risk factor for early death without intervention.[F3] Systemic outflow obstruction at any level, particularly aortic atresia, is also a strong risk factor for early death.

Mitral Atresia

When atresia of the left AV valve coexists with a restrictive opening in the atrial septum, such as in mitral atresia (atrial situs solitus, ventricular D-loop, right ventricular main

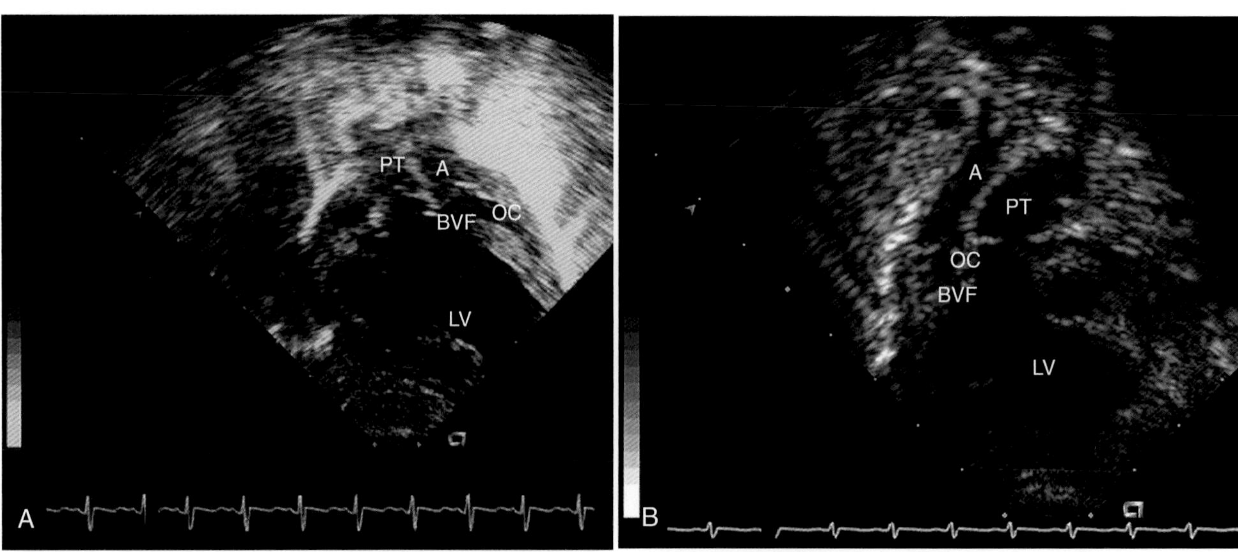

Figure 56-11 Echocardiogram from heart with S,L,L double inlet left ventricle. **A,** Subcostal coronal image demonstrating a somewhat more anterior region (compared with that shown in Fig. 56-10). This image shows pulmonary trunk and aortic connections to heart. Aorta is left sided and anterior in relation to pulmonary trunk and arises from incomplete outlet ventricular chamber. Bulboventricular foramen is visible. Inlets to dominant left ventricle and atrioventricular valves are not visualized because of the anterior image. **B,** Lateral projection. Note anterior position of aorta arising from the anterior incomplete ventricle, and posterior position of pulmonary trunk arising without obstruction from dominant left ventricle. Bulboventricular foramen is very small, causing severe subaortic obstruction. Key: *A,* Aorta; *BVF,* bulboventricular foramen, or ventricular septal defect; *LV,* left ventricle; *OC,* outlet ventricular chamber, or incomplete right ventricle; *PT,* pulmonary trunk.

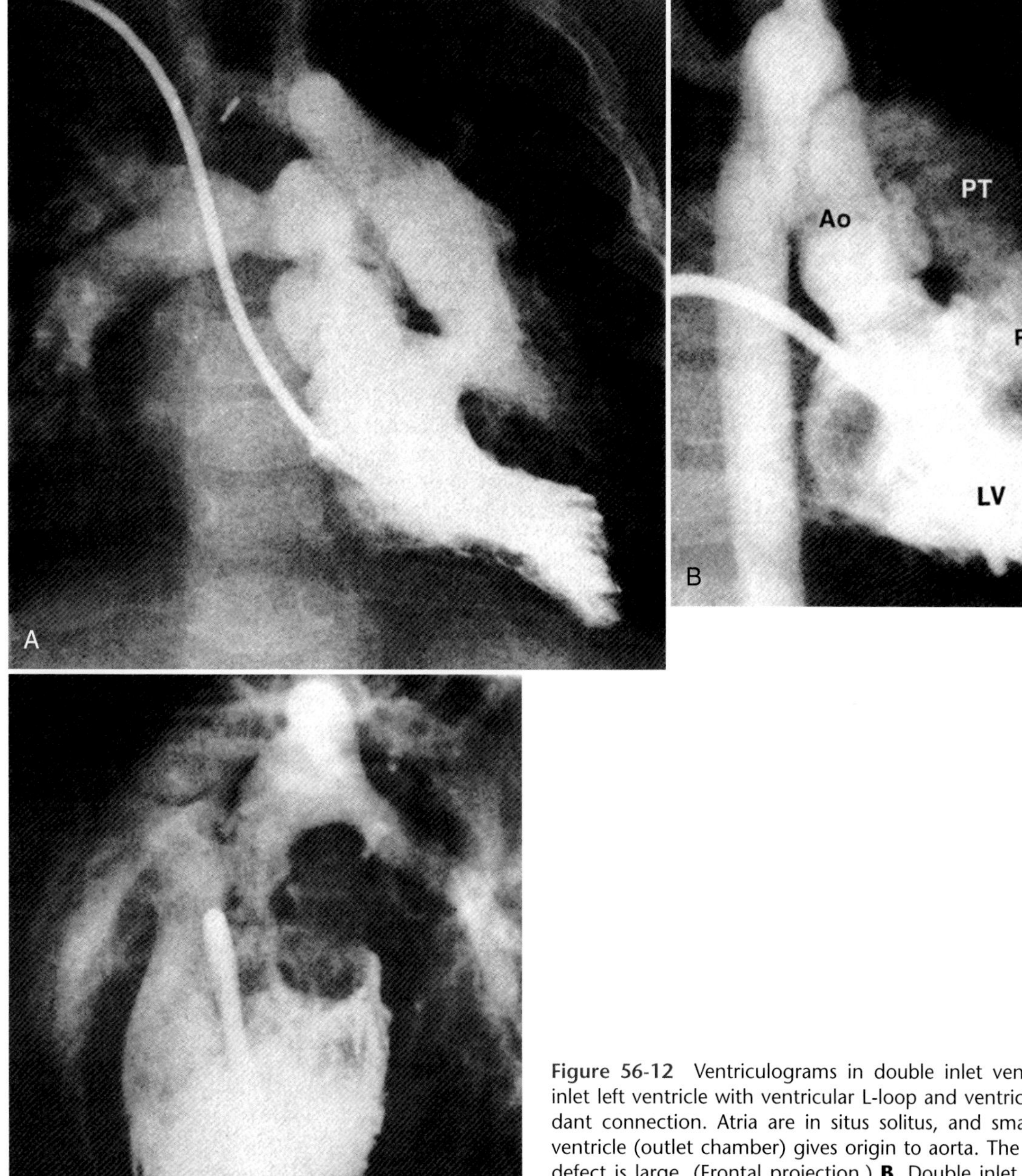

Figure 56-12 Ventriculograms in double inlet ventricle. **A,** Double inlet left ventricle with ventricular L-loop and ventriculoarterial discordant connection. Atria are in situs solitus, and small left-sided right ventricle (outlet chamber) gives origin to aorta. The ventricular septal defect is large. (Frontal projection.) **B,** Double inlet left ventricle (LV) with ventricular L-loop and ventriculoarterial concordant connection. Atria are in situs solitus, and small left-sided right ventricle (RV) gives origin to pulmonary trunk (PT). (Frontal projection.) **C,** Double inlet LV with ventricular D-loop and ventriculoarterial discordant connection. Atria are in situs solitus, and small right-sided RV gives origin to aorta (Ao). (Long axial view.) *Continued*

chamber, and absent or imperforate left AV valve), the situation is rapidly fatal; death usually occurs within the first few months of life. Prognosis is the same in patients with ventricular L-loop and left-sided AV valve atresia (i.e., left-sided tricuspid atresia). Even when the foramen ovale is not restrictive in early life, in this condition there is a strong tendency for it to become restrictive later in infancy or in early childhood.[S13]

Subaortic Stenosis

The tendency to develop subaortic stenosis when the aorta arises from the incomplete ventricle (outlet chamber) poses a serious threat. This category includes patients with (1) double inlet left ventricle and VA discordant connection, (2) tricuspid atresia and VA discordant connection, and (3) mitral atresia and VA concordant connection. The

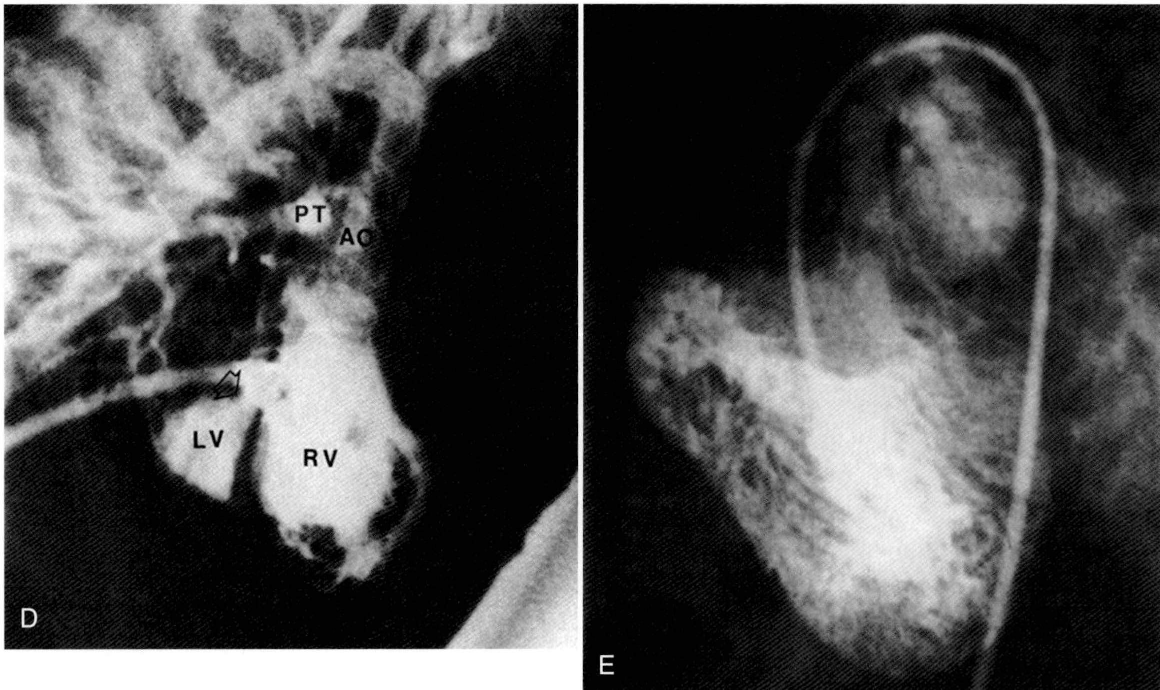

Figure 56-12, cont'd **D,** Double inlet RV with ventricular L-loop and double outlet RV. Atria are in situs solitus, and rudimentary LV lies "in the hip pocket" posteriorly *(arrow)* (elongated right anterior oblique view). Other projections demonstrated coarse trabeculations in right ventricle. **E,** Double inlet indeterminate ventricle, with double outlet and severe subpulmonary stenosis. There is an azygos extension of inferior vena cava, which accounts for catheter course. (From Soto and colleagues.[S12])

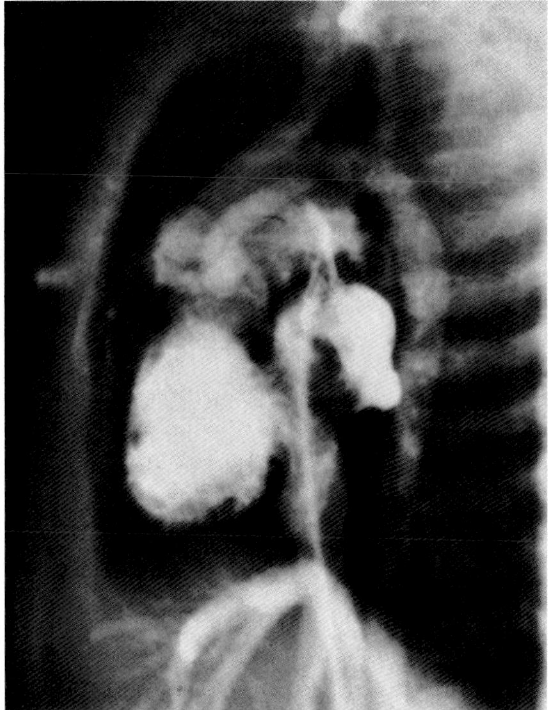

Figure 56-13 Cineangiogram in mitral (left atrioventricular valve) atresia with ventricular D-loop and double outlet right ventricle.

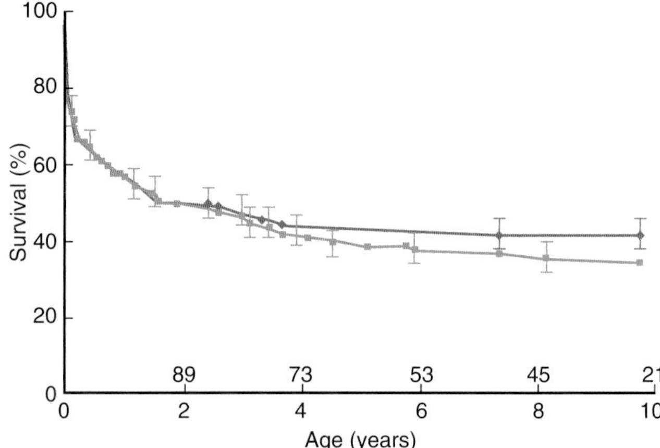

Figure 56-14 Survival without treatment of patients born with double inlet ventricle. Kaplan-Meier estimates are based on 191 patients, with vertical bars representing 70% confidence limits. Numbers represent patients still being followed. Solid line depicts overall survival, including any definitive repair (septation or Fontan operation). Dashed line represents survival before definitive repair (patients censored at time of definitive surgery; see "Competing Risks" in Section IV of Chapter 6). (From Franklin and colleagues.[F3])

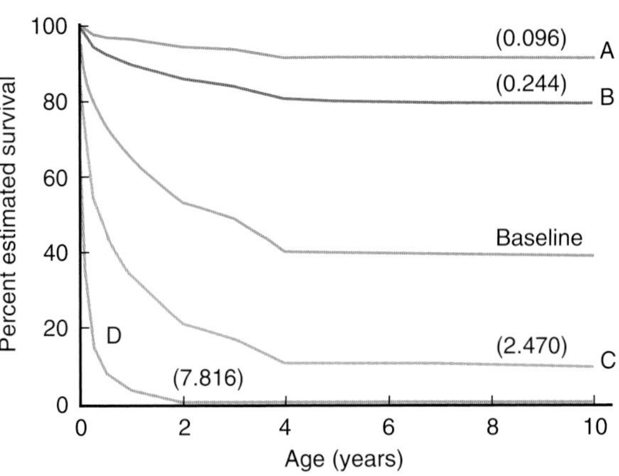

Figure 56-15 Estimated survival without definitive repair (septation or Fontan operation) of patients born with double inlet left ventricle, left-sided subaortic outlet chamber (ventricular L-loop with discordant ventriculoarterial connection) with sufficient pulmonary stenosis that pulmonary-to-systemic flow ratio $\dot{Q}p/\dot{Q}s$ was 1 to 2, presenting at 14 to 60 days of age *(line A)*, or with $\dot{Q}p/\dot{Q}s$ less than 1 *(line B)*. Line C depicts the same morphology, but with pulmonary atresia. Line D depicts patients with right atrial isomerism, double inlet and double outlet right ventricle, a common atrioventricular orifice, anomalous pulmonary venous connection, and low pulmonary blood flow, presenting at less than 14 days of age. Numbers in parentheses are calculated relative risks with respect to fictitious baseline patient *(dotted curve)* (see Fig. 56-14). (From Franklin and colleagues.[F3])

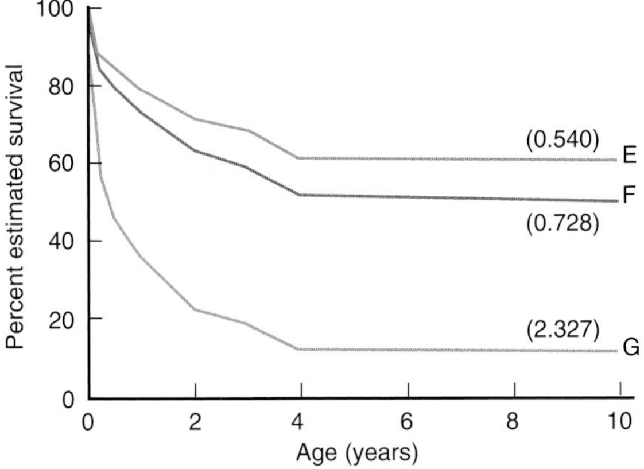

Figure 56-16 Estimated survival without definitive repair of patients with double inlet ventricle (format same as Fig. 56-15). Line E represents patients with usual atrial situs solitus, double inlet left ventricle, discordant ventriculoarterial connection, and high pulmonary blood flow, presenting between age 14 and 60 days. Line F represents same form of double inlet left ventricle but with a common atrioventricular valve. Line G represents same form of double inlet left ventricle but with systemic arterial obstruction (a form of hypoplastic left heart physiology; see under Morphology in Section I of Chapter 49) and high pulmonary blood flow. (From Franklin and colleagues.[F3])

subaortic obstruction is usually caused by a restrictive VSD; however, sometimes muscle within the incomplete subaortic ventricle is the cause, not a small VSD per se. The three morphologic variants have a similar natural history, which is discussed in detail for tricuspid atresia and VA discordant connection in Chapter 41.

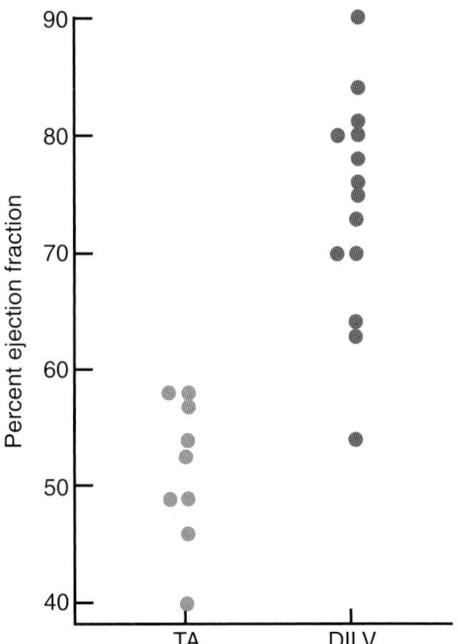

Figure 56-17 Left ventricular ejection fraction in tricuspid atresia compared with that in double inlet left ventricle. Ejection fraction is lower in tricuspid atresia. Key: *DILV,* Double inlet left ventricle; *TA,* tricuspid atresia. (From Redington and colleagues.[R3])

TECHNIQUE OF OPERATION

Fontan Operation

Patients are commonly managed clinically as "single ventricle" physiology. This approach usually results in a definitive Fontan operation, but one or more staging operations done before the Fontan procedure are usually required. These include various forms of pulmonary trunk banding (see "Pulmonary Trunk Banding" in Section I of Chapter 35 and in Section II of Chapter 41), systemic-to–pulmonary artery shunting (see "Techniques of Shunting Operations" in Section I of Chapter 38 and in Section II of Chapter 41), and superior cavopulmonary anastomosis[B7] (see Chapter 41). Timing, number, and appropriate application of these staging operations, and details of the Fontan operation itself, are described under Technique of Operation in Section IV of Chapter 41. Table 56-4 lists the palliative procedures performed in 225 patients with double inlet left ventricle prior to the Fontan operation.[E1]

Closure of Right Atrioventricular Valve

When one AV valve is regurgitant and the other is more or less normal in size and function, the regurgitant valve is closed, either before or as part of the Fontan operation. When both valves are competent and of adequate size, there has been concern that leaving both open will permit flow through each to be only half normal, and that this may encourage thrombosis in and around the valve. There is no strong support for this concern, however, and it appears reasonable at present to leave both open.

If one AV valve is closed surgically, it is usually the right-sided AV valve. Technique of closure must be secure and not produce heart block. Both criteria are met by polyester patch closure of the area occupied by the valve, sewing the patch in place with a continuous whipstitch of 4-0 polypropylene suture in a way that avoids heart block (Fig. 56-18). This can

Table 56-4 Palliative Procedures Performed before Fontan Operation in 225 Patients with Double Inlet Left Ventricle

Procedure	No.
Pulmonary artery band	92
Blalock-Taussig shunt	77
Cavopulmonary shunt	24
Subaortic resection	14
Waterson shunt	11
Central shunt	11
Atrial septectomy	11
Potts shunt	4
Coarctation of aorta repair	4
Placement of permanent pacemaker	4
Other	3
TOTAL	255

From Earing and colleagues.[E1]

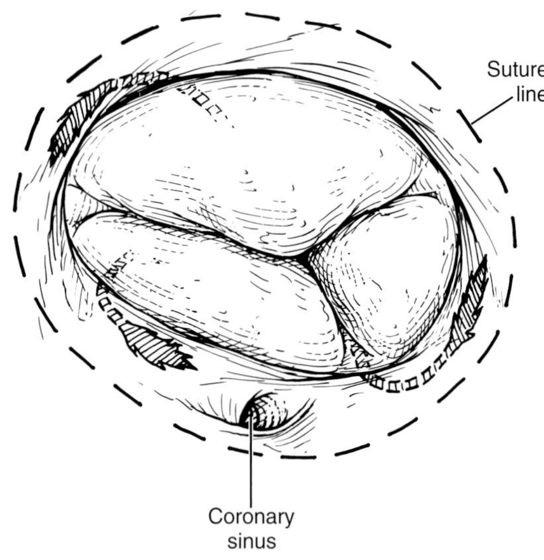

Figure 56-18 Right atrioventricular (AV) valve may be closed as part of Fontan-type repair in double inlet left ventricle. Several possible locations of AV node and proximal bundle of His are shown. Because the location in a given patient is not known precisely, suture line for patch closure of right-sided AV valve is 5 mm outside anulus all the way around.

be achieved by sewing the patch as shown in the figure, or by sewing it precisely to the valve anulus itself. Because the underlying AV valve can open and close beneath the patch, and because thrombi might form between patch and valve, a stitch is placed through the midpoint of the free edge of each leaflet and then through the center of the patch and tied on the atrial side. This is most conveniently done after placing the posterior half of the patch suture line. Simpler techniques of suturing together the free edges of the leaflets, or suturing the patch to the leaflets themselves inside the hinge line, have been associated with more dehiscences than the technique described.

Septation

The septation operation can be performed in either one or two stages. Both procedures are performed exactly the same way as described in text that follows, with the exception that in the two-stage procedure, after the main septation patch is placed, a large hole is made in the center of the patch to create a nonrestrictive VSD. A pulmonary artery band is also placed if there is absence of pulmonary stenosis. At the second stage, performed 6 to 12 months later, the created VSD is closed with a second patch sewn to the first one, and the pulmonary artery band is removed and pulmonary artery reconstructed. The two-stage procedure tends to be performed in smaller patients, particularly those with relatively small ventricular chamber size.[M4]

Although septation occasionally can be applied under appropriate circumstances to several types of double inlet left ventricular main chamber and anterior outlet chamber (and possibly a few with double inlet right ventricle), it is most commonly applied to double inlet left ventricle, ventricular L-loop, and small left-sided subaortic right ventricle. Thus, it is described for this situation. In the series of 11 patients reported by Margossian and colleagues, nine had double inlet left ventricle, one double inlet right ventricle, and one double inlet indeterminate ventricle. Of the nine patients, five had L-transposition of the great arteries, three had normally related great arteries, and one had D-transposition of the great arteries.[M4]

Preparation, draping, incision, and preliminaries to cardiopulmonary bypass (CPB) are the same as for most operations (see "Preparation for Cardiopulmonary Bypass" in Section III of Chapter 2). The aortic purse-string suture may be awkward to place and is most easily done as described for corrected transposition (see Technique of Operation in Section I of Chapter 55).

Cardiac morphology is examined, particularly to identify anomalies of pulmonary or systemic venous return or of AV valve regurgitation. The ventricular mass is frequently enlarged. Interestingly, the right atrium does not usually appear to be as large as it is in patients with isolated VSD, atrial septal defect, or tetralogy of Fallot, but this should not discourage use of the atrial approach.

The approximate size of the septation patch is determined before CPB. This is done by noting the external dimensions of the ventricular mass and subtracting estimated wall thickness.[M7] An appropriate-sized patch is cut from a polyester tube (see "Grafts for Use in Aortic Surgery" under Special Situations and Controversies in Chapter 24) or alternatively, polytetrafluoroethylene.[M4] Although the patch usually seems too small, this size is appropriate because if it is made too large, it bulges into the right ventricle with each systole and impairs cardiac function.[S4] If it is made too small, there is an increased tendency toward dehiscence.

CPB is established by the usual techniques (see "Preparation for Cardiopulmonary Bypass" in Section III of Chapter 2), using direct caval cannulation. Myocardial management is by cold cardioplegia and controlled reperfusion (see "Cold Cardioplegia, Controlled Aortic Root Reperfusion, and [When Needed] Warm Cardioplegic Induction" under Methods of Myocardial Management during Cardiac Surgery in Chapter 3) or by simple single-dose cold crystalloid cardioplegia (see "Single-Dose Cold Cardioplegia in Neonates and Infants" in Chapter 3). The patient is usually cooled to

18°C to 20°C so that periods of circulatory arrest can be used when needed to improve exposure. A small right atriotomy is made and a pump-oxygenator sump sucker passed across a natural or surgically created foramen ovale. The atriotomy is extended into the usual long oblique atriotomy, and stay sutures are applied (Fig. 56-19).

The interior of the left ventricular main chamber is examined through the right-sided AV valve. The subpulmonary area is visualized, as are the VSD, left-sided AV valve, and the relation between these structures. A determination is made whether the repair can be made through the intact right AV valve or whether a radial incision needs to be made in its base. Such an incision (see Fig. 55-15, *B* in Chapter 55) gives a direct approach to the area between the tension apparatus of the left-sided and right-sided AV valves where the sutures for septation must be placed.

A few marking sutures are placed to outline the proposed septation suture line (see Fig. 56-19, *A-B*). Goals are to (1) partition the two ventricles about equally; (2) provide unobstructed pathways from right atrium through the right-sided AV valve to pulmonary trunk, and from left atrium through the left-sided AV valve to VSD, outlet chamber (right ventricle), and aorta; and (3) avoid damage to coronary arteries by placing all sutures from within the ventricle. As McGoon and colleagues emphasized, position of the suture line is predetermined by anatomy of the tension apparatuses of the AV valves posteriorly and inferiorly and by location of semilunar valves and VSD superiorly.[M5] Therefore, only anteriorly can the surgeon select the suture siting in an attempt to partition the ventricle equally.

Pledgeted 2-0 polyester mattress sutures are placed and held individually by small hemostatic forceps. The most difficult area is the heavily trabeculated diaphragmatic surface. Suturing is begun here, if necessary invaginating the ventricular wall with a finger outside the heart as the stitches are placed. Suture placement is then carried posteriorly and superiorly between the tension apparatuses of right-sided and left-sided AV valves. Starting again at the diaphragmatic surface, suture placement is carried to the left and anteriorly and then superiorly along the anterior left ventricular wall along the previously determined line. The suture line passes over the VSD and then swings posteriorly and to the right beneath the subpulmonary area (see Fig. 56-19, *A-B*). Sutures must be placed close together; 20 to 30 sutures are usually required. As they are individually clamped and set aside, care is taken to maintain their proper order. Alternatively, a running suture can be used.[M4]

Size and shape of the previously trimmed patch are inspected and altered if needed. Sutures are passed through the patch, the patch slid into position, and the sutures tied. If a two-stage approach is used, the hole in the patch is made at this time (Fig. 56-20). If the right-sided AV valve has been incised, it is repaired with continuous 6-0 polypropylene sutures (see Fig. 55-15 in Chapter 55).

Cardiac reperfusion is begun, and remainder of procedure is completed as described previously (see "Completing Cardiopulmonary Bypass" in Section III of Chapter 2). A groove or indentation can usually now be seen in the ventricular wall along part of the suture line. Two temporary right atrial and two temporary ventricular epicardial wires are placed, and AV sequential pacing is begun. Usual de-airing procedures are carried out (see "De-airing the Heart" in Section III of Chapter 2).

After hemostasis has been secured, two permanent pacing electrodes are placed on the right atrium and two on the ventricle. Their ends are brought subcutaneously into the right upper quadrant, and in most patients an appropriate pacemaker is inserted a day or two later (see "Permanent Pacing after Intracardiac Surgery" under Technique of Intervention in Section I of Chapter 16).

Cardiac Transplantation

Cardiac transplantation can usually be accomplished, no matter how complex the coexisting venous and arterial anomalies (see Technique of Operation in Chapter 21).[M2]

Procedures for Subaortic Obstruction

Operations designed to address subaortic stenosis are detailed in Chapter 41. Arguments have been developed both in favor of routinely addressing real or potential subaortic stenosis using the DKS anastomosis, Norwood procedure, or rarely the arterial switch in the neonatal period, and in favor of selective use of neonatal pulmonary artery banding with early follow-up and surgical management of subaortic stenosis, if and when it develops.[H3,I1,J1,J2,K1,S6,T2,W2]

If subaortic stenosis is to be surgically approached by direct VSD enlargement, an incision is made in the free wall of the incomplete ventricular chamber. This exposes the VSD, aortic valve, and internal dimensions of the incomplete ventricle. From this perspective, the conduction pathway is always posterior and inferior in relation to the VSD (Fig. 56-21), regardless of whether the heart is L-looped or D-looped. Based on this relationship, the VSD is enlarged as depicted in Figs. 56-22 to 56-24. The ventriculotomy is always closed with a patch (see Fig. 56-24).

SPECIAL FEATURES OF POSTOPERATIVE CARE

Fontan Operation

Care after a Fontan-type procedure is discussed under Special Features of Postoperative Care in Section IV of Chapter 41.

Septation Operation

Usual protocols are followed postoperatively (see Chapter 5). Following septation, right atrial pressure is usually a few mmHg higher than left and should be maintained around 12 to 14 mmHg in the early hours after operation.

Other Operations

Special features of postoperative care after pulmonary trunk banding, atrial septectomy, shunting operations, and operations for subaortic stenosis are described in Chapter 41.

RESULTS

Fontan Operation

Results of the Fontan operation are discussed in detail under Results in Section IV of Chapter 41. Note, however, that several studies have examined the effect of ventricular hypertrophy on outcome following the Fontan operation. In those

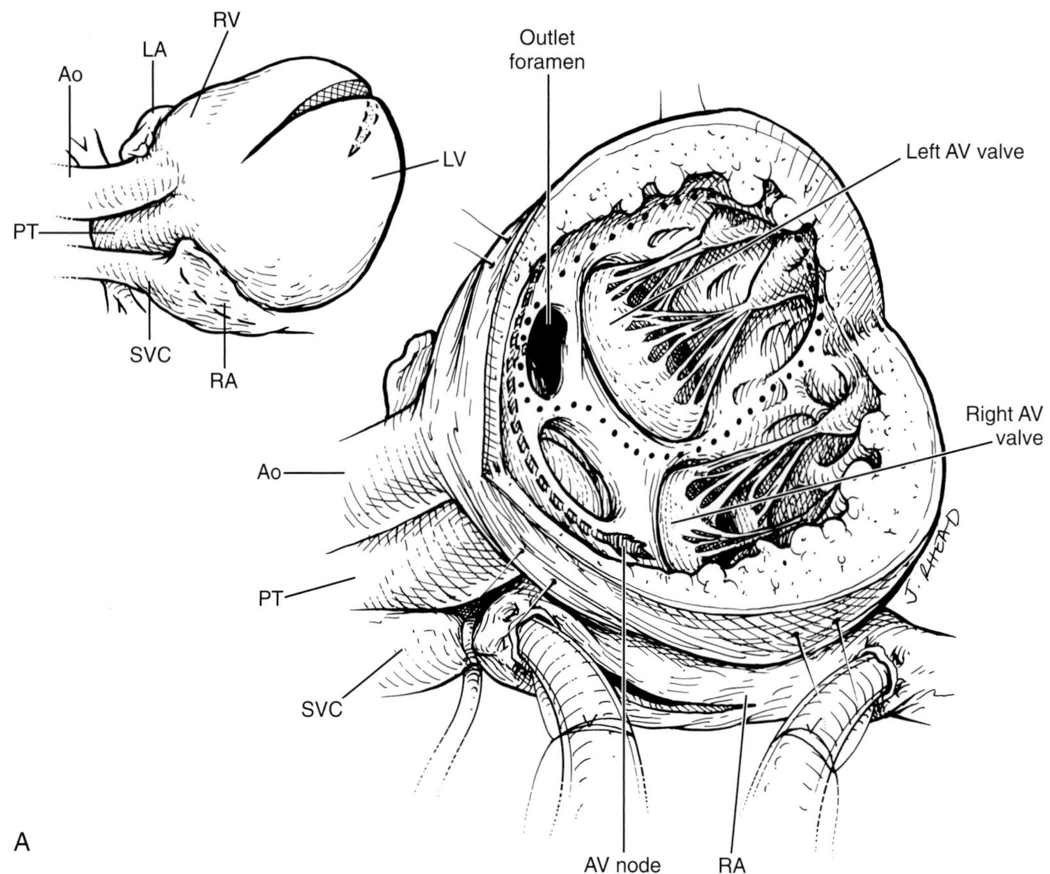

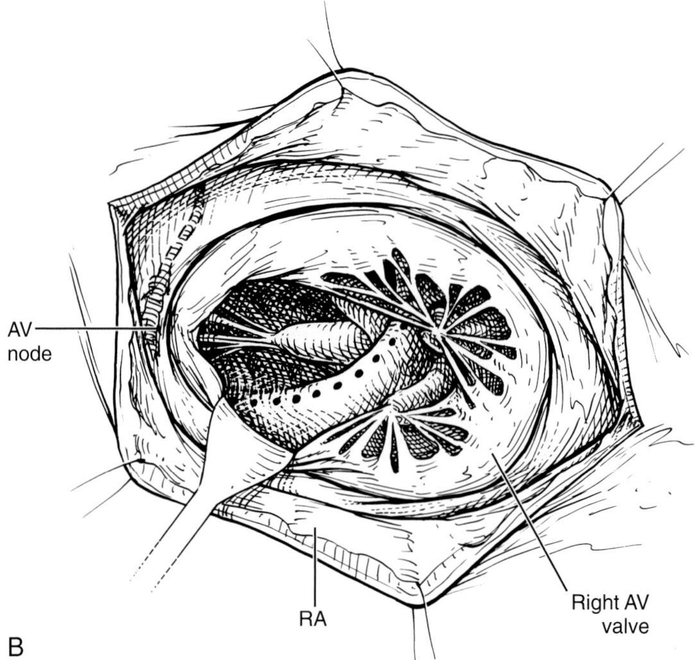

Figure 56-19 Septation operation for double inlet left ventricle and left-sided, small subaortic right ventricle in a patient with atrial situs solitus. **A,** Septation operation is performed through a right atrial approach, but it is best illustrated through the alternative fishmouth incision in the ventricular main chamber. Positions of atrioventricular (AV) node and bundle of His are shown by dashed lines. Note that AV node is anterior, in the right atrial wall at the junction of right atrial roof and atrial septum. The bundle of His penetrates the junction of right AV valve and pulmonary valve to pass over subpulmonary area along anterior left ventricular free wall. **B,** As viewed through right atrium, as it passes along the interventricular septum, it courses anterior to ventricular septal defect (VSD) (or outlet foramen), as seen from this perspective, and divides into left and right bundle branches (see Figs. 56-20 to 56-23 to appreciate the posterior relationship of conduction system to the VSD when viewed from the perspective of an incision in the free wall of the incomplete ventricle). Septation operation usually results in heart block when performed in one stage. Dots indicate suture placement for inserting septation patch. Key: *Ao,* Aorta; *AV,* atrioventricular; *LA,* left atrium; *LV,* right-sided morphologic left ventricle; *PT,* pulmonary trunk; *RA,* right atrium; *RV,* left-sided morphologic right ventricle; *SVC,* superior vena cava.

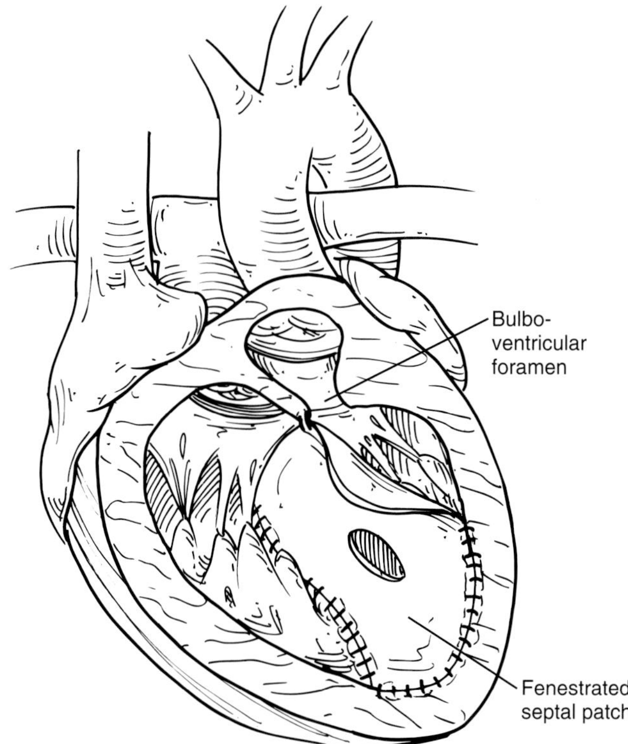

Figure 56-20 Illustration of septation patch fenestration in two-stage repair of double inlet left ventricle with left-sided small sub-aortic right ventricle in situs solitus. Hole in septation patch (created "VSD," fenestration) is placed in a convenient spot in middle of patch for easy access at second-stage procedure. It must be made large enough to create a nonrestrictive communication. (Modified from Margossian and colleagues.[M4])

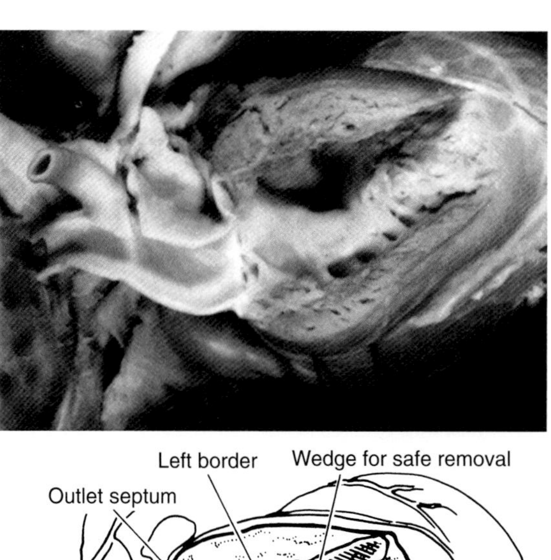

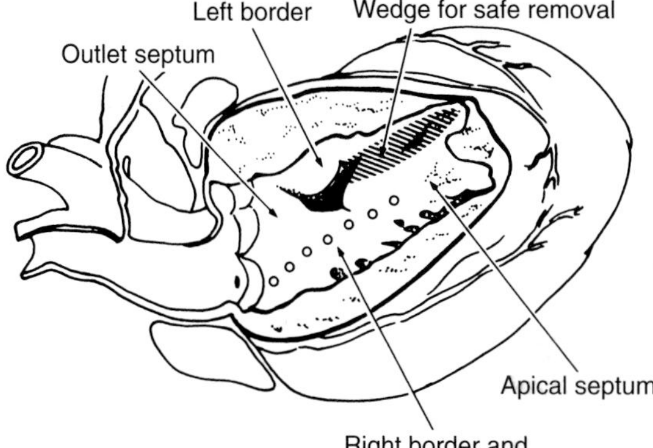

Figure 56-22 Direct relief of subaortic stenosis in double inlet left ventricle with left-sided subaortic incomplete right ventricle. A portion of apical ventricular septum is removed by wedge resection, as illustrated in upper panel. Lower panel shows resection to be clear of conduction tissue (pathway depicted by line of small circles). (From Cheung and colleagues.[C2])

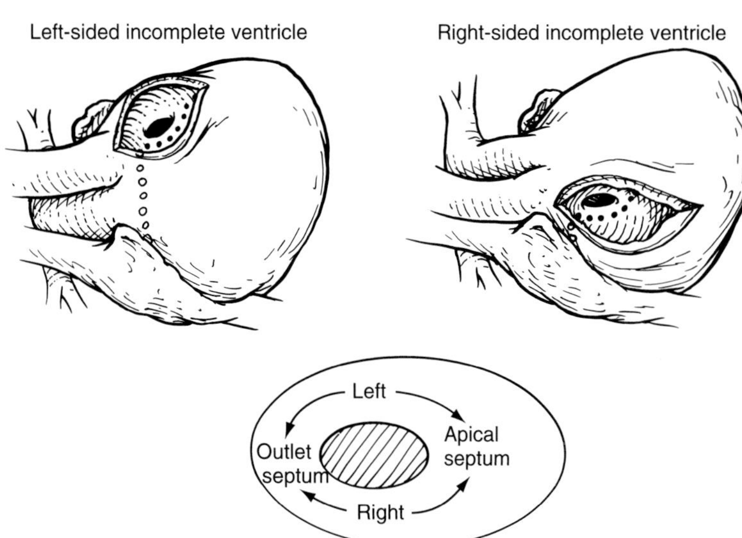

Figure 56-21 Relationship of course of conduction system to ventricular septal defect in hearts with double inlet left ventricle, as viewed from the incomplete (rudimentary) ventricle, which is the same whether the incomplete subaortic ventricle is left sided (left depiction) or right sided (right depiction). Line of tiny circles illustrates course of conduction system. (Modified from Cheung and colleagues.[C2])

studies, the populations were either predominantly or exclusively patients with double inlet left ventricle with subaortic obstruction. Ventricular hypertrophy was shown to be a risk factor for death and poor outcome at and following the Fontan operation, and attempted relief of subaortic stenosis at the time of, or anytime following, the Fontan operation was attended by an increased risk of death at the time of the procedure.[A1,C4,R8]

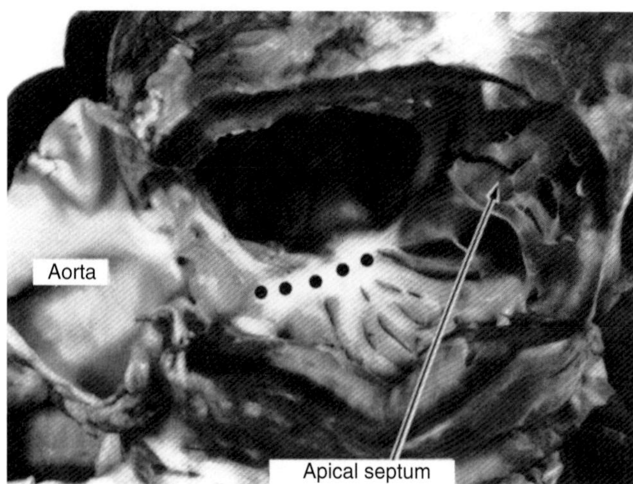

Figure 56-23 Autopsy specimen, viewed after opening incomplete right ventricle and aorta, from a patient who died after enlarging ventricular septal defect as described in Fig. 56-22. Sinus rhythm had been present throughout the postoperative period. A large opening has been created that is clear of conduction tissue, the path of which is demonstrated by black dots. (From Cheung and colleagues.[C2])

Septation Operation

Early (Hospital) Death

In a 1984 report, overall hospital mortality after septation operation was high, about 30% to 40%[S14] (Table 56-5). However, among patients with moderate enlargement of the left ventricular main chamber without concomitant AV valve replacement or an extracardiac conduit, hospital mortality has been about 5%, but confidence limits are wide (Table 56-6 and Fig. 56-25). In a more recent report (1997), overall hospital mortality was less than 10%.[N1] In the series by Margossian and colleagues, 2 of 11 (18%; CL 6.3%-38%) patients died. One death occurred in a two-stage repair that included an arterial switch, and the other in a one-stage repair. This improvement may reflect general progress in the field but may also be influenced by patient selection.

Time-Related Survival

So few patients have survived the early postoperative period after septation operation that estimates of long-term survival have wide CLs, but intermediate survival is reported to be about 60% when all deaths, including those in hospital, are accounted for (see Fig. 56-25).[M7] Remarkably, the single slowly declining hazard function is low after about 5 years. In a more recent study of a 23-patient experience, midterm follow-up (3-11 years) showed an overall survival of 78%.[N1] In the 11-patient series of Margossian and colleagues, there was one late death with median follow-up of 2.3 years, with survival documented up to 8 years.[M4] There are two single-patient case reports of survival of 9 and 12.5 years.[N2,O3]

Modes of Death

Hospital deaths have usually been in acute heart failure, and late deaths sudden or after reoperation (usually for AV valve replacement).[M7]

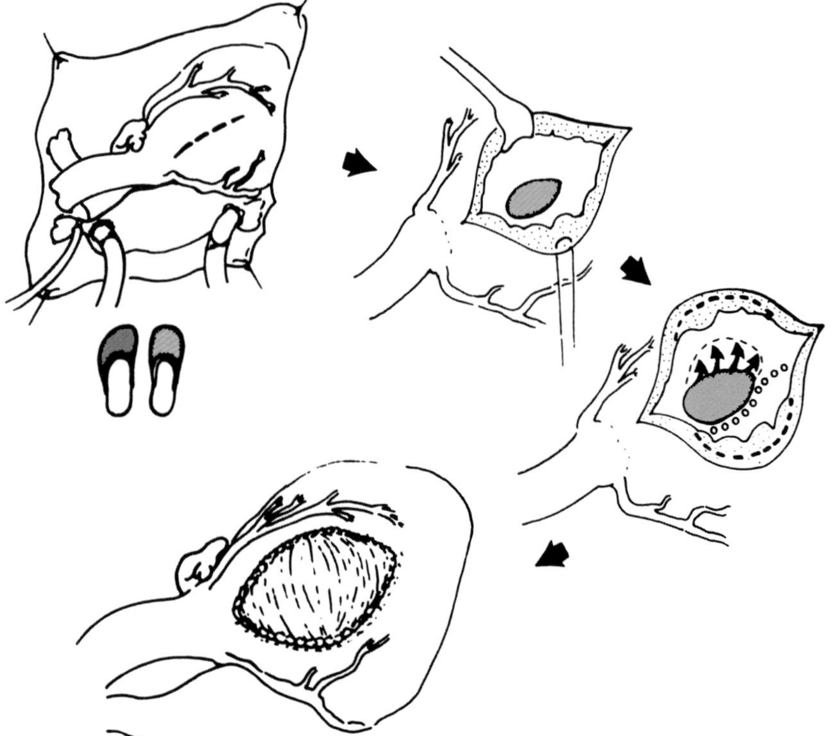

Figure 56-24 Sketches of operative procedure for enlarging ventricular septal defect as described in Figs 56-21 and 56-22. Note enlarging patch that has been used to close ventriculotomy. (From Cheung and colleagues.[C2])

Table 56-5 Hospital Mortality after Septation Operation for Double Inlet Ventricle

Morphology[a]	n	Hospital Deaths No.	%	CL
Ventricular L-loop, two ventricles with dominant and double inlet LV and rudimentary and leftward RV, discordant VA connection, L-malposition of aorta	28	10	36	25-47
Solitary ventricle[b]	5	2	40	14-71
Ventricular L-loop, two ventricles with dominant and double inlet and double outlet RV, superior-inferior ventricles, D-malposition of aorta[c]	1	1	100	15-100
Ventricular D-loop, two ventricles with dominant and double inlet LV, concordant VA connection, more or less normally positioned great arteries	1	0	0	0-85
Ventricular D-loop, two ventricles with dominant and double inlet and double outlet LV, more or less normally positioned great arteries[d]	1	0	0	0-85
TOTAL	36	13	36	27-46

Data from Stefanelli and colleagues.[S14]
[a]No patients with atrial situs inversus had septation; cases are with or without pulmonary stenoses.
[b]One patient, who lived after operation in 1983, had ventricular L-loop, essentially AV and VA discordant connections with essentially two ventricles, an absent septum, right-sided LV morphology, and left-sided RV morphology; another patient, who also lived after operation in 1983, had ventricular D-loop, essentially AV and VA concordant connections with essentially two ventricles, an absent septum, right-sided RV morphology, and left-sided LV morphology (common ventricle); the other three patients had an indeterminate, primitive ventricle.
[c]Severely overriding right-sided left ventricular AV valve.
[d]Severely overriding right-sided ventricular AV valve with right ventricular hypoplasia.
Key: *AV,* Atrioventricular; *CL,* 70% confidence limits; *LV,* left ventricle; *RV,* right ventricle; *VA,* ventriculoarterial.

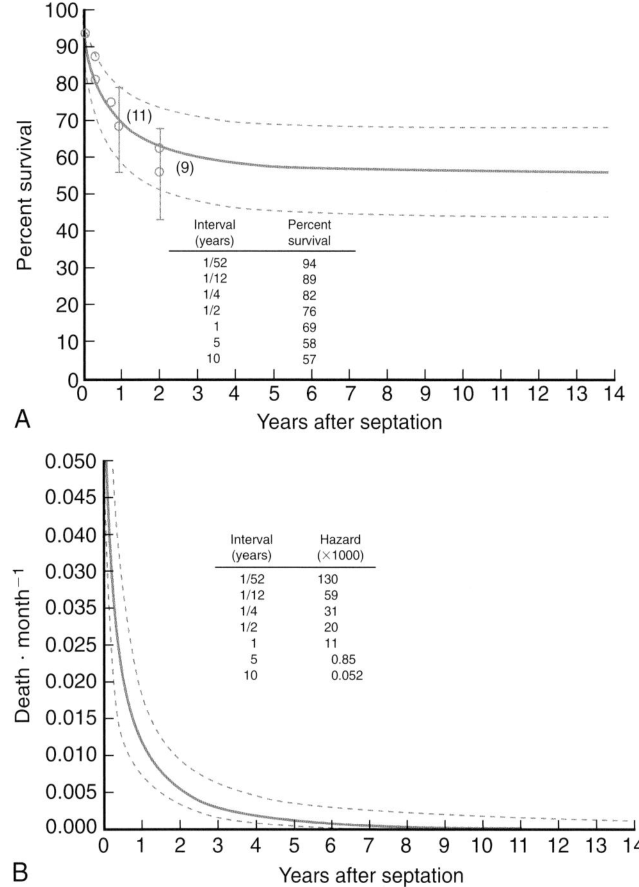

Figure 56-25 Survival after septation operation for double inlet ventricle without atrioventricular valve replacement and without valved extracardiac conduit, in patients with main chamber enlargement greater than grade II (patients are described in Table 56-6). Open circles represent deaths and vertical bars 70% confidence limits (CLs). Solid line represents parametrically estimated survival, and dashed lines enclose 70% CLs. Values in the table are from parametrically determined survival. Numbers in parentheses indicate number of patients available for further follow-up at the interval shown. **A,** Survival. **B,** Hazard function. There is only a single slowly declining hazard phase, which reaches a low level 5 years after septation. (Data, except for subsequently updated follow-up, from McKay and colleagues.[M7])

Table 56-6 Hospital Mortality and Age Distribution in Septation for Single Ventricle[a]

≤	Age Years <	n	No. of Hospital Deaths
	2	16	1
2	4	1	0
4	8	4	0
8	16	7	0
16		3	0
TOTAL		16	1 (6%; CL 0.8%-20%)

Data from McKay and colleagues.[M7]
[a]Data from patients with main chamber enlarged grade 3 or more without concomitant atrioventricular valve replacement or use of a valved extracardiac conduit.
Key: *CL,* 70% confidence limits.

Incremental Risk Factors for Death

Within the group that currently is considered for septation (double inlet left ventricle, ventricular L-loop, left-sided incomplete right ventricle with VA discordant connection, atrial situs solitus), no risk factors have been identified. However, unusual forms of double inlet ventricle, a small ventricular main chamber, concomitant AV valve replacement, and placement of a valved extracardiac conduit have been risk factors.[M7] Aside from morphologic factors, increasing age and ventricular hypertrophy have been identified as risk factors.[N1]

Functional Status

Functional status is generally good after septation. This might be expected from the experimental study by Seki, Tsakiris, and McGoon, which showed no demonstrable detrimental hemodynamic effect of replacing the dog's ventricular septum (and tricuspid valve) with a prosthesis.[S5] It is also supported by detailed hemodynamic study of two patients late after septation by Shimazaki and colleagues.[S8] In one patient 8 years post-septation, both right and left ventricular ejection fractions were normal, as was hemodynamic response to exercise. Kurosawa and colleagues found cardiac indices to be higher after septation than after a Fontan operation.[K8]

However, late after a septation or Fontan operation, cardiorespiratory function by objective measurements at rest and during exercise is depressed compared with normal.[D3] Evidence is contradictory as to whether septation provides better cardiorespiratory function than the Fontan operation. In one study, objectively measured postoperative exercise tolerance, compared with that preoperatively, was more improved after the Fontan operation than after septation,[D3] but in a later study, superior cardiorespiratory function was found after septation.[O1] In a more recent study of double inlet left ventricle patients comparing Fontan or septation, septation patients with native AV valves demonstrated superior cardiopulmonary response to exercise compared with either Fontan patients or septation patients with prosthetic AV valves.[O2]

Heart Block

Complete heart block is not inevitable after septation. It occurred after most septation operations in one series from 1982.[M7] However, in a series from 2002, only 1 of 11 patients (9.1%; CL 1.5%-28%) developed it.[M4] The difference may be that a running suture technique was used in the series with a low occurrence of heart block, rather than interrupted pledgeted mattress sutures that penetrate deeper into the myocardium.

Cardiac Transplantation

Results of cardiac transplantation are discussed in detail under Results in Section II of Chapter 21.

Other Operations

Results for systemic–pulmonary artery shunts, pulmonary trunk banding, operations to relieve systemic outflow obstruction, coarctation repair, atrial septectomy, bidirectional superior cavopulmonary anastomosis, and hemi-Fontan are reported in Chapter 41.

Outcome Related to Specific Morphology

In a multicenter analysis of 150 patients with double inlet left ventricle who were younger than 3 months of age at diagnosis, overall survival was 88% at 1 month and 76% at 10 years. By multivariable analysis, the only risk factor for premature death was a neonatal operation of any kind.[T3]

Outcome for the Fontan in double inlet left ventricle patients is excellent, with a 3% early mortality in patients operated on after 1989, and 20-year actuarial survival of about 70% in one large series.[E4]

Pass and colleagues reported a series of bulboventricular foramen (VSD) enlargement for systemic outflow obstruction in eight patients, five with S,L,L double inlet left ventricle and three with left AV valve atresia. Patients ranged in age from 2 months to 27 years. There was one early and one late death. Gradient relief was complete initially in seven, with one persistent gradient. Two patients developed recurrent obstruction following initial complete relief. All three patients with recurrent or persistent gradients underwent reoperation with relief of the gradient. At mean follow-up of 22 months, all patients were unobstructed. One patient in the series developed new-onset heart block; there was no new-onset aortic regurgitation.[P3]

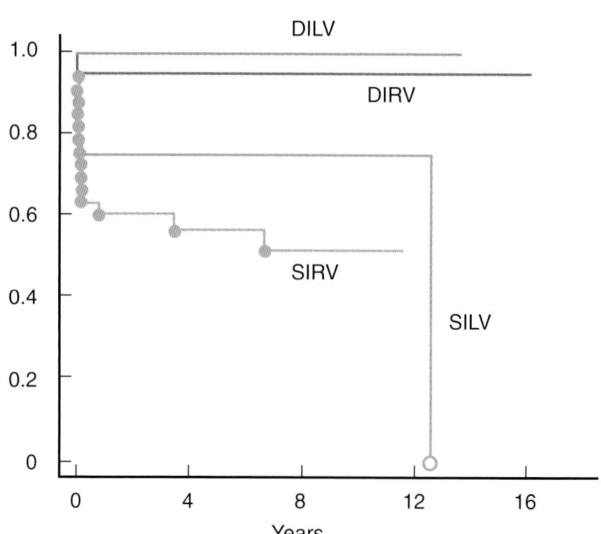

Figure 56-26 Survival after Fontan procedure for various double and single inlet ventricle patients. Survival at 10 years was 95% for patients with double inlet right ventricle (DIRV), 100% for those with double inlet left ventricle (DILV), 75% for those with single inlet left ventricle (SILV), and 51% for those with single inlet right ventricle (SIRV) (*P*[log-rank] = .002). (Modified from Kawahira and colleagues.[K2])

Clarke and colleagues reported a 4% early mortality for interval DKS operation in a series of 15 S,L,L double inlet left ventricle patients initially managed as neonates with pulmonary artery banding and arch reconstruction.[C3] These excellent results are more expected in a favorable population of patients that did not have severe neonatal obstruction of the bulboventricular foramen. In contrast, Lan and colleagues noted a higher mortality when the DKS operation was performed in neonates, as did Lotto and colleagues for the Norwood operation in neonates.[L1,L5]

Kawahira and colleagues reported on a series of 31 double inlet right ventricle patients. Compared with patients having double inlet left ventricle and common inlet ventricle, the prevalence of pulmonary atresia and discontinuous pulmonary arteries was higher in double inlet right ventricle, resulting in more frequent systemic-to–pulmonary artery shunt procedures in this subgroup. Overall outcomes for double inlet right ventricle were similar to those for double inlet left ventricle, however, and were superior to outcomes for common inlet ventricle[K2] (Fig. 56-26).

INDICATIONS FOR OPERATION

Primary considerations in managing patients with double inlet ventricle of any type are first and foremost assessment of, and correction of, important neonatal and infant hemodynamic abnormalities, using the palliative operations described in this chapter. Thereafter, considerations become (1) patients' suitability for septation, Fontan operation, or cardiac transplantation and (2) preventing additional

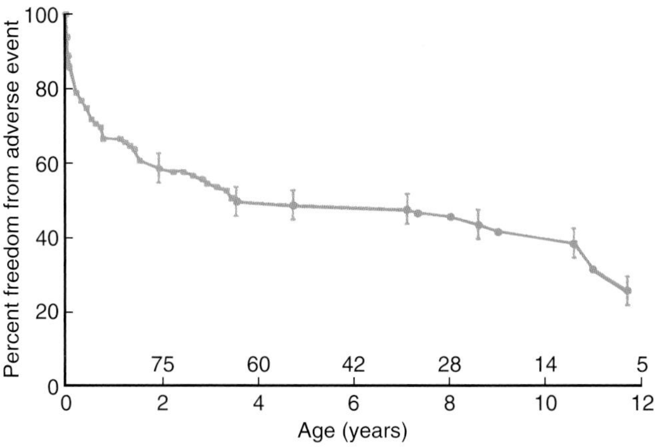

Figure 56-27 Freedom from death or adverse events in patients judged at diagnosis to be suitable for a Fontan operation. This is essentially time-related suitability for Fontan operation. Patients were censored at time of definitive procedure. Depiction is as in Fig. 56-14. (From Franklin and colleagues.[F4])

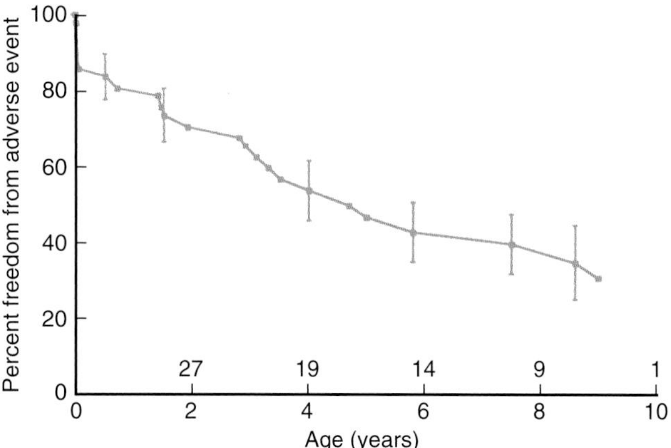

Figure 56-28 Freedom from death or other adverse events in patients judged at diagnosis to be suitable for septation operation. This is essentially time-related suitability for septation operation. Patients were censored as alive at time of definitive procedure. Depiction is as in Fig. 56-14. (From Franklin and colleagues.[F4])

complicating conditions such as subaortic stenosis or pulmonary arterial stenoses.

Fontan Operation

All patients suitable for septation are suitable for a Fontan operation (except those with elevated pulmonary vascular resistance). Some 70% to 80% of patients with various types of double inlet ventricle or atretic AV valve appear at birth to be suitable at a later date,[F4] but nearly 50% of those become unsuitable by about age 2 years (Fig. 56-27). Thus, when in early life a Fontan operation is considered feasible and advisable, an appropriate staged surgical management approach as outlined in Chapter 41 is planned.

Septation Operation

In the past, a septation operation was considered the most desirable of the three if intracardiac morphology was suitable. However, outcomes following the Fontan operation have improved markedly; currently, Fontan operation is generally considered the procedure of choice, possibly even in many cases with suitable morphology for septation.

Apparently, 20% to 25% of patients born with double inlet ventricle are suitable at birth for septation.[F4] By 2 years of age, 30% of those with the malformation are either dead or no longer suitable for septation, and this proportion increases as time passes (Fig. 56-28). A common reason for *developed* lack of suitability is subaortic stenosis.[F4]

To be suitable for septation, the patient must have a somewhat, but not severely, enlarged dominant ventricle (Fig. 56-29) into which enter two reasonably competent and nonstenotic AV valves with little or no overriding or straddling.[F4,M7,P1,S14] Success with a single common AV valve has been reported.[K8] The VA connection must be concordant with the AV valve connections projected for the septated ventricle. There should be little or no pulmonary or systemic outflow obstruction.

Because of the age-related declining proportion of patients suitable for septation, resulting from the adverse effect of increasing hypertrophy of the dominant (main) chamber, and

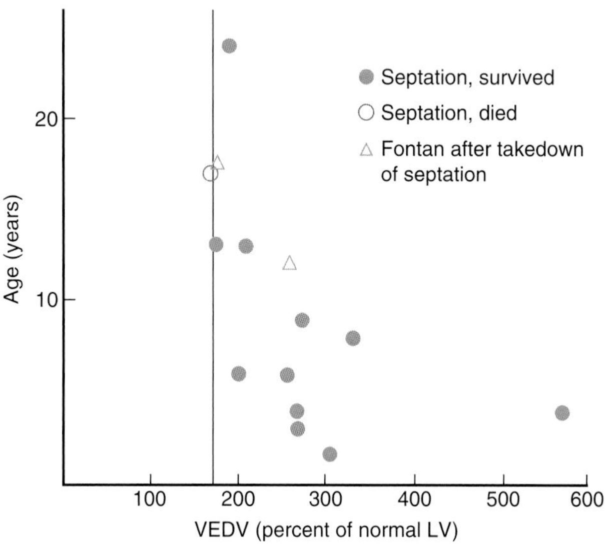

Figure 56-29 End-diastolic ventricular volume before septation was performed for double or single inlet left ventricle and age. Vertical line represents 170% normal left ventricular volume. Note that larger volumes are associated with younger age. Key: *LV,* Left ventricle; *VEDV,* ventricular end-diastolic volume. (From Kurosawa and colleagues.[K8])

the strong tendency for development of pulmonary vascular disease unless there is natural or produced (by banding) pulmonary stenosis, septation should be performed during the first year or two of life. Consideration should be given to a two-stage approach to minimize the probability of producing complete heart block (see "Staged Septation" under Special Situations and Controversies).

Cardiac Transplantation

At birth, 25% to 30% of patients are already unsuitable for either septation or a Fontan operation.[F3] Only about 30% survive the first year of life (Fig. 56-30). The place of cardiac transplantation is arguable for this group of patients, but if

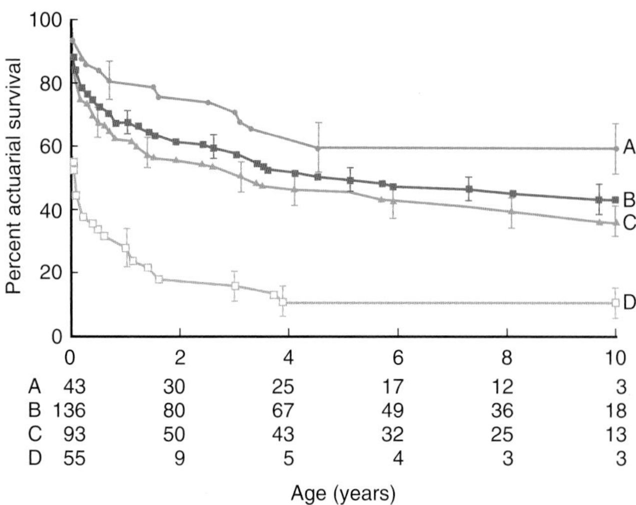

Figure 56-30 Survival according to suitability at diagnosis for *(line A)* patients suitable for septation operation (or a Fontan operation); *(line B)* all patients suitable for a Fontan operation; *(line C)* patients suitable only for a Fontan operation and not for septation operation; *(line D)* patients suitable for neither. Depiction is as in Fig. 56-14. (From Franklin and colleagues.[F4])

anything is to be done for them, transplantation would appear to be appropriate. It should be performed in the first month if possible (see "Indications for Cardiac Transplantation" in Section II of Chapter 21).

Therapeutic Plan in Older Patients

Some patients come for decision making and therapy after infancy, frequently after various palliative procedures. Each case represents a special situation, but some guidelines can be followed.

Unless pulmonary trunk banding has been performed, septation is often contraindicated because of pulmonary vascular disease, severe ventricular hypertrophy, or AV valve regurgitation. Fontan operation is possible when AV valve regurgitation has developed in one of two valves, but at Fontan operation, or as a separate preliminary operation, the valve needs to be perfectly repaired or closed (see "Closure of the Right Atrioventricular Valve" under Technique of Operation earlier in this chapter).[M8]

If pulmonary trunk banding was performed in early life, probability of subaortic stenosis is considerable. It should be suspected, even if no gradient is demonstrable, if the VSD is small or only moderate sized. If subaortic stenosis is severe, consideration should be given to treating this before undertaking the Fontan operation[N4] In this setting, direct enlargement of the VSD is a better option than in neonates, but the DKS anastomosis or arterial switch operation can still be considered.

SPECIAL SITUATIONS AND CONTROVERSIES

Staged Septation

Ebert reported a two-stage approach to septation in a subset of patients.[E2] At the first stage, performed in infancy, a partially septating patch was placed at the apex of the ventricle and a second superiorly between the AV valves, using widely spaced interrupted sutures. A pulmonary trunk band was placed. Septation was completed with a third patch 6 to 18 months later. The other patches were by then completely sealed into position. The band was removed. All patients survived, and all were in sinus rhythm. Margossian and colleagues have also reported success with this approach,[M4] as have McKay and colleagues.[M6]

REFERENCES

A

1. Akagi T, Benson LN, Williams WG, Freedom RM. The relation between ventricular hypertrophy and clinical outcome in patients with double inlet left ventricle after atrial to pulmonary anastomosis. Herz 1992;17:220.
2. Anderson RH. Weasel words in paediatric cardiology. Int J Cardiol 1983;2:425.
3. Anderson RH, Arnold R, Thapar MK, Jones RS, Hamilton DI. Cardiac specialized tissue in hearts with an apparently single ventricular chamber (double inlet left ventricle). Am J Cardiol 1974; 33:95.
4. Anderson RH, Becker AE. Historical review. In Anderson RH, Crupi G, Parenzan L, eds. Double inlet ventricle. 2nd Ed. New York: Elsevier, 1987, p. 29.
5. Anderson RH, Becker AE, Macartney FJ, Shinebourne EA, Wilkinson EA, Tynan MJ. Is tricuspid atresia a univentricular heart? Pediatr Cardiol 1979;1:51.
6. Anderson RH, Lenox CC, Zuberbuhler JR, Ho SY, Smith A, Wilkinson JL. Double-inlet left ventricle with rudimentary right ventricle and ventriculoarterial concordance. Am J Cardiol 1983; 52:573.
7. Anderson RH, Macartney FJ, Tynan M, Becker AE, Freedom RM, Godman MJ, et al. Univentricular atrioventricular connection: single ventricle trap unsprung. Pediatr Cardiol 1983;4:273.
8. Anderson RH, Tynan M, Freedom RM, Quero-Jimenez M, Macartney FJ, Shinebourne EA, et al. Ventricular morphology in the univentricular heart. Herz 1979;4:184.
9. Anderson RH, Wilkinson JL, Gerlis LM, Smith A, Becker AE. Atresia of the right atrioventricular orifice. Br Heart J 1977; 39:414.
10. Arai T, Sakakibara S, Ando M, Takao A. Intracardiac repair for single or common ventricle, creation of a straight artificial septum. Singapore Med J 1973;14:187.
11. Atik E, Ikari NM, Aiello VD, Albuquerque AM, Iwahashi ER, Ebaid M, et al. Atresia of the left atrioventricular valve with patency of the aorta: anatomico-functional analysis of 23 patients. Int J Cardiol 1991;32:281.

B

1. Beardshaw JA, Gibson DG, Pearson MC, Upton MT, Anderson RH. Echocardiographic diagnosis of primitive ventricle with two atrioventricular valves. Br Heart J 1977;39:266.
2. Becker AE, Wilkinson JL, Anderson RH. Atrioventricular conduction tissues in univentricular hearts of left ventricular type. Herz 1979;4:166.
3. Bevilacqua M, Sanders SP, Van Praagh S, Colan SD, Parness I. Double-inlet single left ventricle: echocardiographic anatomy with emphasis on the morphology of the atrioventricular valves and ventricular septal defect. J Am Coll Cardiol 1991;18:559.
4. Bharati S, Lev M. The course of the conduction system in single ventricle with inverted (L-) loop and inverted (L-) transposition. Circulation 1975;51:723.
5. Bharati S, Lev M, Kirklin JW. Cardiac surgery and the conduction system. 2nd Ed. Mount Kisco, N.Y.: Futura, 1992.
6. Blalock A, Taussig HB. The surgical treatment of malformations of the heart in which there is pulmonary stenosis or pulmonary atresia. JAMA 1945;128:189.
7. Bridges ND, Jonas RA, Mayer JE, Flanagan MF, Keane JF, Castaneda AR. Bidirectional cavopulmonary anastomosis as interim palliation for high-risk Fontan candidates. Early results. Circulation 1990;82:IV170.

C

1. Chesler E, Joffe HS, Beck W, Schrire V. Echocardiography in the diagnosis of congenital heart disease. Pediatr Clin North Am 1971;18:1163.
2. Cheung HC, Lincoln C, Anderson RH, Ho SY, Shinebourne EA, Pallides S, et al. Options for surgical repair in hearts with univentricular atrioventricular connection and subaortic stenosis. J Thorac Cardiovasc Surg 1990;100:672.
3. Clarke AJ, Kasahara S, Andrews DR, Cooper SG, Nicholson IA, Chard RB, et al. Mid-term results for double inlet left ventricle and similar morphologies: timing of Damus-Kaye-Stansel. Ann Thorac Surg 2004;78:650-7; discussion 7.
4. Cohen AJ, Cleveland DC, Dyck J, Poppe D, Smallhorn J, Freedom RM, et al. Results of the Fontan procedure for patients with univentricular heart. Ann Thorac Surg 1991;52:1266.

D

1. Doherty A, Ho SY, Anderson RH, Rigby ML. Morphological nature of the atrioventricular valves in hearts with double inlet left ventricle. Pediatr Pathol 1989;9:521.
2. Doty DB, Schieken RM, Lauer RM. Septation of the univentricular heart: transatrial approach. J Thorac Cardiovasc Surg 1979;78:423.
3. Driscoll DJ, Feldt RH, Mottram CD, Puga FJ, Schaff HV, Danielson GK. Cardiorespiratory response to exercise after definitive repair of univentricular atrioventricular connection. Int J Cardiol 1987;17:73.

E

1. Earing MG, Cetta F, Driscoll DJ, Mair DD, Hodge DO, Dearani JA, et al. Long-term results of the Fontan operation for double-inlet left ventricle. Am J Cardiol 2005;96:291-8.
2. Ebert PA. Staged partitioning of single ventricle. J Thorac Cardiovasc Surg 1984;88:908.
3. Edie RN, Ellis K, Gersony WM, Krongrad E, Bowman FO Jr, Malm JR. Surgical repair of single ventricle. J Thorac Cardiovasc Surg 1973;66:350.
4. Elliott LP, Anderson RC, Edwards JE. The common cardiac ventricle with transposition of the great vessels. Br Heart J 1964;26:289.
5. Essed CE, Ho SY, Hunter S, Anderson RH. Atrioventricular conduction system in univentricular heart of right ventricular type with right-sided rudimentary chamber. Thorax 1980;35:123.
6. Essed CE, Ho SY, Shinebourne EA, Joseph MC, Anderson RH. Further observations on conduction tissues in univentricular hearts—surgical implications. Eur Heart J 1981;2:87.

F

1. Felner JM, Brewer DB, Franch RH. Echocardiographic manifestations of single ventricle. Am J Cardiol 1976;38:80.
2. Fontan F, Baudet E. Surgical repair of tricuspid atresia. Thorax 1971;26:240.
3. Franklin RC, Spiegelhalter DJ, Anderson RH, Macartney FJ, Rossi Filho RI, Douglas JM, et al. Double-inlet ventricle presenting in infancy. I. Survival without definitive repair. J Thorac Cardiovasc Surg 1991;101:767.
4. Franklin RC, Spiegelhalter DJ, Rossi Filho RI, Macartney FJ, Anderson RH, Rigby ML, et al. Double-inlet ventricle presenting in infancy. III. Outcome and potential for definitive repair. J Thorac Cardiovasc Surg 1991;101:924.
5. Freedom RM, Williams WG, Fowler RS, Trusler GA, Rowe RD. Tricuspid atresia, transposition of the great arteries, and banded pulmonary artery. Repair by arterial switch, coronary artery reimplantation, and right atrioventricular valved conduit. J Thorac Cardiovasc Surg 1980;80:621.

G

1. Gibson DG, Traill TA, Brown DJ. Abnormal ventricular function in patients with univentricular heart. Herz 1979;4:226.
2. Gittenberger-de Groot AC, Wenink AC. Mitral atresia. Morphological details. Br Heart J 1984;51:252.

H

1. Holmes AF. Case of malformation of the heart. Trans Med Chir Soc Edinb 1824;1:252.
2. Ho SY, Milo S, Anderson RH, Macartney FJ, Goodwin A, Becker AE, et al. Straddling atrioventricular valve with absent atrioventricular connection. Report of 10 cases. Br Heart J 1982;47:344.
3. Huddleston CB, Canter CE, Spray TL. Damus-Kaye-Stansel with cavopulmonary connection for single ventricle and subaortic obstruction. Ann Thorac Surg 1993;55:339.
4. Huhta JC, Seward JB, Tajik AJ, Hagler DJ, Edwards WD. Two-dimensional echocardiographic spectrum of univentricular atrioventricular connection. J Am Coll Cardiol 1985;5:149.

I

1. Ilbawi MN, DeLeon SY, Wilson WR Jr, Quinones JA, Roberson DA, Husayni TS, et al. Advantages of early relief of subaortic stenosis in single ventricle equivalents. Ann Thorac Surg 1991;52:842.
2. Ionescu MI, Macartney FJ, Wooler GH. Intracardiac repair of single ventricle with pulmonary stenosis. J Thorac Cardiovasc Surg 1973;65:602.

J

1. Jacobs ML, Rychik J, Donofrio MT, Steven JM, Nicolson SC, Murphy JD, et al. Avoidance of subaortic obstruction in staged management of single ventricle. Ann Thorac Surg 1995;60:S543.
2. Jensen RA Jr, Williams RG, Laks H, Drinkwater D, Kaplan S. Usefulness of banding of the pulmonary trunk with single ventricle physiology at risk for subaortic obstruction. Am J Cardiol 1996; 77:1089.

K

1. Karl TR, Watterson KG, Sano S, Mee RB. Operations for subaortic stenosis in univentricular hearts. Ann Thorac Surg 1991;52:420.
2. Kawahira Y, Uemura H, Yoshikawa Y, Yagihara T. Double inlet right ventricle versus other types of double or common inlet ventricle: its clinical characteristics with reference to the Fontan procedure. Eur J Cardiothorac Surg 2001;20:228-32.
3. Keeton BR, Macartney FJ, Hunter S, Mortera C, Rees P, Shinebourne EA, et al. Univentricular heart of right ventricular type with double or common inlet. Circulation 1979;59:403.
4. Kitamura S, Kawashima Y, Shimazaki Y, Mori T, Nakano S, Beppu S, et al. Characteristics of ventricular function in single ventricle. Circulation 1979;60:849.
5. Kiraly L, Hubay M, Cook AC, Ho SY, Anderson RH. Morphologic features of the uniatrial but biventricular atrioventricular connection. J Thorac Cardiovasc Surg 2007;133:229-34.
6. Kreutzer G, Galindez E, Bono H, de Palma C, Laura JP. An operation for the correction of tricuspid atresia. J Thorac Cardiovasc Surg 1973;66:613.
7. Kreutzer G, Schlichter A, Laura JP, Suarez JC, Vargas JF. Univentricular heart with low pulmonary vascular resistances: septation vs. atriopulmonary anastomosis. Arq Bras Cardiol 1981;37:301.
8. Kurosawa H, Imai Y, Fukuchi S, Sawatari K, Koh Y, Nakazawa M, et al. Septation and Fontan repair of univentricular atrioventricular connection. J Thorac Cardiovasc Surg 1990;99:314.

L

1. Lan YT, Chang RK, Laks H. Outcome of patients with double-inlet left ventricle or tricuspid atresia with transposed great arteries. J Am Coll Cardiol 2004;43:113-9.
2. Leung MP, Mok CK, Hui PW, Lo RN, Lau KC, Li CK, et al. Cross-sectional and pulsed Doppler echocardiography of the atrioventricular junction of hearts with univentricular atrioventricular connexion. Int J Cardiol 1987;15:215.
3. Lev M. Pathologic diagnosis of positional variations in cardiac chambers in congenital heart disease. Lab Invest 1954;3:71.
4. Lev M, Liberthson RR, Kirkpatrick JR, Eckner FA, Arcilla RA. Single (primitive) ventricle. Circulation 1969;39:577.
5. Lotto AA, Hosein R, Jones TJ, Barron DJ, Brawn WJ. Outcome of the Norwood procedure in the setting of transposition of the great arteries and functional single left ventricle. Eur J Cardiothorac Surg 2009;35:149-55; discussion 55.

M

1. Macartney FJ, Partridge JB, Scott O, Deverall PB. Common or single ventricle. An angiocardiographic and hemodynamic study of 42 patients. Circulation 1976;53:543.
2. Macoviak JA, Baldwin JC, Ginsburg R, Fowler M, Valentine H, Oyer PE, et al. Orthotopic cardiac transplantation for univentricular heart. Ann Thorac Surg 1988;45:85.
3. Mann JD. Cor triloculare biatriatum. Br Med J 1907;1:614.

4. Margossian RE, Solowiejczyk D, Bourlon F, Apfel H, Gersony WM, Hordof AJ, et al. Septation of the single ventricle: revisited. J Thorac Cardiovasc Surg 2002;124:442-7.
5. McGoon DC, Kanielson GK, Ritter DG, Wallace RB, Maloney JD, Marcelletti C. Correction of the univentricular heart having two atrioventricular valves. J Thorac Cardiovasc Surg 1977;74:218.
6. McKay R, Bini RM, Wright JP. Staged septation of double inlet left ventricle. Br Heart J 1986;56:563.
7. McKay R, Pacifico AD, Blackstone EH, Kirklin JW, Bargeron LM Jr. Septation of the univentricular heart with left anterior subaortic outlet chamber. J Thorac Cardiovasc Surg 1982;84:77.
8. Moak JP, Gersony WM. Progressive atrioventricular valvular regurgitation in single ventricle. Am J Cardiol 1987;59:656.
9. Moodie DS, Ritter DG, Tajik AJ, O'Fallon WM. Long-term follow-up in the unoperated univentricular heart. Am J Cardiol 1984;53:1124.
10. Muller WH Jr, Damman JF Jr. Treatment of certain congenital malformations of the heart by the creation of pulmonic stenosis to reduce pulmonary hypertension and excessive pulmonary blood flow (a preliminary report). Surg Gynecol Obstet 1952; 95:213.

N

1. Nagashima M, Imai Y, Takanashi Y, Hoshino S, Seo K, Terada M, et al. Ventricular hypertrophy as a risk factor in ventricular septation for double-inlet left ventricle. Ann Thorac Surg 1997;64:730.
2. Naito Y, Fujiwara K, Komai H, Uemura S. Midterm results after ventricular septation for double-inlet left ventricle in early infancy. Ann Thorac Surg 2001;71:1344-6.
3. Neches WH, Park SC, Lenox CC, Zuberbuhler JR, Bahnson HT. Tricuspid atresia with transposition of the great arteries and closing ventricular septal defect. Successful palliation by banking of the pulmonary artery and creation of an aorticopulmonary window. J Thorac Cardiovasc Surg 1973;65:538.
4. Newfeld EA, Nikaidoh H. Surgical management of subaortic stenosis in patients with single ventricle and transposition of the great vessels. Circulation 1987;76:III29.

O

1. Ohuchi H, Arakaki Y, Yagihara T, Kamiya T. Cardiorespiratory responses to exercise after repair of the univentricular heart. Int J Cardiol 1997;58:17.
2. Ohuchi H, Watanabe K, Kishiki K, Nii M, Wakisaka Y, Yagihara T, et al. Comparison of late post-operative cardiopulmonary responses in the Fontan versus ventricular septation for double-inlet left ventricular repair. Am J Cardiol 2007;99:1757-61.
3. Ottenkamp J, Hazekamp MG. Double-inlet left ventricle: successfully staged ventricular septation with 12.5 years follow-up (comment). Ann Thorac Surg 2002;73:699.

P

1. Pacifico AD. Surgical treatment of double inlet ventricle ("single ventricle"). J Cardiac Surg 1986;1:105.
2. Park SC, Siewers RD, Neches WH, Zuberbuhler JR, Mathews RA, Fricker FJ, et al. Surgical management of univentricular heart with subaortic obstruction. Ann Thorac Surg 1984;37:417.
3. Pass RH, Solowiejczyk DE, Quaegebeur JM, Liberman L, Altmann K, Gersony WM, et al. Bulboventricular foramen resection: hemodynamic and electrophysiologic results. Ann Thorac Surg 2001; 71:1251-4.
4. Penkoske PA, Freedom RM, Williams WG, Trusler GA, Rowe RD. Surgical palliation of subaortic stenosis in the univentricular heart. J Thorac Cardiovasc Surg 1984;87:767.

Q

1. Quaegebeur J, Wenink AC, Anderson RH. Anatomical potential for septation. In Anderson RH, Crupi G, Parenzan L, eds. Double inlet ventricle. New York: Elsevier, 1987, p. 98.
2. Quero-Jimenez M, Cameron A, Acerete F, Quero-Jimenez C. Univentricular hearts: pathology of the atrioventricular valves. Herz 1979;4:161.

R

1. Rao PS, Sissman NJ. Spontaneous closure of physiologically advantageous ventricular septal defects. Circulation 1971;43:83.
2. Rastelli GC, Ongley PA, Titus JL. Ventricular septal defect of atrioventricular canal type with straddling right atrioventricular valve and mitral valve deformity. Circulation 1968;37:816.
3. Redington AN, Knight B, Oldershaw PJ, Shinebourne EA, Rigby ML. Left ventricular function in double inlet left ventricle before the Fontan operation: comparison with tricuspid atresia. Br Heart J 1988;60:324.
4. Redo SF, Engle MA, Ehlers KH, Farnsworth PB. Palliative surgery for mitral atresia. Arch Surg 1967;95:717.
5. Restivo A, Ho SY, Anderson RH, Cameron H, Wilkinson JL. Absent left atrioventricular connection with right atrium connected to morphologically left ventricular chamber, rudimentary right ventricular chamber, and ventriculoarterial discordance. Problem of mitral versus tricuspid atresia. Br Heart J 1982;48:240.
6. Rokitansky CF von. Die Defecte der Scheidewande des Herzens. Vienna: Wilhelm Braumuller, 1875, p. 27.
7. Rowlatt UF. Coronary artery distribution in complete transposition. JAMA 1962;179:269.
8. Rychik J, Murdison KA, Chin AJ, Norwood WI. Surgical management of severe aortic outflow obstruction in lesions other than the hypoplastic left heart syndrome: use of a pulmonary artery to aorta anastomosis. J Am Coll Cardiol 1991;18:809.

S

1. Saalouke MG, Perry LW, Okoroma EO, Shapiro SR, Scott LP 3rd. Primitive ventricle with normally related great vessels and stenotic subpulmonary outlet chamber. Angiographic differentiation from tetralogy of Fallot. Br Heart J 1978;40:49.
2. Sakakibara S, Tominaga S, Imai Y, Uehara K, Matsumuro M. Successful total correction of common ventricle. Chest 1972;61:192.
3. Saleeb SF, Juraszek A, Geva T. Anatomic, imaging, and clinical characteristics of double-inlet, double-outlet right ventricle. Am J Cardiol 2010;105:542-9.
4. Seki S, McGoon DC. Surgical techniques for replacement of the interventricular septum. J Thorac Cardiovasc Surg 1971;62:919.
5. Seki S, Tsakiris A, McGoon DC. The effect of a prosthetic ventricular septum on canine cardiac function. Surgery 1972;71:241.
6. Serraf A, Conte S, Lacour-Gayet F, Bruniaux J, Sousa-Uva M, Roussin R, et al. Systemic obstruction in univentricular hearts: surgical options for neonates. Ann Thorac Surg 1995;60:970.
7. Shimazaki Y, Kawashima Y, Mori T, Kitamura S, Matsuda H, Yokota K. Ventricular volume characteristics of single ventricle before corrective surgery. Am J Cardiol 1980;45:806.
8. Shimazaki Y, Kawashima Y, Mori T, Matsuda H, Kitamura S, Yokota K. Ventricular function of single ventricle after ventricular septation. Circulation 1980;61:653.
9. Shinebourne EA, Lau K, Calcaterra G, Anderson RH. Univentricular heart of right ventricular type: clinical, angiographic and electrocardiographic features. Am J Cardiol 1980;46:439.
10. Shinebourne EA, Macartney FJ, Anderson RH. Sequential chamber localization: logical approach to diagnosis in congenital heart disease. Br Heart J 1976;38:327.
11. Soto B, Bertranou EG, Bream PR, Souza A Jr, Bargeron LM Jr. Angiographic study of univentricular heart of right ventricular type. Circulation 1979;60:1325.
12. Soto B, Pacifico AD, Di Sciascio G. Univentricular heart: an angiographic study. Am J Cardiol 1982;49:787.
13. Starc TJ, Gersony WM. Progressive obstruction of the foramen ovale in patients with left atrioventricular valve atresia. J Am Coll Cardiol 1986;7:1099.
14. Stefanelli G, Kirklin JW, Naftel DC, Blackstone EH, Pacifico AD, Kirklin JK, et al. Early and intermediate-term (10-year) results of surgery for univentricular atrioventricular connection ("single ventricle"). Am J Cardiol 1984;54:811.

T

1. Taussig HB. A single ventricle with a diminutive outlet chamber. J Tech Methods 1939;19:120.
2. Tchervenkov CI, Beland MJ, Latter DA, Dobell AR. Norwood operation for univentricular heart with subaortic stenosis in the neonate. Ann Thorac Surg 1990;50:822.
3. Tham EB, Wald R, McElhinney DB, Hirji A, Goff D, Del Nido PJ, et al. Outcome of fetuses and infants with double inlet single left ventricle. Am J Cardiol 2008;101:1652-6.
4. Thiene G, Daliento L, Frescura C, De Tommasi M, Macartney FJ, Anderson RH. Atresia of left atrioventricular orifice. Anatomical investigation in 62 cases. Br Heart J 1981;45:393.

U

1. Uemura H, Ho SY, Adachi I, Yagihara T. Morphologic spectrum of ventriculoarterial connection in hearts with double inlet left ventricle: implications for surgical procedures. Ann Thorac Surg 2008;86:1321-7.

V

1. Van Praagh R, David I, Gordon D, Wright GB, Van Praagh S. Ventricular diagnosis and designation. In Godman MJ, ed. Paediatric cardiology, Vol. 4. Edinburgh: Churchill Livingstone, 1982, p. 153.
2. Van Praagh R, Ongley PA, Swan HJ. Anatomic types of single or common ventricle in man. Morphologic and geometric aspects of 60 necropsied cases. Am J Cardiol 1964;13:367.
3. Van Praagh R, Plett JA, Van Praagh S. Single ventricle. Herz 1979;4:113.

W

1. Wang JK, Lue HC, Wu MH, Chiu IS, Hung CR. Double-inlet ventricle in Chinese patients. Am J Cardiol 1993;72:85.
2. Webber SA, Sett SS, LeBlanc JG. Univentricular atrioventricular connection with subaortic stenosis: a staged surgical approach. Ann Thorac Surg 1992;54:344.
3. Wenink AC. The conducting tissues in primitive ventricle with outlet chamber: two different possibilities. J Thorac Cardiovasc Surg 1978;75:747.
4. Wilkinson JL, Anderson RH, Arnold R, Hamilton DI, Smith A. The conducting tissues in primitive ventricular hearts without an outlet chamber. Circulation 1976;53:930.
5. Wilkinson JL, Becker AE, Tynan M, Freedom R, Macartney FJ, Shinebourne EA, et al. Nomenclature of the univentricular heart. Herz 1979;4:107.
6. Wilkinson JL, Dickinson D, Smith A, Anderson RH. Conducting tissues in univentricular heart of right ventricular type with double or common inlet. J Thorac Cardiovasc Surg 1979;77:691.

Y

1. Yacoub MH, Radley-Smith R. Use of a valved conduit from right atrium to pulmonary artery for "correction" of single ventricle. Circulation 1976;54:III63.

57 Anatomically Corrected Malposition of the Great Arteries

DEFINITION

Anatomically corrected malposition is an anomaly in the position of the great arteries but not in cardiac connections. Thus, there is atrioventricular (AV) and ventriculoarterial (VA) concordant connection as in the normal heart, but the aortic origin lies to the left and usually anterior to the pulmonary trunk origin when there is situs solitus (Van Praagh's S,D,L; see "Symbolic Convention of Van Praagh" in Chapter 1) and to the right of the pulmonary trunk origin when there is situs inversus (I,L,D). The circulatory pathways remain in series.

HISTORICAL NOTE

Anatomically corrected malposition of the great arteries was first reported by Theveanin in 1895 (cited by Van Praagh and Van Praagh[V2]) and was first termed *anatomically corrected transposition of the great arteries* by Harris and Farber in 1939.[H1] It is possible similar cases were described earlier under a variety of names. This confusion is exemplified by the case of Raghib and colleagues, described in 1966 with the phrase *isolated bulbar inversion in corrected transposition*.[R1] The Van Praaghs, who had doubted its existence, described three cases in 1967 using the term *anatomically corrected transposition of the great arteries*.[V2] At that time, Abbott's influential 1927 definition of transposition, according to which any abnormality in the relationship of the great arteries or between the great arteries and the ventricles was called *transposition*, was still accepted.[A1] This confusion was clarified when Van Praagh and colleagues redefined *transposition* in 1971 as the origin of the aorta from the morphologically right ventricle and the pulmonary trunk from the morphologically left ventricle (i.e., VA discordant connection) and proposed that other positional and connection abnormalities be included in the definition of *malposition*.[V2] The present condition was thus renamed *anatomically corrected malposition of the great arteries*.[V1,V3]

MORPHOLOGY AND MORPHOGENESIS

Morphology

When there is situs solitus of the atria, usually the right atrium is connected to the right ventricle[1] (D-loop), which lies to the right, and the left atrium is connected to the left ventricle, which lies to the left (S,D,L arrangement). Structure of the sinus portions of both ventricles is normal. However, although the aorta arises from the left ventricle and the pulmonary trunk from the right ventricle, there are abnormalities of the outlet, or infundibulum, in both ventricles. The left ventricle probably always exhibits a subaortic conus (infundibulum) with a well-formed conal septum, and muscle exists between aortic and mitral valve anuli.[V1] Aortic origin is accordingly displaced superiorly and anteriorly. The right ventricle may also have an infundibulum, but it may be less well developed than normal and in some cases is absent.[V2] In the latter case, there is pulmonary-tricuspid fibrous continuity. The aorta lies to the left and usually anterior to the pulmonary trunk, and both arteries are parallel. Rarely, there may be situs inversus with an I,L,D arrangement.[A2]

Hearts with similar types of infundibular development but AV discordant connection, although originally included in this category by both the Van Praaghs and Anderson and colleagues, are not called *anatomically corrected malposition* in this text but are included as variants of isolated ventricular inversion (see Section II of Chapter 55).[A2,V2]

Morphogenesis

Van Praagh argues that all forms of abnormally related great arteries relate to maldevelopment of the subsemilunar conal free walls—an abnormality of what he terms the *embryonic*

[1]The adjectives *left* and *right* used to modify atrium or ventricle mean *morphologically* left or right. *Position* of the chamber is referred to as *right-sided* or *left-sided*.

aortic switch procedure.[V1] In anatomically corrected malposition of the great arteries, the ventricles have looped in one direction, which the great arteries have twisted in the opposite direction, carrying with them the subsemilunar conal free wall. Although the great arteries are normally related (aligned), Van Praagh notes that the VA connection is very abnormal because of the abnormality in subsemilunar conal resorption.

Associated Anomalies

All reported cases of anatomically corrected malposition have been associated with other congenital cardiac anomalies.[D1,F1,R2] A large ventricular septal defect (VSD) is commonly present, usually conoventricular but occasionally elsewhere, as would be anticipated with abnormal subarterial conal connections to the ventricles; VSDs may be multiple. When the VSD is subpulmonary, the pulmonary trunk may override onto the left ventricle such that the condition merges with double outlet left ventricle (see Morphology in Chapter 54).[K1] When the VSD is subaortic, the aorta may override onto the right ventricle such that the condition merges with double outlet right ventricle (see Morphology in Chapter 53).[K1] In a recent report of six cases from one institution, VSD was absent in three,[D1] although a literature review of 53 cases reported absence of VSD in only three.[O1]

Pulmonary stenosis is usual, often infundibular in association with the subpulmonary conus, but occasionally valvar. Subaortic stenosis may occur from narrowing of the muscular subaortic conus.[D1] Tricuspid atresia or tricuspid valve hypoplasia has been noted in half the reported cases, accompanied by right ventricular hypoplasia. A right aortic arch is common, as is leftward juxtaposition of the atrial appendages and dextrocardia.

Aortic coarctation and arch hypoplasia has been reported in five cases. Two of these had associated severe subaortic stenosis and left ventricular hypoplasia, and three had no physiologic left ventricular outflow tract obstruction and a normally developed left ventricle.[N1]

CLINICAL FEATURES AND DIAGNOSTIC CRITERIA

Clinical features depend on associated anomalies such as VSD or pulmonary stenosis. Correct diagnosis may first be suspected from the characteristic appearance of L-malposition in the chest radiograph (Fig. 57-1). Two-dimensional echocardiography usually establishes the diagnosis, confirming abnormalities of ventricular outflow tracts, concordant AV and VA connections, situs, positions of cardiac chambers and great vessels, and associated intracardiac defects.[C3] Additional studies such as cineangiography (Fig. 57-2), magnetic resonance imaging[C2] (Fig. 57-3), or computed tomography[C1] (Fig. 57-4) are confirmatory or diagnostic if echocardiography fails to fully characterize the lesion. Occasionally, correct diagnosis is made only at operation. The diagnosis may remain ambiguous when there is a conoventricular VSD and one of the great arteries is overriding.

Possible diagnoses other than anatomically corrected malposition in patients with atrial situs solitus and L-malposition of the aorta include complete transposition with L-malposition (see Chapter 52), AV concordant connection with double outlet right ventricle and L-malposition (see Chapter 53), AV concordant connection with double outlet left ventricle (see

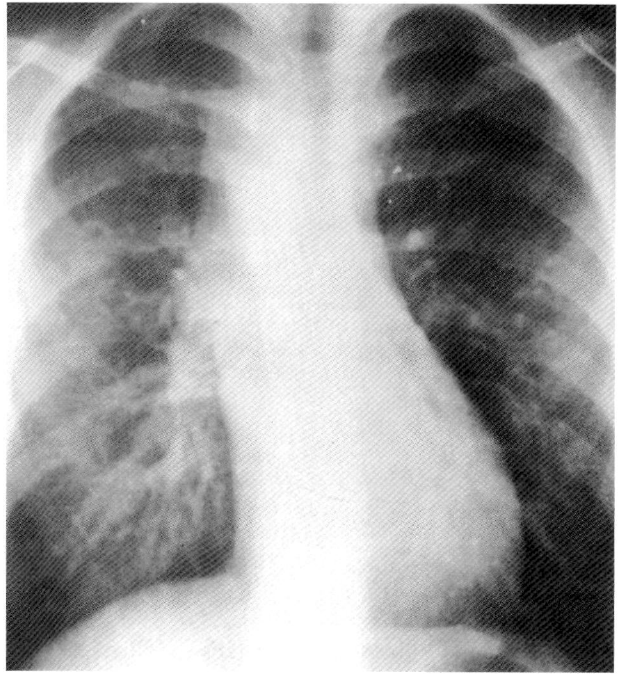

Figure 57-1 Posteroanterior radiograph of anatomically corrected malposition of the great arteries and ventricular septal defect. The ascending aorta is the border-forming structure in the upper left cardiac silhouette. (From Kirklin and colleagues.[K1])

Chapter 54), congenitally corrected transposition of the great arteries (see Chapter 55), AV discordant connection with double outlet right or left ventricle (see Chapter 55), and several forms of univentricular AV connection, most commonly those associated with double inlet left ventricle, rudimentary left-sided right ventricle, and VA discordant connection (see Chapter 56).

NATURAL HISTORY

The simple positional anomaly of anatomically corrected malposition per se has no impact on the natural history of patients. Rather, natural history is affected as typical for the associated cardiac anomalies.

TECHNIQUE OF OPERATION

Surgical treatment of anatomically corrected malposition is determined by associated cardiac anomalies.[K1] The few special problems imposed on aortic cannulation by L-malposition are discussed under surgical treatment of congenitally corrected transposition of the great arteries (see Technique of Operation in Section I of Chapter 55).

When there is tricuspid atresia or important right ventricular hypoplasia, a Fontan-type procedure is performed (see Technique of Operation in Section IV of Chapter 41). When both ventricles are of adequate size, the VSD (if present) is closed, and pulmonary stenosis is treated. This may be accomplished as simply as possible, preferably by valvotomy, infundibular resection, or both. When necessary, a more complex solution is required, such as a transanular patch, an allograft-valved extracardiac conduit, a Lecompte intraventricular repair (*réparation à l'étage ventriculaire* [REV]) (see

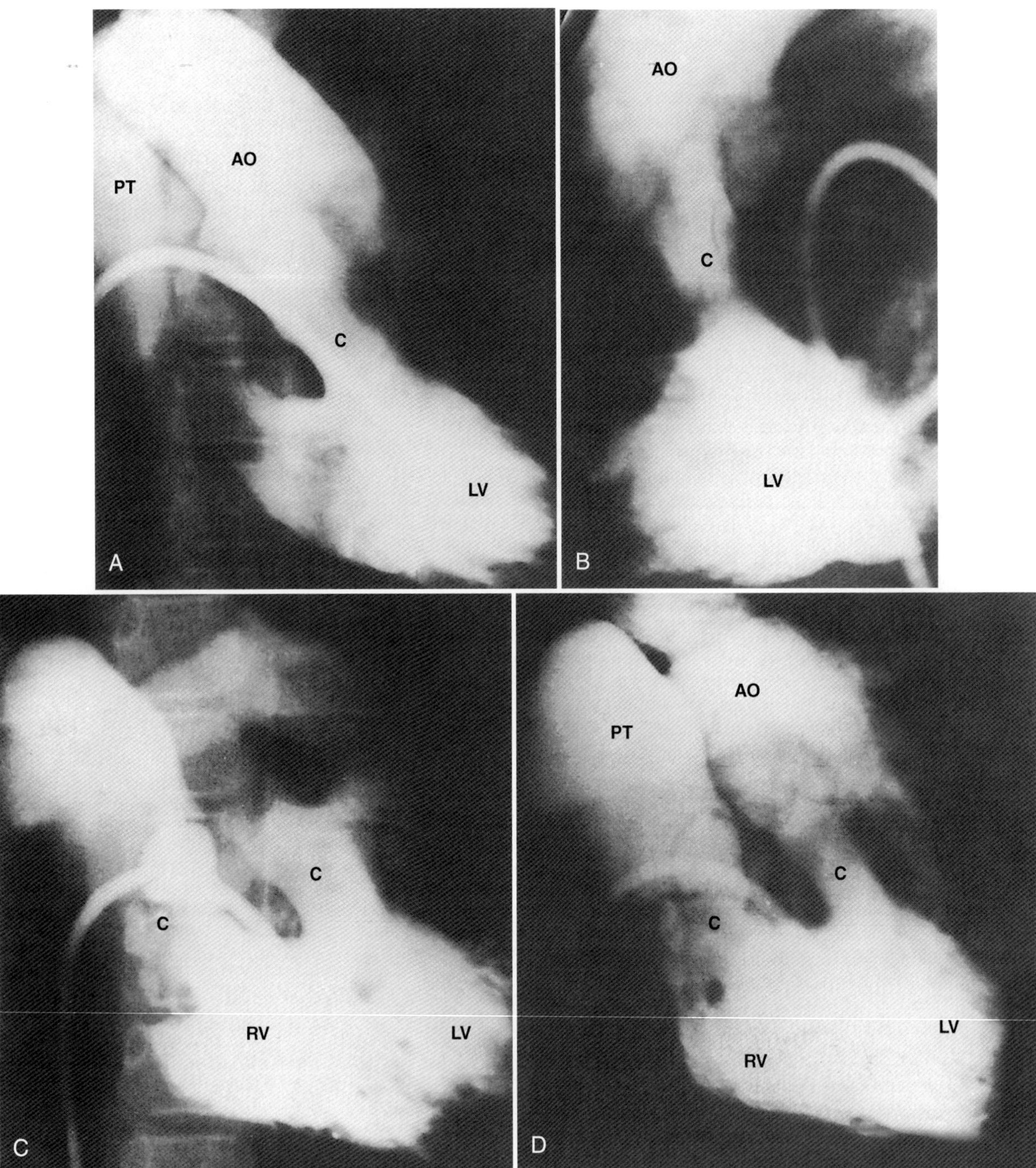

Figure 57-2 Left ventriculograms of anatomically corrected malposition of the great arteries and ventricular septal defect. There is an infundibulum beneath both aorta and pulmonary trunk. The aorta is to the left of the pulmonary trunk, and they are parallel. There is subvalvar pulmonary stenosis. **A,** Anteroposterior projection. **B,** Lateral projection. **C-D,** Later sequences. Key: *AO,* Aorta; *C,* infundibulum (conus); *LV,* left ventricle; *PT,* pulmonary trunk; *RV,* right ventricle. (From Kirklin and colleagues.[K1])

"Lecompte Intraventricular Repair" under Technique of Operation in Chapter 53), or translocation in continuity of the pulmonary trunk and valve to the right ventricle.

RESULTS

Because the anomaly is rare and the associated anomalies that determine indication for operation are variable, no meaningful statements can be made regarding outcomes. Patients undergoing biventricular repair can reasonably be expected to have outcomes similar to those of patients with double outlet right or left ventricle. Those treated as having single-ventricle physiology can reasonably be expected to have outcomes similar to those of patients undergoing various staged procedures leading to and including the Fontan operation (see Chapter 41). In one series, three of four patients survived biventricular repair at midterm follow-up, with one patient dying at reoperation for an obstructed conduit.[C3] In another

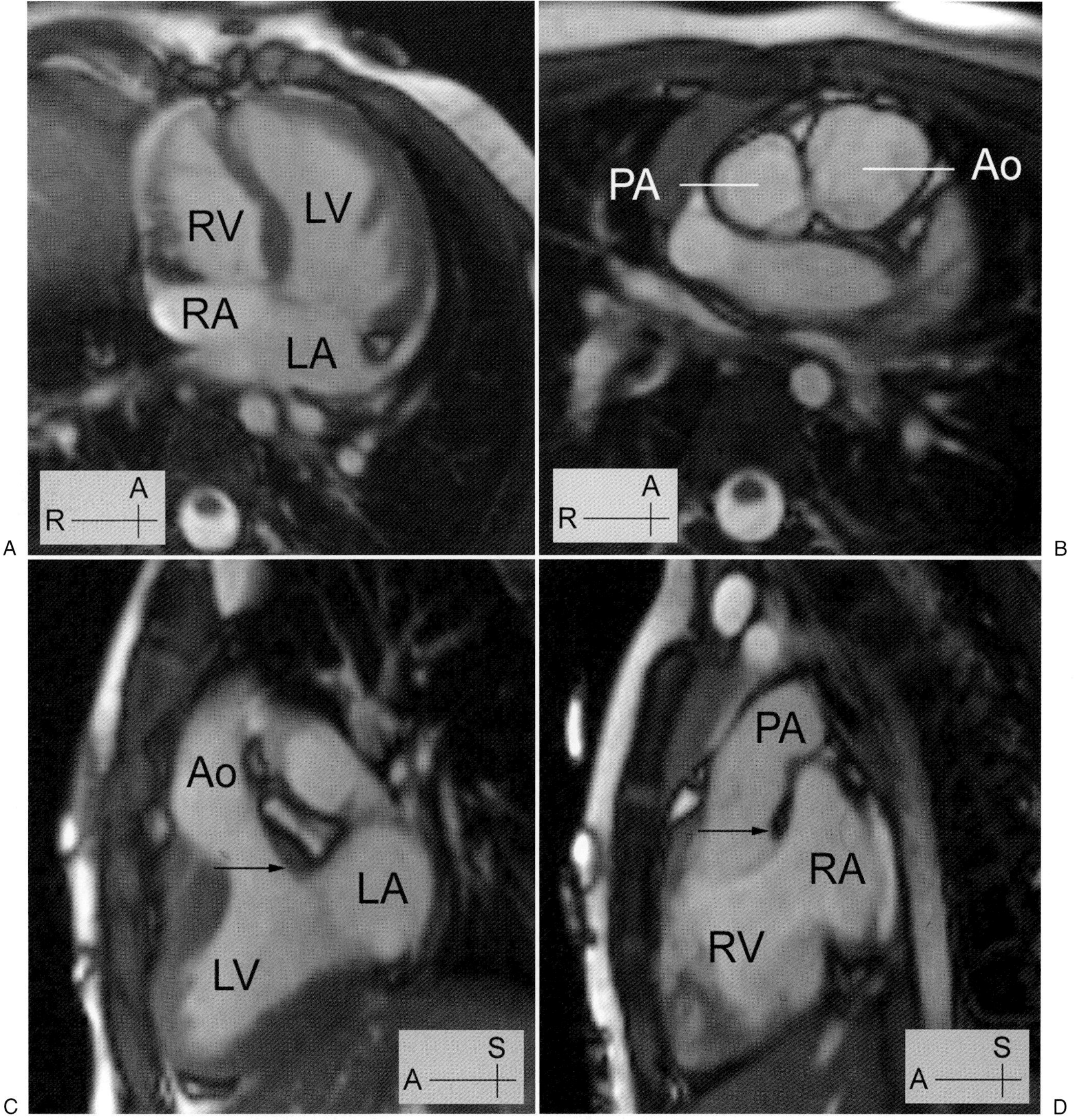

Figure 57-3 Cardiac magnetic resonance images (MRI) of a patient with anatomically corrected malposition of the great arteries. Steady-state free precession cardiac MRI. **A,** Four-chamber view demonstrating mesocardia, atrial situs solitus, and D-looped ventricles. **B,** Axial view demonstrating an abnormal great artery relationship, with the aorta arising slightly more anterior and to the left of the pulmonary trunk. **C-D,** Two-chamber views demonstrating left- and right-sided atrioventricular and ventriculoarterial concordant connections, as well as bilateral conal tissue *(arrows)* resulting in aortic-mitral and pulmonary-tricuspid discontinuity. Key: *A,* Anterior; *Ao,* aorta; *LA,* left atrium; *LV,* left ventricle; *PT,* pulmonary trunk; *R,* right; *RA,* right atrium; *RV,* right ventricle; *S,* superior. (From Clarke and colleagues.[C2])

Continued

report, two patients undergoing VSD closure and right ventricular outflow tract conduit placement survived operation.[R2] Kirklin and colleagues reported two patients, both of whom survived following VSD closure and procedures to relieve right ventricular outflow obstruction.[K1] In the largest single institution report to date (six cases), two patients underwent surgical correction, both successfully.[D1] Beyond these reports, only isolated case reports exist. Two separate cases of associated aortic coarctation with VSD report repair with staged operations.[C3,N1] The first had arch repair with pulmonary artery banding followed by VSD closure and debanding. Both patients survived.

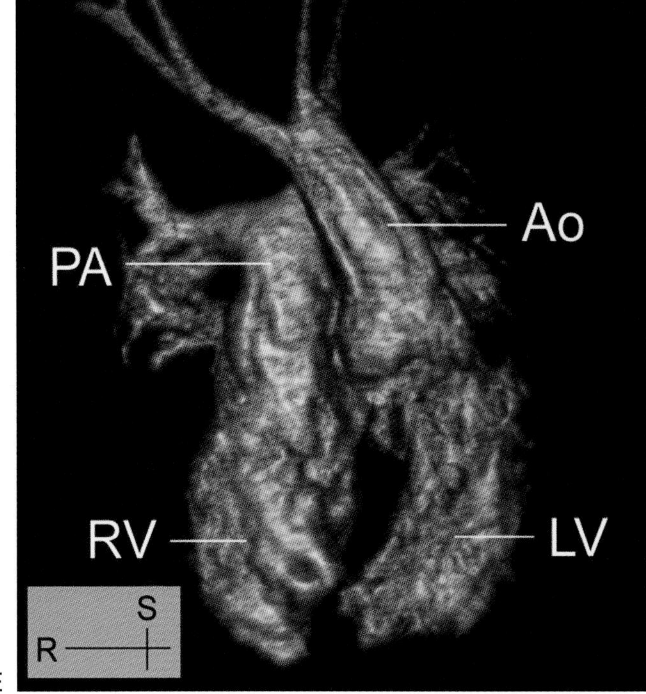

Figure 57-3, cont'd **E,** Three-dimensional reconstruction of a gadolinium-enhanced magnetic resonance angiogram demonstrating an abnormal great artery relationship. The aorta arises slightly more anterior and to the left of the pulmonary trunk. Each great artery arises from the appropriate ventricle, resulting in ventriculoarterial concordance.

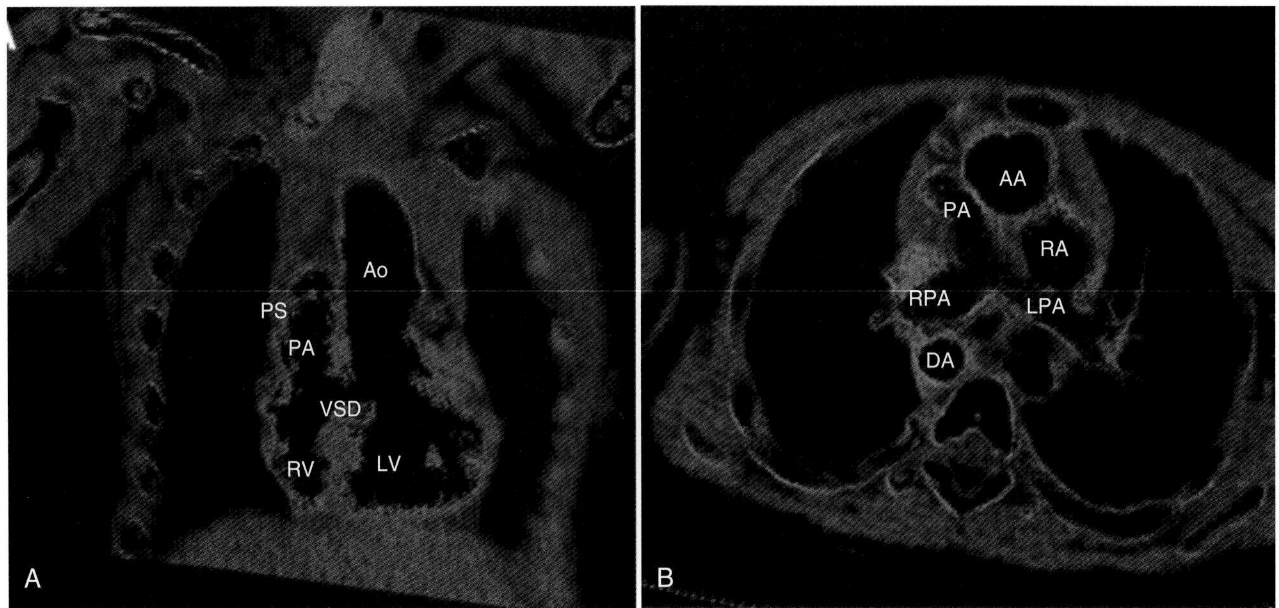

Figure 57-4 Computed tomography images of anatomically corrected malposition of the great arteries. **A-B,** Coronal and axial views showing left anterior position of the ascending aorta to the pulmonary trunk; pulmonary valve stenosis was also noted. Key: *AA* and *Ao,* ascending aorta; *DA,* descending aorta; *LPA,* left pulmonary artery; *LV,* left ventricle; *PA,* pulmonary artery; *PS,* pulmonary valve stenosis; *RPA,* right pulmonary artery; *RV,* right ventricle; *VSD,* ventricular septal defect.

INDICATIONS FOR OPERATION

Anatomically corrected malposition of the great arteries is not an indication for operation. Coexisting cardiac anomalies may present an indication for operation. Most frequently these are VSD and obstruction to right ventricular outflow.

SPECIAL SITUATIONS AND CONTROVERSIES

Several special morphologic concerns warrant emphasis. A transanular patch may be difficult or impossible to place in some cases of right ventricular outflow obstruction, because the right coronary artery passes across the free wall of the

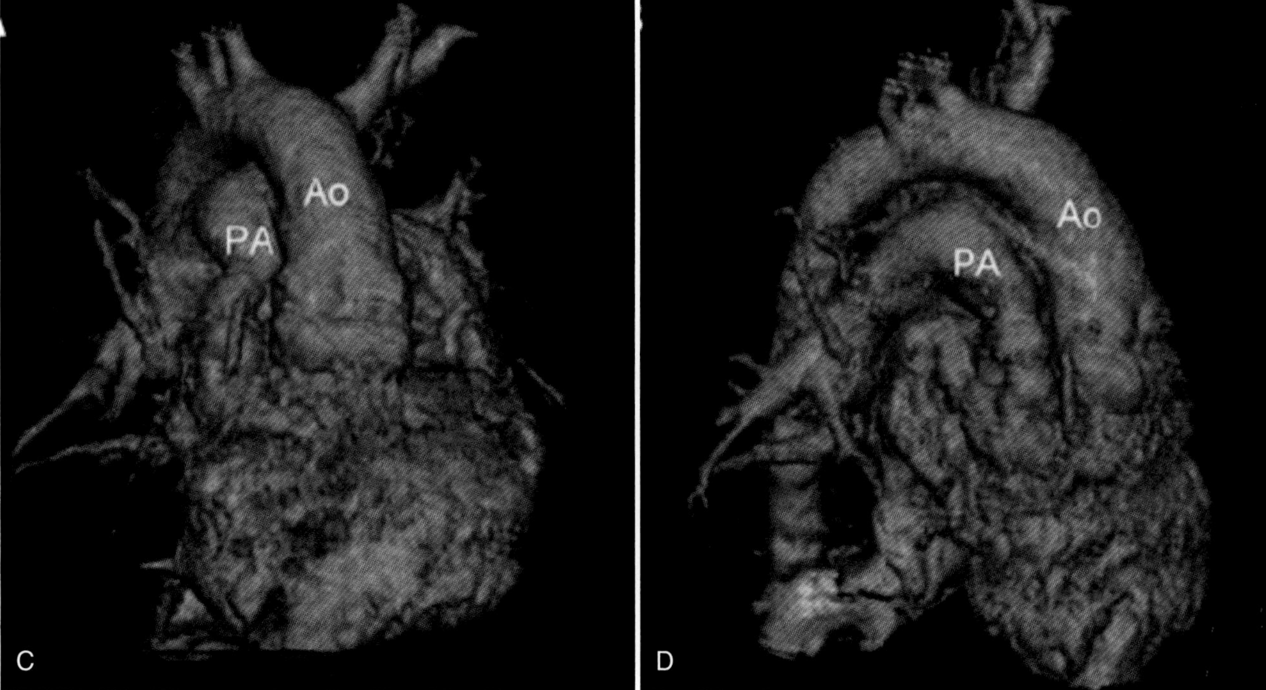

Figure 57-4, cont'd C-D, Three-dimensional reconstruction with true anterior-posterior view and right anterior oblique view showing relation of great arteries. (From Chen and colleagues.[C1])

right ventricular infundibulum. Not unexpectedly, coronary artery abnormalities are common, including abnormalities of the origins and surface course along the ventricles.[O1] These variations make the coronary arteries unreliable guides when planning ventriculotomy.

REFERENCES

A

1. Abbott ME. Congenital cardiac disease. In Osler W, McCrae T, eds. Modern medicine, Vol. 4, 3rd Ed. Philadelphia: Lea & Febiger, 1927, p. 162.
2. Anderson RH, Becker AE, Losekoot TG, Gerlis LM. Anatomically corrected malposition of great arteries. Br Heart J 1975;37: 993.

C

1. Chen MR. Anatomically corrected malposition of the great arteries. Pediatr Cardiol 2008;29:467-8.
2. Clarke CJ, Jayakumar KA, Hoyer AW. Anatomically corrected malposition of the great arteries. Pediatr Cardiol 2010;31:562-3.
3. Colli AM, de Leval M, Somerville J. Anatomically corrected malposition of the great arteries: diagnostic difficulties and surgical repair of associated lesions. Am J Cardiol 1985;55:1367-72.

D

1. Dalvi B, Sharma S. Anatomically corrected malposition: report of six cases. Am Heart J 1993;126:1229.

F

1. Freedom RM, Harrington DP. Anatomically corrected malposition of the great arteries. Report of 2 cases, one with congenital asplenia; frequent association with juxtaposition of atrial appendages. Br Heart J 1974;36:207.

H

1. Harris JS, Farber S. Transposition of the great cardiac vessels with special reference to the phylogenetic theory of Spitzer. Arch Pathol 1939;28:427.

K

1. Kirklin JW, Pacifico AD, Bargeron LM Jr, Soto B. Cardiac repair in anatomically corrected malposition of the great arteries. Circulation 1973;48:153.

N

1. Nagashima M, Takano S, Yamamoto E, Higaki T. Anatomically corrected malposition of the great arteries with tubular hypoplasia of the aortic arch. J Card Surg 2010;25:410-15.

O

1. Oku H, Shirotani H, Yokoyama T, Kawai J, Nishioka T, Noritake S, et al. Anatomically corrected malposition of the great arteries—case reports and a review. Jpn Circ J 1982;46:583.

R

1. Raghib G, Anderson RC, Edwards JE. Isolated bulbar inversion in corrected transposition. Am J Cardiol 1966;17:407.
2. Rittenhouse EA, Tenckhoff L, Kawabori I, Mansfield PB, Hall DG, Brown JW, et al. Surgical repair of anatomically corrected malposition of the great arteries. Ann Thorac Surg 1986;42:220.

V

1. Van Praagh R. Normally and abnormally related great arteries: what have we learned? World J Pediatr Congen Heart Surg 2010; 1:364-85.
2. Van Praagh R, Van Praagh S. Anatomically corrected transposition of the great arteries. Br Heart J 1967;29:112.
3. Van Praagh R, Perez-Trevino C, Lopez-Cuellar M, Baker FW, Zuberbuhler JR, Quero M, et al. Transposition of the great arteries with posterior aorta, anterior pulmonary artery, subpulmonary conus and fibrous continuity between aortic and atrioventricular valves. Am J Cardiol 1971;28:621.

58 Atrial Isomerism

DEFINITION

Atrial isomerism is a condition in which the right-sided and left-sided atria, normally morphologically different, are morphologically similar.[1] Thus, left atrial isomerism and right atrial isomerism can occur. Atrial isomerism is a specific phenotypic feature highly associated with generalized somatic laterality disorders characterized by abnormal arrangement of thoracic and abdominal viscera, including important structural cardiovascular anomalies. The terms *situs ambiguus* and *heterotaxy* are used to describe these laterality disorders. Attempts to classify specific constellations of the many clinical and phenotypic features that can occur with heterotaxy have resulted in descriptive terms such as *asplenia syndrome* and *polysplenia syndrome*.[V2] Experience shows that although there is some tendency for certain constellations to occur, exceptions are frequent or even the rule. About 3% of all congenital heart anomalies occur in the context of heterotaxy.[S10] The various cardiac anomalies found in heterotaxy are shown in Table 58-1.[C4]

In this chapter, individual cardiovascular anomalies and commonly recognized constellations of cardiovascular anomalies that occur with heterotaxy are discussed. These complex associations are analyzed from a perspective that uses left atrial isomerism and right atrial isomerism as reference points or starting points for analysis.

[1]The adjectives *left* and *right* used to modify atrium or ventricle mean *morphologically* left or right. *Position* of a chamber or valve is referred to as *right-sided* or *left-sided*.

HISTORICAL NOTE

Anomalies of right and left sidedness related to asymmetry of the body were recognized at least by the 15th century with Leonardo da Vinci's drawing of situs inversus. In the early 17th century, Marco Aurelio Severino described this anatomic variant, but it was Matthew Baille, a student of John Hunter, who is credited with scientifically describing anomalies of sidedness and their associated lesions in the latter part of the 18th century.[B1] In 1933 Kartagener drew attention to the association of situs inversus with sinusitis (Kartagener syndrome), providing an important clue to the possible morphogenesis of all anomalies of sidedness,[K1] although this had been suggested by Siewert in 1904.[S6] Biorn Ivemark in 1955 identified the syndrome of right atrial isomerism, asplenia, symmetry of thoracic organs, and conotruncal anomalies during his studies at Children's Hospital Boston.[I2]

Subsequently, general interest in the asymmetry of many bilateral animals, from snails to humans (the science related to chiral [asymmetric] bodies), has led to the hypothesis that left-right patterning is related to genetic factor processes that become reflected in midline left-right ciliary structure and function during embryogenesis.[O1,S10] In the 1986 first edition of this book, Kirklin presented the UAB surgical experience with heterotaxy patients, consisting of 28 complete repairs and 28 palliative operations (including two Fontan operations).

MORPHOLOGY AND MORPHOGENESIS

Morphology

Atrial Isomerism

In atrial isomerism, both atria have similar internal, external, and appendage configuration. They are considered either morphologically bilaterally right atria or bilaterally left atria.[M6,R4,V2] Validity of the concept of atrial isomerism, at least from the perspective of the purist, has been questioned.[C4,V3]

Atrial situs is most usefully determined by morphology of the atrial appendages,[C1,M1,S4] because all other studies provide indirect information. Right atrial appendage morphology is present when the appendage is blunt and has a broad junction with a smooth-walled atrium. This type of junction is accompanied by protrusion of the crista terminalis into the atrial cavity.[M1] Left atrial appendage morphology is present when the atrial appendage is long and thin with constrictions along its length. Such appendages have a rather constricted junction with a smooth atrium, within which a crista terminalis is not identifiable.[M1] Rarely, atria and their appendages have mixed right and left atrial morphology.

Atrial isomerism (right or left) commonly corresponds to thoracic isomerism; however, disharmony between atrial morphology and pulmonary and bronchial morphology occurs.[C1,P5,S4,U1] Atrial and thoracic isomerism (i.e., bilateral atrial and thoracic right- or left-sidedness) usually corresponds to bilateral right-sidedness (asplenia) or left-sidedness (polysplenia) of the abdominal viscera, but there are exceptions to this correspondence.[L2,U1] Abdominal asplenia or polysplenia may occasionally exist without atrial isomerism, so splenic state does not always predict atrial morphology.[S5] Because of this variability, Anderson prefers the term *heterotaxy* to denote presence of any of the numerous possible lateralization abnormalities, and then recommends describing the morphologic details for each patient.[A2]

Among 58 consecutive newborn cases of heterotaxy within a single institution, 25 had asplenia and 20 had polysplenia.[L6] In surgical series, left atrial isomerism is more common than right, in one surgical experience with 41 patients, 23 had left and 18 had right atrial isomerism.[S7] Several heterotaxy studies performed in Asian populations show a strong predilection (80% of cases) for right atrial isomerism, suggesting there may be racial differences in the expression of left and right atrial isomerism.[L5,Y1]

Table 58-1 Prevalence of Major Anatomic Cardiac Variables in 81 Patients with Prenatal and Postnatal Diagnosis of Heterotaxy Syndrome

Anatomic Variables	Prenatal Diagnosis ($n = 43$) N (%)	Postnatal Diagnosis ($n = 38$) N (%)
Isomerism of left atrial appendages	17 (39.5)	13 (34.2)
Isomerism of right atrial appendages	26 (60.5)	25 (65.8)
Right-sided heart	14 (32.5)	14 (36.8)
Interrupted inferior vena cava	15 (34.9)	8 (21.0)
Totally anomalous pulmonary venous return (extracardiac)	14 (43.8)	8 (21.0)
Common atrioventricular junction/ common atrioventricular canal	31 (72.1)	30 (78.9)
Hypoplastic left heart syndrome	9 (20.9)	3 (7.9)
Double outlet right ventricle	13 (30.2)	17 (44.7)
Double outlet right ventricle with pulmonary atresia	13 (30.2)	13 (34.2)
Pulmonary outflow obstruction	33 (76.7)	28 (73.7)
Systemic outflow obstruction	9 (20.9)	6 (15.8)
Complete heart block	8 (18.6)	3 (7.9)

Modified from Cohen and colleagues.[C4]

Conduction System

Right atrial isomerism is usually accompanied by bilateral sinus nodes, one in each atrium.[B3,D3,V2] Two atrioventricular (AV) nodes may be present, with a sling of conduction tissue between them. In left atrial isomerism, the sinus node is absent in the majority of cases, but when present is unusually positioned and often hypoplastic.[H5]

The AV node may be normally situated when ventricular architecture is right-handed (D-loop); when it is left-handed (L-loop), two AV nodes and a sling may be present.[D3] Other more severe conduction system abnormalities may also be present, because complete heart block occurs in some neonates with left atrial isomerism.[G1,H4,M5]

Supraventricular atrial tachycardias occur in right atrial isomerism in up to 25% of patients, whereas abnormal axis P waves with slow atrial or junctional rates are the rule in left atrial isomerism.[W3]

Anomalies of Systemic Venous Connection

Anomalies of systemic venous connection are common. The inferior vena cava often does not connect directly to the atrium from below, but instead passes superiorly along the right-sided paravertebral gutter (azygos extension of inferior vena cava) or left-sided gutter (hemiazygos extension of inferior vena cava), emptying into a right-sided or left-sided superior vena cava[U2] (Table 58-2). Azygos extension of the inferior vena cava occurs exclusively in patients with left atrial isomerism, in whom it occurs in about 75% of cases (see Table 58-2).

Table 58-2 Patterns of Inferior Vena Cava Drainage (n = 183)

	Atrial Connection Present		Interrupted		
Atrial Appendage Isomerism	**To Right-Sided Atrium (%)**	**To Left-Sided Atrium (%)**	**Via Right-Sided Azygos Vein (%)**	**Via Left-Sided Azygos Vein (%)**	**Other Patterns**
Right	48	52	0	0	0
Left	12	12	34	40	2

Data from Uemura and colleagues.[U2]

Table 58-3 Patterns of Superior Vena Cava Drainage (n = 183)

	Unilaterally Present			Bilaterally Present	
Atrial Appendage Isomerism	**To Right-Sided Atrial Roof (%)**	**To Left-Sided Atrial Roof (%)**	**Other Patterns (%)**	**Both to Atrial Roof (%)**	**One via Coronary Sinus (%)**
Right	29	19	1	51	0
Left	22	14	2	38	24

Data from Uemura and colleagues.[U2]

Table 58-4 Patterns of Hepatic Vein Drainage (n = 183)

	Confluence Present		Via Independent Channels		
Atrial Appendage Isomerism	**Via IVC (%)**	**Via Common Channel (Interrupted IVC) (%)**	**Unilaterally to Atrium (%)**	**Bilaterally to Atria (%)**	**Other Patterns (%)**
Right	76	0	6	18	0
Left	14	43	8	33	2

Data from Uemura and colleagues.[U2]
Key: *IVC,* Inferior vena cava.

Table 58-5 Patterns of Drainage of Pulmonary Veins (n = 183)

	Direct Connections of All Pulmonary Veins to Atrial Chambers				Via Sump Outside Heart (Confluence of All Pulmonary Veins Present)			Others (Confluence of Pulmonary Veins Incomplete)	
Atrial Appendage Isomerism	**To Left-Sided Atrium (%)**	**To Right-Sided Atrium (%)**	**Bilaterally to Chambers (%)**	**Other Patterns (%)**	**Via Superior Vena Cava (%)**	**Via Portal Vein (%)**	**Atresia of Alternative Channel (%)**	**Some via Systemic Veins and Others Directly to Atrium (%)**	**Via Multiple Channels Outside Heart (%)**
Right	19	19	0	3[a]	27	21	1	5	5
Left	26	14	60	0	0	0	0	0	0

Data from Uemura and colleagues.[U2]
[a]Via central confluence.

Bilateral superior venae cavae occur frequently: in half of patients with right atrial isomerism and in two thirds of patients with left atrial isomerism[U2] (Table 58-3). When present, each typically connects to the top corner of the corresponding atrium; however, in left atrial isomerism, one may connect to the coronary sinus.[M1]

When the inferior vena cava connects directly to the atria from below, it may connect to either the left- or right-sided atrium (see Table 58-2). Hepatic veins connect directly to the atria from below, usually to one atrium but sometimes to both or to both sides of a common atrium.[M1] Such a direct hepatic vein connection is present in all patients with an azygos extension of the inferior vena cava, but it also occurs in patients whose inferior vena cava connects to the atria from below (Table 58-4).

Uemura and colleagues report that the coronary sinus orifice is absent in about 40% of patients with left and in 100% of patients with right atrial isomerism.[U1] Other series, however, show substantial variation from these percentages.[P2,P4,V3] Anomalies of systemic venous connection do not occur exclusively in patients with atrial isomerism.[M4]

Anomalies of Pulmonary Venous Connection

Extracardiac total anomalous pulmonary venous connection (TAPVC) is usually seen in patients with right atrial isomerism (Table 58-5). When pulmonary veins connect to an atrium, pattern of connection is variable. Importantly, there is usually the normal wide area of posterior atrial wall between the pulmonary veins when the heart is viewed from behind.[M1] Pulmonary venous obstruction may be present in up to 40% of patients with right atrial isomerism, especially when the connection is extracardiac.[C3,H2,R3] Pulmonary venous obstruction in left atrial isomerism is much less common.[H2] Atresia of the common pulmonary vein has been reported in right atrial isomerism.[D1]

Atrioventricular Connections

About 75% of patients with left atrial isomerism have biventricular AV connections that are ambiguous.[C3,D2] However, there is a univentricular AV connection in about 50% to 75% of patients with right atrial isomerism, a considerably higher percentage than in any other type of atrial situs, and most of these patients have a solitary ventricular chamber[C3,H3,S7,U1] (Table 58-6).

Atrioventricular Septal and Other Atrial Septal Defects

The complexities of pulmonary and systemic venous connections, variability in the position and nature of AV valves through which the atria empty, and anomalous muscle bands that sometimes traverse the atria often make it difficult to apply conventional terms describing atrial septal defects (ASDs). However, a common atrium (see "Common Atrium"

Table 58-6 Summary of Anatomic Findings (n = 93)

	Right Isomerism (n = 61)		Left Isomerism (n = 32)	
	No.	%	No.	%
UVH	39	64	9	28
Two ventricles	22	36	23	72
CAVV	56	92	18	56
Two AV valves	2	3	10	31
MA or TA	3	5	4	13
VA concordant connection (Ao from LV)	6	10	12	38
VA discordant connection (Ao from RV)	55	90	20	62
Pulmonary atresia	20	33	3	9
Pulmonary stenosis	36	59	17	53
Bilateral SVC	33	54	17	53
Right SVC	24	39	10	31
Left SVC	4	7	5	16
Right IVC	43	70	11	34
Left IVC	17	28	0	—
IVC absence	1	2	21	66
TAPVC	37	61	2	6
PAPVC	1	2	1	3

Data from Hirooka and colleagues.[H3]
Key: *Ao,* Aorta; *AV,* atrioventricular; *CAVV,* common atrioventricular valve; *IVC,* inferior vena cava; *LV,* left ventricle; *MA,* mitral atresia; *PAPVC,* partial anomalous pulmonary venous connection; *RV,* right ventricle; *SVC,* superior vena cava; *TA,* tricuspid atresia; *TAPVC,* total anomalous pulmonary venous connection; *UVH,* univentricular heart; *VA,* ventriculoarterial.

under Morphology in Chapter 34) is present in nearly half the cases.[P4,S3] AV septal defect is present in about 80% of patients, with a higher prevalence in right than in left atrial isomerism[H3] (see Table 58-6). Most patients with atrial isomerism and AV septal defects have a common AV orifice (see “Complete Atrioventricular Septal Defect” under Morphology in Chapter 34) rather than two AV valve orifices. Rarely the atrial septum is well formed and intact or has only a probe-patent foramen ovale.[P4,S3]

Ventricular Morphology and Ventricular Septal Defects
Complexities of AV valves and connections and frequent occurrence of solitary ventricular chambers make it difficult to apply conventional terms. Only rarely is the ventricular septum intact; about 80% of patients with a VSD have an AV septal defect, and in the remainder with intact AV septal structures, various types of VSD are present.

Pulmonary Outflow
Unobstructed pulmonary outflow is rare in right, but more frequent in left, atrial isomerism. In right atrial isomerism, pulmonary stenosis is present in slightly more than half of patients, and pulmonary atresia in about one third. In left atrial isomerism, pulmonary stenosis is present in about half and pulmonary atresia in less than one tenth[H3] (see Table 58-6).

Ventriculoarterial Connections
In surgical series, ventriculoarterial connections are most commonly discordant, and an unusually high proportion (33%) of patients have double outlet right ventricle.[R2] In autopsy series, about 75% to 90% of specimens with right atrial isomerism have discordant ventriculoarterial connection (transposition) or double outlet right ventricle; in left atrial isomerism, this is true in about 20% to 65% of specimens[H3,P4,S7] (see Table 58-6). In some cases, such as double outlet from an indeterminate ventricle, the ventriculoarterial connection cannot be easily characterized.

Other Coexisting Cardiac Anomalies
Anomalies other than those inherent in atrial isomerism are infrequent in surgically treated patients. In autopsy series, obstructive lesions on the left side of the heart, excluding left ventricular hypoplasia and mitral stenosis, are common.[P2]

Summary
In the surgically more common left atrial isomerism, anomalies of systemic venous connection are common, as are abortive forms of cor triatriatum, but extracardiac TAPVCs are not. Common atrium and other types of AV septal defects occur in about half the cases. Univentricular AV connections are uncommon, as are solitary ventricular chambers, but double outlet right ventricle is common. Pulmonary stenosis is present in about half of cases.

In surgical patients with right atrial isomerism, anomalies of systemic venous connection are less common, as are abortive forms of cor triatriatum, but extracardiac forms of TAPVC occur more frequently. Common atrium and other forms of AV septal defect occur in more than 90% of patients, and solitary ventricular chamber occurs in nearly half. The fact that cardiac anomalies are more complex and numerous in hearts with right rather than left atrial isomerism probably explains the higher prevalence of left atrial isomerism in surgical series than in autopsy series.

Morphogenesis

The genetic basis of heterotaxy is thought to be related to genetics of ciliary dysfunction on the embryologic midline node.[C4]

CLINICAL FEATURES AND DIAGNOSTIC CRITERIA

There are no clinical features absolutely specific to atrial isomerism, because there is no specific functional derangement uniformly associated with the atrial morphology. The clinical sign most intimately related to the atrial morphology itself is presence of abnormal P-wave morphology and slow atrial rhythm associated with left atrial isomerism. Asplenia, commonly associated with right atrial isomerism, is associated with an increased number of Howell-Jolly bodies in the routine blood smear in newborns, or persistent Howell-Jolly bodies in older infants. Clinical features depend, therefore, on the specific cardiac anomalies and the many possible noncardiac anomalies and disorders that may be present, including intestinal malrotation, absence of splenic function, primary ciliary dyskinesia, biliary atresia, central nervous system anomalies, craniofacial anomalies, intraabdominal vascular anomalies such as congenital extrahepatic portosystemic shunt, and musculoskeletal anomalies.[C4,N5,S10]

Atrial situs is best diagnosed preoperatively by determining thoracic situs, because atrial and thoracic situs are nearly always the same.[P1,S8,V1] Thoracic situs is best indicated by bronchial anatomy, which does not always correspond to

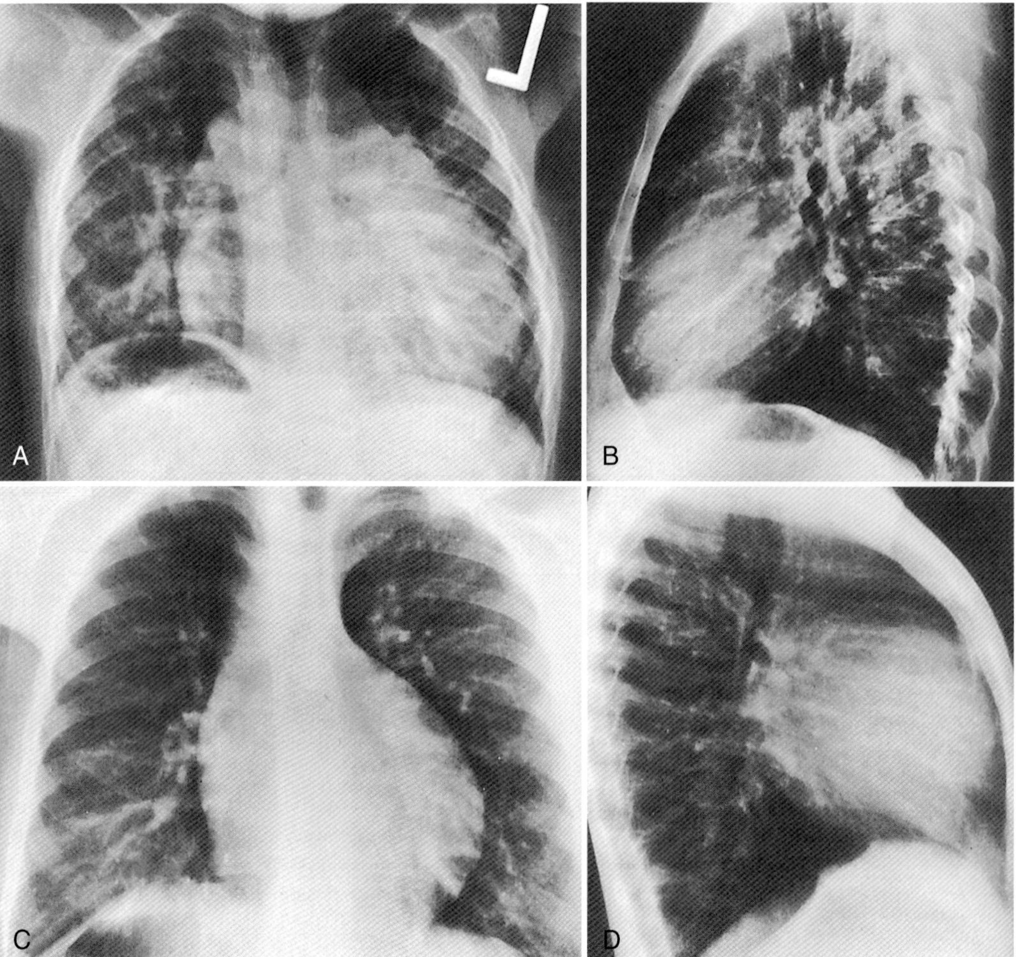

Figure 58-1 Chest radiographs in atrial isomerism. **A,** Left isomerism, frontal chest film. Each bronchus has a similar length. **B,** Lateral view. Pulmonary arteries are superior and posterior to tracheobronchial tree. **C,** Right isomerism, frontal chest film. Each bronchus has a similar length. **D,** Lateral view. Pulmonary arteries are anterior and inferior to bronchi.

lung lobulation.[L2,L3,V1] The length of each mainstem bronchus and its relationship to its respective pulmonary artery provide the most reliable clinical prediction of thoracic situs.[L1,P1,S5] The normal right mainstem bronchus is relatively short, and the right pulmonary artery is anterior and inferior to the bronchus; the normal left mainstem bronchus is relatively long, and the left pulmonary artery is posterior and superior to the bronchus.

Determining these relationships, and thus diagnosis of thoracic situs, is reliably accomplished from plain frontal and lateral chest radiographs, although meticulous attention must be paid to radiologic technique.[B4,P1,S8] If the ratio of the length of the shorter (normally right) bronchus divided by that of the longer (normally the left) is 2 or greater, there is thoracic lateralization; if the ratio is 1.5 or less, thoracic and usually atrial isomerism is present. Also, right isomerism is usually present when each pulmonary artery is anterior to its respective bronchus; left isomerism is usually present when each pulmonary artery is superior and posterior to its respective bronchus (Fig. 58-1).

Prenatal diagnosis of heterotaxy can often be made by echocardiography, but prenatal diagnosis has no impact on survival.[C5,P3] Echocardiography after birth can reliably identify the typical constellations of morphologic abnormalities associated with both left and right atrial isomerism and as a result can strongly suggest the diagnosis[H7] (Figs. 58-2 and 58-3). Echocardiography, however, is limited in delineating all morphologic details related to atrial isomerism, particularly when complex pulmonary artery and pulmonary venous anomalies are present (e.g., pulmonary atresia with discontinuous branch pulmonary arteries, mixed TAPVC). Specific characteristics of the atrial appendages cannot usually be identified with certainty, and the relationship of bronchi to pulmonary arteries cannot be determined. Complex pulmonary artery and pulmonary vein anomalies, and the extracardiac thoracic and abdominal features of left and right atrial isomerism, can best be determined by computed tomography and cineangiography (Figs. 58-4 and 58-5). Specific hemodynamic data can only be obtained by cardiac catheterization.

Almost all children with *right* atrial isomerism are in sinus rhythm, and most have a normal P-wave axis.[W1] Complete AV block coexists in about 10% of patients with *left* atrial isomerism but is rare in right atrial isomerism.[W1]

At operation, the surgeon must make direct observations of the atrial appendages and atrial walls to confirm or deny the preoperative diagnosis of right or left atrial isomerism.

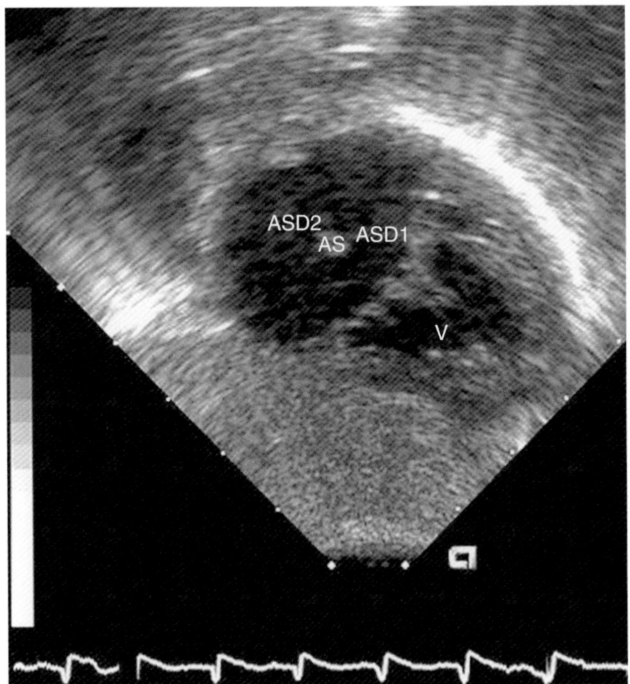

Figure 58-2 Atrial isomerism with asplenia (probably bilateral right-sidedness). Echocardiography can reliably identify most cardiovascular defects associated with the various atrial isomerism (heterotaxy) syndromes. Because the constellation of findings is variable and complex, multiple echocardiographic views are required. This subcostal coronal view demonstrates enlarged atrial chamber. Almost complete absence of atrial septum is evident, with only a central band present. There is a large ostium primum defect and a large ostium secundum defect. The single atrioventricular valve and ventricular mass are also seen. Key: *AS,* Atrial septum; *ASD1,* ostium primum defect; *ASD2,* secundum atrial septal defect; *V,* ventricle.

NATURAL HISTORY

Natural history of patients with atrial isomerism is determined primarily by details of cardiac structures and nature of coexisting cardiac anomalies. However, atrial isomerism itself may contribute to natural history because of its association with neonatal complete heart block and sometimes neonatal death.[G1,M5]

Right atrial isomerism is often accompanied by asplenia, a condition believed to render the patient susceptible to infection, particularly pneumococcal. Left atrial isomerism is often accompanied by polysplenia and a high prevalence of extrahepatic biliary atresia[C2,D5]; the polysplenia is also accompanied by splenic incompetence.

TECHNIQUE OF OPERATION

Cardiopulmonary Bypass

In patients with atrial isomerism, cardiopulmonary bypass (CPB) often presents venous cannulation problems because of systemic venous anomalies. Basic venous cannulation techniques are used, as well as those for situations involving three venae cavae (see "Venous Cannulation" under Preparation for Cardiopulmonary Bypass and "Left Superior Vena Cava" under Special Situations and Controversies in Section III of Chapter 2). Direct caval cannulation is particularly advantageous because of complex intraatrial repairs that are often required.

In patients with left atrial isomerism and two superior venae cavae, it must be remembered in selecting venous cannula size that one of the superior cavae is probably returning the entire inferior vena caval flow by way of the azygos continuation as well as its usual flow, and that a larger than usual cannula is required. In such situations, blood returning from hepatic veins connected directly to an atrium is picked up by a pump-oxygenator sump-sucker placed in the depths of the atrium. The hepatic veins, especially if they become confluent before entering the atrium, may also be directly cannulated. Occasionally, patients with right atrial isomerism will have bilateral superior venae cavae as well as hepatic veins that drain to the atrium separate from the inferior vena cava; in this situation, four venous cannulae may be necessary.

In all of these situations, complexity of the cannulation arrangement (and accompanying complexity of the intracardiac repair in many cases) is such that cooling to moderate to deep hypothermia (20°C-24°C) and using aortic clamping and cold cardioplegia are advised to allow maximum visibility and flexibility of the perfusion flow rate. For example, if a complex atrial baffle is required, one or more of the multiple venous cannulae may be temporarily removed and replaced with a cardiotomy suction device to enhance visibility and ensure the baffle is placed without distortion.

One solution to the venous cannulation problem is to use hypothermic circulatory arrest, cooling and rewarming the patient with a single venous cannula through an atrial appendage. (Advantages and disadvantages of this technique are described in Section IV of Chapter 2.) This method is more likely to be chosen for infants.

Intracardiac Repair

A wide variety of intracardiac repairs are required in patients with atrial isomerism, and repair in individual patients may require two or three procedures. These are described under Technique of Operation in chapters on the specific anomaly encountered. Procedures used in repair of AV septal defects, including common atrium (see Technique of Operation in Chapter 34), are particularly important.

Complex Atrial Baffle

In repairing anomalies of pulmonary or systemic venous connections that are frequently part of the cardiac anomaly, a complex atrial baffle is often required. The first step is usually excising remnants of the atrial septum, except for the anterior limbus, which, if present, may contain the AV node or bundle of His. The temptation to retain part of the septum as a flap should generally be resisted because it tends to increase complexity. When a coronary sinus is present, it is usually cut down, as in the Senning or Mustard repair (see Fig. 52-32 in Chapter 52).

Fig. 58-6 shows a complete AV septal defect with bilateral superior vena cavae, interrupted inferior vena cava with azygos continuation to the right superior vena cava, and two separate hepatic venous connections. Spatial arrangements of the orifices of the pulmonary veins, left-sided superior vena cava in the upper left corner of the atrium, right-sided superior vena cava in the upper right atrial corner, and hepatic

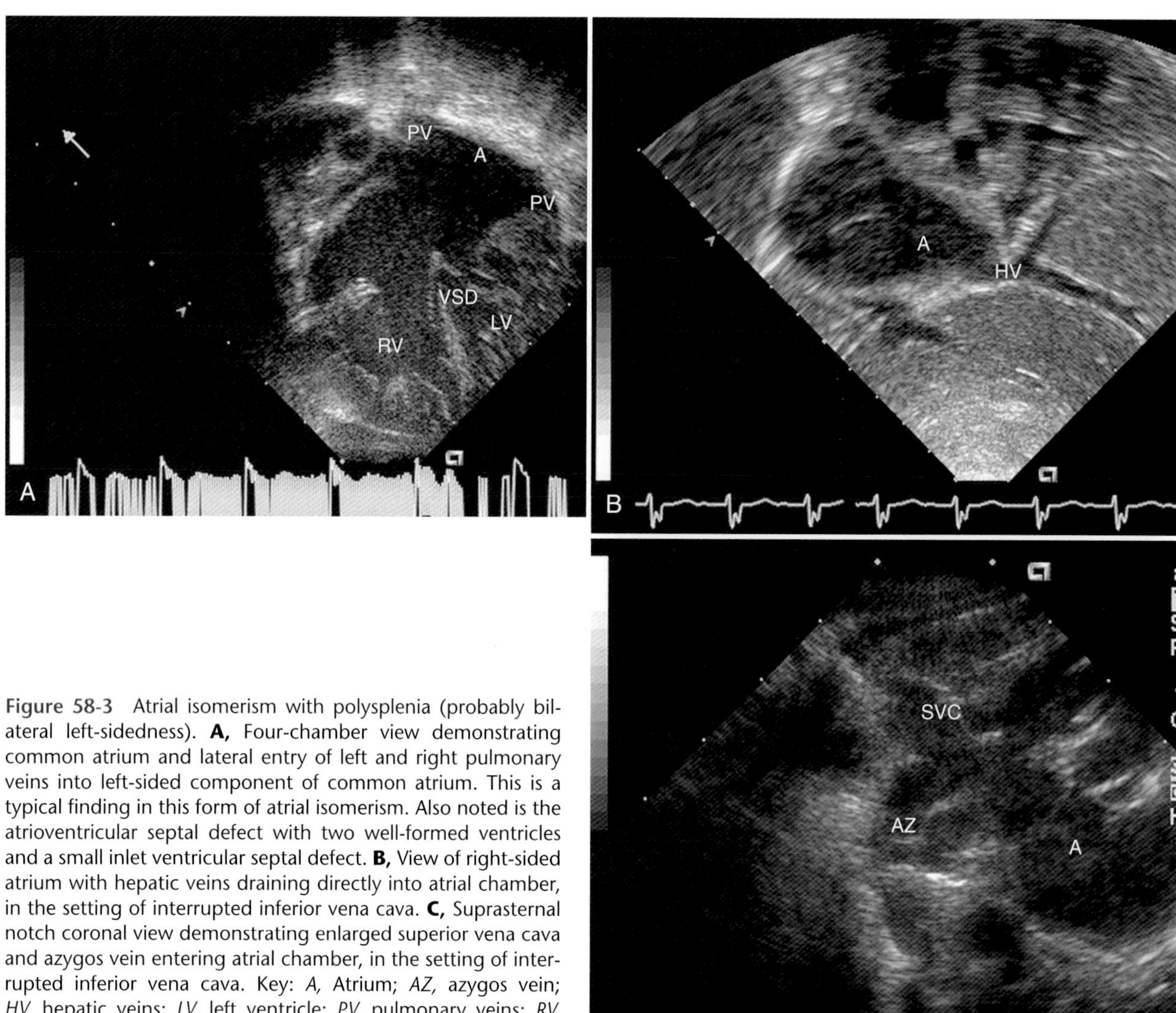

Figure 58-3 Atrial isomerism with polysplenia (probably bilateral left-sidedness). **A,** Four-chamber view demonstrating common atrium and lateral entry of left and right pulmonary veins into left-sided component of common atrium. This is a typical finding in this form of atrial isomerism. Also noted is the atrioventricular septal defect with two well-formed ventricles and a small inlet ventricular septal defect. **B,** View of right-sided atrium with hepatic veins draining directly into atrial chamber, in the setting of interrupted inferior vena cava. **C,** Suprasternal notch coronal view demonstrating enlarged superior vena cava and azygos vein entering atrial chamber, in the setting of interrupted inferior vena cava. Key: *A,* Atrium; *AZ,* azygos vein; *HV,* hepatic veins; *LV,* left ventricle; *PV,* pulmonary veins; *RV,* right ventricle; *SVC,* superior vena cava; *VSD,* ventricular septal defect.

veins lying inferiorly must be visualized in three dimensions and clearly understood (Fig. 58-6, *A*). Also, the superior vena cava receiving venous drainage from the lower body must be recognized as requiring a larger pathway to the AV valve than usual if flow is to be unimpeded. The relationship of these orifices to left-sided and right-sided AV valves must be clarified, because proper positioning of the atrial baffle depends on this knowledge. Presence of an intact inferior vena cava with separate hepatic venous drainage to the atrium, not shown in this figure, would add further complexity.

In planning the baffle and potential drainage pathways to AV valves, ventriculoarterial connections that will exist at the end of the repair must also be clearly visualized. In this regard, the ventricular situs (handedness or loop) per se is not important, because in what will ultimately be a two-ventricle system, pulmonary venous return must be routed to the ventricle that does (or will) connect to the aorta, regardless of whether it is morphologically right or left. Similarly, systemic venous return must be routed to the ventricle connected to the pulmonary trunk.

After these structures and relationships have been visualized clearly, the proposed suture line of the baffle is marked with four to six interrupted suture markers, and the pericardium that was taken initially and set aside is trimmed to a proper shape and size and sutured into place (Fig. 58-6, *B*). This complex atrial baffle is similar to that used for repair of simple unroofed coronary sinus syndrome (see Fig. 33-3 in Chapter 33).

Frequent association of anomalies of venous connection with AV septal defects in patients with atrial isomerism often necessitates combining baffle repair with repair of a complete AV septal defect. In such a procedure, extension of the atrial baffle toward the AV valves is best thought of as simply the intraatrial portion of the two-patch technique used in the repair of complete AV septal defects (see "Two-Patch Technique" under Technique of Operation in Chapter 34).

Techniques have been developed that reduce complexity of the atrial baffle in some circumstances. When bilateral superior venae cavae are present with unroofed coronary sinus, extracardiac connection of the left to the right superior

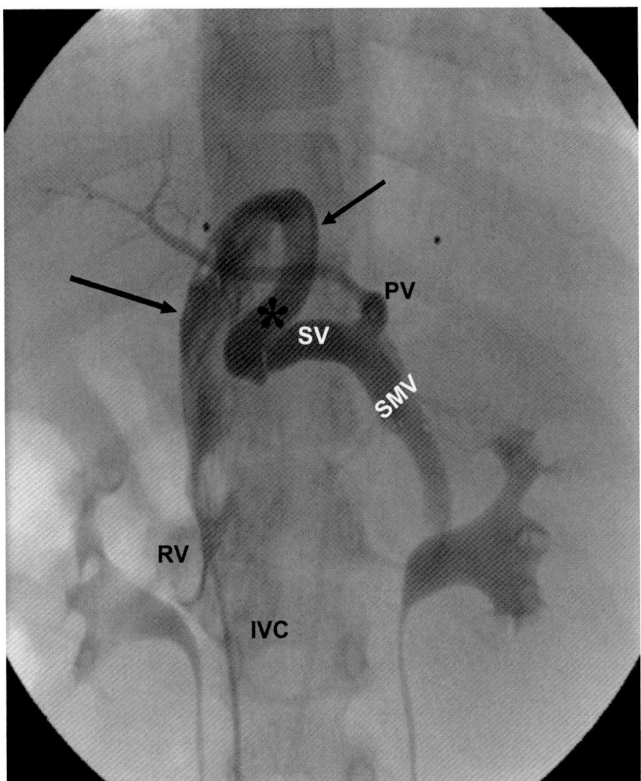

Figure 58-4 Conventional angiogram (posteroanterior view) demonstrates injection of the right splenorenal shunt *(arrows)* via the right femoral vein to inferior vena cava catheter. The catheter has passed through the shunt, with the catheter tip *(*)* in the shunt near the splenic vein connection. The large tortuous shunt is seen extending from the midsplenic vein to the right renal vein at its junction with inferior vena cava–azygos vein junction. The more proximal splenic vein on the right is not filled. There is faint filling of the right renal vein. The portal vein (right branches fill better than left branches) and superior mesenteric vein are patent. Key: *PV,* Portal vein; *RV,* right renal vein; *SMV,* superior mesenteric vein; *SV,* midsplenic vein. (From Newman and colleagues.[N5])

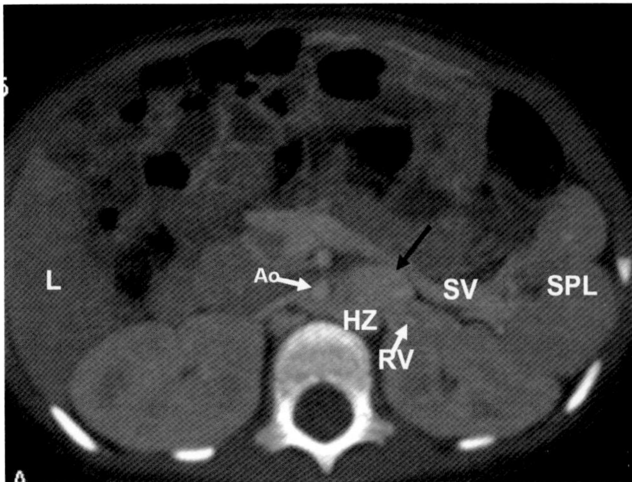

Figure 58-5 Two-year-old with polysplenia syndrome. Axial slice from a contrast-enhanced abdominal computed tomography venogram demonstrates right liver and left polysplenia. There is a splenorenal shunt connecting splenic vein with left renal vein *(arrow)* behind the more proximal splenic vein. This drains posteriorly to hemiazygos vein. The entire course of the shunt cannot be seen on a single image. There is partial visualization of a retroaortic right renal vein, also draining to hemiazygos vein. Key: *Ao,* Abdominal aorta; *HZ,* hemiazygos vein; *L,* liver; *RV,* left renal vein; *SPL,* polyspenia; *SV,* splenic vein. (From Newman and colleagues.[N5])

vena cava can be performed, making partitioning of a common atrium much simpler.[R1]

Fontan Type of Repair

Frequent occurrence of complex cardiac anomalies means that a Fontan type of repair must sometimes be used. Usual techniques of operation as practiced in the current era (see Technique of Operation in Section IV of Chapter 41) serve well. In most instances, some form of extracardiac conduit or lateral tunnel total cavopulmonary shunt operation is useful (see "Persistent Left Superior Vena Cava with Hemiazygos Extension of Inferior Vena Cava" under Special Situations and Controversies in Section IV of Chapter 41).[K2] Several variations of these basic techniques can be used when the hepatic veins enter the atria separately.[N1,N3]

Atrioventricular Valve Repair

Repair of a common atrioventricular valve is an important consideration in heterotaxy patients with single ventricle physiology. Valve regurgitation is a consistently cited risk factor for poor outcome (see Results section). Ota and colleagues[O2] have identified characteristics of valve repair that increase the likelihood of success. Multiple techniques were used, primarily including direct leaflet apposition at clefts, scallops, or prolapsing leaflet edges and various forms of reduction anuloplasty. Additional techniques used were the Alfieri suture and chordal shortening.

Palliative Operations

Standard techniques are used for shunting procedures (see "Technique of Shunting Operations" under Technique of Operation in Section I of Chapter 38 and "Systemic–Pulmonary Arterial Shunt" under Technique of Operation in Section II of Chapter 41) and pulmonary trunk banding (see "Pulmonary Trunk Banding" under Technique of Operation in Section II of Chapter 41). Coexisting juxtaductal pulmonary arterial stenosis, not uncommon in these patients, should be corrected at the time of the shunting operation. Occasionally, discontinuous branch pulmonary arteries arising from bilateral ductus arteriosus, in association with pulmonary atresia, must be reconstructed at the time of the shunting procedure. In one series, this morphology was present in 7 of 28 patients (25%) having pulmonary atresia with right atrial isomerism.[F2]

If a superior cavopulmonary shunt is being considered, careful consideration must be given to presence of bilateral superior venae cavae or of interrupted inferior vena cava. Bilateral bidirectional superior cavopulmonary shunts are discussed in Section III of Chapter 41. The considerations are purely technical, with no physiologic implications different from those of unilateral bidirectional superior cavopulmonary shunt. In contrast, creating a bidirectional cavopulmonary shunt in the setting of interrupted inferior vena cava has important physiologic implications. Because of azygos vein continuation associated with interrupted inferior vena cava,

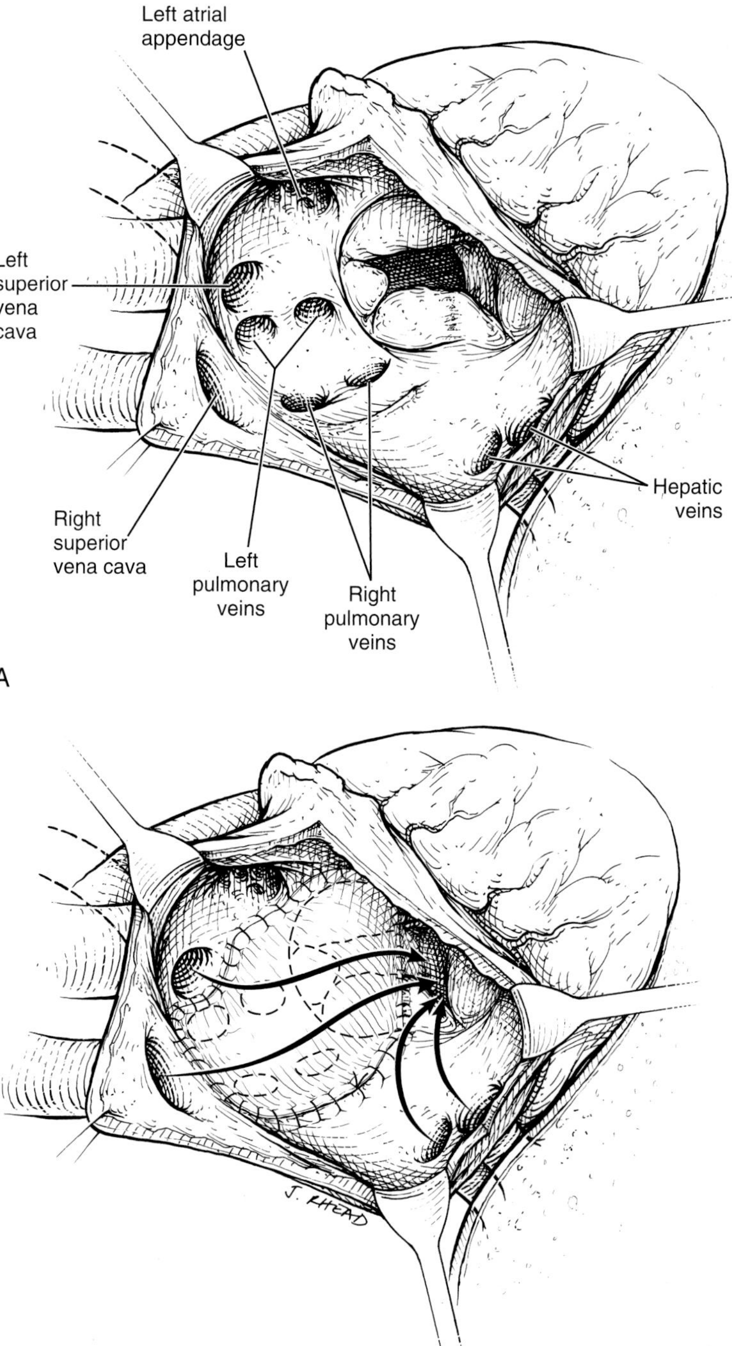

Figure 58-6 Use of a complex atrial baffle in intracardiac repair of atrial isomerism with bilateral superior venae cavae and common atrioventricular (AV) valve orifice (complete AV septal defect). **A,** Appearance of atria after completely excising atrial septum. **B,** Pericardial baffle has been sewn into place to divert pulmonary venous blood to the left side of the partitioned, once common, AV valve orifice and systemic venous blood from multiple sources to the right side. Baffle should not be redundant but taut, and care is taken to ensure that it does not restrict any pathway.

a bidirectional cavopulmonary shunt will deliver all systemic venous return, except for splanchnic blood flow, to the pulmonary circulation. As a result, systemic oxygen saturation and pulmonary artery pressure can both be higher than with a bidirectional cavopulmonary shunt in the setting of intact inferior vena cava. There are also long-term physiologic implications as discussed in the text that follows.

SPECIAL FEATURES OF POSTOPERATIVE CARE

Usual measures of postoperative care are employed after repair of cardiac anomalies in patients with atrial isomerism (see Chapter 5). Special measures used after the Fontan type of procedure are described under Special Features of Postoperative Care in Section IV of Chapter 41.

When a bidirectional cavopulmonary shunt is created in the setting of interrupted inferior vena cava, careful mid- and long-term follow-up is critical to monitor development of pulmonary arteriovenous malformations. These pulmonary vascular abnormalities can develop under various conditions of altered pulmonary blood flow, but their development is particularly rapid and aggressive in this setting. The first sign of pulmonary arteriovenous malformations may be decreased $Sa{O_2}$, although contrast echocardiography may document arteriovenous malformations well before that. At catheterization, angiographic evidence of arteriovenous malformations

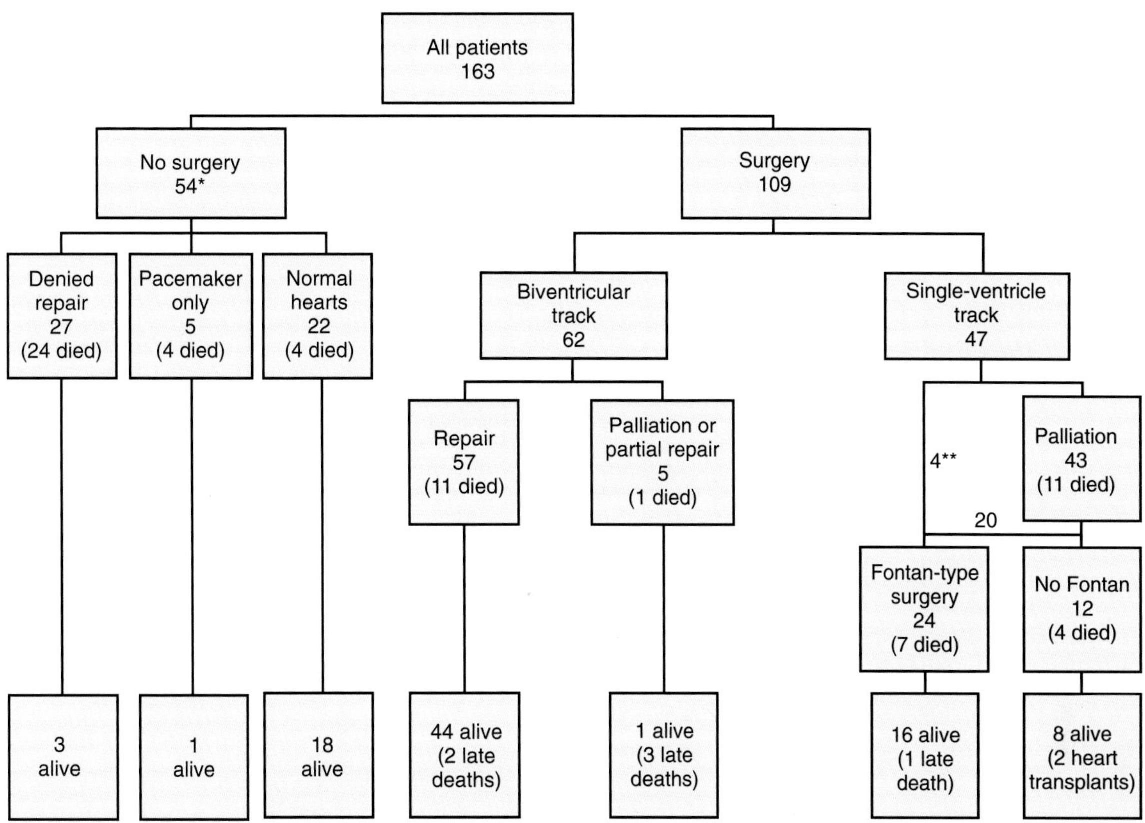

Figure 58-7 Flow chart of interventions in 163 patients with left atrial isomerism. *Comprising 9 patients with biventricular hearts, 23 with single ventricle, and 22 with normal hearts. **Four patients had Fontan-type surgery without prior interventions. Fontan-type includes bidirectional cavopulmonary shunt, right atrium to pulmonary artery anastomosis, and hepatic vein to pulmonary artery rerouting. (From Gilljam and colleagues.[G2])

and desaturated blood in the pulmonary veins confirm the diagnosis. There is evidence that incorporating splanchnic venous blood into the pulmonary circulation along with the remainder of systemic venous return may reverse pulmonary arteriovenous malformations.[I1,M2,W2]

Lack of splenic function in heterotaxy patients increases the risk of nosocomial infection and demands exquisite attention to preoperative sterile technique. In a series of 29 heterotaxy patients, seven (24%; CL 15%-35%) developed sepsis during treatment. Six of the seven were on appropriate antibiotic therapy when sepsis developed. Underscoring the fact that polysplenia patients as well as asplenia patients have splenic dysfunction, five of the seven patients with sepsis had polysplenia. Bacterial sepsis was associated with a 44% mortality.[P6]

RESULTS

Because of wide morphologic variability in patients with atrial isomerism, it is difficult to summarize overall outcomes. However, several general points can be made. First, overall survival is better with left, compared with right, atrial isomerism (94% vs. 79% at 3 years in one series, and 94% vs. 53% at 1 year in another).[A3,T1] Second, in most series survival is better when a biventricular repair is undertaken compared with a management plan that leads to a Fontan procedure[G2,H1,V4] (Figs. 58-7 and 58-8). In the large series reported by Serraf and colleagues, however, mortality in these two categories was similar[S2] (Fig. 58-9). Points one and two above are somewhat related; in all series of heterotaxy, most biventricular repairs are performed in patients with left atrial isomerism morphology. Third, overall results have improved substantially over time, with current-era outcomes suggesting 7% to 15% early mortality, and long-term survival of 75%[A1,A3,D4,M3,S2,T2] (Fig. 58-10). In one large series, all mortality beyond that related to initial neonatal management was due to interstage loss in single-ventricle patients.[A1]

Left Atrial Isomerism Outcomes

In left atrial isomerism, several large series suggest that about one third of patients received a biventricular repair.[A1,G2] The remainder underwent surgical palliation[A1] or did not undergo surgical intervention.[G2] Of those not undergoing operation, death was almost certain if important cardiac defects were present. In earlier series, even in patients with normal hearts there was 18% mortality within the first few years of life because of important noncardiac abnormalities,[G2] and in those patients undergoing some form of surgical intervention, both short- and long-term outcomes were substantially better in those undergoing biventricular repair (Fig. 58-11; see also Fig. 58-7).[G2]

In more recent series, patients undergoing surgical palliation have had excellent survival, as have those undergoing biventricular repair, with no differences noted between these two groups.[A1] In fact, these recent outcomes in patients

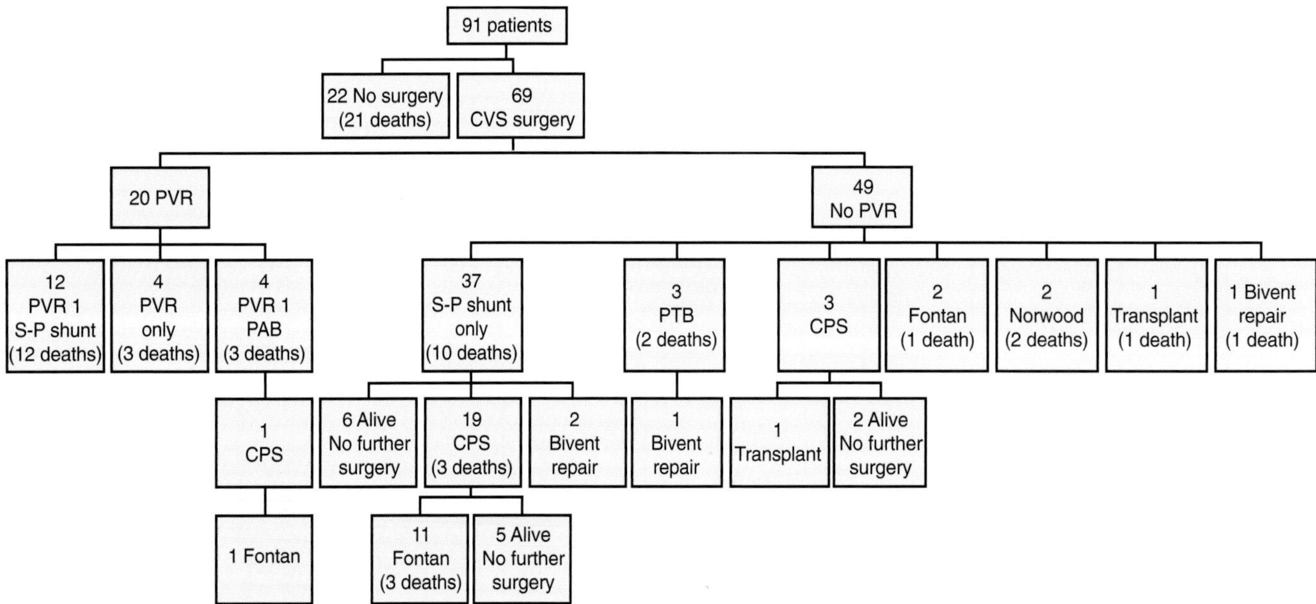

Figure 58-8 Flow chart showing surgical interventions and deaths in patients with right atrial isomerism. Key: *Bivent,* Biventricular; *CPS,* cavopulmonary shunt; *CVS,* cardiovascular surgery; *PTB,* pulmonary trunk band; *PVR,* pulmonary vein repair; *S-P,* systemic to pulmonary; *Transplant,* heart transplantation. (From Hashmi and colleagues.[H1])

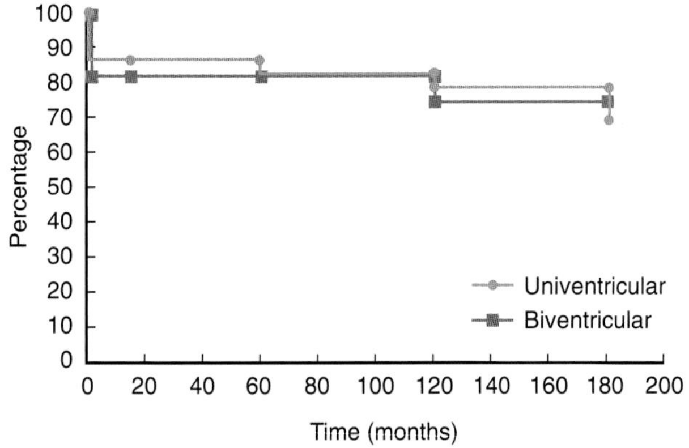

Figure 58-9 Actuarial survival selected by type of surgical management (univentricular repair or biventricular repair) in a group of 139 heterotaxy patients undergoing operation between 1989 and 2008. (From Serraf and colleagues.[S2])

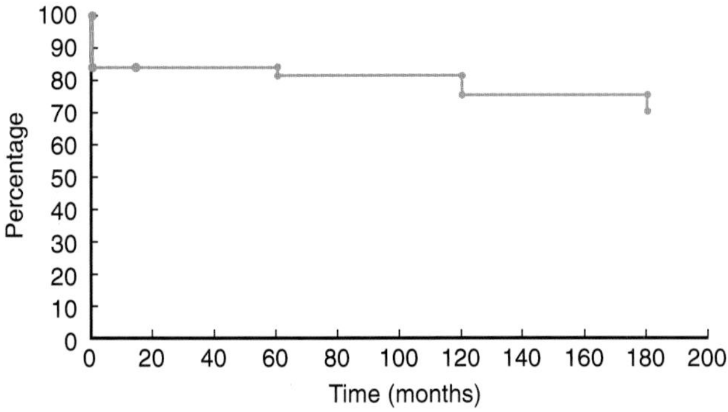

Figure 58-10 Actuarial survival in an unselected group of 139 heterotaxy patients undergoing operation between 1989 and 2008. (From Serraf and colleagues.[S2])

undergoing surgical intervention are substantially better than the 18% mortality in left atrial isomerism patients with normal hearts from older series. Thus, it can be inferred that noncardiac management of heterotaxy patients has also improved. This inference is supported by the fact that noncardiac as well as cardiac risk factors for death were identified in older series (Table 58-7). More recent series show almost no mortality, and understandably: case volumes are small with no identifiable risk factors.[A1,V4] One study of 91 biventricular repairs suggests that attempting biventricular repair in the setting of unbalanced AV septal defect is associated with increased mortality.[L4]

Right Atrial Isomerism Outcomes

In right atrial isomerism, both short- and long-term outcomes are worse than for left atrial isomerism. Although outcomes have improved in recent series, they still remain worse than in left atrial isomerism.[A1,Y2] Risk factors in recent series include presence of AV valve regurgitation, obstructed TAPVC, and mixed TAPVC, similar to those identified in earlier series[A1,F1,N4,Y2] (Table 58-8 and Fig. 58-12). Occurrence of secondary pulmonary vein obstruction after repair of obstructed TAPVC is frequent, adding to the poor prognosis of this association[F1,N4] (Table 58-9). Biventricular repair is possible in few patients with right atrial isomerism (see Fig. 58-7).[H1,L4] In patients not receiving surgical intervention, death is almost a certainty (Fig. 58-13; see also Fig. 58-8).

In patients undergoing surgical palliation, presence of TAPVC requiring operation creates substantial problems in the setting of single-ventricle physiology. The common occurrence of obstructed outflow into the pulmonary circulation and obstructed pulmonary veins makes management of such infants particularly challenging[H1] (see Table 58-8; see also Fig. 58-13).

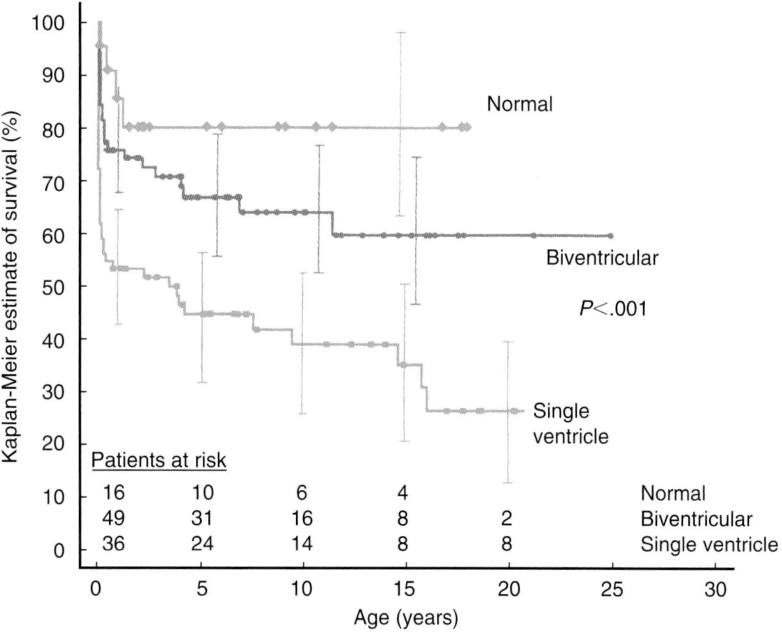

Figure 58-11 Survival of 163 patients with left atrial isomerism and a normal heart (n = 22), a heart suitable for biventricular repair (n = 71), and a heart suitable for single-ventricle surgery (n = 70). Survivors are denoted by dots. Vertical bars represent 95% confidence limits. Differences between groups were analyzed using the log-rank and Wilcoxon tests. (From Gilljam and colleagues.[G2])

Table 58-7 Incremental Risk Factors for Time-Related Mortality in Left Atrial Isomerism

	Including Birth Weight (n = 122)		Excluding Birth Weight (n = 162[a])	
	Relative Hazard (95% CL)	***P***	**Relative Hazard (95% CL)**	***P***
Lower birth weight	0.40 (0.27-0.58)	<.001	—	—
Single ventricle	2.31 (1.37-3.89)	.02	2.79 (1.72-4.54)	<.001
Gastrointestinal malformations[b]	—	—	2.19 (1.21-3.96)	.002
Biliary atresia	—	—	2.76 (1.10-5.46)	.002
Congenital AV block	—	—	4.57 (2.12-9.60)	.001
Coarctation of aorta	3.40 (1.86-6.22)	<.001	3.38 (1.87-6.12)	<.001

Data from Gilljam and colleagues.[G2]
[a]From Cox's proportional hazard modeling. Because of the number of patients with missing values for the variable birth weight, the analysis was repeated excluding this variable, with resultant entry of three additional variables.
[b]Other than biliary atresia.
Key: *AV*, Atrioventricular; *CL*, confidence limits.

Table 58-8 Incremental Risk Factors for Time-Related Mortality in Patients with Right Atrial Isomerism (Cox Proportional Hazards Modeling)[a]

Variable	Coefficient ± SE	*P*	HR (95% CL)
Absence of pulmonary outflow obstruction	−0.80 ± 0.37	.03	2.2 (1.08-4.6)
Presence of major AV valve anomaly	1.65 ± 0.73	.03	5.2 (1.25-22)
Presence of obstructed pulmonary veins	1.69 ± 0.34	.0001	5.4 (2.8-10.5)

Data from Hashmi and colleagues.[H1]
[a]Final model based on 84 observations with nonmissing values.
Key: *AV*, Atrioventricular; *CL*, confidence limits; *HR*, hazard ratio; *SE*, standard error.

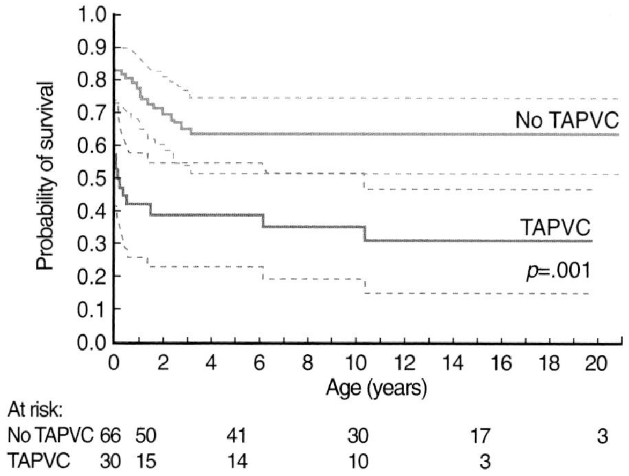

Figure 58-12 Kaplan-Meier survival of 102 patients with right atrial isomerism, stratified by presence of total anomalous pulmonary venous connection (TAPVC). (From Foerster and colleagues.[F1])

Table 58-9 Death and Recurrent Pulmonary Vein Stenosis in 36 Patients with Total Anomalous Pulmonary Venous Connection, According to Type of Connection and Presence of Native Pathway Obstruction

Type of Connection	*n*	Death	No Surgery	Pulmonary Vein Stenosis
Infradiaphragmatic				
Obstructed	9	9	2	3 (3 died)
Unobstructed	1	1	0	0
Mixed				
Obstructed	4	3	1	0
Unobstructed	1	1	1	2 (1 died)
Supracardiac				
Obstructed	8	6	2	3 (2 died)
Unobstructed	13	4	0	6 (3 died)
		24/36	6/36	14/36 (9 died)
		67%; CL 57%-75%	17%; CL 10%-26%	39%; CL 30%-49%

From Foerster and colleagues.[F1]

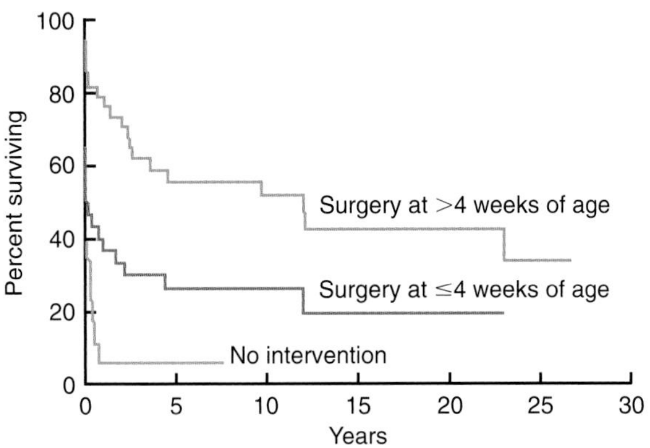

Figure 58-13 Survival estimates for patients with right atrial isomerism with no intervention, first surgical intervention during neonatal period, and first surgical intervention after age 4 weeks. Differences in risk for the three groups were unlikely to be due to chance ($P = .0001$) (Wilcoxon and log-rank tests). (From Hashmi and colleagues.[H1])

Other series support the observation that biventricular repair, when possible, can be performed with low mortality, that surgery in the neonatal period for pulmonary venous obstruction in combination with outflow obstruction to the pulmonary circulation in right atrial isomerism carries a dismal prognosis, and that outcomes following surgical intervention are generally better in left, compared with right, atrial isomerism.[A1,K3,S1,S7]

Fontan Outcomes

In several studies, one multicenter, functional outcome and survival after the Fontan operation were similar in heterotaxy and non-heterotaxy patients.[A4,B2,H6,S9] Heterotaxy patients, however, did undergo their procedure at an older age, were more likely to receive an extracardiac conduit Fontan, had more previous operations, had a higher prevalence of sinus node dysfunction and atrial dysrhythmias, and had more AV valve regurgitation.

Atrioventricular Valve Repair Outcomes

Successful repair can be achieved in two thirds of patients[N2,O2] The technique of leaflet apposition (see "Atrioventricular Valve Repair" under Technique of Operation) was associated with successful repair. Successful repair was associated with improved survival.[O2]

INDICATIONS FOR OPERATION

Need for surgical treatment is dictated by associated cardiac anomalies, not by atrial isomerism. Atrial isomerism, particularly right atrial isomerism and asplenia, strongly suggests the presence of complex cardiac anomalies and a higher-than-usual surgical risk, but coexisting anomalies are usually severe and the natural history unfavorable. Therefore, indications for operation are usually clear.

REFERENCES

A

1. Anagnostopoulos PV, Pearl JM, Octave C, Cohen M, Gruessner A, Wintering E, et al. Improved current era outcomes in patients with heterotaxy syndromes. Eur J Cardiothorac Surg 2009;35:871-8.
2. Anderson RH, Webb S, Brown NA. Defective lateralisation in children with congenitally malformed hearts. Cardiol Young 1998;8:512.
3. Ando F, Shirotani H, Kawai J, Kanzaki Y, Setsuie N. Successful total repair of complicated cardiac anomalies with asplenia syndrome. J Thorac Cardiovasc Surg 1976;72:33-8.
4. Atz AM, Cohen MS, Sleeper LA, McCrindle BW, Lu M, Prakash A, et al. Functional state of patients with heterotaxy syndrome following the Fontan operation. Cardiol Young 2007;17(suppl 2): 44-53.

B

1. Bailie M. Of a remarkable transposition of the viscera. Philos Trans R Soc London 1785-1790;16:483.
2. Bartz PJ, Driscoll DJ, Dearani JA, Puga FJ, Danielson GK, O'Leary PW, et al. Early and late results of the modified Fontan operation for heterotaxy syndrome 30 years of experience in 142 patients. J Am Coll Cardiol 2006;48:2301-5.
3. Bharati S, Lev M. The course of the conduction system in dextrocardia. Circulation 1978;57:163.
4. Brandt HM, Liebow AA. Right pulmonary isomerism associated with venous, splenic, and other anomalies. Lab Invest 1958;7:469.

C

1. Caruso G, Becker AE. How to determine atrial situs? Considerations initiated by 3 cases of absent spleen with a discordant anatomy between bronchi and atria. Br Heart J 1979;41:559.
2. Chandra RS. Biliary atresia and other structural anomalies in the congenital polysplenia syndrome. J Pediatr 1974;85:649.
3. Chiu IS, How SW, Wang JK, Wu MH, Chu SH, Lue HC, et al. Clinical implications of atrial isomerism. Br Heart J 1988; 60:72.
4. Cohen MS, Anderson RH, Cohen MI, Atz AM, Fogel M, Gruber PJ, et al. Controversies, genetics, diagnostic assessment, and outcomes relating to the heterotaxy syndrome. Cardiol Young 2007;17(suppl 2):29-43.
5. Cohen MS, Schultz AH, Tian ZY, Donaghue DD, Weinberg PM, Gaynor JW, et al. Heterotaxy syndrome with functional single ventricle: does prenatal diagnosis improve survival? Ann Thorac Surg 2006;82:1629-36.

D

1. Deshpande JR, Kinare SG. Atresia of the common pulmonary vein. Int J Cardiol 1991;30:221.

2. De Tommasi S, Daliento L, Ho SY, Macartney FJ, Anderson RH. Analysis of atrioventricular junction, ventricular mass, and ventriculoarterial junction in 43 specimens with atrial isomerism. Br Heart J 1981;45:236.
3. Dickinson DF, Wilkinson JL, Anderson KR, Smith A, Ho SY, Anderson RH. The cardiac conduction system in situs ambiguus. Circulation 1979;59:879.
4. Di Donato R, di Carlo D, Squitieri C, Rossi E, Ammirati A, Marino B, et al. Palliation of cardiac malformations associated with right isomerism (asplenia syndrome) in infancy. Ann Thorac Surg 1987; 44:35.
5. Dimmick JE, Bove KE, McAdams AJ. Extrahepatic biliary atresia and the polysplenia syndrome. J Pediatr 1975;86:644.

F

1. Foerster SR, Gauvreau K, McElhinney DB, Geva T. Importance of totally anomalous pulmonary venous connection and postoperative pulmonary vein stenosis in outcomes of heterotaxy syndrome. Pediatr Cardiol 2008;29:536-44.
2. Formigari R, Vairo U, de Zorzi A, Santoro G, Marino B. Prevalence of bilateral patent ductus arteriosus in patients with pulmonic valve atresia and asplenia syndrome. Am J Cardiol 1992;70:1219.

G

1. Garcia OL, Metha AV, Pickoff AS, Tamer DF, Ferrer PL, Wolff GS, et al. Left isomerism and complete atrioventricular block: a report of 6 cases. Am J Cardiol 1981;48:1103.
2. Gilljam T, McCrindle BW, Smallhorn JF, Williams WG, Freedom RM. Outcomes of left atrial isomerism over a 28-year period at a single institution. J Am Coll Cardiol 2000;36:908.

H

1. Hashmi A, Abu-Sulaiman R, McCrindle BW, Smallhorn JF, Williams WG, Freedom RM. Management and outcomes of right atrial isomerism: a 26-year experience. J Am Coll Cardiol 1998; 31:1120.
2. Heinemann MK, Hanley FL, Van Praagh S, Fenton KN, Jonas RA, Mayer JE Jr, et al. Total anomalous pulmonary venous drainage in newborns with visceral heterotaxy. Ann Thorac Surg 1994;57:88.
3. Hirooka K, Yagihara T, Kishimoto H, Isobe F, Yamamoto F, Nishigaki K, et al. Biventricular repair in cardiac isomerism. Report of seventeen cases. J Thorac Cardiovasc Surg 1995;109:530.
4. Ho SY, Fagg N, Anderson RH, Cook A, Allan L. Disposition of the atrioventricular conduction tissues in the heart with isomerism of the atrial appendages: its relation to congenital complete heart block. J Am Coll Cardiol 1992;20:904.
5. Ho SY, Seo JW, Brown NA, Cook AC, Fagg NL, Anderson RH. Morphology of the sinus node in human and mouse hearts with isomerism of the atrial appendages. Br Heart J 1995;74:437.
6. Hoashi T, Ichikawa H, Fukushima N, Ueno T, Kogaki S, Sawa Y. Long-term clinical outcome of atrial isomerism after univentricular repair. J Card Surg 2009;24:19-23.
7. Huhta JC, Smallhorn JF, Macartney FJ. Two-dimensional echocardiographic diagnosis of situs. Br Heart J 1982;48:97.

I

1. Ichikawa H, Fukushima N, Ono M, Kita T, Matsushita T, Miyamoto Y, et al. Resolution of pulmonary arteriovenous fistula by redirection of hepatic venous blood. Ann Thorac Surg 2004; 77:1825-7.
2. Ivemark BI. Implications of agenesis of spleen on pathogenesis of conotruncus anomalies in childhood; analysis of heart malformations in splenic agenesis syndrome, with fourteen new cases. Acta Paediatr 1955;44(suppl. 104):7-110.

K

1. Kartagener M. Zur Pathogenese der Bronchiektasien: Bronchiektasien bei Situs viscerum inversus. Beitr Klin Tuberk 1933;83: 489-501.
2. Kawashima Y, Kitamura S, Matsuda H, Shimazaki Y, Nakano S, Hirose H. Total cavopulmonary shunt operation in complex cardiac anomalies. J Thorac Cardiovasc Surg 1984;87:74.
3. Kawashima Y, Matsuda H, Naito Y, Yagihara T, Kadoba K, Matsuki O. Biventricular repair of cardiac isomerism with common atrioventricular canal with the aid of an endocardial cushion prosthesis. J Thorac Cardiovasc Surg 1993;106:248.

L

1. Landing BH, Lawrence TY, Payne VC Jr, Wells TR. Bronchial anatomy in syndromes with abnormal visceral situs, abnormal spleen and congenital heart disease. Am J Cardiol 1971;28:456.
2. Lev M, Liberthson RR, Eckner FA, Arcilla RA. Pathologic anatomy of dextrocardia and its clinical implications. Circulation 1968;37:979.
3. Liberthson RR, Hastreiter AR, Sinha SN, Bharati S, Novak GM, Lev M. Levocardia with visceral heterotaxy isolated levocardia: pathologic anatomy and its clinical implications. Am Heart J 1973;85:40.
4. Lim HG, Bacha EA, Marx GR, Marshall A, Fynn-Thompson F, Mayer JE, et al. Biventricular repair in patients with heterotaxy syndrome. J Thorac Cardiovasc Surg 2009;137:371-9.
5. Lin JH, Chang CI, Wang JK, Wu MH, Shyu MK, Lee CN, et al. Intrauterine diagnosis of heterotaxy syndrome. Am Heart J 2002; 143:1002-8.
6. Lin AE, Ticho BS, Houde K, Westgate MN, Holmes LB. Heterotaxy: associated conditions and hospital-based prevalence in newborns. Genet Med 2000;2:157.

M

1. Macartney FJ, Zuberbuhler JR, Anderson RH. Morphological considerations pertaining to recognition of atrial isomerism: consequences for sequential chamber localization. Br Heart J 1980; 44:657.
2. Mahle WT, Rychik J, Rome JJ. Clinical significance of pulmonary arteriovenous malformations after staging bidirectional cavopulmonary anastomosis. Am J Cardiol 2000;86:239-41.
3. Marcelletti C, Di Donato R, Nijveld A, Squitieri C, Bulterijs AH, Naeff M, et al. Right and left isomerism: the cardiac surgeon's view. Ann Thorac Surg 1983;35:400.
4. Mazzucco A, Bortolotti U, Stellin G, Gallucci V. Anomalies of the systemic venous return: a review. J Cardiac Surg 1990;5:122.
5. Mehta AV, Sanchez GR. Left isomerism (polysplenia syndrome) and complete atrioventricular block. Am J Cardiol 1983;52:429.
6. Moller JH, Nakib A, Anderson RC, Edwards JE. Congenital cardiac disease associated with polysplenia: a developmental complex of bilateral "left-sidedness." Circulation 1967;36:789.

N

1. Naito Y, Aoki M, Matsuo K, Nakajima H, Aotsuka H, Fujiwara T. Intracardiac Fontan procedure for heterotaxy syndrome with complex systemic and pulmonary venous anomalies. Eur J Cardiothorac Surg 2010;37:197-203.
2. Nakata T, Fujimoto Y, Hirose K, Tosaka Y, Ide Y, Tachi M, et al. Atrioventricular valve repair in patients with functional single ventricle. J Thorac Cardiovasc Surg 2010;140:514-21.
3. Nakata T, Fujimoto Y, Hirose K, Osaki M, Tosaka Y, Ide Y, et al. Fontan completion in patients with atrial isomerism and separate hepatic venous drainage. Eur J Cardiothorac Surg 2010;37: 1264-70.
4. Nakata T, Fujimoto Y, Hirose K, Osaki M, Tosaka Y, Ide Y, et al. Functional single ventricle with extracardiac total anomalous pulmonary venous connection. Eur J Cardiothorac Surg 2009;36: 49-56.
5. Newman B, Feinstein JA, Cohen RA, Feingold B, Kreutzer J, Patel H, et al. Congenital extrahepatic portosystemic shunt associated with heterotaxy and polysplenia. Pediatr Radiol 2010;40:1222-30.

O

1. Oliverio M, Digilio MC, Versacci P, Dallapiccola B, Marino B. Shells and heart: are human laterality and chirality of snails controlled by the same maternal genes? Am J Med Genet Part A 2010;152A:2419-25.
2. Ota N, Fujimoto Y, Hirose K, Tosaka Y, Nakata T, Ide Y, et al. Improving results of atrioventricular valve repair in challenging patients with heterotaxy syndrome. Cardiol Young 2010;20:60-5.

P

1. Partridge JB, Scott O, Deverall PB, Macartney FJ. Visualization and measurement of the main bronchi by tomography as an objective indicator of thoracic situs in congenital heart disease. Circulation 1975;51:188.

2. Peoples WM, Moller JH, Edwards JE. Polysplenia: a review of 146 cases. Pediatr Cardiol 1983;4:129.
3. Pepes S, Zidere V, Allan LD. Prenatal diagnosis of left atrial isomerism. Heart 2009;95:1974-7.
4. Phoon CK, Neill CA. Asplenia syndrome: insight into embryology through an analysis of cardiac and extracardiac anomalies. Am J Cardiol 1994;73:581.
5. Pipitone S, Calcaterra G, Grillo R, Thiene G, Sperandeo V. Bronchoatrial discordance. A clinically diagnosed case. Int J Cardiol 1985;9:374.
6. Prendiville TW, Barton LL, Thompson WR, Fink DL, Holmes KW. Heterotaxy syndrome: defining contemporary disease trends. Pediatr Cardiol 2010;31:1052-8.

R

1. Reddy VM, McElhinney DB, Hanley FL. Correction of left superior vena cava draining to the left atrium using extracardiac techniques. Ann Thorac Surg 1997;63:1800.
2. Rose V, Izukawa T, Moes CA. Syndromes of asplenia and polysplenia: a review of cardiac and non-cardiac malformations in 60 cases with special reference to diagnosis and prognosis. Br Heart J 1975;37:840.
3. Rubino M, Van Praagh S, Kadoba K, Pessotto R, Van Praagh R. Systemic and pulmonary venous connections in visceral heterotaxy with asplenia. Diagnostic and surgical considerations based on seventy-two autopsied cases. J Thorac Cardiovasc Surg 1995; 110:641.
4. Ruttenberg HD, Neufeld HN, Lucas RV Jr, Carey LS, Adams P Jr, Anderson RC, et al. Syndrome of congenital cardiac disease with asplenia: distinction from other forms of congenital cyanotic cardiac disease. Am J Cardiol 1964;13:387.

S

1. Sadiq M, Stumper O, De Giovanni JV, Wright JG, Sethia B, Brawn WJ, et al. Management and outcome of infants and children with right atrial isomerism. Heart 1996;75:314.
2. Serraf A, Bensari N, Houyel L, Capderou A, Roussin R, Lebret E, et al. Surgical management of congenital heart defects associated with heterotaxy syndrome. Eur J Cardiothorac Surg 2010;38: 721-7.
3. Sharma S, Devine W, Anderson RH, Zuberbuhler JR. Identification and analysis of left atrial isomerism. Am J Cardiol 1987;60:1157.
4. Sharma S, Devine W, Anderson RH, Zuberbuhler JR. The determination of atrial arrangement by examination of appendage morphology in 1842 heart specimens. Br Heart J 1988;60:227.
5. Shinebourne EA, Macartney FJ, Anderson RH. Sequential chamber localization: logical approach to diagnosis in congenital heart disease. Br Heart J 1976;38:327.
6. Siewert AK. Ueber einen Fall von Bronchiektasie bei einem Patienten mit Situs inversus viscerum. Berl Klin Wochenschr 1904; 41:139-41.
7. Sinzobahamvya N, Arenz C, Brecher AM, Urban AE. Atrial isomerism: a surgical experience. Cardiovasc Surg 1999;7:436.
8. Soto B, Pacifico AD, Souza AS Jr, Bargeron LM Jr, Ermocilla R, Tonkin IL. Identification of thoracic isomerism from the plain chest radiograph. Am J Roentgenol 1978;131:995.
9. Stamm C, Friehs I, Duebener LF, Zurakowski D, Mayer JE Jr, Jonas RA, et al. Improving results of the modified Fontan operation in patients with heterotaxy syndrome. Ann Thorac Surg 2002; 74:1967-78.
10. Sutherland MJ, Ware SM. Disorders of left-right asymmetry: heterotaxy and situs inversus. Am J Med Genet C Semin Med Genet 2009;151C:307-17.

T

1. Takeuchi K, Murakami A, Hirata Y, Kitahori K, Doi Y, Takamoto S. Surgical outcome of heterotaxy syndrome in a single institution. Asian Cardiovasc Thorac Ann 2006;14:489-94.
2. Turley K, Tarnoff H, Snider R, Ebert PA. Repair of combined total anomalous pulmonary venous connection and anomalous systemic connection in early infancy. Ann Thorac Surg 1981;31:70.

U

1. Uemura H, Ho SY, Devine WA, Anderson RH. Analysis of visceral heterotaxy according to splenic status, appendage morphology, or both. Am J Cardiol 1995;76:846.
2. Uemura H, Ho SY, Devine WA, Kilpatrick LL, Anderson RH. Atrial appendages and venoatrial connections in hearts from patients with visceral heterotaxy. Ann Thorac Surg 1995;60:561.

V

1. Van Mierop LH, Eisen S, Schiebler GL. The radiographic appearance of the tracheobronchial tree as an indicator of visceral situs. Am J Cardiol 1970;26:432.
2. Van Mierop LH, Wiglesworth FW. Isomerism of the cardiac atria in the asplenia syndrome. Lab Invest 1962;11:1303.
3. Van Praagh R, Van Praagh S. Atrial isomerism in the heterotaxy syndromes with asplenia, or polysplenia, or normally formed spleen: an erroneous concept. Am J Cardiol 1990;66:1504.
4. Vodiskar J, Clur SA, Hruda J, Bokenkamp R, Hazekamp MG. Left atrial isomerism: biventricular repair. Eur J Cardiothorac Surg 2010;37:1259-63.

W

1. Wren C, Macartney FJ, Deanfield JE. Cardiac rhythm in atrial isomerism. Am J Cardiol 1987;59:1156.
2. Wu IH, Nguyen KH. Redirection of hepatic drainage for treatment of pulmonary arteriovenous malformations following the Fontan procedure. Pediatr Cardiol 2006;27:519-22.
3. Wu MH, Wang JK, Lin JL, Lai LP, Lue HC, Young ML, et al. Supraventricular tachycardia in patients with right atrial isomerism. J Am Coll Cardiol 1998;32:773.

Y

1. Yan YL, Tan KB, Yeo GS. Right atrial isomerism: preponderance in Asian fetuses. Using the stomach-distance ratio as a possible diagnostic tool for prediction of right atrial isomerism. Ann Acad Med Singapore 2008;37:906-12.
2. Yun TJ, Al-Radi OO, Adatia I, Caldarone CA, Coles JG, Williams WG, et al. Contemporary management of right atrial isomerism: effect of evolving therapeutic strategies. J Thorac Cardiovasc Surg 2006;131:1108-13.

Index

Note: Page numbers followed by "f" indicate figures, "t" indicate tables, and "b" indicate boxes.

B

C

D

E

J

K

M

N

O

P

Q

R

S

T

W

X

Y

Z